QM Library
23 1355055 9

D1582259

PRINCIPLES AND PRACTICE OF PET AND PET/CT

SECOND EDITION

PRINCIPLES AND PRACTICE OF PET AND PET/CT

SECOND EDITION

EDITOR

RICHARD L. WAHL, MD

Professor of Radiology and Oncology, Henry N. Wagner Jr Professor of Nuclear Medicine
Director, Division of Nuclear Medicine and PET
Vice Chairman for Technology and New Business Development
The Russell H. Morgan Department of Radiology and Radiological Sciences
The Johns Hopkins University School of Medicine
Baltimore, Maryland

ASSOCIATE EDITOR: CARDIOVASCULAR PET SECTION

ROBERT S.B. BEANLANDS, MD, FRCPC, FACC

Professor of Medicine (Cardiology)/Radiology
Chief, Cardiac Imaging
Director, National Cardiac PET Centre
University of Ottawa Heart Institute
Ottawa, Ontario

Wolters Kluwer | Lippincott Williams & Wilkins
Health

Philadelphia • Baltimore • New York • London
Buenos Aires • Hong Kong • Sydney • Tokyo

Acquisitions Editor: Lisa McAllister
Managing Editor: Kerry Barrett
Project Manager: Rosanne Hallowell
Manufacturing Manager: Benjamin Rivera
Marketing Manager: Angela Panetta
Art Director: Risa Clow
Production Services: Aptara, Inc.

Second Edition

530 Walnut Street
Philadelphia, PA 19106
LWW.com

Printed in China

Library of Congress Cataloging-in-Publication Data

Principles and practice of PET and PET/CT / editor, Richard L. Wahl, Henry N. Wagner Jr. ; associated editor, cardiovascular PET section, Robert Beanlands. — 2nd ed.

p. ; cm.

Rev. ed. of: Principles and practice of positron emission tomography / editor, Richard L. Wahl ; associate editor, Julia W. Buchanan. c2002.

Includes bibliographical references and index.

ISBN 978-0-7817-7999-9

1. Tomography, Emission. I. Wahl, Richard L. II. Wagner, Henry N., 1927– III. Principles and practice of positron emission tomography.

[DNLM: 1. Positron-Emission Tomography—methods. 2. Tomography, X-Ray Computed—methods. WN 206 P9568 2009]

RC78.7.T62P75 2009

616.07'575—dc22

2008031561

Care has been taken to confirm the accuracy of the information presented and to describe generally accepted practices. However, the authors, editors, and publisher are not responsible for errors or omissions or for any consequences from application of the information in this book and make no warranty, expressed or implied, with respect to the currency, completeness, or accuracy of the contents of the publication. Application of this information in a particular situation remains the professional responsibility of the practitioner.

The authors, editors, and publisher have exerted every effort to ensure that drug selection and dosage set forth in this text are in accordance with current recommendations and practice at the time of publication. However, in view of ongoing research, changes in government regulations, and the constant flow of information relating to drug therapy and drug reactions, the reader is urged to check the package insert for each drug for any change in indications and dosage and for added warnings and precautions. This is particularly important when the recommended agent is a new or infrequently employed drug.

Some drugs and medical devices presented in this publication have Food and Drug Administration (FDA) clearance for limited use in restricted research settings. It is the responsibility of health care providers to ascertain the FDA status of each drug or device planned for use in their clinical practice.

The publishers have made every effort to trace copyright holders for borrowed material. If they have inadvertently overlooked any, they will be pleased to make the necessary arrangements at the first opportunity.

To purchase additional copies of this book, call our customer service department at (800) 638-3030 or fax orders to (301) 223-2320. International customers should call (301) 223-2300.

Visit Lippincott Williams & Wilkins on the Internet at LWW.com. Lippincott Williams & Wilkins customer service representatives are available from 8:30 am to 6 pm, EST.

10 9 8 7 6 5 4 3 2 1

To my wife Sandy and my children, whose generous patience and support during my many hours of work on this book were essential to its genesis and completion. The current state of PET/CT as a broadly applicable method, as reflected in this text, lies squarely on the shoulders of pioneers in nuclear medicine research, ambitious trainees, skilled technologists, and study participants.

CONTENTS

CONTRIBUTING AUTHORS

Anissa Abi-Dargham, MD
Professor, Departments of Psychiatry and Radiology
Columbia University College of Physicians and Surgeons
Chief, Division of Translational Imaging
Department of Psychiatry
New York State Psychiatric Institute
New York, New York

Gerald Antoch, MD
Associate Professor, Department of Diagnostic and Interventional Radiology and Neuroradiology
University at Duisburg-Essen
Vice Chairman, Department of Diagnostic and Interventional Radiology and Neuroradiology
University Hospital Essen
Essen, Germany

Richard P. Baum, Professor Dr. med
Chairman and Director, Department of Nuclear Medicine/Centre for PET/CT
Zentralklinik Bad Berka
Bad Berka, Germany

Robert S. B. Beanlands, MD, FRCPC, FACC
Professor of Medicine (Cardiology)/Radiology
Chief, Cardiac Imaging
Director, National Cardiac PET Centre
University of Ottawa Heart Institute
Ottawa, Ontario

Ambros J. Beer, PhD
Assistant Professor, Department of Nuclear Medicine
Technische Universitat München
Resident, Department of Nuclear Medicine
Klinikum rechts der Isar der TU München
Munich, Germany

Frank M. Bengel, MD
Associate Professor of Radiology and Medicine
Director of Cardiovascular Nuclear Medicine
Division of Nuclear Medicine, Department of Radiology
The Johns Hopkins Medical Institutions
Baltimore, Maryland

Todd M. Blodgett, MD
Assistant Professor
Chief of Cancer Imaging
Department of Radiology
University of Pittsburgh Medical Center
Pittsburgh, Pennsylvania

Andreas Bockisch, MD, PhD
Professor and Director
Department of Nuclear Medicine
University Hospital Essen
Essen, Germany

Nicholas I. Bohnen, MD, PhD
Associate Professor of Radiology and Neurology
Department of Radiology, Division of Nuclear Medicine
University of Michigan Medical Center
Ann Arbor, Michigan

Barton F. Branstetter IV, MD
Associate Professor and Director of Head and Neck Imaging
Departments of Radiology, Otolaryngology, and Biomedical Informatics
University of Pittsburgh School of Medicine
Pittsburgh, Pennsylvania

Michele E. Brenner, MD
Chief Nuclear Medicine Resident, Department of Radiology
Johns Hopkins University
Baltimore, Maryland

Robert Bristow, MD
Professor, Departments of Gynecology and Obstetrics and Oncology
The Johns Hopkins Medical Institutions
Director, Kelly Gynecologic Oncology Service
The Johns Hopkins Hospital
Baltimore, Maryland

Jerry M. Collins, PhD
Associate Director for Developmental Therapeutics
Division of Cancer Treatment and Diagnosis
National Cancer Institute
Rockville, Maryland

Leonard P. Connolly, MD
Assistant Professor
Division of Nuclear Medicine
Children's Hospital Boston, Harvard Medical School
Boston, Massachusetts

Jean DaSilva
Associate Professor, Department of Medicine (Cardiology)
University of Ottawa
Head Radiochemist
Department of PET Centre
University of Ottawa Heart Institute
Ottawa, Ontario

Farrokh Dehdashti, MD
Professor of Radiology, Division of Nuclear Medicine
Edward Mallinckrodt Institute of Radiology
St. Louis, Missouri

Rob deKemp, PhD
Associate Professor, Department of Medicine and Engineering
University of Ottawa
Head Imaging Physicist, Department of Cardiac Imaging
Ottawa Heart Institute
Ottawa, Ontario

Dominique Delbeke, MD, PhD
Professor and Director of Nuclear Medicine and PET
Department of Radiology and Radiological Sciences
Vanderbilt University Medical Center
Nashville, Tennessee

Yu-Shin Ding, PhD
Professor
Co-Director of Yale PET Center
Director of Radiochemistry, Department of Diagnostic Radiology
Yale University School of Medicine
New Haven, Connecticut

Janet F. Eary, MD
Professor, Department of Nuclear Medicine
University of Washington School of Medicine
Seattle, Washington

Sukru Mehmet Erturk, MD
Attending Radiologist
Department of Radiology
Sisli Etfal Training and Research Hospital
Istanbul, Turkey

Hedieh Khalatbari Eslamy, MD
PET/CT Fellow in Clinical Oncology, Department of Radiology
Stanford University Medical Center
Stanford, California

Frederic H. Fahey, DSc
Associate Professor, Department of Radiology
Harvard Medical School
Director of Nuclear Medicine Physics
Division of Nuclear Medicine
Children's Hospital Boston
Boston, Massachusetts

Ronald D. Finn, PhD
Chief, Radiopharmaceutical Chemistry Service
Director, Cyclotron Core Facility
Departments of Radiology and Medical Physics
Memorial Sloan-Kettering Cancer Center
New York, New York

Joanna S. Fowler, PhD
Senior Chemist
Brookhaven National Laboratory
Upton, New York

Michael J. Fulham, MBBS, FRACP
Professor, Faculty of Medicine
Adjunct Professor, School of Information Techologies
University of Sydney
Director, Department of Molecular Imaging
Royal Prince Alfred Hospital
Clinical Director of Medical Imaging Services
Sydney South West Area Health Service
Camperdown, Australia

Perry W. Grigsby, MD
Professor, Department of Radiation Oncology; Obstetrics and Gynecology
Division of Nuclear Medicine
Mallinckrodt Institute of Radiology
Washington University School of Medicine and Alvin J. Siteman Cancer Center
St. Louis, Missouri

Uwe Haberkorn, MD
Professor, Department of Nuclear Medicine
University Hospital
University of Heidelbert
Head, Department of Clinical Cooperation Unit Nuclear Medicine
German Cancer Research Center
Heidelberg, Germany

Rodney P. Hicks, MB BS(Hons), MD, FRACP
Professor, Department of Medicine and Radiology
The University of Melbourne
Parkville, Australia
Director and Co-chair
Translational Research Centre for Molecular Imaging and Translational Oncology
The Peter MacCallum Cancer Centre
East Melbourne, Australia

Ora Israel, MD
Professor, B. and R. Rappaport School of Medicine
Technion-Israel Institute of Technology
Chief, Department of Nuclear Medicine
Rambam Health Care Campus
Haifa, Israel

Hossein Jadvar, MD, PhD, MPH, MBA
Associate Professor, Department of Radiology and Biomedical Engineering
Director, Radiology Research, Keck School of Medicine
University of Southern California
Los Angeles, California

Gary J. Kelloff, MD
National Institutes of Health, National Cancer Institute
Division of Cancer Treatment and Diagnosis
Rockville, Maryland

William E. Klunk, MD, PhD
Professor, Department of Psychiatry
University of Pittsburgh School of Medicine
Pittsburgh, Pennsylvania

Robert A. Koeppe, PhD
Professor, Department of Radiology–Nuclear Medicine
University of Michigan Medical School and Medical Center
Ann Arbor, Michigan

Marc A. Laruelle, MD
Professor, Department of Neurosciences
Imperial College
Vice President, Molecular Imaging
Clinical Pharmacology and Discovery Medicine
GlaxoSmithKline
London, England
Adjunct Professor, Department of Psychiatry and Radiology
Columbia University
New York, New York

Brian J. Lopresti, MD
Department of Radiology
University of Pittsburgh School of Medicine
Pittsburgh, Pennsylvania

Val J. Lowe, MD
Associate Professor and Consultant, Department of Radiology
Mayo Clinic
Rochester, Minnesota

Michael P. MacManus, MD
Associate Professor, Department of Pathology
University of Melbourne
Melbourne, Australia
Radiation Oncologist, Department of Radiation Oncology
Peter MacCallum Cancer Centre
East Melbourne, Australia

Jamshid Maddahi, MD
Clinical Professor, Department of Pharmacology and Medicine–Cardiology
University of Los Angeles School of Medicine
Los Angeles, California

Mahadevappa Mahesh, MS, PhD, FAAPM
Assistant Professor of Radiology and Medicine
The Russell H. Morgan Department of Radiology and Radiological Sciences
Chief Physicist, Department of Radiology
The Johns Hopkins University School of Medicine
Baltimore, Maryland

William B. Mathews, PhD
Research Associate, Department of Radiology
Division of Nuclear Medicine
The Johns Hopkins University
Baltimore, Maryland

Chester A. Mathis, PhD
Professor, Department of Radiology, Pharmacology, and Pharmaceutical Sciences
University of Pittsburgh
Director, PET Facility, Department of Radiology
UPMC Presbyterian Hospital
Pittsburgh, Pennsylvania

Ichiro Matsunari, MD, PhD
Director, Department of Clinical Research
The Medical and Pharmacological Research Center Foundation
Hakui, Japan

Charles R. Meyer, PhD
Professor, Department of Radiology
University of Michigan
Ann Arbor, Michigan

Satoshi Minoshima, MD, PhD
Professor and Vice Chair, Research, Department of Radiology
University of Washington
Seattle, Washington

Armin Mohamed, MBBS, BSc, FRACP
Associate Professor, Faculty of Medicine
University of Sydney
Sydney, Australia
Senior Staff Specialist, Department of Molecular Imaging
Royal Prince Hospital
Camperdown, Australia

Patrick J. Peller, MD
Assistant Professor, Department of Radiology
Mayo Clinic
Rochester, Minnesota

Eric C. Petrie, MD, MS
Associate Professor, Department of Psychiatry and Behavioral Sciences
University of Washington
Staff Physician, Psychiatry
Mental Health Service and Mental Illness Research Education and Clinical Center
Veterans Affairs Puget Sound Health Care System
Seattle, Washington

Morand Piert, MD, PhD
Associate Professor and Director, Department of Radiology
Division of Nuclear Medicine
University of Michigan Health System
Ann Arbor, Michigan

Vikas Prasad. MD
Clinical Research Associate and Assistant Doctor
Department of Nuclear Medicine and Centre for PET/CT
Zentralklinik Bad Berka
Bad Berka, Germany

Sven N. Reske, MD
Professor and Director, Department of Nuclear Medicine
University of Ulm
Ulm, Germany

Jennifer Rodriguez-Ferrer, MD
Division of Nuclear Medicine
Russell H. Morgan Department of Radiology and Radiological Sciences
The Johns Hopkins University School of Medicine
Baltimore, Maryland

Terrence D. Ruddy, MD, FRCPC
Professor, Department of Medicine (Cardiology) and Radiology (Nuclear Medicine)
University of Ottawa
Division Head, Department of Medicine (Cardiology) and Radiology (Nuclear Medicine)
University of Ottawa Heart Institute and the Ottawa Hospital
Ottawa, Canada

Alexander Ryan, MD
Resident, Department of Radiology
University of Pittsburgh
Pittsburgh, Pennsylvania

Takahiro Sasaki, MD, PhD
Instructor, Department of Neurology
Keio University School of Medicine
Tokyo, Japan

David J. Schlyer , PhD
Senior Scientist, Department of Medicine
Brookhaven National Laboratory
Upton, New York

Heiko Schöder, MD
Associate Professor, Department of Radiology
Weill Cornell Medical College
Associate Attending Physician, Department of Radiology/Nuclear Medicine
Memorial Sloan Kettering Cancer Center
New York, New York

Markus Schwaiger, MD
Professor and Chief, Department of Nuclear Medicine
Klinikum r.d. Isar d. Tum
Munich, Germany

Anthony F. Shields, MD, PhD
Professor, Department of Medicine and Oncology
Wayne University School of Medicine
Associate Center Director for Clinical Research
Karmanos Cancer Institute
Detroit, Michigan

Paul Shreve, MD
Medical Director, Department of Radiology
PET Medical Imaging Center and Spectrum Health
Grand Rapids, Michigan

Barry L. Shulkin, MD, MBA
Chief, Department of Radiologic Sciences
Division of Nuclear Medicine
St. Jude's Children's Research Hospital
Memphis, Tennessee

Caroline C. Sigman, PhD
President
CCS Associates
Mountain View, California

Hans C. Steinert, MD
Professor, Department of Medical Radiology
Division of Nuclear Medicine
University Hospital of Zürich
Zürich, Switzerland

Zsolt Szabo, MD, PhD
Professor and Attending Physician of Nuclear Medicine, Department of Radiology
The Johns Hopkins Medical Institutions
Baltimore, Maryland

Nagara Tamaki, MD, PhD
Professor and Director, Department of Nuclear Medicine
Hokkaido University Graduate School of Medicine
Chairman, Department of Nuclear Medicine
Hokkaido University Hospital
Sapporo, Japan

Richard J. Tetrault, RT (N), CNMT, PET
Chief Technologist, Department of Radiology
Dana-Farber Cancer Institute
Boston, Massachusetts

Stephanie Thorn, Msc
PhD Candidate, Department of Cellular and Molecular Medicine
Department of Cardiac Imaging
University of Ottawa
University of Ottawa Heart Institute
Ottawa, Ontario

Timothy G. Turkington, PhD
Associate Professor, Department of Radiology, Medical Physics, and Biomedical Engineering
Duke University
Durham, North Carolina

Heikki Ukkonen, MD, PhD
Assistant to Chief, Department of Cardiology
Turku, Finland

Annick D. Van den Abbeele, MD
Associate Professor, Department of Radiology
Harvard Medical School
Chief and Founding Director, Department of Radiology
Center for Bioimaging in Oncology
Dana-Farber Cancer Institute
Boston, Massachusetts

Richard L. Wahl, MD
Professor, Department of Radiology and Oncology
Henry N. Wagner Jr Professor of Nuclear Medicine
Director, Division of Nuclear Medicine and PET
Vice Chairman for Technology and New Business Development
The Russell H. Morgan Department of Radiology and Radiological Sciences
The Johns Hopkins University School of Medicine
Baltimore, Maryland

Wolfgang A. Weber, MD
Professor and Director, Department of Nuclear Medicine
University of Freiburg
Freiburg, Germany.

Hans-Jürgen Wester, MD
Department of Nuclear Medicine
Technische Universität München
München, Germany

Jinsong Xia, MD, PhD
Postdoctoral Fellow, Department of Radiology
Division of Nuclear Medicine
The Johns Hopkins Medical Institutions
Baltimore, Maryland

Keiichiro Yoshinaga, MD, PhD
Associate Professor, Department of Molecular Imaging
Hokkaido University Graduate School of Medicine
Sapporo, Japan

PREFACE

In the 6 years since the first edition of this comprehensive multiauthored textbook on PET was published, there has been remarkable progress. Progress has been sufficiently transformative that the title of the textbook has been changed to *Principles and Practice of PET **and PET/CT***. This title change is reflective of the major alteration in practice patterns and technology for PET imaging since the introduction of commercial PET/CT systems around the turn of the century. The updated text includes many PET/CT images as well as new chapters specifically dealing with CT scanning and strategies to optimally integrate CT and PET to a "one-stop" diagnosis for cancer, heart disease, and other conditions.

In 1993, Chuck Meyer, my colleagues, and I described the fusion of PET metabolic images with high-quality CT or MRI using software as "Anatomolecular Imaging." While clearly useful, the fusion approach was not routinely practiced because it was time consuming and not uniformly reliable for non-CNS applications. Routine whole-body PET/CT fusion was not the norm in practice until the introduction of dedicated hardware approaches leading to the current "in line" PET/CT, by the instrumentation group at the University of Pittsburgh led by David Townsend. The important contributions of the late Dr. Bruce Hasegawa to SPECT/CT and coincidence PET/CT fusion imaging must be recognized as well. PET/CT technology changed the PET world in the course of only a few years. At present, essentially every new PET scanner is a PET/CT scanner with improved performance of PET/CT as compared to PET in nearly all clinical settings in body imaging.

It is very gratifying to have the opportunity to observe and participate in such a transformative technology. I recall vividly observing the coincidence detecting probes and early PET scanners when I was a student and then a resident/fellow at Washington University School of Medicine in St. Louis, from the mid-1970s to the early 1980s. Drs. Ter-Pogossian and Siegel attempted to teach me the value of the PET method. At that time, I had only a limited concept of the vast potential of noninvasively imaging many aspects of human biology in all organ systems, repeatedly, quantitatively, and nondestructively.

Some of the vast potential of PET has been transformed to practice as PET/CT, now performed on several million patients per year worldwide. PET/CT technology is clearly here to stay. But in the next several years, it is anticipated that more changes are in store. PET/MRI has been developed and is in early stages of deployment. Further, increased scrutiny of radiation doses from CT and nuclear methods, as well as uncertainty regarding and the need for intravenous contrast must be kept in mind, given concerns regarding radiation, carcinogenesis, and renal toxicity. Dedicated PET imaging of small body areas or with positron-sensitive probes and imaging systems, PET-guided biopsies, and more sophisticated quantitation will likely evolve as important. Rapid readout of treatment response to adapt the therapies is expected to have a major role in cancer treatments. New PET tracers, many discussed in this text, will be applied more broadly in research and clinical practice. The realities of health care expenses and real limitations in the resources society can devote to health care spending may be greater limitations than the technologies we can develop.

I am confident the readers will find this text a valuable resource. My co-authors and I have tried to provide a comprehensive, but not exhaustive, clinically focused text that presents sufficiently detailed basic science information for understanding the key aspects of the major clinical and research applications of PET and PET/CT. I would particularly like to thank Dr. Rob Beanlands, who served as the Associate Editor on the updated section on cardiac PET and PET/CT imaging. The efforts of Julia W. Buchanan in providing thoughtful editing of many of the chapters are also greatly appreciated. In addition, the support and encouragement of Kerry Barrett of Lippincott Williams & Wilkins was essential to completing this comprehensive text.

Hopefully, you will keep this book near your PET/CT reading workstation and refer to it often in the coming years. It should, like the first edition, serve as a useful starting point and reference tool for your clinical or research work.

Richard L. Wahl, MD

PREFACE TO THE FIRST EDITION

Our purpose in writing this book is to present a comprehensive guide to how positron emission tomography (PET) works, but more critically, how to use PET to enhance the care of patients. The basic principles of the technique are presented first and discuss how PET radionuclides are produced and incorporated into useful compounds to measure a specific molecular process *in vivo*. Once in the human body, these compounds are detected with specialized and ever-evolving equipment, such as PET/CT scanners. Quantification of PET data requires sophisticated processing of the data sets to produce the displayed images. While much of the focus of the book is clinical, research applications of PET across a wide range of organ systems are also presented.

For nearly 20 years, PET was a potent research tool, but it was available only at select academic institutions. Large teams of investigators from diverse disciplines were needed to handle the complexities involved in the production of short-lived isotopes with balky cyclotrons, the performance of rapid radiochemistry to generate suitable human tracers, and to produce and analyze the often "fuzzy" images resulting from these efforts. Several scans a week represented a "busy" PET operation. The possibility that the "complex" PET technique could become a routine diagnostic method throughout the world by the turn of the century seemed exceedingly unlikely in the late 1970s and early 1980s. However, through the persistence of many investigators and advances in computer technology, cyclotrons, and chemistry are now computer-controlled and substantially automated. Instead of an entire floor of computers that was required to process images, now a single small console sitting on a desk does the task. A single outpatient PET scanner can now perform 10 to 20 scans per day, and scanners are becoming faster.

In the late 1980s, it became apparent that the PET technique and 2-[^{18}F]-fluoro-2-deoxy-D-glucose (FDG) had huge clinical potential. Pilot studies in animals and humans showed FDG PET's ability to image lung, breast, and other cancers—in addition to its known ability to image function in the brain and heart. By the mid 1990s, it became clear to those working with PET that it was clinically effective, but its dissemination was delayed largely due to concerns about health care costs and the prevailing enthusiasm for CT and magnetic resonance imaging (MRI) at that time. Compelling scientific data, reimbursement for PET, involvement of large medical equipment manufacturers in PET, and acceptance of PET by referring physicians due to the excellent clinical results have moved the field rapidly forward in the last few years.

Nearly 5 years before the publication of this book, we felt there was a very large gap in the PET literature and saw a critical need for a textbook that would provide a comprehensive guide to the rapidly evolving field of PET, from the fundamental physics and chemistry, to details on how to implement and interpret clinical PET images.

PET is used to study most organ systems of the body and has contributed to our understanding of the basic physiology and pathophysiology of oncological disorders, the brain, the heart, and other organ systems. PET is also playing a major role in the development of new stable (nonradioactive) drugs and is an ideal tool to image phenotypic alterations resulting from the altered genotype. To date, the greatest application of PET in routine clinical studies has been in patients with cancer, where PET images functional alterations caused by molecular changes in contrast to the traditional anatomic methods of imaging cancer like CT.

The increased metabolism of malignant cells makes it possible to image a wide variety of tumors with the glucose analog, FDG. In this book we have chosen authors who have made major contributions in establishing FDG PET as an accurate, sensitive, and useful technique for evaluating and monitoring patients with numerous types of cancer. The validation of the clinical findings, combined with the current speed at which a study, can be completed and the fact that third-party payers will now provide reimbursement for many studies, has made FDG PET a modality that medical centers cannot be without. The recent addition of PET/CT is further adding to the refinement of these studies by combining precise fusion of anatomic information with the molecular image data as "anatomolecular" images. Referring physicians can quickly relate to images that fuse form and function, and they now routinely wish to have PET or PET/CT to enhance the care for their patients. A variety of other PET radiotracers are discussed, which will further expand the use of clinical PET beyond FDG.

At present, PET is the most rapidly growing area of medical imaging because of its considerable power, and it has now reached a new plateau of widespread, worldwide distribution. We hope this book, which reviews all aspects of PET, will serve as a useful starting point and reference tool to all who use PET in their clinical or research work.

Richard L. Wahl
Julia W. Buchanan

PRINCIPLES AND PRACTICE OF PET AND PET/CT

SECOND EDITION

Production of Radionuclides for PET

RONALD D. FINN AND DAVID J. SCHLYER

Coupled with the advancement in noninvasive cross-sectional imaging techniques to identify structural alterations in diseased tissues, there have been significant advances in the development of *in vivo* methods to quantify functional metabolism in both normal and diseased tissues. Positron emission tomography (PET) is an imaging modality that yields physiologic information necessary for clinical diagnoses based on altered tissue metabolism.

One of the most widely recognized advantages of PET is the use of the positron-emitting biologic radiotracers (carbon-11 [^{11}C], oxygen-15 [^{15}O], nitrogen-13 [^{13}N], and fluorine-18 [^{18}F]) that mimic natural substrates. These radionuclides have well-documented nuclear reaction cross sections appropriate for "baby" cyclotron energies, and the corresponding "hot atom" target chemistries are reasonably well understood. A disadvantage these biologic radionuclides possess is their relatively short half-lives, which means they cannot be transported to sites at great distances from the production facility.

Currently, there are four PET drugs officially recognized by the U.S. Food and Drug Administration (FDA) and approved for intravenous injection. They are sodium fluoride (^{18}F) (previously FDA approved and currently United States Pharmacopeia [USP] listed), rubidium-82-chloride (^{82}Rb), ^{13}N-ammonia and fluorodeoxyglucose (^{18}F-FDG). In 1972, ^{18}F (New Drug Application [NDA] 17-042) was approved as an NDA for bone imaging to define areas of altered osteogenic activity, but the manufacturer ceased marketing this product in 1975. Rubidium-82-chloride (NDA 19-414) was approved in 1989 and is indicated for assessment of regional myocardial perfusion in the diagnosis and localization of myocardial infarction. Most recently, ^{18}F-FDG (NDA 20-306) was recognized in 1994 for identification of regions of abnormal glucose metabolism initially associated with foci of epileptic seizures, but it is now mostly used and approved for its application to various primary and metastatic malignant diseases (1). Nitrogen-13-ammonia is approved for assessment of myocardial blood flow.

Over the past few decades, PET studies with radiolabeled drugs have provided new information on drug uptake, biodistribution, and various kinetic relationships. A critique on the design and development of PET radiopharmaceuticals has been published (2), as well as several articles involving the future of PET in drug research and development and the production targetry available from various manufacturers of cyclotrons (3). Growth in clinical PET applications has led to increased interest in and demand for new PET radiopharmaceuticals.

PRODUCTION

Definition of Nuclear Reaction Cross Section

A nuclear reaction is one in which a nuclear particle is absorbed into a target nucleus, resulting in a very short-lived compound nucleus. This excited nucleus will decompose along several pathways and produce various products. A wide variety of nuclear reactions are used in an accelerator to produce artificial radioactivity. The bombarding particles are usually protons, deuterons, or helium particles. The energies used range from a few million electron volts to hundreds of million electron volts. One of the most useful models for nuclear reactions is the compound nucleus model originally introduced by Bohr in 1936. In this model, the incident particle is absorbed into the nucleus of the target material and the energy is distributed throughout the compound nucleus. In essence, the nucleus comes to some form of equilibrium before decomposing and then emitting particles. These two steps are considered to be independent of each other. Regardless of how the compound nucleus got to the high-energy state, the decay of the radionuclide will be independent of the way in which it was formed. The total amount of excitation energy contained in the nucleus will be given by the following equation:

$$U = \frac{M_A}{M_A + M_a} T_a + S_a$$

where U equals excitation energy, M_A equals the mass of the target nucleus, M_a equals the mass of the incident particle, T_a equals kinetic energy of the incident particle, and S_a equals the binding

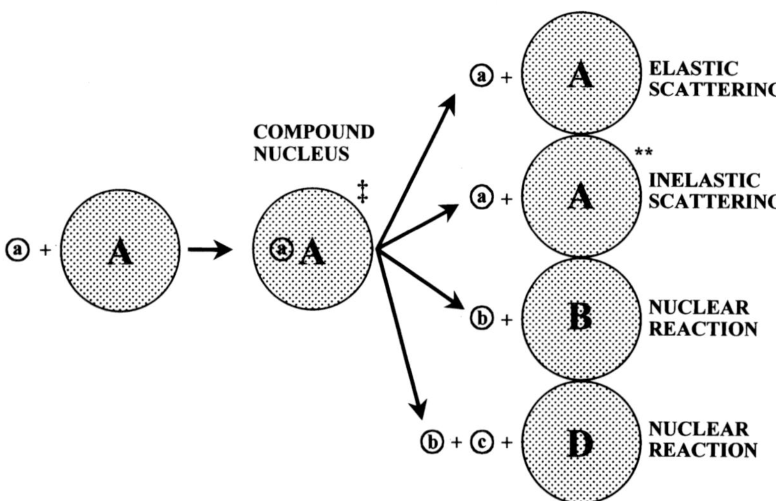

FIGURE 1.1. Formation and disintegration of the compound nucleus.

energy of the incident particle in the compound nucleus. The nucleus can decompose along several channels, as shown in Fig. 1.1.

When the compound nucleus decomposes, the kinetic energy of all the products may be either greater or less than the total kinetic energy of all the reactants. If the energy of the products is greater, the reaction is said to be exoergic. If the kinetic energy of the products is less than that of the reactants, the reaction is said to be endoergic. The magnitude of this difference is called the Q *value*. If the reaction is exoergic, Q values are positive. An energy-level diagram of a typical reaction is shown in Fig. 1.2.

The nuclear reaction cross section represents the total probability that a compound nucleus will be formed and that it will decompose in a particular channel. There is a minimum energy below which a nuclear reaction will not occur except by tunneling effects. The incident particle energy must be sufficient to overcome the coulomb barrier and to overcome a negative Q value of the reaction. Particles with energies below this barrier have a very low probability of reacting. The energy required to induce a nuclear reaction increases as the Z of the target material increases. For many low-Z materials it is possible to use a low-energy accelerator, but for high-Z materials it is necessary to increase the particle energy (4).

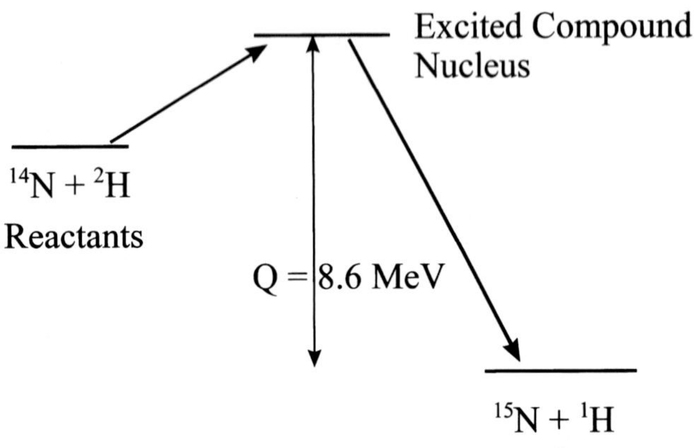

FIGURE 1.2. Energy level diagram for a nuclear reaction. The Q value is the difference in the energy levels of the reactants and the products.

The following relationship (4) gives the number of reactions occurring in 1 second:

$$dn = I_0 N_A ds\sigma_{ab}$$

where dn is the number of reactions occurring in 1 second, I_0 is the number of particles incident on the target in 1 second, N_A is the number of target nuclei per gram, ds is the thickness of the material in grams per centimeter squared, and σ_{ab} is the parameter called the cross section expressed in units of centimeters squared. In practical applications, the thickness ds of the material can be represented by a slab of thickness Δs thin enough that the cross section can be considered as constant. N_A ds are then the number of target atoms in a 1-cm^2 area of thickness Δs. If the target material is a compound, rather than a pure element, then the number of nuclei per unit area is given by the following expression:

$$N_A = \frac{F_A C \Im}{A_A}$$

where N_A is the number of target nuclei per gram, F_A is the fractional isotopic abundance, C is the concentration in weight, $\Im$ is the Avogadro number, and A_A is the atomic mass number of nucleus A.

This leads to one of the basic facts of life in radioisotope production. It is not always possible to eliminate the radionuclidic impurities even with the highest isotopic enrichment and the widest energy selection. An example of this is given in Fig. 1.3 for the production of iodine-123 (^{123}I) with a minimum of iodine-124 (^{124}I) impurity (5–8).

As can be seen from Fig. 1.3, it is not possible to eliminate the ^{124}I impurity completely during the ^{123}I production since the ^{124}I is being concurrently formed at the same energy. To minimize the ^{124}I impurity, irradiation of the target at an energy where the production of ^{124}I is near a minimum becomes an option. In this case a proton energy higher than 20 MeV will give a minimum of ^{124}I impurity.

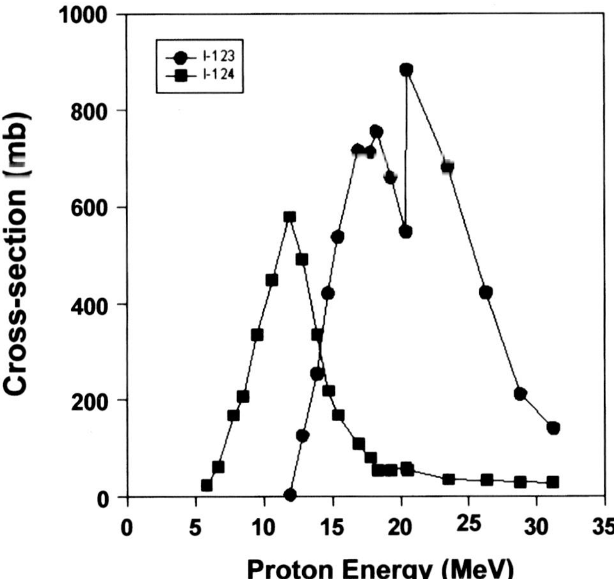

FIGURE 1.3. Plot of yield from the $^{124}Te(p,n)^{124}I$ and the $^{124}Te(p,2n)^{123}I$ nuclear reactions as a function of energy on target.

Enriched Targets

Although they generally play a supplementary role to the applications in the production of radionuclides, stable isotopically labeled compounds find widespread use in pharmacologic and toxicologic investigations. Their use as internal standards in such sensitive and specific analytical techniques as gas chromatography-mass spectroscopy and high-pressure liquid chromatography coupled with mass spectroscopy is of great benefit in the assay of body fluids. Paramagnetic stable nuclides such as carbon-13 (^{13}C) offer opportunities for nuclear magnetic resonance (NMR) analyses of biological samples and possibly whole-body NMR in metabolic studies (9–11).

Stable isotopes have for many years been the foundation for the production of radionuclides when pure radionuclides are necessary. Since the invention of the "cyclotron" by Professor E.O. Lawrence in 1929 and proof of acceleration by M.S. Livingston in 1931, the accelerators have provided unique radionuclides for numerous applications.

In the past decade there has been a significant increase in the acquisition and use of "small" cyclotrons devoted principally to operation by chemists for the production of the biomedically useful radiolabeled compounds or radiopharmaceuticals. The primary impetus has been the acceptance of the potential of PET as a dynamic molecular imaging technique applicable to clinical diagnoses while providing the opportunity to evaluate novel radiotracers and radioligands for monitoring *in vivo* biochemical or physiologic processes with exquisite sensitivity.

Concurrent with the growth of PET/cyclotron facilities has been an emphasis on the production of larger amounts of the short-lived radionuclides in a chemical form suitable for efficient synthetic application. The radionuclidic purity of the final nuclide is an important concern. Targetry and target chemistry continue to be factors for the synthetic chemist's consideration and appreciation of material science and radiation chemistry effects.

With energy constraints imposed by the various accelerators chosen for installation in imaging facilities, the availability and the application of stable enriched target materials for the production of the biologically equivalent radionuclides is of paramount concern. The calutrons at Oak Ridge National Laboratory are no longer in service to prepare and provide the numerous stable enriched nuclides needed for the variety of radionuclides being evaluated for clinical applications. These concerns still plague many investigators who have experienced the lack of or shortages in availability of such important target materials. A current example involves $H_2{}^{18}O$ for ^{18}F production. The $H_2{}^{18}O$ target is the choice of most centers for the production of ^{18}F-labeled fluoride anion used in most ^{18}F-labeled radiopharmaceutical production (12,13). Fortunately, other sources have come forward to provide the $H_2{}^{18}O$ target as use of ^{18}F has increased.

TARGETS AND IRRADIATION

Traditional PET Radioisotopes

There are four positron-emitting radioisotopes that are considered the biologic tracers and their clinical and investigational uses are extensive. The radionuclides are ^{18}F, ^{11}C, ^{13}N, and ^{15}O. The reason these are so commonly used is that they can be easily substituted directly onto biomolecules. Carbon-11, ^{13}N, and ^{15}O are the "elements of life." Substitution of ^{11}C for carbon-12 (^{12}C) does not significantly alter the reaction time or mechanisms of a molecule. A similar situation exists for ^{13}N and ^{15}O. Fluorine-18 can often be substituted for a hydroxy group in a molecule or placed in a position where its presence does not significantly alter the biological behavior of the molecule. When the nucleus decays, the positron emitted will slow to thermal energies and annihilate upon interaction with an electron to produce two 511 keV gamma rays emitted at nearly 180 degrees to each other. The decay characteristics of the positron-emitting radionuclides allow the physiologic processes occurring *in vivo* to be quantitated by detectors outside the body. Physiologic modeling can be carried out using this information, and quantitative assessments of the biologic function can be made.

Target Irradiation

The positron-emitting radionuclides are produced during the target irradiation and converted to a synthetic precursor, either in the target or immediately after exiting the target. The precursor is next converted into the molecule of interest. This chapter covers only the targetry and the formation in the target of the chemical compound. The formation of precursors outside the target and the conversion of these precursors to the desired radiotracer are covered in Chapter 2. Most of the targets for the production of the biologic radionuclides have been either gases or liquids, although several solid targets have also been developed.

The number and type of products that are obtained in a target are a function of the irradiation conditions, the mixture of gases or liquids in the target, and the presence of any impurities in the target or gas mixture. Changing the chemical composition or physical state of the target during irradiation can alter the chemical form of the final product (14). These are all results of the "hot atom" chemistry and radiolysis occurring in the target during the irradiation. *Hot atom* is the term used to identify atoms with excessive thermal or kinetic energy or electronic excitation. When an atom undergoes a nuclear transformation, it usually has a great deal of excess energy imparted from the incident bombarding particle and perhaps from the nuclear reaction. This energy can be manifested in any or all of the normal modes of excitation, including rotational, translational, or electronic. In nearly all cases, the amount of energy present is sufficient to break all the existing chemical bonds to the atom and to send the newly transformed atom off with high kinetic energy. This energy is called the recoil energy, and as the atom slows down, it imparts this energy to the surrounding environment. After the atom has transferred most of its excess energy to the surroundings and slowed to near thermal energies, it usually reacts chemically with the surroundings to form a compound. This compound may be stabilized or may undergo further reactions to form other chemical products.

Several distinguishing characteristics set these types of reactions apart from other chemical reactions. These include reactions that are (a) insensitive to the temperature of the surroundings, (b) independent of the phase of the reaction, (c) dependent on the radical scavengers present in the medium, and (d) dependent on moderators in the medium, such as inert gases (15). There have been several excellent reviews concerning the topic of hot atom chemistry (16–18).

Specific Activity

Another topic of importance in the preparation of radioisotopes is that of specific activity. It is important in several applications, and particularly important in PET, where the radionuclide is incorporated into a radiotracer that is used to probe some physiologic process in which very small amounts of the biomolecule are being used. PET is basically a tracer method, and the goal of the PET experiment is to probe the physiologic process without perturbing that process. If the amount of radiotracer is very small in comparison to the amount of the native compound or its competitor, then the process will be perturbed very little. When carrying out studies such as probing the number of receptors or probing the concentration of an enzyme, either of which may be present in very small quantities, these considerations become even more important (19).

The usual way to express the concept of specific activity is in terms of the amount of radioactivity per mole of compound. There is, of course, an ultimate limit, which occurs only when the radioactive atoms or radiolabeled molecules exist. Table 1.1 lists the characteristics of the PET radionuclides presented in this chapter (20).

As an example, typical specific activities for ^{11}C-labeled molecules being reported are on the order of 10 Ci/μmol (370 GBq/μmol). Therefore, it can be appreciated that only 1 in 1,000 of the radiotracer molecules is actually labeled with ^{11}C. The rest contain stable ^{12}C. The specific activity is important in probing areas such as receptor binding, enzyme reaction, gene expression, and, in some settings, antigen binding with radiolabeled monoclonal antibodies.

In the area of monoclonal antibody labeling, there is the problem of the incorporation of the label into the molecule. If there is excessive carrier, then a smaller amount of the radiolabel will be incorporated into the molecule. This means that a diagnostic radioisotope may be more difficult to visualize or the dose of a therapeutic radioisotope to the target organ may be less than could be achieved. In addition, too many substitutions on the antibody molecule may reduce its immunological functionality. The specific activity of other PET tracers has been explored extensively. Some recent issues are the specific activity of radiotracers produced from the stable species (21), bromine-76 (^{76}Br) (22), and ^{13}N-labeled ammonia (23).

The radionuclide on which more effort has been expended in attempts to control specific activity is ^{11}C, and we use it here as an example of the things that may be done to maximize the specific activity. Carbon-11 is a challenging radioisotope for achieving high specific activity because carbon is so ubiquitous in the environment. There can never be a truly carrier-free radiotracer labeled with ^{11}C, but only one in which no carrier carbon has been added and steps have been taken to minimize the amount of carbon that can enter the synthesis from outside sources. There can never be less carbon incorporated into the molecule than there is carbon present in the target during the irradiation to produce ^{11}C. It is critical to use the highest possible purity of nitrogen gas in the target and to ensure that the target is absolutely as gas tight as possible.

The walls of the target can also influence the specific activity because many alloys used to fabricate targets contain traces of carbon from the manufacturing process. During irradiation, these traces of carbon can make their way out of the target walls and into the gas phase where they will be incorporated into the final product. A correlation between the target surface area and the mass of carbon introduced into the synthesis has been observed and documented (24,25). Solvents used to clean the metal surfaces or oils left

TABLE 1.1 Decay Characteristics for Specific PET Radionuclides

Nuclide	Half-life (min)	Decay Mode	Maximum Energy	Mean Energy	Maximum Range in Water	Maximum Specific Activity (theoretical)
Carbon-11	20.4	100% β^+	0.96 MeV	0.386 MeV	4.1 mm	9,220 Ci/μmol
Nitrogen-13	9.98	100% β^+	1.19 MeV	0.492 MeV	5.4 mm	18,900 Ci/μmol
Oxygen-15	2.03	100% β^+	1.7 MeV	0.735 MeV	8.0 mm	91,730 Ci/μmol
Fluorine-18	109.8	97% β^+	0.69 MeV	0.250 MeV	2.4 mm	1,710 Ci/μmol
Copper-62	9.74	99.7% β^+	2.93 MeV	1.314 MeV	14.3 mm	19,310 Ci/μmol
Gallium-68	68.0	89% β^+	1.9 MeV	0.829 MeV	9.0 mm	2,766 Ci/μmol
Bromide-75	96.0	75.5% β^+	1.74 MeV	0.750 MeV	8.2 mm	1,960 Ci/μmol
Rubidium-82	1.25	95.5% β^+	3.36 MeV	1.5 MeV	16.5 mm	150,400 Ci/μmol
Iodine-122	3.62	75.8% β^+	3.12 MeV	1.4 MeV	15.3 mm	51,950 Ci/μmol
Iodine-124	6019.2	23.3% β^+	2.13 MeV	0.8 MeV	10.2 mm	31 Ci/μmmol

over from the fabrication process can also serve as sources for carbon in the targets. The input and output lines can also have the same or similar contaminants, and such equipment as valves, connectors, insulators, regulators, and flow controllers all can contribute to the carrier carbon, and care must be taken to minimize the carbon added from these sources.

All the chemical reagents used in the synthesis may also add carrier carbon and must be scrutinized to minimize this contribution.

Fluorine-18

Fluorine-18 has a 109.8-minute half-life and decays 97% by positron emission. The other 3% is by electron capture. It forms very strong covalent bonds with carbon compounds and can be incorporated into a wide variety of organic molecules. It can be substituted for a hydroxy group, as in the case of deoxyglucose, or can be substituted for a hydrogen atom. The van der Waals radius of the fluorine atom is similar to that of the hydrogen atom; therefore, substitution of fluorine for hydrogen causes very little steric alteration of the molecule. The concern with the fluorine for hydrogen substitution is that the electronegative nature of fluorine can alter the electron distribution in a way that will alter the binding properties of a molecule. In some ways, however, fluorine is the most attractive of the four positron emitters commonly used in organic synthesis. The low energy of the positron gives the highest potential resolution for PET imaging. The range of the positrons with average energy in water is much less than 2 mm. The nearly 2-hour half-life allows for a more complex synthesis to be carried out within the decay time of the radioisotope. The electronic perturbation has also sometimes resulted in a molecule that has more physiologically desirable properties than the original compound.

The most widely used radiotracer in PET by far is 2-[^{18}F]-fluoro-2-deoxyglucose (^{18}FDG). It has proven to be of great utility in the measurement of the "rate" of glycolytic metabolism in a wide variety of organs and disease states in humans.

Production Reactions for Fluorine-18

There are a number of nuclear reactions that can be used to produce ^{18}F. The major routes are the ^{18}O(p,n)^{18}F reaction (26), usually carried out on oxygen-18 (^{18}O)-enriched water or oxygen gas, and the ^{20}Ne(d,α)^{18}F reaction (27). A number of other reactions are being used, but these two are the principal routes to ^{18}F.

The cross sections for these reactions have been explored extensively and the values are well characterized. The most common reaction in routine applications is the proton reaction on enriched ^{18}O. The yield is significantly higher than the other reactions, and the availability of low-energy proton accelerators has made this the reaction of choice, even in the face of the cost of the enriched ^{18}O target material. The other common reaction, particularly for the production of electrophilic fluorine, is the ^{20}Ne(d,α)^{18}F reaction on natural neon. The yield from this reaction is substantially less, but the ability to add other chemical constituents and the natural abundance of the target material are advantages (28–30).

Targetry for Fluorine-18

The number and types of targets that have been designed and fabricated for the production of ^{18}F are very large. There have been several reviews of the types of targets (28–32). For descriptive purposes, the targets can be divided into three basic categories: (a) the gas target primarily used for the production of electrophilic fluorine, (b) the liquid target, usually used for production of ^{18}F-fluoride, and (c) the solid targets, which are not commonly used for the production of ^{18}F.

For gaseous targets, there are two basic considerations. The first is the neon gas target. This target was used for many years for the production of F_2^{18}F from the ^{20}Ne(d,α)^{18}F reaction (27,28). In this target, a small amount of fluorine gas, typically 0.1% to 0.2%, is added to the neon gas before irradiation. The design of the target has undergone significant changes from the first targets to the current design. Early targets were made of nickel or nickel alloys. The reason for this choice was because it was known that nickel parts would withstand a fluorine atmosphere, and most fluorine handling systems were made from nickel or alloys such as Inconel or Monel (Special Metals Corp, Huntington, West Virginia), which have a high nickel content. It was later shown that any surface that could be passivated by fluorine could be used in the fluorine target (33). This discovery introduced the possibility of using aluminum target bodies for the production of elemental fluorine. The activation properties of aluminum are vastly superior to those of nickel or steel in terms of avoidance of the long-lived activities, which are produced within the target body during the bombardment. Target bodies constructed of aluminum significantly reduce the radiation dose received by the technical staff during the cleaning and maintenance of the target. A more extensive investigation of the properties of the surface has been made (30,34). It was shown that aluminum, copper, and nickel form fluoride layers and therefore passivate. The metal surfaces may also contain oxide layers. Only gold does not form a fluoride layer. Exposure to air after passivation does not alter the surface layer (33,34).

The direct addition of fluorine to the neon before irradiation was one method for the recovery of the fluorine in elemental form. The other method was developed by Nickles et al. (35) and is called the *two shoot method*. In this method, the fluorine is allowed to stick to the walls of the target during the irradiations and is then removed by creating a plasma containing elemental fluorine, which reacts with the ^{18}F on the walls and brings it into the gas phase. The usual gas for this target is the ^{18}O-enriched O_2 gas. Other methods for converting the ^{18}F in other chemical forms such as hydrogen fluoride (HF) to F_2 outside the target have also been attempted, but with limited success (36,37). In this latter case, the neon or ^{18}O-enriched oxygen gas is irradiated and the fluorine allowed to stick to the walls. In some cases, hydrogen is added to the target gas during irradiation. After irradiation, the target gas is removed, and then the target is heated and flushed with hydrogen to bring the fluorine out in the form of HF (3). The production of other fluorinating intermediates has also been described by using in-target chemistry, but these are not currently in widespread use (38).

A high-energy reaction of protons on neon can also be used in the same way as the deuterons on neon (39,40). The fluorine can be brought out of the target in the form of fluoride ion if the target is washed after irradiation with an aqueous solution (29,31), or the glass liner of the target can be used directly as the reaction vessel (35). In all cases, the fluorine is recovered from the surface in relatively high yields (more than 70%). Whether the protons on ^{18}O or neon, or the deuterons on neon reaction, is used, the result and methodology are essentially the same.

By far the most commonly used target compound for the production of ^{18}F in the form of fluoride ion is the H_2^{18}O target. The basic design is relatively straightforward and similar to most of the targets being used routinely. There are wide variations, however, in

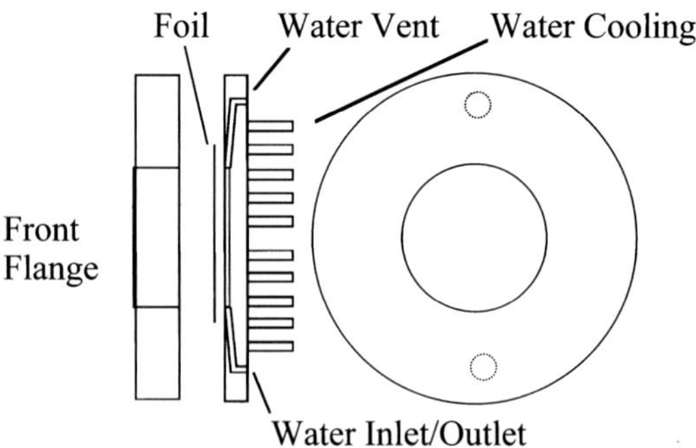

FIGURE 1.4. Typical water target for the production of fluorine-18 from oxygen-18–enriched water.

the details of the design and the construction materials (41–53). The primary constraint is to use as little of the $H_2{}^{18}O$ as possible while leaving enough volume to take maximum advantage of the cross section and to absorb or transfer the heat created by the passage of the beam. A typical target is shown in Fig. 1.4.

There are several considerations in the operation of the target. The first is the fact that the water would boil due to high temperatures generated by irradiation unless the pressure in the target is increased to diminish or inhibit the boiling (54–56). To reduce this problem, the target may be run under elevated pressure of helium, nitrogen, or some other inert gas, or the target may be valved off and allowed to find its own pressure level. In this case, pressure can exceed 40 atm, particularly if the water has not been completely degassed before use. Because a relatively thin foil contains the pressure, there is a limit to the beam current that can be applied in this situation.

The decision to operate at low or high pressure will also have an impact on the target fabrication and the materials chosen for the target. The radiolysis products of the water will have different effects depending on the conditions inside the target. The materials used to construct the target can also have an effect on the chemical reactivity of the fluoride obtained from the target (57–59). If the target is operated at low pressure, there will be some loss of the water out of the beam strike area due to bubble formation (45,54).

There have been some unique designs for the water target using spherical targets (60) or flowing targets (46) or frozen ^{18}O-enriched carbon dioxide targets (61). The helium-3 or α-reaction on natural water has also been used to produce ^{18}F for synthesis (8,62,63). These targets work exactly the same way as the proton on water targets, except that the level of heat deposition is higher with the heavier particles. These targets are not commonly used because the yields are substantially lower.

Radioisotope Separation for Fluorine-18

There are two separate scenarios for recovery of ^{18}F from the target, which depend on the mode of production. In the case of the gas target, the fluorine (with the carrier F_2) is removed from the target as a gas mixture and can be used in the synthesis from there. In the case of the water target, the activity is removed in the aqueous phase. There are two general methods after that. The first is to use the $H_2{}^{18}O$-containing ^{18}F-fluoride ion directly in the synthesis. This method is used by several investigators who have small-volume water targets, and the cost of losing the $H_2{}^{18}O$ is minor compared with the cost of the cyclotron irradiation. The other method is to separate the fluoride from the $H_2{}^{18}O$, either by distillation or by using a resin column (64–66). When the resin is used, it also separates the metal ion impurities from the enriched fluoride solution. This resin purification generally increases the reactivity of the fluoride.

Carbon-11

Carbon-11 has a 20.4-minute half-life and decays 99.8% by positron emission and only 0.2% by electron capture. It decays to stable boron-11. Carbon-11 offers the greatest potential for the synthesis of radiotracers that track specific processes in the body. The short half-life of ^{11}C limits processes that can be adequately studied. The chemical form of ^{11}C can vary depending on the environment during irradiation. The usual chemical forms of ^{11}C obtained directly from the target are carbon dioxide and methane.

Production Reactions for Carbon-11

There are several reactions used to produce ^{11}C. By far the most common reaction is the $^{14}N(p,\alpha)^{11}C$ reaction on nitrogen gas (67,68). This reaction produces a high yield of ^{11}C, and with the addition of trace amounts of oxygen, ^{11}C is almost exclusively in the chemical form of carbon dioxide.

Targetry for Carbon-11

Carbon-11 targets can be either gases or solids. The basic design of the gas target has not changed a great deal since the first targets were developed (69,70). The basic body design is an aluminum cylinder, which can be held at a high enough pressure to stop the beam or at least degrade the energy below the threshold of the reaction being used. A typical gas target is shown in Fig. 1.5.

The choice of aluminum for the target body is a result of its excellent activation properties. The activation products are produced in relatively small amounts or have a short half-life. This aids in the maintenance of the target because the radiation dose to the chemist handling the target is greatly reduced. The usual labeled products from the gas target are carbon dioxide (18,69,71,72) and methane, but other products have been attempted (71–73).

Some recent advances in the design of gaseous targets for the production of ^{11}C are the realization (a) that carrier carbon was being added by the surface of the aluminum (24), (b) that the target was more efficient if it was conical, taking into consideration the

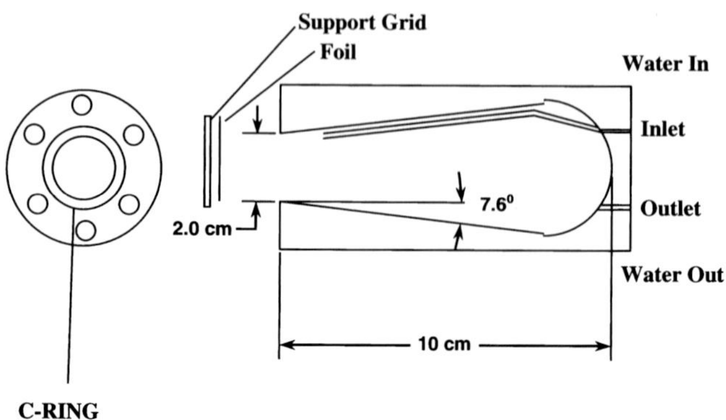

FIGURE 1.5. Typical gas target for the production of radioisotopes from gaseous targets.

fact that the beam was undergoing multiple scattering through the foil window and in the gas (74,75), and (c) that the density of the gas was significantly reduced at high beam currents (76–78).

The foil material used on these targets is also important for several reasons. If the beam energy is high enough, a relatively thick aluminum foil may be used to contain the gas. If the beam energy is lower, then a thinner foil must be used and aluminum does not have sufficient tensile strength to withstand the pressures that are built up inside the target during irradiation. In this case, a thin foil of Havar (Goodfellow Cambridge Ltd, Huntingdon, England) or other high-tensile strength material can be used to withstand the pressures. It is also possible to place grids across the foils to increase the burst pressure of the foils (79,80).

Some solid targets have been used for the production of ^{11}C. These are, for the most part, boron oxide either enriched or natural abundance. A typical target for this would be a stepped plate similar to the inclined plane target used for various isotopes. The difference is that here the powder is pressed into the groves of the target plate and irradiated (70). The difficulty of removing the carbon from the matrix in comparison to the ease of separation in the gas target has made the solid target less widely used.

Radioisotope Separation for Carbon-11

The separation of ^{11}C in the gas target is a simple matter, because the ^{11}C is usually in the form of carbon dioxide when it comes out of the target. The nitrogen gas used as the target material is usually inert in chemical reactions, so the target gas can be passed through a solution for reaction. The carbon dioxide can also be removed by trapping, either in a cold trap or on an adsorbent substrate such as molecular sieves. From there, the ^{11}C can be used to produce a wide variety of precursors.

The separation of the carbon dioxide from the solid matrix of the boron oxide is a more difficult problem but can be accomplished under the correct conditions. The target containing the boron oxide is contained in a gas-tight box (70). A sweep gas is passed through the box during irradiation. The beam heating is sufficient to cause the boron oxide to melt and the carbon dioxide is released into the sweep gas. The labeled gas is trapped downstream, and the irradiation is continued until sufficient ^{11}C has been collected for use in the synthesis. The advantage of this type of target is that, once made, it can be used repeatedly without further maintenance.

Nitrogen-13

Nitrogen-13 decays by pure positron emission (100%) to stable ^{13}C. As with ^{11}C, the short half-life of 9.98 minutes somewhat restricts the potential utility of this radionuclide. Several compounds incorporating ^{13}N have been made, but the time for accumulation in the body is short and the physiologic processes that may be studied must be rapid (81,82). By far the most widely used compound of ^{13}N for PET is in the chemical form of ammonia. It is used as a blood-flow tracer and has found utility in cardiac studies to determine areas of ischemic or infarcted tissue.

Production Reactions for Nitrogen-13

Several reactions lead to the production of ^{13}N. The reactions that are commonly used are the $^{13}C(p,n)^{13}N$ reaction (83,84), the $^{12}C(d,n)^{13}N$ reaction (83), and the $^{16}O(p,\alpha)^{13}N$ reaction (85,86).

The proton on ^{13}C reaction has an advantage in that it requires a low-incident proton energy but suffers from the disadvantage of requiring isotopically enriched material. The most common reaction is the $^{16}O(p,\alpha)^{13}N$ reaction on natural water (87–90).

Targetry for Nitrogen-13

The target for the production of ^{13}N can either be solids, liquids, or gases, depending on the chemical form of the nitrogen that is desired. The chemical form can also be changed by a number of other factors such as the dose and dose rate to the target, the pH level of the liquid targets, and the physical state.

The first target for the production of ^{13}N was a solid target of boron that was bombarded by an α-beam by Joliot and Curie (91). Solid targets have been used for the production of ^{13}N, particularly in the form of either nitrogen gas or ammonia (24,92,93). Solids mixed with liquids have also been used, particularly in the production of ammonia (34,94,95). Solid targets of frozen water have also been used to produce ammonia (14).

Liquid targets are by far the most popular and widely used. The reaction of protons on natural water produces nitrate and nitrite ions, which can be converted to ammonia by reduction (82, 87–89,96). The water target can also be used to form ammonia directly with the addition of a reducing agent or with a radical inhibitor (90,97–101). The chemistry involved in the production of the final product distribution in the water target has been a topic of interest and debate (14,87,102,103). It has been found that high-dose irradiation of liquid water results in the formation of oxidized species, while the same irradiation of frozen water maintains the initial distribution of reduced products (14).

Gas targets have also been used, particularly in the production of nitrogen gas, and there have also been attempts to use the gas target for the production of ammonia (17,104,105).

Radioisotope Separation for Nitrogen-13

The separation of the ^{13}N from the solid target is usually accomplished by burning or heating the solids (93,106,107). The water target with no additives usually produces ^{13}N in the chemical form of nitrates and nitrites. The conversion of the nitrogen, nitrates, or nitrites to other chemical forms requires rapid radiopharmaceutical synthesis techniques.

Oxygen-15

Oxygen-15 is the longest lived of the positron-emitting isotopes of oxygen. The half-life is 122 seconds and it decays 99.9% by positron emission. It decays to stable nitrogen-15 (^{15}N). It was one of the first artificial radioisotopes produced with low-energy deuterons using a cyclotron (108). Oxygen-15 is used to label gases for inhalation such as oxygen, carbon dioxide, and carbon monoxide, and it is used to label water for injection. The major purpose of these gases and liquids is to measure the blood flow, blood volume, and oxygen consumption in the body.

Production Reactions for Oxygen-15

There are several reactions for the production of ^{15}O. The most common are the $^{14}N(d,n)^{15}O$ reaction (109–111), the $^{15}N(p,n)^{15}O$ reaction (112), and the $^{16}O(p,pn)^{15}O$ reaction (113). Of these reactions, the ones that are used commonly are the deuterons on natural nitrogen gas, the protons on enriched ^{15}N nitrogen gas, and the protons on natural oxygen when specific activity is not an issue, as in the case of oxygen gas or labeled water.

Targetry for Oxygen-15

The targets for these compounds are, for the most part, gaseous targets. The ^{15}O-containing compound can be made either directly in the target (114–116) or outside the target in a separate recovery module. The gas targets are usually nitrogen gas bombarded with either protons or deuterons, depending on the accelerator characteristics.

Solid targets have been explored as a source for producing ^{15}O-ozone (117). In this target, irradiating quartz microfibers and allowing the nucleogenic atoms that exit the fibers to react with the surrounding gas produces the ^{15}O.

Radioisotope Separation for Oxygen-15

The radioisotopes can be separated or, in some circumstances, the target gas can be used with a minimum of processing (113,118,119). An example of this is the production of $H_2{}^{15}O$. It can be made directly in the target by adding 5% hydrogen to the nitrogen gas in the target (114). In this case, the water is produced directly. Ammonia is concurrently produced in the target as a radiolytic product of the nitrogen and hydrogen, and it must be removed. The other option is to produce ^{15}O-labeled oxygen gas in the target and then process it to water outside the target. The water has also been produced by bombarding water using the $^{16}O(p,pn)^{15}O$ reaction with a final cleanup on an ion-exchange column (120).

Novel Solid Targets for PET Radiopharmaceutical Preparation

The most well-known medical application of cyclotrons is the production of radionuclides for diagnostic studies applied to nuclear medicine and the nuclear sciences. Yields of most of the medically used radionuclides produced with cyclotrons using various nuclear reactions and energies have been reported (32,121–123).

The increasing amount of clinically relevant data available from PET studies involving the biologic tracers has contributed to the expanding interest in additional positron-emitting radionuclides for both basic research studies and additional clinical applications. The spectrum of physiologic processes that could potentially be studied grows as the number of "alternative" positron-emitting radionuclides that can be prepared increases (121). With the introduction of the new generation of cyclotrons that are capable of delivering hundreds of microamperes of beam current, the potential for increased amounts of numerous radionuclides can no longer be considered limited by the beam fluence, but rather by the optimal thermal performance of the particular target materials and target backings. This is particularly true in the case of the cooling-water/target-backing interface and beam profile considerations for solid target stations now becoming available on some of the "baby" cyclotrons.

Iodine-124, a radionuclide that has potential for both diagnostic and therapeutic applications, is an important example. This nuclide was often viewed as an unwanted radionuclidic impurity in the production of ^{123}I from the energetic proton irradiation of tellurium targets at cyclotron facilities engaged in the commercial production of ^{123}I. Iodine-124 has a half-life of 4.18 days and decays by positron emission (23.3%) and electron capture (76.7%). Although several nuclear reactions have been suggested for its production, the precise measurement of the excitation function for the $^{124}Te(p,n)^{124}I$ reaction indicates its suitability for use on low-energy cyclotrons (124,125). A detailed preparation of this radionuclide via the $^{124}Te(p,n)^{124}I$ nuclear reaction using low-energy cyclotrons has recently been published (126). It uses a reusable target composed of windowless aluminum oxide and an enriched tellurium-124 oxide solid solution matrix. The radioiodide is effectively recovered using a dry distillation process with the volatile iodine species being trapped on a thin Pyrex glass tube coated with a minute amount of sodium hydroxide. Although recovery of the radioiodine from the tube was nearly quantitative, the recovery of the radioiodine from the target was somewhat less (65% to 75%) and appears to be a function of the crystal structure of the tellurium oxide that was irradiated (126).

Another element within the halogen family that possesses several radioisotopes of potential clinical use is bromine. In particular, bromine-75 (^{75}Br) ($t_{1/2}$ = 1.6 hours, $I_{\beta+}$ = 75.5%, $E_{\beta+}$ = 1.74 MeV) has several nuclear reactions reported for its production, but only the proton irradiation processes appear suitable for medium-energy cyclotrons (more than 25 MeV) (i.e., $^{76}Se[p,2n]^{75}Br$). The major impurity associated with the proton process is ^{76}Br. The optimal production conditions for ^{75}Br proton irradiation of enriched selenium-76 (^{76}Se) targets used an incident energy of 30 MeV degraded within the target to 22 MeV and had a reported production rate of ^{75}Br of 100 μCi/μA, with an impurity level for the ^{76}Br reported at 0.9% (127). Several selenides such as those of silver or copper have been found as suitable targets for irradiation at low-beam currents (128,129), and an external rotating target system was reported for preparation of radiobromine from the low melting elemental selenium target (130). Losses of ^{76}Se were approximately 1% after a 1-hour irradiation period at 20 μA for this target system.

As in the case of radioiodine, the separation of the radiobromine from the ^{76}Se-irradiated target material was effected by thermochromographic evolution at 300°C, followed by dissolution of the bromine in a small volume of hot water. The radiochemical yield for the overall process was not exceedingly high, and this as well as the difficulties associated with targetry using highly enriched selenium nuclides may be part of the reason that the application of this procedure for the preparation of ^{75}Br is not more widely employed.

The more widely used method for the production of ^{75}Br requires the acceleration of helium-3 particles of energies, nominally 36 MeV, onto arsenic target materials (131,132). Bromine positron emitters may become more important for PET imaging over the coming years.

The radioisotopes of copper are also finding application in imaging and radiotherapy. Copper-61 (^{61}Cu) has a 3.4-hour half-life and decays 61% of the time with a 1.2 MeV end point energy positron. The other decay mode is electron capture, which results in gamma rays predominately at 283 and 656 keV (133). The production route is through a proton reaction on nickel-61 (134) or an α-reaction on cobalt-59 (135). The proton reaction has a reasonable nuclear reaction cross section. The only drawback is that the isotopically enriched nickel-61 has a 1.1% natural abundance and therefore can be somewhat expensive. There is also a proton reaction on natural zinc, which has been used to produce copper-61 (136).

Copper-64 (^{64}Cu) is a unique radionuclide as it decays with a 12.7-hour half-life by electron capture (44%), positron emission (17%), and β-emission (39%). Thus Cu-64 can be imaged by positron emission tomography in addition to having therapeutic potential associated with its β-particles. Copper-64 has become of great interest in the past few years as a potential PET tracer because of its half-life, because it is a positron emitter, and because it can be incorporated into complex molecules through chelating chemistry

TABLE 1.2 Examples of Generators Yielding Positron-Emitting Daughter Radionuclides of Clinical Interest

Parent (half-life)	Decay Mode (%)	Daughter (half-life)	Decay Mode (%)	Characteristic Gamma Energy (%)
Strontium-82 (25 d)	EC (100)	Rubidium-82 (76 sec)	β^+(96), EC (4)	0.78 MeV (9)
Germanium-68(278 d)	EC (100)	Gallium-68 (68 min)	β^+(88), EC (12)	1.078 (3.5)
Zinc-62 (9.13 hr)	β^+(18), EC (82)	Copper-62 (9.8 min)	β^+(98)	1.17 (0.5)
Xenon-122 (20.1 hr)	EC (100)	Iodine-122 (3.6 min)	β^+(77), EC (23)	0.56 (18.4)

previously developed for ^{67}Cu. The chemistry continues to be developed because the original cages were not capable of holding the copper in place *in vivo*. Smith (137) provides an extensive review of the production and use of ^{64}Cu with an excellent bibliography.

The direct (p,n) reaction on highly enriched nickel-64 leads to large amounts of no carrier added (NCA) ^{64}Cu (134,138,139). A relatively high current target has been produced by electroplating enriched target material on a water-cooled gold backing (140). After irradiation the target material is dissolved off the target holder in hydrochloric acid (HCl) and then placed on an anion exchange column. The nickel fraction is eluted with 6.0 N HCl and the copper radioisotopes are eluted with water (138). Alternatively mixtures of ethanol and HCl may be used to separate ^{64}Cu from an enriched nickel target (139). The use of this target system leads to the coproduction of ^{61}Co contaminant, which can also be removed via anion exchange chromatography with ethanol/HCl mixtures (139). Enriched ^{64}Ni is very expensive due to its naturally occurring low abundance (0.926%), thus, recycling of the target material is necessary, which is relatively simple with these methods.

Generator-Produced Positron-Emitting Radionuclides

The molybdenum-99/technetium-99m (^{99}Mo/^{99m}Tc) generator remains the dominant source for radionuclide availability in nuclear medicine departments and is usually applied to prepared commercially available kits for radiopharmaceutical formulation. However, the impetus for change caused by the expanded application of PET radiopharmaceutical agents, including the equipment fusion of PET with computed tomography or PET with magnetic resonance imaging tomographs, will ensure the continued growth and radiopharmaceutical development of short-lived positron-emitting diagnostic and potentially therapeutic agents. Generator systems for specific PET radionuclides remain a potential resource for further development of the role of PET.

Radionuclide generator systems consist of a parent radionuclide, usually a relatively long-lived nuclide that decays to a daughter nuclide, itself radioactive but with a shorter half-life. The system requires an efficient technique to separate the daughter nuclide from the parent. Conventionally, the parent is adsorbed onto a solid support and decays by particle emission. A solvent in which the daughter complex is soluble is employed to elute (i.e., separate) the desired radionuclide. Unlike the ^{99}Mo/^{99m}Tc generator developed at Brookhaven National Laboratory (141,142), which revolutionized the practice of nuclear medicine, the generator systems currently being applied to PET studies are still primarily research sources for radiopharmaceutical development.

For those research centers and clinical facilities without the luxury of a cyclotron, several generator systems for production of positron-emitting radionuclides have been proposed. Their production routes have been reviewed (143–148). Of the systems proposed, copper-62 (^{62}Cu), gallium-68 (^{68}Ga), and rubidium-82 (^{82}Rb) radionuclides continue to find applications. The decay characteristics of these three generator systems are included in Table 1.2. A great deal of effort has been expended on the production and construction of these generator systems, including investigations into solid support materials and elution characteristics.

The production routes for the parent radionuclide zinc-62 (^{62}Zn) include the irradiation of a copper disc or copper-electroplated alloy to use the ^{63}Cu(p,2n)^{62}Zn irradiation at an optimal proton energy of 26–21 MeV (149–152). The copper is dissolved in hydrochloric acid and the solution is transferred to an anion-exchange resin column (AG 1 × 8, 100 to 200 mesh, Cl^- form). Copper is effectively eluted from the resin with 3 M HCl, and ^{62}Zn is eluted effectively with water. After evaporation to dryness, the zinc is dissolved in 2 M HCl and adsorbed onto an anion-exchange column for periodic elution of the ^{62}Cu. Alternative routes to the preparation of the ^{62}Zn via irradiation of enriched nickel targets or zinc targets have been proposed but have found only limited application (153–155).

Gallium-68 is used to assess blood-brain barrier integrity, as well as tumor localization. It is widely used as a source for the attenuation correction of most PET scanners. The parent germanium-68 is long-lived ($t_{1/2}$ = 271 days), and its production is generally not attempted on medium-energy accelerators due to the low production yields (156,157). The primary sources for the parent radionuclide are the spallation processes available at large energy accelerators where parasitic position and operation are available (158,159). The recovery of the germanium-68 involves several multistep chemical processes.

The earlier generator systems provided the gallium product in a complexed form as a result of either using solvent/solvent extraction techniques or chromatographic supports of alumina or antimony oxide. Refinements made to elute the ^{68}Ga in an ionic form were compromised by solubility problems of the oxide in the eluant and therefore slowed the potential for direct clinical use. Many of the limitations of previous chromatographic systems were overcome with the report of a tin oxide/HCl generator (160). The negative pressure generator consisted of tin oxide (0.16 to 0.25 mm in diameter) contained in a glass column (10 mm in diameter) between glass wool plugs atop a sintered glass base. One normal HCl, with flow rate controlled by a valve at the base of the column, serves as eluant. Results indicate a radiochemical yield approaching 80% in roughly 2 minutes using 5 mL of eluant. The generator performance remains high in spite of accumulated dose delivered to the solid support.

There are two types of chromatographic nuclide generator systems: positive or negative pressure. As is customary in all systems, the parent is adsorbed onto a column support, commonly an organic exchanger or mineral exchanger, which is contained within a borosilicate glass cylinder. The ends of the cylinder are terminated with a filter to ensure that a minimum of particulate materials are eluted from the column and that terminal sterilization by filtration will be possible if the radionuclide is to be used without further modification.

As the half-lives of the daughter nuclides become shorter, the opportunity for chemical manipulation before clinical administration is reduced to such an extent that the eluant must be physiologically acceptable, and quality assurance for parent breakthrough or exchanger breakdown becomes increasingly important. The column is housed within a lead or tungsten shield for radiation protection of the personnel using the system. For efficient elution, attempts are made to minimize both the number of fittings and joints involved in preparing the system and the internal diameter and overall length of the cylindrical tubing.

Rubidium-82 is a myocardial blood-flow agent that has found clinical application. The application of ^{82}Rb-chloride in the diagnosis of ischemic heart disease and location of myocardial infarcts is an active area of application for this generator system (161). The short half-life (1.27 minutes) of ^{82}Rb and its similarity to potassium in biologic transport and distribution suggest that this generator-produced radionuclide might find a clinical role in thrombolytic therapy monitoring. The myocardial uptake of ^{82}Rb is flow limited, being linear up to 2.5 times normal flow rates, giving rise to underestimation and overestimation of values (162,163). The production methods for the preparation of the parent radionuclide strontium-82 have been studied quite extensively (164–167). For this nuclide also, the spallation of molybdenum with high-energy protons is the production route of choice (159,168).

The most commonly used generator system is the strontium/rubidium system for the production of ^{82}Rb. It consists of an alumina column and uses 2% saline as an eluent to achieve 85% to 95% elution efficiency. The generator system has a life span of approximately 3 to 4 months and requires periodic quality assurance for sterility, apyrogenicity, and measurement of breakthrough concentrations. Clinically applied systems are typically not used for more than 1 month to maintain sufficient tracer activity for high-quality clinical images. The generator is a positive pressure system with operating pressures of 50 to 100 psi, and it can function in both the bolus mode and the constant infusion mode. In the latter case, the activity yield is a function of the flow rate (169).

Radionuclide Generator Equations

A synopsis of the equations to allow the calculation of the maximal concentrations of daughter nuclide from a particular generator or the determination of the appropriate time to elute a generator is given through the following expressions (144).

Considering a simple radionuclide generator system of parent daughter in which the half-life of the parent is longer than that of the daughter, the pair will eventually enter a state of transient equilibrium. This can be represented schematically as:

$$\mathrm{A} \rightarrow \mathrm{B} \rightarrow \mathrm{C}$$

where A is the parent radionuclide, which decays to the radioactive daughter B, which in turn decays to the daughter nuclide C. The ratio of decay of each radionuclide is described by the following equation:

$$\frac{dN}{dt} = \lambda N \quad \text{or} \quad N = N_0 e^{-\lambda t}$$

where N is the number of radioactive atoms at a specific time t and λ is the decay constant for the radionuclide and is equivalent to $(\ln(2)/t_{1/2})$.

Considering a generator system, the parent is generally adsorbed onto a solid support and serves as the sole source for the daughter radionuclide production. However, the number of daughter atoms present at any time t is described in a slightly more involved expression:

$$\frac{dN_B}{dt} = \lambda_A N_A - \lambda_B N_B$$

Because the daughter is decaying as well as being produced, the net rate of change on N_B with time is indicated by the decay of A to B minus the decay of B to C. Substitution of the integral of the expression for A yields the net rate of change for B as follows:

$$\frac{dN_B}{dt} = \lambda_A N_A^0 e^{-\lambda_A t} - \lambda_B N_B$$

Integrating this equation to calculate the number of atoms of B at time t gives the following expression:

$$N_B = \left(\frac{\lambda_A}{(\lambda_B - \lambda_A)}\right) N_A^0 (e^{-\lambda_A t} - e^{-\lambda_B t}) + N_B^0 e^{-\lambda_B t}$$

The first term on the right side of the equation represents the growth of the daughter nuclide B from the parent A decay and the loss of B through decay. The second term represents the decay of B atoms, but because the parent A is generally considered a pure parent radionuclide at the time the generator is manufactured, this term is zero. The equation can be rewritten in terms of activities and results as follows:

$$A_B = \left(\frac{\lambda_A}{(\lambda_B - \lambda_A)}\right) A_A^0 (e^{-\lambda_A t} - e^{-\lambda_B t})$$

There are two general conditions for parent-daughter pairs: transient equilibrium in which the parent half-life is greater than the daughter half-life, or secular equilibrium in which the parent half-life is much greater than the daughter half-life. Naturally if the decay should involve branching ratios, the equation above must be appropriately modified.

Further, in the case of the PET generators, it is often useful to calculate the time when the daughter activity is at the maximum value t_{max}. Differentiation of the equation with respect to time gives the following result:

$$t_{max} = \ln\left(\frac{\left(\frac{\lambda_A}{\lambda_B}\right)}{(\lambda_B - \lambda_A)}\right)$$

The role of generators for the future of clinical PET remains uncertain. The initial supposition that generators have potential for PET imaging at sites without a cyclotron or accelerator is being re-evaluated due to the costs associated with the procurement and scheduled availability of the parent radionuclide. Further, any supplementary equipment, such as that of the infusion system required for the strontium/rubidium generator, may result in low demand or choice of alternative radionuclides (148). Nevertheless, the strontium/rubidium generator is in routine clinical use in various medical centers in the United States and elsewhere, and the gallium generator systems are being applied to a limited extent in several centers.

SUMMARY

During recent years, research efforts in nuclear medicine have concentrated on the decay characteristics of particular radionuclides and the design of unique radiolabeled tracers necessary to achieve time-dependent molecular images. The specialty is expanding with specific PET and single photon emission computed tomography radiopharmaceuticals, allowing for an extension from functional process imaging in tissue to pathologic processes and radionuclide-directed treatments. PET is an example of a technique that has been shown to yield the physiologic information necessary for multiple diagnoses, including those in cancer-based on altered-tissue metabolism.

Most PET radiopharmaceuticals are currently produced using a cyclotron at locations that are in close proximity to the hospital or academic center at which the radiopharmaceutical will be administered. In November 1997, the Food and Drug Administration Modernization Act of 1997 was enacted in the United States. It directed the FDA to establish appropriate procedures for the approval of PET drugs in accordance with section 505 of the Federal Food, Drug, and Cosmetic Act and to establish current good manufacturing practice requirements for such drugs. At this time, the FDA is considering adopting special approval procedures and Current Good Manufacturing Practice regulations (C GMP) for PET drugs. The evolution of PET radiopharmaceuticals has introduced a new class of "drugs" requiring production facilities and product formulations that must be closely aligned with the scheduled clinical utilization. The production of the radionuclide in the appropriate synthetic form is one of the critical components in the manufacturing of the finished positron-emitting radiopharmaceutical.

ACKNOWLEDGMENTS

This research was supported in part by grants at Memorial Sloan-Kettering Cancer Center from the U.S. Department of Energy (DE-F02-86-E60407) and the Cancer Center Support Grant (NCI-P30-CA08748) and at Brookhaven National Laboratory under contract DE-AC02-98CH10886 with the U.S. Department of Energy and its Office of Biological and Environmental Research, and by the National Institutes of Health (National Institutes of Neurological Diseases and Stroke [grant NS-15380]).

REFERENCES

1. Dotzel MM. PET drug products; safety and effectiveness of certain PET drugs for specific indications. *Fed Regist* 2000;65:12999–13010.
2. Crouzel C, Clark JC, Brihaye C, et al. Radiochemistry automation for PET. In: Stocklin G, Pike VW, eds. *Radiopharmaceuticals for positron emission tomography.* Dordrecht: Kluwer Academic Publishers, 1993:45–90.
3. Satyamurthy N, Phelps ME, Barrio JR. Electronic generators for the production of positron-emitter labeled radiopharmaceuticals: where would PET be without them? *Clin Positron Imaging* 1999;2:233–253.
4. Deconninick G. *Introduction to radioanalytical physics, nuclear methods monographs*, no 1. Amsterdam: Elsevier Scientific Publishing, 1978.
5. Guillaume M, Lambrecht RM, Wolf AP. Cyclotron production of ^{123}Xe and high purity ^{123}I: a comparison of tellurium targets. *Int J Appl Radiat Isot* 1975;26:703–707.
6. Lambrecht RM, Wolf AP. Cyclotron and short-lived halogen isotopes for radiopharmaceutical applications. In: *New developments in radiopharmaceuticals and labelled compounds,* vol 1. Vienna: IAEA, 1973: 275–290.
7. Clem RG, Lambrecht RM. Enriched ^{124}Te targets for production of ^{123}I and ^{124}I. *Nucl Instruments Methods* 1991;A303:115–118.
8. Qaim SM, Stocklin G. Production of some medically important short-lived neutron deficient radioisotopes of halogens. *Radiochimica Acta* 1983;34:25–40.
9. Newman E. Sources of separated isotopes for nuclear targetry. In: Jaklovsky J, ed. *Preparation of nuclear targets for particle accelerators.* New York: Plenum Publishing, 1981:229–234.
10. Meese CO, Eichelbaum M, Ebner T, et al. ^{13}C and ^{2}H NMR as ex-vivo probe for monitoring human drug metabolism. In: Buncel E, Kabalka GW, eds. *Synthesis and applications of isotopically labelled compounds 1991.* Amsterdam: Elsevier Science, 1992:291–296.
11. Browne TR, Szalio GK. Stable isotope tracer studies of pharmacokinetic drug interaction. In: Buncel E, Kabalka GW, eds. *Synthesis and applications of isotopically labelled compounds 1991.* Amsterdam: Elsevier, 1992:397–402.
12. Finn RD, Johnson R. The radionuclide: an endangered resource? In: Buncel E, Kabalka GW, eds. *Synthesis and applications of isotopically labelled compounds 1991.* Amsterdam: Elsevier Science, 1992:291–296.
13. Finn RD. The search for consistency in the manufacture of PET radiopharmaceuticals. *Ann Nucl Med* 1999;13:379–382.
14. Firouzbakht ML, Schlyer DJ, Ferrieri RA, et al. Mechanisms involved in the production of nitrogen-13 labeled ammonia in a cryogenic target. *Nucl Med Biol* 1999;26:437–441.
15. Helus F, Colombetti, eds. *Radionuclide production.* Boca Raton, FL: CRC Press, 1983.
16. Wolf AP. The reactions of energetic tritium and carbon atoms with organic compounds. In: Gold V, ed. *Advances in physical organic chemistry,* vol 2. New York: Academic Press, 1964:201–277.
17. Welch MJ, Wolf AP. Reaction intermediates in the chemistry of recoil carbon atoms. *Chem Commun* 1968;3:117–118.
18. Ferrieri RA, Wolf AP. The chemistry of positron emitting nucleogenic (hot) atoms with regard to preparation of labelled compounds of practical utility. *Radiochimica Acta* 1983;34:69–83.
19. Dannals RF, Ravert HT, Wilson AA, et al. Special problems associated with the synthesis of high specific activity carbon-11 labeled radiotracers. In: Emran A, ed. *New trends in radiopharmaceutical synthesis, quality assurance, and regulatory control.* New York: Plenum Publishing, 1991:21–30.
20. Fowler JS, Wolf AP. *The synthesis of carbon-11, fluorine-18, and nitrogen-13 labeled radiotracers for biomedical applications.* Washington, DC: U.S. Department of Energy; Nuclear Science Series National Technical Information Services, 1982 (NAS-NS-3201).
21. Link JM, Krohn KA, Weitkamp WG. In-target chemistry during the production of ^{15}O and ^{11}C using ^{3}He reactions. *Radiochimica Acta* 2000;88(03/04):193.
22. Forngren BH, Yngve U, Forngren T, et al. Determination of specific radioactivity for ^{76}Br-labeled compounds measuring the ratio between ^{76}Br and ^{79}Br using packed capillary liquid chromatography mass spectrometry. *Nucl Med Biol* 2000;27(8):851–853.
23. Suzuki K, Haradahira T, Sasaki M. Effect of dissolved gas on the specific activity of N-13 labeled ions generated in water by the $^{16}O(p,\alpha)^{13}N$ reaction. *Radiochimica Acta* 2000;88(03/04):217.

24. Ferrieri RA, Alexoff DA, Schlyer DJ, et al. Target design considerations for high specific activity [^{11}C]CO_2. In: Proceedings of the Fifth Workshop on Targetry and Target Chemistry, September 19–23, 1993; Upton, New York. 1993:140–149.
25. Suzuki K, Yamazaki I, Sasaki M, et al. Specific activity of [^{11}C] CO_2 generated in a N_2 gas target: effect of irradiation dose, irradiation history, oxygen content and beam energy. *Radiochimica Acta* 2000;88 (03/04):211.
26. Ruth TJ, Wolf AP. Absolute cross-section for the production of ^{18}F via the ^{18}O(p,n)^{18}F reaction. *Radiochimica Acta* 1979;26:21–24.
27. Casella V, Ido T, Wolf AP, et al. Anhydrous F-18 labeled elemental fluorine for radiopharmaceutical preparation. *J Nucl Med* 1980;21:750–757.
28. Guillaume M, Luxen A, Nebeling B, et al. Recommendations for fluorine-18 production. *Appl Radiat Isot* 1991;42:749–762.
29. Helus F, Maier-Borst W, Sahm U, et al. F-18 cyclotron production methods. *Radiochem Radioanalytical Lett* 1979;38:395–410.
30. Helus F, Uhlir V, Wolber G, et al. Contribution to cyclotron targetry, II: testing of target construction materials for ^{18}F production via ^{20}Ne(d,α)^{18}F, recovery of ^{18}F from various metal surfaces. *J Radioanalytical Nucl Chem* 1994;182:445–450.
31. Blessing G, Coenen HH, Franken K, et al. Production of [^{18}F]F_2, H^{18}F and $^{18}F^-_{aq}$ using the ^{20}Ne(d,α)^{18}F process. *Appl Radiat Isot* 1986;37: 1135–1139.
32. Qaim SM. Target development for medical radioisotope production at a cyclotron. *Nucl Instruments Methods Phys Res* 1989;A282:289–295.
33. Bishop A, Satyamurthy N, Bida GT, et al. Metals suitable for fluorine gas target bodies-first use of aluminum for the production of [^{18}F]F_2. *Nucl Med Biol* 1996;23:181–185.
34. Alvord CW, Cristy S, Meyer H, et al. Surface-sensitive analysis of materials used in [F-18] electrophilic fluorine production, II: effects of post-passivation exposure. In: Proceedings of the Seventh Workshop on Targetry and Target Chemistry, June 8–11, 1997; Heidelberg, Germany. 1997:92–98.
35. Nickles RJ, Hichwa RD, Daube ME, et al. An ^{18}O-target for the high yield production of ^{18}F-fluoride. *Int J Appl Radiat Isot* 1983;34: 625–629.
36. Straatmann MG, Schlyer DJ, Chasko J. Conversion of HF to F_2 from an O-18 O_2 gas target. Un: Proceedings of the 4th International Symposium on Radiopharmaceutical Chemistry, 1982, Julich, West Germany. 1982:103.
37. Clark JC, Oberdorfer F. Thermal characteristics of the release of fluorine-18 from an Inconel 600 gas target. *J Labelled Compounds Radiopharm* 1982;29:1337–1339.
38. Lambrecht RM, Neirinckx R, Wolf AP. Cyclotron isotopes and radiopharmaceuticals, XXIII: novel anhydrous ^{18}F-fluorinating intermediates. *Int J Radiat Isot* 1978;29:175–183.
39. Lagunas-Solar MC, Carvacho OF. Cyclotron production of PET radionuclides: no-carrier-added fluorine-18 with high energy protons on natural neon gas targets. *Appl Radiat Isot* 1995;46:833–838.
40. Ruth TJ. The production of ^{18}F-F_2 and ^{15}O-O_2 sequentially from the same target chamber. *Appl Radiat Isot* 1985;36:107–110.
41. Wieland BW, Wolf AP. Large scale production and recovery of aqueous [F-18] fluoride using proton bombardment of a small volume [O-18] water target. *J Nucl Med* 1983;24:122.
42. Kilbourn MJ, Hood JT, Welch MJ. A simple ^{18}O water target for ^{18}F production. *Int J Radiat Isot* 1985;36:327–328.
43. Kilbourn MJ, Jerabek PA, Welch MJ. An improved ^{18}O water target for ^{18}F production. *Int J Radiat Isot* 1985;35:599–602.
44. Keinonen J, Fontell A, Kairento A-L. Effective small volume water target for the production of [^{18}F] fluoride. *Appl Radiat Isot* 1986;37: 631–632.
45. Berridge MS, Tewson TJ. Effects of target design on the production and utilization of [F-18]-fluoride from [O-18]-water. *J Labelled Compounds Radiopharm* 1986;23:1177–1178.
46. Iwata R, Ido T, Brady F, et al. [^{18}F] Fluoride production with a circulating [^{18}O] water target. *Appl Radiat Isot* 1987;38:979–984.
47. Mulholland GK, Hichwa RD, Kilbourn MR, et al. A reliable pressurized water target for F-18 production at high beam currents. *J Labelled Compounds Radiopharm* 1989;26:192–193.
48. Huszar I, Weinreich R. Production of ^{18}F with an ^{18}O-enriched water target. *J Radioanalytical Nucl Chem* 1985;93:349–354.
49. Vogt M, Huzar I, Argentini M, et al. Improved production of [^{18}F] fluoride via the [^{18}O]H_2O(p,n)^{18}F reaction for no-carrier-added nucleophilic synthesis. *Appl Radiat Isot* 1986;37:448–449.
50. O'Neil JP, Hanarahan SM, VanBrocklin HF. Experience with a high pressure silver water target system for [^{18}F] fluoride production using the CTI RDS-111 cyclotron. In: Proceedings of the 7th Workshop on Targetry and Target Chemistry, June 8–11, 1997, Heidelberg, Germany. 1997:232.
51. Gonzales-Lepera CE. Routine production of [^{18}F] fluoride with a high pressure disposable [^{18}O] water target. In: Proceedings of the 7th Workshop on Targetry and Target Chemistry, June 8–11, 1997, Heidelberg, Germany. 1997:234.
52. Steel CJ, Dowsett K, Pike VW, et al. Ten years experience with a heavily used target for the production of [^{18}F] fluoride by proton bombardment of [^{18}O] water. In: Proceedings of the 7th Workshop on Targetry and Target Chemistry, June 8–11, 1997, Heidelberg, Germany. 1997:55.
53. Roberts AD, Daniel LC, Nickles RJ. A high power target for the production of [^{18}F] fluoride. *Nucl Instruments Methods* 1995;B99: 797–799.
54. Heselius S-J, Schlyer DJ, Wolf AP. A diagnostic study of proton-beam irradiated water targets. *Int J Appl Radiat Isot* 1989;40[Pt A]:663–669.
55. Pavan RA, Johnson RR, Cackette M. A simple heat transfer model of a closed, small-volume, [^{18}O] water target. In: Proceedings of the 7th Workshop on Targetry and Target Chemistry, June 8–11, 1997, Heidelberg, Germany. 1997:226.
56. Steinbach J, Guenther K, Loesel E, et al. Temperature course in small volume [^{18}O] water targets for [^{18}F] F^- production. *Appl Radiat Isot* 1990;41:753–756.
57. Schlyer DJ, Firouzbakht ML, Wolf AP. Impurities in the [^{18}O] water target and their effect on the yield of an aromatic displacement reaction with [^{18}F] fluoride. *Int J Appl Radiat Isot* 1993;44:1459–1465.
58. Solin O, Bergman J, Haaparanta M, et al. Production of ^{18}F from water targets: specific radioactivity and anionic contaminants. *Appl Radiat Isot* 1988;39:1065–1071.
59. Zeisler SK, Helus F, Gaspar H. Comparison of different target surface materials for the production of carrier-free [^{18}F] fluoride. In: Proceedings of the 7th Workshop on Targetry and Target Chemistry, June 8–11, 1997, Heidelberg, Germany. 1997:223.
60. Becker DW, Erbe D. A new high current spherical target design for ^{18}O(p,n)^{18}F with 18 MeV protons. In: Proceedings of the 7th Workshop on Targetry and Target Chemistry, June 8–11, 1997, Heidelberg, Germany. 1997:268.
61. Firouzbakht ML, Schlyer DJ, Gately SJ, et al. A cryogenic solid target for the production of [^{18}F] fluoride from enriched [^{18}O] carbon dioxide. *Appl Radiat Isot* 1993;44:1081–1084.
62. Nozaki T, Iwamoto M, Ido T. Yield of ^{18}F for various reactions from oxygen and neon. *Int J Appl Radiat Isot* 1974;25:393–399.
63. Fitschen J, Beckmann R, Holm U, et al. Yield and production of ^{18}F by ^{3}He irradiation of water. *Int J Radiat Isot* 1977;28:781–784.
64. Schlyer DJ, Bastos MAV, Alexoff D, et al. Separation of F-18 fluoride from O-18 water using anion exchange resin. *Int J Appl Radiat Isot* 1990;41[Pt A]:531–533.
65. Mock BH, Vavrek MT, Mulholland GK. Back-to-back "one-pot" [^{18}F] FDG syntheses in a single Siemens-CTI Chemistry Process Control Unit. *Nucl Med Biol* 1996;23:497–501.
66. Pascali C, Bogni A, Remonti F, et al. A convenient semi-automated system for optimizing the recovery of aqueous [^{18}F] fluoride from target. In: Proceedings of the 7th Workshop on Targetry and Target Chemistry, June 8–11, 1997, Heidelberg, Germany. 1997:60.
67. Bida GT, Ruth TJ, Wolf AP. Experimentally determined thick target yields for the ^{14}N(p,α)^{11}C reaction. *Radiochimica Acta* 1980;27:181–185.

68. Casella VR, Christman DR, Ido T, et al. Excitation function for the $^{14}N(p,\alpha)^{11}C$ reaction up to 15 MeV. *Radiochimica Acta* 1978;25;17–20.
69. Christman DR, Finn RD, Karlstrom KI, et al. The production of ultra high activity ^{11}C-labelled hydrogen cyanide, carbon dioxide, carbon monoxide and methane via the $^{14}N(p,\alpha)^{11}C$ reaction. *Int J Appl Radiat Isot* 1975;26:435–442.
70. Clark JC, Buckingham PD. Carbon-11. In: Clark JC, Buckingham PD, eds. *Short-lived radioactive gases for clinical use.* London: Butterworth, 1975:215–260.
71. Finn RD, Christman DR, Ache HJ, et al. The preparation of cyanide-^{11}C for use in the synthesis of organic radiopharmaceuticals. *Int J Appl Radiat Isot* 1971;22:735–744.
72. Helus F, Hanisch M, Layer K, et al. Yield ratio of [^{11}C] CO_2, [^{11}C] CO, [^{11}C] CH_4 from the irradiation of N_2/H_2 mixtures in the gas target. *J Labelled Compounds Radiopharm* 1986;23:1195–1198.
73. Buckley KR, Huser J, Jivan S, et al. ^{11}C-methane production in small volume, high pressure gas targets. *Radiochimica Acta* 2000:88:201–205.
74. Schlyer DJ, Plascjak PS. Small angle multiple scattering of charged particles in cyclotron target foils-a comparison of experiment with simple theory. *Nucl Instruments Methods* 1991;B56/57:464–468.
75. Helmeke HJ, Hundeshagen H. Design of gas targets for the production of medically used radionuclides with the help of Monte Carlo simulation of small angle multiple scattering of charged particles. *Appl Radiat Isot* 1995;46:751–757.
76. Wieland BW, Schlyer DJ, Wolf AP. Charged particle penetration in gas targets designed for accelerator production of radionuclides used in nuclear medicine. *Int J Appl Radiat Isot* 1984;35:387–396.
77. Heselius S-J, Lindblom P, Solin O. Optical studies of the influence of an intense ion beam on high pressure gas targets. *Int J Appl Radiat Isot* 1982;33:653–659.
78. Heselius S-J, Malmborg P, Solin O, et al. Studies of proton beam penetration in nitrogen gas targets with respect to production and specific radioactivity of carbon-11. *Int J Appl Radiat Isot* 1987;38:49–57.
79. Hughey BJ, Shefer RE, Klinkowstein RE, et al. Design considerations for foil windows for PET radioisotope targets. In: Proceedings of the 4th Workshop on Targetry and Target Chemistry, September 9–12, 1991. Villigen, Switzerland: PSI, 1991:12.
80. Schlyer DJ, Firouzbakht ML. Correlation of hole size in support windows with calculated yield strengths. In: Proceedings of the 6th Workshop on Targetry and Target Chemistry, August 17–19, 1996, Vancouver, BC, Canada. 1996:142–143.
81. Straatmann MG, Welch MJ. Enzymatic synthesis of nitrogen-13 labeled amino acids. *Radiat Res* 1973;56:48–56.
82. Tilbury RS, Emran AM. [^{13}N] Labeled tracers, synthesis and applications. In: Emran A, ed. *New trends in radiopharmaceutical synthesis, quality assurance, and regulatory control.* New York: Plenum Publishing, 1991:39–51.
83. Firouzbakht ML, Schlyer DJ, Wolf AP. Cross-section measurements for the $^{13}C(p,n)^{13}N$ and $^{12}C(d,n)^{13}N$ nuclear reactions. *Radiochimica Acta* 1991;55(1):1–5.
84. Austin SM, Galonsky A, Bortins J, et al. A batch process for the production of ^{13}N-labeled nitrogen gas. *Nucl Instruments Methods* 1975;126:373–379.
85. Sajjad M, Lambrecht RM, Wolf AP. Cyclotron isotopes and radiopharmaceuticals, XXXVII: excitation functions for the $^{16}O(p,\alpha)^{13}N$ and $^{14}N(p,pn)^{13}N$ reactions. *Radiochimica Acta* 1986;39:165–168.
86. Parks NJ, Krohn KA. The synthesis of ^{13}N labeled ammonia, dinitrogen, nitrite, nitrate using a single cyclotron target system. *Int J Appl Radiat Isot* 1978;29:754–757.
87. Tilbury RS, Dahl JR. ^{13}N Species formed by the proton irradiation of water. *Radiat Res* 1979;79:22–33.
88. Tilbury RS, Dahl JR, Marano SJ. N-13 Species formed by proton irradiation of water. *J Labelled Compounds Radiopharm* 1977;13:208.
89. Helmeke HJ, Harms T, Knapp WH. Home-made routinely used targets for the production of PET radionuclides. In: Proceedings of the 7th Workshop on Targetry and Target Chemistry, June 8–11, 1997, Heidelberg, Germany. 1997:241.
90. Mulholland GK, Kilbourn MR, Moskwa JJ. Direct simultaneous production of [^{15}O] water and [^{13}N] ammonia or [^{18}F] fluoride ion by 26 MeV proton irradiation of a double chamber water target. *Appl Radiat Isot* 1990;41:1193–1199.
91. Joliot F, Curie I. Artificial production of a new kind of radio-element. *Nature* 1934;133:201–202.
92. Shefer RE, Hughey BJ, Klinkowstein RE, et al. A windowless ^{13}N production target for use with low energy deuteron accelerators. *Nucl Med Biol* 1994;21:977–986.
93. Dence CS, Welch MJ, Hughey BJ, et al. Production of [^{13}N] ammonia applicable to low energy accelerators. *Nucl Med Biol* 1994;21:987–996.
94. Bida G, Wieland BW, Ruth TJ, et al. An economical target for nitrogen-13 production by proton bombardment of a slurry of C-13 powder on ^{16}O water. *J Labelled Compounds Radiopharm* 1986;23:1217–1218.
95. Zippi EM, Valiulis MB, Grover J. Synthesis of carbon-13 sulfonated poly(styrene/divinylbenzene) for production of a nitrogen-13 target material. In: Proceedings of the 6th Workshop on Targetry and Target Chemistry, August 17–19, 1995, Vancouver, BC, Canada. 1995: 185–188.
96. Wieland BW, McKinney CJ, Coleman RE. A tandem target system using $^{16}O(p,pn)^{15}O$ and $^{16}O(p,\alpha)^{13}N$ on natural water. In: Proceedings of the Sixth Workshop on Targetry and Target Chemistry, August 17–19, 1995, Vancouver, BC, Canada. 1995:173–179.
97. Berridge MS, Landmeier BJ. In-target production of [^{13}N] ammonia: target design, products and operating parameters. *Appl Radiat Isot* 1993;44:1433–1441.
98. Korsakov MV, Krasikova RN, Fedorova OS. Production of high yield [^{13}N] ammonia by proton irradiation from pressurized aqueous solutions. *J Radioanalytical Nucl Chem* 1996;204:231–239.
99. Medema J, Elsinga PH, Keizer H, et al. Remote controlled in-target production of [^{13}N] ammonia using a circulating target. In: Proceedings of the 7th Workshop on Targetry and Target Chemistry, June 8–11, 1997, Heidelberg, Germany. 1997:80–81.
100. Wieland BW, Bida G, Padgett H, et al. In-target production of [^{13}N] ammonia via proton irradiation of dilute aqueous ethanol and acetic acid mixtures. *Appl Radiat Isot* 1991;42:1095–1098.
101. Bida G, Satyamurthy N. [^{13}N] Ammonia production via proton irradiation of CO_2/H_2O: a work in progress. In: Proceedings of the 6th Workshop on Targetry and Target Chemistry, August 17–19, 1995, Vancouver, British Columbia, Canada. 1995:189–191.
102. Patt JT, Nebling B, Stocklin G. Water target chemistry of nitrogen-13 recoils revisited. *J Labelled Compounds Radiopharm* 1991;30:122–123.
103. Sasaki M, Haradahira T, Suzuki K. Effect of dissolved gas on the specific activity of N-13 labeled ions generated in water by the $^{16}O(p,\alpha)^{13}N$ reaction. *Radiochimica Acta* 2000;88:217–220.
104. Mikecz P, Dood MG, Chaloner F, et al. Glass target for production of [^{13}N] NH_3 from methane, revival of an old method. In: Proceedings of the Seventh Workshop on Targetry and Target Chemistry, June 8–11, 1997, Heidelberg, Germany. 1997:163–164.
105. Straatmann MG. A look at ^{13}N and ^{15}O in radiopharmaceuticals. *Int J Appl Radiat Isot* 1977;28:13–20.
106. McCarthy TJ, Gaehle GG, Margenau WH, et al. Evaluation of a commercially available heater for the rapid combustion of graphite disks used in the production of [^{13}N]NO and [^{13}N]NO_2. In: Proceedings of the 7th Workshop on Targetry and Target Chemistry, June 8–11, 1997, Heidelberg, Germany. 1997:205.
107. Ferrieri RA, Schlyer DJ, Wieland BW, et al. On-line production of ^{13}N-nitrogen gas from a solid enriched ^{13}C-target and its application to ^{13}N-ammonia synthesis using microwave radiation. *Int J Appl Radiat Isot* 1983;34:897–900.
108. Livingston MS, McMillian E. The production of radioactive oxygen. *Phys Rev* 1934;46:439–440.
109. Del Fiore G, Depresseux JC, Bartsch P, et al. Production of oxygen-15, nitrogen-13 and carbon-11 and of their low molecular weight derivatives for biomedical applications. *Int J Appl Radiat Isot* 1979;30: 543–549.

110. Retz-Schmidt T, Weil JL. Excitation curves and angular distributions for $^{14}N(d,n)^{15}O$. *Phys Rev* 1960;119:1079–1084.
111. Vera-Ruiz H, Wolf AP. Excitation function of ^{15}O production via the $^{14}N(d,n)^{15}O$ reaction. *Radiochimica Acta* 1977;24:65–67.
112. Sajjad M, Lambrecht RM, Wolf AP. Cyclotron isotopes and radiopharmaceuticals, XXXIV: excitation function for the $^{15}N(p,n)^{15}O$ reaction. *Radiochimica Acta* 1984;36:159–162.
113. Beaver JE, Finn RD, Hupf HB. A new method for the production of high concentration oxygen-15 labeled carbon dioxide with protons. *Int J Appl Radiat Isot* 1976;27:195–197.
114. Vera-Ruiz H, Wolf AP. Direct synthesis of oxygen-15 labeled water of high specific activity. *J Labelled Compounds Radiopharm* 1978;15: 186–189.
115. Votaw JR, Satter MR, Sunderland JJ, et al. The Edison lamp: O-15 carbon monoxide production in the target. *J Labelled Compounds Radiopharm* 1986;23:1211–1213.
116. Harper PV, Wickland T. Oxygen-15 labeled water for continuous intravenous administration. *J Labelled Compounds Radiopharm* 1981; 18:186.
117. Wieland BW, Russel ML, Dunn WL, et al. Quartz micro-fiber target for the production of O-15 ozone for pulmonary applications-computer modeling and experiments. In: Proceedings of the 7th Workshop on Targetry and Target Chemistry, June 8–11, 1997, Heidelberg, Germany. 1997:114–119.
118. Strijckmans K, VandeCasteele C, Sambre J. Production and quality control of $^{15}O_2$ and $C^{15}O_2$ for medical use. *Int J Appl Radiat Isot* 1985; 36:279–283.
119. Wieland BW, Schmidt DG, Bida G, et al. Efficient, economical production of oxygen-15 labeled tracers with low energy protons. *J Labelled Compounds Radiopharm* 1986;23:1214–1216.
120. Van Naeman J, Monclus M, Damhaut P, et al. Production, automatic delivery and bolus injection of [^{15}O] water for positron emission tomography studies. *Nucl Med Biol* 1996;23:413–416.
121. Pagani M, Stone-Elander S, Larsson SA. Alternative positron emission tomography with non-conventional positron emitters: effects of their physical properties on image quality and potential clinical applications. *Eur J Nucl Med* 1997;24:1301–1327.
122. Chaudhir MA. Yields of cyclotron produced medical isotopes: a comparison of theoretical potential and experimental results. *IEEE Trans Nucl Sci* 1979;26:2281–2286.
123. Qaim SM. Nuclear data relevant to cyclotron produced short-lived medical radioisotopes. *Radiochimica Acta* 1982;30:147–162.
124. Qaim SM, Hohn A, Nortier FM, et al. Production of ^{124}I at small and medium size cyclotrons. In: *Programs and abstracts of the 8th International Workshop on Targetry and Target Chemistry*, 1999; St. Louis, Missouri. Abstract p. 131–133.
125. Scholten B, Kovacs Z, Tarkanyi F, et al. Excitation functions of $^{124}Te(p,xn)^{124,123}I$ reactions from 6 to 31 MeV with special reference to the production of ^{124}I at a small cyclotron. *Appl Radiat Isot* 1995;46: 255–259.
126. Sheh Y, Koziorowshi J, Balatoni J, et al. Low energy cyclotron production and chemical separation of "no carrier added" ^{124}I from a reusable, enriched tellurium-124 dioxide/aluminum oxide solid solution target. *Radiochimica Acta* 2000;88:169–173.
127. Qaim SM. Recent developments in the production of ^{18}F, $^{75,76,77}Br$ and ^{123}I. *Int J Appl Radiat Isot* 1986;37:803–810.
128. Paans AMJ, Welleweerd J, Vaalburg W, et al. Excitation functions for the production of ^{75}Br: a potential nuclide for the labeling of radiopharmaceuticals. *Int J Appl Radiat Isot* 1980;31:267–272.
129. Vaalburg W, Paans AMJ, Terpstra JW, et al. Fast recovery by dry distillation of ^{75}Br induced in reusable metal selenide targets via the $^{76}Se(p,2n)^{75}Br$ reaction. *Int J Appl Radiat Isot* 1985;36:961–964.
130. Kovacs Z, Blessing G, Qaim SM, et al. Production of ^{75}Br via the $^{76}Se(p,2n)^{75}Br$ reaction at a compact cyclotron. *Int J Appl Radiat Isot* 1985;36:635–642.
131. Blessing G, Qaim SM. An improved internal Cu_3As-alloy cyclotron target for the production of ^{75}Br and ^{77}Br and separation of the byproduct ^{67}Ga from the matrix activity. *Int J Appl Radiat Isot* 1984; 35:927–931.
132. Blessing G, Weinreich R, Qaim SM, et al. Production of ^{75}Br and ^{76}Br via the $^{75}As(^{3}He,3n)^{75}Br$ and $^{75}As(\alpha,2n)^{77}Br$ reactions using Cu_3As-alloy as a high-current target material. *Int J Appl Radiat Isot* 1982;33:333–339.
133. Grütter A. Cross sections for reactions with 593 and 540 MeV protons in aluminum, arsenic, bromine, rubidium and yttrium. *Int J Appl Radiat Isot* 1982;33(9):725–732.
134. Szelecsenyi F, Blessing G, Qaim SM. Excitation functions of proton induced nuclear reaction on enriched Ni-61 and Ni-64: possibility of production of no-carrier-added Cu-61 and Cu-64 at a small cyclotron. *Appl Radiat Isot* 1993;44:575.
135. Homma Y, Murakami Y. Production of ^{61}Cu by α and ^{3}He bombardments on cobalt target. *Chem Lett Chem Soc Jpn* 1976:397–400.
136. Rowshanfarzad P, Sabet M, Jalilian AR, et al. An overview of copper radionuclides and production of ^{61}Cu by proton irradiation of $^{(nat)}Zn$ at a medical cyclotron. *Appl Radiat Isot* 2006;64(12):1563–1573.
137. Smith SV. Molecular imaging with copper-64. *J Inorg Biochem* 2004;98(11):1874–1901.
138. McCarthy DW, Shefer RE, Klinkowstein RE, et al. Efficient production of high specific activity ^{64}Cu using a biomedical cyclotron. *Nucl Med Biol* 1997;24:35–43.
139. Hou X, Jacobson U, Jorgensen JC. Separation of no-carrier-added ^{64}Cu from a proton irradiated ^{64}Ni enriched target. *Appl Radiat Isot* 2002;57:773–777.
140. Obata A, Kasamatsu S, McCarthy DW, et al. Production of therapeutic quantities of ^{64}Cu using a 12 MeV cyclotron. *Nucl Med Biol* 2003;30: 535–539.
141. Richards P. *Tc99m: production and chemistry* [Report BNL-9032]. Upton, NY: Brookhaven National Laboratory, 1965.
142. Richards P. *The Tc-99m generator* [Report BNL-9061]. Upton, NY: Brookhaven National Laboratory, 1965.
143. Lambrecht RM. Radionuclide generators. *Radiochimica Acta* 1983; 34:9–24.
144. Finn RD, Molinski VJ, Hupf HB, et al. *Radionuclide generators for biomedical applications.* Springfield: National Technical Information Service, 1983.
145. Knapp FF Jr, Butler TA, eds. *Radionuclide generators* [ACS Symposium series 241]. Washington, DC: American Chemical Society, 1984.
146. Guillaume M, Brihaye C. Generators for short-lived gamma and positron emitting radionuclides: current status and prospects. *Nucl Med Biol* 1986;13:89–100.
147. Qaim SM. Cyclotron production of generator radionuclides. *Radiochimica Acta* 1987;41:111–117.
148. Welch MJ, McCarthy TJ. The potential role of generator-produced radiopharmaceuticals in clinical PET. *J Nucl Med* 2000;41:315–317.
149. Robinson GD Jr, Zielinski FW, Lee AW. The $^{62}Zn/^{62}Cu$-generator: a convenient source of ^{62}Cu for radiopharmaceuticals. *Int J Appl Radiat Isot* 1980;31:111–116.
150. Fujibayashi Y, Matsumoto K, Yonekura Y, et al. A new $^{62}Zn/^{62}Cu$ generator as a copper-62 source for PET radiopharmaceuticals. *J Nucl Med* 1989;30:1838–1842.
151. Green MA, Mathias CJ, Welch MJ, et al. Copper-62-labeled pyruvaldehyde bis(N^4-methylthiosemicarbazonato) copper, II: synthesis and evaluation as a positron emission tomography tracer for cerebral and myocardial perfusion. *J Nucl Med* 1990;31:1989–1996.
152. Zweit J, Goodall R, Cox M, et al. Development of a high performance zinc-62/copper-62 radionuclide generator for positron emission tomography. *Eur J Nucl Med* 1992;19:418–425.
153. Neirinckx RD. Excitation function for the $^{60}Ni(\alpha,2n)^{62}Zn$ reaction and production of ^{62}Zn bleomycin. *Int J Appl Radiat Isot* 1977;28:808–809.
154. Yagi M, Kondo K. A ^{62}Cu generator. *Int J Appl Radiat Isot* 1979;30: 569–570.

155. Piel H, Qaim SM, Stocklin G. Excitation functions of (p,xn)-reactions on ^{nat}Ni and highly enriched ^{62}Ni: possibility of production of medically important radioisotope ^{62}Cu at a small cyclotron. *Radiochimica Acta* 1992;57:1–5.
156. Pao PJ, Silvester DJ, Waters SL. A new method for the preparation of ^{68}Ga-generators following proton bombardment of gallium oxide targets. *J Radioanalytical Chem* 1981;64:267–272.
157. Loc'h C, Maziere B, Comar D, et al. A new preparation of germanium-68. *Int J Appl Radiat Isot* 1982;33:267–270.
158. Grant PM, Miller DA, Gilmore JS, et al. Medium-energy spallation cross sections, I: RbBr irradiation with 800-MeV protons. *Int J Appl Radiat Isot* 1982;33:415–417.
159. Robertson R, Graham D, Trevena IC. Radioisotope production via 500 MeV proton-induced reactions. *J Labelled Compounds Radiopharm* 1982;19:1368(abst).
160. Loc'h C, Maziere B, Comar D. A new generator for ionic gallium-68. *J Nucl Med* 1980;21:171–173.
161. Gould KL. Clinical positron imaging of the heart with Rb-82. In: *PET/SPECT: instrumentation, radiopharmaceuticals, neurology and physiological measurement.* Washington, DC: American College of Nuclear Physicians, 1988:122–133.
162. Goldstein RA, Mullani NA, Fisher DJ, et al. Myocardial perfusion with rubidium-82, II. effects of metabolic and pharmaceutical interventions. *J Nucl Med* 1983;24:907–915.
163. Selwyn AP, Allan RM, L'abbate A, et al. Relation between regional myocardial uptake of rubidium-82 and perfusion: absolute reduction of cation uptake in ischemia. *Am J Cardiol* 1982;50:112–121.
164. Waters SL, Coursey BM, eds. The ^{82}Sr/^{82}Rb generator. *Appl Radiat Isot* 1987;38:171–240.
165. Tarkanyi F, Qaim SM, Stocklin G. Excitation functions of ^{3}He- and α-particle induced nuclear reactions on natural krypton: production of ^{82}Sr at a compact cyclotron. *Appl Radiat Isot* 1988;39:135–143.
166. Tarkanyi F, Qaim SM, Stocklin G. Excitation functions of high-energy ^{3}He- and α-particle induced nuclear reactions on natural krypton with special reference to the production of ^{82}Sr. *Appl Radiat Isot* 1990;41:91–95.
167. Mausner LF, Prach T, Srivastava SC. Production of ^{82}Sr by proton irradiation of RbCl. *Appl Radiat Isot* 1987;38:181–184.
168. Thomas KE. Strontium-82 production at Los Alamos National Laboratory. *Appl Radiat Isot* 1987;38:175–180.
169. Yano Y, Cahoon JL, Budinger TF. A precision flow controlled Rb-82 generator for bolus or constant-infusion studies of the heart and brain. *J Nucl Med* 1981;22:1006–1010.

CHAPTER 2

Radiotracer Chemistry

JOANNA S. FOWLER AND YU-SHIN DING

Over the past 35 years, advances in radiotracer chemistry and positron emission tomography (PET) instrumentation have merged to make PET a powerful scientific tool for studying biochemical transformations and the movement of drugs in the human brain and other organs in the body. With advances in the sequencing of the human genome, we can anticipate the identification of many new genes and their protein products. This, in turn, will create the need for new radiotracers to characterize the functional activity of these new proteins in living systems, and ultimately in humans. In addition, new knowledge on progenitor cells and their promise in treating human disease calls for expanding radiotracer development so that imaging can be used to study cell trafficking as well as the molecular processes involved in stimulating these cells to differentiate *in vivo*.

Radiotracer chemistry is a subfield of chemistry underpinning the development of radiotracers labeled with the short-lived positron emitters, and there have been many chapters, monographs, and review articles on this PET radiotracer development (1–8). Of special utility is a recent compilation with references and compound structures of most of the PET labeled compounds classified according to compound type (9).

This chapter will update the chapter on chemistry in the first edition of this book (10), providing background on the design and synthesis of PET radiotracers and giving examples that illustrate general principles, rather than providing a comprehensive survey. This chapter will substantially focus on carbon-11 (^{11}C) and fluorine-18 (^{18}F), the two positron emitters at the heart of molecular imaging and medical application. There are several other important tracers that are emerging in their application, which are also briefly discussed. This chapter is organized by sections on different classes of labeled compounds designed to bind to and map specific molecular targets such as receptors, transporters, and enzymes. This chapter will conclude with a section on future outlook and needs.

RAPID RADIOTRACER CHEMISTRY

Time dominates all aspects of a PET study, particularly the synthesis of the radiotracer. PET radiotracers must be synthesized and imaged within a time frame compatible with the half-life of the isotope (11). For ^{11}C, this is typically about 10 minutes for isotope production (cyclotron bombardment), 40 minutes for radiotracer synthesis, and up to about 90 minutes for PET imaging. Thus the entire study from the end of cyclotron bombardment to the end of an imaging session must be orchestrated and carried out within about 2.5 hours. Large amounts of radioactivity need to be used initially in order to compensate for radioactive decay and for the sometimes low synthetic yields. Shielding, remote operations, and automation are integrated into the experimental design (12,13). It is ideal to introduce the radioactivity at the last step in the synthesis, which may require multistep syntheses of suitably protected substrates into which the ^{11}C or ^{18}F can be introduced. When protective groups are used, they must be stable to the labeling conditions, and the deprotection conditions must be rapid. The crude reaction mixture is usually purified by high-performance liquid chromatography or a combination of solid phase extraction and high-performance liquid chromatography. Since radiotracers are typically administered intravenously, procedures must be developed to yield radiotracers that are not only chemically and radiochemically pure but also sterile and free from pyrogens (14). One of the exciting new advances is the integration of microfluidics into radiotracer research and routine production (15,16).

Carbon-11 and Fluorine-18 Production

Basic research in hot atom chemistry provided some of the knowledge to understand the chemistry that takes place during the production of the short-lived positron emitters, and it set the stage for

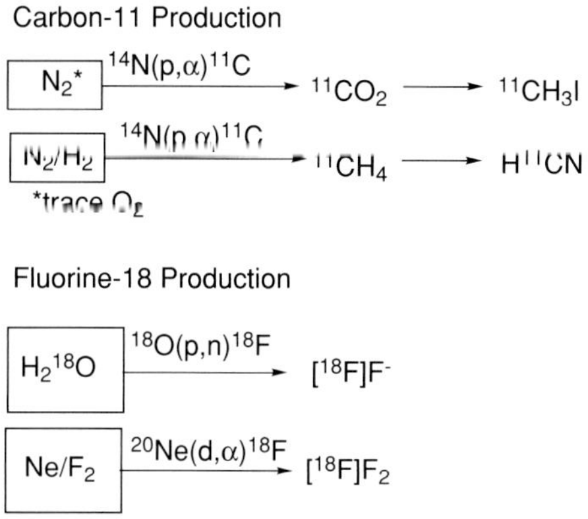

Carbon-11 Production

N_2* $^{14}N(p,\alpha)^{11}C$ → $^{11}CO_2$ → $^{11}CH_3I$

N_2/H_2 $^{14}N(p,\alpha)^{11}C$ → $^{11}CH_4$ → $H^{11}CN$

*trace O_2

Fluorine-18 Production

$H_2{}^{18}O$ $^{18}O(p,n)^{18}F$ → $[^{18}F]F^-$

Ne/F_2 $^{20}Ne(d,\alpha)^{18}F$ → $[^{18}F]F_2$

FIGURE 2.1. Common nuclear reactions and target materials for carbon-11 and fluorine-18 production.

producing the short-lived positron emitters in chemical forms, which were useful for the synthesis of complex radiotracers (for a review see Wolf and Redvanly (17)). Because of the short half-lives of ^{11}C and ^{18}F, each radiotracer synthesis requires the production of the isotope and its conversion to a useful labeled precursor molecule either directly or via some postirradiation synthesis. Production involves bombarding appropriate stable (and sometimes enriched) isotopes with charged particles such as protons and deuterons, which are most commonly and conveniently produced using a cyclotron. Three nuclear reactions, the $^{14}N(p,\alpha)^{11}C$, the $^{18}O(p,n)^{18}F$, and the $^{20}Ne(d,\alpha)^{18}F$ reactions are most commonly used for ^{11}C and ^{18}F production (Fig. 2.1)(2).

An important point is that the substrate that is used for the nuclear reaction (referred to as the target) is usually a different element than the radioisotope produced. Carbon-11, for example, is usually produced from the cyclotron bombardment of stable nitrogen ($^{14}N(p,\alpha)^{11}C$). In principle, at the end of cyclotron bombardment, the only isotope of carbon present would be ^{11}C. However, because stable carbon is ubiquitous in nature, it is not possible to remove it completely from the target and from the reagents used in the synthesis. Even with this unavoidable dilution, the specific activity (units of radioactivity/unit of mass) of PET radiotracers is quite high (Table 2.1). Thus it is typical that the ^{12}C:^{11}C ratio is about 5,000:1, which generally produces radiotracers of sufficiently high specific activity for tracer studies.

Fluorine-18 is most commonly produced by bombarding oxygen-18 enriched water with protons to yield [^{18}F]fluoride (18). As is the case with ^{11}C, it is not possible to remove all stable fluoride ions from the target materials and from the reagents used in the synthesis so that the isotope is always diluted with stable fluoride ion. In contrast to [^{18}F]fluoride, which is always produced without the *intentional* addition of stable fluoride, [$^{18}F]F_2$ is always deliberately diluted with unlabeled F_2. In general, for equal amounts of radioactivity, the chemical mass associated with an [$^{18}F]F_2$ derived radiotracer (carrier-added) exceeds that of an [^{18}F]fluoride ion derived radiotracer (no-carrier-added) by a factor of 1,000 (3). However, there has been progress in achieving high specific activity ^{18}F labeled elemental fluorine by mixing no carrier added (NCA) ^{18}F labeled methyl fluoride (synthesized from aqueous [^{18}F]fluoride ion) with a small amount of elemental fluorine in an inert neon matrix and subjecting it to an electrical discharge (19). The resulting labeled elemental fluorine has a specific activity of up to 55 GBq/μmol, which is sufficiently high for tracer studies of the dopamine transporter (20). Although [$^{18}F]XeF_2$ has been prepared and used in labeling, most labeling requires the use of [$^{18}F]F_2$ (3). Recently it has been reported that XeF_2 exchanges with [^{18}F]fluoride under mild conditions (21); however, specific activity has not been optimized.

High specific activity radiotracers provide the opportunity for imaging biological targets such as neurotransmitter receptors at tracer concentrations (22). However, the chemical mass that constitutes a tracer dose depends on the process being measured. For example, biological targets such as neurotransmitter receptors occur at much lower concentrations than enzymes, and thus higher specific activities are required for neurotransmitter or steroid hormone receptor studies. Typically specific activity is expressed by one of the following terms (23,24):

Carrier free (CF) should mean that the radionuclide or stable nuclide is not contaminated with any other radio or stable nuclide of the same element. This has probably never been achieved with ^{11}C or ^{18}F tracers.

No carrier added (NCA) should apply to an element or compound to which no carrier of the same element or compound has been

TABLE 2.1 Physical Properties of the Short-Lived Positron Emitters

Isotope	Half-life (min)	Specific Activity (Ci/mmol)[a]	Maximum Energy (MeV)	Range (mm) in H_2O[b]	Decay Product
fluorine-18	110	1.71×10^6	0.635	2.4	oxygen-18
carbon-11	20.4	9.22×10^6	0.96	4.1	boron-11
oxygen-15	2.1	9.08×10^7	1.72	8.2	nitrogen-15
nitrogen-13	9.96	1.89×10^7	1.19	5.4	carbon-13

[a]Theoretical maximum; in reality the measured specific activities of ^{11}C, ^{15}F, ^{13}N, and ^{18}F are about 5,000 times lower because of unavoidable dilution with the stable element.
[b]Maximum linear range.

intentionally or otherwise added during its preparation. This applies to most radiotracers.

Carrier added (CA) should apply to any element or compound to which a known amount of carrier has been added.

Because the reporting of specific activities has ambiguities especially in the older literature, other descriptive terms have been introduced to describe radiotracer specific activities, (3) including the term *effective specific activity*, which refers to the value of specific activity measured by biological or biochemical assay and takes into account the presence of species that have biological effects similar to the parent compound. The factors influencing the values of specific activities of compounds that are determined physicochemically and by radioreceptor techniques have been discussed elsewhere (25).

The high specific activity of ^{11}C and ^{18}F labeled precursors influences the stoichiometry and the scale of the reaction. For example, in a NCA synthesis with Na[^{11}C]N (specific activity: 2,000 Ci/mmol), the quantity of NaCN used if one starts with 100 mCi is 50 nmol. With this small quantity of Na[^{11}C]N, all other substrates or reactants used in the synthesis are necessarily in large excess, which is problematic when an excess of a given reagent cannot be tolerated. One must consider that the substrate that will undergo reaction with the labeled precursors must be in a sufficient concentration to react both with the labeled precursors and with other competing reactants that may be present in the reaction mixture.

With such high specific activity ^{11}C and ^{18}F labeled precursors, syntheses are always carried out on a micro or a semimicro scale, and typical chemical masses associated with NCA PET radiotracers are a few micrograms or less. The small scale is advantageous in terms of the relative ease and speed with which one can handle small quantities of reagents and solvents, in minimizing the amounts of substances to be removed in the final purification, and in avoiding the unintentional introduction of impurities that may negatively influence the course of the reaction. However, losses caused by surface-to-volume effects, by adsorption properties of vessels, and of materials used for purification can impact heavily on yields.

Carbon-11 Labeled Compounds

The advantages of ^{11}C as a label are many, including that it can substituted for stable carbon in an organic compound without changing the properties of the molecule. This is of particular importance for the use of PET in drug research and development (26,27). In addition, PET studies can be repeated at 2-hour intervals with a ^{11}C labeled tracer, allowing baseline and experimental studies to be carried out in a single individual within a short time frame. However, there are large experimental hurdles imposed by the 20.4-minute half-life and the limited number of labeled precursors available for synthesis. More specifically, only [^{11}C]O_2 and [^{11}C]H_4 come directly from the cyclotron target using properly adjusted radiation conditions (Fig. 1.1). A number of other precursor molecules are synthesized from labeled carbon dioxide or methane, but all require some synthetic manipulation during or after cyclotron bombardment (2).

Some of the earliest syntheses with ^{11}C depended directly on labeled carbon dioxide and hydrogen cyanide (28). Today, however, alkylation with [^{11}C]methyl iodide is the most widely used method for introducing ^{11}C into organic molecules (29). Alkylations are generally straightforward as in the case of the synthesis of [^{11}C]raclopride, a widely used radiotracer for imaging dopamine D_2 receptor, which is synthesized by alkylating the nor-compound with [^{11}C]methyl iodide (30). (eq. 1)

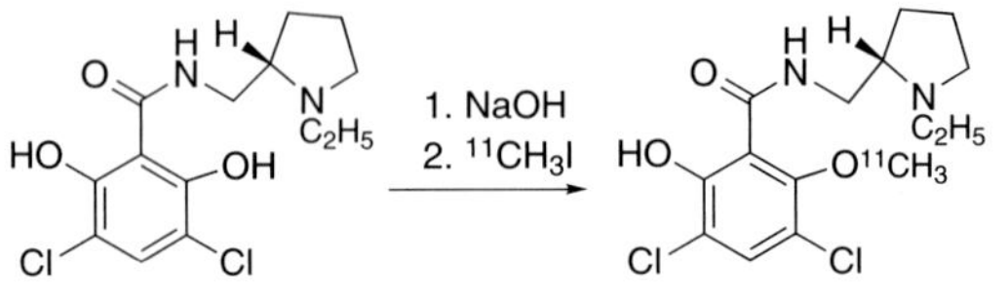

1. NaOH
2. $^{11}CH_3I$

[^{11}C]raclopride [1]

Frequently, however, reactive centers on the reaction substrate must be masked with protective groups that can be rapidly removed. This is illustrated by the synthesis of [^{11}C]*d-threo* (or *l-threo*-methylphenidate) from labeled methyl iodide and a protected derivative of *d-* or *l-threo* ritalinic acid (31). (eq. 2)

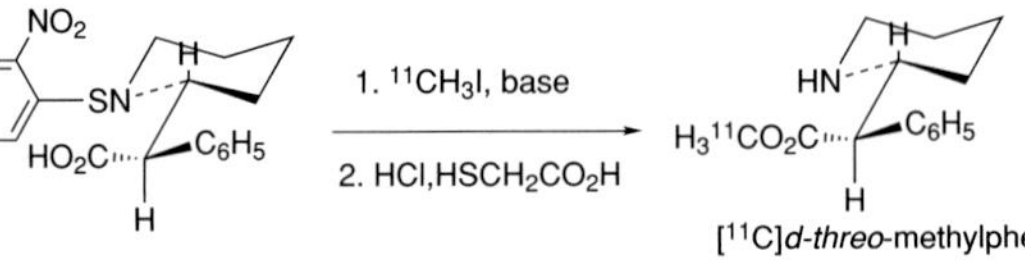

1. $^{11}CH_3I$, base
2. HCl,$HSCH_2CO_2H$

[^{11}C]*d-threo*-methylphenidate [2]

In the case of relatively sensitive compounds like deuterium-substituted [^{11}C]phenylephrine, alkylation can be carried out under milder conditions using [^{11}C]methyl triflate (32,33). (eq. 3)

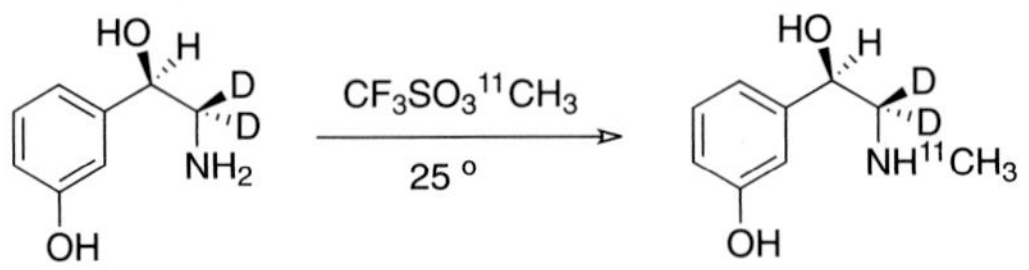

$CF_3SO_3{}^{11}CH_3$
25 °

[^{11}C]-a,a-dideutero-phenylephrine [3]

The introduction of an online gas phase synthesis to give high specific activity [^{11}C]H_3I from labeled methane is a major advance (34,35). Other precursors from [^{11}C]methyl iodide include [^{11}C]methyl magnesium iodide (36) and the Wittig reagent [^{11}C]methylenetriphenylphosphorane (37).

Many useful ^{11}C tracers cannot be synthesized simply by either O- or N-alkylating the nor-compound with [^{11}C]methyl iodide. For examples, the synthesis of PHNO and NPA, potential radiotracers for *in vivo* imaging of the dopamine D_2 high-affinity state, requires the N-alkylation with ^{11}C-labeled propionyl chloride (prepared from [^{11}C]O_2 and ethyl magnesium bromide), followed by reduction with lithium aluminum hydride (38,39). The synthesis of ^{11}C GR89696 or its active enantiomer GR103545 (k-opioid receptor ligand) requires the N-alkylation with a ^{11}C-labeled methylcarbonyl group, which is prepared by the reaction of ^{11}C methanol and phosgene (40).

Carbon-11 synthesis is frequently complicated by the need for chiral-labeled products. In the case of radiotracers like [^{11}C]*d-threo*-methylphenidate described above (eq. 2), this is readily accomplished because the chiral center is present in the substrate (*d*-ritalinic acid) and the reaction conditions preserve the chirality. Chiral high-performance liquid chromatography can also be used to separate the desired labeled enantiomer from a labeled racemic mixture. Asymmetric syntheses have been developed to directly obtain the desired enantiomer. For example, enantiomerically enriched 3-[^{11}C]L-alanine was synthesized from [^{11}C]O_2 (via methyl iodide) (41). (eq. 4)

Labeled methane is also very useful in synthesis because it is available in large quantities and can be readily converted to H[^{11}C]N by passing the target gas (N_2/H_2 plus a small quantity of ammonia) over platinum wool at 1,000°C (28). It has been used in the synthesis of labeled amines, ketones, aldehydes, acids, and amino acids (3).

A special problem in ^{11}C (and ^{18}F) synthesis is the need to design synthetic routes to precursor molecules that are amendable to rapid labeling. Frequently, a new synthetic strategy must be developed for these molecules. The synthesis of [carboxyl-^{11}C]-γ-vinyl-γ-amino-butyric acid ([^{11}C]GVG) required the development of a new five-step synthetic strategy to prepare a suitably protected labeling precursor for the displacement reaction (42). (eq. 5)

In another example, the palladium catalyzed coupling of labeled cyanide to an aromatic ring was used in the synthesis of a radioligand [^{11}C]NAD-299 for evaluation of binding to the 5-HT1A receptor (43). (eq. 6)

Labeled methane has also been converted to [^{11}C]phosgene, which has been used in the synthesis of many compounds including a ring-labeled monoamine oxidase inhibitor befloxatone (44). (eq. 7)

Labeled carbon monoxide ([^{11}C]O) has also been used in the photoinitiated carbonylation reaction to produce carbonyl-^{11}C-labeled amides (45). (eq. 8)

1. TMP/BuLi; -72°
2. $^{11}CH_3I$
hydrolysis
3-[^{11}C]alanine [4]

5 steps
1. $^{11}CN^-$
2. HCl
[^{11}C]GVG [5]

[^{11}C]CN$^-$
[$Pd_2(dba)_3$].$CHCl_3$
H_2O_2/NaOH
[^{11}C]NAD 299 [6]

[^{11}C]OCl_2
[^{11}C]befloxatone
(* = ^{11}C) [7]

^{11}CO
TEA/ hv
1-cyclohexane [^{11}C]carbonyl-4-phenyl-piperazine [8]

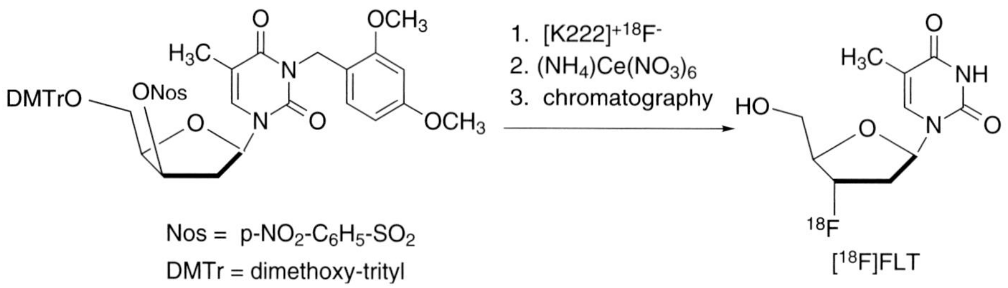

1. $[K222]^{+18}F^{-}$
2. $(NH_4)Ce(NO_3)_6$
3. chromatography

Nos = $p\text{-}NO_2\text{-}C_6H_5\text{-}SO_2$
DMTr = dimethoxy-trityl

$[^{18}F]FLT$

[9]

Problems in ^{11}C synthesis generally include rigorously excluding stable carbon in order to maximize the specific activity of the product, optimizing reaction rates, and developing rapid methods to separate the labeled product from the starting materials and by-products. Reaction times have been reduced and yields have been increased for many labeled compounds by applying microwave technology (46).

Fluorine-18 Labeled Compounds

In contrast to the 20-minute half-life of ^{11}C, which requires that the entire synthesis be accomplished in about 40 minutes, the half-life of ^{18}F at 110 minutes allows more time for relatively complex synthetic manipulations and for more lengthy biological studies. An additional advantage is that ^{18}F has a low positron energy, and thus its maximum range (2.4 mm) allows for the sharpest imaging with a high-resolution PET (Table 2.1). Moreover, as has been exemplified by the successful distribution of 2-deoxy-2-[^{18}F]fluoro-D-glucose (^{18}FDG) from regional production centers, ^{18}F, when tagged to well-designed and validated radiotracers, offers the potential for distribution from a regional production center to clinical and research institutions without a cyclotron and chemistry group. Disadvantages of ^{18}F relative to ^{11}C include the fact that fluorine is not normally present in biological molecules or drugs and the fact that the 110-minute half-life precludes the performance of multiple studies on the same subject on the same day.

There are two simple labeled forms of ^{18}F (fluoride ion and elemental fluorine) that are directly available for radiotracer synthesis. Fluoride ion is the more desirable of the two because it can be produced in higher yield and without added carrier. In principle, 100% of the isotope can be incorporated into the tracer. An example is synthesis of 3'-deoxy-3'-[^{18}F]fluorothymidine ([^{18}F]FLT) based on the [^{18}F]fluoride displacement of a protected nosylate precursor (47). (eq. 9)

In another example, 16-α-[^{18}F]fluoro-estradiol-17-β has been synthesized by the displacement of a triflate with [^{18}F]fluoride and the effect [^{18}F]fluoride solubilization conditions has been studied (48).

In contrast to [^{18}F]fluoride displacement, the maximum radiochemical yield when [$^{18}F]F_2$ is used as a precursor is usually only 50%, because only one of the fluorine atoms in the fluorine molecule is labeled and typically only one atom of fluorine is incorporated into the final product after electrophilic fluorination. This loss of 50% of the label also applies when labeled fluorine is converted to other precursors like labeled acetyl hyprofluorite (3). ^{18}FDG, which is used to measure glucose metabolism, exemplifies the evolution and improvement of a synthesis through time (Fig. 2.2) (for review see Fowler and Ido. [49]). ^{18}FDG was first synthesized by the electrophilic fluorination with [$^{18}F]F_2$ and an improved synthesis from [^{18}F]acetylhypofluorite was reported a few years later (50). However, the synthesis of ^{18}FDG via a nucleophilic substitution with [^{18}F]fluoride was a major breakthrough (51). It gave significantly higher yields and has largely replaced the electrophilic route. ^{18}FDG, the most widely used PET tracer, is currently synthesized via a nucleophilic substitution, followed by acid or base hydrolysis (49). Automated ^{18}FDG synthesis modules produce ^{18}FDG efficiently in research labs or commercial entities and allow it to be widely distributed to other research institutes for carrying

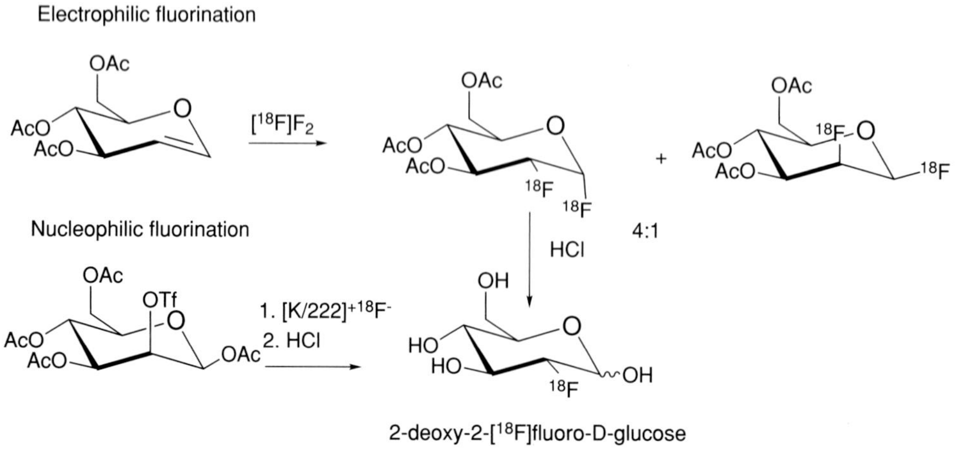

Electrophilic fluorination

$[^{18}F]F_2$

4:1

HCl

Nucleophilic fluorination

1. $[K/222]^{+18}F^{-}$
2. HCl

2-deoxy-2-[^{18}F]fluoro-D-glucose

FIGURE 2.2. Electrophilic and nucleophilic routes to 2-deoxy-2-[^{18}F]fluoro-D-glucose (^{18}FDG).

out basic and clinical research in humans. Although some radiotracers such as [^{18}F]fluorodopa (6-[^{18}F]fluoro]-3,4-dihydroxyphenylalanine) (52) are still conveniently synthesized from [^{18}F]F_2 or [^{18}F]acetylhypofluorite (53), most ^{18}F-labeled radiotracers including [^{18}F]fluorodopa can now be prepared from [^{18}F]fluoride ion (54,55).

The most successful approach for preparing high specific activity ^{18}F-substituted aromatic compounds is the nucleophilic aromatic substitution reaction (56). The minimal structural requirements for efficient nucleophilic aromatic substitution are the presence of an electron withdrawing, activating substituent such as RCO, CN, NO_2 and so forth, as well as a leaving group, such as nitro- or trimethylammonium. This approach is used for the high-yield one pot, two-step synthesis of 6-[^{18}F]fluoro-A85380, a radiotracer with high specificity for nicotinic acetylcholine receptors (57–59). (eq. 10)

In addition to simple fluorine-substituted aromatic compounds, there are important radiotracers with electron donating substituents on the aromatic ring that can impede the nucleophilic aromatic substitution reaction. Recent mechanistic studies have established that nucleophilic aromatic substitution can be carried out in the presence of suitably protected electron donating groups, thus extending the utility of the nucleophilic aromatic substitution to the synthesis of 6-[^{18}F]fluorodopa as well as 6-[^{18}F]fluorodopamine (60), (+)- and (−)-6-[^{18}F]fluoronorepinephrine (61). (eq. 11)

The use of the nucleophilic aromatic substitution reaction produced 6-[^{18}F]fluorodopamine in sufficiently high specific activity for tracer studies without producing hemodynamic effects (62), which are observed when low specific activity 6-[^{18}F]fluorodopamine is used.

In another example of nucleophilic aromatic substitution on an electron-rich ring, 2-[^{18}F]fluoroestradiol was synthesized by the displacement of a trimethylammonium group on the carbon-2 (^{2}C) of an estrogen derivative, with additional activation being provided by a 6-keto group, which was subsequently removed by reduction (63). (eq. 12)

Simple, no-carrier-added [^{18}F]fluoroarenes have also been synthesized via the reaction of [^{18}F]fluoride with diaryliodonium salts (64).

RADIOTRACER DESIGN AND MECHANISMS

Radiotracer design refers to the process of choosing priority structures for labeling in order to image a specific molecular target. For this purpose, it is essential to consider the affinity and selectivity of the compound for the molecular target as well as the concentration of the molecular target itself (for a discussion see Eckelman et al. [65]). However, a chemical compound with high affinity and high selectivity for a specific molecular target that is present in high concentration will not necessarily guarantee high binding specificity and appropriate kinetics *in vivo*. This is due to the fact that the human and animal body presents a complex set of barriers that compete with specific binding and with radiotracer delivery to the target organ. These include plasma protein binding (for examples see Yu et al. [66] and Ding et al. [67]) sequestration in cells, low affinity and nonspecific binding, metabolism, the blood–brain barrier, and probably many others.

For most radiotracers, the physicochemical properties of the compounds, such as their size, charge, solubility, and lipophilicity, are useful parameters and are particularly important in the design of tracers that penetrate the blood–brain barrier (68–70). Thus, the literature of medicinal and pharmaceutical chemistry is a valuable resource for the design and evaluation process of radiotracers (71).

The design of ^{18}FDG is a good example of radiotracer design that benefited a great deal from information that was in the literature at the time. ^{18}FDG was modeled after carbon-14 labeled 2-deoxy-glucose (^{14}C-2DG), a tracer used to measure brain glucose metabolism in animals using autoradiography (Fig. 2.3) (72). The requirements for a positron emitter labeled version of 2-deoxyglucose were:

D-glucose 2-deoxy-D-glucose 2-deoxy-2-fluoro-D-glucose

FIGURE 2.3. Structures of glucose, 2-deoxy-D-glucose and 2-deoxy-2-fluoro-D-glucose.

1. The resulting molecule must contain a positron emitter.
2. The resulting molecule must be a substrate for the glucose transporter, which facilitates the transport of glucose from blood to brain.
3. The resulting molecule must be a substrate for hexokinase the pivotal enzyme in glycolysis.
4. The resulting molecule must *not* undergo metabolism past the point of phosphorylation, allowing the phosphorylated product to be trapped at the site of phosphorylation.

As was reported in 1954, the hydroxyl group on ^{2}C-2 on the glucose skeleton is the only hydroxyl group on glucose that can be removed and still retain the ability of the molecule to be a substrate for hexokinase (typically the rate-limiting enzyme in glycolysis) (73). For this reason, ^{2}C-2 was selected for fluorine substitution. Moreover, the glucose transporter is not sensitive to substitution on ^{2}C-2, and the metabolism beyond the hexokinase step requires the hydroxyl group in ^{2}C-2. Thus ^{18}FDG, in which the ^{18}F is on ^{2}C-2, undergoes carrier mediate transport into the brain where it is phosphorylated to ^{18}FDG-6-phosphate by hexokinase. However, because the hydroxyl group in ^{2}C-2 is missing, no further metabolism occurs and ^{18}FDG-6-phosphate is trapped in the cell where metabolism has occurred (Fig. 2.4). When imaged, metabolically trapped ^{18}FDG-6-phosphate provides a map of glucose metabolism in all brain regions simultaneously. [1-^{11}C]2-deoxy-D-glucose was also labeled with ^{11}C shortly after the development of ^{18}FDG and provided an opportunity to do multiple studies on the same subject in a single scanning session (74,75).

Although ^{18}FDG was initially developed for imaging brain metabolism, early studies showed that it was concentrated in animal tumors (76) due to enhanced glycolysis in cancer cells (77). Consequently, ^{18}FDG has had a profound impact on the management of patients with cancer (78). The success of ^{18}FDG in the detection of human cancers also relates in part to the replacement of the hydroxyl on ^{2}C-2 rather than on another carbon atom. Because the hydroxyl group on ^{2}C-2 is required for active transport of glucose and because the active transport of glucose across the renal tubule is required for glucose resorption (79), ^{18}FDG, in contrast to glucose, is excreted. This, in effect, it lowers the body background after the injection of ^{18}FDG, creating the high contrast for imaging metabolically active tumors.

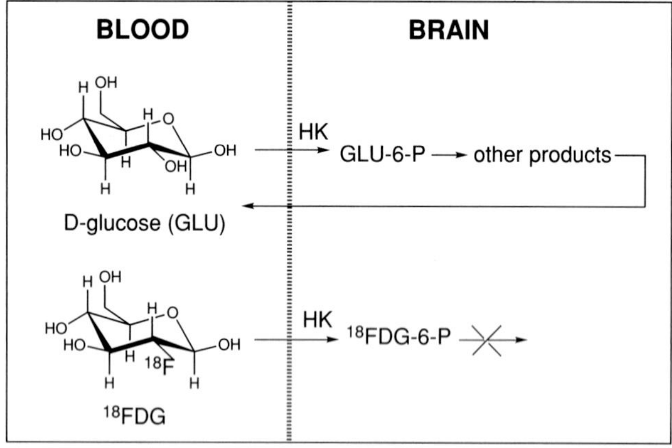

FIGURE 2.4. Simplified diagram comparing the behavior of glucose and 2-deoxy-2-[^{18}F]fluoro-D-glucose (^{18}FDG) in the brain. Glucose crosses the blood–brain barrier by facilitated transport and enters a cell. There it enters the glycolytic cycle where it is first phosphorylated by hexokinase (HK) and eventually produces adenosine triphosphate and metabolites that can leave the cell. Like glucose, ^{18}FDG also undergoes facilitated transport into the brain and is phosphorylated by hexokinase to produce ^{18}FDG -6-phosphate (^{18}FDG-6-P). However ^{18}FDG-6-P does not undergo further metabolism and is trapped in the cell.

RADIOTRACER VALIDATION

A key step in the development of a new radiotracer is to characterize its binding *in vitro* and more important, *in vivo*. Since the PET image itself originates from the annihilation photons produced by positron decay, it provides no information about the chemical compound(s), giving rise to the image or on the cellular or subcellular localization or binding site or on binding specificity. One way to ensure specificity and saturability is to compare the distribution and kinetics of the radiotracer before and after treatment with a pharmacologically specific drug or with a pharmacological dose of the tracer molecule. Another tool for assessing specificity is to compare the binding of the labeled compound in wild type and knockout animals in which the gene for a specific molecular target (receptor, transporter, enzyme) is removed (80). Other approaches include examining the behavior of the same labeled compound in different positions, the comparison of labeled stereoisomers, and, in limited cases, the use of deuterium isotope effects to probe specific reactions (81). Radiotracer kinetics can also be a limiting factor in quantification, therefore, they must be critically examined and appropriate kinetic models developed to calculate parameters that can be related to receptor concentration, enzyme activity, or some other factor (82–88). Some examples are given for illustration.

Comparative Studies of the Same Molecule Labeled in Different Positions

Frequently the position of the label can be adjusted to simplify the profile of labeled metabolites contributing to the image or to determine the localization mechanism. For example, high pancreas uptake of ^{11}C was observed after the injection of [^{11}C]L-dopa (89). To determine the mechanism by which ^{11}C concentrates in the pancreas, a comparison of the radiotracer labeled in the carboxyl group and in the β position was made in the same subject. Only the radiotracer labeled in the β position was retained in the pancreas. This demonstrated that aromatic amino acid decarboxylase (AAADC) (which would result in the loss of the ^{11}C in the carboxyl position, but not the β position) was responsible for the retention of [^{11}C]L-dopa in pancreas and pancreatic tumors. A similar comparative study of [^{11}C]5-hydroxytryptophan (5-HP) labeled in the β position and in the carboxyl position demonstrated tumor uptake and decarboxylation and also provided the means for quantitating AAADC activity. A PET study of [^{11}C]dimethylphenethylamine labeled in two different positions (N-methyl vs. α-methylene) also illustrates the profound difference in ^{11}C kinetics depending on the position of the label, illustrating the importance of label position for probing enzyme activity (90). [^{11}C]WAY-100,635 which has been developed as a radiotracer for the 5-HT_{1A} receptor, was initially labeled in the methoxy position but was subsequently labeled in the carbonyl position to reduce the contribution of labeled metabolites (91). Structures of some of these labeled compounds are shown in Fig. 2.5.

Comparison of Labeled Stereoisomers

Biological targets (enzymes, receptors, etc.) are chiral molecules, and frequently chiral ligands and drugs show binding selectivity for one enantiomer over the other. In some cases, this is useful in assessing binding specificity. For example, methylphenidate (Ritalin) is a racemic drug that binds to the dopamine transporter, and it is used in the treatment of attention deficit hyperactivity disorder and narcolepsy. Comparative PET studies of two enantiomers, [^{11}C]*d-threo*-methylphenidate and [^{11}C]*l-threo*-methylphenidate, provided confirmatory evidence that the pharmacological activity of the drug resides in the *d-threo*-enantiomer, which binds to the human striatum, in contrast to [^{11}C]*l-threo*-methylphenidate, which shows no specific retention (92). [^{11}C]*d-threo*-methylphenidate proved to be an excellent radiotracer for measuring dopamine transporter availability in the human brain (93). A comparison of labeled enantiomers has also been applied in the study of radiotracers for the muscarinic cholinergic system, [^{11}C]dexetimide and [^{11}C]levetimide (94). Another example applies to the development of radiotracers for studies of the serotonin transporter. In one case comparative studies of [^{11}C](+)McN5652 and [^{11}C](−)McN5662 in both mice and humans showed the expected retention of the (+)-enantiomer and clearance of the (−)-enantiomer (95).

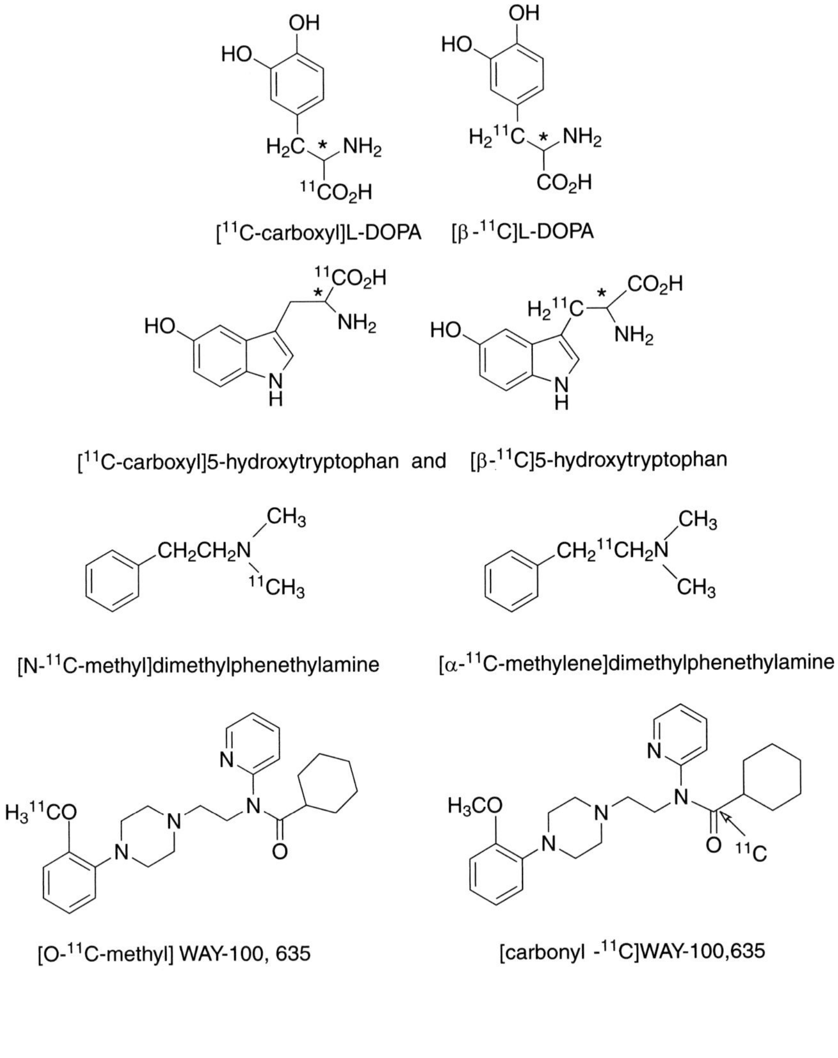

[^{11}C-carboxyl]L-DOPA [β-^{11}C]L-DOPA

[^{11}C-carboxyl]5-hydroxytryptophan and [β-^{11}C]5-hydroxytryptophan

[N-^{11}C-methyl]dimethylphenethylamine [α-^{11}C-methylene]dimethylphenethylamine

[O-^{11}C-methyl] WAY-100, 635 [carbonyl -^{11}C]WAY-100,635

FIGURE 2.5. Structures of labeled compounds in which different label positions have been synthesized and compared either to obtain mechanistic information or to simplify the interpretation of the PET image.

Although the comparison of active and inactive enantiomers *in vivo* is potentially a powerful mechanistic tool, there are pitfalls. This was encountered in the comparison of the active and inactive enantiomers of cocaine (– and + cocaine) to assess cocaine's binding specificity to the dopamine transporter. Instead of demonstrating stereoselective binding in the brain, as was anticipated, the comparison of ^{11}C labeled negative and positive cocaine revealed an extraordinarily rapid metabolism of [^{11}C](+)-cocaine by butyrylcholinesterase, which prevented its penetration into the brain (96). Thus, in this case, rapid peripheral metabolism, rather than stereospecific binding to the dopamine transporter, was responsible for the observed behavior *in vivo*.

DEUTERIUM ISOTOPE EFFECTS

A carbon–hydrogen (C-H) bond is more easily cleaved than a carbon–deuterium bond. If a specific C-H bond in a radiotracer is cleaved in the rate limiting or rate contributing step of a chemical or biochemical reaction, its substitution with deuterium will reduce the rate of reaction and the rate of accumulation in tissue. Deuterium isotope effects have been used as a mechanistic tool in radiotracer studies of monoamine oxidase (MAO), an enzyme known to exhibit strong isotope effects due to the cleavage of the C-H bond α to the nitrogen atom where oxidation is occurring (97). There are several examples in the radiotracer literature, including [^{11}C]L-deprenyl and deuterium-substituted [^{11}C]L-deprenyl (98); [^{11}C]clorgyline and deuterium substituted [^{11}C]clorgyline (99); [^{13}N]phenethylamine and deuterium substituted [^{13}N]phenethylamine (100); [^{11}C]phenylephrine and deuterium substituted phenylephrine (101); and 6-[^{18}F]fluorodopamine and deuterium substituted 6-[^{18}F]fluorodopamine (102). The binding of these radiotracers in tissue (and the PET images) show deuterium isotope effects consistent with MAO catalyzed cleavage of a specific bond. In the case of 6-[^{18}F]fluorodopamine, a comparison of deuterium substitution in the α and in the β positions was used to determine that MAO and not dopamine-β-hydroxylase was responsible for the kinetic profile of 6-[^{18}F]fluorodopamine in the heart (102). In the case of [^{11}C]L-deprenyl, the slower rate of trapping of the deuterium substituted molecule in brain facilitated kinetic modeling in humans (103). Although the deuterium isotope effect is dramatic in these cases, it is important to note that this *only* is useful in mechanistic studies in special cases such as MAO where C-H bond cleavage occurs in the rate-limiting step. Radiotracer structures are shown in Fig. 2.6.

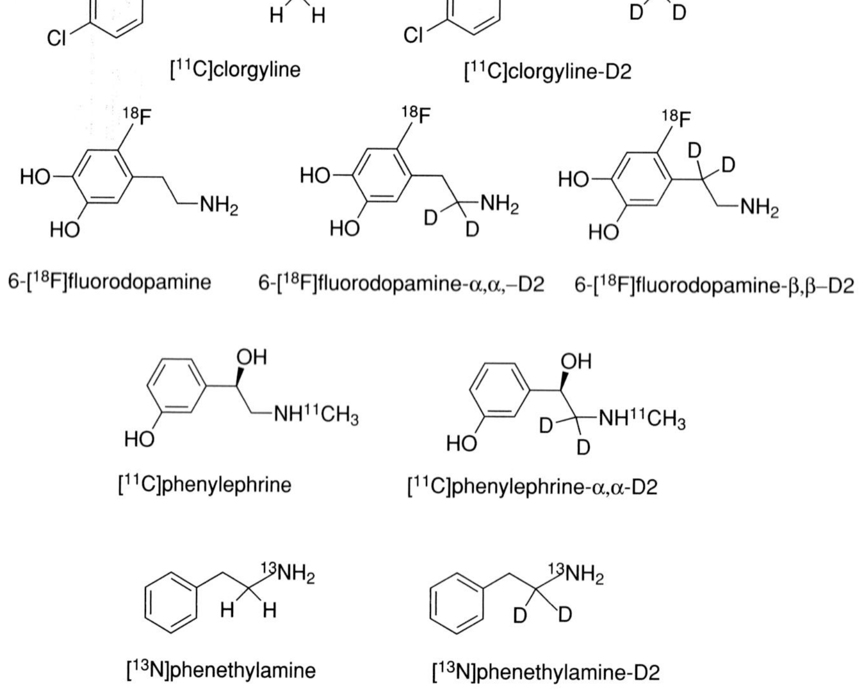

[^{11}C]L-deprenyl [^{11}C]L-deprenyl-D2

[^{11}C]clorgyline [^{11}C]clorgyline-D2

6-[^{18}F]fluorodopamine 6-[^{18}F]fluorodopamine-α,α,–D2 6-[^{18}F]fluorodopamine-β,β–D2

[^{11}C]phenylephrine [^{11}C]phenylephrine-α,α-D2

[^{13}N]phenethylamine [^{13}N]phenethylamine-D2

FIGURE 2.6. Structures of labeled compounds substituted with deuterium to obtain mechanistic information and/or to improve radiotracer kinetics.

RADIOTRACERS FOR NEUROTRANSMITTER SYSTEMS

The development of radiotracers for imaging neurotransmitter systems (including their receptors, plasma membrane, vesicular transporters, the enzymes that synthesize and degrade them, and the processes involved in signal transduction) has dominated radiotracer research over the past several decades (104). The reasons for this are obvious when one considers that brain function is driven by the complex interplay of neurotransmitter systems and that their disruption underlies many diseases of the central nervous system (105). Indeed PET has made it possible to visualize many different aspects of neurotransmitter activity in living systems. Radiotracers for some of the major neurotransmitters will be highlighted in the following sections.

The Brain Dopamine System

Dopamine plays a pivotal role in the regulation of movement, motivation, and cognition. It is also closely linked to reward and reinforcement addiction and is a major molecular target of stimulant drugs and drugs to treat Parkinson disease and schizophrenia. Drugs abused by humans also elevate brain dopamine, although by a variety of different mechanisms. Because of its importance, the study of the brain dopamine system has been a major focus in the basic and clinical neurosciences, and it is by far the most widely studied neurotransmitter system in PET research (106,107).

Dopamine is synthesized in the dopaminergic neurons in the substantia nigra, the ventral tegmental area, and the retrorubral area of the mesencephalon. It is stored within vesicles to protect it from oxidation by MAO. It is released into the synapse in response to an action potential and interacts with dopamine receptors that are present on both postsynaptic sites (where they function in cell-to-cell communication) and on presynaptic sites (where they regulate exocytotic release and dopamine synthesis). There are five subtypes of dopamine receptors that are grouped in two major families: those that stimulate adenyl cyclase (D_1, D5) and those that inhibit it (D_2, D3, D4) (108). The dopamine D_1 and D_2 receptors have significantly higher concentrations than the other subtypes and have highest density in the striatum. Quantitative PET studies of the brain dopamine system are facilitated by the high concentration of dopamine receptors and dopamine transporters in the basal ganglia and an absence of these elements in the cerebellum.

The synaptic concentration of dopamine is regulated primarily by reuptake. Dopamine release is regulated by presynaptic autoreceptors as well as by other neuroanatomically distinct neurotransmitters through interactions with the dopamine neuron. Dopamine is also removed by oxidation by MAO and methylation by catechol-O-methyltransferase (COMT).

Dopamine Metabolism

Dopamine does not cross the blood–brain barrier, and thus the investigation of brain dopamine metabolism with PET required a labeled derivative of L-dopa, the amino acid precursor of dopamine, which is transported into the brain via the large neutral amino acid carrier. [^{18}F]Fluorodopa was the first radiotracer developed to probe brain dopamine metabolism (109). 6-[^{18}F]fluorodopa crosses the blood–brain barrier and is accumulated in dopamine terminals and converted to 6-[^{18}F]fluorodopamine (110). Decreased [^{18}F]fluorodopa accumulation is associated with the loss of dopaminergic neurons (111). Because the metabolism of [^{18}F]fluorodopa is complex, ^{18}F-labeled m-tyrosine, which has simpler metabolism, has also been developed to improve quantification (112). Nonetheless, [^{18}F]fluorodopa is the more widely used of the two. [^{11}C]L-dopa has also been synthesized with the label in two positions and represents a labeled version of the native amino acid (Fig. 2.5) (113).

Dopamine Receptors

Although there are five dopamine receptor subtypes, only radiotracers with specificity for dopamine D_2 and D_1 receptors have been developed, although promising candidates for the D3 receptor subtype have recently been identified (see Fig. 2.7 for structures of some of these compounds). Dopamine D_1 and D_2 receptors are highly concentrated in the striatum with lower concentrations occurring in extrastriatal regions. High-affinity radiotracers are required for imaging extrastriatal receptors because of their low density. Although most of the radiotracer development work has focused on labeled dopamine receptor antagonists, agonists are also of interest because of the potential to image the high-affinity state of the receptor.

Dopamine D_2 receptor availability has been examined with PET using ^{11}C and ^{18}F labeled antagonists to the D_2 receptor. For example, N-methylspiroperidol has been labeled with ^{11}C and with ^{18}F and used to measure dopamine receptor availability and absolute concentration in the normal and diseased brain and to probe dopamine receptor occupancy by antipsychotic drugs (114–117). 3-(2'-[^{18}F]fluoroethyl)spiperone and N-(3-[^{18}F]fluoropropyl)spiperone have also been used for the quantitative estimation of D_2 receptor sites (118,119), and the ethyl derivative has also been used as a reporter in gene-expression studies (120). The irreversible or near-irreversible binding of the spiroperidol derivatives has been a limitation in terms of quantitation because the receptor-binding parameter may be influenced by radiotracer delivery.

[^{11}C]raclopride is the most widely used PET radiotracer for studies of dopamine D_2 receptor availability (121,122) and for measuring changes in extracellular dopamine brought about by drugs and other stimulants. Drug-induced changes in synaptic dopamine have also been measured with [^{11}C]raclopride, since its moderate affinity for the dopamine D_2 receptor and reversible binding allow it to compete with dopamine in the synapse (123,124). Repeated measures with [^{11}C]raclopride with an intervening challenge with dopamine-enhancing drugs like methylphenidate and amphetamine have been successfully used to assess dopaminergic function (125–127). High-affinity reversibly binding benzamide radiotracers such as [^{18}F]fallypride (128,129) and [^{11}C]FLB 457 have also been developed in order to have a longer scanning period and higher striatum:cerebellum ratios and to image extrastriatal dopamine D_2 receptors that are present in low concentration.

The development of radiotracers to probe the high-affinity state of the dopamine D_2/D3 receptor has been approached by a number of investigators (130–132). In particular, recent PET studies with (–)-N-(^{11}C)propyl-norapomorphine show that it is a promising tracer for high affinity states of the D_2/D3 receptor (133,134). Another D_2/D3 receptor agonist, [^{11}C]-(+)-PHNO (4-propyl-9-hydroxynaphthoxazine) has also been synthesized and shown to be more sensitive to changes in dopamine than [^{11}C]raclopride (38,39).

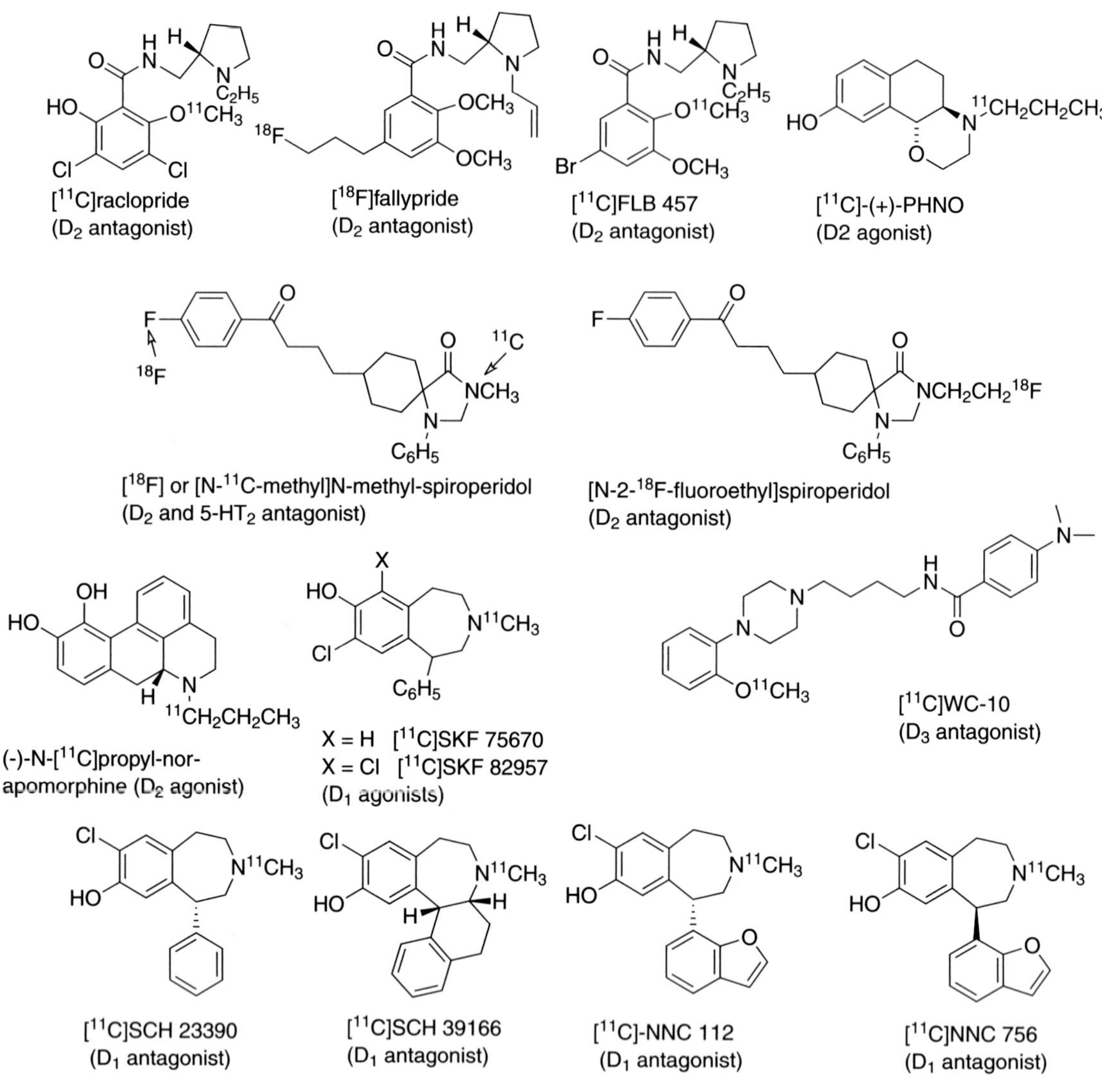

FIGURE 2.7. Structures of some of the radioligands developed for studies of dopamine receptors.

The D_1 receptor antagonists, SCH23390 and SCH39166, have also been labeled with ^{11}C and used to study the central nervous system D_1 receptor (135,136). A high-affinity ligand ^{11}C labeled NNC112 has been developed for imaging extrastriatal D_1 receptors in humans (137). The (+) enantiomer of NNC112 binds selectively and reversibly while the (–) enantiomer did not show appreciable binding. Studies with [^{11}C]NNC112 in humans have shown that kinetic analysis of uptake provides an appropriate method with which to derive dopamine D_1 receptor parameters both in regions of high- and low-receptor density (138).

The dopamine D3 receptor system has been implicated in a number of central nervous system disorders. It is also a new target in drug research and development (139). There has been recent effort and progress in radiotracer development (140). This has been a challenge due to the high concentrations of D_2 receptors relative to D3 receptors among other factors. Recently the N-(2-methoxyphenyl)piperazine derivative WC-10 has been labeled with ^{11}C and shown to have regional distribution consistent with binding to D3 receptors in the central nervous system (141,142).

An attempt to visualize the D4 receptor with [^{11}C]N-[2-[4-(4-chlorophenyl)piperazin-1-yl]ethyl]-3-methoxybenzamide ([^{11}C]PB12) was unsuccessful probably due to the low concentration of dopamine D4 receptors, insufficient binding affinity of the ligand, and high background nonspecific binding (143). Other candidate ligands have also been evaluated (144).

Dopamine and Vesicular Transporters

The plasma membrane dopamine transporter (DAT) has been studied using [^{11}C]nomifensine (145), [^{11}C]cocaine (146), [^{11}C]*d-threo*-methylphenidate (147), cocaine analogues (148–153) and [^{18}F]GBR13119 (154) (Fig. 2.8). These tracers and others have been applied in studies of neurodegeneration, aging, and dopamine transporter occupancy by drugs including cocaine and methylphenidate (155–159). [^{11}C]Cocaine is worthy of mention. Although it was initially developed to measure cocaine pharmacokinetics in the human brain, its rapid reversible kinetics have also served to measure dopamine transporter availability using a graphical analysis for reversible systems (87). A new ligand, [^{11}C]PE2I,

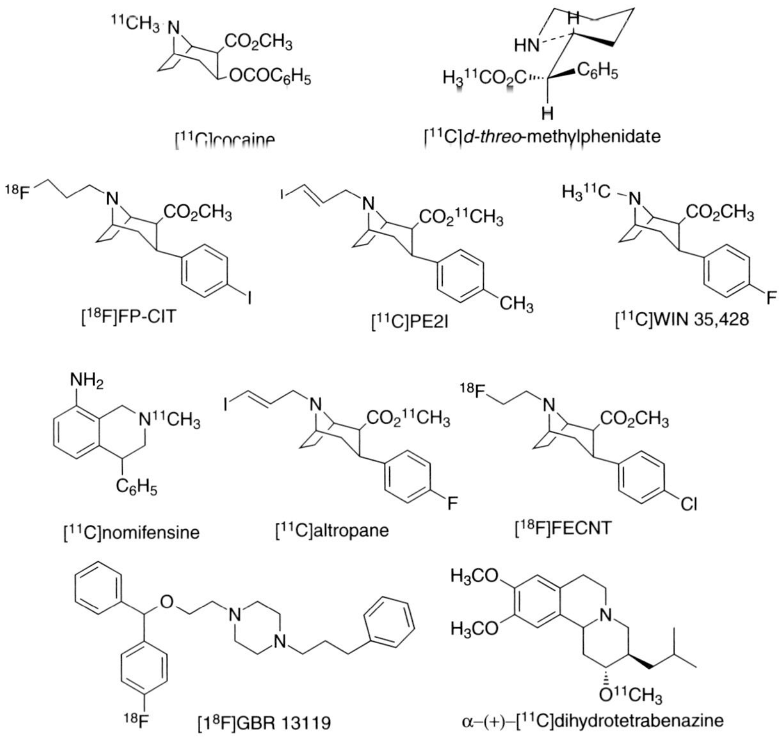

[^{11}C]cocaine
[^{11}C]*d-threo*-methylphenidate
[^{18}F]FP-CIT
[^{11}C]PE2I
[^{11}C]WIN 35,428
[^{11}C]nomifensine
[^{11}C]altropane
[^{18}F]FECNT
[^{18}F]GBR 13119
α–(+)–[^{11}C]dihydrotetrabenazine

FIGURE 2.8. Structures of some of the labeled compounds developed for imaging the dopamine transporter and the vesicular monoamine transporter.

with high affinity toward dopamine transporter has been developed (160). Studies in human subjects showed radioactivity ratios of 10 and 1.8 for the striatum and *substantia nigra* to the cerebellum, respectively, suggesting an advantageous approach for PET examination of DAT binding in the midbrain, a region from which dopaminergic innervation originates (161). Unfortunately, the presence of the pharmacologically active metabolite confounded its kinetic analysis (162).

Vesicular (mono)amine transporters (VMAT2) remove monoamines like dopamine from the cytosol into intracellular vesicles where they are protected from intracellular enzymes like MAO and stored for eventual exocytotic release. Studies have shown that VMAT2 is not altered by regulatory responses to nigrostriatal lesions, changes in dopamine synthesis, or turnover (163,164). Thus, VMAT2 is a useful molecular target for dopamine terminal density. Accordingly, $\alpha(+)$-[^{11}C]dihydrotetrabenazine ([^{11}C]DTBZ) has emerged as an excellent radiotracer, devoid of lipophilic metabolites, and shows stereoselectivity and kinetics amenable to modeling (165,166). Recently, it has been shown that VMAT2 are expressed in human islet β cells as well as in tissues of the central nervous system. Diabetes results from an absolute or relative reduction in pancreatic β cell mass, leading to insufficient insulin secretion and hyperglycemia. [^{11}C]DTBZ can be used to measure VMAT2 density and consequently provide a noninvasive measurement of β cell mass that could be used to study the pathogenesis of diabetes and to monitor therapeutic interventions (167).

Monoamine Oxidase

Monoamine oxidase (for review see Fowler et al. [168]) is a flavin-containing enzyme that exists in two subtypes: MAO A and B (see Fig. 2.9 for structures). MAO oxidizes amines including dopamine and other neurotransmitters (169). Medical interest in MAO stems from the utility of MAO inhibitor drugs in the treatment of depression and Parkinson disease. The first images of functional MAO activity in the human brain were made with ^{11}C labeled suicide enzyme inactivators [^{11}C]clorgyline and [^{11}C]L-deprenyl, which covalently label the enzyme *in vivo* (170). Mechanistic PET studies with deuterium substituted [^{11}C]L-deprenyl demonstrated that the C-H bond in the propargyl group was involved in the rate limiting step for the formation of the PET image and provided a means of selectively controlling the rate of trapping of tracer in the brain to improve quantitation (103). [^{11}C]L-deprenyl and the deuterium substituted derivative have been used to directly examine the effects of MAO B inhibitor drugs, lazabemide and L-deprenyl in the human brain (171,172).

[^{11}C]Clorgyline and [^{11}C]L-deprenyl-D_2 and PET have also revealed a reduction in MAO A and B in brain and peripheral organs in smokers (173–176). This is a pharmacologic effect of smoke, as former smokers have normal MAO levels. Interestingly, the MAO B inhibitory constituent(s) in smoke is not nicotine. In fact, an MAO inhibitory compound was recently isolated from tobacco leaves (177). Reduced brain MAO in smokers may be an important neurochemical link to smoking epidemiology, including the documented decreased risk of Parkinson disease in smokers (178).

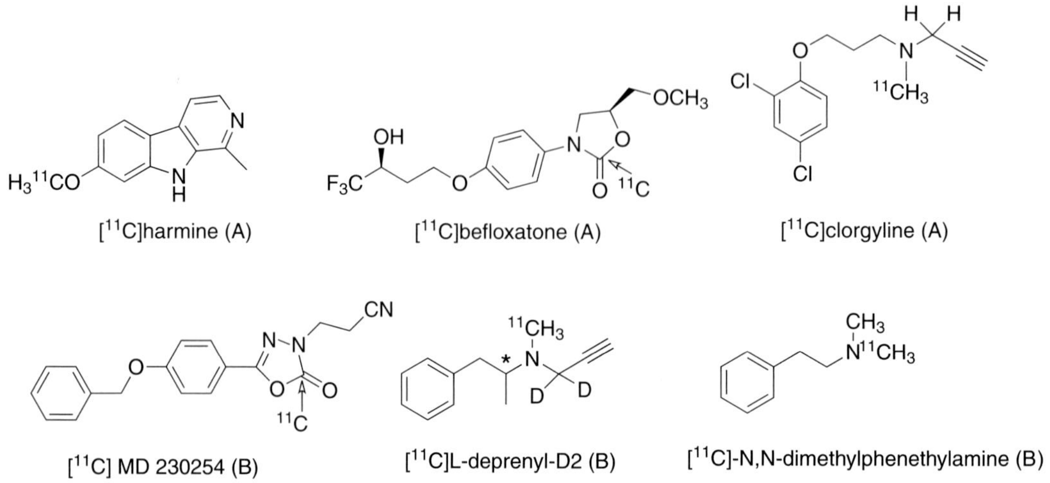

[^{11}C]harmine (A) [^{11}C]befloxatone (A) [^{11}C]clorgyline (A)

[^{11}C] MD 230254 (B) [^{11}C]L-deprenyl-D2 (B) [^{11}C]-N,N-dimethylphenethylamine (B)

FIGURE 2.9. Radiotracers for PET studies of monoamine oxidase. Subtype specificity is in parentheses.

A number of labeled selective, reversible inhibitors of MAO A including [^{11}C]harmine, [^{11}C]methylharmine, [^{11}C]harmaline, [^{11}C]MD230254, and [^{11}C]befloxatone have also been developed and evaluated for their specificity as MAO tracers *in vivo* (44,179–181).

The Brain Serotonin System

The cells that produce serotonin are located in the dorsal raphe nucleus, which extensively innervate neocortical regions (Figs. 2.10 and 2.11). Abnormalities in the brain serotonin system have been implicated in a variety of neuropsychiatric disorders such as anxiety, depression, sleep disorders, eating disorders, and violence. Drugs that change serotonin levels have been widely used in the treatment of depression, anxiety, and obesity. The physiological actions of serotonin are mediated through its interactions with serotonin receptors. These are now assigned to one of seven families, 5HT1–7, comprising a total of 14 structurally and pharmacologically distinct mammalian 5-HT receptor subtypes (182). Thus far, most of the effort in PET radiotracer development has been focused on the 5-HT$_{2A}$ and the 5-HT$_{1A}$ receptor subtypes as well as the serotonin transporter. Recently, [^{11}C]SB-207145 as a potential PET ligand for studying 5-HT$_4$ receptor has been reported (183). The ability of [^{11}C]GSK215083 and [^{11}C]GSK224558 to delineate 5-HT$_6$ receptors has also been evaluated *in vivo* (184).

Progress in the development of radiotracers for the 5-HT$_{2A}$ receptors was reviewed (185,186). [^{11}C]N-methylspiroperidol labeled with ^{11}C and with ^{18}F binds both to the dopamine D$_2$ receptor in the striatum and to the 5-HT$_{2A}$ receptor in the frontal cortex and has been used to image the 5-HT$_{2A}$ receptor (187,188). Other more selective 5-HT$_{2A}$ radiotracers including [^{18}F]altanserin (189), [^{18}F]setoperone (190), and [^{11}C]MDL100,907 (191,192) have been

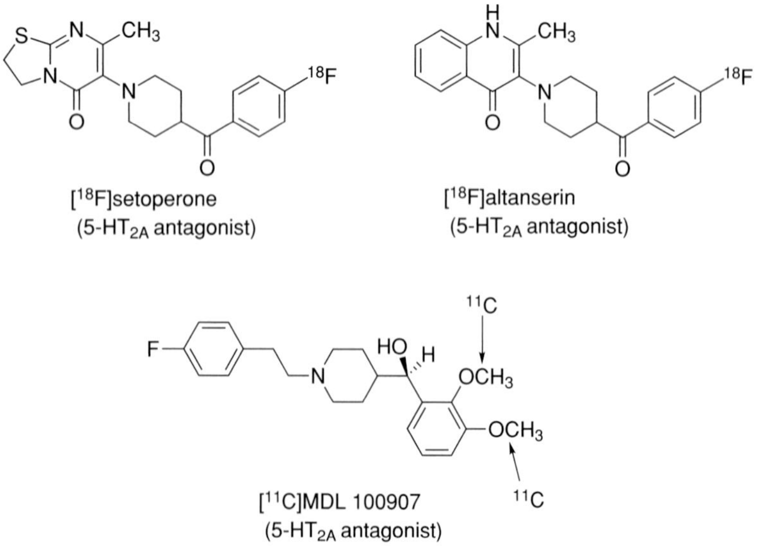

[^{18}F]setoperone (5-HT$_{2A}$ antagonist) [^{18}F]altanserin (5-HT$_{2A}$ antagonist)

[^{11}C]MDL 100907 (5-HT$_{2A}$ antagonist)

FIGURE 2.10. Radiotracers for PET studies of the 5-HT$_{2A}$ receptor.

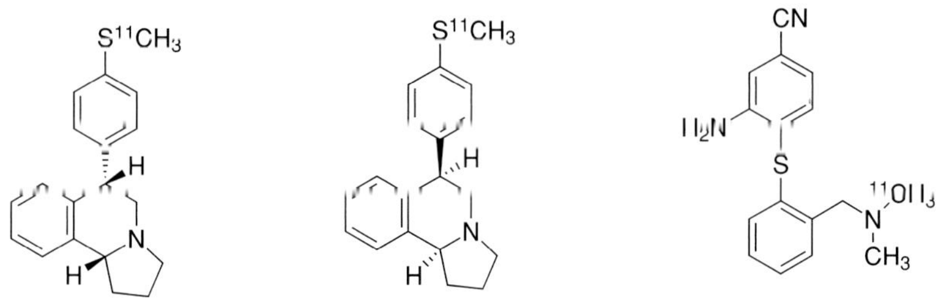

FIGURE 2.11. Structures of some of the radiotracers for studies of the serotonin transporter.

developed and applied in human studies. As with most PET radiotracers, none of these is perfect, each having problems with lipophilic metabolites, nonspecific binding, binding to other neurotransmitter receptors, or kinetics, making their quantification susceptible to blood flow artifacts. The quantification of 5-HT_{2A} receptors with [^{18}F]altanserin in the human brain has been examined using a constant infusion paradigm to reduce the difficulties associated with lipophilic radiolabeled metabolites (193).

5-HT_{1A} receptors are concentrated on cell bodies of the raphe nuclei and serve as autoreceptors, mediating serotonin release. They occur both pre- and postsynaptically. There is a high density of 5-HT_{1A} postsynaptic receptors in the neocortex. The presynaptic sites have been proposed to mediate drug treatment of anxiety and depression, while postsynaptic sites have been found to be elevated in schizophrenic brains postmortem. Radiotracer studies of the 5-HT_{1A} receptor have used the WAY100635 structure as a template. WAY100635 was first labeled with ^{11}C in the O-methyl group (194). This radiotracer was metabolized rapidly and produced a lipophilic-labeled metabolite, WAY100634, via loss of the cyclohexanecarbonyl group (195,196). Unfortunately, this metabolite also has a high affinity for the 5-HT_{1A} receptor and crosses the blood–brain barrier, which limits accurate quantitation. For this reason WAY100635 was later labeled in the carbonyl group (91) to avoid the formation of the [^{11}C]WAY100634 (Fig. 2.5). Human studies with both labeled versions of WAY100635 have been carried out, and delineation of 5-HT_{1A} receptors was improved with the [^{11}C]carbonyl compound (197). Initial human studies have also been carried out with [^{11}C]CPC222, a compound similar in structure to WAY100635, with a bicyclo-octyl group replacing the cyclohexyl group. This structurally modified compound is not metabolized to WAY100634 and thus labeling in the N-methyl group (which is simpler) does not carry the disadvantage as with carbonyl-labeled WAY100635 (198). The synthesis and *in vitro* evaluation of [^{11}C]-(R)-3-N,N-dicyclobutylamino-8-fluoro-3,4-dihydro-2H-benzopyran-5-carboxamide ([^{11}C]NAD-299) in human brain indicated that it is also a promising ligand for the 5-HT_{1A} receptor (Eq. 6) (43). An ^{18}F-labeled radiotracer for the 5-HT_{1A} receptor, p-[^{18}F]MPPF, has also been prepared and used in human studies (199,200). A special issue of *Nuclear Medicine and Biology* has been dedicated to the imaging of 5-HT_{1A} receptors (201).

Radiotracers have also been developed to image the serotonin transporter that removes serotonin from the synapse and are also the molecular target for the selective serotonin reuptake inhibitor (SSRI) class of antidepressant drugs. This is an important area in radiotracer development because of the need to assess toxicity to serotonergic neurons by compounds such as methylenedioxymethamphetamine (MDMA). Accordingly, the pyrrolo isoquinoline McN 5652 was labeled with ^{11}C by S-methylation of the normethyl precursor (202). McN 5652 has a chiral center. The (+) enantiomer is active, while the (–) enantiomer is inactive (Fig. 2.11). PET studies in humans have compared the two enantiomers using the (–) enantiomer to assess nonspecific binding . Although the distribution of (+)-[^{11}C]McN5652 parallels the known distribution of serotonin transporters, there are data that show that it underestimates nonspecific binding in some brain regions (203,204). [^{11}C]N,N-dimethyl-2-(2-amino-4-cyanophenylthio) benzylamine ([^{11}C]DASB) has been shown to have very good properties to image and quantify the serotonin transporter in human studies (205). Several serotonin transporter ligands, such as nortropane analogues and DASB analogues (206,207), have shown promising results as well. [^{11}C]Fluoxetine, [^{11}C]citalopram, and [N-^{11}C]methylparoxetine all have low target-to-nontarget ratios (154,208,209).

The possibility of measuring the rate of serotonin synthesis has also been probed by [^{11}C]-α-methyltryptophan (210,211), although recent PET studies in monkeys report that [^{11}C]-α-methyltryptophan is acting predominantly as a tracer of tryptophan uptake (212).

The Brain Opiate System

Opiate receptors mediate the effects of endogenous and exogenous opioids, including respiratory depression, analgesia, reward, and sedation (Fig. 2.12). There are three major opiate receptor subtypes: μ, δ, and κ with subclasses of these subtypes. The first PET tracer for the opiate receptor was [^{11}C]carfentanil l, a high affinity μ opiate agonist (213). [^{11}C]Carfentanil localizes in opiate receptor-rich regions of the human brain, such as the basal ganglia and the thalamus (214). Its uptake can be reduced by pretreatment with the opiate antagonist naloxone. PET studies with [^{11}C]carfentanil suggest that both age and gender are variables to consider in the interpretation of measures of brain opioid function (215). Another nonsubtype-specific opiate agonist [^{11}C]diprenorphine has been synthesized using [1-^{11}C]cyclopropanecarbonyl chloride (216). Buprenorphine, a compound with a combination of agonist and antagonist properties, has been labeled with ^{11}C in two different positions, the O-methyl position (217–219) and the cyclopropylmethyl position (220). Comparison between [^{11}C]buprenorphine and [^{11}C]diprenorphine in the baboon shows that [^{11}C]diprenorphine

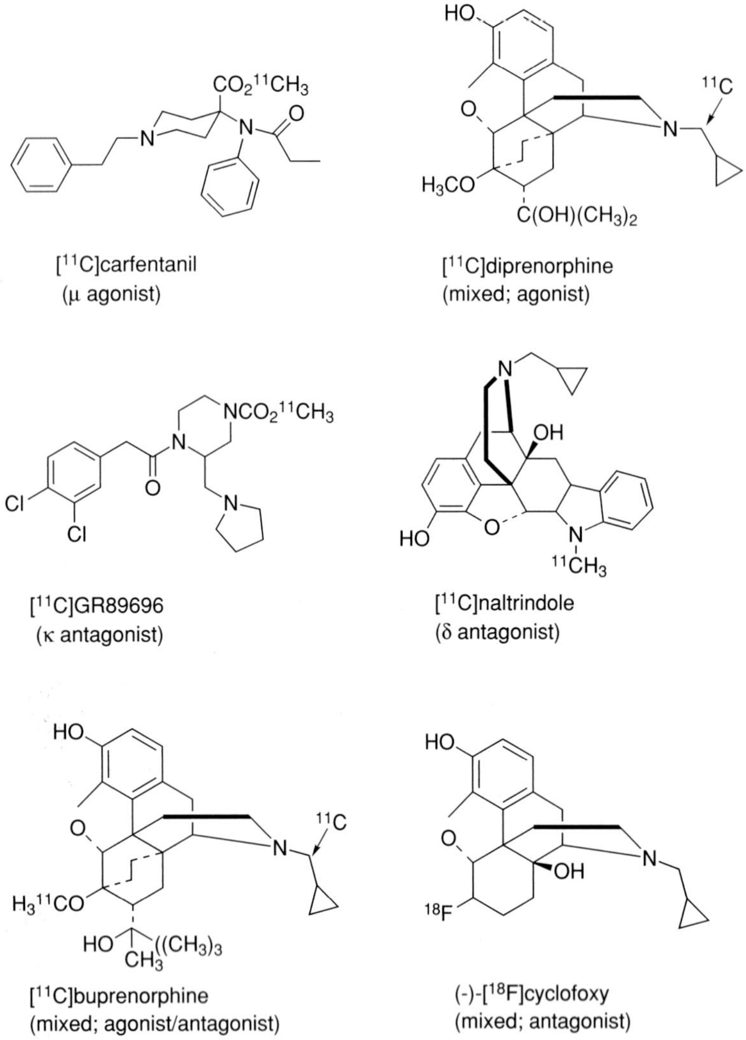

[^{11}C]carfentanil
(μ agonist)

[^{11}C]diprenorphine
(mixed; agonist)

[^{11}C]GR89696
(κ antagonist)

[^{11}C]naltrindole
(δ antagonist)

[^{11}C]buprenorphine
(mixed; agonist/antagonist)

(-)-[^{18}F]cyclofoxy
(mixed; antagonist)

FIGURE 2.12. Structures of some of the radiotracers developed for PET studies of opioid receptors. Receptor subtype is indicated in parentheses.

may be superior for PET studies due to its more rapid clearance from the cerebellum. However, buprenorphine has low toxicity, and it is an approved analgesic drug that could facilitate translation to humans. The high affinity opiate antagonist cyclofoxy binds to both μ and κ sites. It has been labeled with ^{18}F for opiate receptor imaging with PET (221,222). Recently a high-affinity κ-selective compound, GR89696, was labeled with ^{11}C and shows promise in mice for *in vivo* binding to κ sites (223). The regional specific to nonspecific partition coefficient values of ^{11}C-GR103545, the active enantiomer of GR89696, were approximately double those for ^{11}C-GR89696, whereas those for (+)-^{11}C-GR89696 were negligible, demonstrating the enantiomeric selectivity of the binding and the advantage of using the pure active enantiomer for PET studies of κ-opioid receptors (40). The κ-opioid receptors have been imaged in the human brain with [^{11}C]naltrindole and PET (224).

The Benzodiazepine System

Benzodiazepines are a class of chemical compounds that are potent anxiolytics, anticonvulsants, and hypnotics (Fig. 2.13). Binding sites for the benzodiazepines have been subdivided into central and peripheral types. Central types are thought to constitute one of the subunits on the $GABA_A$ (γ-aminobutyric acid) receptor complex and are responsible for the anxiolytic actions of this class of drugs through facilitation of the inhibitory actions of GABA (225). Peripheral binding sites are not associated with GABA and have very low affinity for the central type (226); however, they display high affinity for the isoquinoline derivative PK11195, which is inactive at the central site. Peripheral binding sites occur in the kidneys, liver, and lungs as well as mast cells and macrophages. However, they also occur in the central nervous system on nonneuronal elements such as glial and ependymal cells.

Radiotracers for PET imaging of both the central and peripheral benzodiazepine receptors have been developed and progress has been reviewed (227,228). For the central site, the most well-studied radiotracer is [^{11}C]Ro-15-1788 ([^{11}C]flumazenil), a benzodiazepine antagonist that shows a clear dose-dependent binding with PET (229). [^{11}C]Ro15-1788 also has excellent kinetic properties for the quantitative measurement of the central site, permitting parametric images of flow and benzodiazepine receptor availability from a single tracer injection (230).

Peripheral benzodiazepine receptors have been imaged and quantified with the isoquinoline [^{11}C]PK11195 as a marker for activated microglia in the human brain (231). There have also been

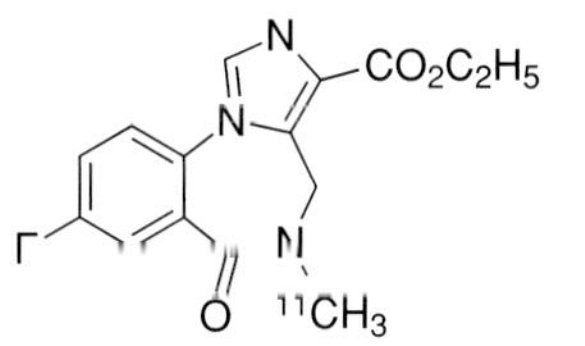

[11C]Ro15 1788
(central)

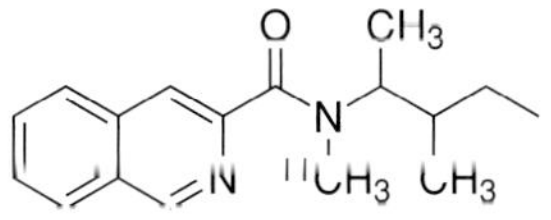

[11C]PK-11195
(peripheral)

FIGURE 2.13. Structures of labeled compounds for PET studies of central and peripheral benzodiazepine receptors.

recent efforts to develop improved radiotracers for the peripheral benzodiazepine receptor (232).

The Cholinergic System

There are two major classes of receptors for the neurotransmitter acetylcholine (ACh): the muscarinic-cholinergic receptors (mAChR) and the nicotinic acetylcholine receptors (nAChR). Because of the importance of acetylcholine in learning and memory and mounting evidence of cholinergic deficits in Alzheimer disease (233), the receptors mediating cholinergic neurotransmission as well as enzymes such as cholineacetyltransferase (ChAT), which mediates its synthesis, and acetylcholinesterase (AChE), which terminates its action, are of intense interest and prime targets for radiotracer development.

Muscarinic Cholinergic Receptors

The mAChR can be divided into four pharmacologically distinct subtypes (M1 to M4) and into five genetically distinct subtypes (m1 to m5) (234) (Fig. 2.14). The development of radiotracers suitable for imaging this system, particularly the M_2 subtype has been pursued for many years because this subtype is involved in Alzheimer disease (235). PET tracers [^{11}C]scopolamine (236), [^{11}C]tropanylbenzilate (237), and [^{11}C]N-methyl-3- and 4-piperidinyl benzilate (238,239), levetimide (94), and benztropine (240) have been developed and evaluated. Human studies have focused on the investigation of normal aging and Alzheimer disease (241–243).

In general, tracers for the muscarinic cholinergic receptors have been limited by low subtype selectivity as well as very rapid binding and slow dissociation, which limit the resolution of blood flow effects from receptor binding (244). In a recent development, an M2 selective agonist 3-(3-(3-[^{18}F]fluoropropyl)thio-1,2,5-thiadiazol-4-yl)-1,2,5,6-tetrahydro-1-methylpyridine ([^{18}F]FP-TZTP) was synthesized (245). PET studies in six rhesus monkeys showed a binding pattern consistent with the distribution of M2 sites, and more recently [^{18}F]FP-TZTP binding was compared in wild type and in M2 knockout animals where binding was unequivocally shown to be M2 specific (80). In addition pretreatment with the acetylcholinesterase inhibitor physostigmine caused a reduction in [^{18}F]FP-TZTP binding, indicating that the tracer is sensitive to drug-induced changes in acetylcholine. The degree of reduction is smallest in the striatum, which has high levels of acetylcholinesterase (246). Because the cholinergic system, and specifically the M2 receptor, has been shown to be lost in aging and degeneration, [^{18}F]TZTP PET studies were carried out to compare young and old subjects and to compare subjects bearing the apolipoprotein E-ε_4 allele with age matched controls who did not carry the apolipoprotein E-ε_4 (247). [^{18}F]TZTP binding was *higher* in older than younger subjects and it was also *higher* in the apolipoprotein E-ε_4 positive subjects than in the control group (248). The authors speculate that with age and with the apolipoprotein E ε_4 allele, there is a decrease in acetyl choline (the neurotransmitter involved in memory) and that this would be expected to decrease occupancy of the M2 sites by endogenous acetylcholine. This, in turn, would elevate the number of unoccupied receptors as well as radiotracer binding. Thus [^{18}F]TZTP offers promise as a tool for evaluating the efficacies of various therapies designed to elevate acetylcholine similar to the use of [^{11}C]raclopride to measure changes in synaptic dopamine. In addition, pending more studies, [^{18}F]TZTP could be use to identify subjects at risk for degenerative disease who would benefit from early acetylcholine enhancing therapy or other drug treatment.

Acetylcholinesterase

Acetylcholinesterase hydrolyzes ACh and thus it is crucial for ACh regulation (Fig. 2.14). The consequences of its inhibition are of great importance both in toxicology and in therapeutics. Because Alzheimer disease is characterized by a deficiency in cholinergic activity, cholinesterase inhibitors represent the most extensively developed class of compounds for its treatment. Similar to the mAChR, the development of radiotracers for quantitation of AChE offers the potential of gaining more insight into the pathophysiology of Alzheimer disease as well as a tool for the design, development, and evaluation of cholinergic therapy.

There have been two approaches to radiotracer development for studies of AChE: the synthesis of labeled inhibitors of AChE such as [^{11}C]physostigmine ([^{11}C]PHY), which measures the number of binding sites, and the synthesis of labeled substrates of AChE such as [N-^{11}C–methyl]-4-piperidinyl acetate ([^{11}C]AMP) and [N-^{11}C-methyl]4-piperidinyl propionate ([^{11}C]PMP), which measures enzyme activity. Physostigmine has been synthesized from [^{11}C]methylisocyanate and eseroline and inhibits AChE by covalent attachment of the carbamate moiety to the enzyme (249). The label is on the carboxyl carbon atom. This ensures covalent binding of ^{11}C with the serine residue of the enzyme's active site so that the retention of ^{11}C after the injection of [^{11}C]physostigmine would, in principle, represent AChE activity. Human studies with [^{11}C]physostigmine showed a retention pattern of ^{11}C typical of AChE activity with a striatum to cortex ratio of 2 (250). Another approach to measuring the number of binding sites of AChE uses a ^{11}C-labeled substrate for AChE, such as [^{11}C]AMP or [^{11}C]PMP, also called [^{11}C]MP4A and [^{11}C]MP4A. These radiotracers are labeled in the N-methyl position such that when they are hydrolyzed by AChE, the labeled hydrophilic product (which has limited ability to diffuse out of the brain) is trapped at the site of AChE activity in proportion to AChE activity and cerebral blood flow (251). Because of the need to optimize the rate of trapping of radiotracer so that the concentration of radioactivity in a volume element of tissue is not limited by radiotracer delivery into the brain, different esters have been evaluated and used to investigate the involvement of this system in normal aging and in Alzheimer disease (252,253). These radioligands can also be used to assess the efficacy of the various anticholinesterases used therapeutically and to determine the doses required to achieve optimal inhibition (254). Fluorine-18-labeled derivatives of acetylcholinesterase substrates have also been synthesized and evaluated to explore the possibility to prepare

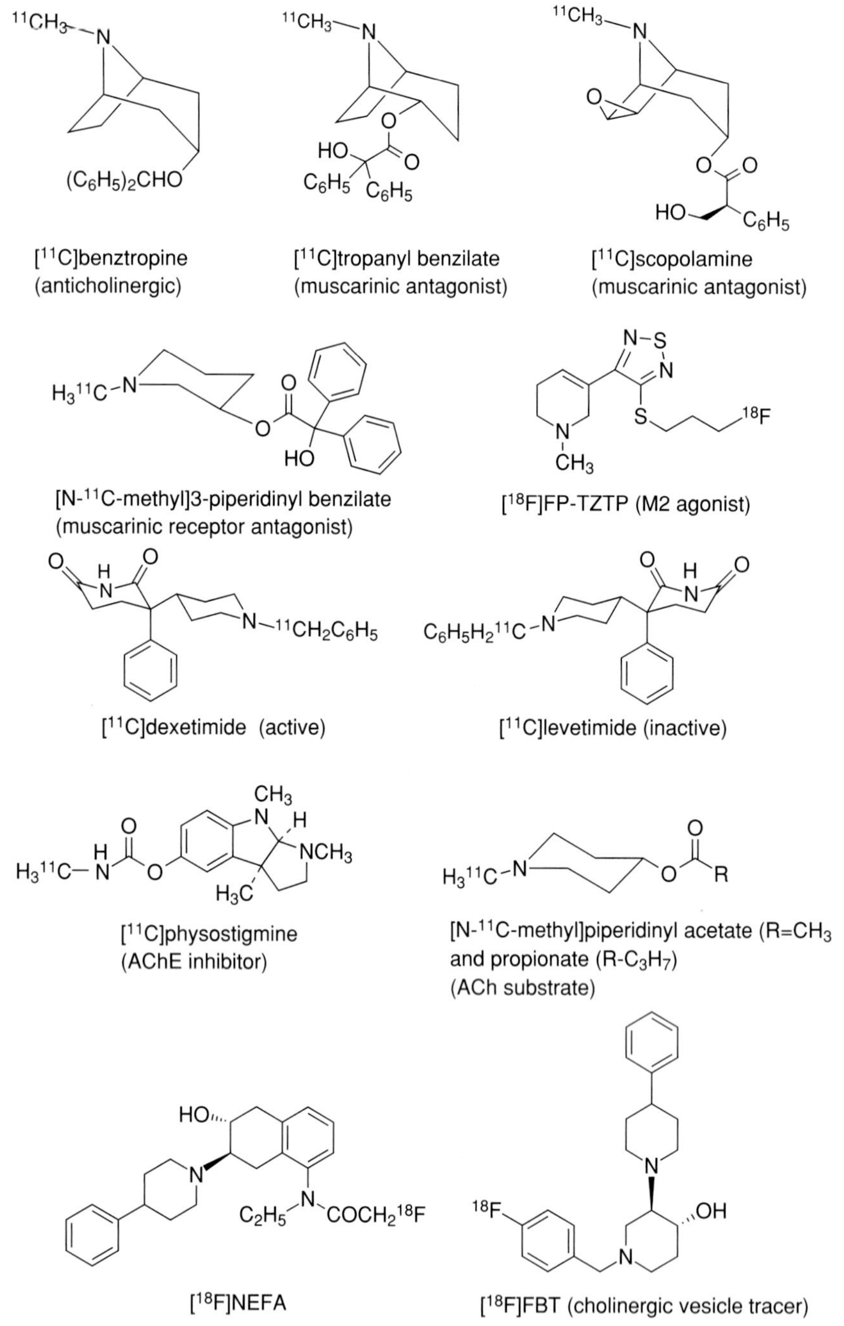

FIGURE 2.14. Structures of labeled compounds for PET studies of muscarinic-cholinergic receptors and for acetylcholinesterase.

batches of radiotracer for multiple patients and delivery of tracer from a central facility to institutions without a cyclotron and chemistry expertise (255,256).

Radiotracers have also been developed to image cholinergic terminals. One of these, [^{18}F]NEFA, an aminobenzovesamicol, was studied in primates with PET to probe striatal dopamine D_2/acetylcholine interactions (257). The measurement of cholinergic terminal density through imaging of the vesicular ACh transporter with [^{18}F](+)-4-flluorobenzyltrozamicol has recently been studied (258). One of the difficulties in radiotracer development in this area is the high toxicity of model compounds.

Nicotinic Acetylcholine Receptors

The nAChR are the major molecular targets for nicotine and important targets for pharmaceutical drug discovery (264) (Fig. 2.15). They are also believed to mediate nicotine's effects on cognition and behavior and play a central role in tobacco addiction. nAChR receptors are associated with the axons and cell bodies of neurons that comprise several major neurotransmitter systems, including the dopamine, norepinephrine, acetylcholine, GABA, and glutamate neurons (259). They exist as pentamers comprised of α and β subunits, leading to considerable diversity. The most abundant subtypes in the mammalian brain

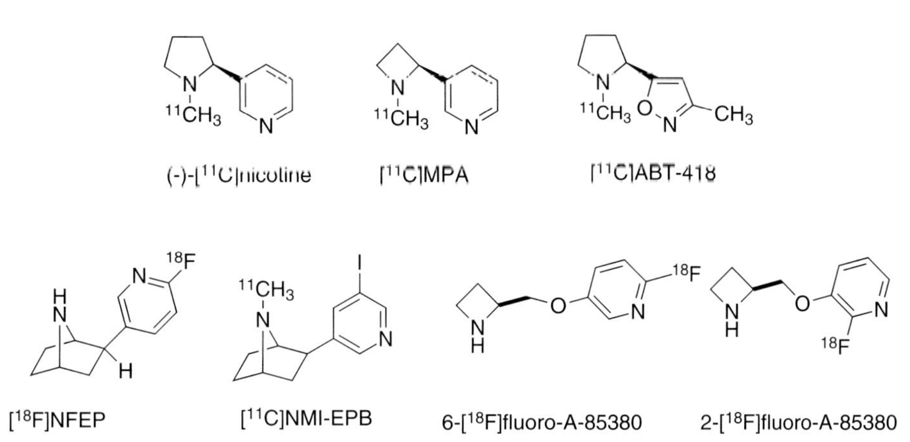

(-)-[^{11}C]nicotine [^{11}C]MPA [^{11}C]ABT-418

[^{18}F]NFEP [^{11}C]NMI-EPB 6-[^{18}F]fluoro-A-85380 2-[^{18}F]fluoro-A-85380

FIGURE 2.15. Structures of labeled compounds for PET studies of nicotinic acetylcholine receptors.

are the $\alpha_4\beta_2$ and the α_7 nAChR. Studies with β_2 knockout mice suggest a role for the β_2-containing nicotinic receptors in nicotine reinforcement (260). Studies in human brain postmortem have documented losses in nAChR with normal aging, which is accentuated in Alzheimer disease (261). In contrast, nAChR are *elevated* in smokers (262). The nAChR are also being investigated as a molecular target for the development of therapeutic drugs for a number of neurodegenerative and neuropsychiatric disorders and pain (263–265).

Three general classes of compounds have been investigated as potential radiotracers for nAChR: nicotine and its derivatives; epibatidine and its derivatives; and 3-pyridyl ether derivatives (266). Although [^{11}C]nicotine's distribution and pharmacokinetics have been measured in the human brain, images are dominated by nonspecific binding (267,268). Although [^{11}C]nicotine is not suitable as a tracer for nAChR, its pharmacokinetics, which show rapid brain entry and efflux that are characteristic of drugs that are highly reinforcing, are of intrinsic interest. Two other nicotinic agonists, (R,S)-1-[^{11}C]methyl-2(3-pyridyl)azetidine ([^{11}C]MPA) and (S)-3-methyl-5-(1-[^{11}C]methyl-2-pyrrolidinyl)isoxazole ([^{11}C]ABT-418), were compared to (S)(–)[^{11}C]nicotine (269). Although [^{11}C]MPA showed a small degree of specific binding relative to [^{11}C]nicotine and [^{11}C]ABT 418, the magnitude was low. A breakthrough in the development of nicotinic tracers with high specific binding *in vivo* came with the discovery of epibatidine, which was isolated from the Ecuadoran poison frog (270), and the demonstration of potent analgesic properties that are mediated through the nAChR (271). The reported specificity of epibatidine for central nervous system nicotinic receptors stimulated the development of methods to label epibatidine with ^{18}F, where fluorine is substituted for the chlorine atom that is present in the natural product to produce [^{18}F]norchlorofluoroepibatidine ([^{18}F]NFEP) (272). Although the ^{18}F-labeled epibatidine derivatives proved to be good radiotracers for the central nAChR and have been used in measuring nAChR occupancy by nicotine (273) as well as interactions between the nicotinic and dopamine systems (274), application in humans is not possible because of the high toxicity of epibatidine and derivatives (275,276).

The development of 3-pyridyl ether derivatives that had higher selectivity for the $\alpha_4\beta_2$ subtype and significantly lower toxicity provided an attractive alternative for radiotracer development (277). Both 2-fluoro-A-85380 and 6-fluoro-A-85380 are nicotinic agonists that have high affinity for neuronal nAChR but are less toxic than epibatidine (278). Fluorine-18-labeled analogues, 2-[^{18}F]fluoro-A-85380 and 6-[^{18}F]fluoro-A-85380, were promising radioligands for PET studies. Several research groups have reported the radiosynthesis of 2-[^{18}F]fluoro-A-85380 (279–281) and 6-[^{18}F]fluoro-A-85380 (282,283) using either iodo or nitro as a leaving group, although the use of a trimethylammonium precursor to 6-[^{18}F]fluoro-A-85380 offers an advantage over other leaving groups (57). Human studies have been carried out with both the 2-[^{18}F]fluoro-A-85380 (284,285) and the 6-[^{18}F]fluoro-A-85380 (58). Interestingly, *specific* binding in white matter is observed for 6-[^{18}F]fluoro-A-85380 (58). A recent important development has been the synthesis and ^{11}C labeling of an *$\alpha_4\beta_2$ antagonist* [^{11}C]NMI-EPB, which shows high specific binding in the baboon brain *in vivo*. The molecule also contains an iodine atom, making it a candidate for labeling for both PET and single-photon emission computed tomography studies (286). There is a need to develop other subtype selective tracers for the nAChR, particularly the α_7 subtype (for which there is evidence of an association with amyloid accumulation in Alzheimer disease) (287).

Signal Transduction Pathways

The effects of neurotransmitter binding to monoamine receptors are mediated by intracellular signal transduction cascades (Fig. 2.16). The second messenger signals transduction pathways (cAMP, diacylglycerol, inositol triphosphate, Ca^{+2}) mediate the actions of many monoamine receptors. This regulation occurs via G proteins that couple receptors to effectors such as adenylate cyclase and phospholipase C that catalyze cAMP and inositol triphosphate formation, respectively. These second messengers regulate the action of second-messenger-dependent protein kinases. All aspects of neuronal functioning that are fundamental to the ability of the brain to respond and to adapt to pharmacological and environmental input are controlled by these pathways (288).

Radiotracers for imaging different aspects of the signal transduction pathways are under development. For example

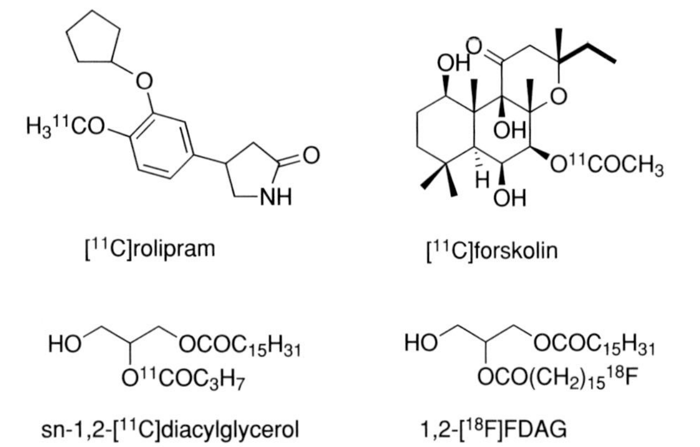

[11C]rolipram

[11C]forskolin

sn-1,2-[11C]diacylglycerol

1,2-[18F]FDAG

FIGURE 2.16. Structures of labeled compounds for PET studies of signal transduction.

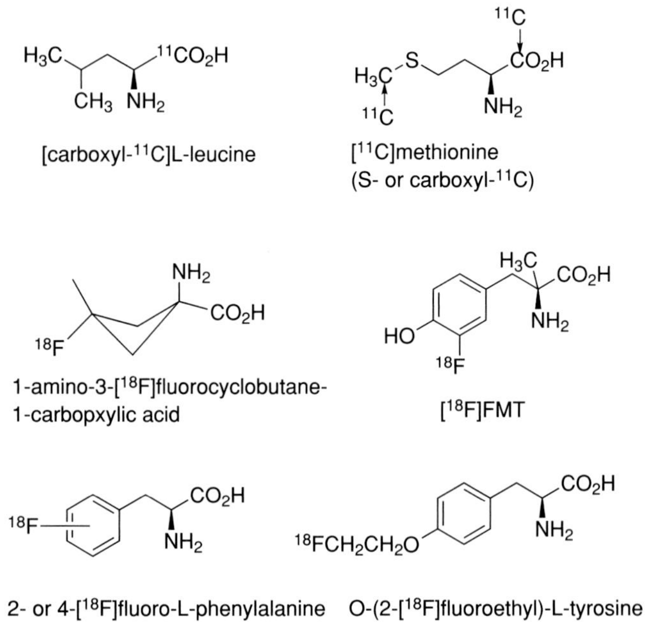

[carboxyl-11C]L-leucine

[11C]methionine (S- or carboxyl-11C)

1-amino-3-[18F]fluorocyclobutane-1-carbopxylic acid

[18F]FMT

2- or 4-[18F]fluoro-L-phenylalanine

O-(2-[18F]fluoroethyl)-L-tyrosine

FIGURE 2.17. Structures of labeled amino acids for PET studies of protein synthesis and amino acid transport.

[^{11}C]-1,2-diacylglycerol and [^{11}C]forskolin have been synthesized and evaluated as probes for signal transduction in tumor cells and in a glioma patient with PET (289,290). After [^{11}C]-1,2-diacylglycerol, ^{11}C was incorporated into the phosphoinositide pool and another phospholipid pool in the proliferative state. When the proliferative state was inhibited by (−)-3D-3-deoxy-3-fluoro-myo-inositol, incorporation into the phosphoinositide pool decreased selectively. A PET study in a human glioma patient showed promise for visualizing the proliferation signal in a human glioma patient (289). Fluorine-18 labeled diacylglycerols (1,2-[^{18}F]FDAG) are also being investigated (291).

The selective phosphodiesterase IV inhibitor rolipram has also been labeled with ^{11}C and shown to have high uptake in the rat brain in regions (i.e., cortex and olfactory system) known to show high expression of phosphodiesterase IV enzymes (292). The first studies in humans with [^{11}C]rolipram showed high radioactivity retention in all regions representing gray matter, which is consistent with suitability for imaging phosphodiesterase IV and possibly cAMP signal transduction in humans (293).

AMINO ACID TRANSPORT AND PROTEIN SYNTHESIS

Protein synthesis, like energy metabolism, is one of the fundamental processes supporting growth and development (Fig. 2.17). Many positron emitter–labeled amino acids and amino acid derivatives have been synthesized over the past 30 years (294,295). This was undertaken with a view to develop a method to quantitatively measure protein synthesis rate similar to the ^{18}FDG method for measurement of brain glucose metabolism. This would offer the opportunity to assess how protein synthesis rates change with brain development, regeneration and repair, neurodegenerative disease, cancer, learning and memory, and in response to therapeutic drugs and drugs of abuse.

One approach to the measurement of protein synthesis rate uses [^{11}C-carboxyl]L-leucine, where the products of amino acid metabolism (loss of [^{11}C]O_2) are not labeled, but the proteins of interest are labeled (296,297). The quantification of protein synthesis rate using this approach has been limited by recycling of amino acids derived from the degradation of proteins, which must be taken into account in the estimation of the precursor pool specific activity in tissue from measurements in plasma (298). However, a kinetic approach has recently been used to correct for recycling of tissue amino acids (299).

[^{11}C-S-methyl]L-methionine and [1-^{11}C]L-methionine have also been examined as substrates for protein synthesis (300,301). With [^{11}C-S-methyl]L-methionine the behavior *in vivo* is complicated by the fact that it can undergo both protein synthesis and transmethylation, which would produce unwanted labeled metabolites. Labeled methionine has been used extensively to delineate tumor tissue, although the mechanism for sequestration has not been fully characterized. [^{11}C]-D- and L-methionine have been compared to show that methionine transport into some tumors is nonselective (302). However, [^{11}C]L-methionine shows irreversible trapping in some tumors and shows a high signal-to-noise ratio (303).

Because most *in vivo* PET studies and kinetic modeling of labeled amino acid uptake in tumors indicate that the accumulation of radioactivity is dominated by transport rather than protein synthesis, the search for an amino acid whose uptake and retention reflects protein synthesis rate has been largely replaced by the search for an amino acid that fulfills the following characteristics: (a) easy high-yield synthesis with ^{18}F so that it could be distributed from a central radiopharmacy; (b) high transport rate into tumors; (c) low uptake in normal brain and peripheral tissues to provide high signal to background; and (d) high metabolic stability. A rapid, high-yield synthesis of O-(2-[^{18}F]fluoroethyl)-L-tyrosine was developed (304) and evaluated in animals and humans. It provides a high signal-to-noise ratio in human cancer patients along with ease of synthesis. Other amino acids developed for brain tumor imaging include 2-[^{18}F]fluorotyrosine (305,306), L-[2-^{18}F]fluorophenylalanine (307), L-[3-^{18}F-fluoro]-α-methyl tyrosine ([^{18}F]FMT) (308), and the unnatural,

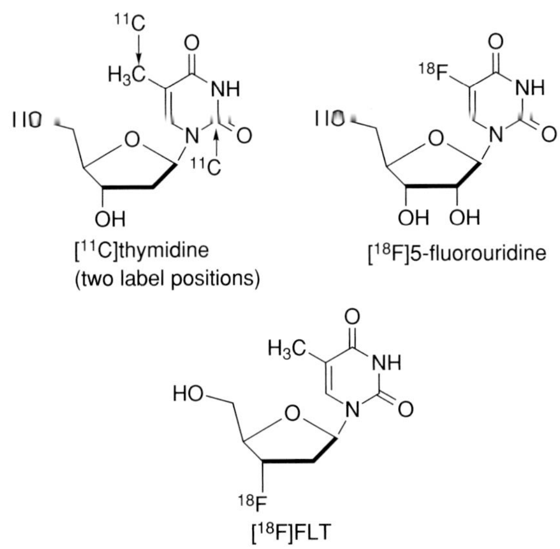

FIGURE 2.18. Structures of labeled compounds for PET studies of DNA synthesis.

nonmetabolized amino acid 1-amino-3-[^{18}F]fluorocyclobutane-1-carboxylic acid (309).

DNA SYNTHESIS

The incorporation of labeled thymidine (tritium or carbon-14 labeled) into cells has long been the gold standard for measuring tissue proliferation and growth kinetics (310,311) (Fig. 2.18). The extension of this approach to the measurement of DNA synthesis in humans using PET was explored in the early 1970s prior to the availability of modern PET instrumentation (312). [^{18}F]Fluorouridine was also synthesized and shown to be taken up by proliferating cells and incorporated into both DNA and RNA (313). More recent research with labeled thymidine has focused on characterizing the biochemistry and kinetics of [^{11}C]thymidine in tumors (314,315) as well as imaging with PET (316–319). Although, in principle, [^{11}C]thymidine should be the gold standard for measuring cellular proliferation, its rapid metabolism leads to interference from labeled metabolites and has been a limiting factor. This has led to the search for a metabolically stable thymidine-like compound labeled with ^{11}C or ^{18}F, but preferably with ^{18}F (320). Ideally, such a tracer would share the following characteristics with thymidine: cellular transport; phosphorylation by thymidine kinase; incorporation into DNA; and limited *in vivo* catabolism. The most promising candidate to date is 3′-deoxy-3′-[^{18}F]fluorothymidine ([^{18}F]FLT; Eq. 9) (47). [^{18}F]FLT is metabolically stable with 90% to 97% of the plasma ^{18}F being in the parent compound at 50 minutes postinjection. PET studies show high contrast images of normal bone marrow and some tumors in canine and human subjects (321). In humans [^{18}F]FLT also shows high uptake in liver (possibly due to glucuronidation in hepatocytes), which limits its use in imaging tumors within the liver and those near marrow. Low tumor uptake would be expected in tumors that proliferate slowly. Development of a model for quantification and further improvement in the synthetic yield are current needs.

Radiotracers Having a High Affinity for Aggregated Amyloid

Alzheimer disease affects 35% of the population over the age of 85. This high incidence, the lack of knowledge as to its causes, and the lack of effective treatments have stimulated the development of radiotracers that bind specifically to aggregated amyloid, an early marker in the pathogenesis of the disease. A number of radiotracers of different chemical classes have been developed and evaluated (Fig. 2.19).

[^{18}F]FDDP, a malononitrile derivative, has been synthesized and evaluated for the *in vitro* and *in vivo* detection of neurofibrillary tangles and β-amyloid plaques, neuropathological lesions found in the brains of the Alzheimer disease patients (322). PET imaging shows greater [^{18}F]FDDP accumulation and longer residence time in plaque-rich cortical regions in patients with Alzheimer disease than in control subjects. [^{18}F]FDDP accumulation is correlated with cognitive impairment and also shows the expected inverse relationship with brain glucose metabolism (323).

Lipophilic, a neutral thioflavin T-derivatives, are another class of compounds that have a high affinity for aggregated amyloid (324). One of these compounds, [^{11}C]PIB (also called 6-OH-BTA), shows high accumulation in cortical brain regions in Alzheimer disease (325). The binding specificity of 6-OH-BTA to plaque was verified in submicrometer resolution in a transgenic mouse model of Alzheimer disease during peripheral administration using multiphoton microscopy, exemplifying the power of multimodality imaging to demonstrate specificity (326). With the growing appreciation that optimal radiotracer quantification requires optimal kinetics, a series of neutral thioflavin T-derivatives with high affinities for aggregated amyloid and a wide range of lipophilicities was studied in mice and in baboons in order to determine the relationship

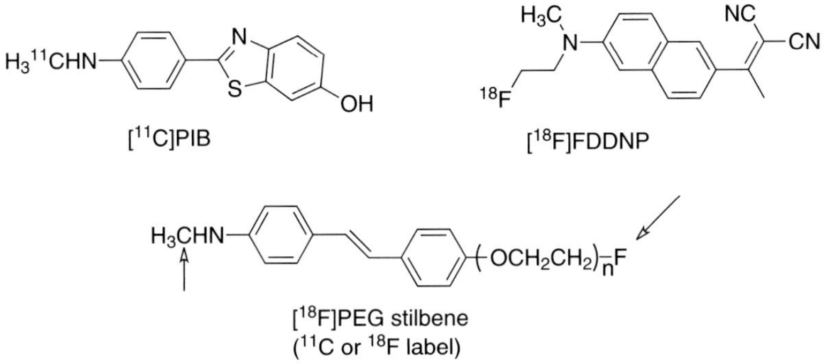

FIGURE 2.19. Structures of labeled compounds for aggregated amyloid.

of lipophilicity to brain uptake and clearance (327). Although lipophilicity is typically used as a predictor of radiotracer uptake, this study points out the importance of lipophilicity as a predictor of radiotracer *clearance* from nonspecific sites to enhance the signal-to-noise ratio. This and structure–activity relationship studies for other radiotracers binding to plaque (328) provide important new knowledge that can be expected to improve the selection of lead structures for further development.

Still another class of compounds that have high binding affinity to aggregated amyloid are the stilbene derivatives (329). Recently, these have been structurally optimized by incorporation of a polyethylene glycol moiety to decrease lipophilicity and improve bioavailability, while also retaining high-binding affinity for plaque. Fluorine-18 can be readily incorporated into the polyethyleneglycol moiety, and a number of these compounds offer the potential for either ^{11}C or ^{18}F labeling (330).

Radioligands for Other Molecular Targets

Some of the radioligands for other molecular targets are listed in the sections to follow (Fig. 2.20).

Norepinephrine Transporter

The development of a radiotracer for visualizing and quantifying the norepinephrine transporter (NET) in the central nervous system (331,332), a major molecular target in the treatment of depression and attention deficit hyperactivity disorder, has long eluded radiotracer chemists. Recent studies in mice (333) and in baboons (334,335) showed that the active enantiomer of the ^{11}C-labeled methyl analogue of the antidepressant drug reboxetine ((S,S-[^{11}C]-methylreboxetine, (S,S)-[^{11}C]MRB) is a promising new radiotracer that binds to NET-rich brain regions such as the thalamus and cerebellum. Studies in peripheral organs also reveal stereoselective binding in the heart (334). Modeling studies in the baboon along with measures of lipophilicity and plasma protein binding have also been carried out for this and other candidate radioligands for the NET (336,337). These studies demonstrate the potential use of (S,S)-[^{11}C]MRB for visualizing and quantifying the NET in brain and in heart (332).

Cannabinoid Receptors

The main psychoactive substance of marijuana is delta-9-tetrahydrocannibinol (THC), which has been postulated to exert its psychoactive effects through interactions with cannabinoid receptors (reviewed in Lindsey et al. (338)), which are highly localized in the cerebellum and hippocampus (339). Although the first images of the cannabinoid receptor in the baboon brain were done with single-photon emission computed tomography (340), the development of suitable PET radioligands has been hampered by the high lipophilicity of these compounds. However, recent progress has

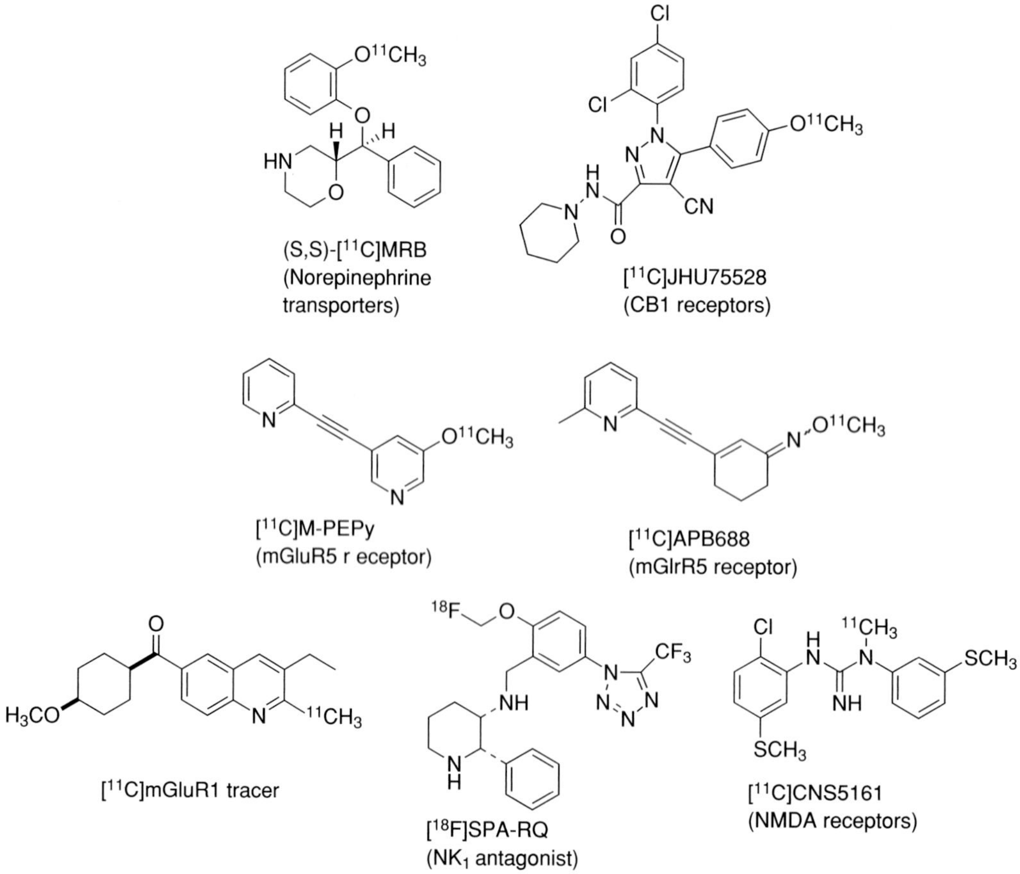

(S,S)-[^{11}C]MRB (Norepinephrine transporters)

[^{11}C]JHU75528 (CB1 receptors)

[^{11}C]M-PEPy (mGluR5 r eceptor)

[^{11}C]APB688 (mGlrR5 receptor)

[^{11}C]mGluR1 tracer

[^{18}F]SPA-RQ (NK_1 antagonist)

[^{11}C]CNS5161 (NMDA receptors)

FIGURE 2.20. Structures of labeled compounds for PET studies of other molecular targets (norepinephrine transporter, cannabinoid receptors, glutamate receptors, and annexin).

been made with the synthesis of [^{11}C]JHU75528, which shows specificity for the CB1 receptor in mouse and baboon brain *in vivo* (341,342).

The Brain Glutamate System

NMDA (*N*-methyl-D-aspartate) receptors play a key role in excitatory neurotransmission and are linked to learning and memory as well as degenerative disorders. A new radioligand for the NMDA receptor, [^{11}C]CNS5161, has been synthesized and characterized and is highly promising as a new investigational tool for studies of excitatory neurotransmission (343).

The Brain Glutamate System

Metabotropic glutamate receptors (mGluR) are G-protein coupled receptors that regulate synaptic transmission in the central nervous system. They occur in three major groups with eight subtypes (344). Radiotracers for imaging this class of receptors are of interest as investigational tools for mGluR and for drug research and development. A ^{11}C-labeled subtype selective metabotropic glutamate 1 receptor (mGluR1) antagonist has been recently synthesized and shown with microPET imaging to have high selectivity *in vivo* (345). Radiotracers for the mGluR5 subtype have also been synthesized and shown to have selectivity *in vivo* (346,347).

Substance P and Neurokinin-1 Receptors

Substance P is a neurotransmitter that interacts with neurokinin-1 receptors in the brain and is of medical interest for the role it plays in mood and anxiety, pain and inflammation, and in the mediation of nausea, an emesis secondary to chemotherapy (348–350). Because substance-P antagonists are of interest as molecular targets in drug development, small molecules have been developed and evaluated for their clinical effects and a number of these have been labeled with ^{11}C and ^{18}F for evaluation for PET imaging (351,352). One of these, [^{18}F]SPA-RQ, has been particularly useful at quantifying NK1 receptor binding sites and has recently been used to determine the receptor occupancy by aprepitant, a selective NK1 antagonist which is used to treat chemotherapy induced nausea (353). Moreover, it was found that NK1 receptor occupancy correlated with plasma levels of aprepitant, validating the use of plasma drug levels to guide dose determination for clinical studies of NK1 receptor antagonist drugs in central therapeutic applications.

Labeled Annexin V to Image Apoptosis

Apoptosis, or programmed cell death, is a genetically controlled process that occurs in a number of diseases, including autoimmune and neurodegenerative diseases, cardiac ischemia, tumor growth, and tumor therapy. During apoptosis, phosphatidylserine, a membrane phospholipid that is normally restricted to the inner surface of the plasma cell, is translocated to the outer surface. Annexin V, a human protein (36 kd) that has nanomolar affinity for phosphatidylserine bound to the outer membrane, has recently been radiolabeled with ^{18}F using N-succinimidyl-4-[^{18}F]-fluorobenzoic acid chemistry and shown to bind specifically to apoptotic tissues in a model of chemically induced apoptosis in rat liver (354,355).

OTHER PET RADIOISOTOPES

Fluorine-18 and ^{11}C radioisotopes are by far the most commonly used radioisotopes in PET radiotracer synthesis. However, ^{15}O ($t_{1/2}$ = 2.1 minutes) and ^{13}N ($t_{1/2}$ = 9.96 minutes) both have important applications (Table 2.1). By virtue of their short half-lives, only limited chemistry can be performed with these radioisotopes. Oxygen-15 and its production method are described in detail in Chapter 1. The production of ^{13}N is also discussed in Chapter 1. Nitrogen 13 is used most commonly in the form of ^{13}N-ammonia, which is an excellent tracer for imaging myocardial blood flow. The U.S. Food and Drug Administration has approved this radiopharmaceutical for blood-flow measurements as well. The requirements for producing sterile ^{13}N-ammonia for injection are described in detail in a recent United States Pharmacopeia monograph (356). Additional PET isotopes and their modes of production are also reviewed in Chapter 1 and in a recent text (357). In addition to these PET, iodine-124, a PET isotope of iodine having a 4.2-day half-life, is gaining use because it offers the opportunity to extend the quantitative aspects of PET to radioimmunotherapy with radioiodinated antibodies and other radioiodinated molecules (358–360). Copper-64 ($t_{1/2}$ = 12.7 hour) is another PET isotope that is extremely useful particularly when paired with copper-67, which is useful for therapy and more recently for imaging hypoxic regions of tumors (361,362). Still another largely unexplored PET radionuclide for radiopharmaceutical research and development is gallium-68 ($t_{1/2}$ = 68 minutes), which is accessible from the germanium-68/gallium-68 generator (363).

OUTLOOK

In spite of the increasing reliance of the biomedical sciences on molecular imaging, the development of new radiotracers remains a slow and even rate-limiting process. Even the familiar radiopharmaceuticals that are the backbone of imaging sciences are the product of enormous effort and even serendipity. Yet the value of radiopharmaceuticals in almost every area of clinical research is of such enormous importance that it justifies a more focused effort in identifying the impediments and in setting scientific and medical priorities. There are a number of urgent requirements to be able to develop labeled molecules that can visualize and quantify a single biochemical process in the human body where all of the chemical reactions of life are occurring.

1. *Deliberate incorporation of functional groups that can be labeled in the drug design and medicinal chemistry.* PET is a sufficiently important tool in drug research and development and in medicinal chemistry to be considered in the drug discovery and molecular design process. For example, the *deliberate* incorporation of a fluorine atom into a drug or ligand molecule for eventual ^{18}F labeling for PET studies and/or the design of drug molecules and ligands that could be labeled with ^{11}C labeling would greatly facilitate imaging for those molecules that show promising *in vitro* characteristics. This, in turn, would facilitate drug evaluation and approval and translation into the practice of medicine.
2. *Access to lead compounds.* A specific limitation in radiotracer research and development has been limited access to lead compounds already developed and tested by pharmaceutical companies but that do not have immediate commercial value as drugs. Efforts to develop mechanisms by which companies could share their compound libraries and still have their intellectual property protected need to be supported (364).
3. *Molecular targeting.* In spite of decades of experience, the ability to predict which chemical compounds will have the bioavailability, specificity, and kinetics required to image and quantify specific molecular targets in the brain and

other organs remains limited. Research is needed to build a foundation of knowledge to increase the probability that the molecules that are chosen for labeling will have a higher chance to succeed. Moreover, the study of series of compounds having minor structural modifications using the modern tools of imaging such as PET and microPET as well as classical methods such as autoradiography will enhance our ability to predict *in vivo* behavior based on the physicochemical and pharmacological properties of the molecule. More informed choices will not only help to advance radiotracer development, but this knowledge may also expedite drug research and development, where the issue of drug bioavailability has received less attention than molecular interactions on the microscale (365).

4. *Nonspecific binding.* High nonspecific binding that masks specific binding is at the heart of many failures in radiotracer research and development. This has given rise to a number of questions: What is "nonspecific" binding? Are there different types of nonspecific binding? A better characterization of nonspecific binding may make it possible to identify common features, which would allow researchers to steer clear of these nonproductive directions in radiotracer synthesis.
5. *Translational research.* Translating a new radiotracer from preclinical research to human studies is difficult and expensive, particularly if the compound has never been tested in humans. It typically requires expensive toxicology studies, even for those radiotracers with a very high safety margin based on animal studies. There is also a need for uniformity in requirements and appreciation by regulatory agencies as to the difference between tracer studies and therapeutic drug studies, as well as the resources to perform these tests.
6. *Attracting and training future radiotracer chemists.* Chemistry is the core discipline underpinning the development of radiotracers for PET. A major current and future concern is the ability to attract and train chemists in this field, in which advances in chemistry are often the rate-limiting step in advancing new knowledge in biology and medicine (366). It is essential to realize that a large portion of the chemists who are trained in the United States are not U.S. citizens and are not eligible for some of the federally sponsored training grants and other prestigious fellowships. This is a serious limitation. Steps need to be taken to remove these restrictions with the knowledge that they, rather than being protective, restrict the ability to recruit the scientific talent that is so badly needed.

ACKNOWLEDGMENT

Much of this work was carried out at Brookhaven National Laboratory under contract DE-AC02-76CH00016 with the U.S. Department of Energy and supported by its Office of Health and Environmental Research and by the National Institutes of Health grant K05 DA02000. Parts of this chapter were excerpted with permission from Fowler and Wolf (8) and Fowler et al. (7).

REFERENCES

1. Fowler JS, Wolf AP. *The synthesis of carbon-11, fluorine-18 and nitrogen-13 labeled radiotracers for biomedical applications.* Nuclear Science Series, National Academy of Sciences, National Technical Information Service, 1982; NAS-NS-3201.
2. Fowler JS, Wolf AP. Positron emitter-labeled compounds: priorities and problems. In: Phelps M, Mazziotta J, Schelbert H, eds. *Positron emission tomography and autoradiography: principles and applications for the brain and heart.* New York: Raven Press, 1986:391–450.
3. Kilbourn MR. *Fluorine-18 labeling of radiopharmaceuticals.* Nuclear Science Series, National Academy of Sciences, National Academy Press, 1990; NAS-NS-3203.
4. Langstrom B, Antoni G, Bjurling P, et al. Synthesis of compounds of interest for positron emission tomography with particular reference to synthetic strategies for ^{11}C labeling. *Acta Radiol Suppl* 1990;374: 147–151.
5. Firnau G, Chirakal R, Nahmias K. New ^{18}F tracers for the investigation of brain functions. *Acta Radiol Suppl* 1990;374:37–40.
6. Tewson TJ, Krohn KA. PET radiopharmaceuticals: state-of-the-art and future prospects. *Sem Nucl Med* 1998;28:221–234.
7. Fowler JS, Ding Y-S, Volkow ND. Radiotracers for positron emission tomography. *Sem Nucl Med* 2003;33:14–27.
8. Fowler JS, Wolf AP. Working against time. Rapid radiotracer synthesis and imaging the human brain. *Acc Chem Res* 1997;30:181–188.
9. Iwata R. Reference book for PET radiopharmaceuticals. World Wide Web URL; http://kakuyaku.cyric.tohoku.ac.jp/public/preface2004.html. Accessed .
10. Fowler JS, Ding Y-S. Chemistry. In: Wahl RL, ed. *Principles and practice of positron emission tomography.* Philadelphia: Lippincott Williams & Wilkins, 2002.
11. Langstrom B, Kihlberg T, Bergstrom M, et al. Compounds labelled with short-lived beta(+)-emitting radionuclides and some applications in life sciences. The importance of time as a parameter. *Acta Chimica Scand* 1999;53:651–669.
12. Brodack J, Kilbourn M, Welch M. Automated production of several positron-emitting radiopharmaceuticals using a single laboratory robot. *Appl Radiat Isot* 1988;39:689–698.
13. Alexoff DL. Knowledge-based automated radiopharmaceutical manufacturing for positron emission tomography. In: Emran E, ed. *New trends in radiopharmaceutical manufacturing for positron emission tomography.* New York: Plenum, 1991:339–353.
14. Vera-Ruiz H, Marcus CS, Pike VW, et al. Report of an International Atomic Energy Agency's Advisory Group meeting on "Quality control of cyclotron-produced radiopharmaceuticals." *Int J Radiat Appl Instrum* 1990;17[Pt B]:445–456.
15. Lee CC, Sui G, Elizarov A, et al. Multistep synthesis of a radiolabeled imaging probe using integrated microfluidics. *Science* 2005;310(5755): 1793–1796.
16. Gillies JM, Prenant C, Chimon GN, et al. Microfluidic reactor for the radiosynthesis of PET radiotracers. *Appl Radiat Isot* 2006;64:325–332.
17. Wolf AP, Redvanly CS. Carbon-11 and radiopharmaceuticals. *Int J Appl Radiat Isot* 1977;28:29–48.
18. Guillaume M, Luxen A, Nebeling B, et al. Recommendations for fluorine-18 production. *Appl Radiat Isot* 1991;42:749–762.
19. Bergman J, Solin O. Fluorine-18 labeled fluorine gas for synthesis of tracer molecules. *Nucl Med Biol* 1997;24:677–683.
20. Laakso A, Bergman J, Haaparanta M, et al. [^{18}F]CFT([^{18}F]WIN 35,428), a radioligand to study the dopamine transporter with PET: characterization in human subjects. *Synapse* 1998;28:244–250.
21. Constantinou MJ, Aigbirhio FI, Smith RG, et al. Xenon difluoride exchanges fluoride under mild conditions: a simple preparation of [18F]xenon difluoride for PET and mechanistic studies. *J Am Chem Soc* 2001;123:1780–1781.
22. Eckelman WC, Reba RC, Gibson RE, et al. Receptor-binding radiotracers: a class of potential radiopharmaceuticals. *J Nucl Med* 1979;20: 350–357.
23. Wolf AP. Synthesis of organic compounds labeled with positron emitters and the carrier problem. *J Labelled Compounds Radiopharm* 1981;18:1–2(abstr). [Reply Wolf AP. *J Nucl Med* 1981;22: 392–393].

24. Wolf AP, Fowler JS. Organic radiopharmaceuticals—recent advances. In: *Radiopharmaceuticals II*. New York: Society of Nuclear Medicine, 1979:73–92.
25. Venturino A, Rivera ES, Bergoc RM, et al. A simplified competition data analysis for radioligand specific activity determination. *Nucl Med Biol* 1990;17:233–237.
26. Fowler JS, Volkow ND, Wang GJ, et al. PET and drug research and development. *J Nucl Med* 1999;40:1154–1163.
27. Bergstrom M, Langstrom B. Pharmacokinetic studies with PET. *Prog Drug Res* 2005;62:279–317.
28. Christman DR, Finn RD, Karlstron K, et al. The production of ultra high activity ^{11}C-labeled hydrogen cyanide, carbon dioxide and methane via the ^{14}N(p,a)^{11}C reaction. *Int J Appl Radiat Isot* 1975;26: 435–442.
29. Langstrom B, Lundqvist H. The preparation of ^{11}C-methyl iodide and its use in the synthesis of ^{11}C-methyl-L-methionine. *Int J Appl Radiat Isot* 1976;27:357–363.
30. Ehrin E, Gawell L, Hogberg T, et al. Synthesis of [methoxy-3H]- and [methoxy-^{11}C]-labeled raclopride. Specific dopamine-D_2 receptor ligands. *J Labelled Compounds Radiopharm* 1987;24:931–940.
31. Ding Y-S, Sugano Y, Fowler JS, et al. Synthesis of the racemate and individual enantiomers of [^{11}C]methylphenidate for studying presynaptic dopaminergic neurons with positron emission tomography. *J Labelled Compounds Radiopharm* 1994;34:989–997.
32. Jewett DM. A simple synthesis of [^{11}C]methyl triflate. *Int J Rad Appl Instrum [A]* 1992;43:1383–1385.
33. Del Rosario RB, Wieland DM. Synthesis of [^{11}C]-α,α-dideuteriophenylephrine for *in vivo* kinetic isotope studies. *J Labelled Compounds Radiopharm* 1995;36:625–630.
34. Larsen P, Ulin J, Dahlstrom K, et al. Synthesis of [^{11}C]iodomethane by iodination of [^{11}C]methane. *Appl Radiat Isot* 1997;48:153–157.
35. Link JM, Krohn KA, Clark JC. Production of [^{11}C]CH_3I by single pass reaction of [^{11}C]CH_4 with I_2. *Nucl Med Biol* 1997;24:93–97.
36. Elsinga PH, Keller E, De Groot TJ, et al. Synthesis of [^{11}C]methyl magnesium iodide and its application to the introduction of [^{11}C]-N-tert-butyl groups and [^{11}C]-sec-alcohols. *Appl Radiat Isot* 1995;46: 227–231.
37. Kihlberg T, Gullberg P, Langstrom B. [^{11}C]Methylenetriphenylphosphorane, a new ^{11}C-precursor used in a one-pot Wittig synthesis of [β-^{11}C]styrene. *J Labelled Compounds Radiopharm* 1990;28:1116–1120.
38. Wilson AA, McCormick P, Kapur S, et al. Radiosynthesis and evaluation of [^{11}C]-(+)-4-propyl-3,4,4a,5,6,10b-hexahydro-2H-naphtho [1,2-b][1,4]oxazin-9-ol as a potential radiotracer for in vivo imaging of the dopamine D_2 high-affinity state with positron emission tomography. *J Med Chem* 2005;48:4153–4160.
39. Ginovart N, Galineau L, Willeit M, et al. Binding characteristics and sensitivity to endogenous dopamine of [^{11}C]-(+)-PHNO, a new agonist radiotracer for imaging the high-affinity state of D_2 receptors *in vivo* using positron emission tomography. *J Neurochem* 2006;97: 1089–1103.
40. Talbot PS, Narendran R, Butelman ER, et al. ^{11}C-GR103545, a radiotracer for imaging-opioid receptors *in vivo* with PET: synthesis and evaluation in baboons. *J Nucl Med* 2005;46:484–494.
41. Fasth KJ, Hörnfeldt K, Langström B. Asymmetric synthesis of ^{11}C-labelled L- and D-amino acids by alkylation of imidazolidinone derivatives. *Acta Chem Scand* 1995;49:301–304.
42. Zhang Z, Ding Y-S, Studenov AR, et al. Novel synthesis of [1-^{11}C]g-vinyl-g-aminobutyric acid ([1-^{11}C]GVG) for pharmacokinetic studies of addiction treatment. *J Labeled Compound Radiopharm* 2001;45: 199–211.
43. Sandell J, Halldin C, Hall H, et al. Radiosynthesis and autoradiographic evaluation of [^{11}C]NAD-299, a radioligand for visualization of the 5-HT1A receptor. *Nucl Med Biol* 1999;26:159–164.
44. Dolle F, Bramoulle Y, Bottlaender M, et al. [^{11}C]Befloxatone, a novel highly potent radioligand for *in vivo* imaging monoamine oxidase A. *J Labelled Compounds Radiopharm* 1999;42(Suppl 1):S608–S609.
45. Itsenko O, Kihlberg T, Langstrom B. Photoinitiated carbonylation with [^{11}C]carbon monoxide using amines and alkuyl iodides. *J Org Chem* 2004;69:4356–4360.
46. Stone-Elander SA, Elander N, Thorell J-O, et al. Microwaving in F-18 chemistry: quirks and tweaks. *Ernst Schering Res Found Workshop* 2007;62:243–269.
47. Grierson JR, Shields AF, Early JF. Radiosynthesis of 3'-[^{18}F]fluoro-3'-deoxynucleosides. *J Labelled Compounds Radiopharm* 1997;40:60–62.
48. Brodack JW, Kilbourn MR, Welch MJ, et al. NCA 16 alpha-[^{18}F]fluoroestradiol-17 beta: the effect of reaction vessel on fluorine-18 resolubilization, product yield, and effective specific activity. *Int J Rad Appl Instrum [A]* 1986;37(3):217–221.
49. Fowler JS, Ido T. Initial and subsequent approach for the synthesis of 18FDG. *J Nucl Med* 2002;32:6–12.
50. Ido T, Wan C-N, Casella V, et al. Labeled 2-deoxy-D-glucose analogs. ^{18}F-labeled 2-deoxy-2-fluoro-D-glucose, 2-deoxy-2-fluoro-D-mannose and ^{14}C-2-deoxy-2-fluoro-D-glucose. *J Labelled Compounds Radiopharm* 1978;14:175–183.
51. Hamacher K, Coenen HH, Stocklin G. Efficient stereospecific synthesis of no-carrier-added 2-[^{18}F]-fluoro-2-deoxy-D-glucose using aminopolyether supported nucleophilic substitution. *J Nucl Med* 1986;27:235–238.
52. Firnau G, Garnett ES, Chirakal R, et al. [^{18}F]fluoro-L-dopa for the *in vivo* study of intracerebral dopamine. *Appl Radiat Isot* 1986;37: 669–675.
53. Luxen A, Guillaume M, Melega WP, et al. Production of 6-[^{18}F]fluoro-L-dopa and its metabolism *in vivo*—a critical review [review]. *Nucl Med Biol* 1992;19:149–158.
54. Ding Y-S, Shiue CY, Fowler JS, et al. No-carrier-added (NCA) Aryl[^{18}F]fluorides via the nucleophilic aromatic substitution of electron rich aromatic rings. *J Fluorine Chem* 1990;48:189–206.
55. Lemaire C, Damhaut P, Plenevaux A, et al. Enantioselective synthesis of 6-[fluorine-18]-fluoro-L-dopa from no-carrier-added fluorine-18-fluoride. *J Nucl Med* 1994;35:1996–2002.
56. Attina M, Cacace F, Wolf AP. Displacement of nitro group by ^{18}F-fluoride ion. A new route to high specific activity aryl fluorides. *J Chem Soc Chem Commun* 1983;31:107–109.
57. Ding Y-S, Liu N, Wang T, et al. Synthesis of 6-[^{18}F]fluoro-3-(S)-(azetidinylmethoxy)pyridine for PET studies of nicotine acetylcholine receptors. *Nucl Med Biol* 2000;27:381–389.
58. Ding Y-S, Fowler JS, Logan J, et al. 6-[^{18}F]Fluoro-A-85380, a new PET tracer for the nicotinic acetylcholine receptor: studies in the human brain and in vivo demonstration of specific binding in white matter. *Synapse* 2004;53(3):184–189.
59. Ding Y-S, Gatley SJ, Fowler JS, et al. Mapping nicotinic acetylcholine receptors with PET. *Synapse* 1996;24:403–407.
60. Ding Y-S, Fowler JS, Gatley SJ, et al. Synthesis of high specific activity 6-[^{18}F]fluorodopamine for positron emission tomography studies of sympathetic nervous tissue. *J Med Chem* 1991;34:861–863.
61. Ding Y-S, Fowler JS, Gatley SJ, et al. Synthesis of high specific activity (+)- and (–)-6-[^{18}F]fluoronorepinephrine via the nucleophilic aromatic substitution reaction. *J Med Chem* 1991;34:767–771.
62. Ding Y-S, Fowler JS, Dewey SL, et al. Comparison of high specific activity (–) and (+)-6-[^{18}F]fluoronorepinephrine and 6-[^{18}F]fluorodopamine in baboons: heart uptake, metabolism and the effect of desipramine. *J Nucl Med* 1993;34(4):619–629.
63. Hostetler ED, Jonson SD, Welch MJ, et al. Synthesis of 2-[^{18}F]fluoroestradiol, a potential diagnostic imaging agent for breast cancer: strategies to achieve nucleophilic substitution of an electron-rich aromatic ring with [^{18}F]F^-. *J Org Chem* 1999;64:178–185.
64. Shah A, Widdowson DA, Pike V. Synthesis of substituted diaryliodonium salts and investigation of their reactions with no-carrier-added [^{18}F]fluoride. *J Labelled Compounds Radiopharm* 1997;40:65–67.
65. Eckelman WC, Kilbourn MR, Mathis CA. Discussion of targeting proteins *in vivo*: *in vitro* guidelines. *Nucl Med Biol* 2006;33(4):449–451.
66. Yu DW, Gatley SJ, Wolf AP, et al. Synthesis of carbon-11 labeled iodinated cocaine derivatives and their distribution in baboon brain

measured using positron emission tomography. *J Med Chem* 1992;35: 2178–2183.

67. Ding Y-S, Gatley SJ, Fowler JS, et al. Mapping catechol-O-methyl-transferase *in vivo* initial studies with [^{18}F]Ro41-0960. *Life Sci* 1996;58(3):195.
68. Dischino DD, Welch MJ, Kilbourn MJ, et al. Relationship between lipophilicity and brain extraction of C-11 labeled radiopharmaceuticals. *J Nucl Med* 1983;24:1030–1038.
69. Abbott NJ, Chugani DC, Zaharchuk G, et al. Delivery of imaging agents into brain. *Adv Drug Deliv Rev* 1999;37(1–3):253–277.
70. Pajouhesh H, Lenz GR. Medicinal chemical properties of successful central nervous system drugs [review]. *NeuroRx* 2005;2(4):541–553.
71. Lin JH. Applications and limitations of interspecies scaling and *in vitro* extrapolation in pharmacokinetics. *Drug Metab Dispos* 1998;26: 1202–1212.
72. Sokoloff L. Mapping of local cerebral functional activity by measurement of local cerebral glucose utilization with [^{14}C]deoxyglucose. *Brain* 1979;102:653–668.
73. Sols A, Crane RA. Substrate specificity of brain hexokinase. *J Biol Chem* 1954;210:581–595.
74. MacGregor RR, Fowler JS, Wolf AP, et al. A synthesis of ^{11}C-2-deoxy-D-glucose for regional metabolic studies. *J Nucl Med* 1981;22:800–803.
75. Volkow ND, Brodie JD, Wolf AP, et al. Brain organization in schizophrenics. *J Cereb Blood Flow Metab* 1986;6:441–446.
76. Som P, Atkins HL, Bandoypadhyay D, et al. A fluorinated glucose analog, 2-fluoro-2-deoxy-D-glucose (F-18): nontoxic tracer for rapid tumor detection. *J Nucl Med* 1980;21(7):670–675.
77. Weber G. Enzymology of cancer cells. *N Engl J Med* 1977;296:541–551.
78. Coleman RE. FDG imaging. *Nucl Med Biol* 2000;27:689–690.
79. Silverman M. Specificity of monosaccharide transport in the dog kid ney. *Am J Physiol* 1970;218:743–750.
80. Jagoda EM, Kiesewetter DO, Shimoji K, et al. Regional brain uptake of the muscarinic ligand, [^{18}F]FP-TZTP, is greatly decreased in M2 receptor knockout mice but not in M1, M3 and M4 receptor knockout mice. *Neuropharmacology* 2003;44:653–661.
81. Langstrom B, Andersson Y, Antoni G, et al. Design of tracer molecules with emphasis on stereochemistry, position of label and multiple isotopic labeling. An important aspect in studies of biologic function using positron emission tomography. *Acta Radiol Suppl* 1991;376: 31–35.
82. Mintun MA, Raichle ME, Kilbourn MR, et al. A quantitative model for the *in vivo* assessment of drug binding sites with positron emission tomography. *Ann Neurol* 1984;15:217–227.
83. Wong DF, Gjedde A, Wagner HN, et. al. Quantification of neuroreceptors in the living human brain. II. Inhibition studies of receptor density and affinity. *J Cereb Blood Flow Metab* 1986;6:147–153.
84. Logan J, Wolf AP, Shiue C-Y, et al. Kinetic modeling a receptor-ligand binding applied to positron emission tomographic studies with neuroleptic tracers. *J Neurochem* 1987;48:73–83.
85. Carson RE. Parameter estimation in positron emission tomography. In: Phelps M, Mazziotta J, Schelbert H, eds. *Positron emission tomography and autoradiography: principles and applications for the brain and heart.* New York: Raven Press, 1986:347–390.
86. Patlak CS, Blasberg RG, Fenstermacher JD. Graphical evaluation of blood-to-brain transfer constants from multiple-time uptake data. *J Cereb Blood Flow Metab* 1983;3:1–7.
87. Logan J, Fowler JS, Volkow ND, et. al. Graphical analysis of reversible radioligand binding from time-activity measurements applied to [N-^{11}C-methyl]-(−)-cocaine PET studies in human subjects. *J Cereb Blood Flow Metab* 1990;10:740–747.
88. Logan J. A review of graphical methods for tracer studies and strategies to reduce bias. *Nucl Med Biol* 2003;30:833–844.
89. Bergstrom M J, Eriksson B, Oberg K, et al. *In vivo* demonstration of enzyme activity in endocrine pancreatic tumors. Decarboxylation of carbon-11 DOPA to carbon-11 dopamine. *J Nucl Med* 1996;37: 32–37.
90. Halldin C, Burling P, Stalnacke C-G, et al. ^{11}C-Labeling of dimethylphenethy-lamine in two different positions and biodistribution studies. *Appl Radiat Isot* 1989;40:557–560.
91. Pike VW, McCarron JA, Lammertsma AA, et al. Exquisite delineation of 5-HT1A receptors in human brain with PET and [carbonyl-^{11}C]WAY-100635. *Eur J Pharmacol* 1996;301:R5–R7.
92. Ding Y-S, Fowler JS, Volkow ND, et al. Chiral drugs: comparison of the pharmacokinetics of [^{11}C]*d-threo* and *l-threo*-methylphenidate in the human and baboon brain. *Psychopharmacology* 1997;131:71–78.
93. Volkow ND, Ding Y-S, Fowler JS, et al. A new PET ligand for the dopamine transporter: studies in the human brain. *J Nucl Med* 1995;36:2162–2168.
94. Dannals RF, Langstrom B, Ravert HT, et al. Synthesis of radiotracers for studying muscarinic cholinergic receptors in the living human brain using positron emission tomography: [^{11}C]dexetimide and [^{11}C]levetimide. *Int J Rad Appl Instrum [A]* 1988;39:291–295.
95. Szabo Z, Kao PF, Scheffel U, et al. Positron emission tomography imaging of serotonin transporters in the human brain using [^{11}C](+)McN5652. *Synapse* 1995;20:37–43.
96. Gatley SJ, MacGregor RR, Fowler JS, et al. Rapid stereoselective hydrolysis of (+)-cocaine in baboon plasma prevents its uptake in the brain: implications for behavioral studies. *J Neurochem* 1990;54(2):720–723.
97. Belleau B, Moran J. Deuterium isotope effects in relation to the chemical mechanisms of monoamine oxidase. *Ann NY Acad Sci* 1963;107: 822–839.
98. Fowler JS, Wolf AP, MacGregor RR, et al. Mechanistic positron Emission tomography studies. Demonstration of a deuterium isotope effect in the MAO catalyzed binding of [^{11}C]L-deprenyl in living baboon brain. *J Neurochem* 1988;51:1524–1534.
99. Fowler JS, Logan J, Ding Y-S, et al. Non-MAO A binding of clorgyline in white matter in human brain. *J Neurochem* 2001;79(5):1039–1046.
100. Tominaga T, Inoue O, Suzuki K, et al. [^{13}N]β-phenethylamine ([^{13}N]PEA): a prototype tracer for measurement of MAO B activity in heart. *Biochem Pharmacol* 1987;36:3671–3675.
101. Raffel DM, Corbett JR, del Rosario RB, et al. Sensitivity of [^{11}C]phenylephrine kinetics to monoamine oxidase activity in normal human heart. *J Nucl Med* 1999;40:232–238.
102. Ding Y-S, Fowler JS, Gatley SJ, et al. Mechanistic PET studies of 6-[^{18}F]fluorodopamine in living baboon heart: selective imaging and control of radiotracer metabolism using the deuterium isotope effect. *J Neurochem* 1995;65:682–690.
103. Fowler JS, Wang G-J, Logan J, et al. Selective reduction of radiotracer trapping by deuterium substitution: comparison of [^{11}C]L-deprenyl and [^{11}C]L-deprenyl-D_2 for MAO B mapping. *J Nucl Med* 1995;36: 1255–1262.
104. Heiss WD, Herholz K. Brain receptor imaging. *J Nucl Med* 2006;47(2):302–312.
105. Deutsch A, Roth RH. Neurochemical systems in the central nervous system. In: Charney DS, Nestler EJ, Bunney BS, eds. *Neurobiology of mental illness.* New York: Oxford University Press, 1999:10–25.
106. Volkow ND, Fowler JS, Gatley SJ, et al. PET evaluation of the dopamine system of the human brain [review]. *J Nucl Med* 1996;37(7): 1242–1256.
107. Stoessl J, Ruth T. Neuroreceptor imaging: new developments in PET and SPECT imaging of neuroreceptor binding (including dopamine transporters, vesicle transporters and postsynaptoic receptor sites). *Curr Opin Neurol* 1998;11:327–333.
108. Neve KA, Seamans JK, Trantham-Davidson H. Dopamine receptor signaling [review]. *J Recept Signal Transduct Res* 2004;24:165–205.
109. Garnett ES, Firnau G, Nahmias C. Dopamine visualized in the basal ganglia in living man. *Nature* 1983;305:137–138.
110. Firnau G, Sood S, Chirakal R, et al. Cerebral metabolism of 6-^{18}F-fluoro-L-3,4-dihydroxy-phenylalanine in the primate. *J Neurochem* 1987;48: 1077–1082.
111. Perlmutter JS. New insights into a pathophysiology of Parkinson disease: the challenge of positron emission tomography. *Trends Neurosci* 1988;11:203–208.

112. DeJesus OT, Endres CJ, Shelton SE, et al. Evaluation of fluorinated m-tyrosine analogs as PET imaging agents of dopamine nerve terminals: comparison with 6-fluorodopa. *J Nucl Med* 1997;38:630–636.
113. Bjurling P, Antoni G, Watanabe Y, et al. Enzymatic synthesis of carboxy-^{11}C-labeled L-tyrosine, L-dopa, L-tryptophan and 5 hydroxy-L-tryptophan. *Acta Chem Scand* 1990;44:178.
114. Arnett CD, Wolf AP, Shiue C-Y, et al. Improved delineation of human dopamine receptors using [^{18}F]-N-methylspiroperidol in PET. *J Nucl Med* 1986;27:1878–1882.
115. Smith M, Wolf AP, Brodie JD, et al. Serial [^{18}F]-N-methylspiroperidol PET studies to measure changes in antipsychotic drug D_2 receptor occupancy in schizophrenic patients. *Biol Psychiatry* 1988;23:653–663.
116. Wagner HN Jr, Burns HD, Dannals RF, et al. Assessment of dopamine receptor densities in the human brain with carbon-11-labeled N-methylspiperone. *Ann Neurol* 1984;15(Suppl):S79–S84.
117. Wong DF, Wagner HN Jr, Tune LE, et al. Positron emission tomography reveals elevated D_2 dopamine receptors in drug-naive schizophrenics. *Science* 1986;234:1558–1563.
118. Satyamurthy N, Barrio JR, Bida G, et al. 3-(2'-[^{18}F]fluoroethyl)spiperone, a potent dopamine antagonist: synthesis, structural analysis and in-vivo utilization in humans. *Appl Radiat Isot* 1990;41:113–129.
119. Welch MJ, Katzenellenbogen JA, Mathias CJ, et al. N-(3-[^{18}F]fluoropropyl)-spiperone: The preferred ^{18}F labeled spiperone analog for PET studies of the dopamine receptor. *Nucl Med Biol* 1988;15:83–97.
120. Gambhir SS, Barrio JR, Herschman HR, et al. Assays for noninvasive imaging of reporter gene expression. *Nucl Med Biol* 1999;26:481–490.
121. Farde L, Ehrin E, Eriksson L, et al. Substituted benzamides as ligands for visualization of dopamine receptor binding in the human brain by positron emission tomography. *Proc Natl Acad Sci U S A* 1985;82: 3863–3867.
122. Moerlein S, Perlmutter JS, Welch MJ. USP standards for raclopride C11 injection. *Pharmacopeial Forum* 1995;21:172–176.
123. Dewey SL, Smith GS, Logan J, et al. Striatal binding of the PET ligand ^{11}C-raclopride is altered by drugs that modify synaptic dopamine levels. *Synapse* 1993;13(4):350–356.
124. Volkow ND, Wang G-J, Fowler JS, et al. Imaging endogenous dopamine competition with [^{11}C]raclopride in the human brain. *Synapse* 1994;16:255–262.
125. Volkow ND, Wang GJ, Fowler JS, et al. Decreased striatal dopaminergic responsiveness in detoxified cocaine-dependent subjects. *Nature* 1997;386(6627):830–833.
126. Breier A, Su TP, Saunders R, et al. Schizophrenia is associated with elevated amphetamine-induced synaptic dopamine concentrations: evidence from a novel positron emission tomography method. *Proc Nat Acad Sci U S A* 1997;94:2569–2574.
127. Laruelle M. Imaging synaptic neurotransmission with *in vivo* binding competition techniques: a critical review. *J Cereb Blood Flow Metab* 2000;20:423–451.
128. Halldin C, Farde L, Hogberg T, et al. Carbon-11-FLB 457: a radioligand for extrastriatal D_2 dopamine receptors. *J Nucl Med* 1995;36(7): 1275–1281.
129. Olsson H, Halldin C, Farde L. Differentiation of extrastriatal dopamine D_2 receptor density and affinity in the human brain using PET. *Neuroimage* 2004;22(2):794–803.
130. Halldin CJ, C-G Swahn, Neumeyer JL, et al. Preparation of two potent and selective dopamine D_2 receptor agonists: R-[propyl-^{11}C]-2-OH-NPA and R-[methyl-^{11}C]-2-OCH_3-NPA. *J Labelled Compounds Radiopharm* 1993;32:S265–S266.
131. Zilstra S. Synthesis and in vivo distribution in the rat of several fluorine-18 labeled N-fluoroalkylporphines. *Appl Radiat Isot* 1993;44: 651–658.
132. Shi B, Narayanan TK, Yang ZY, et al. Radiosynthesis and in vitro evaluation of 2-(N-alkyl-N-1-^{11}C-propyl)amino-5-hydroxytetralin analogs as high affinity agonists for dopamine D_2 receptors. *Nucl Med Biol* 1999;26:725–735.
133. Hwang DR, Kegeles LS, Laruelle M. (–)-N-[^{11}C]propyl-norapomorphine: a positron-labeled dopamine agonist for PET imaging of D(2) receptors. *Nucl Med Biol* 2000;27(6):533–539.
134. Narandren R, Hwang DR, Slifstein M, et al. Measurement of the proportion of D_2 receptors configured in state of high affinity for agonists in vivo: a positron emission tomography study using [^{11}C]N-propyl-norapomorphine and [11C]raclopride in baboons. *J Pharmacol Exp Ther* 2005;315(1):80–90.
135. Ravert HT, Wilson AA, Dannals RF, et al. Radiosynthesis of a selective dopamine D_1 receptor antagonist: R(+)-7-chloro-8-hydroxy-3-[^{11}C]methyl-1-phenyl-2,3,4,5-tetrahydro-1H-3 -benzazepine ([^{11}C] SCH 23390). *Int J Rad Appl Instrum [A]* 1987;38(4):305–306.
136. Halldin C, Farde L, Barnett A, et al. Synthesis of carbon-11 labelled SCH 39166, a new selective dopamine D_1 receptor ligand, and preliminary PET investigations. *Int J Rad Appl Instrum [A]* 1991;42(5): 451–455.
137. Halldin C, Foged C, Chou YH, et al. Carbon-11-NNC 112: a radioligand for PET examination of striatal and neocortical D_1-dopamine receptors. *J Nucl Med* 1998;39:2061–2068.
138. Abi-Dargham A, Martinez D, Mawlawi O, et al. Measurement of striatal and extrastriatal dopamine D_1 receptor binding potential with [^{11}C]NNC 112 in humans: validation and reproducibility. *J Cereb Blood Flow Metab* 2000;20:225–243.
139. Sokoloff P, Diaz J, Le Foll B, et al. The dopamine D3 receptor: a therapeutic target for the treatment of neuropsychiatric disorders [review]. *CNS Neurol Disord Drug Targets* 2006;5(1):25–43.
140. Leopoldo M, Lacavia E, DeGeorgio P, et al. Design, synthesis, and binding affinities of potential positron emission tomography (PET) ligands for visualization of brain dopamine D3 receptors. *J Med Chem* 2006;49:358–365.
141. Chu W, Tu Z, McElveen E, et al. Synthesis and in vitro binding of N-phenyl piperazine analogs as potential dopamine D3 receptor ligands. *Bioorg Med Chem* 2005;13(1):77–87.
142. Mach RH, Tu Z, Chu W, et al. Synthesis and *in vivo* evaluation of a [^{11}C]WC-10: a novel radiotracer for imaging dopamine D3 receptors. *J Nucl Med* 2006;47:27P(abst).
143. Langer O, Halldin C, Chou Y, et al. Carbon-11 pb-12: an attempt to visualize the dopamine d(4) receptor in the primate brain with positron emission tomography. *Nucl Med Biol* 2000;27:707–714.
144. Oh SJ, Lee KC, Lee SY, et al. Synthesis and evaluation of fluorine-substituted 1H-pyrrolo[2,3-b]pyridine derivatives for dopamine D4 receptor imaging. *Bioorg Med Chem* 2004;12:5505–5513.
145. Salmon E, Brooks DJ, Leenders KL, et al. A two compartment description and kinetic procedure for measuring regional cerebral [^{11}C]nomifensine uptake using positron emission tomography. *J Cereb Blood Flow Metab* 1990;10:307–316.
146. Fowler JS, Volkow ND, Wolf AP, et al. Mapping cocaine binding in human and baboon brain *in vivo*. *Synapse* 1989;4:371–377.
147. Ding Y-S, Fowler JS, Volkow ND, et al. Pharmacokinetics and *in vivo* specificity of [^{11}C]*dl-threo*-methylphenidate for the presynaptic dopaminergic neuron. *Synapse* 1994;18:152–160.
148. Frost JJ, Rosier AJ, Reich SG, et al. Positron emission tomographic imaging of the dopamine transporter with ^{11}C-WIN 35,428 reveals marked declines in mild Parkinson disease. *Ann Neurol* 1993;34: 423–431.
149. Wong DF, Yung B, Dannals RF, et al. *In vivo* imaging of baboon and human dopamine transporters by positron emission tomography using ^{11}C-WIN 35,428. *Synapse* 1993;15:130–142.
150. Brownell AL, Elmaleh DR, Meltzer PC, et al. Cocaine congeners as PET imaging probes for dopamine terminals. *J Nucl Med* 1996;37:1186–1192.
151. Chaly T, Dhawan V, Kazumata K, et al. Radiosynthesis of [^{18}F]N-3-fluoropropyl-2-β-carbomethoxy-3-*β*-(4-iodophenyl)nortropane and the first human study with positron emission tomography. *Nucl Med Biol* 1996;23:999–1004.
152. Deterding TA, Votaw JR, Wang CK, et al. Biodistribution and radiation dosimetry of the dopamine transporter ligand [^{18}F]FECNT. *J Nucl Med* 2001;42:376–381.
153. Fischman AJ, Bonab AA, Babich JW, et al. [^{11}C, ^{127}I]Altropane: a highly selective ligand for PET imaging of dopamine transporter sites. *Synapse* 2001;39:332–342.

154. Kilbourn MR, Haka MS, Mulholland GK, et al. Synthesis of radiolabeled inhibitors or presynaptic monoamine uptake systems: [^{18}F]GBR 13119 (DA), [^{11}C]nisoxetine (NE), and [^{11}C]fluoxetine (5-HT). *J Labelled Compounds Radiopharm* 1989;26:412–414.
155. Volkow ND, Fowler JS, Wang G-J, et al. Decreased dopamine transporters with age in healthy human subjects. *Ann Neurol* 1994;36: 237–239.
156. Tedroff J, Aquilonius S-M, Hartvig P, et al. Monoamine reuptake sites in the human brain evaluated *in vivo* by means of ^{11}C nomifensine and positron emission tomography: the effect of age and Parkinson disease. *Acta Neurol Scand* 1988;77:92–101.
157. Volkow ND, Wang G-J, Fischman M, et al. Relationship between subjective effects of cocaine and dopamine transporter occupancy. *Nature* 1997;386:827–830.
158. Volkow ND, Wang G-J, Fowler JS, et al. Dopamine transporter occupancies in the human brain induced by therapeutic doses of oral methylphenidate. *Am J Psychiatry* 1998;155:1325–1331.
159. Volkow ND, Wang GJ, Fowler JS, et al. The slow and long-lasting blockade of dopamine transporters in human brain induced by the new antidepressant drug radafaxine predict poor reinforcing effects. *Biol Psychiatry* 2005;57(6):640–646.
160. Halldin C, Erixon-Lindroth N, Pauli S, et al. [(11)C]PE2I: a highly selective radioligand for PET examination of the dopamine transporter in monkey and human brain. *Eur J Nucl Med Mol Imaging* 2003;30:1220–1223.
161. Pauli S, Halldin C, Farde L. Quantitative analyses of regional [11C]PE2I binding to the dopamine transporter in the human brain: a PET study. *Eur J Nucl Med Mol Imaging* 2006;33(6): 657–668.
162. Shetty HU, Zoghbi SS, Liow JS, et al. Identification and regional distribution in rat brain of radiometabolites of the dopamine transporter PET radioligand [(11)C]PE2I. *Eur J Nucl Med Mol Imaging* 2006;34:667–678.
163. Kilbourn MR, Frey KA, Vander Borght T, et al. Effects of dopaminergic drug treatments on *in vivo* radioligand binding to brain vesicular monoamine transporters. *Nucl Med Biol* 1996;23:467–471.
164. Vander Borght T, Kilbourn M, Desmond T, et al. The vesicular monoamine transporter is not regulated by dopaminergic drug treatments. *Eur J Pharmacol* 1995;294:577–583.
165. Frey KA, Koeppe RA, Kilbourn MR. Imaging the vesicular monoamine transporter [review]. *Adv Neurol* 2001;86:237–247.
166. Kilbourn MR. *In vivo* tracers for vesicular neurotransmitter transporters. *Nucl Med Biol* 1997;24:615–619.
167. Souza F, Simpson N, Raffo A, et al. Longitudinal noninvasive PET-based β cell mass estimates in a spontaneous diabetes rat model. *J Clin Invest* 2006;116(6):1506–1513.
168. Fowler JS, Logan J, Volkow ND, et al. Translational neuroimaging: positron emission tomography studies of monoamine oxidase [review]. *Mol Imaging Biol* 2005;7(6):377–387.
169. Singer T. Monoamine oxidases: old friends hold many surprises. *FASEB J* 1995;9:605–610.
170. Fowler JS, MacGregor RR, Wolf AP, et al. Mapping human brain monoamine oxidase A and B with ^{11}C-suicide inactivators and positron emission tomography. *Science* 1987;235:481–485.
171. Fowler JS, Volkow ND, Logan J, et al. Monoamine oxidase B (MAO B) inhibitor therapy in Parkinson disease: the degree and reversibility of human brain MAO B inhibition by Ro19 6327. *Neurology* 1993;43:1984–1992.
172. Fowler JS, Volkow ND, Logan J, et al. Slow recovery of human brain MAO B after L-deprenyl withdrawal. *Synapse* 1994;18:86–93.
173. Fowler JS, Volkow ND, Wang GJ, et al. Brain monoamine oxidase A inhibition in cigarette smokers. *Proc Natl Acad Sci U S A* 1996;93: 14065–14069.
174. Fowler JS, Volkow ND, Wang GJ, et al. Inhibition of monoamine oxidase B in the brains of smokers. *Nature* 1996;379:733–736.
175. Fowler JS, Logan J, Wang GJ, et al. Comparison of monoamine oxidase A in peripheral organs in nonsmokers and smokers. *J Nucl Med* 2005;46:1414–1420.
176. Fowler JS, Logan J, Wang GJ, et al. Low monoamine oxidase B in peripheral organs in smokers. *Proc Natl Acad Sci U S A* 2003;100: 11600–11605.
177. Khalil AA, Steyn S, Castagnoli N. Isolation and characterization of a monoamine oxidase inhibitor from tobacco leaves. *Chem Res Toxicol* 2000;13:31–35.
178. Morens DM, Grandinetti A, Reed D, et al. Cigarette smoking and protection from Parkinson disease: false association or etiological clue. *Neurology* 1995;45:1041–1051.
179. Bergstrom M, Westerberg G, Kihberg T, et al. Synthesis of some ^{11}C-labeled MAO A inhibitors and their *in vivo* uptake kinetics. *Nucl Med Biol* 1997;24:381–388.
180. Bernard S, Fuseau C, Schmid L, et al. Synthesis and *in vivo* studies of a specific monoamine oxidase B inhibitor 5-[4-benzyloxy)phenyl]-3-(2-cyanoethyl)-1,3,4-oxadiazo-[^{11}C]-2(3H)-one. *Eur J Nucl Med* 1996;23: 150–156.
181. Ginovart N, Meyer JH, Boovariwala A, et al. Positron emission tomography quantification of [^{11}C]-harmine binding to monoamine oxidase-A in the human brain. *J Cereb Blood Flow Metab* 2006;26(3): 330–344.
182. Barnes NM, Sharp T. A review of central 5-HT receptors and their function. *Neuropharmacology* 1999;38:1083–1152.
183. Comley R, Parker C, Wishart M, et al. *In vivo* evaluation and quantification of the 5HT4 receptor PET ligand [^{11}C []SB-207145. *Neuroimaging* 2006;31(Suppl 2):T23.
184. Mickael Huiban J, Passchier L, Martarello VJ, et al. [^{11}C[]GSK224558 as a potential PET ligand for the delineation of 5HT6 receptors. *Neuroimaging* 2006;31(Suppl 2):T13.
185. Crouzel C, Guillaume M, Barre L, et al. Ligands and tracers for PET studies of the 5-HT system—current status. *Int J Rad Appl Instrum B* 1992;19(8):857–870.
186. Pike VW. Radioligands for PET studies of central 5-HT receptors and re-uptake sites—current status [review]. *Nucl Med Biol* 1995;22(8): 1011–1018.
187. Wong DF, Wagner HN, Dannals RF, et al. Effects of age on dopamine and serotonin receptors measured by positron tomography in the living human brain. *Science* 1984;226:1393–1396.
188. Wang G-J, Volkow ND, Logan J, et al. Evaluation of age-related changes in serotonin 5-HT_2 and dopamine D_2 receptor availability in healthy human subjects. *Life Sci* 1995;56:249–253.
189. Biver F, Goldman S, Luxen A, et al. Multicompartmental study of fluorine-18 altanserin binding to brain 5-HT2 receptors in humans using positron emission tomography. *Eur J Nucl Med* 1994;21:937–946.
190. Blin J, Sette G, Fiorelli M, et al. A method for the in vivo investigation of the serotonergic 5-HT_2 receptors in the human cerebral cortex using positron emission tomography and ^{18}F-labeled setoperone. *J Neurochem* 1990;54:1744–1754.
191. Ito H, Nyberg S, Halldin C, et al. PET imaging of central 5-HT2A receptors with carbon-11-MDL 100,907. *J Nucl Med* 1998;39(1): 208–214.
192. Mathis CA, Mahmood K, Simpson NR, et al. Synthesis and preliminary *in vivo* evaluation of [^{11}C]MDL 100907: a potent and selective radioligand for the 5-HT_{2A} receptor system. *Med Chem Res* 1996;6:1–10.
193. Van Dyck CH, Tan PZ, Baldwin RM, et al. PET quantification of 5-HT_{2A} receptors in the human brain; a constant infusion paradigm with [^{18}F]altanserin. *J Nucl Med* 2000;41:234–241.
194. Mathis CA, Simpson NR, Mahmood K, et al. [^{11}C]WAY 100635: a radioligand for imaging 5-HT1A receptors with positron emission tomography. *Life Sci* 1994;55(20):PL403–407.
195. Osman S, Lundkvist C, Pike VW. Characterization of the radioactive metabolites of the 5-HT_{1A} receptor radioligand, [O-methyl-^{11}C]WAY-100635, in monkey and human plasma by HPLC: comparison of the behaviour of an identified radioactive metabolite with parent radioligand in monkey using PET. *Nucl Med Biol* 1996;23:627–634.
196. Osman S, Lundkvist C, Pike VW, et al. Characterisation of the appearance of radioactive metabolites in monkey and human plasma from the 5-HT1A receptor radioligand, [carbonyl-1^{11}C]WAY-100635—explanation of high signal contrast in PET and an aid to biomathematical modelling. *Nucl Med Biol* 1998;25:215–223.

197. Farde L, Ito H, Swahn CG, et al. Quantitative analyses of carbonyl-carbon-11-WAY-100635 binding to central 5-hydroxytryptamine-1A receptors in man. *J Nucl Med* 1998;39:1965–1971.
198. Houle S, Wilson AA, Inaba T, et al. Imaging 5-HT1A receptors with positron emission tomography: initial human studies with [^{11}C]CPC-222. *Nucl Med Commun* 1997;18:1130–1134.
199. Plenevaux A, Weissmann D, Aerts J, et al. Tissue distribution, autoradiography, and metabolism of 4-(2′-methoxyphenyl)-1-[2′-[N-2′-pyridinyl)-p-[(18)F]fluorobenzamido-ethyl]piperazine (p-[(18)F] MPPF), a new serotonin 5-HT(1A) antagonist for positron emission tomography: an *in vivo* study in rats. *J Neurochem* 2000;75:803–811.
200. Kepe V, Barrio JR, Huang SC, et al. Serotonin 1A receptors in the living brain of Alzheimer disease patients. *Proc Natl Acad Sci U S A* 2006;103(3):702–707.
201. Entire issue dedicated to imaging of 5-HT$_{1A}$. *Nucl Med Biol* 2000;27(5).
202. Suehiro M, Ravert HT, Dannals RF, et al. Synthesis of a radiotracer for studying serotonin uptake sites with positron emission tomography: [^{11}C]McN-5652-Z. *J Labelled Compounds Radiopharm* 1992;31: 841–848.
203. Suehiro M, Scheffel U, Ravert HT, et al. [^{11}C](+)McN5652 as a radiotracer for imaging serotonin uptake sites with PET. *Life Sci* 1993;53:883–892.
204. Buck A, Gucker PM, Schönbächler RD, et al. Evaluation of serotonergic transporters using PET and [^{11}C](+)McN-5652: assessment of methods. *J Cereb Blood Flow Metab* 2000;20:253–262.
205. Frankle WG, Slifstein M, Gunn RN, et al. Estimation of serotonin transporter parameters with ^{11}C-DASB in healthy humans: reproducibility and comparison of methods. *J Nucl Med* 2006;47: 815–826.
206. Stehouwer JS, Jarkas N, Zeng F, et al. Synthesis, radiosynthesis, and biological evaluation of carbon-11 labeled 2-beta-carbomethoxy-3beta-(3'-((Z)-2-haloethenyl)phenyl)nortropanes: candidate radioligands for *in vivo* imaging of the serotonin transporter with positron emission tomography. *J Med Chem* 2006;49(23):6760–6767.
207. Huang Y, Hwang D-R, Bae S-A, et al. A new positron emission tomography imaging agent for the serotonin transporter: synthesis, pharmacological characterization, and kinetic analysis of [^{11}C]2-[2-(dimethylaminomethyl)phenylthio]-5-fluoromethylphenylamine ([^{11}C]AFM). *Nucl Med Biol* 2004;31:543–556.
208. Scheffel U, Dannals RF, Suehiro M, et al. Evaluation of ^{11}C-citalopram and ^{11}C-fluoxetine as *in vivo* ligands for the serotonin uptake site. *J Nucl Med* 1990;31:883–884.
209. Dannals RF. Synthesis of a radiotracer for studying serotonin-2 receptors: carbon-11 labeled N-methylparoxetine. *J Labelled Compounds Radiopharm* 1989;26:205–206.
210. Diksic M, Tohyama Y, Takada A. Brain net unidirectional uptake of α-methyltryptophan. *Neurochem Res* 2000;25:1537–1546.
211. Diksic M, Nagahiro S, Sources TL, et al. A new method to measure brain serotonin synthesis *in vivo*. Theory and basis data for a biological model. *J Cereb Blood Flow Metab* 1990;10:1–12.
212. Shoaf SE, Carson RE, Hommer D, et al. The suitability of [^{11}C]-α-methyl-L-tryptophan as a tracer for serotonin synthesis: studies with dual administration of [^{11}C] and [^{14}C] labeled tracer. *J Cereb Blood Flow Metab* 2000;20:244–252.
213. Dannals RF. Synthesis of an opiate receptor binding radiotracer: [^{11}C]carfentanil. *Int J Applied Radiat Isot* 1985;36:303–306.
214. Frost JJ, Wagner HN Jr, Dannals RF, et al. Imaging opiate receptors in the human brain by positron tomography. *J Comp Assist Tomog* 1985;9:231–236.
215. Zubieta JK, Dannals RF, Frost JJ. Gender and age influences on human brain mu-opioid receptor binding measured by PET. *Am J Psychiatry* 1999;156:842–848.
216. Luthra AK, Pike VW, Brady F. The preparation of carbon-11 labeled diprenorphine: a new radioligand for the study of the opiate receptor system *in vivo*. *J Chem Soc Chem Comm* 1985;20:1423–1425.
217. Luthra SK, Pike VW, Brady F, et al. Preparation of [^{11}C]buprenorphine—a potential radioligand for the study of opiate receptor system *in vivo*. *Appl Radiat Isot* 1987;38:65–66.
218. Lever, JR, Mazza SM, Dannals RF, et al. Facile synthesis of [^{11}C]buprenorphine for positron emission tomographic studies. *Appl Radiat Isot* 1990;41:745–752.
219. Galynker I, Schlyer D, Dewey SL, et al. Opioid receptor imaging and displacement studies with [6-O-[11C] methyl]buprenorphine in baboon brain. *Nucl Med Biol* 1996;23: 325–331.
220. Shiue CY, Bai LQ, Teng RR, et al. A comparison of the brain uptake of N-(cyclopropyl[^{11}C]methyl)norbuprenorphine ([^{11}C]buprenorphine) and N-(cyclopropyl[^{11}C]methyl)nordiprenorphine ([^{11}C]diprenorphine) in baboon using PET. *Nucl Med Biol* 1991;18:281–288.
221. Channing M, Eckelman WC, Bennett JM, et al. Radiosynthesis of [^{18}F] 3-acetylcyclofoxy: a high affinity opiate antagonist. *Int J Appl Radiat Isot* 1985;36:429–433.
222. Carson RE, Blasberg RG, Channing MA, et al. Tracer infusion for equilibrium measurements: applications to ^{18}F-cyclofoxy opiate receptor imaging with PET. *J Cereb Blood Flow Metab* 1989;9(Suppl 1):S203.
223. Ravert HT, Mathews WB, Musachio JL, et al. [^{11}C]-methyl 4-[(3,4-dichlorophenyl)acetyl]-3-[(1-pyrrolidinyl)-methyl]-1- piperazinecarboxylate ([^{11}C]GR89696): synthesis and *in vivo* binding to kappa opiate receptors. *Nucl Med Biol* 1999;26:737–741.
224. Madar I, Lever JR, Kinter CM, et al. Imaging of delta opioid receptors in human brain by N1'-[^{11}C]methylnaltrindol and PET. *Synapse* 1996;24:19–28.
225. Barnard EA, Skolnick P, Olsen RW, et al. International Union of Pharmacology. XV. Subtypes of gamma-aminobutyric acid A receptors: classification on the basis of subunit structure and receptor function [review]. *Pharmacol Rev* 1998;50(2):291–313.
226. Gavish M, Bachman I, Shoukrun R, et al. Enigma of the peripheral benzodiazepine receptor [review]. *Pharmacol Rev* 1999;51(4): 629–650.
227. Pike VW, Halldin C, Crouzel C, et al. Radioligands for PET studies of central benzodiazepine receptors and PK (peripheral benzodiazepine) binding sites—current status [review]. *Nucl Med Biol* 1993;20: 503–525.
228. Katsifis A, Kassiou M. Development of radioligands for in vivo imaging of GABA(A)-benzodiazepine receptors [review]. *Mini Rev Med Chem* 2004;4:909–921.
229. Persson A, Ehrin E, Eriksson, et al. Imaging of [11C]-labelled RO 15-1788 binding to benzodiazepine receptors in the human brain by positron emission tomography. *J Psychiatry Res* 1985;19:609–622.
230. Koeppe RA, Holthof VA, Frey KA, et al. Compartmental analysis of [^{11}C]flumazenil kinetics for the estimation of ligand transport rate and receptor distribution using positron emission tomography. *J Cereb Blood Flow Metab* 1991;11:735–744.
231. Kropholler MA, Boellaard R, Schuitemaker A, et al. Development of a tracer kinetic plasma input model for (R)-[^{11}C]PK11195 brain studies. *J Cereb Blood Flow Metab* 2005;25:842–851.
232. Cappelli A, Matarrese M, Moresco RM, et al. Synthesis, labeling, and biological evaluation of halogenated 2-quinolinecarboxamides as potential radioligands for the visualization of peripheral benzodiazepine receptors. *Bioorg Med Chem* 2006;14:4055–4066.
233. Coyle JT, Price DL, DeLong MR. Alzheimer disease: a disorder of cortical cholinergic innervation. *Science* 1983;219:1184–1190.
234. Volpicelli LA, Levey AL. Muscarinio acetylcholine subtypes in cerebral cortex and hippocampus. *Prog Brain Res* 2004;145:59–66.
235. Flynn DD, Farrari-DiLeo G, Mash DC, et al. Differential regulation of molecular subtypes of muscarinic receptors in Alzheimer disease. *J Neurochem* 1995;64;1881–1891.
236. Frey KA, Koeppe RA, Mulholland GK. *In vivo* muscarinic cholinergic receptor imaging in human brain with [^{11}C]scopolamine and positron emission tomography. *J Cereb Blood Flow Metab* 1992;12:147–154.
237. Mulholland GK, Otto CA, Jewett DM, et al. Radiosynthesis and comparisons in the biodistribution of carbon-11 labeled muscarinic antagonists: (+)2U-tropanyl benzilate and N-methyl-4-piperidyl benzilate. *J Labelled Compounds Radiopharm* 1989;26:202.

238. Mulholland GK, Kilbourn MR, Sherman P, et al. Synthesis, *in vivo* biodistribution and dosimetry of [^{11}C]N-methylpiperidyl benzilate ([^{11}C]NMPB), a muscarinic acetylcholine receptor antagonist. *Nucl Med Biol* 1995;22(1):13–17.
239. Tsukada H, Takahashi K, Miura S, et al. Evaluation of novel PET ligands (+)N-[^{11}C]methyl-3-piperidinyl benzilate ([^{11}C](+)3-MPB) and its stereoisomer [^{11}C](–)3-MPB for muscarinic cholinergic receptors in the conscious monkey brain: a PET study in comparison with [^{11}C]4-MPB. *Synapse* 2001;39:182–192.
240. Yoshida T, Kuwabara Y, Ichiya Y, et al. Cerebral muscarinic acetylcholinergic receptor measurement in Alzheimer disease patients on [^{11}C]-N-methyl-4-piperidinyl benzilate—comparison with cerebral blood flow and cerebral glucose metabolism. *Ann Nucl Med* 1998;12:35–42.
241. Lee KS, Frey KA, Koeppe RA, et al. *In vivo* quantification of cerebral muscarinic receptors in normal human aging using positron emission tomography and [^{11}C]tropanyl benzilate. *J Cereb Blood Flow Metab* 1996;16:303–310.
242. Zubieta JK, Koeppe RA, Frey KA, et al. Assessment of muscarinic receptor concentrations in aging and Alzheimer disease with [^{11}C]NMPB and PET. *Synapse* 2001;39:275–287.
243. Dewey SL, Volkow ND, Logan J, et al. Age-related decreases in muscarinic cholinergic receptor binding in the human brain measured with positron emission tomography (PET). *J Neurosci Res* 1990;27:569–575.
244. Buck A, Mulholland GK, Papadopoulos SM, et al. Kinetic evaluation of positron-emitting muscarinic ligands employing direct carotid injection. *J Cereb Blood Flow Metab* 1996;16:1280–1287.
245. Kiesewetter DO, Lee J, Lang L, et al. Preparation of ^{18}F-labled muscarinic agonist with M2 selectivity. *J Med Chem* 1995;38:5–8.
246. Carson RE, Kiesewetter DO, Jagoda E, et al. Muscarinic cholinergic receptor measurements with [^{18}F]FP-TZTP: control and competition studies. *J Cereb Blood Flow Metab* 1998;18(10):1130–1142.
247. Podruchny TA, Connolly C, Bodke A, et al. *In vivo* muscarinic 2 receptor imaging in cognitively normal young and older volunteers. *Synapse* 2003;48:39–44.
248. Cohen RM, Podruchny TA, Bokde ALW, et al. Higher *in vivo* muscarinic-2 receptor distribution volumes in aging subjects with an apolipoproetin E-*4 allele. *Synapse* 2003;49:150–156.
249. Bonnot-Lours S, Crouzel C, Prenant C, et al. Carbon-11 labelling of an inhibitor of acetylcholinesterase. *J Labelled Compounds Radiopharm* 1993;33:277–284.
250. Pappata S, Tavitian B, Traykov L, et al. *In vivo* imaging of human cerebral acetylcholinesterase. *J Neurochem* 1996;67:876–879.
251. Irie T, Fukushi K, Akimoto Y, et al. Design and evaluation of radioactive acetylcholine analogs for mapping brain acetylcholinesterase (AChE) *in vivo*. *Nucl Med Biol* 1994;21:801–808.
252. Kuhl DE, Koeppe RA, Minoshima A, et al. *In vivo* mapping of cerebral acetylcholinesterase in aging and Alzheimer disease. *Neurology* 1999;52:691–699.
253. Herholz K, Weisenbach S, Zundorf G, et al. *In vivo* study of acetylcholine esterase in basal forebrain, amygdala, and cortex in mild to moderate Alzheimer disease. *Neuroimage* 2004;21(1):136–143.
254. Shiraishi T, Kikuchi T, Fukushi K. Estimation of plasma IC50 of donepezil hydrochloride for brain acetylcholinesterase inhibition in monkey using N-[^{11}C]methylpiperidin-4-yl acetate ([^{11}C]MP4A) and PET. *Neuropsychopharmacology* 2005;30(12):2154–1261.
255. Kikuchi T, Zhang MR, Ikota N, et al. N-[^{18}F]fluoroethylpiperidin-4-yl-methyl acetate, a novel lipophilic acetylcholine analogue for PET measurement of brain acetylcholinesterase activity. *J Med Chem* 2005;48:2577–2583.
256. Shao X, Koeppe RA, Butch ER, et al. Evaluation of ^{18}F-labeled acetylcholinesterase substrates as PET radiotracers. *Bioorg Med Chem* 2005;13(3):869–875.
257. Ingvar M, Stone-Elander S, Rogers GA, et al. Striatal D_2/acetylcholine interactions: PET studies of the vesamicol receptor. *Neuroreport* 1993;4:1311–1314.
258. Gage HD, Voytko ML, Ehrenkaufer RL, et al. Reproducibility of repeated measures of cholinergic terminal density using [^{18}F](+)-4-fluorobenzyltrozamicol and PET in Rhesus monkey brain. *J Nucl Med* 2000;41:2069–2076.
259. Domino EF. Tobacco smoking and nicotine neuropsychopharmacology: some future research directions. *Neuropsychopharmacology* 1998;18:456–468.
260. Picciotto MR, Zoli M, Rimondini R, et al. Acetylcholine receptors containing the beta2 subunit are involved in the reinforcing properties of nicotine. *Nature* 1998;391:173–177.
261. Nordberg A. Human nicotinic receptors-their role in aging and dementia. *Neurochem Int* 1994;25:93–97.
262. Perry DC, Davila-Garcia MI, Stockmeier CA, et al. Increased nicotinic receptors in brains from smokers: membrane binding and autoradiography studies. *J Pharm Exp Therap* 1999;289:1545–1552.
263. Gopalakrishnan M, Donnelly-Roberts DL. Nicotine: therapeutic prospects? *Pharm News* 1998;5:16–20.
264. Gotti C, Riganti L, Vailati S, et al. Brain neuronal nicotinic receptors as new targets for drug discovery [review]. *Curr Pharm Des* 2006;12(4): 407–428.
265. Arneric SP, Sullivan JP, Williams M. Neuronal nicotinic acetylcholine receptors—novel targets for central nervous system therapeutics. In: Bloom FE, Kupfer DJ, eds. *Psychopharmacology: the fourth generation of progress*. New York: Raven Press, 1995;95–110.
266. Sihver W, Nordberg A, Langstrom B, et al. Development of ligands for *in vivo* imaging of cerebral nicotinic receptors. *Behav Brain Res* 2000;113:143–157.
267. Nyback H, Nordberg A, von Holst H, et al. Attempts to visualize nicotinic receptors in the brain of monkey and man by positron emission tomography. *Prog Brain Res* 1989;79:313–319.
268. Muzik RF, Berridge MS, Friedland RF, et al. PET quantification of specific binding of carbon-11-nicotine in human brain. *J Nucl Med* 1998;39:2048–2054.
269. Sihver W, Fasth J, Ogren M, et al. *In vivo* positron emission tomography studies on the novel nicotinic receptor agonist [^{11}C]MPA compared with [^{11}C]ABT-418 and (S)-(–)[^{11}C]nicotine in rhesus monkeys. *Nucl Med Biol* 1999;26:633–642.
270. Spande TF, Garraffo HM, Edwards MW, et al. Epibatidine: a novel (chloropyridyl)azabicycloheptane with potent analgesic activity from the Equadoran poison frog. *J Amer Chem Soc* 1992;114:3475–3478.
271. Qian C, Li T, Shen TY, et al. Epibatidine is a nicotinic analgesic. *Eur J Pharmacol* 1993;250:R13–14.
272. Horti A, Ravert HT, London ED, et al. Synthesis of a radiotracer for studying nicotinic acetylcholine receptors: (±)-exo-2-(2-[^{18}F]fluoro-5-pyridyl)-7-azabicyclo[2.2.1]heptane. *J Labelled Compounds Radiopharm* 1996;38:355–365.
273. Ding Y-S, Volkow ND, Logan J, et al. Occupancy of brain nicotinic acetylcholine receptors by nicotine doses equivalent to those obtained when smoking a cigarette. *Synapse* 2000;35:234–237.
274. Ding Y-S, Logan J, Bermel R, et al. Dopamine receptor-mediated regulation of striatal cholinergic activity: PET studies with [^{18}F]norchlorofluoroepibatidine. *J Neurochem* 2000;74:1514–1521.
275. Ding Y-S, Molina PE, Fowler JS, et al. Comparative studies of epibatidine derivatives [^{18}F]NFEP and [^{18}F]N-methyl-NFEP: kinetics, nicotine effect and toxicity. *Nucl Med Biol* 1999;26:139–148.
276. Molina PE, Ding Y-S, Carroll FI, et al. Fluoro-norchloroepibatidine: preclinical assessment of acute toxicity. *Nucl Med Biol* 1997;24:743–747.
277. Abreo MA, Lin N-H, Garvey DS, et al. Novel 3-pyridyl ethers with subnanomolar affinity for central neuronal nicotinic acetylcholine receptors. *J Med Chem* 1996;39:817–825.
278. Valette H, Bottlaender M, Dolle F, et al. Imaging central nicotinic acetylcholine receptors in baboons with [^{18}F]fluoro-A-85380. *J Nucl Med* 1999;40:1374–1380.
279. Horti AG, Koren AO, Ravert HT, et al. Synthesis of a radiotracer for studying nicotinic acetylcholine receptors: 2-[^{18}F]fluoro-3-(2(S)-azetidinylmethoxy)pyridine (2-[^{18}F]A-85380). *J Labelled Compounds Radiopharm* 1998;41:309–318.

280. Dolle F, Valette H, Bottlaender M, et al. Synthesis of 2-[^{18}F]fluoro-3-[2(S)-2-azetidinylmethoxy]pyridine a highly potent radioligand for in vivo imaging central nicotinic acetylcholine receptors. *J Labelled Compounds Radiopharm* 1998;41:451–463.
281. Dolle F, Dolci L, Valette H, et al. Synthesis and nicotinic acetylcholine receptor in vivo binding properties of 2-fluoro-3-[2(S)-2-azetidinylmethoxy]pyridine: a new positron emission tomography ligand for nicotinic receptors. *J Med Chem* 1999;42:2251–2259.
282. Koren AO, Horti AG, Mukhin AG, et al. Synthesis and *in vitro* characterization of 6-[^{18}F]fluoro-3-(2(S)-azetidinylmethoxy)pyridine, a high-affinity radioligand for central nicotinic acetylcholine receptors. *J Labelled Compounds Radiopharm* 1999;42:S409.
283. Scheffel U, Horti AG, Koren AO, et al. 6-[^{18}F]Fluoro-A-85380: an *in vivo* tracer for the nicotinic acetylcholine receptor. *Nucl Med Biol* 2000;27:51–56.
284. Kimes AS, Horti AG, London ED, et al. 2-[^{18}F]F-A-85380: PET imaging of brain nicotinic acetylcholine receptors and whole body distribution in humans. *FASEB J* 2003;17(10):1331–1333.
285. Brody AL, Mandelkern MA, London ED, et al. Cigarette smoking saturates brain $\alpha_4\beta_2$ nicotinic acetylcholine receptors. *Arch Gen Psychiatry* 2006;63:907–915.
286. Ding Y-S, Kil KE, Lin KS, et al. A novel nicotinic acetylcholine receptor antagonist radioligand for PET studies. *Bioorg Med Chem Lett* 2006;16(4):1049–1053.
287. D'Andrea MR, Nagele RG. Targeting the alpha 7 nicotinic acetylcholine receptor to reduce amyloid accumulation in Alzheimer disease pyramidal neurons [review]. *Curr Pharm Des* 2006;12(6): 677–684.
288. Duman RS, Nestler EJ. Signal transduction pathways for catecholamine receptors. In: Meltzer H, ed. *Psychopharmacology: the fourth generation*. New York: Raven Press, 1995;303–320.
289. Imahori Y, Ohmori Y, Fujii R, et al. Rapid incorporation of carbon-11 labeled diacylglycerol as a probe of signal transduction in glioma. *Cancer Res* 1995;55:4225–4229.
290. Sasaki T, Enta A, Nozaki T, et al. Carbon-11-forskolin: a ligand for visualization of the adenylate cyclase-related second messenger. *J Nucl Med* 1993;34:1944–1948.
291. Takahashi T, Ootake A. [^{18}F]Labeled 1,2-diacylglycerols: a new tracer for imaging second messenger system. *J Labelled Compounds Radiopharm* 1994;35:517–519.
292. Lourenco CM, DaSilva J, Warsh JJ, et al. Imaging of cAMP-specific phosphodiesterase-IV: comparison of [^{11}C]rolipam and [^{11}C]Ro 20-1724 in rats. *Synapse* 1999;31:41–50.
293. DaSilva JN, Lourenco CM, Meyer JH, et al. Imaging cAMP-specific phosphodiesterase-4 in human brain with R-[^{11}C]rolipram and positron emission tomography. *Eur J Nucl Med Mol Imag* 2002;29(12): 1680–1683.
294. Vaalburg W, Coenen HH, Crouzel C, et al. Amino acids for the measurement of protein synthesis *in vivo* by PET. *Nucl Med Biol* 1992;19:227–237.
295. Varagnolo L, Stokkel MPM, Mazzi U, et al. ^{18}F-labeled radiopharmaceuticals for PET in oncology, excluding FDG. *Nucl Med Biol* 2000;27:103–112.
296. Hawkins RA, Huang SC, Barrio JR, et al. Estimation of local cerebral protein synthesis rates with L-[1-^{11}C]leucine and PET: methods, model, and results in animals and humans. *J Cereb Blood Flow Metab* 1989;9(4):446–460.
297. Smith CB, Davidsen L, Deibler G, et al. A method for the determination of local rates of protein synthesis in man. *Trans Am Soc Neurochem* 1980;11:94.
298. Smith CB, Deibler GE, Eng N, et al. Measurement of local cerebral protein synthesis *in vivo*: influence of recycling of amino acids derived from protein degradation. *Proc Natl Acad Sci U S A* 1988;85: 9341–9345.
299. Smith CB, Schmidt KC, Qin M, et al. Measurement of regional rates of cerebral protein synthesis with L-[1-^{11}C]leucine and PET with correction for recycling of tissue amino acids: II. Validation in rhesus monkeys. *J Cereb Blood Flow Metab* 2005;25(5):629–640.
300. Ishiwata K, Vaalburg W, Elsing PH, et al. Comparison of L-[1-^{11}C]methionine and L-methyl-[^{11}C]methionine for measuring *in vivo* protein synthesis rates with PET. *J Nucl Med* 1988;29:1419–1427.
301. Bolster JM, Vaalburg W, Elsinga PH, et al. The preparation of ^{11}C-carboxyl labeled L-methionine for measuring protein synthesis. *J Labelled Compounds Radiopharm* 1986;23:1081–1082.
302. Schober O, Duden C, Meyer G-J, et al. Nonselective transport of [^{11}C]methyl]-L- and D-methionine into a malignant glioma. *Eur J Nucl Med* 1987;13:103–105.
303. Bergstrom M, Muhr C, Lundberg PO, et al. Amino acid distribution and metabolism in pituitary adenomas using positron emission tomography with D-[^{11}C]methionine and L-[^{11}C]methionine. *J Comp Assist Tomog* 1987;11:384–389.
304. Langen KJ, Hamacher K, Weckesser M, et al. O-(2-[^{18}F]fluoroethyl)-L-tyrosine: uptake mechanisms and clinical applications. *Nucl Med Biol* 2006;33(3):287–294.
305. Coenen HH, Kling P, Stocklin G. Cerebral metabolism of L-2-[^{18}F]fluorotyrosine, a new PET tracer for protein synthesis. *J Nucl Med* 1989;30:1367–1372.
306. Ishiwata K, Kubota K, Murakami M, et al. Re-evaluation of amino acid PET studies: can the protein synthesis rates in brain and tumor tissues be measured *in vivo*? *J Nucl Med* 1993;34(11):1936–1943.
307. Ogawa T, Miura S, Murakami M, et al. Quantitative evaluation of neutral amino acid transport in cerebral gliomas using positron emission tomography and fluorine-18 fluorophenylalanine. *Eur J Nucl Med* 1996;23:889–895.
308. Tomiyoshi K, Amed K, Muhammed S, et al. Synthesis of a new fluorine-18 labeled amino acid radiopharmaceutical: L-^{18}F-alpha-methyl tyrosine using separation and purification system. *Nucl Med Comm* 1997;18:169–175.
309. Shoup TM, Olson JMH, Votaw J, et al. Synthesis and evaluation of [^{18}F]1-amino-3-fluorocyclobutane-1-carboxylic acid to image brain tumors. *J Nucl Med* 1999;40:331–338.
310. Shields AF. Positron emission tomography measurement of tumor metabolism and growth: its expanding role in oncology. *Mol Imaging Biol* 2006;8(3):141–150.
311. Cronkite EP, Fliedner TM, Bond VP, et al. Dynamics of hemopoietic proliferation in man and mice studied by ^{3}H-thymidine incorporation into DNA. *Ann N Y Acad Sci* 1959;77:803.
312. Christman DR, Crawford EJ, Friedkin M, et al. Detection of DNA synthesis in intact organisms with positron-emitting methyl ^{11}C-thymidine. *Proc Natl Acad Sci U S A* 1971;69:988–989.
313. Crawford EJ, Friedkin M, Wolf AP, et al. ^{18}F-5-fluorouridine, a new probe for measuring the proliferation of tissue *in vivo*. *Adv Enzyme Regul* 1982;20:3–22.
314. Shields AF, Coonrod DV, Quackenbush RC, et al. Cellular sources of thymidine nucleotides: studies for PET. *J Nucl Med* 1987;28: 1435–1440.
315. Shields AF, Larson SM, Grunbaum Z, et al. Short-term thymidine uptake in normal and neoplastic tissues: studies for PET. *J Nucl Med* 1984;25:759–764.
316. Mankoff DA, Dehdashti F, Shields AF. Characterizing tumors using metabolic imaging: PET imaging of cellular proliferation and steroid receptors. *Neoplasia* 2000;2:71–88.
317. Shields AF, Mankoff DA, Link JM, et al. Carbon-11-thymidine and FDG to measure therapy response. *J Nucl Med* 1998;39:1757–1762.
318. Mankoff DA, Shields AF, Link JM, et al. Kinetic analysis of 2-[^{11}C]thymidine PET imaging studies: validation studies. *J Nucl Med* 1999;40:614–624.
319. Eary JF, Mankoff DA, Spence AM, et al. 2-[C-11]thymidine imaging of malignant brain tumors. *Cancer Res* 1999;5:615–621.
320. Shields AF, Grierson JR, Kozawa SM, et al. Development of labeled thymidine analogs for imaging tumor proliferation. *Nucl Med Biol* 1996;23:17–22.
321. Shields AF, Grierson JR, Dohmen BM, et al. Imaging proliferation *in vivo* with [F-18]FLT and positron emission tomography. *Nat Med* 1998;4:1334–1336.
322. Agdeppa ED, Kepe V, Liu J, et al. 2-Dialkylamino-6-acylmalononitrile substituted naphthalenes (DDNP analogs): novel diagnostic and

therapeutic tools in Alzheimer disease [review]. *Mol Imaging Biol* 2003;5(6):404–417.
323. Shoghi-Jadid K, Small GW, Agdeppa ED, et al. Localization of neurofibrillary tangles and beta-amyloid plaques in the brains of living patients with Alzheimer disease. *Am J Geriatr Psychiatry* 2002;10: 24–35.
324. Mathis CA, Klunk WE, Price JC, et al. Imaging technology for neurodegenerative diseases: progress toward detection of specific pathologies [review]. *Arch Neurol* 2005;62(2):196–200.
325. Engler H, Nordberg A, Blomqvist G, et al. First human study with a benzothiazole amyloid-imaging agent in Alzheimer disease and control subjects. *J Neurobiol Aging* 2002;23:S149.
326. Bacskai BJ, Hickey GA, Skoch J, et al. Four dimensional multiphoton imaging of brain entry, amyloid binding and clearance of an amyloid-β ligand in transgenic mice. *Proc Natl Acad Sci U S A* 2003;100: 12462–12467.
327. Mathis CA, Wang Y, Holt DP, et al. Synthesis and evaluation of ^{11}C-labeled 6-substituted 2-arylbenzothiazoles as amyloid imaging agents. *J Med Chem* 2003;46:2740–2754.
328. Zhuang ZP, Kung MP, Wilson A, et al. Structure activity relationship of imidazo[1,2a]pyridines as ligands for detecting beta-amyloid plaques in brain. *J Med Chem* 2003;46:237–243.
329. Zhang W, Oya S, Kung MP, et al. F-18 stilbenes as PET imaging agents for detecting beta-amyloid plaques in the brain. *J Med Chem* 2005;48(19):5980–5988.
330. Zhang W, Oya S, Kung MP, et al. F-18 Polyethyleneglycol stilbenes as PET imaging agents targeting A beta aggregates in the brain. *Nucl Med Biol* 2005;32(8):799–809.
331. Ding Y-S, Fowler J. New-generation radiotracers for nAChR and NET [review]. *Nucl Med Biol* 2005;32:707–718.
332. Ding Y-S, Lin K-S, Logan J. PET imaging of norepinephrine transporters. *Curr Pharm Des* 2006;12:3831–3845.
333. Wilson AA, Johnson DP, Mozley D, et al. Synthesis and *in vivo* evaluation of novel radiotracers for the *in vivo* imaging of the norepinephrine transporter. *Nucl Med Biol* 2003;30:85–92.
334. Ding Y-S, Lin KS, Garza V, et al. Evaluation of a new norepinephrine transporter PET ligand in baboons, both in brain and peripheral organs. *Synapse* 2003;50:345–352.
335. Ding Y-S, Lin KS, Logan J, et al. Comparative evaluation of positron emission tomography radiotracers for imaging the norepinephrine transporter: (S,S) and (R,R) enantiomers of reboxetine analogs ([^{11}C]methylreboxetine, 3-Cl-[^{11}C]methylreboxetine and [^{18}F]fluororeboxetine), (R)-[^{11}C]nisoxetine, [^{11}C]oxaprotiline and [^{11}C]lortalamine. *J Neurochem* 2005;94:337–351.
336. Logan J, Ding Y-S, Lin KS, et al. Modeling and analysis of PET studies with norepinephrine transporter ligands: the search for a reference region. *Nucl Med Biol* 2005;32(5):531–542.
337. Lin KS, Ding Y-S, Kim SW, et al. Synthesis, enantiomeric resolution, F-18 labeling and biodistribution of reboxetine analogs: promising radioligands for imaging the norepinephrine transporter with positron emission tomography. *Nucl Med Biol* 2005;32(4):415–422.
338. Lindsey KP, Glaser ST, Gatley SJ. Imaging of the brain cannabinoid system [review]. *Handb Exp Pharmacol* 2005;168:425–443.
339. Herkenham M, Lynn AB, Little MD, et al. Cannabinoid receptor localization in brain. *Proc Natl Acad Sci U S A* 1990;87(5):1932–1936.
340. Gatley SJ, Lan R, Volkow ND, et al. Imaging the brain marijuana receptor: development of a radioligand that binds to cannabinoid CB1 receptors *in vivo*. *J Neurochem* 1998;70(1):417–423.
341. Willis PG, Pavlova OA, Chefer SI, et al. Synthesis and structure-activity relationship of a novel series of aminoalkylindoles with potential for imaging the neuronal cannabinoid receptor by positron emission tomography. *J Med Chem* 2005;48(18):5813–5822.
342. Horti AG, Fan H, Ravert HT, et al. PET imaging of central cannabinoid receptors with [^{11}C]JHU75528. *J Nucl Med* 2006;47:136P.
343. Zhao Y, Robins E, Turton D, et al. Synthesis and characterization of N-(2-chloro-5-methylthiophenyl)-N'-(3-methylthiophenyl)-N-[^{11}C]methylguanidine [^{11}C]CNS 5161 a candidate PET tracer for functional imaging of NMDA receptors. *J Labelled Compounds Radiopharm* 2006;49:163–170.
344. Pin JP, Duvoisin R. The metabotropic glutamate receptors: structure and functions. *Neuropharmacology* 1995;34:1–26.
345. Huang Y, Narendran R, Bischoff F, et al. A positron emission tomography radioligand for the in vivo labeling of metabotropic glutamate 1 receptor: (3-ethyl-2-[^{11}C]methyl-6-quinolinyl)(cis- 4-methoxycyclohexyl)methanone. *J Med Chem* 2005;48(16):5096–5099.
346. Ametamey SM, Kessler LJ, Honer M, et al. Radiosynthesis and preclinical evaluation of ^{11}C-ABP688 as a probe for imaging the metabotropic glutamate receptor subtype 5. *J Nucl Med* 2006;47(4):698–705.
347. Yu M, Tueckmantel W, Wang X, et al. Methoxyphenylethynyl, methoxypyridylethynyl and phenylethynyl derivatives of pyridine: synthesis, radiolabeling and evaluation of new PET ligands for metabotropic glutamate subtype 5 receptors. *Nucl Med Biol* 2005;32 (6):631–640.
348. Czeh B, Fuchs E, Simon M. NK1 receptor antagonists under investigation for the treatment of affective disorders [review]. *Expert Opin Investig Drugs* 2006;15:479–486.
349. Hill RG, Oliver KR. Neuropeptide and kinin antagonists [review]. *Handb Exp Pharmacol* 2007;(177):181–216.
350. Warr D. The neurokinin 1 receptor antagonist aprepitant as an antiemetic for moderately emetogenic chemotherapy [review]. *Expert Opin Pharmacother* 2006;7:1653–1658.
351. Bergstrom M, Fasth KJ, Kilpatrick G, et al. Brain uptake and receptor binding of two [^{11}C]labelled selective high affinity NK1-antagonists, GR203040 and GR205171—PET studies in rhesus monkey. *Neuropharmacology* 2000;39:664–670.
352. Solin O, Eskola O, Hamill TG, et al. Synthesis and characterization of a potent, selective, radiolabeled substance-P antagonist for NK1 receptor quantitation: ([18F]SPA-RQ). *Mol Imaging Biol* 2004;6:373–384.
353. Bergstrom M, Hargreaves RJ, Burns HD, et al. Human positron emission tomography studies of brain neurokinin 1 receptor occupancy by aprepitant. *Biol Psychiatry* 2004;55(10):1007–1012.
354. Grierson JR, Yagle KJ, Eary JF, et al. Production of [F-18]fluoroannexin for imaging apoptosis with PET. *Bioconjug Chem* 2004;15(2): 373–379.
355. Yagle KJ, Eary JF, Tait JF, et al. Evaluation of ^{18}F-annexin V as a PET imaging agent in an animal model of apoptosis. *J Nucl Med* 2005;46(4):658–566.
356. *The United States Pharmacopeia: the national formulary: 2000.* Rockville, MD: U.S. Pharmacopeial Convention, 2000.
357. Qaim SM. Cyclotron production of medical radionuclides. In: Rosch F, ed. *Handbook of nuclear chemistry*, Vol. 4. *Radiochemistry and radiopharmaceutical chemistry in life sciences.* Dordrecht: Kluwer, 2003:47–76.
358. Pentlow KS, Graham MC, Lambrecht RM, et al. Quantitative imaging of iodine-124 with PET. *J Nucl Med* 1996;37(9):1557–1562.
359. Robinson MK, Doss M, Shaller C, et al. Quantitative immuno-positron emission tomography imaging of HER2-positive tumor xenografts with an iodine-124 labeled anti-HER2 diabody. *Cancer Res* 2005;65:1471–1478.
360. Berding G, Schneider U, Gielow P, et al. Feasibility of central cannabinoid CB1 receptor imaging with [^{124}I]AM281 PET demonstrated in a schizophrenic patient. *Psychiatry Res* 2006;147:249–256.
361. Smith SV. Molecular imaging with copper-64. *J Inorg Biochem* 2004;98:1874–1901.
362. Lewis MR, Wang M, Axworthy DB, et al. *In vivo* evaluation of pretargeted ^{64}Cu for tumor imaging and therapy. *J Nucl Med* 2003;44:1284–1292.
363. Rosch F, Knapp F. Radionuclide generators. In: Rosch F, ed. *Handbook of nuclear chemistry*. Vol. 4. *Radiochemistry and radiopharmaceutical chemistry in life sciences.* Dordrecht: Kluwer, 2003:81–98.
364. World Wide Web URL: http://www.acnp.org/Docs/BulletinPdfFiles/May2006Bulletin.pdf. Accessed .
365. Duyk G. Attrition and translation. *Science*. 2003;302:603–605.
366. Advancing nuclear medicine through innovation. The National Academic Press 2007;120–122.

CHAPTER 3

PET Physics and PET Instrumentation

TIMOTHY G. TURKINGTON

Positron emission tomography (PET) quantitatively measures the biodistribution of positron emitting radiotracers *in vivo*. Positrons emitted from positron-emitting radioisotopes radiotracers, which travel a short distance in tissue, subsequently annihilate and form two 511 keV photons that may be detected by a ring of detectors. Images are produced from the detection of such coincidence counts in a spatially relevant manner. This chapter discusses the basics of positron physics, coincidence detection, PET scanner design, phenomena that degrade PET images, and the union of PET and computed tomography (CT). More extensive information on PET instrumentation can be found in Wernick and Aarsvold (1).

POSITRON PHYSICS

Positron Decay

A nuclide is a specific combination of protons and neutrons in a nucleus. The number of protons (which is called the atomic number, or Z) dictates which chemical element the nuclide is, since it gives the total charge on the nucleus, which in turn dictates the nature of the electron structure of the atom. The number of neutrons plus the number of protons is the mass number. Only certain combinations of neutrons and protons lead to stable nuclides. Those that are not stable, referred to as radionuclides, decay, releasing energy in the form of radiation. The most common way to designate a particular nuclide is to specify the element, which in turn specifies the number of protons and the mass number, which specifies the sum of protons and neutrons. Isotopes are defined as multiple nuclides that share the same atomic number, but it is common in nuclear medicine and physics to use the term *isotope* interchangeably with *nuclide.*

Radionuclides that are not stable due to an abundance of protons can decay via the emission of a positron:

$$ {}^{A}_{Z}X_{N} \rightarrow {}^{\;\;\;A}_{Z-1}Y_{N+1} + e^{+} + \nu + Energy, \qquad [3.1]$$

where X is the original nuclide, with Z protons, N neutrons, and mass number A, Y is the new nuclide, with one more neutron, one fewer proton, and the same mass number, e^+ symbolizes the positron and ν is a neutrino, which has very little mass and interacts extremely weakly with matter. Energy is released in the decay in the form of kinetic energy of the released particles. The positron is the antiparticle counterpart to the electron, and it is opposite to the electron in all ways that there is an opposite (such as charge) and the same in all ways that there is not a known opposite (such as mass).

The kinetic energy of the annihilation is shared between the electron and the neutrino. Unlike gamma decays, in which the emission is always at a particular energy for a particular decay scheme, the positron and neutrino share the energy in variable proportions, so that the positron can have any amount of energy from zero up to the maximum available in the decay.

In addition to the decay energy that differs from one positron emitting radionuclide to the next, the other important variable is half-life. Radioactive decay is a random process, and the number of atoms in a sample that will decay over some time interval is proportional to the number in the sample. This characteristic makes the decay process an exponential one, that is, the number of atoms in a sample that have not decayed is an exponentially decreasing function of time and a constant specific to the radionuclide. It is typical to represent the decay as a half-life, that being the time in which half of a sample will decay. Several PET radionuclides are listed in Table 3.1.

Of the radionuclides listed, the first four are cyclotron-produced, and rubidium-82 [^{82}Rb] comes from a generator that can be purchased. Of the currently commonly used cyclotron-produced radionuclides, only fluorine-18 [^{18}F] has a long enough half-life to be transported; the first three must be produced on site and therefore require an on-site accelerator. Iodine-124 [^{124}I] and certain radioisotopes of copper also have sufficiently long half-lives to be transported, but are not in widespread use.

Positron Annihilation

When a positron is created in tissue, it travels a short distance, undergoing the same interactions as an electron (β particle) would, giving up energy to ionize and excite nearby atoms. When the

TABLE 3.1 Radionuclides Used for PET

Radionuclide	Half-life (min)
oxygen-15	2.1
nitrogen-13	10
carbon-11	20.3
fluorine-18	110
rubidium-82	1.25

positron has lost almost all its energy, it interacts with a nearby electron, resulting in the creation of two photons (Fig. 3.1) This annihilation reaction obeys conservation of energy and conservation of momentum, which dictate that the two photons will leave the annihilation site in opposite directions, each with an energy of 511 keV (the energy corresponding to the mass of the electron).

Coincidence Detection

The generation of two back-to-back photons of known energy provides much more information than does the generation of a single photon. Fig. 3.2 depicts the generation of annihilation photon pairs at multiple locations relative to a pair of radiation detectors. If the annihilation occurs within the column that connects the detectors, there is a possibility (depending on the direction of the photons) that both photons will be detected. Likewise, if an annihilation leads to the detection of both photons, it can only have happened if the annihilation was in the column connecting the detectors. Also depicted in Fig. 3.2, are two pulses representing the electronic pulses that would come simultaneously from two detectors if hit by photons from the same annihilation. (For conventional PET, the difference in arrival time of the two photons to their respective detectors, due to different path lengths, is considered small enough to be negligible.)

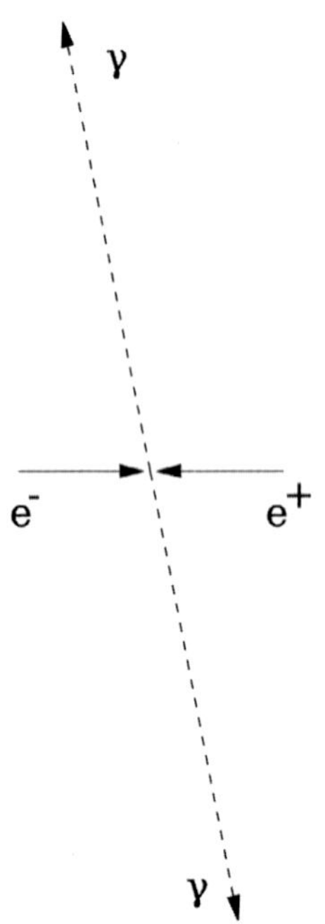

FIGURE 3.1. Positron annihilation. A positron and electron join together, resulting in the back-to-back emission of two 511 keV photons.

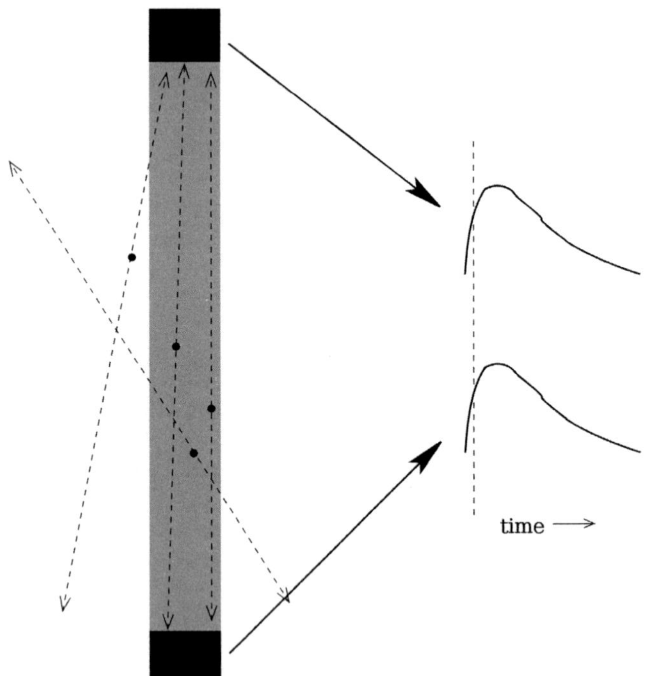

FIGURE 3.2. Coincidence detection. When two detectors are simultaneously hit by an annihilation photon pair, a simultaneous pair of electronic pulses is generated. Most annihilations within the column will not be detected due to photon trajectories that do not interact with the detectors. No annihilation events outside the column can be detected (at most one photon will be detected).

BASIC PET SCANNER

In a basic PET scanner, a section of the patient is surrounded by a ring of detectors, as depicted in Fig. 3.3. Any photon pairs leaving the body in the plane of the detector ring can be detected, and the particular detector pair subsequently registering the detection of 511 keV photons defines a column in which the annihilation must have occurred. Fig. 3.3 depicts one particular photon pair's trajectory and the corresponding detector pair and column. This is but one of a whole continuum of possible emission angles that would be detected by the ring. Unfortunately, far more photon pairs will leave the body undetected because they are not in the plane of the detector ring. In any case, even a small amount of radioactivity in a small region of the body will emit enough positrons, and therefore photon pairs, that radiation will be detected along many of the columns (also called lines of response [LORs]). For example, a cubic centimeter of tumor tissue may contain 1 μCi or more of radioactivity, which corresponds to 37,000 decays per second.

During a PET scan, the system is counting the number of times each detector pair is hit in coincidence, referred to as a *coincidence event*, so the raw data from a PET scan are simply the list of counts obtained along each line of response.

Fig. 3.4 depicts a simple body cross section with a uniform distribution of radioactivity plus a lesion with more concentrated radioactivity. Also depicted are the vertical lines of response. The

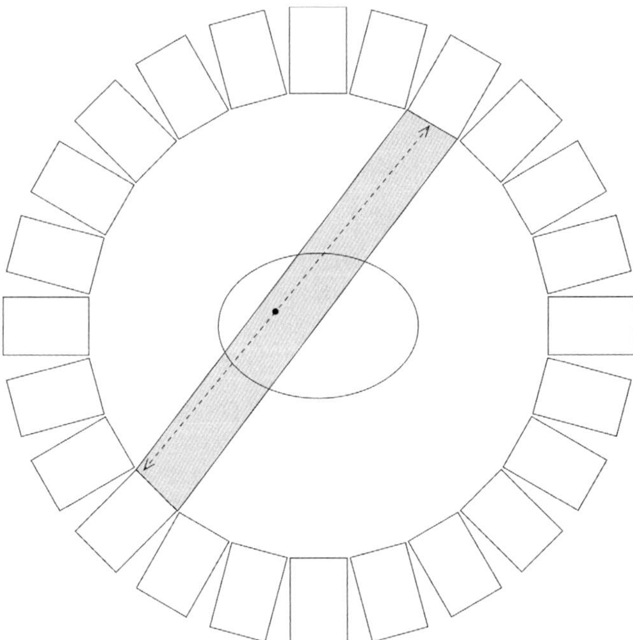

FIGURE 3.3. Simple PET ring. When any two detectors in the ring are hit simultaneously it indicates that an annihilation occurred within the column connecting the detectors.

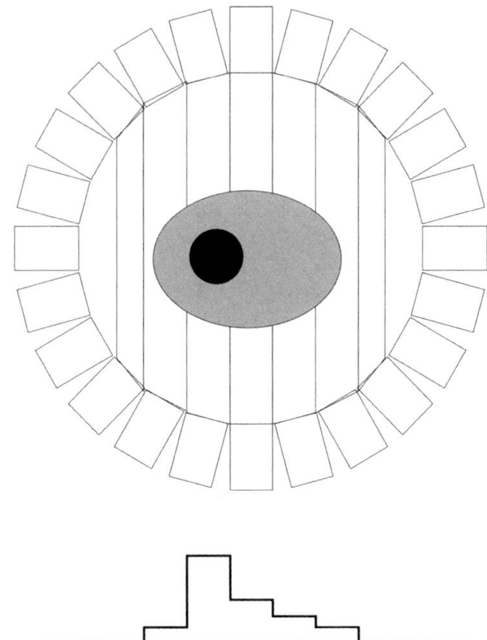

FIGURE 3.4. PET projection. With a radioactivity distribution presented (hot lesion in warm background) in a very coarse detector ring, counts measured along the vertical lines of response might be as shown in the histogram (**below**). This set of measurements is a projection of the radioactivity distribution. Each measurement represents a sum of the radioactivity between the corresponding detectors.

profile at the bottom represents the relative number of counts that might be expected along the vertical lines of response, with more counts coming from thicker sections of the body and even more coming from the lesion region. The distribution of counts along one direction is a projection of the distribution of radioactivity. Although only one projection angle is depicted, the PET scanner is simultaneously measuring all possible projection angles. This is in contrast to SPECT (single-photon emission computed tomography) acquisition, in which the gamma camera obtains only one projection angle at a time and orbits around the body to obtain the full set of projection angles needed to produce cross-sectional slices.

Scanner Design

Multiple factors of image quality have driven the design of PET scanners. A fundamental requirement is to have as much sensitivity for detecting true events as possible. Spatial resolution should also be good. Limiting background counts is another goal that will be discussed later.

Spatial resolution in PET has two fundamental limits. The first is that the positron goes a short distance in tissue before it annihilates. It is the location of the decay that is of interest, but the scanner sees the annihilation site. There is, therefore, a small blurring due to the average positron range. Fortunately, this range is small (<1 mm for [^{18}F] positrons). An additional limit is that the photons are not actually emitted at exactly 180 degrees from one another due to the momentum of the positron. This factor has a larger effect for larger diameter detector rings, but is still relatively small.

An additional factor that can be controlled is the size of the individual radiation detectors. With smaller detectors, each coincidence event can be localized to a smaller column, leading to better spatial resolution. All current commercial human PET systems use detectors composed of scintillation crystals and photomultiplier tubes (PMTs). The 511 keV photons interact in the crystal, producing light. Some of the light is then collected in the PMT and converted into an electronic pulse.

Early PET systems used detectors that coupled a single crystal to a single PMT. This led to count and resolution limitations. The desire for smaller detectors lead to the block design (2). In this design, a small array (from 6×6 up to 13×13) of crystals, or a block of crystal with an array cut into one end, is coupled either to four PMTs or to a single square PMT with four separate quadrants on its face. This unit functions similarly to a small gamma camera, with the sum of all PMT signals representing the energy of an impinging photon, and with the differences in signals being used to determine which of the crystals was hit. This design allows for more than 10,000 very small crystals (currently $\sim 4 \times 4$ mm^2 to $\sim 6 \times 6$ mm^2) without the corresponding size and number requirements for the PMTs, which would be cost prohibitive. Systems that use block detectors currently use three or four rings of these blocks, resulting in 18 to 52 rings of individual crystals. A block-based PET ring is shown in Fig. 3.5.

Although all PET images reflect the three-dimensional (3D) location of radioactivity throughout the body, all PET scanners operate in one of two modes: two-dimensional (2D) or 3D. Fig. 3.6 illustrates the two modes. In the simplest 2D PET operation, only those pairs in which both photons are detected in the same ring are recorded, and data are stored and reconstructed independently, plane by plane. Additional planes are formed by photon pairs that are detected in adjacent rings. Higher sensitivity is achieved in 2D PET by including additional photon trajectories as shown, but all are recorded as if they came from the central plane.

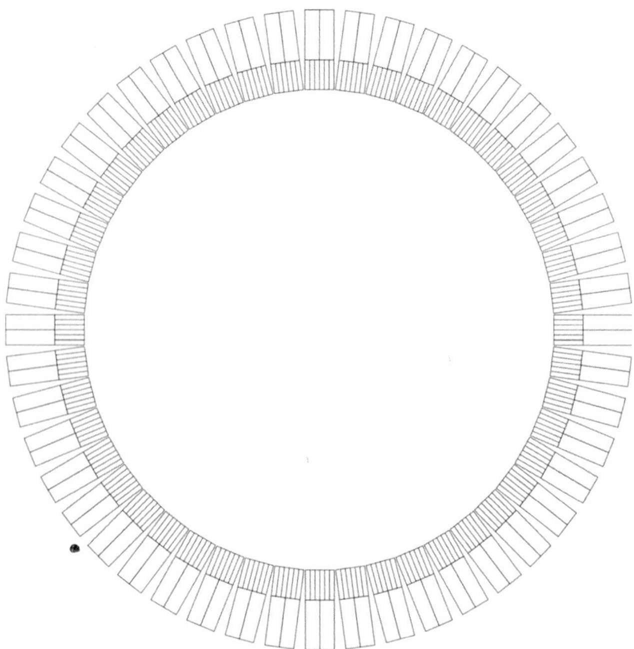

FIGURE 3.5. Block-based ring. Detector units (*blocks*) in many PET systems comprise a small number of photomultipliers reading an array of many small scintillator crystals. Blocks in this ring have a dimension of six crystals in the visible (tangential) direction.

In 3D PET, all photon pairs that are detected are recorded, regardless of which rings the detectors are in. This mode leads to greatly increased sensitivity for true events, particularly at the axial center of the field of view.

DEGRADING FACTORS

Background Events

Two types of background events can be recorded in PET: scattered events and random events. A scattered event is one in which one or both of the photons undergoes Compton scattering before being detected. Possible scattered trajectories are illustrated in Fig. 3.7. The two detected photons define an LOR that does not contain the original annihilation point. Therefore, the detected count is added in the wrong location. Unlike single-photon emission imaging and transmission imaging, scattered PET events can appear to come from outside the body. For a given total number of scattered events, it is desirable that some come from outside the body, since they do not then corrupt the interesting part of the image, and they also serve as a basis for scatter estimation and correction.

The scatter fraction, which is the ratio of scattered events to the sum of scattered and true events ($S/(S+T)$), varies widely, depending on the patient, the section of the body being imaged, the scanner, and the mode (2D or 3D) in which the scanner is operating. Larger body cross sections lead to higher scatter fractions. Better energy resolution in the detectors allows a higher threshold to be placed on detected photons, which in turn rejects more scatter photons.

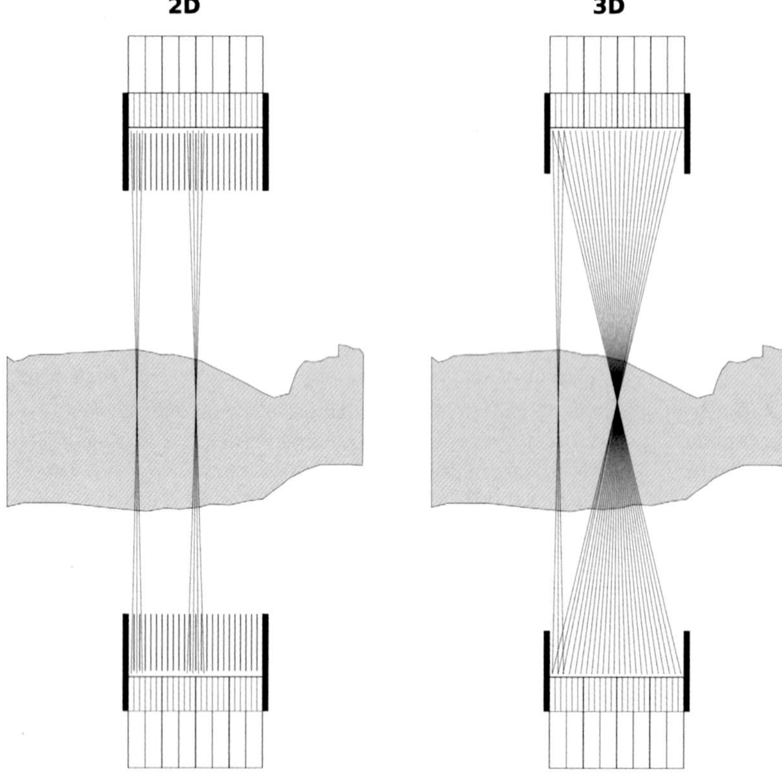

FIGURE 3.6. Side view-2D and -3D. At left is the side view of a multiring system operating in 2D mode. Coincidences are restricted by the septa and by electronics to be within a transaxial plane. A plane is defined for each detector ring (direct planes) and for each detector ring interface (cross planes). In the 3D mode (**right**), the septa are removed, and all photon pairs are recorded, regardless of which rings the photons hit. Radiation from the center of the field of view is more likely to be detected than that from the edge.

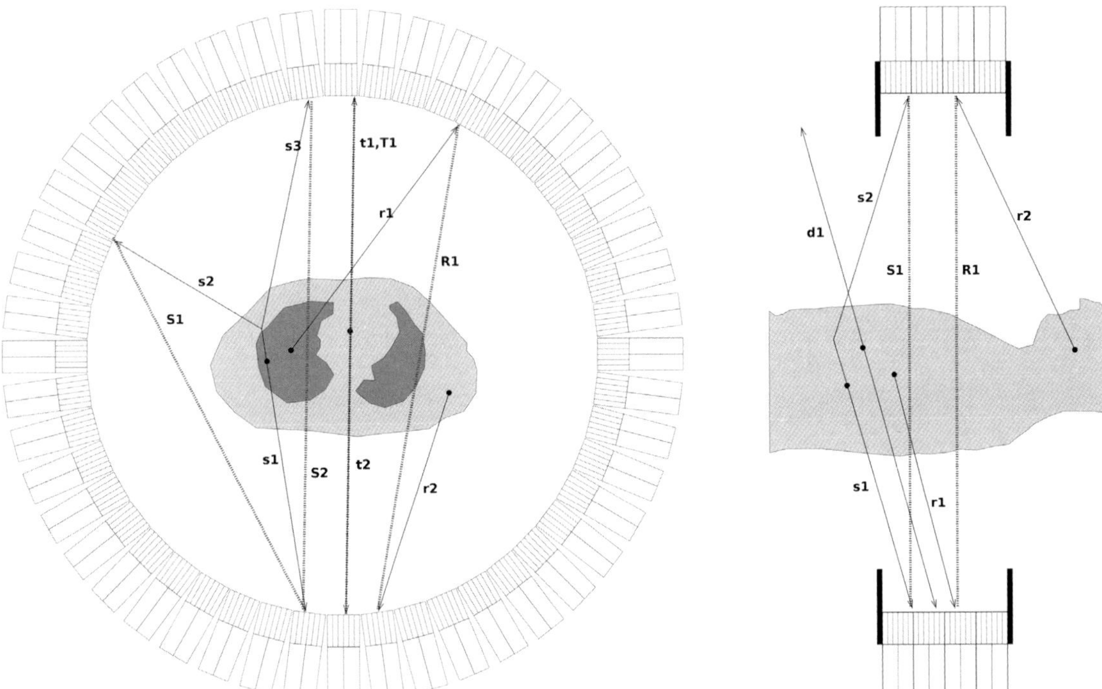

FIGURE 3.7. Background events, transaxial (**left**) and side (**right**) views. The transaxial view of different event types is shown. Annihilation photon pair t1 and t2 form a true coincidence, along line T1. Photons s1 and s2 (which have scattered) form a coincidence, which is incorrectly labeled by the system as coming from line of response S1, outside the body. s3 is a different possible scattered trajectory for the same annihilation, resulting in line of response S2, inside the body. Photons r1 and r2, from different annihilations, form a random coincidence and are recorded along the line R1. Similar events are shown in the side view at right. It can be seen that the use of septa in 2D mode (not shown) would preclude the detection of any of the scattered or random events shown here. In addition, the photon labeled d1, which would not be detected as a coincidence, would still lead to detector dead time unless stopped by septa.

Random coincidences occur when two unrelated photons (from different positrons) are detected simultaneously. In the strict sense, no two unrelated photons would ever be detected at *exactly* the same time. However, *at the same time* on a PET scanner simply means that the photons arrived within some small interval (typically 2 to 5 ns) of each other. That is, when one photon is detected, any other photon detected within time τ of that photon is considered to be in coincidence. This "timing window" is necessary because of the imprecision in the timing; the times measured for the two pulses from a true event will differ by a small amount (due to both the timing imprecision and the differences in corresponding photon paths). Better timing resolution leads to less difference and allows a smaller timing window to be used.

The rate at which random events are recorded between two detectors A and B is:

$$R_R = 2\tau R_A R_B, \qquad [3.2]$$

where R_A is the rate at which detector A is recording individual photons, R_B is the rate at which detector B is recording individual photons, and 2τ is the size of the timing window. The number of random events is therefore directly proportional to the size of the timing window and to the individual rates at which the detectors are being hit. Note that most factors that would influence the count rate on one detector in a scanner ring would also affect the other detectors. For example, doubling the dose to the patient would double R_A and R_B, thereby quadrupling the random rate but only doubling the true event rate. If removing the septa used for 2D imaging increases the individual detector rates by a factor of 10, the random rate goes up by a factor of 100. For these, and other reasons, random events can be negligible in some PET applications and can be the majority of detected events in other cases.

For a given line of response, there is a total number of *prompt* events counted during the scan. The *prompt* total consists of true events (T), scattered events (S), and random events (R):

$$P = T + S + R. \qquad [3.3]$$

It is desirable to reconstruct images free from the additive effects of random and scattered events, and it is common to do a correction:

$$T' = P - S' - R', \qquad [3.4]$$

where S' is an estimate of the number of scattered events, R' is an estimate of the number of random events, and T' is the resulting estimate of T events. It is beyond the scope of this chapter to discuss scatter and random correction techniques that would provide the estimates S' and R', but random corrections have always been quite accurate and scatter corrections, while less straight-forward, have developed substantially, even for 3D PET where scatter fractions can be high.

Even with accurate corrections, the presence of background events has a negative impact from a statistical perspective. For example, a system that yields 10 counts, background free, is better than one that yields 20 counts (10 signal and 10 background) even if the latter can accurately estimate that 10 are background.

PET scanner design and operation is done to maximize the number of true events acquired while minimizing the number of background events. The comparison of 2D and 3D modes (on a scanner that allows both) is interesting, since the sensitivity to true events is much higher in 3D, but the fraction of background events is also higher in 3D. (There are additional effects, such as dead time, which, for a given injected dose, may lead to more true events being lost in 3D than in 2D.) In any case, a useful metric for evaluating the statistical quality of raw PET data, and which loosely translates into the image signal-to-noise ratio squared, is noise equivalent counts (NEC) (3), defined as:

$$\mathrm{NEC} = \frac{T}{1 + S/T + (2)R/T}, \qquad [3.5]$$

where T, S, and R are defined above. An important refinement is that S and T used to calculate NEC (if used for all counts collected in a scan) should exclude those counts that are not on lines of response pointing through the body (which would therefore not influence the image). If S and R are zero, then NEC reduces to T. If they are greater than zero, NEC is less than T. The optional factor of 2 before the random term is used if the random event estimate comes from a count-based estimate, which adds even more noise.

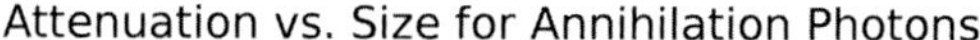

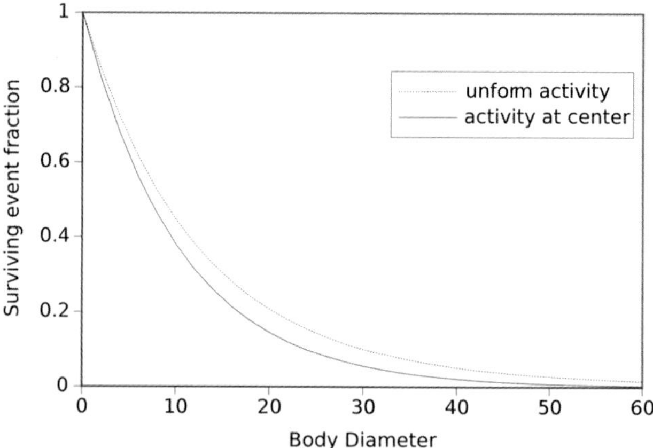

FIGURE 3.8. Attenuation as a function of body size. This plot shows the fraction of photon pairs that would survive body attenuation, as a function of body diameter, assuming a cylindrical body. One curve assumes a uniform distribution of radioactivity throughout the cylinder. The other (the worst case) assumes all activity as at the middle. For the head, approximately 25% of photons pairs survive. For a small body, approximately 10%. For a very large body, 1% to 2%.

ATTENUATION

When one (or both) of the annihilation photons scatters in the body, it is prevented from being detected appropriately, which is called *attenuation*. (It may be detected by a different detector, and this constitutes a scattered coincidence, discussed previously. Only a small fraction of attenuated events are detected as scattered events, though.) The probability of attenuation for annihilation photons is high. The fraction of photon pairs that *are not* attenuated is:

$$e^{-\int \mu dx}, \qquad [3.6]$$

where μ is the linear attenuation coefficient as a function of position in the body and the integral is over the trajectory of *both* photons. For a constant body density (e.g., soft tissue), this expression is:

$$e^{-\mu d}, \qquad [3.7]$$

where d is the total path length through the body. For soft tissue, this exponential introduces a loss of about 10% of photons for each additional centimeter of tissue traversed. The magnitude of the attenuation effect as a function of body size is illustrated in Fig. 3.8.

The loss of true coincidences due to attenuation has several negative effects. First, the overall loss of events leads to increased image noise, and larger bodies lose more counts to attenuation. Second, without accurate attenuation correction, measurements of radioactivity cannot be quantitatively accurate. Finally, attenuation does not affect all areas the same. The position-dependent aspects of attenuation are depicted in Fig. 3.9.

Although the statistical impact (image noise) of losing photons cannot be recovered, the quantitative accuracy and qualitative integrity of PET images can be restored with attenuation correction. Attenuation correction in PET relies on a measurement or estimate of the attenuation probability ($e^{-\int \mu dx}$) along each line of response. This can be calculated if the tissue is uniform and the outer contour is known. Although this is never true in the body, it is a good enough approximation for some brain applications. For nonuniform attenuation, a transmission scan must be performed. Traditional methods involved orbiting radionuclide (mostly positron-emitting) sources around the body and measuring the fraction transmitted through the body along each line of response. Such methods were accurate but involved a substantial increase in total scan time, with the transmission scan typically taking as much time as the emission scan. In addition, because of the limited transmission counts obtained, the corrected images had additional noise. The long total scan duration, motion (either during the transmission or the emission scan), or between the two can add artifacts to the images. The dominant method for correcting attenuation on current PET scanners is to use x-ray CT images. CT-based attenuation correction will be discussed in the PET/CT section.

PET/CT

Since the initial combination of PET and CT into a single device (4), the world of PET instrumentation has changed to the point that nearly all PET systems being purchased now are actually hybrid PET/CT. The benefits of adding CT to PET are multiple, including using the CT images for attenuation correction, using the CT to provide anatomic detail for PET interpretation (image fusion), and allowing two clinical examinations to be performed in one session. Although performed in one imaging session, the two examinations are by no means performed at the same exact time. Rather, it is typical for the CT scan to be performed first, with the PET scan performed immediately after the CT scan has concluded (or vice versa). The PET scanner table generally must index (move) the patient the distance separating the PET and CT rings so the PET

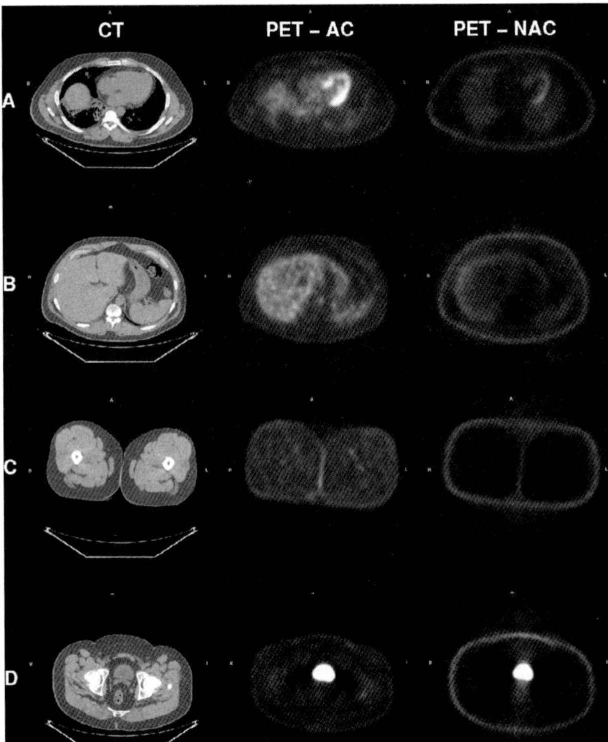

FIGURE 3.9. Qualitative attenuation effects. Images are shown from the four body sections. For each slice, CT, PET with attenuation correction (PET-AC), and PET with no attenuation correction (PET-NAC) are shown. In slice **B**, including the liver, it can be seen that the true uptake in the liver is uniform, but attenuation effects lessen the apparent uptake closer to the body center. In all slices, the artificially prominent body surface is seen, due to the nonattenuated tangential trajectory. In **A** (thorax) the lungs appear to have higher uptake than surrounding tissues, even thought the opposite is true. In **C**, the concave areas between the legs are artificially filled with activity. Finally, in **D**, the hot bladder, elongates in the lower-attenuation superior-anterior direction, while depleting the surrounding tissue in the lateral direction.

and the CT are correctly aligned. Obviously, any patient motion between the PET and CT scans would lead to inaccurate attenuation correction being applied.

In addition to the individual challenges of producing high-quality PET images and high-quality CT images, hybrid systems must also provide good alignment between the resulting PET and CT images so that attenuation correction will be accurate and fusion will be reliable. Accurate alignment of the resulting images has both hardware and software implications. For example, a differential, weight-dependent bed deflection between CT and PET imaging of a given body section would cause a vertical shift between image sets. Photos of the CT and PET components of a PET/CT system are shown in Fig. 3.10.

The need to do PET attenuation correction is one of several advantages of putting PET and CT systems together (5). Advantages of using CT images for attenuation correction include speed and low noise. There are several issues in using x-ray CT for PET attenuation correction. One is that the PET photons are 511 keV, while the CT attenuation map is generated with a spectrum of much lower energy photons, typically 120 to 140 kV(p) (kilovolt peak). A scheme for translating Hounsfield scale pixel values into 511 keV linear attenuation coefficients is presented in Fig. 3.11. Although an accurate translation is possible for air, water, bone, and mixtures thereof, other materials such as iodine-base contrast media and metals confound the process (6).

Another issue is that PET scans are relatively slow, with several minutes being spent per bed position. PET images therefore represent an average over respiratory and cardiac cycles. CT images, each of which represents a fraction of a second, are snapshots of a particular respiratory (and even cardiac) phase. A good match is needed between PET and CT for both the attenuation correction purposes and for fusion. Multiple approaches have been suggested and taken. The most technically advanced and complicated approach is to produce respiratory-gated PET and CT image sets separately, resulting in phase-matched image sets. In addition to matching PET and CT, this approach has the benefit of freezing the motion during PET that otherwise ends up as a blur. A simpler but

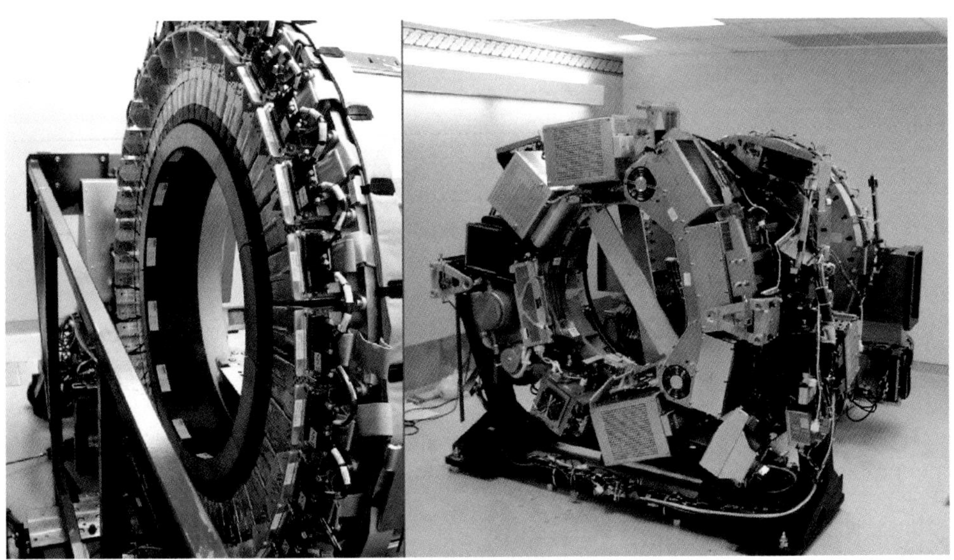

FIGURE 3.10. PET/CT system. PET (**left**) and CT (**right**) components of a PET/CT system during installation. In the PET, the individual blocks can be seen forming a ring. The retractable septa are also visible, in 2D position.

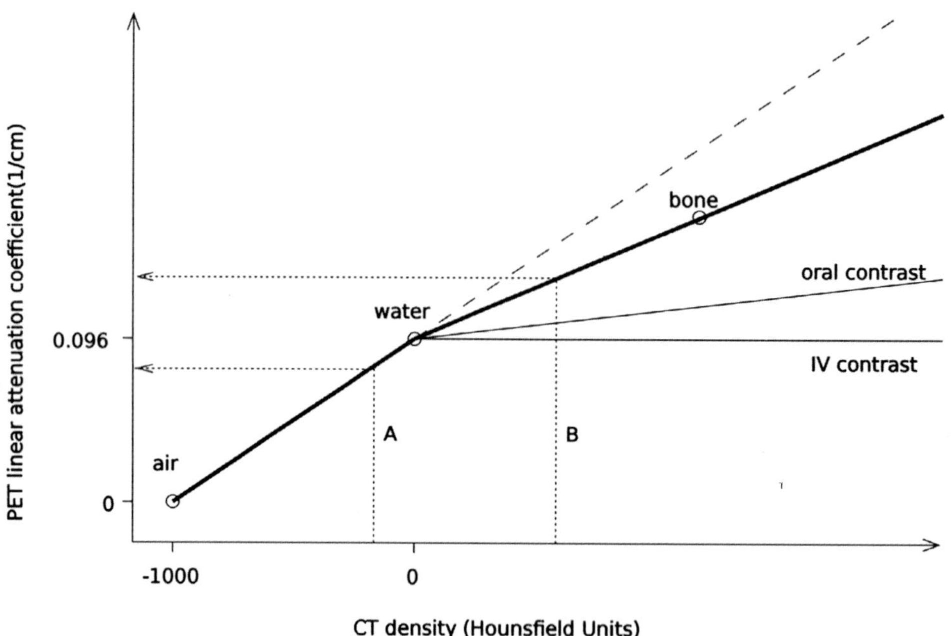

FIGURE 3.11. CT attenuation curves (CTAC). Three points (air, water, cortical bone) define the bilinear transformation for converting CT numbers (horizontal axis) to 511 keV attenuation coefficients (vertical axis) for PET attenuation correction. All CT pixels are assumed to be air, water, bone, or some combination of two of them, due to image noise or blurring. When high-Z contrast media are used, high-density areas may be filled with contrast or bone, so a single transformation will either undercorrect bone, overcorrect contrast areas, or both. Some systems use a different correction when contrast is present during the CT. In the case of intravenous contrast, the contrast is not even present in the same areas during the PET.

often effective approach is to acquire CT at end expiration, or nearly end expiration, and acquire the PET with no instruction. Coronal images shown in Fig. 3.12 illustrate two studies, one where there is a good match between PET and end expiration CT, and one where the match is not good (likely because the CT state was not actually end expiration).

Image Quality and Quantitation

PET image quality is determined by several factors. One factor is the statistical quality of the raw data. As discussed earlier, it is desirable to have as many true counts as possible, with background (random and scatter) fractions that are as low as possible. Although it may not be perfect, NEC is a good start for estimating image quality based on raw data. Higher NEC translates into lower image noise. Independent of scanner differences, more counts will also be obtained with a longer scan. Increased radiotracer dose may or may not lead to increased image quality, depending on the starting point dose, the patient, and the scanner. Dead time and random events are both factors that prevent NEC (and image quality) from increasing linearly with injected dose.

The other important factor in image quality is spatial resolution. Scanners are characterized by their intrinsic spatial resolution, which is actually a set of numbers representing the blurring of a point source at different locations within the field of view. Current systems yield values from 4.2 to 6.8 mm. The first number comes from a system with 4 mm crystals, measured near the scanner center, and the second comes from a system with 6.2 mm crystals, measured 10 cm from center. The general trends are the smaller crystals, measurements nearer the scanner center, and measurements in the tangential direction (as opposed to radial), all of which improve spatial resolution numbers. In addition to these effects there are two other fundamental physical effects. First, the positron travels some range in tissue before annihilating. Second, the annihilation photons do not travel exactly 180 degrees apart. Both effects are relatively small for human PET imaging.

The spatial resolution of PET images is almost never as good as the measured intrinsic spatial resolution numbers. The prime reason is that limited counts translate into image noise. There is always some tradeoff that can be made between image resolution and noise, either through filtering or limiting iterations of the reconstruction algorithm. Since most PET imaging situations are count-limited, image processing tradeoffs generally lead to resolutions that are worse (in some cases considerably worse) than the intrinsic resolution. In fact, the need to process images to lower resolution to be viewable *defines* the situation as count-limited. Several image acquisition, processing, and quality points are illustrated in Fig. 3.13.

Quantitation

When all corrections (attenuation, scatter, random, dead time, sensitivity, etc.) are performed, PET image pixel values represent regional radioactivity concentration. Although the tracer concentration itself is not fundamental to a biological process (e.g., injecting more tracer would lead to higher uptake in the tissue), the concentration serves as the starting point for more physiologically meaningful measures, such

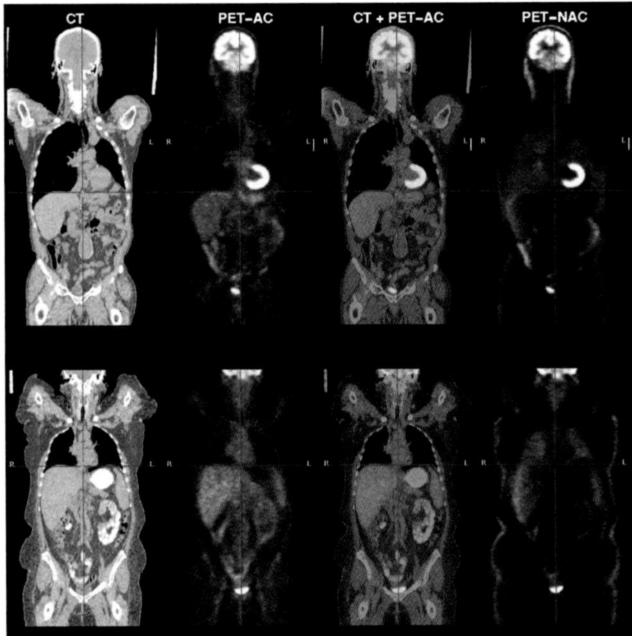

FIGURE 3.12. PET/CT breathing. Two studies obtained with end-expiration breath hold for CT. From left to right in both studies are: CT, PET with attenuation correction (AC), CT fused with AC PET, and PET without attenuation correction. A light line is drawn on both studies to help compare the position of the diaphragm in each image set. At the top is a study where there is a good match between diaphragm positions in the PET and CT. In the lower study, the match is not good. It is misleading to evaluate the match based on the AC PET, since it is heavily influenced by the CT. Although it is harder to discern the lung/liver boundary in the PET without attenuation image (because the lungs are artificially hot, as usual), it appears that the diaphragm is higher in the PET. The clue in the PET-AC image is the dark artifact across what appears to be the base of the lung. This area was lung during the CT, but liver during the PET, so the attenuation correction process under-corrected it.

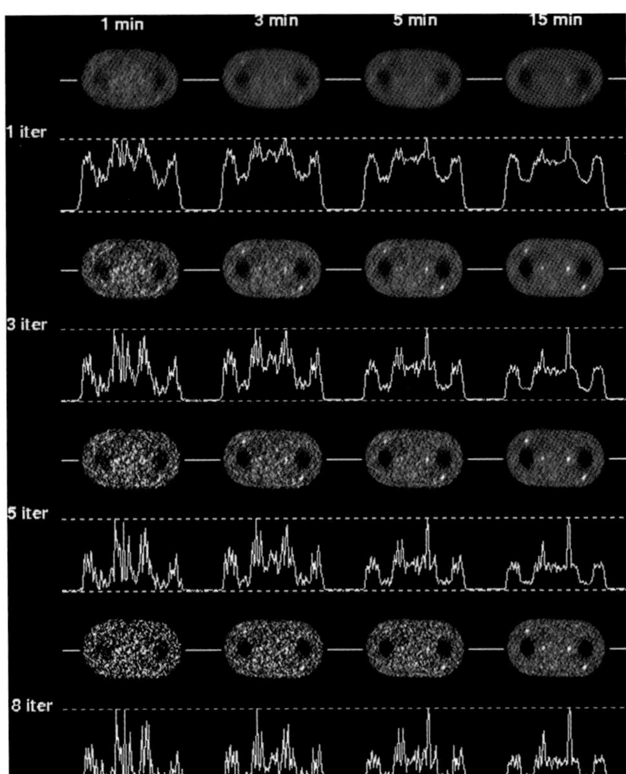

FIGURE 3.13. PET image quality. A phantom with 1 cm hot spheres with eight times the activity concentration of the background. In addition, there is a 5-cm diameter cold area on each side. Each image has a corresponding profile (**below**) that depicts pixel intensities for the row indicated by the white ticks. The columns represent different scan durations (1, 3, 5, 15 minutes). The rows represent different numbers of iterations of a reconstruction algorithm (ordered subsets expectation-maximization [OS-EM] with five subsets). Generally, longer scans have less noise (random variations from one pixel to the next). More iterations lead to better spatial resolution and recovery of hot and cold areas, but more noise.

as glucose metabolic rate and blood flow, obtained by kinetic modeling of the data. Short of kinetic modeling, the standardized uptake value (SUV) is frequently used as an index of tracer uptake:

$$\text{SUV} = \frac{(\text{radiotracer concentration})}{(\text{injected dose})/(\text{body mass})}. \qquad [3.8]$$

Typical units for expressing the SUV are g/mL (density), which is essentially unitless when applied to the body. This index normalizes the activity measured in a pixel (or region of interest) to the average radioactivity throughout the body (ignoring urination).

The accuracy of PET quantitation depends on all the degrading factors that have been discussed, including attenuation, detection of scattered and random events, and dead time. More precisely, it depends on the accuracy of the corrections for these effects. In addition, there is an effect based on the size of the object and the image resolution. The rule of thumb is that if an object size is not at least three times the image resolution, the measured uptake will be too low (for a hot object). For object sizes comparable to or smaller than the image resolution, the effect is quite large. Fig. 3.14 illustrates the effect of object size and resolution for hot sphere imaging.

Accuracy requirements depend on the task at hand. If the task is to track the uptake of tracer in the same patient over time, then some sources of error (such as scatter correction) may be similar enough (since the patient size and shape are not likely to vary too much) that the change in the measurement can be measured more accurately than the absolute measurement.

Time of Flight PET

Since most body imaging PET applications are count-limited, there is a strong desire to improve the noise (or signal-to-noise) of images without compromising spatial resolution. Time of flight (TOF) PET provides such a possibility.

Conventional PET measurements determine the origin of each event to be somewhere within the column between the associated detectors. If the timing precision of the detectors is good enough, the origin can be better pinpointed along the column, as illustrated in Fig. 3.15. The different path lengths of the two photons translate into different detection times, determined by the speed of light. Working backward, a difference in detection times can be translated into a position along the line. Although the principle is sound, the

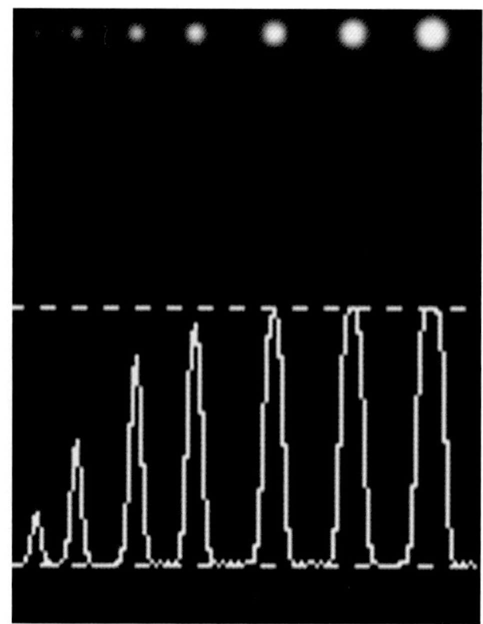

FIGURE 3.14. Object size. Spheres with diameter 2, 3, 4, 5, 6, 7, and 8 (arbitrary units) were simulated and blurred with a 3D Gaussian function with width 2 and are displayed from left to right, respectively. From the images (**top**) and from the count profiles (**bottom**), it is seen that the activity in the six-unit sphere is barely recovered. Smaller spheres do not reach full recovery. The two-unit sphere has a maximum that is only 20% its original intensity.

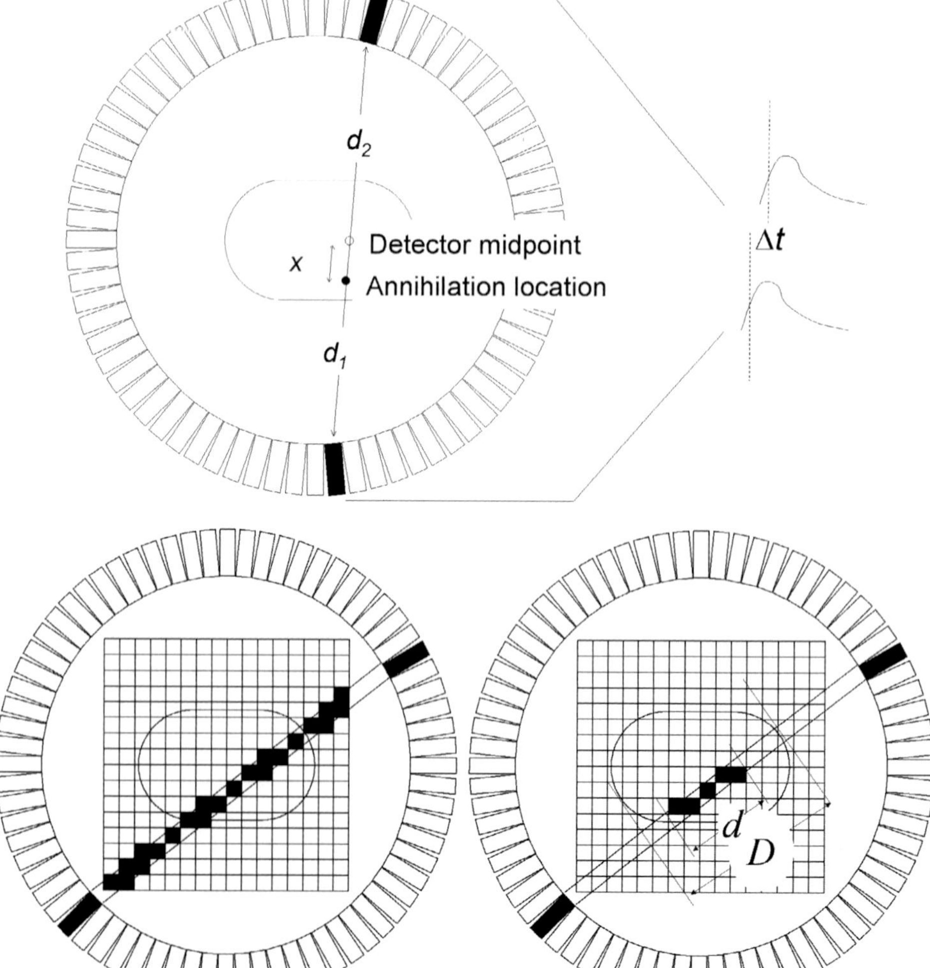

FIGURE 3.15. Time of flight PET. At top, an annihilation occurs a distance x from the center of the detector pair, resulting in paths d_1 and d_2 for the two photons. The path length difference leads to a detection time difference $\Delta t = (d_2 - d_1)/c = 2x/c$. If the system has good enough timing resolution, it can measure (with limited precision) the difference Δt. At the bottom left is depicted the pixels that a traditional reconstruction algorithm would populate with counts from this detector pair. At bottom right is a time-of-flight reconstruction, which can constrain the event to a short segment. Such increased information leads to an improvement in image quality (signal-to-noise).

problem is that timing precision in typical PET detectors has not been high enough to make meaningful measurements of timing differences. For example, if photons are traveling 30 cm/ns, a timing resolution worse than 2 ns would provide no information that is better than the size of the body. Detector materials with very fast pulses were used in first generation TOF PET. These materials were compromised in other qualities, which lead to good PET imaging, including stopping power. Now, certain lutetium-based crystals have good overall PET properties (good stopping power for 511 keV photons, good energy resolution, good timing resolution for random rejection, low dead time) and good enough timing resolution that the annihilation location can be resolved better than the body size. The improvements from TOF PET are expected to be greatest when imaging large bodies (a situation that is unfavorable by most PET standards). More directly, the TOF improvement is expected to be related to the body size divided by the TOF resolution (the length of the segment to which each event can be constrained).

Commercial systems are now available and are being characterized for the improvements made to PET imaging (7).

The process of producing images from the count measurement described here is more fully described in Chapter 4.

REFERENCES

1. Wernick MW, Aarsvold JN, eds. *Emission tomography: the fundamentals of PET and SPECT*. San Diego: Elsevier, 2004.
2. Casey ME, Nutt R. A multicrystal 2-dimensional BGO detector system for positron emission tomography. *IEEE Trans Nucl Sci* 1986;33:460–463.
3. Strother SC, Casey ME, Hoffman EJ. Measuring PET scanner sensitivity: relating count rates to image signal-to-noise rations using noise equivalent counts. *IEEE Trans Nucl Sci* 1990;3:783–788.
4. Beyer T, Townsend DW, Brun T, et al. A combined PET/CT scanner for clinical oncology. *J Nucl Med* 2000;41:1369–1379.
5. Kinahan PE, Townsend DW, Beyer T, et al. Attenuation correction for a combined 3D PET/CT scanner. *Med Phys* 1998;25:2046–2053.
6. Beyer T, Townsend DW. Dual-modality PET/CT imaging: CT-based attenuation correction in the presence of CT contrast agents. *J Nucl Med* 2001;42:210.
7. Surti, Kuhn A, Werner ME, et al. Performance of Philips Gemini TF PET/CT scanner with special consideration for its time-of-flight imaging capabilities. *J Nucl Med* 2007;48(3):471–480.

Fundamentals of CT in PET/CT

MAHADEVAPPA MAHESH

Imaging modalities are commonly differentiated as functional or anatomical in nature. However, both categories of information are complementary and when combined allow integration of data for the diagnosis, planning, and evaluation of cancer therapy. The explosive growth of positron emission tomography (PET) and computed tomography (CT) imaging in the past several years, with an estimated 1.5 million scans per year performed in 2007, attests to the value of fusing form and function into anatometabolic or anatomolecular images (1–3). At the time of the first edition of this textbook, PET/CT had only recently been introduced, and most PET scans were being performed using PET only devices. Now, most clinical PET studies are performed as PET/CT scans for cancer imaging, and nearly all PET scanners sold currently are PET/CT scanners, not dedicated PET devices.

The advantages of combining a CT scanner with a PET scanner are multiple. Both the PET and the CT scans are fully registered, if performed with correct technique without patient motion, which allows online fusion of two sets of volumetric images of different types. PET provides functional images of radiopharmaceutical distribution. CT provides anatomical images used for localizing radiopharmaceutical update and also supply attenuation maps that allow for attenuation correction to be performed and for more quantitatively accurate PET reconstructions (4). CT also provides intrinsically useful anatomical information that is of clear diagnostic value, even if the CT is not performed at the conventional highest diagnostic performance level (5,6).

The advantages of using a CT scanner with a PET scanner in the so-called hybrid imaging systems are that the CT data improve anatomical landmarks for localization of radiotracer uptake. This is due to high photon flux, which improves accuracy and reduced noise levels of attenuation measurements and much higher quality images than those from radionuclide sources. CT also provides high spatial resolution images that can generate highly accurate localization maps and accurate attenuation correction maps. Since the average CT energy is less than 100 keV and the PET energy is in the range of 511 keV, there is little cross talk between the transmission and emission images. Of course, with all current PET systems, these images are obtained sequentially and not simultaneously. PET/CT scanners are designed so that the hybrid scanner is neither PET only nor CT only; it is truly a new imaging tool. It combines two major medical imaging technologies: x-ray CT for anatomical imaging and attenuation corrections, with PET for functional imaging. The PET/CT scanner can operate as a single or a dual modality system, which can be used to acquire only CT scans, only PET scans, or PET/CT scans. Fig. 4.1 shows a schematic drawing of a typical PET/CT scanner. The CT gantry is positioned parallel to the PET gantry. Both the CT gantry and the PET gantry are assembled such that they are positioned in line, so the two components, PET scanner and CT scanner, can relatively easily be separated to allow for repairs or maintenance services on individual scanners, and in line so that the scanners image the same portion of each patient if the table is properly incremented between the devices. The fact that the devices are next to each other, albeit closely integrated, means that each component, the CT and the PET, can advance at its own rate in terms of improvements in technology. In practice, many manufacturers offer several choices of CT scanner performance (slice number, rotational speed, number of x-ray tubes, etc.) that can be paired with the same (or varying) PET scanner performance characteristics (7–9). Thus, very high slice number scanners for CT scanning may be most appropriate for the CT component of PET/CT scanners used in the management of cardiovascular disease, where assessment of the coronary arteries may be a part of the PET/CT, while lower CT slice numbers and slower rotational speeds may be quite adequate for most oncological applications.

Since the PET and the CT scanners adjoin each other closely, but do not perform the PET scan and the CT scan at the same time (or at exactly the same place) on the patient, it is critical that they be aligned carefully. Further, to have the patient imaged at the same exact point with both modalities in all current systems, the imaging table must be advanced between the PET and the CT a distance equal to the separation between the gantries in order to image the same region of the patient. Thus, the table must be "in line" and the PET and CT components of the scanner must be aligned properly in multiple dimensions.

An initial challenge in the development of clinical PET/CT scanners was the stability of the patient table. When the table was extended such that the head of the table is positioned all the way inside the PET gantry, even a minimal flexion or bending of the

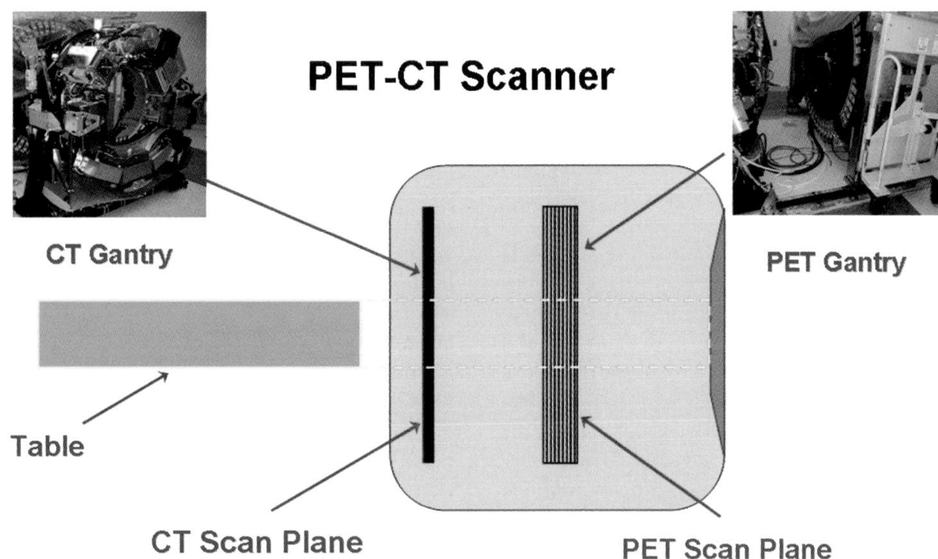

FIGURE 4.1. Schematic diagram of CT (**left**) and PET gantry (**right**) in a PET/CT scanner.

table could result in a significant error in the image fusion processes as the patient would be more posterior on the table that has been flexed posteriorly. Hence, the stability of the patient table when positioned with maximum extension was an initial challenge in the design of these systems. In some early designs, if the table was cantilevered over varying distances, especially with heavy patients, the patient's weight would force the table downward if extended further. Thus, there could be a misregistration with the patient more posterior on the PET image than the CT. Manufacturers avoid this in a variety of ways in current models. However, installation of a PET/CT scanner requires very careful attention to the floor position, so that the floor is flat where the scanner and bed are installed, so the table moves seamlessly and without deviation through the gantry.

A typical PET/CT protocol includes moving the patient first into the CT gantry to perform a CT scan of the region of interest (often much of the body) and then moving the patient further into the PET gantry to acquire the PET scan of a similar region. For example, in one approach to PET scanning, during a whole-body PET/CT scan, the patient is scanned with CT scanner from midear to midthigh, and then the patient is positioned at different location/fields under PET gantry to acquire PET images. The distance of separation is equal to the separation between the CT and the PET image. With such an approach, high-quality, but not perfect, registration of the CT and PET images can be obtained, typically with well less than 1 cm of difference between the lesion location on the CT versus its location on the PET (10,11). Perfect registration is difficult to achieve as the PET images are acquired over a longer period of time than the CT images, meaning that respiratory motion is an intrinsic component of the PET image, which can lead to blurring. Further, the CT may be obtained at a different position than the PET, as the CT is a "snapshot" image. This can be managed, but minor misregistrations between PET and CT are still not uncommon on PET/CT studies.

In this chapter, the fundamentals of CT as applied to PET/CT scanners are discussed. Also discussed are the radiation doses for typical PET/CT scans, particularly from the CT scan portion of the study. The other topics discussed include the scan parameters for typical PET/CT protocols, pitch, and image artifacts. Given that CT scanner technology is changing rapidly and CT protocols of a diagnostic quality with full intravenous and oral contrast are increasingly being applied, a full discussion of all clinical CT protocols is clearly beyond the scope of this review and frankly is in flux. The reader is referred to any of several full textbooks dealing with CT imaging for such guidance but should be aware of potential artifacts induced in quantitation of PET images in the presence of intravenous contrast, although they are often only modest if only relatively low concentrations of intravenous contrast are used, but can be substantial if high Hounsfield Units are present during the CT scan used for attenuation correction (12).

FUNDAMENTALS OF CT

CT is a method of acquiring and reconstructing an image of thin cross sections of the body on the basis of measurements of attenuation of x-ray photons projected from multiple angles. In comparison with conventional radiographs, CT images are substantially free of superimposed tissues and are capable of much higher contrast due to elimination, or at least a major reduction, of scatter. Fundamentally, a CT scanner makes many measurements of attenuation through the plane of a finite thickness of a cross section of the body. The system uses these data to reconstruct a digital image of the cross section, with each pixel in the image representing a measurement of the mean attenuation of a boxlike element called voxel (three-dimensional pixel element) that extends through the thickness of the section. A CT image is based on the measurement of the x-ray attenuation through the section plane using many different positions. This is achieved by rotating both the x-ray tube and the detectors around the patient. An attenuation measurement quantifies the fraction of radiation removed in passing through a given amount of specific material of thickness. Attenuation is expressed as shown in Equation 4.1, where I_t is the x-ray intensity measured with the material of thickness Δx in the x-ray beam, I_o is the x-ray intensity measured without the material in the x-ray beam tag, and the μ is the linear attenuation coefficient of the specific material.

$$I_t = I_o e^{-\mu \Delta x} \quad [4.1]$$

Characteristics of an unknown material can be determined, and given its physical thickness Δx, one can then measure I_o and I_t and derive the characteristic of the material by using the above equation. The image reconstruction is basically a process of determining the attenuation values for each voxel by using many x-ray projections obtained by scanning from different angles. The CT signal is basically acquired because of the tissue discrimination, which is due to attenuation of radiation between voxels, which depends on differences in tissue density, atomic number of elements presented in the voxel, and the detected mean photon energy.

The other fundamental of CT imaging is that the attenuation values are scaled to a more convenient scale and are normalized to voxels containing water and are expressed as CT numbers in Hounsfield units. The CT number of a material is defined as in Equation 4.2, where μ_w is the attenuation coefficient of water, μ_m is the attenuation coefficient of material of interest and k is a scaling factor.

$$CT\# = k\left[\frac{\mu_m - \mu_w}{\mu_w}\right] \quad [4.2]$$

With the scaling factor of 1,000, the CT number of water is always 0, and the CT number of air is 1,000. Tissues denser than water have positive CT numbers, and tissues less dense than water have negative CT numbers. The CT numbers are represented or mapped onto a grayscale that is visible as a CT image.

The other fundamental in CT is the CT gantry. Although the CT gantry has a physical aperture of approximately 60 to 70 cm in diameter, the actual sampling area where the attenuation measurements are made is smaller than the physical opening; the actual sampling area is usually 50 to 55 cm in diameter (although sometimes larger in scanners designed for the obese). Because the sampling area is smaller than the physical gantry opening, the CT image can be degraded, resulting in failure to image appropriately part of patient's shoulder or hip that lies outside the sampling area (truncation artifact). The plane of the gantry opening is called the transaxial plane (x-y plane) and the longitudinal direction that is in and out of the gantry is noted as z-direction.

CT Scanners

PET/CT became practical with helical CT and more recently with multiple-row detector CT (MDCT). The principle behind helical CT or spiral CT is that the patient is transported continuously through the gantry while data are acquired continuously during the several 360-degree rotations. Helical CT was made possible because of three major technological advances: (a) rhe development of the slip-ring gantry, which allowed the x-ray tube to rotate around the patient without having to stop to unwind the wires; (b) the development of interpolation algorithms, which allowed interpolation of data from adjacent helix during helical scan; and (c) development of high-powered x-ray tubes, which allowed continuous data acquisition.

In the 1990s, the introduction of helical CT revolutionized the field of CT diagnosis because it allowed for continuous volumetric data acquisition. In the late 1990s the introduction of MDCT revolutionized the field even further. With the introduction of MDCT the single row of detectors were replaced by multiple rows of detectors. This automatically increased scan volume per rotation. Also, it enabled such scanners to acquire multiple thin sections providing higher z-axis resolution.

The key differences between a single-row detector CT (SDCT) and a MDCT are the number of multiple-row detectors in the longitudinal direction. Also, the x-ray beam width is larger with the MDCT than in SDCT. For the same scan time of the gantry rotation one could acquire four times the scan volume with the MDCT compared to the SDCT. The evolution of MDCT introduced many new clinical applications and is increasing at a rapid pace. The early commercial PET/CT scanners installed in 2001 consisted of an MDCT scanner assembled next to a PET gantry. It is important to examine the multiple-row detector array design in order to understand the various scan acquisition approaches possible for PET/CT.

Multiple-Row Detector Design Arrays

PET/CT became practical with helical CT and more recently with MDCT. Although the first PET/CT scanners included the possibility of single-slice scanning devices, this approach was not used for long. By late 1998 all major CT manufacturers launched MDCT scanners capable of yielding at least four-transaxial slices per x-ray tube rotation. The key difference between the MDCT and SDCT is in the number of row detectors in the longitudinal or z direction, which enabled for increased scan volume per tube rotation and improved z-axis resolution, both of which are key to improving the three-dimentional reconstructed image. The number of transaxial slices that can be obtained per gantry rotation is determined by the data acquisition system (DAS) channels and not by the available number of physical detectors present in the system. When the number of DAS channels is less than the number of physical detector elements, the output of the elements is summed prior to sampling by the DAS channels. For example, as shown in Fig. 4.2A, on a four DAS channel scanner (mistakenly called a four detector scanner), employing a detector with 16 equal detector elements, sampling the inner four elements results in the acquisition of 4 × 1.25 mm slices per rotation. Summing the elements in groups of two, three, or four prior to sampling, results in 4 × 2.5 mm slices (Fig. 4.2B), 4 × 3.75 mm slices, or 4 × 5.0 mm slices respectfully. The number of detectors or the number of slices obtained per rotation has dramatically increased from 4 slices to 16 slices per rotation to 64 slices and beyond per gantry rotation. Fig. 4.3A shows the detector element design in a four-slice MDCT scanner. The detector array design is often categorized as uniform, nonuniform, or hybrid. In a hybrid design, thin detectors are present in the center, and thick detectors are adjacent to them. Four-slice MDCT scanners are still in use, but they have been increasingly replaced by scanners capable of obtaining 16 slices per gantry rotation. As shown in Fig. 4.3B, the detector elements in a 16-section MDCT scanner all have thin sections in the center and thick detectors in the adjacent scanner, each enabling 16 simultaneous slices per gantry rotation. Fig. 4.3C shows the detector array design of 64-slice MDCT scanners capable

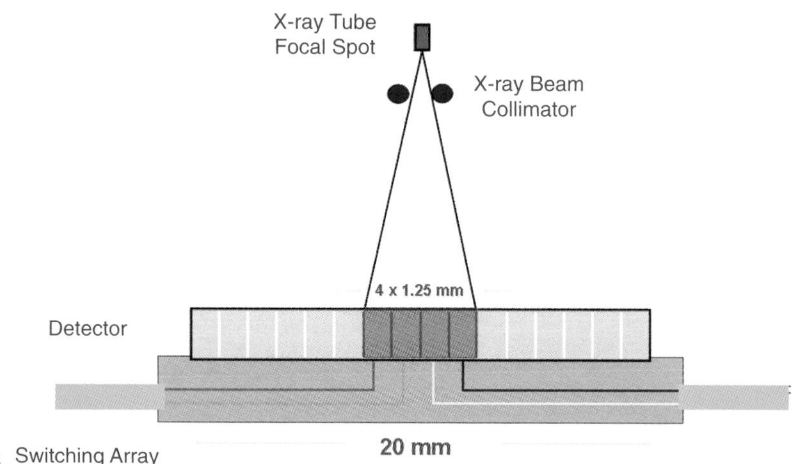

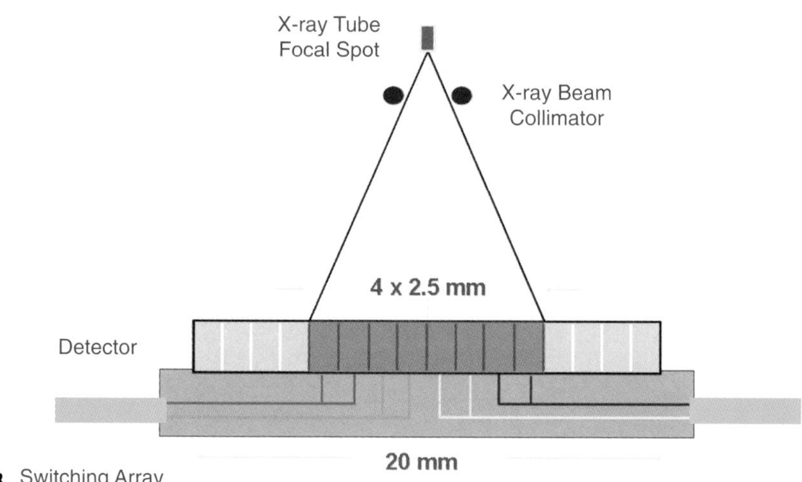

FIGURE 4.2. Schematic diagram showing the detector configuration for the various multiple-row detector CT (MDCT) scan acquisition mode. **A:** Detector configuration for 4 × 1.25 mm scan acquisition. **B:** Detector configurations for 4 × 2.5 mm scan acquisition.

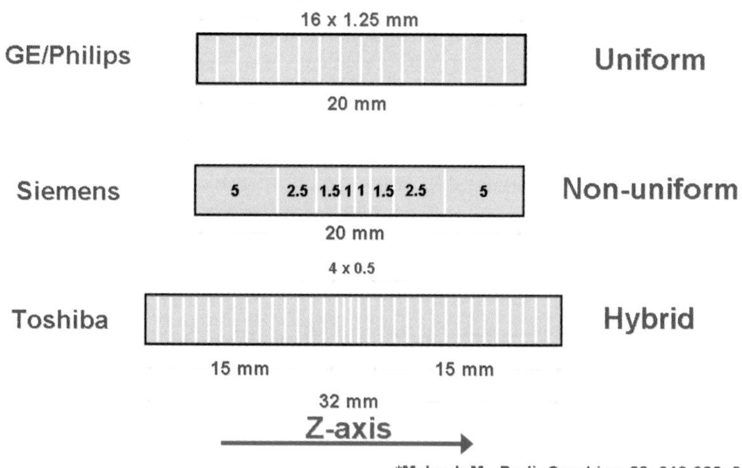

FIGURE 4.3. Various detector array designs used in (**A**) four-section, (*continued*)

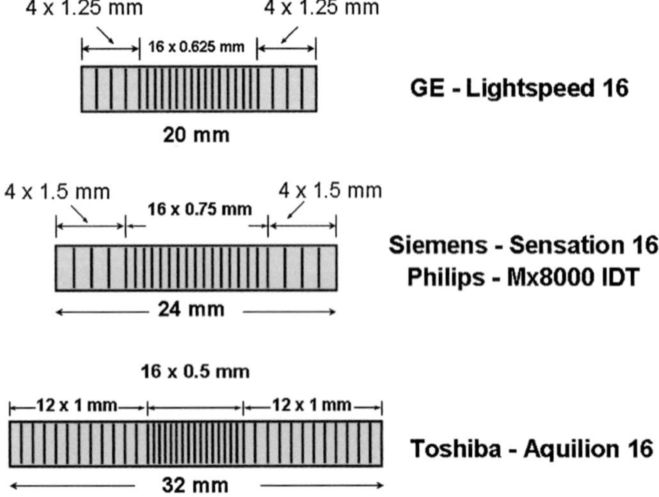

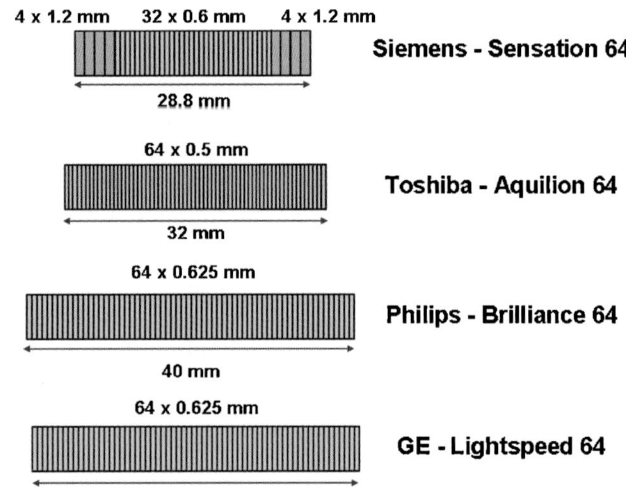

FIGURE 4.3. (*Continued*) (**B**) 16-section, and (**C**) 64-section multiple-row detector CT scanner.

of yielding 64 thin slices per gantry rotation. At present, 64-slice MDCT systems integrated with PET scanners have been installed in a variety of clinical sites by several manufacturers (13). Larger slice numbers also have been developed, and this technology continues to evolve rapidly. Such devices often have rapid rotation speeds and are well suited to demanding tasks such as noninvasive assessments of the coronary arteries, which can now be integrated with PET in the form of PET/CT.

Pitch

The concept of pitch was introduced with helical CT scanners. The understanding of pitch and its impact on the CT image is key, since it impacts both radiation dose and image quality. The pitch is defined as the ratio of the table feed per gantry rotation to the total x-ray beam width (Fig. 4.4). The total x-ray beam width is the product of the number of active DAS channels and width of a single DAS channel. The radiation dose to the patient is inversely proportional to the pitch and directly proportional to the milliamperes per rotation. Typical pitch ratios are 0.5, 1.0, 1.5, and others. A pitch greater than one implies extended imaging with the reduced patient dose and with lower axial resolution, but, a pitch less than one implies overlapping and higher patient dose with higher axial resolution (14). For routine CT scans, a pitch greater than one is quite sufficient. In PET/CT, since the CT image is reconstructed to match the PET slice thickness, a pitch greater than one is quite sufficient for many applications. However, generalizations about the CT chosen for PET are difficult, as a wide range of approaches can be applied in performing the CT as part of PET imaging, ranging from a relatively simple low powered high-pitched scan for attenuation correction and rudimentary lesion localization anatomically to a fully diagnostic thin section assessments of the coronary arteries (high-powered, low-pitch scans). One CT scan protocol increasingly does not fit all clinical situations, and the referring physician may need to vary the CT protocol based on the diagnostic question raised (15).

Pitch† - Radiation Dose

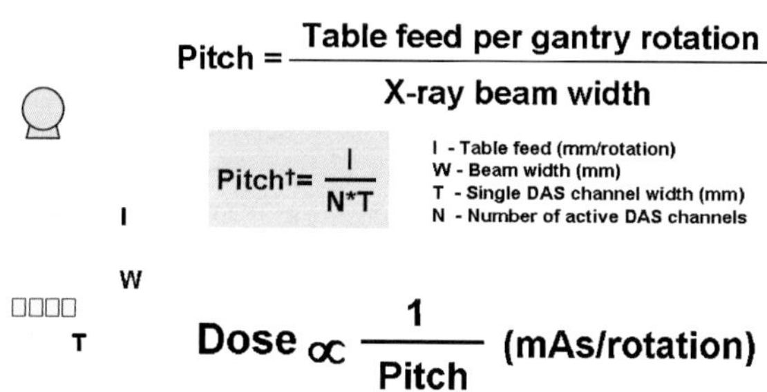

Typical Pitch Ratio - 0.5, 1.0, 1.5

† IEC Part 2-44, 2003

FIGURE 4.4. Pitch is defined as the ratio of the table feed per gantry rotation to the total x-ray beam width. In multiple-row detector CT (MDCT), the total x-ray beam width is the product of the number of active data acquisition system (DAS) channels and width of a single DAS channel.

Effect of attenuation correction on PET images

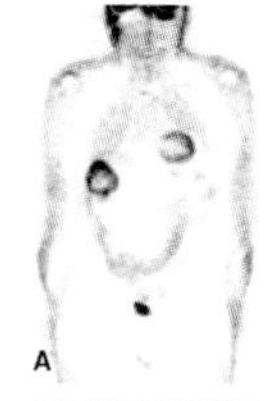

Uncorrected PET scan exhibit characteristic outer rim of apparently increased activity along periphery of body and relatively lower tracer uptake in organs in center of body

Patient specific attenuation map to correct bias in emission data

CT images serves dual purpose
- provides structural information
- attenuation map for PET image

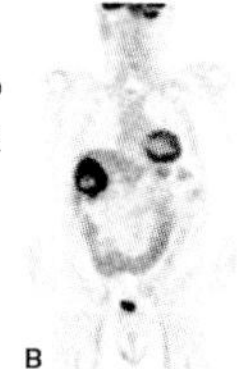

FIGURE 4.6. The effect of attenuation correction on PET images. An uncorrected PET scan (**upper**) exhibits characteristic outer rim of increased activity along the periphery of the body and relatively lower tracer uptake in organs in the center of body. Postattenuated corrected PET image (**lower**), where the uptake more accurately reflects the true radioactivity level within the body.

Scan Parameters for PET/CT

In a PET/CT scanner, CT and PET scanners are assembled adjacently. The patient is transported through the x-ray CT gantry on a carefully aligned and controlled imaging table, where CT scan is generally performed initially and is followed by a PET scan. A typical PET/CT protocol is shown in Fig. 4.5, wherein a patient initially underwent a CT scan followed by a PET scan on the same area. The CT information is then used for two purposes. First, it is used to register the anatomical images obtained with CT fused with the PET images to display as PET/CT images, and if a diagnostic quality CT is performed, for purposes of diagnosis. Second, the CT information is used for scatter correction or attenuation correction, which is used in the PET reconstruction. PET/CT images are displayed for the user's convenience as an axial, coronal, sagittal, or a fused image, and both PET and CT images can be displayed side by side and in any format the user wishes. This enables the clinicians to evaluate both the CT and the PET images to make a suitable diagnosis.

The effect of attenuation correction on PET images is clearly shown in Fig. 4.6. The upper section of Fig. 4.6 shows an uncorrected PET scan, which exhibits a characteristic outer rim of apparently increased activity along the periphery of body and relatively

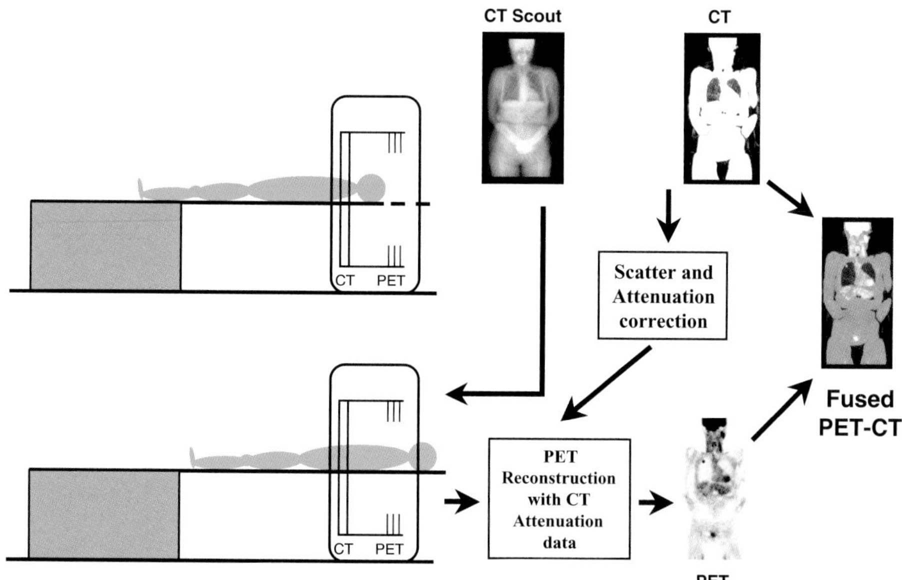

FIGURE 4.5. A typical PET/CT protocol. Patients initially undergo a CT scan followed by a PET scan on the same region. The CT information is then used (a) to register anatomical images with PET images to display fused PET/CT images, and (b) CT information is also used for scatter or attenuation correction on PET scans prior to reconstruction PET images. Figure: Showing typical PET/CT protocol

lower tracer uptake in organs in the center of the body. The lower section of Fig. 4.6 shows a postattenuated corrected PET image wherein the uptake more realistically displays the true radioactivity distribution, as compared to the upper image of Fig. 4.6. Overall CT images serve a dual purpose: (a) it provides structural information that may be fully suitable for diagnosis, and (b) it provides an attenuation map for the PET image.

Typical whole-body PET/CT scan parameters are as follows. This protocol is one used in many outpatient centers in which no intravenous contrast is administered. Such a protocol does not provide the highest quality "diagnostic CT" examination, but does provide important anatomic information, which when combined with PET can result in highly accurate diagnoses. Normally a higher tube voltage (140 kVp) is used for better penetration through the thicker portion of the body such as the pelvis or shoulder, although this can vary by center and scanner. Some centers use 120 kVp x-rays, as they deliver a lower radiation dose and are often used in diagnostic CT. Also a weight-based tube current (milliampere) is typically used at some centers to minimize the radiation dose from CT. Other centers choose to use automated dose-adjustment algorithms provided by the manufacturers, although these are variable in their performance and not uncommonly have difficulty adequately penetrating the thicker portions of the shoulders or the region of the hips. The typical milliampere settings for a whole-body PET/CT along with other scan parameters are shown in Table 4.1. Again, these parameters are not those used with fully diagnostic CT scans, which vary greatly depending on the part of the body being evaluated. It is certainly possible to combine a fully diagnostic CT scan with PET/CT, and this is done in more and more academic centers.

The other key technical features for the PET/CT protocols are that a uniform large field of view is used for all patients and for all parts of the body, and the CT slice is reconstructed to a thickness similar to PET slice thickness in order to facilitate fusion. More modern PET/CT scanners allow "zoomed" settings with reconstruction of smaller field of vision than the full possible field of vision of the scanner. This is not uncommonly applied at our center in the setting of imaging of the head and neck, where a 2X zoom is typically used.

Also, it is important to make sure that the CT reconstruction interval matches PET slice spacing for accurate image fusion. Although the MDCT can provide the highest patient resolution, when the scanner is used in conjunction with the PET/CT scanners, the CT images are basically reconstructed to the slice thicknesses of the PET images in order to enable proper fusion of the PET and CT images. However, newer scanners and software allow for display of thinner, higher resolution CT images than the PET, with fusion to interpolated PET images. Early PET/CT scanners only offered essentially the same CT and PET slice thickness. Typical PET/CT examinations, such as a whole body, involve scanning of a subject from midear region to midthigh. The CT scan typically takes from 15 to 35 seconds, while a PET scan of the same region can take from 15 to 30 minutes. Generally, to achieve the most accurate quantitative PET imaging results, no contrast is used for the CT part during PET/CT scan since introduction of contrast can affect attenuation maps. Typically shallow breathing is allowed to match the breathing nature during the PET scans. Although MDCT scanners have faster gantry rotation time (less than 0.4 seconds), the scan time chosen during PET/CT protocol can be lengthened slightly greater than half a second in order to minimize motion artifacts, although this remains somewhat unproven, and a slower CT scan can degrade CT quality, especially if free tidal breathing is allowed. With tidal breathing the "match" of intra-abdominal organs between PET and CT is typically quite high in quality (10). The CT axis scans are reconstructed so as to match the PET section for accurate attenuation correction.

Transmission Scans with Germanium Rods

In the absence of CT, germanium rod transmission scans are done in PET scan to obtain information regarding attenuation corrections. CT scans in PET/CT provide a much improved statistical quality attenuation correction map. Although the CT images are used for attenuation corrections and fusion, some of the early PET/CT scanners also came with germanium (Ge-68) rods for transmission measurements, and the scanners offered a choice as to whether CT or Ge-68/Ga-68 sources would be used for the attenuation correction. The germanium-68 decays to Ga-68 (a positron emitter) rod transmission images and may be advantageous for attenuation correction in cases where the patients have metal implants, which can result in severe artifacts and can affect fusion images. In those cases, germanium transmission images can be used for attenuation correction. Although some scanners have been shipped with such rods, it is much more common in the newest scanners for only CT attenuation correction to be available. Most of the new MDCTs come with a metal artifact correction program, as well as a CT with contrast program, so germanium transmission

TABLE 4.1 Typical CT Parameters for a Whole-Body PET/CT Scan in Which No Intravenous Contrast is Used (i.e., Attenuation Correction and Localization Scan) and CT approach Can Vary Widely from Center to Center

Scan Parameters	Techniques
Tube voltage	140 (to penetrate uniformly through thick portion of the body)
Tube current (weight-based techniques)	80 mA for 150–200 lb 60 mA for 100–150 lb 40 mA for <100 lb 120 mA for >200 lb
CT gantry rotation time	1 sec rotation
Pitch	1.0 to 1.5

images are used infrequently or not at all in most centers. When used, germanium transmission images typically add an additional 10 to 30 minutes for scan time depending on the extent of the body imaged. An advantage of such images' long duration is that they quite accurately mimic the respiratory blurring and organ position seen on the PET images. They also have the same high-energy photons as positron emitters (in contrast to the lower energy of the CT attenuation maps), which can lead to challenges due to high-density materials such as intravenous or oral contrast. Some artifacts have been attributed to both contrast and organ motion in the bowel, which can be confusing if one is not aware of them (16,17).

Quality Control and Shielding Requirements

Although the quality control of PET scanners is discussed elsewhere in this book and is quite well established, the use of PET/CT has added a requirement for a regular quality control program for the CT scanners that are part of PET. The daily quality control for CT scanners involves scanning a water phantom. The water phantom is positioned in the center of the CT gantry and a single section is obtained through the center of the water bottle of the phantom. The CT number at the center is measured and is compared on a day-to-day basis. The CT number of distilled water is zero and it should not vary more than three to five CT numbers. If the CT number of water is not within the set limits, it warrants the need for air calibration of the CT scanner. If the air calibration is not successful or if the CT number of water does not match or does not fall within the allowed limits, there is a need for a service call before scanning patients. On an annual basis, depending on regulatory requirements applicable to that site, there are rigorous quality controls to be performed by a qualified medical physicist. It is also essential to have a qualified medical physicist perform acceptance testing at the start of the installation. This provides an opportunity to examine the scanner capability and how it is performing compared to its specifications. The tests also provide data that can be compared with scanner performance at a later date. More detailed tests are recommended for an annual evaluation of the CT scanner according to American College of Radiology practice standards and accreditation programs. There are some quality control procedures unique to integrated PET/CT systems. Most notably, the alignment of the PET and CT scanners must be correct. There are a variety of phantom systems that allow for visualization of both radioactive and radiopaque spheres. The alignment provides assurance that the spheres are properly aligned when imaged by both PET and CT. These need to be checked periodically, but most critically, if there is any manipulation of the scanners or the bed as a part of camera service.

Before a PET/CT scanner is installed clinically, a careful analysis of the required regulations of that particular region (city, state, or country) is needed. The location where the CT scanner is intended for installation needs to be analyzed closely for lead shielding of the room housing the scanner. Depending on the type of the regulations existing in the particular state or country, it requires careful analysis from a qualified medical physicist to examine the requirement of shielding for a particular PET/CT scanner. The most significant radiation is usually observed in the uptake room adjacent to the PET/CT scanner, where the patient may spend an hour or more prior to the PET scan. The uptake room shielding requirements are commonly more stringent than those of the room housing the PET/CT scanner. In the PET/CT scanner room, the major contributor is scatter radiation from the CT scanner; whereas in the uptake room the patient acts as a radiation source for which the room has to be well shielded to protect the adjacent areas.

The manufacturers of the PET/CT scanner usually provide a scatter diagram of the radiation present during a CT scan under typical scanning condition. The scatter profile can then be used to determine the lead requirement for all the surrounding walls of a PET/CT scanner. Depending on the location of the PET/CT scanner room it is important to analyze the thickness of the floor and the ceiling to make sure the adjacent areas are well protected. A qualified medical physicist can assist in the evaluation of shielding requirement and also perform acceptance testing of a PET/CT scanner.

Radiation Dose

The number of diagnostic CT procedures performed in the United States and the world has dramatically increased over the past few years. For the past 10 years, the number of CT procedures in United States alone has been increasing at a rate greater than 10% every year. This dramatic increase in CT procedures is raising concerns about the increased risk for radiation-induced cancer for the whole population. In general, the average risk of radiation-induced cancer in the general population is 5% per Sv or 5% per 0.01 rem. Although the risk is exhibited uniform across the age, children are at two to three times higher risk than others, as high as 15% per Sv. For persons aged greater than 50 years, risk falls to one fifth to one tenth of that for younger adults. Therefore, the CT dose in the PET/CT scanner needs to be careful evaluated to reduce the overall radiation dose to the patient. A patient undergoing PET/CT receives a radiation dose from both PET and CT. Since the CT part of PET/CT does not invariably require the very highest diagnostic image quality, the technical factors can be set such that the radiation dose is according to the "as low as reasonably achievable" principle. With the typical PET/CT scan parameters for a whole-body PET/CT scan, such as 140 kVp, 80 mA (average-sized patient) and pitch of 1.5, can yield a CT dose 10 mSv (5 to 15 mSv range). This is in addition to a PET dose of approximately 15 mSv (10 to 20 mSv, depending on the quantity of injected isotope). Together it results in approximately 25 mSv (15 to 35 mSv range) per PET/CT scan, which classifies a PET/CT scan as a relatively high-dose procedure. Table 4.2 shows the effective dose values for typical diagnostic CT

TABLE 4.2 Typical Effective Dose Values from CT Scan

CT Procedure	Effective Dose (mSv)[a]
Head CT	1–2
Chest CT	5–7
Abdomen CT	5–7
Pelvis CT	3–4
Abdomen and pelvis CT	8–11
PET/CT[b]	5–15

[a]Average U.S. background radiation per year is approximately 3.0 mSv.
[b]PET/CT scan includes scanning from midear to midthigh on an average-sized adult. The effective dose values listed above are for the CT scan only. The effective dose for the PET scan with 25 mCi fluoro-D-glucose (FDG) is approximately 15 mSv. Therefore, for a typical PET/CT scan, the effective dose can range from 20 to 40 mSv.

Respiratory motion artifact

PET image

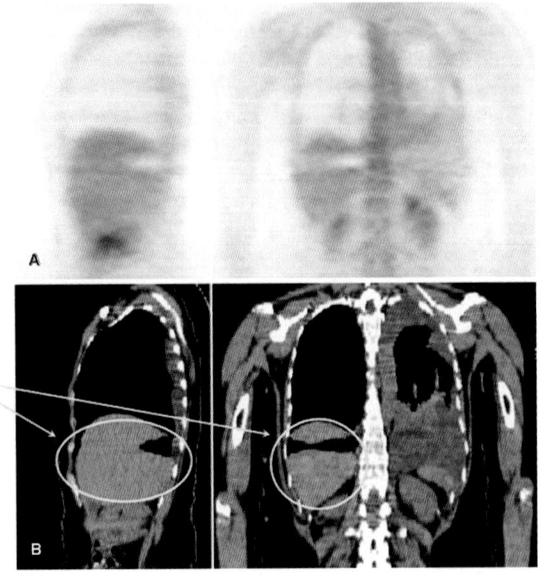

CT at same position indicates partially detached liver

FIGURE 4.7. Variation in respiratory motion between CT and PET data acquisition can yield respiratory motion artifact on the PET image. **Top:** PET image shows the dome of the liver sliced. **Bottom:** CT scan indicate partially detached liver due to respiratory motion.

scans along with the PET/CT scans. Although the CT doses from the described noncontrast PET/CT protocol are lower than a typical diagnostic CT, the CT dose can contribute to nearly 40% of the PET/CT dose.

Examining the results of the radiation doses in an oncologic fluorodeoxyglucose (FDG) PET/CT protocol, the CT dose accounted for nearly 60% of the PET dose for a protocol that included base of the skull to midthigh, 61% from the vertex of skull to midthigh, and 65% from head to toe scan. The CT dose as a percentage of total PET/CT dose was typically 37% for a skull base to midthigh protocol, 38% for vertex of skull to midthigh protocol, and nearly 40% for head to toe protocol (18). The CT doses in PET/CT are typically lower than the typical diagnostic CT of the same region because of the lower tube current and the higher pitch values. Overall, the effective dose from CT ranges from 5 to 15 mSv and accounts for approximately 40% of the total effective dose during PET/CT.

Image Artifacts in PET/CT

There are unique image artifacts observed during PET/CT scans. As CT and PET scans are obtained sequentially and not simultaneously, misregistrations may occur due to patient motion and deep breathing (19). Lateral attenuation increases with arms at side. Lateral streak artifacts are common with reduced tube current. The best images, at least in terms of registration between the PET and the CT, are obtained with shallow breathing or with a near full expiratory breath-hold for the CT scan. An example of a typical image artifact is shown in Fig. 4.7. It is a classic respiratory motion artifact. The top of Fig. 4.7 is the PET image, which shows the dome of the liver sliced, and in the lower image of Fig. 4.7, the CT at the same position indicates a partially detached liver, which is due to motion artifact during the CT acquisition. This results in propagating an artifact into the PET image as well. Fig. 4.8 is an attenuated corrected PET image showing decreased tracer uptake

Head Motion Artifact

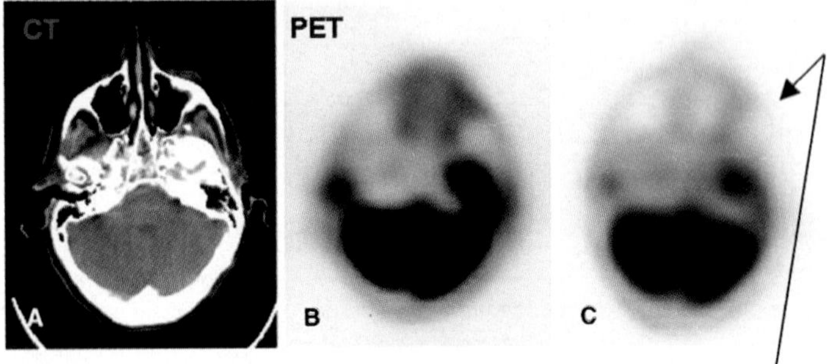

Attenuated corrected PET image show decreased tracer uptake in left side of face

This is due to under-correction of photon attenuation

FIGURE 4.8. Motion artifact can mislead diagnosis on PET scan, as shown in this figure. PET image with attenuation correction from CT data shows decreased tracer uptake in the left side of the face. Upon examining the CT figure, it appears the head was in a different direction during CT scan (**A**). This can lead to undercorrection of photon attenuation, which results in decreased uptake on PET image (**C**), however, preattenuated corrected PET image (**B**) shows uniform uptake on the left side of the face.

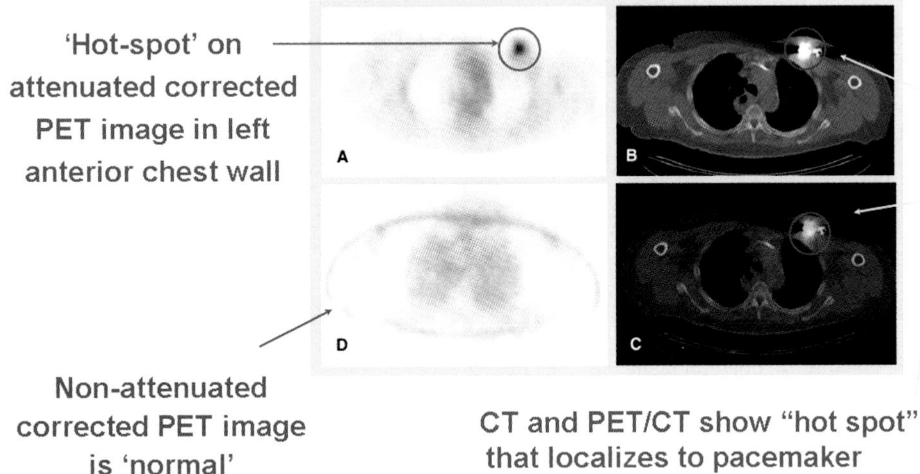

FIGURE 4.9. Pacemaker artifact, visible on CT attenuation corrected PET image in left anterior chest wall on PET, CT, and fused PET/CT image (**A, B, C**) but not visible on preattenuated corrected PET image (**D**).

in the left side of the face (20). This can be misdiagnosed, however, when looking at the CT scan image, where there is a head motion artifact and because of this there is an undercorrection of photon attenuation that resulted in a decreased facial uptake in the left side of the face. Another classic artifact is a pacemaker/metallic artifact, which is visible on the attenuation-corrected PET and fusion images (Fig. 4.9) (21). One can see a hot spot on the attenuated corrected PET image in the left anterior chest wall both on the PET and also on the CT image. However, on examining a nonattenuated corrected PET, the image appears to be normal. Therefore, it is important to examine both the nonattenuated corrected PET image and the attenuated-corrected PET image to eliminate some of these artifacts from the CT attenuation. Similarly in Fig. 4.10, the artifact is due to dense barium contrast. There is an increased FDG uptake throughout the colon on attenuated-corrected PET image. The corresponding CT slices show dense barium in the colon, which resulted in the error in the attenuation correction mass, which automatically translates to the increased FDG uptake. A nonattenuated-corrected PET image shows normal bowel activity. Currently, PET/CT scanners have 64-slice CT scanners, enabling cardiac CTs. Although the CT portion is used a lesser fraction of time than the PET/CT, independent cardiac CTs can be done if needed.

FUTURE DEVELOPMENTS

We continue to see improvement in the CT technology, enabling faster scanners and much thinner slice CT scanners. Although the faster scanners and the thinner slices may not invariably be required or necessarily always be preferred for PET/CT images, when examined independently the thin slice CT scanners with the fastest acquisition are equally important when doing cardiac CT. The other developments include fast scintillators, such as LSO and GSO, for PET might reduce imaging time from 35 minutes to less than

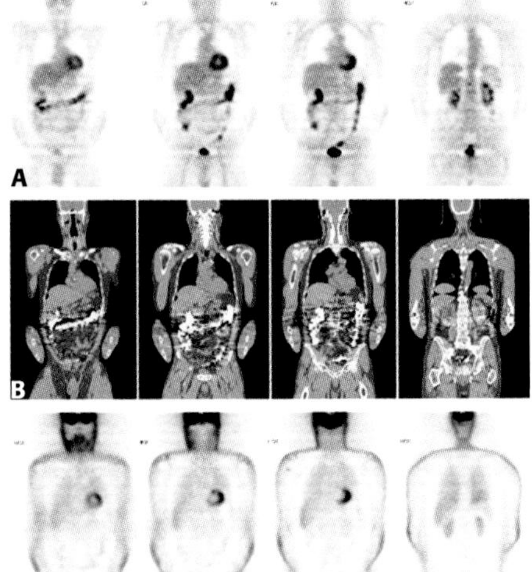

FIGURE 4.10. Image artifact due to barium contrast agent can mislead diagnosis. Increased fluorodeoxyglucose (FDG) uptake throughout colon on CT attenuated corrected PET image (**A**) due to barium contrast agent accumulation in colon (**B**). Preattenuated PET image shows normal bowel activity (**C**).

15 minutes, allowing dynamic whole-body scans and the use of short-lived isotopes.

CONCLUSION

PET/CT is changing; not just the use of PET but also the use of CT. A wide range of studies across diverse disease types have demonstrated consistent advantages to the PET/CT method as compared to PET or CT alone (22–26). Precise localization of pathology can drastically change the patient's management and prognosis. PET/CT has the potential to become the ultimate imaging and treatment planning device for cancer patients. The proper use of CT scanners to address the clinical question at a reasonable radiation dose remains in evolution, and the approach may differ markedly in terms of CT technique depending of the diagnostic question raised. Thus, one CT protocol does not fit all, but must be tailored to the specific patient for best outcomes.

REFERENCES

1. Wahl RL, Quint LE, Cieslak RD, et al. "Anatometabolic" tumor imaging: fusion of FDG PET with CT or MRI to localize foci of increased activity. *J Nucl Med* 1993;34(7):1190–1197.
2. Wahl RL, Quint LE, Greenough RL, et al. Staging of mediastinal non-small cell lung cancer with FDG PET, CT, and fusion images: preliminary prospective evaluation. *Radiology* 1994;191:371–377.
3. Townsend DW. A combined PET/CT scanner: the choices. *J Nucl Med* 2001;42:533–534.
4. Kinahan PE, Townsend DW, Beyer T, et al. Attenuation correction for a combined 3D PET/CT scanner. *Med Phys* 1998;25:2046–2053.
5. Cohade C, Osman M, Leal J, et al. Direct comparison of ^{18}F-FDG PET and PET/CT in patients with colorectal carcinoma. *J Nucl Med* 2003;44:1797–1803.
6. Kamel E, Hany TF, Burger C, et al. CT vs 68Ge attenuation correction in a combined PET/CT system: evaluation of the effect of lowering the CT tube current. *Eur J Nucl Med Mol Imaging* 2002;29:346–350.
7. Townsend DW, Beyer T. A combined PET/CT scanner: the path to true image fusion. *Br J Radiol* 2002;75:S24–S30.
8. Townsend DW. Physical principles and technology of clinical PET imaging. *Ann Acad Med Singapore* 2004;33:133–145.
9. Blodgett TM, Meltzer CC, Townsend DW. PET/CT: form and function. *Radiology* 2007;242:360–385.
10. Nakamoto Y, Tatsumi M, Cohade C, et al. Accuracy of image fusion of normal upper abdominal organs visualized with PET/CT. *Eur J Nucl Med Mol Imaging* 2003;30:597–602.
11. Cohade C, Osman M, Marshall LN, et al. PET-CT: accuracy of PET and CT spatial registration of lung lesions. *Eur J Nucl Med Mol Imaging* 2003;30(5):721–726.
12. Nakamoto Y, Chin BB, Kraitchman DL, et al. Effects of nonionic intravenous contrast agents at PET/CT imaging: phantom and canine studies. *Radiology* 2003;227(3):817–824.
13. Mahesh M. Search for isotropic resolution in CT from conventional through multiple-row detector. *Radiographics* 2002;22:949–962.
14. Mahesh M, Scatarige JC, Cooper J, et al. Dose and pitch relationship for a particular multislice CT scanner. *Am J Roentgenol* 2001;177:1273–1275.
15. Blodgett TM, Casagranda B, Townsend DW, et al. Issues, controversies, and clinical utility of combined PET/CT imaging: what is the interpreting physician facing? *AJR Am J Roentgenol* 2005;184:S138–S145.
16. Cohade C, Osman M, Nakamoto Y, et al. Initial experience with oral contrast in PET/CT: phantom and clinical studies. *J Nucl Med* 2003;44:412–416.
17. Nakamoto Y, Chin BB, Cohade C, et al. PET/CT: artifacts caused by bowel motion. *Nucl Med Commun* 2004;25:221–225.
18. Friedman K, Mahesh M, Wahl R. *Additional radiation exposure associated with PET/CT compared to PET alone.* Presented at: 52nd Annual Meeting of the Society of Nuclear Medicine Meeting, Toronto, 2005.
19. Osman MM, Cohade C, Nakamoto Y, et al. Respiratory motion artifacts on PET emission images obtained using CT attenuation correction on PET-CT. *Eur J Nucl Med Mol Imaging* 2003;30:603–606.
20. Schoder H, Erdi YE, Larson SM, et al. PET/CT: a new imaging technology in nuclear medicine. *Eur J Nucl Med Mol Imaging* 2003;30:1419–1437.
21. Cohade C, Wahl RL. Applications of positron emission tomography/computed tomography image fusion in clinical positron emission tomography-clinical use, interpretation methods, diagnostic improvements. *Semin Nucl Med* 2003;33:228–237.
22. Ha PK, Hdeib A, Goldenberg D, et al. The role of positron emission tomography and computed tomography fusion in the management of early-stage and advanced-stage primary head and neck squamous cell carcinoma. *Arch Otolaryngol Head Neck Surg* 2006;132:12–16.
23. Khandani AH, Wahl RL. Applications of PET in liver imaging. *Radiol Clin North Am* 2005;43:849–860.
24. Tatsumi M, Cohade C, Mourtzikos KA, et al. Initial experience with FDG-PET/CT in the evaluation of breast cancer. *Eur J Nucl Med Mol Imaging* 2006;33:254–262.
25. Wahl RL. Why nearly all PET of abdominal and pelvic cancers will be performed as PET/CT. *J Nucl Med* 2004;45[Suppl 1]:82S–95S.
26. Zimmer LA, McCook B, Meltzer C, et al. Combined positron emission tomography/computed tomography imaging of recurrent thyroid cancer. *Otolaryngol Head Neck Surg* 2003;128:178–184.

CHAPTER

5 Data Analysis and Image Processing

ROBERT KOEPPE

The goal of positron emission tomography (PET) is to make use of tracers labeled with positron-emitting radionuclides for the purposes of diagnostic imaging. PET, a nuclear medicine imaging procedure, differs from standard radiological x-ray procedures in that the radiation detected by the imaging device originates and is emitted from within the subject's body rather than originating from an external source and being transmitted through the body. PET studies, like all nuclear medicine radioisotope emission procedures, yield images that represent the distribution of the radiotracer within the body. This distribution or pattern of uptake and incorporation depends on the physiologic, pharmacologic, and/or biochemical state of the individual's body. In contrast, images produced by conventional x-ray procedures reflect x-ray attenuation and are governed by the physical composition of the body. Thus, nuclear medicine procedures in general and PET procedures in particular are capable of providing information concerning how the body is functioning at a physiologic or biochemical level, while x-ray procedures such as computed tomography (CT) primarily depict human anatomy. Although PET does provide limited anatomic information and some functional information can be derived from CT, each technique is useful in its own way. As we will see later in this and other chapters, recent advances in both hardware and software allow the combination of functional and anatomic information, improving both the ability to answer scientific questions and the overall diagnostic utility of tomographic imaging methods.

PET procedures have the additional potential for providing quantitative measures of radiotracer concentration in a living biological system at spatial resolutions of a few millimeters and with subminute temporal resolution. Methods for obtaining quantitative images of radiotracer concentration from PET involve a technique called image reconstruction from projections. For many PET applications, these quantitative measures of radiotracer concentration can be extended to yield more pertinent measures of biological function through the use of compartmental analysis and tracer kinetic modeling. Analysis of a *temporal sequence* of radiotracer images allows estimates of parameters representing specific physiologic processes such as blood flow, glucose metabolism, protein synthesis, neurotransmitter or enzyme levels, and receptor or binding site density. The production of different positron-emitting radionuclides and the synthesis of a variety of PET radiopharmaceuticals described in Chapters 1 and 2 allow one to study many distinct aspects of organ systems within the functioning human body.

The purpose of this chapter is to discuss the basic principles involved in the production and processing of PET images and to describe various methods used to analyze the quantitative data produced by PET. The goal of image reconstruction and its associated steps is to produce the most accurate images of radiotracer concentration possible, with the highest signal-to-noise (SNR) and at the highest spatial resolution. The primary goal of compartmental modeling is to provide more valuable information related to the functional state of the subject than can be provided by images of radioactivity distribution alone. The overall goal of image display techniques is to provide both spatial and functional information in a visually optimal manner. The following sections describe the theoretical concepts of and methods for (a) image reconstruction from projections, including the additional steps and corrections specific to PET data; (b) compartmental modeling, including data acquisition requirements, curve fitting, parameter estimation, and model validation; and (c) methods for combining and displaying both functional and/or anatomic information for multiple imaging studies (although this is expanded upon in a subsequent chapter).

IMAGE RECONSTRUCTION FROM PROJECTIONS

In conventional nuclear medicine gamma camera imaging or in simple x-ray imaging, information from the three dimensions of a human subject gets collapsed onto a two-dimensional (2D) image. There is ambiguity in such images as all information from one dimension is represented by a single point or pixel of the 2D image. For gamma camera images, radioactivity from different locations within the body appears overlaid upon itself. Tomography, or slice imaging, is a method that allows a three-dimensional (3D) object to be depicted as a series or stack of thin 2D cross-sectional images. Each image of the series represents only two dimensions of object, while information on the third dimension is contained in the different images of the series. Although this appears simple in concept, imaging devices have the inherent problem of recording information from three dimensions on 2D detector surfaces. Thus, each acquired data point recorded still represents information integrated along one dimension of the object. These integrals or weighted sums are referred to as projections or projection rays. Image reconstruction from projections is the mathematical technique or groups of techniques that allow the construction of the set of cross-sectional images, each representing only two dimensions of information.

Historical Background

The beginnings of image reconstruction from projections occurred with a 1917 paper published by the Austrian mathematician J. Radon (1). In this work, he proved that a 2D or 3D object can be reconstructed exactly from the full set of its projections, a projection again representing the object integrated along one dimension. It was not until the 1950s to 1970s when this result was rediscovered by people in several different fields including mathematics (2,3), radio astronomy (4), and electron microscopy (5), in addition to medical imaging (6–8), that applications for image reconstruction from projections began to be found. Although the first suggestions of using positron-emitting radionuclides for medical imaging arose in the 1950s (9–12) and the first positron tomographic imaging devices appeared in the 1960s (13) and 1970s (14), the practical application of PET imaging followed that of single-photon emission computed tomography (15,16) (SPECT) and did not occur until the mid- to late 1970s.

As the field exploded throughout the 1970s, hundreds of papers relating to image reconstruction from projections were published in prominent journals from the fields of mathematics, physics, engineering, and biomedicine. Several reviews of reconstruction algorithms were written (17–19) summarizing the few different general approaches and the many different specific implementations of image reconstruction algorithms.

Reconstruction Algorithms

Although reconstruction algorithms can be categorized in several different ways, most algorithms for PET can be classified into two general approaches: reconstruction by filtered back projection and iterative reconstruction. Before discussing these approaches we will review some concepts common to both.

Projection Data

As described in Chapter 3, the data acquired directly by the PET scanner represents the sum or integral of radioactivity along the lines connecting any given pair of detectors, often referred to as lines of response (LOR). This is true for both 2D and 3D data acquisition. The following paragraphs describe the basics of 2D-image

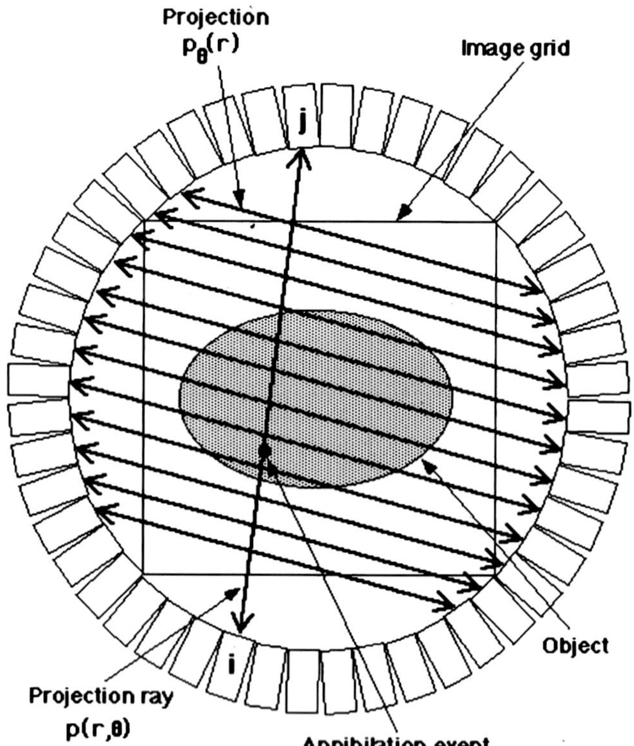

FIGURE 5.1. Projection data for two-dimensional PET acquisition. The diagram represents a single detector ring containing 48 detectors. A coincidence line of response between a given pair of detectors *i* and *j* is called a projection ray, $p(r,\theta)$, and can be defined in terms of an angle 0 and the distance *r* that the line passes from the center of the field of view. The projection ray data give the sum or integral of radioactivity along the line connecting the two detectors. A set of all projection rays having the same angle θ is referred to as a projection and is denoted by $p_\theta(r)$. Each projection P_θ represents one complete view of the object.

reconstruction, most of which applies to 3D reconstruction as well. Specific issues related to 3D-image reconstruction will be discussed in the section "Image Reconstruction for Three-Dimensional PET."

Assume the true 2D radiotracer distribution that we are imaging is given by the function $f(x, y)$, where x and y are standard Cartesian coordinates. The measured PET data, as depicted in Fig. 5.1, can be represented by:

$$p_\theta(x') \equiv p(x',\theta) = \int f(x,y)dy', \quad [5.1]$$

where (x', y') are the coordinates in a Cartesian system rotated by the angle θ.

$$\begin{aligned} x' &= \cos(\theta)x + \sin(\theta)y \\ y' &= \cos(\theta)y - \sin(\theta)x \end{aligned} \quad [5.2]$$

Each (x', θ) pair of the projection data represents a single line integral that in turn corresponds to a specific pair of detectors (line of response). A given $p(x', \theta)$ often is called a projection ray. The collection of projection rays with the same angle θ is referred to as a projection. Thus, we also can define $p_\theta(x')$ as an equivalent representation of the projection data, but one used when referring to the collection of projection rays as a whole rather than the individual rays, $p(x', \theta)$. All the rays of a given projection $p_\theta(x')$ are parallel, where x' is a simple linear measure of the position of each ray within the projection. It is important to note that each projection p_θ of the 2D object has only *one* dimension. Thus, the 2D projection data defined by $p(x', \theta)$ can also be thought of as a *set* of one-dimensional projections, $p_\theta(x')$. Each individual member of this set of projections is defined by a single angle (θ) and represents one complete view of the object. By a complete view, it is meant that each point of the object $f(x, y)$ is included in one and only one ray of each projection. Thus, in a perfect noise-free system, the sum over all rays of a given projection is the same for all projections and is proportional to the total radioactivity in the object:

$$\sum_{x'} p_\theta(x') = \iint f(x, y)\, dx\, dy \quad \text{for all } \theta. \qquad [5.3]$$

The entire collection of projection data when plotted as θ versus x' is called a sinogram since a point source in the object traces a sinusoidal pattern, as shown in Fig. 5.2. It is not mandatory to group the projection rays into parallel collections, as described here, but one can choose other groupings such as all rays that contain a common detector. For 2D data, this particular grouping of projection rays would create a fan-shaped projection, and thus is referred to as fan-beam geometry (x-ray CT terminology). Note though that a single projection still consists of a complete view of the object. Specific groupings may be beneficial for specific applications, however, throughout this chapter the parallel-ray geometry will be retained.

Filtered Back-Projection

One method of reconstructing images from their projections is called filtered back-projection (FBP). As the name implies, this involves two principal steps: filtering the projections and then back-projecting them to create the reconstructed image. The operation of back-projection in terms of the projection data, $p(x', \theta)$, from our 2D object, $f(x, y)$, is given by:

$$b(x, y) = \int_0^{2\pi} p(x', \theta)\, d\theta. \qquad [5.4]$$

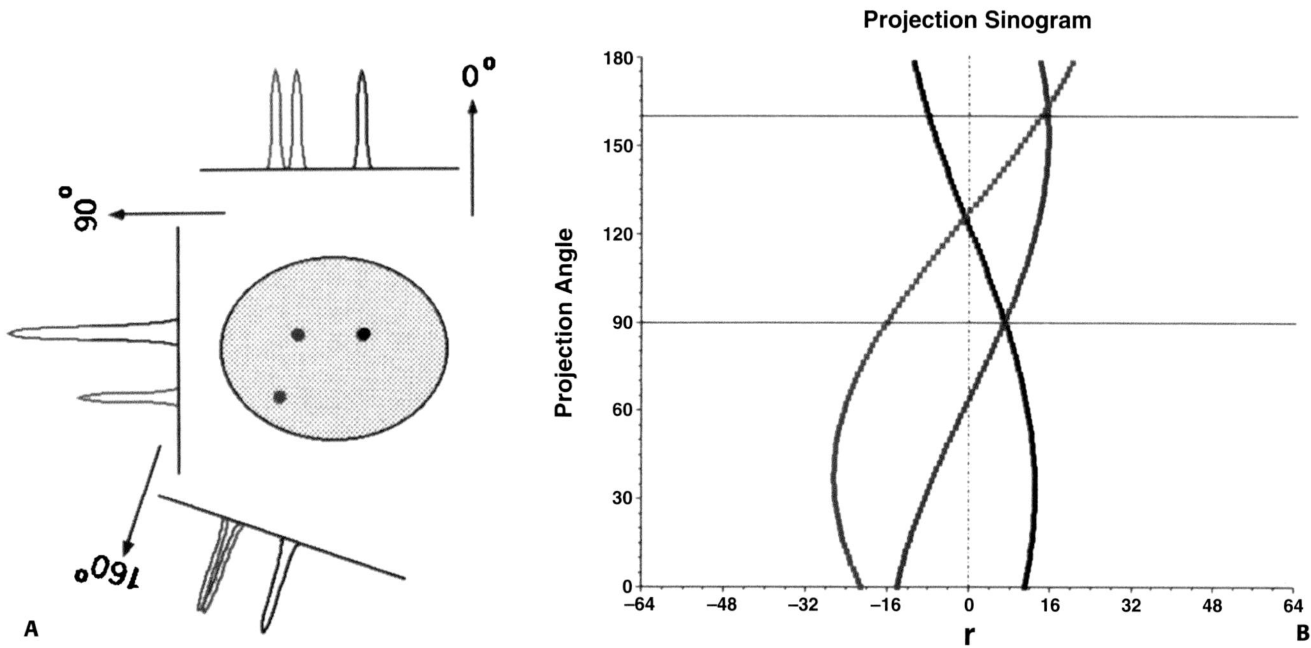

FIGURE 5.2. Two-dimensional projections and projection sinogram. **A:** The top of the illustration depicts an elliptical two-dimensional object containing three discrete points of equal radioactivity (*red, blue, and black dots*). A full set of projections covers angles from 0 degrees to 180 degrees. Three sample projections are shown at 0 degrees, 90 degrees, and 160 degrees. Due to the finite resolution of a PET system, point sources appear within a projection roughly as Gaussian distributions (*red, blue, and black curves*). If the points fall along different rays within a projection as in $p_{0°}$, the resultant curves in the projection are of equal magnitude and are separated spatially. If two of the points fall along the same ray, as seen in $p_{90°}$, only two curves are seen, the red curve representing radioactivity from one point, and the blue/black curve having twice the magnitude, representing radioactivity from the other two points. The 160-degree projection shows a case where two of the points are slightly offset. The resolution of the PET system determines how large a difference in r or θ is necessary to distinguish between two points within an object. Part **B** shows the projection sinogram for this object. A sinogram is a plot of all the projection rays $p(r, \theta)$, sorted as projection angle θ versus r. Note that each point of the object traces out a sinusoidal pattern in this plot, hence the name sinogram. Compare the three projections in **A** with the three horizontal lines in **B** corresponding to projection angles at 0 degrees, 90 degrees, and 160 degrees. Note that the blue and black traces intersect at 90 degrees, while the red and blue traces nearly overlap at 160 degrees.

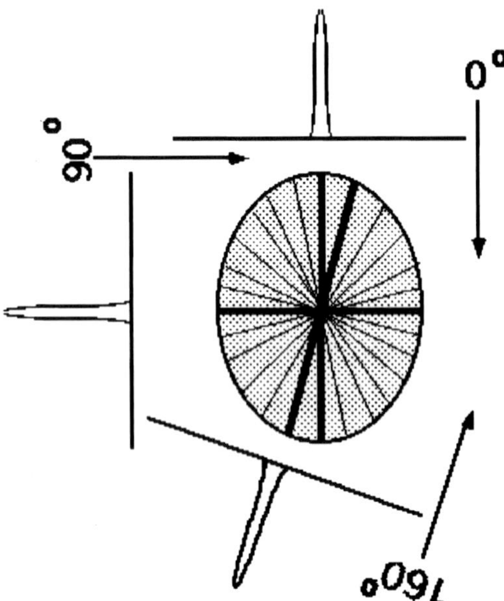

FIGURE 5.3. Two-dimensional back-projection. Depicted is an object containing a single point of radioactivity located at the center of the field of view. Each projection contains a single peak representing the radioactivity from this point. Back-projection (without filtering) consists of taking the data from each projection and "smearing" them back along the rays of the projection. Note that the arrows are shown in the opposite direction, representing the operation of back-projection, than those of Fig. 5.2 that represent the inherent forward-projection operation of data acquisition. The dark lines correspond to the back-projections along three angles—0, 90, and 160 degrees. The lighter lines correspond to back-projections along other projection angles. The resultant back-projected image, however, is not a single point, but a starlike pattern centered on the location of the point. This result demonstrates why "filtering" the projections is necessary before the back-projection step.

Back-projection in one sense is the converse operation to the forward-projection that occurs naturally during PET data acquisition. That is, the act of PET data acquisition itself transforms a 2D array of values into sets of projections or line integrals, while back-projection converts the projection set back to a 2D array. Note, however, that forward-projection followed by simple back-projection does not yield the original object. As shown in Fig. 5.3, an object consisting of a single point source is represented by projection data having a single nonzero value at each projection angle. As these data are back-projected, each angle θ creates a line in the reconstructed image. Thus, a point source object yields an image with a starlike pattern. To arrive back at the true object, the projection data must be modified or filtered prior to back-projection.

Before describing the filtering step, the concept of the Fourier transform must be introduced. A one-dimensional Fourier transform of a one-dimensional function $f(x)$ is a *frequency space* representation of $f(x)$. By this we mean that any function $f(x)$ can be described as the sum of *sin* or *cos* functions having varying frequencies and magnitudes, $F(\nu)$. The value of $F(\nu)$ gives the magnitude of the sinusoidal function with frequency ν. The Fourier transform is defined mathematically as:

$$F(\nu) = \int_{-\infty}^{+\infty} f(x)e^{-i2\pi x\nu}d\nu. \quad [5.5]$$

The Fourier transform of $F(\nu)$ yields the original function $f(x)$. This transform from $F(\nu)$ back to $f(x)$ is called an inverse Fourier transform, although the mathematical formulas for both transforms are identical.

From Radon's work, it can be shown that if the Fourier transform of the projection data at angle θ:

$$P_\theta(\nu) = \int_{-\infty}^{+\infty} p(x',\theta)e^{-i2\pi x'\nu}d\nu, \quad [5.6]$$

is multiplied by ν,

$$P_\theta^F(\nu) = |\nu|P_\theta(\nu), \quad [5.7]$$

then the inverse Fourier transform of P_θ^F

$$p^F(x',\theta) = \int_{-\infty}^{+\infty} P_\theta^F(\nu)e^{-i2\pi\nu x'}dx' \quad [5.8]$$

yields a filtered projection, $p^F(x',\theta)$, which under noise-free conditions yields the true object when back-projected:

$$f(x,y) = b^F(x,y) = \int_0^{2\pi} p^F(x',\theta)d\theta. \quad [5.9]$$

The frequency-space filter, ν, is commonly known as a "ramp" filter. To summarize, image reconstruction by FBP consists of four steps applied to each projection θ from 0 to 2π: (a) Fourier transform the projection, (b) filter the transformed projection in frequency space, (c) inverse Fourier transform the filtered frequency space projection, and (d) back-project the filtered projection.

A major limitation of PET image reconstruction using filtered back-projection is statistical noise. The distribution of spatial frequencies (the power spectrum) of the actual (i.e., noise-free) radiotracer distribution tends to decline at higher frequencies, while statistical noise tends to have a fairly uniform frequency distribution, close to "white" noise. The multiplication in frequency space by a ramp filter amplifies the higher frequencies that tend to be dominated by noise, thus causing decreased SNR in the reconstructed images. To control noise, a postreconstruction smoothing filter can be applied, or more commonly, the ramp filter is modified to preferentially reduce higher frequencies in the projection data. Although many different filter functions have been employed (Butterworth, Hamming, Parzen), all have the same general property that they "roll off" at higher frequencies as shown in Fig. 5.4. Although filters that have a sharper roll off suppress more noise, they also reduce high-frequency signal, thus creating an inherent tradeoff between noise and spatial resolution. In practice, projection data are not continuous but discrete. Shannon's sampling theorem states that the maximum frequency that can be represented by the data, called the Nyquist frequency (ν_N), equals 1 divided by twice the sampling frequency, $\nu_N = 1/(2x')$. Trying to recover higher frequencies produces errors in the reconstruction images called aliasing artifacts. Thus, the frequency space filter extends from 0 to the Nyquist frequency.

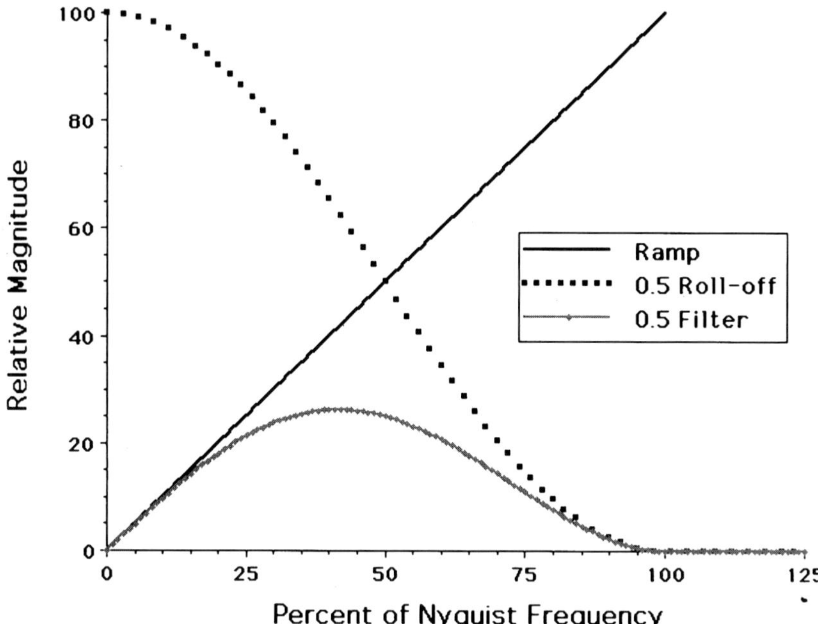

FIGURE 5.4. Back-projection filters. For noise-free data, a linearly increasing "ramp" function in Fourier space gives the appropriate filter necessary for exact reconstruction of the object. The noise in PET data, however, has a fairly uniform frequency distribution; thus, a ramp filter amplifies the high-frequency noise and results in noisy-looking images. To limit noise propagation, the ramp filter is rolled off at higher frequencies. The roll-off function (shown for a Hamming 0.5 filter) is multiplied by the ramp filter to yield the final filter function.

Fourier transforms, while useful, are not essential for FBP. This is because of an equivalence between the convolution of two functions and the product of their Fourier transforms.

$$g(x) \otimes h(x) = \int_{-\infty}^{+\infty} g(u)h(x-u)du = G(\nu) \times H(\nu) \quad [5.10]$$

By applying this principle to Equations 5.7 and 5.8, the filtered projection, $p^F(x', \theta)$, can be obtained by taking the inverse Fourier transform of the frequency space filter $W(\nu)$ and convolving it with the raw projection data $p(x', \theta)$:

$$F^{-1}\{P_\theta^F(\nu)\} = F^{-1}\{[W(\nu) \times P_\theta(\nu)]\}, \quad [5.11]$$

and thus

$$p^F(x', \theta) = [F^{-1}\{W(\nu)\}] \otimes [p(x', \theta)], \quad [5.12]$$

where F^{-1} represents the inverse Fourier transform.

The noise properties of filtered back-projection for low count studies, such as occur in many whole-body fluorine-18-fluorodeoxyglucose ([^{18}F]-FDG) scans, plus the additional noise and significant artifacts associated with transmission scanning and patient movement (see the section "Attenuation" below) have prompted much effort in the development alternative algorithms for image reconstruction. The vast majority of these techniques fall into the category of iterative reconstruction techniques.

Iterative Reconstruction

Iterative reconstruction techniques are not a recent development, but have been available and used for PET as long as filtered back-projection. The main limitation in the past has been the greater computational requirements for iterative methods than for FBP. This section outlines the basic steps of iterative reconstruction. The following section describes advances that have made iterative techniques readily available for routine use.

Rather than using an analytic solution to produce an image from the projection data, iterative reconstruction makes a series of estimates of the image, compares forward-projections of these estimates to the measured data, and refines the estimates by optimizing an objective function until a satisfactory result is obtained. Iterative methods have several advantages over FBP. They allow more accurate modeling of the data acquisition system than the line-integral model used by FBP and more accurate modeling of the statistical noise in emission and transmission images. An additional advantage is that iterative methods can incorporate *a priori* information about the object being scanned into the reconstruction process. For example, since radiotracer concentration is being imaged, all image values must be greater than or equal to zero. Thus, a nonnegativity constraint can be included in the optimization. Another use of *a priori* information is the incorporation of anatomic boundaries from coregistered CT or magnetic resonance (MR) scans with a constraint designed to allow differences across boundaries but penalize differences within boundaries.

The three key steps of an iterative algorithm are: (a) determination of a model describing the data acquisition system (including noise), (b) a calculation using the objective function that quantifies how well the image estimate matches the measured data, and (c) an algorithm that determines the next estimate of the image. The model for the measured data takes the general form $\mathbf{p} = \mathbf{Af}$, where $\mathbf{p} = \{p_j, j = 1, \ldots, m\}$ is a vector containing all m values of the measured projection ray data (i.e., $p(x', \theta)$ for all (x', θ) pairs), $\mathbf{f} = \{f_i, i = 1, \ldots, n\}$ is a vector containing the values of all image voxels (i.e., $f(x, y)$ for all (x, y) pairs), and $\mathbf{A} = \{A_{ij}\}$ is a forward-projection matrix for mapping $\mathbf{f}$ into $\mathbf{p}$. Matrix $\mathbf{A}$ is often called the system, design, or transition matrix. The elements of the matrix A_{ij} contain the probabilities of a positron annihilation event occurring in voxel

i being detected in projection ray j. Several additional unwanted processes, such as random and scattered coincidences, which will be discussed below, affect the measured projection data, thus complicating the general model. These can be incorporated into a system model of the form $\mathbf{p} = \mathbf{Af} + \mathbf{r} + \mathbf{s}$, where $\mathbf{r}$ and $\mathbf{s}$ are vectors representing the random and scattered events included in the measured projection data $\mathbf{p}$, although a discussion of more complex system models is beyond the scope of this chapter. The objective function includes any *a priori* constraints such as nonnegativity and smoothness. Typical objective functions include the Poisson likelihood and the chi-square error (the Gaussian likelihood). The iterative algorithm must ensure that successive estimates of the image converge toward a solution that maximizes (or minimizes) the objective function. The algorithm must also have an exiting criterion that defines when to terminate the iteration process.

The most extensively studied iterative algorithm is the maximum-likelihood expectation-maximization (MLEM) (20), which seeks to maximize the logarithm of the Poisson likelihood:

$$L(\mathbf{p} \mid \mathbf{f}) = \sum_{j=1}^{n} \left[\ln\left(\sum_{i=1}^{n} A_{ij} f_i \right) - \sum_{i=1}^{n} A_{ij} f_i \right] \quad [5.13]$$

In practice, the logarithm of the likelihood function is maximized instead of the likelihood function itself for computation reasons, and since they both are maximized for the same image, $\mathbf{f}$.

The EM algorithm updates the voxel values (f_i) by:

$$f_i^{k+1} = \frac{f_i^k}{\sum_{j=1}^{m} A_{ij}} \sum_{j=1}^{m} \left[A_{ij} \frac{p_j}{\sum_{j=1}^{n} A_{i'j} f_i^k} \right] \quad [5.14]$$

where f^k and f^{k+1} are the image estimates from iteration k and $k + 1$, respectively. Note the double summations over i and j. It is these steps that make the algorithm computationally demanding.

Reduction in Computational Load

As mentioned earlier, the main limitation of iterative reconstruction is its high computational load. For many algorithms, one iteration requires about twice the time of FBP. Thus, considerable effort has been directed not only toward maximizing algorithm performance with respect to image quality, but also toward the development of schemes that converge rapidly. If sufficient quality image estimates can be obtained in 5 instead of 50 iterations, the computation time of iterative routines might well be acceptable.

A significant breakthrough in iterative reconstruction speed occurred with the introduction of reconstruction using ordered subsets (OS) of projection data (21). The concept of ordered subsets can be applied to any iterative algorithm; however, the initial paper and the majority of implementations have paired OS with the EM algorithm, thus yielding the common acronym OSEM. For OSEM, the projection data are grouped into subsets. A standard EM algorithm is then applied to one of the subsets using the appropriate rows of the system matrix. The resulting reconstruction becomes the starting value to be used with the next subset. A single iteration of OSEM is completed when each of the subsets has been used once. Assuming mutually exclusive and exhaustive subsets (i.e., each projection ray is a member of one and only one subset), a single OSEM iteration requires approximately the same computation time as one standard EM iteration. However, "convergence" is much faster. Further iterations can be performed by making additional passes through the same "ordered" subsets. Results from Hudson and Larkin's study show that one or two iterations with either 32 or 16 subsets yield images with lower chi-square and mean-square error than images with 20 or 30 iterations with standard EM (21). Reconstructed images appear visually similar as well. In general, to achieve a reconstruction with a given error level, the number of iterations required is inversely proportional to the number of subsets used.

For implementation with PET, each subset may include several projection angles (a projection being the complete set of parallel projection rays at one angle). The order that the projections are processed is arbitrary from the standpoint of the algorithm; however, particular orders improve image quality and accelerate convergence. For example, selecting projections that are widely and evenly spaced, hence containing substantially different information, is better than selecting projections that are close in angle and do not vary considerably from one another. For the detector configuration of the ECAT Exact scanner, (CTI, Inc., Knoxville, TN) a single 2D sinogram consists of 192 projections, 168 rays per projection. A 32-subset implementation of OSEM uses only six projections per subset (192 projections per 32), with 30 degrees between each projection of the subset.

A problem with the OSEM algorithm is that, except for noise-free data, the solution does not converge to the maximum likelihood solution. Other rapid statistical algorithms, including row-action maximum-likelihood and space-alternating generalized maximum likelihood have been developed that also make application of iterative techniques routinely possible but do converge to the true maximum-likelihood solution. Another potential problem with OSEM, as with the original EM and many other iterative algorithms, is that they produce images with high variance at large numbers of iterations. Such images have a grainy appearance and are visually unappealing. The process to control this is called regularization. Regularization can be accomplished be various means including stopping after a limited number of iterations, postreconstruction smoothing, or incorporation of constraints, penalties, or other *a priori* information, as described earlier.

With faster computers and with the improvements made in the implementation of the algorithms, as described in the proceeding paragraphs, iterative reconstruction for 2D projection sets became practical on a routine basis by the mid-1990s. With a clear advantage in signal-to-noise over filtered back-projection, iterative techniques have become the method of choice for 2D PET image reconstruction. This advantage is greater in lower count whole-body imaging than in higher count brain studies. However, at about the same time, 3D PET acquisition also became readily available, increasing the computation demands on reconstruction algorithms by more than an order of magnitude, and thus a new set of challenges was encountered.

Image Reconstruction for Three-Dimensional PET

The introduction of 3D data acquisition marked a tremendous advance in PET imaging. Although not without its own unique set of problems, 3D acquisition with the interslice septa removed increases scanner sensitivity by a factor of 6 to 8 or more depending on the axial field of view (FOV) of the scanner, thereby increasing the noise equivalent counts (NEC) typically by a factor of 3 to 5. With this large increase in SNR, particularly in high statistical quality brain studies, the advantages that iterative techniques have over FBP are not as pronounced. Furthermore, the computational load of 3D reconstruction is much greater than that for 2D. Therefore, analytic techniques, which have a speed advantage over iterative ones, once again appear more attractive. However, with the recent dramatic increase in clinical PET using [^{18}F]-FDG, particularly whole-body oncology imaging, minimizing scan time is essential both for patient comfort and cooperation and for efficient patient throughput. Thus, the statistical quality of clinical scans is limited even with 3D acquisition, and therefore iterative algorithms will continue to provide a means of improving image SNR. In this section alternatives for reconstruction of projection data from 3D PET are summarized. A more thorough discussion of 3D acquisition and image reconstruction methods as well as other topics can be found in a recent book covering both theoretical and practical aspects of 3D PET (22).

Three-Dimensional Projection Data

Assuming the true 3D radiotracer distribution this is being imaged is given by the function $f(x, y, z)$, then the measured 3D PET data, considering a spherical geometry, can be represented by:

$$p_{\theta,\phi}(x', y') \equiv p(x', y', \theta, \phi) = \int f(x, y, z)dz', \quad [5.15]$$

where x', y', and z' are the coordinates within the rotated plane that is perpendicular to a line with in-plane angle θ and azimuthal (out-of-plane) angle ϕ. There is no perfect correspondence to the 2D case where the projection data $p(x', \theta)$ can be thought of as a set of *one*-dimensional projections $p_\theta(x')$, where the different members of the set are defined by a *single* angle, θ. Three-dimensional projection data need to be thought of as a set of *two*-dimensional projections $p_{\theta,\phi}(x', y')$, where the members of the set are defined by a *two* angles, θ and ϕ. This concept is easily visualized by thinking of a radiographic chest film as being a *2D* projection of the 3D chest, with two angles needed to define its orientation (anteroposterior vs. lateral and superior vs. inferior).

Reconstruction of a 3D object from a complete set of its 2D projections can be performed analytically by 3D FBP in a manner analogous to the use of 2D FBP for reconstructing a 2D object from a complete set of its one-dimensional projections. However, unlike the 2D case where a full ring of PET detectors (which completely encircle a 2D object) can provide the complete set of projections, it is not practical to construct a PET scanner that has full solid angle coverage of a 3D object, the human body. Thus, one cannot acquire the complete set of 2D projections necessary for 3D FBP. Many projections are either truncated or missing entirely. Applying 3D FBP to incomplete projection data can result in severe image artifacts.

Three-Dimensional Filtered Back-projection with Reprojection

To address this problem, an algorithm referred to as 3D back-projection with reprojection (23) was developed that produces estimates of the missing or truncated projection data. With these estimates of projection data for the unmeasured angles, 3D FBP can then be applied to the completed set of 2D projections. The estimates of the missing projections are calculated as follows. First, the projections that would be acquired from 2D acquisition, that is, the complete set of one-dimensional projections for each transverse slice, are extracted from the entire set of measured projection data. These one-dimensional projection sets are reconstructed by standard 2D reconstruction to form a first-pass estimate of the 3D object. Next the line integrals for all missing or incomplete projections are calculated by forward-projection through the first-pass estimate of the 3D volume. These calculated projections are then merged with the measured projections to obtain the complete projection set, which are then used to reconstruct a final 3D image using the standard 3D FBP algorithm. The computation time to reconstruct a 3D data set using 3D FBP with reprojection is more than an order of magnitude greater than the comparable 2D data sets. This is due simply to the tremendous number of projection rays that need to be back-projected. Typical 3D data sets from today's commercial scanners contain as many as 50 to 250 million or more projection rays. Therefore, there continues to be considerable effort put into the development of methods to reduce computational loads and reconstruction time.

One simple means of reducing reconstruction time that is commonly provided by commercial vendors is data reduction by combining neighboring projections. For 3D acquisition, this has been accomplished by averaging projections across both the in-plane polar angles (θ) and, in addition, the azimuthal angles (ϕ) now present due to removal of the septa. This reduction is sometimes called mashing. With current scanners, an in-plane mashing factor of 2 is typical, which reduces the number of polar angles by two. The azimuthal angle data reduction is somewhat more complex, but follows the same general principle of making the angular projection grid coarser. Reconstruction performance needs to be assessed to ensure that this combining of projections does not cause artifacts that result from undersampling projection space. Three- to eightfold reductions in the number of lines of response are usually possible without degrading imaging quality significantly. Three-dimensional data sets can thus be reduced to a much more manageable size of around 10 to 50 MB per scan on current systems.

Rebinning Algorithms

Other analytic approaches have been introduced for 3D reconstruction (24–27), and although they provide satisfactory performance, none have reduced reconstruction time relative to 3D FBP with reprojection by more than a factor of 2. Thus, alternative approaches to the problem have received considerable attention. Since 2D reconstructions are more than an order of magnitude faster than 3D, methods that convert the projections from 3D data into approximations of projections from 2D data (one sinogram per transverse slice) are very attractive. A method for converting 3D to 2D data is commonly referred to as a rebinning algorithm. It is easier to understand rebinning if we consider the 3D projection data as coming from a cylindrical geometry instead of the spherical geometry used for Equation 5.15.

$$[p(x', y', \theta, \phi)]_{spherical} \Leftrightarrow [p(x', \theta, z, \delta)]_{cylindrical}, \quad [5.16]$$

where z is the distance along the axial extent of the scanner and δ is a measure of off-axis tilt. For a scanner with detectors in a cylindrical geometry, consider a plane perpendicular to the long axis of the scanner. All the projection rays within this plane are defined by x' and θ just as in the 2D case. Since all these rays are perpendicular to the scanner's axis, the off-axis tilt δ is 0, and if this plane goes through the center of the axial FOV, z also is 0. This projection set can be reconstructed by a 2D algorithm to yield an image of the transverse slice running through the middle of the axial FOV. Other projection sets that exist in different but parallel planes to this set still would have $\delta = 0$, but have different values of z. Two-dimensional reconstruction of the additional sets yields images of other transverse slices. However, the majority of the projection rays in 3D PET acquisition are not perpendicular to the long axis of the scanner ($\delta \neq 0$) and thus the job of rebinning is to convert data for all projection rays with nonzero δ to rays with zero δ. These data can then be sorted in sets of projections, one for each transverse slice of the scanner, z:

$$p(x', \theta, z, \delta) \Rightarrow p(x', \theta, z) \equiv p_z(x', \theta), \quad [5.17]$$

which can then be reconstructed by a rapid 2D algorithm. In practice, the z value of a given projection ray is defined simply by the average z coordinate of the two detectors represented by this ray. The value of $\delta = \tan(\phi)$, the angle between the projection ray and the transaxial plane, and can be calculated from the ring offset and the physical distance between the two detectors.

Rebinning methods need to be fast, accurate, and must incorporate the entire 3D data set to maintain the advantage of increased sensitivity provided by 3D acquisition. Rebinning can be approximate or exact; however, approximate methods can be implemented more efficiently and thus offer a speed advantage. One very rapid and simple method of rebinning is single-slice rebinning (SSRB) (28), where any projection ray at a given azimuthal (out of plane) angle is rebinned into the transverse slice that is located halfway axially between the two detectors (i.e., merely setting δ to 0). Thus, using SSRB, the conversion of Equation 5.17 becomes:

$$p(x', \theta, z, \delta) \approx p(x', \theta, z, 0) = p_z(x', \theta). \quad [5.18]$$

Although fast, this method is not very accurate for events that occur a large distance from the central axis. If the azimuthal angle of the accepted projection rays is not too large, this method can provide improved SNR for regions located near the center of the FOV. It should be pointed out that this general technique is in fact used in all standard 2D acquisitions. Even in the very first multislice scanners, a cross plane was produced by rebinning the projection rays that came from detectors that are one ring apart (a small but nonzero δ). Current generation scanners typically operate under the SSRB principle by accepting rays from detectors that are offset from one another by 0, ±2, ±4, and ±6 rings for "true" planes and ±1, ±3, ±5 and ±7 rings for cross planes.

Fourier Rebinning

A significant advance in 3D reconstruction came with the introduction of a new rebinning technique based on taking 2D Fourier transforms of the projection data called Fourier rebinning (FORE) (29). The 2D Fourier transform of each oblique projection with respect to x' and θ is given by:

$$P(\nu_{x'}, k, z, \delta) = \int_{-\infty}^{+\infty} dx' \int_{0}^{2\pi} d\theta \, (e^{-i2\pi x'\nu_{x'}}) p(x', \theta, z, \delta) \quad [5.19]$$

The Equation 5.17 conversion using FORE is accomplished in Fourier space instead of projection space:

$$P(\nu_{x'}, k, z, \delta) \cong P(\nu_{x'}, k, z - \frac{k\delta}{\nu_{x'}}, 0) = P(\nu_{x'}, k, z', 0). \quad [5.20]$$

Following the FORE approximation, the inverse 2D Fourier transform yields:

$$p_{z'}(x', \theta) = p(x', \theta, z', 0) = F^{-1}[P(\nu_{x'}, k, z', 0)]. \quad [5.21]$$

Two-dimensional reconstructions are then performed on each set of projections (defined by z') to yield the stack of transverse images defining the 3D volume. The 2D reconstructions can be either filtered back-projection or iterative. Many groups have applied FORE and shown that the method produces images comparable to 3D FBP with reprojection, but with computational savings of greater than an order of magnitude when following FORE with 2D FBP.

The introduction of FORE made the job of processing large numbers of 3D PET scans, such as are needed for repeat oxygen-15-water ([^{15}O]-water) scans or long multiframe dynamic studies much easier. The next logical step was to combine the advantages of the increased sensitivity of 3D scanning with the noise-reduction properties of iterative reconstruction through the use of both rebinning methods, such as FORE, and computation reduction techniques, such as ordered subsets. Several papers have been published recently using FORE+OSEM. Reconstruction performance of the combined FORE+OSEM technique has been compared to 3D FBP with reprojection (30), to FORE+2D FBP and FORE+PWLS (31) (penalized weighted least-squares (32), an alternative to MLEM optimization), and to fully 3D OSEM (33). FORE+OSEM was found to outperform 3D FBP with reprojection in terms of contrast and SNR while requiring less time to perform. FORE+OSEM outperformed FORE+2D FBP. FORE+PWLS was found to be superior to FORE+OSEM when attenuation correction (AC) was not incorporated into the system matrix. However, FORE+OSEM with AC incorporated into the system matrix performed very similarly to FORE+PWLS but is faster computationally. FORE+OSEM was found to perform nearly as well as 3D OSEM, but with a time savings of greater than a factor of 10.

Fully Three-Dimensional Iterative Approaches

It has been shown that reconstruction techniques, including iterative approaches, are now available to handle heavy loads of 3D PET data. This does not mean that current day reconstruction methodology should be considered fully mature. In one sense the quest for better image reconstruction may never end. As new scanners are developed that have higher and higher intrinsic resolution, such as the many recently developed small animal scanners, more detected events are needed per unit volume in order to approach this resolution in the reconstructed images. This in turn requires better models for describing data acquisition and for characterizing the noise properties of the PET data. To this end, work continues on the implementation of fully 3D iterative techniques that avoid even the relatively minor problems associated with techniques such as FORE+OSEM. Qi et al. (34,35) have implemented fully 3D iterative techniques for human and for animal imaging, attempting to obtain the highest quality images possible. In 2000, Leahy and Qi (36) published a review of the current state of the art in regard to statistical approaches to image reconstruction in PET.

Time of Flight

The concept of using time-of-flight (TOF) information as a means of improving PET images was recognized even before PET scanning became a reality (37,38). Simply put, if the detection time of the measured photon interactions can be measured precisely enough, the difference in the detection times between the two coincident photons contains information about where the positron decay occurred along the LOR connecting the two scintillation crystals. The location of the positron decay is nearer to whichever crystal records the earlier detection time. Based on the velocity of the 511 keV photons, a timing uncertainty of 500 picoseconds translates to a position uncertainty of the positron decay of about 7.5 cm along the LOR. Although this restriction in the location of the positron decay is not nearly good enough to improve spatial resolution, the information can be used by the reconstruction algorithm to reduce the effective noise in reconstructed images. At a timing resolution of 500 picoseconds, the effective number of detected events is approximately two to four times higher depending on the size of the object being imaged (39).

Once the first PET scanners were developed in the 1970s it was not long before TOF scanning systems were investigated. By the early 1980s, tomographs using either CsF (cesium fluoride) or BaF_2 (barium fluoride) scintillation crystals had been built (40–42). However, the signal-to-noise gain in the early TOF systems was not fully realized because of the lower stopping power and hence lower inherent sensitivity of these detector materials relative to BGO (bismuth germanate). BGO offered a better combination of resolution and sensitivity and hence became the dominant detector material in PET scanners for nearly two decades, during which time TOF systems nearly disappeared from the scene entirely.

Beginning in the late 1990s the advent of new detector materials such as LSO (cerium activated lutetium orthosilicate; Lu_2SiO_5:Ce), LYSO (lutetium yttrium orthosilicate; $Lu_{(2-x)}Y_xSiO_5$:Ce), or others including $LaBr_3$ (lanthium bromide) presented new possibilities for TOF. These crystals offer fast timing as well as stopping power much better than CsF or BaF_2, approaching that of BGO. In fact, the three major PET scanner manufacturers all offer tomographs with LSO or LYSO detector crystals.

Although the timing properties of LSO had been investigated and shown to have TOF potential (43,44), Moses and Derenzo (45) investigated this potential in a realistic PET setting using LSO detector crystals of a size and shape similar to those found in actual PET scanners. Although their results showed promise, the coincidence timing resolution was about 475 picoseconds, noticeably worse than the 300 picoseconds predicted from first principles due to multiple reflections of light within the scintillation crystal. Continued work on TOF in the present decade has yielded improvements in timing and shows TOF as a realistic proposition for implementation on present day scanners (46). Recently, TOF information has been included in the reconstruction process and used for actual human scans acquired with LSO and LYSO scanners. Reports of the signal-to-noise advantage of TOF are beginning to appear in the literature (47,48).

Inclusion of TOF information adds complexity to the reconstruction process. Image reconstruction for TOF PET was originally implemented for 2D data in the early 1980s when the first TOF scanners were constructed (49,50). Many of the same concerns regarding the speed of the algorithm have been studied for TOF as for conventional PET reconstruction, trying to make the methods rapid enough to use with iterative techniques. As was the case for extending 2D iterative algorithms to 3D PET data, extending 2D TOF algorithms to 3D TOF is relatively straightforward conceptually; however, the challenge again is handling the increased data loads. Two recent papers by Defrise et al. (51) and Vandenberghe et al. (52) have proposed reconstructions for 3D TOF using angular compression of data (mashing) and axial rebinning methods as described previously in this chapter for non-TOF data. Although implementation of TOF with full 3D PET data as well as routine use of TOF in either research or clinical PET has not yet been realized, the potential of TOF clearly has been demonstrated. This is especially the case for whole-body imaging of large patients, and hence research is likely to continue over the next 5 to 10 years, with the expectation that TOF will become a standard part of the image reconstruction process in the foreseeable future.

Data Corrections

Accurate quantitative images of radiotracer concentration are not obtained by direct reconstruction of the raw projection data acquired from a PET scanner. To ensure optimal quantification, several corrections need to be made to the projections prior to or during the reconstruction process. These corrections are important and require as much attention as is given to the reconstruction algorithms.

Normalization

With thousands of detectors in current PET scanning systems, it is unreasonable to assume that all detectors will respond uniformly to a given number of incident radiation events. Some detectors will have a lower response than average, while others will have a higher response. Furthermore, the geometry between a pair of detectors in coincidence is not fixed but varies for several reasons, and thus there are inherent differences in detector responses due to geometric considerations. Even if all the detectors did respond with the same efficiency to a fixed radiation source, the coincidence pair responses (the projection rays) would vary. Therefore, the entire set of projection data for each acquired PET scan needs to be normalized for differences in detector response throughout the scanner. As suggested above, the components of the normalization can be separated into two categories: those related to the relative efficiencies of the individual detectors and those related to the physical or geometric arrangement of the detectors. Thus, although a major portion of the normalization correction accounts for variations in *individual* detector responses, the overall correction is applied on a ray-by-ray basis.

There are two general approaches for determining the correction factors used for normalization. The first is a direct measurement of the factors. In this approach, a low radioactivity source (typically a rotating germanium-68 [^{68}Ge] rod) is used to generate or measure a correction factor for each coincidence pair by acquiring a scan in the same manner as one acquires a "blank" scan. For the 2D case, this correction takes the form:

$$N(r, \theta) = \frac{[\sum_{r=1}^{j} \sum_{\theta=1}^{k} P_N(r, \theta)] / [j \times k]}{P_N(r, \theta)}, \qquad [5.22]$$

where $N(r, \theta)$ is the normalization factor for projection ray sum r of angle θ, $P_N(r, \theta)$ is the uncorrected projection data from the normalization scan, and the summations are over all k projection angles and all j projection rays per angle. The normalized projection data are simply:

$$P_{corr}(r, \theta) = N(r, \theta) \times P(r, \theta), \qquad [5.23]$$

where $P(r, \theta)$ is the uncorrected projection ray measured from any arbitrary PET scan, $N(r, \theta)$ is the correction factor for this ray determined from the normalization scan as given by Equation 5.22, and $P_{corr}(r, \theta)$ is the corrected projection raw value. This approach, in a single measurement, accounts for both the individual detector efficiencies and the differences in geometry between the various detector pairs.

A second correction technique separates the individual detector efficiencies from the geometric effects. In this approach a set of normalization factors for the individual detectors (instead of coincidence pairs) is generated, and then the product of any two detectors efficiencies yields an estimate of the coincidence pair sensitivity. This value is then corrected further for differing geometric effects based the physical locations of the two detectors. This method can be considered an indirect or calculated correction. There are at least two geometric effects that need to be taken into account. One is the differential response depending on how closely the LOR for the two detectors passes to the center of the FOV. For 3D acquisition this effect has both transverse and axial components. A second effect is based on the block detectors in use on current PET systems, where many detector crystals are coupled to a few photomultiplier tubes. The location of a particular detector crystal within a block (center or edge) is important. The overall normalization factor for a detector pair using an indirect or calculated approach takes the form:

$$N(i_m, j_n) = \frac{1}{E(i_m) \times E(j_n) \times G(r, \theta, m, n) \times B(k_{ij}, r, \theta, m, n)}, \quad [5.24]$$

where $N(i_m, j_n)$ is the normalization factor for the projection ray between detector i of ring m and detector j or ring n, $E(i_m)$ and $E(j_n)$ are the individual efficiencies for those two detectors, $G(r, \theta, m, n)$ is the geometric efficiency between two detectors and $B(k_{ij}, r, \theta, m, n)$ is the block-related correction factors with k_{ij} defining the relative positions within a block of detectors i and j.

Current PET scanners are more stable than early scanners, and thus normalization typically needs to be performed only weekly to monthly. A directly measured normalization determines the entire set of normalization factors every time. For an indirect or calculated normalization, however, the individual detector efficiencies, $E(i_m)$, are measured weekly to monthly, while the geometric factors, G and B, can be carefully measured once and stored, then retrieved each time to calculate the normalization factors for a given PET scan.

The relative advantages and disadvantages of the two general approaches, the additional considerations for 3D versus 2D normalization, and the interaction between this correction and other corrections (particularly scatter) are beyond the scope of this chapter. Bailey et al. (53) present an excellent and more detailed discussion of normalization.

Detector Dead Time

During the time a detector is processing a detected event, it is unable to process any additional events. If an event occurs during this time it goes unprocessed and is lost. Such losses are referred to as dead-time losses. As count rate increases, the probability of having a lost event increases and scanner "dead time" increases. These losses are not simply related to the single and the coincidence count rates, but also are dependent on the analog and digital electronics of the system. Dead time is further complicated by the block detector design of current scanners. It is extremely difficult to calculate dead time for PET scanners entirely from first principles. In practice, one can assess dead time by plotting the measured count rate of a decaying source over time. Assuming the source is a single radionuclide, one can calculate the "true" count rate from the half-life of the nuclide and plot this versus the actual measured count rate. At low activity and hence low count rates, the plot will be linear. At higher count rates, a nonlinearity arises as the expected number of events exceeds the measured number. The ratio of the measured to the expected events yields an estimate of scanner dead time. For the majority of present-day scanners, an empirical relationship between count rate and dead time is provided by the manufacturer as part of the software package. Typically, corrections are fairly accurate up to at least 50% and as high as 75% to 80% dead time. For current scanners, dead-time corrections are accurate to better than $\pm$5% for count rates up to at least 5 μCi/mL (in a 20 cm diameter phantom) for 2D acquisitions and up to at least 1 μCi/mL for higher sensitivity 3D acquisition.

Random and Multiple Coincidences

As described in Chapter 3, the detection of the two nearly colinear 511 keV photons within a specified amount of time, τ, called the coincidence window or coincidence resolving time, forms the basis for PET imaging. The near simultaneous ($\leq$10 nanoseconds) detection of two photons is called a coincidence event. Remembering that it is highly likely that only one of the two annihilation photons is detected, usually only a single event is recorded by the scanner during a given time interval τ. Therefore, as the detected count rate increases, the probability that one event is detected from each of two separate positron annihilations within the coincidence window increases as well. This type of event is defined as random coincidence, sometimes also called an accidental coincidence. As shown in Fig. 5.5, the line connecting the two detectors for a random coincidence gives erroneous information about the position of the positron decay, causing image reconstruction artifacts if not accounted for. Since the scanner cannot distinguish "true" coincidences from "random" coincidences on an event-by-event basis, an alternative scheme is required.

Two distinct methods have been used for random coincidence correction. The first requires that the singles detection rates be recorded for each detector of the scanner. The random coincidence rate for a given projection ray of PET scan i, $C_R(i)$ is given by the product of twice the coincidence resolving time, τ, multiplied by the singles rates of the two detectors, $C_{S1}(i)$ and $C_{S2}(i)$:

$$C_R(i) = 2\tau C_{S_1}(i) C_{S_2}(i) \quad [5.25]$$

Note that since the singles count rates increase linearly with the amount of radioactivity in the FOV, and the randoms count rates increase as the square of the amount of radioactivity. Thus, at low count rates randoms are insignificant, while at high count rates the randoms rates easily can exceed the true coincidence rates. This method of correction is applied to each projection ray separately, but only once per scan:

$$C_T(i) = C_M(i) - C_R(i), \quad [5.26]$$

where $C_M(i)$ and $C_T(i)$ are the measured and corrected true coincidence count rates, respectively.

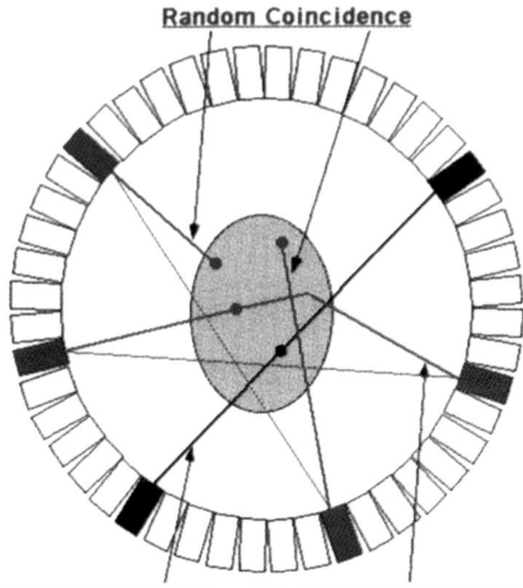

FIGURE 5.5. Random and scattered coincidences. One would like each detected coincidence event to correctly identify a line of response passing through the point of positron decay. For this to occur both 511 keV photons need to be detected and neither photon can be scattered in tissue. The black dot, detectors, and connecting line of response depict such a "true" coincidence event. If only one photon is detected from each of two positron decays and these are detected with the coincidence resolving time, a "random" or accidental coincidence is said to have occurred. This is depicted by the two blue dots and detectors. The two thicker blue lines indicate the path of the two detected photons, while the thinner blue line corresponds to the line of response that is recorded for this "random" coincidence event. Note that this line does not pass through either of the two points and therefore causes misplacement of the coincidence event and hence error in the reconstructed image. If both photons from a single decay are detected but one (or both) photons are scattered in the body prior to detection, the coincidence event also is misplaced as shown by the red dot, detectors, and lines. The two thicker red lines indicate the actual paths taken by the two photons, while the thinner red line indicates the line of response that is recorded for this "scattered" coincidence event. Again, the line does not pass through the point of decay and causes error in the reconstructed image.

The second method involves setting up two distinct coincidence windows. The first window is the standard coincidence window of width τ. As before, both true and random coincidences are recorded in this window, which for this approach is called the *prompt* coincidence window. A second coincidence circuit is set up, but with one of the two inputs being delayed by a time considerably greater than the resolving time, τ. Rather than searching for two events that occur within a single 10-nanosecond window (as is done in the prompt circuit), this circuit, in effect, searches for events that occur in two separate 10-nanosecond windows offset by, for example, 100 nanoseconds. This offset window produces what are called *delayed* coincidence events. The probability that a true coincidence occurs in the delayed window is zero, while the probability that a random coincidence occurs is the same as in the prompt window. Thus, the prompt window records true plus random coincidences, while the delayed window records only randoms. Subtracting delayed from prompt coincidences yields an estimate of *true* coincidences. The advantage of this approach is that it can be implemented online and requires no postacquisition processing. During data acquisition, a memory location exists for each detector pair whose projection ray subtends the FOV. For every prompt coincidence event detected, the memory location representing the appropriate projection ray is incremented by 1. For each delayed event detected, the memory location is decremented by 1. This commonly used decrementing procedure ruins the Poisson statistical model that is the theoretical basis for Equation 5.13 and the MLEM (and OSEM) iterative reconstruction algorithms. Alternative reconstruction methods have been proposed for PET measurements that are precorrected for random coincidences (54,55).

Scattered Coincidence Events

At 511 keV energies, two types of photon interactions occur: Compton scattering and photoelectric absorption. As discussed in Chapter 3, scintillation detectors are designed to maximize the number of photoelectric interactions, while minimizing the probability of Compton scattering. This is accomplished by a material with a high effective atomic number and high density. However, due to the lower effective atomic number in the body, most interactions in human tissue occur via Compton scattering, as depicted in Fig. 5.5. As was the case for random coincidence events, detection of events where one or both of the photons have undergone at least one Compton scatter causes the location of the annihilation to be misplaced. Inclusion of scattered events causes a relatively uniform background, decreasing image contrast and reducing SNR. Naturally we would like to record only unscattered photon events, but is not possible to identify with complete certainty whether a particular event is scattered. Scintillation detectors with higher light output do, however, have better energy resolution and thus are better able to distinguish unscattered from scattered events.

Accurate correction for Compton scattered photons is extremely complex with hundreds of papers having been written on quantifying its effects as well as developing and testing methods for correction. For 2D acquisition, scatter was only moderately important with 15% to 20% of the detected events being scattered. Image quality was not affected greatly, hence scatter correction was often ignored without major impact. With 3D scanning, 35% to 50% of the detected events may be scattered, and correction has become much more critical. Current scatter corrections fall into three basic groups: (a) those using multiple energy windows; (b) those based on direct calculation from analytic formulas for Compton scatter or on Monte Carlo calculations; and (c) methods involving a variety of techniques such as convolution, deconvolution, or the fitting of analytic functions to areas of the image void of radioactivity (thus representing only scattered events).

Although each of these three general techniques has its own advantages and limitations, details of such methods are beyond the scope of this chapter. The reader is referred to Bailey et al. (56) for a more thorough discussion of scattered events and correction methods to account their occurrence. This chapter describes briefly only the direct calculation approach. It is assumed that the true radioactivity distribution can be reconstructed accurately when the measured PET data, emission and transmission, contain only unscattered events. The measured PET data, however, include both true and scattered events. The correction is performed iteratively. The original measured data are reconstructed as an initial estimate of the true radioactivity distribution. From these images and the analytic formulas for Compton scatter, the scatter component to the raw projection data is estimated. This scatter component is subtracted from the measured PET data as the next approximation to the scatter-free projection data. This new projection set is reconstructed as the next approximation to the true radioactivity distribution. These steps are repeated until the images reconstructed from the current estimate of the scatter-free projection data yield predicted scatter that when added to the scatter-free data equal the measured projection data. In practice, successive approximations to the scatter-free distribution can be made during the normal iterations of the OSEM reconstruction algorithm.

Attenuation

A final but extremely important correction to the projection data is that which accounts for the effects of photon attenuation in the body. For a true coincidence event to be detected, both photons must exit the body. This is less likely for annihilations located deep within the body than for ones occurring near the body's surface. One convenient aspect of PET imaging is that the attenuation correction factor for any given projection ray is the same for a positron annihilation occurring anywhere along the ray. The net attenuation is simply the product of the probabilities that each photon escapes without interacting:

$$e^{-\mu x_1} e^{-\mu x_2} = e^{-\mu(x_1+x_2)}, \qquad [5.27]$$

where μ is the linear attenuation coefficient for 511 keV photons in tissue, and $x_{1,2}$ are the distances the two photons must travel through tissue. Since the sum $x_1 + x_2$ always equals the total path length, l, through the body, the attenuation correction factor is given by $e^{+\mu l}$. Independence of the position of the annihilation along the ray is true even if the attenuation coefficient varies across the path due to multiple tissue types (lung, soft tissue, and bone).

Again, there are two general approaches used to account for photon attenuation. First is a calculated or analytic method, where the path length for each projection ray is estimated in some fashion and the value for μ is assumed. The attenuation correction factor, as indicated above, is simply $e^{+\mu l}$. The two main limitations of this approach are: (a) it is not always easy to determine the path length of all projection rays, and (b) variations in μ are not easily accounted for. A major advantage is there is no statistical noise associated with the correction. This approach has been used for brain imaging where the shape of the head can be approximated by an ellipse and the attenuation is uniform except for a thin rim of skull.

A second method is to measure the attenuation factors directly. This approach typically uses external rod sources that are rotated around the FOV, until recently being replaced by CT scanning approaches (see Chapter 2). Most sources contain the positron-emitter ^{68}Ge, which has a 0.75-year half-life. Two scans are acquired as shown in Fig. 5.6, a blank scan, which is acquired with nothing in the FOV (similar in nature to the normalization scan described above), and a transmission scan, where the subject is in the FOV in the identical position as the emission scan. After appropriate corrections, the ratio of the measured projection data from the blank scan divided by the transmission scan yields a correction factor for the emission data. If a particular projection ray has 400 counts in the blank scan, but only 50 counts in the transmission scan, the correction factor for the emission data will be 8.

Although measured attenuation avoids the problems associated with the analytic approach, several other potential problems arise. Statistical uncertainty in the blank and particularly the transmission scan propagates into the reconstructed emission images. This problem is particularly bad in the abdomen (especially with large abdomens) where attenuation is high and thus detected transmission events low. Subject motion between the times of the transmission and emission scans can cause significant errors in the correction factors for particular projection rays, resulting in severe artifacts when motion is substantial. Such artifacts are considerably worse for filtered back-projection than for iterative approaches. Transmission scans also take considerable time. If a subject can reasonably be expected to remain still for 1 to 2 hours, we would want to spend the entire time acquiring emission data. For body scans, however, nearly as much time is required for transmission as emission imaging. Furthermore, for clinical FDG scans that have a 50-minute or longer tracer-uptake period, it becomes problematic to perform all transmission scanning prior to injection of the radiotracer. This is due to both subject motion and study duration issues. If transmission scans are performed postinjection, then the contribution of the FDG events to transmission data must be taken into account.

Over the past decade much work has been done to improve attenuation correction. The two most significant advances are described here. The first was to provide the capability of performing postinjection transmission scans. Prior to this advance, a typical clinical protocol might include 30 minutes of transmission scanning, injection of [^{18}F]-FDG, and then a 50-minute uptake period

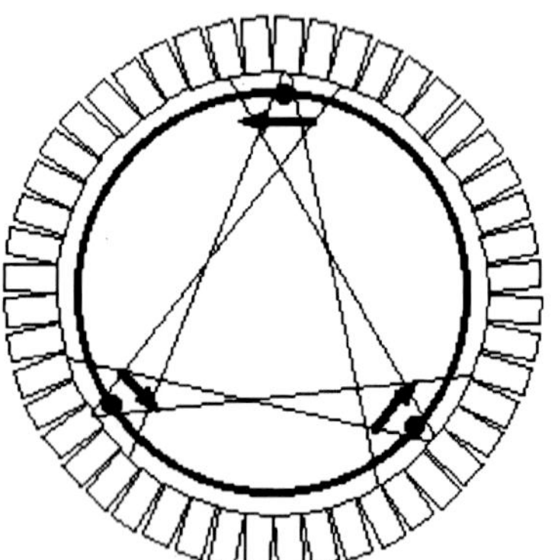

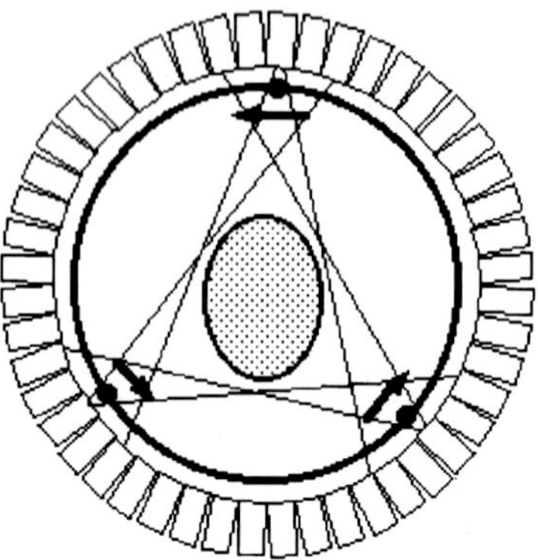

FIGURE 5.6. Schematic for measured attenuation correction. As described in the text, measured attenuation is performed by acquiring two scans: a "blank" scan and a "transmission" scan. Both scans are performed using radioactive sources that are rotated around the gantry in front of the detectors. The blank scan measures the coincidence rate from the sources when nothing is in the field of view. The transmission scan measures the coincidence rate when the object being imaged is in the field of view. The ratio between these two measures is used, ray by ray, to correct the emission projection data.

followed by 30 to 60 minutes or more of emission imaging. Thus, a subject would have to lie still for more than 2 hours. This is both difficult on the patient and it occupies the scanner for long periods of time even when no data are being acquired. Furthermore, registration between transmission and emission scans may be jeopardized by the length of time between the acquisitions. Through the use of rotating rod sources instead of a continuous ring of radioactivity, postinjection transmission scanning is possible. For discrete rod sources, only a small fraction of the projection rays contain valid transmission coincidences at any given time. Only rays that pass through one of the rod sources can have coincidences that originate from within the rod. All other events come from FDG decay. Thus, the majority of emission coincidences that occur at any given time are rejected based on the known positions of the rods.

The second major advance was the development of a combination calculated/measured attenuation correction that makes use of the advantages of each approach. A transmission scan is acquired, but rather than performing the correction based on the ray-by-ray difference between blank and transmission data, this scan is reconstructed into a map of attenuation coefficients. Although individual rays are noisy, the reconstructed transmission image allows segmentation into different tissue types. Each pixel of the image is *assigned* an attenuation coefficient based on the segmentation. The segmented images, in practice, are smoothed and then used to calculate attenuation factors for the emission data. This process greatly reduces noise propagation from the transmission measurements into the reconstructed emission images. Fig. 5.7 shows a 2D whole-body transaxial slice reconstructed with measured attenuation (left) and with segmented attenuation correction (right). Clearly demonstrated is the noise propagation from the transmission data into the emission image when attenuation correction is performed without segmentation. In addition, reconstructions were performed with both FBP (top) and with an iterative OSEM algorithm (bottom). The better noise properties of iterative reconstruction are demonstrated clearly. In particular, notice the reduction in streak artifacts with OSEM that plague back-projection techniques. Keeping in mind that both images are derived from the identical projection data, the improvement from the upper left image to the lower right image (which has both segmented attenuation correction and iterative reconstruction) truly is impressive. A variety of additional issues arise when determining attenuation corrections for 3D PET. A major difficulty is that the radioactivity level of the rod sources required for adequate statistics in 2D studies causes excessive dead time and random coincidence

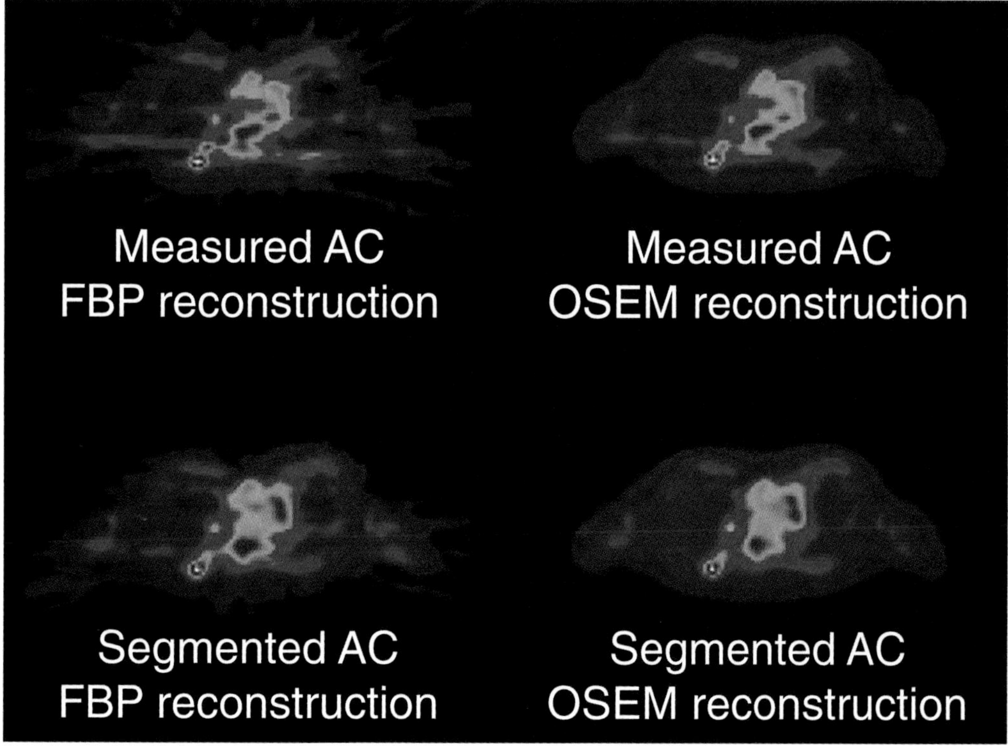

FIGURE 5.7. Effects of segmented attenuation correction and iterative reconstruction on whole-body images. Shown are four different reconstructions of the same set of two-dimensional emission data. The **left image** is reconstructed using measured attenuation correction and filtered back-projection. The **right image** is reconstructed using measured attenuation correction and the iterative OSEM algorithm. The **lower left image** is reconstructed using segmented attenuation correction and filtered back-projection. Finally, the **lower right image** is reconstructed using both segmented attenuation correction and OSEM. The streak artifacts caused by back-projection are seen clearly in the upper left image. These streaks are reduced considerably either by using an iterative algorithm or by using segmented attenuation, which eliminates the majority of the noise associated with the transmission scan. The improvement when using both segmented attenuation correction and iterative reconstruction is striking.

rates in 3D studies. Currently, transmission scans are performed in 2D mode, reconstructed, and then forward projected into the full set of 3D projection rays. Considerable work by Erdogan and Fessler et al. (57,58) has been performed to maximize the quality of the reconstructed transmission data.

The advent of PET/CT has drastically altered the method of correcting for photon attenuation of the measured PET emission data. In combined PET/CT systems the need for rotating rod or point sources is alleviated altogether (although a rotating source remains in some systems to allow evaluation of detector uniformity). The CT scan serves a dual purpose not only in providing high-resolution coregistered anatomy for localizing tracer-avid structures, but in providing the anatomic information needed to calculate the photon attenuation correction factors to be applied to the emission projections. CT images are of much higher statistical quality than rod or point source images, thus almost no statistical noise is introduced by the correction. In addition, since CT scans require much less time to acquire, 30% to 40% of the total scan time that is needed for transmission imaging in PET-only systems is unnecessary and can be used either to shorten the duration of the study or for additional emission imaging. Kinahan et al. (59) first reported the efficacy of CT-based attenuation for PET/CT scanners. Despite the proven utility of CT-based attenuation correction, this procedure is not without its own challenges. These fall into two main categories: (a) the accurate conversion of CT x-ray attenuation coefficients into the attenuation coefficients for 511 keV photons, and (b) errors introduced by misregistration of CT and PET projection data.

Since the effective photon energy of CT is much lower than 511 keV, a calculation is required to convert "CT" attenuation coefficients to 511 keV equivalent "PET" attenuation coefficients. The conversion from x-ray to PET coefficients is relatively straightforward for lung, soft tissue, and bone in the case when no contrast agent is present. Segmentation of the CT into soft tissue (including lung) and bone is followed by applying two separate scale factors to the x-ray attenuation coefficients to yield the appropriate PET attenuation correction factors. However, in the presence of either oral or intravenous contrast, or in the presence of metal implants, the mapping between CT and PET attenuation is not unique and additional correction factors are required. Considerable work has gone into assessing the possible effects that contrast-induced attenuation correction errors have on clinical PET images, as well as work to develop methods to minimize these errors in the attenuation correction factors themselves. Studies by Carney et al. (60) and Nehmeh et al. (61) are examples of efforts to reduce artifacts induced by oral-contrast. Similar correction efforts have been developed for reducing intravenous contrast (62,63) and metal-based (64) attenuation artifacts.

The second category of artifact relates to motion. Although motion problems are not unique to CT-based attenuation correction, they tend to be more pronounced than for the radioisotope transmission scan-based attenuation correction of PET-only systems. The motion can be of two types: gross patient motion, which will be mentioned briefly here, and motion of internal structures caused by the cardiac and respiratory cycles, which will be discussed in the following section. Since the CT and PET acquisitions are not simultaneous, there is the possibility of motion between the two scans, and hence misregistration of the CT attenuation and PET emission projections. Not surprisingly, this can cause very noticeable artifacts when the patient motion is pronounced. For body imaging, the largest artifacts appear in areas near lung/soft-tissue boundaries. Care must be taken to ensure accurate registration of CT and PET data in studies where the areas of interest are near such boundaries. It is still common practice at many PET centers to reconstruct images both with and without attenuation correction to be certain that any areas of increased or decreased radioactivity uptake are not attenuation correction-induced artifacts.

A recent cardiac perfusion investigation reports a series of 28 patients with coronary artery disease who had undergone nitrogen-13-tritium ($^{13}NH_3$) rest-stress PET/CT examinations (65). Six patients had defect sizes that changed by greater than 10% following manual registration of CT with PET prior to applying the attenuation correction. In five of the subjects, total disappearance of the deficit (15% to 46% of the left ventricle) occurred, indicating these apparent deficits were due entirely to emission-transmission misregistration.

Gating

In addition to gross patient motion, both cardiac and respiratory motion cause degradation of PET images. Measurements of and corrections for cardiac motion in nuclear cardiology studies have been around for a long time. The acquisition of PET data can be gated by the patient's own electrocardiogram (ECG) signal and binned into the different portions of the cardiac cycle. In addition to the other clinical uses of cardiac gating in nuclear cardiology, gating improves image resolution by accounting for motion of the heart throughout the PET acquisition.

The problem of motion throughout the respiratory cycle is also a source of image degradation, but until recently this has been studied much less than the problems related to cardiac motion. In PET/CT, however, respiratory motion has proven to be a greater problem than was seen previously in PET-only systems. Besides image degradation due simply to the motion of internal structures, there are possible image artifacts related to the fact that the CT scan is acquired in a relatively short time compared to PET. In PET-only systems, both transmission and emission scans are acquired across many respiratory cycles, and thus in the absence of gross patient motion, the average position of the diaphragm and hence the surrounding internal structures is the same for both scans. In PET/CT, the CT is acquired rapidly enough so that the individual slices may be imaged for only a portion of the respiratory cycle. This portion could vary from subject to subject and represent the anatomical condition at maximum expiration, maximum inspiration, or anywhere in between. With the higher resolution of CT, this can cause artifacts in the attenuation correction at image levels near the diaphragm due to a misalignment of transmission and emission data similar to those described above for gross patient motion.

Over the past few years, the effects of respiratory motion have been examined and the feasibility and utility of respiratory gating has been shown (66–70). Similar to the demonstrated utility of TOF, which may become more widely available over the next decade, respiratory gating is now offered as a software option by all of the major scanner manufacturers and is an area that will continue to receive much attenuation over the next several years. Gating is not yet routinely utilized by many PET centers because not all of the practical issues for easy use have been addressed. For example, if a PET scan is binned into four image sets throughout the respiratory cycle, the image quality of each set, although less affected by internal motion, has poorer signal-to-noise properties than the single ungated image. In this case, the ability to detect small lesions may not be improved. If software becomes available that makes it easy to display not only the individual frames of the gated study in a cine loop, but to provide the ability to coregister and warp the different image sets of the respiratory cycle so they can be summed back into a single set, then respiratory gating of PET studies in the chest and abdomen may become part of standard practice.

The next decade of PET should see a maturing of the PET/CT field and the melding of the many new techniques described in this section, resulting in scanners and software that provide higher resolution, improved signal-to-noise characteristics, more robust and reliable images, and images that are more resistant to artifacts such as those induced by motion.

COMPARTMENTAL MODELING

Image reconstruction in conjunction with the appropriate corrections to the measured projection data yields quantitative measures of a PET tracer's spatial radioactivity distribution within the human body. However, this distribution is not static over the course of the study, but varies with time depending on the different processes that govern its uptake and subsequent biological fate in the body. By acquiring a dynamic sequence of PET measurements information is obtained about the *in vivo* behavior of the particular radiotracer being imaged, which can be used to provide measurements of specific biological functions. This is accomplished through the use of an analysis process commonly referred to as compartmental or tracer kinetic modeling. Compartmental modeling techniques are mathematical constructs that involve the concept of different spaces or compartments in which the tracer can reside plus a set of model rate constants or parameters that describe how rapidly the tracer moves between compartments. With some knowledge of the radiotracer and the biologic properties that govern its *in vivo* behavior, these rate constants are then assumed to represent specific physiologic or biochemical processes such as blood flow, glucose metabolism, protein synthesis, neurotransmitter level, enzyme activity, and receptor or binding site density. The following sections describe the fundamentals of compartmental modeling and tracer kinetic techniques. The steps required for selection, implementation, and validation of a compartmental model are discussed, including consideration of practical issues that affect the use of compartmental model strategies. Models for two specific applications—measurement of blow flow and glucose metabolism—will be reviewed in more detail. Also included in this discussion are examples of applications for neurological, cardiac, and oncological studies.

Fundamentals of Compartmental Modeling

Radiotracers allow for the investigation of physiologic and biochemical processes *without altering* the normal functions of the biologic system. The mathematical description of the movement of radioactive tracer material within the system is known as tracer kinetics. Biologic systems can be represented or modeled as a collection of compartments, sometimes referred to as pools or spaces, linked by kinetic processes that provide a mechanism for exchange of tracer between adjoining compartments. A compartmental model consists of a finite number of compartments, each of which

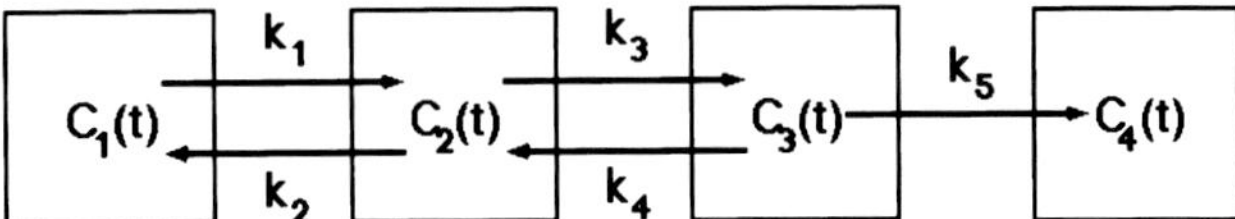

FIGURE 5.8. Generalized compartmental model. The system described by this hypothetical model consists of four compartments that contain a given radiotracer at concentrations C_1, C_2, C_3, and C_4. The radiotracer is exchanged or transferred between compartments at rates proportional to the five rate constants k_1 through k_5. Exchange between compartments 1 and 2 and between compartments 2 and 3 is reversible, whereas exchange of radiotracer between compartments 3 and 4 is irreversible.

is assumed to behave as a single homogeneous, well-mixed, distinct component of the overall biologic system (71). Different compartments may represent either *distinct* physical spaces, such as blood plasma versus brain tissue, or different chemical forms (FDG vs. FDG-6-PO_4) or pharmacological states (bound vs. unbound) of the radiotracer that occupy the *same* physical space.

The various compartments of a tracer kinetic model are linked by a set of parameters commonly called rate constants as seen in Fig. 5.8. The values of these parameters represent the rates at which the radiotracer is exchanged between the various compartments. In the case where two compartments represent different distinct physical spaces, the parameters that link them represent the rates of flow or transport across that particular physical boundary. In the case where two compartments share the same physical space but represent different chemical forms or pharmacological states, the parameters represent the rates of transformation from one chemical form or state of the substance to the other.

The amount or concentration of the radiotracer in the model compartments can be described as a function of time by a set of first-order differential equations in terms of the model parameters. The basis for the differential equations is derived from the law of conservation of mass, or mass balance. Mass balance, for tracer applications, means that the amount of radioactive tracer that enters a compartment per unit time (the influx) minus the amount of tracer that leaves the compartment per unit time (the efflux) is equal to the amount of tracer accumulated in the compartment per unit time. The amount of radiotracer typically is measured in either microcuries or becquerels. Under steady-state or equilibrium conditions, the influx of radiotracer is equal to the efflux, and the net change in the amount or concentration of radiotracer over time is zero.

Fig. 5.8 depicts a hypothetical compartmental system consisting of four compartments and a total of five rate constants. In some fields of compartmental modeling, a rate constant is written with two subscripts depicting both compartments that it links. For example, the rate constant describing transfer of material from compartment 1 to compartment 2 is written as k_{21}, while the rate constant describing transfer of material from compartment 3 to compartment 1 is written as k_{13}. In the field of nuclear medicine it has been more common to use a single subscript as presented in this figure, with transfer from compartment 1 to compartment 2 being referred to as k_1 and transfer from compartment 2 to compartment 1 being referred to as k_2. Rate constants representing transfer between subsequent model compartments are referred to as k_3, k_4, k_5, and so on. In this chapter the nuclear medicine convention using only single subscripts is used. The differential equations describing the concentration of material in each compartment are written in the same form as the mass balance equation and appear as follows:

$$dC_1(t)/dt = k_2C_2(t) - k_1C_1(t)$$
$$dC_2(t)/dt = [k_1C_1(t) + k_4C_3(t)] - [k_2C_2(t) + k_3C_2(t)]$$
$$dC_3(t)/dt = k_3C_2(t) - [k_4C_3(t) + k_5C_3(t)]$$
$$dC_4(t)/dt = k_5C_3(t), \quad [5.28]$$

where dC_i/dt is the rate of change in concentration of radiotracer in compartment i; the positive terms describe influx, and the negative terms describe efflux. Note that the amount of radiotracer leaving a compartment by any route is proportional to the concentration in that compartment. The proportionality constants between the quantities of radiotracer leaving and the concentrations in the compartments are the model rate constants. These rate constants appear as the coefficients for the efflux and influx terms in Equation 5.28. A rate constant generally has units of inverse time (min^{-1}) and describes the fraction of radiotracer leaving a compartment in a given amount of time. For example, a rate constant of 0.1 min^{-1} indicates that an amount of tracer equal to 10% of that in the compartment will be transported out of the compartment every minute. For this model since all the rate constants appear to the first power, all processes governing radiotracer exchange between the model compartments are first order and thus the system is said to obey first-order kinetics.

Steps Required for Design and Implementation of a Compartmental Model

Although there are many ways to group the steps required for using compartmental models, the general procedures common to all PET applications are summarized briefly here. Examples given in this section are specific to the application of [^{15}O] labeled water for the measurement of blood flow. Subsequent sections in the chapter will go into more detail about some of these steps and give examples of how other compartmental models are applied for PET radiotracers designed to measure other biologic functions.

Define the Dynamic Process to be Measured

The first step is to be clear about which specific biologic process or processes are to be measured. For "blood flow," the mass specific rate of tissue perfusion is being measured, that is, the amount of blood supplied to a given volume of tissue per unit time, typically in units of milliliters (blood) $min^{-1}mL^{-1}$ (tissue).

Select an Appropriate Radiotracer

Selecting an appropriate radiotracer is obviously a crucial step in the overall process. The entire field of PET radiochemistry research (Chapter 2) is devoted to developing radiotracers for measuring a vast array of biologic processes. Many PET tracers have been developed for measuring blood flow, including $H_2{}^{15}O$, $^{15}CO_2$, $CH_3{}^{18}F$, ^{11}C-butanol, ^{15}O-butanol, $^{13}NH_3$ and ^{62}Cu-PTSM. Of these, [^{15}O]-water has been used most often.

Understand the Physiology and Biochemistry of the Radiotracer

Application of a compartmental model requires adequate knowledge of the *in vivo* behavior of the radiotracer and should include understanding of (a) the mechanism of transport between blood and tissue (diffusion, carrier-mediated transport); (b) possible trapping, metabolism, synthesis, or breakdown of the tracer; (c) possible reversal of any trapping or metabolic processes; (d) distribution in blood (e.g., binding to plasma proteins, red blood cells); (e) possible creation and presence of radiolabeled metabolites in the blood; and (f) possible creation and presence of radiolabeled metabolites in the tissue. The following is the pertinent information for [^{15}O]-water. [^{15}O] has a half-life of 122 seconds. This requires short scans and thus high counting rates, but allows multiple scans to be performed easily. Water is transported across the plasma membrane into the body tissues by passive diffusion. Water is not trapped or metabolized. This means that a single tissue compartment representing free [^{15}O]-water should suffice for describing the *in vivo* distribution of water in the body. Blood vessels are highly permeable to water, and thus water can diffuse rapidly into and out of tissue and therefore is said to be "freely" diffusible. Plasma proteins do not bind water. Water does diffuse into red cells, but red cells equilibrate very rapidly with plasma, and thus radioactivity in the red cells can be considered to be available for transport in tissue. The body produces no labeled metabolites of water. Similar information needs to be obtained for any other tracer proposed for use with PET.

Develop a Workable Compartmental Model

With knowledge concerning the *in vivo* behavior of [^{15}O]-water, a single-tissue compartment model is proposed, sometimes called a two-compartment model when arterial plasma is considered as a separate compartment. Fig. 5.9 depicts this simple model containing the blood pool, a single tissue compartment, and two rate constants describing the exchange of [^{15}O]-water between the plasma and tissue. C_T represents the concentration of [^{15}O]-water in tissue (μCi mL^{-1} of tissue), C_P represents the concentration of [^{15}O]-water in arterial plasma (μCi mL^{-1} of blood), K_1 is the rate constant for transport of [^{15}O]-water from plasma across the blood–brain barrier to brain (mL blood $min^{-1}mL^{-1}$ tissue), and k_2 is the rate constant for back diffusion from tissue back to blood (min^{-1}). The rate constant K_1 is written in uppercase to denote the difference in units from those of k_2 or other rate constants. This is because the units of C_P are μCi mL^{-1} of blood and not mL^{-1} of brain like the concentration of the tissue compartment.

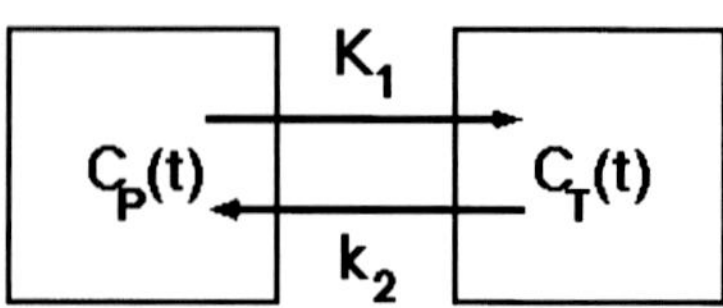

FIGURE 5.9. Compartmental model for $H_2{}^{15}O$. The model consists of a compartment representing arterial plasma and a single tissue compartment representing $H_2{}^{15}O$ in tissue. Other tissue compartments are not required because water is neither trapped nor metabolized in tissue. C_p and C_T represent the concentration of radiotracer in arterial plasma and tissue, respectively. K_1 and k_2 are the rate parameters describing transport of the radiotracer across the capillary membrane.

Understand Model Assumptions

Most compartmental model applications involve a certain number of assumptions that must be valid if the measures obtained about the biological system are to be correct. These assumptions separate into two categories: (a) those that relate to the biologic system and to the radiotracer used; and (b) those that relate to the specific experimental procedures employed to make the measurements. The former will be discussed here, while later sections of the chapter that describe particular applications will contain examples of those in the latter group.

All processes of the biological system that influence the kinetic behavior of the radiotracer are assumed to be in steady state throughout the duration of the experiment. This does not mean that the radiotracer concentration has to be in the steady state. Before continuing, it is important to distinguish between the terms steady state and equilibrium. For radiotracer applications, the existence of steady state means that the concentration of radiotracer in each compartment remains constant over time. This does not necessitate the existence of an equilibrium condition, where there is zero net transfer of radiotracer between compartments, but only that the net rate at which a substance enters a compartment must equal the net rate at which it leaves. Steady state refers to a change in concentration of radiotracer *within* a compartment that has one or more inputs and one or more outputs. Equilibrium refers to the exchange of radiotracer *across* the interface *between* compartments, and exists only when the exchange is equal in both directions. Thus, a *single* compartment can be at (or not at) steady state, while *two* compartments can be in (or not in) equilibrium with each other. In practice, the requirement of steady state means that the concentration or amount of *parent* substance in any compartment must remain constant during the experiment and consequently that the rates of transport or metabolism of the parent substance also must remain constant during the time frame of the study. It is important to note again that the steady-state requirement applies only to the biologic system and not to the radiotracer. For example, the concentration of systemic glucose in the capillaries and tissue, and the concentration of glucose-6-phosphate in tissue must remain constant throughout the PET study, thus keeping the net rates of the processes attempted to be measured, glucose transport and phosphorylation, constant. Note that although a steady state is required for the systemic substance glucose, glucose is not in equilibrium, as there is always a net flux of glucose from blood to tissue and from free glucose to glucose-6-phosphate. In contrast, the concentration of radiotracer (the glucose analogue [^{18}F]-FDG) in the various model compartments varies freely over time.

In most applications the concentration of radiotracer introduced into the system is assumed to be negligible such that it does not effect or perturb the system by its presence in any way. If this assumption is violated, then the measurement may provide information about effects induced by the presence of the radiotracer instead of the systemic process that is being measured. Compliance with this assumption ensures that the processes that govern the kinetic behavior of the radiotracer remain first order and that the conservation laws of mass transport are valid.

Each compartment of the system must be *spatially* homogeneous with respect to the concentrations of both tracer and any systemic substances (in addition to the *temporal* homogeneity requirements described above). To accommodate this, one assumes complete and instantaneous mixing of all materials within a compartment. Although mixing obviously is not instantaneous, in practice it must be rapid compared to the exchange rates between compartments.

Write/Solve the Differential Equations Describing Tracer Exchange Between Model Compartments

From Fig. 5.9, while following the format of Equation 5.28, the linear first-order differential equation for the single-tissue compartmental model is:

$$dC_T(t)/dt = K_1C_P(t) - k_2C_T(t), \qquad [5.29]$$

where $dC_T(t)/dt$ is the first derivative of the [^{15}O]-water time course in tissue with respect to time and represents the rate of change in radiotracer concentration.

The solution to a first-order linear differential equation of this form is:

$$C_T(t) = K_1C_P(t) \otimes e^{-k_2t}, \qquad [5.30]$$

where $\otimes$ denotes the mathematical operation of convolution. Since a PET scanner cannot measure radiotracer instantaneously, Equation 5.20 requires integration of the duration of the scan, yielding:

$$PET_i = \int_{t-start_i}^{t-stop_i} C_T(t)dt = K_1 \int_{t-start_i}^{t-stop_i} C_P(t) \otimes e^{-k_2t}\,dt, \qquad [5.31]$$

where PET_i represents the ith frame of the dynamic PET study and $t\text{-}start_i$ and $t\text{-}stop_i$ are the scan start and stop times for frame i, respectively. The sequence of i PET measurements for any given region describes the time course of the radioactivity in that tissue and is commonly referred to as a time-activity curve (TAC). Note that the tissue concentration is linearly scaled by the uptake rate constant K_1. This means that if the net uptake of a radiotracer is doubled, the entire PET TAC is doubled. Only the parameter k_2 affects the shape of the TAC. This is true for more complex PET models as well. The parameter K_1 always describes the overall *scale* of the measured PET data, while the remaining rate constants (k_2, k_3, k_4, etc.) describe the *shape* of the measured data.

Define the Measured Quantities and Unknown Parameters

Equation 5.31 has two measured quantities, the tissue radioactivity concentration estimated from the dynamic data, PET_i, and the arterial plasma radioactivity concentration, usually estimated from discrete arterial blood samples, and two unknowns to be estimated, K_1 and the clearance exponential coefficient, k_2. More detailed discussion of the measurement of arterial plasma curves and the methods for estimating the model parameters from the measured data are described in later sections of this chapter.

Understand Biological Significance of Model Parameters

Compartmental modeling applications become useful only when a relationship can be made between the mathematical parameters (model rate constants) and the physiologic or biochemical parameters associated with the particular function under investigation. For example, the essential information to be obtained from a [^{15}O]-water

PET study is not actually the value of K_1 or k_2, but is the rate of tissue perfusion.

The physiological definition and hence significance of K_1 can be derived as shown by Gjedde (72) and is the same for most compartmental model applications with PET:

$$K_1 = f(1 - e^{-PS/f}) = f\,E_o \text{ (mL blood min}^{-1}\text{mL}^{-1}\text{ brain)}, \quad [5.32]$$

where f is blood flow (called mass or volume specific flow since it is given per unit mass or volume) with the same units as K_1, mL blood min^{-1}mL^{-1} tissue, PS is the capillary permeability surface area product with permeability in units of cm min^{-1} and surface area in cm^2 mL^{-1}. Since cm^3 is equivalent to mL, the PS product has the appropriate units of mL blood min^{-1}mL^{-1} tissue. The term $(1 - e^{-PS/f})$ ranges from near zero if PS is much smaller than f to near unity if PS is much larger than f. This term is often referred to as the single-pass extraction fraction and is designated by E_0. E_0 gives the fraction of radiotracer in the arterial plasma that crosses the plasma membrane and enters the tissue during a single capillary transit. The radiotracer does not have to remain in the tissue, but may cross back into the blood during the same capillary transit, or may even cross the plasma membrane several times during a single transit. K_1 therefore is equal to the mass specific blood flow multiplied by the fraction of radiotracer that is extracted during a capillary transit. Since the total rate of passage of radiotracer through a capillary is given by $f\,C_P$, and the rate of uptake by tissue is given by K_1C_P, the fraction of radiotracer that is carried into the tissue from the blood, E_0, is given by $K_1C_P/f\,C_P$ (i.e., the uptake rate divided by the total rate of radiotracer passage through the capillary). This equals K_1/f and is consistent with the definition of E_0 given in Equation 5.32. Typically, the rate constant K_1 is referred to as the uptake rate constant, and it describes the unidirectional rate of transfer of the radiotracer from blood to tissue. The value of K_1 is dependent on both blood flow and capillary membrane permeability. For [^{15}O]-water, which is considered to be freely diffusible, K_1 can be interpreted further by making the assumption that the permeability-surface area product is large enough relative to blood flow that the extraction fraction term of K_1 is equal to 1 ($E_0 = 1$). Therefore, for [^{15}O]-water, K_1 is equal to blood flow. Although mass specific flow is commonly given in units of milliliters of blood per minute per 100 g of tissue (mL min^{-1}100g^{-1}), PET measurements yield tissue concentrations in microcuries per unit volume, not per unit mass as the definitions given above reflect this fact. However, multiplying flow values given in mL blood min^{-1}mL^{-1} tissue by the density of tissue (mL g^{-1}), which is only slightly greater than unity, then multiplying by 100 converts flow estimates into the familiar units of mL min^{-1}100 g^{-1}.

The coefficient k_2 is a pure rate constant in that it has units of min^{-1} and describes the rate of clearance of radiotracer or parent substance from tissue back to blood. As discussed previously, a pure rate constant gives the fraction of radioactivity that is removed from tissue per unit time. Typically, the rate constant k_2 is referred to as the clearance rate constant and, like K_1, is also related to both blood flow and capillary membrane permeability. The mean transit time in tissue, τ_m, of water or other nontrapped or metabolized radiotracers is given by the inverse of the clearance rate constant, k_2. Similarly, the *biological* half-clearance time, $\tau_{1/2}$, of a tracer in a compartment (not to be confused with the *physical* half-life of the radioisotope $t_{1/2} = \ln 2/\lambda$) is defined as the time it takes to clear out one half of the tracer from the compartment and is given by τ_m multiplied by the natural log of 2.

Not only do individual rate constants have physiological meaning, but often ratios of certain rate constants have significance. Consider Equation 5.29 under steady-state conditions for water. By definition (no net change in concentration over time), the term $dC_P(t)/dt$ equals zero and thus:

$$K_1[C_P(t)]_{ss} = k_2[C_T(t)]_{ss}, \quad [5.33]$$

or rearranging:

$$K_1/k_2 = [C_T(t)/C_P(t)]_{ss}. \quad [5.34]$$

This steady-state ratio of the concentration in tissue to blood is defined as the volume of distribution, V_d, or the tracer's tissue-to-blood partition coefficient, p. Formally, the volume of distribution is given in units of mL blood mL^{-1} tissue, while the partition coefficient is given in mL blood g^{-1} tissue (73), the difference being only that of the density of tissue. In Equation 5.34 the ratio K_1/k_2 is equal to the steady-state distribution volume of water. Therefore, by using dynamic PET measurements and compartmental modeling it is possible to estimate the volume of distribution of a radiotracer by estimating the rate constants K_1 and k_2, while *never* achieving steady-state conditions for the radiotracer at any time during the PET study.

For the single-tissue compartment model for [^{15}O]-water, Equations 5.29 through 5.31 can be rewritten using the physiologic meanings for the rate constants. Since K_1 equals flow and K_1/k_2 equals the distribution volume of water, the clearance rate constant k_2 can be expressed as f/V_d, yielding:

$$dC_T(t)/dt = fC_P(t) - (f/V_d)C_T(t), \quad [5.35]$$

$$C_T(t) = fC_P(t) \otimes e^{-(f/V_d)t}, \quad [5.36]$$

and finally:

$$PET_i = \int_{t-start_i}^{t-stop_i} C_T(t)dt = f\int_{t-start_i}^{t-stop_i} C_P(t) \otimes e^{-(f/V_d)t}\,dt \quad [5.37]$$

noting that the influx or uptake is determined entirely by blood flow, while the efflux or clearance rate is determined both by blood flow and the tissue distribution volume of the radiotracer. Translating Equation 5.37 back into words, the measured PET data are equal to the blood flow multiplied by the integral of the arterial plasma radioactivity input time course (commonly called an input function) convolved with the exponential clearance or "washout" of activity from tissue:

$$PET_i = CBF\int_i Input\ Function \otimes Clearance. \quad [5.38]$$

Develop Mathematical Schemes for Estimating Model Parameters

Once all of the data have been acquired, images reconstructed, and a compartmental model selected, a method to obtain estimates of the model parameters from the dynamic data must be employed in order to translate *kinetic* information into *physiologically* and/or *biochemically meaningful* information. This step and the following two (sensitivity analysis/model optimization and model validation) are linked. Together, they are used to ensure that estimates of a parameter assumed to reflect a particular biologic process is indeed a good measure or index of that process. As stated before, a compartmental model is a mathematical description of a biologic system. The job of the parameter estimation algorithm is to determine what *values* of the parameters of this mathematical description, when entered into the compartmental model, optimally describe the measured tissue time activity curves. One aspect of parameter estimation is the assessment of the goodness of fit, which quantifies how well the model describes the measured data. Such measures help to determine the appropriateness of a particular model configuration and to compare the performance of different configurations, thus aiding in the determination of the optimal implementation of a tracer kinetic model. The entire process of estimating model parameters to describe a measured data set is often referred to as curve fitting. A thorough discussion of parameter estimation techniques and curve fitting for PET applications by Carson (74) provides further information on this subject. The criteria used for optimization and the methods employed for determining the parameter values will be discussed in more detail in the section "Parameter Estimation."

Sensitivity Analysis/Model Optimization

Analysis of model sensitivity is a crucial step in compartmental modeling applications for PET. The goal of this analysis is to quantify the effects that statistical noise and compartmental model assumptions have on the estimated parameters. Sensitivity analysis uses a combination of simulated data and when possible measured PET data. Typically, a comprehensive model more complex than the actual model that will be implemented is used to derive the mathematical relationships and equations that are best thought to describe the *in vivo* kinetic behavior of the radiotracer. By using a range of values covering those typically expected for the model parameters, the equations of the *comprehensive* model are used to calculate "noise-free" radiotracer concentrations across the duration of the study. Statistical noise and/or biases from potential violations in model assumptions are then added to the noise-free data. Finally, the *practical* model that will be used with the measured PET data is applied to the simulated "noisy" and/or "biased" data, and estimates of the model parameters are obtained. When many sets of simulated data are generated for the same "true" conditions, the mean, standard deviation, bias, uncertainty, and overall accuracy for the estimates of each model parameter can be calculated. Sensitivity analysis not only can predict how well a particular PET radiotracer and proposed compartmental model will perform, but is helpful in optimizing the specific model implementation, the parameter estimation technique used, and the experimental design and acquisition protocols.

Model Validation

When a compartmental model is finally applied to human PET studies, one must validate that the model can accurately predict the measured concentration time course of the radiotracer. In addition, one also must validate that the parameter estimation technique can provide accurate quantitative values for the physiologic parameters that are of interest in the study. It may be the case that more than one model configuration can describe the measured data sufficiently well, yet different configurations will yield different estimates of the same parameter. Care must be taken to ensure that the model is not only mathematically appropriate, but physiologically appropriate. One must ask whether the model is capable of providing *meaningful* estimates of the biological process or processes being measured. More specifically, one needs to address the following two questions: when the biological process of primary interest in the study changes, does the compartmental model yield changes in the parameter or combination of parameters that are interpreted as reflecting that process (i.e., is the model sensitive); and conversely, when another biological process changes, one which is not of interest, does the compartmental model yield unchanged estimates of the parameter of interest (i.e., is the model specific)? Modeling results should be compared with more direct measures of the parameter under investigation whenever possible. Many of these more direct measures may come from studies in animals or an isolated human study where more invasive procedures are performed. Measures that are widely accepted can serve as gold standards for comparison with newly proposed techniques. Examples of such validation studies include (a) measuring cerebral blood flow using a diffusible radiotracer simultaneously with a well-accepted microsphere method, and (b) comparison of neurotransmitter or enzyme activity levels measured with PET to levels determined by direct chemical assay. More detailed examples of validation studies for two particular radiotracers are given in the section "Model Validation."

Practical Considerations

The best-designed experiments with a perfect radiotracer, a state-of-the-art PET scanner and image reconstruction, a validated compartmental model, and a thorough sensitivity analysis still can yield meaningless data if certain practical issues are overlooked. The length of study that can be tolerated by some patients is one very important consideration. If two or more hours of data are required to obtain results with an acceptable degree of accuracy, patients who are very ill may not be able to complete the procedure. Only a certain degree of motion within a study can be accounted for before results are rendered useless. The probability of being able to obtain a useful data set should be considered. Another consideration relates to the amount of data that may need to be acquired, worked-up, and stored. Consider a case where a sensitivity analysis indicates that scans should be acquired every 10 seconds for the first few minutes of the study, and a total of 40 frames is needed to provide optimal results. However, a model simplification is possible that requires only 10 frames, but decreases the accuracy of the estimated parameters by a few percentage points. This most likely is a good practical tradeoff. Sometimes by simplifying a procedure and reducing the work and cost associated with acquiring and processing the data, additional subjects can be studied, and with a greater probability of success per subject, thus improving the power of the experiment by an increase in sample size.

Tracer Models with Multiple Tissue Compartments

The information derivable from radiotracers that can be modeled by a single tissue compartment is limited to the transport rate constants and to simple volumes of distribution. Although these may be sufficient for some applications, they may limit the study of more complex biologic systems. When models with multiple tissue compartments are employed, then the solution to the differential equations, describing the model, the parameter estimation routine, and in addition, the interpretation of the physiological significance of the rate parameters, naturally become more complex. Here the implementation and interpretation of data from multitissue compartment models, using [^{18}F]-FDG as the primary example of a two-tissue compartment model, is discussed.

The solution to the set of differential equations derived from more complex models such as that for FDG becomes increasing complicated as the number of compartments increases. This solution takes the general form:

$$PET_i = \int_i Input\ Function \otimes Tissue\ Impulse\ Response, \quad [5.39]$$

where the measured tissue data (PET_i) equals the integral of the arterial plasma input curve convolved with a term called the tissue impulse response function. The tissue impulse response is what the measured PET concentration curve or *tissue response would be* if the arterial plasma input function were a perfect bolus or delta function *impulse.* This can be seen from Equation 5.39 and the fact that a delta function is the identity function for mathematical convolution; that is, for any arbitrary function $g(t) \otimes \delta(t) = g(t)$. The physiologic parameters to be estimated are contained in the tissue impulse response. The actual arterial plasma input function is never a perfect bolus, and thus the measured PET data are never equivalent to the impulse response function. Since the radiotracer input to the tissue is spread over time, the measured PET data are a "spread out" or "smeared" transformation of the impulse response. The more blunted the arterial input, the more smeared the measured PET data. The form of the impulse response is defined by the specific configuration of the compartmental model. For example from Equation 5.30 we see that the general form of the impulse response for a single-tissue model is $K_1e^{-k_2t}$. The parameters of the impulse response function are linked to the model rate constants and can be estimated from the input function and PET data by a general technique referred to as deconvolution. By deconvolution, it is meant that if $A(t) = B(t) \otimes C(t)$, then $B(t)$ deconvolved from $A(t)$ $= C(t)$. In other words, if we take the PET data and deconvolve the measured input function from it, an estimate of the tissue impulse response is obtained. Deconvolution methods are described in more detail in the section "Parameter Estimation."

The complexity of the impulse response function is governed by the complexity of the compartmental model. For a two-tissue compartment model, such as that used for [^{18}F]-FDG (Fig. 5.10), the general form of the impulse response I_r becomes:

$$I_r(t) = A_1e^{-\alpha_1 t} + A_2e^{-\alpha_2 t}. \quad [5.40]$$

Note that unlike the single-tissue model, where the I_r parameters corresponded directly to the compartment model parameters, the four parameters of the two-tissue I_r (A_1, A_2, α_1, α_2) do not correspond exactly to the compartmental model parameters, but they can be converted easily:

$$\alpha_1 = \frac{\sqrt{(k_2 + k_3 + k_4) - [(k_2 + k_3 + k_4)^2 - 4k_2k_4]}}{2}$$

$$\alpha_2 = \frac{\sqrt{(k_2 + k_3 + k_4) + [(k_2 + k_3 + k_4)^2 - 4k_2k_4]}}{2} \quad [5.41]$$

$$A_1 = \frac{K_1(k_3 + k_4 - \alpha_1)}{(\alpha_2 - \alpha_1)}; \qquad A_2 = \frac{K_1(\alpha_2 - k_3 - k_4)}{(\alpha_2 - \alpha_1)}$$

Volumes of Distribution for Multicompartment Models

Before examining the compartmental model for FDG, the physiological meaning of various combinations of rate constants needs to be revisited. At this time it is necessary to introduce the concepts of reversible and irreversible models. Consider a model with two tissue compartments and rate constants K_1 through k_4 as shown in Fig. 5.10. Note that the exchange across all compartment boundaries is bidirectional. This model configuration is termed reversible. In this case, it is possible for a radiotracer that exists in any compartment to reverse its steps and clear from the tissue. On the other hand, consider a radiotracer that undergoes a metabolic process represented by k_3 that is *ir*reversible. In this case, there would be no process represented by k_4 (i.e., $k_4 = 0$), and an radiotracer that enters the second tissue compartment becomes irreversibly trapped in the tissue. Thus, a model configuration where exchange across at least one compartment boundary is unidirectional is said to be an irreversible model. The differential equations for the two-tissue compartments of a reversible model become:

$$dC_f(t)/dt = K_1C_p(t) - k_2C_f(t) - k_3C_f(t) + k_4C_m(t)$$
$$dC_m(t)/dt = k_3C_f(t) - k_4C_m(t), \quad [5.42]$$

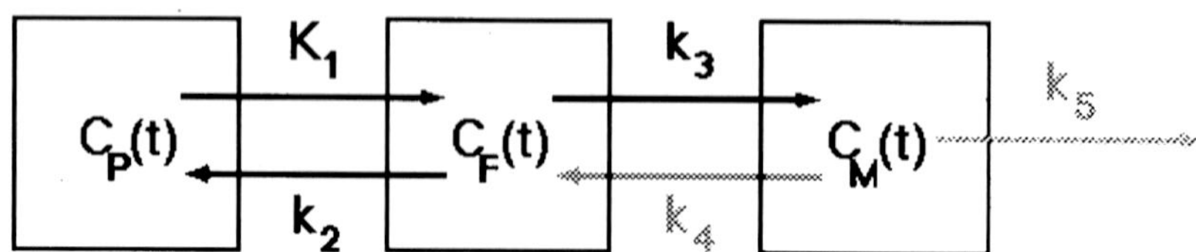

FIGURE 5.10. A two-tissue compartmental model for fluorine-18-fluorodeoxyglucose ([^{18}F]-FDG). The model consists of a compartment representing arterial plasma and two tissue compartments, representing free (unmetabolized FDG) and trapped (FDG-6-P0$_4$; the chemical form of FDG after the first step of metabolism). C_P, C_F, and C_M represent the concentrations of radiotracer in the arterial plasma, the free pool, and the trapped pool, respectively; k_1 and k_2 are the rate parameters describing transport of the radiotracer across the blood–brain barrier, and k_3 and k_4 are the parameters describing rates of the processes of trapping and possible release (phosphorylation and dephosphorylation for FDG). For [^{18}F]-FDG, the rate of dephosphorylation is very slow and is sometimes ignored (the lighter gray arrow and rate constant k_4). Also for [^{18}F]-FDG, no further metabolism occurs past phosphorylation, so k_5 is zero. However, for the parent substance that FDG traces, namely glucose, further metabolism does occur and is irreversible (striped light gray arrow and rate constant k_5).

which simplify to the following equations for an irreversible two-tissue compartment model:

$$dC_f(t)/dt = K_1C_p(t) - k_2C_f(t) - k_3C_f(t)$$
$$dC_m(t)/dt = k_3C_f(t) \quad [5.43]$$

For a single-tissue compartment model there is only one route of clearance from tissue, and thus when steady state occurs (i.e., when $dC_T(t)/dt = 0$), the net exchange between tissue and blood is also zero and thus conditions for equilibrium are satisfied also. Therefore, for a single tissue compartment model, steady-state and equilibrium conditions are satisfied simultaneously, and thus, the equilibrium and steady-state distribution volumes are identical. Similarly, for two-tissue compartment models that are reversible, steady-state and equilibrium conditions are satisfied simultaneously. However, for irreversible two-tissue compartment models, steady-state and equilibrium conditions may not occur simultaneously. The compartments representing free and metabolized radiotracer, C_f and C_m, can never reach equilibrium unless k_3 is zero. Although the metabolized compartment also cannot be in steady state unless k_3 is zero, the free compartment can reach *steady-state* if K_1C_P equals $(k_2+k_3)C_f$. Rearranging, it is clear that this occurs when the ratio of radiotracer concentration in the free compartment relative to that in plasma equals $K_1/(k_2+k_3)$. Note, however, that the free compartment is in *equilibrium* with the blood when K_1C_P equals k_2C_f. This occurs when free radiotracer concentration relative to that in plasma equals K_1/k_2. The steady-state and equilibrium distribution volumes of the free compartment are given by:

$$[V_{d(f)}]_{ss} = K_1/(k_2 + k_3)$$
$$[V_{d(f)}]_{eq} = K_1/k_2. \quad [5.44]$$

In practice, equilibrium is never achieved unless k_3 is zero and then $[V_d]_{ss}$ would equal $[V_d]_{eq.}$ When k_3 is nonzero, however, the steady-state volume is always lower than the equilibrium volume due to the continual removal of the radiotracer by the irreversible pathway.

Returning to the reversible model, by similar logic, the distribution volume for the free compartment (either equilibrium or steady state) is equal to K_1/k_2. If, in addition, the free and metabolic compartments are in equilibrium, then $dC_m(t)/dt = 0$, and $k_3C_f(t)$ must equal $k_4C_m(t)$, and, therefore, the equilibrium ratio of the metabolized to free concentration equals k_3/k_4. Since the equilibrium ratio of the free to plasma concentration is K_1/k_2, then the distribution volume of the metabolized compartment relative to plasma is $(K_1/k_2) \times (k_3/k_4)$.

The total distribution volume would be the sum of the volumes of distribution and, therefore, the distribution volumes for the individual compartments as well as the total are given by:

$$V_{d(f)} = K_1/k_2$$
$$V_{d(m)} = (K_1/k_2) \times (k_3/k_4) \quad [5.45]$$
$$V_{d(tot)} = V_{d(f)} + V_{d(m)} = (K_1/k_2) \times (1 + k_3/k_4).$$

As we will see later, distribution volume estimates can be used as an index for many biochemical and pharmacological processes.

Compartmental Model for Fluorine-18 Fluorodeoxyglucose

The most commonly used and successful PET radiotracer to date has been the glucose analogue [^{18}F]-FDG. This tracer is used routinely to provide local measures of glucose utilization for metabolic studies of the brain and heart and for localization of tumors that readily incorporate [^{18}F]-FDG. The general model for [^{18}F]-FDG is the two-tissue compartment model presented in Fig. 5.10. As defined in the original work using carbon-14-deoxyglucose ([^{14}C]-DG) by Sokoloff et al. (75) and later using [^{18}F]-FDG (76–78), the metabolic rate of glucose (MR_{glc}) is the net rate at which glucose is converted to glucose-6-phosphate:

$$MR_{GLC} = C_P[K_1k_3/(k_2 + k_3)] \qquad (\text{mg min}^{-1}\,100\text{g}^{-1}), \quad [5.46]$$

where C_P is the arterial plasma concentration of stable glucose (mg mL^{-1}) and K_1, k_2, and k_3 are the rate constants for *glucose.* Note that the net rate of utilization is dependent both on the transport rates (K_1 and k_2) and the rate of phosphorylation (k_3).

In practice, the rate constants for glucose are not measured, but instead, the steady-state arterial plasma glucose concentration and the rate constants for FDG can be measured, and, thus, Equation 5.46 can be rewritten as:

$$MR_{GLC} = (C_P/\text{LC})[K^*K_1k_3^*/(k_2^* + k_3^*)] \qquad (\text{mg min}^{-1}100\text{g}^{-1}), \quad [5.47]$$

where K_1^* through k_3^* are the rate constants for ^{18}F-FDG and *LC*, referred to as the lumped constant, is a combination of terms representing the ratio of the metabolic rates of FDG and glucose. The lumped constant takes into account the relative rates of transport and phosphorylation for FDG and glucose, which in turn are dependent on the steady-state distribution volumes and on the Michaelis-Menton constants (V_{max}, K_m) of FDG and glucose.

From Equation 5.47 it is clear that a measurement of the cold glucose level in plasma, an assumed value for the lumped constant, and estimates of K_1*, k_2*, and k_3* from a dynamic sequence of PET scans, provides a measure of the metabolic rate of glucose. However, one of the reasons that [^{18}F]-FDG has been so widely used in PET is that a simplified approach can be used that provides reliable estimates of the rate of metabolism. As first described for animal autoradiography using [^{14}C]-DG by Sokoloff et al. (75) and as later adapted to PET, an approximation of MR_{GLC} can be derived from a set of data acquired at a relatively late time postinjection. This was extremely important for autoradiographic studies, where only one data point can be obtained (since the animal is sacrificed), but also allows for human PET studies to be accomplished more conveniently.

This approach works because of the kinetics of DG and FDG. The rate of phosphorylation is reasonably high, while the rate of dephosphorylation is very low, and thus the radiotracer essentially is trapped once phosphorylated. The fraction of radiotracer residing in the trapped pool increases throughout the study. Since the clearance from tissue is relatively rapid, by 40 to 50 minutes the majority of radiotracer in tissue has been phosphorylated and a single "late" static image closely reflects the relative metabolic rate of glucose, as seen in Fig. 5.11. By assuming "population" average values for the individual rate constants for [^{18}F]-FDG (dropping the asterisks) and given a value for the cold glucose concentration

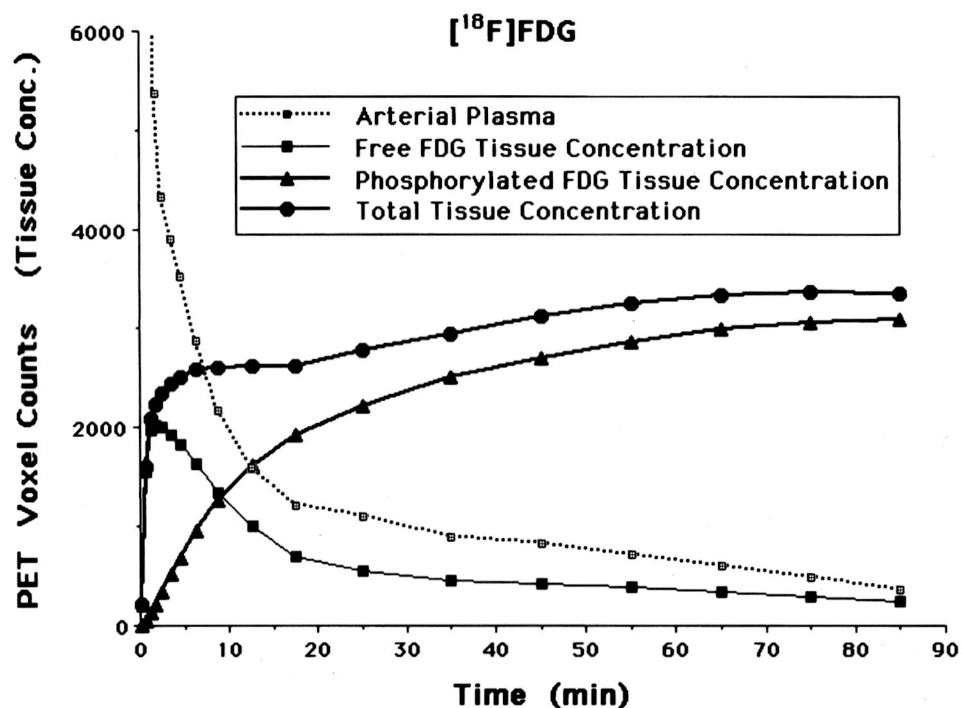

FIGURE 5.11. Time courses for free, phosphorylated, and total fluorine-18-fluorodeoxyglucose ($[^{18}F]$-FDG). Shown is the arterial plasma input function measured from discrete samples (*dashed line*), the calculated time courses for the radioactivity concentration in the free (*squares*) and phosphorylated (*triangles*) compartments, and the total tissue concentration measured by PET (*circles*). Note that the fraction of total measured radioactivity that is in the phosphorylated tissue compartment increases as time progresses. Because the activity in this compartment is metabolized FDG, a "late": PET scan 40 to 60 minutes or more after the injection, serves as a reliable index of glucose metabolism.

in plasma, a calculation for a "*population*" average MR_{GLC} can be obtained:

$$[MR_{GLC}]_{pop} = (C_p/LC)\ [(K_{1pop}\, k_{3pop})/(k_{2pop} + k_{3pop})]. \quad [5.48]$$

MR_{GLC} for an *individual* is then calculated by "correcting" the population average metabolic rate based on the static PET and arterial plasma input function measurements. The method assumes that the best correction factor for estimating an individual's regional metabolic rate is given by the ratio of the regional $[^{18}F]$-FDG concentration in the phosphorylated compartment for the individual, $[C_m]_{ind}$, to the population average, $[C_m]_{pop}$. Since $[C_m]_{ind}$ cannot be determined directly, it is best estimated by subtracting a calculation of the expected free concentration, $[C_f]_{pop}$, from the measured PET value, $[C_{tot}]_{ind}$:

$$[MR_{GLC}]_{ind} = [MR_{GLC}]_{pop} \times [\ \{[C_{tot}]_{ind} - [C_f]_{pop}\}/[C_m]_{pop}\ ]. \quad [5.49]$$

Note that $[C_{tot}]_{ind}$ is the measured PET data for the individual, while $[C_f]_{pop}$ and $[C_m]_{pop}$ are the calculated values of the free and phosphorylated compartments, respectively, based on *population* average rate constants, but the *individual's* arterial input function. $[C_f]_{pop}$ and $[C_m]_{pop}$ can be estimated from the solutions to their differential equations given in Equation 5.42 and the relationships described in Equation 5.41:

$$C_f(t) = [K_1/(\alpha_2 - \alpha_1)]\ [(k_4 - \alpha_1)e^{-\alpha_1 t} + (\alpha_2 - k_4)e^{-\alpha_2 t}] \otimes C_P(t)$$
$$C_m(t) = [K_1 k_3/(\alpha_2 - \alpha_1)][e^{-\alpha_1 t} - e^{-\alpha_2 t}] \otimes C_P(t), \quad [5.50]$$

where $\alpha_{1,2}$ are defined in Equation 5.41 and all *k*'s are *population* average rate constants for $[^{18}F]$-FDG.

Two alternative formulations (79,80) have been proposed for the correction factor in Equation 5.49. It should be emphasized that both the original and these alternative calculations are approximations of the true metabolic rate. Which approximation works best is dependent on how the individual's rate constants differ from the population average values. Propagation of errors for each of the methods differs and depends on several factors as discussed these two articles. It should also be emphasized that although there are some errors in each of these approximations, each has been shown to be relatively small in magnitude under the majority of conditions, and the general FDG method has proven to be an excellent technique for the measurement of glucose metabolism.

An example of how the concept of the steady-state volume of distribution is applied to PET is seen in the use of $[^{18}F]$-FDG for measuring glucose metabolism. The rate at which glucose is transferred from the free to the 6-PO_4 tissue compartment is equal to the rate of phosphorylation of glucose and is given by k_3C_f, as seen in Equation 5.43. Thus, if measuring the metabolic rate of glucose using kinetic modeling is of interest, estimating not only the rate constant for phosphorylation, k_3, but also the concentration of parent glucose in the free tissue compartment is needed. However, C_f is not known or easily measured. Since glucose is assumed to be in the steady state during the study, the steady-state volume of distribution of glucose in the free tissue compartment is given by Equation 5.44 and is equal to $K_1/(k_2 + k_3)$. Multiplying the arterial plasma concentration of glucose, C_P, by the steady-state volume of distribution yields an estimate of C_f for glucose. Therefore, k_3C_f, the rate at which glucose is metabolized, is given by k_3 times the plasma glucose concentration multiplied by the volume of distribution volume for free glucose, or $k_3C_P[K_1/(k_2 + k_3)]$ just as given in Equation 5.46.

Model Complexity: Trade-Off in Bias versus Precision

The *in vivo* behavior of many PET radiotracers is complex. A comprehensive model describing the kinetics of a tracer may require a compartmental configuration with many compartments and many rate parameters. Because of the statistical limits of the data and since PET measures only the *sum* of the radioactivity across all compartments, the actual models used for analysis must be simplified. Most PET radiotracers can support models with two to at most six parameters under the best of circumstances. When one attempts to estimate a large number of model parameters from a single dynamic PET study, parameter variance tends to be high. Variability in parameter estimates may be too high to permit reliable interpretation of the data, and thus the most accurate model descriptions become impractical to implement with PET. However, as less complex models are employed, parameter estimates may become biased and thus also may yield useless information. A tradeoff exists between bias and uncertainty in the model estimates that is controlled largely by the complexity of the model configuration. Methods of reducing model complexity include combining or lumping compartments (assuming that the compartments equilibrate rapidly) and assuming that values for certain model parameters are known. The optimal degree of model complexity needs to be considered carefully for each application.

The appropriate level of model complexity is dependent on what parameter is of greatest interest. The uncertainty in a model parameter that is of little physiological interest can be high as long as the error in its estimate does not propagate into the parameter of interest. Validity of the simplifying assumptions is also important. If, for example, a parameter is held at a fixed value in the model and the value may be in error by ± 50% but causes only a ± 5% bias in the parameter of interest, then this reduction in complexity is acceptable. However, if failure of a simplifying assumption is found to cause a 50% bias in the parameter of interest, then the model simplification is inappropriate. One should also consider whether the biases introduced by a given assumption are of approximately the same magnitude (and direction) across both regions and subjects. If so, then this model reduction may well be acceptable, while if not, the simplification should not be made. The ability to find the optimal level of model complexity is extremely important for successful interpretation of PET data. An analysis of model sensitivity can be used in conjunction with *a priori* knowledge of the expected parameter values and the particular hypotheses being investigated to determine the compartmental configuration with the optimal level of complexity. Other discussions on this topic are available for further reference (81–83).

Compartmental Models for Pharmacological Studies

Fig. 5.12A depicts the general compartmental model for pharmacological studies consisting of the arterial plasma compartment C_P and three tissue compartments representing free ligand in tissue (C_F), nonspecifically bound ligand (C_{NS}), and specifically bound ligand (C_{SP}). Six rate parameters describe exchange between the

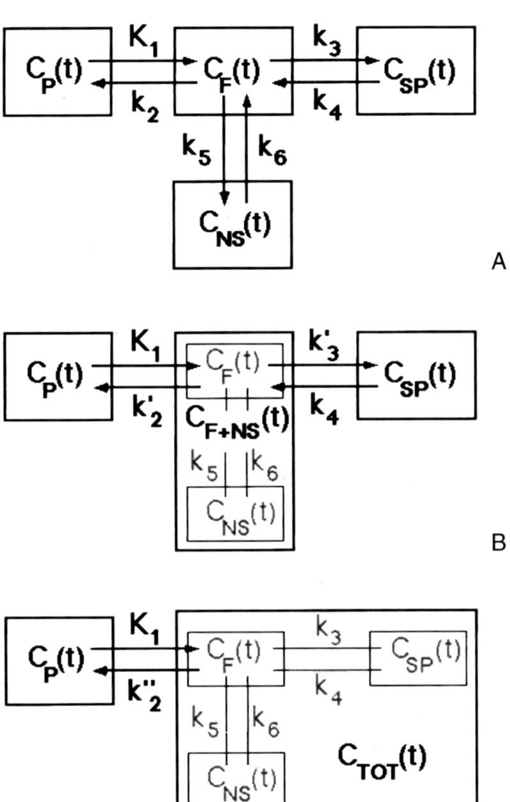

FIGURE 5.12. Compartmental model configurations for pharmacologic PET studies. **A:** A generalized model configuration describing many of the radioligands designed as pharmacologic markers. The model consists of the arterial plasma compartment C_P and three tissue compartments representing free ligand in tissue (C_F), nonspecifically bound ligand (C_{NS}), and specifically bound ligand (C_{sp}). In most applications, the statistical quality of the data cannot support estimation of the six rate constants; thus, simpler configurations are required for practical implementation. **B:** The most common simplification of combining free and nonspecific compartments is by assuming they equilibrate rapidly with one another. The kinetics of four rate constants k_2, k_3, k_5, and k_6 are approximated by two new parameters k_2' and k_3', which are equivalent to $k_2/(1 + k_5/k_6)$ and $k_3/(1 + k_5/k_6)$, respectively. The prime notation is used to indicate the lumping of two compartments into one. Note that the ratio k_5/k_6 is equivalent to the ratio of distribution volumes of the nonspecific to the free compartment as described in Equation 5.51. **C:** A model configuration that can be used when all tissue compartments equilibrate rapidly. In this scenario, a single tissue "clearance" constant k_2'' approximates five rate constants k_2 through k_6 by the relationship $k_2'' = k_2/(1 + k_3/k_4 + k_5/k_6)$. The ratio k_1/k_2'' yields the total tissue distribution volume $V_{d(TOT)}$. This approach may be useful when the ratio k_3/k_4 is the dominating component of the term $(1 + k_3/k_4 + k_5/k_6)$. This is equivalent to saying that the specific distribution is the dominating component of the total distribution volume ($V_{d(TOT)} = V_{d(F)} + V_{d(NS)} + V_{d(sp)}$).

model compartments. As discussed in the preceding section, the statistical quality of PET data usually is not sufficient for estimating this number of parameters, and thus the complexity of the model needs to be reduced. The first simplifying assumption made in most pharmacological applications is that the free and nonspecific binding compartments equilibrate rapidly. This allows combining them into a single compartment (C_{F+NS}). This two-tissue compartment configuration (Fig. 12B) has rate parameters defined as:

$$\begin{aligned} K_1 &= f(1 - e^{-PS/f}) = fE_o \\ k_2' &= K_1/V_{d(F+NS)} = (K_1/V_{d(F)})/(1 + V_{d(NS)}/V_{d(F)}) \\ k_3' &= (k_{on}B_{max})/(1 + V_{d(NS)}/V_{d(F)}) \\ k_4 &= k_{off} \end{aligned} \quad [5.51]$$

and thus:

$$\begin{aligned} k_3'/k_4 &= (k_{on}B_{max}/k_{off})/(1 + V_{d(NS)}/V_{d(F)}) \\ &= (B_{max}/K_D)/(1 + V_{d(NS)}/V_{d(F)}), \end{aligned} \quad [5.52]$$

where $V_{d(F)}$, $V_{d(NS)}$, and $V_{d(F+NS)}$ are the steady-state tissue distribution volumes of free ligand, nonspecifically bound ligand, and their sum, respectively, k_{on} is the bimolecular association rate between ligand and receptor (g pmol^{-1}min^{-1}), B_{max} is the binding site density or concentration of unoccupied binding sites (pmol g^{-1}), k_{off} is the dissociation rate of ligand from the binding site complex (min^{-1}), and K_D is the equilibrium dissociation constant for the specific binding site (pmol g^{-1} or nM). The prime symbols on k_2' and k_3' are used to differentiate these rate constants from the true k_2 and k_3 that describe rates of exchange from the compartment containing only free ligand. The ratio B_{max}/K_D is commonly called the binding potential, while the term $(1+V_{d(NS)}/V_{d(F)})$ reflects the apparent increase in the volume of the binding precursor pool when combining free and nonspecific compartments. Thus, $1/(1 + V_{d(NS)}/V_{d(F)})$ [$= V_{d(F)}/(V_{d(F)} + V_{d(NS)})$] describes the fraction of radiolabel available ("free") either for transport back to plasma or binding and is equivalent to the term f_2 often used to designate the free fraction in tissue. The distribution volumes of free plus nonspecific, specific, and total binding sites are defined in the same manner as those in Equation 5.45:

$$\begin{aligned} V_{d(F+NS)} &= K_1/k_2' \\ V_{d(SP)} &= (K_1/k_2') \times (k_3'/k_4) = (K_1/k_2) \times (k_3/k_4) \\ &= V_{d(F)}(B_{max}/K_D) \\ V_{d(TOT)} &= V_{d(F+NS)} + V_{d(SP)} = (K_1/k_2') \times (1 + k_3'/k_4) \\ &= V_{d(F+NS)} + V_{d(F)}(B_{max}/K_D). \end{aligned} \quad [5.53]$$

An additional model simplification can be made if the rates of association and dissociation from the specific binding site are rapid compared to the transport parameters, K_1 and k_2, reducing the model to a single tissue compartment (Fig. 5.12C), described by K_1 and only an additional rate constant k_2'' giving the *net* clearance from tissue. The total volume of distribution $V_{d(TOT)}$ ($= K_1/k_2''$) has the same definition as in the two-tissue compartment configuration given by Equation 5.53. How closely the $V_{d(TOT)}$ estimates from the two-model configurations agree will depend on how rapidly free and bound compartments equilibrate (i.e., the validity of the simplifying assumption).

The primary goal of a pharmacological study is to provide a reliable index of binding site density or whatever other pharmacological parameter is being studied. In the ideal this would be a direct quantitative measure of B_{max}, the density of available binding sites; however, for practical reasons this may not be possible. As defined in Equations 5.51 through 5.53, other parameters or combinations of parameters relate to binding density, which might provide more reliable measures of binding density. These include k_3 ($= k_{on}B_{max}$), k_3/k_4 ($= B_{max}/K_D$), k_3'/k_4 ($= f_2B_{max}/K_D$), $V_{d(SP)}$ ($= V_{d(F)}[B_{max}/K_D]$), and $V_{d(TOT)}$ ($= V_{d(F+NS)} + V_{d(F)}[B_{max}/K_D]$). The distribution volume estimates, particularly $V_{d(TOT)}$, are functions of more than just binding site density and therefore contain additional intrinsic bias compared to either k_3 or k_3/k_4. However, the precision of distribution volume estimates typically is much better than that of individual rate constants. For every radiotracer, one needs to determine which measure yields the optimal tradeoff between bias and precision and the greatest sensitivity to changes in binding site density.

Data Acquisition Considerations for Compartmental Modeling

In general, compartmental modeling and tracer kinetic analysis require the acquisition of two sets of data—the radioactivity time courses in blood and tissue—in order to yield estimates of physiologic parameters. This section discusses the methodological issues related to measuring these two sets of data. It is very obvious that the quality of the PET data directly affects the reliability of the estimated model parameters. It should be stressed that for compartmental modeling applications that require arterial input functions, equal attention should be paid to obtaining accurate estimates of the arterial plasma concentration curves.

Measurement of the Radiotracer Concentration in Arterial Plasma

Interpretation of the kinetic behavior of a radiotracer, as indicated by Equation 5.39, requires knowledge of the amount of radiotracer being supplied to the tissue. In other words, the level of radioactivity in a particular tissue at any given time is dependent both on the amount of radioactivity delivered to the tissue (the input function) and by what happens to the radiotracer once in the tissue (the tissue response function). Measurement of the amount of radioactivity delivered to the tissue typically is accomplished by acquiring discrete arterial plasma samples, usually from a radial artery, and measuring the radioactivity in a well counter. For cardiac applications, it is possible to derive the input function from PET imaging of the heart blood pool. Although this is relatively straightforward, several additional issues need to be considered.

Red Blood Cell Radioactivity

For many PET radiopharmaceuticals, the radioactivity in arterial plasma is the portion of the total blood-borne radioactivity that is available for transport into the tissue. This is not the case for all radiotracers. If the radiotracer can diffuse rapidly between plasma and red cells, then radioactivity in red cells is available for transport into the tissue. However, if the equilibration time between red cells and plasma is much longer than a single capillary transit, then only radiotracer in the plasma is available for transport, and thus the concentration time course in plasma alone should be used as the input function.

Binding to Plasma Proteins

Another consideration is whether the radiotracer binds to plasma proteins. If this is the case, as occurs with many highly lipophilic tracers, there will be a decreased amount of radiotracer available for transport resulting in a decreased extraction fraction and hence apparent decrease in blood–brain barrier permeability. As with red cells, the possibility of tracer bound to plasma proteins being able to dissociate and cross the capillary membrane during a single capillary transit needs to be considered.

Radiolabeled Metabolites

Another consideration for determining the arterial input function is the possibility of the radiolabel being converted to a chemical form different from that of original radiotracer. This is an issue in many neuroreceptor studies where radiolabeled metabolites of the authentic ligand are found in blood. Since radiolabeled metabolic by-products are formed *in vivo*, the fraction of metabolites in the blood generally increases with time, necessitating a time-dependent correction. This correction is often possible by chromatographic analysis of each or selected blood samples to determine the fraction of plasma radioactivity that is in the form of the authentic ligand (84). There is, however, a requirement that the labeled metabolites are not transported from blood into tissue. Any labeled metabolites that can enter tissue would require inclusion in the compartmental model, necessitating a second input function for the radiolabeled metabolite and a second set of rate constants describing the kinetic behavior of the metabolite in tissue. The statistical quality of PET data generally does not support the estimation of these additional parameters, and thus PET ligands that produce metabolites that cross the capillary membrane are poor candidates for success.

Fig. 5.13 shows a typical input function obtained from a radioligand study of the benzodiazepine receptor system using

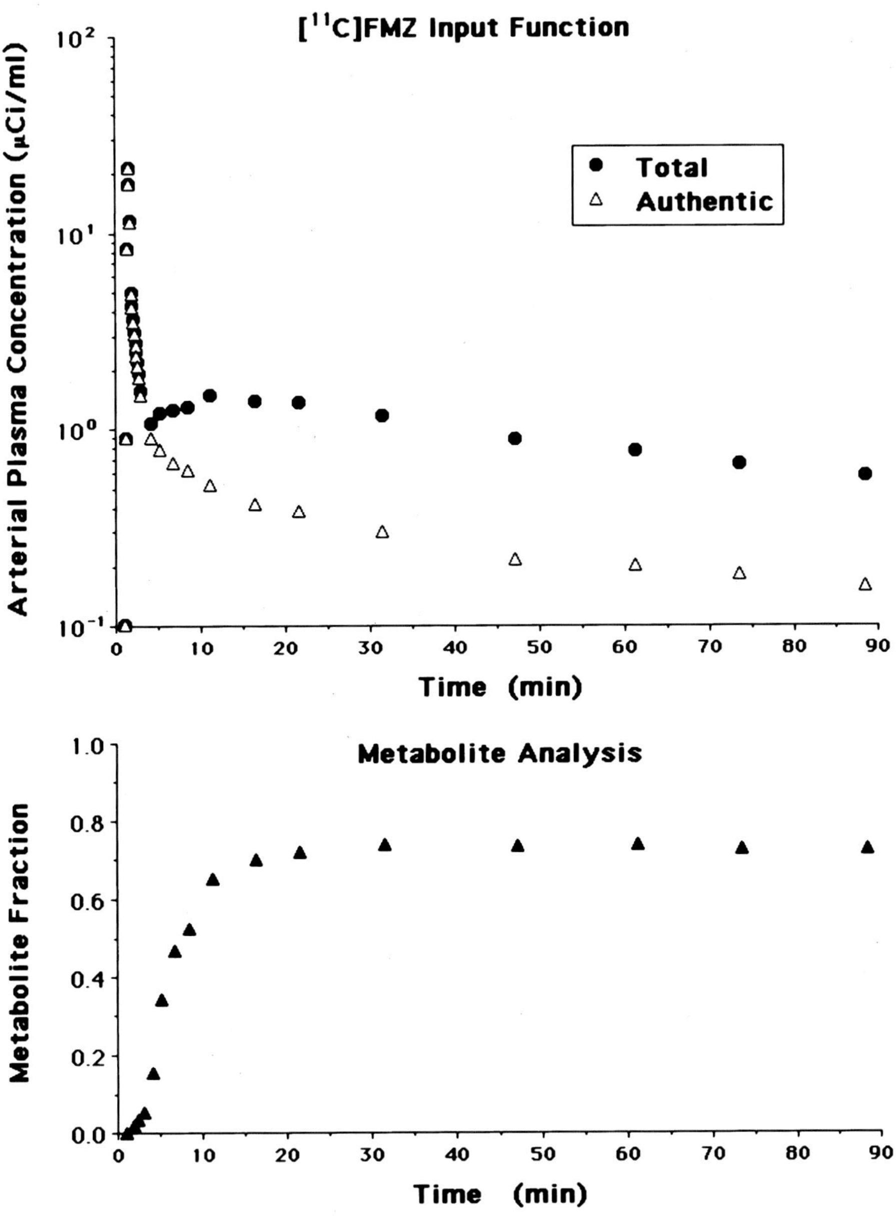

FIGURE 5.13. Arterial input function measurement. A measured input function (**top**) for the radiotracer carbon-11-flumazenil ([^{11}C]-FMZ), a benzodiazepine antagonist. Shown is the total radioactivity concentration (*filled circles*) measured by a sodium iodide well counter from discrete blood samples acquired from the radial artery and spun in a centrifuge separating plasma from red blood cells. As with many PET ligands, radiolabeled metabolites may form in the blood or peripheral tissues and must be accounted for. The relative amounts of authentic and metabolized radiotracer can be determined by chromatographic techniques. Shown are the results (**bottom**) of such a determination, plotting the fraction of total radioactivity in the plasma that is in the form of labeled metabolites over the duration of the study. [^{11}C]-FMZ metabolites are seen to increase rapidly after administration and appear to equilibrate rather quickly at a fraction of about 75%. The metabolite component is then removed from the measure of total radioactivity, to yield just the concentration of authentic [^{11}C]-FMZ (*open triangles in the top*). This curve is used as the input function for compartmental analysis.

[^{11}C]-flumazenil (FMZ). The top panel is a semilog plot showing both total radioactivity in the arterial plasma (filled circles) and the level of authentic [^{11}C]-FMZ only (open triangles). The bottom panel shows the fraction of total activity in the plasma that arises from radiolabeled metabolites. Note that the metabolite fraction monotonically increases, with most rapid production of metabolites early after administration of [^{11}C]-FMZ followed by an apparent equilibration between metabolites and authentic ligand pools at a ratio of about three or four to one. The corrected input function shown in the top panel equals the total plasma radioactivity multiplied by one minus the metabolite fraction.

Measurement of the Tissue Time Activity Curves

The second set of data required for kinetic modeling is the tissue concentration time course measured by the PET scanner. For quantitative modeling studies, it is assumed that all appropriate corrections were made to the acquired PET data and that the image reconstruction algorithms have provided the best possible estimate of the radiotracer's concentration in tissue. In addition, the sensitivity analysis can be used to help determine the scanning sequence required for kinetic analysis. Radiotracers having more rapid kinetics require shorter duration scan frames. Fig. 5.14 shows typical PET time activity curves in the brain for four different radiotracers: [^{15}O]-water (upper left); [^{11}C]-FMZ a benzodiazepine antagonist for measuring receptor density (upper right); [^{13}N]-ammonia for measuring myocardial perfusion (lower left); and [^{11}C]-acetate for measuring oxidative metabolism (lower right). Note that due to the different half-lives of the tracers, the range of scan times can vary dramatically. Some tracers, such as [^{15}O]-water and [^{11}C]-FMZ, enter and leave the tissue rapidly, some, such as [^{11}C]-acetate, enter and leave much more slowly, and while others, such as [^{13}N]-NH_3, are trapped in tissue for long periods of time.

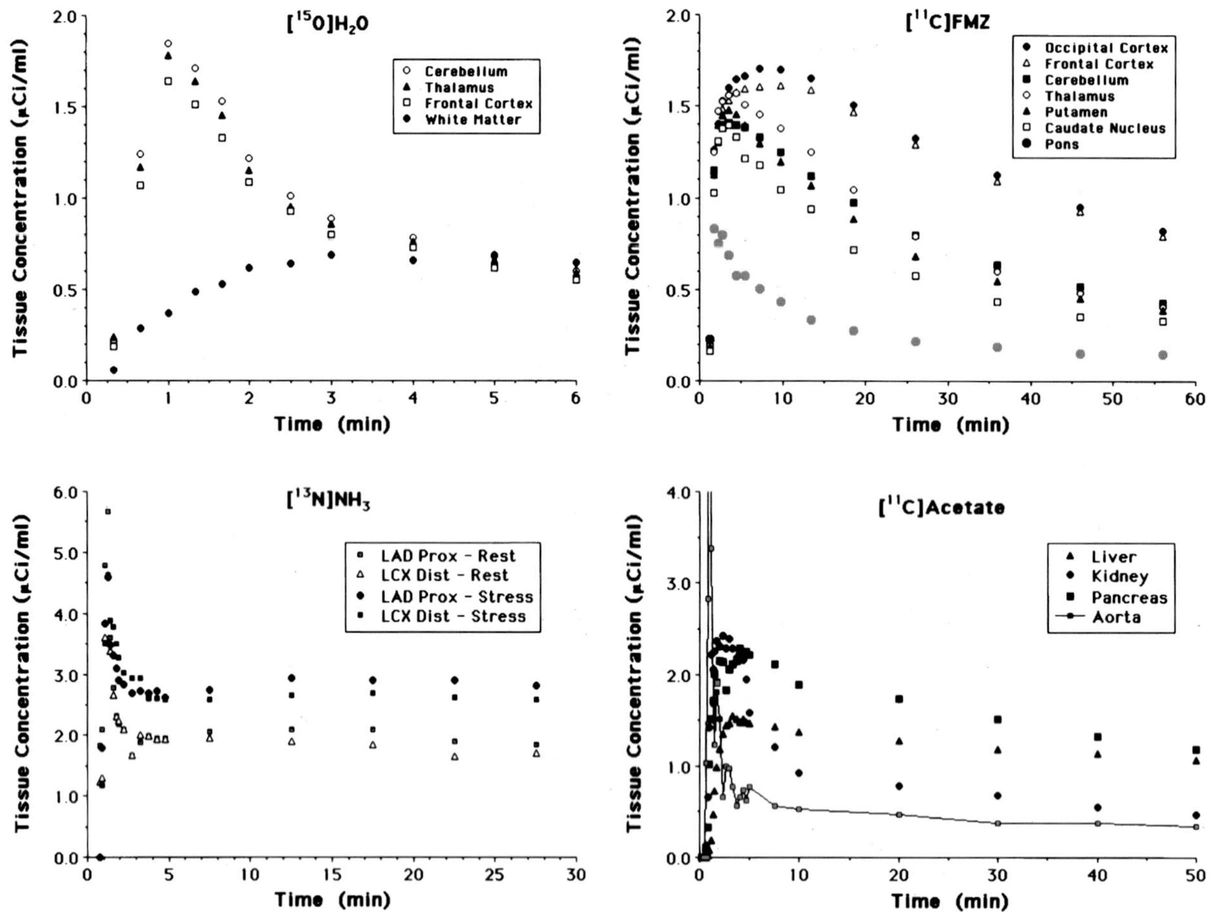

FIGURE 5.14. PET time-activity curves (TACs). Shown are typical PET TACs for four different radiotracers: $H_2{}^{15}O$ used for measuring blood flow (**upper left**); carbon-11-flumazenil for measuring receptor density (**upper right**); [^{13}N]-ammonia for measuring myocardial blood flow (**bottom left**); and [^{11}C]-acetate for measuring oxidative metabolism (**bottom right**). The two sets of curves on the top are from brain studies. Cerebral blood flow is seen to be high in gray matter structures and low in white matter. Benzodiazepine receptor density is high in cortical structures, moderate in cerebellum, deep gray nuclei, and very low in pons and other brainstem structures. The cardiac ammonia study shows curves for both rest and dipyridamole (a coronary vasodilator) stress studies in the regions of the proximal left anterior descending artery (*LAD prox*) and the distal left circumflex artery (*LCX dist*). There is increased uptake of [^{13}N]-ammonia during the stress study, indicating increased flow. Very different tissue kinetics are observed between kidney, liver, and pancreas for the oxidative metabolism study using [^{11}C]-acetate.

Contribution of Blood-Borne Radioactivity

An important issue not addressed to this point is that the measured PET data include detected events from any body component that happens to be in the FOV. Although as previously stated a PET scan measures the radiotracer concentration in *tissue*, every region imaged, whether it is heart, brain, tumor, or another organ, is composed of a mixture of *tissue* and *blood* since these cannot be separated completely at PET resolution. Unless the tissue and blood concentrations are identical, the tissue concentration cannot equal exactly the concentration measured by the tomograph. For example, shortly after a bolus administration, the blood concentration is much higher than the tissue concentration. Thus, although only a small fraction of the space being imaged is blood, the detected events coming from blood-borne radioactivity may comprise a considerable portion of the total signal (85). This is a considerable problem for cardiac studies where the volumes of interest are directly adjacent to large blood pools and it is hard to obtain data without vascular contamination, made even more difficult by heart motion due to both the cardiac and respiratory cycles.

The blood-borne component is more important for radiotracers with low extraction fractions since the tissue concentration rises more slowly. PET measurements, rather than being a direct estimate of the radiotracer concentration in tissue $C_T(t)$, are given by:

$$PET_i = CBV \int_i C_{blood}(t) + (1 - CBV) \int_i C_T(t), \quad [5.54]$$

where $C_{blood}(t)$ is the mean concentration in the blood pool within the region and *CBV* is the cerebral blood volume given as a fraction of the total imaging volume (mL blood mL^{-1} imaging volume). It should be emphasized that the total blood concentration time course, $C_{blood}(t)$, is not the same as the input function $C_P(t)$, since blood consists of red cell, plasma, and plasma protein components; arterial, capillary, and venous components; and may include radiolabeled metabolites. The appropriate model equations for the tissue concentration $C_T(t)$, such as those for single or two compartment models, are inserted into Equation 5.51. *CBV* can be considered as an additional model parameter that can be either (a) estimated in the fitting procedures, (b) estimated by some additional measurement, or (c) assumed to be known and fixed at a constant value.

Parameter Estimation

Parameter estimation routines should provide optimal estimates of the model parameters. In order to be "optimal" there must be a particular criterion that is used as a measure of goodness of fit. This criterion is often called the cost function or optimization function. Values for the parameters are adjusted so that the cost function is either minimized or maximized depending on the function. The most commonly used optimization criterion in PET studies is least squares, where the cost function is defined as the squared discrepancy between the measured PET data and the values predicted by the compartmental model equations summed over the temporal sequence of scans. The optimal parameter values are defined to be those that yield the minimum sum of squared discrepancies, or as the name implies, the least-squares fit to the data. Included in calculation is appropriate weighting of the data based on the known or measured variances in the reconstructed image values. The weighted sum of squared discrepancies is termed the chi-squared value (χ^2). Another optimization criterion is maximum likelihood, as is commonly used in iterative reconstruction, where parameter values are selected such that the measured data values are statistically the most probable to have occurred. The cost function for maximum likelihood estimation varies depending on the assumptions about the data. Least-squares estimation provides the maximum likelihood estimation under the conditions that the errors in the measured data are independent, uncorrelated, follow a Gaussian distribution, and have uniform error variance across the measurements. In practice, however, some or all of these conditions are not met, and the least-squares solution is only an approximation of the maximum likelihood solution.

Nonlinear Regression Techniques

The most common methods for obtaining least-squares estimates from kinetic PET studies fall into the category of regression techniques. Both linear and nonlinear regression methods are used. Although the majority of PET studies require nonlinear regression, simpler linear regression methods can be applied in some cases. A model is said to be linear and thus linear techniques can be applied if the model equation consists only of terms that are linear with respect to each of the model parameters to be estimated. Linear regression has the advantage of being a very rapid means for estimating parameters since there is an analytic solution that provides the least-squares solution to the regression equations.

Most PET radiotracers are not described by linear models and thus require nonlinear regression. In general, nonlinear regression cannot be performed analytically but must be approached in an iterative manner, which, as was noted for image reconstruction, is far more computationally intensive. The standard procedure is to provide initial estimates of each of the unknown model parameters. From this guess, an initial chi-square value is calculated. Consider an n-dimensional set of χ^2 values comprising all numerical combinations of the n parameters. The goal is now to search this n-dimensional space for the global minimum. This location specifics the optimal or best fit set of model parameters (K_1, k_2, ... k_n). There are several possible routines to "search" χ^2 space for the minimum. One common approach, referred to as a gradient search, as described by Marquardt (86) and Bevington (87), updates all parameters simultaneously. The local gradient in χ^2 space is calculated at the point specified by the current set of parameter values. The direction in the n-dimensional parameter space, along which the value of χ^2 changes most rapidly, is determined. The magnitudes of the parameter values are adjusted so that the travel on the χ^2 surface is along the direction of steepest descent. An updated χ^2 value is calculated for the new point in parameter space and is compared to the previous value. This procedure is repeated until the difference between the current and previous χ^2 value is less than some prespecified limit.

The methods of linear and nonlinear regression analysis are designed to provide the least-squares or optimal estimates for the parameters of a given model. However, this does not guarantee that the model applied was appropriate or, even if appropriate, that the optimal values provide stable and reproducible estimates of the model parameters. The χ^2 value also can be used to assess how well the predicted data values describe the actual measured results. The reduced chi-squared, χ^2_ν, is defined as chi-squared divided by the number of degrees of freedom, which is given by the number of independent observations (data points) minus the number of parameters estimated from the data minus 1. It can be shown that χ^2_ν is equivalent to the ratio of the estimated variance of the fit to the estimated true variance in the data. The estimated variance of the fit is dependent on both the dispersion of the data and the accuracy of the fit, while the true variance is dependent only on the dispersion of the data. Thus, the reduced chi-square provides a useful measure of goodness of fit. If the fitting function for the compartmental model contributes no additional variance, then χ^2_ν will have a value of 1. Therefore, if the model describing the measured data is appropriate, the χ^2_ν value will be close to unity; however, if the model does not fit the data well, the estimated variance increases and χ^2_ν values will be significantly greater than 1.

An additional use of the reduced chi-squared value is to assess the relative performance of two different model configurations, as when testing whether a single tissue compartment model is sufficient to describe the kinetics of a radiotracer or whether two tissue compartments are required. The ratio of two χ^2_ν distributions can be shown to follow an F distribution. The F-statistic is used to assess if inclusion of additional model parameters significantly improves the goodness of fit.

Another method of assessing the goodness of fit is to examine a plot of the difference between the measured and predicted data values, termed the residuals. If the model configuration accurately describes the measured data, then the residuals from the least-squares fit will be distributed randomly about zero. The plots of the residuals versus time shown in Fig. 5.15 demonstrate the utility of visual examination. The upper panels show a data set and the least-squares fit for a single tissue compartment model on the left and the plot of the residuals from this fit on the right. The lower panels show the same data set with the least-squares fit for a model with two tissue compartments (*left*) and the plot of its residuals (*right*). Note that while the goodness of fit for the two models are visually similar, with the more complex model yielding only a modestly better fit (as can be seen from the points around the peak concentration), examination of the residuals clearly indicates the superiority of a model with two tissue compartments for describing the data.

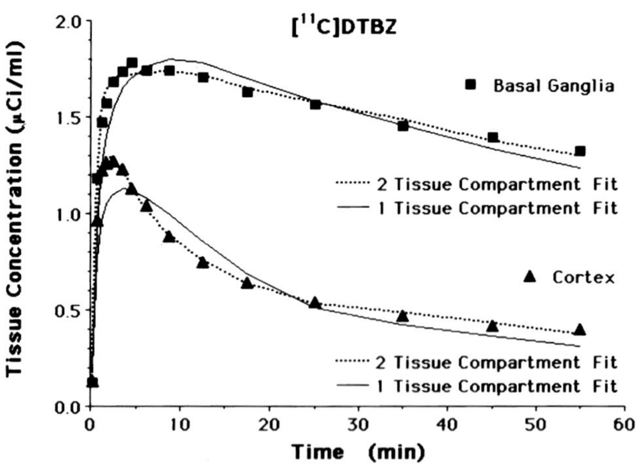

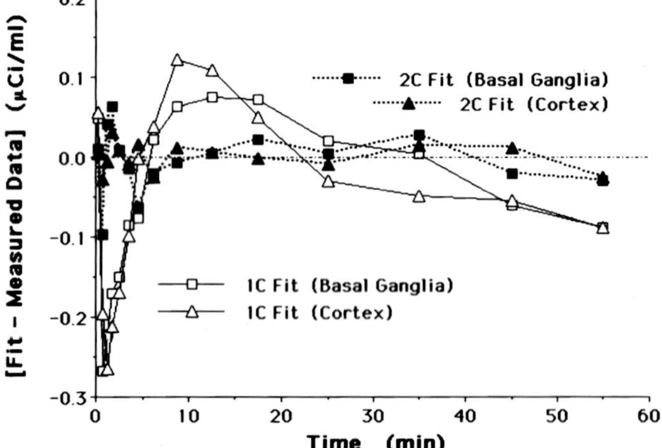

FIGURE 5.15. Least-square fits and residuals for model configurations with one- and two-tissue compartments. Shown are the time activity curves (**top plot**) for the vesicular monoamine transporter marker carbon-11-dihydrotetrabenazine ([^{11}C]-DTBZ) and best-fit model solutions using least-squares optimization. Shown are fits to basal ganglia (*squares*) and cortex (*triangles*) using both a single-tissue compartment with two rate parameters (*solid lines*) and a two-tissue compartment with four rate parameters (*dashed lines*). Although the appearance of the fits for the two model configurations is similar, analysis of the residuals indicates that goodness of fit is superior for the more complex model, particularly at time points near the peak radioactivity concentration. These differences can be seen more clearly in the residuals (**bottom plot**). The residuals give the difference between the best-fit model prediction and the measured data. There are large negative errors shortly after injection for the one-compartment fits. These fits then consistently overestimate the measured data between 5 and 25 minutes after injection and finally again underestimate the later time points. This is compared with the relatively small and random errors resulting from fits using a model configuration with two tissue compartments (*dashed lines*).

Specialized Graphical Approaches

There are certain applications where a simplified graphical or linear approach can be used to provide estimates of the quantity of interest. Although the compartmental model may not be linear with respect to all model parameters, it is sometimes possible to reformulate the model equations so that a linear relationship exists between the data and the primary quantity being measured. Two such approaches deserve mention as they have been used for analysis in hundreds of PET studies. One approach is used with irreversible radiotracers and is called a Patlak plot, while the other is used with reversible radiotracers and is called a Logan plot. For both methods, the linear fitting procedure provides excellent stability against the noise from the dynamic PET measurements.

Patlak analysis estimates the net rate of radiotracer accumulation in an irreversible compartment (88). This approach was applied initially for estimation of glucose metabolic rate from dynamic data rather than from a static scan requiring assumptions about the population average rate constants. Patlak analysis yields an estimate of $K_1k_3/(k_2 + k_3)$, which is the combination of parameters needed to calculate MR_{GLC} as given in Equation 5.47. This is accomplished by performing linear regression on the tissue concentration divided by the plasma concentration as a function of the integral of the plasma concentration divided by the plasma concentration:

$$\frac{C_T(T)}{C_P(T)} = [K_1k_3/(k_2 + k_3)]\frac{\int_0^T C_P(t)dt}{C_P(T)} + [K_1k_2/(k_2 + k_3)^2]. \quad [5.55]$$

This plot, the Patlak plot, becomes linear over time with a slope of $K_1k_3/(k_2+k_3)$ (sometimes written as K) and an intercept of $K_1k_2/(k_2+k_3)^2$. Visual examination of a Patlak plot provides an indication of whether the irreversibility assumption is valid. Although this approach is excellent for measuring *net* incorporation, that is, $K_1k_3/(k_2+k_3)$, one should not assume that every radiotracer that yields a linear Patlak plot should be analyzed by this approach. In many applications, such as receptor studies using irreversible ligands, binding-site density is the biologic function of interest. The parameter k_3 and not the combination of parameters $K_1k_3/(k_2+k_3)$ yields an index of binding. The Patlak slope is dependent both on the binding or trapping rate and on the transport rate constants, K_1 and k_2. This is appropriate for estimating MR_{GLC} but not receptor density. When the value of k_3 is high relative to the transport parameters, $k_3/(k_2+k_3)$ approaches 1 and the slope reflects K_1, not binding. Under such conditions, uptake is said to be flow or delivery limited. It is interesting to note this is the exact principle that radiolabeled microsphere flow measurements are based on. One measures the *net* trapping of the microspheres, yet since trapping is instantaneous ($k_3 \rightarrow \infty$), the rate of trapping directly reflects flow.

Logan analysis provides a related approach for analysis of reversible radiotracers (89). The Logan plot is based on the relationship:

$$\frac{\int_0^T C_T(t)dt}{C_T(T)} = [V_{d(TOT)}]\frac{\int_0^T C_P(t)dt}{C_T(T)} + [INT], \quad [5.56]$$

where $V_{d(TOT)}$ is determined by linear regression of the integral of the tissue activity divided by the instantaneous activity versus the integral of the plasma activity divided by the tissue activity. What is especially useful is that this approach is applicable for models with any number of serial compartments as long as each is reversible. The plot eventually becomes linear with a slope equal to the total radiotracer volume of distribution. For a tracer that can be described by a single-tissue compartment, the plot is linear over all time. As additional compartments are required, the time to reach linearity increases. The intercept (INT) has physiological meaning and for a single-compartment model is approximately equal to k_2^{-1}. Thus, the slope divided by the negative of the intercept yields an estimate of the transport parameter, K_1.

Parameter Estimation without Arterial Input Functions

Another group of specialized parameter estimation techniques are those that avoid the need for arterial plasma sampling. Since arterial sampling is somewhat invasive, is often labor intensive, and can increase errors in the parameter estimates if not performed properly, an approach that does not require blood samples appears very attractive. Although there have been several different strategies for avoiding blood sampling, the most common has been the use of "reference regions" for the analysis of neuroreceptor binding studies. The focus on this particular strategy in this section gives examples of three specific reference region approaches. A reference region is defined as a region within the image FOV that contains no specific binding sites. For each of these approaches it is assumed that the reference region has the same free plus nonspecific volume of distribution as all other regions. Thus, the reference region can be used as a measure of the amount of free plus nonspecific uptake to subtract from the $V_{d(TOT)}$ to arrive at an estimate of the *specific* binding.

Logan et al. (90) developed a reference region method based on an extension of their work described in the preceding section. In the reference region Logan plot, the ratio of distribution volumes (DVR) between a given tissue region and the reference region is determined from the slope of the straight-line portion of a plot of the following relationship:

$$\frac{\int_0^T C_T(t)dt}{C_T(T)} = [DVR]\frac{[\int_0^T C_{RR}(t)dt + C_{RR}(T)/k_2]}{C_T(T)} + [INT], \quad [5.57]$$

where C_{RR} is the PET measure for reference region and $DVR = V_{d(TOT)}/V_{d(RR)}$. The ratio of the slope over the negative of the intercept is related to the ratio of transport rate constants (K_1R) between target and reference volumes. The binding potential (BP) is then given by:

$$BP = V_{d(SP)}/V_{d(RR)} = (V_{d(TOT)} - V_{d(RR)})/V_{d(RR)} = DVR - 1, \quad [5.58]$$

and is equal to the estimate of the slope of the plot, DVR, minus 1.

The reference tissue model (RTM) of Lammertsma and Hume (91) has several similarities to the Logan approach. The RTM equation is derived from the differential equations describing the time rate of change in the tracer's concentration in both tissue and reference regions based on a common arterial plasma input. The simultaneous solution to those equations, eliminating the blood term yields:

$$\int_0^T C_T(t)dt = [K_1R]\int_0^T C_{RR}(t)dt + [k_2 - K_1R\,k_2/(1 + BP)]\int_0^T C_{RR}(t)dt \otimes e^{-[k_2/(1+BP)]t}. \quad [5.59]$$

This model has three parameters, K_1R, k_2, and BP. Standard nonlinear least-squares analysis yields estimates of the three terms in square brackets and hence the three model parameters.

The final reference region approach is to use estimates of the equilibrium ratio of the radiotracer's tissue concentrations in the tissue and in the reference region. BP is given simply by:

$$BP = (C_{T[eq]} - C_{RR[eq]})/C_{RR[eq]}, \quad [5.60]$$

where the concentrations are measured directly by PET under equilibrium conditions, thus requiring a continuous infusion protocol rather than a simple bolus injection of the radiotracer.

Model Validation

Once parameters have been estimated, one should quantify the overall performance of the kinetic model. One should establish not only how well the model configuration describes the kinetics of the radiotracer and how accurately the parameters can be estimated, but that the final results make sense and are consistent with known information about the system being measured.

Besides comparison to other direct or accepted measures, as mentioned previously, another means of physiologic validation is to show that as biological processes change, the compartmental analysis can detect these changes and also to show that these changes are specific to the appropriate parameters of the model. For example, if a compartmental model is used to measure the brain uptake and binding density of a particular ligand, then the compartmental model should be able to distinguish between changes in the delivery of ligand to the brain and the density of binding. Two experiments are performed to validate this specificity: (a) an intervention that changes delivery but not binding, and (b) an intervention that changes binding density. An example of a pair of such experiments for [^{11}C]-flumazenil, a rapidly reversible benzodiazepine antagonist analyzed using a single-tissue compartment model, is shown in Figs. 5.16 and 5.17. The first intervention was performed using an eyes closed/eyes open paradigm to change cerebral blood flow and hence tracer delivery (92). Fig. 5.16 shows that K_1 increased 30% in the visual cortex during the stimulus scan, while $V_{d(TOT)}$ was unchanged. For the second intervention, scans were acquired before and after a partial blocking dose of 0.012 mg/Kg cold FMZ. This was administered 40% by bolus just prior to the second study and 60% by constant infusion over the duration of the scan. Fig. 5.17 shows that specific binding estimates were decreased by about 40% throughout the brain.

A similar validation study was performed using the radiotracer N-[^{11}C]-methylpiperidinyl propionate (PMP), a substrate for hydrolysis by the enzyme acetylcholinesterase (AChE). [^{11}C]-PMP is irreversibly hydrolyzed by AChE and thus a two-tissue compartment three-parameter model is used to analyze the data (93). Two PET studies were acquired, pre- and postadministration of a dose of the AChE inhibitor physostigmine (94), designed to inhibit approximately 50% of the AChE activity. Compartmental estimates of the model parameter k_3, the index for AChE enzyme activity, are shown in Fig. 5.18 and are seen to be 40% to 50% decreased following physostigmine.

COREGISTRATION OF THREE-DIMENSIONAL DATA SETS

Many scientific and clinical questions can be answered better through the use of *multiple* sets of 3D image data. For applications involving PET this includes many scenarios: (a) a dynamic sequence of scans following the injection of a single radiotracer, as is acquired for most compartmental modeling studies;(b) a scan following each of several injections of the same radiotracer, as is acquired for functional activation studies using repeat injections of [^{15}O]-water; (c) scans following the injection of different radiotracers, such as the use of both [^{11}C]-raclopride and [^{11}C]-DTBZ to image multiple aspects of the dopamine system, or both [^{11}C]-methionine and [^{18}F]-FDG in a clinical study on a brain tumor patient; (d) scans from different modality imaging techniques in

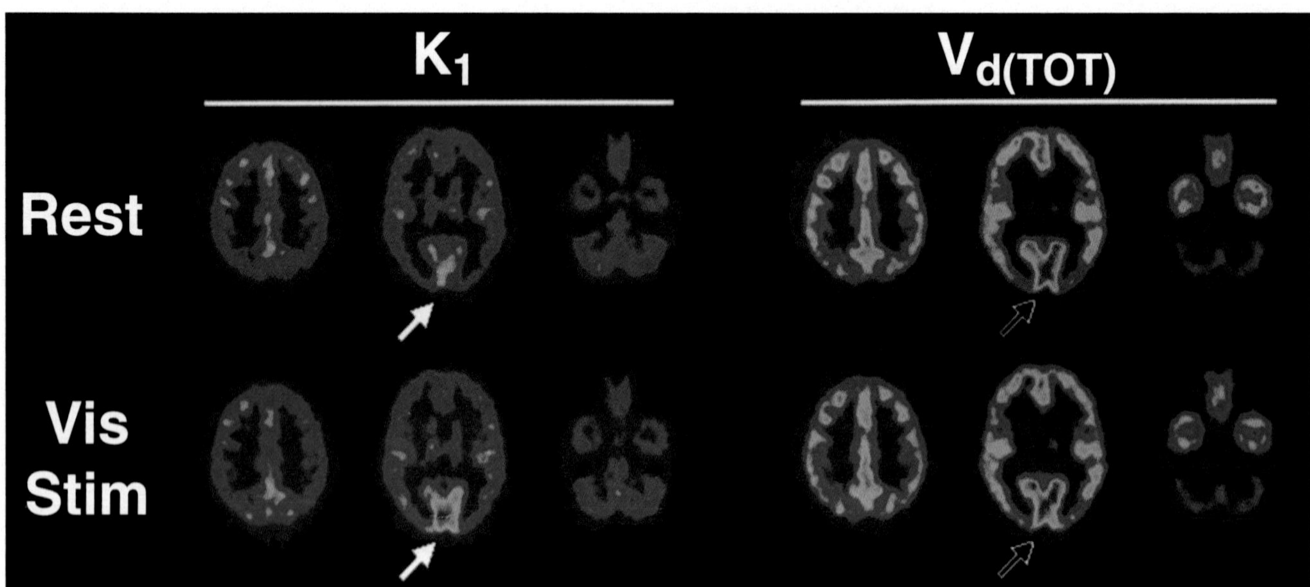

FIGURE 5.16. Model validation: specificity of parameter estimates. Shown are functional images of two parameters, K_1 (**left**) and $V_{d(TOT)}$ (**right**), for carbon-11-flumazenil ([^{11}C]-FMZ) estimated using a single tissue compartment model at three transverse levels of the brain. Calculations were performed voxel by voxel. The top set of images was acquired during a study with the eyes closed. The bottom set of images are from a second study on the same subject, but with visual stimulation and the eyes open. The large increase in tracer uptake due to increased flow is seen clearly in the visual cortex region of the K_1 image (*solid arrows*). In the corresponding slice there was no change in the estimate of $V_{d(TOT)}$, the index of receptor density (*open arrows*). This validation study demonstrates the specificity of the receptor density measure, $V_{d(TOT)}$, due to its insensitivity to changes in flow.

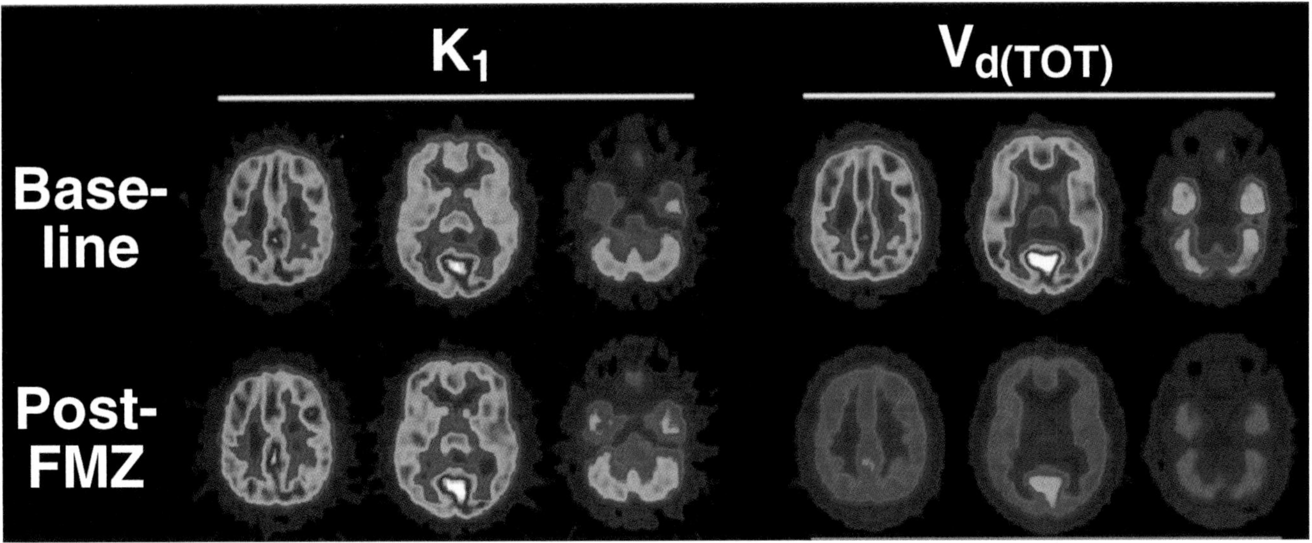

FIGURE 5.17. Model validation: sensitivity of parameter estimates; single-tissue compartment model. Shown are a similar set of functional images from a pair of carbon-11-flumazenil ([^{11}C]-FMZ) studies on another individual, but with the two scans being performed before and following administration of a partial blocking dose of unlabeled FMZ. The transport estimate is nearly identical before and after administration of cold FMZ, while a global decrease of 35% to 40% is seen in the receptor density measure $V_{d(TOT)}$. This validation study demonstrates the sensitivity of the receptor measure to changes in binding site availability.

addition to PET, such as or SPECT, MR, or x-ray CT, the latter two providing the capability of matching function with structure; and (e) scans across different individuals.

In order to make the best use of these multiple 3D images sets, one needs to be certain that extraction (either visual or quantitative) of information from the different data sets is accomplished in a consistent manner. An important first step is to be able to coregister the various image sets to one another: both intra- and intermodality and intra- and intersubject. Coregistration may involve only rigid-body transformation (translate, rotate) for intrasubject applications, but

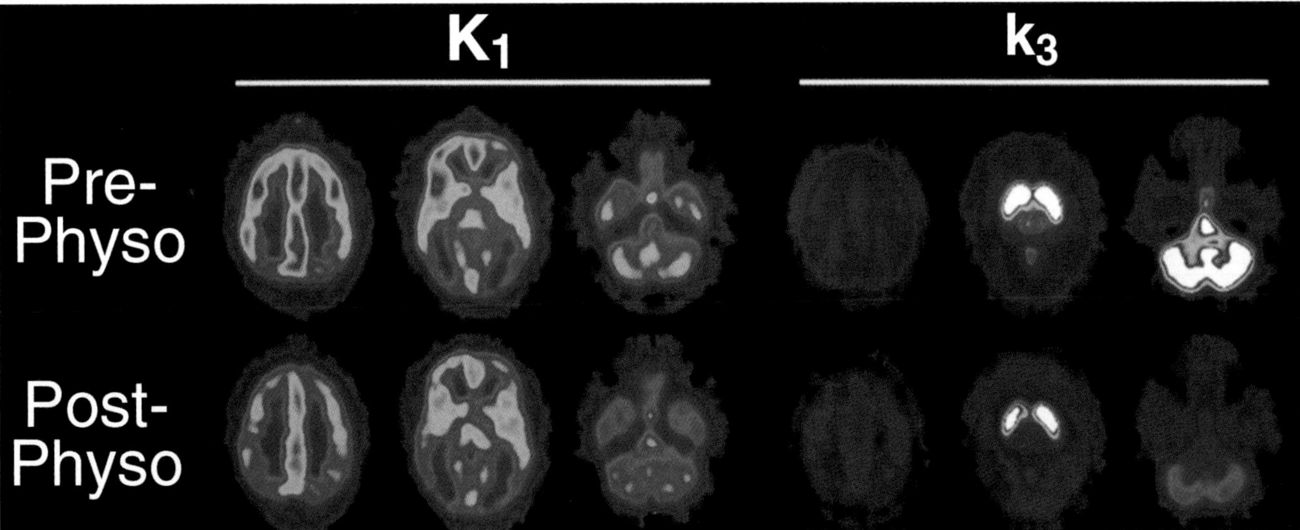

FIGURE 5.18. Model validation: sensitivity of parameter estimates; two-tissue compartment model. Shown are functional images from a pair of scans using N-carbon-11-methylpiperidinyl propionate (PMP), a substrate for the enzyme acetylcholinesterase (AChE). The top images were acquired at baseline, while the bottom images were acquired following administration of 1.5 mg physostigmine (Physo), an AChE inhibitor. The distribution of AChE is seen to vary widely across the brain with enzyme activity, being 20 to 25 times higher in basal ganglia than in cortex (making visual display of the k_3 images difficult). The brain uptake as measured by K_1 is seen to have decreased slightly, while the index of AChE activity is decreased by approximately 50% in all brain regions (most easily seen in cerebellum and brainstem). This validation study demonstrates the sensitivity of the index of AChE activity, k_3, to changes in the concentration of the enzyme.

may also involve nonlinear deformations to register images to a standardized coordinate system.

Intrasubject, Intramodality Registration

The simpler of the above scenarios are the ones involving multiple PET data sets acquired from a single subject. All scans from a single subject have the same underlying anatomy, and all scans acquired using the same modality have many additional similarities, such as resolution. The early strategies to ensure coregistration of multiple scans from the same subject involved physical restraints. Even with such devices, the small amount of movement that occurs cannot be ignored (95). Another early strategy was to use external positron-emitting markers (96). This approach worked reasonably well for brain studies; however, application of external marker methods to whole-body imaging proved problematic. There is greater physiological motion and variation in patient positioning during imaging, and it soon became evident that skin surface anatomy did not always accurately reflect the location of internal structures. Even for brain studies, the skin is not rigidly fixed to the skull, and, therefore, registration accuracy is limited. Although external landmark methods were very fast, they were not sufficiently accurate.

The next step in registration involved user defined landmarks within the image sets. This approach relies on the ability of an expert user identifying a series of points that represent identical locations in each image set. For rigid body registration only three points are needed in each image set, while for nonlinear deformation many more points are needed. The obvious limitation of such approaches, even for rigid-body registration, is that specification of such points cannot be accomplished with perfect accuracy. One way found to improve accuracy of rigid-body registration involves selecting more than three landmarks and using a fitting routine known as the Procrustes algorithm to minimize the sum of the squared discrepancies between homologous landmarks (97). It was demonstrated empirically that approximately 15 landmarks provided registration accuracy of about 0.5 mm (98). These methods, while providing reasonably accurate rigid-body registration, are not as practical for registration that requires nonlinear deformations. Furthermore, the time required for the user to accurately specify the landmarks is substantial.

The limitations encountered in the above approaches prompted work on registration algorithms that are fully or near fully automated. A variety of automated registration routines were proposed in the early 1990s, all based on image similarity but with several different criteria or cost functions used to optimize registration of the two image sets. These have included maximizing the cross correlation between image sets (99), minimizing the variance in the ratio of image sets (100), minimizing either the absolute or squared difference between images (101), and maximizing the number of voxels within a fixed difference between two image sets (102). All of these techniques are robust, work well with PET data, are easy to implement, and are rapid to perform. Registration of multiple [^{15}O]-water scans can be accomplished with an accuracy of better than 0.5 mm for translations and 0.5 degrees for rotations. The final criterion uses an adjustable threshold instead of just the random noise properties and thus is less sensitive to the noise level in the images.

For the image sets that differ greatly from one another, registration strategies not relying on image similarity become necessary. One such method is based on mutual information (MI) or relative entropy (103,104). Such routines are applicable for intramodality registration, but are especially useful for intermodality registration, and thus will be discussed below.

Intrasubject, Intermodality Registration

Accurate registration of PET with other modalities is becoming increasingly valuable. For brain studies, registration of functional and anatomic images has been used to correct for atrophy and as a means to define volumes of interest for subsequent data analyses. Both in research and more recently in clinical practice, there has been great interest in registering whole-body [^{18}F]-FDG PET with CT images from oncology patients, then overlaying the image sets for accurate viewing of the correspondence between regions of high FDG uptake and the underlying anatomic structure. There has also been considerable interest in using coregistered PET/CT images to aid in radiation-therapy planning for lung and other cancers. The push for the ability to display multimodal or "fused" images showing both functional and structural information is such that combined PET/CT systems have recently been introduced by major medical imaging companies. Although having both PET and CT devices within the same gantry will greatly aid this cause, it still is essential to ensure that registration between the image sets is extremely accurate. Small misregistration of PET and MR causes large errors in tissue atrophy measures. Similarly, accurate registration of PET and CT is essential if PET is to be useful in radiotherapy treatment planning for oncology patients. This section reviews briefly the methods, both historical and current, for functional/ structural image registration.

Early registration methods used external contrast markers (radioactive sources for PET, gadolinium for MR, iodine for CT). These methods provide a reasonable first-order registration, but for the same reasons as for intramodality registration, their usefulness is limited. Another general approach for PET-MR/CT registration is based on surface matching. Segmentation defining the body surface is performed on the transmission (or sometimes emission) PET data sets and on the MR or CT images. The two image sets are aligned by minimizing the sum of the distances or squared distances between corresponding points on the two 3D surfaces (105,106). This method has been shown to work reasonably well, but still yields only 1 to 3 mm accuracy. Another method has been a user-driven interactive approach (107). This technique uses superimposed PET and MR (or CT) data sets, displayed simultaneously as transverse, coronal, and sagittal cuts through the body at user-selected levels. The user has full control over the three translation and the three rotational degrees of freedom. This approach is reproducible and again fairly accurate with errors typically less than 2 mm. However, it requires considerable user expertise and time to register a pair of image sets. The Procrustes approach also has been used for cross-modality registration, but suffers from the same problem related to time and user expertise.

As with intramodality registration, fully (or near fully) automated routines have become the standard. These are user independent, reproducible, and more accurate. The two most commonly used approaches for registration of PET data sets with either CT or MR are (a) a method referred to as automated image registration (AIR) (108,109), based on the matching of voxel intensities, and (b) methods based on maximization of mutual information (110,111) as mentioned previously.

AIR is included as part of the SPM (statistical parametric mapping) packages widely used for functional neuroimaging applications and are available over the Internet (e.g., SMP99; Wellcome Department of Cognitive Neurology: http://www.fil.ion.ucl.ac.uk/spm). The voxel intensity approach used by AIR requires segmentation of the anatomic image set into tissue types and some degree of image preprocessing prior to registration. Accuracy is dependent on the quality of both functional and anatomic data, but with current systems, errors are on the order of 1 mm.

Mutual information has proven to be a very usual approach to multimodality image registration. MI is a basic information theory concept that measures the statistical dependence between two random variables or, for this application, two image sets. Thus, MI quantifies the amount of information that an image set from one modality contains about the image set from the other modality. Because no assumptions are made regarding the relationship between the voxel values of the two sets, the method is general and can be applied automatically. For these reasons, MI offers greater flexibility than AIR. The algorithm requires little or no preprocessing and minimal user interaction (user removal of external body tissues is not required).

The mutual information between two variables (or image sets) X and Y is define as:

$$I(X, Y) = \sum_x \sum_y p_{XY}(x, y) \log \left(\frac{p_{XY}(x, y)}{p_X(x) p_Y(y)} \right), \quad [5.61]$$

where p_X and p_Y are the probability density functions of X and Y, respectively, and $p_{X,Y}$ is their joint probability function. MI is also related to entropy by:

$$I(X, Y) = H(X) + H(Y) - H(X, Y), \quad [5.62]$$

where $H(X)$ and $H(Y)$ give the entropy of X and Y, respectively, and $H(X,Y)$ gives their joint entropy:

$$\begin{aligned} H(X) &= -\sum_x p_X(x) \log (p_X(x)) \\ H(Y) &= -\sum_y p_Y(y) \log (p_Y(y)) \quad [5.63] \\ H(X, Y) &= -\sum_x \sum_y p_{XY}(x, y) \log (p_{XY}(x, y)) \end{aligned}$$

The implementation of MI at the University of Michigan by Meyer et al. (111) (MiamiFuse) allows for either affine or nonlinear warping registration via thin-plate splines (112) (TPS). The basic routine consists of the following steps. Approximate control points are selected in each image set. From these points, the geometric mapping from one image set (homologous) to the other (reference) is computed. This transform is then applied to the entire homologous data set to obtain data set pairs for this current estimate of the coregistration. From these data pairs, the joint 2D histogram is created and the MI calculated. Next, an optimizing algorithm adjusts the coordinates of the control points from the homologous image set with the goal of maximizing the resultant MI between the reference and the transformed homologous image set. From the adjusted control points for the homologous image set and the original control points of the reference set, a new mapping is computed. This process is repeated until the MI is maximized.

Figs. 5.19 and 5.20 demonstrate two applications of intermodality registration. Fig. 5.19 shows results from a research study

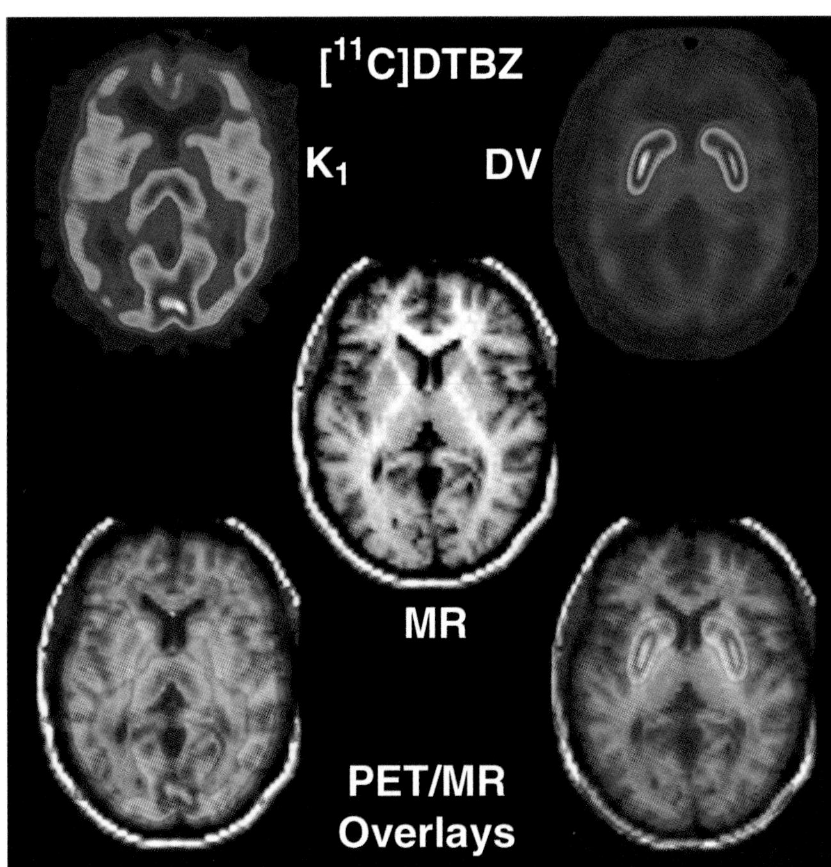

FIGURE 5.19. Functional and anatomic image registration: PET and magnetic resonance (MR). Shown for a single transverse level of the brain are functional images of the two model parameters for carbon-11-dihydrotetrabenazine ($[^{11}C]$-DTBZ), K_1, and $V_{d(TOT)}$ (**top left and right,** respectively), and the coregistered image of the corresponding brain level from an MR scan of the same subject (**middle**). The overlays of the two functional images are seen superimposed on the coregistered structural MR image in the bottom corners. PET and MR data sets were registered by maximization of their mutual information (see text).

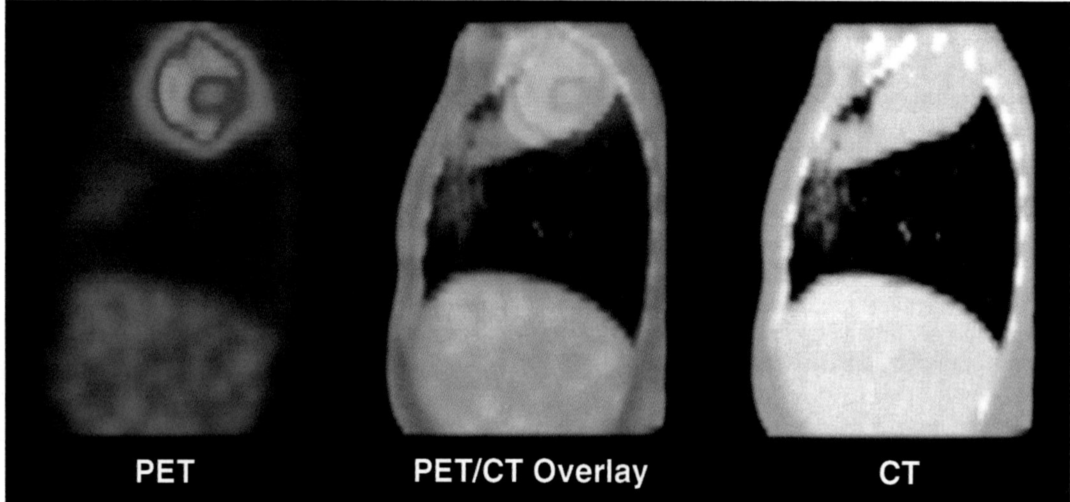

FIGURE 5.20. Functional and anatomic image registration: PET and CT. Shown for a single sagittal section of the body are a functional image of glucose metabolism using fluorine-18-fluorodeoxyglucose ([^{18}F]-FDG) (**left**), the corresponding coregistered image from a CT scan of the same subject (**right**), and the overlay of functional and anatomic information (**middle**). PET and CT data sets were registered by maximization of their mutual information and includes nonlinear warping by thin-plate splines (see text) to account for different body positions of the subject in the PET and CT gantries.

using [^{11}C]-DTBZ to measure VMAT2 binding site density. Two parametric image sets are obtained from the dynamic sequence of PET scans. One represents the transport rate (K_1) of radioligand into the brain (*upper left*) and the second represents its total tissue distribution volume ($V_{d(TOT)}$), an index of the vesicular transporter density (*upper right*). These were estimated by kinetic analysis following intermodality coregistration of the dynamic PET data set. The center image shows the comparable slice from an MR study on the same subject after coregistration by MI maximization. Overlays of both functional PET parameters on the coregistered MR are shown in the bottom images.

Fig. 5.20 shows images of a coregistered [^{18}F]-FDG PET scan with x-ray CT for a cancer patient. Two different transaxial levels of the PET study are shown (*left*), and the corresponding levels of the CT, after registration by MI, are also shown (*right*). The middle pair of images present the fusion of functional and anatomic information.

Intersubject Registration

This section concludes with a brief description of methods to register data sets across subjects. Intersubject registration is important when assessing the same PET measures across one or more groups of subjects. Standardized coordinate systems have been used for a variety of imaging applications for more than a decade with the vast majority focused on the brain. The first PET study attempting to coregister different individuals into a standardized coordinate system (113) employed the stereotactic atlas of Talairach and Tournoux (114), thus the use of the term stereotactic coordinates. In this original approach, transformation of the PET data set into stereotactic coordinates was based on the use of both a PET scan and a lateral skull x-ray for determining the line connecting the anterior and posterior commissures (AC-PC line). Subsequently, routines have been developed that require only the PET data, first an interactive routine (115) and then a completely automated approach (116,117). Initial implementations used only linear scaling of the image sets and did not include nonlinear warping. It was soon understood that nonlinear warping was needed to improve registration across subjects. The first fully automated method for nonlinear warping of PET images used a 3D thin-plate spline approach (118). Other "standardized" coordinate systems have been introduced, such as the brain atlas developed by the International Consortium on Human Brain Mapping (ICBM) (119). A current typical procedure for registering brain scans across subjects starts by intrasubject, intermodality affine registration of each subject's PET and MR (or CT) scans. This is followed by nonlinear warping of the subject's MR image set (since MR has better anatomic detail than PET) to the ICBM standard brain via TPS and MI. The same mapping is then applied to the subject's coregistered PET data to transform the functional images into ICBM coordinates.

The introduction of functional MR has been responsible for a tremendous increase in the amount of work done in the area of registration and nonlinear warping. Currently, much of the work related to intersubject registration and nonlinear deformation of data occurs outside the field of PET. A more detailed discussion of these endeavors is outside the scope of this chapter.

REFERENCES

1. Radon J. Über die Bestimmung von Funktionen durch ihre integralwere längs gewisser Mannigfaltigkeiten [On the determination of functional from their integrals along certain manifolds]. *Ber Saechs Akad Wiss Leipzig Math-Phys Kl* 1917;69:262–277.
2. Cormack A. Representation of a function by its line integrals, with some radiological applications. *J Appl Phys* 1963;34:2722–2727.
3. Cormack A. Representation of a function by its line integrals, with some radiological applications II. *J Appl Phys* 1963;35:2908–2913.

4. Bracewell RN. Strip integration in radio astronomy. *Aust J Phys* 1956;9:189–217.
5. DeRosier DJ, Klug A. Reconstruction of three-dimensional images from electron micrographs. *Nature* 1968;217:130–134.
6. Oldendorf WH. Isolated flying spot detection of radiodensity discontinuities—displaying the internal structural pattern of a complex object. *IRE Trans Biomed Electronics BME* 1961;8:68–72.
7. Kuhl DE, Edwards RQ. Image separation radioisotope scanning. *Radiology* 1963;80:653–661.
8. Hounsfield GN. Computerized transverse axial scanning (tomography): part 1. Description of system. *Br J Radiol* 1973;46:1016–1022.
9. Wrenn FR, Good ML, Handler P. The use of positron-emitting radioisotopes for the localization of brain tumors. *Science* 1951;113: 525–527.
10. Sweet WH. Uses of nuclear disintegrations in the diagnosis and treatment of brain tumors. *N Engl J Med* 1951;245:875.
11. Brownell GL, Sweet WH. Localization of brain tumors with positron emitters. *Nucleonics* 1953;11:52.
12. Anger HO, Rosenthal DJ. Scintillation camera and positron camera. In: *Medical radioisotope scanning*. Vienna: International Atomic Energy Agency and the World Health Organization, 1959:59–82.
13. Rankowitz S, Robertson JS, Higinbotham WA. Positron scanner for locating brain tumors. *IRE Int Conv Rec* 1962;9(10):49–56.
14. Robertson JS, Marr RB, Rosenblum B, et al. 32-crystal positron transverse section detector. In: Freedman GS, ed. *Tomographic imaging in nuclear medicine*. New York: Society of Nuclear Medicine, 1973: 142–153.
15. Kuhl DE, Edwards RQ. The Mark 3 scanner: a compact device for multiple-view and section scanning of the brain. *Radiology* 1970;96: 563–770.
16. Kuhl DE, Edwards RQ, Ricci AR, et al. The Mark IV system for radionuclide computed tomography of the brain. *Radiology* 1976;121:405–413.
17. Gordon R. Herman GT. Three-dimensional reconstruction from projections: a review of algorithms. *Int Rev Cytol* 1974;38:111–151.
18. Brooks RA, DiChiro G. Principles of computer assisted tomography (CAT) in radiographic and radioisotopic imaging. *Phys Med Biol* 1976;21:689–732.
19. Budinger TF, Gullberg GT. Three dimensional reconstruction in nuclear medicine emission imaging. *IEEE Trans Nucl Sci* 1974;21:20.
20. Shepp LA, Vardi Y. Maximum likelihood reconstruction for emission tomography. *IEEE Trans Med Imaging* 1982;2:113–122.
21. Hudson HM, Larkin RS. Accelerated image reconstruction using ordered subsets of projection data. *IEEE Trans Med Imaging* 1994;13:601–609.
22. Defrise M, Kinihan PE. Data acquisition and image reconstruction for 3D PET. In: Townsend DW, ed. *The theory and practice of 3D PET*. Dordrecht: Kluwer, 1998:1–53.
23. Kinihan PE, Rogers JB. Analytic 3D image reconstruction using all detected events. *IEEE Trans Nucl Sci* 1989;36:964–968.
24. Cho ZH, Ra JB, Kilal SK. True three-dimensional reconstruction—application of algorithm towards full utilization of oblique rays. *IEEE Trans Med Imaging* 1983;2:6–18.
25. Stearns CW, Chesler DA, Brownell GL. Accelerated image reconstruction for a cylindrical positron tomograph using Fourier domain methods. *IEEE Trans Nucl Sci* 1990;37:773–777.
26. Defrise M, Townsend DW, Clack R. FAVOR: a fast reconstruction algorithm for volume imaging in PET. In: *Conference Recording of the IEEE 1991 Nuclear Science Symposium*. Santa Fe, New Mexico. 1992: 1919–1923.
27. Stazuk MW, Rogers JG, Harrop R. Full data utilization in PVI using the 3D radon transform. *Phys Med Biol* 1992;37:689–704.
28. Daube-Witherspoon ME, Muehllehner G. Treatment of axial data in three-dimensional PET. *J Nucl Med* 1987;28:1717–1724.
29. Defrise M, Kinihan PE, Townsend DW, et al. Exact and approximate rebinning algorithms for 3D PET data. *IEEE Trans Med Imaging* 1997;16:145–158.
30. Kinihan PE, Defrise M, Townsend DW, et al. Fast iterative image reconstruction of 3D PET. In: *Conference Recording of the IEEE 1996 Nuclear Science Symposium*. Santa Fe, New Mexico. 1997:1918–1922
31. Comtat C, Kinihan PE, Defrise M, et al. Fast reconstruction of 3D data with accurate statistical modeling. *IEEE Trans Nucl Sci* 1998;45:1083-1089.
32. Fessler JA. Penalized weighted least-squares image reconstruction for positron emission tomography. *IEEE Trans Med Imaging* 1994;13: 290–300.
33. Liu X, Comtat C, Michel C, et al. Comparison of 3D reconstruction with 3D-OSEM and with FORE-OSEM for PET. *IEEE Trans Med Imaging* 2001;20:804–814.
34. Qi J, Leahy RM, Cherry SR, et al. High-resolution 3D Bayesian image construction using the microPET small-animal scanner. *Phys Med Biol* 1998;43:1001–1013.
35. Qi J, Leahy RM, Hsu C, et al. Fully 3D Bayesian image reconstruction for the ECAT EXACT HR+. *IEEE Trans Nucl Sci* 1998;45:1096–1103.
36. Leahy RM, Qi J. Statistical approaches in quantitative positron emission tomography. *Stat Comput* 2000;10:147–163.
37. Anger HO. Survey if radioisotope cameras. *Trans ISA* 1966;5:331–334.
38. Brownell GL, Burnham CA, Wilenski, S, et al. New developments in positron scintigraphy and the application of cyclotron-produced positron emitters. In: *Medical radioisotope scintigraphy*. Vienna: International Atomic Energy Agency, 1969:163–176.
39. Budinger TF. Time-of-flight positron emission tomography: status relative to conventional PET. *J Nucl Med* 1983;24:73–78.
40. Allemand R, Gresset C, Vacher J. Potential advantages of a cesium fluoride scintillator for a time-of-flight positron camera. *J Nucl Med* 1980;21:153–155.
41. Mullani NA, Ficke DC, Hartz R, et al. System design of a fast PET scanner utilizing time-of-flight. *IEEE Trans Nucl Sci* 1981;28:104–107.
42. Ter Pogossian MM, Ficke DC, Yamamoto M, et al. Super-PETT I: a positron emission tomograph utilizing time-of-flight information. *IEEE Trans Med Imaging* 1982;1:179–187.
43. Ludziejewski T, Moszynska M, Moszynski M, et al. Advantages of LSO scintillator in nuclear physics experiments. *IEEE Trans Nucl Sci* 1995;42:328–336.
44. Moszynski M, Ludziejewski T, Wolksi D, et al. Timing properties of GSO, LSO and other Ce doped scintillators. *Nucl Instr Meth* 1996;A372:51–58.
45. Moses WW, Derenzo SE. Prospects for time-in-flight PET using LSO scintillator. *IEEE Trans Nucl Sci* 1999;46:474–478.
46. Moszyński M, Kapusta M, Nassalski A, et al. New prospects for time-of-flight PET with LSO scintillators. *IEEE Trans Nucl Sci* 2006; 53(5):2484–2488.
47. Surti S, Kuhn A, Daube-Witherspoon M, et al. Measurements for TOF image quality gain in 3D PET and its implications for clinical imaging. *J Nucl Med* 2006;47:196P.
48. Casey M, Panin V, Bendriem B. Early clinical experience with time-of-flight PET. *J Nucl Med* 2006;47:184P.
49. Tomitani T. Image reconstruction and noise evaluation in photon time-of-flight assisted positron emission tomography. *IEEE Trans Nucl Sci* 1981;NS28:4582–4589.
50. Snyder DL, Thomas LJ, Ter-Pogossian MM. Early clinical experience with time-of-flight PET. *J Nucl Med* 2006;47:184P.
51. Defrise M, Casey ME, Michel C, et al. Fourier rebinning of time-of-flight PET data. *Phys Med Biol* 2005;50:2749–2763.
52. Vandenberghe S, Daube-Witherspoon ME, Robert M, et al. Fast reconstruction of 3D time-of-flight PET data by axial rebinning and transverse mashing. *Phys Med Biol* 2006;51:1603–1621.
53. Bailey DL, Grootoonk S, Kinahan PE, et al. Quantitative procedure in 3D PET. In: Townsend DW, ed. *The theory and practice of 3D PET*. Dordrecht: Kluwer, 1998:88–98.
54. Yavuz M, Fessler JA. Penalized-likelihood estimators and noise analysis for random-precorrected PET transmission scans. *IEEE Trans Med Imaging* 1999;18:665–674

55. Yavuz M, Fessler JA. Maximum likelihood emission image reconstruction for random-precorrected PET scans. In: *Conference Recording of the 2000 IEEE Nuclear Science Symposium Medical Imaging Conference.*
56. Bailey DL, Grootoonk S, Kinahan PE, et al. Quantitative procedure in 3D PET. In: Townsend DW, ed. *The theory and practice of 3D PET.* Dordrecht: Kluwer, 1998:57–87.
57. Erdogan H, Fessler JA. Monotonic algorithms for transmission tomography. *IEEE Trans Med Imaging* 1999;18:801–814.
58. Erdogan H, Fessler JA. Ordered subsets algorithms for transmission tomography. *Phys Med Biol* 1999;44:2835–2851.
59. Kinahan PE, Townsend DW, Beyer T, et al. Attenuation correction for a combined 3D PET/CT scanner. *Med Phys* 1998;25(10):2046–2053.
60. Carney J, Beyer T, Brasse D, et al. CT-based attenuation correction for PET/CT scanners in the presence of contrast agent. In: *IEEE Nuclear Science Symposium Conference Record.* 2003:1443–1446.
61. Nehmeh SA, Erid YE, Halaigian H, et al. Correction for oral contrast artifacts in CT attenuation-corrected PET images obtained by combined PET/CT. *J Nucl Med* 2004;44:1940–1944.
62. Berthelsen AK, Holm S, Loft A, et al. PET/CT intravenous contrast can be used for PET attenuation correction in cancer patients. *Eur J Nucl Med Mol Imaging* 2004;32:1167–1175.
63. Qiao F, Yue U, Pan T, et al. Segmentation of contrast enhanced CT images for attenuation correction of PET/CT data. In: *IEEE Nuclear Science Symposium Conference Record.* 2004:2686–2689.
64. Nuyts J, Stoobants S. Reducation of attenuation correction artifacts in PET/CT. In: *IEEE Nuclear Science Symposium Conference Record.* 2005:1895–1899.
65. Martinez-Möller, Souvatzoglou M, Navab N, et al. Artifacts from misaligned CT in cardiac perfusion PET/CT studies: frequency, effects, and potential solutions. *J Nucl Med* 2007;48:188 193.
66. Nehmeh SA, Erdi YE, Ling CC, et al. Effect of respiratory gating on reducing lung motion artifacts in PET imaging of lung cancer. *Med Phys* 2002;29(3):366–371.
67. Beyer T, Antoch G, Blodgett T, et al. Dual-modality PET/CT imaging: the effect of respiratory motion on combined image quality in clinical oncology. *Eur J Nucl Med Mol Imaging* 2003;30:1333–1338.
68. Boucher L, Rodrigue S, Lecomte R, et al. Respiratory gating for 3-dimensional PET of the thorax: feasibility and initial results. *J Nucl Med* 2005;45:214–219.
69. Pan T, Mawlawi O, Nehmeh SA, et al. Attenuation correction of PET images in respiration-averaged CT imaged in PET/CT. *J Nucl Med* 2005;46:1481–1487.
70. Beyer T, Antoch G, Blodgett T, et al. Respiratory gating of cardiac PET data in list-mode acquisition. *Eur J Nucl Med Mol Imaging* 2006;33: 584–588.
71. Godfrey K. *Compartmental models and their application.* New York: Academic Press, 1983.
72. Gjedde A. Calculation of cerebral glucose phosphorylation from brain uptake of glucose analogs in vivo: a re-examination. *Brain Res Rev* 1982;4:237–274.
73. Lassen NA, Perl W. *Tracer kinetic methods in medical physiology.* New York: Raven Press, 1979.
74. Carson RE. Parameter estimation in positron emission tomography. In: Phelps ME, Mazziotta JC, Schelbert HR, eds. *Positron emission tomography and autoradiography, principles and applications for the brain and heart.* New York: Raven Press, 1986:347–390.
75. Sokoloff L, Reivich M, Kennedy C, et al. The (C-14) deoxyglucose method for the measurement of local cerebral glucose utilization: theory, procedure and normal values in the conscious and anesthetized albino rat. *J Neurochem* 1977;28:897–916.
76. Reivich M, Kuhl D, Wolf A, et al. The [^{18}F] fluorodeoxyglucose method for the measurement of local cerebral glucose utilization in man. *Circ Res* 1977;44:127–137.
77. Phelps ME, Huang SC, Hoffman EJ, et al. Tomographic measurement of local cerebral glucose metabolic rate in humans with (F-18)2-Fluoro-2-Deoxy-D-Glucose: validation of method. *Ann Neurol* 1979;6:371–388.
78. Huang S-C, Phelps ME, Hoffman EJ, et al. Non-invasive determination of local cerebral metabolic rate of glucose in man. *Am J Physiol* 1980;238:E69–E82.
79. Brooks RA. Alternative formula for glucose utilization using labeled deoxyglucose. *J Nucl Med* 1982;23:540–549.
80. Hutchins GD, Holden JE, Koeppe RA, et al. Alternative approach to single-scan estimation of cerebral glucose metabolic rate using glucose analogs, with particular application to ischemia. *J Cereb Blood Flow Metab* 1984;4:35–40.
81. Huang S-C, Phelps ME. Principles of tracer kinetic modeling in positron emission tomography and autoradiography. In: Phelps ME, Mazziotta JC, Schelbert HR, eds. *Positron emission tomography and autoradiography, principles and applications for the brain and heart.* New York: Raven Press, 1986:287–346.
82. Graham MM. Model simplification: complexity versus reduction. *Circulation* 1985;72[Suppl IV]:63–68.
83. Koeppe RA. Compartmental modeling alternatives for kinetic analysis of PET neurotransmitter/receptor studies. In: Kuhl DE, ed. *Frontiers in nuclear medicine: in vivo imaging of neurotransmitter functions in brain, heart, and tumors.* Washington, DC: American College of Nuclear Physicians, 1990:113–139
84. Frey KA, Koeppe RA, Mulholland GK, et al. Parametric *in vivo* imaging of benzodiazepine receptor distribution in human brain. *Ann Neurol* 1991;30:663–672.
85. Koeppe RA, Hutchins GD, Rothley JM, et al. Examination of assumptions for local cerebral blood flow studies in PET. *J Nucl Med* 1987;28:1695–1703.
86. Marquardt DW. An algorithm for least-squares estimation of nonlinear parameters. *J Soc Ind Appl Math,* 1963;11(2):431–441.
87. Bevington PR. *Data reduction and error analysis for the physical sciences.* New York: McGraw-Hill, 1969:232–241.
88. Patlak C, Blasberg RG, Fenstermacher JD. Graphical evaluation of blood-to-brain transfer constants from multiple-time uptake data. *J Cereb Blood Flow Metab* 1983;3:1–7.
89. Logan J, Fowler JS, Volkow ND, et al. Graphical analysis of reversible radioligand binding from time-activity measurements applied to [N-^{11}C-methyl]-(–)-cocaine PET studies in human subjects. *J Cereb Blood Flow Metab* 1990;10:740–747.
90. Logan J. Fowler JS, Volkow ND, et al. Distribution volume ratios without blood sampling from graphical analysis of PET data. *J Cereb Blood Flow Metab* 1996;16:834–840.
91. Lammertsma AA, Hume SP. Simplified reference tissue model for PET receptor studies. *Neuroimage* 1996;4:153–158.
92. Holthoff VA, Koeppe RA, Frey KA, et al. Differentiation of radioligand delivery and binding in the brain: validation of a two-compartment model for [C-11]flumazenil. *J Cereb Blood Flow Metab* 1991;11(5): 745–752.
93. Koeppe RA, Frey KA, Snyder SE, et al. Kinetic modeling of N-[^{11}C]methylpiperidinyl propionate: alternatives for analysis of an irreversible PET tracer for measurement of acetylcholinesterase activity in human brain. *J Cereb Blood Flow Metab* 1999;19: 1150–1163.
94. Kuhl DE, Koeppe RA, Minoshima S, et al. *In vivo* mapping of cerebral acetylcholinesterase activity in aging and Alzheimer's disease. *Neurology* 1999;52:691–699.
95. Phillips RL, London ED, Links JM, et al. Program for PET image alignment: effects on calculated differences in cerebral metabolic rates for glucose. *J Nucl Med* 1990;31:2052–2057.
96. Wilson MW, Mountz JM. A reference system for neuroanatomical localization on functional reconstructed cerebral images. *J Comput Assist Tomogr* 1989;13:174–178.
97. Schonemann PH. A generalized solution to the orthogonal Procrustes problem. *Psychometrica* 1966;31:1–10.
98. Evans AC, Merritt S. Anatomical-functional correlation analysis of the human brain using three dimensional imaging systems. *SPIE Med Imag III Image Proc* 1989;1092:264–274.

99. Junck L, Moen JG, Hutchins GD, et al. Correlation methods for the centering, rotation, and alignment of functional brain images. *J Nucl Med* 1990;31(7):1220–1226.
100. Woods RP, Cherry SR, Mazziotta JC. Rapid automated algorithm for aligning and reslicing PET images. *J Comput Assist Tomogr* 1992;16:620–633.
101. Eberl S, Kanno I, Fulton RR, et al. Automatic 3D spatial alignment for correcting interstudy patient motion in serial PET studies. In: Uemura K, Lassen NA, Jones T, et al., eds. *Quantification of brain function—tracer kinetics and image analysis in brain PET*. International Congress Series 1030. Tokyo: Excepta Medica, 1993:419–428.
102. Minoshima S, Koeppe RA, Fessler JA, et al. Integrated and automated data analysis method for neuronal activation studies using O-15 water PET. In: Uemura K, Lassen NA, Jones T, et al., eds. *Quantification of brain function—tracer kinetics and image analysis in brain PET*. International Congress Series 1030. Tokyo: Excepta Medica, 1993:409–418.
103. Vajda I. *Theory of statistical inference and information*. Dordrecht: Kluwer, 1989.
104. Cover TM, Thomas JA. *Elements of information theory*. New York: Wiley, 1991.
105. Levin DN, Pelizzari CA, Chen GTY, et al. Retrospective geometric correlation of MR, CT, and PET images. *Radiology* 1988;169:817–823.
106. Pelizzari CA, Chen GTY, Spelbring DR, et al. Accurate three-dimensional registration of CT, PET, and or MR images of the brain. *J Comput Assist Tomogr* 1989;13:20–26.
107. Pietrzyk U, Herholz K, Heiss WD. Three-dimensional alignment of functional and morphological tomograms. *J Comput Assist Tomogr* 1990;14:51–59.
108. Woods RP, Mazziotta JC, Cherry SR. MRI-PET registration with automated algorithm. *J Comput Assist Tomogr* 1993;17:536–456.
109. Woods RP, Grafton ST, Holmes CJ, et al. Automated image registration: I. General methods and intrasubject, intramodality validation. *J Comput Assist Tomogr* 1998;22:139–152.
110. Maes F, Collignon A, Vandermeulen D, et al. Multimodality image registration by maximization of mutual information. *IEEE Trans Med Imaging* 1997;16:187–198.
111. Meyer CR, Boes JL, Kim B, et al. Demonstration of accuracy and clinical versatility of mutual information for automatic multimodality image fusion using affine and thin plate spline warped geometric deformations. *Med Image Anal* 1997;3:195–206.
112. Bookstein FL. *Morphometric tools for landmark data: geometry and biology*. Cambridge, UK: Cambridge University Press, 1991.
113. Fox PT, Perlmutter JS, Raichle ME. A stereotactic method of anatomical localization for positron emission tomography. *J Comput Assist Tomogr* 1985;9:141–153.
114. Talairach J, Tournoux P. *Co-planar stereotaxic atlas of the human brain*. New York: Thieme Medical Publishers, 1988.
115. Friston KJ, Passingham RE, Nutt JG, et al. Localisation in PET images. Direct fitting of the intercommissural (AC-PC) line. *J Cereb Blood Flow Metab* 1989;9:690–695.
116. Minoshima S, Berger KL, Lee KS, et al. An automated method for rotational correction and centering of three-dimensional functional brain images. *J Nucl Med* 1992;33:1579–1585.
117. Minoshima S, Koeppe RA, Mintun MA, et al. Automated detection of the intercommissural line for stereotactic localization of functional brain images. *J Nucl Med* 1993;34:322–329.
118. Minoshima S, Koeppe RA, Frey KA, et al. Anatomic standardization: linear scaling and nonlinear warping of functional brain images. *J Nucl Med* 1994;35:1528–1537.
119. Mazziotta JC, Toga AW, Evans A, et al. A probabilistic atlas of the human brain: theory and rationale for its development. The International Consortium for Brain Mapping (ICBM). *Neuroimage* 995;2: 89–101.

Standardized Uptake Values

RICHARD L. WAHL

Positron emission tomography (PET) and PET/CT (computed tomography) are inherently quantitative techniques. Properly performed attenuation-corrected images from well-calibrated scanners accurately reflect radioactivity concentrations in each voxel of the image. There is, admittedly, variability due to statistical noise, meaning larger regions of interest are likely more statistically robust than tiny regions. Although partial volume effects result in underestimation of the radiotracer uptake in small "hot" lesions, the quantitative capabilities of PET are by now quite well understood and for objects over about twice the size as the reconstructed resolution of the PET images (typically objects of 2 cm and larger), the radioactivity concentration in the lesion is accurately represented. This unique quantitative capability of PET images was significantly drawn upon in the preceding chapter on data analysis and processing. Accurate quantitation of radioactivity by PET is required for kinetic modeling of dynamic PET images to provide information about varying aspects of biological processes. PET coupled with kinetic modeling methods is a powerful research tool and its applications are discussed in several locations in this text, including the preceding chapter, the oxidative metabolism (Chapter 11.3), and several others. Kinetic modeling methods can be quite complex, requiring a variety of simplifying assumptions, are subject to variability in part due to the region of interest placement, which requires long dynamic acquisitions and can be degraded by motion, and are only relatively infrequently used in the clinical practice of PET imaging.

A practical challenge with kinetic modeling approaches are that they require the patient to be in the PET scanner for moderately long periods of time to allow for dynamic imaging to be acquired to determine the time activity curves in a variety of tissues. For carbon-11 (^{11}C) or fluorine-18 (^{18}F) images, 60 to 90 minutes of data acquisition, from the time of tracer injection until well into the radioactive decay of the tracers, is required as an imaging period. This length of acquisition is typically not a problem in the research setting, although patient motion is clearly a concern and will degrade, if uncorrected, in such modeling. But the long acquisition times are additionally concerning as they require valuable scanner time. Further, the kinetic modeling approaches are far from routine. Thus, modeling is used much more in research than in routine clinical practice. In clinical practice, the logistical requirements of shorter imaging periods, greater resistance to patient motion, along with qualitative methods of analysis or more simple quantitative methods are much more commonly applied.

In most practice settings, qualitative analysis is the main approach to PET image interpretations, including common oncologic, cardiac, and brain fluorodeoxyglucose (FDG) PET imaging approaches. Qualitative imaging has the inherent challenge of being user, or interpreter, dependent. Readers can apply differing thresholds for positivity and negativity. Although several studies have shown reasonably good reproducibility in qualitative interpretations for both diagnosis and treatment response assessment, these data are limited (1,2). Thus, there is typically a desire for image quantitation. The simple quantitative measurement, the standardized uptake value (SUV), is used in several situations and is growing in application as more use of PET in early treatment response assessment occurs. Some have called the SUV a semiquantitative parameter. This is probably linguistically incorrect since it is a numerical figure and it is really a quantitative metric (3). This parameter is available as a function on virtually any PET/CT device and can be applied to a wide variety of radiotracers. This measurement is used most commonly in the assessment of FDG PET oncology images, and the discussion in this chapter focuses on FDG PET, for the most part.

The SUV value has been called the differential absorption ratio, but this term is not as commonly used as SUV (4). The SUV is defined as:

$$\text{SUV} = [\text{mCi/mL (decay corrected) in tissue}]/[\text{mCi of tracer injected into the patient/body weight in grams}].$$

The value becomes unitless if it is assumed that 1 g of body weight is equal to 1 mL. The SUV calculated in this manner is also known as SUV_{bw}, where bw represents body weight.

The SUV would equal 1 if the injected tracer was completely and uniformly distributed throughout the body after injection and if there was no excretion. In fact, the most commonly used radiotracer for clinical PET is FDG, which does not distribute evenly throughout the body. In the fasting state, little FDG goes to fat or muscle, so these tissues have low SUVs, less than 1, in most instances. By contrast, liver and blood SUVs are often higher than 1.

In general, cancers have elevated glucose metabolism and concordant increases in FDG uptake versus background tissues. Thus, the higher the SUV, in simplistic terms, the more probable it is that a given lesion is malignant. The SUV can be helpful and in some studies has been able to separate malignant from benign tissues quite well (e.g., in lung nodules with an SUV higher than 2.5, cancer is more probable than in low SUV lesions). High SUV may be associated with more aggressive tumors, as well as with sarcoma, lymphomas, and some lung cancers. Similarly, the SUV can be very helpful in a given patient in monitoring the response of a cancer to therapy.

If the patient has been fed, or insulin is present, the fat and muscle can have more FDG uptake due to the activation of their insulin-sensitive glucose transporters (5). In general, FDG PET for tumor imaging is performed in the fasting state, so high muscle uptake is not typically too problematic. Since the FDG reaches the tumor from the

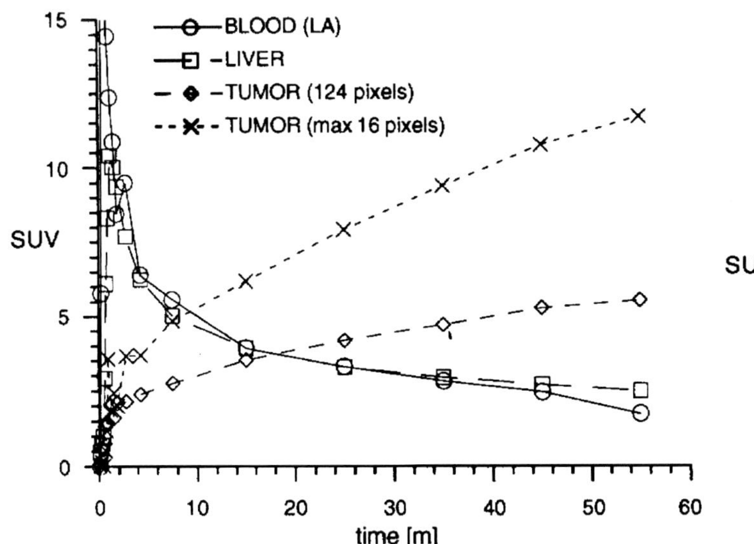

FIGURE 6.1. The standard uptake value (SUV) in normal tissues declines in the 60 minutes postinjection. The SUV in the tumor rises over the same time period. The SUV in the small region of interest (SI) (4 × 4) is much higher than the SUV in the larger region of interest. (From Wahl RL, Zasadny K, Helvie M, et al. Metabolic monitoring of breast cancer chemohormonotherapy using positron emission tomography: initial evaluation. *J Clin Oncol* 1993;11:2101–2111, with permission.)

blood stream, high activity levels in muscle can potentially divert FDG from reaching the tumor and lower the tumor SUV. Thus, uniform patient preparation is very important. Chapter 8.1 of this text additionally details the importance of uniform preparation of patients for PET studies. For oncology studies, a metabolic state of low serum glucose levels and low serum insulin levels is most desirable. This is typically achieved with several hours, commonly 4 or more, of fasting. Some advocate the last meal before the PET scan be a high protein, low carbohydrate meal. Avoiding intense exercise for 24 or more hours prior to PET is probably reasonable as well. Some of the considerations for a reproducible PET study were reported in a recent National Cancer Institute workshop document and in the introductory chapter on tumor imaging in this text, Chapter 8.1 (6).

It is very important to have a consistent time from the injection of the radiotracer until the imaging is performed, if SUV values are to be reproducible from study to study. As is shown in Fig. 6.1 in a patient with untreated breast cancer injected with FDG and imaged continuously over the thorax for 60 minutes, the tumor SUV rises continuously through the first hour of imaging (7). Indeed, it has been shown that in most untreated tumors, the SUV continues to rise through 60 minutes postinjection and can continue to rise though 90 minutes or more postradiotracer injection (6,7). One report showed tumor concentrations of [^{18}F]-FDG did not reach a plateau within the 90 minutes of imaging in any of the pretreatment studies and only in one case posttreatment. Further, the average time to reach 95% of the plateau value pretreatment was 298 +/− 42 minutes (range: 130 to 500 minutes); in posttreatment, it was 154 +/− 31 minutes (range: 65 to 240 minutes). The difference between the plateau drug uptake ratio and the 60-minute value was 46% +/− 6% pretreatment and 17% +/− 5% posttreatment (8). Thus, if one day a patient has a PET scan at 45 minutes postinjection and another day has a scan at 90 minutes postinjection, it is very probable that the tumor SUV will be much higher on the study performed at the later time point, even if there has been no interval treatment (Fig. 6.1). This is in considerable contrast to the tracer behavior in normal tissues, as most of them, such as liver, blood, lung, muscle, and so forth fall over the same period of time (7). So, tumor/background ratios generally increase with time, and this must be realized if there are major differences in the timing of the PET scans from day to day. Without such controls, some have referred to the SUV as a "silly useless value" (9). However, it was also shown that if the time from injection to imaging is kept constant, the SUV values are very consistent from study to study on test retest imaging (10). Thus, for determining SUV it is for critical patients to have the same time from injection until imaging. With such controls the SUV may be more of a "supremely useful value."

The region of interest (ROI) size can have an impact on the SUV calculation. Large ROIs produce lower SUVs than small regions placed over maximal tumor activity. In Fig. 6.1, a small, approximately 1.2 × 2 cm region of interest 0.675 mm in the Z axis (i.e., nonisotropic) had a much higher SUV in the same tumor than an ROI covering a much larger plane of the tumor (7). Thus, it is critical that the same size region of interest be used from study to study. This is particularly important if there are small or heterogeneous structures in which the maximal areas of tumor FDG uptake are small relative to the total tumor size. Some choose to select only the maximal tumor voxel(s). Others have used automated methods to select a 50% threshold volume of the maximum SUV. It must be realized that the same approach should be used from study to study to have optimal results.

The single maximal pixel value in the tumor is often used as a metric and is quite reproducible. In a given center, it is important to be consistent with the way the ROIs are drawn to achieve optimal reproducibility. One approach is to determine the maximum SUV in a tumor and note the maximum SUV average in the "hottest" 1.2-cm square ROI. It has been argued that SUV multiplied by the volume of the lesion is a critical value. This value may be of considerable relevance in treatment-response assessment. This parameter is quite reproducible in experienced hands.

With careful attention to all technical details, at least two studies have shown the SUV to be reproducible from study to study, typically with a 95% confidence level of less than 20% (10,11). This is more precise than some of the parameters used in kinetic modeling, such as the k_3, which estimates the phosphorylation of FDG and is far more variable when evaluated in a test-retest setting (11). This is not, however, to say that this reproducibility is consistently achieved in the nonresearch setting. In addition, it does not mean that the same patient studied at one imaging center and restudied in another center will have the identical SUV result with no intervening therapy.

The two studies examining test/retest behavior of FDG uptake reflected as SUV used relatively large PET volumes for the ROI selection and were performed mainly on untreated tumors with similar results. In one study, PET slices of 6 to 7 mm thickness with either 1.2 cm square ROIs were used (11). In the other, a variable ROI was selected over a whole tumor volume, specifically sized to include a 50% threshold of the maximal pixel value, providing an average SUV for the volume (10). The mean tumor SUV in the two studies was relatively high, about 5.5 in the study of Weber et al. (10) and 8.3 in the study by Minn et al. (11). Variability of 15% to 20% was seen (95% confidence intervals) in the SUV determined from the large ROIs in these relatively hot tumors. Of interest is that other sizes of ROI have shown good reproducibility. For example, smaller, single voxel ROIs have also shown good reproducibility when examined (12). Nakamoto et al. (12) reported on ten patients with lung cancer who underwent two PET examinations within a week with no intervening treatment. The reproducibility of three parameters—(a) maximal SUV of 1 × 1 pixel anywhere in the tumor, calculated on the basis of predicted standard uptake of lean body mass (SULmax); (b) highest average SUV at 4 × 4 pixels in the tumor adjusted by predicted lean body mass (SULmean); and (c) effective glycolytic volume (EGV) calculated by multiplying SUL by tumor volume—using PET images obtained at 50 to 60 minutes postinjection were examined. Plasma glucose, insulin, and free fatty acid levels were also monitored. The SULmax, SULmean, and EGV were measured with a mean +/− standard deviation difference of 11.3% +/− 8.0%, 10.1% +/− 8.2%, and 10.1% +/− 8.0%, respectively. By multiplying SUL by plasma glucose concentration, the mean differences were slightly, but not significantly, reduced to 7.2% +/− 5.8%, 6.7% +/− 6.2%, and 9.5% +/− 8.2%, respectively. These data indicate that commonly used semiquantitative indices of glucose metabolism on PET show high reproducibly, including the more recent single pixel values as well as the EGV (12). The EGV term has also been called the Larson-Ginsburg index (2). This index is the summation of all glycolytically active tumor volumes times the average SUV of that volume. Thus, this value reflects tumor volume as well as the overall glycolytic rate. This supports the potential for use of several kinds of SUV-related parameters in the sequential quantitative analysis of PET, such as in treatment response monitoring.

Some have argued that a volumetric ROI is most appropriate, such as a 1 cm ROI, either spherical or cubic. The 50% cutoff value of untreated tumors used by Weber et al. (10) to study reproducibility of PET included a tumor volume of 17 mL average, but ranged from 0.8 to 111 cc. The study by Minn et al. (11) had a consistent ROI size of 1.2 cm X-Y, with 0.675-mm thick PET slices. Regardless of the approach taken, it is critical to avoid large variability in ROI size from study to study. Thus, if a very small ROI is used in the baseline study, the same small ROI should probably be used in follow-up. If the tumor has decreased in size, use of an ROI larger than the whole tumor could obviously result in underestimation of the true SUV in the tumor. Both reproducibility studies used automated analyses, which may differ from a manual ROI selection.

The use of a single maximal SUV has the attractive characteristic of always having the same size on a given scanner with a given reconstruction matrix, and there is in most systems an automated read out of the maximal pixel value. Thus, a large ROI can be selected and within it, a single pixel can automatically be detected. Thus, this approach is widely applied by many manufacturers. It must be realized, however, that it may be subject to statistical variability, potentially greatest for very small voxels, and some level of caution must be given to such measurements. Most centers use a small ROI, but consistency is key. It is also important to realize that ROI size may make SUV cutoff values differ from study to study based simply on technical parameters mainly related to ROI selection.

In practice, it is not likely that the SUV is as reproducible in practice as it has been in carefully controlled research studies in part because the time from injection until imaging is difficult to exactly control in the routine clinic. Most critical is that test-retest studies be done with exactly the same technique. Thus, with the operational approach, it is important to be cautious in interpreting changes in SUV of less than 25% to 30% as significant. When such changes are seen, comparison of tumor SUV to the SUV in other normal structures, such as the liver or the blood pool, is important. In general, most experienced readers of PET view the SUV as an adjunct to qualitative image assessment. In general, major changes in SUV are visible qualitatively as well as measurably. A list of some factors that can affect SUV are noted in Table 6.1. In practice, among the more common factors are a nonstandard uptake time, a partly extravasated dose, a varying serum glucose level, or an incomplete dose injection for reasons such as an intravenous line problem.

Although the SUV formula considers body weight and adjusts for it, the SUV is not independent of body mass or body size. The SUV rises in blood and normal tissues with increasing body weight and body mass index. Thus, obese patients have higher SUVs in normal blood and liver than do slim patients. This is most likely

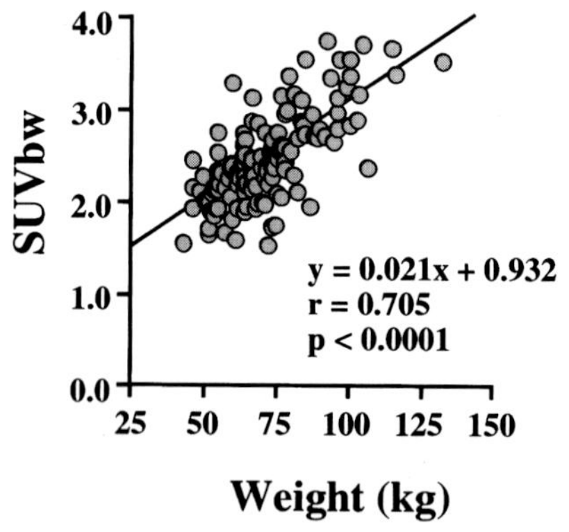

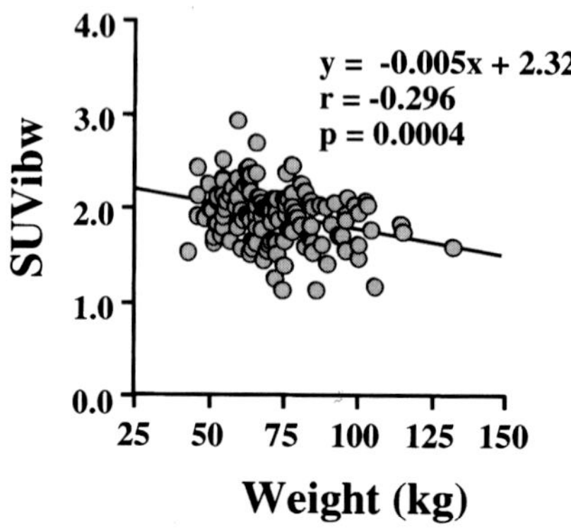

FIGURE 6.2. Standard uptake value (SUV) relationship with weight. SUV (**left**) calculated based on total body mass (SUV_{bw}) is higher in normal blood in heavy patients. SUV (**right**) corrected to ideal body weight (SUV_{ibw}) is less dependent on weight but does show dependence and is an overcorrection. (From Sugawara Y, Zasadny KR, Neuhoff AW, et al. Reevaluation of the standardized uptake value for FDG: variations with body weight and methods for correction. *Radiology* 1999; 213(2): 521–525, with permission.)

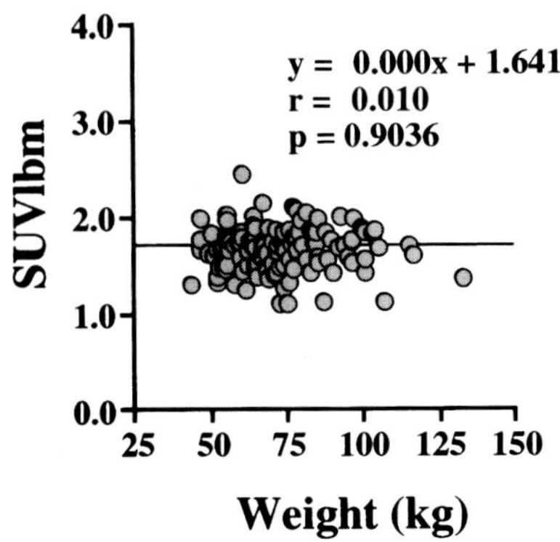

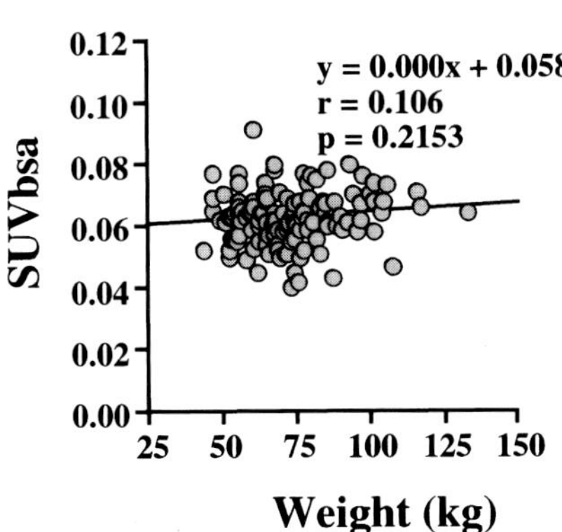

FIGURE 6.3. Standard uptake values (SUVs) corrected for lean body mass (SUV_{lbm}) (**left**) or body surface area (SUV_{bsa}) (**right**) are independent of patient weight. These are the preferred parameters. Because of the small units for SUV_{bsa}, most use SUV_{lbm} (**left**) if patients are obese. (From Sugawara Y, Zasadny KR, Neuhoff AW, et al. Reevaluation of the standardized uptake value for FDG: variations with body weight and methods for correction. *Radiology* 1999;213(2):521–525, with permission.)

because FDG does not distribute into fat in the fasting state, and obese patients have a disproportionate fraction of their body mass in the form of fat (3,12–14). This means that SUVs for tumors and healthy tissue are higher, sometimes much higher in the obese patient, and can be misleading (Fig. 6.2). This points to the obvious limitation of a simple parameter like an SUV of 2.5 for separating benign from malignant tissues other than in populations of uniformly slim patients.

A simple correction, using lean body mass (LBM) or body surface area (BSA) in place of body mass in the SUV calculations, can substantially avoid these problems quite effectively. Thus, we use the SUV_{lean} or SUV-LBM (sometimes called the SUL) calculated by replacing the actual weight of the patient with the LBM in the denominator of the SUV calculation (Table 6.1). SUV_{lean} tends to be lower than SUV, in general. SUV_{bsa} is a valuable index, but the conversion factor leads to numbers far from the typical SUV (Fig. 6.3). Methods for calculating LBM and BSA are shown in Table 6.2, which includes a recent method of LBM calculation (13).

SUV can be used in other tracer studies as well, such as fluorothymidine PET, where it has shown the ability to simplify analysis of PET studies versus full kinetic analyses. There have been efforts to create partial volume correct PET images, which include measurements of tumor size and correction for inadequate count recovery from the small tumor foci. Although such methods can be applied for small tumors, there are large resultant corrections, which means variability may be great from study to study given the considerable variability in measuring tumor size. Thus, it is not normally recommended to determine tumor size for partial volume corrections, although they have been beneficially applied by some (15).

Thus, the SUV, and especially the SUL in larger patients, can be very helpful in treatment-response assessment. A summary of factors that can affect SUV is shown in Table 6.2, and these must be monitored closely. However, the clinical value of the SUV can only be realized if there is careful attention to patient preparation, study conduct, and region of interest selection, to ensure the SUV is indeed "standardized" in its use from study to study. With such control, the SUV is a useful adjunct to qualitative image interpretation. Improvements in software and standardization across manufacturer platforms would be a highly desirable outcome in the coming years for the SUV parameter. In the meantime, standardized consistent practice in a given center is essential for consistent use of the SUV method.

TABLE 6.1 Formulas Used in the Calculation of Standardized Uptake Values

Parameter for Denominator	Calculation
SUV_{bw} (using only body weight)	Weight of the patient
SUV_{ibw} (using ideal body weight)	IBW = 45.5 + 0.91 (height − 152) or IBW + weight if IBW > weight
SUV_{lbm} (using lean body mass)	LBM = 1.07 height − 148 (weight/height)^2
SUV_{bsa} (using body surface area)	BSA = (weight)$^{0.425}$ × (height)$^{0.725}$ × 0.007184

BSA, body surface area; IBW, ideal body weight; LBM, lean body mass; SUV, standardized uptake value.

TABLE 6.2 Technical Factors Affecting Measurements of Standardized Uptake Values with Fluorodeoxyglucose

Factor	Effect
Uptake period after tracer injection	Longer generally results in higher SUV than shorter
Size of ROI	Smaller ROI gives higher SUV
Pixel size of PET image	Higher pixel images typically give higher maximum SUV values
Reconstructed resolution of PET images	Higher resolution produces higher SUV for small ROIs
Body mass index	Obese patients have higher tumor and normal SUVs than thin patients
Serum glucose level	In fasting state, higher glucose levels reduce tumor FDG uptake
Quality of tracer injection	Partly extravasated doses reduce SUV

FDG, fluorodeoyglucose; ROI, region of interest; SUV, standardized uptake value.

REFERENCES

1. Wahl RL, Siegel BA, Coleman RE, et al. Prospective multicenter study of axillary nodal staging by positron emission tomography in breast cancer: a report of the staging breast cancer with PET Study Group. *J Clin Oncol* 2004;22:277–285.
2. Larson SM, Erdi Y, Akhurst T, et al. Tumor treatment response based on visual and quantitative changes in global tumor glycolysis using PET-FDG imaging. The visual response score and the change in total lesion glycolysis. *Clin Positron Imaging* 1999;2:159–171.
3. Zasadny KR, Wahl RL. Standardized uptake values of normal tissues at PET with 2-[fluorine-18]-fluoro-2-deoxy-D-glucose: variations with body weight and a method for correction. *Radiology* 1993;189(3): 847–850.
4. Strauss LG, Clorius JH, Schlag P, et al. Recurrence of colorectal tumors: PET evaluation. *Radiology* 1989;170:329–332.
5. Torizuka T, Fisher SJ, Wahl RL. Insulin-induced hypoglycemia decreases uptake of 2-[F-18]fluoro-2-deoxy-D-glucose into experimental mammary carcinoma. *Radiology* 1997;203:169–172.
6. Shankar LK, Hoffman JM, Bacharach S, et al. Consensus recommendations for the use of ^{18}F-FDG PET as an indicator of therapeutic response in patients in National Cancer Institute trials. *J Nucl Med* 2006;47:1059–1066.
7. Wahl RL, Zasadny K, Helvie M, et al. Metabolic monitoring of breast cancer chemohormonotherapy using positron emission tomography: initial evaluation. *J Clin Oncol* 1993;11:2101–2111.
8. Hamberg LM, Hunter GJ, Alpert NM, et al. The dose uptake ratio as an index of glucose metabolism: useful parameter or oversimplification? *J Nucl Med* 1994;35:1308–1312.
9. Keyes JW Jr. SUV: standard uptake or silly useless value? *J Nucl Med* 1995;36:1836–1839.
10. Weber WA, Ziegler SI, Thodtmann R, et al. Reproducibility of metabolic measurements in malignant tumors using FDG PET. *J Nucl Med* 1999;40:1771–1777.
11. Minn H, Zasadny KR, Quint LE, et al. Lung cancer: reproducibility of quantitative measurements for evaluating 2-[F-18]-fluoro-2-deoxy-D-glucose uptake at PET. *Radiology* 1995;196:167–173.
12. Nakamoto Y, Zasadny KR, Minn H, et al. Reproducibility of common semi-quantitative parameters for evaluating lung cancer glucose metabolism with positron emission tomography using 2-deoxy-2-[18F]fluoro-D-glucose. *Mol Imaging Biol* 2002;4:171–178.
13. Sugawara Y, Zasadny KR, Neuhoff AW, et al. Reevaluation of the standardized uptake value for FDG: variations with body weight and methods for correction. *Radiology* 1999;213(2):521–525.
14. Kim CK, Gupta NC, Chandramouli B, et al. Standardized uptake values of FDG: body surface area correction is preferable to body weight correction. *J Nucl Med* 1994;35:164–167.
15. Vesselle H, Grierson J, Muzi M, et al. *In vivo* validation of 3'deoxy-3'-[(18)F]fluorothymidine ([(18)F]FLT) as a proliferation imaging tracer in humans: correlation of [(18)F]FLT uptake by positron emission tomography with Ki-67 immunohistochemistry and flow cytometry in human lung tumors. *Clin Cancer Res* 2002;8:3315–3323.

CHAPTER 7

Image Fusion

CHARLES R. MEYER AND RICHARD L. WAHL

Functional imaging with positron emission tomography (PET) is normally performed as a tomographic technique designed to trace a specific biological process with a process-specific radiotracer. The tomographic images, as well as the whole-body projection images provided by PET, are generally diagnostically valuable on their own. However, PET imaging evolved initially as a "stand alone" nuclear method capable of visualizing this important functional information but displaying relatively little anatomic information. Although PET imaging devices display functional information in an anatomically correct context, the visualization of normal anatomy is substantially limited. As PET radiotracers became more and more specific for a given process, often only that process accumulated a disproportionately large amount of the radiotracer relative to background, making lesion detection easily possible, but lesion localization a much more approximate undertaking. For example, the highly targeted PET agents like fluorodeoxyglucose (FDG) accumulate so avidly to lesions that it can sometimes be difficult to determine precisely where the tracer-avid lesion is located anatomically. In some instances, precise anatomic localization is not possible as there is not sufficient radiotracer uptake into surrounding normal tissues. Thus, the ability to perform diagnostic imaging is compromised by the lack of anatomic correlative data. The use of image fusion, in the form of "anatometabolic" images for PET fused with magnetic resonance imaging (MRI) or computed tomography (CT) was shown feasible using software techniques in early studies of PET oncologic imaging (1). Software approaches to image fusion are quite valuable and are in widespread utilization, but can be limited if there is substantial patient motion between studies in nonrigid areas of the body. This type of problem is substantially addressed by obtaining the anatomic and functional images in close temporal proximity, often using dedicated in-line hybrid imaging devices such as PET/CT. This chapter reviews the varying approaches to producing fused anatomic/functional (anatomolecular) images.

PET/CT

Prospective "Hardware" Registration and Motion Artifact

Combined PET/CT came into existence because of the obvious diagnostic value of precisely combining functional and anatomic data for diagnostic purposes, which was first shown by software approaches. In addition, because the number of photons associated with CT far exceeded those available from an isotope source, CT supports both the fast acquisition and the computation of a low noise attenuation map for PET emission data, allowing PET to be quantitatively accurate in most instances. Typically the CT attenuation map is segmented into air, bone, soft tissue, water, fat, and possibly other components such as metal and contrast agents and is then used to attenuation-correct PET emission data, assuming no relative motion between the two data sets (1). As this correction is multiplicative (i.e., the PET emission data are multiplied by the appropriate path length related terms), the results become "baked in" to the resulting emission reconstruction. The process is highly problematic if there is misregistration between the two data sets, CT attenuation and PET emission, typically due to physiological or undetected frank patient motion. Nowhere are the results of such misregistration more visible than in the attenuation-corrected emission scans of older PET/CT machines seen in coronal cross section, where the CT acquisition was slow enough to catch the dome of the liver at two or more separate respiratory positions during the scan (see Chapter 4, Fig. 4.7 lower panel). Due to the multiplicative process it should be no surprise that the resulting attenuation corrected emission PET shows the same disarticulated liver segments as those captured in the CT scan, although we know that the same effects do not exist in the emission data from shallow respiration collected over three 40-minute periods. Such effects are not as visible in the newer scanners primarily due to the higher speed of CT scanning, but the insidious appearance of perfect registration is still omnipresent. Other organ locations are also affected by respiration (e.g., the prostate can move as much as 1 cm cranially caudally between full inspiration and expiration) (2). Undetected patient motion can occur between the CT attenuation and PET emission scans. If a patient repositions his or her head between the two scans, the resulting head and neck emission scan may appear to show high lymph node uptake where the attenuation correction is applied to data collected with little or no actual attenuation. If the interpreting physician suspects a motion-induced intensity artifact in the emission scan he or she can compare the geometry between reconstructions of the CT and *uncorrected* PET emission scan for differences as well as the presence of relative local uptake differences, but unfortunately such comparisons are likely to occur only if there is sufficient suspicion of misregistration. Otherwise misregistration effects, if present, may not be detected by visual inspection of the apparently beautifully registered CT and PET attenuation-corrected emission data sets. Indeed, while the mechanical alignment of PET and CT devices in inline PET/CT scanners allows registration accuracy in the millimeter to submillimeter range, it is not possible to achieve this level of registration accuracy in most living patients due to physiological and voluntary positional differences seen between PET and CT during image acquisitions, which do not occur simultaneously with any of the commercial PET/CT scanners currently manufactured.

Retrospective Registration

Before PET/CT machines, registration of PET and CT data sets as well as those of other modalities occurred through the use of automatic and semiautomatic registration algorithms. There is a continuing need to register multimodal data combinations other than just PET/CT and single-photon emission computed tomography (SPECT)-CT and the number of combinations may be more than just two (e.g., MR-PET-SPECT). Additionally, there may be a need to register multiple interval examinations to carefully describe lesion growth. Because there are several excellent reviews on the genesis of registration (3–5), only superficial highlights will be emphasized here.

Metrics of Registration Accuracy

Before 1995 most registration problems were treated as isomodal (of the same modality) or were made similar by preprocessing to extract surfaces, edges, crest lines, and so forth so that cost functions (so named because they should be minimized), such as sum of square error, could be used. In 1995 three research groups nearly simultaneously gave birth to multimodality registration using image intensities directly via information theoretic objective functions (so named because they should be maximized), such as mutual information, or cost functions, such as entropy (6–8). These information-based theoretic measures proved to be very robust against issues such as missing data or differences in point spread function and are now popular in many registration methods found today. Even in isomodality registration, mutual information-based objective functions play an important role in easily handling unexpected differences in the data sets due to differences in phase of contrast injection and/or presence or absence of oral contrast agents in the gut.

Geometric Degrees of Freedom

Geometric degrees of freedom (DOF) are determined by the morphology of the problem that is trying to be solved. If there is an interest in registering the head of the same patient over multiple interval examinations, the problem is simplified to that of registering a rigid body (i.e., just rotation and translation are required), unless there are suspected temporal differences in the brain structures. For three spatial dimensions (3D) there are three translation and three rotation parameters, for a total of six parameters (i.e., six DOF). If in addition isotropic registration is allowed the DOF become seven. If shearing and scaling on each axis is allowed in addition to rotation and translation, there are now 12 parameters (or 12 DOF) for this linear, often called "affine" transform. Although more than six DOF is no longer a rigid body geometry problem, up to and including 12 DOF is still a linear solution (i.e., straight lines are still straight after this transform). Although little in the human body except bony structures and the effects of gradient shearing encountered in echo planar diffusion MRI acquisitions can be handled exactly by linear transforms (rigid body is a subset of linear transforms), many small regional deformations can be well approximated by full affine transforms (e.g., liver motion as a function of shallow respiration) (9).

In general the solution to registration problems in the human body (i.e., same patient with different poses), and certainly across different patients, requires warping (i.e., more than 12 DOF). In this registration domain there are many approaches as well. Geometric interpolants (i.e., functions that are computed to represent the best warping deformations between two poses of the same object) vary from:

- Solutions to, or approximations of the Navier-Stokes equation for viscous flow where the DOF approach the number of voxels in the reference data set (10,11),
- Harmonic series (e.g., the discrete Fourier or cosine transform where the DOF equals the number of nonzero coefficients) (12),
- Polynomials described by maximum variation order (13),
- Cubic or thin plate splines (14,15), and a
- Multiplicity of locally piecewise, linear solutions (16).

One caution is that the information content of each of the two data sets to be registered must be sufficient to support the DOF of the requested geometric solution. In cases where the DOF of the requested solution exceeds the support of the images' information content, the objective function flattens with respect to change in the variables such that the optimizer cannot find a global solution and spends a great deal of time searching before it stops in a local minimum, usually far from the optimum solution.

Carbon-11-Choline PET and CT

Specifically consider the problem of retrospectively registering carbon-11 ([^{11}C])-choline PET and CT of the pelvis for prostate radiation therapy planning. The patient's position on the two scanners can vary in a number of ways most of which can be easily generalized to the effects of (a) local anisotropic scaling primarily due to differences in phase of respiration, (b) torsion around the vertical axis, and (c) bending in the remaining two planes. Two local affine solutions would then describe the solutions in the upper and lower pelvis with the region between defined by the interpolation between the two local solutions. A very nice approach to this problem is the use of thin plate splines (TPS) with control points that describe two triangles, one in the upper pelvis and one in the lower pelvis, that is, six points at three DOF/point yields 18 DOF (Fig. 7.1). The TPS solution is a minimum bending energy solution between optimized control points and is found by the controller's (Nelder-Mead simplex) movement of the loci of control points in the floating image, the CT data set in this case, to best map onto the reference data set (i.e., the PET attenuation-corrected emission data), as determined by optimizing the mutual information objective function (15); the axial slice displayed in Fig. 7.2 was selected specifically to show registration at the level of the prostate. These kinds of lower DOF solutions are easily, accurately, and robustly computed.

Before the existence of the PET/CT machines, the resolution of a PET FDG study was only about half of what it is currently (i.e., 6 to 7 mm and sometimes with reconstructed resolutions of over 1 cm). Since the resulting registration quality is related to the information

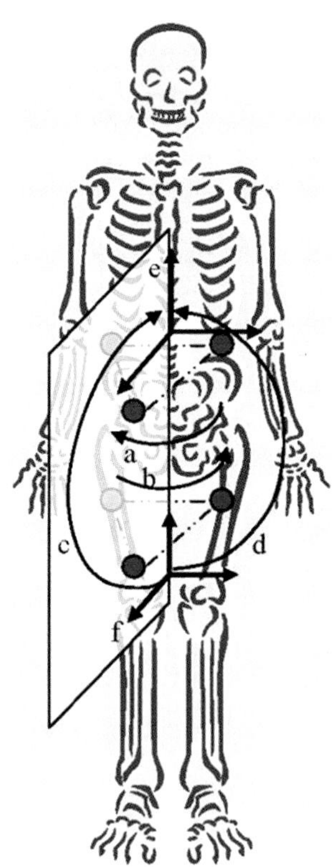

FIGURE 7.1. Pelvic geometry accommodation with six thin plate spline control points.

content of the data having the minimum information, PET/CT registration was compromised by lower information content due to the reduced resolution of PET emission. At least one experiment showed that by registering CT with the PET attenuation scan obtained with a rod source and then applying the computed registration to the attenuation-corrected emission data was more accurate than registering the CT directly to the attenuation-corrected emission scan (17). At today's improved PET resolutions on the order of 3 to 4 mm that may no longer be a problem.

MR-PET-SPECT

In addition to the multimodality problem posed by PET and CT, it is often the case that other modalities may be needed. In the following case, the clinical question pivoted around the question of whether the new out-pouching from the previously radiated tumor was regrowth of the primary or continuing necrosis. In Fig. 7.3 the T1-weighted MRI shown in green served as the anatomical study of the brain, the FDG PET in red demonstrated metabolism, and the thallium-201 SPECT in blue showed breakdown of the blood–brain barrier and viable tumor perfusion. The lack of metabolism above that of white matter and the break down of the blood–brain barrier indicated the new feature was continuing necrosis. Although these registrations were obtained by registering both the PET and SPECT studies to the MR, newer joint registration techniques support simultaneous registration of all three modalities (18–23); since these are calibrated modalities involving the head of the same patient, the geometric model used was that of rigid body, or just six DOF. Again such registrations are very robust to noise and easily

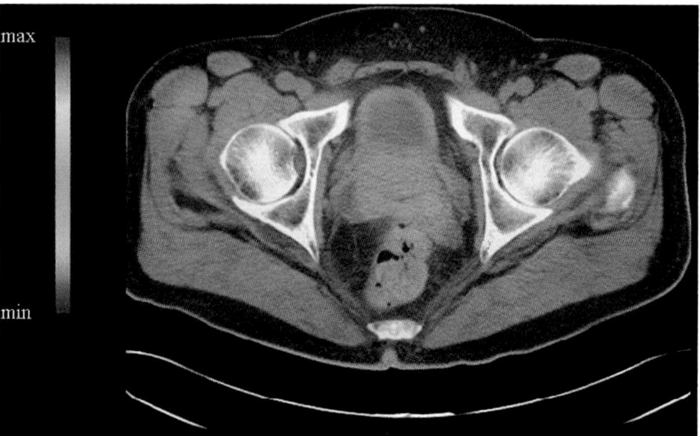

FIGURE 7.2. One slice of retrospective PET/CT registration using six control points (18 degrees of freedom); fluorodeoxyglucose PET in pseudocolor (encoded via sidebar) overlaid on grayscale CT. (Deidentified data from Kettering Memorial Hospital PET Center, Dayton, Ohio, supplied courtesy of Cherry T. Thomas MD, and Martin Jacobs MD. Prostatectomy pathology showed T2c disease, that is, cancer in both lobes.)

computed with accuracies on the order of 0.1 mm at the periphery of the brain.

SPECT-MR

SPECT-MR is another frequently registered pair of modalities. The clinical reasons vary from estimating organ dose from targeted radioactive antibodies in the abdomen, pelvis, or thorax to detecting

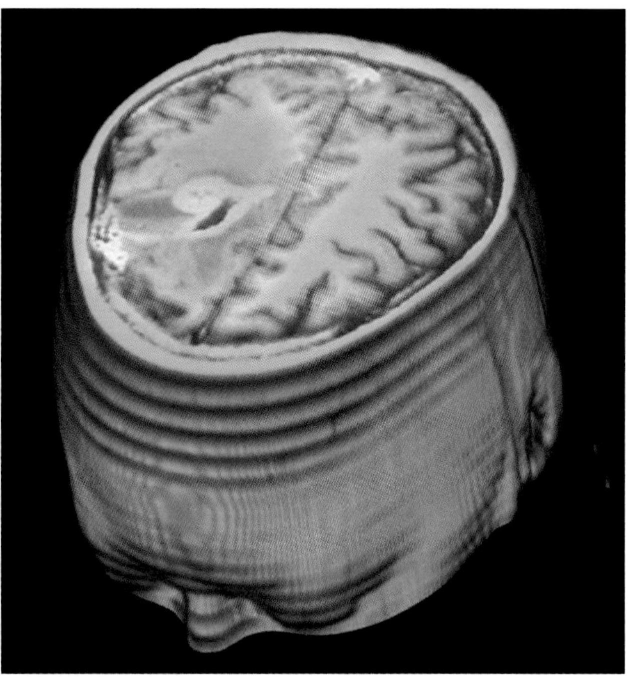

FIGURE 7.3. Retrospective registration of fluorodeoxyglucose PET in red hue onto magnetic resonance in green hue and single-photon emission computed tomography in blue hue onto the same magnetic resonance image.

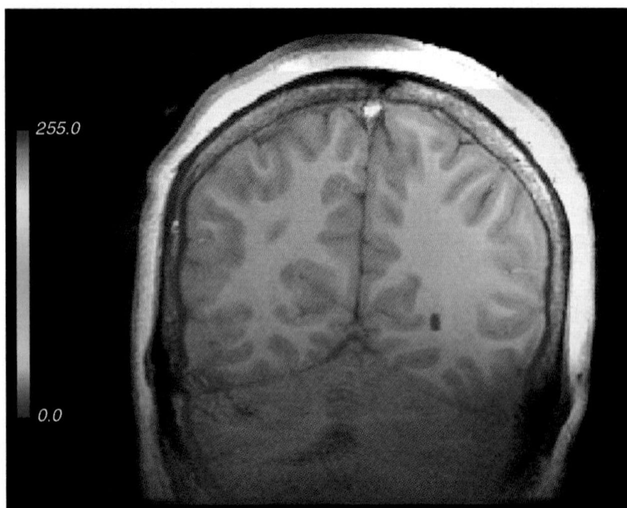

FIGURE 7.4. Retrospective registration of single-photon emission computed tomography in pseudocolor (encoded via sidebar) and grayscale magnetic resonance.

epileptic foci based on ^{99m}Tc ECD (technetium-99m ethylcysteinate dimer; Neurolite, Dupont-Merck Pharmaceutical Co, Billerica, Massachusetts) or HMPAO (hexamethyl propylamine oxime; Ceretec, Amersham, U.K.), blood flow in the brain. In the former case the SPECT data sets have relatively poor spatial resolution if high-energy photons are used due to their penetration of lead septa in the collimator, resulting in restrictions on DOF. In all likelihood for ^{131}I a 15-18 DOF warping (i.e., registration just beyond the linear regime) can be computed at most. In the latter case a ^{99m}Tc ECD or HMPAO study is performed while the patient is having a seizure (ictal SPECT) and another is performed in the period between seizures (interictal SPECT). The two SPECT data sets are registered and then subtracted (ictal minus interictal), while one of the SPECT data sets, for example the ictal study, is registered to the patient's surgical planning MRI. The difference SPECT data set is then displayed against the MRI for the surgeon and neurologist to plan surgical removal of the ictus or to drive decisions on surgical grid placement for electrophysiological validation of the ictus before surgical removal. Again these studies are from calibrated modalities and thus only require rigid body geometry resulting in robust, accurate registrations (Fig. 7.4).

Mapping Histology Back to *In Vivo* Imaging

Correlating *in vivo* imaging with histology is an elusive generic problem that has at least two major components that must be addressed by all methods: (a) correcting for 2D distortions in the preparing and cutting of the histology specimen from the tissue block, and (b) restoring the 3D geometry of the tissue block back to its *in vivo* state. Almost always both steps require warping. Previous published papers demonstrate a wide variety of methods. In 1997 Kim et al. (24) demonstrated an automatic method for warping neuroautoradiographic slices back to their geometry in the tissue block and then one final 3D warping from the geometry of the tissue block to its geometry in the *in vivo* brain MRI image using mutual information (6,8) as the objective function and thin plate splines as the geometric warping interpolants (25). In 1999 Jacobs et al. (26) described a sequential technique first using the automatic surface fitting method from Pelizzari et al. (27) for rigid structures, followed by manually defined warping using thin plate splines to

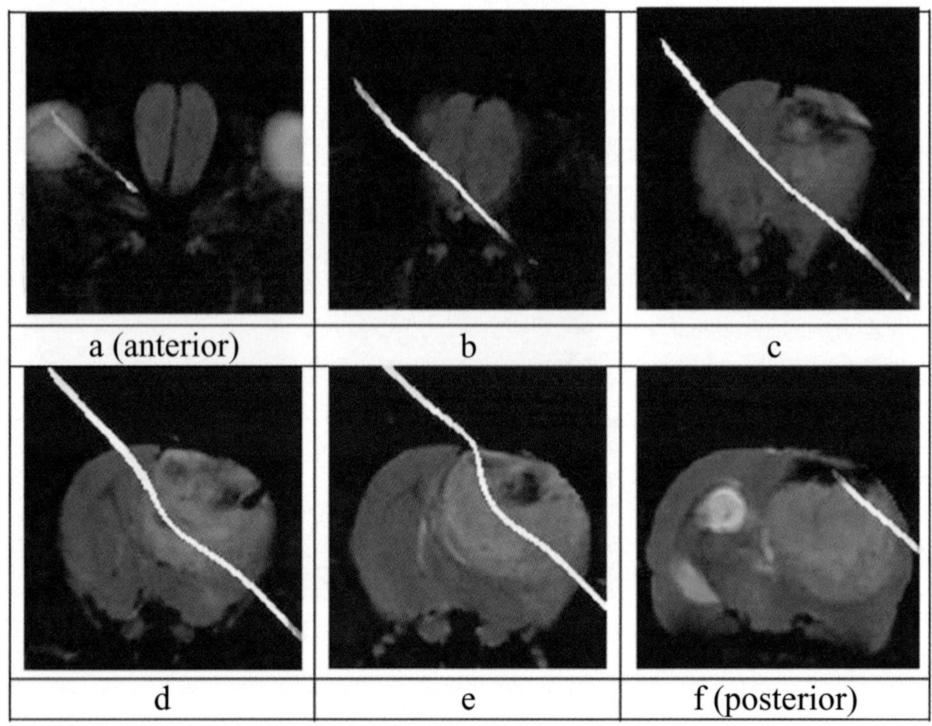

FIGURE 7.5. Intersections of two-dimensional histology manifold (*bright curved lines*) mapped onto *in vivo* magnetic resonance imaging planes as determined by optimizing mutual information between magnetic resonance image and the histology section restored to its presectioning block face geometry.

MR slices obtained by manual reformation of the *in vivo* MR data set to look like the histology slide. In 2003 to 2004 several papers were published describing the use of manually inserted needle tracks and the iterative closest point method (28) to register *in vivo* MRI with tissue slices in 3D followed by the use of manually chosen homologous points augmented with points on contours to warp the 2D histology slices back into the geometry of the tissue slices (29–31). In 2004 Zarow et al. (32) described postmortem MRI and brain tissue registration obtained using the Pearson cross-correlation coefficient first and mutual information last as two separately and sequentially applied objective functions and an *n*th order polynomial as a 2D (only) geometric warping interpolant, again assuming that the appropriate MR slice can be obtained by manual reformation of the MR volume. Building on the early work of Kim et al., Meyer et al. (33) described a method that recognizes that the *in vivo* MRI is a weak link in the registration chain to map histology back to the *in vivo* image due to lower information content necessitated by a short scanning interval. An intermediate approach of obtaining a high resolution and high signal-to-noise (SNR) MRI of the *ex vivo* sample in paraformaldehyde where scanning time is of little consequence is used as an alternative to map 2D geometry restored histology specimens back into their 2D manifold in the 3D volume. Given all the deformations in the specimen extraction and preparation the likelihood seems infinitesimally small that a 2D histology sample maps directly back onto a 2D ***plane*** in the *in vivo* image volume (Fig. 7.5).

In summary, accurate multimodality fusion imaging underlies much of current PET/CT. Although hardware fused PET/CT is adequate for many aspects of clinical practice, this approach does not address patient motion and organ deformations adequately. Further, it is not adequate for registration with some other imaging methods in many instances. Thus, continued work in the field of image fusion will be required to achieve more precise fusions beyond those now available clinically and for research purposes.

REFERENCES

1. Bai C, Kinahan P, Brasse D, et al. An analytic study of the effects of attenuation on tumor detection in whole-body PET oncology imaging. *J Nucl Med* 2003;44:1855–1861.
2. Morrill S, Langer M, Lane R. Real-time couch compensation for intra-treatment organ motion: theoretical advantages. *Med Phys* 1996;23:1083.
3. van den Elsen PA, Pol MJD, Viergever MA. Medical image matching—a review with classification. *IEEE Engr Med Biol* 1993;12(1):26–39.
4. Pluim J, Maintz J, Viergever M. Mutual-information-based registration of medical images: a survey. *IEEE Trans Med Imaging* 2003;22(8): 986–1004.
5. Maes F, Vandermeulen D, Suetens P. Medical image registration using mutual information. *Proc IEEE* 2003;91(10):1699–1722.
6. Collignon A, Vandermeulen D, Suetens P, et al. 3D multimodality medical image registration using feature space clustering. In: Ayache N, ed. *Proceedings of First International Conference on Computer Vision, Virtual Reality and Robotics in Medicine. Lecture notes in computer science.* Berlin: Springer-Verlag, 1995;905:195–204.
7. Studholme C, Hill D, Hawkes D. Multi-resolution voxel similarity measures for MR-PET registration. In: Bizais Y, Barillot C, Di Paola R, eds. *Information processing in medical imaging: Proceedings: International Conference on Information Processing in Medical Imaging.* New York: Springer-Verlag, 1995;3:287–298.
8. Viola P, Wells WM. Alignment by maximization of mutual information. In: *Proceedings of 5th International Conference on Computer Vision.* Washington, DC: IEEE Computer Society 1995;95(744):16–23.
9. Kessler M, Meyer C, Balter J, et al. (2004) A robust system for registration of 3D and 4D image data. In: Yi BY, Choi EK, eds. *Proceedings of the 14th International Conference on the Use of Computers in Radiation Therapy.* Seoul: Jeong, 2004:383–385.
10. Bro-Nielsen M, Gramkow C. Fast fluid registration of medical images. In: Hohne KH, Kikinis R, eds. *Proceedings of Visualization in Biomedical Computing 1996, Hamburg, Germany. Lecture notes in computer science.* Springer, 1996;1131:267–276.
11. Miller MI, Christensen GE, Amit Y, et al. Mathematical textbook of deformable neuroanatomies. *Proc Natl Acad Sci USA* 1993;90(24): 11944–11948.
12. *SPM Statistical Parametric Mapping* [software]. Wellcome Department of Imaging Neuroscience, 2005.
13. Woods R. *Automated image registration (AIR).* 2006.
14. Rueckert D, Sonoda LI, Hayes C, et al. Nonrigid registration using free-form deformations: application to breast MR images. *IEEE Trans Med Imaging* 1999;18(8):712–721.
15. Meyer CR, Boes JL, Kim B, et al. Demonstration of accuracy and clinical versatility of mutual information for automatic multimodality image fusion using affine and thin-plate spline warped geometric deformations. *Med Image Analysis* 1997;1(3):195–206.
16. Collins DL, Peters TM, Evans AC. An automated 3D non-linear image deformation procedure for determination of gross morphometric variability in human brain. In: *Proceedings of Visualization in Biomedical Computing.* Rochester, MN: SPIE 1994;2359:180–190.
17. Skalski J, Wahl RL, Meyer CR. Comparison of mutual information based warping accuracy for fusing body CT and PET by two methods: CT mapped onto PET emission scan, vs. CT mapped onto PET transmission scan. *J Nucl Med* 2002;43(9):1184–1187.
18. Rueckert D, Frangi A, Schnabel J. Automatic construction of 3D statistical deformation models of the brain using nonrigid registration. *IEEE Trans Med Imaging* 2003;22(8):1014–1025.
19. Studholme C, Cardenas V. A template free approach to volumetric spatial normalization of brain anatomy. *Pattern Recognit Lett* 2004;25: 1191–1202.
20. Neemuchwala H, Hero AO, Carson PL, et al. Local feature matching using entropic graphs. In: *Proceedings of International Symposium on Biomedical Imaging (ISBI), Arlington, VA.* IEEE, 2004:704–707.
21. Twining CJ, Cootes T, Marsland S, et al. A Unified Information-Theoretic Approach to Groupwise Non-rigid Registration and Model Building. In: *Proceedings of Information Processing in Medical Imaging (IPMI). Lecture notes in computer science.* 2005;3565:1–14.
22. Zhang J, Rangarajan A. Multimodality image registration using an extensible information metric and high dimensional histogramming. In: Christiansen GE, Sonka M, eds. *Proceedings of Information Processing in Medical Imaging (IPMI). Lecture notes in computer science.* Springer, 2005;3565:725–737.
23. Zollei L, Learned-Miller E, Grimson E, et al. Efficient population registration of 3D data. In: *Proceedings of Computer Vision for Biomedical Image Applications (CVBIA). Lecture notes in computer science.* 2005; 3765:291–301.
24. Kim B, Boes JL, Frey KA, et al. Mutual information for automated unwarping of rat brain autoradiographs. *Neuroimage* 1997;5(1):31–40.
25. Bookstein FL. Principal Warps: Thin-plate splines and the decomposition of deformations. *IEEE Trans Pattern Anal Mach Intell* 1989;11(6): 567–585.
26. Jacobs M, Windham J, Peck D, et al. Registration and warping of magnetic resonance images to histological sections. *Med Phys* 1999;26(8): 1568–1578.
27. Pelizzari CA, Chen GTY, Halpern H, et al. Three dimensional correlation of PET, CT and MRI images. *J Nucl Med* 1987;28(4):683.
28. Besl PJ, McKay ND. A method for registration of 3-D shapes. *IEEE Trans Pattern Anal Mach Intell* 1992;14(2):239–256.
29. Lazebnik R, Lancaster T, Breen M, et al. Volume registration using needle paths and point landmarks for evaluation of interventional MRI treatments. *IEEE Trans Med Imaging* 2003;22(5):653–660.

30. Breen M, Lancaster T, Lazebnik R, et al. Three-dimensional method for comparing in vivo interventional MR images of thermally ablated tissue with tissue response. *J Mag Reson Imag* 2003;18:90–102.
31. Wilson D, Breen M, Lazebnik R, et al. Radiofrequency thermal ablation: 3D MR-histology correlation for localization of cell death in MR lesion images. In: *Proceedings of International Symposium on Biomedical Imaging, Arlington, VA*. 2004;1537–1540.
32. Zarow C, Kim T-S, Singh M, et al. A standardized method for brain-cutting suitable for both stereology and MRI-brain coregistration *J Neuorsci Methods* 2004;139:209–215.
33. Meyer C, Moffat B, Kuszpit K, et al. A methodology for registration of a histological slide and in vivo MRI volume based on optimizing mutual information. *Mol Imaging* 2006;5(1):16–23.

CHAPTER 8.1

Principles of Cancer Imaging with 18-F Fluorodeoxyglucose (FDG)

RICHARD L. WAHL

Anatomic imaging has been the fundamental approach to cancer imaging for more than 100 years. The continued utility of anatomic methods is supported by their daily use in managing individual patients with cancer in the third millennium, with estimates of over 20 million computed tomography (CT) scans for cancer performed annually in the United States. Currently, the most widely used systems for assessing response tumor response to therapy, World Health Organization (WHO) and Response Evaluation Criteria in Solid Tumors (RECIST), are anatomically based, reflecting the continued importance of anatomic imaging. Although widely applied, a major limitation of anatomic imaging is detection of a phenotypic alteration that is sometimes, but not invariably, associated with cancer—a mass. Although a mass may often represent cancer, with anatomic imaging, it cannot be distinguished if masses are due to malignant or benign etiologies, such as can occur in solitary pulmonary nodules or borderline-sized lymph nodes. Small cancers are often undetectable with traditional anatomic methods, as they have not yet formed a mass or the mass is so small it can be visualized, but is indistinguishable from normal tissues in its CT or magnetic resonance imaging (MRI) anatomic characteristics. After surgery or other treatments, it is even more difficult to assess for the presence or absence of recurrent tumor with anatomic methods. Posttreatment anatomic scans are complicated by dependence on comparisons with normal anatomy, often symmetries, to detect altered morphologic findings due to cancer. Anatomic methods do not predict response to treatment and do not quickly reveal those tumors responding to therapy (1–3). Delays in change in tumor size, despite substantial antitumor activity, have been seen with several targeted biological therapies, such as treatment of gastrointestinal stromal tumor with imatinib and other agents. Despite these challenges, anatomic images remain routine in cancer management. Positron emission tomography (PET), a functional imaging method, helps address many of the limitations of anatomic imaging, and when combined with anatomic images in fusion images, especially those generated with dedicated hardware PET/CT systems, is emerging as a particularly valuable—indeed now a standard—tool, providing both anatomic precision and functional information in a single image set (3) (Table 8.1.1).

MOLECULAR AND FUNCTIONAL ALTERATIONS IN CANCER

The molecular etiologies of neoplasia are increasingly being understood. Mutations in genomic DNA typically precede development of overt neoplasia (4). These mutations can be both activating through oncogenes or mutations of tumor suppressor genes. With sufficient alterations in genotype, phenotypic changes occur (Table 8.1.2). These genotypic and phenotypic changes in cancer antedate development of discrete mass lesions and represent potential targets for innovative imaging agents.

The concept of an altered "genome," "proteome," and resulting alterations in metabolism are consistent with an altered "metabolosome" are increasingly recognized as present in cancers. Recently, alterations in methylation of genes have been described in DNA of malignant cells, causing silencing of key genes and contributing to the malignant phenotype. PET, due to its superb sensitivity to low concentrations of radioactivity, is able to detect signals from tracers targeting downstream phenotypic alterations preferentially present in cancer.

With a greater understanding of the causes of cancer, it is appreciated that there are many "hallmarks" of cancer, which are quite commonly seen across tumor types but include the following characteristics as reported by Hanahan and Weinberg (5): (a) self-sufficiency in growth signals; (b) evading apoptosis; (c) insensitivity

TABLE 8.1.1 Limitations of Anatomic Imaging Methods for Cancer Assessment

- Masses adjoining normal structures such as bowel are commonly undetected
- Commonly fail to detect small tumor foci
- Do not define the composition of the mass
- Lymph nodes are detected but not characterized as malignant or benign
- Often impossible to interpret after surgery due to altered anatomy
- Do not predict what therapy should be chosen
- Do not quickly determine whether tumor is responding to therapy
- Often do not provide prognostic information

to antigrowth signals; (d) tissue invasion and metastasis; (e) limitless replicative potential; and (f) sustained angiogenesis. Although these are widely present, it is also true that many of the following characteristics are often present:

Increased rate of proliferation

Over- or underexpression of receptors/tumor antigens (e.g., somatostatin receptors)

Presence of hypoxia in regions of the tumor

Presence of necrosis

Increased metabolism of:

A. Glucose

B. Amino acids

C. Membrane precursors

D. Other substrates such as glutamine, DNA precursors

Accelerated rate of apoptosis

Each of these downstream phenotypic features represents a possible target for tumor imaging with PET tracers, and many of these processes have been targeted with PET tracers. Thus, the PET tracers in current and evolving use to a substantial extent target the tumor biological features that are reasonably common across cancer types. With a few exceptions, the characteristics of cancer that are biologically suitable targets for imaging are not totally specific for cancer. For example, the most commonly used target for tumor imaging at present, increased glucose metabolism, is not a tumor-specific process.

TABLE 8.1.2 Molecular and Functional Alteration in Cancer

Function	Increased	Decreased
Glucose metabolism	X	
Amino acid transport	X	
Protein synthesis	X	
DNA synthesis	X	
Blood flow	X	X
Receptors	X	
Oxygen tension		X
Apoptosis	X	X
Membrane turnover	X	
Signal transduction	X	
Vascular density	X	
Vascular permeability	X	
Oncogene products	X	
Many other genetic markers	X	X

There are also tumor-, or at least tissue-, specific targets on tumor cells. For example, the norepinephrine transporter (NET) is highly specific to neuroblastomas, pheochromocytomas, and neuroendocrine tumors, but the transporter is also expressed on normal tissues like the adrenal glands and brown fat. Similarly, estrogen receptors are very specific markers of a subtype of breast cancer, however, these receptors are clearly not specific for this cancer as they are expressed on many cells from the normal breast and uterus. Another quite specific tracer is the somatostatin receptor family, which can be targeted in certain neuroendocrine tumors like carcinoid, for example. Some of these more specific PET tracers are discussed in selected chapters, such as the chapter on neuroendocrine tumors, thyroid cancer imaging (e.g., iodine-124), hypoxia, and breast cancer. This section mainly focuses on the use of fluorine-18-fluoro-2-deoxy-D-glucose ([^{18}F]-FDG) in cancer imaging as it is by far the most commonly used agent at present in clinical PET, or as in vogue "clinical molecular imaging."

GLUCOSE METABOLISM AS A TARGET

Accelerated glucose metabolism has been known to be present in cancers for about 80 years (6). Increased glucose metabolism is not specific for cancer, however. Indeed, the dominant tracer used in clinical PET imaging to date, [^{18}F]-FDG was developed as a tracer to study the initial steps of glucose metabolism in the brain (7). This tracer is transported into glucose-consuming cells, such as those in the brain or cancers, phosphorylated by hexokinase, typically type II, to FDG 6-phosphate, and then retained mainly as the polar molecule FDG 6-phosphate and can be imaged by PET (Fig. 8.1.1).

The development of FDG as a tumor imaging agent was not as rapid as its use in brain imaging. Although the Brookhaven group and others recognized and showed the promise of FDG for tumor targeting in animal models, this agent achieved only limited application to visceral imaging for many years following its introduction (8,9). As early as 1982, the feasibility of imaging brain tumors and colorectal cancer with PET was shown in humans (10,11). Several other reports of successful tumor imaging with FDG and either planar imaging or PET appeared in small clinical studies in the late 1980s (12–14). Pioneering studies of tumor imaging were also being performed in this time period by investigators in Japan using carbon-11 ([^{11}C])-L-methionine (15). The tumor targeting properties of FDG were further developed in a series of animal studies performed in the late 1980s (16,17). In these studies, the targeting of FDG to a wide variety of human tumor xenografts was evaluated in nude mice and compared with the targeting ability of monoclonal antibodies, which were the more typical agents of that time. The author and his colleagues found that across a very wide range of human tumors, including breast, lung, renal, bladder, ovarian, tes-

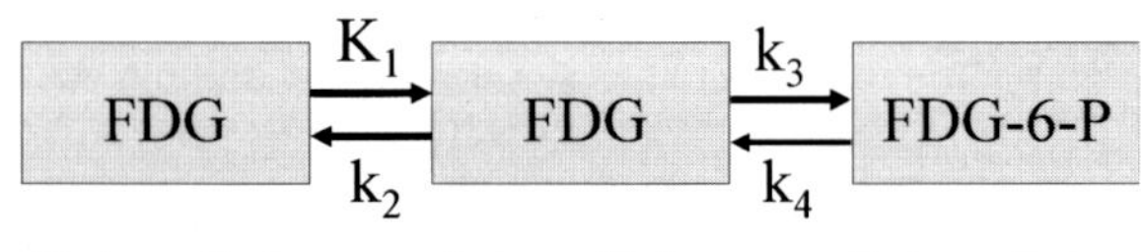

FIGURE 8.1.1. Fluorodeoxyglucose kinetic modeling. K_1 is in part facilitated by GLUT1 glucose transporter molecules. k_3 is due to hexokinase activity. k_4 is due to glucose-6-phosphatase, which is typically at low levels in most cancers.

ticular, head and neck, and lymphoma and melanoma, the uptake of FDG was very much higher (in terms of tumor-to-background uptake ratios) than that which was seen with the higher molecular weight, and in theory, more "specific" monoclonal antibody tracers. Higher tumor/blood uptake ratios were commonly seen within a few hours of intravenous tracer injection. Similarly, targeting to tumor metastases in lymph nodes was very high in comparison to targeting seen with comparable monoclonal antibody agents. These preclinical data strongly suggested that tumor imaging of both primary and metastatic disease would be possible in man.

In brief, in nearly every circumstance in which animal models predicted that FDG would allow for successful imaging of tumors, the human studies showed the same: FDG targeted and imaged well breast cancer, bladder cancer, ovarian cancer, melanoma, lung cancer, germ cell tumors, many renal cancers, and many others (18–23). Many groups made similar observations in humans in a variety of cancers (24–27). It quickly became abundantly clear that FDG PET imaging would be a useful technique for cancer imaging, although the precise roles of PET in a variety of cancers continue to be refined to this day and the limitations of the technique are also increasingly recognized.

UNDERSTANDING THE SIGNAL SEEN WITH FLUORODEOXYGLUCOSE PET

Although superb images of many common kinds of cancer are feasible using FDG PET, it is important to understand the mechanisms of tracer uptake in cancers to fully understand the images and, more practically, the causes of false-positive and false-negative imaging results. In the past 15 years, improved understanding of some of the molecular alterations in glucose metabolism in cancer has been achieved. For example, overexpression of facilitative glucose transporters on the cell surface is common, with the GLUT1 transporter and sometimes GLUT3, overexpressed in many cancers (28–30). Glucose transporters are the molecular species that facilitate FDG transit from outside the cancer cell into the cell. Similarly, some of the hexokinase enzymes, such as hexokinase II, can be overexpressed in cancer (31). These are important proteins in the early phases of glucose metabolism, most notably the transport and phosphorylation of glucose to glucose 6-phosphate. Glucose 6-phosphate is metabolized further, but the tracer [^{18}F]-FDG is not substantially further metabolized after this step of conversion to FDG 6-phosphate. FDG 6-phosphate is a polar molecule and has been shown to be the major species accumulated and imaged within cancers using FDG PET. By contrast, renal and genitourinary activity seen with PET, which can be vexing in image interpretation due to the presence of [^{18}F] activity in the urine and elsewhere, in the form of FDG.

These generally prevalent alterations in glucose metabolism in cancer occur for several reasons. It has been shown that oncogenic transformation of cells, for example, by transforming oncogenes such as *myc*, *sarc*, and *ras*, can result in increased glucose metabolism as a part of the transformation to a malignant phenotype (32,33). There has also been an increased understanding that after malignant transformation, due to a number of key mutations in the cellular DNA, cancer cells will grow, and before they are well vascularized, or possibly after, they are vascularized but outgrow their blood supplies and can reach a state of hypoxia, where they cannot supply their intrinsic energy metabolism via oxidative metabolism (34). In such circumstances, tumor growth can be sustained through glycolytic metabolism, which does not require oxygen and can occur at the hypoxic edge of the growing tumor. Increased FDG uptake in hypoxic cells has been shown in several studies *in vitro* (35).

As cancers often outgrow their blood supply, an adaptive mechanism to hypoxia is activation of the hypoxia-inducible factors, such as HIF-1α and HIF-2α (36–40). These proteins are made more active, under conditions of hypoxia (in the case of HIF-1α, the protein is not destroyed under hypoxic conditions), and this can lead to increases in a variety of key glycolytic enzymes including hexokinase II. Under the influence of HIF-1α, at least some tumors have accelerated glucose metabolism. However, the biological story is more complex because although HIF-1α protein levels are correlated with glucose uptake as measured by PET in some tumors, this is not always the case (30). Indeed, in some instances, HIF-1α levels are not clearly elevated in cancers with high glycolytic rates. Another enzyme of some importance in glycolysis is pyruvate dehydrogenase kinase I. This enzyme inactivates pyruvate dehydrogenase, which is essential for conversion of pyruvate to acetyl Co-A. Acetyl Co-A enters the Krebs cycle, allowing for oxidative metabolism to occur. The enzyme that inactivates pyruvate dehydrogenase, PDK1, tends to prevent pyruvate from entering the mitochondria. With increased levels of PDK1, oxidative glycolysis is not favored (41). It is of interest that up-regulation of vascular endothelial growth factor is also seen in the presence of hypoxia, increasing blood vessel growth and facilitating tumor growth. Thus, considerable interlinkage of glycolysis with the survival advantages of cancer is increasingly appreciated. Preferential glucose metabolism is very likely a survival advantage for rapidly growing tumors under conditions of hypoxia. These tumors also use glucose at high rates even under conditions of normoxia. It has been shown, however, that high FDG uptake in cancers is apparent in the cells that are most hypoxic, consistent with hypoxia's role in the FDG signal.

Although the reasons for increased glucose utilization in cancer are multifactorial, some general observations have been seen in a wide range of cancers as relates to the biological significance of the FDG signal. In general, across a wide range of tumor types, the extent of FDG uptake in tumors seems, at least in untreated tumors, is reasonably well and positively correlated with the viable cell number in that tumor (Figs. 8.1.2 and 8.1.3), both *in vitro* and *in*

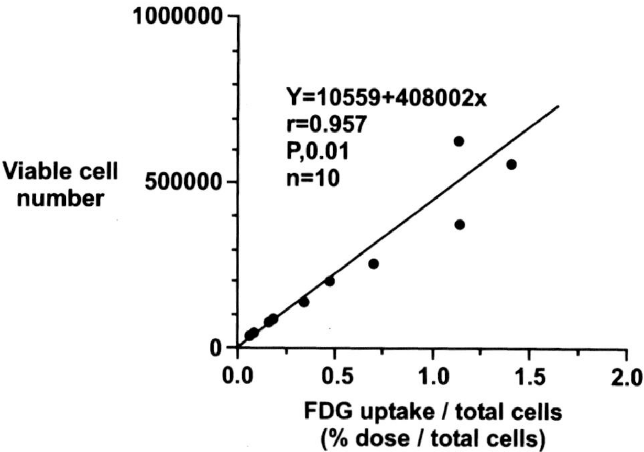

FIGURE 8.1.2. Relationship between viable cell number and fluorodeoxyglucose (FDG) uptake. This is shown in an adenocarcinoma line, but the relationship holds across many cell lines of varying etiologies. Uptake of FDG is more related to living cancer cell numbers than to the cell cycle, thus differing from agents imaging proliferation.

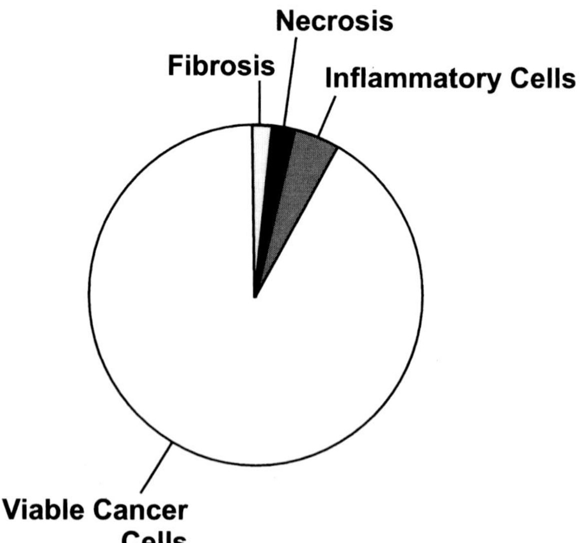

FIGURE 8.1.3. Distribution of fluorodeoxyglucose activity determined with quantitative autoradiographic techniques in breast cancer after intravenous delivery. The bulk of uptake in the untreated tumor is in viable cancer cells, but some uptake occurs into nonmalignant elements.

vivo (28,42–45). In our hands, the number of viable cancer cells expressing GLUT1 on the cell membrane appears best correlated with the extent of FDG uptake in a given type of cancer (Fig. 8.1.4). This association between GLUT1 protein levels and tumor FDG uptake is generally the case, but not invariably present. Strong relationships between GLUT1 membrane expression and FDG uptake have been shown in breast cancer, esophageal cancer, and lung cancer as examples (46,47). Some studies in humans have shown FDG uptake to be correlated with HIF-1α levels and proliferating cell nuclear antigen (PCNA) levels as well. Correlations with PCNA and HIF-1 has been less strong than correlations with GLUT1 expression. In some cancer systems, the uptake of FDG in tumors is strongly and positively correlated with tumor blood flow rates (48). The glycolytic pathway has also been shown to be closely linked to the AKT pathway as well (49–51).

The relationships between cancer cell number, glucose transporters, flow, hexokinase levels, insulin levels, oxygen tension, cell-cycle status, adenosine triphosphate levels, receptor status, and the [^{18}F] signal seen at PET are complex (Table 8.1.3). Of some note is that FDG uptake and GLUT1 expression rise markedly *in vitro* in many types of cancer cells that are made hypoxic. Tumors with low flow and high FDG uptake might well be expected to be hypoxic (52). Some studies have suggested that low blood flow and high FDG uptake in breast cancer is associated with a poor prognosis. Studies have shown high frequencies of GLUT1 positive cancer cells near necrotic regions, suggesting these border-zone cells are hypoxic (35,53). This has been confirmed in animal studies by several groups, who have shown that hypoxic tumors, as evidenced by pimonidazole staining, have higher FDG uptake than non-pimonidazole stained (less hypoxic) tumors (54). Such border zones often have elevated HIF-1α staining as well.

Determining which process—delivery of tracer to the tumor, transport of FDG into the cancer cell, or phosphorylation of the tracer into the form of FDG—is rate limiting has been a topic of some discussion. In the brain, delivery of FDG to brain is excellent. Due to the high blood flow rates, transport across blood vessels to the brain is rapid, and the glucose phosphorylation rate k_3 is generally felt to represent the rate-limiting step in FDG accumulation into normal brain, with the accumulated [^{18}F] activity in the form

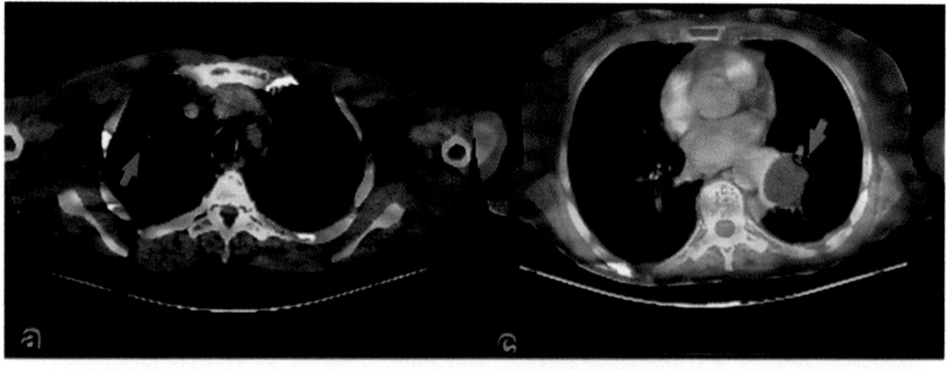

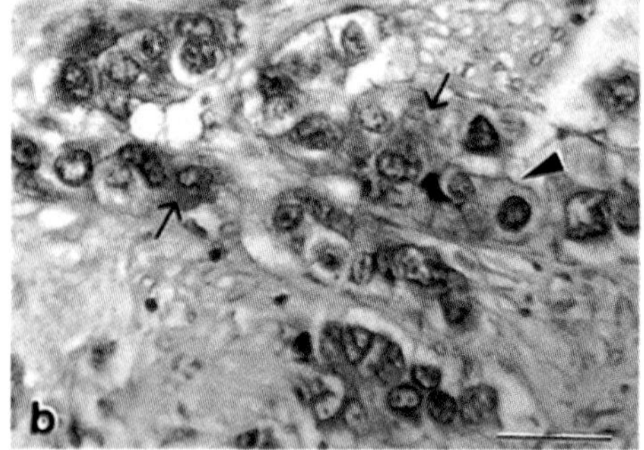

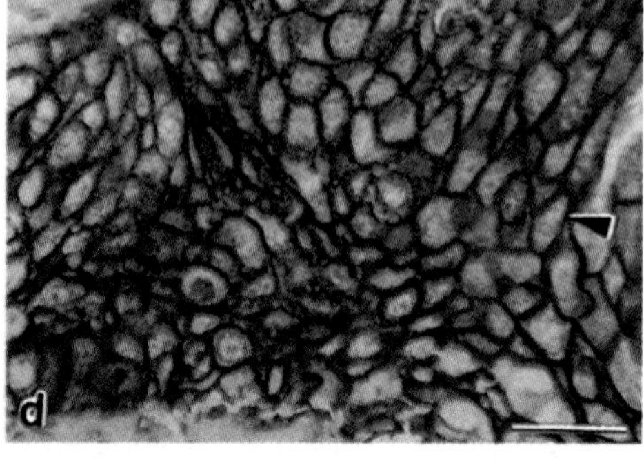

FIGURE 8.1.4. Fluorodeoxyglucose (FDG) uptake on PET (fused with CT using computer methods) into lung cancers in different patients. The FDG-avid tumor on the right has high cellularity and highly GLUT1 positive cancer cells. The tumor on the left has lower FDG uptake and lower GLUT1 positivity.

TABLE 8.1.3 Factors Affecting Fluorodeoxyglucose Uptake in Tumors

Factor	Increased	Decreased
Viable cell number	X	
Tumor perfusion	X	
Hypoxia	X	
Inflammatory cells	X	
Necrosis		X
Hyperglycemia		X
Insulin		X
Adenosine triphosphate levels	X	
Glucose transporter expression	X	
Hexokinase activity	X	
Receptor agonists	X	
Receptor blockade		X
Chemotherapy acute	X	
Chemotherapy effective		X
Radiation acute	X	
Radiation chronic		X

of FDG 6-phosphate (7). Tumors are somewhat different in that their perfusion rate is lower than normal brain, on average, and they have areas of very low perfusion, which are hypoxic in many cases due to continued growth of tumor. Thus, delivery of tracer and transport may be more critical than the phosphorylation rate in some of these tumors (29) or at least in areas of the tumors. This area is quite complex and controversial (55,56).

It is clear that higher levels of transporter molecules alone, such as in transgenic animals with an overexpression of GLUT1, can result in lower serum glucose levels, greater total body glucose utilization, and lesser susceptibility to the development of diabetes. This supports the concept that glucose transport can have important influences on glucose consumption rates, seemingly separate from the influence of the hexokinase levels (56). Using kinetic modeling approaches, some studies in humans have shown that tumors with higher standard uptake values (SUVs) actually had lower k_3 values than a group of tumors with high k_3 values (lung k_3 averaged lower than breast k_3, but lung SUVs were much higher than breast SUVs). This supports the importance of delivery and transport of the tracer to the net [^{18}F] accumulation in tumors (57). Studies have also shown that when flow is measured by H_2[^{15}O](^{15}O-water) and compared with FDG uptake, they correlate reasonably strongly, suggesting tumor [^{18}F] uptake and flow are reasonably well linked. Thus, factors other than GLUT1 positive viable tumor cell number contribute to the net accumulation of FDG in the form of FDG 6-phosphate in tumors, but the signal is clearly correlated with the number of living, glycolytically active cancer cells in the tumor.

Knowing FDG to be a tracer of a general process altered in cancers and not a tumor-specific process helps us understand false-positive results with FDG. Inflammatory cells of several types can accumulate FDG. This high FDG uptake can lead to confusion of infections/inflammation, with cancer in some instances. However, the high tracer uptake in infections can also serve as a useful tool to detect infections and inflammation in some circumstances. Inflammation can cause false-positive results after therapy (58–60). The role of FDG in detecting infections is detailed in Chapter 12.

FDG uptake can rise in tumor cells for other reasons. For example, receptor stimulation by receptor binding of agonists can increase tracer uptake, as can an acute cellular response to irradiation or chemotherapy, with which the cell uses glucose at an increased level in response to the "shock" of treatment in the early phases posttreatment (61). In the presence of certain chemotherapies, FDG uptake in cancers can decline to a greater extent than the number of viable cancer cells. Such "stunning" typically is short lived *in vitro*, but must be considered when FDG is used after chemotherapy. It is generally suggested that the use of FDG PET be delayed until several weeks after a chemotherapy dose has been given to minimize the risk of this "stunning" effect. Otherwise, a major decline in FDG uptake may inappropriately be attributed to successful cancer cell kill. *In vitro*, dissociations of glycolysis rate from viable cell number occur over only a few days, however, and the precise length of time required following chemotherapy to optimally assess for treatment efficacy is not yet fully resolved (62).

The learning process continues about FDG uptake and its mechanisms and alterations relative to specific therapies (63,64). It seems quite clear that caution must be exercised if inflammation is believed to be present or if there has been recent therapy. Obviously, stability in measurements of glucose metabolism will depend on careful attention to detail in replicating study preparation conditions. With careful attention to detail, PET with FDG can serve as an excellent method to monitor response of cancers to therapy (64). Much like high FDG uptake, low FDG uptake in certain tumors can be understood mechanistically. For example, bronchioloalveolar carcinomas often have low tracer uptake, as do mucinous adenocarcinomas (65). Likewise prostate cancer, carcinoid tumors, and lobular and renal cancers can have low FDG uptake. These tumors have much lower cellularity than many other tumors. It is important that the mechanisms of uptake of FDG and other new molecular imaging tracers be well understood at the cellular level to best interpret scans.

FDG is currently the most commonly used and versatile tracer for cancer imaging. It has limitations, however, and although exceedingly useful in answering many common questions in cancer imaging, other tracers currently available or in development may provide additional valuable information. Various processes use glucose, and the results can be confusing, for example, in infection, inflammation, normal brain, the heart, and others. Further, FDG is excreted by the kidneys to a much greater extent than glucose due to lesser renal reabsorption of FDG than glucose. This intense FDG uptake in the genitourinary system and brain can be confusing and make lesion detection difficult. FDG competes with glucose for uptake in tissues, so diabetics can have low FDG uptake in tumors if their serum glucose levels are high. FDG uptake does not vary markedly over the cell cycle, so if proliferation rate imaging is desired, FDG may not be the optimal tracer. Finally, some tumors have low enough FDG uptake that they are sometimes not detectable, such as some prostate cancers (66). Alternative tracers of a variety of types are under study. Choline-based compounds, radiolabeled amino acids, and carbon-11-acetate are showing promise in prostate and other cancers, for example (67–69).

Most cancer cells only modestly—or not at all—depend on insulin for FDG uptake, having little in the way of insulin-sensitive GLUT4 transporters on their cell surfaces. The heart, however, is very dependent on GLUT4. Thus, preparation of patients for oncologic FDG studies is completely different from that for cardiac FDG imaging. Glucose loading and insulin treatment are not generally warranted to achieve optimal cancer imaging in the euglycemic patient for cancer imaging. By contrast, for cardiac imaging, high insulin levels are essential at the time of FDG injection. Preclinical and clinical studies also clearly showed that high glucose levels in the blood reduce tumor targeting with FDG. Thus, close attention to dietary preparation is needed with FDG when the goal is optimal tumor imaging (70–72).

PRACTICAL ISSUES IN PET IMAGING OF THE CANCER PATIENT WITH FLUORODEOXYGLUCOSE

To successfully detect cancer in patients with FDG PET, images of consistently high technical quality must be obtained and consistent interpretation criteria applied by skilled physician interpreters. Excellent interpreters cannot overcome the limitations of poor quality images, but poor interpreters can cause excellent quality images to be misinterpreted. Similarly, it is possible, through a poor choice of imaging parameters and reconstruction methods, to have suboptimal quality images generated with a state of the art PET/CT system. Since nearly all new PET scanners are PET/CT scanners, a strong understanding of CT anatomy, both normal and pathological, is required to optimally interpret PET/CT images.

The determinants of lesion detectability in PET are severalfold and are reviewed, in part, in the physics section of this text and in the clinical chapters. With FDG, as with other tracers, there must be a sufficient signal detected by the PET scanner versus background activity for lesion detection (73). The absolute intensity of the signal is dependent on the biology of the lesion and the injected dose of radiotracer. For example, untreated breast cancer and prostate cancers have lower FDG uptake, on average, than similarly sized untreated small–cell lung cancers or melanomas (57). The images obtained from obese patients have substantially fewer of the usable high-quality counts per millicurie injected than those from thin patients due to the attenuation of the 511 keV photons by the body. Detectability will depend not only on the radioactivity levels in the tumor but also on the background levels in adjoining healthy tissues, the resolution and sensitivity of the scanning device, the reconstruction algorithm chosen, the injected dose, patient motion, and the experience of the interpreting physician.

IMAGING DEVICE

PET imaging devices continue to evolve in terms of their performance capabilities. Dedicated PET devices are typically fairly expensive, in part because of the thick detector materials required to stop the energetic 511 keV photons resulting from positron annihilation. Typically bismuth germanate (BGO) or other materials such as lutetium oxyorthosilicate (LSO), lutetium yttrium orthosilicate (LYSO), or germanium orthosiliate (GSO), and occasionally sodium iodide (NaI) are used. For high sensitivity from a PET scanner, there is presently no substitute for high-quality detector materials. Many high-quality "true" coincidence counts are needed to produce PET images of excellent quality. Since the half-value layer of 511 keV photons in water is just 7 cm, and both photons have to escape from the patient and be detected to have a coincidence event detected, attenuation effects are substantial as are attenuation correction factors.

Attempts to convert thin crystal, such as three eighths- to three-quarter-inch-thick NaI gamma cameras, even dual- and triple-head devices, into collimated gamma cameras for detection of the high-energy 511-keV photons have been disappointing. Their poor performance relative to dedicated PET systems occurs because many counts are rejected by thick collimators and because such devices do not take advantage of coincidence detection. In general, such systems have difficulty detecting small tumors, and when these systems have been compared with dedicated PET imaging, up to half of small lesions, <3 cm, were not detected with the collimated gamma camera but were detected with dedicated PET (74). Although some cancers can be seen with this method, and results in lung nodules of adequate size have been somewhat promising in some studies, collimated FDG single-photon emission computed tomography imaging is not recommended for clinical use due to its insensitivity for small lesions (75). Medicare in the United States will not reimburse for FDG imaging with such a device, practically making the technique unused for tumor imaging. Collimated FDG single-photon emission computed tomography systems are more useful for assessing myocardial viability.

There has been a greater level of interest and substantial progress in modifying dual- or triple-headed gamma cameras with NaI crystals as devices for positron imaging. These devices use coincidence circuitry as in dedicated PET and have spatial resolution comparable to that of high-quality gamma cameras. The cameras have a lower efficiency for detecting true coincidences than dedicated full-ring PET cameras and detect many more scatter events due to their need to use three-dimensional (3D) imaging to have good sensitivity.

The lower efficiency of NaI crystals and the large crystal size result in more potential acceptance of scattered counts. Although these cameras can work reasonably well in thin patients and in the thorax and neck in many clinical studies, they produce significantly inferior lesion detection statistics for lesions <2 to 3 cm, particularly those in the abdomen (76). These cameras may have utility in some limited settings, such as evaluating a large mass for viability; however, if dedicated PET is available, it is the preferred method for imaging.

The technology of these cameras has improved rapidly, and more recent generation scanning devices with thicker crystals, attenuation correction, some septa present (two and a half dimension, not 3D), and sophisticated iterative reconstruction programs have led to improved quality of images. However, the limited amount of detector material and its composition in these devices has generally resulted in images that are inferior to those obtained with traditional two-dimensional (2D) dedicated PET devices (77). Recognition of the lower accuracy of the hybrid devices led U.S. Medicare to substantially limit the use of these devices in PET imaging. This limitation on reimbursement has slowed dissemination of this form of technology. Such dual-purpose scanners can provide some value in imaging but are used with increasing rarity for dedicated PET applications.

Clearly, camera technology continues to evolve, and nearly all PET scans are now performed with dedicated PET scanners with thick detector crystals. Indeed since the introduction of PET/CT technology in commercial scanners, in 2001, virtually all PET sales and the vast majority of clinical PET scans in the United States are performed as PET/CT images. The CT images serve as rapid high photon flux transmission correction images with comparable quantitation to traditional positron-emitting source transmission images.

PATIENT SELECTION FOR PET

The number of indications for PET and PET/CT continue to grow, as evidenced by the many clinical application chapters in this book. In the United States, rather broad availability of PET/CT has been made possible through reimbursement by Centers for Medicare and Medicaid Services with a "coverage with evidence development" methodology. Specific indications in a variety of disease types are discussed. However, it is suggested that PET be used to answer questions it is best capable of answering and to achieve proper but not overutilization. Although specific indications for PET/CT are discussed in multiple sections of this book, a few general principles should apply in patient selection. Issues physicians face often are requests of a referring physician to evaluate a lesion <5 mm in size, either in the thorax or elsewhere in the body. This is asking a lot from PET, because many malignant lesions of this size are not detected on PET, due to resolution and count limitations (73). Although some can be seen, positive scan results are much more useful and reliable than negative scan results when the lesions are small. Such a scan may not be completely unreasonable if there is a concern for other foci of metastatic disease which might be more widely distributed. The issues faced with each patient should be thoroughly considered and if outside the realm of normal indications should be discussed with the referring physician so that expectations from the test are realistic, before the study is performed. If there are clear indications that the data from the PET study will not be helpful in the care of a certain patient, then it is the nuclear medicine physician's responsibility to discourage doing it.

Another frequently asked question is whether there is a tumor present after surgery. Trying to answer such a question a few days after surgery is difficult with PET, because there is normally uptake in surgical wounds and scars. If a wound is infected and whether a tumor is present or not are quite difficult to resolve because PET results are often positive in infections whether a tumor is present or not (60). Again, discussion with the referring physician may result in a postponement of the PET study for several months or until the infection has resolved.

Similarly, claustrophobic patients, patients with severe movement disorders (who cannot lie still for the scan), patients who are morbidly obese, patients who cannot lie on their backs or side, and poorly controlled diabetics are not optimal candidates for FDG PET. Access to all relevant history and correlative information is also quite important for optimal PET imaging. Education and discussion with the referring physician are essential to ensure that PET is used wisely and the risks and benefits of the test are known.

PATIENT PREPARATION

In contrast to cardiac PET imaging, in which insulin levels must be increased to target FDG to the cardiac muscle, in cancer imaging, the goal is to have low insulin levels at the time of FDG injection and a low blood sugar level. This optimizes tumor uptake and minimizes FDG uptake into skeletal muscle. This is typically achieved by making the patient fast for 4 or more hours before the scan. Often, patients are encouraged to drink water to maintain a good hydration level for the scans. This can enhance urinary excretion. Patients are usually instructed to avoid extensive physical activity before the PET scan so there is not FDG uptake into skeletal muscle. Low insulin and low glucose levels are best for PET imaging, however, too low a level of insulin or insulin nonresponsiveness, as is seen in diabetics, can be problematic. Many PET centers will not perform PET images on patients whose glucose levels exceed 200 mg/dL. This level of glucose can interfere with imaging and certainly can lower the SUV. For patients whose blood sugars exceed this level, many centers will reschedule the patients after their blood sugar is better controlled.

Practices vary, and patients with diabetes who are managed with oral hypoglycemics may be scanned early in the morning after an overnight fast. With such an approach, glucose levels can be manageable. Some allow the oral hypoglycemics to be taken pre-PET, others do not. Clearly, high insulin activity will degrade the quality of PET imaging by redirecting the FDG to muscle. If insulin is given to lower blood glucose levels it can degrade PET quality, and it is not recommended that regular insulin be given just before an oncologic PET study. If insulin management is undertaken for patients with hyperglycemia, close attention to serum glucose levels must be present, as such an approach can result in rapid development of dangerous hypoglycemic levels. On some occasions, low doses of regular insulin one or more hours prior to FDG injection may result in sufficiently low serum glucose levels to persist after the period of hyperinsulinemia, which may be suitable for PET imaging. This has been studied most closely in rodent diabetes models and less rigorously in patients with diabetes. Certainly, high serum glucose and directly interfered with FDG uptake, and we recommend it be measured at the time of each PET study.

There can be intense uptake of FDG into brown adipose tissue, which is clearly present in adults and which is even more prevalent in children. Brown adipose tissue (BAT), or "USA-fat" (uptake in the supraclavicular area fat), is a thermogenic structure, and although most is located in the supraclavicular region, there is commonly such fat in the neck, paraspinal regions, and not uncommonly in the upper abdomen near the adrenals and about the kidneys. Efforts should be undertaken to minimize brown fat FDG uptake as it can be confusing on PET and lead to difficulty in detecting small lesions located near brown fat or, in the worst situation, can be mistaken for tumor tissue (78–84). Since brown fat is richly innervated by the β-adrenergic system, β-blockers like propranolol can be effective in decreasing uptake of FDG into brown fat, both in preclinical systems and clinically (85). Although not a randomized trial, a dose of 20 mg orally of propranolol given 60 minutes pre-PET in a group of patients who had already had PET scans with intense FDG uptake present in BAT on a preceding scan had much lower FDG uptake in BAT. In this study, BAT SUVs in 26 patients studied without β-blockers was 5.52+/–2.3. By contrast, postpropranolol SUV_{max} (maximum SUV) was 1.39+/–0.42 (P <.0001). Tumor SUV did not change, however. In children, there is some evidence that stronger analgesics will diminish brown fat uptake. Although diazepam has been used, it has not been rigorously proven that this decreases the uptake of FDG in BAT at low doses. BAT uptake is not reduced in animals using benzodiazepines. Intravenous fentanyl pretreatment has been shown in children to decrease BAT uptake versus no pretreatment controls. Although there is some variability, it appears that cold weather makes brown fat uptake more prominent, or more likely, that exposure to the cold prior to PET scanning can increase FDG uptake into brown fat. Thus, most laboratories will have their uptake rooms quite warm prior to the performance of the PET scan with considerable efforts to keep the patient warm during the uptake phase.

Patient Interview

It is recommended that patients be interviewed by an imaging physician before they are scanned. Sometimes the history supplied in writing by the referring physician is inadequate or limited. Many centers provide a worksheet for the patient to describe any current medications and provide a brief medical history summary. The timing of correlative imaging studies and their availability and results are important issues to securing the proper diagnosis. Particularly important is securing historical information related to whether there have been recent surgical procedures, biopsies, and therapies, as well as regarding the patient's medications. For example, sites of recent biopsies can have increased tracer uptake. Similarly, patients who have just received effective chemotherapy are less likely to have their tumors visualized than patients who have not had recent therapy (e.g., chemotherapy can reduce tumor signal) (64). Bone metastases will be more difficult to detect in patients who have recently received colony-stimulating factors, because these increase the marrow signal (86). Obviously, exclusion of pregnancy in female patients is as important as securing information regarding claustrophobia or difficulty lying stationary for the scans. Thus, as in any nuclear medicine procedure, historical information can be very important. It is very important to be aware of the precise reason the PET scan is requested so that the scan can provide maximal diagnostic information regarding the diagnostic question. Given increasing concerns about radiation exposure, it may be decided that a more limited extent field of view PET/CT be performed to address a specific problem. This can only be known by a careful determination of the patient history, including input from multiple sources including charts, requisitions, correlative imaging data, and the patient interview.

INJECTION AND IMAGING

Various approaches to injected dose size and imaging duration have been studied. One important issue is the simple one of where to inject the dose. FDG is generally given intravenously, but the choice of vein is important. If FDG is extravasated in the arm, it typically accumulates in draining lymph nodes with great avidity (16). Thus, if the goal is to evaluate the right axilla of the patient for possible tumor involvement, injection of the right arm would not be preferred. Either the left arm or a foot vein would be preferable to minimize the possibility of a small amount of tracer extravasating and localizing to the draining regional lymph nodes. Although not commonly done, FDG can be given through central venous lines if there is good attention to flushing. Although this is not preferred, it is likely superior to an extravasated subcutaneous injection. FDG can also be given orally, but it is not specifically approved for this purpose. FDG is absorbed fairly rapidly after oral ingestion, so this approach may be suitable for brain imaging or imaging the thorax. It is more challenging in the abdomen as bowel activity can be intense. However, it is important to note that if given orally, SUV values will likely be lower than those for the intravenous route due to incomplete absorption, and if tumor imaging is the goal, delays from oral administration until imaging may be appropriate. For example, if tumor imaging is normally done at 1 hour postinjection of FDG intravenously, imaging at 2 hours postoral administration may be most appropriate.

The choice of the injected millicurie dose of FDG will be partly dependent on the scanning device chosen. With 2D (septa in use) BGO or 2D LYSO PET scanners, injected doses in the 10- to 15-mCi range are common, with doses of 20 mCi not unusual. Most oncologic PET with BGO scanners perform in the 2D mode to minimize scattered and random event detection. Scattered photons can substantially degrade the quality of whole-body images in some BGO systems, especially in larger patients. The emitted photon flux differs between small and large patients due to attenuation effects. With such systems, an injected dose of about 0.22 mCi/kg has been used and found generally to produce high-quality scans across a moderate range of patient sizes (87). By such approaches, larger patients may need a higher millicurie dose than small patients. With 3D acquisition mode scanners, which are increasingly the norm, lower injected doses can be given, although high-quality images can be achieved more rapidly with lower doses. With NaI detector full-ring scanners, an injected dose of approximately 5 mCi may be completely adequate. Such scanners are not being sold any longer. As time of flight scanners become available, careful attention must also be paid so as not to exceed the count rate capabilities of the scanner and degrade the time of flight capabilities. The injected dose should be adjusted to suit the scanner and its performance. Some centers give the same injected dose to all patients and change the duration of imaging based on patient size. Injected doses in Europe tend to be lower than those used in the United States. Critical in any discussion of injected dose is that most patients having whole-body PET studies have cancer and need an accurate diagnosis. Thus, while injecting a low dose is desirable from a radiation safety standpoint, the diagnostic quality of the study should not be compromised, or the low dose of radiation will have been given to no good end.

The duration of imaging is dependent to some extent on the injected dose. If more millicuries are given, a shorter acquisition will be feasible for comparable statistical quality. Typically 3 to 10 minutes of acquisition per imaging level is performed (emission), although the exact and optimal duration is not well established. The author currently acquires for oncology patients a scan level for 5 minutes based on an average 15-mCi injected dose per patient in 2D or 3D modes. The duration of acquisition in 3D can be shortened versus that of 2D.

If the goal is to detect a very small lesion, a larger injected dose and longer duration may be required. As reimbursement for PET imaging declines, patient throughput is increasingly important to optimize, so the technology can be available more broadly. Scanning smaller, more targeted parts of the body, along with faster acquisitions, is a means to increase patient throughput.

After patients are injected intravenously with FDG, they are asked to remain still and quiet and to not exert themselves, and at the appropriate time, they are asked to void and then imaging is begun. Voiding is done before PET emission imaging to minimize the FDG signal from the bladder and kidneys, where it is excreted. Fluorine-18 has a half-life of <2 hours, so the longer the uptake phase, the fewer the total counts available. Thus, although it is known that FDG uptake in tumors generally rises as a fraction of the injected dose from the time of injection until the time of imaging, emission images are usually begun between 50 and 60 minutes after the tracer is injected. Longer delays can provide better target-to-background ratios, but it is not clear that this results in improved accuracy in most cases, and it clearly results in lower statistical image quality. It has been suggested that delayed FDG imaging can help distinguish malignant and benign processes from one another. However, this ability is imperfect and such an approach is only used occasionally in busy clinics (88). Such an approach may increase the sensitivity of lesion detection in small lesions. Some centers are routinely imaging at 90 to 120 minutes post-FDG injection to take advantage of the higher target/background uptake ratios. Such an approach may increase sensitivity slightly. However, since such good results have been achieved with PET performed at 1 hour after tracer injection, it is the norm in most centers to perform PET at about 1 hour postinjection. It is important that the FDG imaging protocol be followed carefully to achieve reproducible results. Because FDG uptake after injection rises with time, the lesion uptake changes with time. Performing repeated FDG studies at precisely the same time after injection maximizes the chances of achieving reproducible results.

A decision must be made as to whether to perform attenuation correction of images or not. Attenuation correction adds time and noise to the study. There has been a trend toward reducing the duration of time used in acquiring the attenuation correction data and efforts to reduce noise (89). With perfect attenuation correction, PET is a precisely quantitative procedure, but perfect attenuation correction is not achieved due to statistical limitations, and in many instances, precise quantitation is not required diagnostically. For lesion detection, experienced readers can often detect nearly as many lesions with attenuation correction as without, and if there is a motion artifact or a low-quality attenuation scan, the nonattenuation-corrected images can be more diagnostically useful than the attenuation-corrected ones. Many institutions, including the author's, use attenuation correction with a segmented method to minimize noise and time requirements and also reconstruct the nonattenuation-corrected data sets for examination. The availability of quick and accurate attenuation correction from CT scans has made it quite normal for attenuation correction to be performed on each scan (90). Thus, in contrast to the state of affairs in the late 20th century, attenuation correction is the norm in PET today, with most attenuation correction performed using the CT scan and the CT-based attenuation factors. Given that artifacts can be introduced by attenuation correction, including if there is movement between the CT and the PET emission images, it is typically recommended that both the attenuation-corrected and noncorrected images be examined. It is normal to reconstruct both sets of images, attenuation corrected and noncorrected, routinely.

It should be noted that since the energy of the maximum (peak) x-rays in CT is 120 to 140 Kv(p) (thus with an average energy of well <100 KeV), the iodinated contrast and barium will absorb the photon energy to a much greater extent than such contrast absorbs the 511 KeV photons from a positron annihilation source, like germanium-68 or gallium-68, traditionally used in PET scanners in the pre- and to some extent post-, PET/CT eras. This can result in overattenuation correction in some instances where there is high contrast-related Hoonsfield Unit (HU) present on the CT chosen for attenuation correction. Such overcorrection can lead to overestimation of SUV values in the areas of very high contrast (91). However, the overestimates typically occur only where there is very dense contrast present, and such dense contrast is usually not present in most CT scans. It can occur if barium has been given days before the PET and there has been poor or slow reabsorption, or if there is imaging over the injected vein or the heart during the CT for contrast acquisition. However, in general these effects are quite modest and of little clinical significance at least for qualitative analysis purposes (92). Quantitative alterations in practice on PET/CT have been in the 10% to 15% maximum range in terms of tumor SUV. This can occur in lymph node lesions that vigorously enhance, for example (92). Thus, consideration of these contrast effects must be made if the contrast CT is chosen for attenuation correction.

The extent of the body imaged depends on the clinical question. For most cancers, images of the body from the acoustic meatus through the midthigh are viewed as adequate. Imaging of the full brain is not routine in most centers unless the patient has melanoma or known or strongly suspected brain metastases. Imaging of the brain is limited because a significant fraction of metastases do not have intense tracer uptake and may fail to be detected. The lower extremities are generally imaged if there is a specific question related to that portion of the body. For example, in patients with a history of melanoma of the foot, imaging the entire lower extremity is very appropriate. Imaging the entire body takes a long time and may necessitate shorter acquisition protocols per imaging level to be feasible. If a clinical question is focused only on the brain, then brain-only imaging is appropriate. If the clinical question is mainly regarding the head and neck, then more limited imaging for a longer duration may be most rational. For example, a dedicated head and neck PET imaging protocol with magnification and longer duration imaging showed higher SUV and probably detection of more small nodal metastases than was feasible with a whole-body acquisition, although the overall area under the curve for both was comparable (93).

Given that sometimes the question asked of PET is quite regional, such as evaluation of a solitary pulmonary nodule, it is reasonable that the PET/CT scan be tailored to the specific clinical question. Thus, a scan of only the lungs and upper abdomen may be adequate for evaluation of a solitary pulmonary nodule, while a larger field of view scan is appropriate for melanoma or lymphoma, which can arise anywhere.

Image reconstruction algorithms and filters are discussed elsewhere, but their choice is important for optimal imaging. It must be realized that to avoid very noisy appearing images, some image smoothing, or filtering, must take place. This means that the resolution of the scanner in patient studies is not as good as the potential optimal resolution of the scanner using, for example, a ramp filter in phantoms (73). The choice of reconstruction algorithm varies, but in many centers, the venerable filtered back-projection method is still often used in high-count brain PET studies. Iterative algebraic methods, such as the ordered subset expectation maximization, are more commonly used for visceral imaging. These algebraic methods reduce streak artifacts but can produce other distortions such as "hot spots," not "hot lines." The interpreting physician and physicist for the facility must make a rational choice of filter type, filter cutoff and reconstruction algorithms for the camera, and injected dose and use them consistently to maximize reproducibility of PET studies.

Interpretation of PET images requires considerable clinical experience. It is recommended that images be read in an interactive fashion on a computer monitor with the ability to display coronal, sagittal, transverse, and maximum-intensity projection or rotating views. The ability to vary the gray scale is very important. Although images can be read on film, most centers prefer to read soft-copy image sets. A familiarity with normal structures and their variants is important (Chapter 8.3). The quantitation of PET using SUV is discussed in detail elsewhere in this book (Chapter 6) .

Choice of the CT Scan

With the widespread availability of PET/CT there are important protocol choices for not just the PET scan, but also for the CT scan.

The range of CT equipment available is quite extensive, ranging from simple single or 4-slice CT scanners to 8-, 16-, 40-, and 64-slice scanners. It can be expected that the quality of CT scanners deployed as part of PET/CT will continue to improve as the overall quality and performance of CT scanners continues to rise. The range of CT scans performed as part of PET/CT varies considerably depending on the specific diagnostic question. If the PET/CT is designed to be a "one-stop-shop" in which a fully diagnostic CT and a diagnostic PET is performed in the same imaging session, the CT choices would be dictated by the clinical needs for a CT scan. Thus, for a liver question, a multiphase CT of the liver may be considered, which would be a different approach than for a patient with a question of disseminated cancer. A discussion of diagnostic CT protocols is beyond the scope of this chapter, but books on the specific topic and Web sites like (ctisus.com) often have useful information for CT choices.

The extent of the CT scan and the power settings both contribute to the radiation absorbed dose from PET/CT. Thus, a more limited CT scan at low power will be potentially reasonable in some settings. Although adequate attenuation correction can be achieved at tube currents of 10 mA or even less, these provide only limited anatomic information and can compromise diagnostic quality. Some center use radiation doses of 80 mA or more with a relatively high pitch for the whole body area studied, and then do a follow-up more detailed CT of the region in question. For example, contrast might only be used in the head and neck images and not the remaining images.

The proper way to perform the CT of PET/CT will vary, depending on the specific clinical situation. There has been increasing sentiment, even among body imagers, that high-quality contrast CT scans may add little in, for example, the follow-up of patients with lymphoma who are otherwise doing well (Radiological Society of North America Imaging Symposium 2007. Special focus session: PET/CT versus PET alone: Is CT always appropriate?) Clearly, trying to minimize the radiation dose from PET/CT while maximizing diagnostic information from both studies is the goal. There has been a trend in many centers to move from nearly all "noncontrast" low-powered CT scans for attenuation correction and lesion localization to a more fully diagnostic CT. However, it must be recognized that virtually all CT scans carry with them diagnostic information of substantial quality. This information is incremental to that provided by PET in many cases, so that the CT must always be looked at carefully for abnormalities, in addition to the PET images (94).

QUANTITATIVE MEASUREMENTS

Quantitative and semiquantitative methods can be used in PET image interpretation, although most centers use qualitative interpretation techniques as the major part of the diagnostic procedure. The only semiquantitative technique relatively routinely applied is the SUV (95). The SUV is discussed in detail in Chapter 6 and other quantitative approaches are discussed in Chapter 5. The SUV can be normalized to body weight, lean body mass, or body surface area. The author's preference is the SUV normalized to predicted lean body mass, but it is very important to be consistent across patients.

FUSION OF FORM AND FUNCTION

FDG has a high level of targeting to many cancers, which is highly desirable on most counts. However, an early and obvious limitation

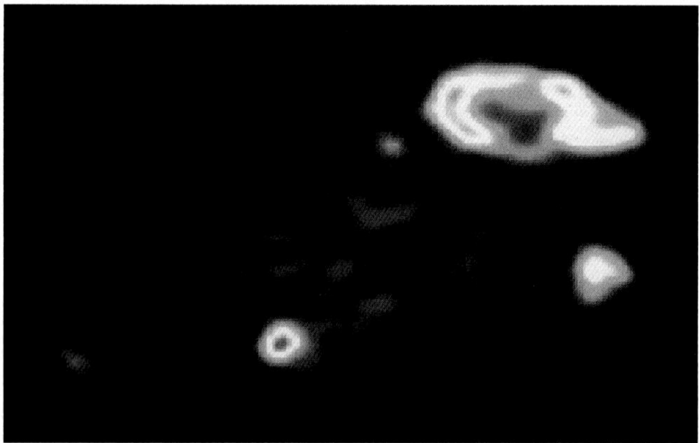

FIGURE 8.1.5. Fluorodeoxyglucose PET scan of a patient with breast cancer, showing the difficulty in anatomically locating "hot spots" representing tumor. This transverse scan shows the large primary tumor on the patient's left, a left axillary node and posterior uptake in the spine or possibly the lung. (From Wahl RL, Cody RL, Hutchins GD, et al. PET imaging of breast cancer with ^{18}F-FDG. *Radiology* 1989;173: 419P, with permission.)

seen in our earliest clinical studies of breast cancer in 1989 showed a disadvantage of being successful, almost too well, in targeting a radiopharmaceutical to cancer. The problem was that the tumors could be seen, but it was difficult to tell precisely where they were located anatomically. An early image obtained of breast cancer shows this clearly (Fig. 8.1.5); there are tumors present, but the exact anatomic location could not be determined. Anatomy is still needed. Working with my colleague Chuck Meyer at Michigan, we developed methods to fuse the anatomic information of CT with PET into "anatometabolic images" (1). These images show what the functional activity is and where. However, they are challenging to generate in some circumstances and are prone to misalignment unless great caution is taken in positioning patients identically between the PET and CT or MRI studies (1). Thus, a need for better fusion is clearly needed.

Although FDG is a potent, but simple, molecular imaging tracer and has been the cornerstone of clinical PET imaging in cancer, PET methods, while anatomically precise, are limited in their accuracy for precisely localizing lesions. A major practical problem has been that PET can find the specific molecular alteration, but it can be very difficult to know what to do about it clinically if it cannot be localized or biopsied to add certainty to the diagnosis. Some years ago, the technique of "anatometabolic fusion imaging" was described by the author and his colleagues, detailing the fusion of PET and CT data sets via software. This ability to use software and more recently dedicated hardware solutions to present PET molecular imaging data in a clear and well-understood anatomic context is key to the progress of molecular imaging. However, software approaches require extreme attention to detail to be successful and are very difficult to use reliably, other than in the brain.

Beyer et al. (90) fused the PET and CT methods using hardware and software, by combining a PET and a CT scanner in the same hybrid device so the patient has both types of scans performed during a single acquisition period. This technology was of obvious utility, and the fusions were of high quality. Several manufacturers were able to see the obvious benefits of this type of approach. Those at Johns Hopkins Hospital are fortunate to have access to the first commercially produced PET/CT scanner in the United States and have used it in diagnosing cancer in many thousands of patients since

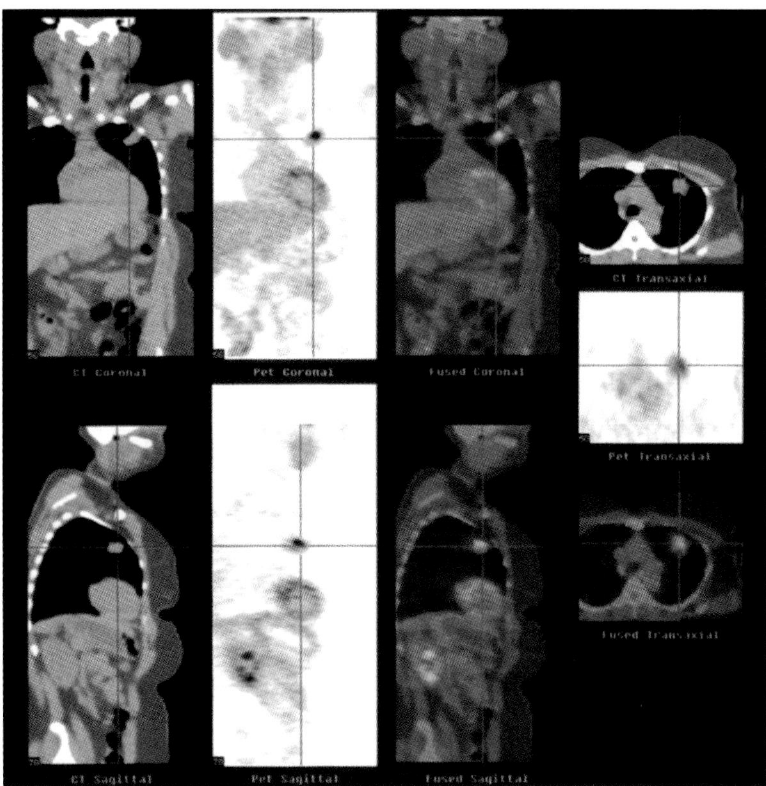

FIGURE 8.1.6. "Anatomolecular" images obtained from a patient with suspected lung cancer using the Discovery LS (GE Healthcare Americas, Waukesha, WI) PET/CT system. Fusion of molecular functional information with CT is achieved and demonstrates intense uptake into a left lung abnormality seen on CT, which indicates primary lung cancer.

mid-2001. The benefits of this technology were immediately apparent to those interpreting studies on a daily basis, but they are being rigorously studied to determine if this technology is clearly cost-effective versus alternative methods. An example of a combined PET/CT scan obtained with this equipment is shown in Fig. 8.1.6. It is estimated that 1 to 1.5 million PET or CT scans per year were performed worldwide in 2007. The vast majority will would have been done with combined PET/CT. Indeed, it is not possible to purchase a PET-only scanner for whole-body imaging in the United States at this time, with only PET/CT scanners commercially available.

Anatomolecular imaging using FDG and PET/CT is a clinical reality, and PET/CT has been adopted as the new clinical standard for noninvasive imaging for many cancer patients.

COST-EFFECTIVENESS

Excellent examples of cost-effectiveness studies and a review of cost-effectiveness with an emphasis on PET have appeared in the literature (96,97). PET appears to be quite cost-effective in a substantial number of cancers including lung, colon, and lymphoma, among others, if used at the time of a key management decision (98). Suffice it to say that in many instances, PET is the most accurate diagnostic test for cancer, and it often costs less than or no more than performing CT scans of multiple levels of the body, with and without contrast. The major cost savings with PET occur, however, when PET provides diagnostic information that reduces the frequency of alternative expensive procedures—for example, avoiding thoracotomy in lung or esophageal cancer or eliminating the need for surgery in patients with colorectal cancer. In the United States, the cost/efficacy ratio of PET has recently improved, as Medicare has continued to lower reimbursement for PET. Lower PET reimbursement serves to make PET more cost-effective. If rates are cut too much, PET could become less available, however. Although PET has been considered an "expensive" imaging test by many, it is clear that the improved quality of decisions resulting from PET and lower costs for PET based on improved throughput have served to make the test one considered effective and necessary by referring physicians, not one in which a careful cost/benefit decision must be made in each case of intended use. With the use of PET to personalize cancer therapy in individual patients, it is clear that we must continue to learn and more rationally apply PET to choose our treatments in a more cost-effective manner, thus amplifying the cost-efficacy of PET.

SUMMARY

Anatomic imaging of cancer using x-rays has proven very useful for more than 100 years but has clear limitations. Anatomic methods reliably show whether a large mass is present or absent, but not what the mass is composed of. Imaging additional phenotypic alterations of the altered genotype of cancers with PET adds clinically valuable information for patient management. Although many molecular alterations are present in cancer, the one by far most exploited in clinical practice and research has been the accelerated glucose metabolism present in most cancers. This process is imaged well with the radiotracer [^{18}F]-FDG. The ability to spatially localize the molecular alterations of cancer, through fused "anatomolecular" image sets generated by PET/CT, is key to optimal use of the imaging methods, as is careful attention to consistency in scan acquisition.

Although a wide range of newer relevant biological targets are available and are discussed elsewhere in this text, for now, in clinical practice, [^{18}F]-FDG is the dominant tracer. A thorough understanding of the use of FDG in PET, as well as how to best integrate it with CT, will allow the vast majority of clinical PET oncologic diagnoses to be made successfully.

REFERENCES

1. Anzai Y, Carroll WR, Quint DJ, et al. Recurrence of head and neck cancer after surgery or irradiation: prospective comparison of 2-deoxy-2-[F-18]fluoro-D-glucose PET and MR imaging diagnoses. *Radiology* 1996;200(1):135–141.
2. Sugawara Y, Zasadny KR, Grossman HB, et al. Germ cell tumor: differentiation of viable tumor, mature teratoma, and necrotic tissue with FDG-PET and kinetic modeling. *Radiology* 1999;211(1):249–256.
3. Wahl RL, Quint LE, Cieslak RD, et al. "Anatometabolic" tumor imaging: fusion of FDG-PET with CT or MRI to localize foci of increased activity. *J Nucl Med* 1993;34(7):1190–1197.
4. Zhang W, Laborde PM, Coombes KR, et al. Cancer genomics: promises and complexities. *Clin Cancer Res* 2001;7(8):2159–2167.
5. Hanahan D, Weinberg RA. The hallmarks of cancer. *Cell* 2000;100 (1):57–70.
6. Warburg O. *The metabolism of tumors.* New York: Richard R. Smith, 1931:129–169.
7. Phelps ME, Huang SC, Hoffman EJ, et al. Tomographic measurement of local cerebral glucose metabolic rate in humans with (^{18}F)2-fluoro-2-deoxy-D-glucose: validation of method. *Ann Neurol* 1979;6(5):371–388.
8. Som P, Atkins HL, Bandoypadhyay D, et al. A fluorinated glucose analog, 2-fluoro-2-deoxy-D-glucose (^{18}F): nontoxic tracer for rapid tumor detection. *J Nucl Med* 1980;21(7):670.
9. Larson SM, Weiden PL, Grunbaum Z, et al. Positron imaging feasibility studies, II: characteristics of 2-deoxyglucose uptake in rodent and canine neoplasms: concise communication. *J Nucl Med* 1981;22(10):875–879.
10. Patronas NJ, Di-Chiro G, Brooks RA, et al. Work in progress: [^{18}F] fluorodeoxyglucose and positron emission tomography in the evaluation of radiation necrosis of the brain. *Radiology* 1982;144(4):885–889.
11. Yonekura Y, Benua RS, Brill AB, et al. Increased accumulation of 2-deoxy-2-[^{18}F]fluoro-D-glucose in liver metastases from colon carcinoma. *J Nucl Med* 1982;23(12):1133–1137.
12. Kern KA, Brunetti A, Norton JA, et al. Metabolic imaging of human extremity musculoskeletal tumors by PET. *J Nucl Med* Feb 1988;29 (2):181–186.
13. Paul R. Comparison of fluorine-18-2-fluorodeoxyglucose and gallium-67 citrate imaging for detection of lymphoma. *J Nucl Med* Mar 1987;28(3):288–292.
14. Strauss LG, Clorius JH, Schlag P, et al. Recurrence of colorectal tumors: PET evaluation. *Radiology* 1989;170(2):329–332.
15. Fujiwara T, Matsuzawa T, Kubota K, et al. Relationship between histologic type of primary lung cancer and carbon 11 L methionine uptake with positron emission tomography. *J Nucl Med* 1989;30(1):33–37.
16. Wahl RL, Kaminski MS, Ethier SP, et al. The potential of 2-deoxy-2[^{18}F]fluoro-D-glucose (FDG) for the detection of tumor involvement in lymph nodes. *J Nucl Med* 1990;31(11):1831–1835.
17. Wahl RL, Hutchins GD, Buchsbaum DJ, et al. ^{18}F-2-deoxy-2-fluoro-D-glucose uptake into human tumor xenografts. Feasibility studies for cancer imaging with positron-emission tomography. *Cancer* 1991;67: 1544–1550.
18. Wahl RL, Cody RL, Hutchins GD, et al. PET imaging of breast cancer with ^{18}F-FDG. *Radiology* 1989;173:419P.
19. Wahl RL, Cody R, Hutchins GD, et al. Primary and metastatic breast carcinoma: initial clinical evaluation with PET with the radiolabeled glucose analog 2-[^{18}F]-fluoro-deoxy-2-D-glucose (FDG). *Radiology* 1991;179:765–770.
20. Wahl RL, Harney J, Hutchins G, et al. Imaging of renal cancer using positron emission tomography with 2-deoxy-2-(^{18}F)-fluoro-D-glucose: pilot animal and human studies. *J Urol* 1991;146(6):1470–1474.
21. Harney JV, Wahl RL, Liebert M, et al. Uptake of 2-deoxy, 2-(^{18}F) fluoro-D-glucose in bladder cancer: animal localization and initial patient positron emission tomography. *J Urol* 1991;145(2):279–283.
22. Wahl RL, Hutchins GD, Roberts J. FDG-PET imaging of ovarian cancer: initial evaluation in patients. *J Nucl Med* 1991;32(5):982.
23. Gritters LS, Francis IR, Zasadny KR, et al. Initial assessment of positron emission tomography using 2-fluorine-^{18}fluoro-2-deoxy-D-glucose in the imaging of malignant melanoma. *J Nucl Med* 1993;34(9):1420–1427.
24. Kubota K, Matsuzawa T, Amemiya A, et al. Imaging of breast cancer with [^{18}F]fluorodeoxyglucose and positron emission tomography. *J Comput Assist Tomogr* 1989;13(6):1097–1098.
25. Dahlbom M, Hoffman EJ, Hoh CK, et al. Whole-body positron emission tomography: part I: methods and performance characteristics. *J Nucl Med* 1992;33:1191–1199.
26. Rosenfeld SS, Hoffman JM, Coleman RE, et al. Studies of primary central nervous system lymphoma with fluorine-18-fluorodeoxyglucose positron emission tomography. *J Nucl Med* 1992;33(4):532–536.
27. Hoh CK, Hawkins RA, Glaspy JA, et al. Cancer detection with whole-body PET using 2-[^{18}F]fluoro-2-deoxy-D-glucose. *J Comput Assist Tomogr* 1993;17(4):582–589.
28. Brown RS, Wahl RL. Over expression of Glut-1 glucose transporter in human breast cancer: an immunohistochemical study. *Cancer* 1993; 72(10):2979–2985.
29. Tian M, Zhang H, Nakasone Y, et al. Expression of Glut-1 and Glut-3 in untreated oral squamous cell carcinoma compared with FDG accumulation in a PET study. *Eur J Nucl Med Mol Imaging* 2004;31(1):5–12.
30. Bos R, van Der Hoeven JJ, van Der Wall E, et al. Biologic correlates of (18)fluorodeoxyglucose uptake in human breast cancer measured by positron emission tomography. *J Clin Oncol* 2002;20(2):379–387.
31. Natsuizaka M, Ozasa M, Darmanin S, et al. Synergistic up-regulation of hexokinase-2, glucose transporters and angiogenic factors in pancreatic cancer cells by glucose deprivation and hypoxia. *Exp Cell Res* 2007;313(15):3337–3348.
32. Dang CV, Lewis BC, Dolde C, et al. Oncogenes in tumor metabolism, tumorigenesis, and apoptosis. *J Bioenerg Biomembr* 1997;29(4):345–354.
33. Shim H, Dolde C, Lewis BC, et al. c-Myc transactivation of LDH-A: implications for tumor metabolism and growth. *Proc Natl Acad Sci U S A* 1997;94(13):6658–6663.
34. Gatenby RA, Gillies RJ. Glycolysis in cancer: a potential target for therapy. *Int J Biochem Cell Biol* 2007;39(7–8):1358–1366.
35. Clavo AC, Brown RS, Wahl RL. Fluorodeoxyglucose uptake in human cancer cell lines is increased by hypoxia. *J Nucl Med* 1995;36(9): 1625–1632.
36. Semenza GL, Roth PH, Fang HM, et al. Transcriptional regulation of genes encoding glycolytic enzymes by hypoxia-inducible factor 1. *J Biol Chem* 1994;269(38):23757–23763.
37. Dang CV, Semenza GL. Oncogenic alterations of metabolism. *Trends Biochem Sci* 1999;24(2):68–72.
38. Semenza GL, Artemov D, Bedi A, et al. "The metabolism of tumours": 70 years later. *Novartis Found Symp* 2001;240:251–260; discussion 260–264.
39. Kim JW, Gao P, Liu YC, et al. Hypoxia-inducible factor 1 and dysregulated c-Myc cooperatively induce vascular endothelial growth factor and metabolic switches hexokinase 2 and pyruvate dehydrogenase kinase 1. *Mol Cell Biol* 2007;27(21):7381–7393.
40. Semenza GL. HIF-1 mediates the Warburg effect in clear cell renal carcinoma. *J Bioenerg Biomembr* 2007;39(3):231–234.
41. Kim JW, Gao P, Liu YC, et al. HIF-1 and dysregulated c-Myc cooperatively induces VEGF and metabolic switches, HK2 and PDK1. *Mol Cell Biol* 2007;27(21):7381–7393.
42. Brown RS, Fisher SJ, Wahl RL. Autoradiographic evaluation of the intra-tumoral distribution of 2-deoxy-D-glucose and monoclonal antibodies in xenografts of human ovarian adenocarcinoma. *J Nucl Med* 1993;34(1):75–82.
43. Higashi K, Clavo AC, Wahl RL. Does FDG uptake measure proliferative activity of human cancer cells? *In vitro* comparison with DNA flow cytometry and tritiated thymidine uptake. *J Nucl Med* 1993;34:414–419.
44. Brown RS, Leung JY, Fisher SJ, et al. Intratumoral distribution of tritiated-FDG in breast carcinoma: correlation between Glut-1 expression and FDG uptake. *J Nucl Med* 1996;37(6):1042–1047.

45. Brown RS, Leung JY, Kison PV, et al. Glucose transporters and FDG uptake in untreated primary human non-small cell lung cancer. *J Nucl Med* 1999;40(4):556–565.
46. Westerterp M, Sloof GW, Hoekstra OS, et al. (18)FDG uptake in oesophageal adenocarcinoma: linking biology and outcome. *J Cancer Res Clin Oncol* 2007;134(2):227–236.
47. van Baardwijk A, Dooms C, van Suylen RJ, et al. The maximum uptake of (18)F-deoxyglucose on positron emission tomography scan correlates with survival, hypoxia inducible factor-1alpha and GLUT-1 in non-small cell lung cancer. *Eur J Cancer* 2007;43(9):1392–1398.
48. Zasadny KR, Tatsumi M, Wahl RL. FDG metabolism and uptake versus blood flow in women with untreated primary breast cancers. *Eur J Nucl Med Mol Imaging* 2003;30(2):274–280.
49. Elstrom RL, Bauer DE, Buzzai M, et al. AKT stimulates aerobic glycolysis in cancer cells. *Cancer Res* 2004;64(11):3892–3899.
50. Plas DR, Thompson CB. AKT-dependent transformation: there is more to growth than just surviving. *Oncogene* 2005;24(50):7435–7442.
51. Bui T, Thompson CB. Cancer's sweet tooth. *Cancer Cell* 2006;9(6): 419–420.
52. Burgman P, Odonoghue JA, Humm JL, et al. Hypoxia-induced increase in FDG uptake in MCF7 cells. *J Nucl Med* 2001;42(1):170–175.
53. Clavo AC, Wahl RL. Effects of hypoxia on the uptake of tritiated thymidine, L-leucine, L-methionine and FDG in cultured cancer cells. *J Nucl Med* 1996;37(3):502–506.
54. Dearling JL, Flynn AA, Sutcliffe-Goulden J, et al. Analysis of the regional uptake of radiolabeled deoxyglucose analogs in human tumor xenografts. *J Nucl Med.* 2004;45(1):101–107.
55. Aloj L, Caraco C, Jagoda E, et al. Glut-1 and hexokinase expression: relationship with 2-fluoro-2-deoxy-D-glucose uptake in A431 and T47D cells in culture. *Cancer Res* 1999;59(18):4709–4714.
56. Hansen PA, Marshall BA, Chen M, et al. Transgenic overexpression of hexokinase II in skeletal muscle does not increase glucose disposal in wild-type or Glut1-overexpressing mice. *Biol Chem* 2000;275(29): 22381–22386.
57. Torizuka T, Zasadny KR, Recker B, et al. Untreated primary lung and breast cancers: correlation between F-18 FDG kinetic rate constants and findings of *in vitro* studies. *Radiology* 1998;207(3):767–774.
58. Kubota R, Yamada S, Kubota K, et al. Intratumoral distribution of fluorine-18-fluorodeoxyglucose *in vivo:* high accumulation in macrophages and granulation tissues studied by microautography. *J Nucl Med* 1992;33(11):1972–1980.
59. Brown RS, Leung JY, Fisher SJ, et al. Intratumoral distribution of tritiated fluorodeoxyglucose in breast carcinoma, I: are inflammatory cells important? *J Nucl Med* 1995;36(10):1854–1861.
60. Sugawara Y, Braun DK, Kison PV, et al. Rapid detection of human infections with fluorine-18 fluorodeoxyglucose and positron emission tomography: preliminary results. *Eur J Nucl Med* 1998;25(9):1238–1243.
61. Higashi K, Clavo AC, Wahl RL. *In vitro* assessment of 2-fluoro-2-deoxy-D-glucose, L-methionine and thymidine as agents to monitor the early response of a human adenocarcinoma cell line to radiotherapy. *J Nucl Med* 1993;34(5):773–779.
62. Engles JM, Quarless SA, Mambo E, et al. Stunning and its effect on 3H-FDG uptake and key gene expression in breast cancer cells undergoing chemotherapy. *J Nucl Med* 2006;47(4):603–608.
63. Minn HR, Zasadny KR, Quint LE, et al. Lung cancer: reproducibility of quantitative measurements for evaluating 2-[F-18]-fluoro-2-deoxy-D-glucose uptake at PET. *Radiology* 1995;196:167–173.
64. Wahl RL, Zasadny KR, Hutchins GD, et al. Metabolic monitoring of breast cancer chemohormonotherapy using positron emission tomography (PET): initial evaluation. *J Clin Oncol* 1993;11(11):2101–2111.
65. Higashi K, Ueda Y, Seki H, et al. Fluorine-18-FDG-PET imaging is negative in bronchioloalveolar lung carcinoma. *J Nucl Med* 1998;39(6): 1016–1020.
66. Shreve PD, Grossman HB, Gross MD, et al. Metastatic prostate cancer: initial findings of PET with 2-deoxy-2-[F-18]fluoro-D-glucose. *Radiology* 1996;199(3):751–756.
67. Kobori O, Kirihara Y, Kosaka N, et al. Positron emission tomography of esophageal carcinoma using ^{11}C-choline and ^{18}F-fluorodeoxyglucose: a novel method of preoperative lymph node staging. *Cancer* 1999;86(9):1638–1648.
68. Oyama N, Miller TR, Dehdashti F, et al. ^{11}C-acetate PET imaging of prostate cancer: detection of recurrent disease at PSA relapse. *J Nucl Med* 2003;44(4):549–555.
69. Schuster DM, Votaw JR, Nieh PT, et al. Initial experience with the radiotracer anti-1-amino-3-^{18}F-fluorocyclobutane-1-carboxylic acid with PET/CT in prostate carcinoma. *J Nucl Med* 2007;48(1):56–63.
70. Wahl RL, Henry CA, Ethier SP. Serum glucose: effects on tumor and normal tissue accumulation of 2-[^{18}F]-fluoro-2-deoxy-D-glucose in rodents with mammary carcinoma. *Radiology* 1992;183(3):643–647.
71. Torizuka T, Fisher SJ, Brown RS, et al. Effect of insulin on uptake of FDG by experimental mammary carcinoma in diabetic rats. *Radiology* 1998;208(2):499–504.
72. Torizuka T, Fisher SJ, Wahl RL. Insulin-induced hypoglycemia decreases uptake of 2-[F-18]fluoro-2-deoxy-D-glucose into experimental mammary carcinoma. *Radiology* 1997;203(1):169–172.
73. Raylman RR, Kison PV, Wahl RL. Capabilities of two- and three-dimensional FDG-PET for detecting small lesions and lymph nodes in the upper torso: a dynamic phantom study. *Eur J Nucl Med* 1999;26(1):39–45.
74. Macfarlane DJ, Cotton L, Ackermann RJ, et al. Triple-head SPECT with 2-[fluorine-18]fluoro-2-deoxy-D-glucose (FDG): initial evaluation in oncology and comparison with FDG-PET. *Radiology* 1995;194(2): 425–429.
75. Mastin ST, Drane WE, Harman EM, et al. FDG SPECT in patients with lung masses. *Chest* 1999;115(4):1012–1017.
76. Shreve PD, Steventon RS, Deters EC, et al. Oncologic diagnosis with 2-[fluorine-18]fluoro-2-deoxy-D-glucose imaging: dual-head coincidence gamma camera versus positron emission tomographic scanner. *Radiology* 1998;207(2):431–437.
77. Delbeke D, Sandler MP. The role of hybrid cameras in oncology. *Semin Nucl Med* 2000;30(4):268–280.
78. Cohade C, Osman M, Pannu HK, et al. Uptake in supraclavicular area fat ("USA-Fat"): description on ^{18}F-FDG PET/CT. *J Nucl Med* 2003; 44(2):170–176.
79. Cohade C, Mourtzikos KA, Wahl RL. "USA-Fat": prevalence is related to ambient outdoor temperature-evaluation with ^{18}F-FDG PET/CT. *J Nucl Med* 2003;44(8):1267–1270.
80. Hany TF, Gharehpapagh E, Kamel EM, et al. Brown adipose tissue: a factor to consider in symmetrical tracer uptake in the neck and upper chest region. *Eur J Nucl Med Mol Imaging* 2002;29(10):1393–1398.
81. Bar-Shalom R, Gaitini D, Keidar Z, et al. Non-malignant FDG uptake in infradiaphragmatic adipose tissue: a new site of physiological tracer biodistribution characterised by PET/CT. *Eur J Nucl Med Mol Imaging* 2004;31(8):1105–1113.
82. Gelfand MJ, O'Hara S M, Curtwright LA, et al. Pre-medication to block [(18)F]FDG uptake in the brown adipose tissue of pediatric and adolescent patients. *Pediatr Radiol* 2005;35(10):984–990.
83. Tatsumi M, Engles JM, Ishimori T, et al. Intense (18)F-FDG uptake in brown fat can be reduced pharmacologically. *J Nucl Med* 2004;45(7): 1189–1193.
84. Yeung HW, Grewal RK, Gonen M, et al. Patterns of (18)F-FDG uptake in adipose tissue and muscle: a potential source of false-positives for PET. *J Nucl Med* 2003;44(11):1789–1796.
85. Soderlund V, Larsson SA, Jacobsson H. Reduction of FDG uptake in brown adipose tissue in clinical patients by a single dose of propranolol. *Eur J Nucl Med Mol Imaging* 2007;34(7):1018–1022.
86. Sugawara Y, Fisher SJ, Zasadny KR, et al. Preclinical and clinical studies of bone marrow uptake of fluorine-1-fluorodeoxyglucose with or without granulocyte colony-stimulating factor during chemotherapy. *J Clin Oncol* 1998;16(1):173–180.
87. Tatsumi M, Clark PA, Nakamoto Y, et al. Impact of body habitus on quantitative and qualitative image quality in whole-body FDG-PET. *Eur J Nucl Med Mol Imaging* 2003;30(1):40–45.

88. Zhuang H, Pourdehnad M, Lambright ES, et al. Dual time point ^{18}F-FDG PET imaging for differentiating malignant from inflammatory processes. *J Nucl Med* 2001;42(9):1412–1417.
89. Wahl RL. To AC or not to AC: that is the question. *J Nucl Med* 1999;40(12):2025–2028.
90. Beyer T, Townsend DW, Brun T, et al. A combined PET/CT scanner for clinical oncology. *J Nucl Med* 2000;41(8):1369–1379.
91. Nakamoto Y, Chin BB, Kraitchman DL, et al. Effects of nonionic intravenous contrast agents at PET/CT imaging: phantom and canine studies. *Radiology* 2003;227(3):817–824.
92. Mawlawi O, Erasmus JJ, Munden RF, et al. Quantifying the effect of IV contrast media on integrated PET/CT: clinical evaluation. *AJR* 2006;186(2):308–319.
93. Yamamoto Y, Wong TZ, Turkington TG, et al. Head and neck cancer: dedicated FDG PET/CT protocol for detection—phantom and initial clinical studies. *Radiology* 2007;244(1):263–272.
94. Osman MM, Cohade C, Fishman EK, et al. Clinically significant incidental findings on the unenhanced CT portion of PET/CT studies: frequency in 250 patients. *J Nucl Med* 2005;46(8):1352–1355.
95. Zasadny KR, Wahl RL. Standardized uptake values of normal tissues at PET with 2-[fluorine-18]-fluoro-2-deoxy-D-glucose: variations with body weight and a method for correction. *Radiology* 1993;189(3):847–850.
96. Park KC, Schwimmer J, Shepherd JE, et al. Decision analysis for the cost-effective management of recurrent colorectal cancer. *Ann Surg* 2001;233(3):310–319.
97. Valk PE. Clinical trials of cost effectiveness in technology evaluation. *Q J Nucl Med* 2000;44(2):197–203.
98. Mansueto M, Grimaldi A, Torbica A, et al. Cost-effectiveness analysis in the clinical management of patients with known or suspected lung cancer: [(18F)]fluorodeoxyglucose PET and CT comparison. *Q J Nucl Med Mol Imaging* 2007;51(3):224–234.

CHAPTER

8.2 How to Optimize CT for PET/CT

GERALD ANTOCH AND ANDREAS BOCKISCH

Dual-modality positron emission tomography plus computed tomography (PET/CT) imaging systems permit the combined acquisition of functional and morphological data within a single session (1). Diagnostic advantages of PET/CT for staging compared to CT alone or PET alone have been reported for many different malignant diseases (2–5). By integration of CT with PET, PET/CT overcomes the major limitation of CT alone, which is the lack of relevant functional data. Compared to PET alone, correlation of function with CT offers the opportunity for accurate location of a lesion in question. However, the question now is, how good must the quality of CT be to optimize anatomical correlation for PET? When comparing CT protocols in use for PET/CT imaging worldwide, a wide variety of imaging protocols have been proposed and applied, and the "correct" way of acquiring the CT portion of the combined examination has been a matter of great debate. Are low-dose and noncontrast enhanced CT data sufficient or does diagnostic PET/CT require contrast-enhanced and full-dose CT? Does the quality of the CT component affect the diagnostic accuracy of the combined imaging procedure? If contrast agents are of benefit, do we need contrast-enhanced CT in every PET/CT or should we decide on a case-by-case basis? To address these questions this chapter will give an overview of currently available CT imaging protocols and will discuss in which clinical situation each protocol may be beneficial. It also must be recognized that this field continues to evolve rapidly, so the final and optimal combination of PET and CT for diagnosis is not yet fully resolved for all clinical situations.

CT CONTRAST AGENTS

Oral Contrast Agents

Nondistended intestinal structures, adjacent organs, and lymph nodes are characterized by similar Hounsfield units, which range from 30 to 60 H, slightly higher than that of water (Fig. 8.2.1). An oral contrast agent is required to differentiate the bowel from adjacent structures and potential pathological findings. Oral contrast agents have been in use for PET/CT imaging for some years, and their value in marking intestinal structures has been accepted by most groups worldwide. There are two oral contrast agents available: positive and water-equivalent (negative) agents.

Positive oral contrast agents lead to an increase in the Hounsfield units of the intestine. By marking the intestinal lumen, the bowel can be differentiated from surrounding structures (Fig. 8.2.2). For positive intestinal contrast, either a barium-based or an iodine-based contrast agent may be applied. Barium is usually administered as a 1.0% to 2.5% suspension in water, while the iodine-based agent is often administered as a 1% to 3% solution in water. The concentration of the contrast agent may differ among institutions. However, the maximal concentration of the positive oral contrast agent is limited by two factors: (a) higher concentrations of the oral contrast agents may lead to artifacts on CT, and (b) artifacts may occur in the PET image if PET attenuation correction is based on the CT data from a PET/CT study (see below). Based on the increase in intraluminal Hounsfield units, positive oral contrast agents are valuable to differentiate the intestine from adjacent structures including pathological lymph nodes. However, intraluminal lesions and the bowel wall cannot be accurately assessed if there is only limited intestinal distension.

Water-equivalent oral contrast agents distend the intestinal lumen. These contrast agents have also been referred to as negative contrast agents because they do not opacify the intestine, although they do make it visible. Since air has been widely known as a negative contrast agent for conventional radiography, the term negative may be somewhat misleading, as water-based agents are used for intestinal distension rather than the ones based on air in PET/CT. The water-based agent leads to intestinal distension with intraluminal Hounsfield units of 0 to 20. To avoid intestinal absorption of water during the PET/CT scan, different substances may be added; currently a combination of 1.5 L of water containing 2.5% mannitol and 0.2% of locust bean gum is used. The osmotic property of mannitol improves bowel distension, and locust bean gum has a gelling quality that avoids water resorption (6). This water-equivalent contrast agent is pharmacy provided within some hospitals, but other water-equivalent oral contrast agents have become commercially available. Hausegger et al. (7) have evaluated a commercially available vegetarian-based negative oral contrast agent for PET/CT.

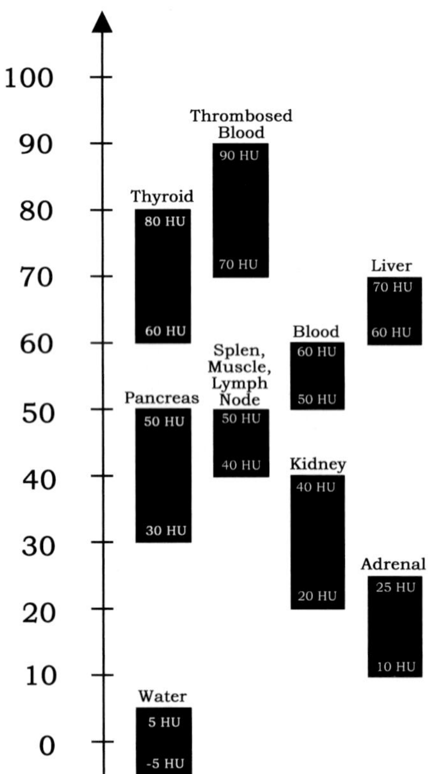

FIGURE 8.2.1. Densities of different organs and of pathology as expressed in Hounsfield (H) units. The most clinically relevant structures have similar Hounsfield units ranging between 10 and 90 H.

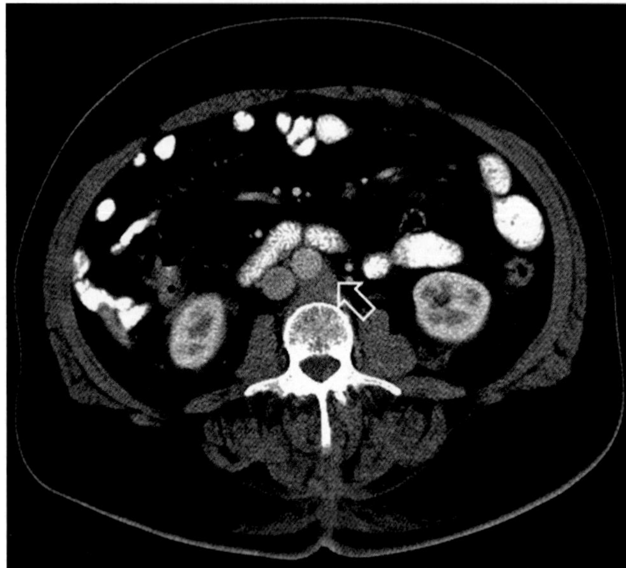

FIGURE 8.2.2. A CT image of the abdomen after administration of oral and intravenous contrast agents. There is a distinct delineation of the bowel from adjacent structures and the surrounding fat tissue. A retroperitoneal lymphoma (*arrow*) is clearly distinguished from the adjacent aorta and from bowel loops. A contrast agent was administered in this study.

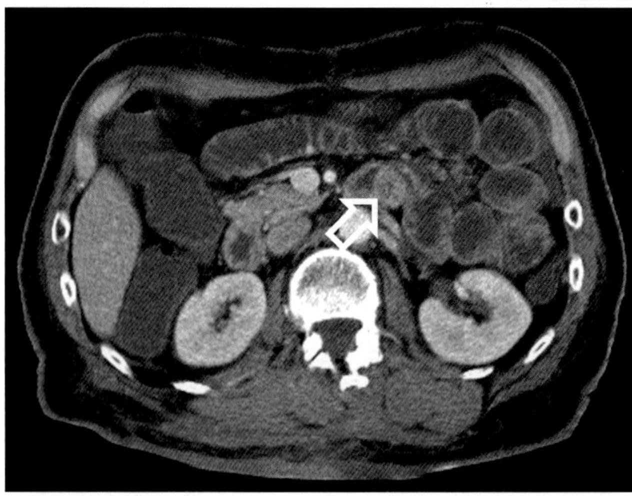

FIGURE 8.2.3. A 62-year-old male with a gastrointestinal stromal tumor of the jejunum. A water-equivalent contrast agent was administered for intestinal distension, and a tumor of the bowel wall prolapsing into the bowel lumen is clearly delineated.

Excellent intestinal distension was reported in 85% of patients in this study.

The intestinal distension provided by water-equivalent oral contrast agents offers a more accurate assessment of the intestinal wall. This can be of benefit over positive oral contrast agents if a tumor adjacent to the bowel is suspected to invade the intestinal wall. Furthermore, the detection of intraluminal tumors may be easier than with positive oral contrast agents (Fig. 8.2.3). A limitation of water-equivalent contrast agents is the differentiation of a distended bowel loop from a centrally necrotic lymph node. In patients with suspected lymph node necrosis, a positive oral contrast agent may be more valuable than a water-equivalent agent. As oral contrast agents are prepared, it is important to avoid using lemonade or other materials that contain glucose as these can raise serum glucose and insulin levels, thus degrading scan quality.

Intravenous Contrast Agents

Parenchymal organs, blood vessels, muscles, and lymph nodes have similar density, as represented by Hounsfield units in the range of 30 to 70 H (Fig. 8.2.1). Even when considering a soft-tissue CT window, differentiation of these anatomical structures from one another often will be limited due to overlapping tissue densities. Parenchymal lesions, such as liver metastases, frequently have similar Hounsfield units as their harboring organ (Fig. 8.2.4). To overcome this limitation of noncontrast enhanced CT data sets, intravenous contrast agents can be applied. Since uptake characteristics of the contrast agents differ in parenchymal organs, in other organs, and in pathological tissue, this leads to more accurate differentiation of anatomical structures (8–10) and to a higher accuracy in lesion detection (11,12). If more than one contrast-enhancing phase is acquired, this can aid in more accurate characterization of a lesion's etiology on CT.

Intravenous contrast agents are iodine-based, nonionic substances with low osmolarity. Compared to former ionic agents, nonionic contrast has been reported to cause fewer adverse events.

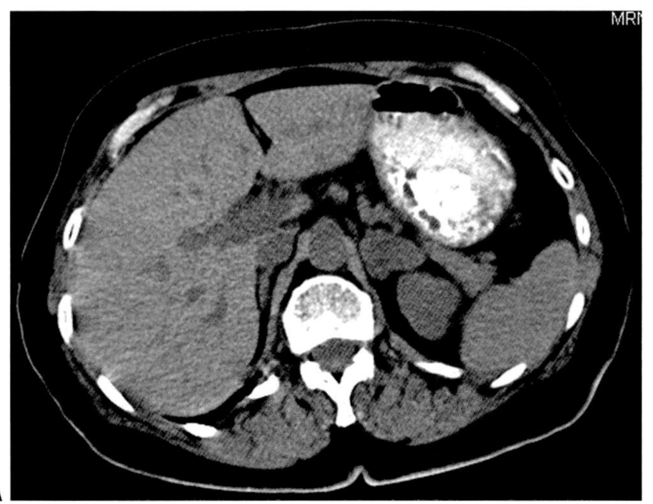

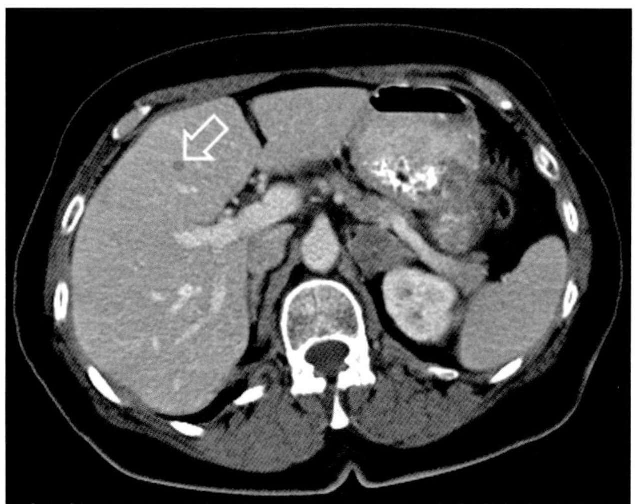

FIGURE 8.2.4. Hepatic metastases from colorectal cancer. The nonenhanced CT **(A)** does not clearly show metastatic disease in the liver. On the contrast-enhanced scan acquired in the portal venous phase **(B)** a small hepatic metastasis is detected in segment four of the liver (*arrow*). Contrast-enhanced CT data increase the sensitivity of PET/CT to detect hepatic metastases.

However, although adverse events are less common than with ionic contrast agents, they may occur with nonionic contrast agents. These may include nephrotoxicity, thyrotoxic effects, and allergic reactions to the contrast material.

Acute adverse reactions have to be differentiated from delayed allergic reactions. Although acute effects occur within the first 30 minutes after the injection of the contrast material, delayed allergic reactions may occur up to 48 hours following the contrast media administration. Based on the contrast agent used, the concentration of iodine may differ between 200 and 370 mg iodine/mL. For most CT studies, as well as for contrast-enhanced PET/CT, a contrast agent with a concentration of 300 mg iodine/mL seems adequate. Higher concentrations are used for special indications such as visualization of hypervascular lesions with CT.

EFFECT OF CT CONTRAST AGENTS ON ATTENUATION-CORRECTED PET DATA

To potentially improve PET image quality and reduce examination times by as much as 30%, the CT data are generally used for attenuation correction purposes in combined PET/CT. Based on the two-step scaling algorithm implemented for attenuation correction in all currently available PET/CT scanners (13), PET attenuation can be overestimated in the presence of positive contrast agents (14–17). A threshold is set to separate soft tissue from bone. To obtain the corresponding attenuation map at 511 keV, CT values are scaled with a scaling factor for either soft tissue or bone. Compared to annihilation photons of 511 keV used in PET, CT and x-rays with energies of 70 to 140 keV are attenuated substantially more by structures containing elements of high atomic numbers such as iodine and barium. If not accounted for, contrast agents may lead to a bias in the estimated attenuation coefficients, which may translate into artifacts in the corrected PET images.

These artifacts are correlated with Hounsfield units on CT images. The higher the Hounsfield units based on positive contrast enhancement, the more distinct the area of apparently increased tracer uptake (18,19). When considering intravenous contrast agents these PET artifacts may be found in coregistration with a contrast-enhanced blood vessel, typically in thoracic veins carrying undiluted contrast following contrast injection (18) (Fig. 8.2.5).

Artifacts associated with intravenous contrast agents in other areas of the body are rare. To avoid false positive interpretation of an area with apparently increased fluorodeoxyglucose (FDG) uptake as pathological, nonattenuation-corrected images should also be read to solve questionable cases. To avoid artifacts associated with the application of intravenous contrast agents, the CT acquisition protocol should be modified with regard to a stand-alone CT. By scanning caudocranially rather than craniocaudally, contrast artifacts caused by a bolus passage in thoracic veins can be avoided. The use of a saline chaser immediately following the contrast injection may serve as another alternative to avoid a contrast-associated artifact in the upper thorax.

Apart from the potential to cause PET artifacts, intravenous contrast agents may, at least theoretically, have an impact on tracer quantification. However, the effect of intravenous contrast agents on quantitative PET has been reported to be clinically insignificant, with the maximal bias in parenchymal organs being 15% for the liver (17). Phantom measurements have shown an overestimation of the PET activity concentration of approximately 20% for clinically used concentrations of oral contrast agents (15,20). However, Dizendorf et al. (16) reported only a 4% overestimation of the related standardized uptake values (SUV) when evaluated in clinical routine. Based on these results, the effect of oral CT contrast agents on the SUV seems to be negligible. In patients with gastrointestinal stenoses, or in patients with compromised gastrointestinal motility, accumulation of the oral contrast agent may cause a more severe increase in Hounsfield units on CT, which can cause higher inaccuracies in PET tracer quantification in these areas (15). A simple solution to avoid artifacts associated with the application of positive oral contrast agents is to use water-equivalent contrast agents, as described above.

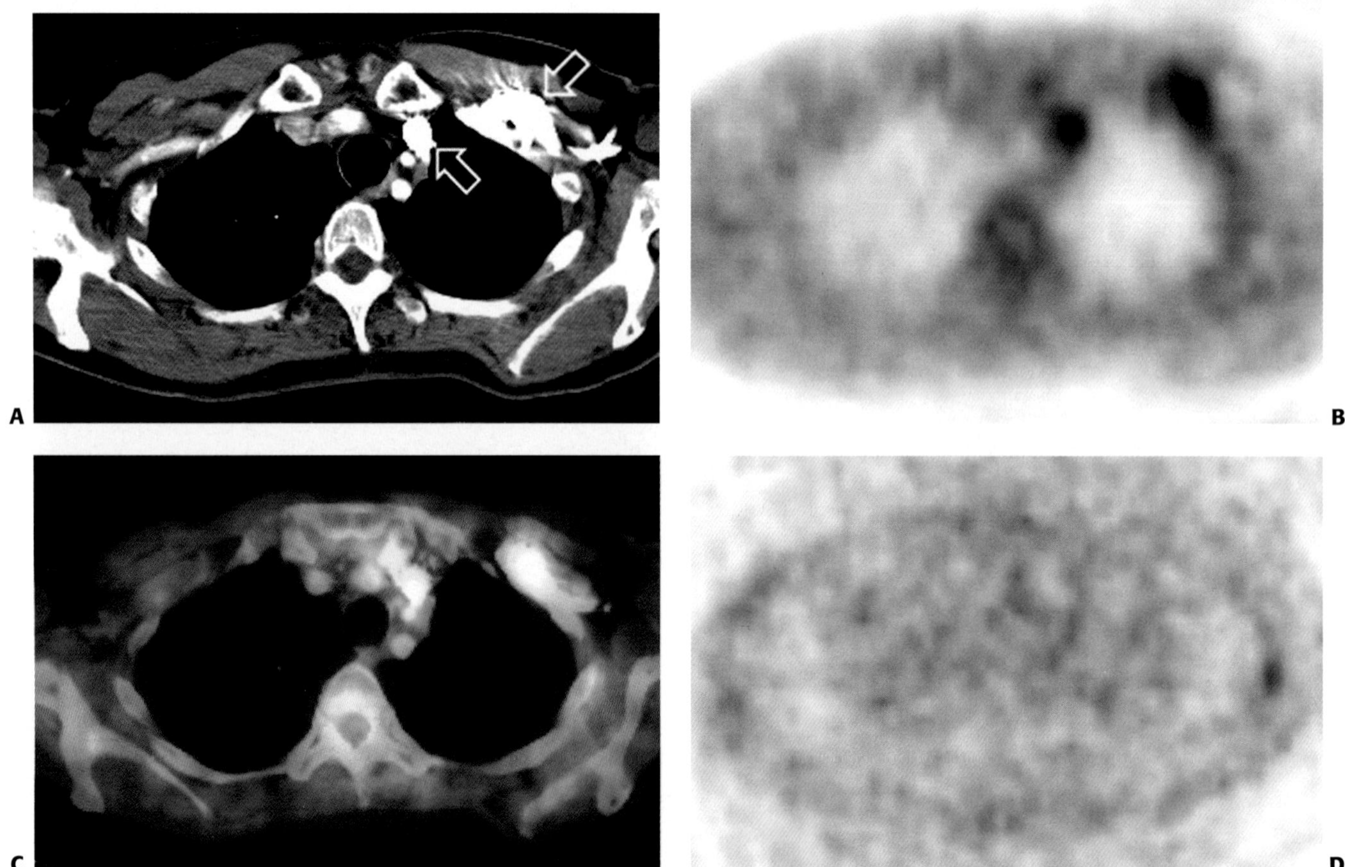

FIGURE 8.2.5. Contrast bolus passage in the left subclavian vein and left brachiocephalic vein. The highly concentrated contrast agent (Hounsfield units greater than 1,000) on CT **(A)** leads to an artifact on PET **(B)**, which appears as an area of apparently increased tracer uptake in coregistration with the contrast-enhanced blood vessel. This artifact is caused by the CT-based attenuation correction of PET. **C:** Demonstrates the fused PET/CT data set. If PET images are reconstructed without attenuation correction the artifact will not be detected **(D)**. It is often very helpful to evaluate both the attenuation corrected and the nonattenuation corrected images.

CT PROTOCOLS FOR TUMOR STAGING WITH PET/CT

Field of View

For tumor staging PET/CT needs to provide information about the local tumor stage (T category), the presence or absence of lymph node metastases (N category) and potentially present distant metastases (M category). A PET/CT staging protocol requires data acquisition of the whole body. Although some institutions define a "whole-body" scan as a field of view from the head to the upper thighs, others report the necessity to acquire PET/CT data from head to toe (21). Preliminary reports have shown that inclusion of the legs in the field of view may help to detect additional metastases over the "limited whole-body approach" and may be beneficial in selected cases for tumor staging. This will require longer examination times compared to the whole-body field of view, including an area from head to the upper thighs. Each institution will have to decide which protocol is best suited for a given indication. Malignant diseases that frequently have metastases to the extremities may be scanned differently from other malignant diseases. At the authors' institution, for example, patients with malignant melanoma are scanned from head to toe, and patients with head and neck tumors are staged from head to the upper thighs.

Some institutions include the brain in PET/CT scanning, while others do not. If FDG is used for tumor staging, FDG uptake will be physiologically present in the brain. This physiologically high tracer uptake in the brain results in low sensitivities for detection of small intracranial metastases with FDG-PET. In this setting, the CT data of PET/CT could be of benefit. However, diagnostic CT of the brain typically requires a higher tube current than scanning the body's trunk. Scanning the whole body with different tube currents has not been available commercially for PET/CT. In addition, the CT gantry should be tilted in cranial CT to avoid artifacts caused by the teeth in the field of view. Since CT and PET are closely aligned, the CT gantry cannot be tilted in PET/CT.

Staging a patient for brain metastases with CT alone is typically performed with contrast enhancement and a delay of at least 10 minutes between contrast administration and CT scanning. The typical delay of image acquisition in the abdomen is the portal venous phase with a delay of 60 seconds. Thus, whole-body PET/CT staging and CT of the brain cannot be performed simply in one session. Based on these limitations, the decision whether to include the brain in the field of view should be decided case by case depending on the patient's type of malignancy, the patient's history, and clinical symptoms. Additional stand-alone CT or MRI of the brain may be an option to completely stage a patient at the cost of an additional examination.

Patient Positioning

The patient is positioned supine for whole-body scanning. To avoid truncation artifacts caused by the patient's arms, the arms have to be positioned outside the field of view of the CT scan or fully contained in the field of view. For whole-body staging of any tumor except head and neck malignancies, this can be accomplished by resting the arms above the head. The whole-body scan is performed in one scanning session in a caudocranial direction. The caudocranial direction is used to avoid contrast-associated artifacts in thoracic veins (see above). Truncation artifacts are avoided in the thorax and abdomen and are only minimal in the head and neck area if the patients are positioned with their arms rested above the head.

To obtain the best-quality CT image of the head and neck the whole-body protocol can be divided into two parts. First, the patient is positioned with his or her arms down (beside the trunk) and the head and neck area is scanned with PET/CT. After scanning the head and neck, the patient's arms can be repositioned above the head and the rest of the body scanned with the arms up to avoid truncation in the remaining areas of the body. The patient's arms should be supported by an armrest. Positioning aids (foam molds or vacuum-lock bags) can be used in addition to the standard armrest to avoid patient motion and ensure more accurate image coregistration. Some patients with severe arthritis cannot have their CT scans performed with their arms above their heads, so compromises in CT technical acquisition standards are sometimes required.

CT Acquisition Parameters

The image quality desired in CT is represented by sufficient spatial resolution with an acceptable signal-to-noise ratio. This mandates the use of an appropriate detector collimation. PET/CT scanners today are typically equipped with a multidetector CT in the range of 2 to 64 detector rows. Thus, image acquisition protocols not only depend on the physician's need for high-quality CT, but also rely on the CT system in use. Based on the CT scanner integrated in the PET/CT, the chosen detector collimation should be large enough (1.5 to 2.5 mm) to enable the acquisition of a whole-body scan within a reasonable time frame. A detector collimation of about 2.5 mm will be chosen for CT scanners with fewer detector rows, whereas smaller collimations may be applied in faster CT systems. The collimation may vary based on the specifications of the imaging protocol. If whole-body coverage is desired in one breath-hold, collimations of 2.5 mm will also be required in a 64-detector row CT to ensure a short CT acquisition time compatible with a single breath-hold. Nevertheless, the collimation should not exceed 2.5 mm to enable reconstruction of data sets at 2.5 mm increments suitable for three-dimensional postprocessing if this is desired. However, some centers performing CT scans for localization purposes use thicker slices.

The use of a full-dose CT versus a low-dose CT as part of the PET/CT examination for tumor staging has been controversial. Although similar staging results have been reported with an 80 mA/sec CT as compared to a 120 mA/sec CT (22), others favor a full-dose CT acquisition to stage different malignant diseases (23). There is a potential advantage of a full-dose CT over a low-dose CT for staging with PET/CT. If used in combination with intravenous contrast agents, the availability of full-dose CT data from combined PET/CT can improve lesion detection and characterization, which will be of benefit in FDG-PET negative tumors or tumors with only a mild increase in FDG-uptake (23). For initial tumor staging a full-dose CT protocol may be desirable for PET/CT. From a practical standpoint, if a full diagnostic quality CT scan can be obtained in the same general imaging session as the PET study, this may add efficiency to health care delivery by not requiring a separate CT with contrast imaging session.

Contrast Agents

Early CT studies comparing contrast-enhanced with nonenhanced CT have demonstrated a substantial benefit of contrast-enhanced protocols over nonenhanced data sets (8,10–12,24–27). Violante and Dean (11) have reported an increase in the accuracy of CT alone for the detection of liver lesions (6 mm in size) from 63% to 90% when applying intravenous contrast agents. Burgener and Hamlin (12) demonstrated an increased accuracy of contrast-enhanced images as compared to nonenhanced data sets when assessing a potential infiltration of pelvic malignancies into adjacent structures. Of course, some authors argue cogently that the radioactive tracer applied leads to tumor detection on PET. Thus, CT will mainly serve for anatomical correlation of the PET data. However, recent studies have reported advantages of contrast-enhanced PET/CT data over nonenhanced PET/CT. Setty et al. (28) demonstrated an increased accuracy in the detection of hepatic lesions when applying intravenous contrast agents in PET/CT as compared to nonenhanced data. This issue remains unsettled, however, and the type of CT scan obtained may vary based on the disease type and the specific diagnostic question asked.

It is a well-known limitation of FDG-PET imaging that small liver metastases may not be detected due to smearing of tracer uptake caused by respiratory motion while acquiring the PET. This limitation may be solved by diagnostic CT data. Apart from a higher accuracy in lesion detection and assessment of the local tumor extent, lesions may be characterized more accurately with contrast-enhanced CT, and anatomical structures will be easier to differentiate from one another. Although delineation of anatomical structures must be considered of interest in most PET/CT staging examinations, lesion detection and characterization with contrast-enhanced CT will be beneficial in PET-negative tumors and tumors with only mild tracer uptake (23).

The use of oral and intravenous contrast agents seems beneficial in PET/CT examinations scheduled for tumor staging of various malignant diseases. Different CT protocols for PET/CT using enhanced and nonenhanced CT data sets have been proposed (29–32). Of course, the contrast agent administration needs to be adjusted to the CT scanner specifications. Patients who have recently undergone contrast-enhanced CT before being referred for PET/CT scanning may not need additional contrast-enhanced PET/CT if the previous data set is available for image correlation. The CT for PET/CT should also be monitored closely for total radiation dose delivery, with a goal to deliver no more dose than necessary to make the optimal diagnosis.

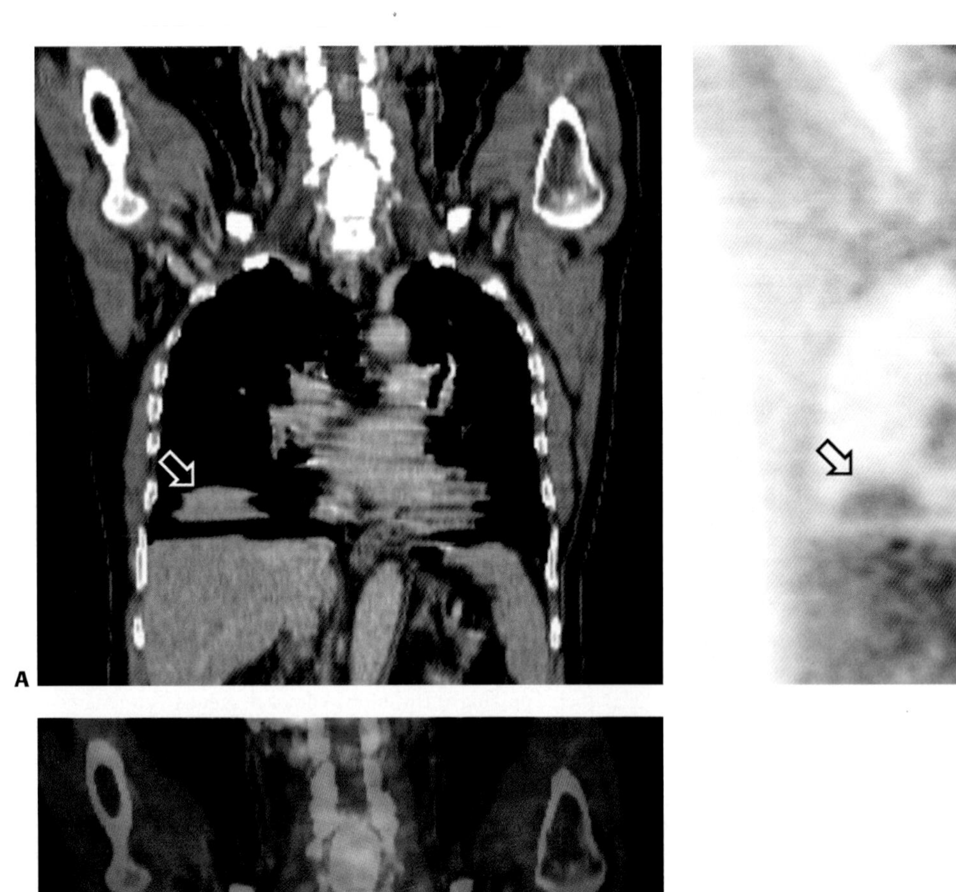

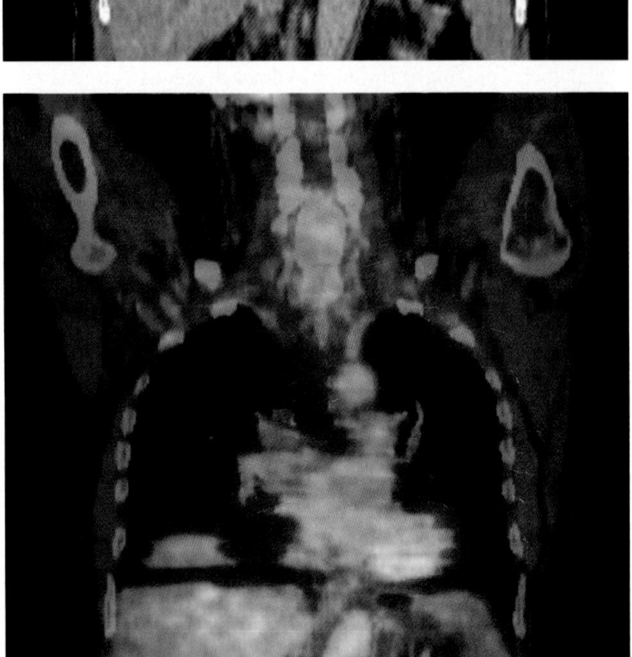

FIGURE 8.2.6. A breathing-associated "mushroomlike" artifact on CT **(A)** showing as a double-contoured right diaphragm. The artifact translates into the attenuation-corrected PET **(B)** and PET/CT (CT-based attenuation correction) **(C)**.

Chest CT for Detection of Pulmonary Nodules

PET has been shown have low sensitivity for detection of small pulmonary lesions due to limitations in its spatial resolution, background tracer activity in the normal lungs, and to pulmonary movement while acquiring the PET data. Adding CT to PET improves the sensitivity for detection of smaller pulmonary lesion over PET alone. To ensure detection of small pulmonary lesions the chest CT needs to be acquired in inspiration. For detection of pulmonary nodules, a chest CT obtained during free breathing or in normal expiration has been reported to be inferior to a chest CT obtained at maximal inspiration (33). Therefore, for tumor staging an additional low-dose CT of the chest following the combined PET/CT scan can be of benefit over the expiration CT scan of the PET/CT. Depending on the scanner in use, 40 mA/sec or even less can be used to perform the low-dose CT of the chest. Although the number of pulmonary lesions detected increases with this imaging protocol, the clinical value of detecting small additional lesions has not yet been determined. Since the PET data cannot always be relied on for differentiation of benign from malignant lesions below 5 mm, the evaluating physician has to cope with the same limitations when assessing small pulmonary lesions as have been documented for CT. Differentiation of malignant nodules from benign nodules will not be possible in some cases and will require further imaging follow-up. It should be noted that the fusion of the PET and CT will typically be much more accurate on the free-breathing PET than on the full inspiratory CT scan.

Respiration Issues

Several studies have evaluated the optimal state of respiration to fuse CT and PET data sets acquired with a hybrid PET/CT scanner. Goerres et al. (34) have documented a more accurate coregistration of CT and PET data sets of pulmonary lesions when acquiring the CT in normal expiration as compared to shallow breathing or inspiration. The mismatch of CT and PET is most distinct if acquiring the CT in maximal inspiration. Shallow breathing during CT scanning leads to a substantial number of breathing-associated artifacts in the area of the diaphragm. These "mushroomlike" artifacts may translate into the PET image if the CT data are used for attenuation correction of PET (35) (Fig. 8.2.6). Therefore, the CT portion of the PET/CT should be acquired in normal expiration. Depending on the CT integrated in the PET/CT imaging system, this can be achieved in a single expiration breath-hold for 64-detector row machines, or may require dedicated breathing protocols for CT scanners with fewer detector rows. For whole-body staging with CT scanners with fewer than 64 detector rows, the CT breathing protocol may include shallow breathing when scanning areas distant from the diaphragm. When the CT spiral approaches the diaphragm, the patient is instructed to hold his or her breath in expiration and will be allowed to continue shallow breathing once the area of the diaphragm has been imaged (36). Use of tidal breathing, which normally is in exhalation as opposed to inhalation, often results in quite satisfactory fusions and is used by many groups.

Radiation Issues

Although radiation exposure in patients with advanced tumor stages can be considered clinically relatively insignificant, the radiation dose from the PET/CT examination will be a more important issue in younger patients with potentially curable diseases. The CT part of the examination contributes a substantial part to the radiation dose from a PET/CT study. Depending on the field of view and the scanning parameters, the radiation dose from the CT component may vary in the range of 3 to 20 mSv. For a whole-body scan with full-dose CT, the radiation dose will be between 15 to 20 mSv from the CT component. Thus, in PET/CT with full-dose CT acquisition, the CT component is responsible for the major part of the radiation dose. With low-dose CT the radiation exposure from the CT component will be approximately 3 to 6 mSv (37).

CT PROTOCOLS FOR THERAPY ASSESSMENT WITH PET/CT

CT imaging protocols for PET/CT differ when comparing staging examinations and PET/CT scans for therapy assessment. Before the start of therapy, a whole-body scan will typically be performed to stage the patient and to provide a baseline for further imaging follow-up. With the knowledge of the extent of the tumor, the field of view for both CT and PET of follow-up examinations can potentially be limited to the body region of interest. When assessing therapy response with FDG-PET/CT (or other tracers) a substantial decrease in tracer uptake will indicate tumor response, while a substantial increase in tracer utilization suggests progressive disease. Since the accurate location of an area of increased tracer uptake has been defined with the staging PET/CT, the CT data for response assessment are less important than for staging. Noncontrast-enhanced and low-dose CT data will be adequate for most clinical questions. However, if PET/CT is indicated to assess tumor recurrence after therapy, a whole-body PET/CT with diagnostic CT data should be considered for reliable detection of tumor recurrence and to reveal new metastases in body regions distant from the primary tumor. Although intravenous contrast typically only has modest effects on SUV, it should be noted that the ideal approach to measuring tumor SUV involves use of CT with identical parameters on subsequent studies to minimize variance. For this reason, some centers routinely perform low milliampere CT scans without contrast when quantitation is desired and then more limited contrast CT studies following the completion of the PET. This allows certainty of quantitation and can limit the radiation dose.

Thus, the optimal choice for CT as part of PET/CT varies. The field of view, quality of the scan (inversely related to the radiation dose), type of contrast, arm position, respiratory status, as well as time from contrast administration must be tailored to the specific patient's clinical problems. One CT scan approach does not fit all patients. It is clear, however, that contrast CT scans are beginning to play a greater role in PET/CT, although the PET using a simple noncontrast CT scan remains a very powerful diagnostic tool.

REFERENCES

1. Beyer T, Townsend DW, Brun T, et al. A combined PET/CT scanner for clinical oncology. *J Nucl Med* 2000;41:1369–1379.
2. Lardinois D, Weder W, Hany TF, et al. Staging of non–small-cell lung cancer with integrated positron-emission tomography and computed tomography. *N Engl J Med* 2003;348:2500–2507.
3. Antoch G, Saoudi N, Kuehl H, et al. Accuracy of whole-body dual-modality FDG-PET/CT for tumor staging in oncology: comparison with CT and PET. *J Clin Oncol* 2004;22:4357–4368.
4. Vansteenkiste JF, Stroobants SG, Dupont PJ, et al. FDG-PET scan in potentially operable non-small cell lung cancer: do anatometabolic PET-CT fusion images improve the localisation of regional lymph node metastases? The Leuven Lung Cancer Group. *Eur J Nucl Med* 1998;25:1495–1501.
5. Wahl RL, Quint LE, Cieslak RD, et al. "Anatometabolic" tumor imaging: fusion of FDG PET with CT or MRI to localize foci of increased activity. *J Nucl Med* 1993;34:1190–1197.
6. Antoch G, Kuehl H, Kanja J, et al. Dual-modality PET/CT scanning with negative oral contrast agent to avoid artifacts: introduction and evaluation. *Radiology* 2004;230:879–885.
7. Hausegger K, Reinprecht P, Kau T, et al. Clinical experience with a commercially available negative oral contrast medium in PET/CT. *Rofo* 2005;177:796–799.
8. Kormano MJ, Goske MJ, Hamlin DJ. Attenuation and contrast enhancement of gynecologic organs and tumors in CT. *Eur J Radiol* 1981;1:307–311.
9. Alfidi RJ, Haaga JR. Computed body tomography. *Radiol Clin North Am* 1976;14:563–570.
10. Albertyn LE. Rationales for the use of intravenous contrast medium in computed tomography. *Australas Radiol* 1989;33:29–33.
11. Violante MR, Dean PB. Improved detectability of VX2 carcinoma in the rabbit liver with contrast enhancement in computed tomography. *Radiology* 1980;134:237–239.
12. Burgener FA, Hamlin DJ. Intravenous contrast enhancement in computed tomography of pelvic malignancies. *Rofo Fortschr Geb Rontgenstr Nuklearmed* 1981;134:656–661.
13. Kinahan PE, Townsend DW, Beyer T, et al. Attenuation correction for a combined 3D PET/CT scanner. *Med Phys* 1998;25:2046–2053.
14. Carney JP, Townsend DW. CT-based attenuation correction for PET/CT scanners. In: Schulthess Gv, ed. *Clinical PET, PET/CT and SPECT/CT: combined anatomic-molecular imaging.* Philadelphia: Lippincott Williams & Wilkins, 2002: .

15. Cohade C, Osman M, Nakamoto Y, et al. Initial experience with oral contrast in PET/CT: phantom and clinical studies. *J Nucl Med* 2003; 44:412–416.
16. Dizendorf E, Hany TF, Buck A, et al. Cause and magnitude of the error induced by oral CT contrast agent in CT-based attenuation correction of PET emission studies. *J Nucl Med* 2003;44:732–738.
17. Nakamoto Y, Chin BB, Kraitchman DL, et al. Effects of nonionic intravenous contrast agents at PET/CT imaging: phantom and canine studies. *Radiology* 2003;227:817–824.
18. Antoch G, Freudenberg LS, Egelhof T, et al. Focal tracer uptake: a potential artifact in contrast-enhanced dual-modality PET/CT scans. *J Nucl Med* 2002;43:1339–1342.
19. Bockisch A, Beyer T, Antoch G, et al. Positron emission tomography/ computed tomography—imaging protocols, artifacts, and pitfalls. *Mol Imaging Biol* 2004;6:188–199.
20. Antoch G, Jentzen W, Freudenberg LS, et al. Effect of oral contrast agents on CT-based PET attenuation correction in dual-modality PET/CT imaging. *Invest Rad* 2003;38:784–789.
21. Osman MM, Khayyat N, Mosley C, et al. Prevalence and patterns of soft tissue metastases from non–small cell lung cancer detected with true whole-body F-18 FDG-PET. *Radiology* 2004;308 (abst).
22. Hany TF, Steinert HC, Goerres GW, et al. PET diagnostic accuracy: improvement with in-line PET-CT system: initial results. *Radiology* 2002;225:575–581.
23. Antoch G, Freudenberg LS, Beyer T, et al. To enhance or not to enhance? 18F-FDG and CT contrast agents in dual-modality 18F-FDG PET/CT. *J Nucl Med* 2004;45[Suppl 1]:56S–65S.
24. Alfidi RJ, Haaga J, Meaney TF, et al. Computed tomography of the thorax and abdomen: a preliminary report. *Radiology* 1975;117:257–264.
25. Garrett PR, Meshkov SL, Perlmutter GS. Oral contrast agents in CT of the abdomen. *Radiology* 1984;153:545–546.
26. Plewes DB, Dean PB. Detectability of spherical objects by computed tomography. *Radiology* 1979;133:785–786.
27. Zatz LM. Iodinated contrast media in cranial tomography. *Invest Radiol* 1980;15:S155–159.
28. Setty BN, Blake MA, Sahani DV, et al. Role of contrast-enhanced CT (CECT) in hybrid PET-CT for liver metastases in patients with colorectal cancer. *Radiology* 2005;452 (abst).
29. Beyer T, Antoch G, Muller S, et al. Acquisition protocol considerations for combined PET/CT imaging. *J Nucl Med* 2004;45[Suppl 1]: 25S–35S.
30. Beyer T, Antoch G, Bockisch A, et al. Optimized intravenous contrast administration for diagnostic whole-body 18F-FDG PET/CT. *J Nucl Med* 2005;46:429–435.
31. Kuehl H, Veit P, Rosenbaum S, et al. Can PET/CT replace separate diagnostic CT for cancer imaging? Optimizing CT protocols for imaging cancers of the chest and abdomen. *J Nucl Med* 2007;48(Suppl 1): 45S–47S.
32. Brechtel K, Klein M, Vogel M, et al. Optimized contrast-enhanced CT protocols for diagnostic whole-body 18-FDG PET/CT: technical aspects of single phase versus multiphase CT imaging. *J Nucl Med* 2006;47:470–476.
33. Allen-Auerbach M, Yeom K, Park J, et al. Standard PET/CT of the chest during shallow breathing is inadequate for comprehensive staging of lung cancer. *J Nucl Med* 2006;47:298–301.
34. Goerres GW, Kamel E, Seifert B, et al. Accuracy of image coregistration of pulmonary lesions in patients with non-small cell lung cancer using an integrated PET/CT system. *J Nucl Med* 2002;43:1469–1475.
35. Osman MM, Cohade C, Nakamoto Y, et al. Clinically significant inaccurate localization of lesions with PET/CT: frequency in 300 patients. *J Nucl Med* 2003;44:240–243.
36. Beyer T, Antoch G, Blodgett T, et al. Dual-modality PET/CT imaging: the effect of respiratory motion on combined image quality in clinical oncology. *Eur J Nucl Med Mol Imaging* 2003;30:588–596.
37. Brix G, Lechel U, Glatting G, et al. Radiation exposure of patients undergoing whole-body dual-modality 18F-FDG PET/CT examinations. *J Nucl Med* 2005;46:608–613.

CHAPTER

8.3 Artifacts and Normal Variants in FDG PET

PAUL SHREVE AND CHUONG DAC HUY BUI

Advances in positron emission tomography (PET) capability and widespread recognition of the value of fluorodeoxyglucose (FDG) PET in oncology and has led to the routine whole-body (CF torso) imaging in most oncologic indications of FDG PET. The high FDG uptake by most malignancies relative to the level of FDG distributed throughout much of the body facilitates identification of malignant neoplasm. Compared to conventional anatomic approaches alone, whole-body FDG PET permits much more rapid and accurate identification of the presence and extent of malignant disease. Focal FDG tracer accumulation due to cancer, however, must be distinguished from normal, normal variant, and benign pathological sources of FDG uptake. This is a principal task in the interpretation of whole-body FDG PET scans applied to oncologic diagnosis.

FDG tracer uptake depicts tissue glucose metabolism. Hence, in addition to the abnormal glucose metabolism associated with malignant neoplasm, both normal variations in glucose metabolism and increased glucose metabolism due to a variety of pathologies are revealed on FDG PET. Interpretation of whole-body FDG PET thus requires knowledge of normal and normal-variant patterns of FDG uptake as well as familiarity with the many benign pathologic causes of increased FDG uptake. Frequently both anatomic and physiologic knowledge is needed to reliably identify sites of FDG uptake as normal, variant, or benign pathological etiologies.

NORMAL WHOLE-BODY FLUORODEOXYGLUCOSE DISTRIBUTION

On whole-body PET performed between 1 and 2 hours following intravenous administration of FDG, the brain, heart, and urinary tract are the most prominent sites of tracer accumulation (Fig. 8.3.1). The brain, an obligate user of glucose, is always prominent relative to the rest of the body. Both supratentorial and infratentorial gray matter are FDG avid, and the level of FDG uptake is in the range typical of FDG-avid malignancies. The myocardium is of similar FDG avidity in the fed state, but with sufficiently long fast (typically greater than 12 hours), the myocardium metabolism shifts to fatty acids as a source of energy, and the myocardial uptake becomes largely indistinguishable from blood pool tracer activity. FDG follows a urinary excretory route, hence in the absence of aggressive hydration, diuretics, and urinary bladder catheterization, FDG is present in the bladder and to varying degrees the upper urinary tract.

Elsewhere, tracer activity is distributed at low levels in recognizable anatomic structures on attenuation-corrected images (Fig. 8.3.1). Cardiac and mediastinal great vessel blood pool is discernable against the very low tracer activity of the lungs (Fig. 8.3.2). Glandular tissue of the breast is associated with low-level uptake, slightly greater than blood pool, in younger women. The liver and spleen are associated with slightly higher FDG activity than blood pool levels and are reliably identified in the abdomen, as are the kidneys. The pancreas is normally not discretely identified. Bowel is seen to varying degrees, as is the stomach due to widely variable levels of FDG uptake in the alimentary tract. Bone marrow normally is associated with FDG accumulation at levels higher than blood pool activity, hence vertebral bodies are reliably identified, as well as in major marrow containing skeletal structures such as the pelvis, hips, and sternum. In the neck lymphoid tissue associated with the palatine tonsils is consistently FDG avid and typically clearly identified (Fig. 8.3.3). The parotid and submandibular salivary glands are discernable by uniform low-level FDG activity. Muscles of vocalization within the larynx, specifically the posterior cricoarytenoid and vocalis muscles, are commonly seen on routine whole-body scans. Musculature at the base of the tongue, just within the lower anterior mandible, is almost always seen. Cervical spinal cord is identifiable with uniform low-level FDG uptake (Fig. 8.3.3).

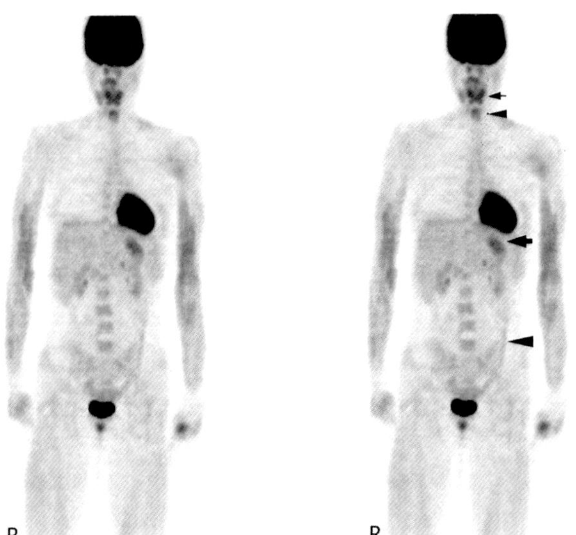

FIGURE 8.3.1. Normal whole-body distribution of fluorodeoxyglucose (FDG) 1 hour following intravenous tracer administration. Attenuation-corrected anterior maximum intensity projection image. Intense tracer activity is present in the brain, heart, and bladder. In the neck, palatine tonsil lymphoid tissue tracer activity (*small arrow*) and minimal laryngeal muscle activity (*small arrowhead*) is seen. Inferior to the heart is low-level gastric tracer activity (*large arrow*) and the outlines of the liver, spleen, and kidneys are discernable. Normal bone marrow tracer activity defines vertebral bodies and the pelvis. Vertical linear tracer activity in the left abdomen and pelvis is the descending colon (*large arrowhead*). Mild increased tracer activity is seen in the arm musculature.

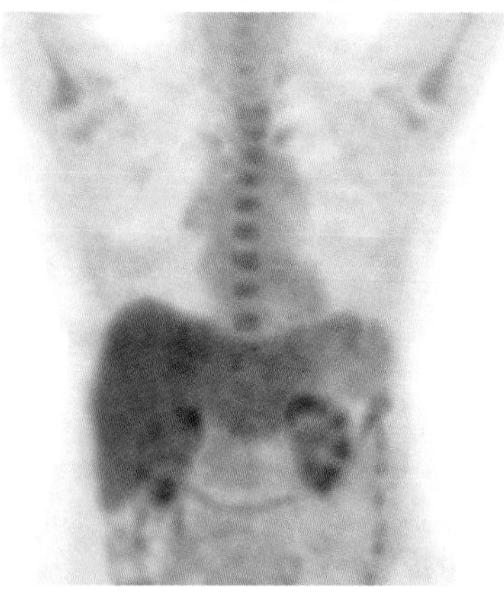

FIGURE 8.3.2. Normal distribution of fluorodeoxyglucose in the chest 90 minutes following intravenous tracer administration. Attenuation-corrected anterior maximum intensity projection image. Blood pool tracer activity in the great vessels defines the contours of the mediastinum. Lung tracer activity is uniform and very low, reflecting blood pool. Normal breast glandular tissue is discernable in this young female. Myocardial uptake in this fasted patient is equivalent to mediastinal background activity. Normal liver and spleen tracer activity is seen in the upper abdomen.

NORMAL VARIANT FLUORODEOXYGLUCOSE DISTRIBUTION

Myocardium

Uptake of FDG in myocardium in patients who have fasted 4 to 18 hours is variable, ranging from uniform and intense, to nearly absent. In the fed state, FDG uptake in intact myocardium is intense, on the order of brain gray matter. With a sufficient fast, myocardium will shift energy metabolism from glucose to fatty acids (1), and demonstrate little FDG uptake; however, in practice, even with overnight fasting, FDG uptake in myocardium is not reliably absent. There is some evidence that an all-protein diet the day before an FDG study enhances the shift of myocardial metabolism to fatty acids. With contemporary dual modality of PET with computed tomography (CT) and image reconstruction algorithms, the presence of intense FDG uptake in the myocardium does not generally present limitations in interpretation of the lungs and mediastinum, except for abnormalities associated with the pericardium or directly adjacent lung. The transition from the intense FDG uptake of dominant glycolytic myocardial metabolism to absent FDG uptake of dominant fatty acid metabolism is frequently nonuniform (Fig. 8.3.4). The base of the left ventricular myocardium tends to be the last portion to lose glucose avidity. Such irregular FDG left ventricular myocardial distribution can be observed in patients who have fasted 4 to 18 hours, yielding apparent discrete foci at the base of the heart that could be misinterpreted as FDG-avid mediastinal lymph nodes if anatomic relationships are not appreciated. In addition, atrial myocardium is sometimes discernable, and again irregular FDG distribution can occur, yielding apparent small focal abnormalities in the mediastinum (Fig. 8.3.5). In the fed state, right ventricular myocardium is typically seen at low levels, but can become as prominent as the left ventricular myocardium in the setting of right ventricular hypertrophy, such as seen with pulmonary hypertension.

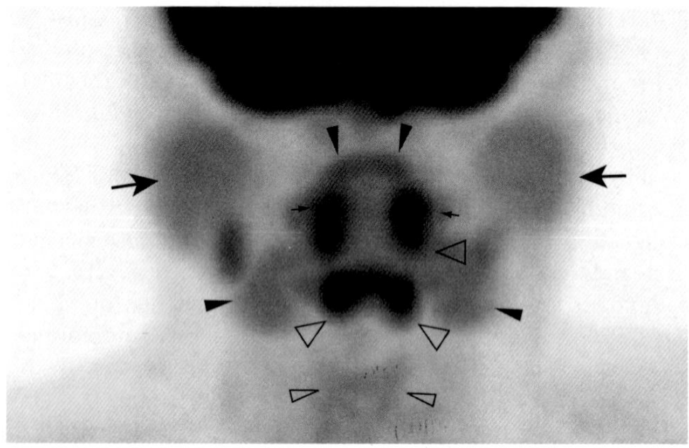

FIGURE 8.3.3. Normal distribution of fluorodeoxyglucose in the neck 90 minutes following intravenous tracer administration. Attenuation-corrected fine matrix anterior maximum intensity matrix image. The parotid glands (*large arrow*) and submandibular glands (*large arrowhead*) are defined by uniform low-level tracer activity. Intense tracer activity in the palatine tonsils (*small arrows*) is nearly always present, while the lingular tonsil portion of the Waldeyer ring is sometimes discernable (*small arrowheads*). Intense tracer uptake is almost always seen in the musculature at the base of the tongue, comprising the genioglossus, hyoglossus, and anterior belly of the digastric muscles (*large open arrowheads*). Usually the muscles of vocalization (posterior cricoarytenoid and vocalis muscles) are also seen (*small open arrowheads*).

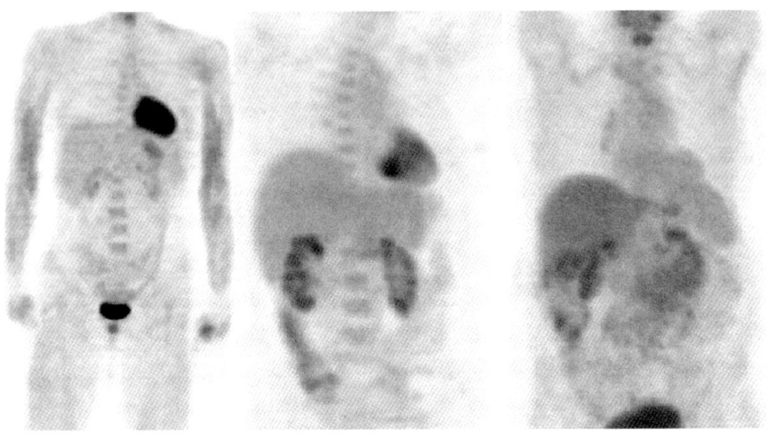

FIGURE 8.3.4. Variable appearance of myocardial tracer activity in fasting patients. Attenuation-corrected anterior maximum intensity projection images. **A:** Fully retained myocardial fluorodeoxyglucose (FDG) tracer uptake with uniform tracer activity throughout the myocardium. **B:** Heterogeneous myocardial FDG tracer activity with relatively preserved tracer activity towards the base of the heart. **C:** When myocardium has fully shifted to fatty acid metabolism in response to fasting, FDG tracer activity is uniformly low, equivalent to mediastinal background activity.

Skeletal Muscle

At rest, skeletal muscle relies on fatty acid oxidative metabolism for energy. With increased energy demand, glycolysis becomes the major source of energy for skeletal muscle depending on relative oxygen delivery and tissue oxidative capacity. Fast twitch muscle fibers, with sparse mitochondria and limited oxidative capacity, are associated with consistent high glucose demand; extraocular muscles routinely demonstrate elevated FDG accumulation (2). Skeletal muscle composed of slow twitch fibers will demonstrate glucose uptake when under active contraction or following glycogen depletion. Hence, skeletal muscle under active contraction during the FDG uptake phase (largely the first 30 minutes after tracer administration) will demonstrate elevated FDG accumulation. Further, skeletal muscle under heavy use prior to injection of FDG may also exhibit FDG uptake, likely related to replenishment of glycogen stores (3). For this reason, patients are typically advised to refrain from heavy exercise the day prior to their FDG PET examination, and following FDG administration, to sit semirecumbent or lie quietly. Since insulin increases muscle uptake of glucose, insulin given prior to, or immediately after, FDG administration will result in diffusely increased muscle uptake (Fig. 8.3.6) (4).

Low-level uptake in the forearm muscles is relatively common (Fig. 8.3.1). Major truncal muscles can be prominent with patients who have been physically active even hours before FDG injection (Fig. 8.3.6). Heavy ventilatory efforts associated with physical exertion or pulmonary disease commonly result in identifiable intercostal muscles and diaphragmatic crura (Fig. 8.3.7) (5). The symmetry and configuration of muscle FDG uptake generally permits correct identification on the FDG PET images alone; however, the FDG uptake does not always involve the entire muscle. Imbalance in muscle groups due to disease or associated treatment such as surgery can result in focal asymmetric FDG uptake, which in certain locations such as the neck, can lead to potential misdiagnosis (6). Asymmetric or isolated major muscle FDG uptake can be confounding in the shoulder girdle musculature. The teres minor is commonly seen when patients are scanned in an arms-by-the-side positioning and should not be confused with metastasis or other pathology in the shoulder region. Identification of the muscle origin of FDG activity is greatly facilitated by review of the registered and aligned images provided on PET/CT acquisitions.

Speech during the uptake phase of FDG increases FDG activity in the laryngeal muscles and the tongue (7). Laryngeal musculature uptake is, in the absence of prior related surgery or unilateral recurrent nerve palsy, nearly always symmetrical and hence readily appreciated as normal. The principal muscles seen are the posterior cricoarytenoid muscles and the vocalis muscles (Fig. 8.3.8). The unilateral absence of FDG activity in the vocalis and cricoarytenoid muscles is a sign of unilateral recurrent laryngeal nerve palsy (Fig. 8.3.9), such as due to tumor mass in the mediastinum or neck.

Tongue uptake varies from mild to intense, typically involves the entire tongue or top of the tongue, and is easily recognizable on maximum intensity projection and sagittal images. Isolated focal uptake can be seen, however. Prior surgery involving the tongue can yield focal asymmetrical muscle uptake, which may be indistinguishable from residual or recurrent malignancy (Fig. 8.3.10). Muscle flaps in the tongue will result in focal tracer uptake indistinguishable from recurrent neoplasm on the FDG PET images. Careful and experienced review of the corresponding CT images (preferably registered and

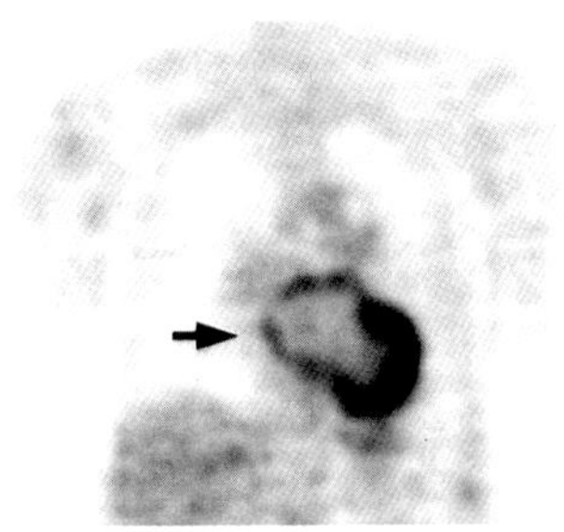

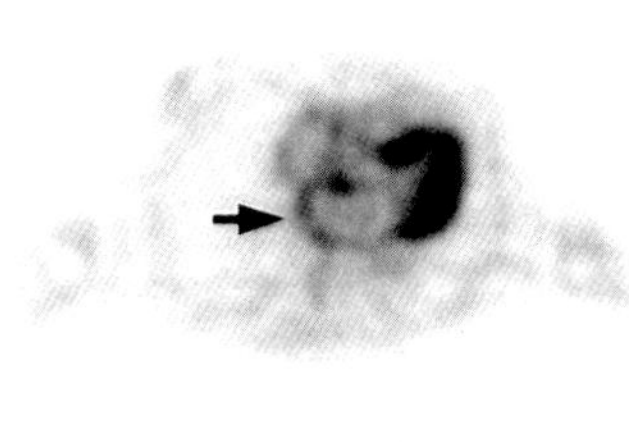

FIGURE 8.3.5. Atrial muscle fluorodeoxyglucose uptake. Attenuation-corrected coronal and transaxial images. Tracer uptake in atrial muscle can be resolved (*arrow*), especially in patients with valvular disease or heart failure, and may appear irregular with somewhat focal regions of tracer activity.

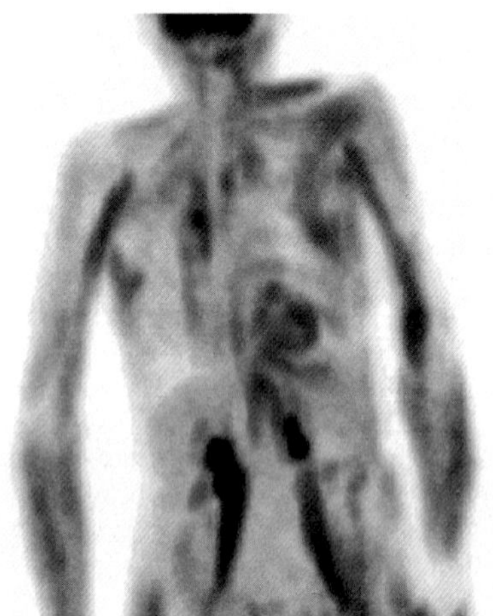

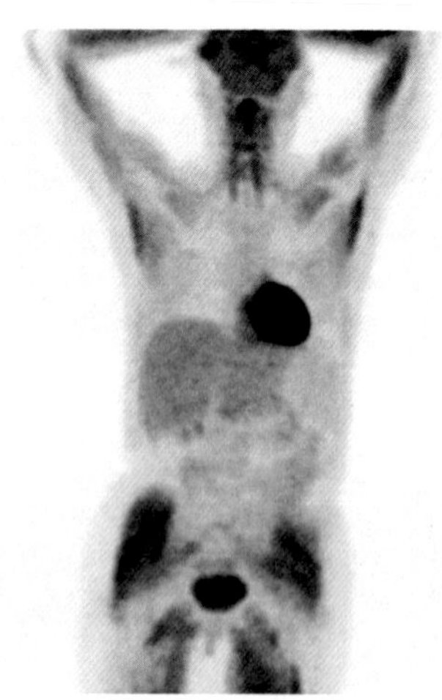

A, B

FIGURE 8.3.6. Skeletal muscle fluorodeoxyglucose (FDG) uptake. **A:** Attenuation-corrected anterior maximum intensity projection image shows major truncal and upper body skeletal muscle FDG uptake in a patient who performed heavy physical labor hours prior to the FDG administration. **B:** Diffuse skeletal muscle uptake due to endogenous insulin response to a sugar-containing meal or beverage just prior to FDG administration. Note intense myocardial activity, reflecting the myocardial shift to glucose metabolism in response to insulin. A similar pattern of skeletal and myocardial muscle FDG uptake occurs when exogenous insulin is given just prior to FDG administration.

aligned from a PET/CT scan) and surgical and treatment history is often essential in distinguishing benign from malignant sources of focal FDG tracer activity in the posttreatment neck.

Brown Adipose Tissue

Brown adipose tissue (BAT) is abundantly present in infancy and diminishes with age. BAT expresses a unique mitochondrial uncoupling protein that permits direct heat generation rather than adenosine triphosphate (ATP) production from fatty acid oxidation in response to cold exposure, ingestion of food, or increased sympathetic activity. This process requires an increased supply of ATP, which in turn is provided by an increase in glycolytic metabolism. With routine use of PET/CT, it is now recognized that surprisingly intense increased FDG activity can localize to adipose tissue (most likely BAT) in the neck, supraclavicular regions, axillae, paravertebral locations at the thoracic spine, mediastinum, and occasionally subdiaphragmatic and perinephric fat (Fig. 8.3.11). This phenomenon is seen more often in young patients, females, and slender patients, appears to occur more frequently in the months with colder outdoor temperatures, and is correlated with patient anxiety (8). Activated BAT may also explain increased FDG uptake in lipomatous hypertrophy of interatrial septum. This rare normal variant can mimic malignancy in the mediastinum, but can usually be

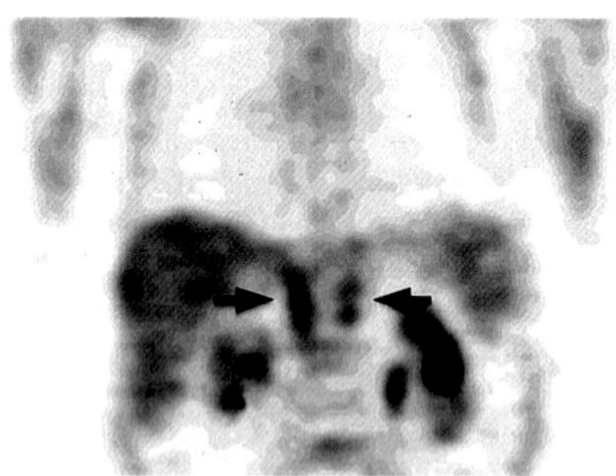

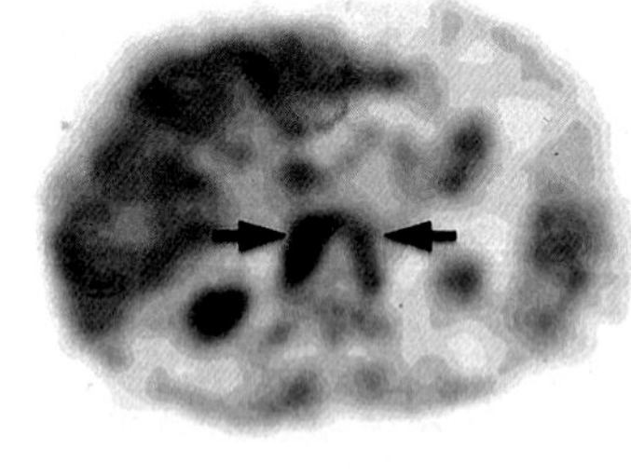

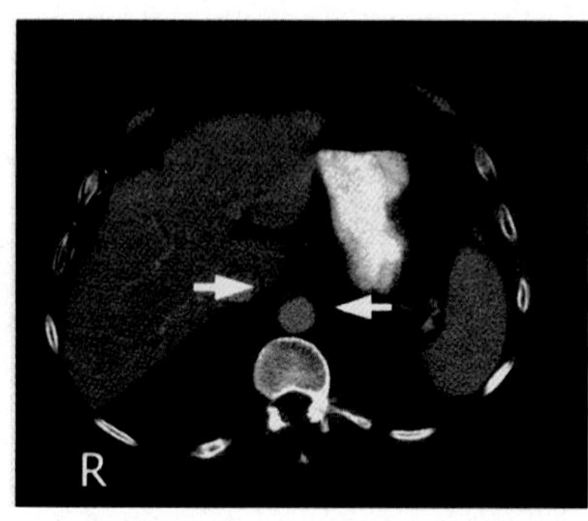

FIGURE 8.3.7. Respiratory muscle fluorodeoxyglucose (FDG) uptake. Coronal and transaxial attenuation-corrected FDG PET images and corresponding transaxial CT image showing tracer uptake in the diaphragmatic crura (*arrow*). Elevated ventilatory efforts during the FDG uptake phase, such as in patients with severe chronic obstructive pulmonary disease, may result in FDG uptake in intercostal and diaphragmatic muscles. Focal tracer uptake in the paraspinous diaphragmatic crura typically will have an elongated configuration on coronal images and is readily localized and identified on registered and aligned CT images.

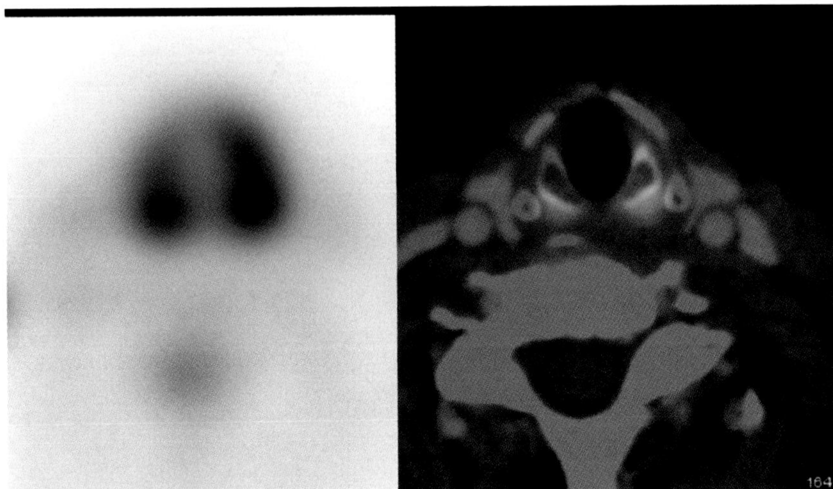

FIGURE 8.3.8. Normal fluorodeoxyglucose (FDG) uptake in the muscles of vocalization. Transaxial attenuation-corrected FDG PET image and PET/CT fusion image reveals symmetrical focal FDG activity posteriorly corresponding to the posterior cricoarytenoid muscles and uniform tracer activity, extending at the level of the true vocal cords corresponding to the vocalis muscles.

correctly identified with PET/CT–generated registered and aligned images. Close attention to controlling the patient's level of anxiety and the environmental temperature (at least 25°C) for 15 minutes to 2 hours before FDG injection as well as during the FDG uptake phase can significantly reduce FDG uptake in brown fat in the neck and paravertebral area (9–11). Drugs such as propranolol and reserpine reduce brown fat uptake by blocking adrenergic receptor–mediated stimulation of BAT (12).

Alimentry Tract

FDG uptake in the alimentary tract, from the esophagus to rectosigmoid colon, is widely variable both in terms of distribution and intensity. The etiology of FDG uptake in the alimentary tract is presently not understood and may reflect different normal and benign pathologic phenomenon in different portions of the alimentary tract. The esophagus occasionally is associated with

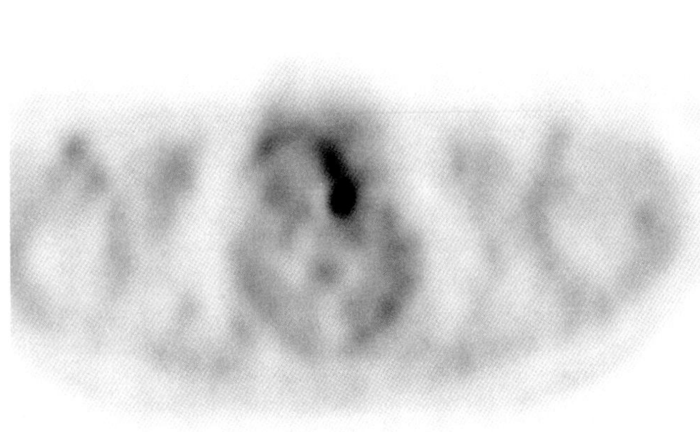

A

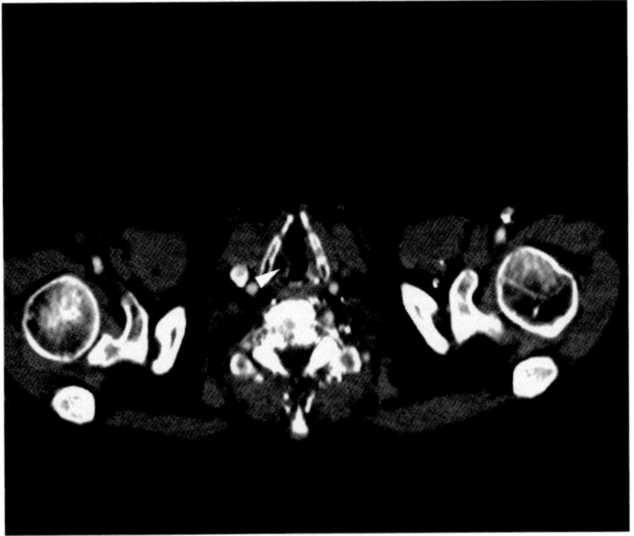

B

FIGURE 8.3.9. Abnormal asymmetric fluorodeoxyglucose uptake in the muscles of vocalization. **A:** Absent tracer activity is observed at the right posterior cricoarytenoid and vocalis muscles, while normal tracer activity is observed in the left posterior cricoarytenoid and vocalis muscles on the transaxial attenuation-corrected PET images. **B:** The registered and aligned CT image also reveals the flaccid right true vocal cord (*white arrowhead*) in this patient with a right-sided mediastinal mass, causing right recurrent laryngeal nerve palsy.

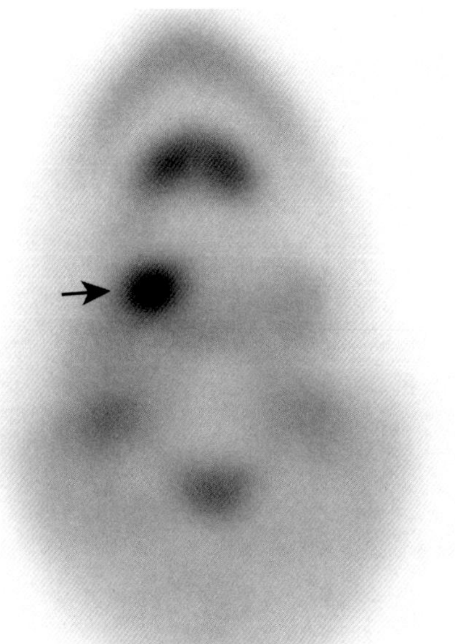
A

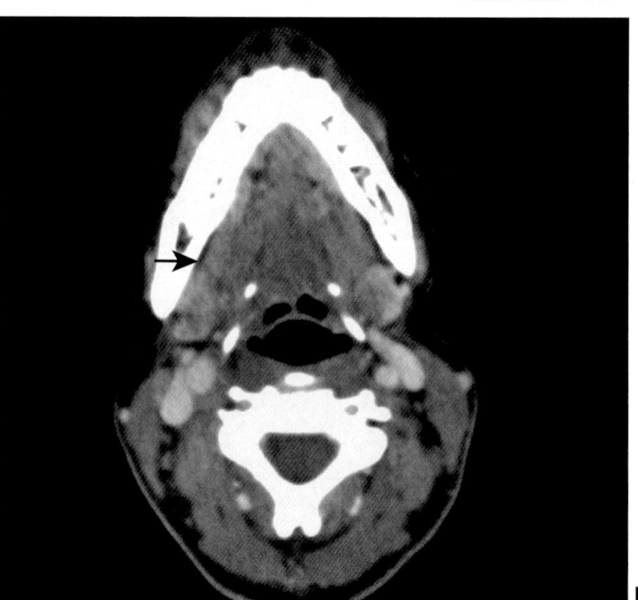
B

FIGURE 8.3.10. Focal fluorodeoxyglucose (FDG) uptake in the tongue. Transaxial attenuation-corrected FDG PET and transaxial CT images of a postoperative tongue reveal a small focus of abnormal FDG tracer activity at the right tongue base (**A**) (*arrow*) with no corresponding mass or abnormal enhancement on the CT images (**B**) (*arrow*). The partial resection of tongue muscle associated with the resection of a primary tongue neoplasm can cause imbalance in tongue musculature, resulting in focal physiologic skeletal muscle FDG tracer uptake.

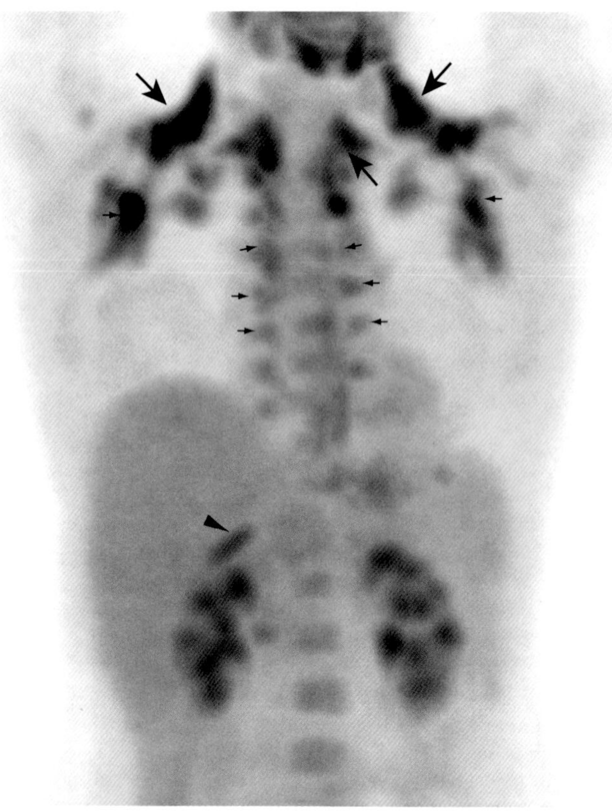
A

FIGURE 8.3.11. Brown adipose tissue (BAT) fluorodeoxyglucose (FDG) uptake. Anterior attenuation-corrected maximum intensity projection FDG PET (**A**) and coronal attenuation-corrected FDG PET (**B**,**D**) and PET/CT fusion images (**C**,**E**). Intense FDG tracer uptake is present in fat at the base of the neck, upper mediastinum (*large arrows*), supraclavicular region, axilla, paravertebral (*small arrows*), and upper abdomen retroperitoneal fat (*small arrowheads*). Properly registered and aligned PET and CT images allow for reliable identification of FDG tracer uptake in brown adipose tissue and distinction from pathologic lymph node tracer uptake, such as in the mediastinum, neck, supraclavicular fossa, and axilla. (*continued*)

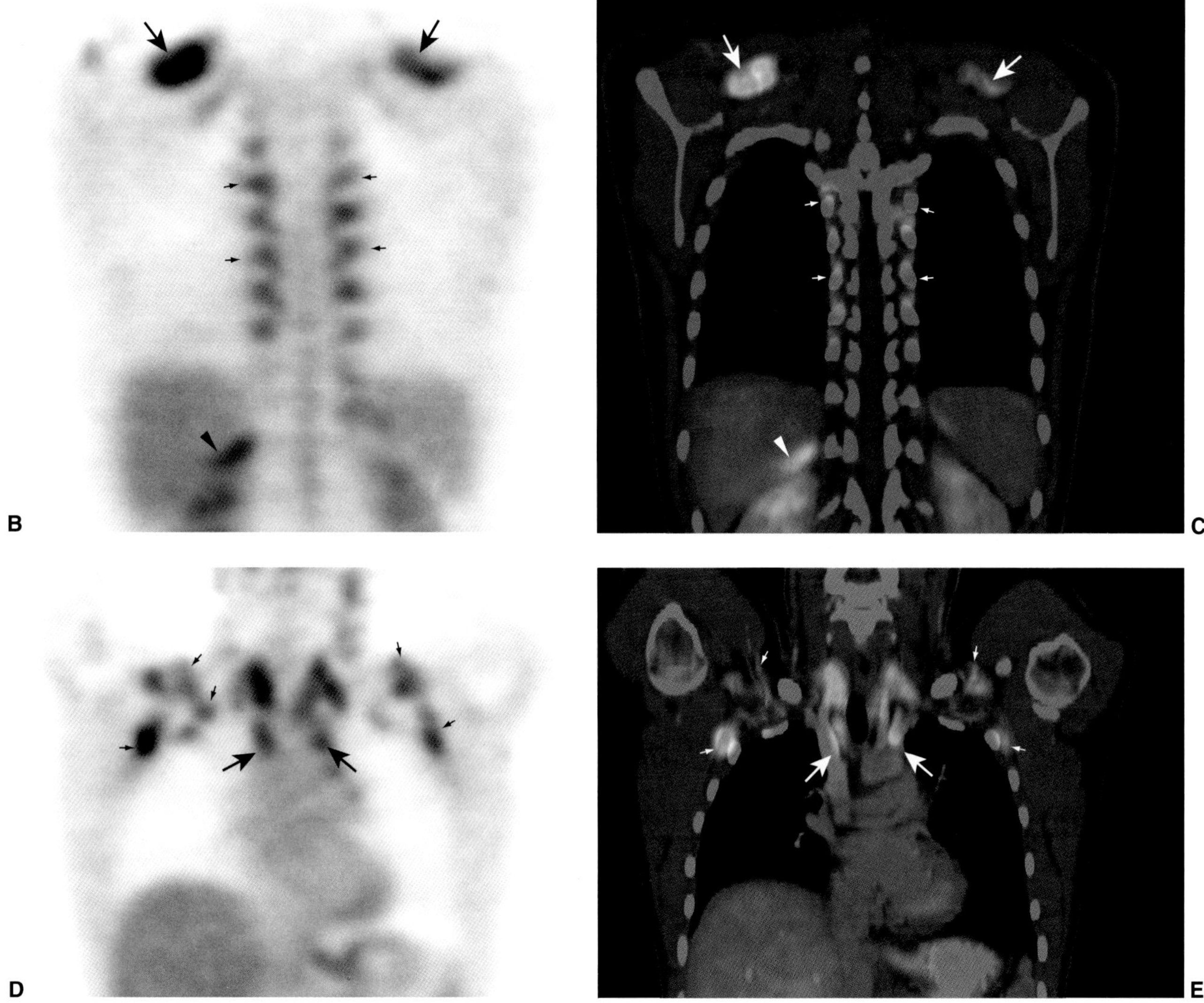

FIGURE 8.3.11. *(Continued)*

low-level activity throughout its extent (Fig. 8.3.12). Relatively intense fusiform and extended FDG uptake occurs in the presence of esophagitis (Fig. 8.3.13), which is indistinguishable from the configurations of esophageal cancer when the cancer has extended along the lymphatic plexus of the esophagus. It should be noted that esophagitis is common and often asymptomatic; hence, FDG uptake in the esophagus, when segmental and even intense, is not specific for esophageal malignancy. A focal area of FDG tracer uptake, especially when seen with focal thickening or asymmetric mass on CT, should be considered suspicious for neoplasm. A small focus of FDG activity is frequently seen at the gastroesophageal junction, probably related to the lower esophageal sphincter, and when no corresponding abnormal thickening or mass on CT is present, generally should not be presumed to be related to malignancy.

The normal stomach commonly shows FDG uptake, usually somewhat greater than FDG activity in the liver, and readily identifiable based on location and configuration (Fig. 8.3.14A). Gastric FDG uptake can be intense and, if the stomach is contracted, appear as an isolated FDG-avid mass. Location and configuration of the stomach, as well as distribution of FDG uptake in the gastric wall, can be variable, in some instances requiring careful reference to registered and aligned CT images to confirm the gastric origin of the FDG uptake. Gastric lymphoma and gastric carcinoma are thus not reliably diagnosed on FDG PET alone. The propensity for gastric FDG uptake is maintained in hiatal hernias, and hence FDG tracer activity in the lower mediastinum must be correlated with CT images.

Bowel, particularly the right colon (Fig. 8.3.14B), commonly demonstrates FDG uptake. The bowel uptake appears to be in the wall, and may reflect to varying degrees active smooth muscle, metabolically active mucosa, bowel wall lymphoid tissue, swallowed secretions, or colonic microbial activity. Tracer uptake is typically segmental or contiguous in the colon, and the appearance on maximum intensity projection images can be reminiscent of radiographic contrast studies of the colon (Fig. 8.3.14B). Small bowel

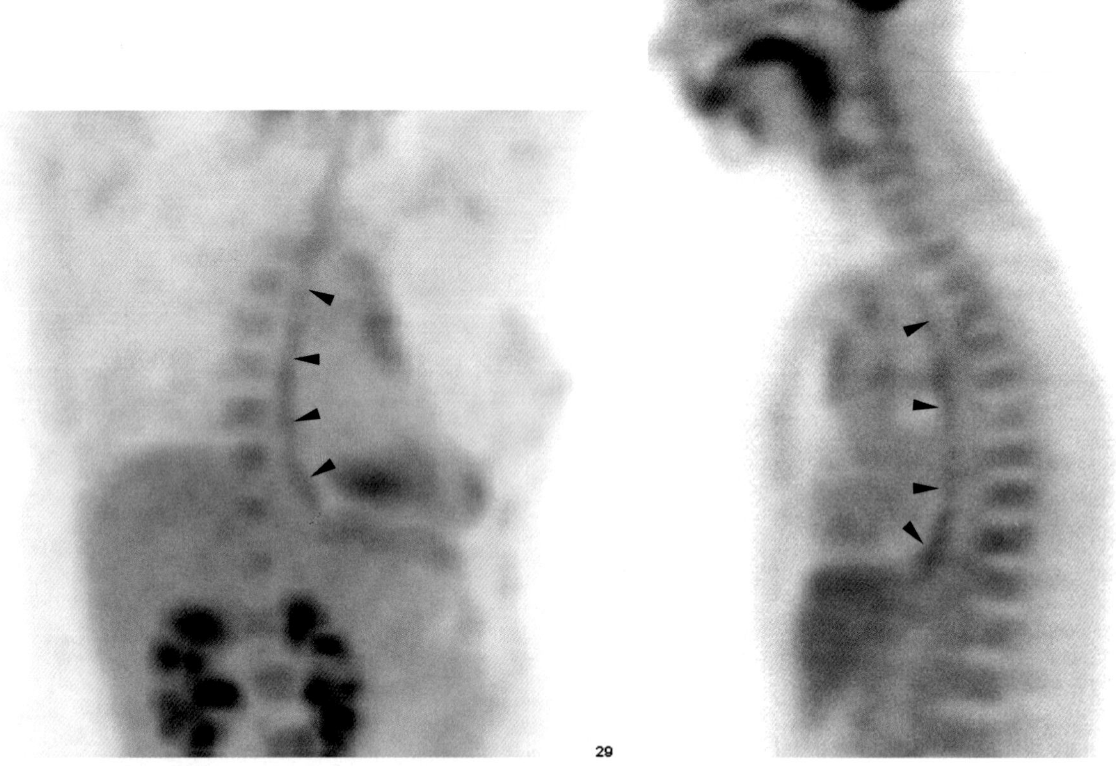

FIGURE 8.3.12. Normal esophageal fluorodeoxyglucose uptake. Attenuation-corrected anterioblique maximum intensity projection (**A**) and sagittal image (**B**) show uniform mild tracer uptake along the course of the esophagus (*arrowheads*).

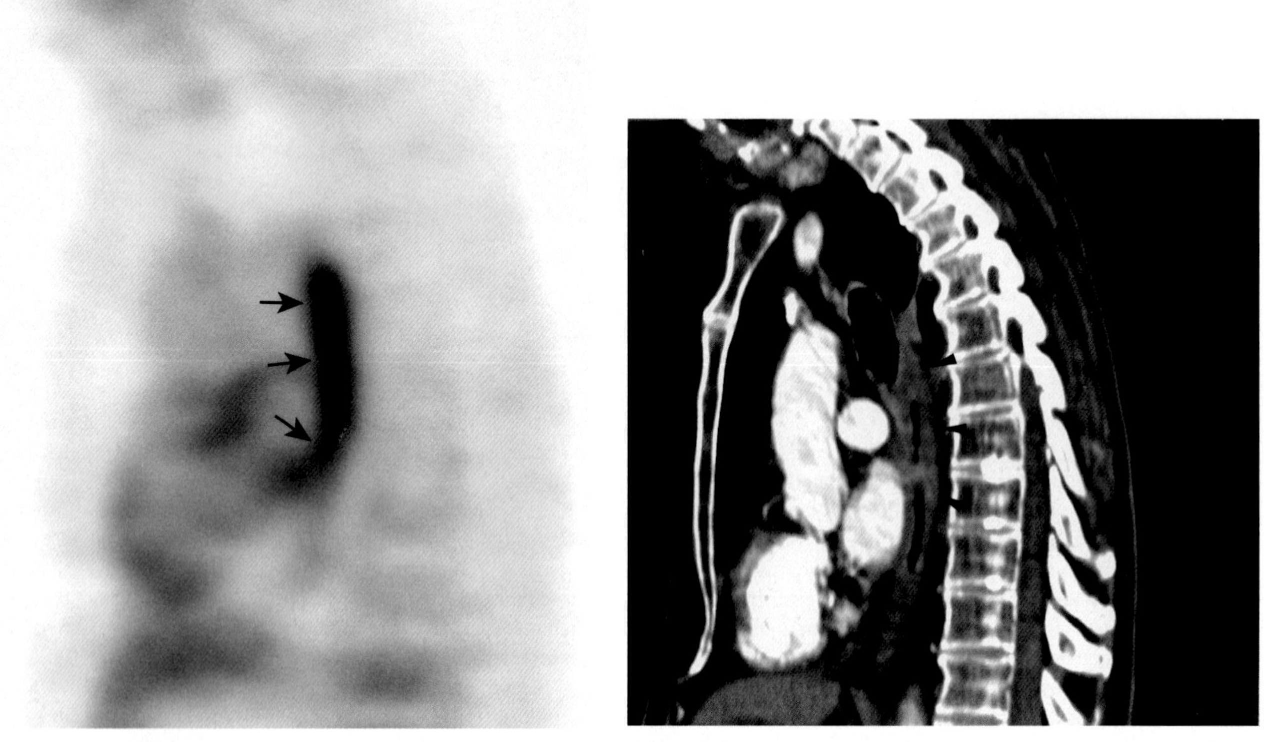

FIGURE 8.3.13. Segmental fluorodeoxyglucose (FDG) uptake due to esophagitis. Attenuation-corrected sagittal FDG PET (**A**) and sagittal reformat CT images (**B**) show an intense segment of tracer uptake in the midesophagus (*small arrows*), corresponding to diffuse esophageal wall thickening (*arrowheads*), due to postradiation treatment of the mediastinum-related esophagitis. Similar segmental FDG tracer uptake in the lower esophagus can occur due to reflux esophagitis. Esophageal cancer, while usually focal, can, however, present as a segment of tracer uptake and esophageal wall thickening.

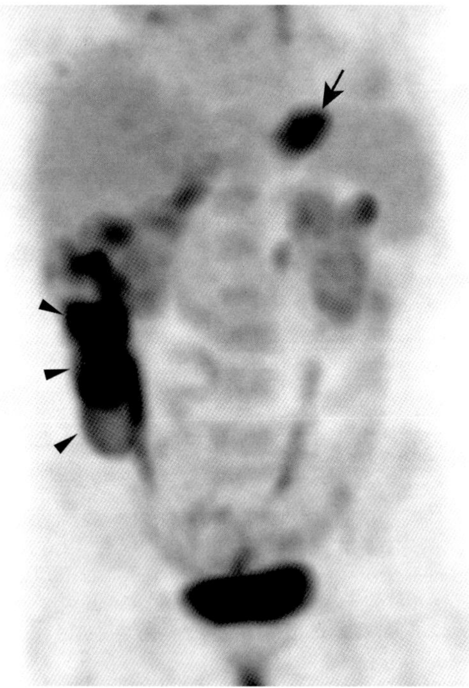

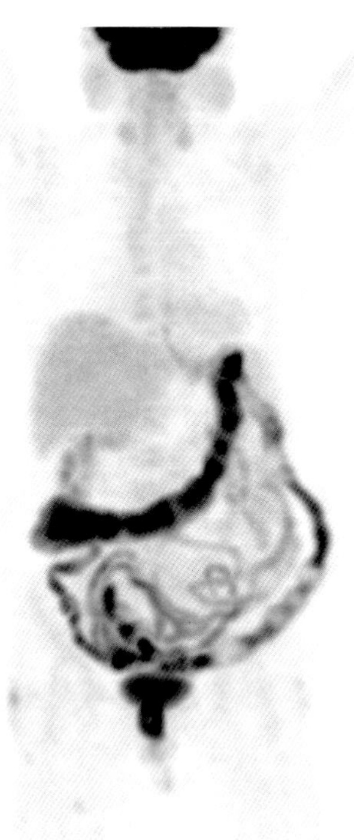

FIGURE 8.3.14. Physiologic fluorodeoxyglucose (FDG) activity in the stomach and bowel. Attenuation-corrected anterior maximum intensity projection images. **A:** Diffuse tracer in the partially contracted stomach (*arrow*) and diffuse tracer activity in the right colon (*arrowheads*). The stomach is usually associated with low-level tracer activity, but tracer uptake can be moderately intense. Physiologic FDG tracer uptake in the colon is variable, with the right colon more commonly seen and with variable intensity. **B:** Extensive physiologic FDG tracer uptake can be present throughout much and large bowel and long segments of small bowel. The relationships and course of tracer-avid bowel loops are best appreciated on rotating maximum intensity projection images, and registered and aligned CT images acquired on PET/CT readily confirm the bowel origin of the tracer activity.

FDG activity is usually lower in intensity than FDG activity observed in the colon and is typically seen in the lower pelvis (Fig. 8.3.14B), with continuous or segmental components to its appearance assisting in proper identification.

Focality of FDG uptake in either large or small bowel can be confounding, as peritoneal metastatic implants or mesenteric lymph node pathology may be entirely indistinguishable. Careful review of registered and aligned CT images can be essential for assigning isolated focal FDG uptake in the abdomen or pelvis to physiologic bowel tracer activity versus adjacent lymph nodes or serosal implants (Fig. 8.3.15). Focal FDG tracer activity, particularly when more intense than background liver activity within the bowel lumen

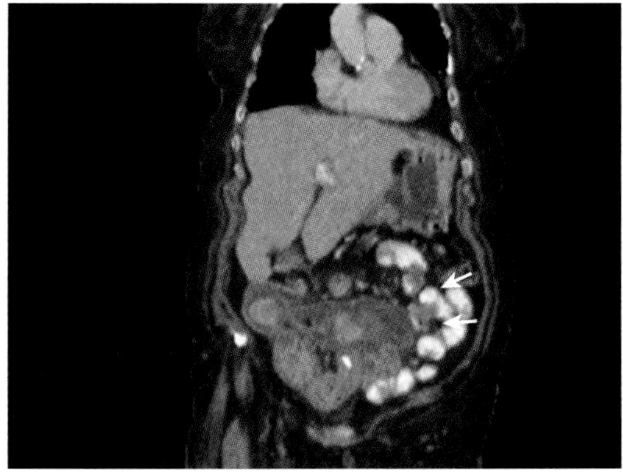

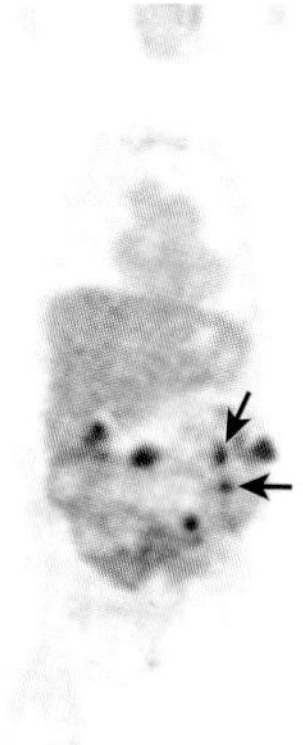

FIGURE 8.3.15. Focal fluorodeoxyglucose (FDG) activity associated with bowel. Attenuation-corrected coronal CT and FDB PET images demonstrate foci of increased tracer activity corresponding to abnormal soft tissue on bowel wall (*arrows*), reflecting serosal implants of metastatic colon cancer.

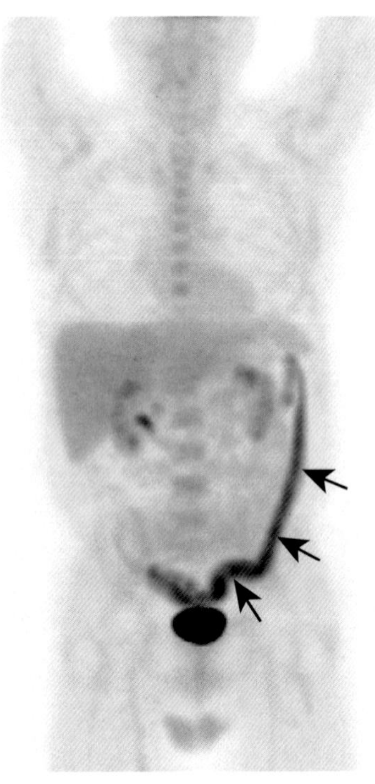

FIGURE 8.3.16. Fluorodeoxyglucose (FDG) activity associated with inflammatory bowel disease. Attenuation-corrected anterior maximum intensity projection image (**A**) shows diffuse featureless increased tracer activity throughout the descending and sigmoid colon (*arrows*). Coronal attenuation-corrected FDG PET (**B**) and CT (**C**) images demonstrate the tracer activity in diffusely thickened bowel wall (*arrows*) and pericolonic inflammatory changes (*arrowheads*). The level of FDG tracer uptake in inflamed bowel is within the range of physiologic bowel uptake, and hence reference to the CT appearance is required for differentiation.

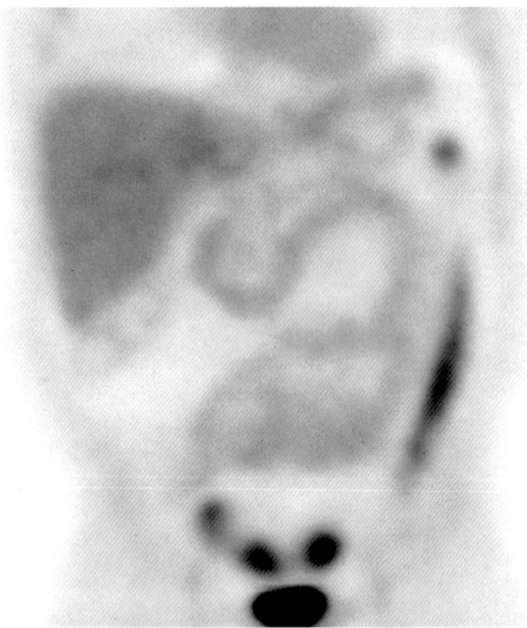

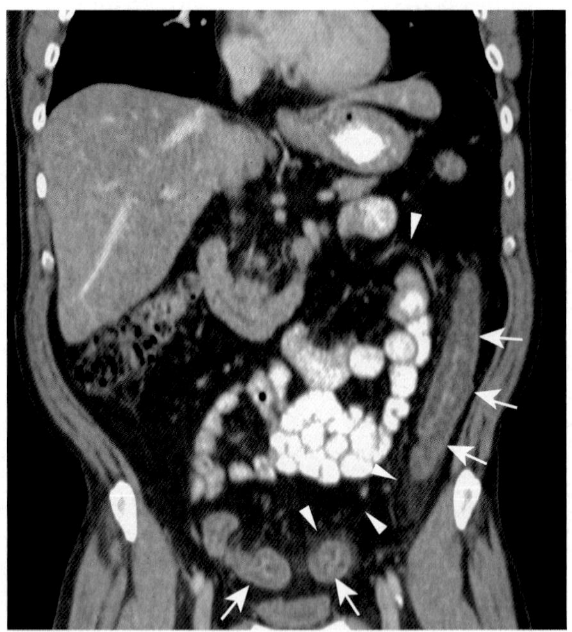

adjacent to colon wall, frequently corresponds to pathology, either villous adenomatous polyp or primary colon cancer, requiring further evaluation such as endoscopic examination (13,14). Sometimes a corresponding nodule can be identified on CT, but often no convincing CT abnormality is identified on routine CT, even with contrast enhancement. Inflammatory bowel disease is known to cause diffuse or segmental FDG uptake (15), and the FDG PET appearance tends to be of a featureless tubular structure, analogous to radiographic depictions (Fig. 8.3.16). Characteristic CT signs of inflammatory bowel disease, when present, allow for reliable distinction between benign physiologic FDG tracer uptake and inflammatory bowel disease (Fig. 8.3.16). Non-distended colon can also appear thickened and demonstrate physiologic FDG uptake. Some centers have reported reduction of bowel FDG uptake using smooth muscle relaxants immediately prior to FDG administration (16) or isosmotic bowel preparations the evening prior to the examination (17), although this is not routinely practiced at most centers.

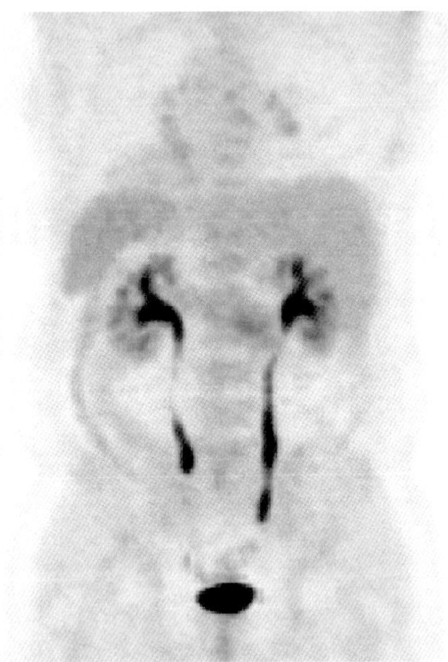

FIGURE 8.3.17. Normal distribution of urinary fluorodeoxyglucose (FDG) tracer activity. Anterior maximum intensity projection image shows excreted urinary FDG tracer in the intrarenal collecting systems, including calyces and pelves of the kidneys, ureters, and the bladder. Urinary tracer activity in the ureters can be continuous, segmental, or focal depending on peristaltic and luminal diameter status of the ureter.

Genitourinary Tract

Unlike glucose, FDG is not resorbed by the tubular cells of the kidney, and consequently the excretory route of FDG in the urine results in intense tracer activity in the intrarenal collecting systems, ureters, and bladder (Fig. 8.3.17). Presence of urinary tracer in the intrarenal collecting systems and ureters is dependent on the degree of hydration and renal function of the patient. Both hydration and use of furosemide can facilitate clearance of urinary tracer from the intrarenal collecting systems and ureters and reduce the intensity of urinary tracer activity in the bladder (18). In most instances, however, the intensity and location of the urinary FDG permits correct identification of the calyces, renal pelvis, and ureters. The dependent location of the upper pole renal calyces in the supine patient frequently results in urinary tracer pooling, which should not be confused with abnormal tracer uptake within or adjacent to the upper pole of the kidney. Small primary renal malignancies and metastases such as from lung cancer can appear quite similar to calyceal urinary tracer activity, and hence careful review of corresponding CT images of the kidneys should be routine (Fig. 8.3.18). Similarly, abnormalities in the upper urinary tract, such as urinary diversions, redundant and dilated ureters, diverticula, or communicating cysts, can result in focal tracer activity that could be confused with an FDG-avid mass (Fig. 8.3.19); correlation with the anatomic imaging is again essential in such circumstances. Occasionally ureteral activity will be limited to a small, isolated focus (Fig. 8.3.20), which can be very difficult to differentiate from a retroperitoneal lymph node. With contemporary image reconstruction algorithms intense urinary tracer activity in the bladder does not significantly compromise assessment of regional structures, and anatomic alterations such as diverticula or transurethral resection of the prostate defects are discernable. Tracer activity in the bladder can be reduced by use of intravenous hydration and diuretics or by direct urinary bladder catheterization and lavage (18).

Uterine endometrium can demonstrate elevated FDG uptake in the ovulatory and menstrual phase in premenopausal women that should not be confused with uterine or presacral neoplasm (Fig. 8.3.21) (19). Increased ovarian FDG uptake is associated with malignancy in postmenopausal women, but may be functional in premenopausal women particularly, and is seen at the midcycle ovulatory phase (Fig. 8.3.22) (19). Moderately intense FDG uptake occurs in the testes (Fig. 8.3.23), which is a consistently normal finding, and tends to decline with advancing age (20).

Thyroid

Normal thyroid tissue is not associated with a level of FDG tracer activity that allows delineation of the thyroid gland on PET images. Diffuse increased FDG tracer activity (Fig. 8.3.24) can be seen and appears to reflect chronic lymphocytic (Hashimoto) thyroiditis (21) or subacute thyroiditis (22). Focal thyroid lesions found on FDG PET (Fig. 8.3.25) carries a significant risk (30% to 40%) of malignancy (particularly if associated with intense FDG uptake), and further imaging (ultrasound) and histopathological evaluation should be considered (23,24).

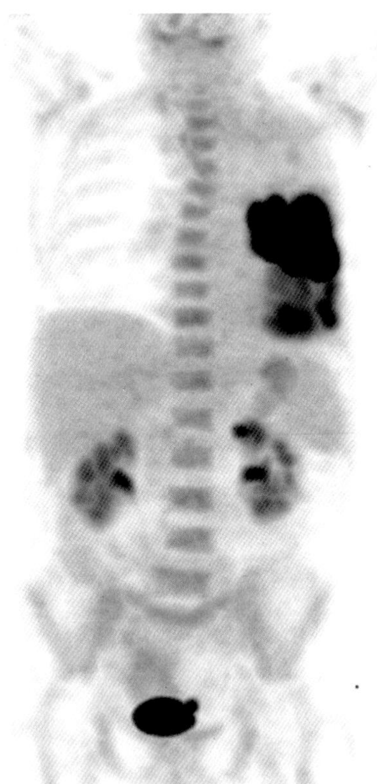

FIGURE 8.3.18. Calyceal urinary fluorodeoxyglucose (FDG) tracer activity. Attenuation-corrected anterior maximum intensity projection image demonstrates focal tracer activity in renal calyces, a common finding (**A**). Large area of intense FDG tracer activity in left hemithorax is primary lung cancer. *(continued)*

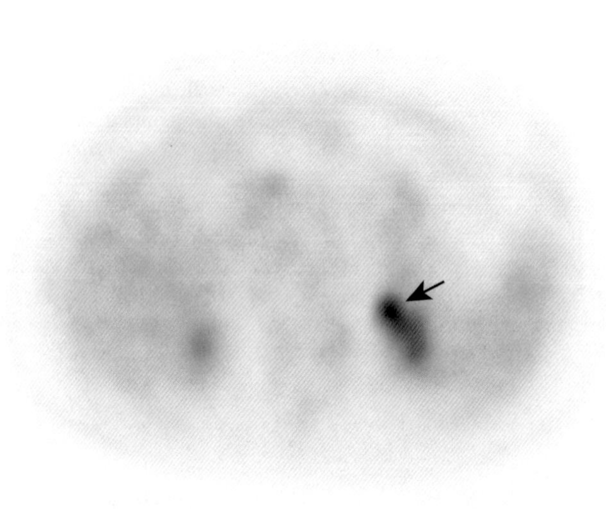

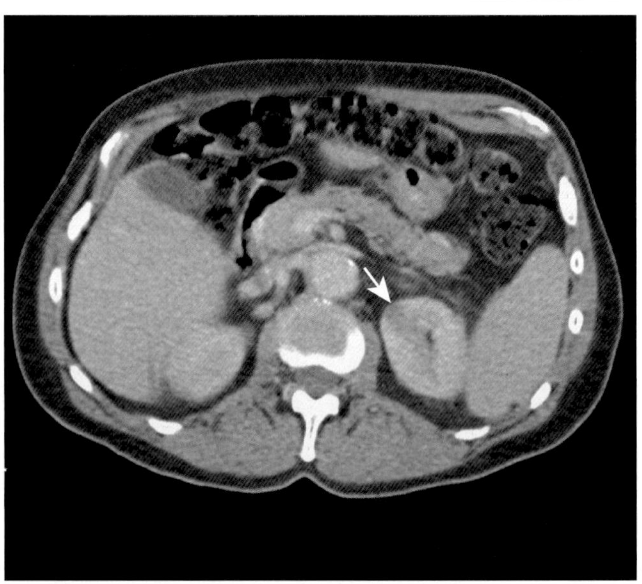

FIGURE 8.3.18. (*Continued*) Review of the transaxial attenuation-corrected FDG PET (**B**) and transaxial contrast-enhanced CT images (**C**) reveals a focus of increased tracer activity in the upper pole of the left kidney (*arrow*), which is not a calyx but rather a small mass corresponding to an isolated renal metastasis of lung cancer (*white arrow*).

Bone Marrow

Bone marrow is normally associated with modest FDG uptake, roughly equivalent to liver. The level of FDG bone marrow uptake in children is higher than in adults. Marrow is commonly identified in the vertebral bodies, pelvis, hips, proximal long bones, and the sternum. Any process disturbing marrow distribution will alter the marrow-related FDG distribution. Radiation therapy will reduce bone marrow FDG activity to background, resulting in apparent absent vertebral bodies, for example (Fig. 8.3.26). Vertebral body marrow FDG activity is also diminished with vertebral body height loss in patients with insufficiency

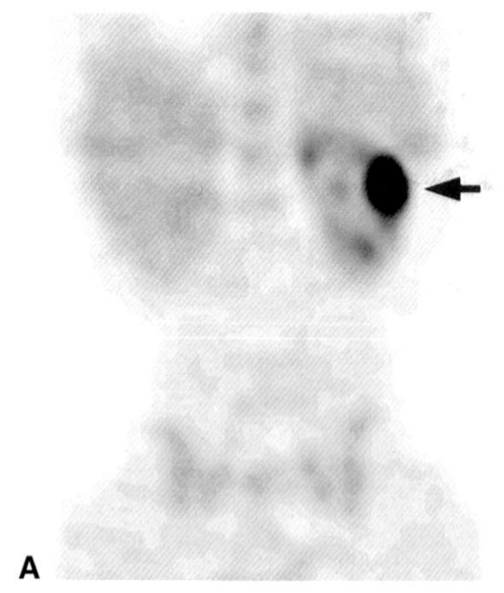

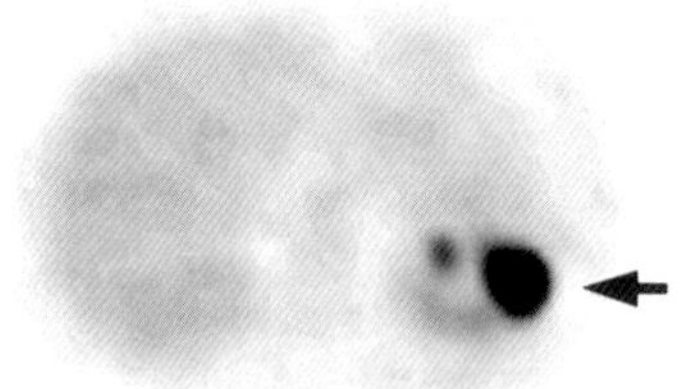

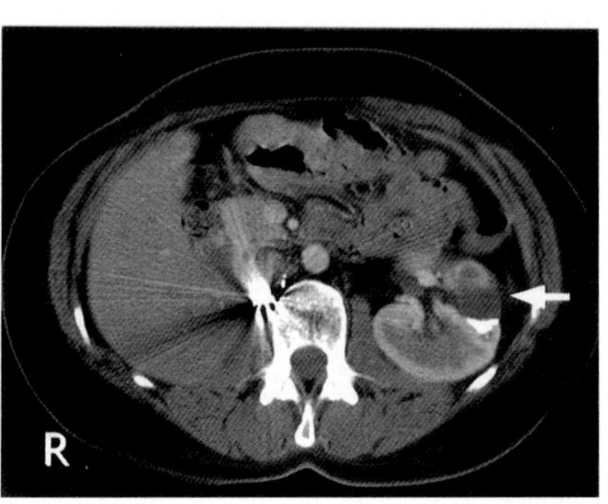

FIGURE 8.3.19. Calyceal diverticulum. Attenuation-corrected coronal (**A**) and axial FDG PET images (**B**) and corresponding transaxial CT image (**C**). Urinary tracer accumulation in a left renal calyceal diverticulum (*arrow*).

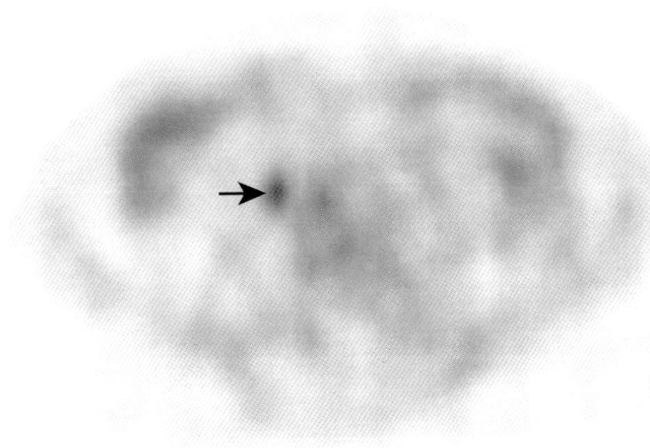

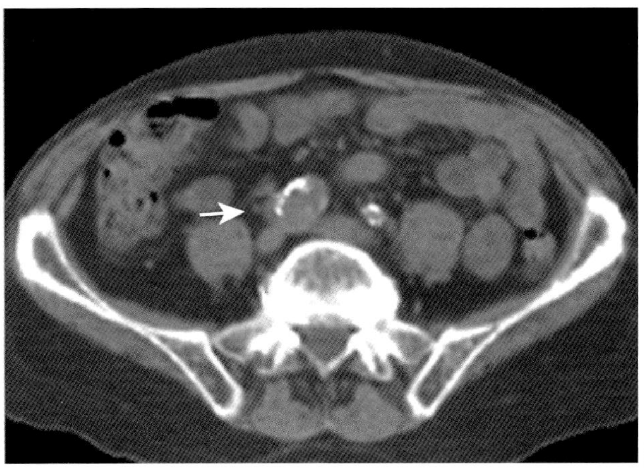

FIGURE 8.3.20. Focal urinary fluorodeoxyglucose urinary activity. Attenuation-corrected anterior maximum intensity projection FDG PET image demonstrated an isolated focus of tracer activity in the right midabdomen (not shown), which on attenuation-corrected transaxial PET image (**A**) is in the retroperitoneum (*arrow*). The registered and aligned CT image (**B**) reveals the focal tracer activity to be in the right ureter (*white arrow*) and not in a retroperitoneal lymph node.

compression deformities or fractures, resulting in apparent relatively "hot" vertebral bodies, which could be misinterpreted as metastatic foci in vertebral bone marrow (Fig. 8.3.27). Patients undergoing treatment with hematopoietic stimulants such as colony stimulating factors will have increased bone marrow FDG uptake (Fig. 8.3.28), which can be intense and extensive (25). This benign phenomenon may be misinterpreted as malignant marrow infiltration, particularly if there are photopenic areas from previously radiation therapy, previously treated malignant vertebral disease, or vertebral hemangioma. Diffuse disease involvement such as lymphoma or breast cancer can be difficult to distinguish from hematopoietic-stimulated normal bone marrow on PET images alone.

Lymphoid Tissue

Lymphoid tissue in certain locations is associated with sufficient FDG uptake to be routinely identified. The palatine tonsils are

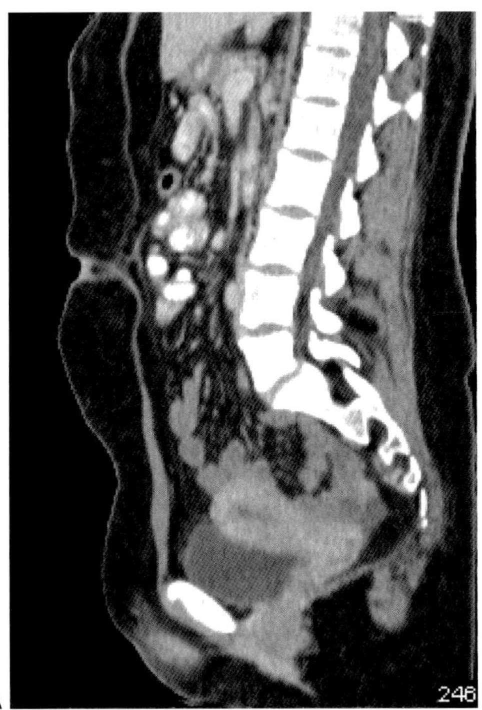

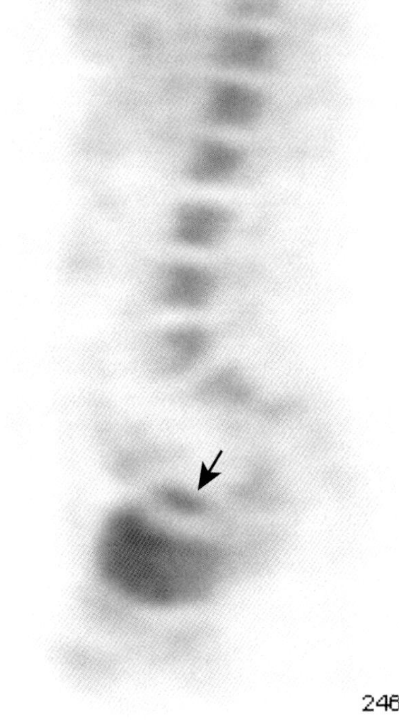

FIGURE 8.3.21. Normal uterine endometrial fluorodeoxyglucose (FDG) tracer activity. Sagittal CT (**A**) and attenuation-corrected sagittal FDG PET image (**B**) of a 38-year-old woman at the ovulatory menstrual phase. Moderate FDG tracer activity (*arrow*) is present in the uterine endometrium.

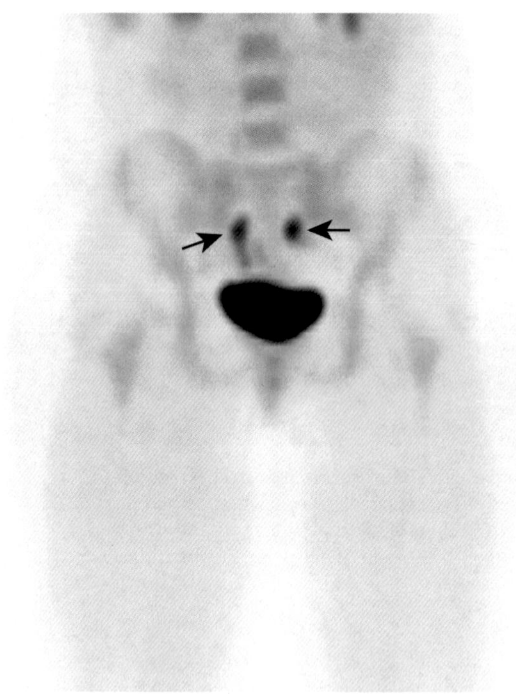

FIGURE 8.3.22. Normal ovarian fluorodeoxyglucose tracer activity. **A:** Attenuation-corrected anterior maximum intensity FDG PET projection image (**A**) of 22-year-old woman in midovulatory cycle demonstrates two intense foci of tracer activity in the midpelvis (*arrows*), which on the transaxial attenuation-corrected PET (**B**) and PET/CT fusion (**C**) images are shown to correspond to normal ovaries.

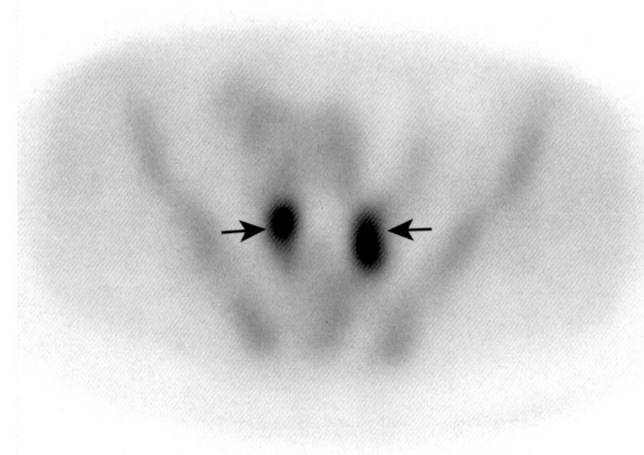

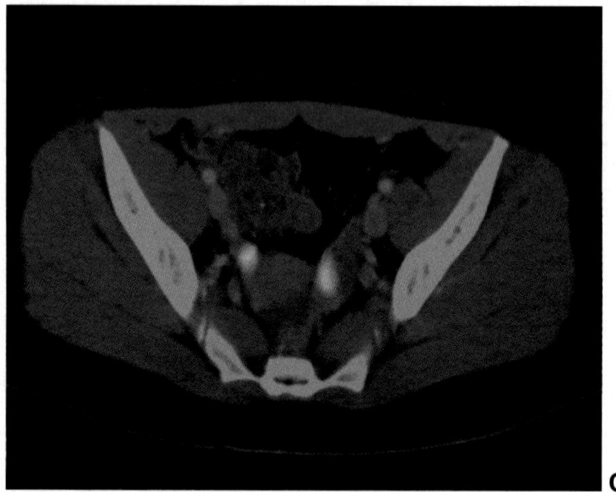

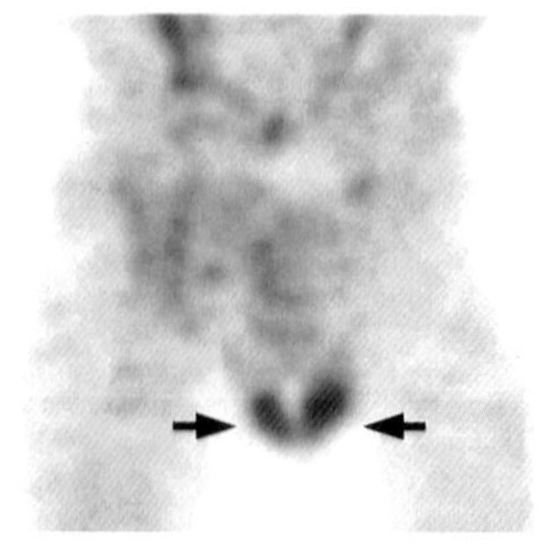

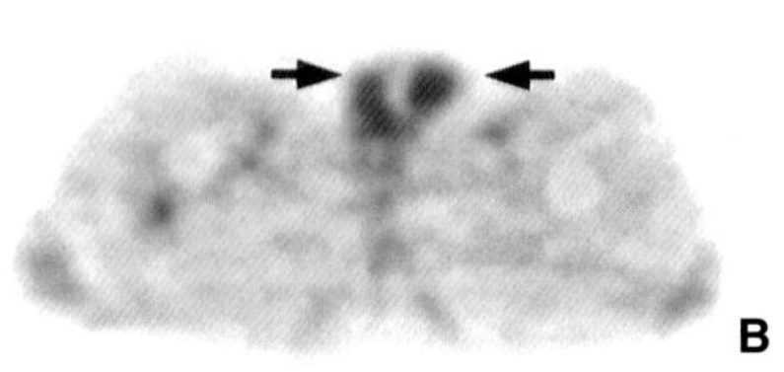

FIGURE 8.3.23. Normal testicular fluorodeoxyglucose activity. Attenuation-corrected FDG PET coronal (**A**) and transaxial images (**B**) show moderate tracer uptake (*arrows*) in the testes, a normal finding.

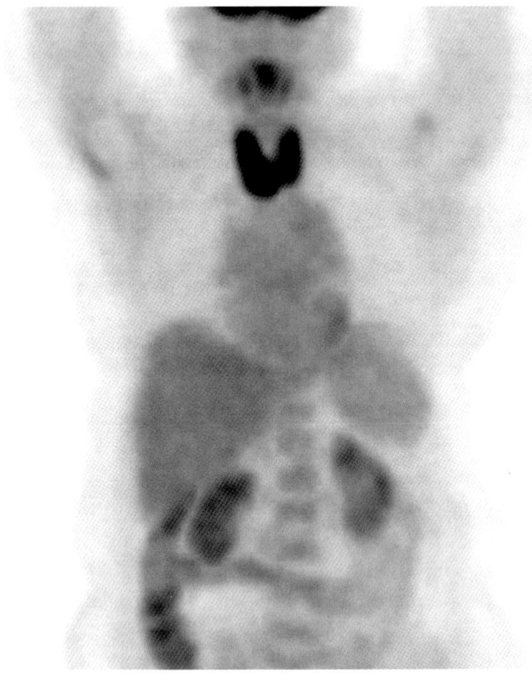

FIGURE 8.3.24. Diffuse elevated fluorodeoxyglucose (FDG) activity in the thyroid gland. Attenuation-corrected anterior maximum intensity projection image demonstrates intense uniform tracer activity, defining an enlarged but otherwise normal configuration thyroid gland. FDG tracer activity in the thyroid gland can be seen at background levels, mildly increased or relatively intense in euthyroid patients. The presence of intense diffuse tracer uptake has been implicated in subclinical thyroiditis.

almost always identified and can be fairly intense and are joined by the lingual tonsils, completing the lymphoid tissue of the Waldeyer ring (Fig. 8.3.3) (2). In young patients adenoid lymphoid tissue will often also demonstrate intense FDG uptake (Fig. 8.3.29). Likewise in young patients the thymus is well delineated, associated with FDG uptake modestly above blood pool, and usually easily identified based on configuration, especially on maximum intensity projection image reformat (Fig. 8.3.30) and in conjunction with correlative CT images. The palatine tonsils can be markedly asymmetric in the setting of prior surgery or unilateral radiation therapy, resulting in an apparent intense focus of FDG activity in the contralateral normal palatine tonsil, which should not be mistaken for a primary tonsilar cancer (Fig. 8.3.31).

FLUORODEOXYGLUCOSE UPTAKE IN NONMALIGNANT TUMORS

The increased glycolysis and cellular glucose uptake associated with malignant transformation underlies cancer detection using FDG PET. Certain benign tumors are also associated with increased FDG uptake, which can be of intensity in the range of malignant neoplasms. Although FDG PET has been reported to have a high level of accuracy in diagnosis of adrenal nodules due to metastatic disease, it should be noted that benign hypertrophy and rarely benign adenoma of the adrenals can yield identifiable FDG uptake (Fig. 8.3.32) (26). Morphologic characterization of the adrenal gland can thus be essential when adrenal FDG uptake is present. In males, gynecomastia can result in unexpected somewhat focal areas of FDG uptake in the chest wall that is readily confirmed as glandular breast tissue on CT images. A variety of benign skeletal tumor or tumorlike lesions, including giant cell tumors, chondroblastomas, fibrous dysplasia, and nonossifying fibromas, can demonstrate increased FDG activity (27). Myositis ossificans

A. B

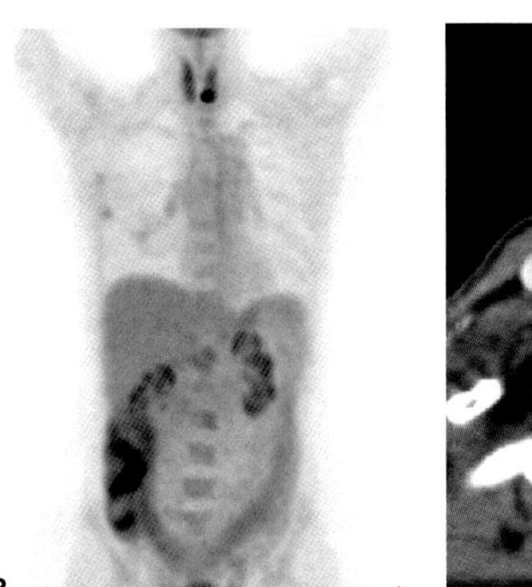

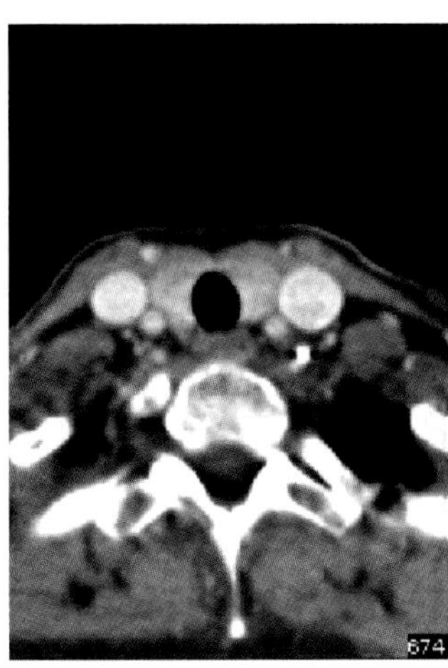

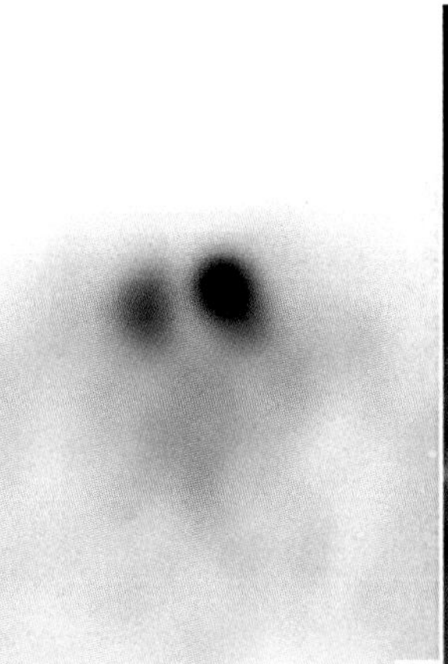

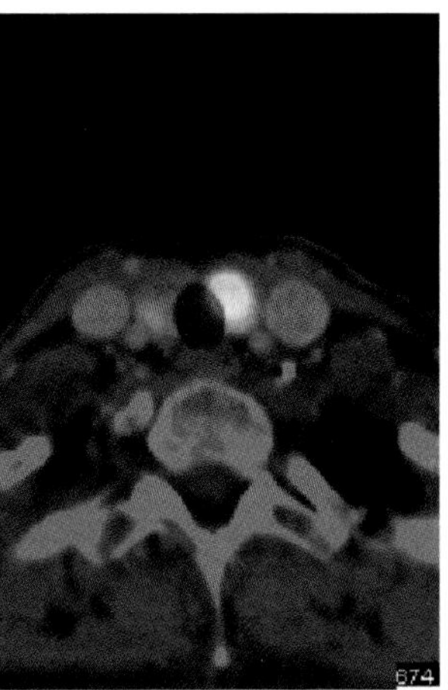

C, D

FIGURE 8.3.25. Focal fluorodeoxyglucose (FDG) uptake in the thyroid gland. Attenuation-corrected anterior maximum intensity projection FDG PET image (**A**) demonstrates an intense focus of FDG tracer activity in the left of midline lower neck, which on the registered and aligned transaxial CT (**B**) and attenuation-corrected FDG PET (**C**) and PET/CT fusion (**D**) corresponds to a thyroid nodule. Such isolated thyroid nodules which are low attenuation or isointense on the contrast enhanced CT with elevated FDG tracer uptake are usually benign nodules, but carry significant risk (30% to 40%) of primary thyroid malignancy and very rarely metastatic disease such as from melanoma or renal cell carcinoma.

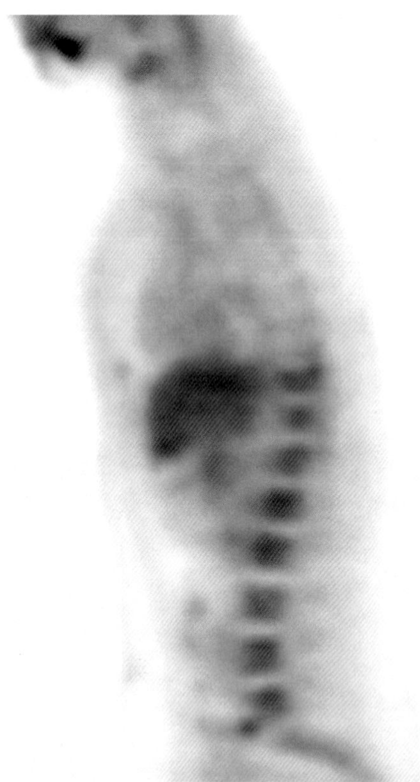

FIGURE 8.3.26. Effect of radiation therapy on bone marrow physiologic fluorodeoxyglucose (FDG) uptake. Attenuation-corrected sagittal FDG PET image of the spine of a patient previously treated with radiation therapy of lung cancer reveals absent FDG tracer uptake in thoracic vertebral body bone marrow.

and active heterotopic bone also can be associated with fairly intense FDG activity (Fig. 8.3.33). Again, morphologic characterization in the first instance is essential in determining the benign etiology of such findings. When the skull base is included on whole-body PET imaging, focal increased FDG tracer activity in the pituitary fossa should not be assumed as a metastasis, as pituitary adenomas, while rare, are associated with elevated FDG tracer uptake of the same degree as malignant neoplasm (28). Benign salivary gland tumors such as Warthin's tumor or pleomorphic adenoma are not an uncommon finding on whole-body FDG PET scans that include the upper neck, as these can be associated with fairly intense focal FDG tracer uptake (Fig. 8.3.34) (29).

BENIGN PATHOLOGIC FLUORODEOXYGLUCOSE UPTAKE DUE TO INFLAMMATION

Inflammation in myriad manifestations is the most significant cause of FDG uptake that can be mistaken for malignant disease. Glycolytic metabolism is elevated in the leukocyte infiltration associated with inflammatory processes, hence, sterile, pyogenic, and granulomatous inflammation is associated with increased FDG uptake. In some instances the configuration and/or location of FDG uptake is easily identified as a manifestation of inflammation. In other instances careful anatomic correlation is required to confirm the benign etiology, and finally in many cases, such as with lymph nodes, it is not possible to distinguish benign inflammatory FDG uptake from malignancy.

Normal wound healing is associated with an inflammatory response, hence, modest FDG uptake is associated with healing wounds (Fig. 8.3.35). Similarly, the inflammatory response associated with tissue resorption results in modest FDG uptake in resolving hematoma or thrombus (30). FDG is quite sensitive to inflammation, with focal uptake readily seen at the entrance site of uncomplicated indwelling percutaneous tubes or lines (Fig. 8.3.36) or even small cutaneous carbuncles (Fig. 8.3.37). Ostomies will show modest FDG uptake. Vascular grafts are associated with moderate FDG uptake and are frequently observed (Fig. 8.3.38), and the uptake appears to persist for months or longer and is not related to initial healing about the graft. The presence of FDG uptake is therefore not specific for infection of a vascular graft, although isolated or superimposed focal FDG uptake in a graft has been reported as a specific sign of infection (31). Major arterial vessels involved with advanced atheromatous disease, such as the abdominal or thoracic aorta, will often be unexpectedly conspicuous (32) due to low-level FDG uptake in the vessel wall (Fig. 8.3.39). Intense uniform increased FDG uptake in large vessel vasculitis such as Takayasu arteritis or temporal arteritis have been described (33). Pleurodesis can demonstrate intense FDG tracer uptake (Fig. 8.3.40) even years after the procedure, presumably due to persistent foreign body response to the talc (34).

Pyogenic infection, such as in abscesses, and pneumonia are associated with intense FDG uptake (35,36). Pneumonia typically causes diffuse, relatively uniform FDG activity that is easily recognized; however, with cavitation, the appearance can be indistinguishable from certain cavitating neoplasms such as squamous cell carcinomas. Likewise, abscesses, which typically are defined by a rim of intense FDG uptake, can have an appearance indistinguishable from a malignant neoplasm mass with a necrotic center (Fig. 8.3.41). Fistulous tracts and sinus tracts are associated with inflammation related to FDG uptake and can appear as focal areas of FDG uptake and be mistaken for metastases or primary bowel neoplasm.

Focal FDG uptake occurs in both in uncomplicated and complicated pancreatitis (37). Diffuse FDG uptake is typically seen in acute pancreatitis, although focality can occur. Complications such as abscess or phlegmonous mass can be associated with intense focal FDG uptake, even in relatively asymptomatic patients, months after initial disease presentation (Fig. 8.3.42).

Healing fractures demonstrate increased FDG uptake weeks into the healing process (38). Healing sternotomy and rib fractures (Fig. 8.3.43) are a common source of FDG uptake in bone that could be misinterpreted as osseous metastatic disease if careful review of CT or other correlative imaging is not performed. Sacral fractures can be quite subtle on CT, but are not uncommon in elderly patients and should not be confused with osseous metastases to the sacrum (Fig. 8.3.44) (39). Acute vertebral body fractures will be associated with increased FDG uptake and vertebral plasty–treated vertebral bodies commonly will demonstrate increased FDG uptake (Fig. 8.3.27). Degenerative or inflammatory joint disease can give rise to elevated FDG uptake.

(*text continues on page 163*)

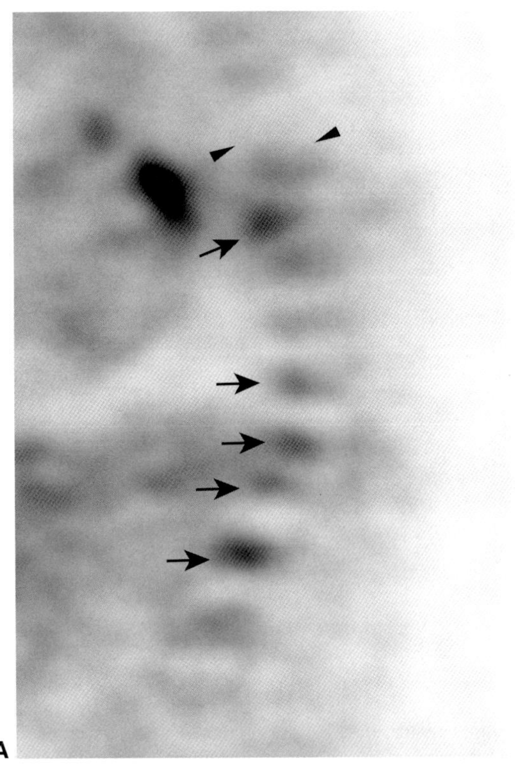

FIGURE 8.3.27. Variable appearance of physiologic bone marrow fluorodeoxyglucose (FDG) activity in setting of degenerative changes and treated and untreated vertebral body compression fractures. Sagittal attenuation-corrected FDG PET (**A**), CT (**B**), and PET/CT fusion images (**C**) demonstrate increased tracer activity at some vertebroplasty sites (*arrows*) and decreased tracer activity in old compression fracture/deformity vertebral bodies (*arrowheads*) as well as normal vertebral body tracer activity. Vertebroplasty treated compression fractures can be FDG avid due to healing bone, or if the vertebroplasty cement is very dense, artifactual apparent increased tracer activity can occur due to attenuation-correction artifact.

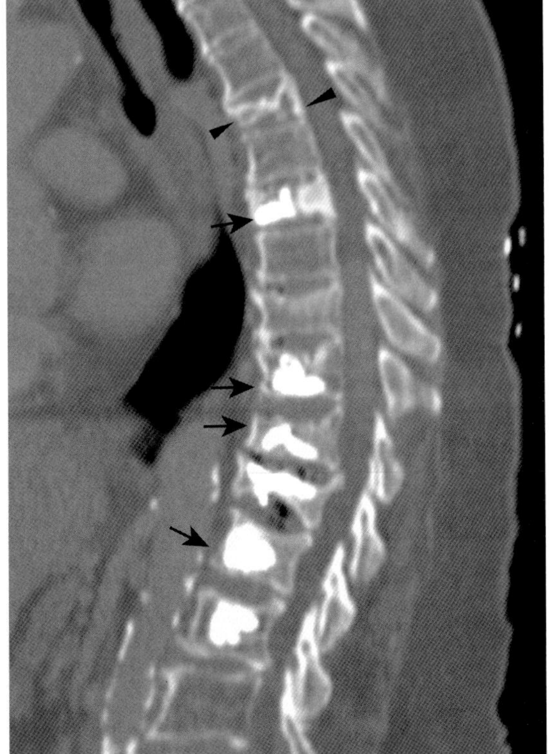

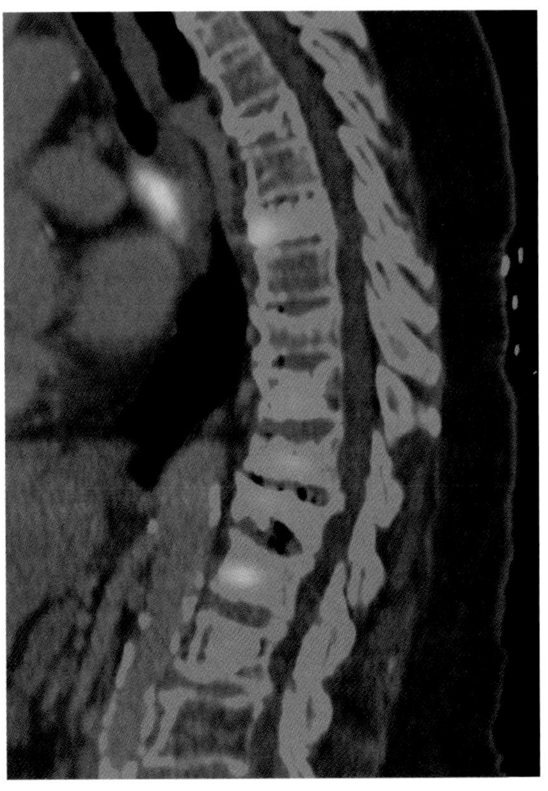

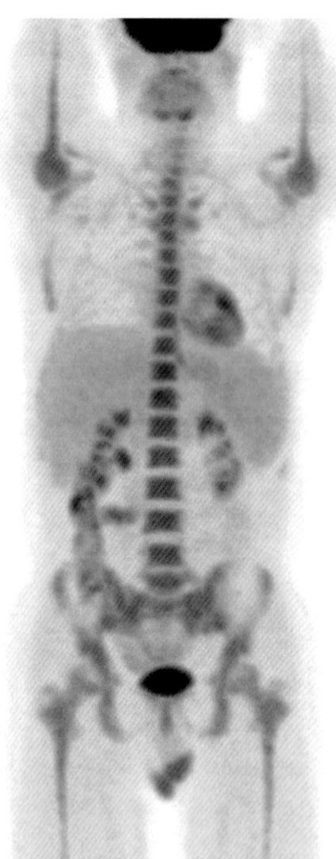

FIGURE 8.3.28. Diffuse increased bone marrow physiologic fluorodeoxyglucose uptake due to hematopoietic stimulation. Attenuation-corrected anterior maximum intensity projection image reveals intense tracer activity throughout bone marrow due to recent or ongoing use of a colony-stimulating factor in the chemotherapy regimen.

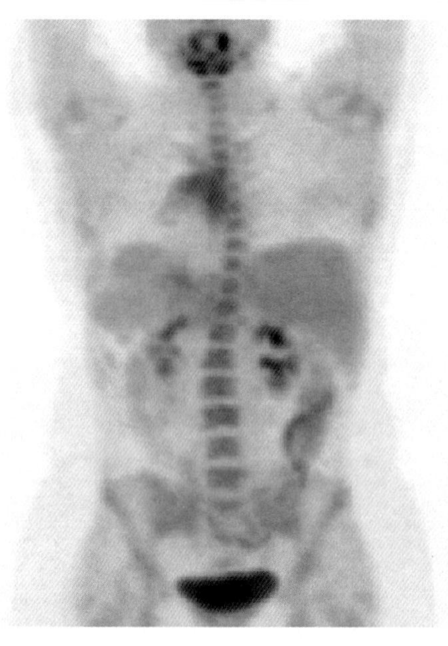

FIGURE 8.3.30. Normal fluorodeoxyglucose (FDG) activity in the thymus gland. Attenuation-corrected anterior maximum intensity projection FDG PET image best reveals the typical configuration of the prominent thymus gland in this young patient. In children and young adults the thymus gland is prominent and readily depicted on FDG PET, while in older adults the thymus tracer activity is absent, except in the setting of completed chemotherapy, where a "rebound" phenomenon can be seen in which the thymus gland increases in size and FDG tracer uptake is increased.

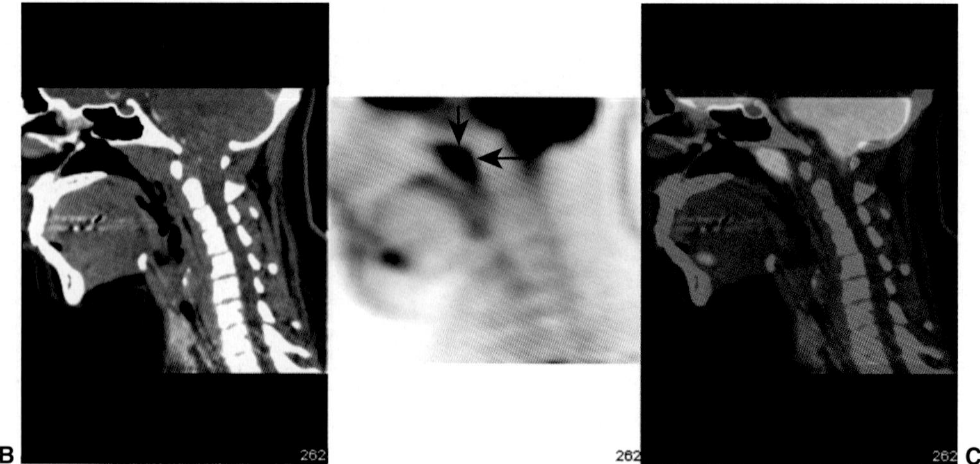

FIGURE 8.3.29. Normal fluorodeoxyglucose (FDG) activity in the adenoid tonsil. Sagittal CT (**A**), attenuation-corrected sagittal FDG PET (**B**) and PET/CT fusion (**C**) show intense tracer activity in the adenoid tissue (*arrows*) in a 16-year-old patient. Such activity is normal in children and young adults, and CT images will typically demonstrate corresponding prominence of adenoid soft tissue.

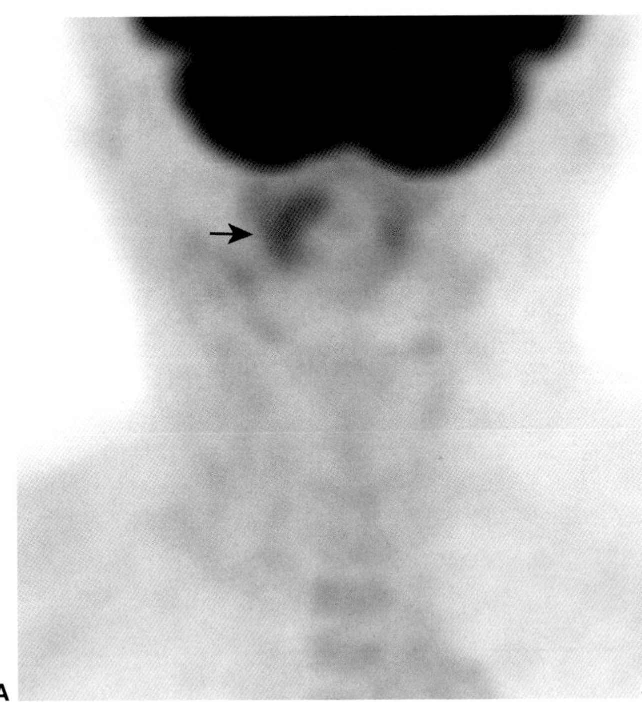

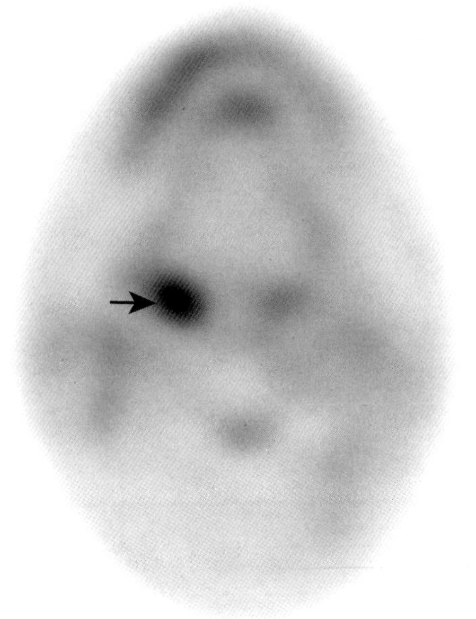

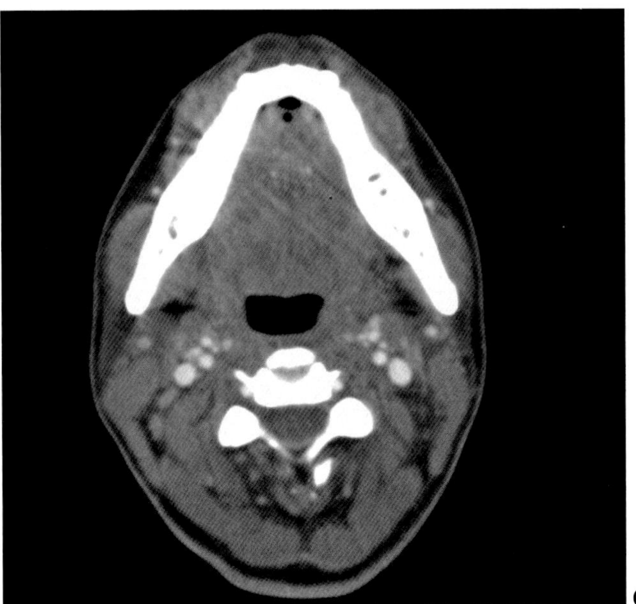

FIGURE 8.3.31. Asymmetric palatine tonsil fluorodeoxyglucose (FDG) activity due to radiation therapy. Attenuation-corrected anterior maximum intensity projection image (**A**) shows intense, apparently focal, FDG tracer activity in the region of the right palatine tonsil (*arrow*) and relative absent tracer activity in the region of the left palatine tonsil. Transaxial attenuation-corrected FDG PET (**B**) and CT (**C**) images show the apparent "hot" right palatine tonsil without corresponding mass or abnormal contrast enhancement. The patient had undergone radiation therapy to the left neck for a left-sided squamous cell carcinoma, resulting in ablation of normal left palatine tonsil lymphoid tissue.

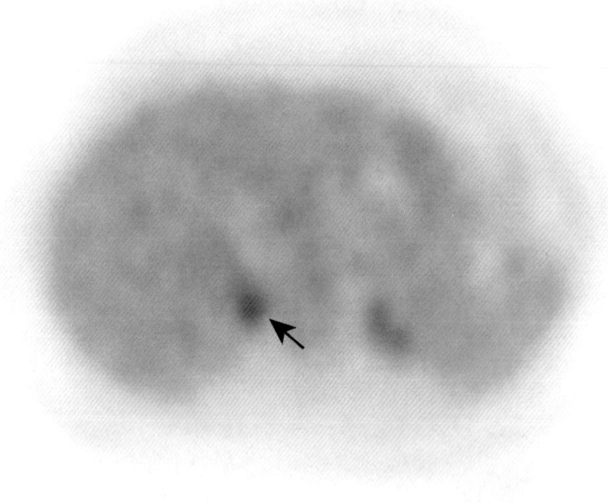

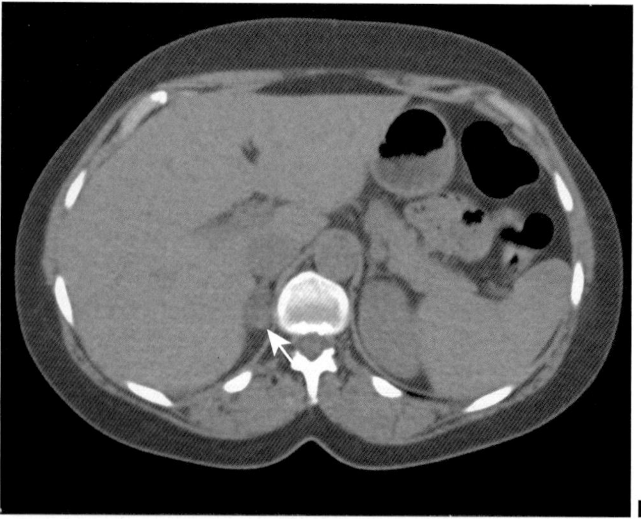

FIGURE 8.3.32. Fluorodeoxyglucose (FDG) activity in benign adrenal adenoma. Attenuation-corrected transaxial FDG PET (**A**) and CT images (**B**) reveal modest FDG tracer uptake, slightly greater than liver background (*arrow*), in a right adrenal nodule (*white arrow*). On the noncontrast-enhanced CT the adrenal nodule is of low attenuation (Hounsfield units = 8), typical of a benign adenoma.

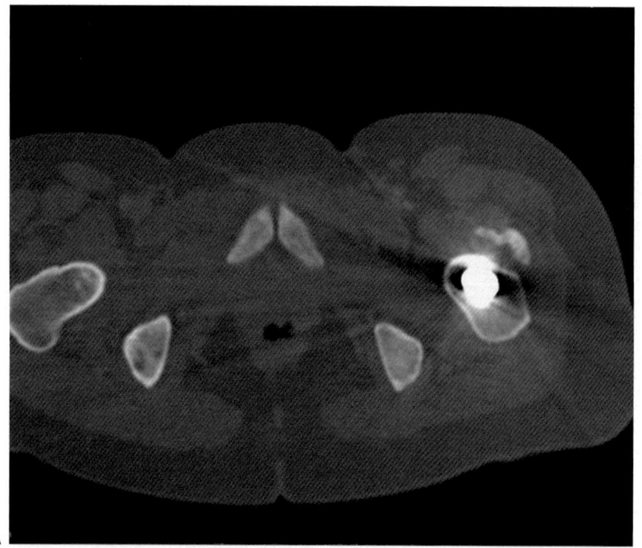

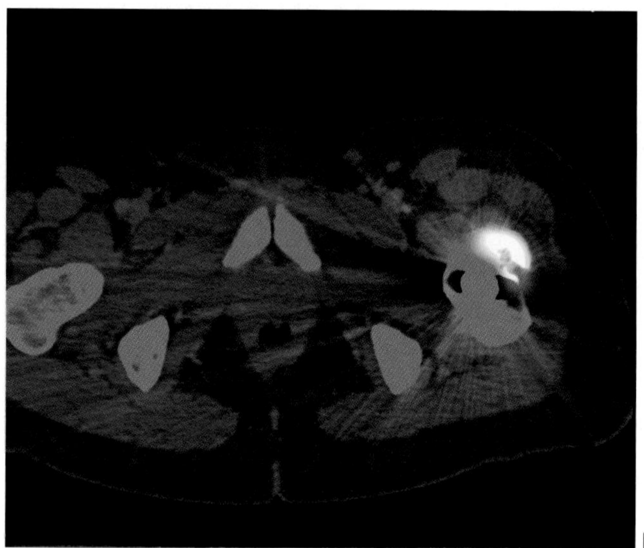

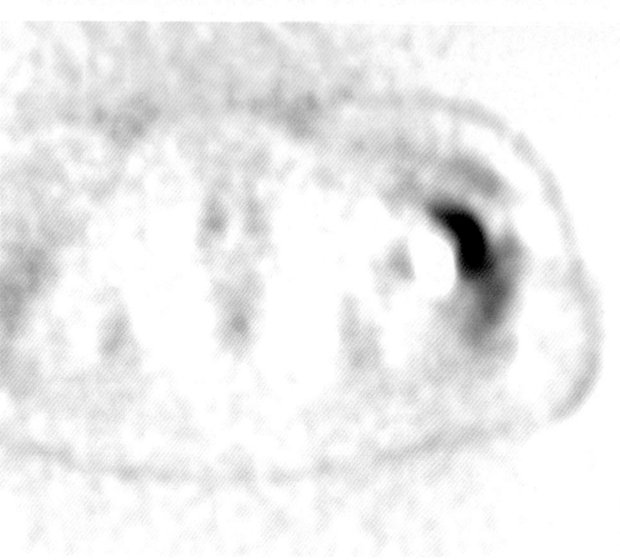

FIGURE 8.3.33. Fluorodeoxyglucose (FDG) activity in myositis ossificans. Transaxial CT (**A**) and PET/CT fusion (**B**) images show intense FDG tracer activity corresponding to myositis ossificans adjacent to the hip, 3 months postrepair of pathologic hip fracture. Nonattenuation-corrected transaxial FDG PET image (**C**) demonstrates the FDG tracer activity is not due to attenuation artifact from the hip prosthesis metallic components. Benign osseous-related pathologies can often be characterized based on the morphologic features seen on the corresponding CT images.

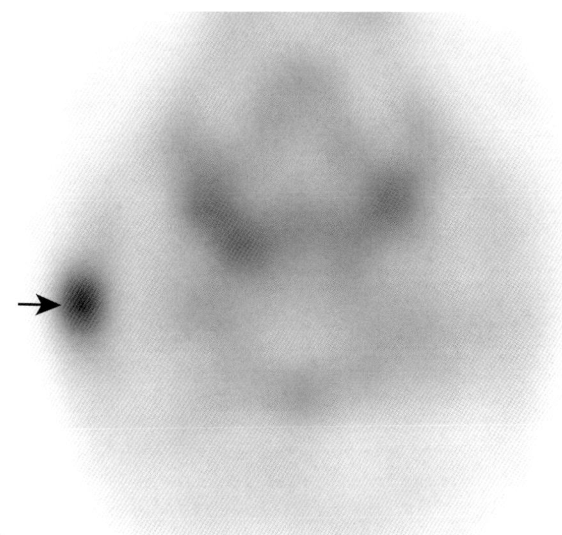

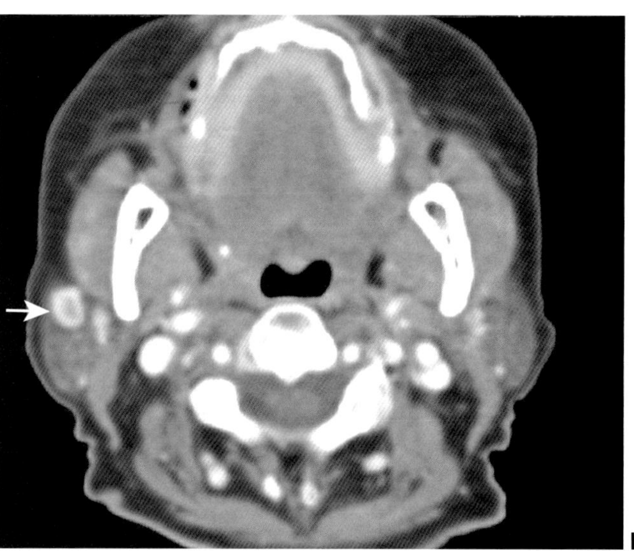

FIGURE 8.3.34. Warthin tumor. Transaxial attenuation-corrected fluorodeoxyglucose (FDG) PET (**A**) and CT images (**B**) reveal focal intense FDG tracer activity in the right anterior parotid gland (*arrow*), corresponding to a small enhancing focus of soft tissue (*arrow*). Benign salivary tumors such as Warthin's tumor and adenomas can be highly FDG avid and should not be mistaken for a primary parotid malignant neoplasm, focus or lymphoma, or a metastatic deposit.

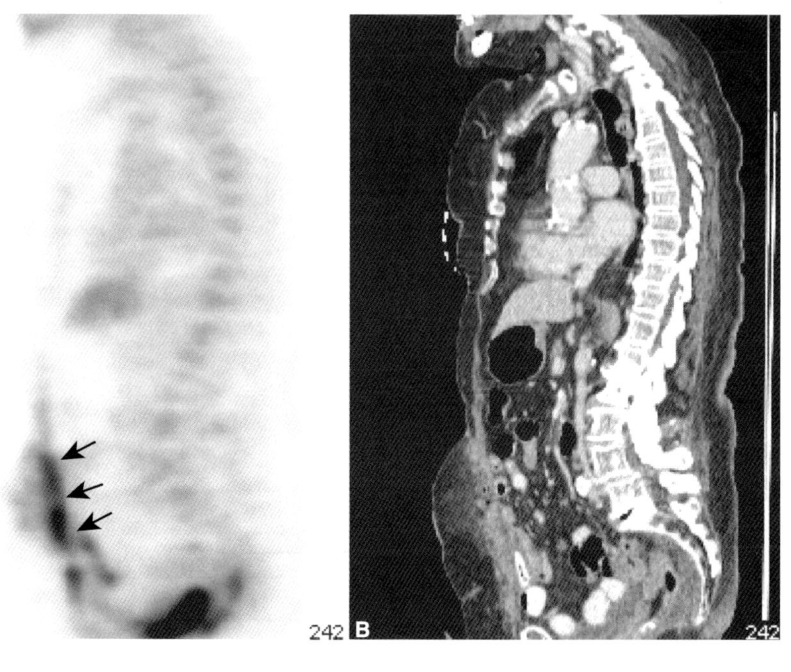

FIGURE 8.3.35. Normal fluorodeoxyglucose (FDG) activity in a healing incision wound. Sagittal attenuation-corrected FDG PET (**A**) and CT (**B**) images reveal linear FDG tracer activity (*arrow*), reflecting the normal inflammatory process in wound healing of a midline incision 3 weeks after surgery. Focal areas of relatively intense FDG tracer activity can reflect abscess formation or even seeded tumor deposits and need to be carefully correlated with the CT depicted morphologic features to provide a complete interpretation.

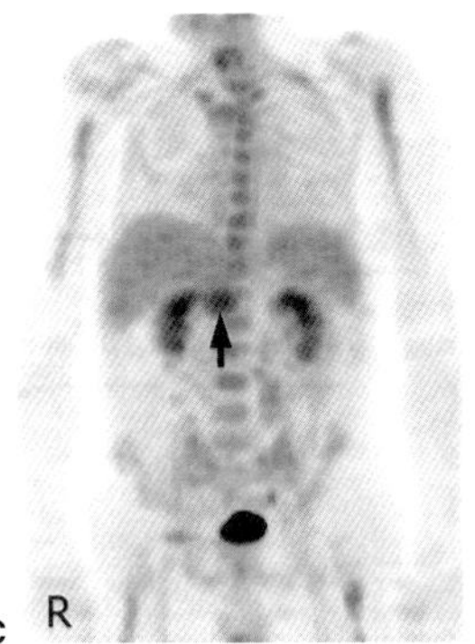

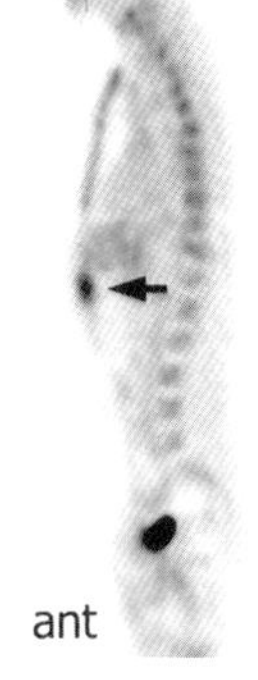

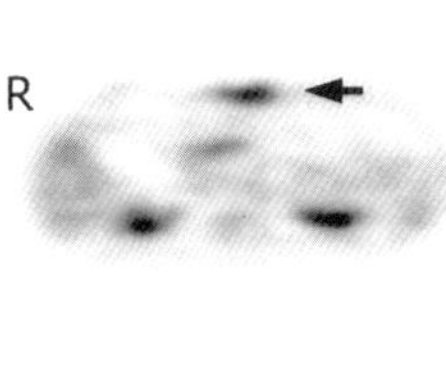

FIGURE 8.3.36. Percutaneous tube insertion. Anterior attenuation-corrected maximum intensity projection image (**A**) and attenuation-corrected sagittal (**B**) transaxial images (**C**) show focal fluorodeoxyglucose tracer activity (*arrow*) at the uncomplicated insertion site of an indwelling percutaneous gastric feeding tube.

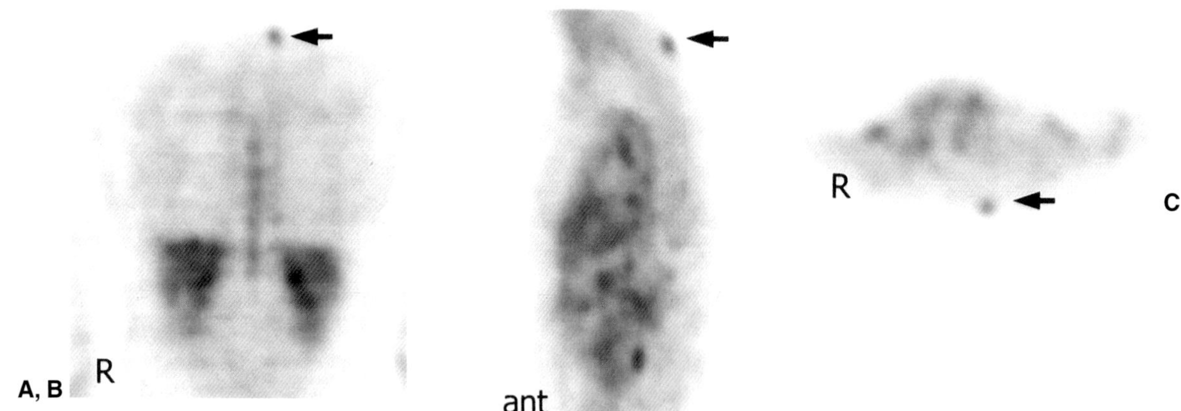

FIGURE 8.3.37. Cutaneous carbuncle. Coronal (**A**), sagittal (**B**), and transaxial (**C**) attenuation-corrected fluorodeoxyglucose (FDG) PET images demonstrate focal increased FDG tracer activity in a carbuncle at the upper back (*arrow*).

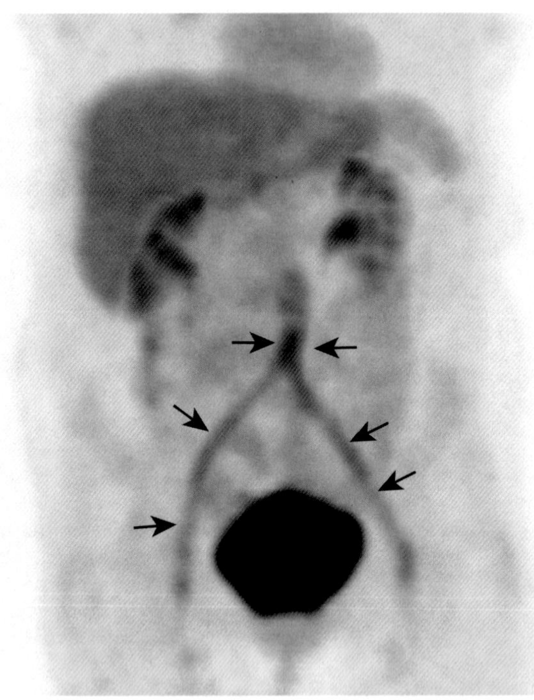

FIGURE 8.3.38. Normal fluorodeoxyglucose (FDG) activity in an aortoiliac graft. Anterior attenuation-corrected maximum intensity projection image shows diffuse increased FDG tracer activity in an aortoiliac graft (*arrows*). Such activity does not imply the graft is infected or recently placed.

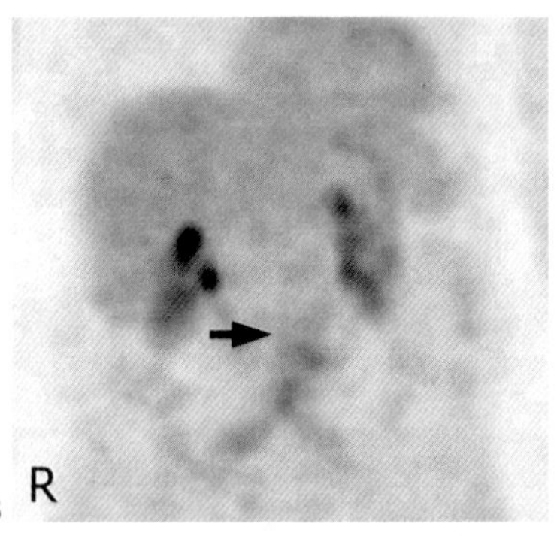

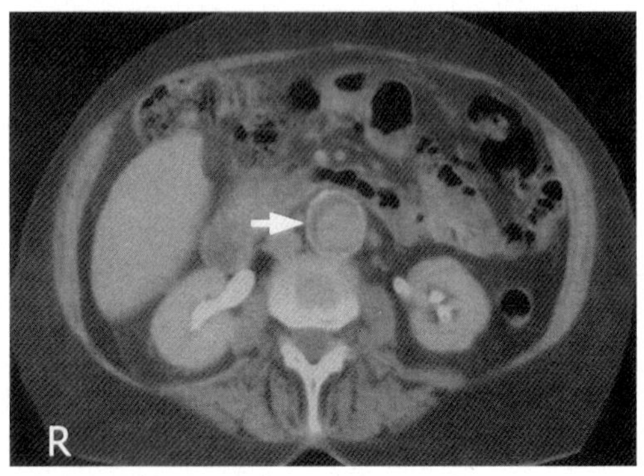

FIGURE 8.3.39. Atherosclerosis. Anterior attenuation-corrected FDG PET maximum intensity projection image (**A**) shows modest but definitely increased fluorodeoxyglucose (FDG) tracer activity in the aorta (*arrow*), reflecting the increased tracer activity in the partially calcified atheromatous plaque (*arrow*) seen on the transaxial CT image (**B**).

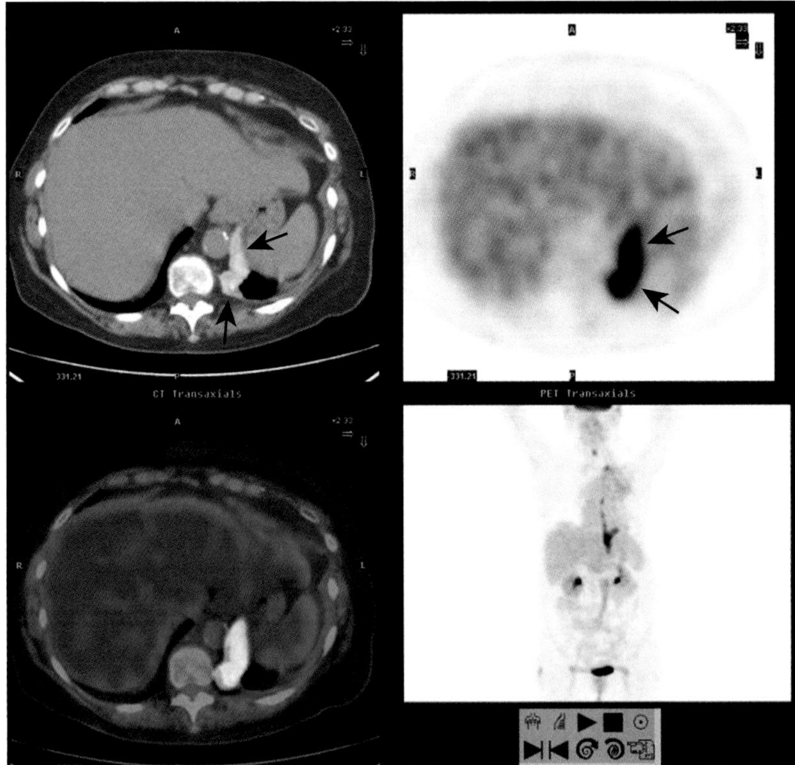

FIGURE 8.3.40. Pleurodesis. Intense fluorodeoxyglucose tracer uptake at the pleural space is seen (*arrows*) projection image corresponding to areas of pleurodesis (*arrows*) performed 8 years prior.

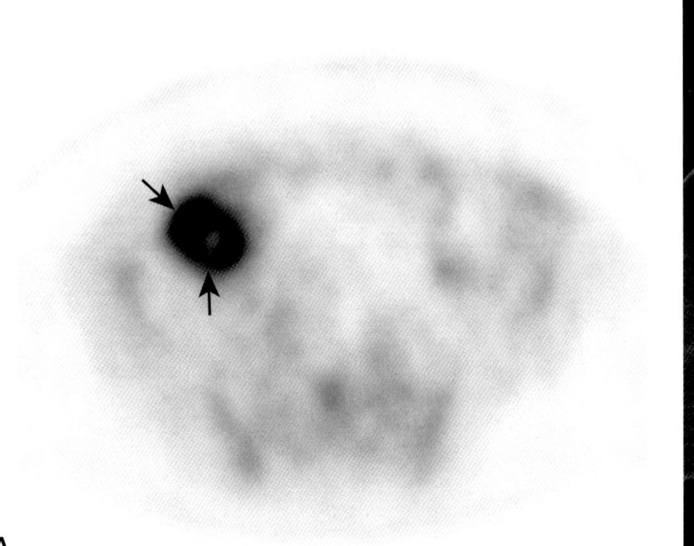

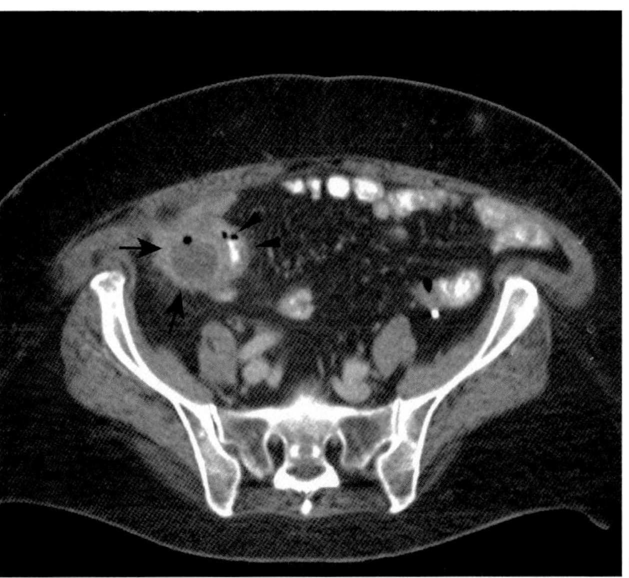

FIGURE 8.3.41. Abscess. Transaxial attenuation-corrected fluorodeoxyglucose PET (**A**) and CT images (**B**) reveal a ring of intense tracer activity (*arrows*) corresponding to a thick walled mass (*arrows*) containing complex fluid with a small air bubble, adjacent to and effacing the cecum (*arrowheads*), reflecting a postoperative abscess.

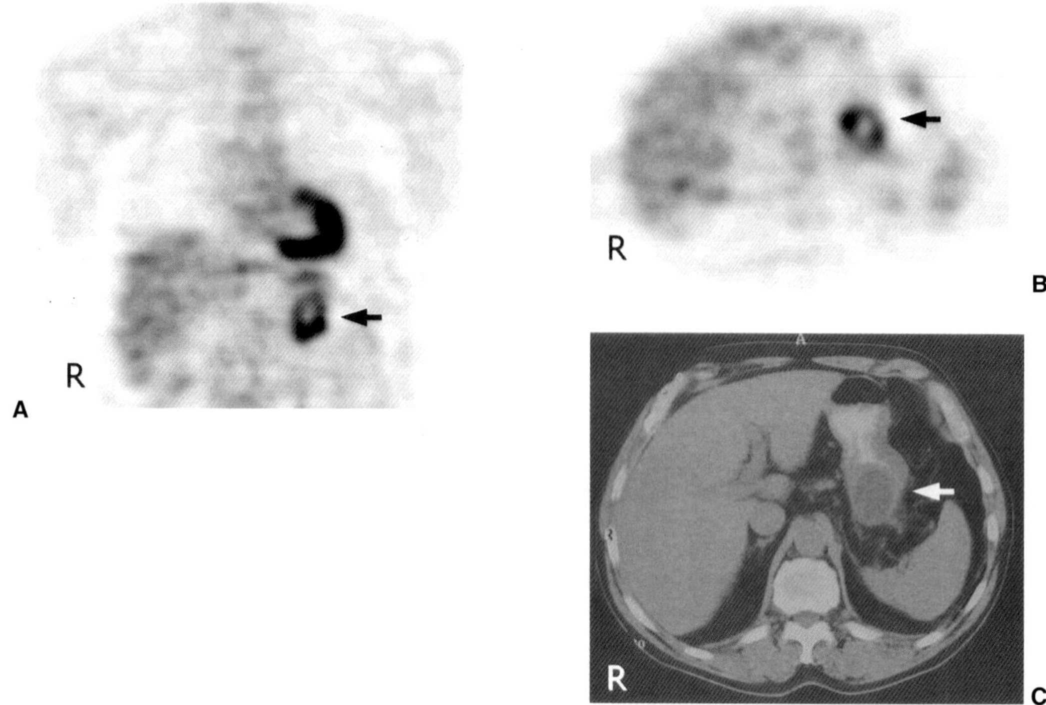

FIGURE 8.3.42. Pancreatitis with pseudocyst formation. Coronal (**A**) and transaxial (**B**) attenuation-corrected fluorodeoxyglucose (FDG) PET and CT (**C**) images show intense FDG tracer activity in phlegmonous changes originating in the tail of the pancreas that had extended to the gastric wall (*arrow*) months after clinical symptoms of pancreatitis had resolved.

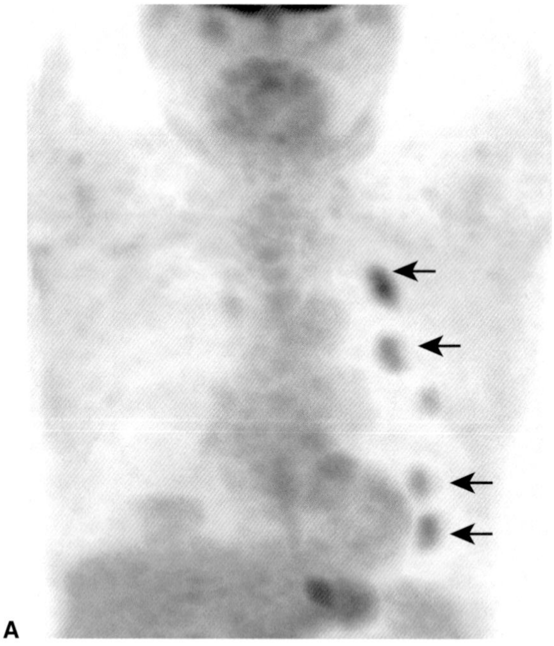

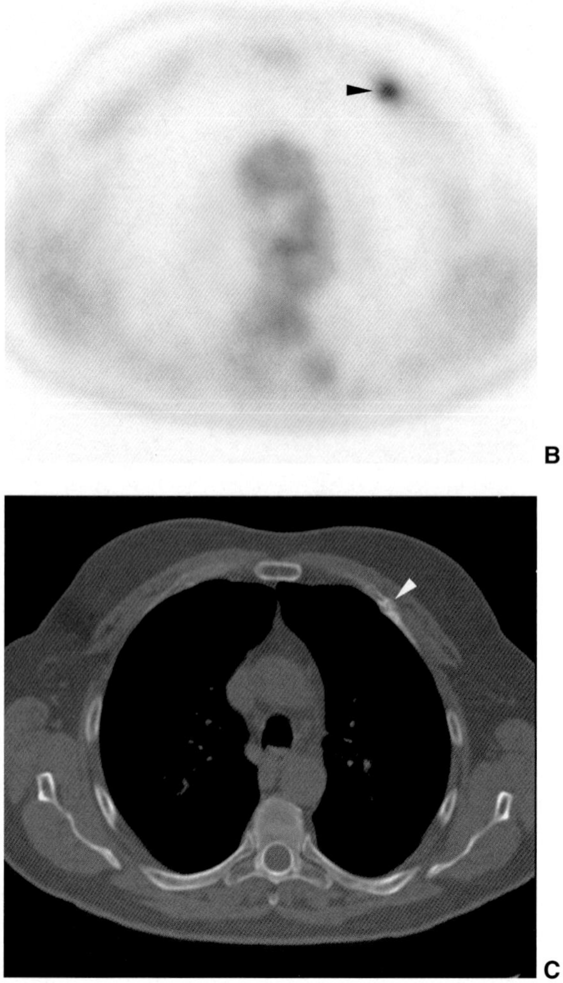

FIGURE 8.3.43. Healing rib fractures. Anterior attenuation-corrected maximum intensity projection image (**A**) demonstrates foci of increased tracer activity in ribs (*arrows*) of this patient who fell 6 weeks prior. Transaxial attenuation-corrected fluorodeoxyglucose PET (**B**) and CT (**C**) images reveal the focal tracer activity is associated with callus formation of a healing fracture (*arrowhead*).

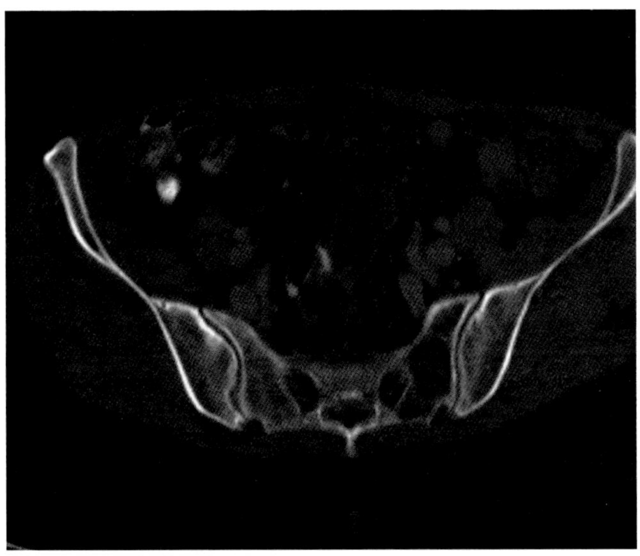

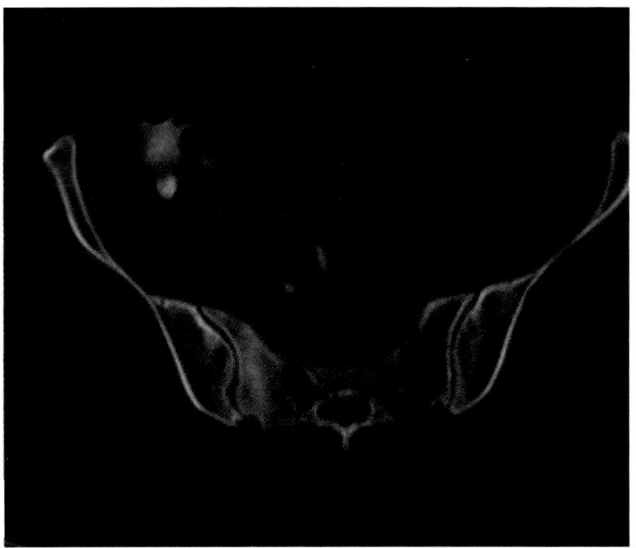

FIGURE 8.3.44. Sacral insufficiency fracture. Transaxial CT (**A**) and PET/CT fusion (**B**) images demonstrate focal fluorodeoxyglucose tracer uptake at the right sacral ala, reflecting an insufficiency fracture, where only subtle sclerosis is seen on the CT image.

Sternoclavicular joints, and to a lesser extent the acromioclavicular joints, which frequently demonstrate elevated tracer uptake on bone scans, far less frequently are seen on FDG scans. Anterior rib ends likewise occasionally demonstrate focal FDG uptake. Costovertebral joints rarely show modest uptake, although this may be difficult to distinguish from paravertebral brown fat or musculature.

Sequela of radiation therapy is associated with FDG uptake (40), usually equivalent to slightly greater than blood pool activity, even months after therapy (Fig. 8.3.45). Radiation pneumonitis can, however, be intense (Fig. 8.3.46) and difficult to differentiate from active infection or neoplasm and is directly related to delivered dose (41).

Although FDG PET is more specific than anatomic criteria in determining the presence or absence of malignancy, the specificity is limited by FDG uptake in lymph nodes secondary to inflammatory changes. Active granulomatous disease, such as tuberculosis and sarcoidosis, frequently cause high FDG uptake (42,43), well into the range of FDG uptake observed with FDG-avid malignancy such as lung cancer (Fig. 8.3.47). Similarly, chronic inflammation

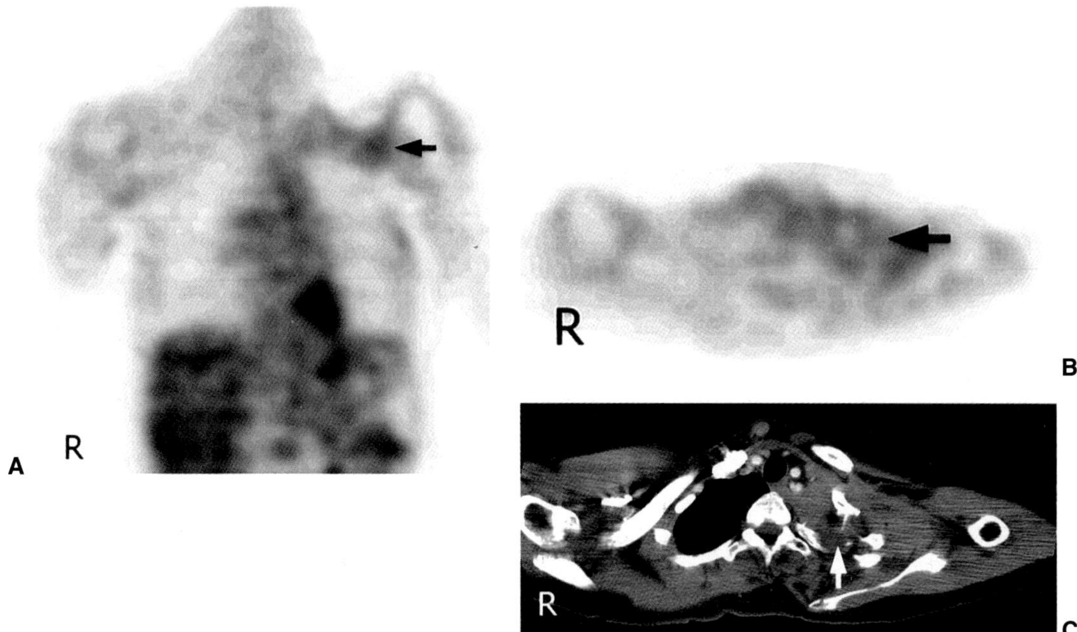

FIGURE 8.3.45. Radiation therapy sequela. Anterior attenuation-corrected maximum intensity projection image (**A**) and transaxial attenuation-corrected fluorodeoxyglucose (FDG) PET (**B**) and CT (**C**) images show modest FDG tracer uptake in the left apical pulmonary parenchymal scarring from radiation therapy completed 2 years prior (*arrows*).

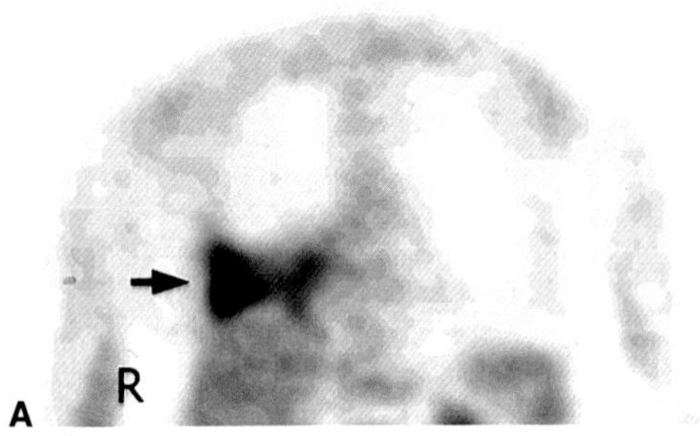

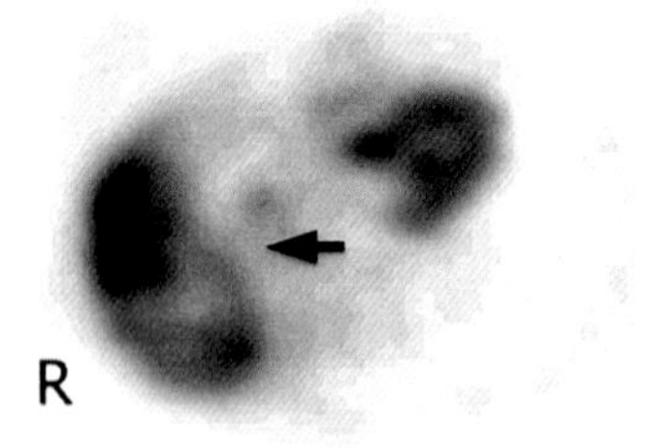

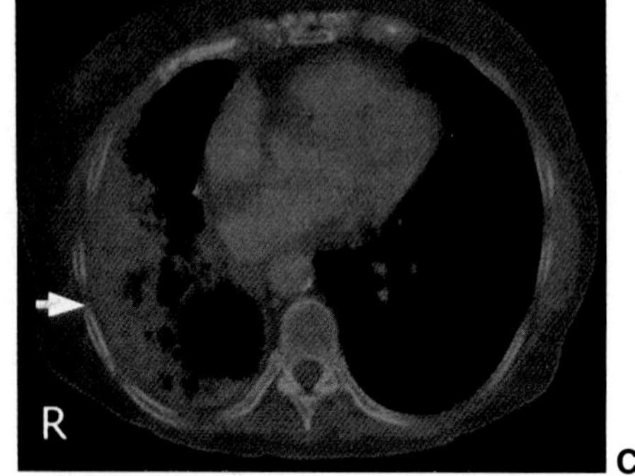

FIGURE 8.3.46. Radiation pneumonitis. Anterior attenuation-corrected FDG PET maximum intensity projection image (**A**) and transaxial attenuation-corrected fluorodeoxyglucose (FDG) PET (**B**) and CT (**C**) images demonstrate intense FDG tracer activity in the lung parenchyma air space opacity (*arrow*), reflecting radiation therapy-induced pneumonitis from radiation therapy completed 8 weeks prior.

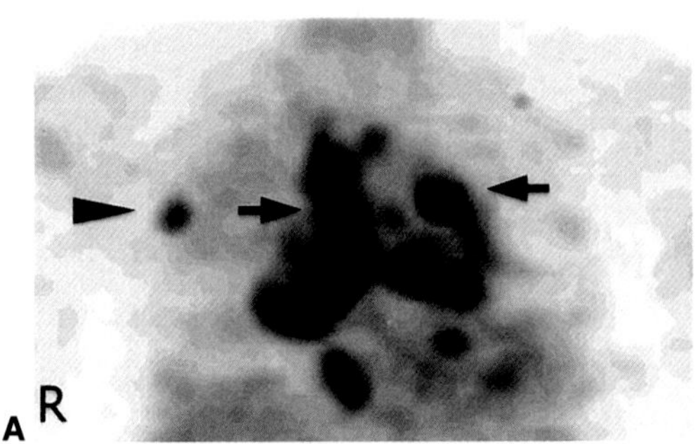

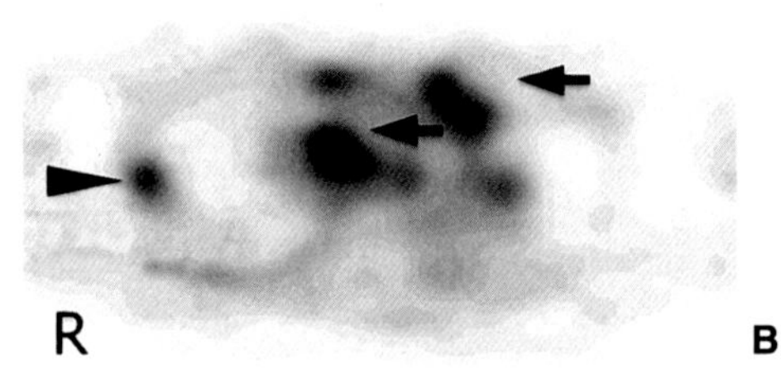

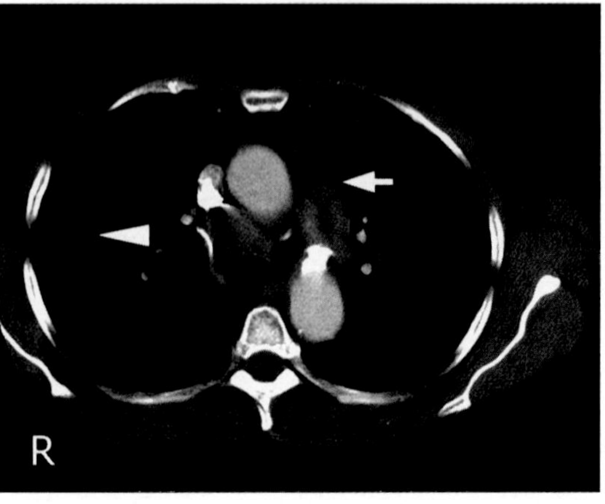

FIGURE 8.3.47. Sarcoidosis. Anterior attenuation-corrected FDG PET maximum intensity projection image (**A**) and transaxial attenuation-corrected fluorodeoxyglucose (FDG) PET (**B**) and CT (**C**) images show intense FDG tracer activity in enlarged mediastinal and hilar lymph nodes (*arrows*) in an asymptomatic patient. The lymph nodes were found to contain granulomatous change on mediastinoscopy biopsy. The subpleural pulmonary nodule (*arrowhead*) was a primary non-small cell carcinoma.

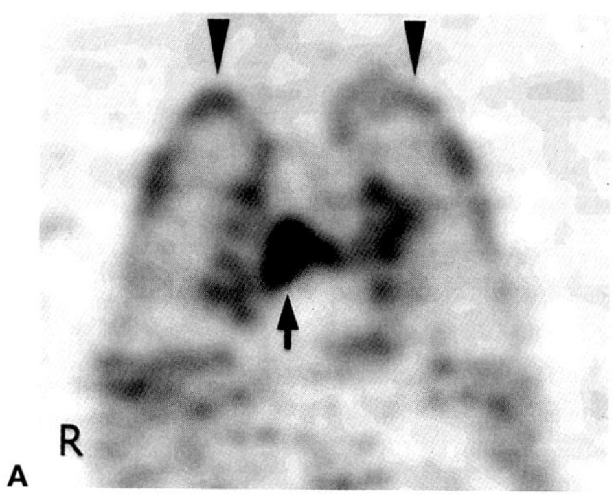

A

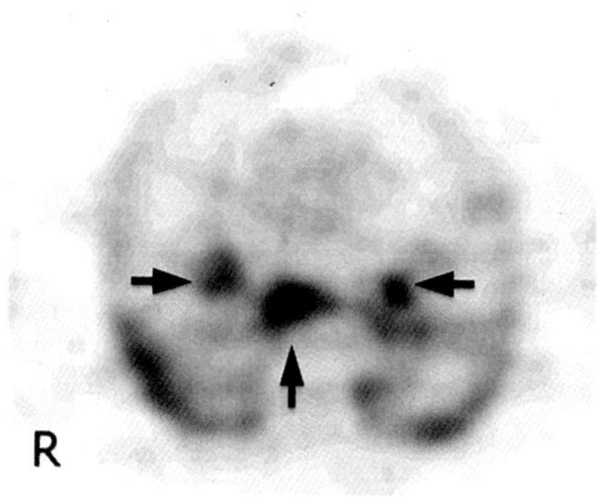

B

C

FIGURE 8.3.48. Occupational lung disease. Anterior attenuation-corrected FDG PET maximum intensity projection image (**A**) and transaxial attenuation-corrected fluorodeoxyglucose (FDG) PET (**B**) and CT (**C**) images reveal moderate FDG tracer activity along the periphery of the lung parenchyma (*arrowheads*) and intense FDG tracer activity in the subcarinal and hilar lymphadenopathy (*arrows*) in a retired quarry worker with known occupational lung disease.

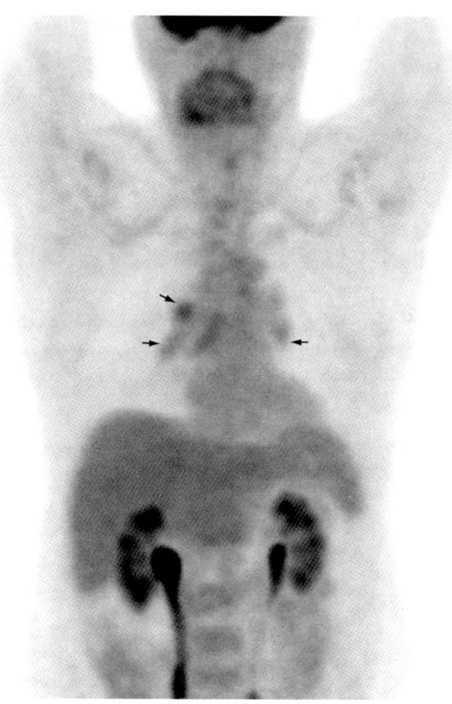

FIGURE 8.3.49. Modest increased fluorodeoxyglucose (FDG) activity in mediastinal and hilar lymph nodes. Attenuation-corrected anterior maximum intensity projection image shows FDG tracer activity in mediastinal and hilar lymph nodes (*arrows*), which is modest, but clearly greater than mediastinal background activity. Such activity distributed symmetrically is commonly seen and reflects low-level benign inflammatory response in the lymph nodes.

associated with occupational lung disease is associated with FDG-avid mediastinal lymph nodes in additional to lung and pleural-based inflammation–associated FDG uptake (Fig. 8.3.48). The generalized inflammatory response of regional lymph nodes to infection or recent instrumentation is a common source of elevated FDG uptake in noncancerous lymph nodes, hence FDG-avid lymph nodes near sites of known infection or recent instrumentation must be interpreted with caution (36). Low-level FDG tracer activity in mediastinal and hilar lymph nodes in a relatively symmetrical pattern is common, reflecting low-level benign inflammatory reaction (Fig. 8.3.49). Inflammatory response of lymph nodes in the chest and neck can be intense, even with no identifiable regional cause, and the level and distribution of abnormal lymph nodes can be entirely indistinguishable from malignancy (Fig. 8.3.50). The immunologic challenge to lymph nodes subserving the aeroepithelium accounts for the generalized false-positive rate of up to 15% for lymph nodes in the neck and mediastinum (44,45). For somewhat similar reasons, false-positive lymph nodes occur, although less frequently, in the axilla and inguinal nodal basins. Although not common, persistent inflammation associated with prior surgery can yield intense abnormal FDG uptake.

ARTIFACTS DUE TO IMAGE RECONSTRUCTION

Due to the current rapid development of PET technology and image reconstruction algorithms, the interpretive pitfalls associated with image reconstruction will vary among equipment and image acquisition and reconstruction protocols. Because present statistical image reconstruction algorithms can yield focal apparent

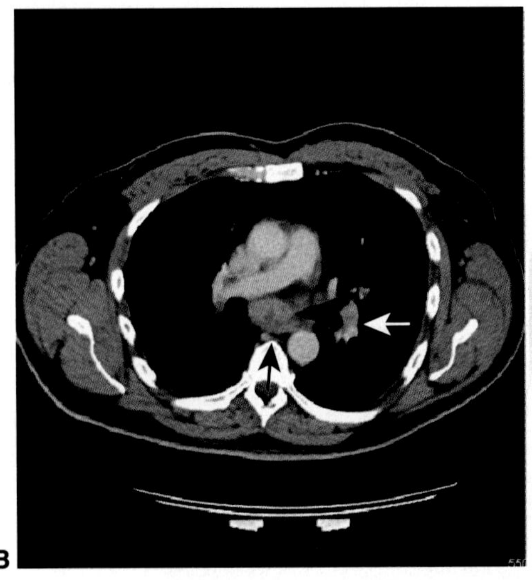

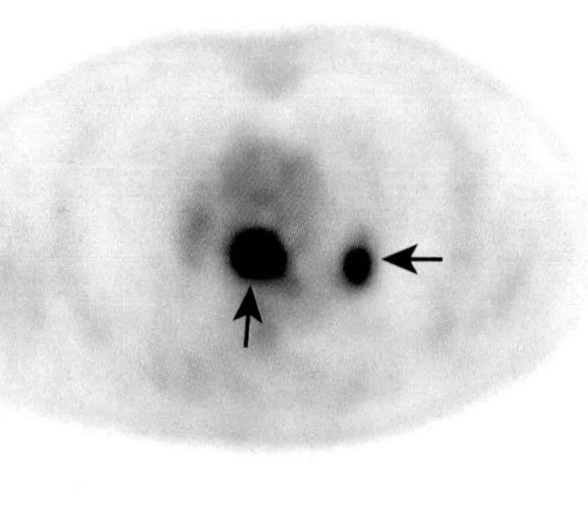

A, B

FIGURE 8.3.50. Intense fluorodeoxyglucose (FDG) activity in lymph nodes due to inflammatory response. Transaxial CT (**A**) and attenuation-corrected transaxial FDG PET (**B**) demonstrate intense FDG tracer activity in an enlarged subcarinal and a left hilar lymph node (*arrows*). Caseating granulomatous changes were found on biopsy.

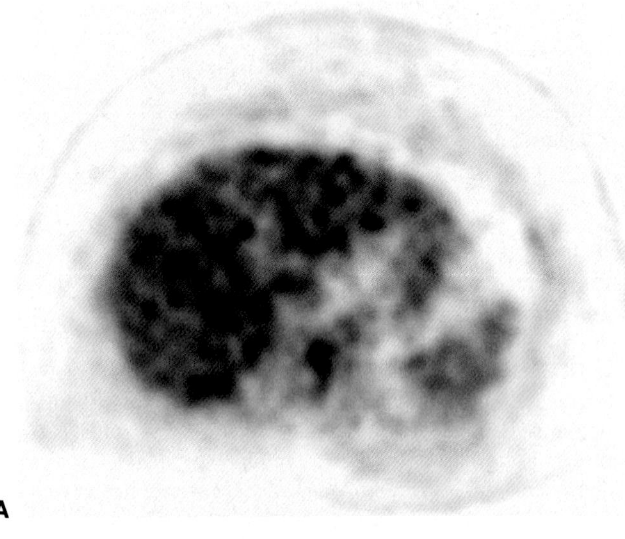

A

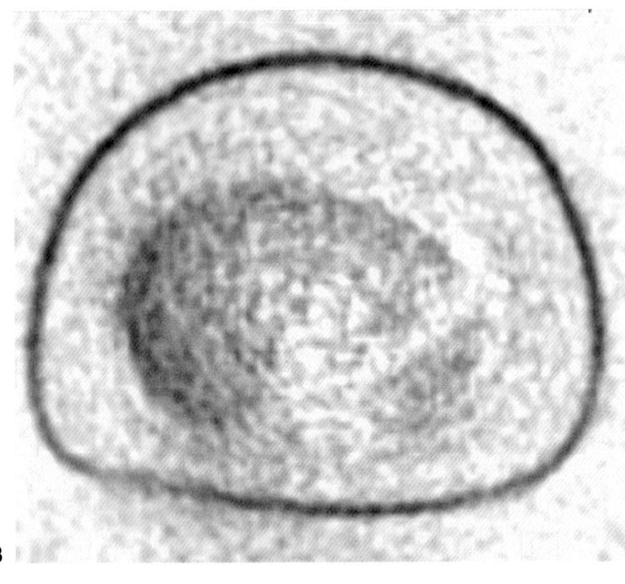

B

FIGURE 8.3.51. Spurious focal fluorodeoxyglucose (FDG) tracer activity due to statistical image reconstruction methods. Transaxial attenuation-corrected image generated using OSEM (ordered-subsets expectation maximization) reconstruction method with three iterations and eight subsets (**A**) shows multiple tiny apparent foci of increased FDG activity in the liver of a large patient. The nonattenuation-corrected filtered back projection reconstructed image (**B**) reveals uniform distribution of tracer throughout the liver, allowing for radial attenuation error. Statistical reconstruction methods depict image noise as foci, rather than lines of projection.

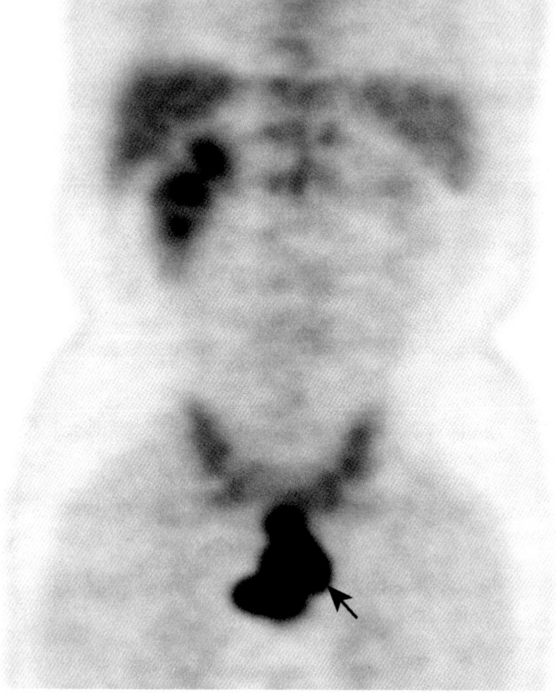

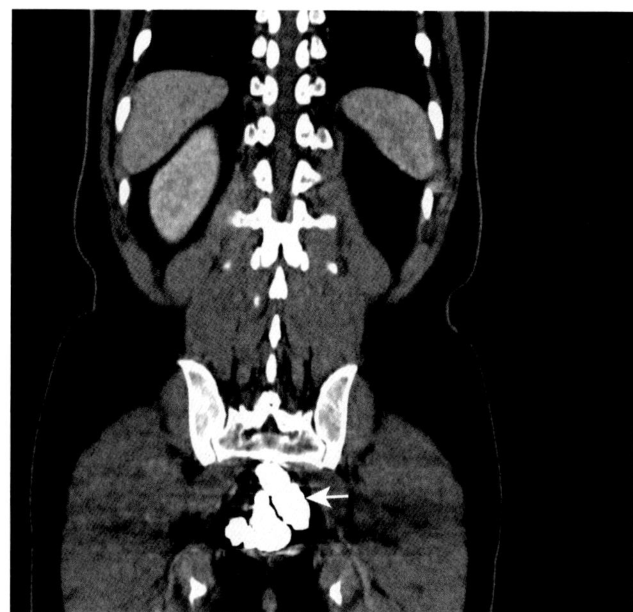

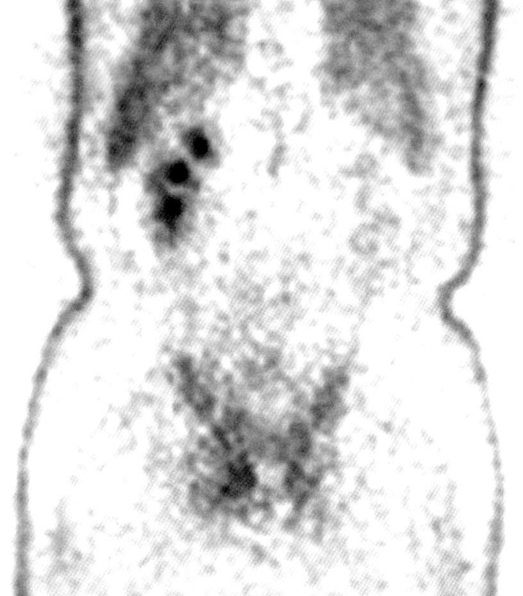

FIGURE 8.3.52. Attenuation artifact on PET/CT. Attenuation-corrected coronal fluorodeoxyglucose (FDG) PET (**A**) shows intense apparent abnormal FDG tracer activity in the sigmoid colon (*arrow*), while the registered and aligned coronal CT image (**B**) reveals dense concentrated barium contrast (*white arrow*), causing some beam-hardening artifact from an upper gastrointestinal radiographic study performed a few days prior. The nonattenuation-corrected coronal FDG PET image (**C**) reconstruction reveals no abnormal tracer activity present in the sigmoid colon. When the CT images are used for the attenuation correction, as is routine in PET/CT imaging, very dense structures can yield artifactually increased apparent tracer activity.

increased activity from movement artifacts or generalized noise, it is advisable to have nonattenuation-corrected filtered back projection images for confirmation of such suspect abnormalities (Fig. 8.3.51). When the CT images are used to perform attenuation correction of the PET projection data, dense objects such as metallic implants and high-density barium alimentary contrast material can cause apparent "hot spot" artifacts on the PET images (Fig. 8.3.52), as well as beam hardening artifact on the CT images. Again the artifactual nature of such findings can be confirmed by review of the nonattenuation-corrected filtered back projection PET images.

REFERENCES

1. Schelbert HL. Myocardial metabolism. Assessment of blood flow and substrate metabolism in the myocardium of the normal human heart. In: Schwaiger M, ed. *Cardiac positron emission tomography*. Norwell: Kluwer, 1996:207–216.
2. Jabour BA, Choi Y, Hoh CK, et al. Extracranial head and neck: PET imaging with 2-[F-18]fluoro-2-deoxy-D-glucose and MR imaging correlation. *Radiology* 1993;186:27–35.
3. Pappas GP, Olcott EW, Drace JE. Imaging skeletal muscle function using (18)FDG PET: force production, activation, and metabolism. *J Am Phys* 2001;90:329–337.

4. Kelley DE, Williams KV, Price JC. Insulin regulation of glucose transport and phosphorylation in skeletal muscle assessed by PET. *Am J Phys* 1999;277:3610–3369.
5. Chander S, Ergun EL, Zak IT, et al. Diaphragmatic and crural FDG uptake in hyperventilating patients: a rare pattern important to recognize. *Clin Nucl Med* 2004;29:296–299.
6. Shreve PD, Anzai Y, Wahl RL. Pitfalls in oncologic diagnosis with FDG PET imaging: physiologic and benign variants. *RadioGraphics* 1999;19: 61–77.
7. Kostakoglu L, Wong JCH, Barrington SF, et al. Speech-related visualization of laryngeal muscles with fluorine-18-FDG. *J Nucl Med* 1996;37: 1771–1773.
8. Yeung HWD, Grewal RK, Gonen M, et al. Patterns of ^{18}F-FDG uptake in adipose tissue and muscle: a potential source of false-positives for PET. *J Nucl Med* 2003;44:1789–1796.
9. Garcia CA, Van Nostrand D, Atkins F, et al. Reduction of brown fat 2-deoxy-2-[F-18]fluoro-D-glucose uptake by controlling environmental temperature prior to positron emission tomography scan. *Mol Imaging Biol* 2006;8:24–29.
10. Christensen CR, Clark PB, Morton KA. Reversal of hypermetabolic brown adipose tissue in F-18 FDG PET imaging. *Clin Nucl Med* 2006;31:193–196.
11. Gelfand MJ, O'Hara SM, Curtwright LA, et al. Pre-medication to block [(^{18})F]FDG uptake in the brown adipose tissue of pediatric and adolescent patients. *Pediatr Radiol* 2005;35:984–990.
12. Tatsumi M, Engles JM, Ishimori T, et al. Intense (^{18})F-FDG uptake in brown fat can be reduced pharmacologically. *J Nucl Med* 2004;45: 1189–1193.
13. Tatldil R, Jadvar H, Bading JR, et al. Incidental colonic fluorodeoxyglucose uptake: correlation with colonoscopic and histopathologic findings. *Radiology* 2002;224:783–787.
14. Israel O, Yefremov N, Bar-Shalom R, et al. PET/CT detection of unexpected gastrointestinal foci of ^{18}F-FDG uptake: incidence, localization patterns, and clinical significance. *J Nucl Med* 2005;46:758–762.
15. Meisner RS, Spier BJ, Einarsson S, et al. Pilot study using PET/CT as a novel, noninvasive assessment of disease activity in inflammatory bowel disease. *Inflamm Bowel Dis* 2007;13:993–1000.
16. Stahl A, Weber W, Avril N, et al. The effect of N-butylscopolamine on intestinal uptake of F-18 fluorodeoxyglucose in PET imaging of the abdomen. *Eur J Nucl Med* 1999;26:1017.
17. Miraldi F, Vesselle H, Faulhaber PF, et al. Elimination of artifactual accumulation of FDG in PET imaging of colorectal cancer. *Clin Nucl Med* 1998;23:3–7.
18. Vesselle HJ, Miraldi FD. FDG PET of the retroperitoneum: normal anatomy, variants, pathologic conditions, and strategies to avoid diagnostic pitfalls. *RadioGraphics* 1998;18:805–823.
19. Lerman H, Metser U, Grisaru D, et al. Normal and abnormal ^{18}F-FDG endometrial and ovarian uptake in pre- and postmenopausal patients: assessment by PET/CT. *J Nucl Med* 2004;45:266–271.
20. Kosuda S, Fisher S, Kison PV, et al. Uptake of 2-deoxy-2[18F]fluoro-D-glucose in the normal testis: retrospective PET study and animal experiment. *Ann Nucl Med* 1997;11:195–199.
21. Karantanis D, Bogsrud TV, Wiseman GA, et al. Clinical significance of diffusely increased ^{18}F-FDG uptake in the thyroid gland. *J Nucl Med* 2007;48:896–901.
22. Meller J, Sahlmann CO, Scheel AK. ^{18}F-FDG PET and PET/CT in fever of unknown origin. *J Nucl Med* 2007;48:35–45.
23. Kang KW, Kim SK, Kang HS, et al. Prevalence and risk of cancer of focal thyroid incidentaloma identified by ^{18}F-fluorodeoxyglucose positron emission tomography for metastasis evaluation and cancer screening in healthy subjects. *J Clin Endocrinol Metab* 2003;88:4100–4104.
24. Choi JY, Lee KS, Kim HJ, et al. Focal thyroid lesions incidentally identified by integrated ^{18}F-FDG PET/CT: clinical significance and improved characterization. *J Nucl Med* 2006;47:609–615.
25. Sugawara Y, Fisher SJ, Zasadny KR, et al. Pre-clinical and clinical studies of bone marrow uptake of fluorine-18-fluorodeoxy-glucose with or without granulocyte colony-stimulating factor during chemotherapy. *J Clin Oncol* 1998;16:173–180.
26. Blake MA, Slattery JM, Karla MK, et al. Adrenal lesions: characteristics with fused PET/CT image in patients with proved or suspected malignancy-initial experience. *Radiology* 2006;238:970–977.
27. Aoki J, Watanabe H, Shlnozaki T, et al. FDG PET of primary benign and malignant bone tumors: standardized uptake value in 52 lesions. *Radiology* 2001;219:774–777.
28. Koo CW, Bhargava P, Rajagopalan V, et al. Incidental detection of clinically occult pituitary adenoma on whole-body FDG PET imaging. *Clin Nucl Med* 2006;31:42–43.
29. Uchida Y, Minoshima S, Kawata T, et al. Diagnostic value of FDG PET and salivary gland scintigraphy for parotid tumors. *Clin Nucl Med* 2005;30:170–176.
30. Wittram C, Scott JA. ^{18}F-FDG PET of pulmonary embolism. *AJR Am J Roentgenol* 2007;189:171–176.
31. Fukuchi K, Ishida Y, Higashi M, et al. Detection of aortic graft infection by fluorodeoxyglucose positron emission tomography: comparison with computed tomographic findings. *J Vasc Surg* 2005;42:919–925.
32. Yun M, Yeh D, Araujo LI, et al. F-18 FDG uptake in the large arteries: a new observation. *Clin Nucl Med* 2001;26:314–319.
33. Webb M, Al-Nahhas A. Molecular imaging of Takayasu's arteritis and other large-vessel vasculitis with ^{18}F-FDG PET. *Nucl Med Commun* 2006;27:547–549.
34. Kwek BH, Aquino SL, Fischman AJ. Fluorodeoxyglucose positron emission tomography and CT after talc pleurodesis. *Chest* 2004;125:2356–2360.
35. Stumpe KDM, Dazzi H, Schaffner A, et al. Infection imaging using whole-body FDG-PET. *Eur J Nucl Med* 2000;27:822–832.
36. Love C, Tomas MB, Tronco GG, et al. FDG PET of infection and inflammation. *Radiographics* 2005;25:1357–1368.
37. Shreve PD. Focal fluorine-18 fluorodeoxyglucose accumulation in inflammatory pancreatic disease. *Eur J Nucl Med* 1998;25:259–264.
38. Zhuang H, Sam JW, Chacko TK, et. al. Rapid normalization of osseous FDG uptake following traumatic or surgical fractures. *Eur J Nucl Med Mol Imaging* 2003;30:1096–1103.
39. Fayad LM, Cohade C, Wahl RL, et al. Sacral fractures: a potential pitfall of FDG positron emission tomography. *AJR Am J Roentgenol* 2003;181: 1239–1243.
40. Lowe VJ, Hebert ME, Anscher MS, et al. Serial evaluation of increased chest wall F-18 fluorodeoxyglucose (FDG) uptake following radiation therapy in patients with bronchogenic carcinoma. *Clin Positron Imaging* 1998;1:185–191.
41. Guerrero T, Johnson V, Hart J, et al. Radiation pneumonitis: local dose versus [(^{18})F]-fluorodeoxyglucose uptake response in irradiated lung. *Int J Radiat Oncol Biol Phys* 2007;68:1030–1035.
42. Goo JM, Im JG, Do KH, et al. Pulmonary tuberculoma evaluated by means of FDG PET: findings in 10 cases. *Radiology* 2000;216:117–121.
43. Yamada Y, Uchida Y, Tatsumi K, et al. Fluorine-18-fluorodeoxyglucose and carbon-11 methionine evaluation of lymphadenopathy in sarcoidosis. *J Nucl Med* 1998;39:1160–1166.
44. Stuckensen T, Kovacs AF, Adams S, et al. Staging of the neck in patient with oral cavity squamous cell carcinomas: a prospective comparison of PET, ultrasound, CT and MRI. *J Craniomaxillofac Surg* 2000;28:319–324.
45. Gupta NC, Tamim WJ, Graeber GG, et al. Mediastinal lymph node sampling following positron emission tomography with fluorodeoxyglucose imaging in lung cancer staging. *Chest* 2001;120:521–527.

CHAPTER

8.4 Monitoring Response to Treatment

ANTHONY F. SHIELDS

Clinical imaging of many types, including x-ray, nuclear, and ultrasound techniques, is widely used to detect and stage cancer. After detection and staging are accomplished, the appropriate therapy must be chosen, and this may include a combination of surgery, radiation, chemotherapy, and biologic therapies. To evaluate the success of such treatment often requires additional imaging studies. As therapy continues to improve and more options are available for patients with cancer, the field of monitoring cancer therapy has burgeoned. For many years, the standard approach has relied on various anatomic imaging techniques to determine if the tumor has recurred, shrunk, or grown. Although cross-sectional imaging with computed tomography (CT) and magnetic resonance imaging (MRI) have become standard in evaluating treatment response, they have a number of limitations. They only evaluate the size of the lesion, not its viability, proliferative rate, or physiologic state.

The major issues that affect the sensitivity and specificity of detecting response by measuring size include delays in shrinking of dying tumors, slow growth of tumors despite unsuccessful treatment, and the persistence of fibrotic or necrotic tumors. Furthermore, new forms of therapy have methods of action that may be more cytostatic than cytocidal. Such treatments are less likely to result in rapid tumor shrinkage, making anatomic response assessment particularly challenging. Positron emission tomography (PET), with its images of many types of physiology, offers a new approach to assess tumor response. Although work in this field is still early in its exploration, studies are already demonstrating that it is becoming the new standard for some tumors and treatments. The optimal imaging approach will depend on the tumor types and treatment and when an answer regarding the success of therapy is needed.

The measurement of the results of treatment is becoming more important as more successful treatment options become available. For example, up until the past few years, it was argued that chemotherapy had little role in the treatment of unresectable non–small cell lung cancer. It has now become accepted that treatment of metastatic disease can prolong survival. Thus, determining if this treatment is successful and whether it should continue has gained importance. Knowing when to discontinue therapy is also of great importance since treatments are toxic and very costly.

Recently, new second- and third-line therapies have been approved for some patients with advanced tumors resistant to first-line treatment. This means that determining that the primary treatment has failed is more critical. New therapies, such as inhibitors of growth factors and tumor vascularity, are being used. Such agents may by cytostatic and slow tumor growth without causing extensive shrinkage in anatomic images. Finally, as therapy becomes more successful, a more common phenomenon is the persistence of fibrotic lesions, which do not contain viable tumor. All of these issues make the development of PET imaging of tumor response an area of growing interest.

The timing of response is certainly a common issue in the assessment of response. The standard approach for patients receiving cytotoxic drugs is to have CT-MRI done every 2 months. The appearance of new lesions or significant growth of old lesions signals that the treatment has failed and that the patient should be offered alternative treatments or supportive care. Even when treatment is successful, it can take months to become evident. How much benefit are patients deriving from stable disease? Recent data, especially those including cytostatic agents, suggest that stable disease provides important benefits, but it is hard to differentiate those with slowly growing tumors where the treatment is not helping from those where the treatment has induced a decrease in the tumor growth rate.

TIMING OF PET IMAGING

A number of small studies have addressed the use of PET in the assessment of response and studied a variety of time lines after the start of therapy. Depending on the tumor type, the treatment, and the goal of the imaging study, one can choose to image as soon as therapy starts to very late after the completion of treatment (Table 8.4.1).

TABLE 8.4.1 Possible Times for Imaging after the Start of Therapy and Rationale

Time After Treatment	Imaging Rationale
IMMEDIATE	
Hours to days	Immediate effects on metabolism/proliferation Drug pathway interference Blood flow changes Receptor blockade
EARLY	
3 to 4 weeks During therapy Cycle one of chemotherapy	Metabolic response Proliferation changes
END	
2 to 6 months (completion of therapy)	Restage Assess residual lesions
LATE	
Months to years	Necrosis vs. recurrence Restage

In assessments done within hours to days after the start of treatment, one is often looking for *immediate* effects on the cellular pathways targeted by the therapy. For example, has an antiangiogenesis agent really interfered with blood flow, or has tamoxifen blocked estrogen retention in the breast tumor? At this point, such uses have generally been limited to gain a better understanding of the treatment as part of a research application. Those involved in new drug development have been particularly interested in this application (see Chapter 13).

In some cases, one is looking for immediate changes in proliferation or metabolism. This use blends into the next category—the *early* evaluation during the treatment—but after sufficient time to allow for a clear response of the tumor to treatment being. As previously discussed, anatomic imaging employed in this setting is often repeated 2 to 3 months after the start of treatment. Studies with PET early in the course of treatment are done to speed the assessment with the idea that those without any metabolic evidence of tumor response should stop the present therapy and consider alternate treatment (1). At this point, there are a limited number of studies that address this use. Furthermore, third-party payers do not consistently reimburse for this use at the present time, although the U.S. National Oncology PET Registry does support this use in the United States.

There have been a larger number of studies using PET at the *end* of a course of treatment or at later times to restage patients and to determine if residual masses represent persistent viable tumor or fibrosis. These uses have found widespread clinical applicability and are leading to the rapidly increasing use of PET in oncology. Recent U.S. government approval of payment for such uses in a number of tumor types is likely to spur this approach further.

Finally, PET is also used in the setting *late* after treatment to assess persistence or regrowth of the tumor compared to necrosis or fibrosis. The best examples are in the evaluation of patients after treatment for brain tumors, lymphoma, and lung cancer (see below).

TRACERS FOR MEASUREMENT OF RESPONSE

Fluorodeoxyglucose and Tumor Glycolysis

A wide variety of tracers have been tested in the measurement of tumor response. Fluorodeoxyglucose (FDG) has become the most widely used agent for use in oncology because of its easy synthesis, moderate half-life, and generally high tumor retention. As a result, it is very useful for the detection and staging of cancer, as well as determining if the tumor is responding to treatment. It has been commercially produced and centrally distributed, thus allowing for centers without cyclotrons to have ready access to the tracer. In many clinical PET centers it is the only tracer used in cancer, attesting to its profound importance in PET.

As with any tracer, FDG does have its limitations. The greatest limitation is that not all tumors readily retain FDG. In some cases this reflects the fact that tumors may have mucinous or cystic areas or a high degree of fibrosis or differentiation, all of which may have limited FDG retention. Although the rapid renal excretion of unmetabolized FDG is generally an advantage, the tracer accumulation in the bladder has limited its use in the lower pelvis. This has made assessment of prostate and bladder cancers more difficult. The introduction of iterative reconstruction techniques has helped in this regard by limiting streak artifacts that could obscure tumors.

Methionine and Protein Synthesis

The next most commonly reported tracer in the assessment of tumor response is carbon-11 ([^{11}C])-L-methionine. Its easy synthesis, a one-step process using methyl iodide, allows for the production of large quantities in PET centers with cyclotrons. It is readily retained in many tumors and provides high-contrast images in many sites. *In vitro* studies demonstrated that there are more rapid declines in protein synthesis than in glucose retention when treatment is successful (2). This has led to a number of promising clinical trials with this agent.

Limitations in the use of labeled methionine include the short half-life of [^{11}C] and the requirement of a cyclotron on site. Although it was originally intended to provide a relative measure of protein synthesis, it has become clear that its retention also reflects the transmethylation reaction and its early signal is related to perfusion and transport into the cancer cell. Because of the complex pathways available for methionine retention, it is difficult to provide a simple model of kinetic analysis. Increased uptake of methionine in the pancreas, due to the high level of protein synthesis, limits its use in that organ. Other protein synthesis tracers continue to be developed, but there have been limited clinical studies to date.

Thymidine and Nucleoside Analogues

One of the central problems associated with cancer is the uncontrolled growth of tumor cells. The study of cell proliferation in the laboratory has been at the heart of cancer research for decades. In the clinic, measuring tumor growth has generally relied on serial size determinations, as previously discussed. More direct measurements of growth parameters have required biopsies to look for histologic evidence of proliferation (mitotic figures), nuclear antigens associated with growth, and flow cytometric measurements (S-phase fraction). In some clinical studies, direct measurements of growth have been done by injecting patients with ^{3}H-thymidine prior to biopsy. The requirement for tissue samples has severely limited the studies one can do with such an approach.

Work on noninvasive imaging of cell proliferation has focused on the use of labeled nucleosides, in particular with thymidine and it analogues. The metabolic restriction of incorporation of thymidine into DNA, rather than RNA, had lead to its routine use in the laboratory. Thymidine has been labeled with [^{11}C], both in the methyl group and ring-2 position. Although a small number of trials have demonstrated the utility of labeled thymidine in clinical studies, the short half-life of [^{11}C] and relatively difficult synthesis of the tracers and its metabolism have limited its widespread use. This has lead investigators to begin to explore an number of analogues that can be labeled with fluorine-18 (^{18}F) such as 3'-fluorothymidine (FLT) and iododeoxyuridine, which can be labeled with iodine-124 (^{124}I) (3,4).

Blood Flow

PET has been widely used to measure blood flow in the brain and heart. Initial work relied on the use of [^{15}O]-labeled water, and many academic PET centers became very adept at using this very short half-life (2 minutes) radiotracer. Repeated brain activation studies have been done allowing just a few minutes for decay between injections.

The recent introduction of tumor antivascular agents into clinical trials has led to a growing interest in the use of [^{15}O]-water blood flow studies. One may not see clear evidence of tumor shrinkage with such agents; therefore, primary disruption of the blood supply is eagerly sought by investigators to demonstrate efficacy.

The optimal dose of the antivascular agents may best be determined by measuring the lowest dose needed to decrease tumor flow. Early trials have found changes in tumor blood flow 30 minutes after the injection of agents such as Combretastatin (A4-phosphate Prodrug; OXiGENE Inc, Waltham, Massachusetts) (5). PET provides data complementary to that obtained with MRI (dynamic contrast enhanced), which measures a combination of permeability and flow. Although it is not likely that this will become a common clinical use, PET is playing a valuable role in helping to develop these new drugs.

Labeled Drugs

One particularly interesting application of PET is in the evaluation of labeled anticancer agents. The injection of such labeled compounds allows one to measure the clearance from the blood, as well as the uptake and retention into tumors. For example, studies have been done comparing the uptake of nitrogen-13 ([^{13}N])-cisplatin into brain tumors and have demonstrated that an intra-arterial injection results in higher tumor uptake than simple intravenous delivery (6).

The uptake of labeled drugs has also been used to predict if a patient is likely to be susceptible to a given agent. That is, low uptake and retention may predict resistance to the drug. This has been demonstrated using [^{18}F]-5-fluorouracil, an agent commonly used to treat patients with colorectal cancer (7). In patients with liver metastases those with low uptake were uniformly nonresponders, while the higher the uptake the greater the likelihood of response.

Overall the number of labeled drugs has been small, and although such compounds are useful in measuring the pharmacology of the drugs, they are generally not useful in monitoring response. Although labeled drugs may provide important information to understand the drugs' distribution and possibly predict therapeutic outcome, there are limited uses so far in monitoring response to treatment.

QUANTITATION OF TUMOR MEASUREMENTS WITH PET

One of the critical issues in using PET to measure treatment response is the issue of how to best quantitate the imaging results (8,9). When FDG PET is used in diagnostic studies many centers routinely evaluate the images visually to determine if there are areas of activity with more intense uptake compared to the background. A similar approach is used in the routine staging of patients. This is often supplemented with the semiquantitative evaluation using the standardized uptake value (SUV), with untreated malignant lesions having a value well over 2.0 to 3.0.

When evaluating the response to therapy more accurate quantitation gains added importance, for although a tumor may still be visible, significant declines in tumor metabolism may indicate a favorable response (1). This has led to the use of kinetic analysis of image data obtained dynamically along with blood input curves. This allows one to measure overall flux of the tracer into tumors along with the individual rate constants. The relative utility of these approaches depends on the clinical setting and is likely to vary with each tumor and treatment.

For the simple answer of determining if a viable tumor is present at the end of therapy or late after the completion of treatment, simple visual assessment has been successfully employed in some studies (10). In such cases persistent tumor may be reported if activity above background for the surrounding tissues is noted. A similar approach has been employed in determining if recurrence is present rather than necrosis.

When one wishes to obtain information immediately after the start or early in the course of therapy, more quantitative approaches

TABLE 8.4.2 Brain Tumors and PET Evaluation after Therapy

Tracer/Pt #	Treatment	Timing of PET Relative to Treatment	PET Analysis	Clinical Evaluation	Result	Author	Year
FDG n = 33	XRT	late after	visual	path & F/U	88% accuracy	Kim	1992
FDG n = 8	chemo	1 wk before ~7 wks after	T:N	MRI	FDG uptake not correl	Vlassenko	2000
FDG n = 9	chemo	19 days after start	kinetic SUV	CT & F/U	Correl PET & response	Brock	2000
FDG n = 18	Radiosurg	6–8 mo after	T:N	MRI	Correl w/ progression	Lee	2003
FDG n = 25	Radiosurg	33 weeks	visual	MRI survival	91% accuracy	Belohlavek	2003
FDG n = 19	chemo or chemo/RT	before 7 weeks	SUV	survival	Correl PET & chemo survival	Charnley	2006
Methionine n = 14	XRT	3, 6, 12, >21 mon	T:N SUV	MRI & F/U	Correl PET & response	Nuutinen	2000
Methionine n = 21	Radiosurg	12 months	T:N SUV		78% sensitive 100% specific for reccur	Tsuyuguchi	2003
Methionine/ FDG n = 30	multiple	late after	T:N		methionine more sensitive	Van Laere	2004

Patient number
Treatment: XRT — radiation therapy; chemo—chemotherapy, radiosurg —radiosurgery,
PET analysis: T:N— tumor to normal tissue ratio; kinetic-metabolic rate calculation
Clinical Evaluation: F/U- follow up
Result: Correl —correlates PET with the indicated evaluation

are more likely to be of value (11). At this point the relative merits of using semiquantitative measurements of SUV and more detailed measurements of kinetic parameters are still open to debate. Some studies have demonstrated benefits for both approaches (12). One issue is clearly the reproducibility of such measurements. Although there are limited data, most trials suggest that repeated measurements made without intervening treatment will vary from 10% to 20% (13). Until the best technique is determined, it has been suggested the data be obtained in a standardized way allowing groups to compare their results and recalculate response values. To this end a recent National Cancer Institute conference has developed recommendations on how to obtain the PET scan and measure the SUV (14).

PET EVALUATION OF TUMOR RESPONSE: CLINICAL AND RESEARCH EXPERIENCE

Brain Tumors

The use of PET in oncology began with the study of brain tumors. There have been a number of studies over the years that have examined the course of treatment with surgery, chemotherapy, and radiation and the changes seen using PET (a sample of such studies is seen in Table 8.4.2). In one of the earliest studies looking at response at the end of treatment Ogawa et al. (15) demonstrated that FDG retention decreased by 1 month after chemoradiotherapy, but they did not see declines in blood flow or oxygen consumption.

For a long time the primary use of PET in oncology was to determine disease persistence versus radionecrosis in patients late after therapy for astrocytomas (16). This is useful in determining patient prognosis and deciding if further surgery is indicated. FDG PET has also been used after radiosurgery for brain tumors and brain metastases, but for the most part imaging has been done months after treatment. FDG PET was found to be useful in assessing the remission status and treatment outcome (17,18). The limitations of this approach are the high FDG retention in the normal brain, which can make interpretation difficult at times, and the limited therapeutic options available with each diagnosis.

On the other hand, a rapid increase in tumor activity was seen 1 day after treatment with stereotactic radiosurgery, but this declined by 1 week later (19). The early increase in tumor metabolism on the day after treatment, often called a *flare reaction*, was shown to correlate with survival in patients treated with carmustine (20). Another pilot study imaged patients 4 hours after radiosurgery and found that the FDG phosphorylation rate rapidly increased in these patients, and this may be a predictor of the ultimate response (21).

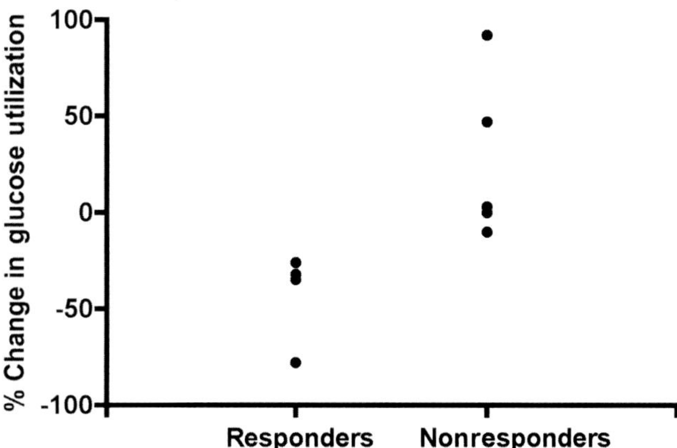

FIGURE 8.4.1. Treatment results in patients with high-grade gliomas treated with temozolomide. The change in metabolic rate of fluorodeoxyglucose (MRFDG) in the highest uptake areas of the tumor was compared to objective response at 8 weeks. PET was able to separate responders from nonresponders ($P < .02$). (Adapted from Brock CS, Young H, O'Reilly SM, et al. Early evaluation of tumour metabolic response using [^{18}F]fluorodeoxyglucose and positron emission tomography: a pilot study following the phase II chemotherapy schedule for temozolomide in recurrent high-grade gliomas. *Br J Cancer* 2000;82(3):608–615, with permission.)

As new drugs are developed for this disease, PET is gaining a role in evaluating response to therapy. In a trial temozolomide was given to nine patients with gliomas and FDG PET repeated 14 days after the start of therapy (12). The change in metabolic rate in the regions with high focal tumor uptake was found to correlate with the anatomic response at 8 weeks (Fig. 8.4.1). This analysis required the study of those areas of tumor with high focal uptake rather than the whole tumor. Although SUV changes also correlated with response, the metabolic rate parameters were a better measure of treatment outcome. On the other hand, a study using a cytostatic agent, imaging done about 7 weeks after the start of treatment, did not find a correlation between outcome and FDG retention (22). This emphasizes the point that the best imaging approach may depend on the type of treatment.

Although FDG has been the primary tracer used for PET studies of the brain, methionine has also been used in some trials. For example, patients with low-grade (13) or anaplastic (1) astrocytomas were imaged with methionine before and 3, 6, 12, or more than 21 months after radiation (23). The SUV ratio in tumor to normal brain rose significantly in those who died of progressive disease, was stable in those alive with disease, and declined slightly in those without evidence of disease. Imaging with methionine was also shown to be more sensitive and specific after radiosurgery, 78% and 100%, respectively (24). One trial comparing FDG and methionine imaging was done in 30 patients with possible recurrence of brain tumors. Although the two approaches were found to be complementary, methionine was better able to delineate the tumors with increased uptake noted in 93% compared with only 57% with FDG (25). Although methionine appears to be a promising tracer, because of its short half-life it is still not readily available.

The high background of normal glucose utilization has made the use of FDG problematic in trying to determine if patients have small areas of persistent or recurrent disease. Tracers of tumor proliferation have also been developed to assist in monitoring brain tumor therapy including thymidine and its analogues. Agents such as thymidine, FLT, or iododeoxyuridine may assist in this assessment (26,27) (Fig. 8.4.2).

Lymphoma

FDG PET imaging of lymphoma is already done clinically in many centers. It is routinely used in staging, but its greatest role at present is in the assessment of treatment response at the end of therapy. Chemotherapy can be curative in a majority of patients with both Hodgkin's lymphoma and non-Hodgkin's lymphoma. A major problem in these patients is that they are often left with residual masses at the end of chemotherapy, and this may represent persistent disease or fibrosis. Knowledge of persistent disease is critical since alternate

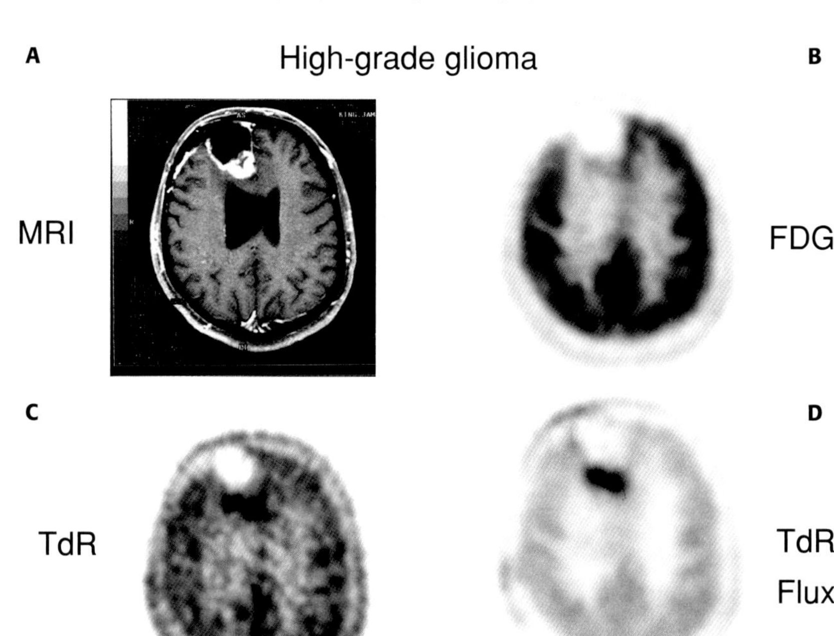

FIGURE 8.4.2. Images of a patient with recurrent glioma as imaged with (**A**) magnetic resonance imaging, (**B**) fluorodeoxyglucose PET, and (**C**) [^{11}C]-thymidine (TdR) PET imaged from 20 to 60 minutes. **D:** Parametric image of thymidine flux constant. The later image best shows the area of recurrent tumor in the area posterior to the previous resection. (From Eary JF, Mankoff DA, Spence AM, et al. 2-[C-11]thymidine imaging of malignant brain tumors. *Cancer Res* 1999;59(3):615–621, with permission.)

TABLE 8.4.3 Lymphoma and PET Evaluation after Chemotherapy

Tracer/Pt #	Disease	Timing of PET Relative to Treatment	PET Analysis	Clinical Evaluation	Result	Author	Year
FDG n = 11	NHL	1 & 6 wk after start	SUV kinetic	F/U & CT	81% PET accuracy	Romer	1998
FDG n = 37	HD	10 weeks after end	visual	F/U & CT	74% PET accuracy	de Wit	2001
FDG n = 54	HD = 19 NHL = 35	1–3 mo after end	visual	F/U & CT	85% PET accuracy	Jerusalem	1999
FDG n = 72	HD = 29 NHL = 41	after completion	visual	F/U & path	85% PET accuracy	Cremerius	1999
FDG n = 54	HD = 43 NHL = 11	after completion	visual	F/U & CT	93% PET accuracy	Stumpe	1998
FDG n = 30	HD & NHL	after 6–8 cycles	visual	F/U & CT	87% PET accuracy	Kostakoglu	2002
FDG n = 48	HD	58 days after	visual	F/U & CT	92% PET accuracy	Guay	2003
FDG n = 101	HD & NHL	2 months after	visual	F/U & CT	88% PET accuracy	Reinhart	2005
FDG n = 90	NHL	after 2 cycles	visual	F/U	66% PET accuracy	Haioun	2005
FDG n = 120	NHL	after 2–3 cycles	visual	F/U & CT	82% PET accuracy	Mikhaeel	2005
FDG n = 108	HD	after 2 cycles	visual	F/U & CT	95% PET accuracy	Gallamini	2006
FDG n = 41	HD & NHL Children	after completion	visual	F/U	91% PET accuracy	Rhodes	2006

#See table 2 for abbreviations.

treatments are available, including radiation, other chemotherapies, and even high-dose therapy with stem cell rescue. Gallium-67 (^{67}Ga)-scintigraphy was used to assist in this problem but has been variable in its acceptance and has significant limitations in the abdomen. Furthermore, trials have demonstrated that FDG PET is superior to gallium single-photon emission computed tomography (SPECT) in the staging of lymphoma (28,29). A number of studies have been completed that demonstrate the utility of FDG PET to evaluate patients during and at the end of their treatment (Table 8.4.3).

Although initial studies concentrated on imaging patients at the conclusion of treatment, Romer et al. (30) imaged patients before and at 1 and 6 weeks after the start of therapy in 11 patients with non-Hodgkin's lymphoma (Fig. 8.4.3). When measured using SUV quantitation, they noted a 60% decrease in tumor FDG uptake at 1 week and an average overall decline of 79% by 6 weeks. Although the decline at 1 week was significant, there was too much overlap between patients attaining a long-term complete response and those who relapsed to be of routine clinical use. In analyzing the 6-week images, an SUV cutoff of 2.5 was able to differentiate those maintaining a complete response (CR) from failing patients with an 81% accuracy (Fig. 8.4.4). In their study all three patients with a high SUV relapsed. The problem in assessment came from patients with apparent CR by PET who went on to relapse (two patients). This is an expected limitation with any imaging technology since it will fail to detect microscopic disease that can lead to eventual relapse.

In more recent studies, patients with non-Hodgkin's lymphoma were imaged after two to three cycles of chemotherapy, and the accuracy of response assessment varied from 66% to 82% (31,32). In the study by Mikhaeel et al. (32) the 5-year progression-free survival was 88.8%, 59.3%, and 16.2% in the patients with PET negative, minimal residual uptake, and PET positive groups, respectively. Another study found that those with negative and positive PET scans achieved a complete remission 83% and 58% of the time, respectively (31). In those with positive scans there was a 43% 2-year event-free survival. Overall, these studies demonstrate that those with positive scans early in the course of treatment generally do poorly, but it is still not clear that if one switched treatment that the outcome would be improved. This must await future trials.

A recent study of 108 patients with Hodgkin's lymphoma repeated FDG PET after two cycles of ABVD (doxorubicin, bleomycin, vinblastine, dacarbazine) chemotherapy (33). The overall accuracy of PET in response assessment was 95%, but more

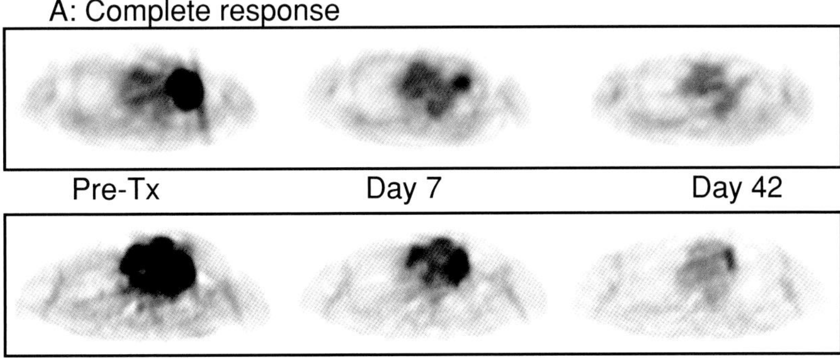

FIGURE 8.4.3. A (*top row*): Patient with high-grade NHL and a large parahilar lesion. This patient had a complete response based on PET and remained in complete response 15 months later. **B** (*bottom row*): A patient with extensive mediastinal involvement with high-grade lymphoma. Although the patient had a partial response to therapy, a lesion with an standardized uptake value of 4.1 was still visible at day 42. The patient relapsed during the third course of chemotherapy. Images were obtained pretreatment and days 7 and 42 after the start of therapy. fluorodeoxyglucose, FDG; TdR, [^{11}C]-thymidine flux. (From Romer W, Hanauske A, Ziegler S, et al. Positron emission tomography in non-Hodgkin's lymphoma: assessment of chemotherapy with fluorodeoxyglucose. *Blood* 1998;91(12):4464–4471, with permission.)

importantly only 2 of 20 (10%) who had positive PET scans after cycle two remained in remission. Again, further work is needed to determine if alternate therapy should be studied in this situation.

More work has been done in imaging patients after the completion of therapy. In a study of 37 patients with HD, imaging with FDG PET at a mean of 10 weeks after treatment had a 74% accuracy in predicting relapse (34). This compared to the accuracy of 32% with CT. Only 1 of 28 patients with a negative PET scan relapsed, while 12 of 22 patients with positive PET scans did not relapse. Some patients had radiation and repeat scans done after chemotherapy. If one takes into account only the PET scans obtained after completing all therapy, the accuracy was 85% and there were only five false-positive scans.

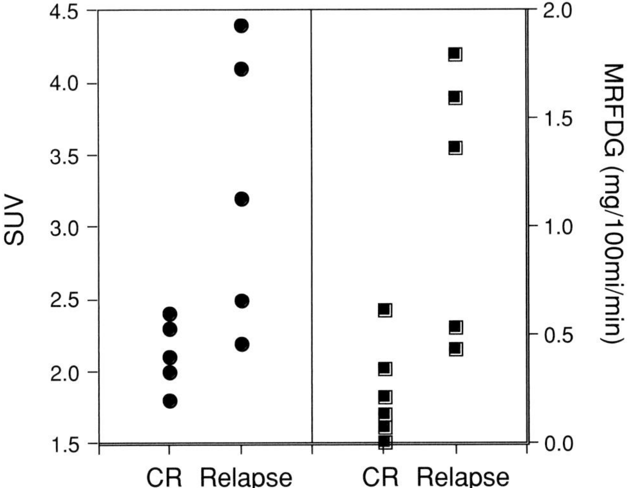

FIGURE 8.4.4. Comparison of fluorodeoxyglucose (FDG) PET and ultimate relapse or complete response (CR) in patients undergoing chemotherapy for non-Hodgkin's lymphoma. PET measurements were obtained as SUVmax (*circles*) and metabolic rate for FDG (MRFDG) (*squares*). (Adapted from Romer W, Hanauske A, Ziegler S, et al. Positron emission tomography in non-Hodgkin's lymphoma: assessment of chemotherapy with fluorodeoxyglucose. *Blood* 1998;91(12): 4464–4471, with permission.)

Jerusalem et al. (35) studied 19 patients with Hodgkin's lymphoma and 35 with non-Hodgkin's lymphoma in the posttreatment evaluation of patients 1 to 3 months after chemotherapy. All six patients with positive posttreatment PET scans progressed as did 8 of 48 patients (17%) with negative scans. The overall accuracy of PET was 85% in predicting relapse, compared with 67% for CT. Although all patients with positive PET relapsed, only 26% (5 of 19) of patients with positive CT and negative PET progressed, and 10% of those with both negative PET and CT progressed.

Similar results were also found by Cremerius et al. (36) who studied 72 patients (29 Hodgkin's lymphoma, 41 with non-Hodgkin's lymphoma, and 2 unclassified) with an accuracy of 85% for PET compared with 54% for CT. The major problem with CT is the low specificity (31%) in those with residual masses. PET was found to be 90% accurate in predicting remission in those with moderate risk for disease, but the negative predictive value of PET was only 50% to 67% in those with a high risk of relapse. A number of other investigators have found that PET was about 80% to 90% accurate in predicting relapse about 2 months after the completion of treatment of Hodgkin's and non-Hodgkin's lymphoma (37–39).

Not all studies have shown such accuracy, however, as demonstrated in a recent report of 41 children imaged after therapy for Hodgkin's and non-Hodgkin's lymphoma (40). Although PET/CT was 95% sensitive and can be useful in ruling out persistent disease, the positive predictive value in this mixed group of patients was only 53%. Positive PET results, therefore, need to be confirmed by other tests or follow-up.

In summary, the data clearly indicate the superiority of FDG PET in the restaging of both Hodgkin's and non-Hodgkin's lymphoma after the completion of therapy. The greatest advantage of PET is in the demonstration that persistent fibrotic lesions are not metabolically active. Such patients may be watched with the likelihood that they will remain in remission. Limitations of PET include that even PET negative areas may harbor microscopic tumor that may recur. Furthermore, the timing of PET is important in that studies done during or shortly after therapy may not have had time to fully resolve. This can be especially problematic in patients who have radiation as part of their treatment. Keeping these limitations in mind PET has been found to be an important addition to the clinical evaluation of patients being treated for lymphoma and is part of standard clinical practice.

Head and Neck Cancer

The treatment of head and neck cancers routinely employs the use of chemotherapy and radiation, often prior to the surgical resection of residual disease. This is a very useful setting to evaluate the ability of PET to measure changes resulting from treatment and to determine if viable tumor remains at the end of therapy (Table 8.4.4). In addition to the routine use of FDG, methionine has also been used in such studies. One of the early studies presented by Chaiken et al. (41) demonstrated that in patients receiving radiation therapy, those with stable or increasing FDG retention (six of seven; 86%) were found to have a persistence of recurrent disease. All patients who achieved remission after radiation therapy had declines in the T:N ratio (tumor:normal tissue). Sakamoto et al. (42) studied 22 patients using FDG with radiation therapy alone or with carboplatin chemotherapy. The mean SUV fell from 7.0 before therapy to 3.8, 3 to 4 weeks after the completion of therapy. In those patients going on to surgery the SUV ranged from 8.3 to 2.9 in those who still had some viable tumor left, while it was 3.3 to 1.9 if no viable tumor was present. Although there was some overlap, at an SUV of about 3.0, PET was clearly superior to conventional imaging techniques and the accuracy of predicting pathologic response was 73%. The results seen with conventional imaging did not correlate with those found with PET or pathologic results. Slevin et al. (43) used PET and MRI at 4 and 8 months after x-ray treatment to assess results. In almost all cases PET and MRI were consistent and both correlated with the status of the disease and final outcome. PET was positive in four patients, of which two eventually died of the disease and two were disease free at almost 2 years. Both PET and MRI each failed to detect one recurrence.

Imaging after treatment with chemotherapy alone has also demonstrated that as early as 1 week after treatment one could see changes in FDG SUV that correlated with changes in tumor size (44). Lowe et al. (45) also obtained images 1 to 2 weeks after chemotherapy, and they were found to correlate with pathologic response to treatment (Fig. 8.4.5). The mean decline in SUV was 34% in those with residual disease and 82% in pathologic CR. PET had a 90% sensitivity for persistent pathologic disease and overall 89% accuracy. Similar results were seen at 4 weeks posttherapy by Berlangieri et al. (46).

TABLE 8.4.4 Head and Neck and PET Evaluation after Therapy

Tracer/Pt #	Treatment	Timing of PET Relative to Treatment	PET Analysis	Clinical Evaluation	Result	Author	Year
FDG n = 15	XRT	during & 2–12 wk after	T:N	F/U	+ PET recur in 6/7 pts	Chaiken	1993
FDG n = 22	XRT +/− Chemo	3–4wk after end	SUV	F/U and path	73% PET accuracy	Sakamoto	1998
FDG n = 21	XRT	4 mo & 8 mo after	T:N	MRI & F/U	result correl	Slevin	1999
FDG n = 11	Chemo	1 wk after start	SUV	CT	Change SUV correl CT	Haberkorn	1993
FDG n = 28	Chemo	1–2 wk after end	Visual SUV	Pathology	89% PET accuracy	Lowe	1997
FDG n = 6	Chemo/XRT	during & 2 yr after	T:N	F/U	All decrease with therapy	Berlangieri	1994
FDG n = 56	Chemo/XRT	3.5 months	visual	F/U	89% accuracy	Yao	2004
FDG n = 28	Chemo/XRT	2 months	visual	F/U	86.7% accuracy	Andrade	2006
Methionine n = 15	XRT	during	SUV	F/U	No correl with outcome	Nuutinen	1999
Methionine n = 15	XRT	3 wk after end	SUV	Pathology	84% PET accuracy	Lindholm	1995

#See table 2 for abbreviations.

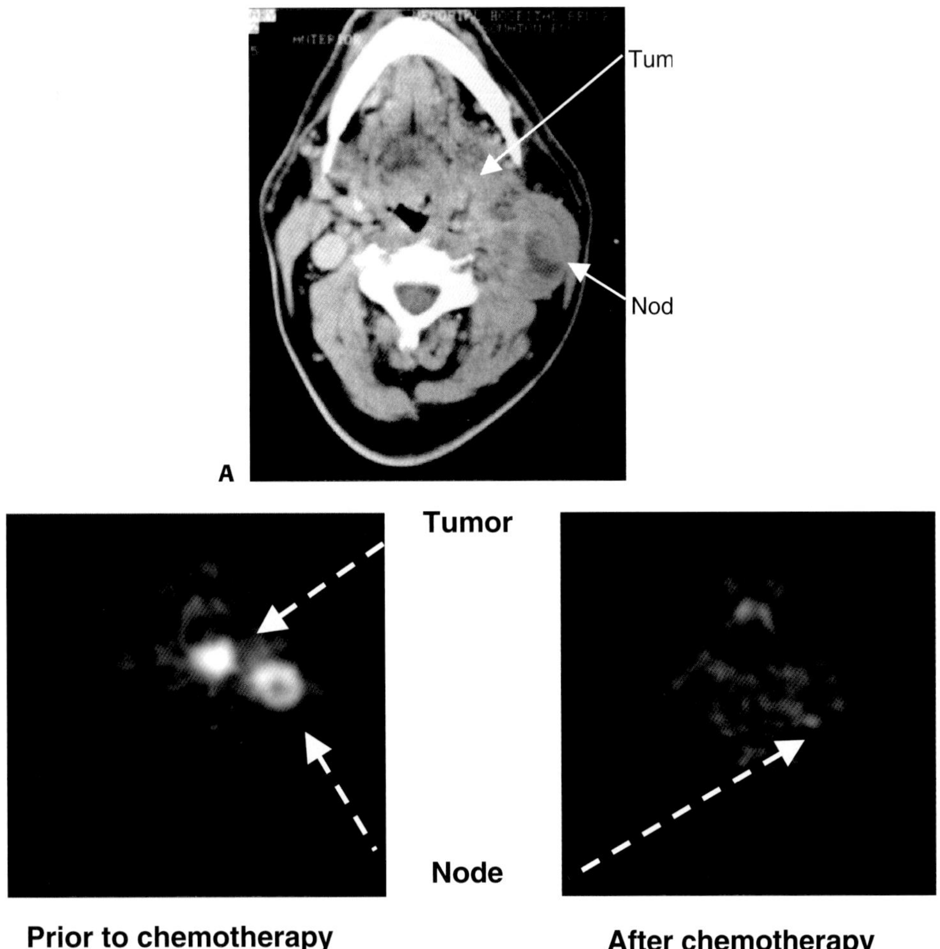

FIGURE 8.4.5. A patient with head and neck cancer imaged with CT before treatment (**A**) and fluorodeoxyglucose (FDG) PET before and after chemotherapy (**B**). The patient had a base of tongue lesion that resolved completely on PET and a nodal lesion with a marked decrease in metabolism. (From Lowe V, Dunphy F, Varvares M, et al. Evaluation of chemotherapy response in patients with advanced head and neck cancer using [F-18]fluorodeoxyglucose positron emission tomography. *Head Neck* 1997;19(8):666–674, with permission.)

PET obtained an average of about 3.5 months after treatment had an overall accuracy of 89% in detecting persistent cancer (47). The use of combined PET/CT scans has been particularly helpful in head and neck cancer because of the complex anatomy. FDG PET/CT was performed at a mean of 8 weeks after completing chemoradiotherapy in 28 patients (48). PET/CT had an overall accuracy of 85.7%, but the only false-negative patients (n = 3) and false-positive cases (1) occurred before 8 weeks, while PET/CT was 100% accurate after 8 weeks. On the other hand, contrast-enhanced CT alone produced a number of false positive results before and after eight weeks.

Methionine PET has also been used in patients treated with radiation alone. Measurements obtained during the first 2 to 3 weeks of therapy showed declines in most of the treated patients (Fig. 8.4.6) (49). Researchers were, however, unable to predict who would eventually relapse or remain in remission. On the other hand, methionine PET SUV measurements obtained a median of 3 weeks after the completion of therapy were found to correlate with pathologic response at resection (50).

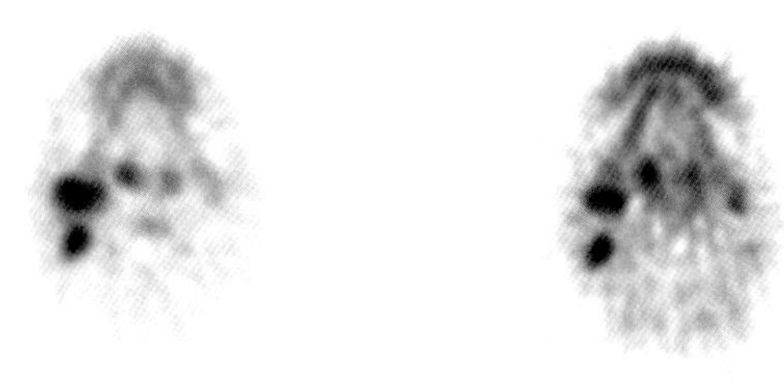

FIGURE 8.4.6. ^{11}C-Methionine PET images of a patient with head and neck cancer metastatic to the lymph nodes. Images were obtained before (**left**) and during radiotherapy (**right**) and the standard uptake value decreased from 9.4 to 5.4 in the larger lymph nodes, while retention in the oral mucosa went up slightly. This patient remained in remission over 27 months after treatment. (From Nuutinen J, Jyrkkio S, Lehikoinen P, et al. Evaluation of early response to radiotherapy in head and neck cancer measured with [^{11}C]methionine-positron emission tomography. *Radiother Oncol* 1999;52(3):225–232, with permission.)

TABLE 8.4.5 Breast Cancer and PET Evaluation after Therapy

Tracer/Pt #	Treatment	Timing of PET Relative to Treatment	PET Analysis	Clinical Evaluation	Result	Author	year
FDG n = 11	chemo-hormone	during cycles 1–3	visual SUV	mammo	Correl PET & mammo	Wahl	1993
FDG n = 16	chemo	during & end	SUV visual	path	76% PET accuracy	Bassa	1996
FDG n = 30	chemo	during & end	SUV kinetic	path	79% PET accuracy	Smith	2000
FDG n = 22	chemo	during cycles 1, 2	SUV	path	88% PET accuracy	Schelling	2000
FDG n = 50	chemo	at end	SUV	path	Correl PET & path	Kim	2004
FDG n = 11	chemo	after cycles 1 & 2	SUV	clinical	Correl PET & clinical	Dose Schwarz	2005
FDG n = 64	chemo	after cycles 1, 2, 3, & 6	SUV	path	87% accuracy after cycle 2	Rousseau	2006
FDG & Methio n = 16	chemo	during cycles 1, 3/4	SUV	CT & clinical	Correl PET & clinical	Jansson	1995
Methioinine n = 8	chemo, hormone, or XRT	during 3–14 wk	SUV kinetic	clinical	Correl PET & clinical	Huovinen	1993
FES n = 7	hormone	2 wk after start	semi-quantitative	clinical	Correl PET & clinical	McGuire	1991
FES & FDG n = 11	hormone	7–10 d after start	semi-quantitative	clinical	FDG 100% accurate	Dehdashti	1999
FLT & FDG n = 14	chemo, hormone	5 weeks after start	SUV	clinical	Correl FLT & clinical	Pio	2005

#See table 2 for abbreviations.

In summary, PET has demonstrated early declines in both radiation and chemotherapy. The clinical value of these images obtained during the course of treatment is unclear at present, given the limited number of patients studied. Images obtained at the conclusion of therapy appear to be predictive of the ultimate outcome.

Breast Cancer

Breast cancer treatment has been assessed using PET both in the treatment of metastatic and locally advanced disease (Table 8.4.5). The evaluation of hormonal therapy with PET has also been of interest. Wahl et al. (51) compared baseline FDG PET with up to four scans obtained during chemohormonal therapy. Metabolic changes in the tumors were documented with PET, as determined visually and with SUV, and with kinetic parameters correlated with response as detected by mammographic shrinkage of the tumors. The response as measured by PET appeared to be more prompt than declines in tumor size. In an early trial, Bassa et al. (52) imaged patients before, during, and at the end of neoadjuvant therapy. Visual analysis of the images obtained just prior to surgery were 76% accurate in determining if residual tumor was present. The greatest failing of PET was in missing small volumes of residual disease after chemotherapy had been administered.

In a study of 30 patients with locally advanced breast cancer, the ultimate pathologic response to therapy could be predicted after the first cycle of therapy using FDG PET (53). Using a 20% decrease in SUV as a cutoff, PET had a sensitivity of 90% and specificity of 74% (overall accuracy 79%) in predicting the pathologic disappearance of all microscopic or macroscopic tumors (Fig. 8.4.7). A similar result was found in the study of Schelling et al. (54) who also studied patients with locally advanced breast cancer before and after the first and second cycles of chemotherapy (Fig. 8.4.8). They determined that the optimal threshold was a decrease of the SUV by at least 45%, and that this had an overall accuracy of 88% in predicting which patients would have minimal residual disease (Fig. 8.4.9).

FDG PET is also gaining use in the evaluation of experimental treatment. One of the larger and more extensive studies of PET included 64 patients who were image before and after 1, 2, 3, and

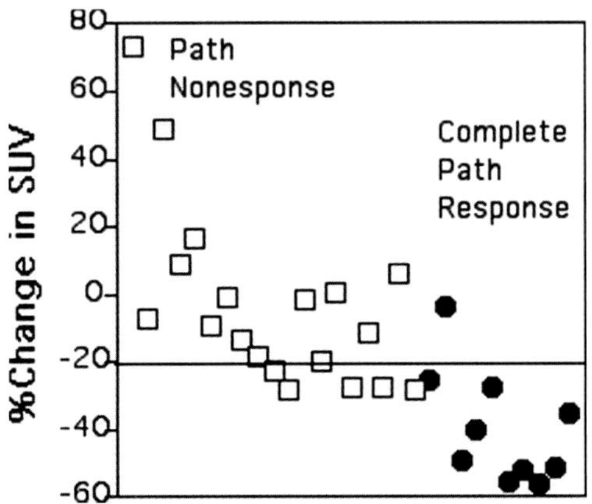

FIGURE 8.4.7. Fluorodeoxyglucose (FDG) PET imaging results after one cycle of treatment for primary breast cancer. The percentage change in standard uptake value (SUV) was compared in those judged nonresponsive by pathology (*open squares*) or to those with at least a macroscopic pathologic response (*closed circles*). (Adapted from Smith IC, Welch AE, Hutcheon AW, et al. Positron emission tomography using [(18)F]-fluorodeoxy-D-glucose to predict the pathologic response of breast cancer to primary chemotherapy. *J Clin Oncol* 2000;18(8):1676–1688, with permission.)

6 cycles of chemotherapy prior to surgery (55). A decline in maximum SUV by greater than 40% after the second cycle of therapy was found to be optimal and had an accuracy of 87%. After the first cycle of therapy, the accuracy was 77%, while the accuracy was 81% after three cycles. It is notable that accuracy declined after six cycles, since many pathologic nonresponders still had large declines in FDG retention by that time. Nevertheless, PET done at that point is still more accurate than conventional imaging. In another study where FDG PET was done before and after the completion of neoadjuvant chemotherapy, a reduction in the peak SUV of greater than 79% was able to separate pathologic responders from nonresponders with an 85.2% sensitivity and 82.6% specificity (56).

In patients with advanced disease, imaging was also studied after the first and second cycles of chemotherapy (57). Those who eventually responded to treatment had an average decline of 28%, versus only a mean decline of 6% in nonresponders. There was an overall survival of only 8.8 months in those judged to be nonresponding by PET, while PET responders had an average survival of 19.2 months.

Methionine has also been used to monitor response to treatment in patients receiving chemotherapy for breast cancer. Jansson et al. (58) studied patients before and after the first and third/fourth cycles of chemotherapy with either FDG or methionine. Seven patients were studied with both tracers before treatment and methionine demonstrated better contrast in five, so it was chosen for further use in repeat studies. The other patients were studied with only FDG or methionine. Nine of 16 patients had repeated methionine studies and 7 had FDG. Eleven of 12 patients with major clinical responses also had decreases in methionine (6) or FDG (5) during the first course of therapy. Methionine was also found to be useful in monitoring response to both hormonal and chemotherapy (59).

The analogue FLT, which can measure tumor proliferation, has also been used to measure treatment response after the first cycle of therapy in patients with advanced disease (60). Changes in FLT retention were found to correlate with more standard clinical measurements, such as CT, obtained later in the course of treatment.

Labeling of estrogens for the measurement of receptor status *in vivo* using PET has been employed by investigators and compared with assay made by receptor assays from pathologic specimens (61). All these studies have found that PET analysis using either labeled [^{18}F]-fluorotamoxifen or 16α[^{18}F]-fluoro-17β-estradiol (FES) was predictive of response to antiestrogen treatment. Imaging done before and after antiestrogen therapy showed a decline in FES uptake in all lesions. In a subsequent study, 11 patients with estrogen receptor–positive breast cancer were imaged with both FDG and FES prior to and 7 to 10 days after the start of tamoxifen therapy (62). The responders had a greater decline in FES retention than the nonresponders, as measured by the change in SUV. Of even more scientific interest was that all the responders had a "metabolic flare" reaction as demonstrated by an average increase in FDG retention by 1.4 SUV (minimum 0.8 in any patient). The greatest increase in FDG retention in nonresponders was 0.4 SUV.

In summary, PET has been demonstrated to be useful in monitoring the response in patients being treated for breast cancer. Such information is increasingly being applied to clinical decision making, although it is clear that more data will be required to enable oncologists to be fully comfortable making clinical decisions based on the scan results.

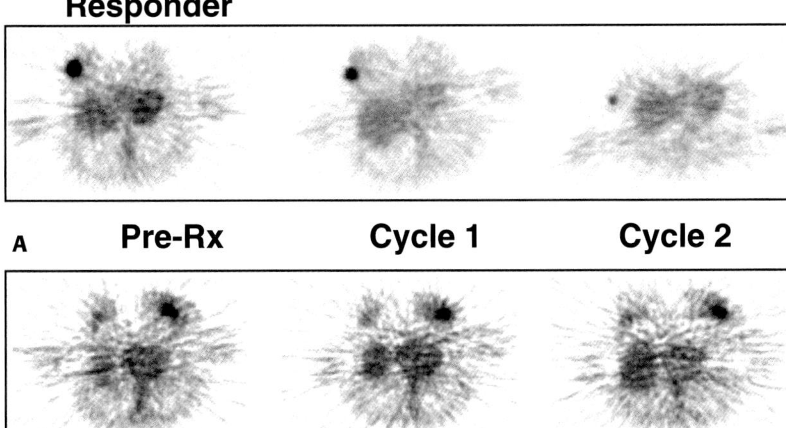

FIGURE 8.4.8. Fluorodeoxyglucose (FDG) PET images in two patients with primary breast cancer. Images were obtained before and after the first and second cycles of therapy. **A** (*top row*): Shows a responding patient who had minimal disease after therapy. **B** (*bottom row*): A nonresponding patient. (From Schelling M, Avril N, Nahrig J, et al. Positron emission tomography using [(^{18})F]fluorodeoxyglucose for monitoring primary chemotherapy in breast cancer. *J Clin Oncol* 2000;18(8):1689–1695, with permission.)

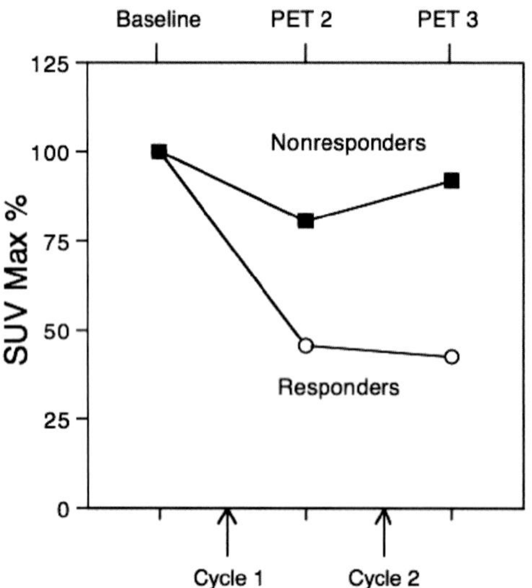

FIGURE 8.4.9. Change in mean maximum standard uptake value (SUVmax) after the treatment of breast cancer with chemotherapy. Nonresponders (17 patients) have gross residual tumor at the end of therapy, while responders (seven patients) had minimal residual disease. (Adapted from Schelling M, Avril N, Nahrig J, et al. Positron emission tomography using [(^{18})F]fluorodeoxyglucose for monitoring primary chemotherapy in breast cancer. *J Clin Oncol* 2000;18(8):1689–1695, with permission.)

Lung Cancer

PET imaging of lung cancer treatment has generally been done after radiation, either alone or in combination with other treatments (Table 8.4.6). In one of the first studies, Kubota et al. (63) imaged patients who had been treated with radiotherapy with PET using [^{11}C]-L-methionine before and 2 weeks after the conclusion of therapy. They measured the change in T:N uptake with PET and change in tumor size on CT scan. Patients were divided into three response groups: those with early progression, late local recurrence, and no local recurrence. Those with no local recurrence or late recurrence had similar decreases in methionine retention (65% and 72%, respectively). This was in contrast to the early progression group with a 22% decline in methionine uptake. The early and late recurrence groups could be differentiated by the lack of tumor shrinkage in the former group.

The study of Hebert et al. (64) compared the results of FDG PET before and after radiation to the local control rate in lung caner. Four patients had complete responses as judged by PET and none recurred locally. Of the eight patients with a partial or no response by PET, four had persistent local disease and another four remained alive and well at least 11 months after treatment. In this study a negative PET scan was very helpful, but a positive scan did not predict whether the patient would relapse. It is notable that the follow-up PET scans were done at variable times after the completion of radiation, with some being as early as 1 month after treatment. It is this experience that has led investigators to allow more time for responses after radiation treatment.

The study of Patz et al. (65) analyzed the follow-up PET scan obtained on 113 patients after treatment, which could include chemotherapy, radiation, surgery, or a combination. Imaging was

TABLE 8.4.6 Lung Cancer and PET Evaluation after Therapy

Tracer/Pt #	Treatment	Timing of PET Relative to Treatment	PET Analysis	Clinical Evaluation	Result	Author	Year
Methionine n = 16	XRT	2 wk after end	T:N	F/U & CT	Correl PET & clinical	Kubota	1993
FDG n = 12	XRT	variable after end	visual SUV	F/U & CT	Correl CR on PET & clinical	Hebert	1996
FDG n = 126	XRT, chemo, surgery	every 6 mo after end	visual SUV	F/U & CT	84% PET accuracy	Bury	1999
FDG n = 113	XRT, chemo, surgery	median 8 mo after end	visual	F/U & CT	Correl PET & clinical	Patz	2000
FDG n = 57	chemo	after cycle 1	SUV	F/U & CT	Correl PET & clinical	Weber	2003
FDG n = 56	chemo, XRT surgery	up to 1 month after end	SUV	path	96% PET accuracy	Cerfolio	2004
FDG n = 88	XRT +/−chemo	10 wk after end	visual	F/U & CT	Correl PET & clinical	MacManus	2005
FDG n = 50	chemo, XRT surgery	end of chemo and XRT	SUV	path	100% PET accuracy	Pottgen	2006
FDG n = 26	chemo, XRT surgery	end of chemo and XRT	SUV	path	85% PET accuracy	Yamamoto	2006

#See table 2 for abbreviations.

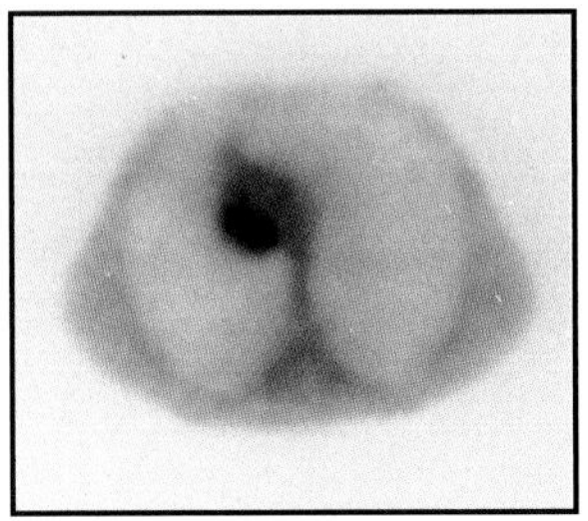

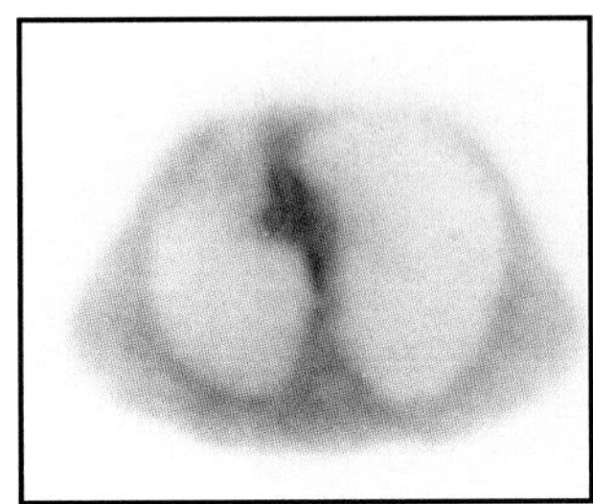

FIGURE 8.4.10. Fluorodeoxyglucose (FDG) PET images of a patient with unresectable non-small cell lung cancer before and 2 months after radiation therapy and carboplatin. Posttreatment the tumor has the same activity level as the normal mediastinal structures and was judged a complete response. (From MacManus M, Hicks R, Wada M, et al. Early F^{-18} FDG PET response to radical chemoradiotherapy correlates strongly with survival in unresectable non-small cell lung cancer. *Proc ASCO* 2000;19:483a, with permission.)

done a median of 8 months after treatment but ranged from 2 days to 9 years. Only 13 patients had negative PET scans, but 11 of these (85%) are alive and disease free a median of 34 months after the PET scan. Of the 101 patients with positive PET scans the median survival was only 12 months (95% confidence interval 9 to 15 months). Bury et al. (66) did a similar study of the follow-up of a mixed group of 126 patients imaged with PET and CT every 6 months after treatment. The accuracy of PET was 96% and CT 84% in detecting residual or recurrent tumor. Although the specificity of both approaches was about equal in this study (92% to 95%), the sensitivity of PET in detecting tumor was 100% and CT only 72%. PET had three false-positive patients due to radiation pneumonitis. In patients receiving chemotherapy alone the PET scan done after the first cycle of treatment was predictive of ultimate response (67). Those with a decrease of FDG SUV greater than 20% had a median survival of 151 days, compared to 54 days in nonresponders.

In a trial of 88 patients imaged before and after radiation (with or without chemotherapy) researchers waited a median of 10 weeks for the second study (Fig. 8.4.10) (68). This was to allow time for inflammation in the lung, pleura, and tumor to decrease. For those visually determined to have a CR by PET the actuarial 2-year survival was 62%, while it was only 30% for those with a poorer response. Even after a multivariate analysis PET was a significant predictor of survival. There was no difference in survival in those judged to have a CR by CT response compared to those without CR, demonstrating the superiority of PET for this use. The inflammatory response that accompanies the radiation therapy may provide benefit and has been shown to correlate with tumor response (69).

Cerfolio et al. (70) studied 56 patients also treated with neoadjuvant chemotherapy (n = 33) or combined chemoradiotherapy (n = 23) and imaged them within 1 month of the completion of treatment and before resection. The change in SUV_{max} correlated with the percentage of nonviable tumor cells at resection, and a complete pathologic response could be predicted with 96% accuracy using a cutoff of SUV_{max} decline by 80%. A more recent study examined 50 patients with locally advanced non–small cell lung cancer. Patients were imaged before therapy, after three cycles of induction chemotherapy (about day 63), and then again after combined chemoradiotherapy (about day 84), and then they underwent resection (71). The mean decline in SUVmax after induction chemotherapy was 67% in those with less than 10% viable or no viable cancer at resection. Patients with greater than 10% tumor viability had a decline that was not as great (mean 34%). Using this approach they were able to separate responding and nonresponding patients. The scans after the completion of radiotherapy showed declines of 73% and 49%, compared to baseline, in responding and nonresponding patients, respectively. Yamamoto et al. (72) studied 26 patients who had PET scans with FDG at 2 hours and using a 65% decline as a cutoff they had an 85% accuracy in predicting pathologic response.

Other tracers have been used to evaluate the biology of tumor response in pilot trials of patients with lung cancer. Patients with small cell lung cancer treated with chemotherapy FDG PET and $[^{11}C]$-thymidine were imaged before and around 1 week into therapy (73). Although both imaging approaches demonstrated rapid declines in tumor metabolism, the measurements of proliferation declined more rapidly in patients with successful treatment. The difficulties encountered with $[^{11}C]$-thymidine are its synthesis, a shorter half-life compared to $[^{18}F]$, and *in vivo* degradation, which have limited the routine use of this approach. The more recent development of metabolically stable proliferation tracers such as FLT may allow for more routine clinical use of this approach.

The role of hypoxia in the measurement of response to treatment of tumors has also been evaluated with tracers such as $[^{18}F]$-fluoromisonidazole (FMISO). In a pilot study, seven patients were imaged repeatedly during the course of radiation for non–small cell lung cancer (Fig. 8.4.11) (74). The fraction of tumor volume that was judged to be hypoxic was shown to decline from a median of 58% pretreatment, to 29% at midtreatment, and 22% at the end of therapy. This approach may be useful in assessing the role of tumor hypoxia on resistance to radiation. With the development of new antivascular agents FMISO and similar compounds may find another role in determining the success of efforts to disrupt vessel perfusion.

In summary, FDG PET is gaining a role in the follow-up of patients with lung cancer, in addition to its use in initial staging. Studies indicate that it is more predictive of eventual outcome after the completion of treatment than conventional anatomic imaging with CT. Further studies are needed to look at its use early after treatment and how one can best incorporate PET imaging to determining when to change therapy.

Gastrointestinal Cancers

FDG PET has been used to evaluate a number of gastrointestinal tumors, but most prominently in studying patients with metastatic colorectal cancer and more recently gastrointestinal stromal tumors (Table 8.4.7). Findlay et al. (75) examined patients before and around 2 and 4 weeks after the start of chemotherapy for colorectal cancer. The measurement of SUV and T:N ratio at these times was compared to the measurements of CT obtained 12 weeks after the start of treatment. They found that a decline of at least 15% at 4 weeks in the T:N ratio was the most predictive of ultimate response (95% accurate) (Fig. 8.4.12). Although a decline was seen at 2 weeks in some patients, four lesions actually increased at 2 weeks before rapidly declining. SUV values also declined significantly by 4 weeks, but it did not separate responders and nonresponders as well as T:N ratios did.

As has been noted in evaluating radiation treatment for other tumors, FDG PET had difficulty assessing response at the end of radiotherapy in patients with colorectal cancer (76). Patients were treated with a course of photon radiation, which was followed by neutron therapy. Imaging was done before, after the photon

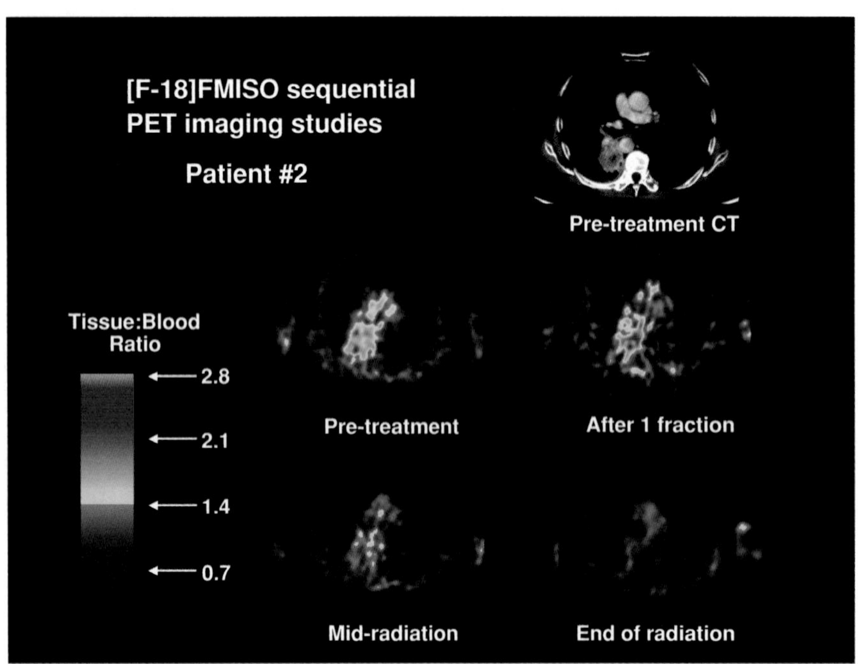

FIGURE 8.4.11. [^{18}F]-Fluoromisonidazole (FMISO) images from a patient with unresectable non-small cell lung cancer. The patient was imaged before, during, and at the end of a 4-week course of neutron radiation. The image intensity scale is set so that areas of hypoxia appear yellow to red and had a FMISO tumor:blood ratio greater than or equal to 1.4. (From Koh WJ, Bergman KS, Rasey JS, et al. Evaluation of oxygenation status during fractionated radiotherapy in human non-small cell lung cancers using [F-18]fluoromisonidazole positron emission tomography. *Int J Radiat Oncol Biol Phys* 1995;33(2):391–398, with permission.)

therapy, and then 6 weeks after completion of neutron treatment. Although all patients had evidence of clinical palliation, only 50% had a decline in FDG SUV values. The authors argue that a longer interval may be needed to assess response in these patients receiving radiation treatment.

Although methionine imaging has found use in other tumor types, it was not very helpful in rectal cancer, where imaging was done before and 4 weeks after neoadjuvant chemoradiotherapy.

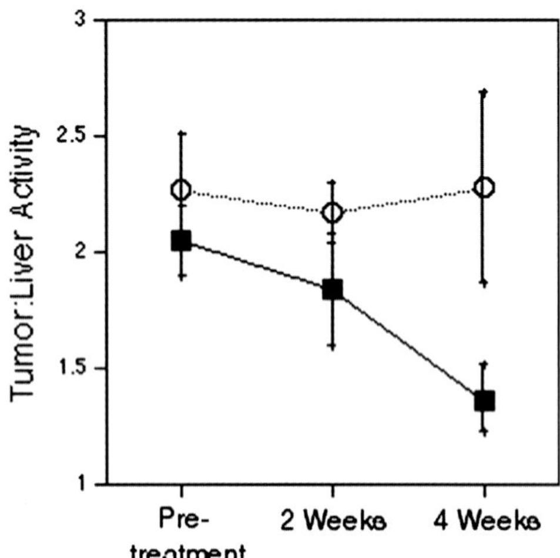

FIGURE 8.4.12. Fluorodeoxyglucose (FDG) PET results in patients with metastatic colorectal cancer in the liver responding (*dark squares*) or not responding (*open circles*) to chemotherapy. Patients were imaged before, and at 1 to 2 weeks, and 4 to 5 weeks after the start of treatment and results are expressed as the tumor:normal liver ratio (mean and 95% confidence intervals). (Adapted from Findlay M, Young H, Cunningham D, et al. Noninvasive monitoring of tumor metabolism using fluorodeoxyglucose and positron emission tomography in colorectal cancer liver metastases: correlation with tumor response to fluorouracil. *J Clin Oncol* 1996;14(3):700–708, with permission.)

Here declines in tracer retention did not correlate with improvements in T category or pathologic response (77). All 15 patients studied had decreases in SUV of about 50%, but this was not helpful in separating those with clinical response.

In a study of 14 patients receiving chemotherapy for esophageal cancer, FDG PET was done before and after 2 or 3 cycles of chemotherapy (8 to 13 weeks) (78). PET results were quantitated by both T:N ratio and calculating the metabolic rate for FDG. The two approaches had a correlation coefficient of 0.87. In the six patients with over 30% decrease in T:N ratio all had clinical evidence of response, while two patients with an increase in T:N had no response. Of the five patients with a 0% to 30% decrease none had CT evidence of response, but three had clinical improvements in dysphagia.

A more recent study of 65 patients with gastroesophageal junction tumors demonstrated that PET performed at 14 days after the start of therapy was a useful measure of response (79). Those with a greater than 35% decline in FDG retention had an improved pathologic response rate (44%) compared to only 5% in PET nonresponders. Three-year survival was 70% and 35% in PET responders and nonresponders, respectively.

Gastrointestinal stromal tumors are uncommon tumors that generally overexpress *ckit* and are thus exceedingly responsive to treatment with new tyrosine kinase inhibitors such as imatinib and sunitinib. Although treatment can provide rapid clinical improvement, these agents are not curative. Standard anatomic imaging can be misleading, since these tumors often do not change dramatically in size because of fibrosis and edema. Changes in the retention of FDG on PET can occur within days and have been reflective of clinical response. In one study 16 patients were imaged before and 1 week after the start of imatinib and the ultimate response was predicted with 93% accuracy (80). The 11 responders and 5 nonresponders had average changes in SUV that declined by 65% or increased by 16%, respectively. Another study found that PET done 8 days after the start of treatment gave results comparable to CT at 2 months 86% of the time (81). But even at 2 months after treatment, PET appears to perform better than CT in assessing

TABLE 8.4.7 Gastrointestinal and Genitourinary Cancer and PET Evaluation after Therapy

Tracer/Pt #	Disease	Treatment	Timing of PET Relative to Treatment	PET Analysis	Clinical Evaluation	Result	Author	Year
FDG n = 18	Colon	chemo	during wk 2 & 4	SUV T:N	CT	95% PET accuracy	Findlay	1996
FDG n = 12	Colon	radiation	during & end	SUV	CT	50% accuracy	Haberkorn	1996
MET n = 15	Rectal	chemo/RT	4 weeks	SUV	path	NOT accurate	Wieder	2002
FDG n = 14	Esophageal	chemo	during wk 13-Aug	T:N kinetics	F/U & CT	Correl PET & clinical	Couper	1998
FDG n = 65	GE junction	chemo	14 days after start	SUV	F/U & path	Correl PET & clinical	Ott	2006
FDG n = 17	GIST	chemo	8 days	SUV	clinical	Correl PET & clinical	Stroobants	2003
FDG n = 16	GIST	chemo	1 week	SUV	clinical	Correl PET & clinical	Jager	2003
FDG n = 49	GIST	chemo	2 months	SUV	symptoms & CT	96% PET accuracy	Gayed	2004
FDG n = 20	GIST	chemo	1, 3, 6 months	SUV	clinical	85% PET accuracy at 1 month	Antoch	2004
FDG n = 18	GIST	chemo	2 months	visual	clinical	100% PET accuracy	Goldstein	2005
FDG n = 21	germ cell	chemo	end	SUV kinetics	path	Correl PET & clinical	Sugawara	1999
FDG n = 30	germ cell	chemo	6 wk	SUV	path	Correl PET & clinical	Stepehens	1996
Methionine n = 15	bladder	chemo	during wk 3 & 9	SUV kinetics	CT	variable	Letocha	1994
FDG n = 33	ovarian	chemo	after 1 & 3 cycles	SUV	clinical	Correl PET & clinical	Avril	2005

#See table 2 for abbreviations.

long-term response, being correct 94% and 75% of the time, respectively (82). Similar results have been found by other investigators (83,84). On the other hand, even when PET shows that the tumor is no longer active, if the lesions are removed after neoadjuvant treatment a small proportion of viable tumor cells are generally found (85).

Soft tissue sarcomas have also been examined using FDG PET after neoadjuvant treatment with chemotherapy (86). Forty-six patients were imaged before and after a median of three cycles of chemotherapy and the change in SUV_{max} measured. Recurrence occurred in only 33% of those with an elevated baseline SUVmax 6.0 or greater and 40% or more decline compared to 85% in those with a smaller decline in SUV_{max}. It is notable that changes assessed by PET were more predictive of long-term outcome than finding little viable tumor on pathology at resection.

Genitourinary

A limited number of studies of prostate cancer have been done with both FDG and other tracers. FDG has been somewhat limited in its use in this disease because of difficulties in detecting tumors adjacent to the bladder (87). Furthermore, even in patients with metastatic disease to the bone FDG PET has had a relatively low sensitivity, but good specificity (88). Early trials have found a correlation between changes in FDG and blood prostate-specific antigen levels after therapy (89). Given the limitations of FDG in prostate cancer, investigators have begun to explore other tracers such as [^{18}F]-fluorocholine (90), which look promising in the pilot studies, to detect and monitor tumor response.

Although chemotherapy is very successful in patients with nonseminomatous germ cell tumors, some patients have viable tumor remaining and these can be salvaged by surgery. A proportion of the patients also have teratoma remaining in the lesions (about 40%), and this should be removed since tumor may eventually recur. Surgery is not needed in those with tumor necrosis (about 40% to 45%), but this is difficult to predict prior to surgery. In patients with germ cell tumors imaging was done with FDG PET after completing chemotherapy and just prior to resection of residual masses (Table 8.4.7) (91). In this study of 30 patients, the mean SUV of patients with viable tumor was 8.8, compared with 2.9 and 3.1 for those with necrosis and teratoma, respectively. Using an SUV cutoff of 5.0 detected all but one of the patients with active germ cell tumors. Unfortunately, PET alone could not differentiate teratoma from necrosis. It is known that those with pathologic evidence of teratoma in the primary tumor and those who have rapid shrinkage of tumor on CT are at lower risk for having remaining teratoma. A negative PET scan in this group of patients may be useful in obviating the need for surgery. Another study of this issue was done by Sugawara et al. (92) with similar results. They found the SUV measurement could differentiate viable tumor from necrosis or teratoma. Although SUV measurements could not distinguish necrosis from teratoma, this was possible using a kinetic analysis of the K1 rate constant for FDG. This study, which was done in a relatively small number of patients, needs confirmation.

Response of ovarian cancer has been assessed with FDG PET in 33 patients treated with chemotherapy (93). Pretreatment images were obtained and repeated after the first and third cycles of treatment and the results compared to survival and clinical responses. A decline of 20% and 55% in SUV was used as a cutoff for response after the first and third cycles. After cycle one, PET responders had a median survival of 38.3 months, while nonresponders survived 23.1 months. PET was found to be a more accurate measure of response than clinical criteria or even histopathologic response at second-look surgery.

Methionine has been used to measure the response in patients receiving neoadjuvant chemotherapy for bladder cancer (94). Patients were studied before and after cycle one of therapy, and again after cycle three for some patients. In the 11 patients studied after one cycle all had declines in the SUV, while those with complete responses had at least a 50% decline in tumor retention and some patients who had declines as high as 78% still only had partial responses. In the four patients also imaged after three cycles of therapy, two had complete responses with SUV decreases of 61% and 100%, while those with lesser declines only had a partial response. This limited data set demonstrates that further study is needed to determine the optimal timing of imaging in this disease.

SUMMARY

The use of PET in assessing treatment response has grown rapidly in the past several years. In a wide variety of cancers, rapid and persistent declines in FDG uptake after therapy have been associated with superior complete response and often in time to disease recurrence and survival data. Although the exact timing and optimal role of PET in a variety of cancers continues to evolve and is somewhat treatment specific, it is clear that FDG PET as well as PET with other tracers such as those of amino acid transport or proliferation will assume a growing role in the early prediction and monitoring of cancers to therapies in the coming years.

REFERENCES

1. Price P, Jones T. Can positron emission tomography (PET) be used to detect subclinical response to cancer therapy? The EC PET Oncology Concerted Action and the EORTC PET Study Group. *Eur J Cancer* 1995;31A(12):1924–1927.
2. Kubota K, Ishiwata K, Kubota R, et al. Tracer feasibility for monitoring tumor radiotherapy: a quadruple tracer study with fluorine-18-fluorodeoxyglucose or fluorine-18-fluorodeoxyuridine, L-[methyl-^{14}C]methionine, [6-^{3}H]thymidine, and gallium-67. *J Nucl Med* 1991;32:2118–2123.
3. Tjuvajev JG, Macapinilac HA, Daghighian F, et al. Imaging of brain tumor proliferative activity with iodine-131-iododeoxyuridine. *J Nucl Med* 1994;35(9):1407–1417.
4. Shields A, Grierson J, Dohmen B, et al. Imaging proliferation in vivo with [F-18]FLT and positron emission tomography. *Nat Med* 1998;4:1334–1336.
5. Anderson H, Jap J, Price P. Measurement of tumor and normal tissue perfusion by positron emission tomography (PET) in the evaluation of antivascular therapy: results in the phase I study of combretastatin A4 phosphate. *Proc Am Soc Clin Oncol* 2000;19:179a.
6. Ginos JZ, Cooper AJL, Dhawan V, et al. [^{13}N]Cisplatin PET to assess pharmacokinetics of intra-arterial versus intravenous chemotherapy for malignant brain tumors. *J Nucl Med* 1987;28:1844–1852.
7. Dimitrakopoulou-Strauss A, Strauss LG, Schlag P, et al. Fluorine-18-fluorouracil to predict therapy response in liver metastases from colorectal carcinoma. *J Nucl Med* 1998;39(7):1197–1202.
8. Hoekstra CJ, Paglianiti I, Hoekstra OS, et al. Monitoring response to therapy in cancer using [^{18}F]-2-fluoro-2-deoxy-D-glucose and positron emission tomography: an overview of different analytical methods. *Eur J Nucl Med* 2000;27(6):731–743.
9. Weber WA, Schwaiger M, Avril N. Quantitative assessment of tumor metabolism using FDG-PET imaging. *Nucl Med Biol* 2000;27(7): 683–687.
10. MacManus M, Hicks R, Wada M, et al. Early F-18 FDG-PET response to radical chemoradiotherapy correlates strongly with survival in unresectable non-small cell lung cancer. *Proc Am Soc Clin Oncol* 2000; 19:483a.
11. Young H, Baum R, Cremerius U, et al. Measurement of clinical and subclinical tumour response using [^{18}F]-fluorodeoxyglucose and positron emission tomography: review and 1999 EORTC recommendations. European Organization for Research and Treatment of Cancer (EORTC) PET Study Group. *Eur J Cancer* 1999;35(13):1773–1782.
12. Brock CS, Young H, O'Reilly SM, et al. Early evaluation of tumour metabolic response using [^{18}F]fluorodeoxyglucose and positron emission tomography: a pilot study following the phase II chemotherapy schedule for temozolomide in recurrent high-grade gliomas. *Br J Cancer* 2000;82(3):608–615.
13. Minn H, Zasadny KR, Quint LE, et al. Lung cancer: reproducibility of quantitative measurements for evaluating 2-[F-18]-fluoro-2-deoxy-D-glucose uptake at PET. *Radiology* 1995;196(1):167–173.
14. Shankar LK, Hoffman JM, Bacharach S, et al. Consensus recommendations for the use of ^{18}F-FDG PET as an indicator of therapeutic response in patients in National Cancer Institute Trials. *J Nucl Med* 2006;47(6):1059–1066.
15. Ogawa T, Uemura K, Shishido F, et al. Changes of cerebral blood flow, and oxygen and glucose metabolism following radiochemotherapy of gliomas: a PET study. *J Comput Assist Tomogr* 1988;12:290–297.
16. Kim EE, Chung SK, Haynie TP, et al. Differentiation of residual or recurrent tumors from post-treatment changes with F-18 FDG PET. *Radiographics* 1992;12:269–279.
17. Belohlavek O, Simonova G, Kantorova II, et al. Brain metastases after stereotactic radiosurgery using the Leksell gamma knife: can FDG PET help to differentiate radionecrosis from tumour progression? *Eur J Nucl Med Mol Imaging* 2003;30(1):96–100.
18. Lee JK, Liu RS, Shiang HR, et al. Usefulness of semiquantitative FDG-PET in the prediction of brain tumor treatment response to gamma knife radiosurgery. *J Comput Assist Tomogr* 2003;27(4):525–529.
19. Rozental JM, Levine RL, Mehta MP, et al. Early changes in tumor metabolism after treatment: the effects of stereotactic radiosurgery. *Int J Radiat Oncol Biol Phys* 1991;20:1053–1060.

20. De Witte O, Hildebrand J, Luxen A, et al. Acute effect of carmustine on glucose metabolism in brain and glioblastoma. *Cancer* 1994;74(10): 2836–2842.
21. Yamamoto T, Nishizawa S, Maruyama I, et al. Acute effects of stereotactic radiosurgery on the kinetics of glucose metabolism in metastatic brain tumors: FDG PET study. *Ann Nucl Med* 2001;15(2):103–109.
22. Vlassenko AG, Thiessen B, Beattie BJ, et al. Evaluation of early response to SU101 target-based therapy in patients with recurrent supratentorial malignant gliomas using FDG PET and Gd-DTPA MRI. *J Neurooncol* 2000;46(3):249–259.
23. Nuutinen J, Sonninen P, Lehikoinen P, et al. Radiotherapy treatment planning and long-term follow-up with [(^{11})C]methionine PET in patients with low-grade astrocytoma. *Int J Radiat Oncol Biol Phys* 2000;48(1):43–52.
24. Tsuyuguchi N, Sunada I, Iwai Y, et al. Methionine positron emission tomography of recurrent metastatic brain tumor and radiation necrosis after stereotactic radiosurgery: is a differential diagnosis possible? *J Neurosurg* 2003;98(5):1056–1064.
25. Van Laere K, Ceyssens S, Van Calenbergh F, et al. Direct comparison of 18F-FDG and ^{11}C-methionine PET in suspected recurrence of glioma: sensitivity, inter-observer variability and prognostic value. *Eur J Nucl Med Mol Imaging* 2005;32(1):39–51.
26. Dohmen B, Shields A, Grierson J, et al. [^{18}F]FLT-PET in brain tumors. *J Nucl Med* 2000;41:216P.
27. Eary JF, Mankoff DA, Spence AM, et al. 2-[C-^{11}]thymidine imaging of malignant brain tumors. *Cancer Res* 1999;59(3):615–621.
28. Kostakoglu L, Leonard J, Coleman M, et al. Comparison of FDG-PET and Ga-67 SPECT in staging of lymphoma. *J Nucl Med* 2000;41:118p.
29. Lin P, Chu J, Pocock N. ^{18}F Fluorodeoxyglucose imaging with coincidence dual-head gamma camera (hybrid-PET) for staging of lymphoma: comparison with Ga-67 scintigraphy. *J Nucl Med* 2000;41:118p.
30. Romer W, Hanauske A, Ziegler S, et al. Positron emission tomography in non-Hodgkin's lymphoma: assessment of chemotherapy with fluorodeoxyglucose. *Blood* 1998;91(12):4464–4471.
31. Haioun C, Itti E, Rahmouni A, et al. [^{18}F]fluoro-2-deoxy-D-glucose positron emission tomography (FDG-PET) in aggressive lymphoma: an early prognostic tool for predicting patient outcome. *Blood* 2005;106(4):1376–1381.
32. Mikhaeel NG, Hutchings M, Fields PA, et al. FDG-PET after two to three cycles of chemotherapy predicts progression-free and overall survival in high-grade non-Hodgkin lymphoma. *Ann Oncol* 2005;16(9):1514–1523.
33. Gallamini A, Rigacci L, Merli F, et al. The predictive value of positron emission tomography scanning performed after two courses of standard therapy on treatment outcome in advanced stage Hodgkin's disease. *Haematologica* 2006;91(4):475–481.
34. de Wit M, Bohuslavizki KH, Buchert R, et al. ^{18}FDG-PET following treatment as valid predictor for disease-free survival in Hodgkin's lymphoma. *Ann Oncol* 2001;12(1):29–37.
35. Jerusalem G, Beguin Y, Fassotte MF, et al. Whole-body positron emission tomography using ^{18}F-fluorodeoxyglucose for posttreatment evaluation in Hodgkin's disease and non-Hodgkin's lymphoma has higher diagnostic and prognostic value than classical computed tomography scan imaging. *Blood* 1999;94(2):429–433.
36. Cremerius U, Fabry U, Kroll U, et al. Clinical value of FDG PET for therapy monitoring of malignant lymphoma—results of a retrospective study in 72 patients. *Nuklearmedizin* 1999;38(1):24–30.
37. Guay C, Lepine M, Verreault J, et al. Prognostic value of PET using ^{18}F-FDG in Hodgkin's disease for posttreatment evaluation. *J Nucl Med* 2003;44(8):1225–1231.
38. Reinhardt MJ, Herkel C, Altehoefer C, et al. Computed tomography and ^{18}F-FDG positron emission tomography for therapy control of Hodgkin's and non-Hodgkin's lymphoma patients: when do we really need FDG-PET? *Ann Oncol* 2005;16(9):1524–1529.
39. Stumpe KD, Urbinelli M, Steinert HC, et al. Whole-body positron emission tomography using fluorodeoxyglucose for staging of lymphoma: effectiveness and comparison with computed tomography. *Eur J Nucl Med* 1998;25(7):721–728.
40. Rhodes MM, Delbeke D, Whitlock JA, et al. Utility of FDG-PET/CT in follow-up of children treated for Hodgkin and non-Hodgkin lymphoma. *J Pediatr Hematol Oncol* 2006;28(5):300–306.
41. Chaiken L, Rege S, Hoh C, et al. Positron emission tomography with fluorodeoxyglucose to evaluate tumor response and control after radiation therapy. *Int J Radiation Oncology Biol Phys* 1993;27:455–464.
42. Sakamoto H, Nakai Y, Ohashi Y, et al. Monitoring of response to radiotherapy with fluorine-18 deoxyglucose PET of head and neck squamous cell carcinomas. *Acta Otolaryngol Suppl* 1998;538:254–260.
43. Slevin NJ, Collins CD, Hastings DL, et al. The diagnostic value of positron emission tomography (PET) with radiolabelled fluorodeoxyglucose (^{18}F-FDG) in head and neck cancer. *J Laryngol Otol* 1999;113(6):548–554.
44. Haberkorn U, Strauss L, Dimitrakopoulou A, et al. Fluorodeoxyglucose imaging of advanced head and neck cancer after chemotherapy. *J Nucl Med* 1993;34:12–17.
45. Lowe V, Dunphy F, Varvares M, et al. Evaluation of chemotherapy response in patients with advanced head and neck cancer using [F-18]fluorodeoxyglucose positron emission tomography. *Head Neck* 1997;19(8):666–674.
46. Berlangieri SU, Brizel DM, Scher RL, et al. Pilot study of positron emission tomography in patients with advanced head and neck cancer receiving radiotherapy and chemotherapy. *Head Neck* 1994;16(4): 340–346.
47. Yao M, Graham MM, Smith RB, et al. Value of FDG PET in assessment of treatment response and surveillance in head-and-neck cancer patients after intensity modulated radiation treatment: a preliminary report. *Int J Radiat Oncol Biol Phys* 2004;60(5):1410–1418.
48. Andrade RS, Heron DE, Degirmenci B, et al. Posttreatment assessment of response using FDG-PET/CT for patients treated with definitive radiation therapy for head and neck cancers. *Int J Radiat Oncol Biol Phys* 2006;65(5):1315–1322.
49. Nuutinen J, Jyrkkio S, Lehikoinen P, et al. Evaluation of early response to radiotherapy in head and neck cancer measured with [^{11}C]methionine-positron emission tomography. *Radiother Oncol* 1999;52(3):225–232.
50. Lindholm P, Leskinen-Kallio S, Grenman R, et al. Evaluation of response to radiotherapy in head and neck cancer by positron emission tomography and [^{11}C]methionine. *Int J Radiat Oncol Biol Phys* 1995;32(3):787–794.
51. Wahl RL, Zasadny K, Helvie M, et al. Metabolic monitoring of breast cancer chemohormonotherapy using positron emission tomography: Initial evaluation. *J Clin Oncol* 1993;11:2101–2111.
52. Bassa P, Kim EE, Inoue T, et al. Evaluation of preoperative chemotherapy using PET with fluorine-18-fluorodeoxyglucose in breast cancer. *J Nucl Med* 1996;37:931–938.
53. Smith IC, Welch AE, Hutcheon AW, et al. Positron emission tomography using [(^{18})F]-fluorodeoxy-D-glucose to predict the pathologic response of breast cancer to primary chemotherapy. *J Clin Oncol* 2000;18(8):1676–1688.
54. Schelling M, Avril N, Nahrig J, et al. Positron emission tomography using [(^{18})F]fluorodeoxyglucose for monitoring primary chemotherapy in breast cancer. *J Clin Oncol* 2000;18(8):1689–1695.
55. Rousseau C, Devillers A, Sagan C, et al. Monitoring of early response to neoadjuvant chemotherapy in stage II and III breast cancer by [^{18}F]fluorodeoxyglucose positron emission tomography. *J Clin Oncol* 2006;24(34):5366–5372.
56. Kim SJ, Kim SK, Lee ES, et al. Predictive value of [^{18}F]FDG PET for pathological response of breast cancer to neo-adjuvant chemotherapy. *Ann Oncol* 2004;15(9):1352–1357.
57. Dose Schwarz J, Bader M, Jenicke L, et al. Early prediction of response to chemotherapy in metastatic breast cancer using sequential ^{18}F-FDG PET. *J Nucl Med* 2005;46(7):1144–1150.
58. Jansson T, Westlin JE, Ahlstrom H, et al. Positron emission tomography studies in patients with locally advanced and/or metastatic breast cancer: a method for early therapy evaluation? *J Clin Oncol* 1995;13(6):1470–1477.
59. Huovinen R, Leskinen-Kallio S, Nagren K, et al. Carbon-11-methionine and PET in evaluation of treatment response of breast cancer. *Br J Cancer* 1993(67):787–791.

60. Pio BS, Park CK, Pietras R, et al. Usefulness of 3'-[F-18]fluoro-3'-deoxythymidine with positron emission tomography in predicting breast cancer response to therapy. *Mol Imaging Biol* 2006;(8):36–42.
61. Mintun MA, Welch MJ, Siegel BA, et al. Breast cancer: PET imaging of estrogen receptors. *Radiology* 1988;169:45–48.
62. Dehdashti F, Flanagan FL, Mortimer JE, et al. Positron emission tomographic assessment of "metabolic flare" to predict response of metastatic breast cancer to antiestrogen therapy. *Eur J Nucl Med* 1999;26(1):51–56.
63. Kubota K, Yamada S, Ishiwata K, et al. Evaluation of the treatment response of lung cancer with positron emission tomography and L-[methyl-^{11}C]methionine: a preliminary study. *Eur J Nucl Med* 1993;20:495–501.
64. Hebert ME, Lowe VJ, Hoffman JM, et al. Positron emission tomography in the pretreatment evaluation and follow-up of non–small cell lung cancer patients treated with radiotherapy: preliminary findings. *Am J Clin Oncol* 1996;19(4):416–421.
65. Patz EF Jr, Connolly J, Herndon J. Prognostic value of thoracic FDG PET imaging after treatment for non–small cell lung cancer. *AJR Am J Roentgenol* 2000;174(3):769–774.
66. Bury T, Corhay JL, Duysinx B, et al. Value of FDG-PET in detecting residual or recurrent non–small cell lung cancer. *Eur Respir J* 1999;14(6):1376–1380.
67. Weber WA, Petersen V, Schmidt B, et al. Positron emission tomography in non-small-cell lung cancer: prediction of response to chemotherapy by quantitative assessment of glucose use. *J Clin Oncol* 2003;21(14): 2651–2657.
68. Mac Manus MP, Hicks RJ, Matthews JP, et al. Metabolic (FDG-PET) response after radical radiotherapy/chemoradiotherapy for non-small cell lung cancer correlates with patterns of failure. *Lung Cancer* 2005;49(1):95–108.
69. Hicks RJ, Mac Manus MP, Matthews JP, et al. Early FDG-PET imaging after radical radiotherapy for non–small-cell lung cancer: inflammatory changes in normal tissues correlate with tumor response and do not confound therapeutic response evaluation. *Int J Radiat Oncol Biol Phys* 2004;60(2):412–418.
70. Cerfolio RJ, Bryant AS, Winokur TS, et al. Repeat FDG-PET after neoadjuvant therapy is a predictor of pathologic response in patients with non–small cell lung cancer. *Ann Thorac Surg* 2004;78(6):1903–1909; discussion 1909.
71. Pottgen C, Levegrun S, Theegarten D, et al. Value of ^{18}F-fluoro-2-deoxy-D-glucose-positron emission tomography/computed tomography in non–small-cell lung cancer for prediction of pathologic response and times to relapse after neoadjuvant chemoradiotherapy. *Clin Cancer Res* 2006;12(1):97–106.
72. Yamamoto Y, Nishiyama Y, Monden T, et al. Correlation of FDG-PET findings with histopathology in the assessment of response to induction chemoradiotherapy in non–small cell lung cancer. *Eur J Nucl Med Mol Imaging* 2006;33(2):140–147.
73. Shields AF, Mankoff DA, Link JM, et al. [^{11}C]Thymidine and FDG to measure therapy response. *J Nucl Med* 1998;39:1757–1762.
74. Koh WJ, Bergman KS, Rasey JS, et al. Evaluation of oxygenation status during fractionated radiotherapy in human non–small cell lung cancers using [F-18]fluoromisonidazole positron emission tomography. *Int J Radiat Oncol Biol Phys* 1995;33(2):391–398.
75. Findlay M, Young H, Cunningham D, et al. Noninvasive monitoring of tumor metabolism using fluorodeoxyglucose and positron emission tomography in colorectal cancer liver metastases: correlation with tumor response to fluorouracil. *J Clin Oncol* 1996;14(3):700–708.
76. Haberkorn U, Strauss LG, Dimitrakopoulou A, et al. PET studies of fluorodeoxyglucose metabolism in patients with recurrent colorectal tumors receiving radiotherapy. *J Nucl Med* 1991;32(8):1485–1490.
77. Wieder H, Ott K, Zimmermann F, et al. PET imaging with [^{11}C]methyl-L-methionine for therapy monitoring in patients with rectal cancer. *Eur J Nucl Med Mol Imaging* 2002;29(6):789–796.
78. Couper GW, McAteer D, Wallis F, et al. Detection of response to chemotherapy using positron emission tomography in patients with oesophageal and gastric cancer. *Br J Surg* 1998;85(10):1403–1406.
79. Ott K, Weber WA, Lordick F, et al. Metabolic imaging predicts response, survival, and recurrence in adenocarcinomas of the esophagogastric junction. *J Clin Oncol* 2006;24(29):4692–4698.
80. Jager PL, Gietema JA, van der Graaf WT. Imatinib mesylate for the treatment of gastrointestinal stromal tumours: best monitored with FDG PET. *Nucl Med Commun* 2004;25(5):433–438.
81. Stroobants S, Goeminne J, Seegers M, et al. ^{18}FDG-Positron emission tomography for the early prediction of response in advanced soft tissue sarcoma treated with imatinib mesylate (Glivec). *Eur J Cancer* 2003;39(14):2012–2020.
82. Gayed I, Vu T, Iyer R, et al. The role of ^{18}F-FDG PET in staging and early prediction of response to therapy of recurrent gastrointestinal stromal tumors. *J Nucl Med* 2004;45(1):17–21.
83. Antoch G, Kanja J, Bauer S, et al. Comparison of PET, CT, and dual-modality PET/CT imaging for monitoring of imatinib (STI571) therapy in patients with gastrointestinal stromal tumors. *J Nucl Med* 2004;45(3):357–365.
84. Goldstein D, Tan BS, Rossleigh M, et al. Gastrointestinal stromal tumours: correlation of F-FDG gamma camera-based coincidence positron emission tomography with CT for the assessment of treatment response—an AGITG study. *Oncology* 2005;69(4):326–332.
85. Goh BK, Chow PK, Chuah KL, et al. Pathologic, radiologic and PET scan response of gastrointestinal stromal tumors after neoadjuvant treatment with imatinib mesylate. *Eur J Surg Oncol* 2006;32(9): 961–963.
86. Schuetze SM, Rubin BP, Vernon C, et al. Use of positron emission tomography in localized extremity soft tissue sarcoma treated with neoadjuvant chemotherapy. *Cancer* 2005;103(2):339–348.
87. Effert PJ, Bares R, Handt S, et al. Metabolic imaging of untreated prostate cancer by positron emission tomography with 18fluorine-labeled deoxyglucose. *J Urol* 1996;155(3):994–948.
88. Kao CH, Hsieh JF, Tsai SC, et al. Comparison and discrepancy of ^{18}F-2-deoxyglucose positron emission tomography and Tc-99m MDP bone scan to detect bone metastases. *Anticancer Res* 2000;20(3B):2189–2192.
89. Kurdziel K, Bacharach S, Carrasquillo J, et al. Using PET ^{18}F-FDG, ^{11}CO, and ^{15}O-water for monitoring prostate cancer during a phase II anti-angiogenic drug trial with thalidomide. *Clin Positron Imaging* 2000;3:144.
90. DeGrado TR, Coleman RE, Wang S, et al. Synthesis and evaluation of ^{18}F-labeled choline as an oncologic tracer for positron emission tomography: initial findings in prostate cancer. *Cancer Res* 2001;61(1):110–117.
91. Stephens AW, Gonin R, Hutchins GD, et al. Positron emission tomography evaluation of residual radiographic abnormalities in postchemotherapy germ cell tumor patients. *J Clin Oncol* 1996;14(5): 1637–1641.
92. Sugawara Y, Zasadny KR, Grossman HB, et al. Germ cell tumor: differentiation of viable tumor, mature teratoma, and necrotic tissue with FDG PET and kinetic modeling. *Radiology* 1999;211(1):249–256.
93. Avril N, Sassen S, Schmalfeldt B, et al. Prediction of response to neoadjuvant chemotherapy by sequential F-18-fluorodeoxyglucose positron emission tomography in patients with advanced-stage ovarian cancer. *J Clin Oncol* 2005;23(30):7445–7453.
94. Letocha H, Ahlstrom H, Malmstrom PU, et al. Positron emission tomography with L-methyl-^{11}C-methionine in the monitoring of therapy response in muscle-invasive transitional cell carcinoma of the urinary bladder. *Br J Urol* 1994;74(6):767–774.

CHAPTER 8.5

PET and PET/CT in Radiation Oncology

MICHAEL P. MAC MANUS AND RODNEY J. HICKS

Most patients with malignant disease require radiation therapy at some point in their illness. At many institutions, more than one half of all radiation therapy treatments are given with "radical" or curative intent (often described as "definitive" radiation therapy in the United States), although the proportion varies widely by country, treatment center, and by disease type (1). Cure rates for cancers treated primarily with definitive radiation or chemoradiation show wide variation according to disease type and stage. For example, more than 80% of patients with early stage nodular lymphocyte predominant Hodgkin lymphoma may be cured with radiation therapy alone (2), whereas, for anaplastic thyroid cancer, fewer than 5% of patients will survive for 5 years despite aggressive concurrent chemoradiation (3).

Long-term survival rates for most cancers treated with definitive radiation therapy fall between these extremes, and appropriate patient selection is essential to ensure that this potentially life-saving but frequently toxic form of therapy is administered only to those who are most likely to benefit from it. Early relapse with metastatic disease after aggressive local therapy is generally the result of a failure of the staging process to identify the true extent of disease prior to treatment. Patients with *a priori* incurable disease are generally better served by palliative therapies, which can often include low-dose radiation therapy for local symptom relief.

When curative or definitive radiation therapy is being considered, most often for patients with a solid tumor that is considered unresectable or where radiation offers the best chance of cure with organ preservation, the radiation oncologist needs to know a number of key pieces of information. These include:

1. Does the patient have distant metastasis that would make curative therapy futile?
2. Does the patient have nodal disease, and if so, is the disease of an extent that can be treated using radiation with curative intent?
3. What is the distribution of all gross tumor in three-dimensional space in relation to the anatomy of normal tissues?

This essential information can often be obtained only by accurate imaging, placing radiologists and nuclear medicine physicians squarely at the center of patient selection and treatment planning for many cancers. Of course, other information such as pathology reports, clinical examination, and endoscopy results may provide crucial additional information, depending on the clinical situation, but imaging is usually the foundation for patient selection and treatment planning.

Every physician knows that high doses of ionizing radiation can cause severe toxicity to normal tissues. The risk of significant treatment-related morbidity or even mortality is determined by the intrinsic radiosensitivity of the organs that are irradiated, by the volume of normal tissue exposed to radiation, and by the dose and fractionation of the radiation that is administered. Modern computed tomography (CT)-based radiation therapy treatment planning systems allow accurate estimates of normal tissue irradiation by providing dose-volume histograms for organs at risk and thereby facilitating the production of treatment plans that minimize unnecessary irradiation of normal tissues.

An ideal treatment plan is one that delivers a killing dose of radiation to the tumor but no dose at all to the normal tissues. The closest approximation to this impossible ideal may be achieved theoretically by using a proton beam to deliver therapy (4), but in conventional clinical practice carefully shaped and modulated photon beams can produce highly conformal treatment plans with acceptable levels of normal tissue irradiation.

Accurate treatment planning is dependent on knowledge of the true tumor location in three-dimensional space. A complex and expensive multifield radiotherapy treatment course is a futile exercise if high-dose radiation is not delivered to the entire tumor volume or if the patient is incapacitated by toxicity resulting from unnecessary irradiation of normal tissues. Unfortunately, in the pre–positron emission tomography (PET) era, many treatments were delivered to volumes that did not include all gross tumor and consequently were doomed to failure from the outset. It is probable that in many of these cases incorporation of PET information into treatment planning might have avoided a catastrophic geographic miss.

Radiation therapy technology has improved vastly in recent years and will continue to do so in the foreseeable future (5). Our ability to quantify dose to volumes of normal tissues is a significant advance (6) and has been accompanied by an increased ability to treat complex three-dimensional shapes. Linear accelerators with independently controlled multileaf collimators can deliver highly conformal treatments to complex target volumes (7), often making use of complex planning methods such as intensity modulated radiation therapy (IMRT) (8), which enable the radiation oncologist to simultaneously increase tumor dose and reduce normal tissue dose. More sophisticated devices with names like tomotherapy and the Gamma Knife (Elekta Corp, Stockholm) or CyberKnife (Accuray, Sunnyvale, California) deliver highly localized radiation doses, but require very precise image-guided direction. This can lead to improvements in local disease control (9) or facilitate maintenance of a high cure rate with a reduction in toxicity (10), as in some head and neck cancers where parotid-sparing techniques can often avoid permanent xerostomia.

Advances in radiation therapy have increased the need for accurate tumor imaging. The advent of clinical PET, with its vastly superior ability to image many common types of cancer, has coincided with these developments in radiation therapy and has opened up new possibilities for the integration of the best available imaging with the best available radiation therapy. The integration of PET into radiation therapy staging and treatment planning paradigms is becoming increasingly commonplace. Lung cancer is the disease for which PET is best characterized both for patient selection and for treatment planning in radiation therapy patients. Therefore, we will often refer to the literature on lung cancer to illustrate general principles of the use of PET in radiation oncology, but these principles may frequently be applied to other cancers, bearing in mind the significant biological and therapeutic differences that exist between different malignancies. It also must be emphasized that this field is in rapid evolution with extension of PET methods into treatment planning for a broad spectrum of cancers.

PET AND PET/CT IN PATIENT SELECTION FOR CURATIVE RADIATION THERAPY

General Principles

For many common cancer types, patient management is determined primarily by the stage of disease at presentation. Demonstration of extensive nodal disease might make surgery inappropriate for a patient and lead to consideration of radical radiation therapy. In turn, demonstration of distant metastatic disease might indicate that radical radiation therapy would be futile. In rare cases, demonstration of a solitary metastasis might lead to an attempt at cure by treating the local and distant disease aggressively.

PET scanning, using fluorine-18-fluorodeoxyglucose ([^{18}F]-FDG) as the tracer, has rapidly acquired a key role in the staging of cancers that are commonly treated with radiation therapy, such as non–small cell lung cancer (NSCLC) (11,12), Hodgkin and non-Hodgkin's lymphomas (13,14), head and neck cancers, esophageal cancers (15,16), and cervical carcinomas (17,18). FDG-PET is also of clear value in selected patients with high-risk malignant melanoma (19,20), breast cancer, soft tissue sarcoma (21), gastrointestinal cancers (22), and a range of less common neoplasms (23,24).

The more recent advent of PET/CT has been a major advance and is of particular value to radiation oncologists because PET/CT displays metabolic activity denoting active tumor in the context of exquisite anatomical detail. PET/CT images are ideal for clinical staging, as they allow appropriate assignment of focal areas of tracer uptake to the correct anatomical structure, thereby facilitating identification of subtle lymph node and distant metastases.

The PET/CT images themselves are often the best available starting points for radiation therapy planning for FDG-avid tumors, provided the images are captured with appropriate patient positioning. Although markedly superior to PET alone, the advent of PET/CT is an incremental advance on stand-alone PET and does not make the large body of clinical information already obtained with PET or PET plus separately acquired CT any less valuable or relevant.

FDG is currently the most generally useful cancer staging pharmaceutical. However, other PET tracers may be valuable in imaging tumors that have a low uptake of FDG or are located within or near organs with high FDG uptake. For example, [^{18}F]-labeled fluoroethylcholine PET may be effective in imaging prostate cancer in patients planned for high-dose radiation therapy. PET may help to identify lesions that are actively proliferating, using [^{18}F]-labeled fluorothymidine (25) and thereby may distinguish between some inflammatory and neoplastic conditions. This may be of great value when planning radiation therapy for patients with coexistent cancers and inflammatory conditions, such as lung cancer and sarcoidosis, but this warrants further study, as proliferation can occur in nonmalignant tissues as well.

Tumors that are hypoxic tend to be more resistant to radiation and may be identified by PET imaging using [^{18}F]-labeled misonidazole or [^{18}F]-fluoro-azomycin arabinoside (FAZA) as tracers (26). In the future PET hypoxia imaging may be used to help select radioresistant tumors for higher total radiation doses or to guide the delivery of higher doses to hypoxic regions (so-called dose painting) or to identify patients who might benefit from hypoxic cell sensitizers or cytotoxins (26). Despite these interesting exceptions, almost all of the useful clinical trials of PET with relevance to radiation therapy relate to FDG as the tracer.

Much of the strongest evidence that is used to support the use of PET in staging prior to radiation therapy comes from clinicopathological studies of surgical candidates who proceeded to surgical staging after PET. These patients had pathological confirmation of the true tumor extent and nodal involvement and were good tests of the accuracy of preoperative PET. Surgical staging studies have uniformly shown that inclusion of PET in the staging work-up makes preoperative evaluation much more accurate, especially for nodal evaluation of common epithelial malignancies such as lung cancer and esophageal cancer.

There are some dangers in directly extrapolating results from imaging studies of patients with surgical resectable tumors (predominantly early stage with relatively low risk of distant metastasis) to patients who are candidates for radiation therapy for unresectable locoregional disease (more advanced disease with a relatively high risk of distant metastases).

Bayesian principles and indeed the available clinical data both show that the probability of upstaging by PET is greatest in patients already known to have more advanced tumors. Surgical studies may actually underestimate the potential value of PET in patients with more advanced disease. In some neoplasms, such as esophageal carcinoma, small nodes close to an intensely FDG-avid primary tumor may be impossible to visualize on PET due to spill over of activity from the primary, thereby reducing the sensitivity and specificity of PET for such nodes. For radiation therapy planning this may not be a significant problem because these nodes would routinely be included in the high-dose volume in any case.

Relatively few PET staging studies have been published that have focused on patients with known unresectable disease who were candidates for radical radiation therapy. This is, in part, because pathological confirmation is usually unavailable in patients considered unsuitable for radical surgery, making it difficult to tell if the pretreatment PET was accurate or not. Indeed, invasive staging procedures are usually considered inappropriate and unethical in such patients if they involve any significant risk. Even demonstration of superior accuracy in surgical patients may not be sufficient to prove the utility of PET in radiation oncology patients with more advanced manifestations of the same disease, to the satisfaction of reviewers tasked with advising governments on the utility of new health technology. Some reviewers may inappropriately apply "evidence-based medicine" assessment techniques designed for therapies rather than imaging, demanding surgical staging as "high-level" evidence in nonsurgical patients. Evidence-based medicine is the gold standard only if the most appropriate types of evidence are considered. There may be reluctance to fund PET for radiation therapy patients who have conditions where surgical staging is not usually carried out because of the circular argument that no surgical staging information is available for this particular patient group to prove that PET is more accurate than standard imaging tests. This issue with PET applications in radiation oncology is quite similar to those faced with moving PET forward to clinical practice in tumor staging and treatment response assessment in the past few years, and likely will be increasingly overcome as the performance characteristics of PET are increasingly appreciated.

In a large prospective study of PET staging in patients with NSCLC who were candidates for radical radiation therapy at the Peter MacCallum Cancer Centre, which is discussed further below in the section "Lung Cancer," the authors attempted to overcome this difficulty by studying survival after PET. The hypothesis of the study was that if PET truly does increase the accuracy of staging, then survival and freedom from progression will be predicted better by a staging work-up that included PET than by conventional staging. In that study the authors found that the overall staging groupings (stage I, II, III, and so forth) determined without PET were a rather poor predictor of survival (27).

Stage groupings determined with the aid of PET were often very different from the CT-based groupings, and PET stage predicted survival much more accurately than CT (P = .0001). These data confirmed that PET could be highly predictive of survival in a large patient population. To show a benefit of PET in such a population, it was irrelevant if the accuracy of any individual lesion was determined by biopsy or not, because the purpose of staging is to predict survival. A confirmatory study was performed at the authors' center in esophageal cancer, again showing that PET-based stage was a much more accurate predictor of survival than CT-based staging (28).

Detection of Distant Metastasis

Solid tumors that have spread beyond the local lymphatics to involve distant sites are almost always considered incurable with radiation therapy, although in rare cases, such as a solitary brain metastasis, patients may experience long-term survival after aggressive treatment of both primary and metastatic disease. Simply by helping to exclude incurable patients with distant metastasis from futile radiation therapy, PET can apparently achieve better outcomes in those patients who proceed to treatment after PET staging (29). This is an effect of stage migration. PET has the greatest impact in cancers, like lung cancer, where most patients present with disease that already appears locoregionally advanced on conventional imaging. These patients have a high probability of being upstaged to incurable locoregionally advanced or distant metastatic disease by PET.

PET identified distant metastases at a significantly greater rate in patients with mediastinal nodal disease compared to those with apparently earlier stage disease in a series of NSCLC patients from the Peter MacCallum Cancer Centre. The incidence of PET-detected metastasis was 7% in those with apparent stage I disease, 18% in apparent stage II, and 24% in apparent stage III. As the majority of candidates for radical radiation therapy have stage III disease, the impact of PET is greatest in radiation therapy patients compared to surgical candidates who mainly have stage I disease and have a rate of detection of distant metastasis of around 5%. PET-detected metastases were associated with relatively short survival, although those with a single distant metastasis had far superior survival to those with two or more (30).

Lymph Node Staging

Lymph node staging is crucial for many cancers treated with radiation therapy, both for patient selection and for treatment planning. Extensive nodal involvement may be impossible to treat safely or may have such a poor prognosis that aggressive radiation therapy would be futile. Historically, CT has been the most widely used noninvasive method for detecting intrathoracic lymph node metastasis in NSCLC and many other cancers. Survival in NSCLC is powerfully correlated with lymph node staging and drops precipitously when mediastinal nodes contain tumor (25). Because reactive lymphadenopathy is common in lung cancer and because tumor is often present in nodes with a short axis smaller than 1 cm, a commonly used criterion for nodes considered to be positive for tumor, CT has low sensitivity and specificity for the detection of thoracic lymph nodes involved by tumor (31).

The accuracy of FDG-PET in staging the intrathoracic lymph nodes in NSCLC has been directly estimated in numerous clinicopathological studies. In all of these studies (32–37), including a meta-analysis (38), PET has been shown to be more accurate than CT for staging the mediastinum. The best noninvasive results have been obtained by correlating the results of both PET and CT images (36). The results of these clinicopathological staging studies are of great importance for radiation oncologists. They conclusively prove that when PET is used in addition to CT to evaluate intrathoracic nodes for malignancy, the accuracy of the assessment is significantly greater than for CT alone.

Although it is impossible to state with certainty that PET is accurate in the assessment of any single node without excisional biopsy, it is clear that in NSCLC, treatment planning based on PET/CT is on average much more likely to be accurate that treatment planning based on CT alone.

Upstaging of nodal disease by PET is also commonly seen in esophageal cancer (39,40), with important implications for radiation therapy when nodes are more distant than the paraesophageal nodal station, as discussed further below, although evaluation for distant metastasis may be even more accurate (41). PET increases the detection rate of gross nodal involvement in locoregionally advanced malignant melanoma (42,43), for which radiation therapy is often an important component of therapy, especially in the head and neck area. However, unlike sentinel node biopsy, PET does not reliably detect microscopic disease (44) in melanoma, and it is therefore rarely useful in stage I or II disease. PET may also provide crucial information on the nodal status of patients with head and neck cancer (45) or breast cancer (46), with implications for the use of radiation therapy.

INTEGRATION OF PET AND PET/CT INTO THE RADIATION THERAPY PLANNING

Process

Complex three-dimensional radiation therapy is conventionally planned using data acquired from a dedicated CT scanner. This provides both essential three-dimensional anatomic information and a three dimensional electron-density map, crucial for calculating radiation absorption and scatter. Although necessary for dose calculation in radiation oncology, CT by itself often provides insufficient information on the anatomic extent of tumor to allow accurate contouring of disease. To image the boundaries of a neoplastic lesion successfully on CT, there must be sufficient contrast between the lesion and normal tissues.

When tumors have similar imaging characteristics to surrounding normal tissues, as is often the case for lesions in the liver or spleen, they may be completely invisible on CT. Consequently, when CT is used to guide curative radiation therapy, geographic miss and ultimate treatment failure may be inevitable. Failure to image the boundary between tumor and atelectatic lung is a common problem for the radiation oncologist relying on CT for treating lung cancer and may lead to unnecessary irradiation of large volumes of collapsed lung in order to avoid a geographic miss.

As discussed above, accurate lymph node staging is also crucial for treating such locoregionally advanced cancers with curative intent (47,48), and CT scanning is often inadequate because of the unreliability of lymph node size as a predictor of involvement (49). In the absence of any better noninvasive method of staging, for many cancers CT has historically been the nearest thing to a gold standard for radiotherapy planning, albeit a flawed one.

In the years since the introduction of clinical PET, its importance as a tool for radiation therapy planning has become increasingly recognized (50). Manufacturers have become aware of the need to accommodate the importation and display of PET information in radiotherapy planning systems. They have produced systems capable of allowing seamless integration of PET/CT information into the radiation therapy (RT) contouring workstation.

When PET and CT imaging are combined for radiotherapy planning, the aim is to produce a biological target volume (BTV) (51), incorporating all available structural and functional imaging. At the authors' center, the PET/CT scanner suite has had identical laser positioning devices fitted to those in our simulator and linear accelerator suite, ensuring reproducibility of patient setup for PET/CT, simulation, and treatment. After a treatment planning PET/CT scan is carried out with the patient in the radiotherapy treatment position with appropriate immobilization devices fitted, CT and PET data are imported into the treatment planning software. For centers without PET/CT, separate acquisitions of PET and CT must be carried out with the same rigorous patient positioning.

After the patient's PET/CT data are loaded into the radiation therapy treatment planning workstation, the next step is the contouring of tumor and normal tissues. Regions of tumor are identified and contoured by the radiation oncologist using a pointing device on individual PET/CT slices. Consultation with a nuclear medicine physician is highly recommended to clarify the tumor extent on the scans. The contouring process generates a gross tumor volume (GTV) (52). To ensure reproducibility, uniform rules for setting of the thresholds for the normal tissue background are applied when contouring, and a consistent approach is taken to determine the involvement of individual nodes.

In lung cancer, for example, small (less than 1 cm) nodes are included within the target volume if they are qualitatively FDG avid, but larger nodes are routinely excluded at the authors' center if they are negative on PET, provided the primary tumor is FDG avid. Some centers include such nodes, thus typically expanding the GTV with PET. Contouring of normal tissues on individual CT slices allows the radiation dose delivered to important dose-limiting organs to be assessed quantitatively.

The volume that actually needs to be irradiated to the prescribed dose in radical radiation therapy is of course greater than the GTV, because additional margins must be applied. These margins allow for a range of factors, including microscopic extension of disease beyond the imaged tumor, variability in the accuracy of patient setup on each day of treatment, and movement of the tumor, for example, with respiration. The margins applied to the GTV are disease and site specific.

The volume that the radiation oncologist decides to treat, which incorporates all of the margins around the GTV, is known as the planning target volume (PTV). The PTV is often an expansion of the GTV, generated automatically by the treatment planning software. An ideal PTV should include all gross and microscopic tumor (or at least microscopic tumor that will not be eliminated by systemic therapy) and be large enough to accommodate movement of the tumor during treatment (internal target volume [ITV]) (53).

A variable number of individually shaped and modulated megavoltage photon beams is then chosen from a virtually infinite range of beam sizes shapes and angles. Often using human trial and error, a treatment plan emerges that aims to treat all parts of the PTV with the prescribed dose, or close to the prescribed dose, while exposing adjacent healthy normal tissues to the minimum radiation dose. The dose delivered to normal tissues is "dumped" in regions where it will do least harm. When IMRT is used, the optimization of the treatment plan is carried out by the computer, after a complex series of parameters are set. Of course, the plan must be approved by the treating physician after all data are processed.

The most important step in the entire process is the determination of the GTV. If the location of gross tumor in three-dimensional space is not accurately known and a geographic miss occurs, then treatment will have been a complex, toxic, and futile exercise. Although it must be acknowledged that PET information is not always accurate and that PET cannot detect microscopic disease, for many tumor types PET provides such a significant increase in the accuracy of assessment of the tumor extent that failure to use it would mean denying the patient the best chance for successful radiation therapy planning.

There are two main approaches to contouring the edges of tumors on PET/CT. The first, which is preferred at the authors' institution, is to use a standardized visual approach, where the radiation oncologist manually draws the contour using uniform window and color settings with a rigorous contouring protocol, as discussed above. This relies on the intelligence, experience, and training of the operator, who has knowledge of the tumor type, probability of significant tumor movement during image acquisition, overall accuracy of PET scanning interpretation at the parent institution, heterogeneity of FDG uptake in the tumor, and a range of other factors that can confound the interpretation of the images.

The second approach to contouring recognizes that visual methods can suffer from unacceptable variability due to human factors and makes use of the quantitative information available

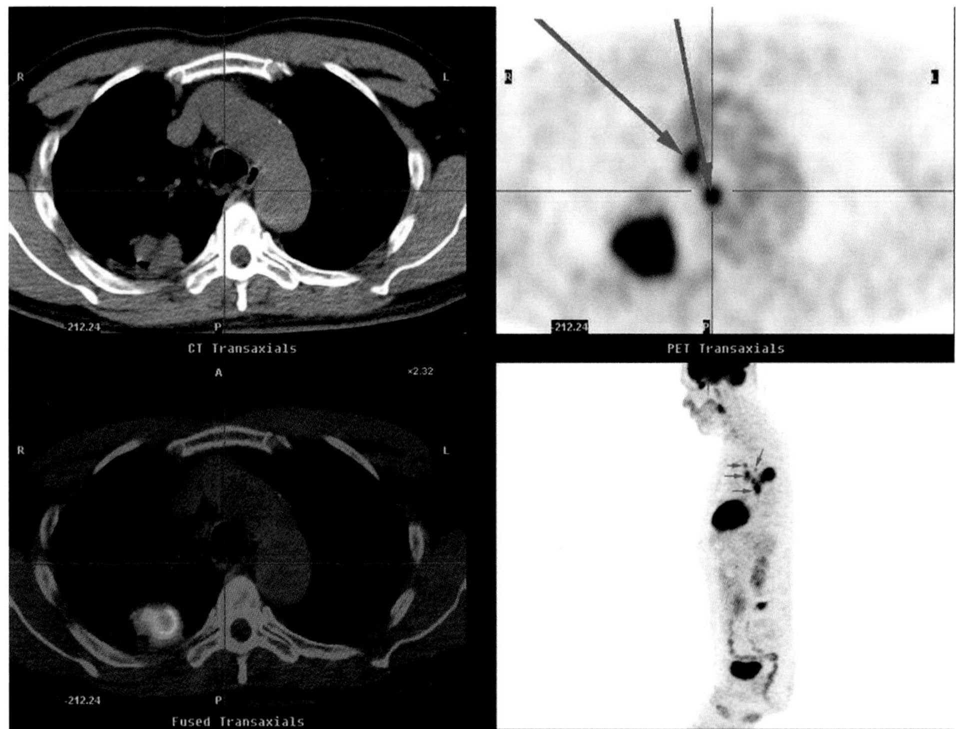

FIGURE 8.5.1. Although less intense than enlarged nodes in the left pulmonary hilum and subcarinal nodal stations, contiguous nodal abnormality in the aortopulmonary window and paratracheal lymph node stations (*large arrows*) at the level of the aortic arch in this case are highly suggestive of malignant nodal involvement. The lower fluorodeoxyglucose uptake (standard uptake value [SUV] <2.5) in these nodes likely reflects partial volume effects and emphasizes the problem with relying on SUV thresholds, rather than pattern recognition, for determining the nature of nodal abnormalities. The transaxial extent of nodal disease is well demonstrated on the lateral MIP image (*small arrows*) and was used for radiotherapy planning in this case. Images show CT alone (upper left), PET alone (upper right), fused PET and CT (lower left) and lateral PET image (lower right).

from PET. Various automated or semiautomated approaches are being tried for tumor contouring (51,54–56). None of these methods has yet proven to be a comprehensive solution to the problem and gained wide acceptance (57). Nevertheless, static phantoms can be effectively contoured using such methods (53). Unfortunately, FDG uptake in humans is not only a consequence of malignant processes, but can result from a range of inflammatory and physiological conditions that no computer software can recognize. Fortunately, the morphology of many of these processes can be readily recognized by an experienced physician (e.g., uptake in brown fat or muscle, sarcoidosis, and so forth).

At the authors' center, given the relatively crude nature of the available automated contouring algorithms, the reliance on a simple computational solution, such as a standard uptake value (SUV) cutoff (58), would guarantee reproducibility only at the expense of a decrease in accuracy (Fig. 8.5.1). To use such a method clinically, each computer-derived tumor contour should be carefully and intelligently analyzed and, if necessary, edited by the radiation oncologist, who bears final responsibility for the integrity of the planning process. In a worst-case scenario, small FDG-avid nodes could be excluded from the target volume because they had low measured SUV due to partial volume effects if a solely SUV-driven algorithm was used.

Movement

The region of three-dimensional space within which a lesion moves can be referred to as the internal target volume (53,56), a feature that is often well appreciated on PET scanning because of its long acquisition time. Metabolically active lesions usually appear qualitatively elongated in the axes of respiratory movement compared to their true dimensions, reflecting temporal blurring of activity, unless the CT image is acquired using some form of gating. FDG activity tends to be less intense at the extremes of movement in those axial planes where the tumor spends proportionally less time. The PET-determined volume thus indicates most clearly the region of space where a tumor spends the most time, although it may not accurately reflect the extremes of movement. This is a better situation than a single randomly acquired CT image, which takes no account of movement whatsoever. A treatment centered on the PET-determined tumor volume is more likely to be aimed correctly (59,60) than one determined using conventional CT planning. In the future, treatments may be further improved by gated acquisition of PET images combined with gated treatment delivery to enhance accuracy and reduce normal tissue radiation exposure (60).

ROLE OF PET IN RADIATION THERAPY PLANNING IN SPECIFIC TUMOR SITES

Lung Cancer

Significantly improved survival has already been demonstrated in patients with NSCLC selected for radical RT using PET compared to a conventionally staged control group (29), largely because patients with PET-detected metastases and advanced locoregional disease were denied futile aggressive therapy. Lung cancer is the malignancy in which PET has had the greatest impact on selection of patients for radiotherapy and on radiotherapy planning (61). This relates both to the clarity of imaging of a metabolically active cancer in a location favorable for PET and to the high rate of incremental abnormal findings seen on PET, compared to conventional imaging (62).

As discussed above, there is an abundance of evidence from surgical series, with systematic clinicopathological correlation, proving that PET is much more accurate than CT in the assessment of thoracic lymph nodes, especially when CT and PET information are combined (38). These data are routinely extrapolated to radiotherapy candidates for whom mediastinoscopy is not usually performed if the patient clearly has unresectable disease on the basis of CT findings or is medically unfit for surgery, although an even higher incidence of true positivity would be expected in those already known to have more advanced disease before PET (63).

Detection of incurable systemic metastatic disease routinely prevents futile aggressive attempts at cure (30).

PET for Selection of Patients with Non–small Cell Lung Cancer for Radical Radiation Therapy

In a large prospective study at the Peter MacCallum Cancer Centre, 153 patients with NSCLC, all of whom were suitable candidates for radical RT on the basis of clinical assessment and conventional imaging, underwent PET scanning (27). PET data were used for patient selection for radical RT and were also used to assist with RT planning in those who remained suitable. In that study, after PET, 30% of patients were considered unsuitable for radical RT because they had distant metastases (20%) or thoracic disease too extensive for radical irradiation (10%). Patients rejected for radical RT after PET were considered suitable only for palliative therapies and had very poor survival, but the remaining patients had very good survival after aggressive therapy.

A comparison of a prospective PET staged cohort treated with radical RT/chemo RT with a comparable group of patients, treated similarly in a phase III trial without PET staging at the same institution, showed that PET staged patients had significantly better survival (29). It is likely that this was primarily an effect of superior patient selection with exclusion of those with distant metastases from radical therapy (64). However, the superior outcomes could also have reflected, in part, superior treatment delivery in those deemed still suitable for treatment with curative intent.

Published Studies of PET in Radiotherapy Planning in Lung Cancer

NSCLC is the malignancy where the effect of PET on RT planning has been most intensively studied and where PET has had the greatest impact. Despite this fact, knowledge in this area is still limited, and no convincing data have yet been published that demonstrate superior outcomes due to incorporation of PET into RT planning, beyond the effects of superior patient selection. This is, however, an area of intensive study, and all published studies indicate that target volumes determined using PET or PET/CT are often very different from those determined using CT alone. The greatest impact arises in patients for whom PET shows different lymph node status from CT, most commonly upstaging the extent of apparent nodal disease (65). A high impact is also seen in patients with atelectasis, where the boundary between tumor and collapsed or consolidated lung may only be identified with the aid of PET (66).

A number have studies have tried to quantify the impact of PET on RT planning in NSCLC. In the authors' earliest study, PET rather that PET/CT was used and there was no ability to coregister images (27). Despite those limitations 22 of 102 patients had a significant increase in RT target volumes to cover new sites of disease seen only on PET. In 16 patients, the target volume was reduced because regions of bland atelectasis could be excluded or enlarged nodes proved not to be FDG avid.

In 1998, Nestle et al. (66) reported that a significant increase in the radiation field was required to cover PET detected disease in 9% of 34 patients, but a significant decrease was seen in 26%, especially those with atelectasis. Munley et al. (67) recorded that 35% of 35 patients had an increase in the RT field as a result of PET. In a larger study of 73 patients, Vanuytzel et al. (68) found that there was an increase in GTV in 22% of patients and a decrease in 40%. Other significant studies include work by Bradley et al. (69) who used coregistered sequential PET and CT scans and reported increased GTV in 46% and reduced GTV in 12%. Brianzoni et al. (70) reported that GTV/CTV was increased in 44% and reduced in 6% of 24 patients with lung cancer when RT was planned using a dedicated PET/CT scanner.

Head and Neck Cancer

Epithelial cancers of the head and neck, the great majority of them squamous carcinomas, are often curable with high-dose radical RT. They are usually metabolically active and therefore can be well imaged by PET (Fig. 8.5.2) in addition to CT and magnetic resonance imaging (MRI). Fusion of PET with MRI is feasible (71) and may have clinical utility in these tumors. In addition to delineating the primary tumor, PET can be very helpful in staging the neck (72,73), especially when there is FDG uptake in normal-sized lymph nodes (74). PET may also detect unsuspected second cancers (75). In patients with locoregionally advanced disease, PET may also detect unsuspected distant metastases, indicating that the disease is incurable.

When PET is used to determine a radiotherapy target volume in head and neck cancer, the situation is complex (76). The boundaries of primary tumors can differ significantly from one another in the same patient when determined using PET, CT, or MRI (77), making it difficult to decide exactly where to draw the GTV for radiotherapy planning, although PET is probably the most accurate single modality (78). In head and neck cancers, this is an especially important issue because very high doses of radiation (70 Gy) are commonly delivered to lesions close to radiosensitive vital structures such as the brainstem or optic chiasm, and consequently radiotherapy margins are often tight around the tumor. Immobilization techniques allow treatment at these sites to be delivered with millimeter accuracy, and it is essential that tumor margins are well appreciated (71).

Careful comparison of FDG-PET, MRI, and CT scans with the histopathology of resected tumor specimens shows that none of these three imaging modalities is completely accurate. PET adds extremely useful incremental information to conventional imaging and clinical assessment, and all available imaging and pathological staging information should be considered when planning target volumes in head and neck cancers. PET may not yet be ready for routinely determining target volumes in RT for head and neck cancer but should remain an area for active research.

PET scanning using bioreductive agents such as [^{18}F]-fluoromisonidazole (FMISO) and FAZA can image hypoxia in a majority of advanced epithelial head and neck cancers. FMISO uptake can be used to predict response to chemoradiation regimens that include the hypoxic cell toxin tirapazamine. Tumors with imageable hypoxia respond better to a tirapazamine-containing regimen, while those without hypoxia may respond better to conventional chemoradiation (26).

Esophageal Cancer

Esophageal cancers are usually locally or regionally advanced at presentation, and only a tiny percentage of patients can be cured by surgery alone. Concurrent platinum-based chemoradiation with or without surgery is commonly used to treat this disease, and it significantly increases overall survival and cure rates compared to radiotherapy alone. As with lung cancer, CT is usually relied on to determine the target volume for radiotherapy, and incorporation of PET data into RT planning has the potential to improve the accuracy of the process (79) (Fig. 8.5.3).

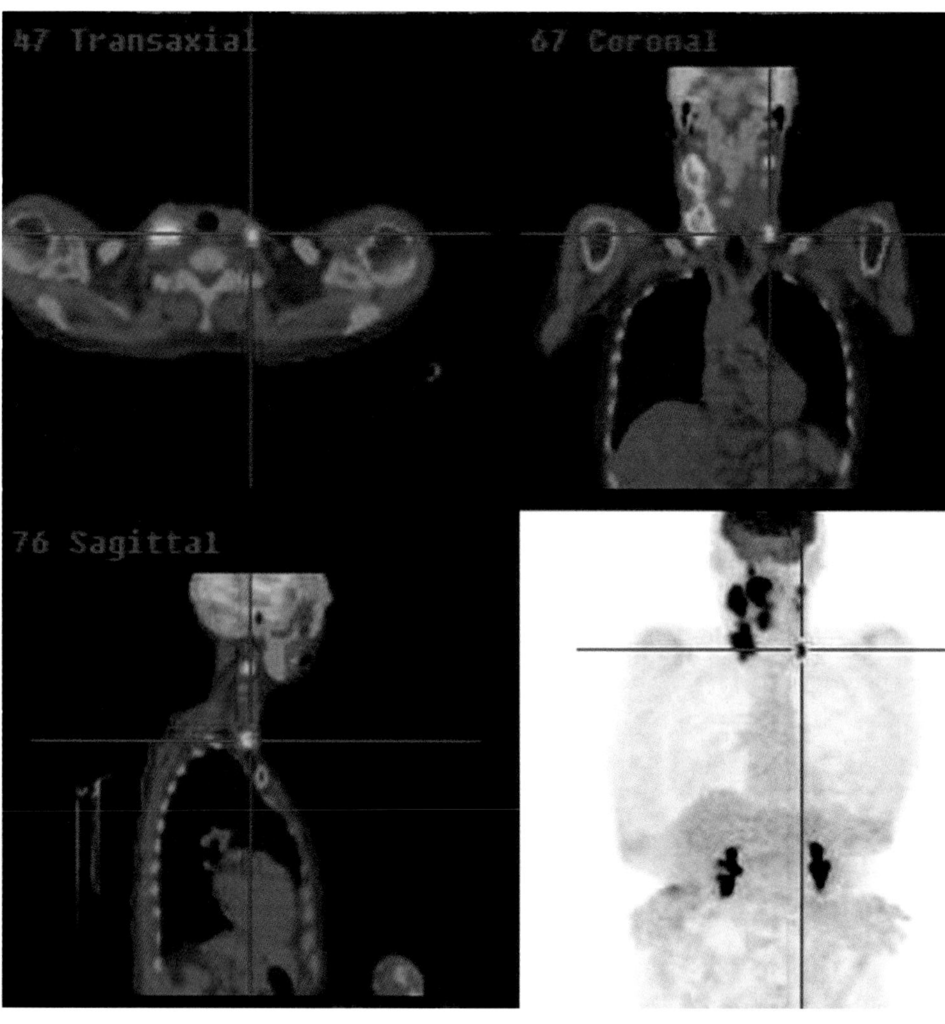

FIGURE 8.5.2. To diagnose metastatic nodal disease in head and neck cancer requires either nodal enlargement on CT scanning or alteration in the enhancement pattern of nodes suggesting necrosis. In this case of advanced right oropharyngeal cancer, clear nodal enlargement was identified on CT in the right neck. However, focal and intense uptake of fluorodeoxyglucose was also present in an ipsilateral parapharyngeal node superior to both the primary tumor and enlarged nodes and in multiple contralateral nodes of normal size. The lower left neck lesion is indicated on a transverse PET/CT image (upper left), coronal PET/CT (upper right), sagittal PET/CT (lower left) and an anterior view showing PET alone. Although the contralateral nodes in the upper cervical chain would have received radiation in parallel, opposed beams used to treat the primary, the left lower cervical node would not have received any radiation based on conventional CT planning. The ispilateral parapharyngeal node would also have been underdosed in an attempt to spare parotid toxicity on this side. As conformal radiotherapy planning becomes more sophisticated, so does the requirement for more accurate delineation of the extent of disease.

CT scanning is very poor at assessing the longitudinal extent of tumor and is often inaccurate when used to estimate the extent of nodal involvement (38). As discussed above, PET is significantly more accurate than CT for the assessment of nodes that are not immediately adjacent to the esophagus and can more accurately delineate the longitudinal extent of tumor than CT. This is especially useful in cases where an endoscope is unable to pass through a stenosed esophagus to visualize the lower boundary of the tumor.

The authors' group has demonstrated that FDG PET has a significant impact on patient management in a multidisciplinary setting, both in selecting patients for neoadjuvant chemoradiation (28) and also following it prior to definitive surgery (80). In both these settings, the findings on FDG-PET were strong predictors of survival irrespective of the management pathway chosen. Results from a prospectively conducted trial of PET in RT planning, also conducted at the authors' center, show that PET has a significant impact of RT target volumes in esophageal cancer, often helping to avoid geographic miss by identifying unsuspected lymph node involvement (81).

Lymphoma

PET is increasingly being used to select patients with lymphoma for RT (13,82) and to help delineate radiation fields (83), although the latter has not yet been studied systematically in a large series. The lymphomas are a large and heterogeneous group of diseases, often with widely varying treatments. In patients with localized disease, RT may be an important component, or indeed the only component, of potentially curative therapy for this especially radiosensitive group of malignancies.

Accurate staging is important in the management of three of the most common disease groups included in the World Health Organization lymphoma classification, namely Hodgkin's lymphoma, the group of "aggressive lymphomas," the most common of which is diffuse large B cell lymphoma (DLBCL) and follicle center lymphoma. In each of these malignancies, early stage disease is commonly treated with "involved-field" radiotherapy, where the treatment volume covers involved extranodal sites and lymph node regions only. More advanced disease is usually treated with more intensive chemotherapy, with RT reserved only for bulky masses or poorly responsive disease sites. RT may be given alone, as in stage I or II follicular lymphoma, or after a number of cycles of chemotherapy, as in stage I or II DLBCL or Hodgkin's lymphoma.

PET scanning has been intensively studied in the aggressive lymphomas (84) and in Hodgkin's lymphoma (85). FDG-PET is significantly more accurate in both staging and assessment of treatment response in these diseases than conventional structural imaging (86). PET data are now routinely incorporated visually into the RT treatment planning process. Because large regions of the body are often irradiated with a relatively low dose, there has been less pressure to minutely shape RT fields by incorporating PET directly into

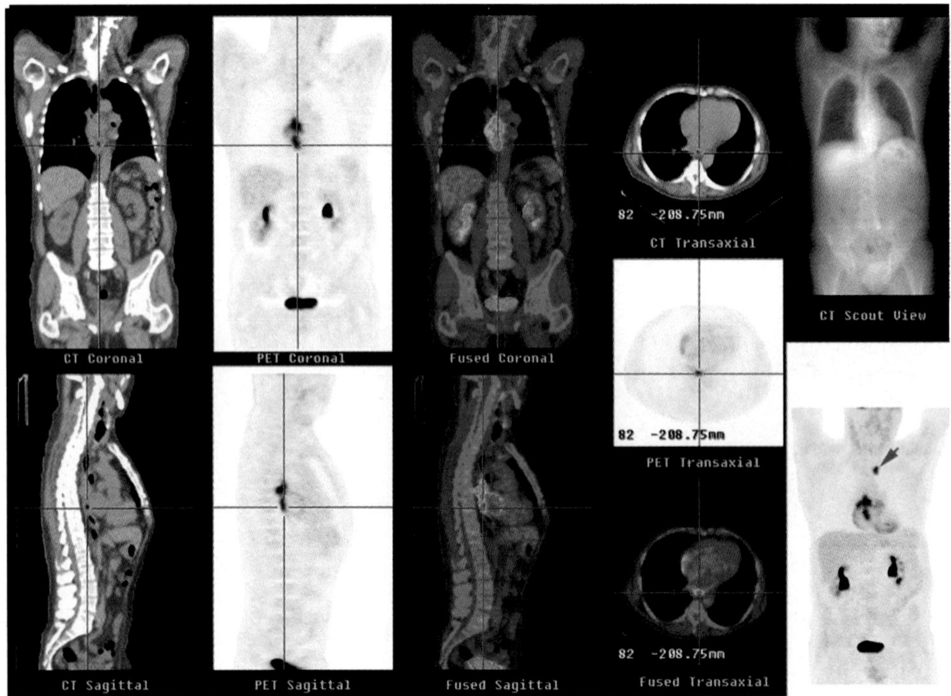

FIGURE 8.5.3. The key issue for radiotherapy planning in esophageal cancer is not the status of peritumoral nodes, for which PET is somewhat insensitive, but rather exclusion of remote nodal and systemic metastatic sites that would render aggressive locoregional therapy futile. In this example an obstructing tumor of the midesophagus (*triangulated* in the first three columns of images) could not be passed by the endoscope, and therefore it was difficult to define the axial extent of the primary. The lesion was poorly imaged by CT (first images on upper and lower rows) but-well seen on PET (alone (second images on upper and lower rows) and PET/CT (third images on upper and lower rows). Endoscopic ultrasound-guided biopsy confirmed subcarinal nodal disease, also seen superior to the primary on PET. This finding was missed on CT (fourth row upper image) but was well seen on PET (fourth row middle image) and PET/CT (fourth row lower image). The key finding in this patient on PET was, however, remote left superior mediastinal/supraclavicular nodal disease (arrowed on lower image last row, upper image shows digitally reconstructed radiograph). This finding has both prognostic and therapeutic planning implications.

the RT planning systems than, for example, lung or head and neck cancers. It is often sufficient to know that a lymph node region contains tumor when RT is being planned because the target volume is often determined by the anatomic boundaries of the involved region rather than the precise distribution of disease within the region.

PET commonly influences RT fields in lymphoma by upstaging small nodes that are negative by structural imaging criteria (87,88) or by demonstrating disease in sites where there is inadequate contrast between lymphoma and normal tissues on CT, such as spleen, liver, salivary glands, and bowel. PET may also be used to assess the response of lymphomas to chemotherapy (89), either definitively at the end of therapy, or as an interim measure, after only one or two cycles of chemotherapy (90). Persistent tumor FDG uptake after several cycles of chemotherapy (91) or at the end of chemotherapy is very highly correlated with prognosis and may assist with the decision to deliver RT.

To date, there is no good evidence to suggest that an excellent interim PET response to chemotherapy can be used in early stage Hodgkin's lymphoma or the aggressive lymphomas to identify patients who do not require RT as part of what would normally be given as combined modality therapy. At the authors' center there have been several cases where isolated relapses have occurred within areas that would have been irradiated but RT was withheld because of an excellent early PET response.

Other Cancers

PET information has the potential to help plan RT or to select patients for RT in an increasing number of malignancies. These include cervical cancer (92), soft tissue sarcomas (93), pediatric cancers (94), malignant melanoma (20), and small cell lung cancer (88). The influence of PET varies significantly among these diseases but shows significant promise in each of them. It is likely that PET information will be given increasing priority by radiation oncologists in these and other malignancies in the future as more information becomes available.

CONCLUSIONS

PET staging is rapidly becoming a standard part of the evaluation of a majority of patients with unresected FDG-avid cancers who are candidates for definitive radiation therapy. In the future PET data will be seamlessly integrated into the treatment planning process. For many cancers, treatment planning with CT alone will be remembered as a historically necessary but notoriously inaccurate means of planning radiation therapy. Nuclear medicine physicians will become increasingly important members of the team of physicians required to optimize the practice of radiation oncology. Finally, it is possible that use of newer tracers, such as those capable of defining hypoxia,

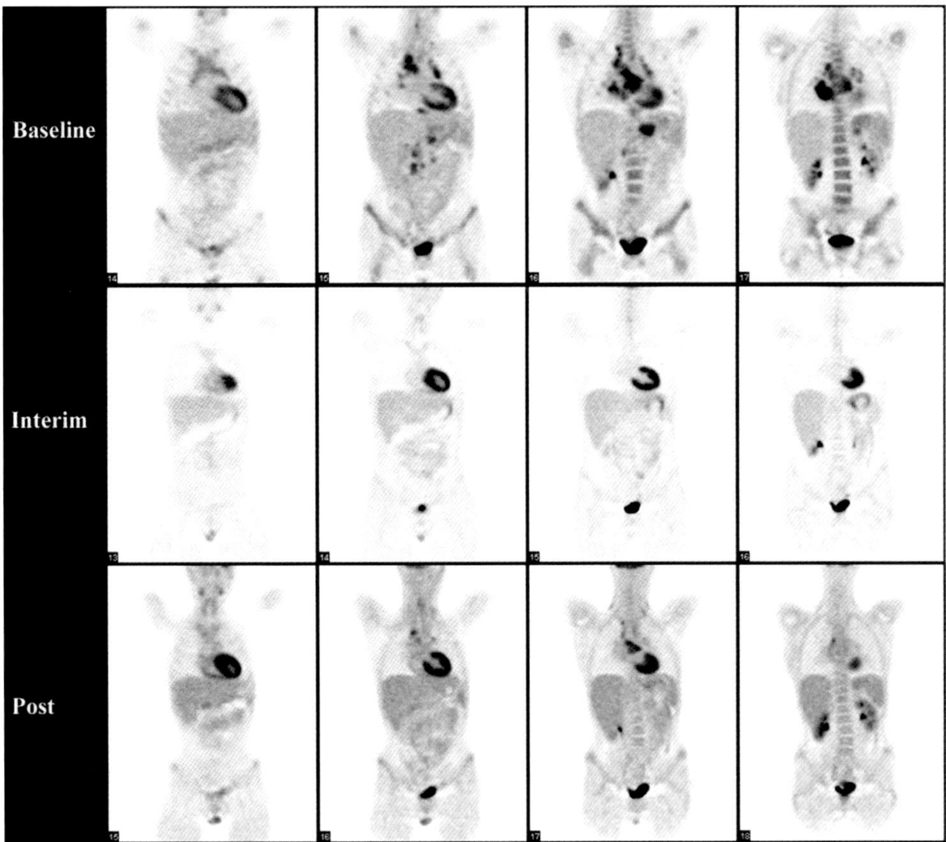

FIGURE 8.5.4. The role of fluorodeoxyglucose (FDG) PET in lymphoma treatment selection, planning, and monitoring is rapidly expanding. Although it is recognized that a positive PET scan early during treatment carries an unfavorable prognosis compared to a negative scan, there is, as yet, no justification for reducing therapy based on a negative interim PET scan result. In this adolescent female with bulky supradiaphragmatic Hodgkin's lymphoma (stage IIa), FDG-PET at staging demonstrated infradiaphragmatic disease in nonenlarged nodes (**upper panel** of coronal images). Due to concerns regarding the risk of radiotherapy, chemotherapy was chosen as the appropriate treatment option. Based on a complete metabolic response early in treatment (**middle panel**), reduced chemotherapy was delivered and radiotherapy consolidation of sites of previous bulk disease was not performed. On routine surveillance PET posttreatment (**lower panel**) demonstrated relapse in the sites of previously bulky disease, although there was continuing reduction in size of previous mediastinal masses on correlative CT. Sites of nonbulky disease remained negative but had never been abnormal on CT and therefore were not amenable to conventional response assessment.

will lead to altered dose delivery within tumors based on the hypoxic tumor volumes or other key biological parameters. Thus, the integration of PET/CT with radiation oncology is an area of both clinical and research opportunity for the foreseeable future.

REFERENCES

1. Lindholm C, Cavallin-Stahl E, Ceberg J, et al. Radiotherapy practices in Sweden compared to the scientific evidence. *Acta Oncol* 2003;42(5–6):416–429.
2. Wirth A, Yuen K, Barton M, et al. Long-term outcome after radiotherapy alone for lymphocyte-predominant Hodgkin's lymphoma: a retrospective multicenter study of the Australasian Radiation Oncology Lymphoma Group. *Cancer* 2005;104(6):1221–1229.
3. Haigh PI. Anaplastic thyroid carcinoma. *Curr Treat Options Oncol* 2000;1(4):353–357.
4. Chang JY, Liu HH, Komaki R. Intensity modulated radiation therapy and proton radiotherapy for non–small cell lung cancer. *Curr Oncol Rep* 2005;7(4):255–259.
5. Svensson H, Moller TR. Developments in radiotherapy. *Acta Oncol* 2003;42(5–6):430–442.
6. Drzymala RE, Mohan R, Brewster L, et al. Dose-volume histograms. *Int J Radiat Oncol Biol Phys* 1991;21(1):71–78.
7. Ling CC, Burman C, Chui CS, et al. Conformal radiation treatment of prostate cancer using inversely-planned intensity-modulated photon beams produced with dynamic multileaf collimation. *Int J Radiat Oncol Biol Phys* 1996;35(4):721–730.
8. Leibel SA, Fuks Z, Zelefsky MJ, et al. Intensity-modulated radiotherapy. *Cancer J* 2002;8(2):164–176.
9. Pickles T, Pollack A. The case for dose escalation versus adjuvant androgen deprivation therapy for intermediate risk prostate cancer. *Can J Urol* 2006;13[Suppl 2]:68–71.
10. Bussels B, Maes A, Hermans R, et al. Recurrences after conformal parotid-sparing radiotherapy for head and neck cancer. *Radiother Oncol* 2004;72(2):119–127.
11. Kalff V, Hicks RJ, Mac Manus MP, et al. Clinical impact of (18)F fluorodeoxyglucose positron emission tomography in patients with non–small cell lung cancer: a prospective study. *J Clin Oncol* 2001;19(1): 111–118.
12. Vansteenkiste JF, Stroobants SG. Positron emission tomography in the management of non–small cell lung cancer. *Hematol Oncol Clin North Am* 2004;18(1):269–288.

13. Wirth A, Seymour JF, Hicks RJ, et al. Fluorine-18 fluorodeoxyglucose positron emission tomography, gallium-67 scintigraphy, and conventional staging for Hodgkin's disease and non-Hodgkin's lymphoma. *Am J Med* 2002;112(4):262–268.
14. Jerusalem G, Beguin Y, Fassotte MF, et al. Whole-body positron emission tomography using ^{18}F-fluorodeoxyglucose for posttreatment evaluation in Hodgkin's disease and non-Hodgkin's lymphoma has higher diagnostic and prognostic value than classical computed tomography scan imaging. *Blood* 1999;94(2):429–433.
15. Pramesh CS, Mistry RC. Role of PET scan in management of oesophageal cancer. *Eur J Surg Oncol* 2005;31(4):449.
16. Lerut T, Flamen P, Ectors N, et al. Histopathologic validation of lymph node staging with FDG-PET scan in cancer of the esophagus and gastroesophageal junction: a prospective study based on primary surgery with extensive lymphadenectomy. *Ann Surg* 2000;232(6):743–752.
17. Grigsby PW, Siegel BA, Dehdashti F. Lymph node staging by positron emission tomography in patients with carcinoma of the cervix. *J Clin Oncol* 2001;19(17):3745–3749.
18. Follen M, Levenback CF, Iyer RB, et al. Imaging in cervical cancer. *Cancer* 2003;98[9 Suppl]:2028–2038.
19. Kalff V, Hicks RJ, Ware RE, et al. Evaluation of high-risk melanoma: comparison of [18F]FDG PET and high-dose 67Ga SPET. *Eur J Nucl Med Mol Imaging* 2002;29(4):506–515.
20. Wagner JD. Fluorodeoxyglucose positron emission tomography for melanoma staging: refining the indications. *Ann Surg Oncol* 2006;13(4): 444–446.
21. Hicks RJ, Toner GC, Choong PF. Clinical applications of molecular imaging in sarcoma evaluation. *Cancer Imaging* 2005;5(1):66–72.
22. Esteves FP, Schuster DM, Halkar RK. Gastrointestinal tract malignancies and positron emission tomography: an overview. *Semin Nucl Med* 2006;36(2):169–181.
23. Gyorke T, Zajic T, Lange A, et al. Impact of FDG PET for staging of Ewing sarcomas and primitive neuroectodermal tumours. *Nucl Med Commun* 2006;27(1):17–24.
24. Franzius C, Schober O. Assessment of therapy response by FDG PET in pediatric patients. *Q J Nucl Med* 2003;47(1):41–45.
25. Yap CS, Czernin J, Fishbein MC, et al. Evaluation of thoracic tumors with 18F-fluorothymidine and 18F-fluorodeoxyglucose-positron emission tomography. *Chest* 2006;129(2):393–401.
26. Rischin D, Hicks RJ, Fisher R, et al. Prognostic significance of [18F]-misonidazole positron emission tomography-detected tumor hypoxia in patients with advanced head and neck cancer randomly assigned to chemoradiation with or without tirapazamine: a substudy of Trans-Tasman Radiation Oncology Group Study 98.02. *J Clin Oncol* 2006;24 (13):2098–2104.
27. Mac Manus MP, Hicks RJ, Ball DL, et al. F-18 fluorodeoxyglucose positron emission tomography staging in radical radiotherapy candidates with non–small cell lung carcinoma: powerful correlation with survival and high impact on treatment. *Cancer* 2001;92(4): 886–895.
28. Duong CP, Demitriou H, Weih L, et al. Significant clinical impact and prognostic stratification provided by FDG-PET in the staging of oesophageal cancer. *Eur J Nucl Med Mol Imaging* 2006;33(7):759–769.
29. Mac Manus MP, Wong K, Hicks RJ, et al. Early mortality after radical radiotherapy for non–small cell lung cancer: comparison of PET-staged and conventionally staged cohorts treated at a large tertiary referral center. *Int J Radiat Oncol Biol Phys* 2002;52(2):351–361.
30. Mac Manus MR, Hicks R, Fisher R, et al. FDG-PET-detected extracranial metastasis in patients with non-small cell lung cancer undergoing staging for surgery or radical radiotherapy—survival correlates with metastatic disease burden. *Acta Oncol* 2003;42(1):48–54.
31. Toloza EM, Harpole L, McCrory DC. Noninvasive staging of non–small cell lung cancer: a review of the current evidence. *Chest* 2003;123[1 Suppl]:137S–146S.
32. Vansteenkiste JF, Stroobants SG, De Leyn PR, et al. Lymph node staging in non-small-cell lung cancer with FDG-PET scan: a prospective study on 690 lymph node stations from 68 patients. *J Clin Oncol* 1998; 16(6):2142–2149.
33. Gupta NC, Graeber GM, Bishop HA. Comparative efficacy of positron emission tomography with fluorodeoxyglucose in evaluation of small (<1 cm), intermediate (1 to 3 cm), and large (>3 cm) lymph node lesions. *Chest* 2000;117(3):773–778.
34. Wahl RL, Quint LE, Greenough RL, et al. Staging of mediastinal non-small cell lung cancer with FDG PET, CT, and fusion images: preliminary prospective evaluation. *Radiology* 1994;191(2):371–377.
35. Pieterman RM, van Putten JW, Meuzelaar JJ, et al. Preoperative staging of non–small cell lung cancer with positron-emission tomography. *N Engl J Med* 2000;343(4):254–261.
36. Vansteenkiste JF, Stroobants SG, Dupont PJ, et al. FDG-PET scan in potentially operable non-small cell lung cancer: do anatometabolic PET-CT fusion images improve the localisation of regional lymph node metastases? The Leuven Lung Cancer Group. *Eur J Nucl Med* 1998;25(11):1495–1501.
37. Poncelet AJ, Lonneux M, Coche E, et al. PET-FDG scan enhances but does not replace preoperative surgical staging in non–small cell lung carcinoma. *Eur J Cardiothorac Surg* 2001;20(3):468–474; discussion 474–475.
38. Dwamena BA, Sonnad SS, Angobaldo JO, et al. Metastases from non–small cell lung cancer: mediastinal staging in the 1990s—meta-analytic comparison of PET and CT. *Radiology* 1999;213(2):530–536.
39. Kim K, Park SJ, Kim BT, et al. Evaluation of lymph node metastases in squamous cell carcinoma of the esophagus with positron emission tomography. *Ann Thorac Surg* 2001;71(1):290–294.
40. Choi JY, Lee KH, Shim YM, et al. Improved detection of individual nodal involvement in squamous cell carcinoma of the esophagus by FDG PET. *J Nucl Med* 2000;41(5):808–815.
41. Buchmann I, Hansen T, Brochhausen C, et al. FDG-PET in the initial staging of squamous cell oesophageal carcinoma. *Nuklearmedizin* 2006;45(6):235–241.
42. Acland KM, O'Doherty MJ, Russell-Jones R. The value of positron emission tomography scanning in the detection of subclinical metastatic melanoma. *J Am Acad Dermatol* 2000;42(4):606–611.
43. Kumar R, Mavi A, Bural G, et al. Fluorodeoxyglucose-PET in the management of malignant melanoma. *Radiol Clin North Am* 2005;43(1):23–33.
44. Acland KM, Healy C, Calonje E, et al. Comparison of positron emission tomography scanning and sentinel node biopsy in the detection of micrometastases of primary cutaneous malignant melanoma. *J Clin Oncol* 2001;19(10):2674–2678.
45. Adams S, Baum RP, Stuckensen T, et al. Prospective comparison of ^{18}F-FDG PET with conventional imaging modalities (CT, MRI, US) in lymph node staging of head and neck cancer. *Eur J Nucl Med* 1998;25(9):1255–1260.
46. Sloka JS, Hollett PD, Mathews M. A quantitative review of the use of FDG-PET in the axillary staging of breast cancer. *Med Sci Monit* 2007;13(3):RA37–46.
47. Mountain CF. Lung cancer staging classification. *Clin Chest Med* 1993;14(1):43–53.
48. Luciani A, Itti E, Rahmouni A, et al. Lymph node imaging: basic principles. *Eur J Radiol* 2006;58(3):338–344.
49. Webb WR, Gatsonis C, Zerhouni EA, et al. CT and MR imaging in staging non-small cell bronchogenic carcinoma: report of the Radiologic Diagnostic Oncology Group. *Radiology* 1991;178(3):705–713.
50. Ling CC, Humm J, Larson S, et al. Towards multidimensional radiotherapy (MD-CRT): biological imaging and biological conformality. *Int J Radiat Oncol Biol Phys* 2000;47(3):551–560.
51. Ciernik IF, Huser M, Burger C, et al. Automated functional image-guided radiation treatment planning for rectal cancer. *Int J Radiat Oncol Biol Phys* 2005;62(3):893–900.
52. Austin-Seymour M, Kalet I, McDonald J, et al. Three dimensional planning target volumes: a model and a software tool. *Int J Radiat Oncol Biol Phys* 1995;33(5):1073–1080.
53. Caldwell CB, Mah K, Skinner M, et al. Can PET provide the 3D extent of tumor motion for individualized internal target volumes? A phantom study of the limitations of CT and the promise of PET. *Int J Radiat Oncol Biol Phys* 2003;55(5):1381–1393.

54. Davis JB, Reiner B, Huser M, et al. Assessment of (18)F PET signals for automatic target volume definition in radiotherapy treatment planning. *Radiother Oncol* 2006;80:43–50.
55. Drever L, Robinson DM, McEwan A, et al. A local contrast based approach to threshold segmentation for PET target volume delineation. *Med Phys* 2006;33(6):1583–1594.
56. Chetty IJ, Fernando S, Kessler ML, et al. Monte Carlo–based lung cancer treatment planning incorporating PET-defined target volumes. *J Appl Clin Med Phys* 2005;6(4):65–76.
57. Yaremko B, Riauka T, Robinson D, et al. Thresholding in PET images of static and moving targets. *Phys Med Biol* 2005;50(24):5969–5982.
58. Hong R, Halama J, Bova D, et al. Correlation of PET standard uptake value and CT window-level thresholds for target delineation in CT-based radiation treatment planning. *Int J Radiat Oncol Biol Phys* 2007; 67(3):720–726.
59. Steenbakkers RJ, Duppen JC, Fitton I, et al. Observer variation in target volume delineation of lung cancer related to radiation oncologist-computer interaction: a "Big Brother" evaluation. *Radiother Oncol* 2005; 77(2):182–190.
60. Jin JY, Ajlouni M, Chen Q, Yin FF, et al. A technique of using gated-CT images to determine internal target volume (ITV) for fractionated stereotactic lung radiotherapy. *Radiother Oncol* 2006;78(2):177–184.
61. Mac Manus MP, Hicks RJ. PET scanning in lung cancer: current status and future directions. *Semin Surg Oncol* 2003;21(3):149–155.
62. Gilman MD, Aquino SL. State-of-the-Art FDG-PET imaging of lung cancer. *Semin Roentgenol* 2005;40(2):143–153.
63. Dendukuri N, Rahme E, Belisle P, et al. Bayesian sample size determination for prevalence and diagnostic test studies in the absence of a gold standard test. *Biometrics* 2004;60(2):388–397.
64. Mac Manus MP, Hicks RJ, Matthews JP, et al. High rate of detection of unsuspected distant metastases by pet in apparent stage III non–small cell lung cancer: implications for radical radiation therapy. *Int J Radiat Oncol Biol Phys* 2001;50(2):287–293.
65. Nestle U, Schaefer-Schuler A, Kremp S, et al. Target volume definition for (18)F-FDG PET-positive lymph nodes in radiotherapy of patients with non-small cell lung cancer. *Eur J Nucl Med Mol Imaging* 2007;34(4)453–462.
66. Nestle U, Walter K, Schmidt S, et al. ^{18}F-deoxyglucose positron emission tomography (FDG-PET) for the planning of radiotherapy in lung cancer: high impact in patients with atelectasis. *Int J Radiat Oncol Biol Phys* 1999;44(3):593–597.
67. Munley MT, Marks LB, Scarfone C, et al. Multimodality nuclear medicine imaging in three-dimensional radiation treatment planning for lung cancer: challenges and prospects. *Lung Cancer* 1999;23(2):105–114.
68. Vanuytsel LJ, Vansteenkiste JF, Stroobants SG, et al. The impact of (18)F-fluoro-2-deoxy-D-glucose positron emission tomography (FDG-PET) lymph node staging on the radiation treatment volumes in patients with non-small cell lung cancer. *Radiother Oncol* 2000;55(3):317–324.
69. Bradley J, Thorstad WL, Mutic S, et al. Impact of FDG-PET on radiation therapy volume delineation in non-small-cell lung cancer. *Int J Radiat Oncol Biol Phys* 2004;59(1):78–86.
70. Brianzoni E, Rossi G, Ancidei S, et al. Radiotherapy planning: PET/CT scanner performances in the definition of gross tumour volume and clinical target volume. *Eur J Nucl Med Mol Imaging* 2005;32(12): 1392–1399.
71. Daisne JF, Sibomana M, Bol A, et al. Evaluation of a multimodality image (CT, MRI and PET) coregistration procedure on phantom and head and neck cancer patients: accuracy, reproducibility and consistency. *Radiother Oncol* 2003;69(3):237–245.
72. Nowak B, Di Martino E, Janicke S, et al. Diagnostic evaluation of malignant head and neck cancer by F-18-FDG PET compared to CT/MRI. *Nuklearmedizin* 1999;38(8):312–318.
73. Murakami R, Uozumi H, Hirai T, et al. Impact of FDG-PET/CT imaging on nodal staging for head-and-neck squamous cell carcinoma. *Int J Radiat Oncol Biol Phys* 2007;68(2):377–382.
74. Schoder H, Carlson DL, Kraus DH, et al. ^{18}F-FDG PET/CT for detecting nodal metastases in patients with oral cancer staged N0 by clinical examination and CT/MRI. *J Nucl Med* 2006;47(5):755–762.
75. Stokkel MP, ten Broek FW, Hordijk GJ, et al. Preoperative evaluation of patients with primary head and neck cancer using dual-head 18fluorodeoxyglucose positron emission tomography. *Ann Surg* 2000;231(2): 229–234.
76. Paulino AC, Koshy M, Howell R, et al. Comparison of CT- and FDG-PET-defined gross tumor volume in intensity-modulated radiotherapy for head-and-neck cancer. *Int J Radiat Oncol Biol Phys* 2005;61(5):1385–1392.
77. Geets X, Daisne JF, Tomsej M, et al. Impact of the type of imaging modality on target volumes delineation and dose distribution in pharyngo-laryngeal squamous cell carcinoma: comparison between pre- and per-treatment studies. *Radiother Oncol* 2006;78(3):291–297.
78. Daisne JF, Duprez T, Weynand B, et al. Tumor volume in pharyngolaryngeal squamous cell carcinoma: comparison at CT, MR imaging, and FDG PET and validation with surgical specimen. *Radiology* 2004; 233(1):93–100.
79. Konski A, Doss M, Milestone B, et al. The integration of 18-fluoro-deoxy-glucose positron emission tomography and endoscopic ultrasound in the treatment-planning process for esophageal carcinoma. *Int J Radiat Oncol Biol Phys* 2005;61(4):1123–1128.
80. Duong CP, Hicks RJ, Weih L, et al. FDG-PET status following chemoradiotherapy provides high management impact and powerful prognostic stratification in oesophageal cancer. *Eur J Nucl Med Mol Imaging* 2006;33(7):770–778.
81. Leong T, Everitt C, Yuen K, et al. A prospective study to evaluate the impact of FDG-PET on CT-based radiotherapy treatment planning for oesophageal cancer. *Radiother Oncol* 2006;78(3):254–261.
82. Hicks RJ, Mac Manus MP, Seymour JF. Initial staging of lymphoma with positron emission tomography and computed tomography. *Semin Nucl Med* 2005;35(3):165–175.
83. Yahalom J. Transformation in the use of radiation therapy of Hodgkin's lymphoma: new concepts and indications lead to modern field design and are assisted by PET imaging and intensity modulated radiation therapy (IMRT). *Eur J Haematol Suppl* 2005(66):90–97.
84. Israel O, Keidar Z, Bar-Shalom R. Positron emission tomography in the evaluation of lymphoma. *Semin Nucl Med* 2004;34(3): 166–179.
85. Hutchings M, Eigtved AI, Specht L. FDG-PET in the clinical management of Hodgkin's lymphoma. *Crit Rev Oncol Hematol* 2004;52(1):19–32.
86. Divgi C. Imaging: staging and evaluation of lymphoma using nuclear medicine. *Semin Oncol* 2005;32[1 Suppl 1]:S11–18.
87. Hueltenschmidt B, Sautter-Bihl ML, Lang O, et al. Whole body positron emission tomography in the treatment of Hodgkin's disease. *Cancer* 2001;91(2):302–310.
88. Blum RH, Seymour JF, Wirth A, et al. Frequent impact of [18F]fluorodeoxyglucose positron emission tomography on the staging and management of patients with indolent non-Hodgkin's lymphoma. *Clin Lymphoma* 2003;4(1):43–49.
89. Juweid ME, Wiseman GA, Vose JM, et al. Response assessment of aggressive non-Hodgkin's lymphoma by integrated International Workshop Criteria and fluorine-18-fluorodeoxyglucose positron emission tomography. *J Clin Oncol* 2005;23(21):4652–4661.
90. Haioun C, Itti E, Rahmouni A, et al. [18F]fluoro-2-deoxy-D-glucose positron emission tomography (FDG-PET) in aggressive lymphoma: an early prognostic tool for predicting patient outcome. *Blood* 2005;106(4):1376–1381.
91. Mikhaeel NG, Hutchings M, Fields PA, et al. FDG-PET after two to three cycles of chemotherapy predicts progression-free and overall survival in high-grade non-Hodgkin's lymphoma. *Ann Oncol* 2005;16(9):1514–1523.
92. Lin LL, Yang Z, Mutic S, et al. FDG-PET imaging for the assessment of physiologic volume response during radiotherapy in cervix cancer. *Int J Radiat Oncol Biol Phys* 2006;65(1):177–181.
93. Hicks RJ. Functional imaging techniques for evaluation of sarcomas. *Cancer Imaging* 2005;5(1):58–65.
94. Krasin MJ, Hudson MM, Kaste SC. Positron emission tomography in pediatric radiation oncology: integration in the treatment-planning process. *Pediatr Radiol* 2004;34(3):214–221.

CHAPTER

8.6 Central Nervous System

MICHAEL J. FULHAM AND ARMIN MOHAMED

Central nervous system (CNS) tumors can be separated into primary brain tumors and cerebral metastases. The main emphasis in this chapter is primary CNS tumors, but for completeness, the role of positron emission tomography (PET) and PET with computed tomography (CT) in the assessment of cerebral metastases is also included.

CNS tumors arise mainly from neuroepithelial, meningeal, hematopoietic, nerve sheath, and germ cells. There is also a miscellaneous group, which includes tumorlike lesions such as epidermoids, dermoids, colloid cysts, Rathke cleft cysts, and others. In adults, more than 90% of the tumors arise from neuroepithelial cells, and they include astrocytomas, oligodendrogliomas, oligoastrocytomas, and ependymomas; they are collectively referred to as gliomas. There are two main peaks in the incidence of gliomas: one in childhood, where CNS tumors are the second leading cause of cancer-related death; and a second in later life, between ages 65 and 79 years. Primary CNS tumors have an incidence of 5 to 10 per 100,000 persons per year, and there is a suggestion that the incidence of malignant gliomas is increasing in the elderly (older than 85 years) (1). The tumor types and their locations also differ in these two age groups. In children, the most common tumor is the primitive neuroectodermal tumor (including medulloblastoma) followed by diffuse infiltrating neuroepithelial tumors, which are much more common in the cerebellum, diencephalon, and brainstem than in the cerebral hemispheres. In adults, neuroepithelial astrocytic tumors are most common and account for over 60% of all primary brain tumors and, of these, glioblastoma multiforme (GBM) accounts for about 60%. These adult neuroepithelial tumors are more likely to occur in the supratentorial compartment in the frontal and temporal lobes, but they can occur in any location in the neuraxis including the brainstem, cerebellum, and spinal cord.

The recent revision of the World Health Organization (WHO) brain tumor classification is used for this chapter (2). The WHO classification uses specific morphological features—nuclear atypia, mitoses, microvascular proliferation, and necrosis—to grade gliomas according to degree of malignancy. Therefore, in order of increasing degree of anaplasia the grades are: grade I pilocytic astrocytoma (PA), grade II diffuse astrocytoma (low grade), grade III anaplastic astrocytoma, and grade IV glioblastoma multiforme. Oligodendrogliomas and ependymomas are classified as WHO grade II, with the anaplastic-equivalent tumors as grade III.

The use of specific morphological criteria has been an important advance in glioma grading, but problems remain in the reliable identification of the different cell types (3–9). Neuropathological interpretation continues to be subjective and based, to some extent, on experience. There is poor reproducibility within and between observers, which is readily apparent to clinicians who participate in multidisciplinary tumor board meetings (10). Partly, in recognition of the shortcomings of the histopathological gold standard and of the developments in molecular and genetic analysis of gliomas, the latest WHO classification has incorporated some of the recent advances in the molecular characterization of the gliomas (2).

It is beyond the scope of this chapter to provide a comprehensive description of the diverse molecular and genetic alterations found in gliomas, but some relevant references are included in the bibliography (11–16). However, it is relevant to briefly note some of the better-characterized alterations in oncogenes and tumor suppressor genes that are found in gliomas. Currently, with the exception of the allelic loss of 1p and 19 q chromosomes in oligodendrogliomas, which identifies a glioma subgroup that has a relatively long natural history and is chemo- and radiosensitive (17–20), molecular analyses of gliomas are not routinely available and tend to be confined to the research setting (21,22). In low-grade gliomas the earliest changes include overexpression of platelet-derived growth factor (PDGF) ligands/receptors and inactivation of the *TP53* gene. The PDGF receptor leads to changes in signal transduction pathways that induce cellular proliferation and perhaps the migration and dissemination of glioma cells, while inactivation of *TP53* promotes cell division and may facilitate anaplastic transformation.

There are two distinct types of GBMs: one arises *de novo* in elderly patients and the other results from the malignant transformation of a low-grade glioma. *De novo* GBMs have amplification and overexpression of epidermal growth factor (EGF) in about 40% to 50% of cases and *TP53* mutations are rare. The EGF ligands and transforming growth factor TGF-α induce cellular proliferation and invasiveness. Meanwhile, *TP53* mutations can be found in the secondary GBM as well as other genetic alterations, including those found in the retinoblastoma-mediated cell-cycle pathway. Other genetic alterations are found in these high-grade gliomas, and there is loss of heterozygosity on chromosome 10q in 80% to 90% of GBMs. Much attention has focused on the *PTEN/MMAC* (phosphatase and tensin homology or mutated in multiple advanced cancer) gene, as a candidate gene in this location because it is mutated in 20% to 30% of primary and secondary GBMs (2,3,15). It is likely that delineation of the molecular characteristics and genetic alterations will become part of the routine evaluation of gliomas in the future.

The common presentations of patients with primary and secondary brain tumors include, in decreasing frequency, focal or generalized seizures, unaccustomed headache, personality and cognitive changes, and focal neurologic signs (23,24). Individual clinical features depend on the location of the tumor, its histologic type, and its rate of growth. *De novo* GBMs typically have a short history, which can be measured in weeks. Unaccustomed headache is usually related to raised intracranial pressure and cerebral edema, and it is often worse in the morning and may be associated with nausea and vomiting; occasionally it is due to acute hemorrhage into the tumor. For low-grade gliomas it is generally impossible to know when these lesions first developed; they have been detected incidentally in asymptomatic subjects without neurological signs when neuroimaging has been done for some other reason. It is not uncommon for a patient with a low-grade glioma to mention having had migraine headaches without aura for many years prior to the diagnosis; the migraine may have been symptomatic of the underlying tumor, but then again migraine is common in the general population.

Low-grade gliomas tend to be detected when imaging is done after a seizure. The high-grade gliomas—GBMs and anaplastic astrocytomas—have a poor prognosis with median survival of 1 year for GBMs and 2 to 3 years for anaplastic astrocytomas. Mean age of onset for GBMs is 53 years when compared to 40 years for anaplastic astrocytomas; men are more commonly affected than women (3 to 2). Low-grade gliomas have a better prognosis, and survival ranges from 12 to 128 months. In the authors' opinion, low-grade gliomas are rarely if ever cured because they tend to infiltrate surrounding brain beyond the macroscopic abnormality that is evident on imaging and at operation. They occur in a younger age group, and the mean age of onset is 35 years for astrocytomas and 45 years for oligodendrogliomas (25–27).

In a patient with a suspected primary brain tumor, the initial step in the evaluation, after a history and neurologic examination, is to perform some form of neuroimaging. This is usually anatomic imaging with CT or magnetic resonance (MR) imaging. Both techniques provide exquisite anatomical detail and can assess the integrity of the blood–brain barrier (BBB) via intravenous contrast. MR imaging can also provide an assessment of tumoral metabolites with MR spectroscopy (MRS), function via echoplanar techniques, vascularity through MR angiography, and diffusion. Ideally, neuroimaging would provide detailed information not only about the site and extent of the lesion, but its grade, cell type, and proliferative capacity. A tissue sample would then be obtained in all cases of suspected primary brain tumors, and this sample would reflect the biological behavior of the tumor and management would then be tailored appropriately. However, in clinical medicine this is not generally the case.

Anatomic imaging has shortcomings, in particular, in relation to tumor characterization. Contrast enhancement is a nonspecific indication of disruption of the BBB and, while the neovascularization of high-grade gliomas leaks contrast because the tumor endothelial cells lack tight junctions and normal endothelium is affected by tumoral humoral agents, not all high-grade tumors enhance and enhancement is also seen after treatment (28–32).

Gliomas are heterogeneous (33) and biopsies are subject to sampling error, notwithstanding the difficulty in morphological assessment mentioned previously. Some gliomas are also inaccessible. Management decisions are based on the grade of the suspected or proven tumor, its size and location, the patient's age, clinical symptoms, performance status (24,34,35), but also, importantly, on the experience and expertise of the managing team. A lesion located in the dominant temporal lobe (eloquent cortex) in a patient who is neurologically intact, with a presumed low-grade glioma, poses different challenges when compared to the aphasic patient who has papilledema and has a similarly placed lesion, which enhances avidly with contrast.

Although [^{1}H]-MRS (proton-MRS), as one of the functional counterparts of MR imaging that allows the depiction of brain metabolites (N-acetylaspartate [NAA], choline, creatine, lactate) (30), has been used in the evaluation of brain tumors for over a decade, it has not gained widespread use. PET and PET/CT provide the opportunity to complement and improve the neuroimaging assessment in this patient group (29). In the authors' opinion, MR imaging and PET/CT, together with conventional CT in particular circumstances, provide the highest quality assessment of brain tumors and should not be regarded as mutually exclusive or competitive. Whereas in other areas of oncology PET/CT could be regarded as a replacement technology for CT, for example, staging and restaging of the lymphomas and recurrent ovarian cancer, in CNS tumors it is a fundamental and complementary component of best-practice management of brain tumors.

The main PET ligand that has been used in this assessment and the most widely used ligand in clinical use today is fluorine-18-fluorodeoxyglucose ([^{18}F]-FDG), an analogue of glucose (30). But whereas in the previous edition of this book the focus of this chapter was imaging with PET-only devices and the examples that were used were from patients who were scanned on a whole-body PET scanner with bismuth germanate detectors, the arrival of clinical PET/CT in 2001 fundamentally changed the neuroimaging landscape for clinicians and PET practitioners. The role of PET/CT and the PET ligands that are used in clinical practice will be covered in the ensuing paragraphs with emphasis on the practical use of the technology to answer the main clinical questions, which are asked by clinicians who care for patients with brain tumor. These questions can be summarized as follows:

1. Is the lesion a high-grade or low-grade tumor? An ancillary question relates to identifying the underlying cell type.
2. What part of the lesion, if only a partial resection is done or if only a biopsy is performed, should be targeted to determine the biological behavior of the tumor?
3. Has this low-grade glioma undergone malignant degeneration?
4. Is there residual tumor after treatment?
5. Is the patient's clinical deterioration due to recurrent tumor or the effects of treatment? Or is the change on the patient's imaging studies due to recurrent tumor or the effects of treatment?
6. How far does the tumor extend into the surrounding tissue?

PET LIGANDS FOR IMAGING BRAIN TUMORS

The largest clinical PET experience in brain tumors is with [^{18}F]-FDG and then carbon-11-methionine ([^{11}C]-MET). More recently there has been interest in [^{18}F]-fluorothymidine ([^{18}F]-FLT) as a tracer to image cellular proliferation. However, over the past two decades a variety of PET ligands have been used to examine aspects of brain tumor biology, and so before expanding on the role of [^{18}F]-FDG, [^{11}C]-MET, and [^{18}F]-FLT it is instructive to review the fate of some of these previous brain tumor PET ligands.

Tumoral glucose and oxygen metabolism, blood flow, pH, BBB, amino acid uptake, hypoxia, receptor binding, and drug delivery/distribution/pharmacokinetics have all been investigated with PET. However, although valuable insights into tumoral biology were obtained, many of the PET ligands that were used have not made the transition into clinical application. Rhodes et al. (36) studied glioma oxygen metabolism and showed that gliomas extract a lower fraction of oxygen than normal brain, suggesting that gliomas are adequately oxygenated. Rottenberg et al. (37) found surprisingly, using [^{11}C]-dimethyl-2,4-oxazolidinedione and later confirmed with phosphorus-31 MRS (38), that brain tumors had an alkaline pH level relative to normal brain. Putrescine serves as a precursor to the polyamines and increased polyamine metabolism is associated with malignancy, so [^{11}C]-putrescine was proposed as a tracer for tumoral DNA synthesis (39); but subsequent studies showed that [^{11}C]-putrescine merely depicted disruption of the BBB (40,41).

Experimental data suggest that benzodiazepines may regulate glial cell proliferation via the peripheral benzodiazepine receptors (PBRs) (42), and it was hoped that PBR ligands might be used as markers of glioma cell density (43,44). PET studies with two PBR ligands, Ro-5-4864 and PK-11195, found that there was no specific binding to astrocytomas with [^{11}C]-Ro-5-4864; and although [^{11}C]-PK-11195 did bind to human gliomas, it did not provide any meaningful data on tumor grading and it also bound to ischemic and inflammatory lesions, thus suggesting it would have limited value in separating recurrent tumor from radiation necrosis, which is essentially a vascular injury (45–47). Interest in altering the tumoral milieu with chemical radiosensitizers and bioreductive agents prior to radiotherapy to eliminate tumor hypoxia and make gliomas more radiosensitive (48–51) resulted in the introduction of [^{18}F]-fluoromisonidazole ([^{18}F]-FMISO) as a hypoxic imaging agent (52). However, since the initial report if Valk et al. (53), where three patients were studied with FMISO, there have been few further data to indicate that it has an impact on patient management (54,55).

Carbon-11-methionine and Amino Acid Transport

The initial hope was that [^{11}C]-MET uptake would reflect incorporation of methionine into tumoral protein and thus provide an index of tumor activity and proliferation. However, several studies have shown that [^{11}C]-MET uptake relates to a saturable carrier-mediated process via an L-type amino acid transporter (56–59). Since the initial reports by the Uppsala group (60,61) of the potential role of [^{11}C]-MET in the evaluation of gliomas, there have been a large number of reports in the literature (62–74). The studies are difficult to compare: some have small patient numbers across the spectrum of gliomas (low- and high-grade astrocytoma, oligodendroglioma, and GBM), the certainty of histopathological diagnosis is unclear for others, scanning and analytical techniques differed, [^{11}C]-MET has been compared to various imaging modalities including [^{18}F]-FDG, thallium-SPECT, and anatomical imaging, and some of the findings have been conflicting. In early work (60,61,70), [^{11}C]-MET was compared with CT and MR, but without gadolinium contrast, and appeared to better delineate the local extension of the tumor into surrounding brain in low-grade gliomas.

Ogawa et al. (71) reported, in 50 patients (32 high- and 18 low-grade gliomas), that although there was a significant difference in [^{11}C]-MET uptake between high-grade and low-grade tumors, in an individual case it was difficult to evaluate the degree of malignancy from [^{11}C]-MET accumulation alone. Kaschten et al. (67) found that although [^{11}C]-methionine uptake was increased in GBMs, it could not separate low-grade from anaplastic astrocytomas. Further, [^{11}C]-MET uptake was increased in oligodendrogliomas but was decreased in anaplastic oligodendrogliomas.

In a larger series of 196 patients where 121 were untreated and there was histopathology in 99, Herholz et al. (66) reported that [^{11}C]-MET uptake could distinguish between different grades of glioma; but high tracer uptake was seen in pituitary adenomas, meningiomas, and ependymomas where there was contrast enhancement and disruption of the BBB. In addition, they reported that steroids reduced [^{11}C]-MET uptake, and intriguingly there was greater [^{11}C]-MET uptake in residual and recurrent tumors when compared to primary tumors. Although these investigators concluded that [^{11}C]-MET uptake was independent of contrast enhancement, some of the conflicting data could be explained if [^{11}C]-MET uptake paralleled disruption of the BBB, which is to be expected in patients with suspected recurrent tumor after initial treatment and which, of course, is influenced by corticosteroids. Indirect support comes from increased [^{11}C]-MET uptake in acute infarction and its inability to separate recurrent tumor from radiation necrosis (75,76).

However, careful work by Derlon et al. (63,65) in two studies has provided some of the answers to the differences in the literature. In 22 untreated patients with low-grade tumors, they found that low-grade astrocytomas had decreased, normal or only moderately increased [^{11}C]-MET uptake, whereas all oligodendrogliomas had high [^{11}C]-MET uptake (63). These findings in low-grade astrocytomas indicate that it would not be possible to identify the extension of tumor into the surrounding brain with [^{11}C]-MET and suggest that investigators in the earlier reports may have studied oligodendrogliomas (60,61,70,71). Then in 47 patients—27 with low-grade oligodendrogliomas and 20 anaplastic oligodendrogliomas—the same investigators showed that these two tumor grades could be separated by degree of [^{11}C]-MET uptake (65).

In recent work where [^{11}C]-MET uptake was compared to microvessel density, measured by immunostaining of excised tissue with factor VIII antibody, there was a direct correlation, and the highest [^{11}C]-MET uptake values and vessel densities were seen in an anaplastic oligodendroglioma (69). The investigators suggested that such data could be used to identify patients who could potentially respond to antiangiogenic therapies. Recently, vascular endothelial growth factor (VEGF), a protein that plays a critical role in tumor angiogenesis, has been targeted by bevacizumab, a recombinant humanized antibody that binds to and inhibits VEGF in clinical trials in brain tumor patients (77).

A number of other PET ligands that use amino acid transporters and have similar characteristics to [^{11}C]-MET have been synthesized and used in similar clinical settings, albeit in small series. These include [^{18}F]-fluorotyrosine, [^{18}F]-fluoroethyltyrosine, [^{18}F]-fluorophenylalanine, [^{11}C]-aminocyclopentane carboxylic acid, and [^{11}C]-methyl-α-aminoisobutyric acid (78,79). Apart from the advantage of an [^{18}F] label over [^{11}C], these ligands have not provided additional major insights into the biology of gliomas or had an impact in the clinical setting; but this may reflect limited opportunities to use these ligands in clinical practice.

Carbon-11-thymidine and Fluorine-18-fluorothymidine: Cellular Proliferation

Although there has been intense interest recently in using PET to measure tumor cell growth and hence response to therapy (80), the first attempts at imaging cellular proliferation date back to the Brookhaven group in the 1970s using [^{11}C]-labeled thymidine ([^{11}C]-Tdr) (81,82). Thymidine is a pyrimidine nucleoside that is rapidly taken up by cells and incorporated into DNA, and not RNA, through thymidine kinase (TK). Animal studies identified that there was a correlation between PET-Tdr uptake and DNA synthesis, and the first human studies were carried out in patients with non-Hodgkin's lymphoma by Martiat et al. (83) in 1988.

In an early brain tumor study, Vander Borght et al. (84) performed dynamic [^{11}C]-Tdr scans in 20 patients with a mixture of untreated low- and high-grade gliomas, recurrent gliomas, and non-gliomas, including meningiomas, lymphomas, and a metastasis. Although the number of patients was small, they reported [^{11}C]-Tdr uptake in gliomas, regardless of grade, but also in benign meningiomas and noted uptake into the choroid plexus; importantly, these investigators did not examine the degree of contrast enhancement on anatomical imaging in their patients. However, [^{11}C]-Tdr is a problematic ligand with its short half-life, rapid degradation *in vivo* to labeled metabolites and the requirement for dynamic scanning, arterial blood sampling, plasma metabolite analysis, and mathematical modeling to accurately assess uptake, which explains the lack of large patient series. However, the development of a fluorinated analogue of thymidine, 3'-deoxy-3'-[^{18}F]-fluorothymidine ([^{18}F]-FLT), which is more practical for clinical studies, rekindled interest in this area (80).

The analogue [^{18}F]-FLT has a high specificity for thymidine kinase 1 in the cytosol and is phosphorylated but then essentially trapped in the cell and not incorporated into DNA because it lacks 3'-hydroxyl (85). Thus, [^{18}F]-FLT labels the intracellular nucleotide pool but is dephosphorylated and ultimately conjugated with glucuronide in the liver before being excreted by the kidneys. Early reports by a number of investigators have suggested that [^{18}F]-FLT shows promise as marker of proliferation in high-grade gliomas (86–91). However, two of these studies also included patients with nontumorous lesions and found that there was increased [^{18}F]-FLT uptake in regions of infarction, demyelination, granuloma, and also in low-grade tumors such as gangliogliomas, germinomas, and dysembryoplastic neuroepithelial tumors (DNETs) (87,90). In addition, Muzi et al. (92) also showed that without contrast enhancement (disruption of the BBB) there was no [^{18}F]-FLT uptake, and that dynamic scanning, with arterial blood sampling and modeling analysis, was needed to separate [^{18}F]-FLT transport (K1) across the BBB from [^{18}F]-FLT incorporation into cells. Although the work of Muzi et al. will need to be replicated, their work suggests that [^{18}F]-FLT may have a limited role in the evaluation of treatment response in gliomas.

Fluorine-18-fluorodeoxyglucose

FDG is an analogue of glucose and is taken up by cells and phosphorylated by hexokinase to fluorodeoxyglucose-6-phosphate (FDG-6-P). However, because it is FDG-6-P it cannot participate in other steps of the glycolytic cycle and so is effectively "trapped" in the cell. The phosphorylation of FDG to FDG-6-P reflects cellular glucose utilization. Glucose enters the cell via a number of different glucose transporter proteins (GLUTs), which are expressed in neurons, glia, and also vascular endothelium in the CNS (93–95).

There is avid FDG uptake into the normal brain as glucose is the only fuel that the brain uses for energy metabolism. The predominant site of energy utilization in mammalian nervous tissue is at synaptic terminals, for excitatory and inhibitory neurotransmission, rather than in the cell body (96). This feature and knowledge of the various synaptic connections in the CNS has important implications for the accurate interpretation of neurologic PET/CT scans (see the section "Diaschisis" below). Thus, a neurologic [^{18}F]-FDG PET image reflects synaptic activity but with two exceptions: (a) high-grade tumors and (b) a seizure focus during the ictus, where somal glucose metabolism predominates.

An underlying principle of [^{18}F]-FDG PET in the assessment of CNS tumors is that the higher the grade of malignancy, the greater the glucose metabolism, which is due in part to greater "anaerobic glycolysis" with increasing grade of malignancy and overexpression of specific glucose transporters (29,97,98). Di Chiro et al. (99) showed in 1982 that increased FDG uptake, relative to white matter, was seen in high-grade tumors (anaplastic astrocytoma, GBM), whereas in low-grade tumors, glucose metabolism was less than, equal to, or only slightly greater than that in normal white matter. Examples, studied with PET/CT, are shown in Figs. 8.6.1 and 8.6.2.

Many other investigators (100–103) subsequently replicated these findings. There have been a few exceptions (104,105) where investigators did not find a correlation between glucose metabolism and tumor grade in small series of patients. However, these investigators compared average, rather than maximum, tumoral FDG uptake to FDG uptake in the contralateral brain (gray and white matter) with early generation PET scanners. The surprisingly low metabolic values for high-grade tumors in their series could be at least partly explained by partial volume error and region of interest placement that included areas of necrosis.

In a large number of patients, Fulham et al. (106) reported that the average value for the ratio of tumor to white matter glucose metabolism is 1.3 for low-grade tumors, 4.2 for anaplastic astrocytomas, and 6.5 for GBM. Independently, Delbeke et al. (102) suggested a "cutoff" ratio of 1.5 tumor/white matter ratio to separate low-grade from high-grade gliomas.

Unfortunately, the Tyler et al. (105) and Oriuchi et al. (104) citations mentioned above and the normal avid FDG uptake into the normal brain continue to be cited in the literature and are used by investigators to identify the limitations of [^{18}F]-FDG in the

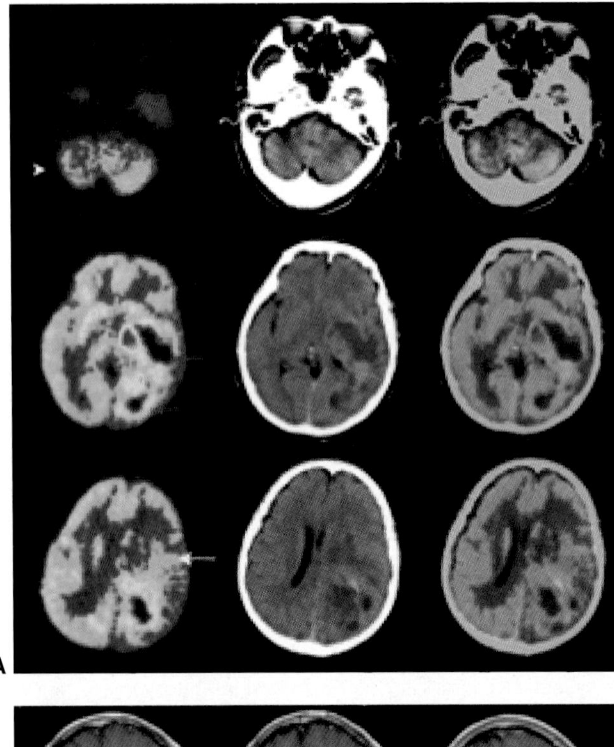

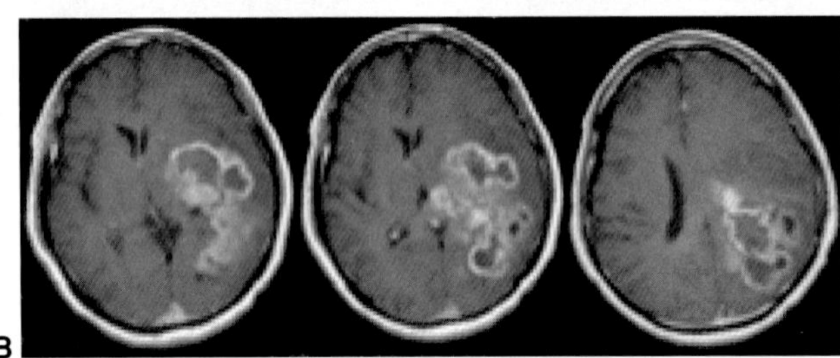

FIGURE 8.6.1. A: Patient TM: A man in his early 60s with a large left-dominant hemisphere glioblastoma multiforme (World Health Organization grade IV) involving the left-temporoinsular, occipital, and parietal lobes. Representative transaxial fluorine-18-fluorodeoxyglucose (^{18}F-FDG) PET, noncontrast CT, and fused PET/CT images (*left to right*) performed on an LSO Biograph Duo PET/CT (Siemens, Hoffman Estates, Illinois). There is mild misregistration between the PET and CT data sets. In the first horizontal panel there is right cerebellar hypometabolism (*white arrowhead*)—crossed cerebellar diaschisis—secondary to the large left hemisphere mass. On CT there are hypo- and hyperdense regions in the L hemisphere associated with mass effect, compression of the left lateral ventricle, and midline shift. On ^{18}F-FDG PET there are multiple, necrotic cavities (*red arrows*) surrounded by heterogeneous increased FDG uptake; the most markedly glucose-avid component is located deep in the left temporal lobe. The superficial cortex is hypometabolic due to deafferentation, although "tongues" of tumor tissue (*white arrows*) are seen extending anteriorly into white matter and cortex of the posterior left frontal lobe. **B:** Transaxial T1-weighted (T1W) gadolinium-enhanced magnetic resonance images (*left to right*) show the large, irregular, ill-defined left hemisphere mass with ragged enhancement surrounding multiple cystic/necrotic lesions throughout the posterior left hemisphere; there is marked mass effect with compression of the left ventricular system and midline shift to the right. The marked heterogeneity in FDG uptake in the rim of the lesions contrasts to the homogeneous, if irregular, gadolinium enhancement.

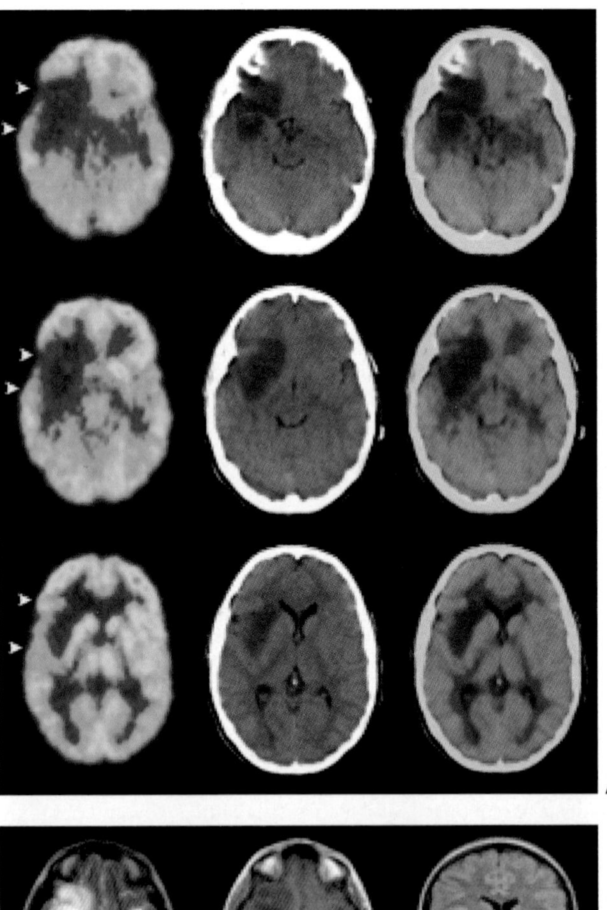

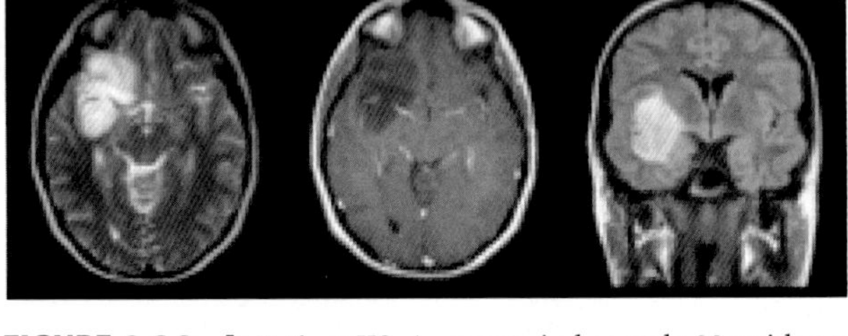

FIGURE 8.6.2. A: Patient KS: A woman in her early 20s with a normal neurological examination and a low-grade astrocytoma (World Health Organization grade II). Representative [^{18}F]-FDG PET/CT (LSO Biograph Duo, Siemens, Hoffman Estates, Illinois) images (*left to right*): There is minimal misregistration between the PET and CT data. Extensive glucose hypometabolism is evident on PET in the right temporal, insula, and frontal white matter, but there is also relatively reduced metabolism in the overlying cortices (*white arrowheads*), probably due to a combination of tumor infiltration and deafferentation. There is mass effect with displacement and relative hypometabolism of the right basal ganglia. The mass lesion envelops the right middle cerebral artery (MCA). There are no regions of increased glucose metabolism to indicate focal anaplasia or malignant change. **B:** Single transaxial T2-weighted (T2W), gadolinium-enhanced T1W, and coronal fluid-attenuated inversion recovery magnetic resonance images show the apparently well-circumscribed abnormality—a hyperintense lesion extending from the right temporal lobe to involve the right insula and posterior right frontal lobes. There is no enhancement; the right MCA is seen in the center of the lesion.

evaluation of gliomas (66,72,86–89,107–109). In the authors' opinion this repetition reflects a fundamental lack of understanding of brain tumor pathophysiology and the interpretation of [^{18}F]-FDG PET and PET/CT scans.

Gliomas arise from glia and may have extensive connections with surrounding glial cells, but they do not have synaptic terminals. Although glia can be found in the gray matter (cortex), they are mainly located in the white matter with the axons of neurons; there is very little energy utilization in axons, less than the cell soma. Thus, white matter [^{18}F]-FDG uptake is a reflection of normal glial glucose metabolism.

To determine if a glial tumor has increased metabolism it is appropriate to compare it to normal white matter; it is illogical to compare metabolism in a glial tumor to cortical glucose metabolism. The authors' practice is to use the white matter of the centrum semiovale of the contralateral cerebral hemisphere; the availability of PET/CT means that there is little problem in identifying contralateral white matter and avoiding the lateral ventricle and the moderate [^{18}F]-FDG uptake in the body of the caudate nucleus (106,110). When there is malignant degeneration of a low-grade glioma, the initial clue is increased metabolism in the white matter, or in cortex, that was previously hypometabolic.

The limitations of the PET device should be considered when interpreting scans. It is not surprising that a PET device with a 5 to 7 mm in-plane and z-axis resolution will have difficulty detecting a 1 to 2 mm thin rim of tumor because of partial volume effects.

Low-grade gliomas characteristically infiltrate the surrounding brain, spreading between axons and normal glia in the white and gray matter. They spread beyond the abnormality identified on T2-weighted MR images and also the macroscopic abnormality that is identified at surgery. In part, this explains why a patient can have a very large low-grade glioma with no neurological findings (Fig. 8.6.2). As the volume of tumor increases there is disturbance of normal synaptic activity, and if afferent axons to the cortex are compressed the overlying cortex may become relatively hypometabolic when compared to the adjacent cortex. When a patient is imaged for the first time, it can be difficult to determine if islands of retained metabolism that are seen in the cortex within an extensive area of glucose hypometabolism are focal areas of anaplastic change or normal cortex, which is infiltrated and compressed by low-grade glioma cells. In such instances serial scans and comparison to MR imaging will resolve the matter; on [^{18}F]-FDG the cortex becomes more and more hypometabolic over time.

DIASCHISIS

As mentioned earlier, a neurologic [^{18}F]-FDG PET scan depicts synaptic activity *in vivo*. It is not uncommon to see reduced glucose metabolism in the cerebellar hemisphere contralateral to a supratentorial glioma, so-called crossed cerebellar diaschisis (CCD) (Fig. 8.6.1). The term CCD was introduced by Baron et al. (111) to describe the reduction of blood flow in the cerebellar hemisphere contralateral ("crossed") to a supratentorial cerebral infarct. Similar findings were confirmed with [^{18}F]-FDG in brain tumor patients (112). "Diaschisis" was first introduced by Von Monakow in 1910 to describe a "state of reduced or abolished function . . . after a brain injury and acting on a neural region remote from the lesion" (113). However, despite the marked reduction in cerebellar glucose metabolism, with CCD there is not a clinical manifestation that can be detected with standard bedside tests of cerebellar function. CCD can accompany any supratentorial process including tumor, extensive unilateral cerebral edema, infarction, gliosis, trauma, and demyelination.

The mechanism for CCD is an interruption to the corticopontocerebellar (CPC) pathway from the cerebral hemispheres to the contralateral cerebellar cortex. The CPC pathway arises from all lobes of the cerebral hemispheres, but the main inputs come from prefrontal, sensorimotor, and occipital cortices (114). The first CPC synapse is in the ipsilateral pons and second-order neurons cross the midline, via the middle cerebellar peduncle, to terminate in the cerebellar cortex. Fulham et al. (115) showed that there is ipsilateral pontine glucose hypometabolism consistent with this hypothesis together with relative preservation of glucose metabolism in the dentate nucleus of the hypometabolic cerebellar hemisphere. Regions of ipsilateral glucose hypometabolism can be found in the frontal or parietal cortices due to the interruption of ipsilateral cortical association fibers and due to loss of afferent input from a lesion in the thalamus. In both these situations the glucose hypometabolism, due to deafferentation, is visually obvious.

EFFECTS OF MEDICATION

Corticosteroids are commonly administered to patients with brain tumor for the symptomatic relief of cerebral edema. Common side effects of prolonged steroid therapy include centripetal obesity, cushingoid facies, abdominal striae, disordered sleep patterns, and neuropsychiatric disturbances, which can range from a mild behavioral change to psychosis (116). Steroids can also reduce cerebral glucose metabolism, and studies typically appear "noisy" with poor delineation of the usual functional landmarks.

Fulham et al. (117) reported a marked reduction in cerebral glucose metabolism in 45 patients with unilateral cerebral gliomas when compared to normal subjects and patients with brain tumor who were not taking steroids. A progressive decline in metabolism was noted in patients as the steroid dose was increased, and cessation of steroids resulted in restoration of metabolism. This effect was independent of radiotherapy, concurrent anticonvulsant medication, transhemispheric functional disconnection (transhemispheric diaschisis), and blood sugar level.

Reduced glucose metabolism can also be seen with sedatives, including barbiturates and major tranquilizers, to a marked extent, and is visually apparent, and with antiepileptic drugs (AEDs) to a lesser extent where region of interest analysis is usually required to detect it (118–121).

TECHNICAL ASPECTS OF BRAIN PET/CT

In this chapter in the previous edition the clinical examples that were used were taken from a bismuth germanate whole-body PET scanner (ECAT 951, Siemens, Hoffman Estates, Illinois). The z-axis field of view was essentially 10 cm, and two data acquisitions were required to cover the entire brain. Hooper et al. (122) used a postinjection transmission method for attenuation correction, and the typical study duration for a two data acquisitions study was approximately 1 hour. There was emphasis on alignment of [^{18}F]-FDG-PET data to CT and MR because of the poor visualization of functional anatomy with PET (123,124). PET/CT has now rendered much of these previous data obsolete. The authors installed our first PET/CT scanner (LSO Biograph Duo; Siemens, Hoffman Estates, Illinois) in 2003 and in December 2006 our second PET/CT, the 64-slice Truepoint Biograph (Siemens, Hoffman Estates, Illinois) with

LSO detectors, was installed. The physics of PET/CT are covered elsewhere in this book (see Chapter 3) and will not be expanded upon here.

This section outlines the practical aspects of performing routine clinical [^{18}F]-FDG PET/CT studies:

- Adult patients are studied after a 6-hour fast; In women of reproductive age the possibility of pregnancy is discussed at the time of interview and if there is doubt, the study is delayed while a pregnancy test is performed;
- In the authors' center, two peripheral venous cannulas are placed prior to the injection of isotope in heated upper limbs; one is used for isotope injection and the other for venous blood sampling for the quantitative measurement of glucose metabolism; the authors use a simplified "arterialized venous" method with three blood samples (125) because the authors believe that it helps study interpretation; many centers only obtain a single sample to assess blood glucose levels;
- A standard amount of [^{18}F]-FDG (350 MBq) is injected into each subject;
- The uptake period is 45 minutes during which the patient rests quietly, the eyes are patched and the ears are plugged from just before the injection of isotope toward the end of the uptake period;
- Sedation is not given as a routine; if patients require sedation the authors' preference is for the patients to be given a short general anesthetic under controlled circumstances at the end of the uptake period and planned to last for the duration of the PET acquisition; with this timing the sedative medication has the least effect on glucose metabolism; occasionally a short acting benzodiazepine is given after the patient is positioned on the scanning bed, but this is not the authors' preferred option;
- Video electroencephalogram (EEG) monitoring is done in all patients; a washable, removable cap with surface electrodes is used; EEG data are acquired prior to the injection of isotope and throughout the uptake period;
- At the end of the uptake period the patient is placed on the scanning bed; at completion of the scan patients are provided with a drink and a sandwich and encouraged to drink fluid over the next 6 hours;
- Scan parameters for:
  - PET/CT Duo: 130 kV; effective mAs—190; slice width—5 mm; collimation 2.5 mm; feed/rotation 7.3 mm; PET data three-dimensional acquisition—7 minutes;
  - PET/CT Truepoint: 120 kV, effective mAs—350; slice width—2 mm; collimation—1.2 mm; feed/rotation—23 mm; PET three-dimensional list mode acquisition—7 minutes;
- Data reconstruction for:
  - PET/CT Duo: reconstructed slice thickness is 3.4 mm for both PET and CT; attenuation correction—CT-based: FORE three-dimensional to two-dimensional rebinning; discrete inverse Fourier transform reconstruction algorithm with zoom 2.7X, 512 × 512 matrix; postreconstruction filter—2 mm FWHM Gaussian;
  - PET/CT Truepoint: reconstructed slice thickness is 2 mm for both PET and CT; attenuation correction—CT based: FORE three-dimensional to two-dimentional rebinning; filtered back projection with zoom 2.7X, 256 × 256 matrix; postreconstruction filter—2.5 mm FWHM Gaussian;
- Radiation exposure for:
  - PET/CT Duo: CT 1.5 mSv and PET 7 mSv;
  - PET/CT Truepoint: CT 2.0 mSv and PET 7 mSv;
- When necessary PET/CT are registered to CT and MR data using an algorithm developed locally (123).

"Noisy" Studies

There are a number of situations where "noisy," poor-quality images are encountered:

- In patients with hyperglycemia the tracer dose of [^{18}F]-FDG competes with serum glucose for the cerebral GLUTs and hexokinase. The result is reduced cerebral [^{18}F]-FDG uptake and "noisy," poor-quality images. Increasing the time for data acquisition will improve the counting statistics in this situation.
- Corticosteroids have a similar effect on image quality, which is independent of the blood sugar level, although steroids can also raise blood glucose levels worsening image quality (see above).
- Head motion during the acquisition period also degrades image quality. Prior to the advent of PET/CT the extent of the problem was probably underrecognized. It was certainly appreciated by experienced PET practitioners because some type of head fixation (e.g., thermoplastic face masks) were widely used for PET scanners. However, unless there was marked movement, many experienced PET physicians were reassured, perhaps falsely, that motion was not a major problem. In addition, some centers had developed algorithms to correct for motion (126,127), but accurate identification of motion was not trivial and required a motion-tracking device before the motion could be corrected (128).

It is the authors' opinion that it is still better to limit motion rather than to correct for it later. In the authors' center, the acquisition time for a PET scan went from 60 minutes to 10 minutes with the introduction of our first PET/CT. The ability to fuse the CT and PET data also identified that head motion was an issue; it was more noticeable in whole-body studies where scan duration was longer, but in neurologic cases where motion occurred it had the potential to introduce errors into reconstruction and interpretation (Fig. 8.6.3). Subtle degrees of misregistration are also identified in some of the accompanying images in this chapter. The authors have noticed a marked reduction in the degree of misregistration with the head holder on our new PET/CT scanner.

THE IMPORTANT CLINICAL QUESTIONS

In any discussion about the role/value of PET/CT in the management of brain tumors it is essential to consider the local clinical practice, as this is the major factor in how PET/CT impacts upon patient care. "Local practice" includes the local expertise, as well as philosophy, in neurosurgery, neurology, neuro-oncology, radiation oncology, neuropathology, PET/CT, and neuroradiology. It is also important to consider the available infrastructure including MR imaging, radiosurgery including Gamma Knife (Elekta Corp, Stockholm) or dedicated radiosurgery devices, type of PET device (PET, PET/CT and type), and intraoperative MR imaging. Although many centers have expertise across some areas, it is often difficult to have excellence across all areas and state-of-the-art technology in every subspecialty. In the authors' center there is a long-standing interest in brain tumor management, and patients are discussed in fortnightly, multidisciplinary tumor board meetings where the clinical, imaging, pathological findings, and management issues are discussed with representation from all the disciplines. The authors do not have access to a dedicated radiosurgery facility at present, but it, together with an intraoperative

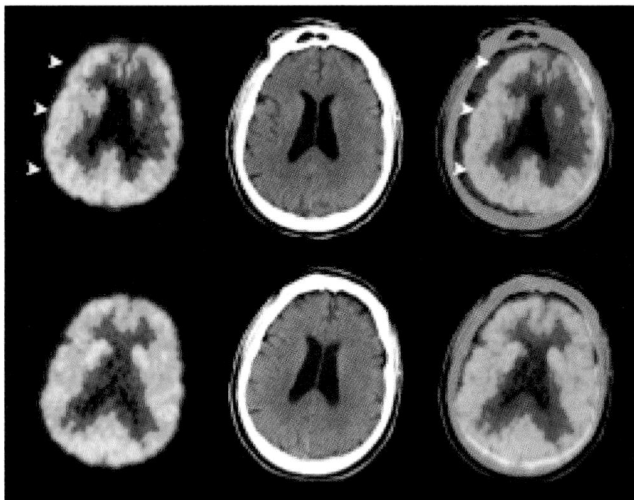

FIGURE 8.6.3. Patient JC: A nearly 40-year-old retarded man scanned on two separate occasions for assessment of his hypoxic brain damage after a drug overdose. Single representative transaxial fluorine-18-fluorodeoxyglucose ([^{18}F]-FDG) PET/CT (LSO Biograph Duo, Siemens, Hoffman Estates, Illinois) images (*left to right*). First study (**top panel**) shows an apparent relative increase in glucose metabolism in the right hemisphere cortex (*white arrowheads*) when compared to the left, which is due to misregistration (*white arrowheads*) and incorrect attenuation correction between the PET and CT data sets seen on fused image. On the second study (**bottom panel**), performed some months later, the patient was more cooperative and was given a short-acting sedative prior to the scan. There is still mild misregistration between PET and CT data on the fused image, and there is now relatively symmetric glucose metabolism in the hemispheres.

1.5T MR device, will be installed later this year and both will influence the brain tumor program and the role of PET/CT.

The following sections discuss some of the important clinical questions that arise in tumor management.

Is the Lesion a High-grade or Low-grade Tumor?

As indicated earlier, the first investigation that is usually performed in the evaluation of a suspected brain tumor is a brain CT or MR scan because they are usually more readily available than PET/CT. It is an accepted general principle that in this clinical context, a mass lesion that enhances after intravenous contrast (iodinated or paramagnetic) agents is considered to be a high-grade tumor. Similarly, a lesion with minimal or no enhancement is regarded as a low-grade tumor with a few notable exceptions (see the section "Special Tumor Types" below) (34,129–135).

Some illustrative clinical examples are cited below. Patient MT (shown previously at Fig. 8.6.1) is a 61-year-old man who developed severe headache and left arm weakness while on a trip in the week prior to admission. According to his family, they had noticed problems with his language in the months preceding his admission, but he was otherwise in good health. There was no other relevant past medical history. On examination, he was right handed, had a right hemiparesis, a moderately severe aphasia, and a Karnofsky performance status (KPS) of 50; medications were dexamethasone 8 mg twice a day. The very extensive, heterogeneous, partly necrotic lesion was partly resected. Unfortunately, the most glucose-avid element deep in the left hemisphere could not be resected. Histopathology revealed a GBM and postoperatively, when the wound was healed, he underwent combined chemoradiotherapy with temozolomide. How does PET/CT help in this setting? PET/CT provided additional valuable information about the tumor. It demonstrated the marked heterogeneity in glucose metabolism in the tumor rim, which surrounded large regions of necrosis, compared to the relatively homogenous enhancement on MR. It also identified that, unfortunately, the most metabolically active part of the tumor was located deep in the left mesial temporal lobe and thus unlikely to be resected. Although initial management did not change, the PET/CT data were used in radiotherapy planning, and an additional radiotherapy boost was given to the deep component in the mesial temporal lobe. Prospective comparisons of [^{18}F]-FDG PET to MR imaging with gadolinium have been reported (136,137). Davis et al. (136) reported findings in 22 gliomas while Melisi et al. (137) analyzed 160 [^{18}F]-FDG PET studies from 113 patients with gliomas. Both studies identified that [^{18}F]-FDG PET and enhanced MR imaging were complementary, but Melisi et al. (137) noted that in 20% of cases, there was a disparity between [^{18}F]-FDG PET and MR. This disparity included patients with primary high-grade tumors that had increased [^{18}F]-FDG uptake on PET but did not enhance on MR. Other investigators reported similar findings; Chamberlain et al. (138) showed that 31% of highly anaplastic and 54% of moderately anaplastic astrocytomas did not enhance on CT. In smaller series, Kondziolka et al. (32) and Kelly et al. (139) noted a similar lack of enhancement with MR imaging (between 47% and 90%) in anaplastic astrocytomas.

However, it is important to appreciate that *de novo* GBMs grow rapidly and, rarely, may not be identified at the initial presentation. Patient ES (Fig. 8.6.4) is a 43-year-old man, previously well, who presented with a generalized tonic/clonic seizure at work. In the minutes prior to losing consciousness he had an aura of being unable to speak and hearing "funny noises." When the first scan was done the KPS was 100 and medication was phenytoin 300 mg per day. Six weeks later he was readmitted to hospital aphasic, with KPS of 50 and complaining of severe headache. The subtle lesion evident in the left temporal lobe was now much larger and necrotic.

At surgery, 1 day later, a GBM was resected. It was initially thought that the patient had a low-grade glioma and serial imaging was planned. However, it is highly likely that the lesion was a GBM from the outset but that the lesion was small. Although it was able to provoke a seizure there was no gadolinium enhancement and minimal edema. Was the tumor rim of increased metabolism missed on [^{18}F]-FDG PET/CT because of surrounding normal glucose metabolism in the cortex? The authors have no doubt that PET/CT missed the very small active tumor component, which was likely to be smaller than the resolution of the scanner. It is arguable whether or not any PET ligand could have made the diagnosis of a GBM.

Although a number of investigators have drawn attention to the avidity of normal cerebral cortical glucose metabolism for [^{18}F]-FDG as a limitation to its use as a clinical tool in identifying high-grade tumors, in the authors' experience instances such as those for patient ES are rare (66,72,86–89,107–109).

The presentation of patient SK is very similar to patient ES. Patient SK (Fig. 8.6.2) had a generalized tonic/clonic seizure in her sleep. For 2 months prior to the witnessed generalized seizure she had had several episodes of *deja vu* and episodes of "unresponsiveness" during classes. Neurological examination was normal. In this case a biopsy was not done initially to prove the suspected diagnosis because it would not have changed management. As shown in Fig. 8.6.2, this lesion is not resectable and it is difficult to imagine

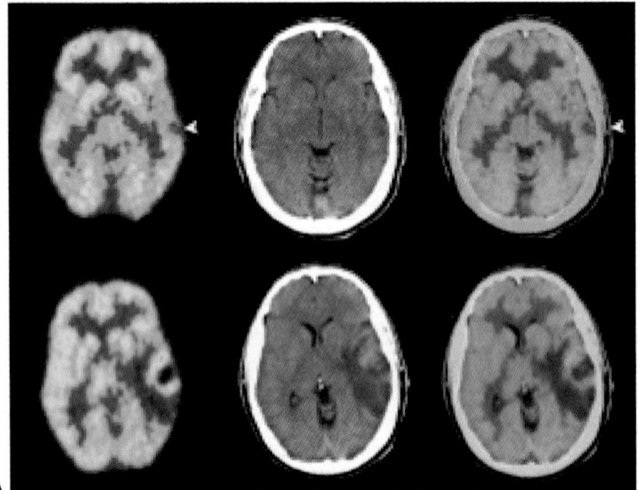
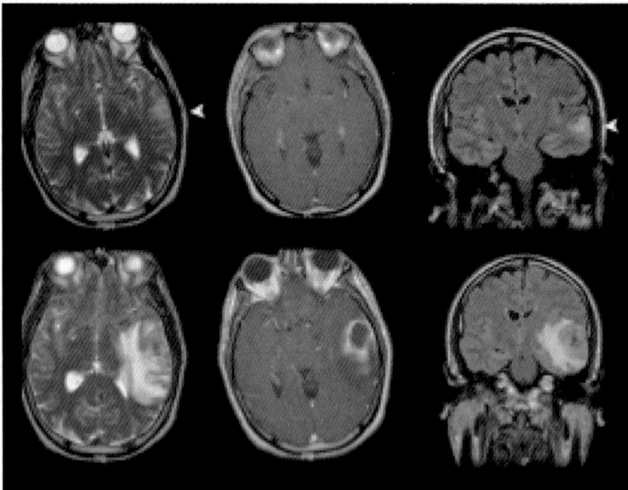

FIGURE 8.6.4. A: Patient ES: A man in his early 40s with a left temporal glioblastoma multiforme. Scans were performed 6 weeks apart. Single representative transaxial [^{18}F]-FDG PET/CT (LSO Biograph Duo, Siemens, Hoffman Estates, Illinois) images (*left to right*). There is good registration between the PET and CT images. First scan (**top panel**) shows a subtle region of glucose hypometabolism in left temporal cortex (*white arrowhead*). The second scan done 6 weeks later (**bottom panel**) shows a large, heterogeneous rim of increased metabolism surrounding an ametabolic (necrotic) center consistent with a high-grade glioma. There is mass effect and surrounding cortical hypometabolism due to marked vasogenic edema seen on CT. **B:** Corresponding magnetic resonance (MR) imaging studies were done a few days before the PET/CT scan on each occasion. Single transaxial T2-weighted (T2W), enhanced T1W, and coronal fluid-attenuated inverse recovery (FLAIR) MR images are shown (*left to right*). The absent gadolinium-enhancement and minimal hyperintensity seen on the T2W and FLAIR images (**top panel**) on first study (*white arrowheads*) contrasts markedly with images from the second scan 6 weeks later (**bottom panel**) where there is extensive edema and contrast enhancement, which surrounds the hypointense center of the lesion.

that even with the latest development in neurosurgical microsurgery and intraoperative imaging (see later) that this lesion could be totally resected.

Low-grade gliomas are typically hyperintense on T2-weighted and flair MR images and do not enhance after contrast. The management of patients with proven or suspected low-grade gliomas is controversial, and there are no randomized trials to support any active approach. Some clinicians advocate attempted gross surgical removal. Others perform a biopsy and if anaplasia is detected it may be followed by radiotherapy. Still others perform a biopsy, and if the pathologic findings are consistent with a low-grade glioma, they may then manage the patient conservatively with serial imaging. Finally, some clinicians do not perform a biopsy in an asymptomatic patient and instead await clinical deterioration before intervention (23,24,140–143).

In the authors' opinion, for a patient with a hypometabolic lesion on [^{18}F]-FDG PET/CT, controlled seizures and no neurological signs, there is a persuasive argument to follow the patient with serial scans, given that the natural history of low-grade gliomas is uncertain and there is no evidence that early intervention alters this natural history. Further, surgical resection/stereotactic and open biopsy cannot make a asymptomatic patients better and rather exposes them to the risk of a neurological deficit regardless of the neurosurgeon's expertise. Additional factors to consider are the sampling error associated with biopsy and the risks associated with both radiotherapy and chemotherapy (144). There is clearly variability in practice patterns in this regard.

Patient A-LL is now nearly 60 years old and continues to work full time in a clerical field (Fig. 8.6.5). At age 42, she had a focal seizure involving her right side and collapsed after getting out of bed. A CT brain scan was performed and was initially reported as showing a left parietal cerebral infarct; the lesion was not calcified and did not enhance with contrast. There were no neurological findings on initial examination, and an open biopsy was performed soon after presentation. The biopsy was reported initially as showing a low-grade astrocytoma. The pathology was then reviewed at the authors' multidisciplinary tumor board meeting and the pathology was revised to a central neurocytoma, despite its location in the periphery of the left parieto-occipital lobe. Over time the lesion became heavily calcified and another pathology review was requested; the patient has remained relatively asymptomatic apart from occasional focal motor and sensory seizures that she manages. She continues to have a normal neurological examination. The pathology was revised to a low-grade oligodendroglioma. She has not had radiotherapy or chemotherapy.

What Is the Cell Type?

The identification of the glioma cell type is beyond the capabilities of current neuroimaging modalities including MR imaging, MRS, and PET/CT. Indirect inferences can be made from the current techniques, but it should be remembered that they are inferences only. For example, a ragged pattern of enhancement seen on MR in an untreated patient is likely to indicate a high-grade tumor, but the

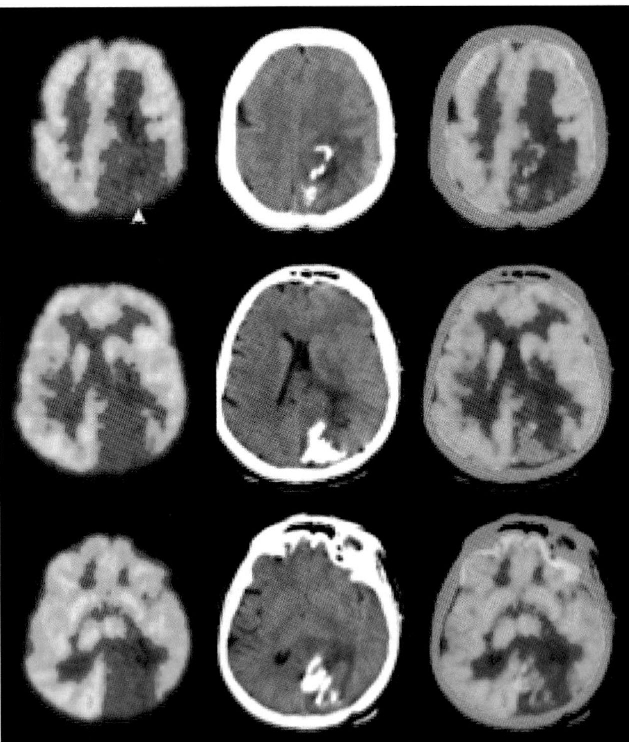

FIGURE 8.6.5. Patient A-LL: A nearly 60-year-old woman with a low-grade oligodendroglioma. The lesion was first identified after a seizure 14 years prior to this scan; the patient continues to work full time. Representative transaxial fluorine-18-fluorodeoxyglucose ([^{18}F]-FDG) PET/CT (LSO Biograph Duo, Siemens, Hoffman Estates, Illinois) images (*left to right, top to bottom*) show the extensive glucose hypometabolism in the left parieto-occipital lobes in the large diffuse mass, which is heavily calcified. There is focal reduced cortical metabolism in the left parietal cortex (*white arrowhead*), which is likely to represent infiltrated cortex because over time it has become more hypometabolic. Gene deletion studies were not done.

underlying tumor may be a cystic anaplastic astrocytoma, a necrotic GBM, or a cystic/necrotic oligodendroglioma. Further, ragged enhancement is nonspecific, and a similar picture can be seen in large regions of demyelination, abscess formation, and in brain tumors after treatment. A GBM, on [^{18}F]-FDG PET/CT, has a typical irregular "doughnut" shape with a rim of heterogeneous increased metabolism surrounding a central region of absent metabolism (necrosis) (Figs. 8.6.1 and 8.6.4). Cystic regions also have absent metabolism, and anaplastic astrocytomas/oligodendrogliomas should also be considered in the differential diagnosis. Calcification, readily identified with PET/CT, can be found in oligodendrogliomas (Fig. 8.6.5), but again this finding does not have the specificity to be clinically valuable because calcification is found in astrocytomas, mixed oligoastrocytomas, as well as in other types of tumors including gangliogliomas and craniopharyngiomas.

Cerebral lymphomas, in the authors' experience, tend to display the most markedly increased [^{18}F]-FDG uptake of all brain tumors, but occasionally a GBM or anaplastic tumor will have a similar degree of uptake. The authors suggest that a combination of imaging findings will improve specificity; for example, a mass lesion that does not enhance on MR, is hypometabolic but partly calcified with [^{18}F]-FDG PET/CT, and displays increased [^{11}C]-MET uptake is more likely to be an oligodendroglioma than an astrocytoma, but ultimately a histopathological/molecular genetic analysis will be the only way to be sure about the cell type.

What Part of the Lesion Should be Targeted?

The ability of [^{18}F]-FDG PET to identify tumor heterogeneity improves the diagnostic yield of stereotactic biopsy (145–147). A number of investigators have shown that when focal hypermetabolism seen with [^{18}F]-FDG PET is targeted, it is more likely that tissue that reflects the tumor biology will be obtained than when anatomic imaging is used alone. Levivier et al. (146) reported improved yields when PET, compared to CT, was used to guide stereotactic biopsy, in 38 patients with supratentorial brain tumors. Massager et al. (147) applied a similar technique to brainstem lesions, but with PET compared with MR imaging, and showed that a combined PET-MR approach improved the accuracy of targeting. The combined approach reduced the number of trajectories needed to obtain representative tissue, thereby limiting the risk for neurologic damage at this eloquent site.

In the authors' center, the neurosurgeons use stereotactic biopsy sparingly and generally only for deep lesions, lesions in the brainstem, and for lesions in eloquent cortex in patients with poor KPS, and in this context [^{18}F]-FDG PET/CT is invaluable.

Has This Low-grade Glioma Undergone Malignant Degeneration?

In the authors' opinion the majority of proven and suspected low-grade gliomas will progress to a more anaplastic tumor over time. However, currently it is impossible to predict when this "malignant degeneration" will occur. In the authors' center, [^{18}F]-FDG PET/CT scans are often performed annually on patients with proven or presumed low-grade gliomas, but the individual patient's wishes are always considered in this determination. The uncertainty of "living with" a low-grade tumor, which may become malignant at some stage in the future, yet cannot be removed, is very difficult to manage; some patients prefer not to know and others are reassured if the scan shows little change. Imaging is done earlier if there are changes in symptoms; for example, an increase in seizure or headache frequency or a change in seizure type occurs, without a clearly identifiable cause, particularly in patients older than 50 years.

When increased glucose metabolism is seen in the lesion on [^{18}F]-FDG PET/CT, regardless of the MR findings, it is then time to reevaluate the options for treatment and consider a tissue sample (148,149). An example is shown in Fig. 8.6.6, patient BF, a 45-year-old man who initially presented in status epilepsy 2 years prior to the latest PET/CT. Neurological examination was normal. A biopsy was not done; he was stabilized on AEDs and then followed with serial imaging. He had remained well until just prior to the latest study, shown in Fig. 8.8.6, when he had another seizure despite adequate AEDs, and there was a short-lived postictal paresis of the left upper limb. Partial resection subsequently revealed a low-grade astrocytoma with focal anaplasia. Patients such as these pose difficult management issues.

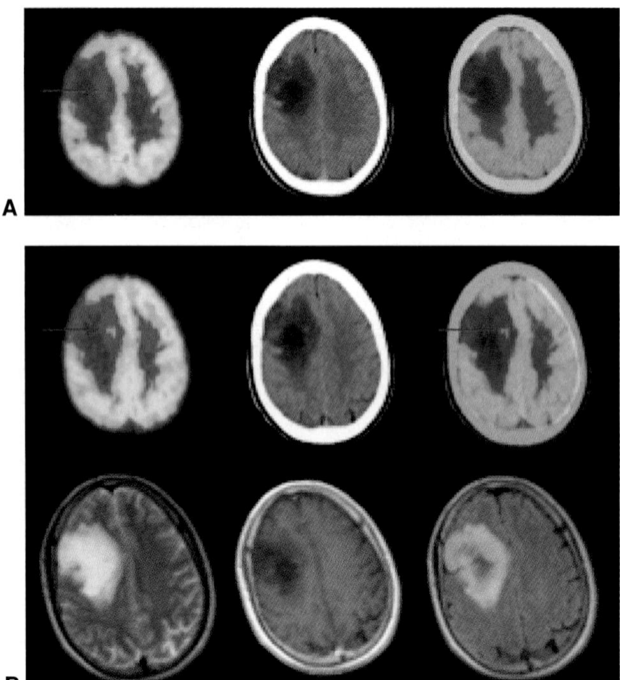

FIGURE 8.6.6. Patient BF: A man in his mid-40s with malignant transformation of a low-grade astrocytoma. He had presented in status epilepsy 2 years earlier. Images shown are studies done 6 months apart. The patient had a normal neurological examination. **A:** Representative transaxial fluorine-18-fluorodeoxyglucose ([^{18}F]-FDG) PET/CT (LSO Biograph Duo, Siemens, Hoffman Estates, Illinois) images (*left to right*) show an extensive region of hypodensity and hypometabolism in the white matter and cortex of the right frontal lobe with mass effect. There is a region of slightly increased metabolism adjacent to the midline (*arrow*), which was suspicious but not definitive for focal anaplasia. **B (top panel)**: Transaxial [^{18}F]-FDG PET/CT (LSO Biograph Duo) images 6 months later show increased metabolism (*arrow*) adjacent to the midline, which is consistent with focal anaplasia. The mass is also larger but essentially remains predominantly hypometabolic. (**Bottom panel**): Transaxial T2-weighted (T2W), enhanced T1W, and coronal fluid-attenuated inverse recovery magnetic resonance images performed just prior to the PET/CT show no evidence of gadolinium enhancement.

Whenever possible in high-grade tumors (grades III and IV) a gross macroscopic resection is performed for symptom relief, to obtain a tissue sample, and because there is some suggestion that median survival is prolonged (150). It has been well documented that patients with glucose hypermetabolism on [^{18}F]-FDG PET have shortened survival (100,151–153). Further, results for high-grade tumors treated with aggressive local therapies such as brachytherapy or radiosurgery are better if the tumor volume is small (154). However, neurosurgeons are influenced by the location of the tumor and the associated risks of surgery, and in the absence of a neurologic deficit they are often reluctant to perform an extensive resection. There is no simple answer to this dilemma. The authors have found that in these circumstances discussion with the patient about the risks/benefits and the other specialists at the multidisciplinary tumor board meeting is valuable.

The patient in Fig. 8.6.7 is a more straightforward case. He has had an oligodendroglioma for over 20 years. The patient was about 30 years old when he had his first generalized seizure, and a cerebral CT showed a left posterior frontal lesion. Seizure control at that time was problematic, but he was followed with serial imaging and biopsy was not done. Imaging was stable until he developed a subacute onset of right hemiparesis, which was associated with worsening of his seizure control. Anatomical imaging showed a mass lesion with some hemorrhage and gadolinium enhancement at the site of the presumed glioma. The patient subsequently had a resection of an anaplastic astrocytoma; 1p and 19q deletions were present. There was improvement in the patient's hemiparesis after surgery. The patient then underwent radiotherapy and chemotherapy.

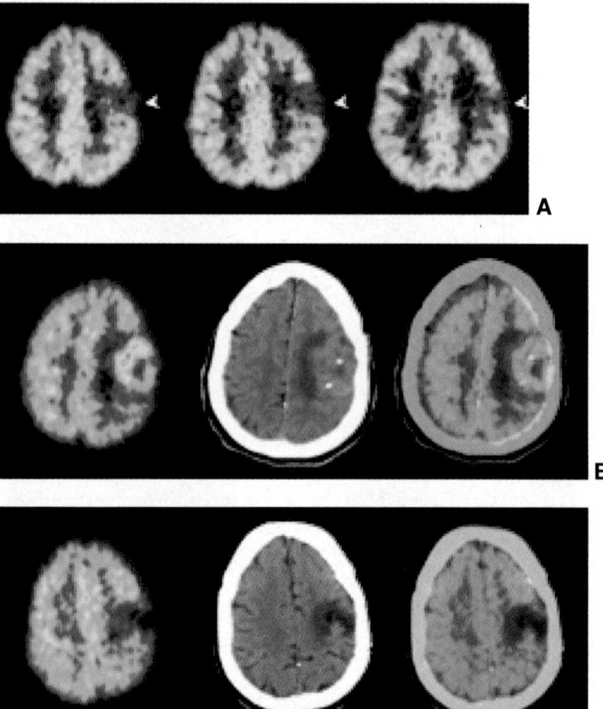

FIGURE 8.6.7. Patient RS: A man in his mid-40s who has had a glioma for 20 years; the tumor underwent malignant degeneration 17 years after the first seizure and the lesion in the left posterior frontal lobe was first detected on CT. **A (top panel)**: Transaxial fluorine-18-fluorodeoxyglucose ([^{18}F]-FDG) PET only scans (performed on an ECAT 951 [Siemens, Hoffman Estates, Illinois] whole-body PET scanner) were done 5 years before the middle panel. Images show focal glucose hypometabolism in left posterior frontal lobe (*arrowheads*). **B (middle panel)**: Transaxial [^{18}F]-FDG PET/CT (LSO Biograph Duo, Siemens, Hoffman Estates, Illinois) images, which are mildly misregistered, at the time of the development the right hemiparesis show the large relatively hyperdense mass lesion that is partly calcified at the site of the previous hypometabolism seen in FIGURE 8.6.7A. There is a heterogeneous rim of increased metabolism surrounding a hypometabolic center. The lesion was resected and was an anaplastic oligodendroglioma. **C (bottom panel)**: Transaxial [^{18}F]-FDG PET/CT (LSO Biograph Duo) images done 18 months after radiotherapy and chemotherapy had been completed. The surgical cavity is smaller than expected and there is surrounding hypodensity and hypometabolism, which is likely to be due to residual low-grade tumor.

Has the Tumor Responded to Treatment?

The imaging gold standard to assess response in brain tumor clinical trials is a measurement of the extent of gadolinium enhancement on MR imaging (155). The same approach is used in the day-to-day management of patients with brain tumors. Perhaps the most compelling evidence that such an approach is limited is that enhancement is nonspecific. Enhancement any time beyond 24 hours after surgery may be due to a combination of residual tumor and the effects of surgery (156). In addition, corticosteroids have a profound effect on the degree of contrast enhancement, peritumoral edema, and to a lesser extent, the apparent volume of enhancing tumor by partial restoration of the BBB (157–160). Up to a 50% reduction in the enhancing volume of anaplastic tumors has been reported to occur after corticosteroid administration (157). Although corticosteroid doses are often rigorously controlled in the clinical trial setting to mitigate this effect, it is often not practicable in routine clinical practice.

It would make sense to use PET to assess response (161). The authors use [^{18}F]-FDG PET/CT to monitor response on a routine basis and have also used it in the trial setting where the changes in glucose utilization predate changes on MR imaging. Two examples of patients who were enrolled in one of the initial clinical trials with temozolomide, at our center, are shown in Fig. 8.6.8. In both cases there were marked changes in the degree of tumoral FDG uptake; in Fig. 8.6.8A there was an early reduction in peak FDG uptake at day 9 and at day 56 when the MR study at the end of two cycles of temozolomide was carried out; there was very little FDG uptake evident but still marked enhancement. In Fig. 8.6.8B, FDG uptake increased at day 9 and there was a new site of disease not evident on the initial MR study; a further increase in FDG uptake was seen at day 29 but at this stage it was accompanied by clinical deterioration. There was very little change in the MR study at the two time points. These patients were part of a group of six, and although the number was small, as a group, a reduction in FDG uptake in the first week identified those patients who responded. As indicated earlier, more work is required with PET ligands to reliably identify tumor proliferation in gliomas, but in the interim, [^{18}F]-FDG appears to be a valuable tool to assess response.

Is the Patient's Clinical Deterioration and Change on the Patient's Imaging Studies Due to Recurrent Tumor or the Effects of Treatment?

Clinical deterioration in a patient with glioma months or years after treatment and new regions of enhancement on anatomic imaging are generally thought to be due to tumor recurrence and sometimes

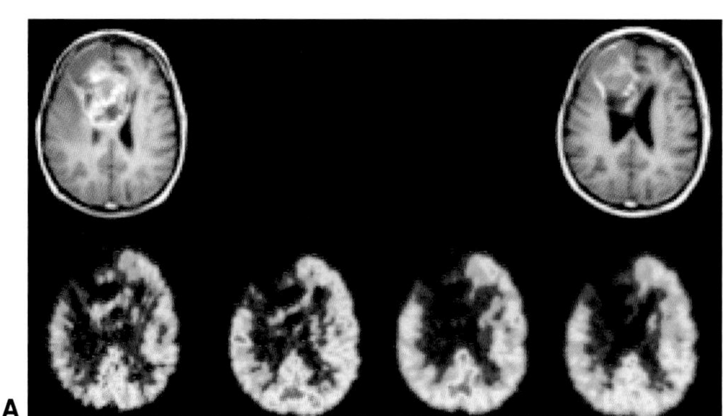

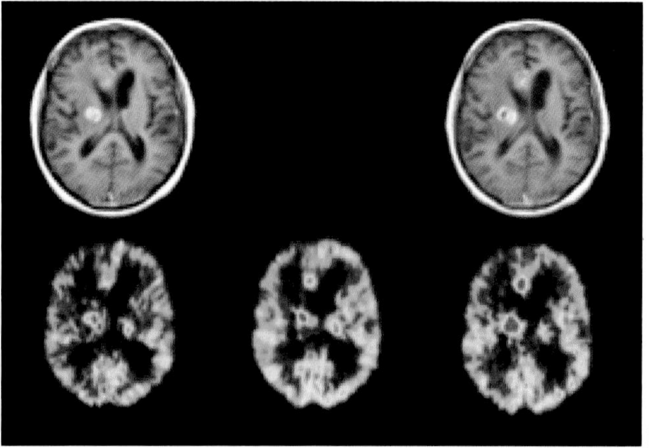

FIGURE 8.6.8. Transaxial early time point fluorine-18-fluorodeoxyglucose ([^{18}F]-FDG) PET scans performed on an ECAT 951 (Siemens, Hoffman Estates, Illinois) whole-body PET scanner in two patients with high-grade gliomas performed before and after treatment. **A:** A man in his early 40s with an anaplastic astrocytoma who relapsed 14 months after radiotherapy. Coregistered enhanced T1-weighted (T1W) magnetic resonance (MR) scans were performed before (**upper left**) and at the completion of two cycles of chemotherapy 2 months later (**upper right**). Coregistered [^{18}F]-FDG PET scans were done before, at day 7, at day 21, and at the same time as the second MR scan. A marked reduction in tumoral glucose metabolism was seen at the end of 1 week, minimal glucose metabolism was seen after 3 weeks, and at 2 months there was almost a complete response. The large enhancing mass lesion was still seen with MR in the right frontal lobe and corpus callosum, and the lesion still enhanced markedly at 2 months and only fulfilled anatomic criteria of a partial response. The patient remained well with a good performance status for a further 8 months. **B:** A nearly 60-year-old man with a glioblastoma multiforme who relapsed 5 months after primary therapy. Coregistered enhanced T1W MR scans were performed before (**upper left**) and 3 weeks later (**upper right**) when the patient continued to deteriorate clinically. Coregistered [^{18}F]-FDG PET scans were done before, and at days 7 and 21 after the commencement of therapy. On MR imaging, there were two enhancing lesions: one in the right frontal lobe and a second in the white matter of the right centrum semiovale; at day 21, the lesions were slightly larger and partly necrotic, but they did not meet the criteria for progressive disease. On [^{18}F]-FDG PET, the lesions did not change significantly at day 7, and at day 21 were larger and more metabolically active, consistent with progressive disease; there was also a third lesion seen on PET, but not MR, adjacent to the body of the left caudate nucleus that also increased in size and glucose avidity but not as rapidly as the right-sided lesions. Chemotherapy was stopped and the patient died 6 weeks later.

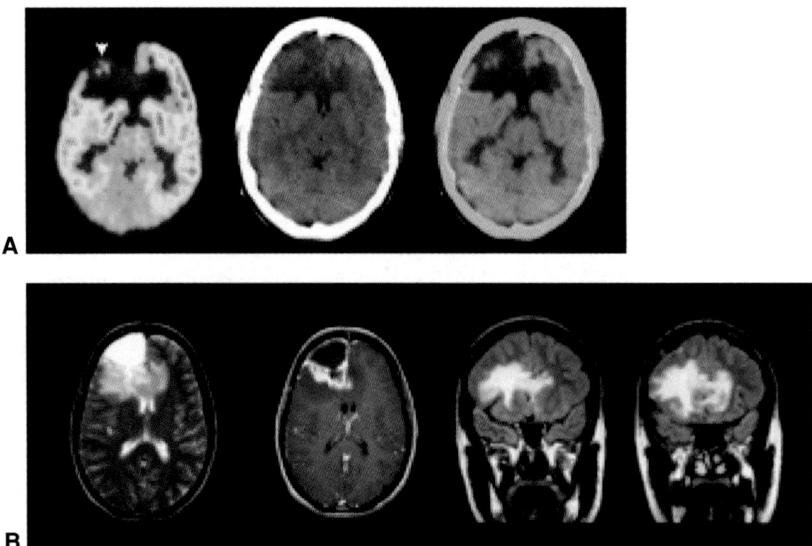

FIGURE 8.6.9. Patient EB: An approximately 30-year-old woman with an anaplastic oligodendroglioma of the right frontal lobe treated with surgery and then combined chemoradiotherapy. The patient was asymptomatic, had no neurological signs, and had a Karnofsky performance status of 90. **A** (**top panel**): Representative transaxial fluorine-18-fluorodeoxyglucose ([^{18}F]-FDG) PET/CT (LSO Biograph Duo, Siemens, Hoffman Estates, Illinois) images. A region of absent metabolism is seen at the right frontal pole at the site of previous surgery. There is glucose hypometabolism consistent with radio/chemonecrosis behind the surgical resection margin where there are hypodense changes on anatomical imaging extending into a swollen corpus callosum. There is a small region of increased glucose metabolism over the right frontal lateral convexity (*arrowheads*) consistent with recurrent tumor. At pathology there was a combination of recurrent tumor at the lateral edge of the previous surgical resection and radiation/chemonecrosis seen more medially close to the callosum. **B** (**bottom panel**): Transaxial T2-weighted (T2W) and gadolinium-enhanced T1W and coronal fluid-attenuated inverse recovery (*left to right*) magnetic resonance images show marked bilateral bifrontal gray and white matter edema and gadolinium enhancement at the resection margin, which also extends into the corpus callosum. These regions correspond to the regions of hypometabolism but also the focal region of increased metabolism seen on PET/CT.

radiation or chemonecrosis. Now that adjuvant concurrent temozolomide and radiotherapy is the standard of care for newly diagnosed GBMs, it is possible that radiation and chemonecrosis may become more prevalent (162). Anatomic imaging may reveal a mass with surrounding edema and marked contrast enhancement. Unfortunately, these radiologic imaging findings are nonspecific and can reflect tumor recurrence, treatment-related necrosis, previous surgery, seizure activity, and any of these combinations. Whenever this question arises it is important to also consider the patient's clinical history and the management options that are available because in some instances, surgical resection may be appropriate for both tumor recurrence and radiation necrosis.

Radiation necrosis generally appears a year or more after irradiation with doses greater than 50 Gy, and it is rare at less than 3 months after completion of standard external beam therapy. Its development is proportional to the dose and is inversely proportional to the number of fractions or time during which the radiation is administered (163,164). Some investigators regard it as an idiosyncratic phenomenon that cannot always be predicted or explained on the basis of dose, distribution, and fractionation of the radiotherapy. However, in the authors' experience, when conventional radiotherapy doses are given (50 to 55 Gy), it is more common in the elderly and in patients with underlying vascular disease, hypertension, and diabetes.

Necrosis is an expected therapeutic effect with aggressive treatment protocols that deliver high doses of radiation locally (e.g., Gamma Knife and brachytherapy) (154). The pathology and pathologic diagnosis of radiation or chemonecrosis is difficult. The main site of injury in radiation necrosis is the white matter, but as with chemonecrosis, the gray matter can also be affected. It is mainly a vascular injury and the affected vessels undergo fibrinoid necrosis (165). Tissue samples removed from radionecrotic areas contain large irregular distorted tumor cells that are regarded as "viable" as well as necrotic cells. But the pathologist is often unable to determine if these "viable" cells are capable of replicating.

Unequivocal evidence for tumor recurrence depends on the presence of pseudopalisading surrounding necrotic areas, but this is generally not the rule (165). Often there is both tumor recurrence and radiation necrosis on the pathologic specimen, and the clinical dilemma is then what to do next (Fig. 8.6.9). The answer depends on the clinical situation and the performance status of the patient. Reoperation and removal of recurrent tumor and radionecrotic tissue may be required; in other cases corticosteroids and additional chemotherapy may be appropriate in the setting of predominant tumor recurrence.

The National Institutes of Health group led by Di Chiro et al. (166) and Patronas et al. (167) were the first to report that [^{18}F]-FDG PET was able to differentiate hypometabolic radiation necrosis and chemonecrosis from recurrent hypermetabolic tumors.

These findings were replicated later by Doyle et al. (168) and Valk et al. (169), with accuracy of 84%, in glioma patients who had been treated with interstitial brachytherapy and others with high-grade gliomas (170–172). These earlier findings were later challenged by Ricci et al. (108) in a retrospective series of 84 patients where there was histological confirmation in 31 by biopsy or surgical resection. These investigators reported that [^{18}F]-FDG PET was correct in only 68% (21 of 31) of cases, and the cases that were misidentified had increased metabolism relative to contralateral white matter. Unfortunately, the main limitations of the study were that clinical and pathological data were sparse. It is surprising, given that seven of the nine cases where radiation necrosis was reported had high-grade gliomas, (GBM = 5; III to IV astrocytoma = 1, III to IV oligodendroglioma) that the pathologists did not identify any evidence of residual tumor.

Finally, for PET practitioners, clinically inapparent seizure activity—nonconvulsive status epilepsy (NCSE)—should be considered in this setting. Seizures are a common accompaniment of brain tumors throughout the course of the illness. Furthermore, the authors believe that NCSE occurs more commonly than it is recognized. Seizures produce glucose hypermetabolism in the cell body as well as at the efferent terminals of the epileptogenic zone. The epileptogenic zone, which is responsible for seizures in patients with brain tumors, is often located in the cortex at the edge of the imaging abnormality. The authors have noted focal glucose hypermetabolism adjacent to the surgical resection margin and also in the cortex overlying the glioma and presumed glioma. An example of NCSE is shown in Fig. 8.6.10.

Patient DB is a businessperson in her late 20s. She had a witnessed generalized seizure in sleep; there were then multiple seizures on the way to the hospital. Upon admission she was stabilized. Anatomical imaging (CT and MR) was done on the day of admission and PET/CT was done 4 days after admission; at the time medications were phenytoin 250 mg per day. There were no focal neurological signs, and she was examined by competent neurosurgery and neurology staff; however, at the time of the PET/CT scan, although "normal," she seemed "stunned," and this was commented on by her twin sister.

This is important to recognize because it may be interpreted, erroneously, as evidence of high-grade tumor recurrence or a high-grade tumor at presentation. MR imaging can also be misleading with T2 hyperintensity and enhancement present. Patients can have focal neurological signs, global neurologic impairment, or be asymptomatic to all but an astute observer as was the case in patient DB (Fig. 8.6.10). Although the authors routinely perform video EEG on all our brain tumor patients prior to the PET/CT scan, it is not always helpful in identifying seizure activity; [^{18}F]-FDG PET provides the clue, and there can be marked improvement in performance status with anticonvulsant medication alone.

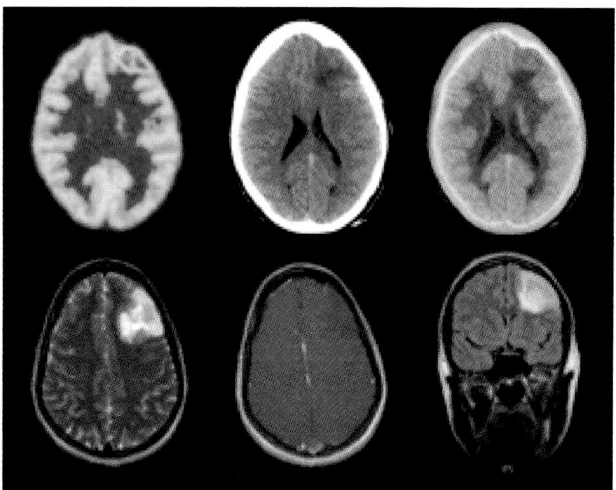

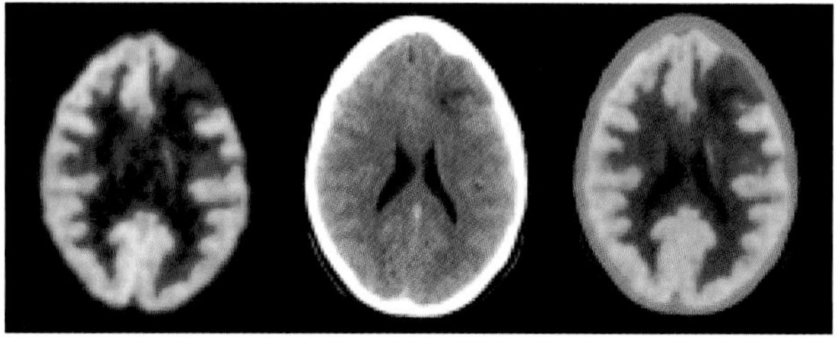

FIGURE 8.6.10. Patient DB: A woman in her late 20s who was admitted after a witnessed generalized convulsion. The fluorine-18-fluorodeoxyglucose ([^{18}F]-FDG) PET/CT scans were performed 5 weeks apart on the LSO Truepoint 64-slice PET/CT Biograph (Siemens, Hoffman Estates, Illinois). There is good registration between the PET and CT images. **A** (**top panel**): Representative transaxial [^{18}F]-FDG PET/CT (LSO Truepoint Biograph) images show an exophytic abnormality of mixed density involving both white and gray matter. This lesion shows markedly increased metabolism relative to white matter and adjacent cortex. The increased metabolism appears to be restricted to the gray matter. (**Bottom panel**): Transaxial T2W, gadolinium-enhanced T1-weighted (T1W) and coronal fluid-attenuated inverse recovery (FLAIR) images performed 3 days before the PET/CT scan show a large heterogeneous hyperintense mass lesion on T2W and FLAIR images, and there is a small white matter focus of gadolinium enhancement but no abnormalities in the cortex. The provisional PET/CT diagnosis was nonconvulsive status epilepsy in a presumed low-grade glioma. **B:** Five weeks later, after a change in antiepileptic drugs, the previous region of increase metabolism involving the gray matter is now hypometabolic. The mass lesion on anatomical imaging is unchanged. The imaging changes coincided with the patient returning to her usual self. Anatomical was not done. The provisional diagnosis is a low-grade glioma and serial imaging is now being carried out.

How Far Does the Tumor Extend into the Surrounding Tissue?

The hypothesis, which underlies this question, is that cure from a glioma is possible if all the neoplastic cells can be excised. This hypothesis remains to be proven, but there are long-term survivors of high-grade tumors, often young patients where small lesions have been radically excised. The problem is delineating the "true" extension of a glioma into the adjacent brain, and microscopic invasion beyond the macroscopic abnormality seen at operation and on anatomic imaging studies has been proven (139,173,174). None of the current imaging technologies—CT, MR, MRS, and PET/CT—is able to reliably provide an answer to the question. Of the PET ligands, [^{11}C]-MET is perhaps the best for delineating the tumor margin for low-grade gliomas, but probably only for oligodendrogliomas (63–65,70). Because low-grade astrocytomas and oligodendrogliomas are hypometabolic with [^{18}F]-FDG PET/CT, the edge of the lesion merges imperceptibly with the normal hypometabolism of the white matter (Figs. 8.6.2, 8.6.5, 8.6.6, and 8.6.10). Notwithstanding these issues there are also other practical considerations.

Neurosurgeons at the authors' center have an inherent reluctance to resect "normal-looking brain" at operation. Despite the cystic appearance and well-demarcated edge that can be seen on MR imaging, this is not the case under the operating microscope where the tumor merges into normal brain, in particular, in low-grade gliomas. Even with intraoperative evoked potential mapping and "awake surgery" it is not possible to entirely remove the macroscopic abnormality in every case. Further, any imaging and coregistration of data sets (MR plus CT plus PET/CT) done prior to surgery is affected once the surgical resection begins; there is brain swelling (brain shift) and surface/anatomical landmarks change. The introduction of intraoperative 1.5T MR scanners and fiber tracking with tensor imaging has overcome the issues of brain shift and seen renewed interest in the more complete resection of low- and high-grade gliomas (175–178). We will await with interest the long-term follow-up of patients after these resections, in particular for low-grade gliomas, to determine if the natural history can be improved.

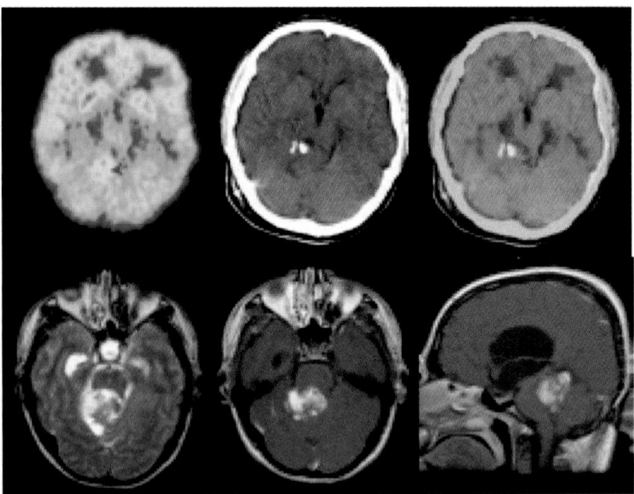

FIGURE 8.6.11. Patient MA: A 20-year-old male builder. He presented with a short history of headache and diplopia and on examination he also had papilledema. On anatomical imaging there was obstructive hydrocephalus due to a large brainstem, fourth ventricular mass and so a ventriculoperitoneal shunt was inserted before further surgery. (**Top panel**): Transaxial fluorine-18-fluorodeoxyglucose ([^{18}F]-FDG) PET/CT (LSO Biograph Duo, Siemens, Hoffman Estates, Illinois) images show increased metabolism (*arrowheads*) in the partly calcified mass in the vicinity of the superior vermis of the cerebellum and the right side of the midbrain/tectum. (**Bottom panel**): T2-weighted (T2W), enhanced T1W transaxial, and gadolinium-enhanced T1W sagittal magnetic resonance images (*left to right*) show the complex mass lesion on T2W images, which has irregular enhancement. The tumor was removed from the tectum and was found to be a pilocytic astrocytoma (World Health Organization grade I).

SPECIAL TUMOR TYPES

Rare primary tumors are also included in the WHO classification, and neuroimaging characteristics have only recently been described. Some of these tumors may be encountered in a clinical PET/CT program, and their features are important to recognize.

Pilocytic Astrocytoma

Pilocytic astrocytomas (PAs) are regarded as a low-grade astrocytoma (WHO grade I) with a good prognosis (2,33). They occur in a younger age group than other low-grade astrocytomas. They enhance avidly on MR imaging (132), and a key feature is their location in midline structures—the midline cerebellum, hypothalamus, and optic chiasm—but they can be found in the cerebral hemispheres when they are usually located in the temporal lobes (33). They also display markedly increased [^{18}F]-FDG uptake on PET, similar to that seen with anaplastic tumors (Fig. 8.6.11) (106).

There is as of yet no clear explanation for the enigmatic [^{18}F]-FDG PET findings reported by Fulham et al. (106); these investigators speculated whether it is related to GLUT expression. They also questioned if the findings invalidated the [^{18}F]-FDG PET assessment of brain tumors and if they violated the general principle that low-grade tumors have reduced glucose metabolism and that high-grade tumors are hypermetabolic. However, it seems that PAs are particularly unusual tumors with a number of atypical and unlikely features for a low-grade astrocytoma: (a) although regarded as benign, they may undergo malignant degeneration and metastasize many years after the original diagnosis (179,180); (b) they can have high proliferative indices, using Ki-67 labeling, pleomorphic cells, mitoses, and chromosomal abnormalities, usually seen in high-grade tumors (181–184); (c) they were deliberately excluded from the Daumas-Duport pathological grading system, where the claim was that the grading system correlated well with clinical outcome, because they would be incorrectly classified as aggressive tumors (6).

The vascular endothelium of PAs has poorly developed tight junctions, which explains the intense enhancement on structural imaging, and vessels of this type are also usually found in malignant tumors (185,186). Thus, it is important that a PA should be considered in the differential diagnosis when on [^{18}F]-FDG PET/CT there is a hypermetabolic lesion seen in a midline structure that enhances avidly on MR imaging, and where there is little surrounding edema in a young patient.

Ganglioglioma

Gangliogliomas are composed of well-differentiated, slow-growing, atypical neuronal elements (ganglion cells) and neoplastic glia; they are WHO grade I and II (2). They may rarely undergo anaplastic change and are then considered WHO grade III (33). They occur at any age and are commonly found in the temporal lobes where they can produce refractory epilepsy, but they may be found anywhere in the neuraxis. The tumors may be solid or cystic and have areas of calcification; temporal lobe tumors are more likely to be solid (130). In a large series reported by Zentner et al. (135), enhancement on MR imaging was found in 16 of 36 patients. In the authors' experience, these tumors are hypometabolic with [^{18}F]-FDG PET, consistent with the findings of Kincaid et al. (187), who reported hypometabolism in 11 patients.

There is one report of increased glucose metabolism in a temporal lobe tumor in a 13-year-old boy with refractory complex partial seizures (188). Unfortunately, there were no details of the scanning protocol; no mention was made of EEG monitoring or the time of the most recent seizure. The tumor was resected and proven to be low grade. Although the authors suggest caution when judging the malignant potential of a tumor with [^{18}F]-FDG PET "in children or young adults with uncharacteristic findings," in the authors' opinion, an alternative and more likely explanation is that the increased glucose hypermetabolism was secondary to unsuspected seizure activity in the uptake or scan period.

Dysembryoplastic Neuroepithelial Tumor

DNETs were first identified in tissue resected from patients with long-standing refractory epilepsy (189). They are WHO grade I and are benign (2). The original pathologic features included a supratentorial cortical location, a multinodular architecture, which may be associated with cortical dysplasia, and a "glioneuronal" element arranged in columns perpendicular to the cortex. This glioneuronal element comprises columns of axons lined by small oligodendroglia-like cells (190). On MR imaging there are characteristic cystlike elements evident on T2-weighted images, and although none of the original tumors described by Daumas-Duport et al. (189) showed contrast enhancement, about one-third will show some enhancement (2). Since the original report it is now apparent that they can be found in sites other than the cortex—the cerebellum and caudate nucleus—although they are commonly found in the mesial temporal lobes, the perirolandic region, and the parietal and occipital lobes (2).

There are limited PET data reported in DNETs; in the authors' center with [^{18}F]-FDG, all DNETs show predominant glucose hypometabolism in the regions of abnormal signal intensity on MR imaging but with islands of preserved or relatively reduced metabolism, which the authors suspect is due to deafferentation or compression (Fig. 8.6.12). The authors have not seen cases with increased glucose metabolism; however, if such cases were to occur, the first consideration would be seizure activity prior to or during the scan. Maehara et al. (191) reported that there was no [^{11}C]-MET uptake in four patients with DNETs and refractory epilepsy; these patients also did not have enhancement on MR imaging.

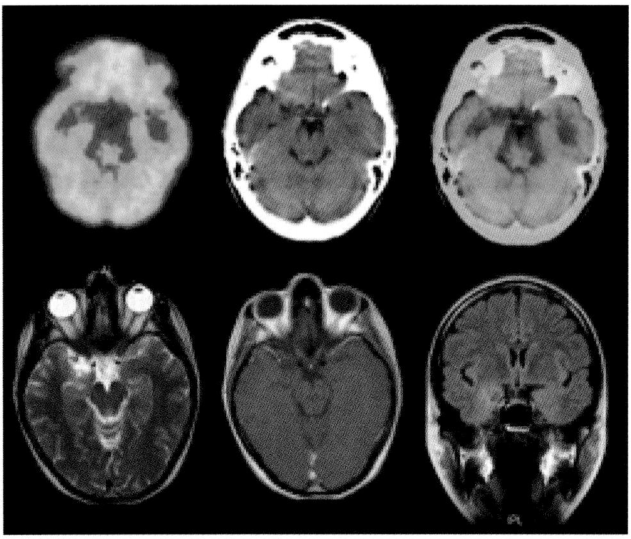

FIGURE 8.6.12. Patient BM: A 30-year-old woman with a 10-year history of refractory epilepsy. (**Top panel**): Representative transaxial fluorine-18-fluorodeoxyglucose ([^{18}F]-FDG) PET/CT (LSO Biograph Duo, Siemens, Hoffman Estates, Illinois) images; there is mild misregistration between the PET and CT images in the vicinity of the orbitofrontal cortex seen on fused images. PET images show glucose hypometabolism in the subtle region of hypodensity seen on CT (*arrowheads*); there is also a small tongue of reduced metabolism in the anterior temporal pole just behind normal glucose metabolism in the right frontal cortex, which is a typical finding in a dysembryoplastic neuroepithelial tumor (DNET). (**Bottom panel**): Transaxial T2W, enhanced T1W, and coronal fluid-attenuated inverse recovery images show the typical hyperintensity in the anatomical lesion on T2W images in a DNET. The "cystic" hyperintense lesions appear to be restricted to the cortex. There is no enhancement with gadolinium. A DNET was removed at surgery and confirmed on pathology.

Pleomorphic Xanthoastrocytoma

The pleomorphic xanthoastrocytomas (PXA) is a rare tumor that was first described in 1979 (192). It is thought to arise from subpial astrocytes, which explains its superficial location where the overlying meninges are often involved. Histologically there are pleomorphic lipid-laden glial fibrillary acid protein-positive neoplastic cells in an abundant reticulin network; there can be mitoses and even necrosis. Despite these histological features PXAs are regarded as having a relatively favorable prognosis and are designated as WHO grade II (2). Nevertheless they can recur after resection and develop behavior and characteristics of an anaplastic tumor and ultimately be indistinguishable from a GBM. They tend to occur in young adults, but are described at any age; they are usually found in the temporal lobes and less commonly in the frontal and parietal lobes (33). Until recently, all tumors that were reported in the literature were located in the supratentorial compartment, but cerebellar tumors were described in two patients (193,194). Interestingly, in both cases, the cerebellar tumors appeared more than a decade after an initial PXA had been removed. PXAs enhance avidly on CT and MR imaging (194–198).

Since the first report of a PET study in a 19-year-old man with a recurrent PXA in 1995 by Bicik et al. (195) there have been additional cases reported using both [^{18}F]-FDG and [^{11}C]-MET (191,198–201). In the case reported with [^{18}F]-FDG PET the tumor recurred 10 and 15 months after the original subtotal resection (195). On each occasion, tumor recurrence was associated with clinical and radiologic deterioration; the tumor showed markedly increased [^{18}F]-FDG uptake relative to white matter and was similar to the degree of uptake seen in anaplastic astrocytomas (106). Subsequent reports have shown reduced (200) and increased (198,199) [^{18}F]-FDG uptake similar to the initial report; increased [^{11}C]-MET uptake has also been reported (191,198,201), but it is unclear if this uptake is also influenced by the enhancement seen in all cases. In the authors' center two additional patients were studied; in both patients, the tumor (Fig. 8.6.13) recurred after an earlier resection many years prior, and in both the tumors showed markedly increased [^{18}F]-FDG uptake.

Gliomatosis Cerebri

Nevin (202) first used the term gliomatosis cerebri in 1938 to describe a diffuse overgrowth of the nervous system with neoplastic glia. The white matter is usually extensively infiltrated with bland neoplastic cells, but occasionally it can be confined to gray matter. Its histogenesis is uncertain and in some cases the abnormal cells resemble astrocytes while in others are characteristically similar to oligodendroglia (2,33). Nevertheless, it is regarded as a malignant WHO grade III tumor (2). It is reported in all age groups, has a peak

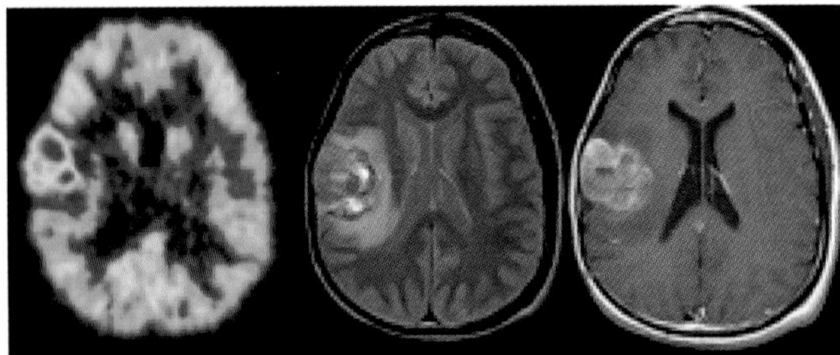

FIGURE 8.6.13. Patient TD: A 25-year-old man with a recurrent pleomorphic xanthoastrocytoma. Original tumor in right parietal lobe was resected at age 7 and patient received postoperative radiotherapy. Transaxial fluorine-18-fluorodeoxyglucose ([^{18}F]-FDG) PET (ECAT 951R, Siemens, Hoffman Estates, Illinois, PET tomograph) (**left**) and proton density (**middle**) and enhanced T1-weighted (T1W) (**right**) magnetic resonance (MR) images show that the tumor is heterogeneous and markedly glucose avid on PET, has mixed signal intensity due to recent hemorrhage on MR, and gadolinium enhancement extends to the cortical surface on MR images.

incidence in the fifth decade, and the prognosis is poor with only 25% of patients alive at 36 months. It is notoriously difficult to diagnose. Initial symptoms are vague or nonspecific. Seizures, headache, and focal neurologic signs typically appear late in the course of the disease. CT and MR imaging underestimate the extent of the disease (203,204). The neoplastic cells have a proliferative potential similar to that of low-grade gliomas (205). There are only a few PET reports in patients with gliomatosis cerebri (206–211). There is some variability in the quality of the reports: the findings and the patients and the PET ligands used were heterogeneous, some included treated and untreated patients (208,209), some used [^{11}C]-MET PET alone (207), [^{18}F]-FDG PET alone (206), and combinations of [^{11}C]-MET PET, [^{18}F]-FDG PET, [^{15}O]-PET, [^{18}F]-methyl tyrosine (^{18}F-FMT), and [^{201}Tl]SPECT (208–211) with differences in scanning technique and uptake periods.

In the better characterized cases it would appear that with [^{11}C]-MET there can be extensive, diffuse, abnormal uptake in the white matter and cortex (207,210); with [^{18}F]-FDG, extensive cortical glucose hypometabolism due to direct involvement of the cortex (206) or deafferentation from white matter involvement (208,209). In all instances where [^{18}F]-FDG was used there was glucose hypometabolism, rather than regions of increased metabolism consistent with low-grade tumor infiltration. The series reported by Sato et al. (209) is the largest with eight patients and the only study to report findings with [^{18}F]-FMT. Four of the eight patients had already been treated, one of whom had survived for 9 years, which was very unusual for gliomatosis cerebri. In seven of eight patients there was abnormal and increased [^{18}F]-FMT, and all patients had extensive glucose hypometabolism with [^{18}F]-FDG.

Spinal Cord Tumors

There is still a paucity of data on the role of PET in the evaluation of patients with proven or suspected spinal cord tumors. Di Chiro et al. (212) studied seven patients with [^{18}F]-FDG, two with an early generation device (ECAT II) and five with the NeuroPET, which was a head-only tomograph used in the early 1980s. There was only one true spinal tumor and it was studied with the ECAT II, which had an in-plane resolution of 17 mm; the remaining tumors were brainstem tumors. There was a single case report of a cervical cord GBM that was assessed after treatment for recurrent tumor versus radiation necrosis, and the [^{18}F]-FDG-PET, done on a PENN PET system with sodium iodide detectors, showed increased metabolism (213).

Wilmhurst et al. (214) reported findings in 14 patients with intramedullary tumors (n = 13) and one schwannoma using a whole-body PET scanner with both [^{18}F]-FDG and [^{11}C]-MET. They compared the PET with the MR findings and found a close correlation in the patients scanned on presentation (n = 8). They also commented that the PET uptake was in keeping with the low-grade histology, meaning low uptake, and PET did not provide additional useful information.

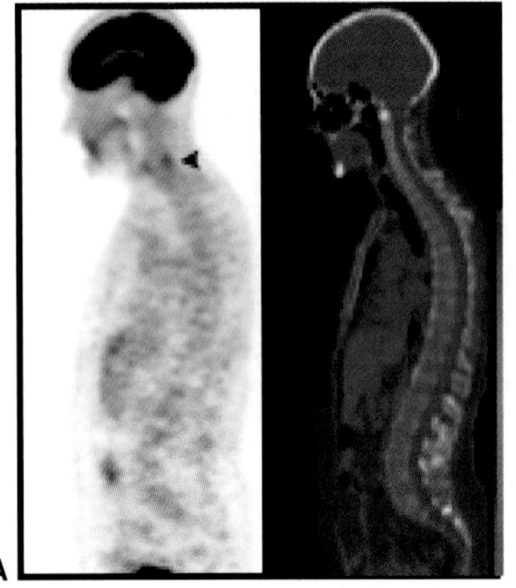

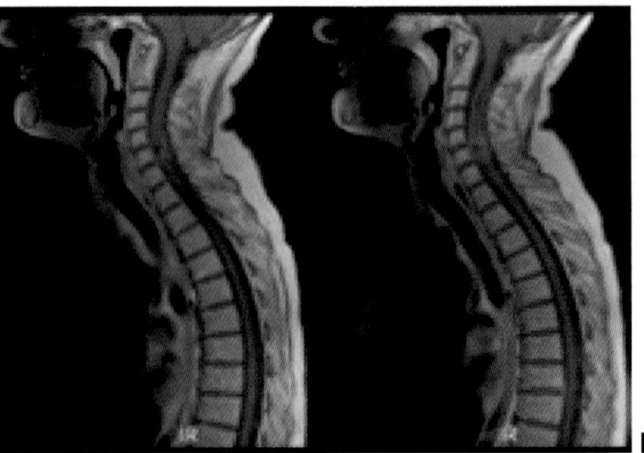

FIGURE 8.6.14. Patient JS: A mid-60-year-old woman with paresthesia in both arms and hands for at least 10 years. The lesion on imaging has slowly enlarged but metabolism has remained static. **A:** Sagittal whole-body fluorine-18-fluorodeoxyglucose ([^{18}F]-FDG) PET/CT (LSO Biograph Duo, Siemens, Hoffman Estates, Illinois) scan shows a small focal region of increased FDG uptake relative to normal cord in the midcervical region (*arrowhead*); CT images show bone window settings. **B:** Sagittal magnetic resonance gadolinium-enhanced T1-wieghted (T1W) magnetic resonance images show irregular enhancement in the cord lesion with a syrinx cavity above and below the exophytic enhancing mass.

In the authors' center, we have had a different experience and have now scanned over 40 patients with a diagnosis of proven spinal cord tumor or suspected spinal cord tumor with both a whole-body PET scanner and PET/CT. The diagnosis was based on neurologic findings compatible with a cord lesion and MR findings that suggested that the likely diagnosis was an intramedullary spinal cord tumor. The authors' findings differ from those of Wilmshurst et al. (214) in that all the low-grade intramedullary spinal cord tumors showed increased FDG uptake relative to the spinal cord (Fig. 8.6.14) and to FDG uptake values obtained in healthy subjects. This finding is in direct contrast to the degree of FDG uptake in low-grade gliomas in the CNS above the foramen magnum. The explanation for these findings is still uncertain. However, [^{18}F]-FDG PET was useful in management in that it was able to differentiate spinal cord infarction, ischemia, and inflammation (demyelination) because these processes were hypometabolic. Shimizu et al. (215) recently reported increased [^{18}F]-FDG uptake in a single patient with a low-grade oligoastrocytoma of the thoracic cord, further supporting the authors' findings.

PET IN THE ASSESSMENT OF CEREBRAL METASTASES

Loeffler et al. (216) suggest that cerebral metastases are up to ten times more common than primary brain tumors. Although cerebral metastases may be detected before or at the same time the primary malignancy is found, in more than 80% of cases, they are found after a diagnosis of systemic cancer is made and they occur in 20% to 40% of these patients. In this clinical setting, a number of scenarios may be encountered.

First, a patient with a known malignant tumor, for example, a melanoma, presents with headache or a seizure. Should a neurologic PET/CT scan be done to determine if the patient has a cerebral metastasis? For most experienced PET practitioners, the answer is generally no. Even the current generation PET/CT does not have the PET spatial resolution to detect small cerebral metastases; the best imaging tool is a contrast-enhanced MR scan.

Does a contrast-enhanced 64-slice CT scanner have the same accuracy in detecting cerebral metastases when compared to MR imaging? The answer to this question is unknown, and while 64-slice CT offers many advantages over earlier generation helical CT, the authors suspect that the answer will still be that MR imaging is superior. Further, there is no radiation from MR imaging.

Most metastases occur at the gray–white junction, and it is often impossible to separate a small hypermetabolic focus of metastatic tumor with little surrounding edema from the normal cortical glucose utilization with [^{18}F]-FDG PET/CT. In addition, in our experience, although many cerebral metastases appear to have homogeneous enhancement on MR imaging, they are often partly necrotic or cystic, and the active metabolic rim is only 1 to 2 mm thick. Although [^{11}C]-MET and [^{18}F]-FLT are not taken up by normal brain to a marked degree, the poorer signal-to-noise ratio of these ligands makes them unlikely diagnostic tools in this situation.

Griffeth et al. (217) reported findings in 19 patients who had 31 metastases; [^{18}F]-FDG PET detected 68% of the metastases. Although many of the patients had already been treated with radiotherapy and/or chemotherapy and an early generation PET scanner had been used, PET was not able to detect four lesions, which were 1.2 cm in diameter. Despite the advances in PET/CT technology the authors believe that PET/CT still does not have a major role in the evaluation of cerebral metastases.

In the setting of a single, large enhancing cerebral lesion in a patient with known cancer, where the differential diagnosis includes a primary brain tumor, the authors may perform a PET/CT scan to aid the neurosurgeon in planning surgery and/or biopsy. However, the main role of PET/CT in patients with cerebral metastases at the authors' center is in cases where a cerebral lesion is removed and then found to be a metastasis at pathology; whole-body PET/CT is then done to identify the underlying malignancy and/or stage it (Fig. 8.6.15).

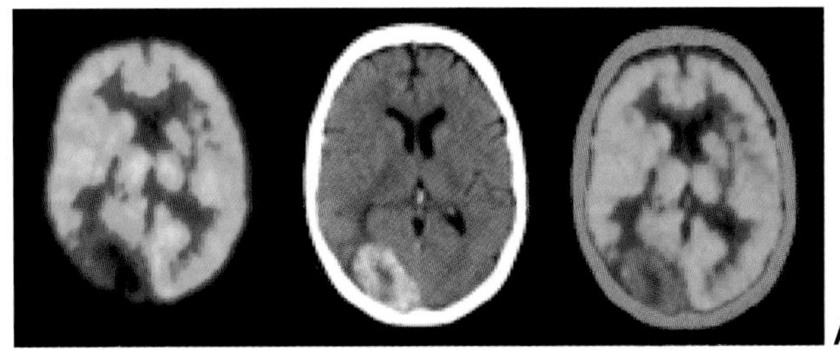

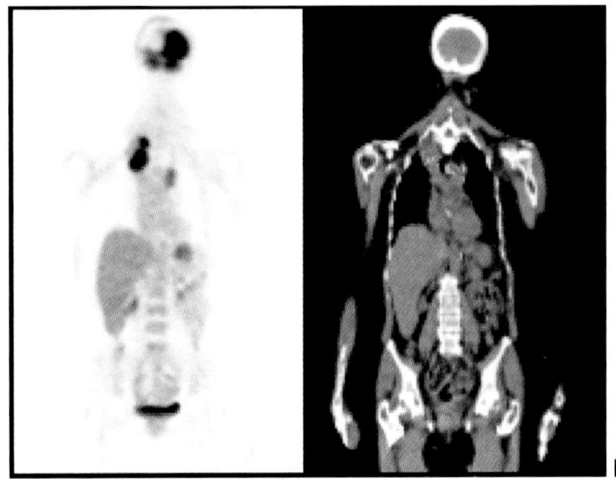

FIGURE 8.6.15. Patient MS: A mid-70-year-old woman with the subacute onset of a left homonymous inferior quadrantanopia. **A:** Transaxial fluorine-18-fluorodeoxyglucose ([^{18}F]-FDG) PET/CT (LSO Biograph Duo, Siemens, Hoffman Estates, Illinois) images show a region of absent and markedly reduced metabolism at the site of the increased density seen on the CT image in the right occipital lobe. There is also mild misregistration between PET and CT data. There were no markedly glucose avid regions identified to indicate an underlying tumor, but nevertheless the provisional PET/CT differential diagnosis was a hemorrhage or a hemorrhagic metastasis. The lesion was resected and pathology showed a partly necrotic, papillary adenocarcinoma, probably of pulmonary origin, but breast and pancreatic primaries were also included. **B:** Coronal whole-body [^{18}F]-FDG PET/CT (LSO Biograph Duo) images (*left*, PET; *right*, CT at soft tissue settings) show glucose-avid masses in both upper lobes of the lungs (left greater than right). The right-sided mass extended into overlying soft tissue and was eroding a rib; the left-sided mass was located adjacent to the aortic arch, and there was a separate lesion identified in left cervical nodes consistent with extrathoracic nodal disease. The right-sided lung primary was proven and the patient was then treated palliatively.

The patient MS (Fig. 8.6.15) developed the subacute onset of a visual field defect. There was remote history of breast cancer—a right mastectomy followed by radiotherapy to chest and axilla was done 20 years prior and a lumpectomy also followed by radiotherapy done 10 years prior to presentation. She was a nonsmoker. Chest CT was abnormal and showed bilateral upper lobe lung masses, which had been noted in a previous chest CT 3 years earlier and were interpreted as being consistent with fibrosis secondary to previous radiotherapy.

After anatomical imaging (CT, MR, and single voxel proton MRS) the radiological diagnosis was thought to be a meningioma. Thus a neurologic PET/CT scan was initially requested. The neurologic PET/CT was not able to identify the increased metabolism in the hemorrhagic adenocarcinoma metastasis, which was removed at surgery. The pathologists could not be certain of the site or origin—lung, breast, or pancreas—and other sites of disease were sought. CT of the chest/abdomen/pelvis only revealed the long-standing changes at the apices of both lungs, and a whole-body PET/CT was requested. Unfortunately, instead of finding a solitary lung tumor, which could have been resected, there were bilateral tumors probably related to previous radiotherapy for breast cancer.

When a cerebral lesion is found in a patient with known systemic cancer (e.g., metastatic melanoma), a staging whole-body PET/CT is done to determine further management.

CONCLUSION

Although PET/CT has limitations, it is the authors' opinion that in combination with PET ligands such as [^{18}F]-FDG, [^{11}C]-MET, and perhaps [^{11}C]-Tdr (or FLT), it is currently and will continue to play a fundamental and complementary role in the quality management of patients with brain tumors. As suggested by Di Chiro (218) over a decade ago, [^{18}F]-FDG is still the most versatile PET ligand in clinical brain tumor work, but a multiligand approach to patient management is becoming part of clinical practice, and it is hoped that such an approach will in the near future include ligands that target tumor angiogenesis, receptors, and gene products.

REFERENCES

1. Legler JM, Ries LA, Smith MA, et al. Cancer surveillance series [corrected]: brain and other central nervous system cancers: recent trends in incidence and mortality. *J Natl Cancer Inst* 1999;91(16):1382–1390.
2. Kleihues P, Cavenee WK, eds. *World Health Organisation Classification of Tumours: pathology and genetics of tumours of the nervous system.* Lyon: IARC Press, 2000.
3. Behin A, Hoang-Xuan K, Carpentier AF, et al. Primary brain tumours in adults. *Lancet* 2003;361(9354):323–331.
4. Burger PC. What is an oligodendroglioma? *Brain Pathol* 2002;12(2): 257–259.
5. Coons SW, Johnson PC, Scheithauer BW, et al. Improving diagnostic accuracy and interobserver concordance in the classification and grading of primary gliomas. *Cancer* 1997;79(7):1381–1393.
6. Daumas-Duport C, Scheithauer B, O'Fallon J, et al. Grading of astrocytomas: a simple and reproducible method. *Cancer* 1988;62:2152–2165.
7. Daumas-Duport C, Varlet P, Tucker ML, et al. Oligodendrogliomas. Part I: patterns of growth, histological diagnosis, clinical and imaging correlations: a study of 153 cases. *J Neurooncol* 1997;34(1):37–59.
8. Fortin D, Cairncross GJ, Hammond RR. Oligodendroglioma: an appraisal of recent data pertaining to diagnosis and treatment. *Neurosurgery* 1999;45(6):1279–1291; discussion 1291.
9. Burger PC, Vogel FS, Green SB. Glioblastoma and anaplastic astrocytoma: pathologic criteria and prognostic considerations. *Cancer* 1985;56:1106–1111.
10. Di Chiro G, Fulham MJ. Virchow's shackles: can PET-FDG challenge tumor histology? *AJNR Am J Neuroradiol* 1993;14(3):524–527.
11. Dehais C, Laigle-Donadey F, Marie Y, et al. Prognostic stratification of patients with anaplastic gliomas according to genetic profile. *Cancer* 2006;107(8):1891–1897.
12. Hesson L, Bieche I, Krex D, et al. Frequent epigenetic inactivation of *RASSF1A* and *BLU* genes located within the critical 3p21.3 region in gliomas. *Oncogene* 2004;23(13):2408–2419.
13. Kujas M, Lejeune J, Benouaich-Amiel A, et al. Chromosome 1p loss: a favorable prognostic factor in low-grade gliomas. *Ann Neurol* 2005;58(2):322–326.
14. Maher EA, Brennan C, Wen PY, et al. Marked genomic differences characterize primary and secondary glioblastoma subtypes and identify two distinct molecular and clinical secondary glioblastoma entities. *Cancer Res* 2006;66(23):11502–11513.
15. Maher EA, Furnari FB, Bachoo RM, et al. Malignant glioma: genetics and biology of a grave matter. *Genes Dev* 2001;15(11):1311–1133.
16. Marie Y, Sanson M, Mokhtari K, et al. OLIG2 as a specific marker of oligodendroglial tumour cells. *Lancet* 2001;358(9278):298–300.
17. Cairncross JG. Aggressive oligodendroglioma: a chemosensitive tumor. *Recent Results Cancer Res* 1994;135:127–133.
18. Cairncross JG, Macdonald DR. Oligodendroglioma: a new chemosensitive tumor. *J Clin Oncol* 1990;8(12):2090–2091.
19. Ino Y, Betensky RA, Zlatescu MC, et al. Molecular subtypes of anaplastic oligodendroglioma: implications for patient management at diagnosis. *Clin Cancer Res* 2001;7(4):839–845.
20. Paleologos NA, Cairncross JG. Treatment of oligodendroglioma: an update. *Neurooncol* 1999;1(1):61–68.
21. Reifenberger J, Reifenberger G, Liu L, et al. Molecular genetic analysis of oligodendroglial tumors shows preferential allelic deletions on 19q and 1p. *Am J Pathol* 1994;145(5):1175–1190.
22. Sonabend AM, Lesniak MS. Oligodendrogliomas: clinical significance of 1p and 19q chromosomal deletions. *Expert Rev Neurother* 2005;5[6 Suppl]:S25–32.
23. Jaeckle KA. Clinical presentation and therapy of nervous system tumors. In: Bradley WG, Daroff RB, Fenichel GM, et al., eds. *Neurology in clinical practice*, 1st ed. Boston: Butterworth-Heinemann, 1991:1008–1030.
24. Wen PY, Black PM. Clinical presentation, evaluation and preoperative preparation of the patient. In: Berger MS, Wilson CB, eds. *The gliomas.* Philadelphia: WB Saunders, 1999:328–336.
25. Bauman G, Lote K, Larson D, et al. Pretreatment factors predict overall survival for patients with low-grade glioma: a recursive partitioning analysis. *Int J Radiat Oncol Biol Phys* 1999;45(4):923–929.
26. Olson JD, Riedel E, DeAngelis LM. Long-term outcome of low-grade oligodendroglioma and mixed glioma. *Neurology* 2000;54(7):1442–1448.
27. Pignatti F, van den Bent M, Curran D, et al. Prognostic factors for survival in adult patients with cerebral low-grade glioma. *J Clin Oncol* 2002;20(8):2076–2084.
28. Byearne TN. Imaging of gliomas. *Semin Oncol* 1994;21(2):162–171.
29. Di Chiro G. Positron emission tomography using [18F]fluorodeoxyglucose in brain tumors: a powerful diagnostic and prognostic tool. *Invest Radiol* 1987; 22:360–371.
30. Fulham MJ, Di Chiro G. Positron emission tomography and ^{1}H-spectroscoic imaging. In: Berger MS, Wilson CB, eds. *The gliomas.* Philadelphia: WB Saunders, 1999:295–317.
31. Gruber ML, Hochberg FH. Systematic evaluation of primary brain tumors [editorial]. *J Nucl Med* 1990;31:969–971.
32. Kondziolka D, Lunsford LD, Martinez AJ. Unreliability of contemporary neurodiagnostic imaging in evaluating suspected adult supratentorial (low-grade) astrocytoma. *J Neurosurg* 1993;79:533–536.
33. Bigner DD, McLendon RE, Bruner JM, eds. *Russell and Rubinstein's pathology of tumours of the nervous system*, 6th ed. London: Arnold, 1998.

34. Jaeckle KA. Neuroimaging for central nervous system tumors. *Semin Oncol* 1991;18(2):150–157.
35. Shapiro WR, Shapiro JR. Primary brain tumors. In: Asbury AK, McKhann GM, McDonald WI, eds. *Diseases of the nervous system: clinical neurobiology*, 2nd ed. Philadelphia: WB Saunders, 1992:1074–1092.
36. Rhodes CG, Wise RJ, Gibbs JM, et al. *In vivo* disturbance of the oxidative metabolism of glucose in human cerebral gliomas. *Ann Neurol* 1983;14:614–624.
37. Rottenberg DA, Ginos JZ, Kearfott KJ, et al. *In vivo* measurement of brain tumor pH using [11C]DMO and positron emission tomography. *Ann Neurol* 1985;17:70–79.
38. Radda G. The use of NMR spectroscopy for the understanding of disease. *Science* 1986;233:640–645.
39. Hiesiger E, Fowler JS, Wolf AP, et al. Serial PET studies of human cerebral malignancy with [1-11C]putrescine and [1-11C]2-deoxy-D-glucose. *J Nucl Med* 1987;28:1251–1261.
40. Hiesiger EM, Fowler JS, Logan J, et al. Is [1-11C]putrescine useful as a brain tumor marker? *J Nucl Med* 1992;33:192–199.
41. Rottenberg DA. Carbon-11-putrescine: back to the drawing board [editorial]. *J Nucl Med* 1992;33:200–201.
42. Pawlikowski M, Kunert-Radek J, Radek A, et al. Inhibition of cell proliferation of human gliomas by benzodiazepines *in vitro*. *Acta Neurol Scand* 1988;77:231–233.
43. Black KL, Ikezaki K, Toga AW. Imaging of brain tumors using peripheral benzodiazepine receptor ligands. *J Neurosurg* 1989;7(1):113–118.
44. Starosta-Rubinstein S, Ciliax BJ, Penney JB, et al. Imaging of a glioma using peripheral benzodiazepine receptor ligands. *Proc Natl Acad Sci U S A* 1987;84:891–895.
45. Bergstrom M, Mosskin M, Ericson K, et al. Peripheral benzodiazepine binding sites in human gliomas evaluated with positron emission tomography. *Acta Radiol* 1986;369:409–411.
46. Junck L, Olson JMM, Ciliax BJ, et al. PET imaging of human gliomas with ligands for the peripheral benzodiazepine binding site. *Ann Neurol* 1989;26:752–758.
47. Pappata S, Cornu P, Samson Y, et al. PET study of carbon-11-PK 1195 binding to peripheral type benzodiazepine sites in glioblastoma: a case report. *J Nucl Med* 1991;32:1608–1610.
48. Bush RS, Jenkins RDT, Allt WC, et al. Definitive evidence for hypoxic cells influencing cure in cancer therapy. *Br J Cancer* 1978;37[Suppl 3]: 302–306.
49. Kayama T, Yoshimoto T, Fujimoto S, et al. Intratumoral oxygen pressure in malignant brain tumors. *J Neurosurg* 1991;74:55–59.
50. Mottram JC. Factors of importance in the radiosensitivity of tumors. *Br J Radiol* 1936;9:606–614.
51. Powers WE, Tolmach LJ. A multi-component x-ray survival curve for mouse lymphosarcoma cells irradiated *in vivo*. *Nature* 1963;197: 710–711.
52. Rasey JS, Koh WJ, Grierson JR, et al. Radiolabelled fluoromisonidazole as an imaging agent for tumor hypoxia. *Int J Radiat Oncol Biol Phys* 1989;17(5):985–991.
53. Valk PE, Mathis CA, Prados MD, et al. Hypoxia in human gliomas: demonstration by PET with fluorine-18-fluoromisonidazole. *J Nucl Med* 1992;33:2133–2137.
54. Bruehlmeier M, Roelcke U, Schubiger PA, et al. Assessment of hypoxia and perfusion in human brain tumors using PET with 18F-fluoromisonidazole and $^{15}O\text{-}H_2O$. *J Nucl Med* 2004;45(11): 1851–1859.
55. Cher LM, Murone C, Lawrentschuk N, et al. Correlation of hypoxic cell fraction and angiogenesis with glucose metabolic rate in gliomas using ^{18}F-fluoromisonidazole, ^{18}F-FDG PET, and immunohistochemical studies. *J Nucl Med* 2006;47(3):410–418.
56. Bergstrom M, Ericson K, Hagenfeldt L, et al. PET study of methionine accumulation in glioma and normal brain tissue: competition with branched chain amino acids. *J Comput Assist Tomogr* 1987;11(2):208–213.
57. Bergstrom M, Lundqvist H, Ericson K, et al. Comparison of the accumulation kinetics of L-(methyl-11C)-methionine and D-(methyl-11C)-methionine in brain tumors studied with positron emission tomography. *Acta Radiol* 1987;28(3):225–229.
58. Christensen HN. Role of amino acid transport and countertransport in nutrition and metabolism. *Physiol Rev* 1990;70(1):43–77.
59. Sanchez del Pino MM, Peterson DR, Hawkins RA. Neutral amino acid transport characterization of isolated luminal and abluminal membranes of the blood–brain barrier. *J Biol Chem* 1995;270(25):14913–14918.
60. Ericson K, Lilja A, Bergstrom M, et al. Positron emission tomography with ([11C]methyl)-L-methionine, [11C]D-glucose, and [68Ga]EDTA in supratentorial tumors. *J Comput Assist Tomogr* 1985;9(4):683–689.
61. Lilja A, Bergstrom K, Hartvig P, et al. Dynamic study of supratentorial gliomas with L-methyl-11C-methionine and positron emission tomography. *AJNR Am J Neuroradiol* 1985;6(4):505–514.
62. Chung JK, Kim YK, Kim SK, et al. Usefulness of ^{11}C-methionine PET in the evaluation of brain lesions that are hypo- or isometabolic on ^{18}F-FDG PET. *Eur J Nucl Med Mol Imaging* 2002;29(2):176–182.
63. Derlon J-M, Petit-Taboue M-C, Chapon F, et al. The *in vivo* metabolic pattern of low-grade brain gliomas: a positron emission tomographic study using ^{18}F-fluorodeoxyglucose and ^{11}C-L-methylmethionine. *Neurosurgery* 1997;40:276–288.
64. Derlon JM, Bourdet C, Bustany P, et al. (11C)L-methionine uptake in gliomas. *Neurosurgery* 1989;25:720–728.
65. Derlon JM, Chapon F, Noel MH, et al. Non-invasive grading of oligodendrogliomas: correlation between *in vivo* metabolic pattern and histopathology. *Eur J Nucl Med* 2000;27(7):778–787.
66. Herholz K, Holzer T, Bauer B, et al. ^{11}C-methionine PET for differential diagnosis of low grade-gliomas. *Neurology* 1998;50:1316–1322.
67. Kaschten B, Stevenaert A, Sadzot B, et al. Preoperative evaluation of 54 gliomas by PET with fluorine-18-fluorodeoxyglucose and/or carbon-11-methionine. *J Nucl Med* 1998;39:778–785.
68. Kim S, Chung JK, Im SH, et al. ^{11}C-methionine PET as a prognostic marker in patients with glioma: comparison with ^{18}F-FDG PET. *Eur J Nucl Med Mol Imaging* 2005;32(1):52–59.
69. Kracht LW, Friese M, Herholz K, et al. Methyl-[11C]-l-methionine uptake as measured by positron emission tomography correlates to microvessel density in patients with glioma. *Eur J Nucl Med Mol Imaging* 2003;30(6):868–873.
70. Mosskin M, Ericson T, Hindmarsh T, et al. Positron emission tomography compared with magnetic resonance imaging and computed tomography in supratentorial gliomas using multiple stereotactic biopsies as reference. *Acta Radiol* 1989;30:225–232.
71. Ogawa T, Shishido F, Kanno I, et al. Cerebral glioma: evaluation with methionine PET. *Radiology* 1993;186:45–53.
72. Sasaki M, Kuwabara Y, Yoshida T, et al. A comparative study of thallium-201 SPET, carbon-11 methionine PET and fluorine-18 fluorodeoxyglucose PET for the differentiation of astrocytic tumours. *Eur J Nucl Med* 1998;25(9):1261–1269.
73. Sato N, Suzuki M, Kuwata N, et al. Evaluation of the malignancy of glioma using ^{11}C-methionine positron emission tomography and proliferating cell nuclear antigen staining. *Neurosurg Rev* 1999;22(4):210–214.
74. Van Laere K, Ceyssens S, Van Calenbergh F, et al. Direct comparison of ^{18}F-FDG and ^{11}C-methionine PET in suspected recurrence of glioma: sensitivity, inter-observer variability and prognostic value. *Eur J Nucl Med Mol Imaging* 2005;32(1):39–51.
75. Jacobs A. Amino acid uptake in ischemically compromised brain tissue. *Stroke* 1995;26(10):1859–1866.
76. Lilja A, Lundqvist H, Olsson Y, et al. Positron emission tomography and computed tomography in differential diagnosis between recurrent or residual glioma and treatment-induced brain lesions. *Acta Radiol* 1989;30:121–128.
77. Pope WB, Lai A, Nghiemphu P, et al. MRI in patients with high-grade gliomas treated with bevacizumab and chemotherapy. *Neurology* 2006;66(8):1258–1260.
78. Popperl G, Gotz C, Rachinger W, et al. Value of O-(2-[18F]fluoroethyl)-L-tyearosine PET for the diagnosis of recurrent glioma. *Eur J Nucl Med Mol Imaging* 2004;31(11):1464–1470.

79. Weber WA, Wester HJ, Grosu AL, et al. O-(2-[18F]fluoroethyl)-L-tyearosine and L-[methyl-11C]methionine uptake in brain tumours: initial results of a comparative study. *Eur J Nucl Med* 2000;27(5): 542–549.
80. Shields AF, Grierson JR, Dohmen BM, et al. Imaging proliferation in vivo with [F-18]FLT and positron emission tomography. *Nat Med* 1998;4(11):1334–1336.
81. Christman D, Crawford EJ, Friedkin M, et al. Detection of DNA synthesis in intact organisms with positron-emitting (methyl-^{11}C)thymidine. *Proc Natl Acad Sci U S A* 1972;69(4):988–992.
82. Crawford EJ, Christman D, Atkins H, et al. Scintigraphy with positron-emitting compounds. I. Carbon-11 labeled thymidine and thymidylate. *Int J Nucl Med Biol* 1978;5(2–3):61–69.
83. Martiat P, Ferrant A, Labar D, et al. *In vivo* measurement of carbon-11 thymidine uptake in non-Hodgkin's lymphoma using positron emission tomography. *J Nucl Med* 1988;29(10):1633–1637.
84. Vander Borght T, Pauwels S, Lambotte L, et al. Brain tumor imaging with PET and 2-[carbon-11]thymidine. *J Nucl Med* 1994;35:974–982.
85. Krohn KA, Mankoff DA, Muzi M, et al. True tracers: comparing FDG with glucose and FLT with thymidine. *Nucl Med Biol* 2005;32(7): 663–671.
86. Chen W, Cloughesy T, Kamdar N, et al. Imaging proliferation in brain tumors with ^{18}F-FLT PET: comparison with ^{18}F-FDG. *J Nucl Med* 2005;46(6):945–952.
87. Choi SJ, Kim JS, Kim JHet al. [18F]3'-deoxy-3'-fluorothymidine PET for the diagnosis and grading of brain tumors. *Eur J Nucl Med Mol Imaging* 2005;32(6):653–659.
88. Jacobs AH, Kracht LW, Gossmann A, et al. Imaging in neurooncology. *NeuroRx* 2005;2(2):333–347.
89. Jacobs AH, Thomas A, Kracht LW, et al. ^{18}F-fluoro-L-thymidine and ^{11}C-methylmethionine as markers of increased transport and proliferation in brain tumors. *J Nucl Med* 2005;46(12):1948–1958.
90. Saga T, Kawashima H, Araki N, et al. Evaluation of primary brain tumors with FLT-PET: usefulness and limitations. *Clin Nucl Med* 2006;31(12):774–780.
91. Yamamoto Y, Wong TZ, Turkington TG, et al. 3′-Deoxy-3′-[F-18]fluorothymidine positron emission tomography in patients with recurrent glioblastoma multiforme: comparison with Gd-DTPA enhanced magnetic resonance imaging. *Mol Imaging Biol* 2006;8(6):340–347.
92. Muzi M, Spence AM, O'Sullivan F, et al. Kinetic analysis of 3'-deoxy-3'-^{18}F-fluorothymidine in patients with gliomas. *J Nucl Med* 2006;47(10):1612–1621.
93. Guerin C, Laterra J, Drewes LR, et al. Vascular expression of glucose transporter in experimental brain neoplasms. *Am J Pathol* 1992;140: 417–425.
94. Guerin C, Laterra J, Hruban RH, et al. The glucose transporter and blood–brain barrier of human brain tumors. *Ann Neurol* 1990;28:758–765.
95. Pessin JE, Bell GI. Mammalian facilitative glucose transporter family: structure and molecular regulation. *Annu Rev Physiol* 1992;54:911–930.
96. Kadekaro M, Vance WM, Terrell ML, et al. Effects of antidromic stimulation of the ventral root on glucose utilization in the ventral horn of the spinal cord in the rat. *Proc Natl Acad Sci* 1987;84: 5492–5495.
97. Warburg O. *Metabolism of tumors.* London: Arnold and Constable, 1930.
98. Warburg O. On the origin of cancer cells. *Science* 1956;123:309–314.
99. Di Chiro G, DeLaPaz R, Brooks RA, et al. Glucose utilization of cerebral gliomas measured by [18F]fluorodeoxyglucose and positron emission tomography. *Neurology* 1982;32:1323–1329.
100. Alavi JB, Alavi A, Chawluk J, et al. Positron emission tomography in patients with glioma: a predictor of prognosis. *Cancer* 1988;62:1074–1078.
101. Coleman RE, Hoffman JM, Hanson MW, et al. Clinical application of PET for the evaluation of brain tumors. *J Nucl Med* 1991;32: 616–622.
102. Delbeke D, Meyerowitz C, Lapidus RL, et al. Optimal cutoff levels of F-18 fluorodeoxyglucose uptake in the differentiation of low grade from high-grade brain tumors with PET. *Radiology* 1995;195: 47–52.
103. Kim CK, Alavi JB, Alavi A, et al. New grading system of cerebral gliomas using positron emission tomography with F-18 fluorodeoxyglucose. *J Neurooncol* 1991;10:85–91.
104. Oriuchi N, Tomiyoshi K, Inoue T, et al. Independent thallium-201 accumulation and fluorine-18-fluorodeoxyglucose metabolism in glioma. *J Nucl Med* 1996;37(3):457–462.
105. Tyler JL, Diksic M, Villemure J-G, et al. Metabolic and hemodynamic evaluation of gliomas using positron emission tomography. *J Nucl Med* 1987;28:1123–1133.
106. Fulham MJ, Melisi JW, Nishimiya J, et al. Neuroimaging of juvenile pilocytic astrocytomas: an enigma. *Radiology* 1993;189:221–225.
107. Olivero WC, Dulebohn SC, Lister JR. The use of PET in evaluating patients with primary brain tumours: is it useful? *J Neurol Neurosurg Psychiatry* 1995;58:250–252.
108. Ricci PE, Karis JP, Heiserman JE, et al. Differentiating recurrent tumor from radiation necrosis: time for re-evaluation of positron emission tomography? *AJNR* 1998;19:407–413.
109. Wong TZ, van der Westhuizen GJ, Coleman RE. Positron emission tomography imaging of brain tumors. *Neuroimaging Clin North Am* 2002;12(4):615–626.
110. Di Chiro G, Brooks RA. PET-FDG of untreated and treated cerebral gliomas. *J Nucl Med* 1988;29:421–422.
111. Baron JC, Bousser MG, Comar D, et al. Crossed cerebellar diaschisis in human supratentorial infarction. *Ann Neurol* 1980;8:128(abst).
112. Patronas NJ, Di Chiro G, Smith BH, et al. Depressed cerebellar glucose metabolism in supratentorial tumors. *Brain Res* 1984;291:93–101.
113. West JR. The concept of diaschisis: a reply to Markowitsch and Pritzel. *Behav Biol* 1978;22:413–416.
114. Brodal A. *The cerebellum. neurological anatomy in relation to clinical medicine.* New York: Oxford University Press, 1981:294–391.
115. Fulham MJ, Brooks RA, Hallett M, et al. Cerebellar diaschisis revisited: pontine hypometabolism and dentate sparing. *Neurology* 1992;42: 2267–2273.
116. Carlstedt-Duke J, Gustafsson J-A. The molecular mechanism of glucocorticoid action. In: Ludecke DK, Chrousos GP, Tolis G, eds. *ACTH, Cushing's syndrome and other hypercortisolemic states.* New York: Raven Press, 1990:7–14.
117. Fulham MJ, Brunetti A, Aloj L, et al. Decreased cerebral glucose metabolism in patients with brain tumors: an effect of corticosteroids. *J Neurosurg* 1995:657–664.
118. Blacklock JB, Oldfield EH, Di Chiro G, et al. Effect of barbiturate coma on glucose utilization in normal brain versus gliomas. Positron emission tomography studies. *J Neurosurg* 1987;67:71–75.
119. Gaillard WD, Zeffiro T, Fazilat S, et al. Effect of valproate on cerebral metabolism and blood flow: an ^{18}F-2-deoxyglucose and ^{15}O water positron emission tomography study. *Epilepsia* 1996;37: 515–521.
120. Leiderman DB, Balish M, Bromfield EB, et al. Effect of valproate on human cerebral glucose metabolism. *Epilepsia* 1991;32:417–422.
121. Pahl JJ, Mazziotta JC, Bartzokis G, et al. Positron-emission tomography in tardive dyskinesia. *J Neuropsychiatry Clin Neurosci* 1995;7: 457–465.
122. Hooper PK, Meikle SR, Eberl S, et al. Validation of post injection transmission measurements for attenuation correction in neurologic FDG PET studies. *J Nucl Med* 1996;37:128–136.
123. Ardekani BA, Braun M, Hutton BF, et al. A fully automatic multimodality image registration algorithm. *J Comput Assist Tomogr* 1995;19(4):615–623.
124. Eberl S, Kanno I, Fulton RR, et al. A general automated inter-study image registration technique for SPECT and PET studies. *J Nucl Med* 1996;37:137–145.
125. Eberl S, Anayat AR, Fulton RR, et al. Evaluation of two population-based input functions for quantitative FDG PET studies. *Eur J Nucl Med* 1997;24(3):299–304.

126. Fulton RR, Eberl S, Meikle SR, et al. A practical 3D tomographic method for correcting patient head motion in clinical SPECT. *IEEE Trans Nucl Sci* 1999;46(3):667–672.
127. Green MV, Seidel J, Stein SD, et al. Head movement in normal subjects during simulated PET brain imaging with and without head movement. *J Nucl Med* 1994;35(9):1538–1546.
128. Fulton RR, Meikle SR, Eberl S, et al. Use of an optical motion tracking system to measure patient head movements in positron emission tomography (PET). *IEEE Trans Nucl Sci* 2002;49(1):116–123.
129. Butler AR, Horii SC, Kricheff II, et al. Computed tomography in astrocytomas. *Radiology* 1978;129:433–439.
130. Castillo M, Davis PC, Takei Y, et al. Intracranial ganglioglioma: MR, CT, and clinical findings in 18 patients. *AJNR* 1990;11(1):109–114.
131. Joyce P, Bentson J, Takahashi M, et al. The accuracy of predicting histologic grades of supratentorial astrocytomas on the basis of computerized tomography and cerebral angiography. *Neuroradiology* 1978;16:346–348.
132. Lee Y-Y, van Tassel P, Bruner JM, et al. Juvenile pilocytic astrocytomas: CT and MR characteristics. *AJR* 1989;152:1263–1270.
133. Leeds NE, Elkin CM, Zimmerman RD. Gliomas of the brain. *Semin Roentgenol* 1984;19:27–43.
134. McCormack BM, Miller DC, Budzilovich GN, et al. Treatment and survival of low-grade astrocytoma in adults—1977–1988. *Neurosurgery* 1992;31:636–642.
135. Zentner J, Wolf HK, Ostertun B, et al. Gangliogliomas: clinical, radiological, and histopathological findings in 51 patients. *J Neurol Neurosurg Psychiatry* 1994;57(12):1497–1502.
136. Davis WK, Boyko OB, Hoffman JM, et al. [18F]2-fluoro-2-deoxyglucose-positron emission tomography correlation of gadolinium-enhanced MR imaging of central nervous system neoplasia. *AJNR* 1993;14(3):515–523.
137. Melisi JW, Fulham MJ, Patronas N, et al. Comparison of Gd-DTPA enhanced MRI with PET-FDG in assessment of gliomas. In: *Congress of Neurological Surgeons, 1991*. Orlando, FL: Congress of Neurological Surgeons, 1991:264–266.
138. Chamberlain MC, Murovic JA, Levin VA. Absence of contrast enhancement on CT brain scans of patients with supratentorial malignant gliomas. *Neurology* 1988;38:1371–1374.
139. Kelly PJ, Daumas-Duport C, Scheithauer B, et al. Stereotactic histological correlations of computerized tomography- and magnetic resonance imaging-defined abnormalities in patients with glial neoplasms. *Mayo Clin Proc* 1987;62:450–459.
140. Cairncross JG. The biology of astrocytomas: lessons learned from chronic myelogenous leukemia—hypothesis. *J Neurooncol* 1987;5:11–27.
141. Cairncross JG. Low grade glioma: to treat or not to treat? *Arch Neurol* 1989;46:1238–1239.
142. Laws ERJ, Taylor WF, Clifton MB, et al. Neurosurgical management of low-grade astrocytoma of the cerebral hemisphere. *J Neurosurg* 1984;61:665–673.
143. Peipmeier JM. Observations on the current treatment of low grade astrocytic tumors of the cerebral hemispheres. *J Neurosurg* 1987;67:177–181.
144. Peterson K, DeAngelis LM. Weighing the benefits and risks of radiation therapy for low-grade glioma. *Neurology* 2001;56:1255–1256.
145. Hanson MW, Glantz MJ, Hoffman JM, et al. FDG-PET in the selection of brain lesions for biopsy. *J Comput Assist Tomogr* 1991;15:796–801.
146. Levivier M, Goldman S, Pirotte B, et al. Diagnostic yield of stereotactic brain biopsy guided by positron emission tomography with [18F]fluorodeoxyglucose. *J Neurosurg* 1995;82:445–452.
147. Massager N, David P, Goldman S, et al. Combined magnetic resonance imaging and positron emission tomography–guided stereotactic biopsy in brainstem mass lesions: diagnostic yield in a series of 30 patients. *J Neurosurg* 2000;93:951–957.
148. Francavilla TL, Miletich RS, Di Chiro G, et al. Positron emission tomography in the detection of malignant degeneration of low-grade gliomas. *Neurosurgery* 1989;24:1–5.
149. Fulham MJ. PET with [18F]fluorodeoxyglucose (PET-FDG): an indispensable tool in the proper management of brain tumors. In: Hubner KF, Collmann J, Buonocore E, et al., eds. *Clinical positron emission tomography*. St Louis: Mosby Year Book, 1992:50–60.
150. Sawaya R. Extent of resection in malignant gliomas: a critical summary. *J Neurooncol* 1999;42(3):303–305.
151. Holzer T, Herholz K, Jeske J, et al. FDG PET as a prognostic indicator in radiochemotherapy of glioblastoma. *J Comput Assist Tomogr* 1993;17(5):681–687.
152. Patronas NJ, Di Chiro G, Kufta C, et al. Prediction of survival in glioma patients by means of positron emission tomography. *J Neurosurg* 1985;62:816–822.
153. Schifter T, Hoffman JM, Hanson MW, et al. Serial FDG PET studies in the prediction of survival in patients with primary brain tumors. *J Comput Assist Tomogr* 1993;17(4):509–516.
154. Gutin PH, Leibel SA, Wara WW, et al. Recurrent malignant gliomas: survival following interstitial brachytherapy with high-activity iodine-125 sources. *J Neurosurg* 1987;67:864–873.
155. Macdonald DR, Cascino TL, Schold SC, et al. Response criteria for Phase II studies of supratentorial malignant glioma. *J Clin Oncol* 1990;8:1277–1280.
156. Cairncross JG, Pexman JHW, Rathbone MP, et al. Postoperative contrast enhancement in patients with brain tumor. *Ann Neurol* 1985;17:570–572.
157. Cairncross JG, Macdonald DR, Pexman JH, et al. Steroid-induced CT changes in patients with recurrent malignant glioma. *Neurology* 1988;38:724–726.
158. Crocker EF, Zimmerman RA, Phelps ME, et al. The effect of steroid on the extravascular distribution of radiographic contrast material and technetium pertechnetate in brain tumors as determined by computed tomography. *Radiology* 1976;119:471–474.
159. Hatam A, Bergstrom M, Yu Z-Y, et al. Effect of dexamethasone treatment on volume and contrast enhancement of intracranial neoplasms. *J Comput Assist Tomogr* 1983;7:295–300.
160. Muller W, Kretzschmar K, Schicketanz K-H. CT-analyses of cerebral tumors under steroid therapy. *Neuroradiology* 1984;26:293–298.
161. Eary JF, Krohn KA. Positron emission tomography: imaging tumor response. *Eur J Nucl Med* 2000;27:1737–1739.
162. Chamberlain MC. Treatment options for glioblastoma. *Neurosurg Focus* 2006;20(4):E2.
163. Marks JE, Wong J. The risk of cerebral radionecrosis in relation to dose, time and fractionation. *Prog Exp Tumor Res* 1985;29:210–218.
164. Sheline GE, Wara WM, Smithe V. Therapeutic irradiation and brain injury. *Int J Radiat Oncol Biol Phys* 1980;6:1215–1228.
165. Burger PC, Boyko OB. The pathology of central nervous system radiation injury. In: Gutin PH, Leibel SA, Sheline GE, eds. *Radiation injury to the nervous system*. New York: Raven Press, 1991:191–210.
166. Di Chiro G, Oldfield E, Wright DC, et al. Cerebral necrosis after irradiation and/or intraarterial chemotherapy for brain tumors: PET and neuropathologic studies. *AJNR* 1987;8:1083–1109.
167. Patronas NJ, Di Chiro G, Brooks RA, et al. Work in progress: [18F]fluorodeoxyglucose and positron emission tomography in the evaluation of radiation necrosis of the brain. *Radiology* 1982;144:885–889.
168. Doyle W, Budinger TF, Valk PE, et al. Differentiation of cerebral radiation necrosis from tumor recurrence by [^{18}F]FDG and ^{82}Rb positron emission tomography. *J Comput Assist Tomogr* 1987;11:563–570.
169. Valk PE, Budinger TF, Levin VA, et al. PET of malignant cerebral tumors after interstitial brachytherapy: demonstration of metabolic activity and clinical outcome. *J Neurosurg* 1988;69:830–838.
170. Glantz MJ, Hoffman JM, Coleman RE, et al. The role of F18 FDG PET imaging in predicting early recurrence of primary brain tumors. *Ann Neurol* 1991;29:347–355.
171. Kim EE, Chung SK, Haynie TP, et al. Differentiation of residual or recurrent tumors from post-treatment changes with F-18 FDG PET. *Radiographics* 1992;12(2):269–279.
172. Ogawa T, Kanno I, Shishido F, et al. Clinical value of PET with ^{18}F-fluorodeoxyglucose and L-methyl-^{11}C-methionine for diagnosis of

recurrent brain tumor and radiation injury. *Acta Radiol* 1991;32(3): 197–202.
173. Burger PC, Dubois PJ, Schold SC. Computerized tomographic and pathologic studies of untreated, quiescent, and recurrent glioblastoma multiforme. *J Neurosurg* 1983;58:159–169.
174. Earnest F, Kelly PJ, Scheithauer BW, et al. Cerebral astrocytomas: histopathologic correlation of MR and CT contrast enhancement with stereotaxic biopsy. *Radiology* 1988;166:823–827.
175. Mandonnet E, Jbabdi S, Taillandier L, et al. Preoperative estimation of residual volume for WHO grade II glioma resected with intraoperative functional mapping. *Neurooncology* 2007;9(1):63–69.
176. Nimsky C, Ganslandt O, Buchfelder M, et al. Intraoperative visualization for resection of gliomas: the role of functional neuronavigation and intraoperative 1.5 T MRI. *Neurol Res* 2006;28(5):482–487.
177. Schneider JP, Trantakis C, Rubach M, et al. Intraoperative MRI to guide the resection of primary supratentorial glioblastoma multiforme—a quantitative radiological analysis. *Neuroradiology* 2005;47(7):489–500.
178. Talos IF, Zou KH, Ohno-Machado L, et al. Supratentorial low-grade glioma resectability: statistical predictive analysis based on anatomic MR features and tumor characteristics. *Radiology* 2006;239(2):506–513.
179. Mishima K, Nakamura M, Nakamura H, et al. Leptomeningeal dissemination of cerebellar pilocytic astrocytoma. *J Neurosurg* 1992;77: 788–791.
180. Obana WG, Cogen PH, Davis RL, et al. Metastatic juvenile pilocytic astrocytoma: a case report. *J Neurosurg* 1991;75:972–975.
181. Germano IM, Ito M, Cho KG, et al. Correlation of histopathological features and proliferative potential of gliomas. *J Neurosurg* 1989;70: 701–706.
182. Jenkins RB, Kimmel DW, Moertel CA, et al. A cytogenetic study of 53 gliomas. *Cancer Genet Cytogenet* 1989;39:253–279.
183. Murovic JA, Nagashima T, Hoshino T, et al. Pediatric central nervous system tumors: a cell kinetic study with bromodeoxyuridine. *Neurosurgery* 1986;19:900–904.
184. Tsanaclis AM, Robert F, Michaud J, et al. The cycling pool of cells within human brain tumors: *in situ* cytokinetics using the monoclonal antibody Ki-67. *Can J Neurol Sci* 1991;18:12–7.
185. Long DM. Capillary ultrastructure and the blood brain barrier in human malignant brain tumors. *J Neurosurg* 1970;32:127–144.
186. Sato K, Rorke LB. Vascular bundles and wickerworks in childhood brain tumors. *Pediatr Neurosci* 1989;15:105–110.
187. Kincaid PK, El-Saden SM, Park SH, et al. Cerebral gangliogliomas: preoperative grading using FDG-PET and 201Tl-SPECT. *AJNR* 1998;19:801–805.
188. Meyer PT, Spetzger U, Mueller HD, et al. High F-18 FDG uptake in a low-grade supratentorial ganglioglioma: a positron emission tomography case report. *Clin Nucl Med* 2000;25(9):694–697.
189. Daumas-Duport C, Scheithauer BW, Chodkiewicz JP, et al. Dysembryoplastic neuroepithelial tumor: a surgically curable tumor of young patients with intractable partial seizures. *Neurosurgery* 1988;23:545–556.
190. Daumas-Duport C. Dysembryoplastic neuroepithelial tumors. *Brain Pathol* 1993;3:283–295.
191. Maehara T, Nariai T, Arai N, et al. Usefulness of [11C]methionine PET in the diagnosis of dysembryoplastic neuroepithelial tumor with temporal lobe epilepsy. *Epilepsia* 2004;45(1):41–45.
192. Kepes JJ, Rubinstein LJ, Eng LF. Pleomorphic xanthoastrocytoma: a distinctive meningcerebral glioma of young subjects with a relatively favorable prognosis: a study of 12 cases. *Cancer* 1979;44:1839–1852.
193. Glasser RS, Rojiani AM, Mickle JP, et al. Delayed occurrence of cerebellar pleomorphic xanthoastrocytoma after supratentorial pleomorphic xanthoastrocytoma removal. *J Neurosurg* 1995;82:116–118.
194. Lindboe CF, Cappelen J, Kepes JJ. Pleomorphic xanthoastrocytoma as a component of a cerebellar ganglioglioma: a case report. *Neurosurgery* 1992;31:353–355.
195. Bicik I, Raman R, Knightly JJ, et al. PET-FDG of pleomorphic xanthoastrocytoma. *J Nucl Med* 1995;36:97–99.
196. Blom RJ. Pleomorphic xanthoastrocytoma. CT appearance. *J Comput Assist Tomogr* 1988;12:351–354.
197. Rippe DJ, Boyko OB, Radu M, et al. MRI of temporal lobe pleomorphic xanthoastrocytoma. *J Comput Assist Tomogr* 1992;16(6): 856–859.
198. Tsuyuguchi N, Matsuoka Y, Sunada I, et al. Evaluation of pleomorphic xanthoastrocytoma by use of positron emission tomography with. *AJNR Am J Neuroradiol* 2001;22(2):311–313.
199. Etzl MM Jr, Kaplan AM, Moss SD, et al. Positron emission tomography in three children with pleomorphic xanthoastrocytoma. *J Child Neurol* 2002;17(7):522–527.
200. Im SH, Chung CK, Kim SK, et al. Pleomorphic xanthoastrocytoma: a developmental glioneuronal tumor with prominent glioproliferative changes. *J Neurooncol* 2004;66(1–2):17–27.
201. Torii K, Tsuyuguchi N, Kawabe J, et al. Correlation of amino-acid uptake using methionine PET and histological classifications in various gliomas. *Ann Nucl Med* 2005;19(8):677–683.
202. Nevin S. Gliomatosis cerebri. *Brain* 1938;61:170–191.
203. Artigas J, Cervos-Navarro J, Iglesias JR, et al. Gliomatosis cerebri: clinical and histological findings. *Clin Neuropathol* 1985;4: 135–148.
204. Koslow SA, Classen D, Hirsch WL, et al. Gliomatosis cerebri: a case report with autopsy correlation. *Neuroradiology* 1992;34:331–333.
205. Hara A, Sakai N, Yamada H, et al. Assessment of proliferative potential of gliomatosis cerebri. *J Neurol* 1991;238:80–82.
206. Dexter MA, Parker GD, Besser M, et al. MR and positron emission tomography with fludeoxyglucose F18 in gliomatosis cerebri. *AJNR* 1995;16:1507–1510.
207. Mineura K, Sasajima T, Kowada M, et al. Innovative approach in the diagnosis of gliomatosis using carbon-11-L-methionine positron emission tomography. *J Nucl Med* 1991;32:726–728.
208. Plowman PN, Saunders CA, Maisey MN. Gliomatosis cerebri: disconnection of the cortical grey matter, demonstrated on PET scan. *Br J Neurosurg* 1998;12(3):240–244.
209. Sato N, Inoue T, Tomiyoshi K, et al. Gliomatosis cerebri evaluated by 18Falpha-methyl tyearosine positron-emission tomography. *Neuroradiology* 2003;45(10):700–707.
210. Shintani S, Tsuruoka S, Shiigai T. Serial positron emission tomography (PET) in gliomatosis cerebri treated with radiotherapy: a case report. *J Neurol Sci* 2000;173(1):25–31.
211. Yaguchi M, Nakasone A, Sohmiya M, et al. Gliomatosis cerebri involving the lumbosacral spinal cord. *Intern Med* 2003;42(7):615–618.
212. Di Chiro G, Oldfield E, Bairamian D, et al. Metabolic imaging of the brain stem and spinal cord: studies with positron emission tomography using ^{18}F-2-deoxyglucose in normal and pathological cases. *J Comput Assist Tomogr* 1983;7(6):937–945.
213. Alavi A, Kramer E, Wegener W, et al. Magnetic resonance and fluorine-18 deoxyglucose imaging in the investigation of a spinal cord tumor. *J Nucl Med* 1990;31:360–364.
214. Wilmshurst JM, Barrington SF, Pritchard D, et al. Positron emission tomography in imaging spinal cord tumors. *J Child Neurol* 2000;15(7):465–472.
215. Shimizu T, Saito N, Aihara M, et al. Primary spinal oligoastrocytoma: a case report. *Surg Neurol* 2004;61(1):77–81.
216. Loeffler JS, Patchell RA, Sawaya R. Treatment of metastatic cancer. In: DeVita VT, Hellman S, Rosenberg SA, eds. *Cancer: principles and practice of oncology*, 5th ed. Philadelphia: Lippincott-Raven, 1997:2523–2536.
217. Griffeth LK, Rich KM, Dehdashti F, et al. Brain metastases from non-central nervous system tumors: evaluation with PET. *Radiology* 1993;186(1):37–44.
218. Di Chiro G. Which PET radiopharmaceutical for brain tumors [editorial]. *J Nucl Med* 1991;32:1346–1348.

CHAPTER

8.7 Use of PET and PET/CT in the Evaluation of Patients with Head and Neck Cancer

TODD M. BLODGETT, ALEXANDER RYAN, AND BARTON BRANSTETTER IV

PROTOCOLS FOR EVALUATION OF HEAD AND NECK CANCER

Combined positron emission tomography (PET) and computed tomography (CT) has several advantages over either CT or PET alone in the evaluation of patients with head and neck cancer. The accurate coregistration of images and improved localization achieved with a combined modality are particularly important in the neck, where there is not only anatomical complexity, but several structures that demonstrate variable physiologic fluorodeoxyglucose (FDG) uptake.

In order to maximize the utility of PET/CT, it is important to optimize the several scan protocol options available when performing PET/CT for the evaluation of patients with head and neck cancer. A typical baseline diagnostic PET/CT for a patient with head and neck cancer is increasingly common to include a full-power CT scan with intravenous contrast in addition to an FDG PET scan acquired during the same imaging session on a hardware combined PET/CT device. Oral contrast may or may not be utilized, depending on the extent of area being scanned. A typical protocol for patients with head and neck cancer might include the skull base through the abdomen; therefore, oral contrast is not routinely utilized in the authors' protocol, but oral contrast is routinely utilized in some centers. FDG must be injected at a consistent time interval prior to the start of patient imaging; a relatively standard protocol would involve injection of FDG 1 hour prior to the commencement of the scan. Longer times from injection until imaging are used by some groups as the tumor/background uptake ratios typically rise with time postinjection; however, about 60 minutes postinjection of tracer is very common to commence imaging.

Neck immobilization is an important protocol consideration with the evaluation of patients with head and neck cancer, as this is the area of interest. A variety of soft collars and external immobilization devices are available to help minimize or eliminate neck movement.

Arm positioning for the examination is also an important consideration. The two most commonly used positions for arm positioning during PET/CT imaging are standard "arms up" and "arms down." In general, the most important determinant of arm positioning in PET/CT is the indication of malignancy that is being evaluated and subsequent areas of interest being scanned. The goal of any arm positioning protocol should be to minimize CT beam-hardening artifacts in the area of interest. Therefore, for patients with head and neck cancer it is usually preferable to scan patients with arms down, at least at the level of the neck. Alternatively, two scans may be performed, one with data acquisition through the chest and abdomen (with or without the pelvis) while the arms are positioned up followed by a more limited second scan acquisition through the neck area with arms positioned down. Care should be taken to ensure adequate overlap of scans at the thoracic inlet, as lower neck structures can shift substantially with the change in arm position.

The most important CT consideration for patients with head and neck cancer is whether, when, and how to use intravenous contrast and whether to use low- or high-dose CT. Because of the anatomical complexity of the neck, if logistically possible, a diagnostic CT with contrast is typically recommended. This will make it easier to differentiate the vascular from nonvascular structures, as well as to distinguish pathology from normal structures more clearly. Vascular structures can contain FDG, and such uptake can sometimes be confused with small nodes in noncontrast studies.

Other options include performing a low-dose, noncontrast CT (40 to 80 mA), which reduces radiation exposure to the patient but may have a lower sensitivity and specificity for the detection of malignancy on its own, although this has not been rigorously studied in a variety of clinical settings. It can be used for simple localization purposes, but is typically more difficult to interpret due to the lack of structural differentiation. The quality of the scan is too poor to charge for reimbursement in most centers for the PET alone. However, since most of the tumor detection is being done with the FDG, the quality of the CT scan may not be as critical to the total diagnostic accuracy as the PET plus the localizing information from the CT. It is possible that for follow-up PET studies, such as those used for tumor surveillance, that there is little benefit from the use of a full-contrast CT scan. Not all noncontrast CT scans are performed the same way. Full-dose, noncontrast CT is another option that may be the best for patients with a significant contrast allergy.

Contrast-enhanced CT offers the most advantages to the interpreting physician, but it does require medical personnel immediately available to respond to unexpected contrast reactions. One potential disadvantage of using contrast in PET/CT imaging is the presence of attenuation-correction artifacts that are unique to PET/CT. These are discussed in detail at the end of this chapter. Although attenuation-correction artifacts generally are easy to recognize and are a valid reason to avoid intravenous contrast for qualitative PET assessments, the interpreting physician must be aware of these artifacts in order to avoid confusion with malignancy. Further, there can be some modest alterations in apparent standardized uptake value (SUV) in the presence of high concentrations of intravenous contrast.

Another approach involves a low-dose noncontrast CT prior to PET imaging (for the purpose of artifact-free attenuation correction) followed by a full-dose contrast CT of diagnostic quality. This is ideal from an imaging point of view but exposes the patient to potentially unnecessary radiation. However, this approach may be acceptable if contrast CT is only needed for a small area of the patient such as the head and neck.

Optimizing arm positioning and intravenous contrast into a single algorithm is a convenient approach. A full CT scan algorithm might include a noncontrast low-dose CT with arms up performed first (this CT will be utilized for attenuation correction) followed by CT performed with contrast after the PET acquisition. During the contrast-enhanced CT acquisition, the arms would be positioned at the side to minimize beam hardening through the area of interest. Another approach is to perform the neck study first with no contrast and the arms down, followed by the CT with contrast. This practice varies somewhat by center, but it is suggested that the use of intravenous contrast be seriously considered in any protocol designed to detect cancer in the head and neck region.

It is not clear whether all patients with a history of head and neck cancer will benefit from a diagnostic CT as part of their PET/CT workup. In general, when patients are suspected of having active disease during their initial evaluation, during therapy, and in the interim following therapy, contrast-enhanced CT is recommended. An exception can be made for patients who have had a contrast-enhanced CT performed recently. Asymptomatic patients with successfully treated malignancies undergoing surveillance with low suspicion of viable cancer and those with a recent diagnostic CT are good candidates for low-dose CT as part of their PET/CT examination.

PHYSIOLOGIC FLUORODEOXYGLUCOSE DISTRIBUTION IN HEAD AND NECK

Several normal structures in the head and neck may demonstrate physiological FDG activity on PET or PET/CT. It is important to be familiar with the appearance of normal, as well as atypical, patterns of physiological FDG uptake. Among the structures that take up FDG normally are the salivary glands, thyroid gland, brown fat, lymphoid tissue, mucosal tissue, and muscles of the neck, pharynx, and face. FDG is taken up by salivary glands and excreted into the saliva to a limited extent (1). The parotid, submandibular, and thyroid glands can demonstrate mild to intense symmetric uptake (Figs. 8.7.1 and 8.7.2).

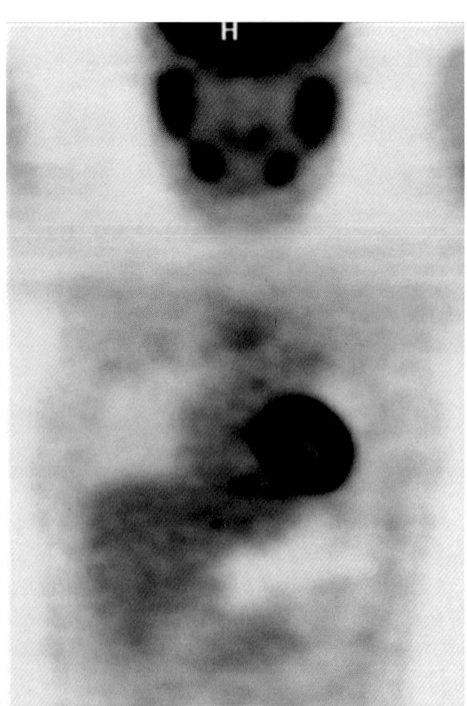

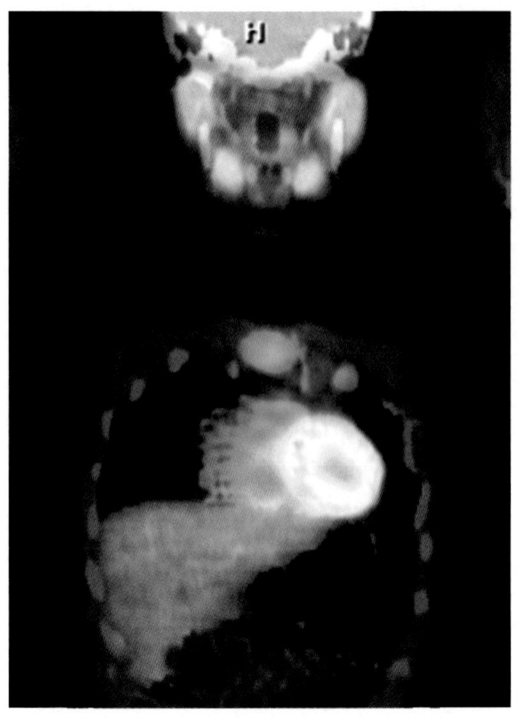

FIGURE 8.7.1. Salivary gland physiologic fluorodeoxyglucose (FDG) activity. Coronal PET (**A**) and fused PET/CT (**B**) images demonstrate intense symmetrical physiologic FDG activity within the parotid and submandibular glands bilaterally.

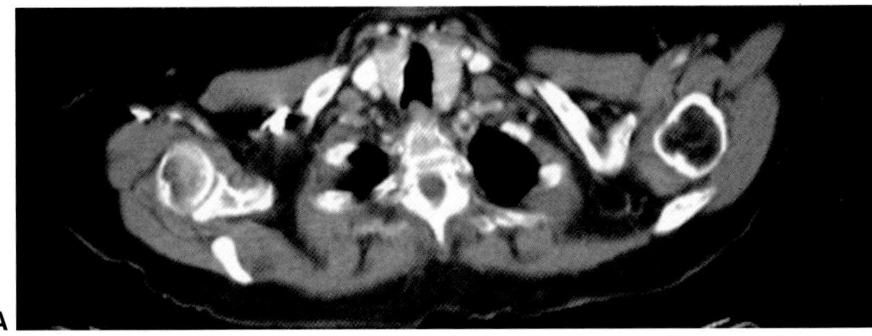

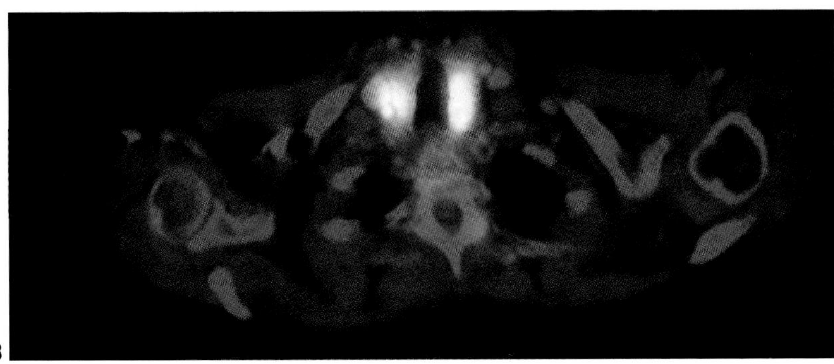

FIGURE 8.7.2. The physiologic thyroid activity. Axial CT (**A**) and fused PET/CT (**B**) images demonstrate intense physiologic activity within both lobes of the thyroid. The differential diagnosis for diffuse fluorodeoxyglucose activity within the thyroid gland also includes inflammatory and infectious processes, making diffuse uptake in the thyroid nonspecific.

Brown fat may be found throughout the neck and thorax as well as outside the neck (Fig. 8.7.3) (2–4). FDG is taken up by macrophages and lymphocytes, therefore, lymphoid structures are also commonly appreciated on FDG PET scans (Fig. 8.7.4). Examples of lymphoid structures include all the structures of Waldeyer's ring (adenoids, palatine, and lingual tonsils), as well as lymph nodes (5–8). Mucosal tissue such as that found in the nasal turbinates and seen throughout the oro- and nasopharynx, commonly shows FDG uptake. Muscles are among the many normal structures commonly seen on FDG PET or PET/CT studies (Fig. 8.7.5). Muscles of mastication, including the pterygoid muscles, and muscles of the oral floor may also be seen (Fig. 8.7.6), as well as the pharyngeal constrictor muscles, muscles controlling the vocal cords, and the vocal cords themselves (Fig. 8.7.7) (9). An in-depth review of the more atypical physiologic FDG uptake patterns and pitfalls is provided at the end of this chapter.

CONVENTIONAL IMAGING MODALITIES

Conventional Imaging

One of the reasons that conventional imaging suffers when assessing nodal metastases is that the CT and magnetic resonance imaging (MRI) characteristics of cancer do not differ sufficiently from one

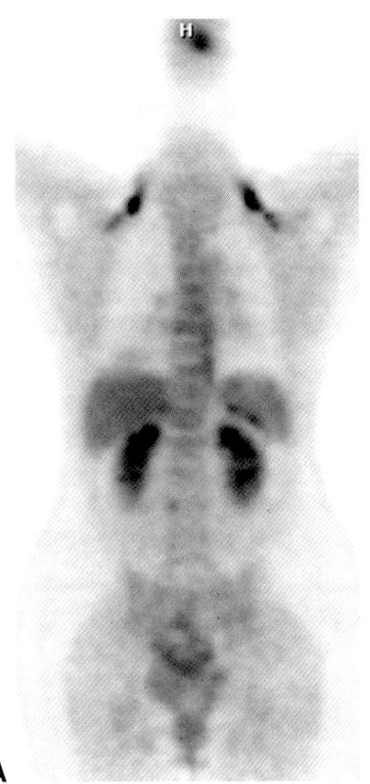

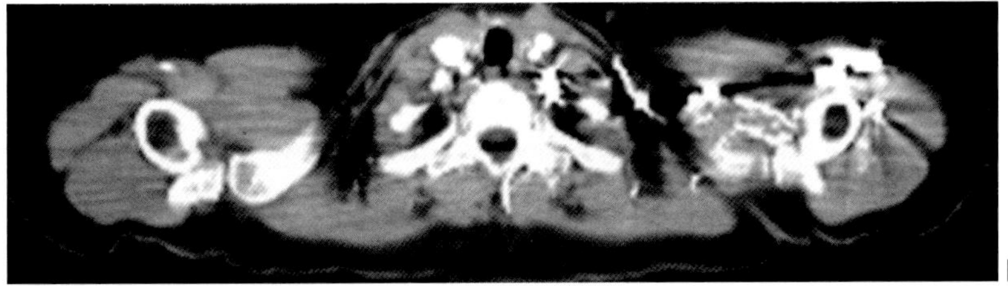

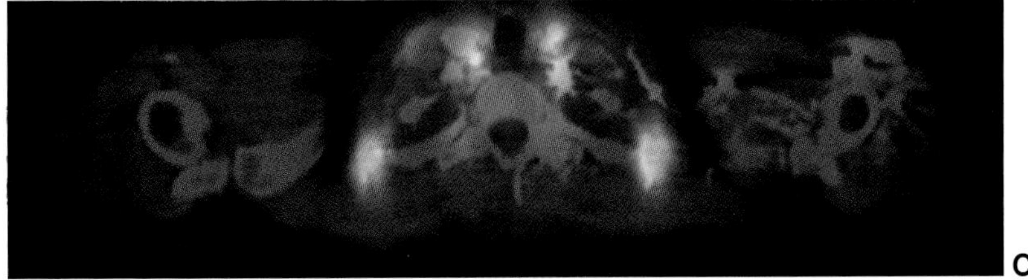

FIGURE 8.7.3. Brown fat. Coronal PET (**A**), axial CT (**B**), and axial fused PET/CT (**C**) images demonstrate symmetrical intense fluorodeoxyglucose activity within areas of fat attenuation on CT compatible with physiologic brown fat uptake.

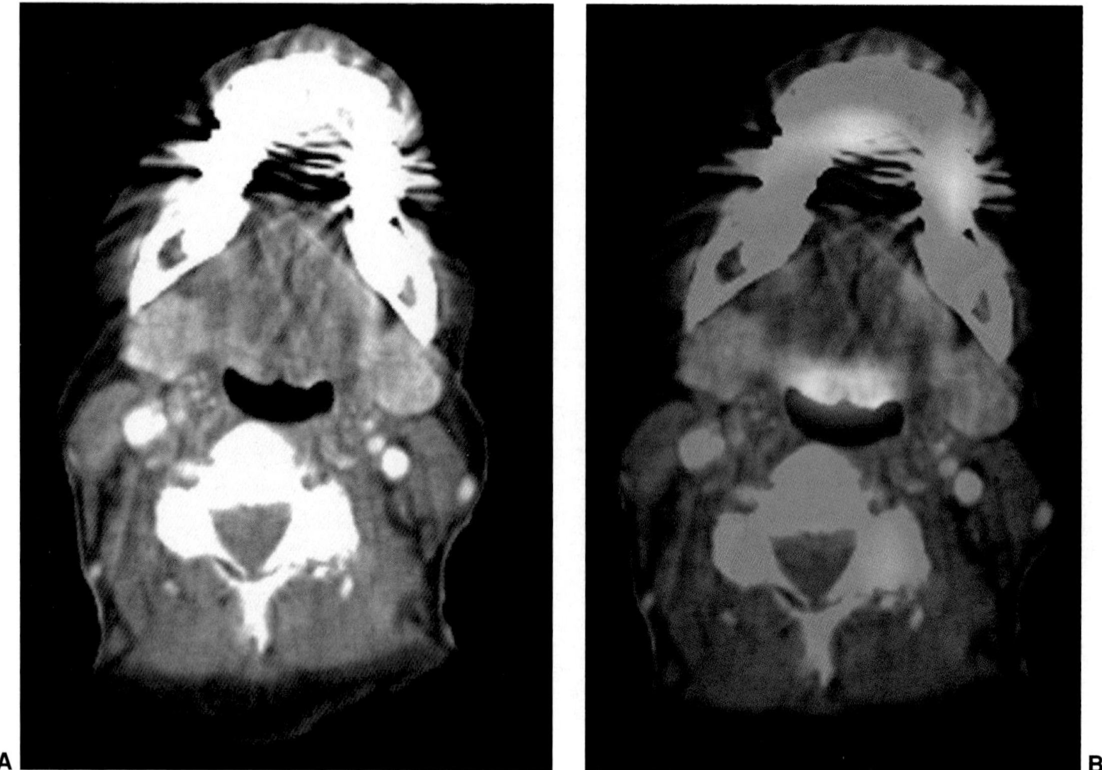

FIGURE 8.7.4. Physiologic lymphoid fluorodeoxyglucose (FDG) uptake. Axial CT (**A**) and fused PET/CT (**B**) images demonstrate intense symmetrical physiologic activity within the lingual tonsils bilaterally. Any lymphoid structure may demonstrate physiologic activity that ranges from minimal activity to very intense. Symmetrical FDG activity is almost always considered physiologic.

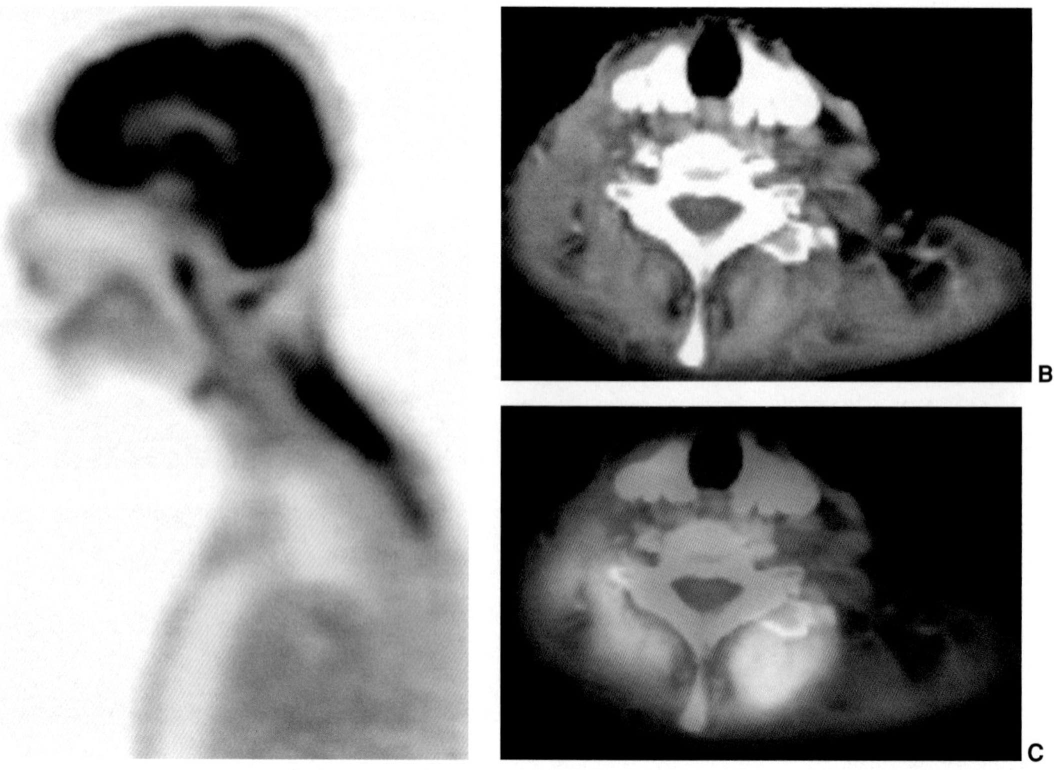

FIGURE 8.7.5. Asymmetrical muscle activity. Sagittal PET (**A**), axial CT (**B**), and axial fused PET/CT (**C**) images demonstrate a symmetrical intense area of fluorodeoxyglucose activity that appears linear on the sagittal images and correlates to the left paraspinal musculature, which is compatible with physiologic activity. Inspection of all three orthogonal planes is important to detect linear activity within most muscles.

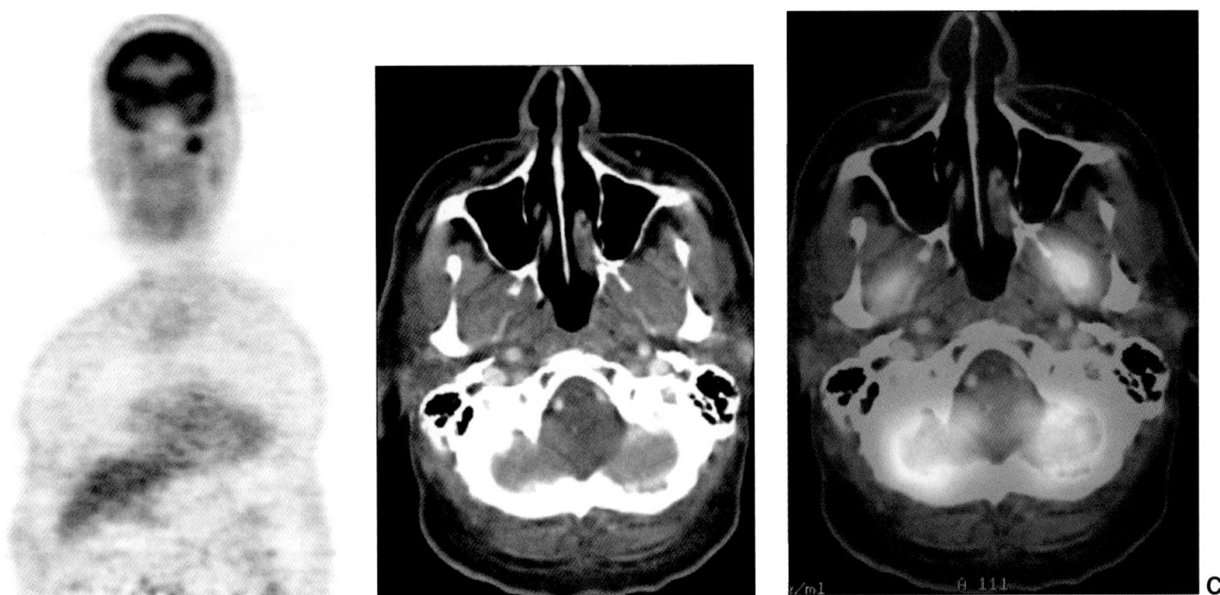

FIGURE 8.7.6. Physiologic pterygoid muscle activity. Coronal PET (**A**), axial CT (**B**), and axial fused PET/CT (**C**) images demonstrate intense physiologic activity within the pterygoid muscles bilaterally. Asymmetrical intense physiologic activity has been reported several times in the literature and needs to be considered as a potential pitfall and a cause of a physiological intense uptake within the neck region.

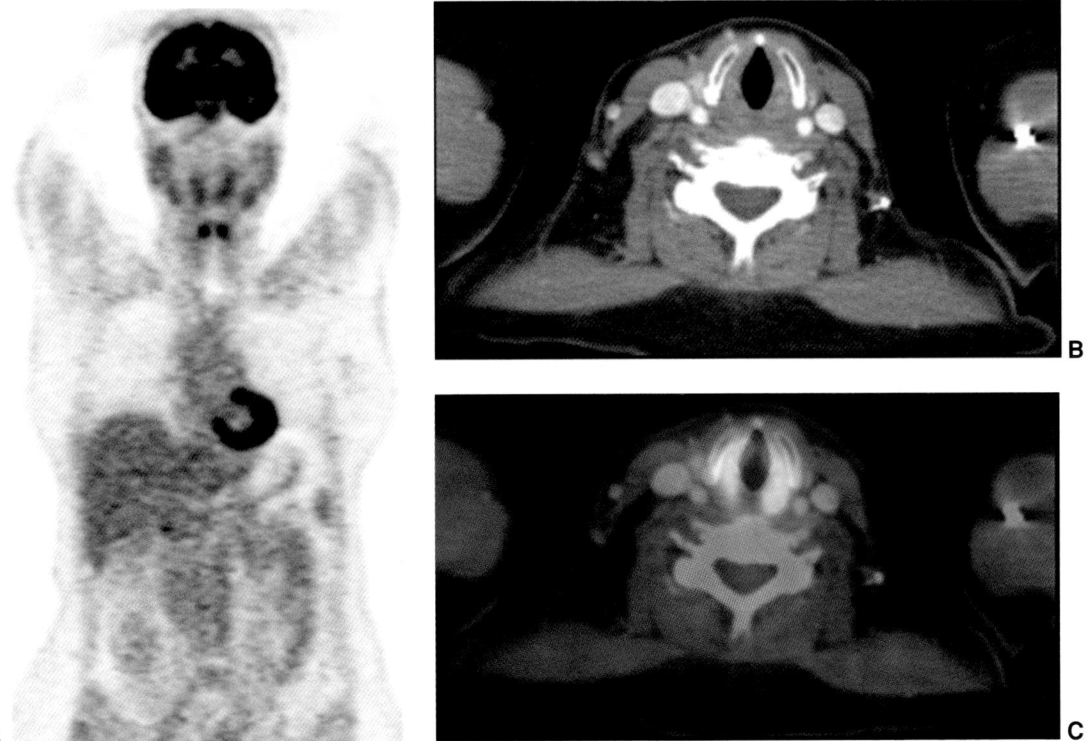

FIGURE 8.7.7. Physiologic vocal cord activity. Coronal PET (**A**), axial CT (**B**), and axial fused PET/CT (**C**) images demonstrate intense symmetrical physiologic activity within the vocal cords. This appearance is seen more frequently when patients talk during the uptake phase after fluorodeoxyglucose injection.

another to offer a truly specific diagnosis. The lack of reliable criteria for identifying metastatic cervical lymph nodes based on size is understandable given the limitations of the techniques applied (10). Size criteria are most commonly reported, but experts cannot even agree on which axis (short or long) is a better determinant of malignancy. Although much of the literature reports use of the short axis, the long axis may correlate better with clinical assessments of the nodes. Different thresholds for lymph node size have been studied, ranging from 5 to 15 mm. As expected, smaller thresholds result in higher sensitivities at the expense of specificity. No single size criterion is sufficient, however, because nodes less than 5 mm can contain foci of malignancy. Similarly, large nodes may be reactive and not contain cancer. Size alone is simply not reliable for detecting cancer in lymph nodes.

Other criteria for malignancy have recently gained favor. The presence of central necrosis is almost always indicative of malignancy in adult patients. Caution should be taken, however, that a central fatty hilum (generally more indicative of benignancy) is not confused with central necrosis (indicative of malignancy). It should also be recognized that some infectious processes can also cause central necrosis of lymph nodes.

Contrast enhancement characteristics are also important. Lymph nodes that enhance earlier and to a greater degree than their counterparts are more likely to contain tumor. The border of a suspicious node may be helpful; an ill-defined border suggests extracapsular spread. Of course, most metastatic nodes will not have progressed to extracapsular extension, so a well-defined border cannot be taken as a sign of benignancy.

Perhaps the best anatomic characteristic for distinguishing benign from malignant nodes is the configuration of the node. Reniform nodes, especially those with an identifiable hilum, are almost always benign. Spherical nodes are more worrisome.

The decision of whether to use CT or MRI for the initial evaluation of a head and neck tumor depends on the referring physician and radiologist's personal preference. Some feel that MRI defines tumor margins better than CT, but others feel that high-resolution CT has bridged the diagnostic gap, so the added expense and inconvenience of MRI is not warranted. Clinical studies show CT to have a small but measurable advantage in the assessment of cervical lymphadenopathy (10).

In a few anatomic areas, the choice between CT and MRI is clearer. Tumors of the skull base and temporal bone are usually first imaged with CT to establish bony extent. MRI is often called on secondarily in these cases. Tumors of the oral tongue are better evaluated with MRI. MRI is far superior for establishing the presence or absence of perineural spread.

Advanced Cross-sectional Techniques

In recent years, researchers in CT and MRI have tried many techniques to conclusively distinguish between benign and malignant cervical lymph nodes. These techniques represent the alternatives to PET/CT. PET has been shown to be superior to CT or MRI in the detection of recurrent tumors. Several studies have shown somewhat superior diagnostic accuracy for PET as compared to CT in the characterization of lymph nodes for the presence or absence of involvement with cancer.

Dynamic contrast techniques have been studied in both CT and MRI (11). These techniques rely on the more rapid contrast enhancement and more rapid contrast washout of malignant nodes. Repeat images are obtained at select cross-sectional levels over the course of a contrast bolus to determine the perfusion patterns of the tissues. These studies, when performed using the CT technique, do impart a higher radiation dose than simple static images.

Novel contrast agents, such as iron oxide particles, have been used in MRI (12). These agents interfere with the magnetic field when taken up by the normal lymphatic system. Lymph nodes replaced by tumor do not take up the contrast agent, and thus fail to drop signal. These techniques are promising, but the most promising contrast agent is not yet approved by the U.S. Food and Drug Administration.

MRI techniques such as magnetization transfer and T1-rho imaging showed initial promise in detecting metastatic nodes, but these techniques have fallen out of favor in recent years (13,14). Doppler sonography has been shown to detect and to some extent distinguish malignant nodes by their increased blood flow, but the inability to assess deep tissues and the strong operator dependence have limited this technique (15).

PET/CT IN EVALUATION OF PATIENTS WITH HEAD AND NECK MALIGNANCIES

General

Studies have been performed over the past few years looking for potential added benefit with PET/CT over PET and CT performed separately. The use of combined PET/CT has reduced the incidence of pitfalls and allows easy differentiation of physiologic FDG uptake from pathologic uptake, more accurate localization of lesions, and detection of lesions that do not produce anatomic distortion (16–23). Physiologic structures such as muscle and brown fat are easily distinguishable from pathology on PET/CT, whereas with PET alone, with or without CT correlation, differentiation can be challenging or impossible and can lead to unnecessary further evaluation.

In terms of the overall added benefit of PET/CT compared to PET and CT interpreted separately in patients with head and neck cancer, a recent study from the University of Pittsburgh Medical Center showed the incremental value of PET/CT over PET and CT interpreted separately. PET/CT had an overall sensitivity of 98%, specificity of 92%, and accuracy of 94% for evaluating patients with known or suspected squamous cell carcinoma (SCC) of the head and neck (24). The study also showed that for all 125 lesions that were examined, CT was inferior to PET and PET was inferior to PET/CT and that 62% of lesions considered equivocal on CT and 41% of lesions equivocal on PET were categorized more definitively when radiologists had access to fused PET/CT images.

Another similar study by Schoder and Yeung (25) comparing PET and PET/CT in patients with any malignant lesion of the head and neck showed that PET/CT had a higher accuracy for depicting cancer than PET alone (96% vs. 90%). In this study 100 of 157 lesions had improved localization with PET/CT than with PET alone and 53% of equivocal lesions were classified more confidently based on PET/CT. These data demonstrate the superiority of PET/CT to PET alone and build on a large number of studies showing the superiority of PET to MRI or CT in several settings in patients with known or suspected head and neck cancers. These were extensively reviewed in the first edition of this book and only the more recent reports are emphasized in this update.

PET/CT in Unknown Primaries

Patients with head and neck SCC will often present with an enlarging neck mass. Fine-needle aspiration of the neck mass will reveal metastatic SCC, but because SCC does not arise *de novo* from lymph nodes, the source of the disease may remain obscure. Usually clinical, radiographic, and endoscopic evaluation will reveal the primary tumor that is the source of the metastatic disease. In some cases, blind random biopsies of likely anatomic areas (tonsils, base of tongue) are used to find the primary tumor. Despite these efforts, unknown primary tumors account for up to 10% of head and neck SCC.

There are several possible reasons for a primary tumor to remain unknown. Tumors less than 5 mm may be difficult to identify with endoscopy and cross-sectional imaging. Tumors embedded deep in the crypts of the palatine tonsils may escape notice. Clinicians accustomed to evaluating the head and neck can easily overlook cutaneous primary tumors and primary tumors outside the head and neck.

It is critically important for a primary tumor to be identified when metastatic SCC is discovered. The treatment of head and neck SCC focuses on surgical removal of the primary tumor and/or directed radiation therapy. If a primary tumor cannot be identified, the patient must undergo radiation of the entire upper aerodigestive mucosa. This results in considerable morbidity, particularly xerostomia and stenoses. More advanced treatment modalities, such as intensity-modulated radiation therapy (IMRT) and CyberKnife (Accuray, Sunnyvale, California) radiation, are not generally an option in patients with an unknown primary.

Many studies have addressed the efficacy of PET in evaluating patients with unknown primary tumors. These studies are difficult to compare because the definition of "unknown primary" varies from only clinical assessment to a full assessment with endoscopy and cross-sectional imaging. PET has been studied in this patient population and a sensitivity ranging from 5% to 60% was found, but larger studies suggested a sensitivity in the range of 25% to 35% (26–33). Preliminary studies suggest that PET/CT may offer a slight increase in overall sensitivity (33% to57%) for detecting unknown primary tumors, but may offer significantly more information regarding biopsy localization information (Fig. 8.7.8) (34,35).

The major pitfall for identifying the primary tumor in the setting of known SCC metastases is the variable physiologic uptake of FDG in the common locations of hidden primary tumors. In particular, the palatine tonsils and the lingual tonsil at the tongue base can have variable (and asymmetric) uptake in normal individuals, and this uptake may mask an underlying lesion. In this situation, PET/CT has an advantage over PET because the presence or absence of a mass on the CT can lend credence to asymmetric FDG uptake. Alternatively, physiologic uptake may be mistaken for tumor.

The role of PET/CT in the assessment of the unknown primary is to lead the surgeon to potential sources of tumor. As such, these examinations should be read with high sensitivity, because the risk of a negative biopsy is worth the potential benefits of identifying the primary lesion.

Role of PET/CT in Staging

Many patients who are candidates for staging PET/CT will have already undergone a CT of the neck. Patients who are seen at primary care hospitals often begin their radiographic work-up at those sites. Also, if a patient's diagnosis is in question, a CT may be performed before it is clear that a PET/CT would have been the better choice.

Not all patients who have already undergone a good quality neck CT require an additional staging PET/CT with a contrast-enhanced CT. Because traditional cross-sectional imaging is usually sufficient to evaluate the primary lesion, typically only patients who are at substantial risk of nodal or hematogenous metastases would benefit from PET/CT. In this patient population, it is not uncommon to find metastases outside of the head and neck (Fig. 8.7.9). Since many of the risk factors for head and neck cancer are also risk factors for lung cancer, the detection of additional primary cancers is also not uncommon when PET/CT is used for tumor staging.

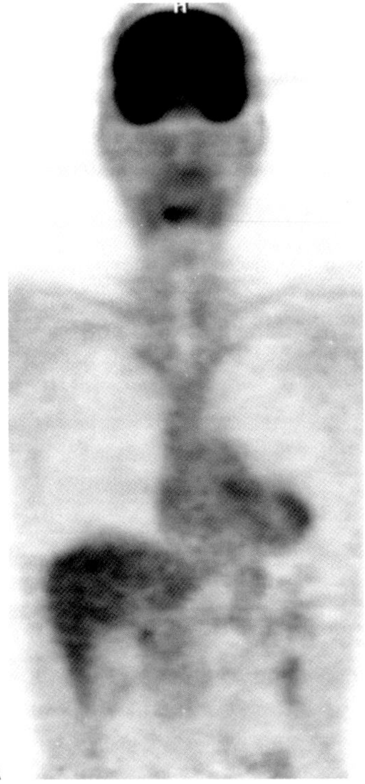
A

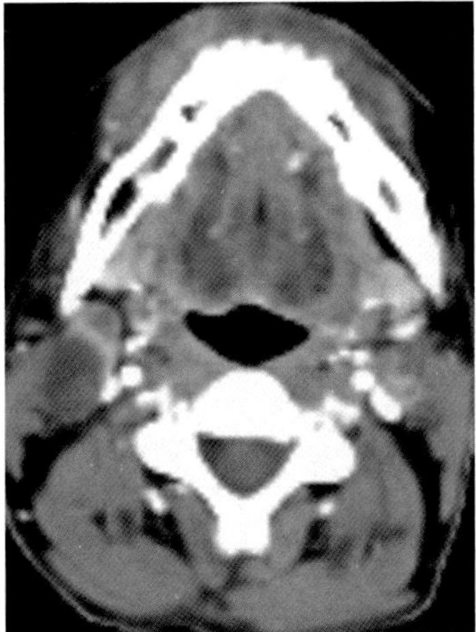

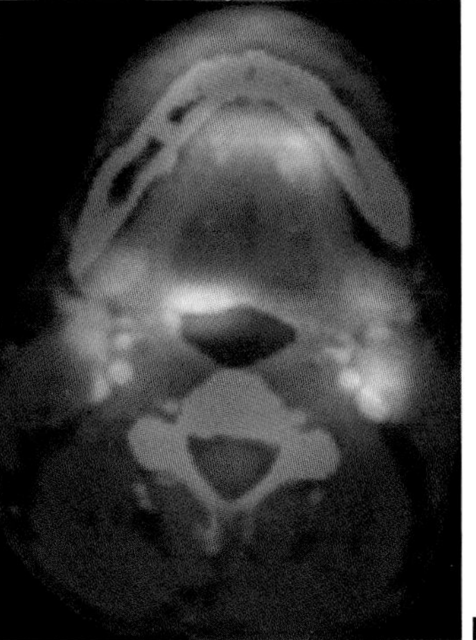
B, C

FIGURE 8.7.8. Detection of unknown primary tumors. Coronal PET image (**A**) shows a focal area of intense fluorodeoxyglucose activity to the right of midline, although accurate localization is not possible. Axial CT image (**B**) demonstrates no definite evidence for a malignant lesion along the mucosal surface. Axial fused PET/CT (**C**) confirms the presence of a mucosal lesion and also allows accurate definitive localization within the right base of tongue. (From Branstetter BF, IV, Blodgett TM, Zimmer LA, et al. Head and malignancy: is PET/CT more accurate than PET or CT alone? *Radiology* 2005;235:580–586, with permission.)

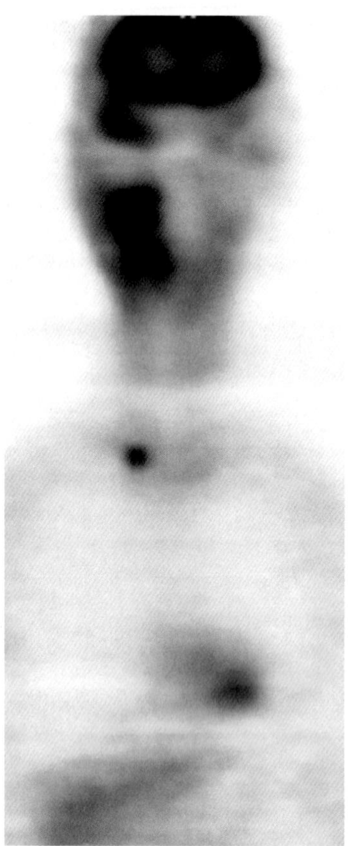

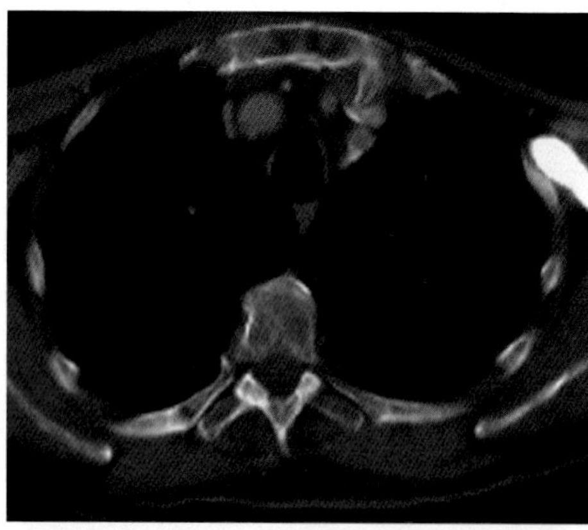

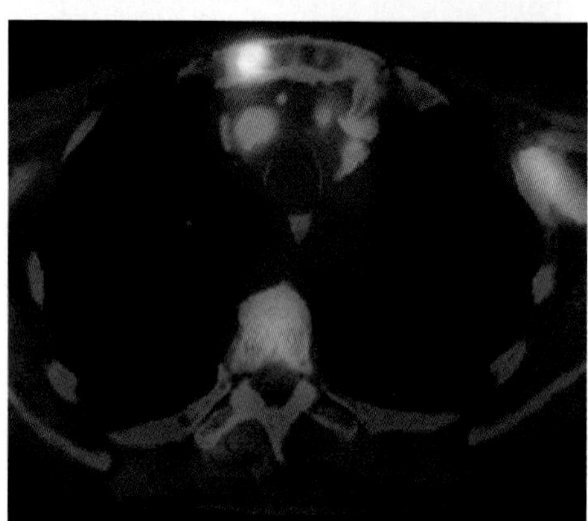

A, B, C

FIGURE 8.7.9. Detection of lesions outside of the neck. Coronal PET image (**A**) demonstrates a focal area of intense fluorodeoxyglucose (FDG) activity in the thorax, but the precise localization cannot be determined. This patient was referred for restaging PET/CT of squamous cell carcinoma of the right oropharynx. Axial CT (**B**) shows no definite abnormalities in the thorax. The fused PET/CT image (**C**) shows a focal area of intense FDG activity in the sternum just to the left of the right sternoclavicular joint, compatible with a metastatic lesion outside of the neck. (From Fukui MB, Blodgett TM, Snyderman CH, et al. Combined PET/CT in the head and neck: part 2. Diagnostic uses and pitfalls of oncologic imaging. *RadioGraphics* 2005;25:913-930, with permission.)

Patients with primary tumors that are prone to bilateral metastases should be evaluated with PET/CT because contralateral metastases are often less conspicuous on conventional imaging (Fig. 8.7.10). Primary tumors of the nasopharynx, tongue base, and supraglottis fit this category.

Patients with T3 or T4 lesions of the oral cavity, oropharynx, or larynx are at substantial risk of metastatic disease, both nodal and hematogenous. Thus, these patients merit pretreatment evaluation with PET/CT. Other tumors that are prone to metastatic disease are well described in the otolaryngology literature, but a complete listing is beyond the scope of this chapter. It is assumed, but not yet proven, that PET/CT has greater sensitivity than conventional modalities for the detection of metastatic lesions in these patients.

Syed et al. (36) also showed that PET/CT significantly increases interobserver agreement and confidence levels in localizing lesions for staging of SCC. Several studies have shown the benefit of PET in evaluating regional nodal spread, particularly when there are normal-sized malignant lymph nodes detected (37–44). PET/CT can add additional localization information, such as the precise nodal levels involved and even which of the nodes within a level are abnormal. For staging of SCC in the head and neck, PET/CT has also been reported to be helpful in delineating perineural spread of disease and can show osseous extension of the primary tumor that may affect the surgical approach (45). PET/CT can be helpful in further characterizing and evaluating additional foci of FDG uptake outside of the neck region, which may represent a second primary malignancy or metastatic spread of the head and neck cancer (46,47).

Treatment Planning

Coregistered contemporaneous functional and anatomical image data appear to be ideally suited to guide treatment planning. The accuracy of brain tumor biopsies has been improved by incorporating PET data into the surgical plan (48). There is now growing evidence that radiation portals, which are typically based on anatomic image data, may be more accurately delineated with PET/CT (38,49–51). The addition of metabolic information with PET can alter these decisions in approximately one third of cases (52,53).

Recently, there has been an increasing expectation that delineation of tumor targets with image-guided radiation therapy must shift toward incorporating biological information (54,55). A prospective phantom study from the University of Pittsburgh Medical Center assessed the impact of PET/CT relative to CT alone on radiation therapy simulation for head and neck cancer (51). Gross tumor volumes and abnormal nodal regions were evaluated with and without the FDG PET information. This work demonstrated larger volumes for primary tumors using CT rather than PET, presumably due to the superior ability of PET to delineate normal tissue and tumor. However, further study is needed to assess the influence of combined imaging on patient outcome.

With the advent of IMRT, precise tumor localization is vital to emphasize dose delivery to the tumor while minimizing radiation-induced damage to neighboring tissues. Schwartz et al. (38) showed the superiority of registered FDG PET and CT images

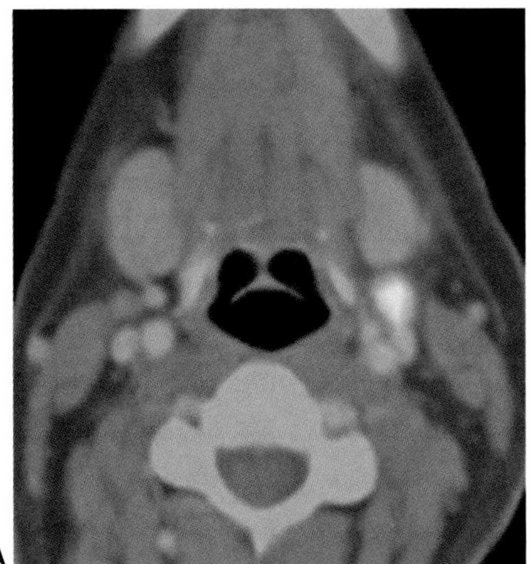

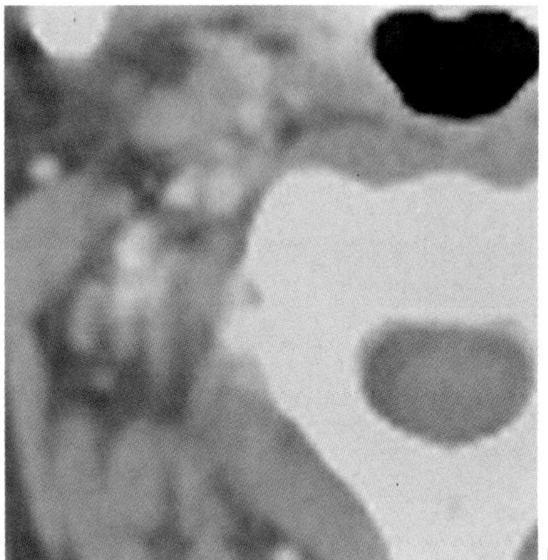

FIGURE 8.7.10. Contralateral lymph node detection. Two axial fused PET/CT images (**A,B**) demonstrate an enlarged left neck node compatible with a malignant lesion in this patient with a left-sided primary squamous cell carcinoma. However, a cluster of normal-sized lymph nodes are also present within the right neck, none of which are pathologic by CT criteria. The second fused PET/CT image confirms the presence of intense activity within one of the lymph nodes, causing this patient to have bilateral radical neck sections.

over CT alone for geographic localization of nodal disease in 63 patients with newly diagnosed SCC of the oral cavity, oropharynx, or hypopharynx. Since the magnitude of FDG uptake reflects, in part, cell proliferation rates and overall patient prognosis, preliminary work has explored the potential for tailoring IMRT dose delivery based on the FDG activity distribution (56–60).

Solberg et al. (61) reported on the feasibility of using combined PET/CT to plan IMRT. Selective areas with FDG-avid tumoral tissue were boosted, while dose delivery to normal structures at risk was minimized, with good results. The authors further emphasized the superiority of combined PET/CT over posthoc registration of PET and CT data sets.

Surveillance and Restaging

Evaluation of the posttherapy neck with CT is complicated by loss of the normal fat planes and distortion of normal structures (Fig. 8.7.11). PET, and more recently PET/CT, has been shown to be more sensitive (88% to 100%) and specific (75% to 100%) than

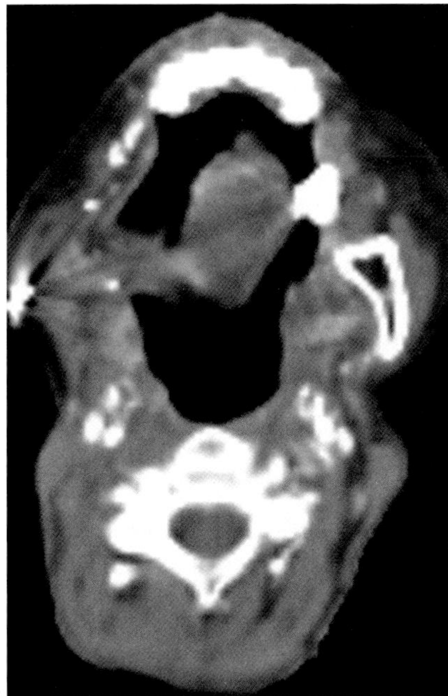

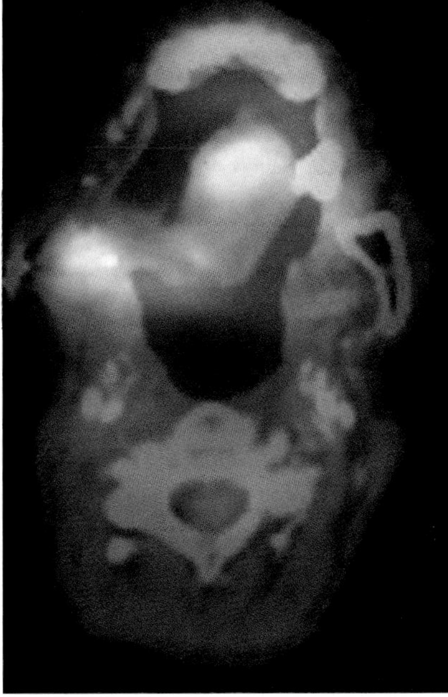

FIGURE 8.7.11. Postoperative PET/CT evaluation. Axial CT with contrast enhancement (**A**) in this patient who had extensive resection demonstrates extensive postoperative changes without definite evidence for residual or recurrent tumor. Axial fused PET/CT image (**B**) confirms the presence as well as the location of definite areas of residual or recurrent tumor. Subsequent biopsies confirm the presence of residual disease at these sites. Biopsy in cases such as this one is critical as these patients can have variable normal levels of tracer uptake in their tongues due to muscle contraction.

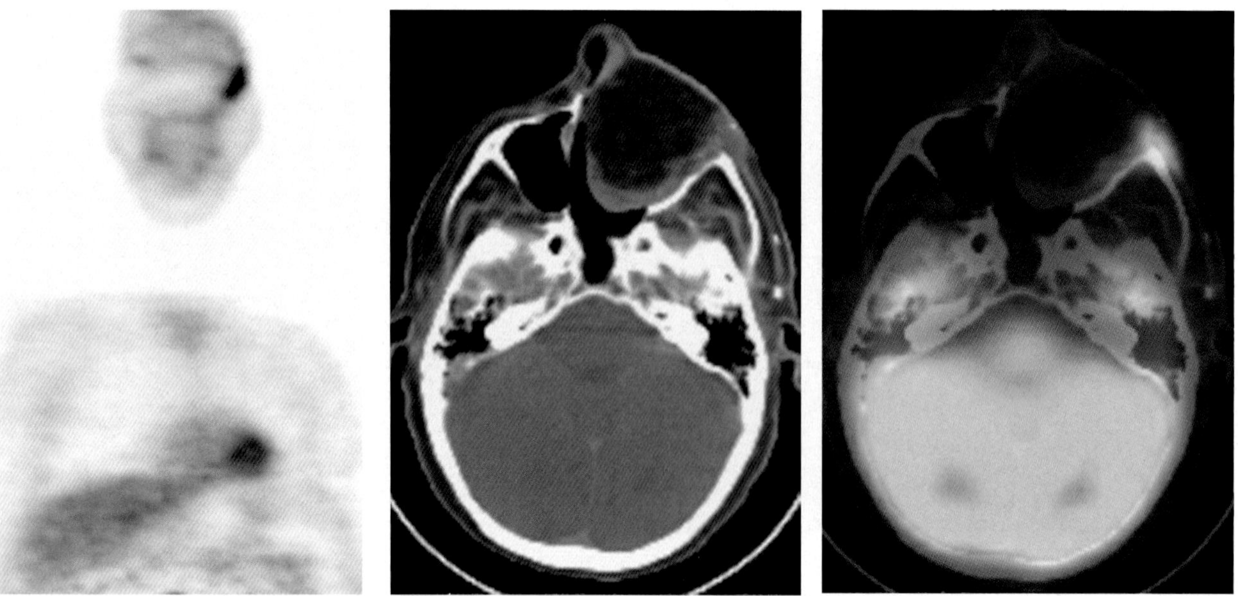

FIGURE 8.7.12. Improved lesion localization. Coronal PET image (**A**) shows a focal area of intense fluorodeoxyglucose activity in this patient who underwent extensive resection for adenocarcinoma and had positive surgical margins along the posterior border. Axial CT (**B**) shows postsurgical changes with no definite residual or recurrent malignancy. However, axial fused PET/CT image (**C**) confirms the presence of residual tumor and localizes it along the lateral, rather than the posterior, flap border. Subsequent resection confirms the presence of tumor along the lateral rather than the posterior flap border. (From Fukui MB, Blodgett TM, Snyderman CH, et al. Combined PET/CT in the head and neck: part 2. Diagnostic uses and pitfalls of oncologic imaging. *RadioGraphics* 2005;25:913–930, with permission.)

CT-MRI (sensitivity 38% to 90% and specificity 38% to 85%) for the detection of recurrent or residual disease both at the primary site as well as for nodal recurrence (8,41,62–74). The added ability of PET/CT to accurately localize disease makes it more appealing than PET alone, which can help determine the presence or absence of disease where the precise localization is often difficult (Fig. 8.7.12). The high rate of second primary tumors in this population further emphasizes the utility of PET/CT for restaging.

PET/CT may also be useful in the surveillance of patients who were definitively treated with chemoradiation. Patients followed with PET/CT may avoid unnecessary adjunctive surgery, such as planned neck dissection, in favor of a high-frequency PET/CT monitoring program.

Prognosis

SUVs using FDG PET have been shown to correlate with tumor-free intervals and overall prognosis, although no studies have been conducted looking at the possible additional prognostic value of PET/CT in the head and neck (72).

Treatment Complications

PET/CT can be used to assess complications of cancer treatment, and, most importantly, to distinguish complications from recurrent or residual tumor. The foremost application in this category is in the assessment of the jaw. An irregular pattern of bone erosion is a nonspecific finding in the jaw of a patient who has been treated for SCC in that vicinity. The differential possibilities include tumor invasion of bone, osteoradionecrosis as a complication of treatment, and infection (osteomyelitis). Patients with radiation-treated SCC are prone to all three of these diseases.

PET/CT is useful for distinguishing osteoradionecrosis, which is typically expected, although not always, to have low FDG avidity from infection (moderate FDG avidity) versus recurrent tumor (high FDG avidity). The distinction between tumor recurrence and infection can be difficult on PET, but the diagnosis (or exclusion) of osteoradionecrosis is helpful clinically. Similar logic can be applied to chondronecrosis of the larynx after radiation therapy. Because osteoradionecrosis often coexists with osteomyelitis, care should be taken when interpreting positive scans, and biopsies are still required, as there can be clear overlap in the scanning patterns.

One of the most frequent complications of radiation therapy to the neck is edema of the laryngeal (and, to a lesser degree, pharyngeal) mucosa. Diffuse thickening of the mucosa is seen on both CT and MRI. Although edema should be distinguishable from tumor on the basis of inherent density and degree of enhancement, laryngeal edema is nonetheless a confusing radiographic finding that may mask a small tumor recurrence.

PET also has difficulty in this setting because it may be hard to decide whether increased uptake in and around the larynx is the result of physiologic uptake in the intrinsic muscles of the larynx or evidence of recurrent disease. The combined modality makes the identification of recurrence within an edematous postradiation larynx more reliable.

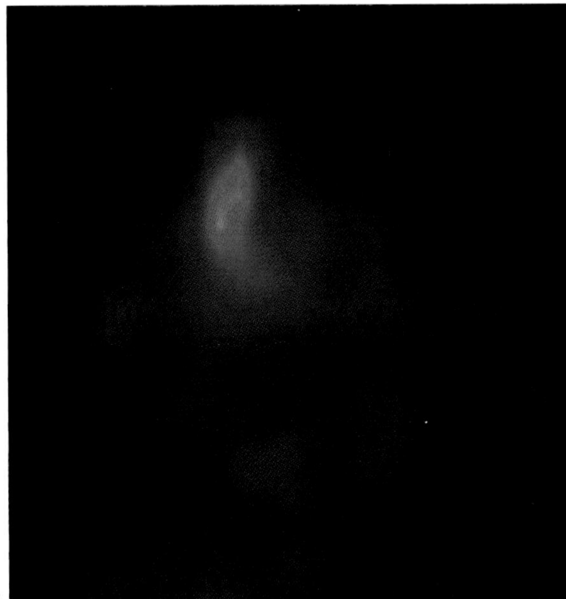

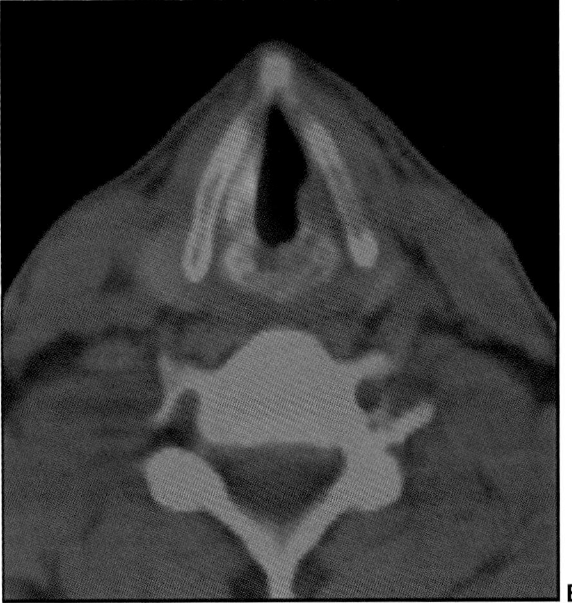

FIGURE 8.7.13. Asymmetrical vocal cord activity. Axial PET image (**A**) demonstrates asymmetrical intense fluorodeoxyglucose (FDG) activity on the right, possibly within the vocal cord in this patient who had a history of left recurrent laryngeal nerve damage from prior thyroidectomy. Axial fused PET/CT image (**B**) confirms the presence of FDG uptake to be within the right vocal cord, compatible with superphysiologic activity within the normal contralateral cord. There is an absence of FDG uptake within the paralyzed left vocal cord. (From Blodgett TM, Fukui MB, Snyderman CH, et al. Combined PET/CT in the head and neck: part 1. Physiologic, altered physiologic, and artifactual FDG uptake. *RadioGraphics* 2005;25:897–912, with permission.)

Vocal cord paralysis, another frequent complication of neck surgery, can be quite confusing on PET imaging. The contralateral vocal cord frequently shows increased FDG avidity, presumably compensatory, while the affected side shows diminished uptake (Fig. 8.7.13). The resulting asymmetry can be striking and may falsely suggest tumor recurrence. The CT portion of a combined PET/CT will demonstrate the paralyzed cord and prevent false-positive PET interpretation in this setting.

SALIVARY GLAND MALIGNANCIES

The evaluation of salivary gland malignancies is a troublesome topic in PET/CT. Unfortunately, the FDG uptake of most salivary malignancies is variable, so PET/CT is unreliable for staging and surveillance. Furthermore, many benign salivary lesions have increased FDG uptake, making the distinction between benign and malignant lesions difficult (Fig. 8.7.14).

The variable uptake of FDG within the parenchyma of the glands of the head and neck only adds to the uncertainty (24). This is an area in which PET/CT has a distinct advantage over PET alone. Even if a tumor has low FDG avidity, it may still be evident on the CT portion of the examination. Also, physiologic uptake is easier to confirm with CT correlation.

In the setting of glandular tumors, patients may benefit from pretreatment PET/CT, so that the FDG avidity of the tumor can be assessed before it is surgically removed. This allows the radiologist to make recommendations on the utility of PET/CT for posttreatment monitoring. Patients with tumors that are not FDG avid can be monitored with CT alone, rather than PET/CT.

Thyroid nodules are sometimes encountered in patients being evaluated for unrelated pathology. Focal uptake in a thyroid nodule is sufficiently suspicious to warrant tissue sampling, even if the lesion does not meet conventional imaging criteria for malignancy.

PITFALLS OF PET/CT IN THE HEAD AND NECK

Atypical Physiologic and Altered Physiologic Structures

Variable FDG uptake in normal structures, such as the nasal turbinates, pterygoid muscles, extraocular muscles, parotid and submandibular glands, and lymphoid tissue in Waldeyer's ring, may confuse interpretation and result in false-positive interpretations of head and neck PET/CT scans (75). Although FDG uptake in primary neoplasms is usually greater than that observed in even the most metabolically active normal structures, overlap between tumor and physiologic uptake may confound interpretation.

Often the interpreting physician relies on symmetry or location to differentiate between physiologic and pathologic FDG accumulations. Unfortunately, symmetry is a good but not completely reliable indicator of physiologic processes. Malignancies can rarely present with symmetrical FDG uptake, and conversely, physiologic uptake will often be asymmetrical (Fig. 8.7.15).

Symmetry is not reliable in postsurgical patients. In patients who have undergone removal of a gland or muscle, for example, FDG uptake in the remaining gland or muscle will typically produce an asymmetric appearance (Fig. 8.7.16).

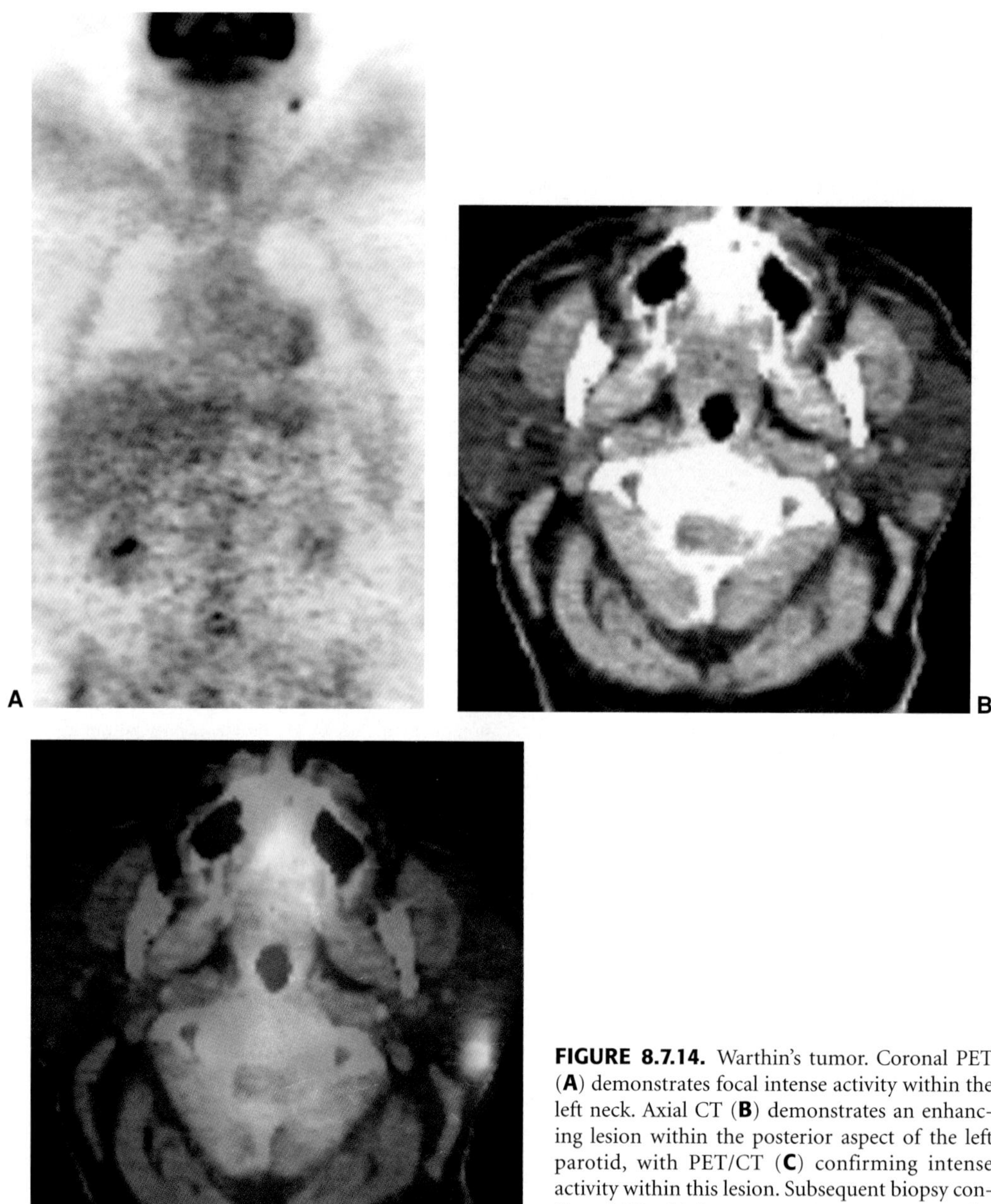

FIGURE 8.7.14. Warthin's tumor. Coronal PET (**A**) demonstrates focal intense activity within the left neck. Axial CT (**B**) demonstrates an enhancing lesion within the posterior aspect of the left parotid, with PET/CT (**C**) confirming intense activity within this lesion. Subsequent biopsy confirmed Warthin's tumor, a common cause of a benign parotid lesion causing intense activity.

Patients are generally instructed to remain quiet during the FDG uptake phase to limit physiologic vocal cord uptake. Other interventions, such as sedation or neck collars, minimize physiological uptake in the head and neck (5,76). These protocols are generally inconvenient for the patient, and they do not eliminate physiologic uptake.

Several limitations of FDG PET scanning in patients with malignancies of the head and neck have been overcome with in-line sequential combined PET/CT scanners. This modality has undoubtedly facilitated the differentiation of physiologic and pathologic processes, but has unfortunately also introduced new artifacts unique to the modality (77,78).

In order to effectively and accurately interpret PET or combined PET/CT scans, a comprehensive knowledge of physiologic and altered physiologic FDG uptake in the head and neck, as well as an awareness of potential modality-specific artifacts, is essential.

FDG taken up by the salivary glands generally produces symmetrical mild to moderate uptake patterns in the parotid and submandibular glands. Asymmetric uptake can be seen in patients who have undergone surgical removal of one of the glands, or in patients with primary or metastatic lesions to the glands. Relatively FDG-avid parotid tumors include Warthin's tumor, some pleomorphic adenomas, and primary parotid lymphoma (79–82). Many benign and malignant salivary tumors (oncocytoma, adenoid cystic carcinoma) have been reported to have varying degrees of FDG uptake. Nonmalignant causes of salivary gland FDG uptake include Warthin's tumor, infectious etiologies, and granulomatous diseases such as sarcoidosis (83).

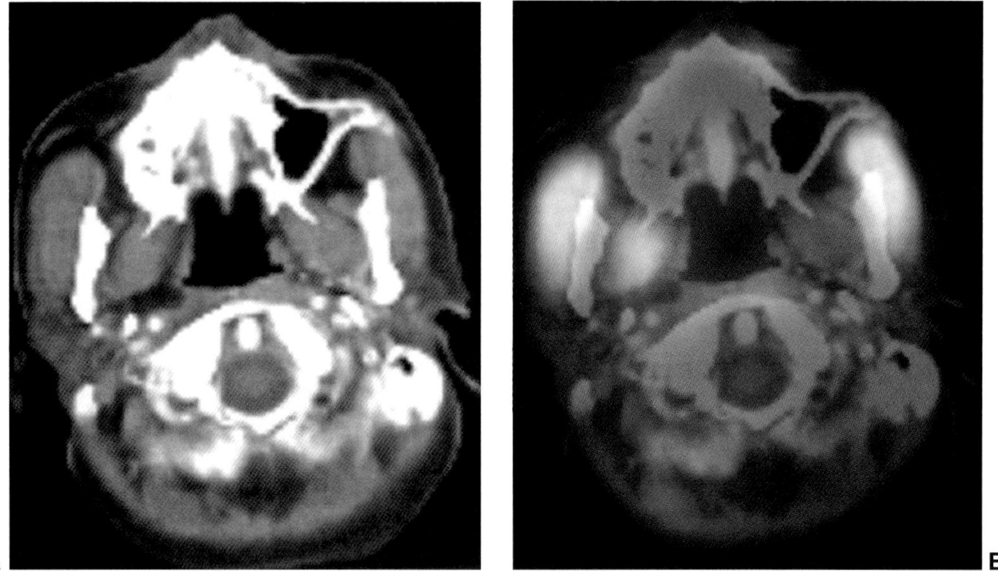

FIGURE 8.7.15. Asymmetrical physiologic muscle activity. Axial CT (**A**) and fused PET/CT (**B**) images demonstrate moderate to intense linear fluorodeoxyglucose activity within the right lateral pterygoid muscle compatible with asymmetrical physiologic activity. There is also intense physiologic activity bilaterally within the other muscles of mastication.

In general, benign or malignant processes can cause both unilateral and bilateral FDG uptake within the salivary glands, and it is necessary to consider all available clinical information, including prior oncologic and surgical history, to make an accurate diagnosis. PET/CT has a definite advantage over PET alone because of the improved surgical and anatomic information, as well as the potential to identify non–FDG-avid tumors.

Physiologic FDG uptake within neck muscles can be a diagnostic dilemma when interpreting PET scans (5,84). Frequently, muscular uptake can be distinguished from malignant nodal uptake by identifying the characteristic pattern of linear symmetric uptake in muscle. Inspection of coronal or sagittal reconstructions may facilitate characterization of muscle uptake by revealing the linearity in one or more reconstruction.

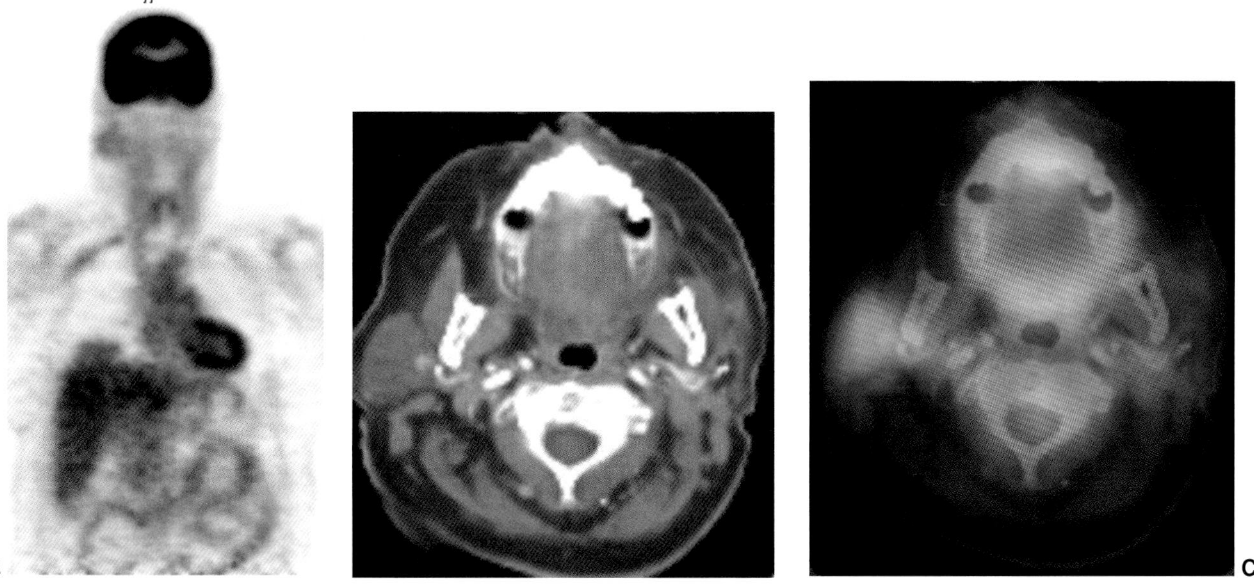

FIGURE 8.7.16. Asymmetrical glandular fluorodeoxyglucose uptake. Coronal PET (**A**) demonstrates mild to moderate asymmetrical activity within the right neck worrisome for a possible neck mass. Axial CT (**B**) and fused PET/CT (**C**) images confirm the activity to be within the right parotid gland. The asymmetrical appearance is due to absence of the left parotid gland from a prior parotidectomy.

Unfortunately, muscles often have more focal uptake patterns, which can be quite confusing on PET alone. Fused PET/CT will confirm the source of the increased uptake in these situations. Increased uptake is most frequently associated with the myotendinous junctions. Common sites of confusing muscle uptake include the sternocleidomastoid muscle, the strap muscles in the anterior neck, and the pterygoid muscles of the jaw.

Another muscle frequently demonstrating asymmetric tracer uptake is the inferior capitis obliquus muscle. Uptake within this muscle may appear focal on coronal images, but its linear nature is evident when viewed in an axial plane. The extreme posterior position of these paraspinal muscles is also often helpful in identifying the source of the FDG uptake. Viewing the fused PET/CT image in the axial plane allows easier identification of inferior obliquus capitis muscle uptake.

The muscles of facial expression may also demonstrate linear FDG uptake. Because most muscles in the neck can display asymmetric FDG uptake, both physiologically and after strain, close inspection of all three orthogonal planes is essential to avoid misdiagnosis.

Although several methods have been used to minimize muscle uptake, including the use of soft collars and benzodiazepines during the tracer uptake period, these techniques are inconvenient to the patient and are often not completely effective (76).

Several muscles of the oropharynx and hypopharynx demonstrate symmetric physiologic FDG uptake, including the pterygoid muscles and the muscles of the floor of the mouth. These may mimic focal areas of malignancy when they are asymmetric. It is critical patients be instructed not to chew gum or other substances during the uptake phase to minimize muscle uptake of radiotracer.

Lingual FDG uptake is also common and may appear as diffuse or as bilateral symmetrical focal uptake. Lingual uptake is often inseparable from the slightly more superior palatal mucosal uptake on PET images alone, but can be differentiated on the fused PET/CT images.

It is well recognized that talking during the FDG uptake period may cause tracer accumulation in the muscles of phonation and vocal cords. Another muscle that can appear as a focal area of FDG uptake is the cricopharyngeus muscle (9). Coughing during the uptake period may produce FDG activity in the pharyngeal constrictor muscles, as well as in the vocal cords. Pronounced uptake in these muscles can interfere with interpretation of PET scans in any patient, but when scans are performed in patients with head and neck malignancies, thyroid cancer, or lymphoma, it can be very difficult to distinguish physiologic muscle uptake from pathologic uptake (85,86). PET/CT is particularly useful in these instances because the lack of a corresponding CT abnormality is reassuring.

Before the use of PET/CT, physiologic linear and focal uptake in the neck was attributed to muscle alone. After the implementation of combined PET/CT imaging, however, it became apparent that uptake previously attributed to muscle had no definite soft tissue or muscle correlate when the fusion images were inspected. Several authors have reported intense FDG uptake within areas with fat attenuation on CT, now known to represent areas of brown fat (2–4). This represents an interesting example of mislocalization of physiologic FDG accumulation resolved by combined PET/CT imaging.

There are many lymphatic structures in the head and neck, including Waldeyer's ring (the adenoids, palatine tonsils, and lingual tonsils), lymph nodes, and lymphatic channels. Physiologic FDG uptake can be seen in any lymphatic structure in the head and neck, due at least in part to accumulation of FDG within macrophages and lymphocytes. Several authors have described physiologic FDG uptake within these structures using dedicated PET (5,6–8). The interpretation is straightforward in most cases, especially when there is symmetric uptake. However, malignancy (particularly lymphoma) or hyperplasia may have a similar symmetric appearance.

It is not uncommon for the FDG uptake in Waldeyer's ring to be asymmetric and caused by benign pathologies such as infection or inflammation, or it may be a normal variant. Malignancy will usually present with asymmetric FDG uptake as well, with or without significant anatomic abnormalities.

When infiltrated into the subcutaneous tissues, FDG can be transported through the lymphatic system and cause a lymphangiogram effect on the PET images. If FDG is infiltrated into the soft tissues of the upper extremity, FDG may accumulate in the lymph nodes of the axilla and supraclavicular area.

PET/CT Artifacts

Several artifacts specific to PET imaging, including prominent "skin" activity on non–attenuation-corrected images and relative photopenic areas due to prosthetic devices, have been described (87). These artifacts are present on PET/CT images as well. However, there are a number of new artifacts that are unique to the PET/CT modality. These are not generated on PET scanners that use point-source based systems for attenuation correction because the artifacts are generated by the CT-based attenuation-correction protocols.

Metallic devices, including dental implants (Fig. 8.7.17), cause areas of photopenia on PET images. When correcting for attenuation with germanium point sources, these areas remain photopenic on the attenuation-corrected images. In contrast, when using current CT-based attenuation-correction algorithms, these areas can demonstrate falsely elevated FDG uptake. This artifact is a limitation of the current CT attenuation protocols, but by using uncorrected images for comparison, misdiagnosis can be avoided.

Intravenous contrast can also cause artifacts on attenuation-corrected images when using CT-based attenuation-correction protocols. Dense contrast material is present in venous structures during the CT acquisition, but not during the PET portion of the examination. This mismatch causes areas of linear artifact (mimicking intense FDG accumulations) on the attenuation-corrected PET images (Fig. 8.7.18). Occasionally, this artifact can appear focal and mimic a metastatic lymph node in the axilla or supraclavicular area (77). Rarely a small malignant lymph node or small soft tissue abnormality can lie within or directly beside a contrast artifact, partially or completely obscuring the abnormality.

Calcium densities can cause artifacts as well (Fig. 8.7.19). Calcified lymph nodes do not reliably cause attenuation-correction artifacts, but when they do they are easy to mistake for malignancy due to their morphology. Areas of sclerotic bone have also been shown to cause this type of artifact. These are less common and this artifact can be overemphasized by looking at fused images only, where the "white" of the CT density is additive to the color from the PET image. Examining PET-only images may help avoid confusion with true increased FDG uptake.

If there is any diagnostic uncertainty regarding the presence of a CT-based attenuation artifact, the emission data set (i.e.,

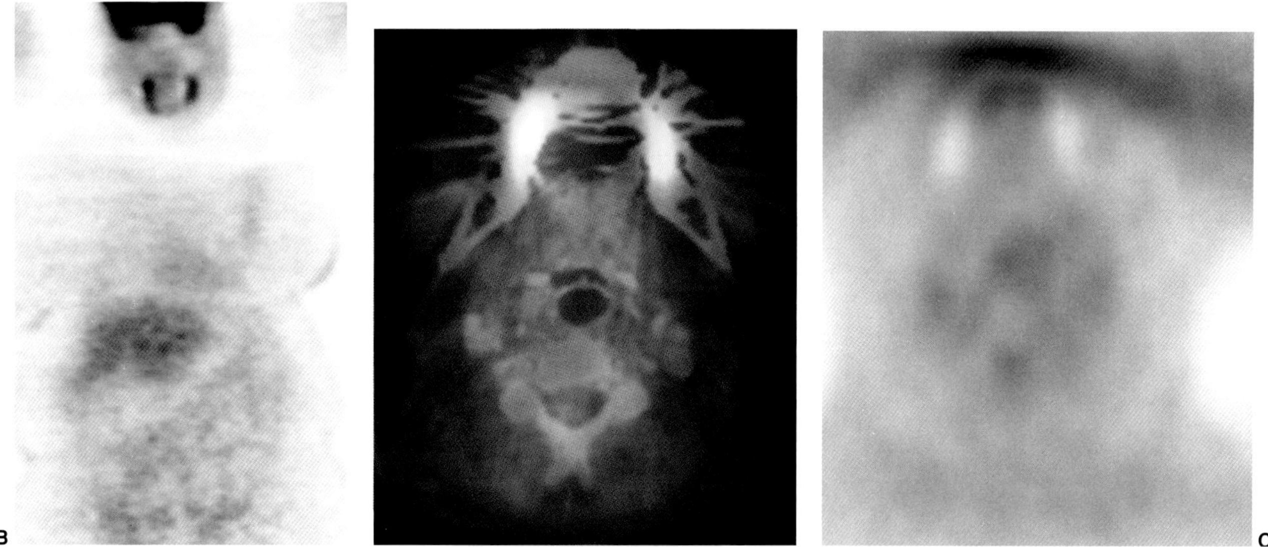

FIGURE 8.7.17. Dental artifact. Coronal PET image (**A**) demonstrates intense bilateral fluorodeoxyglucose activity in the mouth. Axial fused PET/CT image (**B**) using an attenuation-corrected PET image demonstrates the activity to be within the fillings. Inspection of the non–attenuation-corrected PET image (**C**) confirms the absence of activity, proving this to be an attenuation-correction artifact.

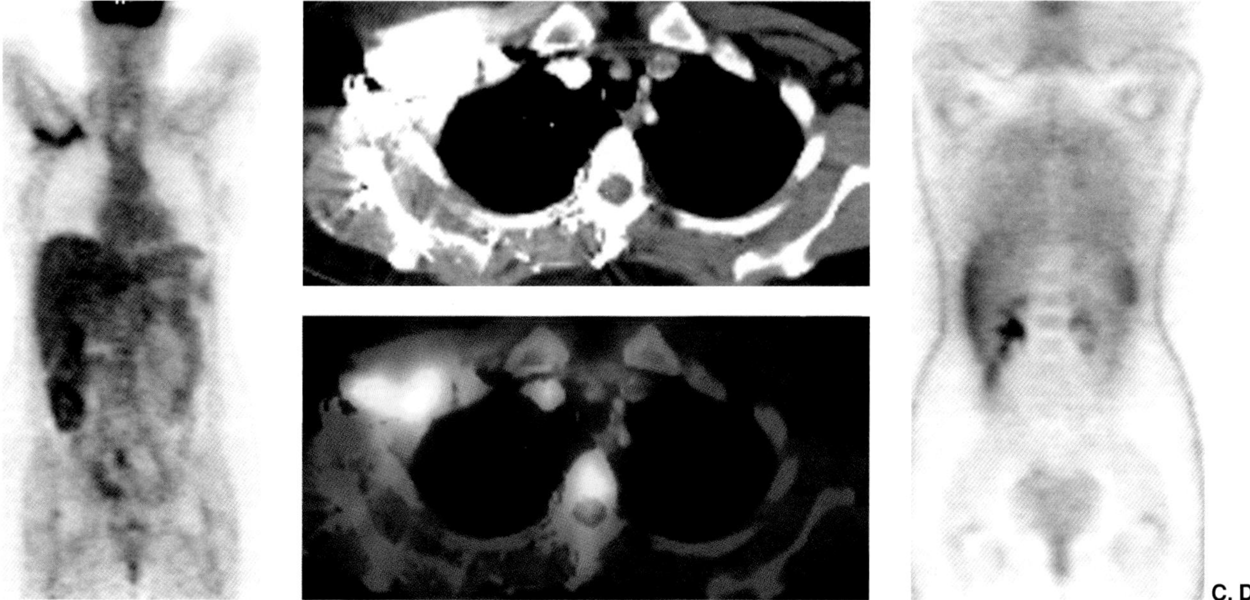

FIGURE 8.7.18. Intravenous contrast attenuation-correction artifact. The coronal attenuation-corrected PET image (**A**) demonstrates a linear apparent intense fluorodeoxyglucose activity in the right supraclavicular area. The axial CT (**B**) and fused PET/CT (**C**) images localize the activity to pooling contrast within the right subclavian vein. The coronal non–attenuation-corrected PET image (**D**) shows the activity to be artifactual, due to high attenuation intravenous contrast material.

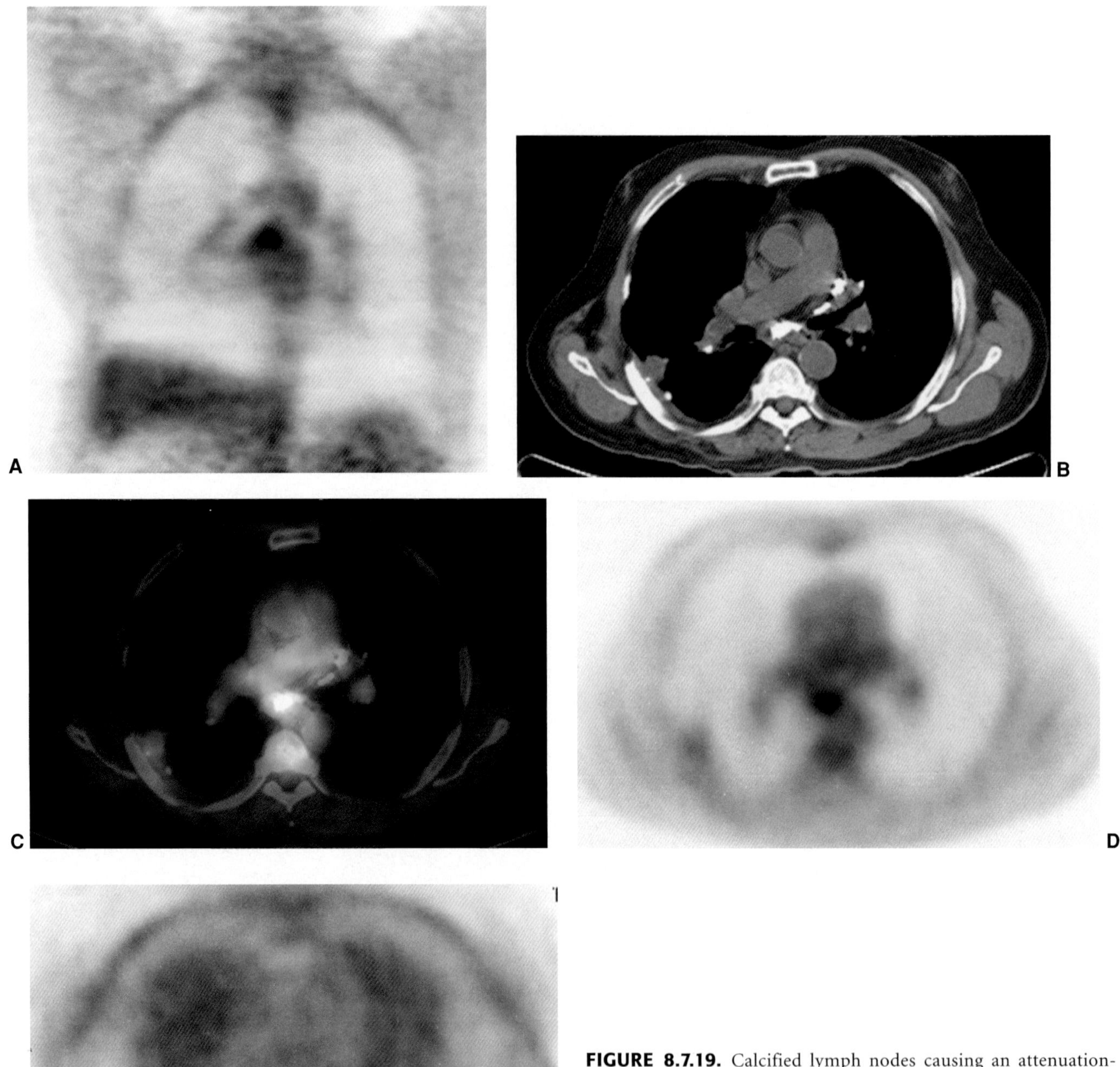

FIGURE 8.7.19. Calcified lymph nodes causing an attenuation-correction artifact. Coronal (**A**) and axial (**D**) PET images demonstrate intense fluorodeoxyglucose activity in the subcarinal area. Axial CT (**B**) and fused PET/CT (**C**) images demonstrate the intense activity to be within heavily calcified subcarinal lymph nodes. However, inspection of the non–attenuation-corrected PET image (**E**) shows no activity within this area, proving the uptake to be artifactual due to an attenuation-correction artifact.

non–attenuation-corrected PET image) should be examined to determine whether the apparent increase in FDG uptake is real.

SUMMARY

PET with FDG has been shown to offer substantial advantages compared to CT or MRI especially in the setting of recurrent tumor detection, treatment response monitoring (see Chapter 8.4) and primary tumor detection and staging. PET/CT, when directly compared to PET, has had superior performance characteristics. The anatomy of the head and neck region is complex and normal structures can have intense, but physiological, tracer accumulation. Through the careful use of PET/CT excellent diagnostic performance can be achieved. Although there are a broad range of possible artifacts, optimized PET/CT protocols, often including the use of intravenous contrast, are assuming a larger role in the management of patients with known or suspected head and neck cancers.

REFERENCES

1. Stahl A, Dzewas B, Schwaiger M, et al. Excretion of FDG into saliva and its significance for PET imaging. *Nuklearmedizin* 2002;41(5):214–216.
2. Cohade C, Osman M, Pannu HK, et al. Uptake in supraclavicular area fat ("USA-Fat"): description on (18)F-FDG PET/CT. *J Nucl Med* 2003;44(2):170–176.
3. Virtanen KA, Peltoniemi P, Marjamaki P, et al. Human adipose tissue glucose uptake determined using [(18)F]-fluoro-deoxy-glucose ([(18)F]FDG) and PET in combination with microdialysis. *Diabetologia* 2001;44(12):2171–2179.
4. Hany TF, Gharehpapagh E, Kamel EM, et al. Brown adipose tissue: a factor to consider in symmetrical tracer uptake in the neck and upper chest region. *Eur J Nucl Med Mol Imaging* 2002;29(10):1393–1398.
5. Shreve PD, Anzai Y, Wahl RL. Pitfalls in oncologic diagnosis with FDG PET imaging: physiologic and benign variants. *Radiographics* 1999; 19(1):61–77; quiz 150–151.
6. Stokkel MP, Bongers V, Hordijk GJ, et al. FDG positron emission tomography in head and neck cancer: pitfall or pathology? *Clin Nucl Med* 1999;24(12):950–954.
7. Kawabe J, Okamura T, Shakudo M, et al. Physiological FDG uptake in the palatine tonsils. *Ann Nucl Med* 2001;15(3):297–300.
8. Hanasono MM, Kunda LD, Segall GM, et al. Uses and limitations of FDG positron emission tomography in patients with head and neck cancer. *Laryngoscope* 1999;109(6):880–885.
9. Kostakoglu L, Wong JC, Barrington SF, et al. Speech-related visualization of laryngeal muscles with fluorine-18-FDG. *J Nucl Med* 1996;37(11):1771–1773.
10. Curtin HD, Ishwaran H, Mancuso AA, et al. Comparison of CT and MR imaging in staging of neck metastases. *Radiology* 1998;207(1):123–130.
11. Fischbein NJ, Noworolski SM, Henry RG, et al. Assessment of metastatic cervical adenopathy using dynamic contrast-enhanced MR imaging. *AJNR Am J Neuroradiol* 2003;24(3):301–311.
12. Anzai Y, Prince MR. Iron oxide-enhanced MR lymphography: the evaluation of cervical lymph node metastases in head and neck cancer. *J Magn Reson Imaging* 1997;7(1):75–81.
13. Markkola AT, Aronen HJ, Paavonen T, et al. T1 rho dispersion imaging of head and neck tumors: a comparison to spin lock and magnetization transfer techniques. *J Magn Reson Imaging* 1997;7(5):873–879.
14. Yousem DM, Montone KT, Sheppard LM, et al. Head and neck neoplasms: magnetization transfer analysis. *Radiology* 1994;192(3):703–707.
15. Eida S, Sumi M, Yonetsu K, et al. Combination of helical CT and Doppler sonography in the follow-up of patients with clinical N0 stage neck disease and oral cancer. *AJNR Am J Neuroradiol* 2003;24(3):312–318.
16. Nakamoto Y, Tatsumi M, Hammoud D, et al. Normal FDG distribution patterns in the head and neck: PET/CT evaluation. *Radiology* 2005;234(3):879–885.
17. Kapoor V, Fukui MB, McCook BM. Role of ^{18}F-FDG PET/CT in the treatment of head and neck cancers: principles, technique, normal distribution, and initial staging. *AJR Am J Roentgenol* 2005;184(2):579–587.
18. Blodgett TM, Fukui M, Snyderman CH, et al. Combined PET-CT in the head and neck part 1. Physiologic, altered physiologic and artifactual FDG uptake. *Radiographics* 2005;25:897–912.
19. Minotti AJ, Shah L, Keller K. Positron emission tomography/computed tomography fusion imaging in brown adipose tissue. *Clin Nucl Med* 2004;29(1):5–11.
20. Kostakoglu L, Hardoff R, Mirtcheva R, et al. PET-CT fusion imaging in differentiating physiologic from pathologic FDG uptake. *Radiographics* 2004;24(5):1411–1431.
21. Jacene HA, Patel PP, Chin BB. 2-Deoxy-2-[18F] fluoro-D-glucose uptake in intercostal respiratory muscles on positron emission tomography/computed tomography: smokers versus nonsmokers. *Mol Imaging Biol* 2004;6(6):405–410.
22. Yeung HW, Grewal RK, Gonen M, et al. Patterns of (18)F-FDG uptake in adipose tissue and muscle: a potential source of false-positives for PET. *J Nucl Med* 2003;44(11):1789–1796.
23. Goerres GW, Von Schulthess GK, Hany TF. Positron emission tomography and PET CT of the head and neck: FDG uptake in normal anatomy, in benign lesions, and in changes resulting from treatment. *AJR Am J Roentgenol* 2002;179(5):1337–1343.
24. Branstetter BFt, Blodgett TM, Zimmer LA, et al. Head and neck malignancy: is PET/CT more accurate than PET or CT alone? *Radiology* 2005;235(2):580–586.
25. Schoder H, Yeung HW. Positron emission imaging of head and neck cancer, including thyroid carcinoma. *Semin Nucl Med* 2004;34(3): 180–197.
26. Regelink G, Brouwer J, de Bree R, et al. Detection of unknown primary tumours and distant metastases in patients with cervical metastases: value of FDG-PET versus conventional modalities. *Eur J Nucl Med Mol Imaging* 2002;29(8):1024–1030.
27. Nieder C, Gregoire V, Ang KK. Cervical lymph node metastases from occult squamous cell carcinoma: cut down a tree to get an apple? *Int J Radiat Oncol Biol Phys* 2001;50(3):727–733.
28. Jungehulsing M, Scheidhauer K, Damm M, et al. 2[F]-fluoro-2-deoxy-D-glucose positron emission tomography is a sensitive tool for the detection of occult primary cancer (carcinoma of unknown primary syndrome) with head and neck lymph node manifestation. *Otolaryngol Head Neck Surg* 2000;123(3):294–301.
29. Bohuslavizki KH, Klutmann S, Kroger S, et al. FDG PET detection of unknown primary tumors. *J Nucl Med* 2000;41(5):816–822.
30. Stokkel MP, Terhaard CH, Hordijk GJ, et al. The detection of unknown primary tumors in patients with cervical metastases by dual-head positron emission tomography. *Oral Oncol* 1999;35(4):390–394.
31. Lassen U, Daugaard G, Eigtved A, et al. ^{18}F-FDG whole body positron emission tomography (PET) in patients with unknown primary tumours (UPT). *Eur J Cancer* 1999;35(7):1076–1082.
32. Greven KM, Keyes JW Jr, Williams DW 3rd, et al. Occult primary tumors of the head and neck: lack of benefit from positron emission tomography imaging with 2-[F-18]fluoro-2-deoxy-D-glucose. *Cancer* 1999;86(1):114–118.
33. Braams JW, Pruim J, Kole AC, et al. Detection of unknown primary head and neck tumors by positron emission tomography. *Int J Oral Maxillofac Surg* 1997;26(2):112–115.
34. MacLaughlin LH, Zimmer L, Blodgett TM, et al. Combined PET/CT in the detection of unknown primary malignancy of the head and neck. *Radiology* 2002;225:599.
35. Freudenberg LS, Fischer M, Antoch G, et al. Dual modality of ^{18}F-fluorodeoxyglucose-positron emission tomography/computed tomography in patients with cervical carcinoma of unknown primary. *Med Princ Pract* 2005;14(3):155–160.
36. Syed R, Bomanji JB, Nagabhushan N, et al. Impact of combined (18)F-FDG PET/CT in head and neck tumours. *Br J Cancer* 2005;92(6):1046–1050.
37. Dammann F, Horger M, Mueller-Berg M, et al. Rational diagnosis of squamous cell carcinoma of the head and neck region: comparative evaluation of CT, MRI, and ^{18}FDG PET. *AJR Am J Roentgenol* 2005; 184(4):1326–1331.
38. Schwartz DL, Ford E, Rajendran J, et al. FDG-PET/CT imaging for preradiotherapy staging of head-and-neck squamous cell carcinoma. *Int J Radiat Oncol Biol Phys* 2005;61(1):129–136.
39. Schwartz DL, Rajendran J, Yueh B, et al. Staging of head and neck squamous cell cancer with extended-field FDG-PET. *Arch Otolaryngol Head Neck Surg* 2003;129(11):1173–1178.
40. Schmid DT, Stoeckli SJ, Bandhauer F, et al. Impact of positron emission tomography on the initial staging and therapy in locoregional advanced squamous cell carcinoma of the head and neck. *Laryngoscope* 2003; 113(5):888–891.
41. Kresnik E, Mikosch P, Gallowitsch HJ, et al. Evaluation of head and neck cancer with 18F-FDG PET: a comparison with conventional methods. *Eur J Nucl Med* 2001;28(7):816–821.
42. Stuckensen T, Kovacs AF, Adams S, et al. Staging of the neck in patients with oral cavity squamous cell carcinomas: a prospective comparison of PET, ultrasound, CT and MRI. *J Craniomaxillofac Surg* 2000;28(6):319–324.

43. Kao CH, Hsieh JF, Tsai SC, et al. Comparison of 18-fluoro-2-deoxyglucose positron emission tomography and computed tomography in detection of cervical lymph node metastases of nasopharyngeal carcinoma. *Ann Otol Rhinol Laryngol* 2000;109(12 Pt 1):1130–1134.
44. Di Martino E, Nowak B, Hassan HA, et al. Diagnosis and staging of head and neck cancer: a comparison of modern imaging modalities (positron emission tomography, computed tomography, color-coded duplex sonography) with panendoscopic and histopathologic findings. *Arch Otolaryngol Head Neck Surg* 2000;126(12):1457–1461.
45. Bhatnagar AK, Heron DE, Schaitkin B. Perineural invasion of squamous cell carcinoma of the lip with occult involvement of the infraorbital nerve detected by PET-CT and treated with MRI-based IMRT: a case report. *Technol Cancer Res Treat* 2005;4(3):251–254.
46. Israel O, Yefremov N, Bar-Shalom R, et al. PET/CT detection of unexpected gastrointestinal foci of ^{18}F-FDG uptake: incidence, localization patterns, and clinical significance. *J Nucl Med* 2005;46(5): 758–762.
47. Ishimori T, Patel PV, Wahl RL. Detection of unexpected additional primary malignancies with PET/CT. *J Nucl Med* 2005;46(5):752–757.
48. Thiel A, Pietrzyk U, Sturm V, et al. Enhanced accuracy in differential diagnosis of radiation necrosis by positron emission tomography-magnetic resonance imaging coregistration: technical case report. *Neurosurgery* 2000;46(1):232–234.
49. Paulino AC, Koshy M, Howell R, et al. Comparison of CT- and FDG-PET-defined gross tumor volume in intensity-modulated radiotherapy for head-and-neck cancer. *Int J Radiat Oncol Biol Phys* 2005;61(5): 1385–1392.
50. Koshy M, Paulino AC, Howell R, et al. F-18 FDG PET-CT fusion in radiotherapy treatment planning for head and neck cancer. *Head Neck* 2005;27(6):494–502.
51. Heron DE, Andrade RS, Flickinger J, et al. Hybrid PET-CT simulation for radiation treatment planning in head-and-neck cancers: a brief technical report. *Int J Radiat Oncol Biol Phys* 2004;60(5): 1419–1424.
52. Rizzo G, Cattaneo GM, Castellone P, et al. Multi-modal medical image integration to optimize radiotherapy planning in lung cancer treatment. *Ann Biomed Eng* 2004;32(10):1399–1408.
53. Gabriele P, Malinverni G, Moroni GL, et al. The impact of ^{18}F-deoxyglucose positron emission tomography on tumor staging, treatment strategy and treatment planning for radiotherapy in a department of radiation oncology. *Tumori* 2004;90(6):579–585.
54. Apisarnthanarax S, Chao KS. Current imaging paradigms in radiation oncology. *Radiat Res* 2005;163(1):1–25.
55. Bujenovic S. The role of positron emission tomography in radiation treatment planning. *Semin Nucl Med* 2004;34(4):293–299.
56. Haberkorn U, Strauss LG, Reisser C, et al. Glucose uptake, perfusion, and cell proliferation in head and neck tumors: relation of positron emission tomography to flow cytometry. *J Nucl Med* 1991;32(8): 1548–1555.
57. Minn H, Clavo A, Grenman R, Wahl R. *In vitro* comparison of cell proliferation kinetics and uptake of tritiated fluorodeoxyglucose and L-methionine in squamous-cell carcinoma of the head and neck. *J Nucl Med* 1995;36:252–258.
58. Pugsley JM, Schmidt RA, Vesselle H. The Ki-67 index and survival in non–small cell lung cancer: a review and relevance to positron emission tomography. *Cancer J* 2002;8(3):222–233.
59. Schwartz DL, Rajendran J, Yueh B, et al. FDG-PET prediction of head and neck squamous cell cancer outcomes. *Arch Otolaryngol Head Neck Surg* 2004;130(12):1361–1367.
60. Das SK, Miften MM, Zhou S, et al. Feasibility of optimizing the dose distribution in lung tumors using fluorine-18-fluorodeoxyglucose positron emission tomography and single photon emission computed tomography guided dose prescriptions. *Med Phys* 2004;31(6):1452–1461.
61. Solberg TD, Agazaryan N, Goss BW, et al. A feasibility study of ^{18}F-fluorodeoxyglucose positron emission tomography targeting and simultaneous integrated boost for intensity-modulated radiosurgery and radiotherapy. *J Neurosurg* 2004;101[Suppl 3]:381–389.
62. Anzai Y, Carroll WR, Quint DJ, et al. Recurrence of head and neck cancer after surgery or irradiation: prospective comparison of 2-deoxy-2-[F-18]fluoro-D-glucose PET and MR imaging diagnoses. *Radiology* 1996;200(1):135–141.
63. Fischbein NJ, Aassar OS, Caputo GR, et al. Clinical utility of positron emission tomography with ^{18}F-fluorodeoxyglucose in detecting residual/recurrent squamous cell carcinoma of the head and neck. *AJNR Am J Neuroradiol* 1998;19(7):1189–1196.
64. Lapela M, Eigtved A, Jyrkkio S, et al. Experience in qualitative and quantitative FDG PET in follow-up of patients with suspected recurrence from head and neck cancer. *Eur J Cancer* 2000;36(7): 858–867.
65. Lapela M, Grenman R, Kurki T, et al. Head and neck cancer: detection of recurrence with PET and 2-[F-18]fluoro-2-deoxy-D-glucose. *Radiology* 1995;197(1):205–211.
66. Li P, Zhuang H, Mozley PD, et al. Evaluation of recurrent squamous cell carcinoma of the head and neck with FDG positron emission tomography. *Clin Nucl Med* 2001;26(2):131–135.
67. Lonneux M, Lawson G, Ide C, et al. Positron emission tomography with fluorodeoxyglucose for suspected head and neck tumor recurrence in the symptomatic patient. *Laryngoscope* 2000;110(9):1493–1497.
68. Lowe VJ, Boyd JH, Dunphy FR, et al. Surveillance for recurrent head and neck cancer using positron emission tomography. *J Clin Oncol* 2000;18(3):651–658.
69. McGuirt WF, Williams DW 3rd, Keyes JW Jr, et al. A comparative diagnostic study of head and neck nodal metastases using positron emission tomography. *Laryngoscope* 1995;105(4 Pt 1):373–375.
70. Stokkel MP, Terhaard CH, Hordijk GJ, et al. The detection of local recurrent head and neck cancer with fluorine-18 fluorodeoxyglucose dual-head positron emission tomography. *Eur J Nucl Med* 1999;26(7): 767-73.
71. Terhaard CH, Bongers V, van Rijk PP, et al. F-18-fluoro-deoxy-glucose positron-emission tomography scanning in detection of local recurrence after radiotherapy for laryngeal/pharyngeal cancer. *Head Neck* 2001;23(11):933–941.
72. Wong RJ, Lin DT, Schoder H, et al. Diagnostic and prognostic value of [(18)F]fluorodeoxyglucose positron emission tomography for recurrent head and neck squamous cell carcinoma. *J Clin Oncol* 2002; 20(20):4199–4208.
73. Yen RF, Hung RL, Pan MH, et al. 18-fluoro-2-deoxyglucose positron emission tomography in detecting residual/recurrent nasopharyngeal carcinomas and comparison with magnetic resonance imaging. *Cancer* 2003;98(2):283–287.
74. Zimmer LA, Snyderman C, Fukui MB, et al. The use of combined PET/CT for localizing recurrent head and neck cancer: the Pittsburgh experience. *Ear Nose Throat J* 2005;84(2):104.
75. Jabour BA, Choi Y, Hoh CK, et al. Extracranial head and neck: PET imaging with 2-[F-18]fluoro-2-deoxy-D-glucose and MR imaging correlation. *Radiology* 1993;186(1):27–35.
76. Barrington SF, Maisey MN. Skeletal muscle uptake of fluorine-18-FDG: effect of oral diazepam. *J Nucl Med* 1996;37(7):1127–1129.
77. Antoch G, Freudenberg LS, Egelhof T, et al. Focal tracer uptake: a potential artifact in contrast-enhanced dual-modality PET/CT scans. *J Nucl Med* 2002;43(10):1339–1342.
78. Goerres GW, Hany TF, Kamel E, et al. Head and neck imaging with PET and PET/CT: artefacts from dental metallic implants. *Eur J Nucl Med Mol Imaging* 2002;29(3):367–370.
79. Horiuchi M, Yasuda S, Shohtsu A, et al. Four cases of Warthin's tumor of the parotid gland detected with FDG PET. *Ann Nucl Med* 1998; 12(1):47–50.
80. Matsuda M, Sakamoto H, Okamura T, et al. Positron emission tomographic imaging of pleomorphic adenoma in the parotid gland. *Acta Otolaryngol Suppl* 1998;538:214–220.

81. Okamura T, Kawabe J, Koyama K, et al. Fluorine-18 fluorodeoxyglucose positron emission tomography imaging of parotid mass lesions. *Acta Otolaryngol Suppl* 1998;538:209–213.
82. Shih WJ, Ghesani N, Hongming Z, et al. F-18 FDG positron emission tomography demonstrates resolution of non-Hodgkin's lymphoma of the parotid gland in a patient with Sjogren's syndrome: before and after anti-CD20 antibody rituximab therapy. *Clin Nucl Med* 2002;27(2): 142–143.
83. Sagowski C, Ussmuller J. [Clinical diagnosis of salivary gland sarcoidosis (Heerfordt syndrome)]. *HNO* 2000;48(8):613–615.
84. Bar-Shalom R. Muscle uptake of 18-fluorine fluorodeoxyglucose. *Semin Nucl Med* 2000;30(4):306–309.
85. Igerc I, Kumnig G, Heinisch M, et al. Vocal cord muscle activity as a drawback to FDG-PET in the followup of differentiated thyroid cancer. *Thyroid* 2002;12(1):87–89.
86. Zhu Z, Chou C, Yen TC, et al. Elevated F-18 FDG uptake in laryngeal muscles mimicking thyroid cancer metastases. *Clin Nucl Med* 2001;26(8):689–691.
87. Cook GJ, Fogelman I, Maisey MN. Normal physiological and benign pathological variants of 18-fluoro-2-deoxyglucose positron-emission tomography scanning: potential for error in interpretation. *Semin Nucl Med* 1996;26(4):308–314.

CHAPTER

8.8 Thyroid Cancer and Thyroid Imaging

MICHELE BRENNER AND RICHARD L. WAHL

This chapter is designed to serve as a guide to clinicians seeking to better understand the role of positron emission tomography (PET) in the management of proven thyroid malignancies as well as providing insights on the role of PET in detecting and characterizing primary thyroid disease processes, both malignant and nonmalignant.

The incidence of thyroid cancer ranges between 4 and 12 cases per 100,000 per year, but it is increasing (1,2). Radiation exposure is one of the risk factors for thyroid cancer. Many aspects in the management of this disease are debated. The use of PET adds an additional topic for debate, but its role in management is becoming increasingly well established. The differentiated cancers, papillary and follicular, constitute approximately 90% of thyroid cancers (3) (Figs. 8.8.1 and 8.8.2). Although differentiated thyroid cancers are highly treatable, they require vigilant follow-up. When indicated, initial therapy consists of a total thyroidectomy and radioiodine ablation therapy (4). Despite this, approximately 20% of patients develop recurrences, most within the first 10 years after diagnosis (1,5). After treatment, patients are monitored clinically, with iodine scans and with measurements of serum thyroglobulin. Serum levels of this protein should be undetectable with effective treatment. An increase in serum thyroglobulin over time is suspicious for recurrent or metastatic disease. In 10% to 15% of patients with an elevated thyroglobulin, a diagnostic iodine-131 (^{131}I) whole-body scintigraphy (WBS) to localize disease is negative (6). Poorly differentiated or progressively dedifferentiated thyroid cancer cells often lose the ability to concentrate radioactive ^{131}I. Furthermore, 50 % of these patients, when retreated empirically, will have uptake on posttreatment WBS scan (7), indicating the diagnostic scan was falsely negative. Although false-negative scans could probably be made less frequently by using a higher dose of radioiodine for the scans, this is probably not desirable as "stunning" of the gland could occur, potentially resulting in less-effective treatments. At the same time, these cells often exhibit increased metabolic activity, as evidenced by enhanced glucose uptake (8). The imaging of these poorly differentiated, noniodine-avid metastases and recurrences is problematic. Radioiodine imaging detects well-differentiated recurrences and metastases with a high specificity but only moderate sensitivity. A 2-fluorine-18-fluoro-2-deoxyglucose (^{18}F-FDG) PET may improve on this sensitivity and has been proposed as a molecular imaging modality for these patients.

For many years, ^{131}I, ^{123}I, and technetium-99m (^{99m}Tc) pertechnetate have had major roles in evaluating thyroid diseases, both malignant and benign. In areas where ^{123}I costs are not prohibitively high, this tracer has assumed a major role in evaluating the thyroid. Although the positron emitter ^{124}I should be able to do most imaging currently done by other isotopes, and perhaps at a higher quality, it is not yet widely available. Further, the dosimetry of ^{124}I is somewhat problematic in that there is substantial radiation dose deposited by the positron annihilation events and the long, 4-plus-day half-life, coupled with the considerable fraction of decay events associated with gamma ray emissions, which are not imaginable with PET.

Thus, this chapter concentrates on the radiotracer most commonly used in PET thyroid cancer imaging, FDG. The [^{18}F]-FDG PET has already been shown to effectively detect various types of cancer by virtue of their increased glucose metabolism (9).

METABOLISM OF GLUCOSE

The ^{18}F label allows visualization of physiologic glucose metabolism. FDG, a structural analogue of glucose, is transported across the cell membrane by glucose transporters, phosphorylated to [^{18}F]-FDG-6-PO_4 by hexokinase 1, and can no longer diffuse out of the cell. Unlike glucose, FDG cannot enter glycolysis; therefore, it becomes trapped within glucose-metabolizing cells. Normal thyrocytes express glucose transporters and concentrate and phosphorylate glucose. Furthermore, expression of the glucose transporter 1 (*GLUT1*) gene is increased in some, although not all, human thyroid cancers (10–12). Planar gamma camera imaging using a specially modified gamma camera was shown capable of imaging metastatic thyroid cancer in a small study performed in the late 1980s (13). In that small study of three patients it was recognized that there were several different metabolic uptake patterns in these cancers including (a) iodine positive, FDG negative; (b) positive for both tracers, and (c) FDG positive, iodine negative, as well as both negative. The authors also recognized that FDG positive lesions appeared to be more aggressive. In addition, these observers recognized that lesions could vary in uptake patterns within the same patient.

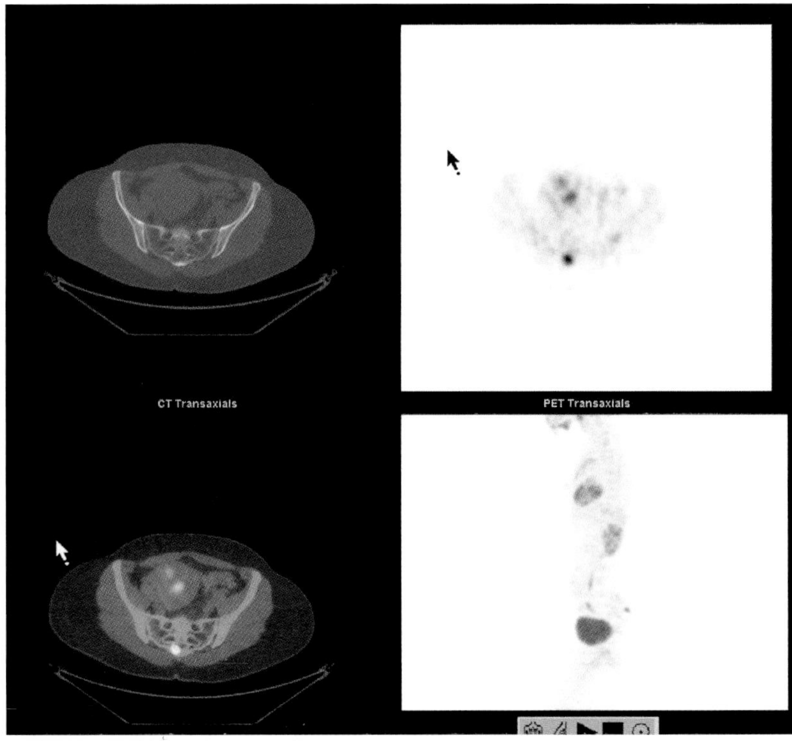

FIGURE 8.8.1. Metastatic follicular variant of papillary thyroid cancer (to sacrum). Arrow indicates right side of image.

This same group using a planar gamma camera was able to demonstrate that in the thyroid gland itself, while thyroid cancers did accumulate FDG, several benign thyroid processes also accumulated FDG. Thus, the accumulation of the FDG was not completely specific for malignant thyroid nodules (14). This background is important in considering the emerging role of FDG PET in thyroid cancer imaging.

18-F FLUORODEOXYGLUCOSE PET

The role FDG PET (or PET/CT) will play in thyroid cancer remains in evolution. However, the role of FDG PET in the follow-up of patients with well-differentiated thyroid cancer, status post–total thyroidectomy and ^{131}I ablation with increasing thyroglobulin levels and negative ^{131}I whole-body scans is increasingly well established. As indicated, early studies have shown that there can be a flip-flop in uptake patterns in thyroid cancers, with them being first iodine positive, FDG negative, and with progression becoming FDG positive, iodine negative (15). It is these latter tumors, those that are iodine negative, in which FDG PET appears to be most potentially beneficial.

Chung et al. (16) demonstrated that FDG PET was most useful in patients with negative ^{131}I scans, detecting cervical lymph node metastasis in 87.9%, lung metastasis in 27.3%, mediastinal metastasis in 33.3%, and bone metastasis in 9.1%. In a study by Hsu et al. (17) 15 patients with posttherapy local invasive or aggressive differentiated thyroid cancer were evaluated. FDG PET was useful for detecting dedifferentiated lesions and was superior to ^{131}I WBS in detecting residual cervical or mediastinal lesions and suspected small metastatic foci in the lung. FDG PET was inferior to ^{131}I WBS in detecting diffuse lung metastases and distant bone metastases. Early prospective studies in small numbers of patients confirm FDG PET's usefulness in correctly detecting recurrence or metastases. Despite the heterogeneity of ^{18}F-FDG techniques; FDG PET correctly detected metastatic disease in 60% to 94% of patients and changed management in 50% to 78% (3,18–24). The reported sensitivity and specificity have varied widely as well. The sensitivity has been reported between 40% and 100% (25), and the specificity between 25% and 95.2% (16,20,26). Two larger studies, Wang et al. (23) and Schulter et al. (24), with 37 and 64 patients, respectively, confirmed the utility of FDG PET to localize residual thyroid cancer lesions and affect management in patients who have negative diagnostic ^{131}I whole-body scans and elevated thyroglobulin levels. The positive predictive value ranged 83% to 92% and the negative predictive value ranged from 25% to 93%. True-positive FDG PET findings were correlated with increasing human thyroglobulin level; FDG PET is most often positive at human thyroglobulin levels of greater than 10 μg/L. Overall, follow-up of these patients should be in conjunction with ^{131}I WBS (1,24) for best overall sensitivity and specificity.

In recent years fusion imaging using PET combined with computed tomography (CT) has been able to increase the diagnostic accuracy, reduce pitfalls, and change therapeutic strategies in a substantial number of patients (1). Nahas et al. (27) conducted a retrospective analysis of 33 patients with suspected recurrent papillary thyroid carcinoma who had undergone PET/CT. In 67% of cases, PET/CT supplied additional information that altered or confirmed the management plan. PET/CT correlated correctly with histopathological findings in 25 of 36 distinct anatomical sites, with an accuracy of 70%. The sensitivity of PET/CT in identifying recurrence was found to be 66%, with a specificity of 100%, a positive predictive value of 100%, and a negative predictive value of 27%. Therefore, a negative finding on PET/CT is not sufficiently reliable to preclude further investigation and treatment. Importantly, in this study a positive PET/CT is a powerful tool for predicting exact

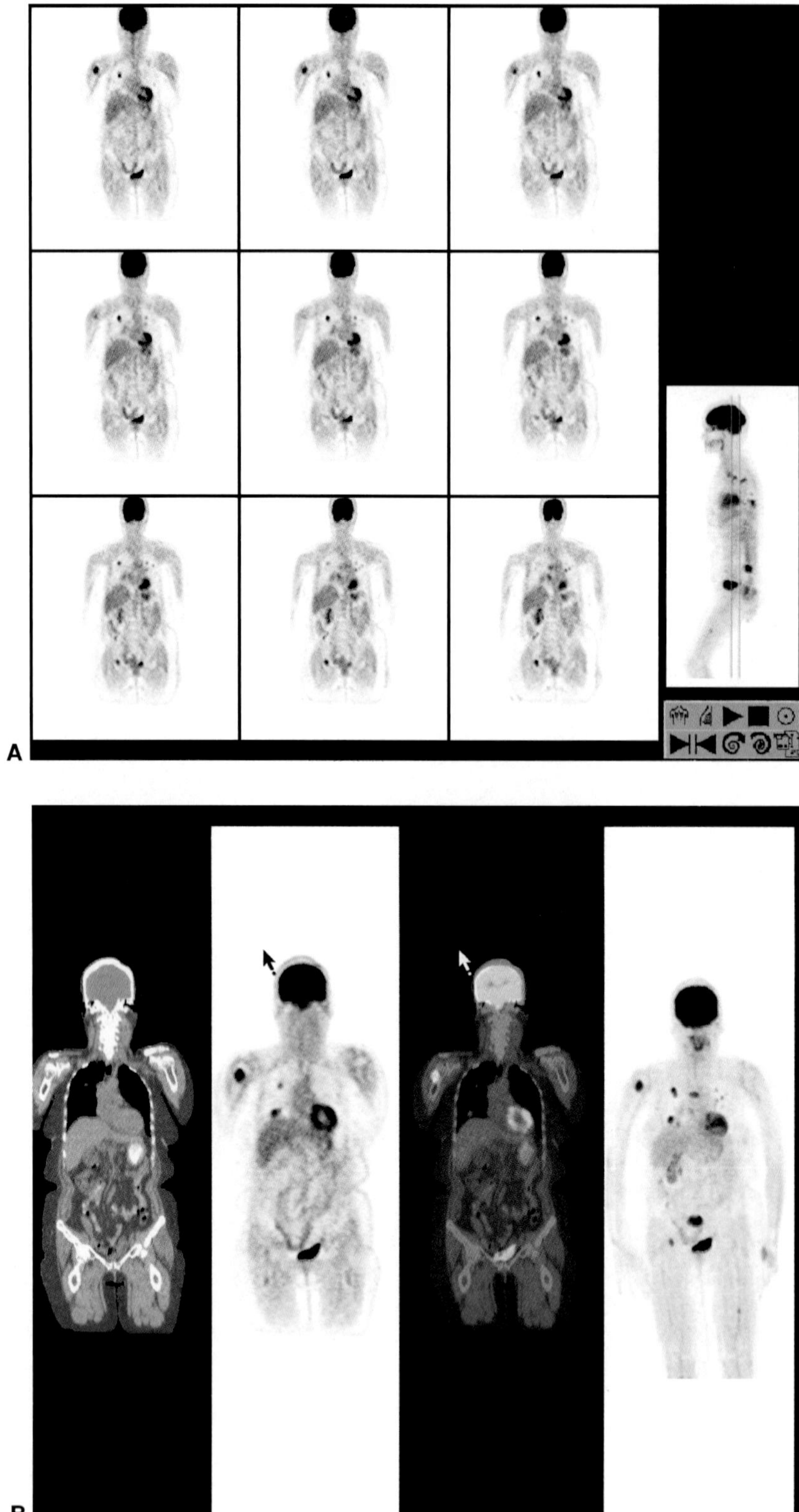

FIGURE 8.8.2. A: Metastatic papillary thyroid cancer with metastasis to bones and lungs (coronal PET images). **B:** Same patient, PET, CT, fused and MIP (R) images show metastases in lungs, bones, and mediastinum. Arrow indicates right side of patient different views.

locations of recurrent papillary thyroid cancer, thus making it a generally reliable guide for surgical planning. Furthermore, the modality was most useful in patients who had average thyroglobulin levels greater than 10 ng/mL and when the tumor no longer concentrated radioactive iodine.

Similar findings were reported by Shammas et al. (9) in a prospective study, with [^{18}F]-FDG PET/CT of 61 consecutive patients who had elevated thyroglobulin levels or a clinical suspicion of recurrent disease after total thyroidectomy followed by radioiodine ablation. Clinical management changed for 27 (44%) of 61 patients, including surgery, radiation therapy, or chemotherapy. Their accuracy (73.8%) was equally high. Furthermore, [^{18}F]-FDG PET/CT can provide precise anatomic localization of recurrent or metastatic thyroid carcinoma, leading to improved diagnostic accuracy, and can guide therapeutic management. In two patients, increased ^{18}F-FDG uptake identified a second primary malignancy. Although not as robust, they report a specificity of 82.4%, with four false positives, and a sensitivity of 68.4%, with 12 false-negative patients. Similarly, the sensitivities of ^{18}F-FDG PET/CT at serum thyroglobulin levels of less than 5, 5 to 10, and more than 10 ng/mL were 60%, 63%, and 72%, respectively. A negative finding on PET/CT is not sufficiently reliable to preclude further investigation and treatment. It is also commonly the case that the number of FDG avid foci seen at PET is fewer than the number of lymph nodes containing tumor removed surgically.

FDG PET may have prognostic value in following patients with thyroid cancer. Wang et al. (8) incorporated ^{18}F-FDG PET into the routine follow-up of a cohort of 125 thyroid cancer patients who had previous thyroidectomies. During 41 months of follow-up, 14 patients died. Univariate analysis demonstrated that survival was reduced in those aged over 45 years, distant metastases, PET positivity, high rates of FDG uptake, and high volume of FDG-avid disease (greater than 125 mL). The 3-year survival probability of patients with FDG volumes of 125 mL or less was 0.96 (95% confidence interval, 0.91 to 1.0) compared with 0.18 (95% confidence interval, 0.04 to 0.85) in patients with FDG volume greater than 125 mL. Multivariate analysis demonstrated that the single strongest predictor of survival was the volume of FDG-avid disease. Patients over 45 years with distant metastases that concentrate FDG are at the highest risk. Of the ten patients with distant metastases and negative PET scans, all were alive and well. Only one death (of leukemia) occurred in the PET-negative group (n = 66). Once distant metastases are discovered in patients with differentiated thyroid carcinoma, FDG PET can identify high and low risk subsets. Subjects with a FDG volume greater than 125 mL have significantly reduced short-term survival. Such findings are consistent with the FDG signal reflecting the total tumor burden, as FDG uptake is often related rather directly to the number of viable cancer cells.

THYROID-STIMULATING HORMONE AND PET IMAGING

The optimal conditions for imaging thyroid cancer are being more fully characterized. Already, FDG PET is taking advantage of the increased glucose metabolism and increased *GLUT1* gene in some human thyroid cancers (10,11). It has been shown that thyroid-stimulating hormone (TSH) stimulates native glucose transport and glycolytic activity in thyrocytes (28–30). The role of TSH stimulation in FDG PET imaging of thyroid cancer is still unclear, but it may enhance FDG uptake based on this principle. In a case study in the early 1990s, Sisson et al. (31) showed that moderating the level of serum TSH affected both FDG and thallous chloride (Tl-201) uptake into thyroid metastases. A higher TSH level was associated with both higher FDG and Tl-201 uptake levels. Thus, this suggested FDG PET could detect thyroid cancers and showed, anecdotally, that FDG uptake could be modified by endogenous elevations in serum TSH levels, even in metastases with appropriate patient stimulation. Although an early study by Wang et al. (23) in 1999 concluded that TSH stimulation had no effect on FDG uptake, later studies have shown that TSH stimulation improves the diagnostic yield of FDG PET to varying extents.

Moog (32), in a prospective study of ten patients using thyroid hormone withdrawal, Van Tol, et al. (33), in a prospective study of eight patients using withdrawal, Petrich et al. (34), in a prospective study of 30 patients using recombinant TSH stimulation, and Chin et al. (35), in a prospective study of eight patients using recombinant TSH stimulation all demonstrated TSH stimulation improves the detectability of occult thyroid metastases with FDG PET, compared with scans performed on TSH suppression (Fig. 8.8.3). In fact, the performance of FDG PET during TSH stimulation was either superior (detecting more lesions or lesions not previously seen) or equal to FDG PET during TSH suppression, but never inferior. Furthermore, lesions demonstrated better target to background contrast and significantly higher FDG uptake. More studies with larger patient populations and uniform FDG PET techniques are needed to further evaluate this question, but the evidence is increasingly clear that for optimal visualization of thyroid cancers with FDG that TSH levels should be elevated.

Furthermore, no studies have compared endogenous verses exogenous TSH stimulation directly. An early prospective study by Saab et al. (36) of 15 patients did include patients prepared for PET/CT imaging with thyroid hormone withdrawal (n = 7) or recombinant human TSH (n = 8) and found a similar impact on FDG uptake, but the study was not designed to directly compare the two methods. It seems that recombinant TSH offers similar benefit and may provide a better quality of life compared to withdrawal for the patient. In any case, it is prudent that follow-up examinations are performed under identical TSH conditions to prevent erroneous interpretation (32). It thus remains unclear if recombinant TSH given exogenously or an endogenous elevation of TSH levels are equivalent nor is it clear precisely what the proper timing of recombinant TSH administration should be. It also is not clear if every thyroid cancer is responsive to recombinant TSH or if this is only a property of some of the cancers. At present, it is typical for PET studies to be performed at about 24 hours after the second dose of recombinant TSH.

FINE-NEEDLE ASPIRATION

The role of fine-needle aspiration in the preoperative evaluation of thyroid nodules is firmly established (37,38). An average of 20% of thyroid nodules may be cytologically diagnosed as suspicious for malignancy, indeterminate, or follicular neoplasm. Approximately 30% of these lesions are malignant; however, histologic examination is necessary for a definitive diagnosis. Therefore, a less invasive examination to further stratify patients for surgery would be welcome. As indicated earlier, planar imaging studies showed there was overlap between malignant and benign thyroid nodules in terms of their FDG avidity with some benign nodules having high FDG

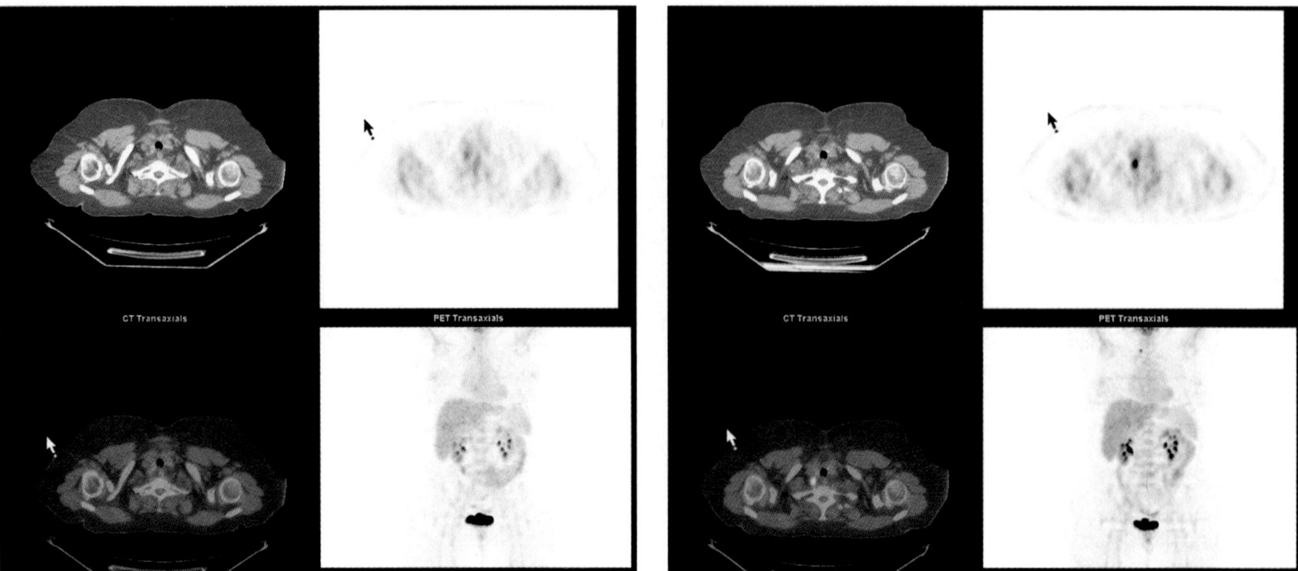

FIGURE 8.8.3. PET/CT recombinant thyroid-stimulating hormone R-TSH increases fluorodeoxyglucose detectability of right neck recurrent papillary thyroid carcinoma. Scans pre (left) and post (right) (Arrow indicates right side of body).

uptake. An early study by Bloom et al. (39) prospectively studied 19 patients for preoperative evaluation of a thyroid nodule with FDG PET. They found the FDG dose uptake ratio (DUR; equivalent to standard uptake value [SUV]) as measured by PET scanning successfully discriminated between all benign and malignant tumors. Subsequent studies have shown that DUR, as with most quantitative measures of FDG uptake, needs to be interpreted cautiously (40). Mitchell et al. (41) prospectively studied 31 patients for preoperative FDG uptake of thyroid nodules with a reported sensitivity of 60%, specificity of 91%, and positive and negative predictive values of 75% and 83%, respectively. Conversely, Kim et al. (42) studied 46 patients with thyroid nodules greater than 1 cm cytologically diagnosed as follicular neoplasm at preoperative evaluation. FDG PET showed hypermetabolism of all nodules; benign thyroid follicular nodules were often as FDG avid as were malignant nodules. These findings suggest that FDG PET has limited value for selecting candidates for surgery among patients cytologically diagnosed as follicular neoplasm. Further studies may be warranted, however, FDG PET does not seem to offer consistent benefit in this arena.

One arena where FDG PET can be used to guide further evaluation is in the finding of an incidental nodule in patients undergoing [^{18}F]-FDG PET/CT for other reasons. The detection of unexpected additional primary malignancies with PET/CT has been established (43). Ishimori et al. (43) reported the incidence of secondary malignancy in patients undergoing [^{18}F]-FDG PET/CT for known or suspected malignant lesions. In this retrospective study of 1,912 patients, they found suspicious, FDG-avid lesions in 79 (4.1%). Of these, 22 (1.2%) were pathologically proven to be malignant. In this same study, the incidence of suspicious thyroid lesions was 0.57% (11 of 1,912). Of these lesions 6 of 11 (54.5%) proved to be malignant by pathology.

Several large, retrospective studies of patients without a history of thyroid disease who underwent FDG PET imaging for the evaluation of known malignancies not associated with the thyroid, including 331 healthy volunteers who underwent voluntary cancer screening, confirmed similar findings. Cohen et al. (44) studied 4,525 subjects, Kang et al. (45) studied 1,330 subjects, Kim et al. (46) studied 4,136 subjects, and Choi et al. (47) studied 1,763 subjects. Incidental focal thyroid FDG uptake ranged from 0.57% to 4%. Within the study that included healthy volunteers (45), there were no significant differences between volunteers and those with known or suspected malignancy. Importantly, when found, the incidence of malignancy in these thyroid lesions is 26.7% to 54.5%. The usefulness of SUV was variable; but malignant lesions may have higher maximum SUV than benign lesions; thus it may be helpful in predicting benign versus malignant histology, but in our hands, the degree of overlap is too large and all FDG-avid thyroid nodules must be considered as potentially malignant and it is currently recommend they be surgically excised.

Although focal FDG uptake in the thyroid is highly concerning for the presence of cancer, diffuse thyroid uptake is also encountered quite commonly. Diffuse uptake of FDG in the thyroid is in practice a much less worrisome finding than the focal intense uptake described above. Karantanis et al. (48) found 138 of 4,732 patients (2.9%) had diffuse thyroid uptake in a clinical PET practice. Data from 133 of the patients showed 63 (47.4%) had a prior diagnosis of hypothyroidism or autoimmune thyroiditis, and 56 were receiving thyroxine therapy. In an age- and sex-matched control group who had no thyroid uptake on PET there were 13 (9.8%) with a prior diagnosis of hypothyroidism and only 11 were receiving thyroxine therapy. Not all patients with increased FDG uptake were investigated, but 19 were found to have autoimmune thyroiditis or hypothyroidism. FDG uptake and TSH levels were not correlated. Thus, this diffuse uptake is seen much more often than focal uptake and is often associated with subclinical Hashimoto disease. It probably should be noted that when visualized on PET, so a modest thyroid work-up can be performed by the referring physician, some patients will be hypothyroid, although possibly not previously recognized as such.

POORLY DIFFERENTIATED FORMS OF THYROID CANCER

The [^{18}F]-FDG PET has been evaluated for the follow-up of the poorly differentiated varieties of thyroid cancer, including medullary, Hurthle cell, and anaplastic thyroid cancer. Medullary thyroid cancer (MTC) is generally a more aggressive, less well-differentiated subtype of the thyroid cancers. It does not concentrate radioactive iodine. The primary treatment is total thyroidectomy and regional lymph node dissection. Persistently elevated or postoperative increases in biomarkers portend residual disease or recurrence. Frequently, anatomic imaging is negative and the best modality for follow-up of these patients is unclear. Early studies suggested that ^{18}F-FDG PET offers a useful option to restage patients with MTC and elevated biomarkers. FDG PET detected 68% of these lesions; with a sensitivity of 78% and a specificity of 79% (49). Mucha et al. (50) examined the diagnostic accuracy of PET for the localization of occult MTC in five patients after surgery with increase levels of calcitonin, in whom conventional imaging failed to identify a source. In four of five patients had PET that detected residual tumor or recurrence confirmed by histopathology. Recently, these findings were confirmed by Iagaru et al. (51) in a retrospective study of 13 patients with histologic diagnosis of MTC who underwent PET after rising levels of calcitonin with negative anatomic imaging. Recurrent or metastatic disease was identified in 7 of 13 (54%) of these patients. The reported sensitivity and specificity of FDG PET was 85.7% and 83.3%, respectively.

Hurthle cell carcinoma is rare (making up about 4% of thyroid cancers) and is only about one fourth as common as follicular cancers. Hurthle cell cancer of the thyroid is usually classified with follicular thyroid cancer, although it really is a distinct kind of tumor. When controlled for age, Hurthle cell tumors behave very similarly (survival) to follicular tumors. Radioactive iodine does not work as well for Hurthle cell cancer as it does for follicular cancer, as they generally have less iodine avidity. Pryma (52) described, in a retrospective analysis, the diagnostic accuracy and prognostic value of [^{18}F]-FDG PET in this disease. The study reported a diagnostic sensitivity of 95.8% and a specificity of 95%. Furthermore, [^{18}F]-FDG PET revealed additional sites of disease, compared with 5 of 11 positive by CT and three of six positive by radioiodine scintigraphy. As well, [^{18}F]-FDG PET correctly classified ten false negatives by radioiodine scintigraphy and three false positives by CT. Increased maximum SUV was an indicator of a poor prognosis. In this single study, [^{18}F]-FDG PET showed excellent diagnostic accuracy, which improved on CT and radioiodine scintigraphy, but further study is warranted.

ANAPLASTIC CARCINOMAS

Anaplastic carcinomas of the thyroid are the most aggressive, lethal, and feared of thyroid cancers. Fortunately, they are also the rarest. They generally do not accumulate any radioiodine as they are so poorly differentiated, but do accumulate FDG. The literature on these tumors is limited, but small case reports and studies have shown them to be suitable targets for PET imaging (53–58).

ALTERNATIVE PET TRACERS

Although this chapter has focused mostly on FDG PET and PET/CT, it must be realized that other tracers can be valuable in PET imaging of thyroid cancer. As an example, ^{124}I PET has been used in imaging thyroid cancer patients for dosimetry and lesion detection by several groups. The use of this tracer can result in promising dose-volume histograms and may provide insights into individual tumor's responses to treatment (58,59). Also ^{124}I can serve as a highly robust predictor for ^{131}I therapy. In addition, ^{124}I PET/CT can be diagnostically useful for thyroid cancer staging. It remains to be seen whether and how ^{124}I will evolve in clinical practice of thyroid cancer imaging. It is somewhat difficult to make ^{124}I with many of the relatively small medical cyclotrons in current use, and it is thus not likely to be too widely available for generalized utilization. Further, if costs in production are high, this may limit availability and dissemination of the agent. Although it is reasonable to believe that other tracers such as carbon-11, L-methionine, carbon-11-choline, and tracers of proliferation could be useful in imaging thyroid cancer, they have not been studied to any significant extent.

SUMMARY

FDG PET performed as PET/CT is the most established PET imaging procedure in head and neck cancer. Evidence of PET's efficacy is greatest in patient populations at risk of increased serum thyroglobulin levels postsurgery. High FDG uptake, especially in a substantial volume of tumor, is associated with poor outcomes. Tumor visualization with FDG is enhanced if serum TSH levels are elevated. FDG uptake in thyroid nodules is seen incidentally, not uncommonly, and warrants additional work-up as cancer is commonly present in such nodules. Diffuse uptake is not as worrisome for cancer but can be seen in patients with thyroiditis. PET is not established as a robust tool in evaluating thyroid nodules; however, ^{124}I is a promising PET tracer and can produce high-quality images, but it is not yet widely available. Its quantitative capabilities make it very attractive as a tool for dosimetry, and it may ultimately provide better lesion detection than currently available using ^{123}I or ^{131}I, but more study is needed.

REFERENCES

1. Lind P, Kohlfurst S. Respective roles of thyroglobulin, radioiodine imaging, and positron emission tomography in the assessment of thyroid cancer. *Semin Nucl Med* 2006;36(3):194–205.
2. Pacini, F, Schlumberger M, Dralle H, et al. European consensus for the management of patients with differentiated thyroid carcinoma of the follicular epithelium. *Eur J Endocrinol* 2006;154(6):787–803.
3. Hundahl SA, Fleming ID, Fremgen AM et al. A National Cancer Data Base report on 53,856 cases of thyroid carcinoma treated in the US, 1985–1995. *Cancer* 1998;83 (12):2638–2648.
4. Lerch H, Schober O, Kuwert T, et al. Survival of differentiated thyroid carcinoma studied in 500 patients. *J Clin Oncol* 1997;15(5):2067–2075.
5. Mazzaferri EL. An overview of the management of papillary and follicular thyroid carcinoma. *Thyroid* 1999;9:421–427.
6. Schlumberger M, Baudin E. Serum thyroglobulin determination in the follow-up of patients with differentiated thyroid carcinoma. *Eur J Endocrinol* 1998;138:249–252.
7. Mazzaferri EL. Empirically treating high serum thyroglobulin levels. *J Nucl Med* 2005;46(7):1079–1088.
8. Wang W, Larson SM, Fazzari M, et al. Prognostic value of [18F]fluorodeoxyglucose positron emission tomographic scanning in patients with thyroid cancer. *J Clin Endocrinol Metab* 2000;85(3):1107–1113.

9. Shammas A, Degirmenci B, Mountz JM, et al. ^{18}F-FDG PET/CT in patients with suspected recurrent or metastatic well-differentiated thyroid cancer. *J Nucl Med* 2007;48(2): 221–226.
10. Lazar V, Bidart JM, Caillou B, et al. Expression of the Na+/I– symporter gene in human thyroid tumors: a comparison study with other thyroid-specific genes. *J Clin Endocrinol Metab* 1999;84: 3228–3234.
11. Schonberger J, Ruschoff J, Grimm D, et al. Glucose transporter 1 gene expression is related to thyroid neoplasms with an unfavorable prognosis: an immunohistochemical study. *Thyroid* 2002;12:747–754.
12. Musholt TJ, Musholt PB, Dehdashti F, et al. Evaluation of fluorodeoxyglucose-positron emission tomographic scanning and its association with glucose transporter expression in medullary thyroid carcinoma and pheochromocytoma: a clinical and molecular study. *Surgery* 1997;122(6):1049–1060.
13. Joensuu H, Ahonen A. Imaging of metastases of thyroid carcinoma with fluorine-18 fluorodeoxyglucose. *J Nucl Med* 1987;28(5): 910–914.
14. Joensuu H, Ahonen A, Klemi PJ. ^{18}F-fluorodeoxyglucose imaging in preoperative diagnosis of thyroid malignancy. *Eur J Nucl Med* 1988; 13(10):502–506.
15. Feine U, Lietzenmayer R, Hanke JP, et al. ^{18}FDG whole-body PET in differentiated thyroid carcinoma. Flipflop in uptake patterns of ^{18}FDG and ^{131}I. *Nuklearmedizin* 1995;34(4):127–134.
16. Chung JK, So Y, Lee JS, et al. Value of FDG PET in papillary thyroid carcinoma with negative ^{131}I whole-body scan. *J Nucl Med* 1999;40(6): 989–992.
17. Hsu CH, Liu RS, Wu CH, et al. Complementary role of ^{18}F-fluorodeoxyglucose positron emission tomography and ^{131}I scan in the follow-up of post-therapy differentiated thyroid cancer. *J Formos Med Assoc* 2002;101(7):459–467.
18. Grunwald F, Schomburg A, Bender H, et al. Fluorine-18 fluorodeoxyglucose positron emission tomography in the follow-up of differentiated thyroid cancer. *Eur J Nucl Med* 1996;23(3):312–319.
19. Muros MA, Llamas-Elvira JM, Ramirez-Navarro A, et al. Utility of fluorine-18-fluorodeoxyglucose positron emission tomography in differentiated thyroid carcinoma with negative radioiodine scans and elevated serum thyroglobulin levels. *Am J Surg* 2000;179(6):457–461.
20. Frilling A, Tecklenborg K, Gorges R, et al. Preoperative diagnostic value of [(18)F] fluorodeoxyglucose positron emission tomography in patients with radioiodine-negative recurrent well-differentiated thyroid carcinoma. *Ann Surg* 2001;234(6):804–811.
21. Helal BO, Merlet P, Toubert ME,. Clinical impact of ^{18}F-FDG PET in thyroid carcinoma patients with elevated thyroglobulin levels and negative ^{131}I scanning results after therapy. *J Nucl Med* 2001;42(10): 1464–1469.
22. Lind P, Kresnik E, Kumnig G, et al. ^{18}F-FDG-PET in the follow-up of thyroid cancer. *Acta Med Austriaca* 2003;30(1):17–21.
23. Wang W, Macapinlac H, Larson SM, et al. ^{18}F-2-fluoro-2-deoxy-D-glucose positron emission tomography localizes residual thyroid cancer in patients with negative diagnostic ^{131}I whole body scans and elevated serum thyroglobulin levels. *Clin Endocrinol Metab* 1999;84(7): 2291–2302.
24. Schluter B, Bohuslavizki KH, Beyer W, et al. Impact of FDG PET on patients with differentiated thyroid cancer who present with elevated thyroglobulin and negative ^{131}I scan. *J Nucl Med* 2001;42(1):71–76.
25. Leboulleux S, Schroeder PR, Schlumberger M, et al. The role of PET in follow-up of patients treated for differentiated epithelial thyroid cancers. *Natl Clin Pract Endocrinol Metab* 2007;3(2):112–121.
26. Choi MY, Chung JK, Lee HY, et al. The clinical impact of ^{18}F-FDG PET in papillary thyroid carcinoma with a negative ^{131}I whole body scan: a single-center study of 108 patients. *Ann Nucl Med* 2006;20(8):547–552.
27. Nahas Z, Goldenberg D, Fakhry C, et al. The role of positron emission tomography/computed tomography in the management of recurrent papillary thyroid carcinoma. *Laryngoscope* 2005;115(2):237–243.
28. Filetti S, Damante G, Foti D. Thyrotropin stimulates glucose transport in cultured rat thyroid cells. *Endocrinology* 1987;120:2576–2581.
29. Hosaka Y, Tawata M, Kurihara A, et al. The regulation of two distinct glucose transporter (*GLUT1* and *GLUT4*) gene expressions in cultured rat thyroid cells by thyrotropin. *Endocrinology* 1992;131:159–165.
30. Russo D, Damante G, Foti D, et al. Different molecular mechanisms are involved in the multihormonal control of glucose transport in FRTL5 rat thyroid cells. *J Endocrinol Invest* 1994;17:323–327.
31. Sisson JC, Ackermann RJ, Meyer MA, et al. Uptake of 18-fluoro-2-deoxy-D-glucose by thyroid cancer: implications for diagnosis and therapy. *J Clin Endocrinol Metab* 1993;77(4):1090–1094.
32. Moog F, Linke R, Manthey N, et al. Influence of thyroid-stimulated hormone levels on uptake of FDG in recurrent and metastatic differentiated thyroid carcinoma. *J Nucl Med* 2000;41(12):1989–1995.
33. Van Tol KM, Jager PL, Piers DA, et al. Better yield of 18-fluorodeoxyglucose-positron emission tomography in patients with metastatic differentiated thyroid carcinoma during thyrotropin stimulation. *Thyroid* 2002;12(5):381–387.
34. Petrich T, Borner AR, Otto D, et al. Influence of rhTSH on [(18)F]fluorodeoxyglucose uptake by differentiated thyroid carcinoma. *Eur J Nucl Med Mol Imaging* 2002;29(5):641–647.
35. Chin BB, Patel P, Cohade C, et al. TSH stimulates recombinant human thyrotropin stimulation of fluoro-D-glucose positron emission tomography uptake in well-differentiated thyroid carcinoma. *J Clin Endocrinol Metab* 2004;89(1): 91–95.
36. Saab G, Driedger AA, Pavlosky W, et al. Thyroid-stimulating hormone-stimulated fused positron emission tomography/computed tomography in the evaluation of recurrence in ^{131}I-negative papillary thyroid carcinoma. *Thyroid* 2006;16(3):267–272.
37. Piromalli D, Martelli G, Del Prato I, et al. The role of fine needle aspiration in the diagnosis of thyroid nodules: analysis of 795 consecutive cases. *J Surg Oncol* 1992;50(4):247–250.
38. Sangalli G, Serio G, Zampatti C, et al. Fine needle aspiration cytology of the thyroid: a comparison of 5469 cytological and final histological diagnoses. *Cytopathology* 2006;17(5):245–250.
39. Bloom AD, Adler LP, Shuck JM. Determination of malignancy of thyroid nodules with positron emission tomography. *Surgery* 1993;114(4): 728–734.
40. Hamberg LM, Hunter GJ, Alpert NM, et al. The dose uptake ratio as an index of glucose metabolism: useful parameter or oversimplification? *J Nucl Med* 1994; 35(8):1308.
41. Mitchell JC, Grant F, Evenson AR, et al. Preoperative evaluation of thyroid nodules with ^{18}FDG-PET/CT. *Surgery* 2005;138(6):1166–1174; discussion 1174–1175.
42. Kim JM, Ryu JS, Kim TY, et al. ^{18}F-Fluorodeoxyglucose positron emission tomography does not predict malignancy in thyroid nodules cytologically diagnosed as follicular neoplasm. *J Clin Endocrinol Metab* 2007;92:1630–1634.
43. Ishimori T, Patel PV, Wahl RL. Detection of unexpected additional primary malignancies with ET/CT. *J Nucl Med* 2005;46(5):752–757.
44. Cohen MS, Arslan N, Dehdashti F, et al. Risk of malignancy in thyroid incidentalomas identified by fluorodeoxyglucose-positron emission tomography. *Surgery* 2001;130(6):941–946.
45. Kang KW, Kim SK, Kang HS, et al. Prevalence and risk of cancer of focal thyroid incidentaloma identified by ^{18}F-fluorodeoxyglucose positron emission tomography for metastasis evaluation and cancer screening in healthy subjects. *J Clin Endocrinol Metab* 2003;88(9):4100–4104.
46. Kim TY, Kim WB, Ryu JS, et al. ^{18}F-fluorodeoxyglucose uptake in thyroid from positron emission tomogram (PET) for evaluation in cancer patients: high prevalence of malignancy in thyroid PET incidentaloma. *Laryngoscope* 2005;15(6):1074–1078.
47. Choi JY, Lee KS, Kim HJ, et al. Focal thyroid lesions incidentally identified by integrated ^{18}F-FDG PET/CT: clinical significance and improved characterization. *J Nucl Med* 2006;47(4):609–615.
48. Karantanis D, Bogsrud TV, Wiseman GA, et al. Clinical significance of diffusely increased ^{18}F-FDG uptake in the thyroid gland. *J Nucl Med* 2007;48(6):896–901.

49. Diehl M, Risse JH, Brandt-Mainz K, et al. Fluorine-18 fluorodeoxyglucose positron emission tomography in medullary thyroid cancer; results of a multicenter study. *Eur J Nucl Med* 2001;28(11):1671–1676.
50. Mucha SA, Kunert-Radek J, Pomorski L. Positron emission tomography (^{18}FDG-PET) in the detection of medullary thyroid carcinoma and metastases. *Endokrynol Pol* 2006;57(4):452–455.
51. Iagaru A, Masamed R, Singer PA. Detection of occult medullary thyroid cancer recurrence with 2-deoxy-2-[F-18]fluoro-D-glucose-PET and PET/CT. *Mol Imaging Biol* 2007;9(2):70–77.
52. Pryma DA, Schoder H, Gonen M, et al. Diagnostic accuracy and prognostic value of ^{18}F-FDG PET in Hurthle cell thyroid cancer patients. *J Nucl Med* 2006;47(8): 1260–1266.
53. Nguyen BD, Ram PC. PET/CT staging and post-theraputic monitoring of anaplastic thyroid carcinoma. *Clin Nucl Med* 2007;32(2):145–149.
54. Iagaru A, McDougall IR. F-18 FDG PET CT Demonstration of an adrenal metastasis in a patient with anaplastic thyroid cancer. 2007;32(1): 13–15.
55. Jadvar H, Fischman AJ. Evaluation of rare tumors with [F-18]fluorodeoxyglucose positron emission tomography. *Clin Positron Imaging* 1999;2: 153–158.
56. Poppe K, Lahoutte T, Everaert H, et al. The utility of multimodality imaging in anaplastic thyroid carcinoma. *Thyroid* 2004;14:981–982.
57. Khan N, Oriuchi N, Higuchi T, et al. Review of fluorine-18-2-fluoro-2-deoxy-D-glucose positron emission tomography (FDG-PET) in the follow-up of medullary and anaplastic thyroid carcinomas. *Cancer Control* 2005;12:254–260.
58. Eschmann SM, Reischl G, Bilger K, et al. Evaluation of dosimetry of radioiodine therapy in benign and malignant thyroid disorders by means of iodine-124 and PET. *Eur J Nucl Med Mol Imaging* 2002;29(6): 760–767.
59. Freudenberg LS, Antoch G, Jentzen W, et al. Value of ^{124}I-PET/CT in staging of patients with differentiated thyroid cancer. *Eur Radiol* 2004;14(11):2092–2098.

CHAPTER

8.9 Lung Cancer

PATRICK J. PELLER AND VAL J. LOWE

Lung cancer is the most common cancer in the United States with an estimated 175,000 new cases and 163,000 deaths annually. Lung cancer death rates have begun to plateau recently in the United States, particularly in men (1). There are more than 600,000 deaths worldwide from lung cancer, and this rate is expected to rise for the next two decades and quite likely even longer (2). Lung cancer deaths in the United States exceed all those in breast, prostate, and colorectal cancer patients combined. In the past 10 years, there has been decreasing mortality in breast, prostate, and colorectal cancer patients due, in part, to increased screening and improved diagnosis and treatment, but no similar significant trend has been seen with lung cancer (3).

Smoking is closely linked to lung cancer, and historically the incidence of lung cancer parallels the availability of mechanically produced cigarettes (4). In the United States today, there are 25.5 million male smokers and 21.5 million female smokers, representing just less than 24% of the population. The incidence of smoking remains higher in Native Americans and black Americans than in the general population. The overall incidence of smoking has declined slowly over the past decade, but in certain populations, especially teenagers and those under the poverty level, there is concern for high and rising smoking rates (5). Prevention of lung cancer and smoking are inexorably tied and continues to be a major health battle.

Significant advances in the management of lung cancer have been seen over the past decade. Traditional computed tomography (CT) has substantially changed with low-dose CT screening and especially with multidetector CT. Surgery remains the mainstay for lung cancer therapy, but multimodality treatment is increasingly common as many cancers are first diagnosed after they are too large or too disseminated for surgical management. New chemotherapy agents and regimens are available, especially targeted treatments such as antiangiogenesis and epidermal growth factor receptor agents. Positron emission tomography (PET) scanning continues to evolve in use as there is increasingly common reimbursement for PET and PET/CT at multiple stages within the course of the disease. Significant technical developments in PET, such as new lutetium oxyorthosilicate (LSO), gadolinium silicate (GSO), and lutetium yttrium orthosilicate (LYSO) detector systems, improved electronics, three-dimensional imaging, time-of-flight PET, respiratory gating, and integration with CT have changed the face of PET imaging in many ways. Widespread availability of commercially prepared fluorodeoxyglucose (FDG) and PET scanners has brought access to PET to most patients with lung cancer in the United States, although patterns of use differ among practitioners. PET has multiple roles in patients with known or suspected lung cancers. Although PET with FDG is the focus of this chapter, it should be realized that PET with carbon-11-L-methionine, used commonly in Japan and in other centers with cyclotrons, also performs quite well in staging and assessing lung cancer.

EVALUATION OF PULMONARY NODULES

Solitary pulmonary nodules (SPN) are a significant clinical problem and are predominantly detected incidentally on chest x-ray or CT. Traditionally, SPNs were nodules 1 to 3 cm in size. More than 75% of the patients are asymptomatic at the time of detection (6). The major clinical question is what is the etiology of this nodule, benign or malignant? This leads to asking if the SPN should be followed or resected. The evaluation becomes risk assessment, which becomes the "cost" of resecting a benign nodule versus the "cost" of missing a malignancy. Multidetector CT has started to make the "solitary" part of SPN a disappearing entity and adds complexity, as the SPN on chest x-ray becomes one of many nodules being detected, although most of the nodules are small (<1 cm). Thus, work-up of nodules less than 1 cm in size is more common than it once was.

Attacking the question of a pulmonary nodule has led to a wide variety of management strategies. All strategies clearly start with establishing the presence or absence of the nodule on a prior chest x-ray or CT; size stability over a 2-year time period is accepted as evidence of benignity. Unfortunately, it is often the case that no prior imaging studies are available, and the stability of lesion size cannot be confirmed. Otherwise, a three-pronged individual risk assessment is employed. Patient risk in terms of age, smoking, prior cancer history, occupational exposure to carcinogens, and the presence of hemoptysis are all weighed as well as the presence of any prior diagnosis of cancer. The pulmonary nodule evaluated by helical, preferably multidetector, CT is assessed for nodule size, calcification, border regularity, density, and cavitation. The individual patient's risk for tissue sampling and surgery is next weighed. This risk assessment requires significant mental calculus for the clinician, often facing discordant information (7). In general, the smaller the nodule, the younger the patient, the less the exposure to carcinogens, the greater the probability that the nodule is benign. However, risk of cancer often falls into an intermediate range, and a decision must be made as to whether to observe the lesion or to secure a histological diagnosis.

A variety of tissue sampling techniques are available: fiberoptic bronchoscopy and biopsy, percutaneous needle aspiration or needle biopsy, video-assisted thoracoscopy, and thoracotomy. Bronchoscopy is least invasive and thoracotomy will yield the most certain histologic opinion. The morbidity and small, but real, risk of death increase with the invasiveness of the tissue sampling procedure. This risk of invasiveness correlates with increased certainty of the yield of biopsy from about 50% to nearly 100% (8–10). The clinician commonly weighs watchful waiting with serial CT scans every 3 months for 2 years versus a tissue sampling procedure and then deciding which procedure. Nodules near the periphery of the lung are better suited to needle biopsy, whereas nodules centrally located near the major airways are often better candidates for bronchoscopic biopsy. Nodules in the middle area of the lung are often quite hard to reach reliably by either methods. Since the nonsurgical approaches have sensitivities less than 100%, a negative study does not exclude the presence of cancer. Thus, some centers often try to move to the most definitive procedure quickly, especially if a negative result will not be sufficient to plan future management.

An FDG PET has proved to be quite sensitive for the detection and evaluation of pulmonary nodules. Gould et al. (11), in a meta-analysis of 40 published studies, demonstrated that the sensitivity of FDG PET was 96.8% and the specificity was 77.8% in 1,474 focal lesions, all greater than 1 cm. FDG PET compared to histology in these published studies was highly sensitive and moderately specific. They stressed the negative predictive value of 97.6% of FDG PET. This suggested that applied to patient populations with 1 cm or larger nodules similar in risk factors to those from the meta-analysis, a patient with a negative FDG PET would have a posttest likelihood of malignancy in the SPN of less than 3% (Fig. 8.9.1). One of the challenges, however, is that the risk is not reduced to 0%, so that some follow-up imaging remains necessary if a choice is made to observe a patient after a negative PET study. Another challenge is that physicians are often asked to perform PET scans in patients with solitary pulmonary nodules less than 1 cm in diameter. In such patients, the diagnostic sensitivity is probably lower due to recovery coefficient limitations of PET scanners and the scan becomes of greatest value when positive.

Many schemas combining PET and biopsy strategies have been proposed. Typically, PET and biopsy provide complementary information (12). In some approaches, tissue sampling is used for greatest certainty, and PET covers those patients where the nodule was inconvenient to biopsy or nondiagnostic. In other schema PET is performed first, and if PET is positive, patients may in some centers go straight to surgery. Even when PET is applied only when the biopsy was nondiagnostic, FDG PET performs well to diagnose lung cancer (13) (Fig. 8.9.2).

Gould et al. (7) used decision analysis to create a management strategy for the physician managing the deployment of the many available diagnostic options for pulmonary nodules. Their analysis found four major roles for PET in evaluating a pulmonary nodule: (a) when a patient's risk of lung cancer and CT findings are not congruent, (b) when the surgical or procedure biopsy risk is high, (c) when a nondiagnostic biopsy occurs, or (d) when the patient is uncomfortable with watchful waiting. The sensitivity analysis demonstrated the broad utility of PET for evaluating pulmonary nodules.

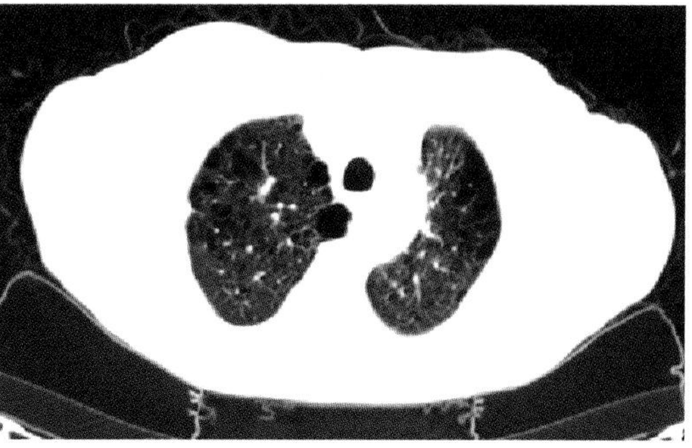

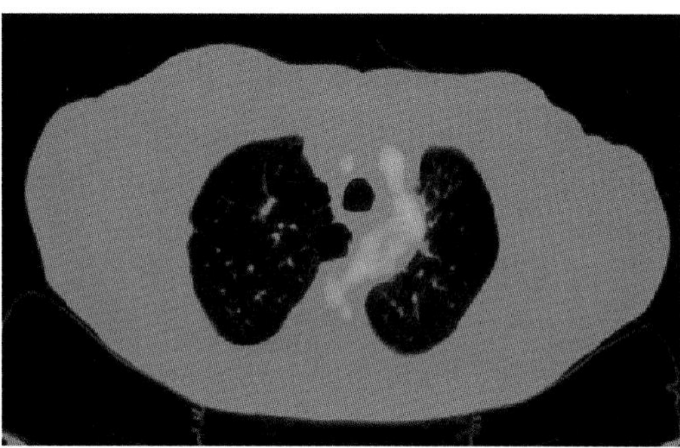

FIGURE 8.9.1. PET/CT evaluation of pulmonary nodule—transaxial CT (**top**), PET (**middle**), and fused images (**lower**). This patient is a 69-year-old man with a long history of smoking enrolled in a CT lung cancer screening study. The patient developed a 15 × 7 mm right upper lobe nodular density during screening. PET and PET/CT images are negative. The patient had subsequent CT scans at 3-month intervals for 18 months that demonstrated slowly changing configuration of this nodule and eventual resolution. Clinical follow-up was typical of a nonmalignant process.

Dynamic contrast enhancement with multidetector CT (MDCT) is more effective in categorizing SPNs as benign or malignant than noncontrast CT. A recent evaluation of integrated PET/CT was compared to dynamic contrast MDCT. FDG PET/CT had a significant advantage in sensitivity (96% vs. 81%) with similar specificity (88% vs. 93%). PET/CT exhibited negative predictive values similar to established PET data, but with improved positive predictive value. In a head-to-head comparison of state-of-the-art

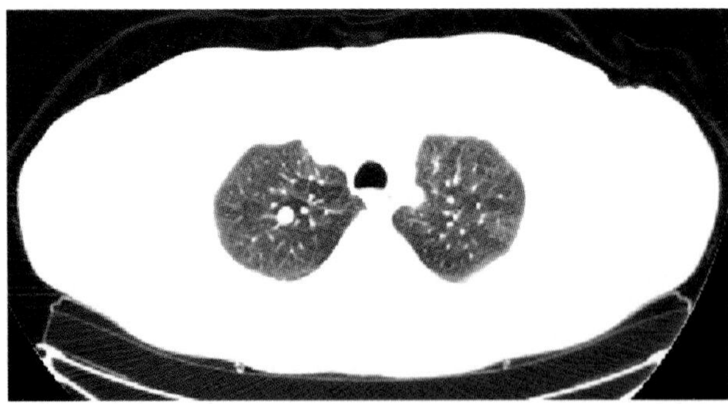

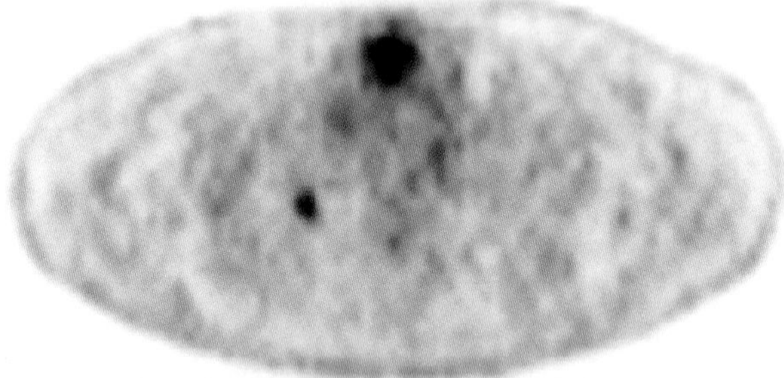

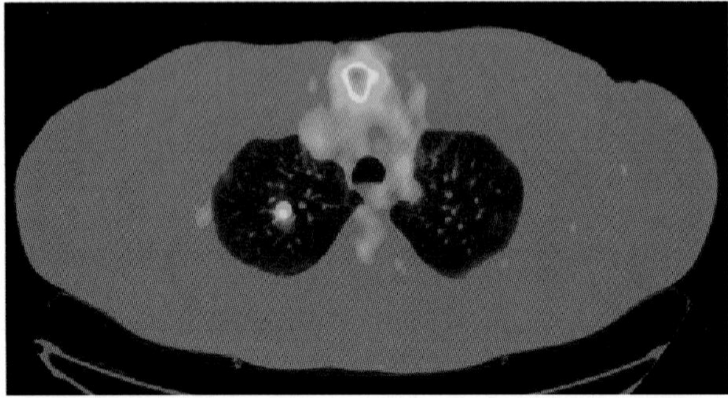

FIGURE 8.9.2. PET/CT evaluation of a pulmonary nodule—transaxial CT (**top**), PET (**middle**), and fused images (**bottom**). This patient is a 59-year-old smoker with a right upper lobe lung nodule detected incidentally on a CT scan performed to evaluate the patient for shortness of breath and a possible pulmonary embolism. The patient underwent a percutaneous needle biopsy of this right upper lobe nodule that was nondiagnostic. PET and PET/CT images demonstrate moderate increased fluorodeoxyglucose accumulation typical of a malignancy (the sternal activity is due to recent surgery). Resection demonstrated a squamous cell carcinoma.

imaging technology, PET/CT provides greater accuracy than MDTC. These techniques may be complementary, but the use of contrast-enhanced CT for characterization of solitary pulmonary nodules does not appear to be as widely adopted as is PET/CT scanning, which seems appropriate based on the performance characteristics of the two methodologies (14).

Integrated PET/CT compared to PET provides somewhat improved or similar nodule resolution, faster scanning times, and CT visualization of SPN. PET/CT technology provides additional methods of evaluating and improving evaluation of a pulmonary nodule. Dual point imaging involves FDG uptake measurements at two different times, typically separated by an hour. The SPN is evaluated by both its intensity of FDG uptake and the change over time. Most lung cancers have a high standardized uptake value (SUV) and the SUV increase is greater than 10% in the 1-hour period. Some, but not all, inflammatory processes have a decline in FDG uptake in this period of observation. However, some inflammatory processes can have rises in FDG uptake with time, and most centers do not currently apply the dual time point technique, in part due to logistical reasons (15). Although virtually all of the literature on PET and PET/CT with FDG has been developed using a 50- to 60-minute uptake period, there are some groups that perform the PET imaging at 90 minutes or more post-FDG injection. Although tumor/background ratios typically rise in this period of time, some caution must be used in interpretation, as interpretation criteria were developed based on the 1-hour uptake period and may differ slightly with a 90-minute uptake period.

The apparent FDG uptake of a nodule is impacted by the partial value effect. The size of the SPN on CT can be used to correct for partial volume effect. Initial research suggests that partial volume correction improves SUV measurements of nodules smaller than 2 cm and increases the sensitivity for malignancy (16). Movement of a SPN with respiration during a PET/CT study causes the counts from the FDG uptake to be distributed over multiple pixels. However, for small nodules, the correction in the SUV is substantial and dependent on lesion size. Measurements of lesion size for small lesions are quite subject to variability, and this variability can be propagated to the SUV assessments. Thus, many interpreting physicians perform a "visual" partial volume correction, in which they use their clinical judgment to realize that modest levels of FDG uptake, sometimes no more than blood pool, in lesions under 1 cm, may be indicative of the presence of a small cancer. Respiratory gating, especially in the lower lobes, corrects for the respiratory excursion of 1 to 3 cm during PET imaging. The apparent activity within the moving nodule may increase between 20% and 36% (17). These techniques show promise but need further investigation before full utilization is likely. It must be realized that some pulmonary nodules that are malignant or behave in a malignant fashion may have relatively low SUVs. Bronchioalveolar carcinoma is very commonly in this category and in the pure state they have SUV values that are much lower than other cancers, sometimes less than 2.5. Carcinoid tumors, both primary and metastatic, can also have low SUVs relative to more typical lung cancers. The CT characteristics of bronchioalveolar carcinoma often are quite suggestive of the presence of this tumor, even if the SUV is low.

When interpreting PET in SPN, a variety of interpretation schemes can be used. Since most PET imaging involves the use of PET/CT, it is important that the CT be examined to determine lesion size. Smaller lesions, less than two times the resolution of the imaging system, will not have all counts recovered, so their apparent SUV will be lower than their true radioactivity concentration. In many centers, a qualitative interpretation is applied in which SPNs with FDG uptake greater than that in blood pool background are called "positive" while those with less than blood pool background are called "negative." Quantitative cutoff values of SUV have been proposed with 2.5 as a good separator of malignant and benign nodules; however, in practice, measurement errors could make a lesion with a true SUV of 2.7 appear to have an SUV of 2.4 (due to variance of the measurement method). Most centers tend to err on the side of sensitivity as opposed to specificity in interpreting PET of SPN to avoid false-negative results. A review of the meta-analysis of Gould et al. (7) shows that although a joint operating sensitivity/

specificity of 91% is possible with PET using FDG in SPN, most readers operate to achieve higher sensitivity at the tradeoff of lower specificity.

NON–SMALL CELL LUNG CANCER

Non–small cell lung cancer (NSCLC) comprises about 80% of all lung cancers, and many patients are smokers or have had significant exposure to secondhand smoke. The most common cell types, in order of occurrence, are adenocarcinoma, including bronchoalveolar variants, squamous cell carcinoma, and large cell. In the past decade, the frequency of adenocarcinomas has grown steadily. Some of the patients with adenocarcinomas are nonsmokers, and a significant fraction are females (18). Surgical resection represents the best opportunity for cure, but recently combination therapy including chemotherapy, radiation therapy, and to some extent biological therapy has been employed with increasing frequency. NSCLC staging is based on the TNM system and requires accurate characterization of the primary tumor (T), regional lymph nodes (N), and distant metastases (M). Staging is important for appropriate selection of treatment and assessment of prognosis.

Non–small Cell Lung Cancer Tumor Stage

Tumors are described as T1 when they are 3 cm or less in greatest dimension arising distal to a main bronchus. A T2 tumor is one that is larger than 3 cm, invades the visceral pleura, or has local atelectasis or obstruction associated with it and is located greater than 2 cm from the carina. A T3 tumor invades the chest wall, diaphragm, mediastinal pleura, or pericardium or is associated with diffuse atelectasis or obstruction, and it can be 0 to 2 cm from the carina without involving the carina. A T4 tumor is one that invades vital mediastinal structures such as heart, great vessels, trachea, carina, or vertebral bodies or has a malignant effusion or separate tumor nodules in the same lobe. These stages are largely intended to distinguish which tumors are and are not resectable—all but T4 being potentially resectable. These tumor stages are components of the TNM staging classification (19).

Traditionally T stage information has been obtained by CT and depends on anatomic abnormalities detectable by CT. This can be most helpful when determining the direct extension and involvement of the tumor into normal structures that can change disease stage. FDG PET alone had played a minor role in T staging due to challenges in measuring tumor size and in determining the precise borders/extent of the FDG uptake. Integrated PET/CT provides improved T staging in the detection of chest wall and mediastinal invasion and for evaluating the degree of atelectasis involved in the CT tumor mass (20). The detection of malignant pleural effusions and pleural metastases is substantially aided by PET/CT evaluation.

Non–small Cell Lung Cancer Node Stage

The presence of metastatic disease in lymph nodes correlates closely with worsening survival. N0 status indicates no nodal metastases. An N1 status implies a metastasis to ipsilateral peribronchial, lobar, or interlobar nodes. N2 implies a metastasis to ipsilateral mediastinal or subcarinal nodes. N3 indicates involvement of contralateral lymph nodes, scalene, or supraclavicular nodes. N0 status correlates with a 56.5% 5-year survival rate, and N1 disease correlates with a 47.5% 5-year survival rate. Only a 10% to 20% survival rate or less is seen once N2-level nodes are involved. Generally, those with N3 lymph node disease do not survive 5 years, and N3 disease is commonly a contraindication to surgery (21).

The noninvasive assessment of mediastinal nodes for tumor involvement is relatively difficult with CT. Because of the possibility of nodal enlargement from reactive or inflammatory lung diseases or even congestive heart disease, there is ample probability that enlarged nodes may not be involved with tumor. The nodal size limit of normality used in CT imaging is about 1 cm for the short axis of the lymph node. Therefore, any lymph node containing tumor that is less than 1 cm in short axis length will not be called abnormal by size criteria. Any lymph nodes that are larger than 1 cm will be called abnormal and are suggestive of a metastasis in a patient with a lung cancer history. Many such enlarged nodes do not contain malignant cells but are enlarged due to other causes.

Alternatively, invasive sampling with mediastinoscopy can be performed to assess lymph node status. This procedure is unable to assess all lymph nodes with a single point of access. Specifically the aortopulmonary lymph nodes cannot be assessed without a different approach to the lymph nodes. The result is that the selection of lymph nodes for biopsy by the mediastinoscopy technique is based on accessibility. This results in a high, albeit imperfect, sensitivity for mediastinal disease of about 90% (22,23). It is unlikely that this will improve due to the limitations of the technique. Transbronchial needle biopsy of lymph nodes is also useful but is limited in sensitivity in part due to its "blind" nature and due to areas that cannot be sampled. This approach can be guided by PET and by ultrasound, but still suffers from sampling errors that lower sensitivity of the method.

Preoperative noninvasive evaluation of hilar and mediastinal adenopathy is a major clinical role of PET imaging. Abnormal FDG uptake in metastatic NSCLC within lymph nodes is readily visualized by PET and well documented in the literature. Multiple reports dating from Wahl's prospective study published in *Radiology* in 1994 have shown FDG PET to be significantly more accurate than CT for staging the mediastinum in patients with NSCLC (24).

Pieterman et al. (25) compared PET and CT to surgical staging of the mediastinum in 102 patients. PET provided a 16% improvement in sensitivity over CT (91% vs. 75%) and a 20% improvement in specificity (86% vs. 66%). FDG PET provides substantial improvement in N staging over CT. Unfortunately, PET alone led to poor anatomical accuracy, which is often sought by pulmonologists and surgeons.

The combined functional and structural data with PET/CT is synergistic for NSCLC N staging. Lardinosis et al. (20) documented this substantial improvement in accuracy. In their study, PET was only 61% accurate versus integrated PET/CT, which was 81% accurate. It is unclear why PET was of such low accuracy in this study, given that the accuracy of PET in many other studies is higher, but it was clear that PET/CT was significantly better than PET alone. Compared to histologic evaluation of the mediastinum, PET/CT was correct 88% of the time, whereas PET only was definitive in 40% and equivocal in 40%. In this study, PET/CT failed to detect three nodal locations, two microscopic and one 5-mm metastases. A reduction in the number of equivocal readings is quite common for PET/CT versus PET.

Accurate nodal staging is imperative for surgical decision making. Cefolio et al. (26) demonstrated that integrated PET/CT predicted stage I and II substantially better than PET alone, and selected those patients where primary surgical therapy would be

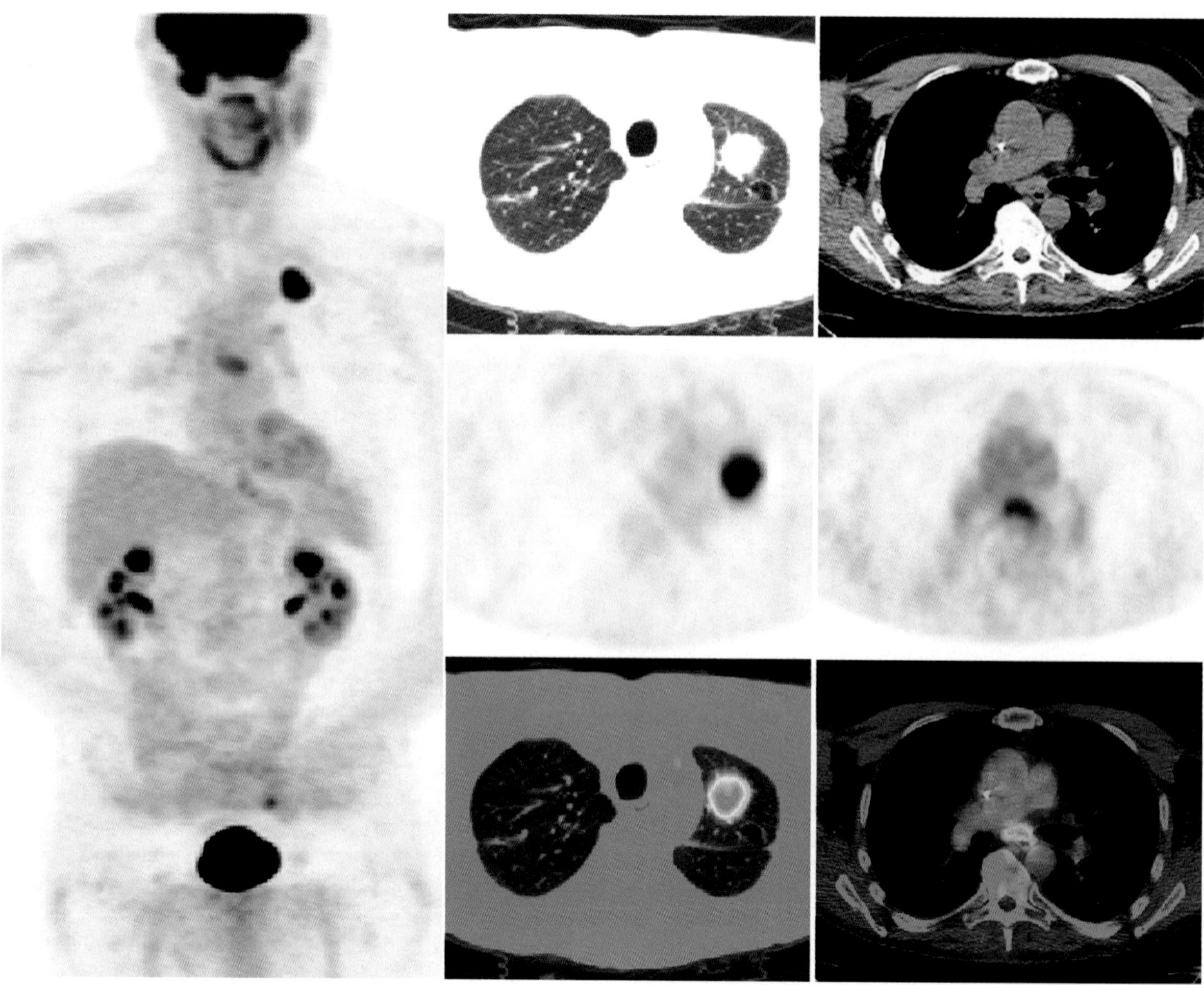

FIGURE 8.9.3. Non–small cell lung cancer staging—maximum intensity projection (MIP) (**left**) and transaxial CT (**top**), PET (**middle**), and fused images (**bottom**). This patient is a 62-year-old man with left-sided pleuritic chest pain. On CT a 3.2 cm soft tissue mass was noted in the left upper lobe. PET/CT images demonstrate intense increased activity within this mass. Moderate activity is present in the enlarged subcarinal lymph node. Transtracheal bronchoscopic directed biopsy confirmed adenocarcinoma in the subcarinal lymph node. The patient was treated with neoadjuvant chemoradiotherapy and is awaiting re-evaluation for surgery.

favored. Correct identification of N1 and N2 disease was observed with reported accuracies of 90% and 96% respectively. When PET and PET/CT nodal staging is used to direct surgical biopsy, the process is more selective and sensitive. Vesselle et al. (27) reported that 25% of surgical biopsies to confirm PET staging in NSCLC were correctly directed away from customary locations (Fig. 8.9.3). Thus, PET/CT is a commonly performed procedure before biopsy is performed in many patients with known or suspected NSCLC.

Non–small Cell Lung Cancer Metastasis Stage

The presence of distant metastases (M1) categorizes the patient as having stage IV NSCLC, which removes the consideration for cure and treatment is nonsurgical and primarily palliative. The most common locations of distant metastases in NSCLC are the adrenal glands, skeleton, brain, and liver (28). Undetected M1 disease is partially responsible for the overall 5-year survival, with "curative" surgery being less than 60%. PET scan coverage of trunk, neck, and proximal extremities is well suited for detection of distant metastases. Sensitivity in the head for PET is less than that for anatomic imaging, however, as many small metastases can fail to be detected due to their location at the gray–white matter interface, where they are less apparent due to the intense tracer activity in the normal brain.

In a recent meta-analysis, Hellwig et al. (29) evaluated 581 patients and demonstrated that the sensitivity of PET for distant metastasis was 94% and the specificity was 97%. The rate of unexpected extrathoracic metastasis in the literature ranges from 6% to 20%. In NSCLC patients evaluated with integrated PET/CT 35% show multiple metastatic lesions. Greater than 50% of solitary extrapulmonary lesions typically are due to metastases. With PET/CT additional malignancies are identified in nearly 10%, but inflammation or other benign causes occur in nearly 40% of

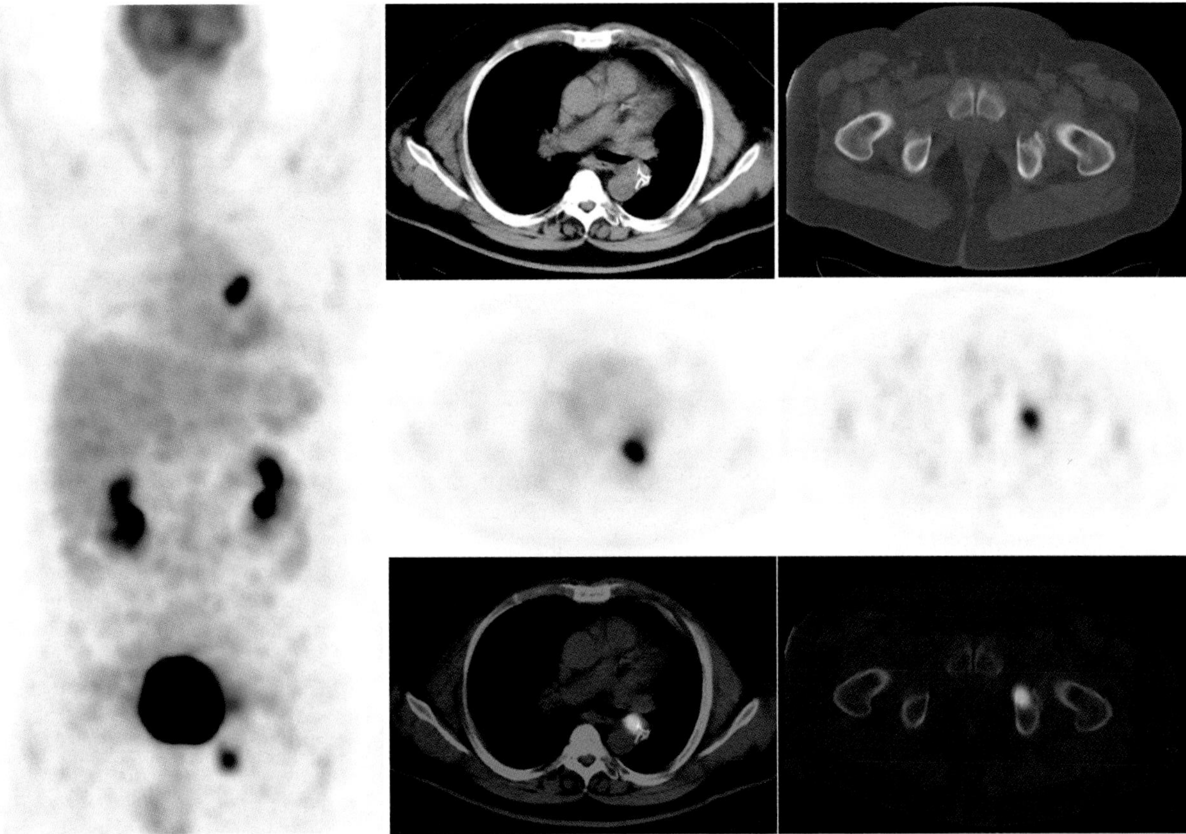

FIGURE 8.9.4. PET/CT non–small cell lung cancer staging—maximum intensity projection (MIP) (**left**) and transaxial CT (**top**), PET (**middle**), and fused images (**bottom**). This patient is a 51-year-old man with a new onset of cough and a CT scan demonstrating a left lower lobe lung nodule and a normal mediastinum. PET/CT images demonstrated intense increased fluorodeoxyglucose accumulation within this nodule. No mediastinal nodal abnormalities were present but an intense abnormality was noted in the right acetabulum. Bone biopsy confirmed metastatic adenocarcinoma corresponding to the bronchoscopic biopsy of the patient's lung nodule. The patient received chemotherapy and radiation therapy to the left lung.

patients (30). The CT portion of the integrated PET/CT not only enhances anatomical localization but allows improved classification and aids specificity in distant metastases. The frequency of detection of metastatic disease at presentation is dependent to a considerable extent on the size of the primary tumor. For early stage I tumors, PET of the whole body has a lower yield than for T2 to T4 primary lesions (Fig. 8.9.4).

For some, SUV stands for "silly useless value" (31). The semiquantitative evaluation of FDG accumulation with SUV is not crucial for most aspects of clinical diagnosis or staging. Accurate and precise SUV determinations require consistent technique: standard time of imaging after FDG administration, completeness of injection, routine entry of accurate patient data such as weight/height, fasting, similar acquisition and reconstruction parameters, and region of interest. A number of authors have suggested that SUV has important prognostic value. In the largest study to date Cerfolio et al. (32) found that patients with maximum SUVs in excess of 10.0 were associated with poorly differentiated malignancies and advanced stage. In an evaluation of 315 patients with surgical resection of NSCLC, an SUV 10.0 or greater in the primary tumor corresponded to poorer disease-free survival. When patients were stratified by stage, the 4-year survival varied significantly depending on maximum SUV. SUV was an independent predictor of outcome regardless of stage. The SUV provided additional prognostic information above and beyond the TNM stage to predict recurrence and survival in NSCLC.

The impact of PET on the management of lung cancer patients has been a source of controversy for the past decade. The authors are aware of more than ten published studies over the 3-year period following Pieterman's article in 1997 that demonstrated proposed changes in management ranging from 10% to 59% with the potential application of PET (25). A variety of methods and measurements were utilized, and many studies were retrospective. The European PET in LUng cancer Staging (PLUS) study enrolled patients in one of two randomized arms adding PET to the evaluation of NSCLC patients in one arm (33). This study demonstrated that the addition of PET produced a 50% drop in futile thoracotomies. Additional analysis showed that the results of adding PET were quite robust. PET information added clinical benefit prior to, during, and after surgery, and in this group lowered total cost, mainly due to a 51% reduction in number of thoracotomies. In the United States the prospective American College of Surgeons Oncology Group trial demonstrated similar findings where unnecessary thoracotomies were avoided in one of five patients (34).

Integrated PET/CT improves detection of T4 and M1 disease. PET/CT is very important in N staging and can provide specific regional node classification as described by Mountain and Dressler (35). The SUV has prognostic implications independent of TNM staging. The FDG uptake provides tumor conspicuity, the CT component provides the anatomic clarity, and the PET/CT fused images yield diagnostic certainty. NSCLC is and should remain a frequent indication for PET and PET/CT.

Non–small Cell Lung Cancer Restaging

Detection of NSCLC recurrence compared to postoperative surgical changes is often quite difficult on clinical grounds and with CT. Hellwig et al. (36) employed PET following lung cancer surgery and demonstrated relapse with PET in 51 patients for a sensitivity of 93%. PET also predicted the absence of relapse in 16 of 18 patients for a specificity of 89%. The intensity of FDG uptake in the recurrent foci had important prognostic implications as a maximum SUV greater than 11.0 was associated with diminished survival regardless of therapy. The identification of relapse by PET allowed selection of patients who were candidates for repeat surgical resection of disease.

The evaluation of patients for residual malignancy at completion of therapy has become an important role of PET. Bury et al. (37) evaluated PET and CT in 126 patients with NSCLC following completion of treatment. PET demonstrated residual disease in 100% versus a sensitivity of 72% with CT scan. Similar specificity was seen with both PET and CT (92% vs. 95%). PET was correct 96% of the time in predicting the patient's response to therapy. PET was substantially better when CT demonstrated residual scar or fibrosis in the area of prior tumor. Of course, PET cannot be expected to detect microscopic disease especially after the FDG uptake is reduced by treatment.

Determining the response to chemotherapy in NSCLC has led investigators to PET for measurement of metabolic response rather than using morphologic response on CT. The advent of neoadjuvant chemotherapy has created a substantial additional role for PET. Eschmann et al. (38) studied 70 patients before and after completing preoperative chemoradiotherapy. PET scanning demonstrated high sensitivity (95%) and moderate specificity (80%) for evaluation of the residual disease. PET detected downstaging of the mediastinum with results validated by mediastinoscopy or surgery. In this group of patients a negative PET scan or a decrease in SUV of greater than 80% was predictive of prolonged survival.

Cerfolio et al. (39) compared PET to CT assessment of neoadjuvant chemotherapy for predicting final pathologic response of resected NSCLC. In 56 patients who had PET and CT performed prior to chemotherapy and immediately prior to surgery, the change in SUV predicted tumor response. The cutoff of greater than 80% decline of maximum SUV predicted a greater than 80% response in tumor. PET sensitivity for response was 90% versus CT sensitivity of 47%. Pottgen et al. (40) evaluated patients with stage III NSCLC undergoing chemotherapy with two serial PET/CT scans, before and after three cycles. A 50% drop in SUV of the primary tumor and N2 nodes indicated histologic response. Disease-free survival was 83% in responders versus 43% in nonresponders. PET/CT response in the primary tumor and mediastinal lymph nodes also had prognostic value.

With the utility of PET in evaluating neoadjuvant chemotherapy prior to surgery and the predictive value of survival supported by data in the literature, Weber et al. (41) chose to evaluate the early prediction of tumor response with PET. Patients were evaluated immediately prior to and after the first cycle of chemotherapy. A SUV decline of 20% was used as the criterion of response. Tumor response was based on Response Evaluation Criteria in Solid Tumor (RECIST) standards blinded to PET results. PET's ability to predict clinical response overall with high sensitivity (96%) and specificity (97%) would allow rapid shift to alternative therapy in PET nonresponders. These encouraging results are being further evaluated in a larger prospective multicenter trial (Fig. 8.9.5).

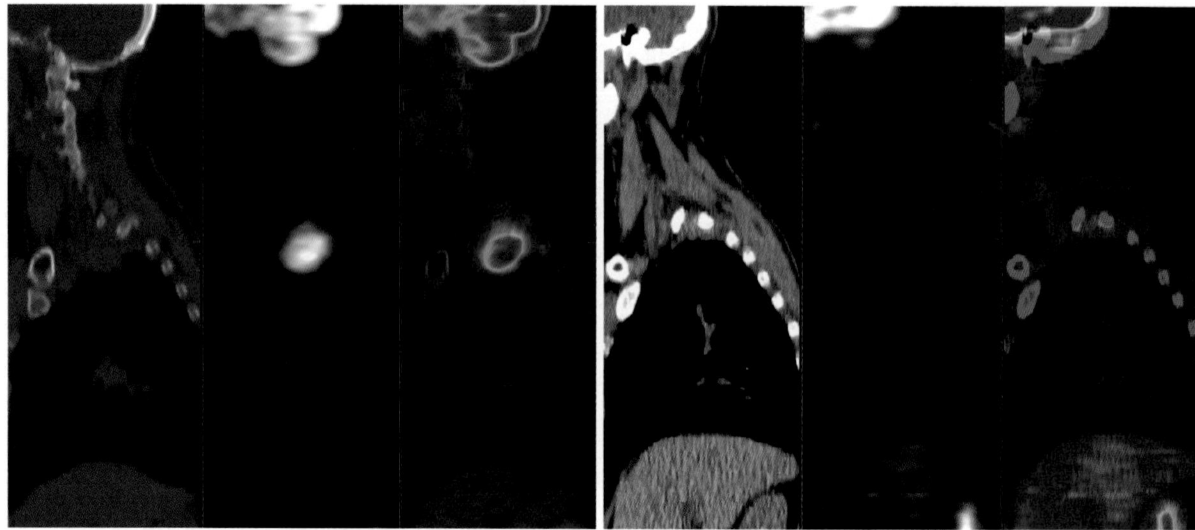

FIGURE 8.9.5. PET–CT restaging of non–small cell lung cancer—sagittal CT, PET, and fused images (**left**) prior to therapy and (**right**) after therapy. This patient is a 63-year-old man with a left Pancoast tumor who had biopsy proven squamous cell carcinoma. Because of the degree of chest wall invasion, the patient underwent chemoradiotherapy with marked shrinkage of the mass. The patient subsequently underwent *en bloc* resection.

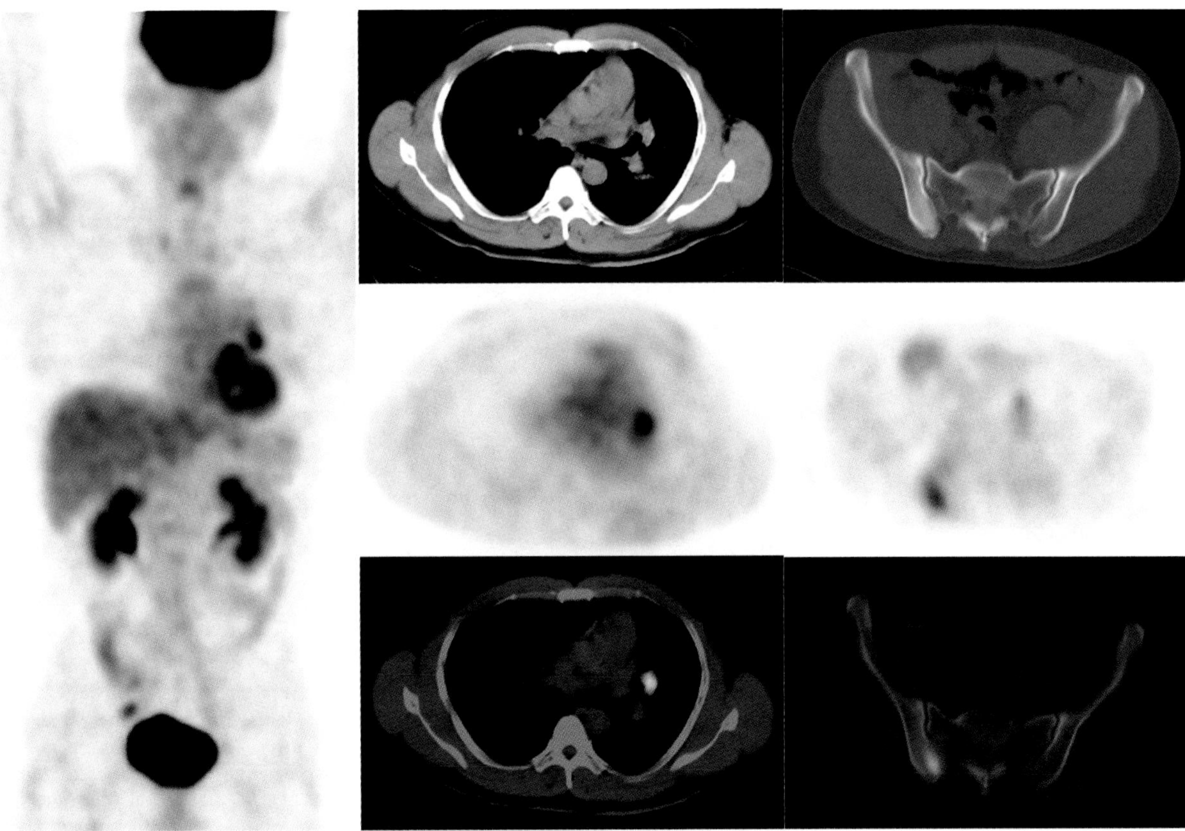

FIGURE 8.9.6. PET/CT small cell lung cancer staging—maximum intensity projection (MIP) (**left**) and transaxial CT (**top**), PET (**middle**), and fused images (**bottom**). This patient is a 56-year-old man with a history of four packs a day smoking. His chest x-ray demonstrated left hilar prominence. A CT scan demonstrated a central 2-cm lung mass. Bronchoscopic biopsy of the endobronchial mass demonstrated small cell lung cancer. Based on the CT scan and bronchoscopy, the patient was initially felt to be limited stage small cell lung cancer. Chemotherapy followed by radiation or possibly surgical resection was originally planned. PET/CT demonstrates intense activity in the left lung mass and similar fluorodeoxyglucose uptake in a right ilium. Bone biopsy confirmed extensive stage small cell lung cancer. Chemotherapy produced complete resolution of these lesions.

SMALL CELL LUNG CANCER

Small cell lung cancer (SCLC) represents about 20% of all lung cancers and is a disease almost exclusively of smokers. SCLC has rapid tumor mass doubling time, high growth fraction, and the early development of distant metastases. Because of these differences from NSCLC a two-stage system is employed: limited stage, defined as disease in only one hemithorax, and extensive stage, defined as disease outside tone hemithorax. At presentation, about 30% to 40% of patients have limited-stage disease, but all are assumed to have dissemination. Limited-stage disease is typically treated with combined chemoradiotherapy therapy, while those with extensive-stage disease receive chemotherapy alone. Although SCLC is highly responsive to chemotherapy and radiotherapy, most patients relapse within 2 years despite aggressive treatment. The overall 5-year survival is only 3% to 8% of all patients with SCLC and is 10% to 13% of those with limited disease (42).

The biology of SCLC leads to high FDG uptake in sites of tumor. The utility of PET for staging SCLC versus conventional CT and magnetic resonance was studied in 120 patients. Concordant staging was found in the majority, but ten were correctly upstaged and three downstaged. For detection of extrathoracic nodal disease PET was more sensitive than CT (100% vs. 70%) with similar specificity (98% vs. 94%). In detection of extracerebral distant metastases, PET was more sensitive and specific (98% vs. 83%, 92% vs. 79%). The sensitivity of PET typically was poor in the brain (46%) compared to magnetic resonance, much as is the case in NSCLC (43). Kamel et al. (44) demonstrated that utilizing PET to evaluate SCLC changed management in 29% of patients. The majority of changes were in modifying the patient's radiotherapy following completion of chemotherapy to ensure inclusion of all known disease. Many patients have persistent positive PET scans following completion of current treatment and have clinical relapses within 12 months at these FDG-avid sites. Blum et al. (45) suggest that patients treated to a complete remission on posttherapy PET have a longer median time to disease remission (Fig. 8.9.6).

PLEURAL DISEASE

The parietal pleura lining the inner surface of the chest wall and the visceral pleura on the outer surface of the lung create a potential

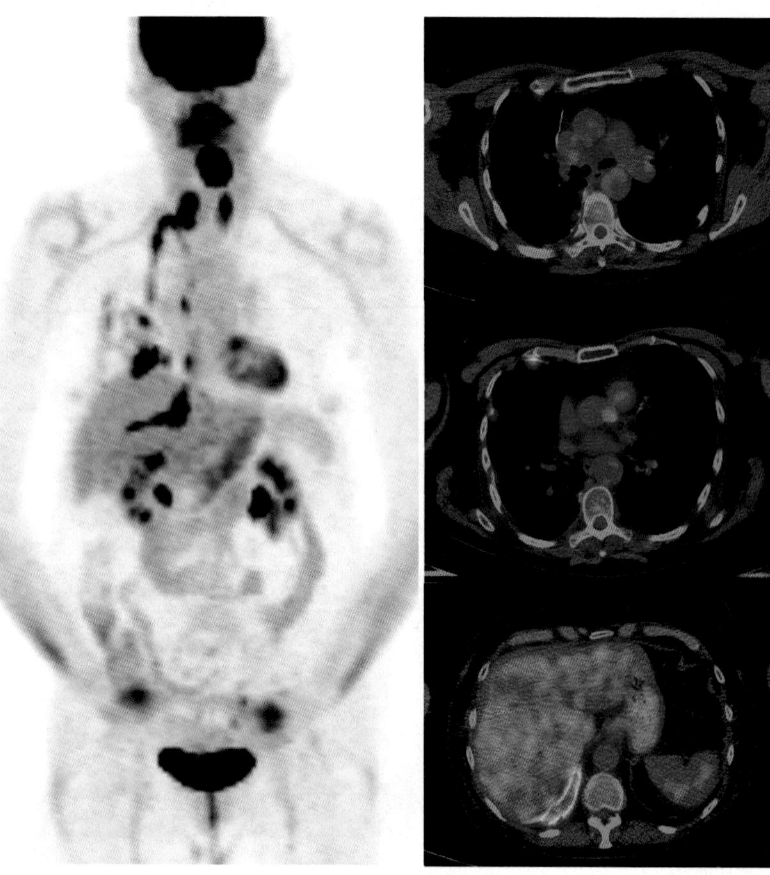

FIGURE 8.9.7. Talc pleurodesis—maximum intensity projection (MIP) (**left**) and transaxial CT, PET, and fused images (**right**). This patient presented for staging of laryngeal cancer. The patient had a persistent right pneumothorax 6 years prior and had undergone talc pleurodesis. There is substantial fluorodeoxyglucose accumulation along the right pleural surfaces where talc remains a chronic irritant.

space where tumor cells can freely migrate. Irritation and alteration of permeability of the pleural layers can increase the fluid in the pleural space dramatically. Pleural effusions are produced by a wide variety of causes. Carcinoma of the lung, breast, and ovary and lymphoma are responsible for inducing about 80% of all malignant effusions. CT scanning demonstrates pleural anatomy and the presence of an effusion, but diagnosis requires fluid analysis via thoracentesis. The cause of a pleural effusion may not be evident following initial diagnostic thoracentesis in up to 25% of patients, and pleural biopsies are not uncommonly required (46).

FDG PET has been used to evaluate pleural masses and pleural effusions for evidence of malignancy. Initial reports by Eramus et al. (47) in 25 patients demonstrated FDG accumulation within malignant pleural effusions. The reported sensitivity and specificity were 95% and 67%, respectively. A high positive predictive value allowed FDG PET to improve staging in NSCLC involving the pleura and in patients with metastatic disease to the pleural surface (48). PET/CT has substantially increased the ability to detect small pleural effusions and small pleural metastases. FDG PET negative pleural effusions are commonly followed as opposed to aggressively investigated, although it should be recognized that both false-positive and false-negative PET studies can be demonstrated, and it is not clear what the precise optimal cutoff value is for intensity of FDG uptake in an effusion to separate tumor-positive from tumor-negative effusions.

Talc pleurodesis is performed for treatment of persistent pneumothorax or a recurrent pleural effusion in patients with cancer and occasionally in patients without malignancies. Malignant pleural effusions are frequently treated with talc to avoid symptoms due to recurrent fluid accumulation. The talc irritates the pleura and creates a persistent, chronic inflammation that leads to fibrosis and obliteration of the pleural space. Talc-induced inflammation typically induces moderate to intense FDG uptake, which might be mistaken as due to tumor. Evaluation of the corresponding CT images will demonstrate increased density due to the talc. The FDG uptake can be focal or diffuse along the pleura, most commonly observed in dependent locations and the costophrenic angles. The activity will often persist on PET for months to years. On serial studies, the abnormal activity from talc pleurodesis will remain stable, whereas a new pleural abnormality is likely a metastasis. Draining lymph nodes can also receive talc and become inflamed and have persistent increased FDG uptake, despite a lack of tumor involvement. It is critical to obtain a careful clinical history in each patient to evaluate for possible talc treatment (49) (Fig. 8.9.7).

Mesothelioma is a rare malignancy, which most commonly arises from the pleural surface. Mesothelioma insidiously grows along the pleural surface and presents with a large pleural effusion. It typically occurs in the fifth to seventh decades of life, and many patients have a history of asbestos exposure. CT is commonly used to diagnose stage and monitor the treatment. Mesothelioma has an extremely poor prognosis, with a mean survival of 4 to 13 months in untreated patients (50).

PET/CT has been employed in the diagnosis and staging of malignant pleural mesothelioma. In 29 patients who by conventional imaging were judged to be candidates for subpleural pneumonectomy and who underwent PET/CT evaluation, integrated PET/CT provided additional staging information in 38% of the patients. T4 unresectable disease was found in 21% and distant metastases were detected in 29%. A total of 40% of patients thought

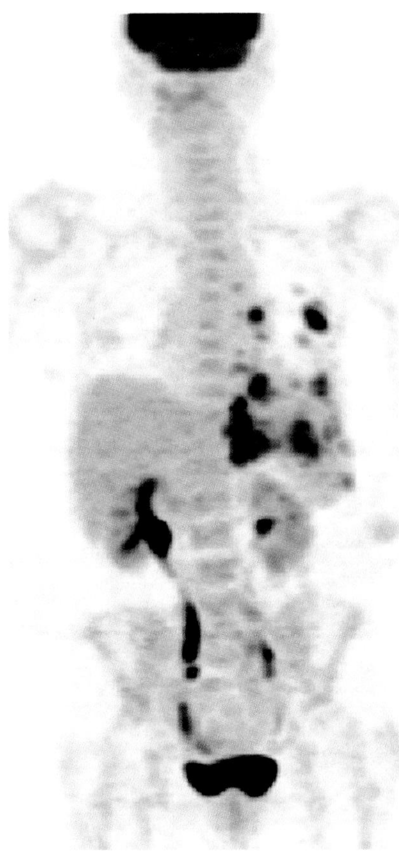
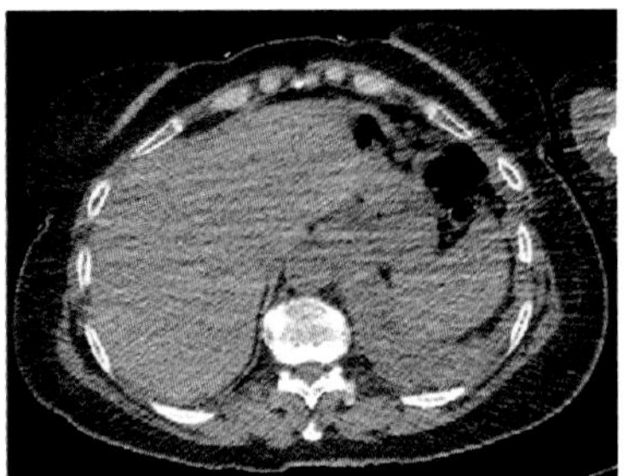
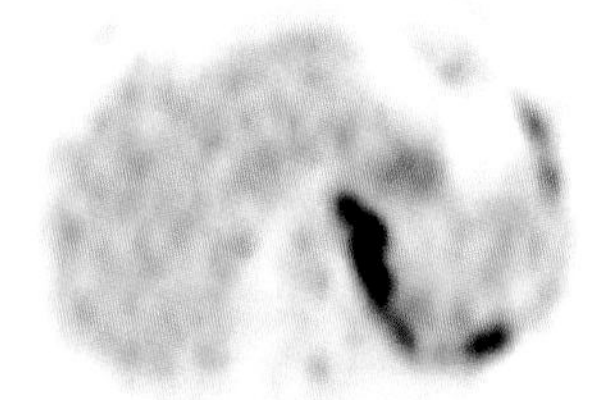
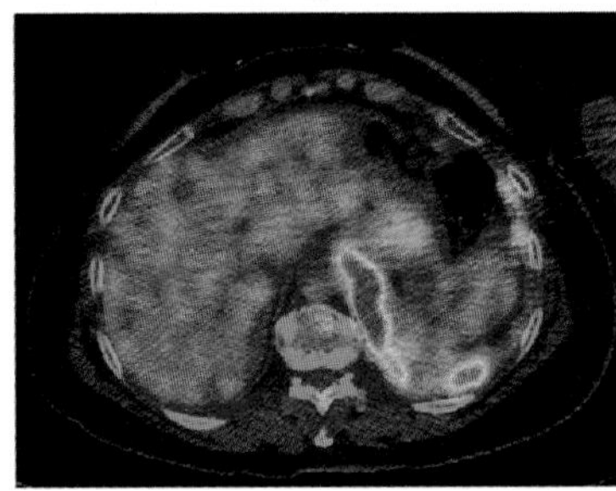

FIGURE 8.9.8. PET/CT mesothelioma staging—maximum intensity projection (MIP) (**left**) and transaxial CT (**top**), PET (**middle**), and fused images (**bottom**). This patient is a 53-year-old man with right pleural thickening who presented for a right pleural effusion. The markedly thickened pleura on the left has patchy but intense hypermetabolism and is typical of mesothelioma. Hypermetabolic adenopathy in the hilum is present and was confirmed to be metastatic disease. The patient received neoadjuvant chemoradiotherapy and underwent an extra pleural left pneumonectomy.

to be potential candidates for curative surgery were found to have local or distant disease with PET/CT, which precluded an attempt to cure (51). A recent publication showed that maximum SUV values greater than 10.0 in malignant mesothelioma predict a poorer prognosis similar to that found in NSCLC. High SUV tumors were associated with 1.9 times the risk of death than lower uptake tumors (52). A multidisciplinary approach to malignant mesothelioma has become common. Patients not uncommonly are receiving chemoradiotherapy prior to attempts at curative surgery. PET measurements of tumor FDG uptake declining more than 25% were used as criterion for a metabolic response to therapy. These patients with metabolic response had twice the median survival of nonresponders (53) (Fig. 8.9.8).

OTHER PET TRACERS

This chapter has focused on the most widely used PET tracer, FDG. This tracer has advanced PET imaging and PET/CT to its current state and is immensely valuable. Although page limitations prevent extensive discussion of other tracers here, it should be realized that tracers of amino acid transport (e.g., carbon-11-L-methionine and proliferation, such as fluorine-18-fluorothymidine) may also be quite useful in lung cancer assessment. Although uptake of fluorothymidine is lower than that of FDG in many tumors, it may be more specific and may have a growing role in therapy assessment (see Chapter 8.4). The carbon-11 amino acid is unlikely to be used in routine practice, but there is considerable effort under way to develop fluorine-18–labeled amino acids for tumor imaging. Similarly, agents targeting hypoxia may also prove useful in evaluating lung cancer, especially when it comes to radiation therapy planning, which is discussed in detail in Chapter 8.5. Thus, while FDG remains the workhorse of PET imaging, other tracers may have a growing role in the coming years (see Chapter 8.25), although it is improbable FDG will be supplanted as the lead tracer in PET lung cancer imaging.

CONCLUSION

Smoking and lung cancer continue to inflict significant morbidity and mortality on patients throughout the world. In the past decade, there has been increased understanding of lung cancer biology, enhancement in PET and CT technology, and improved therapy, including medical, surgical, and radiation treatments. The superb performance characteristics of PET along with marked improvements in FDG availability, reimbursement, access to PET, and PET technology have fueled an explosion in the use of PET. PET and PET/CT with FDG have, in the past 15 years, become firmly established as one of the earliest tests to obtain in patients with known or suspected lung cancer. PET is accurate in characterizing solitary pulmonary nodules as malignant or benign. It is highly accurate in initial nodal and systemic staging. As discussed in Chapter 8.4 and 8.5, it is increasingly applied to plan radiation treatment procedures and is now used to monitor both neoadjuvant and systemic chemotherapy and combined treatments. PET techniques continue to improve, but there are limitations of PET with FDG with both false-positive and false-negative scans. Nonetheless, PET and PET/CT are now firmly established as valuable tools for assessment of lung cancer at many points in the course of disease management.

The authors hope that advancements against the lung cancer epidemic will continue and steadily improve patient care and outcomes.

REFERENCES

1. Jemal A, Siegel R, Ward E, et al. Cancer statistics, 2006. *CA Cancer J Clin* 2006;56:106.
2. Pisani P, Parkin DM, Ferlay J. Estimates of the worldwide mortality from eighteen major cancers in 1985. Implications for prevention and projections of future burden. *Int J Cancer* 1993;55:891.
3. Ginsberg MS. Epidemiology of lung cancer. *Semin Roentgenol* 2005;40(2):83–89.
4. Proctor RN. The global smoking epidemic: a history and status report. *Clin Lung Cancer* 2004;5(6):371–376.
5. Kuper H, Adami HO, Boffetta P. Tobacco use, cancer causation and public health impact. *J Intern Med* 2002;251(6):455–466.
6. Toomes H, Delphendahl A, Manke H-G, et al. The coin lesion of the lung. A review of 955 resected coin lesions. *Cancer* 1983;51:534.
7. Gould MK, Sanders GD, Barnett PG, et al. Cost-effectiveness of alternative management strategies for patients with solitary pulmonary nodules. *Ann Intern Med* 2003;138:724.
8. Herth FJ, Ernst A, Becker HD. Endobronchial ultrasound-guided transbronchial lung biopsy in solitary pulmonary nodules and peripheral lesions. *Eur Respir J* 2002;20:972.
9. Berquist TH, Bailey PB, Cortese DA, et al. Transthoracic needle biopsy: accuracy and complications in relation to location and type of lesion. *Mayo Clin Proc* 1980;55:475.
10. Allen MS, Deschamps C, Lee RE, et al. Video-assisted thoracoscopic stapled wedge excision for indeterminate pulmonary nodules. *J Thorac Cardiovasc Surg* 1993;106:1048.
11. Gould MK, Maclean CC, Kuschner WG, et al. Accuracy of positron emission tomography for diagnosis of pulmonary nodules and mass lesions: a meta-analysis. *JAMA* 2001;285(7):914–924.
12. Chhajed PN, Bernasconi M, Gambazzi F, et al. Combining bronchoscopy and positron emission tomography for the diagnosis of the small pulmonary nodule < or = 3 cm. *Chest* 2005;128(5): 3558–3564.
13. Pitman AG, Hicks RJ, Kalff V, et al. Positron emission tomography in pulmonary masses where tissue diagnosis is unhelpful or not possible. *Med J Aust* 2001;175(6):303–307.
14. Yi CA, Lee KS, Kim BT, et al. Tissue characterization of solitary pulmonary nodule: comparative study between helical dynamic CT and integrated PET/CT. *J Nucl Med* 2006;47(3):443–450.
15. Zhuang H, Pourdehnad M, Lambright ES, et al. Dual time point ^{18}F-FDG PET imaging for differentiating malignant from inflammatory processes. *J Nucl Med* 2001;42(9):1412–1417.
16. Hickeson M, Yun M, Matthies A, et al. Use of a corrected standardized uptake value based on the lesion size on CT permits accurate characterization of lung nodules on FDG-PET. *Eur J Nucl Med Mol Imaging* 2002;29(12):1639–1647.
17. Nehmeh SA, Erdi YE, Pan T, et al. Four-dimensional (4D) PET/CT imaging of the thorax. *Med Phys* 2004;31(12):3179–3186.
18. Gabrielson E. Worldwide trends in lung cancer pathology. *Respirology* 2006;11(5):533–538.
19. Greene FL, Page DL, Fleming ID, et al., eds. *American Joint Committee on Cancer cancer staging manual*, 6th ed. New York: Springer-Verlag, 2002.
20. Lardinois D, Weder W, Hany TF, et al. Staging of non–small cell lung cancer with integrated positron-emission tomography and computed tomography. *N Engl J Med* 2003;348(25):2500–2507.
21. Riquet M, Manac'h D, Le Pimpec-Barthes F, et al. Prognostic significance of surgical-pathologic N1 disease in non–small cell carcinoma of the lung. *Ann Thorac Surg* 1999;67(6):1572–1576.
22. Van Schil PE, Van HRH, Schoofs EL. The value of mediastinoscopy in preoperative staging of bronchogenic carcinoma. *J Thorac Cardiovasc Surg* 1989;97:240–244.
23. Patterson GA, Ginsberg RJ, Poon PY, et al. A prospective evaluation of magnetic resonance imaging, computed tomography, and mediastinoscopy in the preoperative assessment of mediastinal node status in bronchogenic carcinoma. *J Thorac Cardiovasc Surg* 1987;94:679–684.
24. Wahl RL, Quint LE, Greenough RL, et al. Staging of mediastinal non-small cell lung cancer with FDG PET, CT, and fusion images: preliminary prospective evaluation. *Radiology* 1994;191(2):371–377.
25. Pieterman RM, van Putten JW, Meuzelaar JJ, et al. Preoperative staging of non-small-cell lung cancer with positron-emission tomography. *N Engl J Med* 2000;343(4):254–261.
26. Cerfolio RJ, Ojha B, Bryant AS, et al. The accuracy of integrated PET-CT compared with dedicated PET alone for the staging of patients with non–small cell lung cancer. *Ann Thorac Surg* 2004;78(3):1017–1023.
27. Vesselle H, Pugsley JM, Vallieres E, et al. The impact of fluorodeoxyglucose F18 positron-emission tomography on the surgical staging of non–small cell lung cancer. *J Thorac Cardiovasc Surg* 2002;124(3):511–519.
28. Reck M, Gatzemeier U. Chemotherapy in stage-IV NSCLC. *Lung Cancer* 2004;45[Suppl 2]:S217–222.
29. Hellwig D, Ukena D, Paulsen F, et al. Onko-PET der Deutschen Gesellschaft fur Nuklearmedizin [Meta-analysis of the efficacy of positron emission tomography with F-18-fluorodeoxyglucose in lung tumors. Basis for discussion of the German Consensus Conference on PET in Oncology 2000]. *Pneumologie* 2001;55(8):367–377.
30. Lardinois D, Weder W, Roudas M, et al. Etiology of solitary extrapulmonary positron emission tomography and computed tomography findings in patients with lung cancer. *J Clin Oncol* 2005;23(28):6846–6853.
31. Keyes JW Jr. SUV: standard uptake or silly useless value? *J Nucl Med* 1995;36(10):1836–1839.
32. Cerfolio RJ, Bryant AS, Ohja B, et al. The maximum standardized uptake values on positron emission tomography of a non–small cell lung cancer predict stage, recurrence, and survival. *J Thorac Cardiovasc Surg* 2005;130(1):151–159.
33. van Tinteren H, Hoekstra OS, Smit EF, et al. Effectiveness of positron emission tomography in the preoperative assessment of patients with suspected non–small cell lung cancer: the PLUS multicentre randomised trial. *Lancet* 2002;359(9315):1388–1393.
34. Reed CE, Harpole DH, Posther KE, et al. Results of the American College of Surgeons Oncology Group Z0050 trial: the utility of positron emission tomography in staging potentially operable non–small cell lung cancer. *J Thorac Cardiovasc Surg* 2003;126(6):1943–1951.
35. Mountain CF, Dressler CM. Regional lymph node classification for lung cancer staging. *Chest* 1997;111:1718–1723.
36. Hellwig D, Groschel A, Graeter TP, et al. Diagnostic performance and prognostic impact of FDG-PET in suspected recurrence of surgically treated non–small cell lung cancer. *Eur J Nucl Med Mol Imaging* 2006;33(1):13–21.
37. Bury T, Corhay JL, Duysinx B, et al. Value of FDG-PET in detecting residual or recurrent non–small cell lung cancer. *Eur Respir J* 1999;14(6):1376–1380.
38. Eschmann SM, Friedel G, Paulsen F, et al. (18)F-FDG PET for assessment of therapy response and preoperative re-evaluation after neoadjuvant radio-chemotherapy in stage III non–small cell lung cancer. *Eur J Nucl Med Mol Imaging* 2007;34(4):463–471.
39. Cerfolio RJ, Bryant AS, Winokur TS, et al. Repeat FDG-PET after neoadjuvant therapy is a predictor of pathologic response in patients with non–small cell lung cancer. *Ann Thorac Surg* 2004;78(6):1903–1909.
40. Pottgen C, Levegrun S, Theegarten D, et al. Value of ^{18}F-fluoro-2-deoxy-D-glucose-positron emission tomography/computed tomography in non–small cell lung cancer for prediction of pathologic response and times to relapse after neoadjuvant chemoradiotherapy. *Clin Cancer Res* 2006;12(1):97–106.
41. Weber WA, Petersen V, Schmidt B, et al. Positron emission tomography in non–small cell lung cancer: prediction of response to chemotherapy by quantitative assessment of glucose use. *J Clin Oncol* 2003;21(14): 2651–2657.
42. Janne PA, Freidlin B, Saxman S, et al. Twenty-five years of clinical research for patients with limited-stage small cell lung carcinoma in North America. *Cancer* 2002;95:1528.
43. Brink I, Schumacher T, Mix M, et al. Impact of [18F]FDG-PET on the primary staging of small cell lung cancer. *Eur J Nucl Med Mol Imaging* 2004;31(12):1614–1620.

44. Kamel EM, Zwahlen D, Wyss MT, et al. Whole-body (18)F-FDG PET improves the management of patients with small cell lung cancer. *J Nucl Med* 2003;44(12):1911–1917.
45. Blum R, MacManus MP, Rischin D, et al. Impact of positron emission tomography on the management of patients with small-cell lung cancer: preliminary experience. *Am J Clin Oncol* 2004;27(2): 164–171.
46. Collins TR, Sahn SA. Thoracentesis: complications, patient experience, and diagnostic value. *Chest* 1987;91:817.
47. Erasmus JJ, McAdams HP, Rossi SE, et al. FDG PET of pleural effusions in patients with non-small cell lung cancer. *AJR Am J Roentgenol* 2000;175(1):245–249.
48. Schaffler GJ, Wolf G, Schoellnast H, et al. Non–small cell lung cancer: evaluation of pleural abnormalities on CT scans with ^{18}F FDG PET. *Radiology* 2004;231(3):858–865.
49. Kwek BH, Aquino SL, Fischman AJ. Fluorodeoxyglucose positron emission tomography and CT after talc pleurodesis. *Chest* 2004;125(6): 2356–2360.
50. Antman KH. Natural history and epidemiology of malignant mesothelioma. *Chest* 1993;103:373S.
51. Erasmus JJ, Truong MT, Smythe WR, et al. Integrated computed tomography-positron emission tomography in patients with potentially resectable malignant pleural mesothelioma: staging implications. *J Thorac Cardiovasc Surg* 2005;129(6):1364–1370.
52. Flores RM, Akhurst T, Gonen M, et al. Positron emission tomography predicts survival in malignant pleural mesothelioma. *J Thorac Cardiovasc Surg* 2006;132(4):763–768.
53. Ceresoli GL, Chiti A, Zucali PA, et al. Early response evaluation in malignant pleural mesothelioma by positron emission tomography with [18F]fluorodeoxyglucose. *J Clin Oncol* 2006;24(28):4587–4593.

CHAPTER

8.10 Lymphoma and Myeloma

S. N. RESKE

MALIGNANT LYMPHOMA

The use of positron emission tomography (PET) and PET combined with computed tomography (CT) in lymphoma management has shown remarkable growth in the past few years as a wide range of articles have been published showing the generally broad applicability of PET with fluorodeoxyglucose (FDG) in this group of diseases (1–10).

This chapter will summarize the current state of the art for PET and PET/CT in lymphoma, emphasizing the performance, value, and limitations of these technologies. Due to highly increased glycolysis in most malignant lymphomas, FDG is currently the preferred radiopharmaceutical for PET imaging of lymphomas. Interestingly, however, one of the earliest reports of PET imaging in lymphoma used calcium-11-methionine for assessment of viability of a residual mass in non-Hodgkin's lymphoma (NHL) after radiation therapy (11). In a letter to *Lancet* in 1990, Leskinnen-Kallio et al. (11) made the farsighted statement that "PET may be a new way of detecting viable malignant tissue." Since that time, many reports have shown the use and value of PET and more recently of PET/CT imaging of malignant lymphomas for pretherapeutic staging, therapy control, interim response assessment of various combinations of radio-, chemo-, immuno- and radioimmunotherapy (3,12–14), and evaluation of prognosis (10,15,16). Several excellent recent reviews covering these issues have been published (15–19). This chapter will briefly summarize use of FDG PET and PET/CT for (a) initial pretherapeutic staging, (b) relevance of response monitoring, (c) technical considerations, (d) treatment remission assessment, (e) evaluation after completion of chemotherapy and/or radiotherapy, and (f) early response assessment, as well as discuss some novel functional imaging approaches in malignant lymphoma.

Staging

The Ann Arbor classification can be used both for Hodgkin's lymphoma and NHL and differentiates malignant lymphoma distribution into four categories.

Stage I: disease limited to a single lymph node or a single lymph node group;

Stage II: two or more noncontiguous nodal groups or the spleen on the same side of the diaphragma;

Stage III: two or more nodal groups or the spleen on both sides of the diaphragma;

Stage IV: disease in extranodal sides (bone marrow, liver, lung, bone, or other organs/tissues).

Extension from a nodal manifestation into extranodal tissue (S) such as the lung, pleura, pericardium, skin, and so forth may occur in stage I through III and does not increase the stage to stage IV, but is designated by the involved tissue/organ with the subscript "E." Nodal disease greater than 10 cm in the largest diameter is defined as "bulky" and designated with a suffix "X" to the numeric stage (18).

There are several preferred sites of involvement of NHL: compared to Hodgkin's lymphoma, Waldeyer's ring is involved in 5% to 10% of patients with NHL and extremely rarely involved in Hodgkin's lymphoma. Waldeyer's ring involvement by NHL may be associated with involvement of the gastrointestinal tract/stomach or bowel. Mesenteric lymph node involvement is quite common in NHL, but only rarely seen (less than 5%) in Hodgkin's lymphoma. Bone marrow involvement is present in 15% to 40% of patients with NHL (17).

Stage is an important component of a predictive model for untreated patients with intermediate- or high-grade NHL (9). The five important factors at presentation are age (60 years or less vs. greater than 60 years, serum low-density lipoprotein concentration (one or less times normal vs. greater than one times normal), performance status (0 or 1 vs. 2 to 4), stage (I or II vs. III or IV), and extranodal involvement (one or less site vs. more than one site).

FDG PET or more recently FDG PET/CT can be used both for nodal and extranodal staging (14,20–25). Fast and convenient imaging of the whole body or, more practically, the body from the ear to the proximal thigh, within about 30 minutes in conjunction

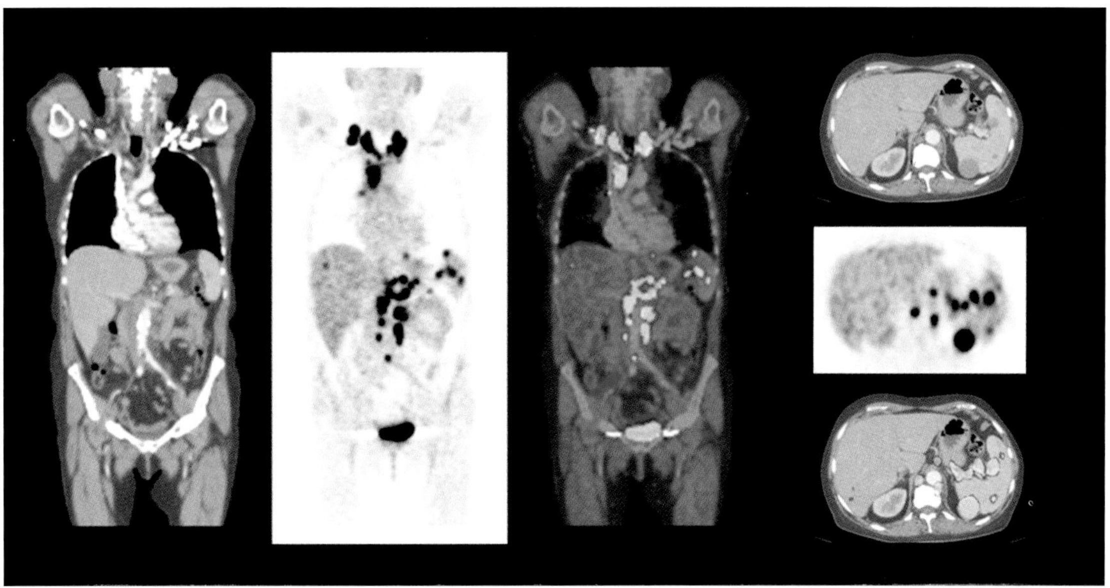

FIGURE 8.10.1. Fluorodeoxyglucose PET-CT staging in non-Hodgkin's lymphoma. The patient has supra- and infradiaphragmatic nodal disease as well as multifocal involvement within the spleen. CT (left), PET (middle), PET/CT (right).

with contrast-enhanced CT provides excellent and precise imaging of virtually all organs and tissues potentially involved by Hodgkin's lymphoma or NHL (Fig. 8.10.1). This approach offers the advantage of both diagnostic CT with the added benefit of the functional imaging of FDG PET with high technical quality and less dependence on size-based criteria, limiting the sensitivity of nodal staging of CT. Thus, increased FDG uptake can be easily measured with FDG PET or FDG PET/CT in nodes less than 1 cm in diameter. In addition, it has been shown that focal involvement of bone marrow can be accurately detected with FDG PET or PET/CT, but is limited with CT. Virtually all nodal groups can be reasonably accurately imaged, with the FDG PET/CT approach in high- and intermediate-grade lymphoma.

Practically all studies comparing FDG PET to CT reported a 10% to 20% higher accuracy of FDG PET for staging of lymphoma and resulted in treatment changes of 10% to 20% (see Hicks et al. [14] for a review). Improved staging in Hodgkin's lymphoma with FDG PET/CT compared to CT was recently demonstrated by Hutchings et al. (26). Many of the lesions detected with PET are in lymph nodes of under 1 cm in size and thus are called normal nodes on CT. Similarly, detection of disease within the spleen is markedly improved using PET versus CT methods.

Limitations of FDG PET or FDG PET/CT for staging are diffuse bone marrow involvement by NHL with less than 10% infiltration of bone marrow with NHL (23), with a reduced sensitivity of FDG PET and probably also FDG PET/CT in some indolent (low-grade) lymphomas (27). The manifestations of FDG uptake in lymphoma vary depending on the histology (28). In a recent study, the sensitivity of FDG PET was excellent (approximately 95%) in grade I to III follicular lymphoma, moderate (74%) in mantle cell lymphoma, and limited (approximately 50%) in B-cell small cell lymphocytic lymphoma (28). A study by Jerusalem et al. (27) reported that FDG PET identified 40% more abnormal lymph node sites then conventional staging in 24 patients with follicular histology, but less than 58% of abnormal nodal sites compared to CT in 11 patients with small lymphocytic lymphoma.

As suggested by studies in a small number of patients, performance of FDG PET is less accurate in patients with mucosa-associated lymphoid tissue lymphoma (29). Sensitivity is probably dependent on histology and limited in low-grade mucosa-associated lymphoid tissue lymphoma (30). With regard to a false-negative case of bronchial wall involvement by NHL reported by Bangerter et al. (31), it is clear that microscopic involvement in any tissue is beyond the detection capabilities of FDG PET or FDG PET/CT. Small tumor volume likely accounts for failure to detect small levels of bone marrow involvement with PET. Unspecific nodal or extranodal FDG uptake due to focal inflammatory disease may be a cause of false-positive results, but this rarely causes problems in the context of initial staging of malignant lymphomas.

Relevance of Response Monitoring

As recently reviewed by Mikhaeel (16), many forms of lymphoma are curable disease, but its treatment is associated with significant short- and long-term toxicity. In the treatment of curable lymphoma (Hodgkin's) and aggressive high-grade NHL the goal of treatment is to achieve a complete response (CR), which is a prerequisite for cure. Patients who do not achieve a CR by the end of treatment are offered various salvage treatment regimens. Accurate assessment of remission after the completion of a planned course of treatment is therefore essential to improve the prognosis of patients with less than CR and to avoid unnecessary treatment-related toxicity and treatment-associated short- and long-term morbidity in those patients who achieve a complete CR.

FDG PET and PET/CT have been very successfully employed for this *posttreatment remission assessment.* Another comparable interesting and potentially more important form of assessment is *early response assessment.* The main goal of this approach is to adjust the intensity and type of treatment to the individual patient's prognosis. Response to treatment is probably the most important single factor determining the prognosis of the individual patient. Response adjusted treatment aims to optimize the balance between the chance of cure and potential toxicity for the individual patient. Early response assessment enables a strategy for minimizing treatment for patients with a good prognosis and intensifying treatment for patients with a poor prognosis (16).

Technical Considerations

The best time for end of treatment evaluation remains unknown, but most investigators suggest waiting at least 1 month after the last day of chemotherapy and 3 months after the last dose of radiotherapy (15,16). It must be kept in mind, that fluorine-18 (^{18}F)-FDG PET or PET/CT cannot exclude minimal residual disease, and it may be indicated to repeat [^{18}F]-FDG PET or PET/CT during routine follow-up to overcome insecurities regarding the potential of residual tumor at the end of treatment (15). Residual lymphoma also may be missed or its extent underestimated because low-grade lymphoma is not FDG avid or has very low uptake. This is, however, relatively uncommon.

Positive findings in PET/CT do not necessarily represent residual disease. Meticulous evaluation of PET images is mandatory to avoid false-positive findings associated with muscle tension or normal intestinal structures. Brown fat can avidly incorporate FDG and is frequently seen in slim young women. Because FDG is not a tumor-specific radiotracer and acute inflammation stimulates glycolytic flux in leucocytes (32), inflammatory lesions may show intense FDG uptake. Documented causes of false-positive PET studies in the assessment of response of lymphoma are shown in Table 8.10.1.

Although not studied in detail in lymphoma, it is well known from studies in various solid tumors that diabetes mellitus and increased blood sugar concentration can reduce the sensitivity of FDG PET considerably (33,34). Therefore, it is the author's institutional practice to examine patients only with a blood sugar concentration below 150 mg/dL and to keep patients fastened at least 5, better 8, hours before the examination. Practice varies by center, but most would not perform PET studies if the serum glucose level exceeds 200 mg/dL. Intravenous furosemide before the PET study in order to flush the renal collecting system and thus to avoid reconstruction artifacts is no longer used by most centers, since powerful iterative reconstruction algorithms and CT-based attenuation correction impressively improve the image quality of PET scans.

Assessment of Treatment Remission

The assessment of remission status commonly involves clinical examination, blood tests, CT scanning, and in some cases histopathological examination of bone marrow and other imaging modalities such as magnetic resonance tomography (16,35). Criteria for response assessment and response categories have been established for lymphoma and are commonly known as the International Workshop Classification (IWC) (35). The IWC predominantly relies on anatomical imaging modalities such as CT scanning or magnetic resonance tomography.

Criteria for response assessment have been recently revised and PET or PET/CT has been implemented (9). The reason for revision was that it had been long recognized that lymphoma masses, especially when bulky on presentation, may not disappear completely if the disease has been eradicated completely (Fig. 8.10.2). These "residual masses" are formed mainly from necrotic or fibrotic tissue and may continue to shrink during follow-up (16,36). Only about 20% of residual masses harbor residual viable malignant cells. Therefore, offering more treatment to all patients with residual masses would involve overtreating many patients unnecessarily (16) (Fig. 8.10.3). Follow-up of these masses to treat only the progressing ones may waste valuable time and compromise the chances of cure.

TABLE 8.10.1 Documented Causes of False-positive Fluorine-18-fluorodeoxyglucose PET Studies in Evaluation of Response

SECOND PRIMARY
Thyroid adenoma
Rebound thymic hyperplasia
INFECTIOUS PROCESS
Toxoplasmosis
Tuberculosis
Pneumonia
Radiotherapy-induced pneumonia/pneumonitis
Inflammatory lung process
Pleural inflammation
Histiocytic reaction
Benign follicular lymph node hyperplasia
Unspecific lymphadenitis
Granulomatous lymphadenitis
Sarcoidosis and sarcoidlike reaction
Epithelioid cell granuloma
Eosinophilic granuloma
Erythema nodosum
Fracture at the site of lymphoma infiltration before treatment
Fistula
Granulation tissue
Nonviable scar tissue
Talc granuloma

(Adapted from Jerusalem G, Hustinx R, Beguin Y, Fillet G. Evaluation of therapy for lymphoma. *Semin Nucl Med* 2005;35(3):186–196, with permission.)

The introduction of functional metabolic imaging using FDG PET or PET/CT has proven to be helpful in accurate assessment of remission posttreatment and in characterizing residual masses. The role of FDG PET in assessing residual masses has been widely accepted (9).

As recently recommended by the imaging subcommittee of the International Harmonization Project in Lymphoma, pretherapy PET is not obligatory for assessment of response after treatment of patients with Hodgkin's lymphoma and those subtypes of NHL that normally have a high glycolytic rate and hence high FDG uptake. These include diffuse large B-cell lymphoma, follicular lymphomas, and mantle cell lymphoma (7). However, FDG PET or PET/CT is indicated in these subtypes as a baseline examination and a reference of lymphoma manifestations for follow-up (7). In contrast, FDG PET or PET/CT is mandatory in those subtypes with variable FDG uptake when FDG PET will be used during follow-up (7). These subtypes include aggressive NHL excepting diffuse large B-cell lymphoma (i.e., T-cell lymphoma) and indolent lymphoma excepting follicular lymphoma (7). In practice, many centers prefer

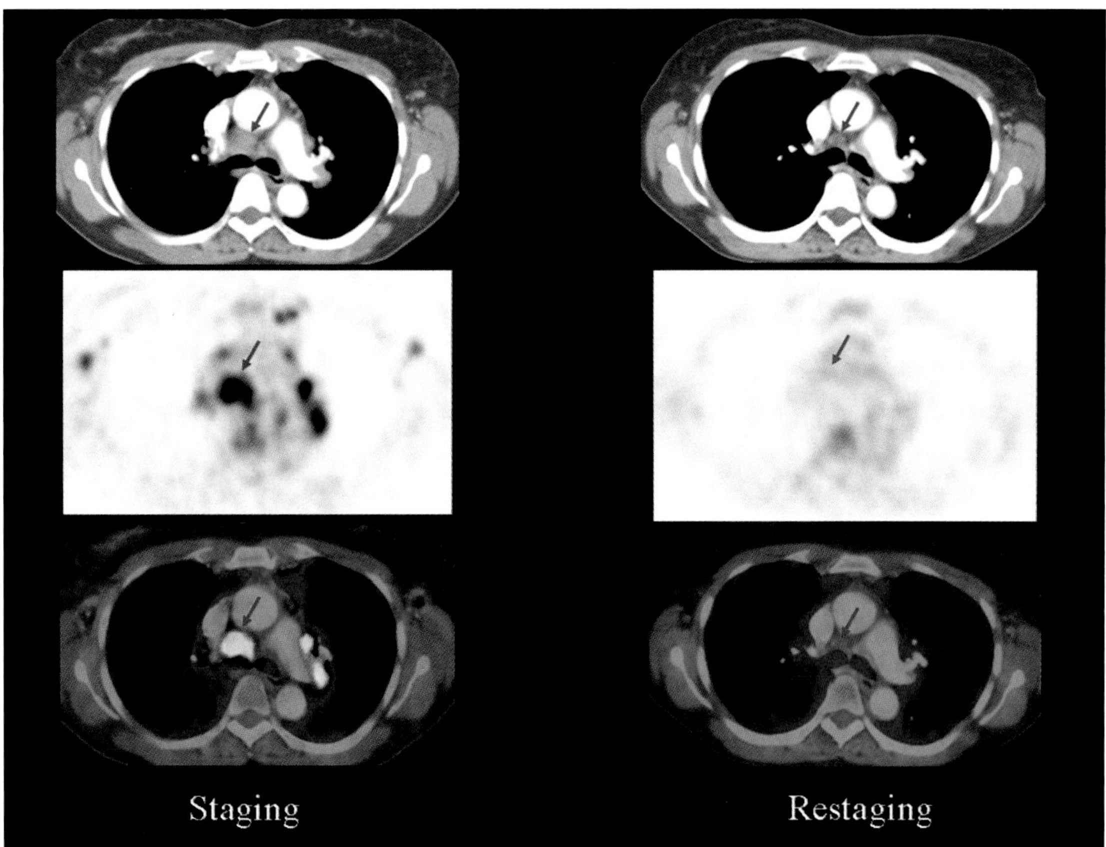

FIGURE 8.10.2. Assessment of remission with fluorodeoxyglucose (FDG) PET/CT after completion of chemotherapy in a patient with Hodgkin's lymphoma. All nodal manifestations with increased FDG uptake (axillary nodes right and left, mammary internal nodes left, mediastinal nodes) show complete normalization (i.e., no residual FDG uptake 4 weeks after completion of chemotherapy). A residual mediastinal mass without FDG uptake in CT (*arrow*) is indicative of scar tissue.

to have a baseline PET study so that tumor burden and starting standard uptake value (SUV) can be determined. Indeed, some investigators feel it is much better to secure a baseline PET/CT study in all patients with lymphoma if at all possible.

Diagnostic Criteria

PET after completion of chemotherapy should be performed at least 3 weeks, preferably 6 to 8 weeks, after chemotherapy or chemoimmunotherapy, and 8 to 12 weeks after irradiation or combined radio- and chemotherapy (7). Mediastinal blood pool activity is recommended as the reference background radioactivity for classification of residual masses either as positive (i.e., viable lymphoma), when their radioactivity concentration is increased over the reference background, or negative (i.e., scar tissue), when their radioactivity is less than the reference background. Visual assessment of potential lymphoma manifestations is regarded as adequate.

Mild and diffusely increased FDG uptake in residual masses 2 cm or greater in diameter with intensity less than or equal to mediastinal blood pool structures should be considered negative for lymphoma. New FDG positive lung nodules should be regarded as inflammatory when all other previously known lymphoma manifestations show complete response. Residual hepatic or splenic lesions greater than 1.5 cm on CT and FDG uptake greater than or equal to that of liver or spleen should be considered positive. Clearly increased multifocal bone marrow uptake should be interpreted as positive for lymphoma. A detailed discussion of FDG imaging criteria was recently published by Juweid et al. (7).

From the published literature, some general conclusions can be drawn (16):

1. FDG PET is more accurate than CT in virtually all studies (except in the relatively low FDG avidity lymphomas noted previously).
2. The accuracy of PET is high enough to be used as a standard measure for assessment of remission, either supplementing or in combination with PET/CT, replacing the "CT only" study in the FDG avid lymphomas.

Evaluation After Completion of Chemotherapy and/or Radiotherapy

Achieving a complete remission is a major objective in patients with Hodgkin's lymphoma or NHL because it is usually associated with a longer progression-free survival than a partial remission (see Jerusalem et al. [15] for a review). However, in as many as 64% of all Hodgkin's lymphoma cases and in 30% to 60% of all NHL cases, CT

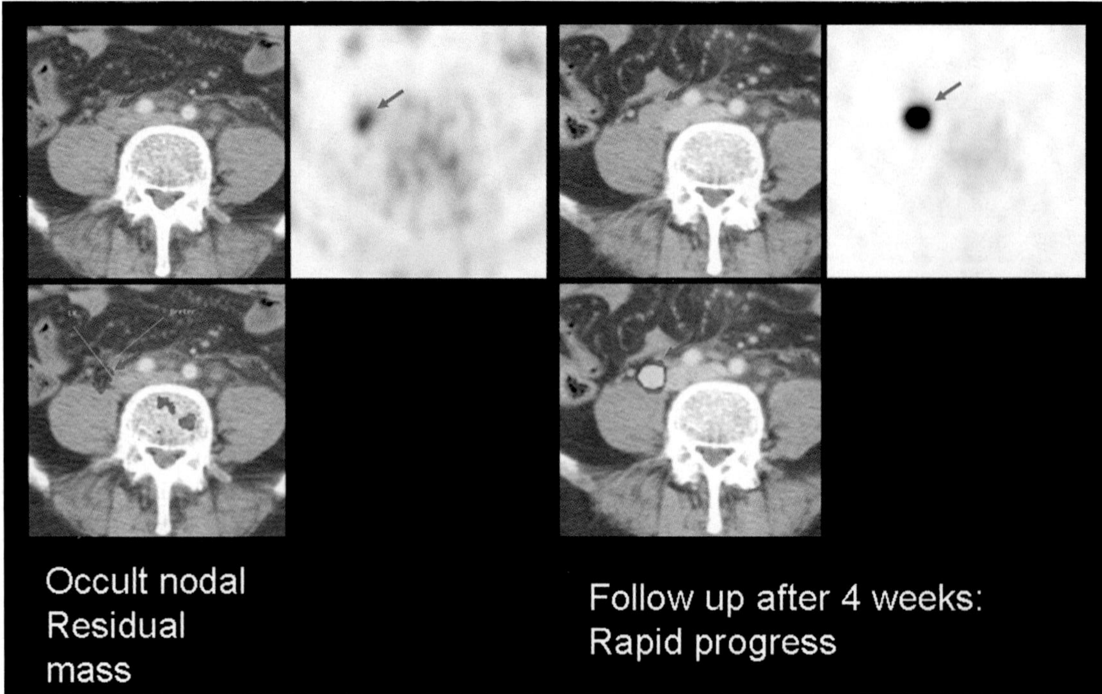

FIGURE 8.10.3. Fluorodeoxyglucose PET/CT of residual occult viable non-Hodgkin's lymphoma 8 weeks after completion of chemotherapy. There is rapid progression of disease at 4-week follow-up.

or magnetic resonance tomography shows abnormalities during restaging (16). Residual masses are observed more frequently in patients with aggressive NHL and with a large tumor mass at diagnosis, as well as in patients suffering from Hodgkin's lymphoma of the nodular sclerosis histologic subtype (15). Unfortunately, conventional anatomic imaging cannot differentiate between benign fibrous tissue and an inflammatory process or persistent malignant disease. A maximum of only 20% of residual masses at the completion of treatment are reported to be positive for lymphoma on biopsy, and they eventually relapse (35,36). If the tumor is easily accessible, such as an enlarged peripheral lymph node, the questionable lesion can be excised and histologically analyzed.

If anatomical access is difficult, noninvasive imaging with FDG PET or PET/CT is of major importance (Fig. 8.10.4). Several recent

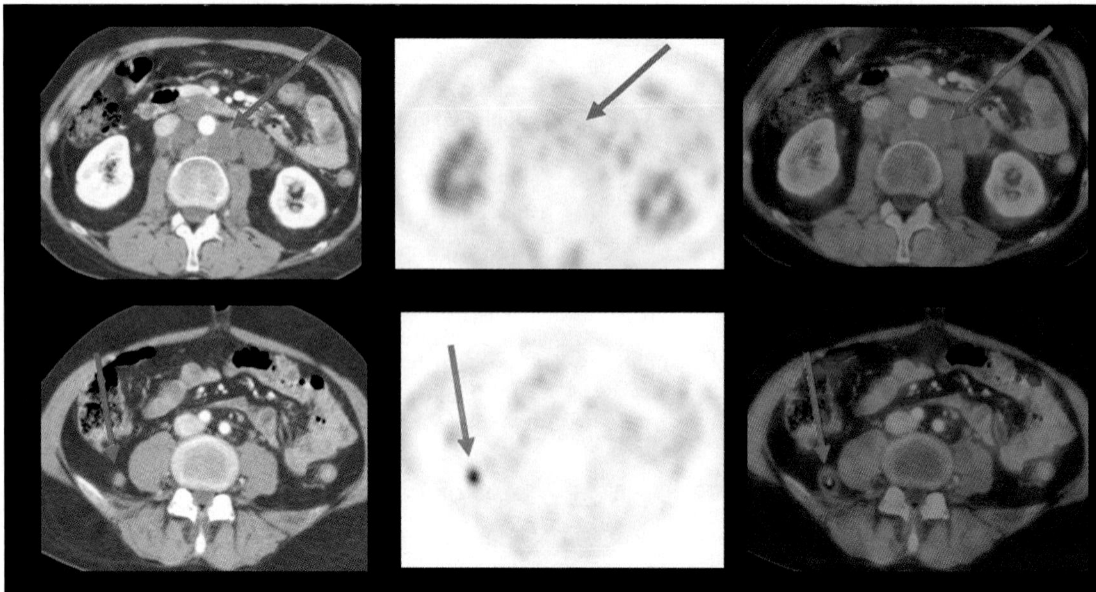

FIGURE 8.10.4. A negative fluorodeoxyglucose PET/CT study of a residual left para-aortic mass 6 months after completion of chemotherapy for non-Hodgkin's lymphoma (**upper row**, *arrows*). There is simultaneous abdominal relapse (*arrow*) in a lymph node near right M. iliopsoas (**lower row**, *arrow*).

TABLE 8.10.2 Predictive Value of Whole-Body Fluorine-18-fluorodeoxyglucose for Posttreatment Evaluation in Non-Hodgkin's Lymphoma

Authors (ref.)	Median Follow-up (mo)	Sensitivity	Specificity	Positive Predictive Value	Negative Predictives Value	Accuracy
Mikhaeel et al. (63)	30	60% (9/15)	100% (30/30)	100% (9/9)	83% (30/36)	87% (39/45)
Spaepen et al. (64)	21	70% (26/37)	100% (56/56)	100% (26/26)	84% (56/67)	88% (82/93)
Overall		67% (35/52)	100% (86/86)	100% (35/35)	83% (86/103)	88% (121/138)

(From Jerusalem G, Hustinx R, Beguin Y, Fillet G. Evaluation of therapy for lymphoma. *Semin Nucl Med* 2005;35(3):186–196, with permission.)

studies demonstrate the value of FDG PET or PET/CT for end-of-treatment response assessment (15). Jerusalem et al. (15) compiled the results of 17 selective studies with a total of 752 patients. In these studies the overall accuracy of PET was 88% to 91%. PET had a better positive predictive value for NHL (100%) than for Hodgkin's lymphoma (74%) and a better negative predictive value (for Hodgkin's lymphoma 93%) than for NHL (83%) (Tables 8.10.2 and 8.10.3). As indicated by Mikhaeel (16), a positive PET after treatment of NHL is strongly predictive of residual disease, but less so in Hodgkin's lymphoma. A negative PET after Hodgkin's lymphoma treatment is predictive of freedom of residual disease, but this is slightly less in NHL. This finding possibly reflects the presence of inflammatory cellular infiltrate in Hodgkin's lymphoma and the higher relapse rate of NHL (16).

Since FDG uptake is not specific for tumor tissue, it may be advisable to be cautious to verify tumor involvement by biopsy or other methods such as close follow-up in lesions occurring outside of normal FDG uptake of initially involved sites, because infectious or inflammatory lesions are much more abundant in these lesions. The importance of the baseline PET, even in the FDG-avid tumors, is particularly apparent in such cases, as lesions that develop during the course of therapy outside other areas that have responded may commonly be false-positive findings.

Early Assessment of Response

About 30% to 40 % of patients with aggressive NHL fail to achieve CR with initial standard chemotherapy, which is a prerequisite for cure. Overall, long-term cure is achieved only in 50% to 60%. This means that a substantial portion of patients may not respond to their initial treatment. Assessment of early response is usually performed with CT after three to four cycles of chemotherapy. PET has been investigated to potentially improve the accuracy of early response assessment through functional metabolic imaging (15–17).

The results of several recent studies have been summarized by Jerusalem et al. (15) (Table 8.10.4). Despite the limitations of some studies, some general conclusions can be drawn (16):

1. CR is evident on a repeated PET or PET/CT after one to three cycles of chemotherapy much earlier than size reduction of lymphoma masses seen on the CT scan.
2. Such an early CR on PET, presumably reflecting high chemosensitivity, correlates with better prognosis.
3. Early PET is a more accurate predictor of outcome than posttreatment PET.

Mikhael et al. (37) and Hutchings et al. (38) introduced the concept of minimal residual uptake (MRU). These authors studied 121 patients with high-grade NHL with FDG PET after two to three cycles of chemotherapy (37) for prediction of progression-free survival (PFS) and overall survival (OS). They reported that early interim PET was an accurate and independent predictor of PFS and OS (37). They could also identify a subgroup of patients with NHL and MRU and an intermediate prognosis between those patients with a negative PET and an excellent prognosis as shown by a PFS of 89%, and for those with a positive PET, a dismal prognosis and a PFS

TABLE 8.10.3 Predictive Value of Whole-Body Fluorine-18-fluorodeoxyglucose PET for Posttreatment Evaluation in Hodgkin's Lymphoma

Authors (ref.)	Median Follow-up (mo)	Sensitivity	Specificity	Positive Predictive Value	Negative Predictive Value	Accuracy
De Wit et al. (65)	26	100% (10/10)	78% (18/23)	67% (10/15)	100% (18/18)	85% (28/33)
Dittmann et al. (66)	6	87% (7/8)	94% (17/18)	87% (7/8)	94% (17/18)	92% (24/26)
Spaepen et al. (67)	32	50% (5/10)	100% (50/50)	100% (5/5)	91% (50/55)	92% (55/60)
Weihrauch et al. (68)	28	67% (6/9)	80% (16/20)	60% (6/10)	84% (16/19)	76% (22/29)
Guay et al. (69)	16	79% (11/14)	97% (33/34)	92% (11/12)	92% (33/36)	92% (44/48)
Friedberg et al. (70)	24	80% (4/5)	85% (23/27)	50% (4/8)	96% (23/24%)	84% (87/32)
Panizo et al. (71)	28	100% (9/9)	85% (17/20)	75% (9/12)	100% (17/17)	90% (26/29)
Overall		80% (52/65)	91% (174/192)	74% (52/70)	93% (174/187)	88% (226/257)

(From Jerusalem G, Hustinx R, Beguin Y, Fillet G. Evaluation of therapy for lymphoma. *Semin Nucl Med* 2005;35(3):186–196, with permission.)

TABLE 8.10.4 Predictive Value of Whole-Body Fluorine-18-fluorodeoxyglucose PET for Assessment of Early Response

Authors (ref.)	No. of Cycles Before Evaluation	Median Follow-up (mo)	Sensitivity	Specificity	Positive Predictive Value	Negative Predictive Value	Accuracy
Mikhaeel et al. (63)	2–4	30	100% (7/7)	94% (15/16)	87% (7/9)	100% (15/15)	96% (22/23)
Jerusalem et al. (72)	3–(2–5)	17	42% (5/12)	100% (14/14)	100% (5/5)	67% (14/21)	73% (19/26)
Kostakoglu et al. (73)	1	19	87% (13/15)	87% (13/15)	87% (13/15)	87% (13/15)	87% (26/30)
Spaepen et al. (74)	3–4	36	85% (33/39)	100% (31/31)	100% (31/37)	84% (31/37)	91% (64/70)
Zijlstra et al. (75)	2	25	64% (9/14)	75% (9/12)	75% (9/12)	64% (9/14)	69% (18/26)
Torizuka et al. (76)	1–2	24	87% (14/16)	50% (2/4)	87% (14/16)	50% (2/4)	80% (16/20)
Friedberg et al. (70)	3	24	80% (4/5)	94% (16/17)	80% (4/5)	94% (16/17)	91% (20/22)
Overall			79% (85/108)	92% (100/109)	90% (85/94)	81% (100/123)	85% (185/217)

(From Jerusalem G, Hustinx R, Beguin Y, Fillet G. Evaluation of therapy for lymphoma. *Semin Nucl Med* 2005;35(3):186–196, with permission.)

of only 16% (37). It was concluded from this study that early interim FDG PET is an accurate and independent predictor of PFS and OS in NHL (37). This study shows also that early interim PET has the potential to improve individualized management of patients with NHL, providing a basis for early identification of non-responding patients to whom an alternative second-line therapy may be offered.

As the authors of the above cited study state, the three group classification system of FDG uptake—class (1): negative; class (2): MRU; class (3): positive—suffers from the limitations of the subjectivity of the MRU designation, which needs a definition producing objective and reproducible results (37).

The same investigators also studied the value of early interim PET (i.e., after two to three cycles of chemotherapy) in 85 patients with Hodgkin's lymphoma (38). After a median follow-up of 3 years, 3 of 63 patients with a negative PET and 1 of 13 patients with MRU relapsed (38). In contrast, 9 of 13 patients with a positive PET progressed and 2 patients died (38). Survival analysis showed a highly significant association between early interim PET and PFS ($P < .0001$) as well as OS ($P < .03$). All advanced-stage patients with a positive early interim PET scan relapsed within 2 years (38).

The time from early interim PET to recognition of progression with conventional methods was 1 to 21 months (mean 9 months) for eight PET-positive patients and 12 to 33 months (mean 24.3 months) for three PET-negative patients (38).

The results of a recent prospective study by Hutchings et al. (39) in 77 patients with Hodgkin's lymphoma confirm these observations. For prediction of PFS, interim PET was as accurate after two cycles as later during treatment and superior to CT at all time points. In regression analysis, interim PET was stronger than the established prognostic factors. Other significant prognostic factors for progression were advanced stage and extranodal disease.

Novel Functional Imaging Approaches in Malignant Lymphoma

Current molecular targets for PET imaging may be divided into principles relying on overexpression of key proteins of important pathways of intermediary metabolism up-regulated in malignant lymphomas and receptors or antigens overexpressed at the cell membrane of lymphoma cells. Glucose transporters and key enzymes of glycolysis are certainly the most abundantly used molecular targets for diagnostic PET imaging in lymphoma. These are discussed elsewhere in this book.

Amino acid utilization is increased in malignant lymphoma as well as in many other malignant tumors or tumor cell lines (40). The molecular targets for this imaging approach are a variety of amino acid transporters, facilitating amino acid cellular influx. Most investigators assume that increased tumoral uptake of, for example, carbon-11-methionine mainly reflects transmembrane amino acid transport and not protein synthesis (41). The author's group found highly increased L-type amino acid transporter expression on the DoHH2 (Epstein-Barr virus–negative B-cell line) lymphoma cell line (42).

Proliferation may be increased in Hodgkin's lymphoma and NHL, depending on the histologic subtype, stage, and biological aggressiveness. Increased proliferation has been linked to an impaired prognosis in NHL. The major metabolic targets for assessment of proliferation *in vivo* with PET are key enzymes of the thymidine salvage pathway (43), particularly thymidine kinase 1 (TK1) and probably also DNA-dependent polymerases, overexpressed in many malignant tumors including malignant lymphoma (44).

Several authors reported mildly overexpressed somatostatin receptors, predominantly subtype 2 and 3 (45,46), in a subgroup of patients with NHL, forming the basis of the first imaging studies with appropriately radiolabeled somatostatin receptor ligands (47).

Clusters of differentiation such as CD20, CD19, CD45, and many other cluster-defined antigens may be abundantly overexpressed in NHL (48). These receptors are addressed by a variety of monoclonal antibodies radiolabeled with "therapeutic isotopes" and have demonstrated considerable therapeutic success (48,49). Since kinetics of most antibodies in blood and tissue are relatively slow and radiolabeling methods of antibodies with appropriate PET isotopes are not widely available, the exquisite antibody mediated targeting approach is currently not used for PET imaging of malignant lymphoma.

Imaging Proliferative Activity in Malignant Lymphoma

Imaging proliferative activity of malignant lymphoma is of considerable interest because proliferative activity of lymphomas is linked to biologic aggressiveness. Imaging of proliferative activity in individual lymphoma manifestations may improve early detection of the development of aggressive transformation of low-grade lymphoma (50). Fluorothymidine (FLT) is the radiopharmaceutical currently most widely used for imaging proliferative activity.

Fluorothymidine

Thymidine is incorporated into DNA in close relation to cellular proliferation and tritium-thymidine uptake in experimental systems is well established for measuring cellular or tissue proliferation rates. Since carbon-11-thymidine is very rapidly degraded *in vivo*, several carbon-11 or fluorine-18 labeled thymidine analogues were developed for evaluating tissue proliferation *in vivo* with PET (43,50). FLT was first described by Shields et al. (51) in 1998 as a PET-imaging probe in a dog lymphoma. FLT is taken up by the cell through passive diffusion and facilitated sodium-positive–dependent nucleoside transporter mediated inward transport (see Been et al. [43] for a review). Within the cell, FLT is phosphorylated by TK1 to FLT monophosphate and to a limited degree also to the di- and triphosphate. Only minor amounts of FLT are incorporated into DNA and result in DNA chain terminations. TK1 is virtually absent in quiescent cells but is up-regulated several fold in proliferating cells during the late G1 and S phase of the cell cycle (43).

Proliferation Imaging with Fluorothymidine

FLT is physiologically taken up into bone marrow and liver and excreted via the urinary tract (52). There is no physiologic uptake of FLT in brain, myocardium, or skeletal muscle. Uptake in the liver is due to glucuronidation of FLT followed by renal excretion. Recent studies from the author's group comparing FDG and FLT in patients with NHL indicated that both tracers detected a comparable number of lesions (53). A close correlation was observed in eight of nine patients. A significant correlation of the Ki67 labeling index and the SUV of FLT in lymphoma manifestations in another study in 26 patients with NHL ($r = 0.76$; $P < .01$) was observed (52) (Fig. 8.10.5).

An attractive approach is the use of *in vivo* markers of lymphoma proliferative activity, the presumed true measure of the malignancy grade of malignant lymphoma (10). Using FLT, the author's group demonstrated excellent separation between aggressive and indolent lymphoma. A high correlation was observed between the SUV of FLT and proliferative activity of lymphomas (50) (Fig. 8.10.6). As stated by Juweid and Cheson (10) in a recent review, the use of FLT might obviate the need for quantitative tracer kinetic methods that are potentially required when other radiotracers such as FDG are used for grading NHL. In fact, lymphoma grading could turn out to become the predominant indication in PET imaging of lymphoma. However, FLT does have the challenge of high-level uptake in the liver and bone marrow, making it likely that lesion detection will be more difficult in these tissues than with FDG. Thus, although FLT is a promising agent, its precise role in lymphoma imaging remains in evolution.

Beyond this diagnostic approach, novel proliferation markers are currently being developed, which are incorporated into DNA and can be used as molecular carriers for Auger electron-mediated cell kill. First experimental results from the author's group indicate that this targeted nano-irradiation of DNA is highly effective in triggering apoptosis in DoHH2 cells with radiation doses as low as 0.1 Gy. PET may represent an excellent means of assessing such forms of therapy as they develop.

MULTIPLE MYELOMA

Plasma cell neoplasms represent a spectrum of diseases characterized by clonal proliferation and accumulation of immunoglobulin-producing terminally differentiated B cells. The spectrum includes clinically benign common conditions such as monoclonal gammopathy of unknown significance, as well as rare disorders such as Castleman's disease and α-heavy-chain disease; indolent conditions such as Waldenström's macroglobulinemia, the more common malignant entity plasma cell myeloma, a disseminated B-cell malignancy; and a more aggressive form, plasma cell leukemia, with circulating malignant plasma cells in the blood. All of these disorders share common features of plasma cell morphology, production of immunoglobulin molecules, and immune dysfunction. A plasma cell neoplasm is considered to originate from a single B cell, with resultant monoclonal protein secretion that characterizes its type (54,55).

Epidemiology

The incidence rate of multiple myeloma is 4 per 100,000 per year. Approximately 15,000 new cases are diagnosed each year in the United States. The current prevalence of myeloma in the United States is about 50,000, and there were 10,800 deaths from the disease reported in 2001. Worldwide, it is estimated that there are at least 32,000 new cases reported and 24,000 deaths each year. Myeloma is twice as common among African Americans as compared to whites and affects men more than women (56).

Clinical Manifestations

Patients with multiple myeloma may be entirely asymptomatic and diagnosed on routine blood testing or may present with myriad symptoms: hematologic manifestations, bone-related problems, infections, various organ dysfunctions, neurologic complaints, or bleeding tendencies. These signs and symptoms result from direct tumor involvement in bone marrow or extramedullary plasmacytomas, the effect of the protein produced by the tumor cells deposited in various organs, production of cytokines by the tumor cells or by the bone marrow microenvironment, and effects on the immune system.

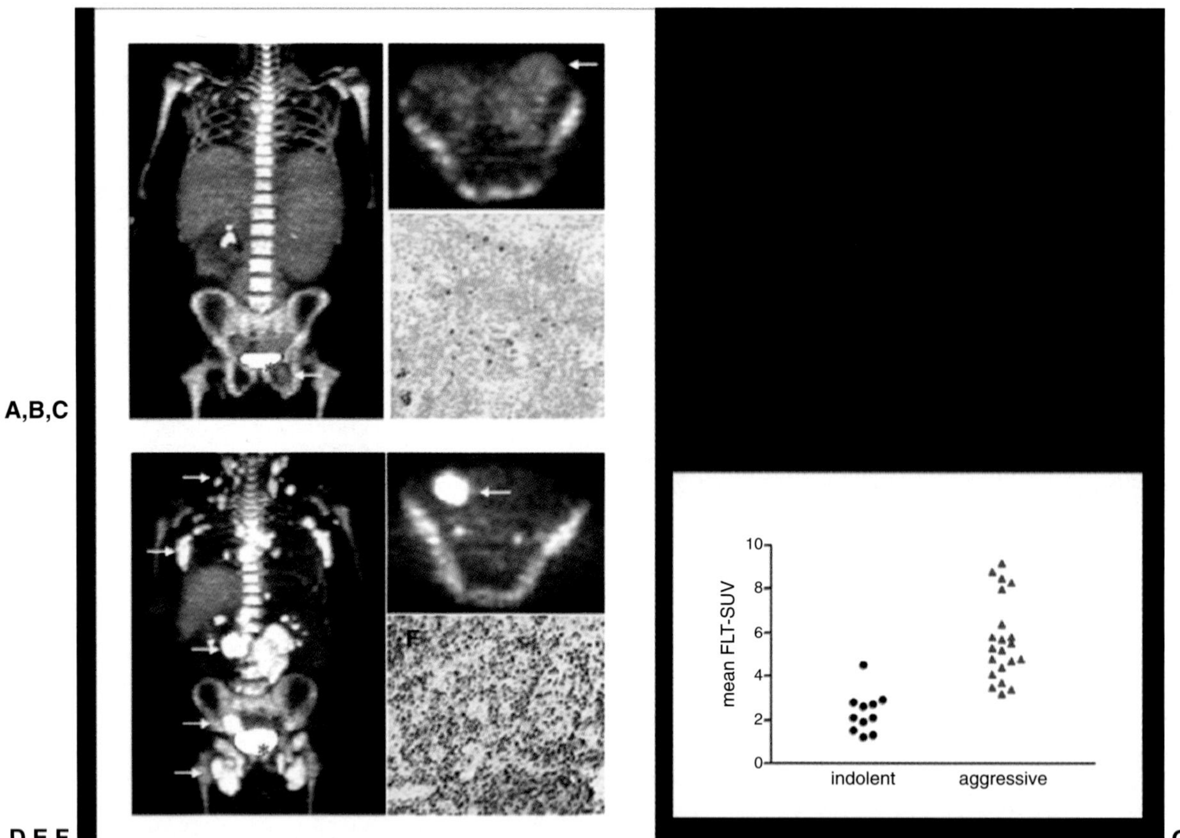

FIGURE 8.10.5. Significantly higher fluorothymidine (FLT) uptake was observed in aggressive compared to indolent lymphoma. **A:** An FLT-PET image (maximum intensity projection) of patient 2 with indolent lymphoma shows low FLT uptake in the enlarged spleen and in para-aortic, iliac, and inguinal bulky lesions (*arrow*). There is physiological intense FLT uptake in proliferating bone marrow and mild FLT uptake in the liver. **B:** A transaxial section of the inguinal region with low FLT uptake in lymphoma (*arrow*). **C:** Anti-Ki-67 immunostaining (MIB-1) indicates a low proliferation fraction of less than 5%. **D:** An FLT-PET image (maximum intensity projection) of patient 14 with aggressive lymphoma. There is intense uptake of FLT in cervical, axillary, mediastinal, para-aortic, iliac, and inguinal lymph nodes (*arrows*). **E:** A transaxial section of the inguinal region shows intense FLT uptake in lymphoma (*arrow*). **F:** Anti-Ki-67 immunostaining. **G:** There is a significantly higher standardized uptake value (SUV) of FLT in aggressive compared to indolent lymphoma. (From Buck A, Bommer M, Pitterle K, et al. Molecular imaging of proliferation in malignant lymphoma. *Cancer Res*, with permission.)

Hypercalcemia and Bone Disease

The mechanism of bone abnormalities in myeloma, especially destruction, is an unbalanced process of increased osteoclast activity and suppressed osteoblast activity. These changes are due to an increase in osteoclast-activating factors produced predominantly by the bone marrow microenvironment but also by myeloma cells. As a result, osteoporosis and lytic bone lesions develop. These bone changes frequently involve the vertebral column and result in compression fractures, lytic bone lesions, and related pain. A new onset of back pain or other bone pain is a frequent presenting symptom in patients with myeloma. Changes in the cytokine milieu and bone destruction may also lead to the development of hypercalcemia, which is observed in approximately 25% of patients at some stage of the disease. Symptoms of high calcium levels can include changes in mental status, lethargy, constipation, and vomiting.

Extramedullary Disease

Extramedullary disease manifestations are uncommon in patients with myeloma at presentation. However, such manifestations have been observed in the setting of advanced-stage disease or relapse after allogeneic transplantation. Solitary or multiple extramedullary plasmacytomas have been described in the liver, spleen, lymph nodes, kidneys, subcutaneous tissues, and brain parenchyma. Extramedullary involvement may be suspected in patients who have more aggressive features of myeloma.

Diagnosis and Staging

Because patients with myeloma present with a variety of symptoms not specific to the disease, the diagnosis of myeloma is quite often delayed. An older patient with a new onset of unexplained back

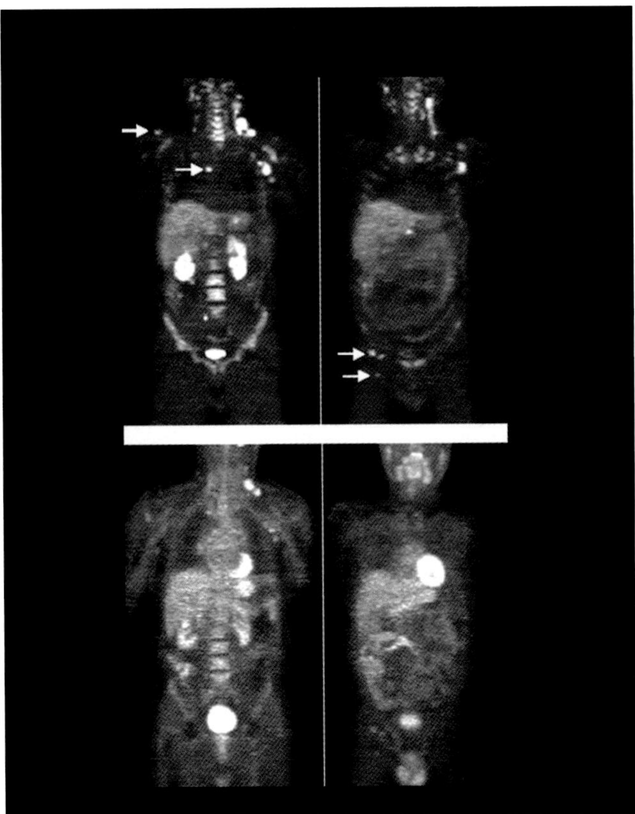

FIGURE 8.10.6. Fluorothymidine PET (**A** top left, **B** top right) shows more extensive nodal involvement compared to fluorodeoxyglucose PET (**C** bottom left, **D** bottom right) in aggressive non-Hodgkin's lymphoma. Lesions not detected with conventional imaging are shown (*arrows*). (From Buck A, Bommer M, Pitterle K, et al. Molecular imaging of proliferation in malignant lymphoma. *Cancer Res*, 2006;66(22): 11055–11061. With permission.)

pain or bone pain, recurrent infection, anemia, or renal insufficiency should be screened for myeloma. Additional findings such as hyperproteinemia or proteinuria, anemia, hypoalbuminemia, low immunoglobulin levels, or marked elevation of the erythrocyte sedimentation rate should prompt a further complete evaluation for diagnosis of plasma cell myeloma.

The initial evaluation includes a hemogram, complete skeletal radiographic survey, serum and urine protein electrophoresis and immunofixation, quantitative immunoglobulin levels, urinary protein excretion in 24 hours, and bone marrow aspiration and biopsy (56,57).

Staging and Risk Assessment

Radiographic Evaluation

The radiographic survey of bone is a standard diagnostic evaluation. It shows osteopenia in an early phase of the disease and, with increasing tumor burden, lytic punched-out lesions. Osteosclerotic lesions are observed in POEMS (*p*olyneuropathy, *o*rganomegaly, *e*ndocrinopathy, *m*onoclonal gammopathy, and *s*kin changes) syndrome. Due to the predominant osteolytic activity with osteoblastic inactivity, bone scans seldom give positive results, unless a recent fracture has occurred, and are therefore not particularly useful in the diagnosis of multiple myeloma.

Functional imaging either with magnetic resonance imaging (MRI) of bone marrow or FDG PET, best performed in conjunction with CT, provides a better assessment of tumor burden and is essential in the work-up of patients with solitary plasmacytomas of bone (56,58). There are typical imaging patterns on MRI: one-third have diffuse involvement of the bone marrow, one-third have focal lesions, and the remaining third have heterogeneous focal and diffused marrow involvement (58). Because myeloma is a macrofocal disease, random bone marrow sampling may not be diagnostic or predictive of disease status.

A focal marrow plasmacytoma can be further analyzed through CT-guided fine-needle aspiration, which allows cytologic diagnosis and further risk assessment based on evaluation of the results of cytogenetic and fluorescence *in situ* hybridization analysis, as well as labeling index (54).

Fluorodeoxyglucose PET and PET/CT

PET has also been evaluated in a small number of studies and may provide a better functional definition of lesions observed on MRI or CT, as well as allowing selection of lesions for biopsy. Durie et al. (59) examined 66 patients, of which there were 14 with monoclonal gammopathy of unknown significance, 16 with active, untreated multiple myeloma, 10 with disease in remission, and 26 with relapsing multiple myeloma. Negative whole-body FDG PET scans reliably predicted stable monoclonal gammopathy of unknown significance. All patients with untreated multiple myeloma had focal or diffuse increased FDG bone marrow uptake, indicative of active multiple myeloma. In particular, 25% of the patients with newly diagnosed multiple myeloma had positive FDG PET findings, despite fully negative skeletal surveys. Another 23% to 25% of newly diagnosed or relapsed multiple myeloma had extramedullary multiple myeloma, which was confirmed by biopsy or other imaging techniques. This extramedullary FDG uptake was a very poor prognostic factor, as indicated by the median survival of only 7 months for these patients with extramedullary, FDG-positive multiple myeloma. Persistent positive findings after induction therapy predicted early relapse. The FDG PET results were especially helpful in identifying focal recurrent disease in patients with nonsecretory or hyposecretory disease amenable to local irradiation therapy.

Bredella et al. (60) reported in a series of 23 patients with sensitivity and specificity of 80% and 92%, respectively, for detecting active myeloma. Two "subcentimeter" lytic lesions detected at skeletal surveys had no or only very mild FDG uptake. There was also one false-positive finding observed 3 weeks after radiotherapy. In this study FDG PET was helpful in differentiating between post-therapeutic changes and residual or recurrent multiple myeloma manifestations. In roughly one third of the patients FDG PET influenced therapeutic management.

Orchard et al. (61) found in a very small series of three patients that FDG PET was particularly useful in showing sites of occult disease and sites of active multiple myeloma in nonsecretory myeloma, solitary plasmacytoma, and relapse following autologous or allogeneic stem cell transplantation.

Schirrmeister et al. (62) confirmed and extended the results of previous authors using FDG PET for staging and restaging multiple myeloma and solitary plasmacytoma. In 28 patients with multiple myeloma and 15 patients with solitary plasmacytoma, they observed focally increased FDG uptake in bone marrow of 38 of 41 patients with known osteolytic bone lesions, resulting in a sensitivity of 93%. In addition, 71 lesions with negative skeletal radiographs were

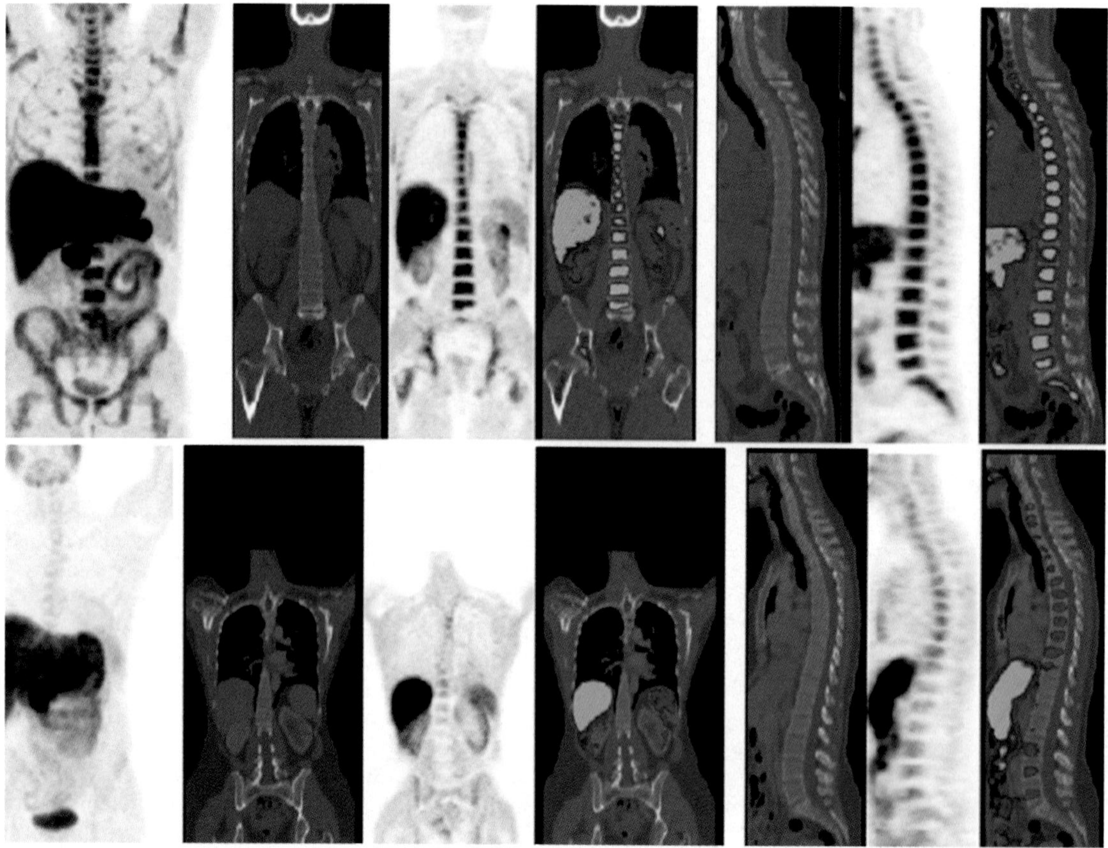

FIGURE 8.10.7. Homogenous and low carbon-11-methionine uptake in a control patient (**upper row**) compared to diffusely increased carbon-11-methionine uptake in the whole vertebral spine (**bottom row**) of a patient with multiple myeloma.

observed. Twenty-six of these 71 lesions were confirmed by biopsy or other imaging techniques in 20 patients. Clinical management was changed in 14% of all patients examined. Sensitivity and specificity of increased diffuse FDG uptake in bone marrow indicative of active disseminated disease was 84% to 92% and 93% to 100%, respectively. Compared to FDG PET, skeletal radiographs underestimated the extent of disease in 61% of the patients examined in this study.

Given the well-known increased synthesis of the monoclonal immunoglobulin in multiple myeloma, it can be reasoned that functional imaging of increased amino acid utilization by multiple myeloma cells may provide a direct approach for imaging, precise localization, and possibly quantitation of multiple myeloma mass *in vivo*. A sixfold increase of sulfur-35-methionine incorporation into CD138+ plasmacytoma cells, freshly isolated from bone marrow of patients with newly diagnosed, untreated multiple myeloma, compared to normal CD138– bone marrow cells confirmed the validity of this novel approach (57). Nineteen patients with multiple myeloma and ten controls without hematological diseases were examined with carbon-11-methionine and imaged 20 minutes post infection with PET/CT. The presence and extent of CT-assessed tumor manifestations and carbon-11-methionine bone marrow (BM) uptake were determined. Carbon-11-methionine BM uptake in normal controls with no known hematological disease was homogeneous and low (Fig. 8.10.7). All patients with multiple myeloma except one with exclusively extramedullary multiple myeloma had carbon-11-methionine positive osteolyses (Figs. 8.10.8 and 8.10.9). Maximal lesional BM carbon-11-methionine SUV_{max} was 10.2 ± 3.4 and significantly higher than that of BM of controls (1.8 ± 0.3; $P < .001$). Extramedullary multiple myeloma was clearly visible in three patients (SUV_{max} 7.2 ± 2.4) (Fig. 8.10.10). Additional carbon-11-methionine positive lesions in normal cancellous bone were found in nearly all patients. Preferentially in pretreated patients, a moderate fraction of osteolyses had no carbon-11-methionine uptake.

Based on increased methionine uptake in myeloma cells, active multiple myeloma could be reliably imaged with carbon-11-methionine PET/CT. This novel approach has a high potential for differentiating active multiple myeloma from inactive scar tissue in radiologically demonstrated osteolyses. In addition, similar to previous findings with FDG PET (62), there were many focal lesions with increased carbon-11-methionine uptake and normal bone structure (Fig. 8.10.10), suggesting the presence of new, metabolically active lesions developing earlier than structural osteolytic bone changes (57).

In summary, FDG PET or PET/CT or alternatively carbon-11-methionine PET/CT can reliably image both solitary and multiple myeloma, nonsecretory myeloma, extramedullary myeloma, and relapsing myeloma. Monoclonal gammopathy of unknown significance can be differentiated from multiple myeloma. Active multiple myeloma presents with multiple, metabolically highly active

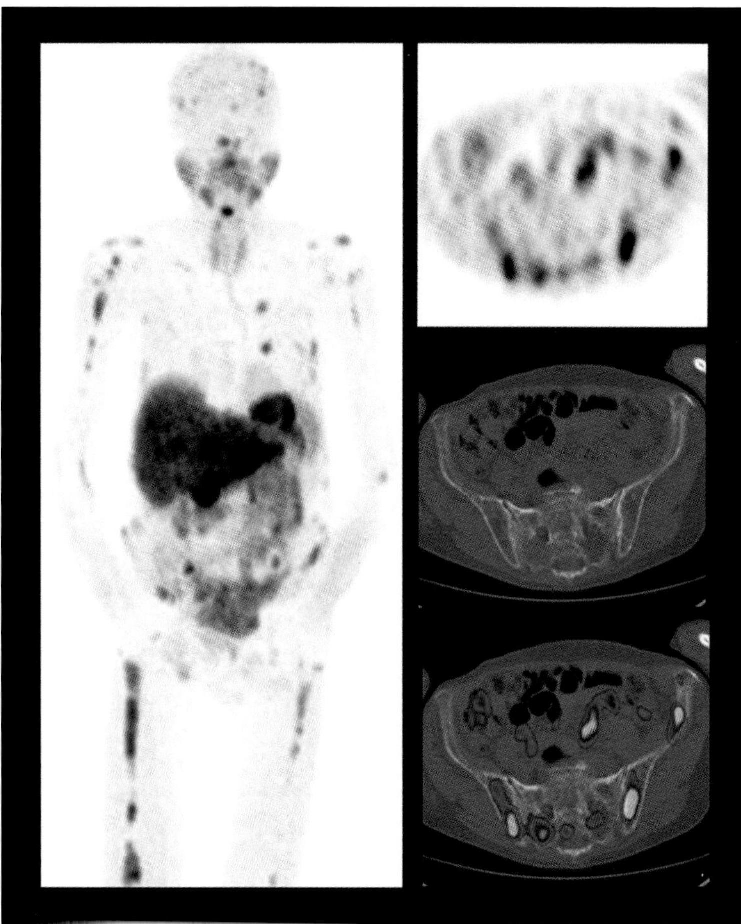

FIGURE 8.10.8. This maximum intensity projection image (trunk & head) shows multiple focal lesions with increased carbon-11-methionine uptake, suggesting widespread disseminated multiple myeloma. The patient with relapsing multiple myeloma has disseminated lesions in the right and left ileum and the sacrum. Some lesions have intense carbon-11-methionine uptake, whereas others have virtually no carbon-11-methionine uptake.

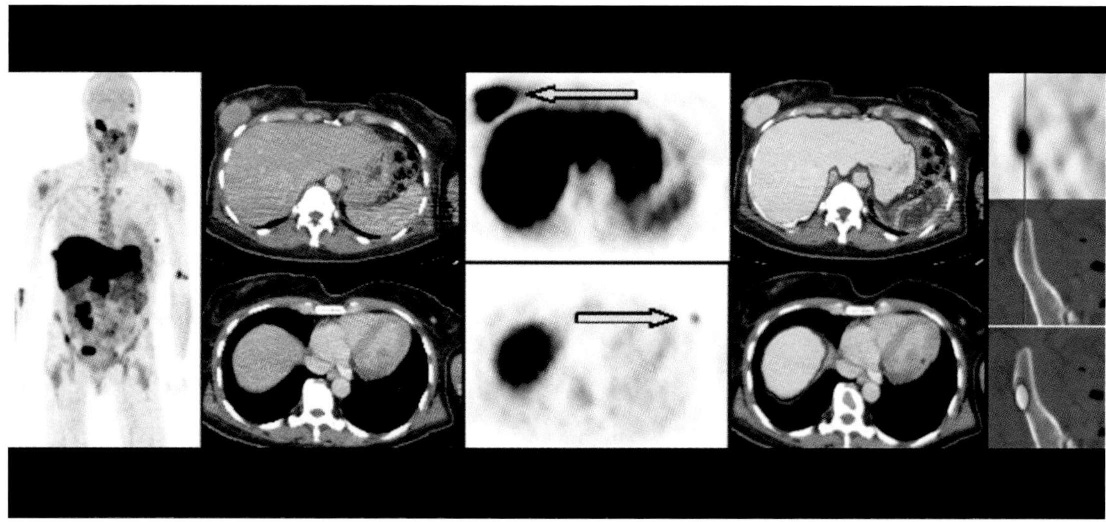

FIGURE 8.10.9. A lytic skull lesion shown by CT has highly increased carbon-11-methionine uptake, which is a typical manifestation of multiple myeloma. An additional lesion with increased carbon-11-methionine uptake was diagnosed in the left humerus shaft.

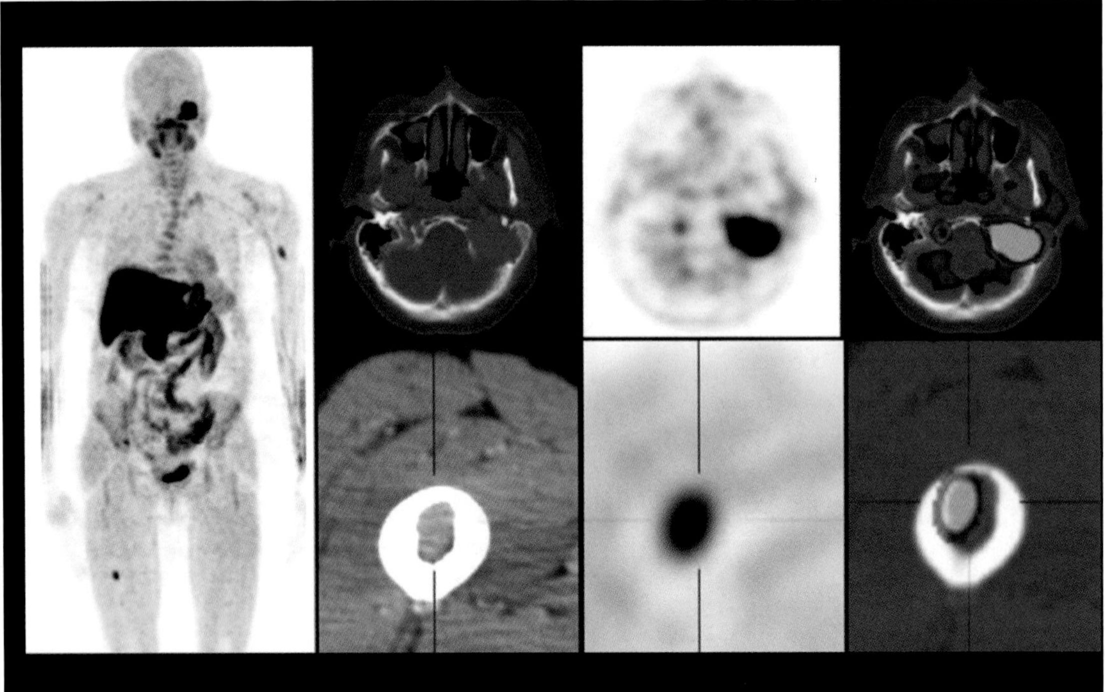

FIGURE 8.10.10. Extramedullary bilateral mammary multiple myeloma lesions (*arrows*) and abdominal bulk manifestation (maximum intensity projection image). There is intense carbon-11-methionine uptake in all of the soft tissue lesions. A further bone lesion (right ileum) without visible change of bone structure in CT is seen with carbon-11-methionine.

lesions, whereas in treated multiple myeloma many inactive osteolytic lesions suggest scar tissue in a considerable fraction of radiologically detectable bone changes. The presence of metabolically active lesions in structurally unchanged cancellous bone suggests metabolically active lesions preceding radiologically detectable structural bone changes. FDG PET or better PET/CT has now been incorporated into the Salmon/Durie PLUS staging system for myeloma staging (56,57).

REFERENCES

1. Juweid ME. Utility of positron emission tomography (PET) scanning in managing patients with hodgkin lymphoma. *Hematol Am Soc Hematol Educ Program* 2006; :259–265.
2. Schiepers C, Filmont J, Czernin J. PET for staging of Hodgkin's disease and non-Hodgkin's lymphoma. *Eur J Nucl Med Mol Imaging* 2003;30 [Suppl 1]:S82–S88.
3. Friedberg JW, Chengazi V. PET scans in the staging of lymphoma: current status. *Oncologist* 2003;8(5):438–447.
4. Lowe VJ, Wiseman GA. Assessment of lymphoma therapy using (18)F-FDG PET. *J Nucl Med* 2002;43(8):1028–1030.
5. Segall GM. FDG PET imaging in patients with lymphoma: a clinical perspective. *J Nucl Med* 2001;42(4):609–610.
6. Reske SN, Kotzerke J. FDG-PET for clinical use. Results of the 3rd German Interdisciplinary Consensus Conference, "Onko-PET III," 21 July and 19 September 2000. *Eur J Nucl Med* 2001;28(11):1707–1723.
7. Juweid ME, Stroobants S, Hoekstra OS, et al. Use of positron emission tomography for response assessment of lymphoma: consensus of the Imaging Subcommittee of International Harmonization Project in Lymphoma. *J Clin Oncol* 2007;25(5):571–578.
8. Cheson BD, Pfistner B, Juweid ME, et al. Revised response criteria for malignant lymphoma. *J Clin Oncol* 2007;25(5):579–586.
9. Juweid ME, Wiseman GA, Vose JM, et al. Response assessment of aggressive non-Hodgkin's lymphoma by integrated international workshop criteria and fluorine-18-fluorodeoxyglucose positron emission tomography. *J Clin Oncol* 2005;23(21):4652–4661.
10. Juweid ME, Cheson BD. Role of positron emission tomography in lymphoma. *J Clin Oncol* 2005;23(21):4577–4580.
11. Leskinen-Kallio S, Minn H, Joensuu H. PET and [11C]methionine in assessment of response in non-Hodgkin lymphoma. *Lancet* 1990;336 (8724):1188.
12. Reske SN. PET and restaging of malignant lymphoma including residual masses and relapse. *Eur J Nucl Med Mol Imaging* 2003;30[Suppl 1]: S89–S96.
13. Israel O, Keidar Z, Bar-Shalom R. Positron emission tomography in the evaluation of lymphoma. *Semin Nucl Med* 2004;34(3):166–179.
14. Hicks RJ, Mac Manus MP, Seymour JF. Initial staging of lymphoma with positron emission tomography and computed tomography. *Semin Nucl Med* 2005;35(3):165–175.
15. Jerusalem G, Hustinx R, Beguin Y, Fillet G. Evaluation of therapy for lymphoma. *Semin Nucl Med* 2005;35(3):186–196.
16. Mikhaeel NG. Use of FDG-PET to monitor response to chemotherapy and radiotherapy in patients with lymphomas. *Eur J Nucl Med Mol Imaging* 2006;33[Suppl 13]:22–26.
17. Jhanwar YS, Straus DJ. The role of PET in lymphoma. *J Nucl Med* 2006;47(8):1326–1334.
18. Lu P. Staging and classification of lymphoma. *Semin Nucl Med* 2005;35(3):160–164.
19. Schröder H, Larson SM, Yeung HWD. PET/CT in oncology: integration into clinical management of lymphoma, melanoma, and gastrointestinal malignancies. *J Nucl Med* 2004;45(1):72–81.

20. Buchmann I, Moog F, Schirrmeister H, et al. Positron emission tomography for detection and staging of malignant lymphoma. *Recent Results Cancer Res* 2000;156:78–89.
21. Moog F, Kotzerke J, Reske SN. FDG PET can replace bone scintigraphy in primary staging of malignant lymphoma. *J Nucl Med* 1999;40(9):1407–1413.
22. Moog F, Bangerter M, Diederichs CG, et al. Lymphoma: role of whole-body 2-deoxy-2-[F-18]fluoro-D-glucose (FDG) PET in nodal staging. *Radiology* 1997;203(3):795–800.
23. Moog F, Bangerter M, Kotzerke J, et al. 18-F-fluorodeoxyglucose-positron emission tomography as a new approach to detect lymphomatous bone marrow. *J Clin Oncol* 1998;16(2):603–609.
24. Moog F, Bangerter M, Diederichs CG, et al. Extranodal malignant lymphoma: detection with FDG PET versus CT. *Radiology* 1998;206(2):475–481.
25. Jerusalem F, Beguin Y, Fassotte MF, et al. Whole-body positron emission tomography using 18F-fluorodeoxyglucose compared to standard procedures for staging patients with Hodgkin's disease. *Haematologica* 2001;86:266–273.
26. Hutchings M, Loft A, Hansen M, et al. Position emission tomography with or without computed tomography in the primary staging of Hodgkin's lymphoma. *Haematologica* 2006;91(4):482–489.
27. Jerusalem G, Beguin Y, Najjar F, et al. Positron emission tomography (PET) with ^{18}F-fluorodeoxyglucose (18F-FDG) for the staging of low-grade non-Hodgkin's lymphoma (NHL). *Ann Oncol* 2001;12(6):825–830.
28. Karam M, Novak L, Cyriac J, et al. Role of fluorine-18-fluoro-deoxyglucose positron emission tomography scan in the evaluation and follow-up of patients with low-grade lymphomas. *Cancer* 2006;107(1):175–183.
29. Hoffmann M, Kletter K, Diemling M, et al. Positron emission tomography with fluorine-18-2-fluoro-2-deoxy-D-glucose (F18-FDG) does not visualize extranodal B-cell lymphoma of the mucosa-associated lymphoid tissue (MALT)-type. *Ann Oncol* 1999;10(10):1185–1189.
30. Rodriguez M, Ahlstrom H, Sundin A, et al. [18F] FDG PET in gastric non-Hodgkin's lymphoma. *Acta Oncol* 1997;36(6):577–584.
31. Bangerter M, Griesshammer M, Binder T, et al. New diagnostic imaging procedures in Hodgkin's disease. *Ann Oncol* 1996;7[Suppl 4]:55–59.
32. Jones HA, Cadwallader KA, White JF, et al. Dissociation between respiratory burst activity and deoxyglucose uptake in human neutrophil granulocytes: implications for interpretation of 18F-FDG PET images. *J Nucl Med* 2002;43(5):652–657.
33. Diederichs C, Staib L, Glatting G, et al. FDG-PET: elevated plasma glucose reduces both uptake and detection rate of pancreatic malignancies. *J Nucl Med* 1998;39:1030–1033.
34. Langen KJ, Braun U, Rota-Kops E, et al. The influence of plasma glucose levels on fluorine-18-fluorodeoxyglucose uptake in bronchial carcinomas. *J Nucl Med* 1993;34(3):355–359.
35. Cheson BD, Horning SJ, Coiffier B, et al. Report of an international workshop to standardize response criteria for non-Hodgkin's lymphomas. NCI Sponsored International Working Group. *J Clin Oncol* 1999;17(4):1244.
36. Canellos GP. Residual mass in lymphoma may not be residual disease. *J Clin Oncol* 1988;6(6):931–933.
37. Mikhaeel NG, Hutchings M, Fields PA, et al. FDG-PET after two to three cycles of chemotherapy predicts progression-free and overall survival in high-grade non-Hodgkin lymphoma. *Ann Oncol* 2005;16(9):1514–1523.
38. Hutchings M, Mikhaeel NG, Fields PA, et al. Prognostic value of interim FDG-PET after two or three cycles of chemotherapy in Hodgkin lymphoma. *Ann Oncol* 2005;16(7):1160–1168.
39. Hutchings M, Loft A, Hansen M, et al. FDG-PET after two cycles of chemotherapy predicts treatment failure and progression-free survival in Hodgkin lymphoma. *Blood* 2006;107(1):52–59.
40. Chillaron J, Roca R, Valencia A, et al. Heteromeric amino acid transporters: biochemistry, genetics, and physiology. *Am J Physiol Renal Physiol* 2001;281(6):F995–1018.
41. Jacobs AH, Thomas A, Kracht LW, et al. ^{18}F-fluoro-L-thymidine and ^{11}C-methylmethionine as markers of increased transport and proliferation in brain tumors. *J Nucl Med* 2005;46(12):1948–1958.
42. Reske SN. PET assessment of lymphoma: beyond ^{18}F-fluorodeoxyglucose. *PET Clin* 2006;1(3):275–281.
43. Been LB, Suurmeijer AJH, Cobben DCP, et al. ^{18}F-FLT-PET in oncology: current status and opportunities. *Eur J Nucl Med Mol Imaging* 2004;31(12):1659–1672.
44. Toyohara J, Wakib A, Takamatsub S, et al. Basis of FLT as a cell proliferation marker: comparative uptake studies with [3H]thymidine and [3H]arabinothymidine, and cell-analysis in 22 asynchronously growing tumor cell lines. *Nucl Med Biol* 2002;29:281–287.
45. Reubi JC, Waser B, Schaer JC, et al. Somatostatin receptor sst1-sst5 expression in normal and neoplastic human tissues using receptor autoradiography with subtype-selective ligands. *Eur J Nucl Med* 2001;28:836–846.
46. Reubi JC. Peptide receptors as molecular targets for cancer diagnosis and therapy. *Endocr Rev* 2003;24(4):389–427.
47. Ferone D, Semino C, Boschetti M, et al. Initial staging of lymphoma with octreotide and other receptor imaging agents. *Semin Nucl Med* 2005;35(3):176–185.
48. Press O, Leonard J, Coiffier B, et al. Immunotherapy of non-Hodgkin's lymphomas. In: *Hematology*. Orlando, FL: American Society of Hematology, 2001:221–240.
49. Witzig TE. Yttrium-90-ibritumomab tiuxetan radioimmunotherapy: a new treatment approach for B-cell non-Hodgkin's lymphoma. *Drugs Today (Barc)* 2004;40(2):111–119.
50. Toyohara J, Hayashia A, Sato M, et al. Development of radioiodinated nucleoside analogs for imaging tissue proliferation: comparisons of six 5-iodonucleosides. *Nucl Med Biol* 2003;30:687–696.
51. Shields AF, Grierson JR, Dohmen BM, et al. Imaging proliferation *in vivo* with [F-18]FLT and positron emission tomography. *Nat Med* 1998;4(11):1334–1346.
52. Buck A, Bommer M, Pitterle K, et al. Molecular imaging of proliferation in malignant lymphoma. *Cancer Res* 2006;66(22):11055–11061.
53. Buchmann I, Neumaier B, Schreckenberger M, et al. (18F)3'-deoxy-3'-fluorothymidine-PET in NHL patients. whole-body biodistribution and imaging of lymphoma manifestations—a pilot study. *Cancer Biother Radiopharm* 2004;19(4):436–442.
54. Munshi NC, Anderson KC. Plasma cell neoplasms. In: DeVita VT, Hellman S, Rosenberg SA, eds. *Cancer: principles and practice of oncology*. Philadelphia: Lippincott Williams & Wilkins, 2005:2155–2188.
55. Richardson P, Hideshima T, Anderson KC. Multiple myeloma and related disorders. In: Abeloff MD, Armitage JO, Niederhuber JE, et al, eds. *Clinical oncology*, 3rd ed. London: Churchill Livingstone, 2004:2955–2984.
56. Durie BG, Kyle RA, Belch A, et al. Myeloma management guidelines: a consensus report from the scientific advisors of the International Myeloma Foundation. *Hematol J* 2003;4(6):379–398.
57. Dankerl A, Liebisch P, Glatting G, et al. Molecular imaging of multiple myeloma with [11C]methionine PET/CT. *Radiology* 2007;242(2):498–508.
58. Angtuaco EJ, Fassas AB, Walker R, et al. Multiple myeloma: clinical review and diagnostic imaging. *Radiology* 2004;231(1):11–23.
59. Durie BG, Waxman AD, D'Agnolo A, et al. Whole-body ^{18}F-FDG PET identifies high-risk myeloma. *J Nucl Med* 2002;43(11):1457–1463.
60. Bredella MA, Steinbach L, Caputo G, et al. Value of FDG PET in the assessment of patients with multiple myeloma. *AJR Am J Roentgenol* 2005;184(4):1199–1204.
61. Orchard K, Barrington S, Buscome J, et al. Fluoro-deoxyglucose positron emission tomography imaging for the detection of occult disease in multiple myeloma. *Br J Haematol* 2002;117(1):133–135.
62. Schirrmeister H, Bommer M, Buck AK, et al. Initial results in the assessment of multiple myeloma using ^{18}F-FDG PET. *Eur J Nucl Med Mol Imaging* 2002;29(3):361–366.
63. Mikhaeel NG, Timothy AR, O'Doherty MJ, et al. 18-FDG-PET as a prognostic indicator in the treatment of aggressive non-Hodgkin's

lymphoma—comparison with CT. *Leuk Lymphoma* 2000;39(5-6): 543–553.
64. Spaepen K, Stroobants S, Dupont P, et al. Prognostic value of positron emission tomography (PET) with fluorine-18 fluorodeoxyglucose ([18F]FDG) after first-line chemotherapy in non-Hodgkin's lymphoma: is [18F]FDG-PET a valid alternative to conventional diagnostic methods? *J Clin Oncol* 2001;19(2):414–419.
65. De Wit M, Bohuslavizki KH, Buchert R, et al. 18FDG-PET following treatment as valid predictor for disease-free survival in Hodgkin's lymphoma. *Ann Oncol* 2001;12(1):29–37.
66. Dittmann H, Sokler M, Kollmannsberger C, et al. Comparison of ^{18}FDG-PET with CT scans in the evaluation of patients with residual and recurrent Hodgkin's lymphoma. *Oncol Rep* 2001;8(6):1393–1339.
67. Spaepen K, Stroobants S, Dupont P, et al. Can positron emission tomography with (18F)-fluorodeoxyglucose after first-line treatment distinguish Hodgkin's disease patients who need additional therapy from others in whom additional therapy would mean avoidable toxicity? *Br J Haematol* 2001;115:272–278.
68. Weihrauch MR, Re D, Scheidhauer K, et al. Thoracic positron emission tomography using 18F-fluorodeoxyglucose for the evaluation of residual mediastinal Hodgkin disease. *Blood* 2001;98(10):2930–2934.
69. Guay C, Lepine M, Verreault J, et al. Prognostic value of PET using ^{18}F-FDG in Hodgkin's disease for posttreatment evaluation. *J Nucl Med* 2003;44(8):1225–1231.
70. Friedberg JW, Fischman A, Neuberg D, et al. FDG-PET is superior to gallium scintigraphy in staging and more sensitive in the follow-up of patients with *de novo* Hodgkin lymphoma: a blinded comparison. *Leuk Lymphoma* 2004;45(1):85–92.
71. Panizo C, Perez-Salazar M, Bendandi M, et al. Positron emission tomography using ^{18}F-fluorodeoxyglucose for the evaluation of residual Hodgkin's disease mediastinal masses. *Leuk Lymphoma* 2004;45(9):1829–1833.
72. Jerusalem G, Beguin Y, Fassotte MF, et al. Persistent tumor ^{18}F-FDG uptake after a few cycles of polychemotherapy is predictive of treatment failure in non-Hodgkin's lymphoma. *Haematologica* 2000;85(6):613–618.
73. Kostakoglu L, Coleman M, Leonard JP, et al. PET predicts prognosis after 1 cycle of chemotherapy in aggressive lymphoma and Hodgkin's disease. *J Nucl Med* 2002;43(8):1018–1027.
74. Spaepen K, Stroobants S, Dupont P, et al. Early restaging positron emission tomography with ^{18}F-fluorodexoxyglucose predicts outcome in patients with aggressive non-Hodgkin's lymphoma. *Ann Oncol* 2002;13: 1356–1363.
75. Zijlstra JM, Hoekstra OS, Raijmakers PG, et al. ^{18}FDG positron emission tomography versus 67Ga scintigraphy as prognostic test during chemotherapy for non-Hodgkin's lymphoma. *Br J Haematol* 2003;123 (3):454–462.
76. Torizuka T, Nakamura F, Kanno T, et al. Early therapy monitoring with FDG-PET in aggressive non-Hodgkin's lymphoma and Hodgkin's lymphoma. *Eur J Nucl Med Mol Imaging* 2004;31(1):22–28.

CHAPTER

8.11 PET and PET/CT of Malignant Melanoma

HANS C. STEINERT

Malignant melanoma is the most aggressive cancer of the skin. The incidence of cutaneous malignant melanoma among whites living in the United States, Australia, and in Western Europe is increasing, but this increase is partly due to improved screening programs, although it seems undeniable the tumor is also occurring with greater frequency for other reasons (1). According to the American Cancer Society, malignant melanoma accounts for 1% to 2% of cancer deaths per year. As with most cancers, the causes of malignant melanoma are multifactorial. Numerous studies have demonstrated that the development and progression of melanoma are based on increasing levels of cutaneous solar exposure, especially to ultraviolet B radiation, in combination with the genotype, phenotype, and immunocompetence of the patient. The risk for a second melanoma is estimated to be about 5% in patients with a previous diagnosis of melanoma.

About 70% of melanomas are of the superficial spreading type. Nodular melanoma is the second most common type and comprises about 20% of melanomas. Lentigo maligna melanoma comprises 5% to 10%, and acral lentiginous melanoma 2% to 8% of melanomas. Cutaneous malignant melanoma can be located anywhere on the body, but lentigo maligna melanoma occurs primarily on the face, and acral lentiginous melanoma occurs primarily on the palms, soles, and nail beds. In women, melanomas most commonly occur on the lower extremities and in men on the back.

Any pigmented lesion with a change in size, configuration, or color should be considered a potential melanoma, and an excisional biopsy should be performed. Fortunately, in most developed countries, most patients are diagnosed early, so that melanoma can generally be cured by surgical excision of the lesion. Nevertheless, late diagnosis in locations that are not visible to the patient such as the scalp, the neck, the back, or in a plantar location are fairly common. The widely varying mortality reports in the literature depend more on the stage at diagnosis than on variations in surgical and treatment technique.

Histologic verification and accurate microstaging of tumor thickness are essential for treatment decisions and to predict the risk of metastases. For microstaging, two methods are used. The Breslow method measures the thickness of the lesion using an ocular micrometer to define the total vertical height of the melanoma, from its surface to the deepest part of the lesion. The Clark method categorizes different levels of invasion that reflect depth of penetration into the dermal layers and the subcutaneous fat (i.e., levels II, III, IV, or V). It has been demonstrated that the Breslow tumor thickness is the most important prognostic factor in clinically localized melanoma and is a highly reproducible parameter (2).

The American Joint Committee on Cancer (AJCC) has developed a four-stage system that allows subclassification of primary localized melanomas according to their malignant potential (3). Important prognostic factors, such as ulceration of the primary, microscopic or macroscopic nodal involvement, the number of positive nodes, the anatomic location of nodal, and distant metastases have been included in this staging system.

Stages I and II refer to localized melanoma and negative lymph nodes. Early malignant melanoma is curable by means of surgical excision. Stage III melanoma includes patients with lymph node metastases, either in regional nodes or as satellite or in-transit metastases. Patients with distant metastases represent stage IV. Despite the enormous progress of modern oncology, the prognosis of metastatic melanoma has remained particularly poor. Patients with regional lymphatic metastasis have a cure rate of approximately 20%, whereas no curative treatment is currently available for generalized metastatic melanoma, although occasional long-term survival has been reported for surgically resected oligometastatic disease.

The Breslow tumor thickness is an important prognostic factor in melanoma and guides treatment decisions. Patients with a Breslow tumor thickness up to 1 mm have an excellent prognosis not differing significantly from that of the general population. Patients with thin melanomas less than 1 mm are usually cured by excision of the primary lesion. Melanomas with a size of 1 to 2 mm are generally treated with wide local excision and are nowadays also commonly evaluated by sentinel lymph node scintigraphy. Patients with an indeterminate melanoma thickness of 2 to 4 mm have an increased risk of occult regional nodal metastases but have a relatively low risk (less than 20%) of distant metastases and are often staged using sentinel node detection methods. Melanomas greater than 4 mm in thickness have a 10-year survival of less than 40%. Once patients develop metastases, other prognostic factors have to be considered. The number of metastatic nodes has a significant prognostic value. Surgical excision of metastatic nodes is the only effective treatment for cure or locoregional disease control. These patients are generally treated by radical lymphadenectomy. High-risk patients with resected regional lymph node metastases may be candidates for various adjuvant chemo- or immunotherapies.

The high mortality of patients with melanoma is due to the early hematogenous spread. The mechanism of hematogenous spread and implantation of melanoma cells is poorly understood, and the location of metastases is unpredictable. The skin, subcutaneous tissue, and distant lymph nodes are the most common sites of distant metastases, but melanoma can metastasize to all organs. Early detection and surgical excision of single distant metastases are important in improving the prognosis. As soon as distant metastases are associated with a poor prognosis, significant factors predicting survival in patients with distant metastases are the number of metastatic sites and the remission duration (less than 12 months versus more than 12 months). The results of vaccine therapies for melanoma suggest that immune and clinical responses are promising in patients with metastatic disease.

For unknown primary melanomas, the distribution of metastases localized to a region or multiple sites at presentation is 43% and 57%, respectively. One must assume that the predominant origin of these unknown primary melanomas arises from a cutaneous melanoma that spontaneously regressed. Spontaneous regression is observed in up to 0.4% of melanomas and is likely mediated by an immune mechanism. The 5-year survival rate is similar to the rate of stage III disease (49%). Several reports have shown that the surgical management of patients with lymph node disease from unknown primary melanomas fared as well as patients with known cutaneous primary sites.

The clinical course of melanoma can be characterized by the risk of recurrent disease and death well beyond 10 years after the initial diagnosis. Twenty-five percent of the patients who survive more than 10 years will experience recurrence. Among patients with stage III disease, about 70% relapse, and two-thirds are at distant locations. Therefore, lifetime annual follow-up has been recommended, and imaging studies are a key to this follow-up.

STAGING OF MALIGNANT MELANOMA

Proper tumor staging is a key prerequisite for choosing the appropriate treatment strategy in melanoma. After resection of the primary melanoma, the analysis of Breslow tumor thickness gives an immediate estimate of the likelihood of regional lymph node metastases and distant metastases. In patients with thin melanomas (Breslow thickness less than 1 mm), the likelihood of metastases is so small that staging with imaging modalities is not cost-effective, although in some centers, for submillimeter lesions, sentinel nodal identification procedures are performed.

Patients with a Breslow thickness of 1 to 4 mm have an increased risk of occult regional nodal metastases but have a relatively low risk of distant metastases. Hafner et al. (4) has demonstrated that sentinel lymph node scintigraphy and biopsy is the most effective examination for staging these patients at baseline. One hundred consecutive patients with malignant melanoma and a tumor thickness greater than 1 mm were enrolled in the study. The patients underwent extensive baseline staging including physical examination, ultrasound of the regional lymph nodes and of the abdomen, sentinel lymph node scintigraphy and biopsy, chest x-ray film, and whole-body fluorodeoxyglucose (FDG) positron emission tomography (PET). Twenty-six percent of patients had a positive sentinel lymph node among 90% with microscopic disease. The macroscopic nodal metastases could be detected by physical examination, ultrasound, or PET. Therefore, in the author's institution, a sentinel lymph node scintigraphy is performed at baseline for microscopic staging. A whole-body PET scan is performed to screen for distant metastases only when a metastatic sentinel lymph node is found. This observation of higher sensitivity of sentinel node imaging/histological assessment as compared to PET for small volume tumor has been shown by several groups.

Patients with melanomas more than 4 mm have a high risk (greater than 30% to 70%) of developing distant metastases. Due to the erratic pattern of distant metastases whole-body staging is recommended. In the past, a combination of conventional imaging modalities have been used for staging of malignant melanoma, such as chest x-ray, ultrasound, computed tomography (CT), magnetic resonance imaging (MRI), and bone scintigraphy. However, specific identification of tumor tissue is difficult with these methods. Cross-sectional imaging methods are generally used to evaluate a specific region, rather than the entire body. Diagnosis of a lymph node metastasis with cross-sectional imaging modalities is mainly based on size, choosing 1 to 1.5 cm in short-axis nodal diameter as a cut-off value between benign and pathologic lymph nodes. However, using these criteria, metastases in small nodes can be missed, and reactively enlarged nodes can cause false-positive results, limiting the value of the methods. CT often misses small metastases, particularly those in bowel and bone. CT is known to have a high rate of false-positive findings if applied as a screening method in patients with malignant melanoma (5).

Due to the limitations of morphological imaging modalities, several radiopharmaceuticals have been used in nuclear medicine to visualize metastases of melanoma. These include gallium-67-citrate (6), immunoscintigraphy with monoclonal antibodies (7), indium-111-pentetreotide (8), technetium-99m-methoxyisobutyl isonitrile (9), iodine-123-methyltyrosin (10), fluorine-18-fluoroethyltyrosine (11), iodine-123-iodobenzufuran (12), fluorine-18-fluoro-dopa (13), bromine-76-bromodeoxyuridine (14), and fluorine-18-fluorodesoxyuridine (15). However, these radiotracers did not offer any significant advantage in diagnostic sensitivity in systemic staging for metastases of malignant melanoma. False-negative scan results were common because of the poor sensitivity. These radiotracers were found to be suitable for systemic staging of melanoma only in exceptional cases. Several carbon-11–labeled radiopharmaceuticals have been used for experimental studies in malignant melanoma. Due to the short half-life of carbon-11, the clinical use of these tracers for whole-body staging remains limited.

WHOLE-BODY PET AND PET/CT IMAGING WITH FLUORODEOXYGLUCOSE

Today, 2-[^{18}F]-fluoro-2-deoxy-D-glucose (FDG) is the most widely used radiopharmaceutical for staging of malignant melanoma. *In vitro* and *in vivo* experiments with tumor cells demonstrated higher FDG accumulation in melanoma than in any other tumors (16). Whole-body PET and integrated PET with CT (PET/CT) with FDG have proven to be highly effective and cost-saving modalities to screen for metastases of malignant melanoma throughout the body (17–26). With the exception of the brain and the lung, whole-body FDG PET and PET/CT scans largely replace the standard battery of imaging tests currently performed on high-risk patients (Fig. 8.11.1).

Due to the erratic pattern of metastases of malignant melanoma, whole-body FDG PET scanning or PET/CT scanning is

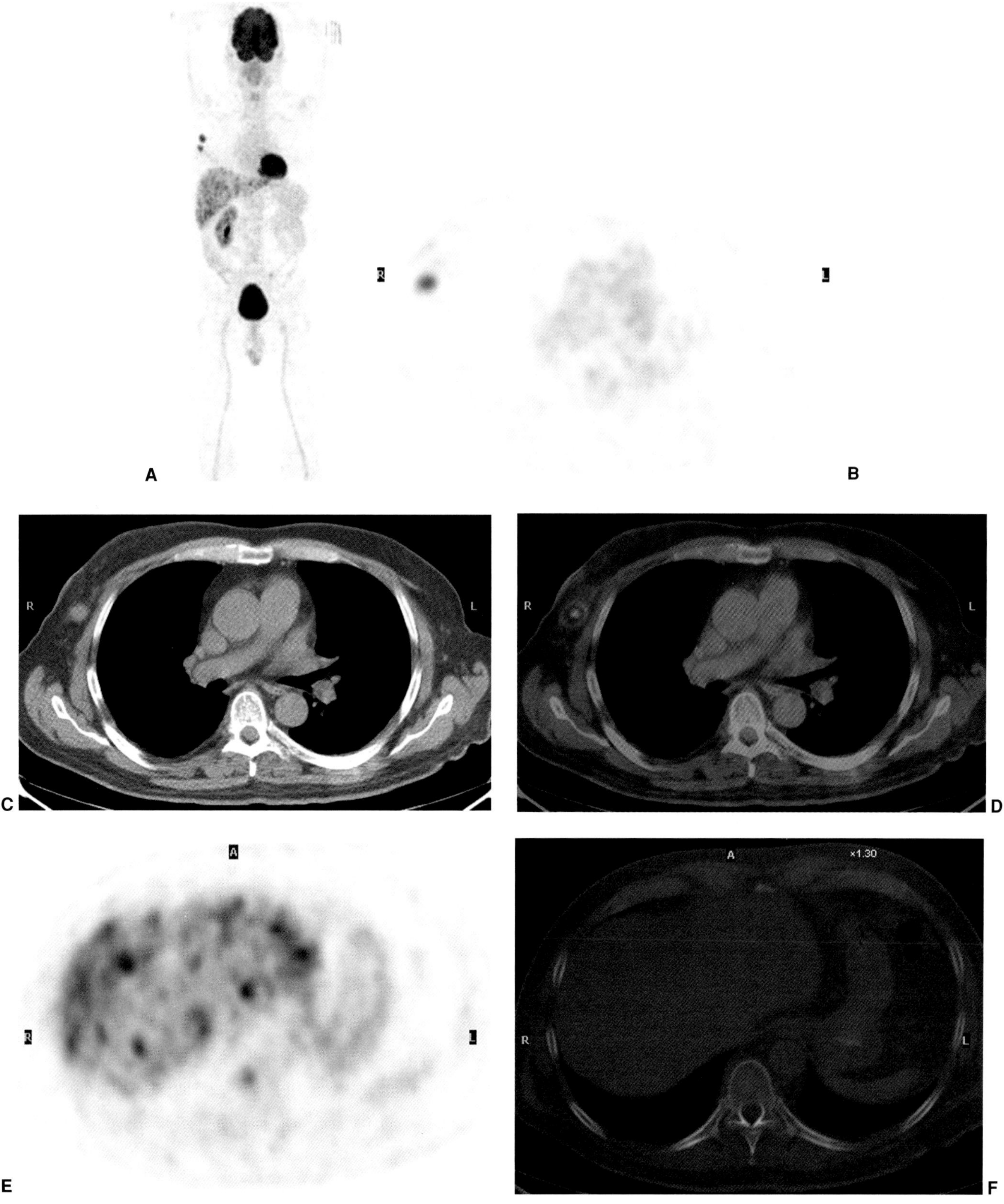

FIGURE 8.11.1. A 49-year-old man with abdominal malignant melanoma excised 1 year ago (Breslow tumor thickness 4.3 mm). There was a suspicion on lymph node metastases in the right axilla. PET/CT was performed for staging and detected in addition to the axillary lymph node metastases unknown metastases in the liver and bone. **A:** Maximum intensity projection (MIP) fluorodeoxyglucose (FDG) PET scan demonstrated two focal lesions in the right axilla, multiple lesions in the liver, and a focal lesion in the left pelvis. Transaxial PET section (**B**), corresponding CT section (**C**), and corresponding PET/CT section (**D**) clearly showed the axillary lymph node metastases. Transaxial PET section (**E**), corresponding CT section (**F**), and corresponding PET/CT section (**G**) of the liver demonstrated multiple FDG-active metastases. (*continued*)

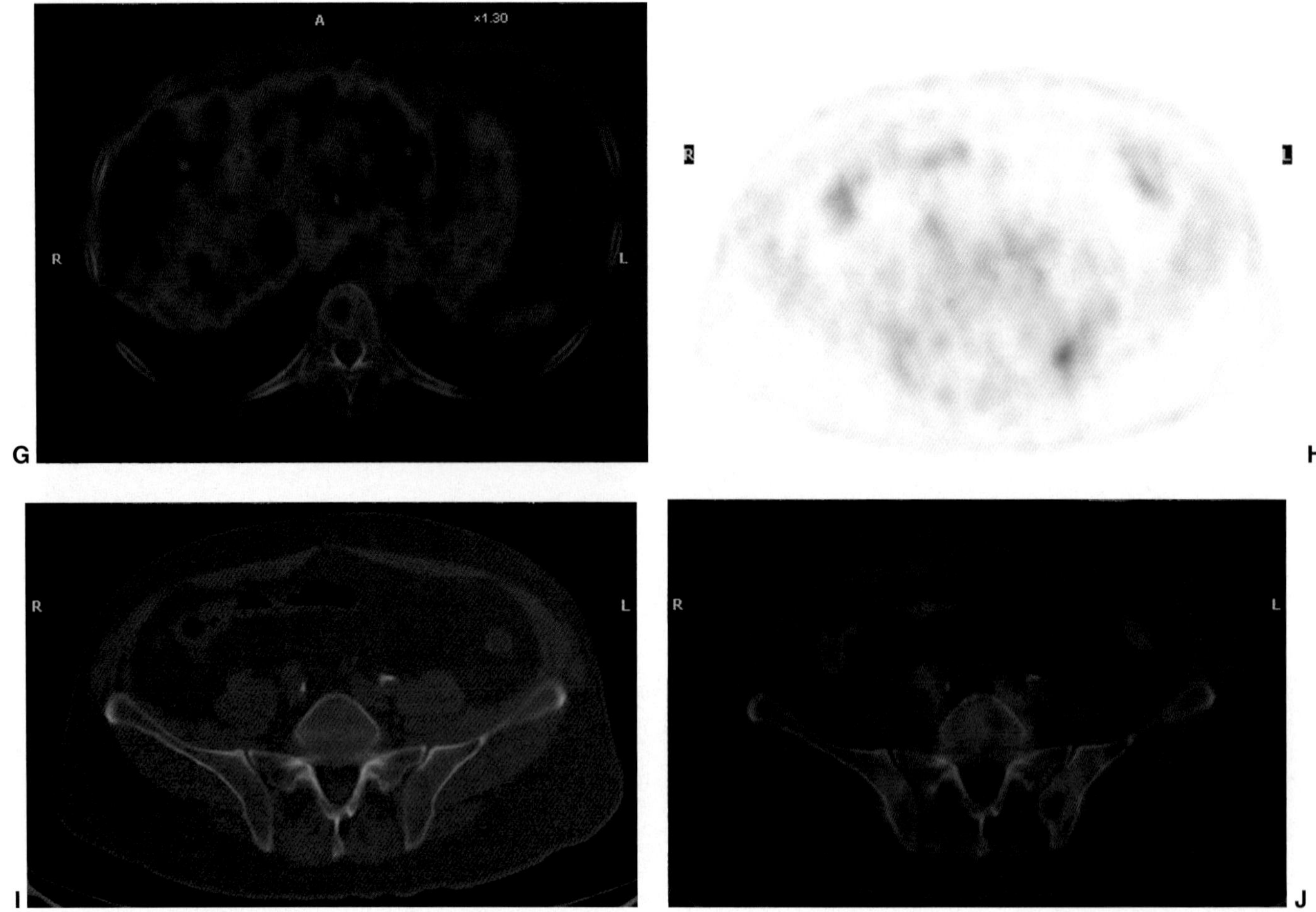

FIGURE 8.11.1. (*Continued*) Transaxial PET section (**H**), corresponding CT section (**I**), and corresponding PET/CT section (**J**) of the pelvis showed an FDG active bone metastasis in the left iliac bone.

required. In the author's institution, only combined PET/CT systems are available. A whole-body PET/CT scan is routinely performed from the head to the knees. If the primary tumor was located in a lower limb, additional PET/CT scanning is performed from the knee to the feet for the detection of satellite lesions or in-transit metastases (N3 stage).

In the author's institution, whole-body PET/CT with FDG is restricted to patients with high-risk malignant melanoma (Breslow tumor thickness greater than 4 mm or a known metastasis). The preselection of patients ensures the high effectiveness of PET/CT imaging. According to the guidelines of the Swiss Society of Dermatology, PET or PET/CT scanning is annually recommended in the first 5 years after the diagnosis of a high-risk melanoma (27). For baseline staging, sentinel lymph node scintigraphy and biopsy are routinely performed in patients with a Breslow tumor thickness from 1 to 4 mm. In cases of microscopic tumor spread to the sentinel lymph node, an additional whole-body PET/CT for screening of distant metastases will be performed.

Whole-body FDG PET or PET/CT should be used to exclude unsuspected occult metastases in patients in whom surgery of a known metastasis is planned. If multiple metastases are present, chemotherapy is the therapy of choice. In extended disease, only palliative therapy is indicated. Whole-body FDG PET or PET/CT plays an important role in the evaluation of patients when immunotherapy is considered. Adjuvant treatment with recombinant interferon α is only indicated in disease-free patients after resection of high-risk melanoma. FDG PET or PET/CT is also useful in evaluating the treatment response.

As early as 1993, Gritters et al. (17) described promising results of FDG PET imaging in melanoma. In this initial study, the sensitivity of PET was 100% for intra-abdominal visceral and lymph node metastases, but it enrolled only 12 patients in the study with known metastatic melanoma on conventional staging. This study clearly demonstrated that melanoma generally has a high FDG accumulation, that PET can detect most lesions seen by conventional imaging with the exception of pulmonary nodules, and that PET also detects occult disease originally missed by CT while correctly excluding morphological false-positive lesions.

Steinert et al. (18) reported in a study of 33 patients a sensitivity of 92% with a specificity of 77% for reading the PET images without clinical information. Specificity improved to 100% when clinical information such as location of biopsy sites or location of subcutaneous injections of interferon were obtained. PET was also highly accurate in differentiating benign from malignant lesions. In six patients (20%), whole-body PET depicted previously unknown metastases. In four of these six patients, the metastases were surgically removed.

A study by Rinne et al. (19) described a per-lesion sensitivity in primary staging of high-risk melanoma of 100%, a specificity of 94%, and an accuracy of 95% based on follow-up and biopsy, compared to an accuracy of only 68% for conventional imaging. Importantly, different sensitivities of PET compared to conventional imaging by body region were observed. Lesion detection was substantially higher by PET in the neck nodes and abdomen but substantially lower in the lung.

The excellent results in staging high-risk melanoma patients with whole-body FDG PET were confirmed in large patient studies in different PET centers worldwide (20–25). PET demonstrated high FDG accumulation by melanoma metastases in the lymph nodes and viscera. Due to the results, whole-body FDG PET and PET/CT are reimbursed by insurance and by government health care agencies for patients with high-risk melanoma in many countries.

Steinert et al. (28) performed a meta-analysis of the literature for staging of high-risk melanoma with FDG PET. In this study, a quality assessment of all articles was applied. PET studies for the microscopic tumor involvement of sentinel lymph node were excluded. Only PET studies with the definitive confirmation of lesions were included. These pooled data were then used for the meta-analysis. A total of 323 lesions could be included for the meta-analysis. An overall sensitivity of 90% (95% confidence level, 86% to 94%) and an overall specificity of 87% (95% confidence level, 79% to 95%) were determined. Other reviews of the FDG PET literature have been published. Since studies for the detection of microscopic tumor involvement of lymph nodes were included in these analyses, the accuracy of FDG PET was lower than our results (29,30). It is clear that lesion size is important in detecting tumor foci with PET and PET/CT so those studies involving small tumor-involved nodes are more likely to produce false-negative results.

It has been demonstrated that FDG PET is superior to CT in detecting melanoma metastases throughout the body. Buzaid et al. (5) analyzed the value of CT in the staging of patients with locoregional metastases of melanoma. The records of 99 patients were recorded. False-positive findings were observed in 22% of patients. Holder et al. (21) compared FDG PET with CT in 76 patients with metastatic melanoma. For the detection of melanoma metastases PET scanning had a sensitivity of 94% compared with 55% for CT scanning. The four false-negative FDG PET scan results were due to smaller lesions (less than 0.3 mm).

FDG PET and PET/CT have a strong role in the evaluation of patients with clinical recurrence. The superiority of PET over conventional staging has been reported (31). In a study by Fuster et al. (32) 156 patients with recurrent melanoma were examined with both PET and CT. The overall accuracy of PET was 81% compared with 52% for other methods.

However, limitations of FDG PET imaging have been recognized. A number of factors may interfere with the accuracy of PET scanning for metastases. It is well known that FDG is not a tumor-specific substance. False-positive results may be caused by an increased FDG accumulation in inflammatory lesions or postoperative changes (33–34). Therefore, the clinical correlation of lesions with increased FDG accumulation is obligatory to exclude tracer uptake in recent sites of surgery or infected or inflamed lesions, or at injection sites, for example. In most cases, these benign causes of FDG uptake can be specifically recognized and properly categorized. Other common benign lesions with a focal FDG uptake are colonic adenomas, inflammatory changes such as villonodular synovitis and tendinitis, Warthin tumors, and acute fractures (35) (Fig. 8.11.2). Sarcoidlike lesions may mimic generalized metastatic melanoma. Therefore, histological confirmation of lesions is recommended, particularly when PET or PET/CT findings might result in a change of treatment.

False-negative results may occur in patients with slow-growing metastases and in metastases with a large necrotic component. Due to the physiological FDG uptake in the cerebral cortex, CT and MRI are generally superior to FDG PET for the detection of brain metastases. However, in the author's institution the brain is always included in the whole-body PET/CT examination, and images have to be carefully analyzed in search of metastases. In some cases clinically occult brain metastases have been detected. In patients with neurological symptoms, MRI of the brain is the reference method to diagnose or exclude brain metastases. Due to the small tumor volume, cutaneous and subcutaneous lesions can be missed by PET imaging (18). Therefore, thorough clinical examination of the patients is mandatory.

In the assessment of pulmonary metastases of melanoma, FDG PET shows a higher specificity but lower sensitivity than CT (19,36). In a more recent study, the sensitivity of CT and PET were 93% and 57%, respectively, in the evaluation of lung nodules (31). In the author's experience, this limitation of PET imaging can be overcome by the use of integrated PET/CT imaging (37). FDG-inactive but solid pulmonary nodules without calcification are highly suspicious for lung metastases. Since the author's institute implemented integrated PET/CT scanning in staging of melanoma patients, it has encountered cases with FDG-inactive lung metastases. An explanation might be the slow proliferating rate of these lesions. Small lesions and lesions near the lung bases with more extensive motion may also be falsely negative on PET. Therefore, dedicated CT analysis is strongly recommended to improve the sensitivity and the accuracy of the integrated PET/CT imaging in the staging of the patients with high-risk melanoma (Fig. 8.11.3).

Recently it has been shown that the diagnostic performance of whole-body PET/CT for staging of distant metastases was significantly superior to CT alone and PET alone (26) (Fig. 8.11.4). In the study by Reinhardt et al. (26), 250 consecutive patients were included. The most significant advantage of combined PET/CT imaging in comparison to the single modalities was the improved detection and differentiation of visceral metastases. The accurate anatomic correlation of areas with increased FDG uptake resulted in a significant reduction of false-positive and false-negative findings by PET/CT. The specificity of PET/CT compared to PET alone was clearly superior for the detection of distant lymph node metastases (97% and 90%, respectively) and visceral metastases (95% and 88%, respectively). As in other reported studies, a significant contribution of CT was the detection of pulmonary metastases, where PET is highly specific but has a limited sensitivity. Even the specificity of CT for the differentiation of pulmonary metastases increased after image fusion with PET from 86% to 96%.

Although malignant melanoma is one of the most avidly FDG-accumulating tumors, the spatial resolution of 5 mm of dedicated PET scanners is limited. Resolution is further degraded near the edges of the scanner field of view and with the filtering methods typically applied to smooth the PET images for interpretation. The smallest metastases detected with dedicated PET scanners were 4 to 5 mm. Micrometastatic disease cannot be reliably detected with any noninvasive imaging modality. Sentinel lymph node scintigraphy and biopsy is the most effective examination for microscopic

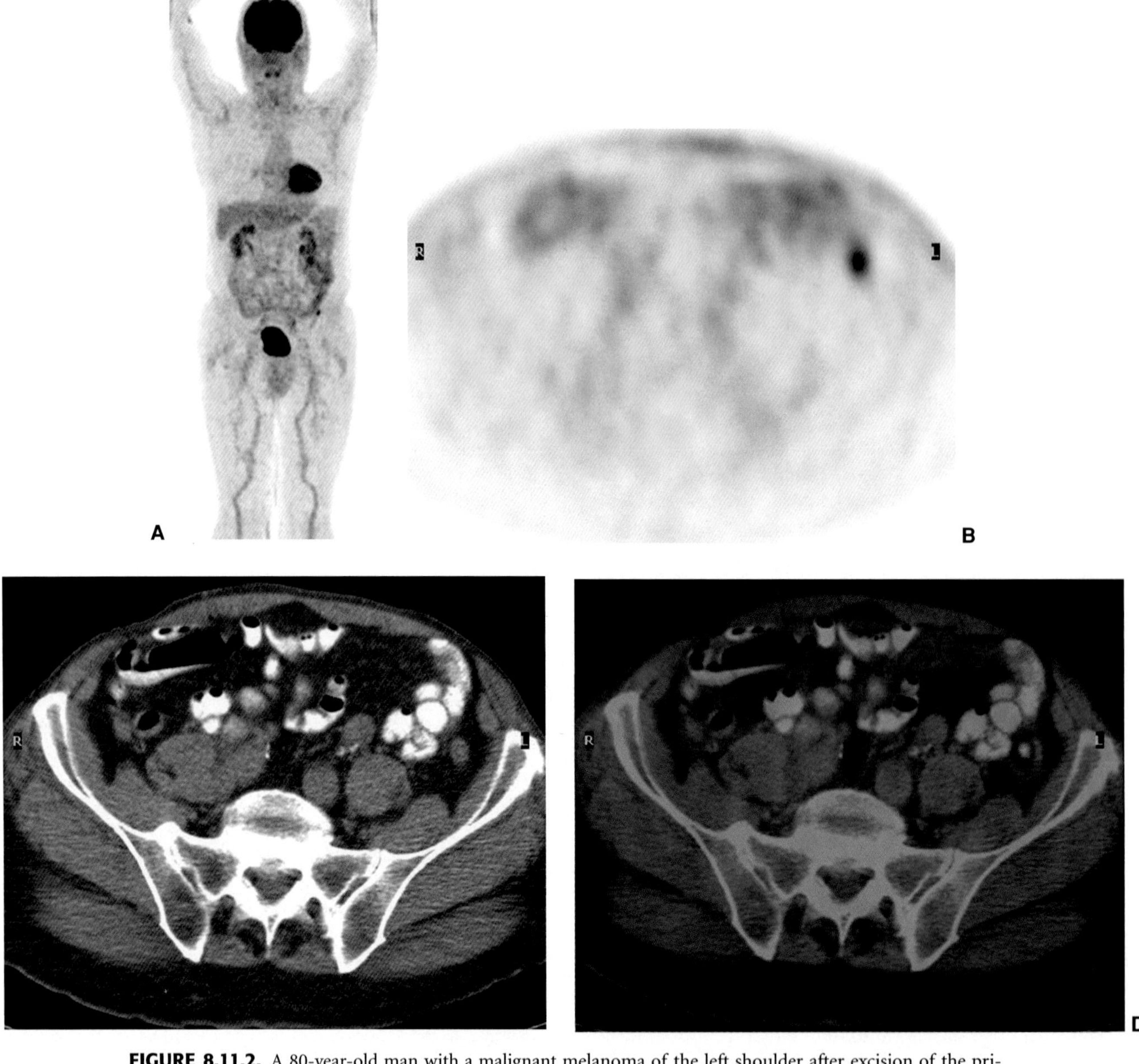

FIGURE 8.11.2. A 80-year-old man with a malignant melanoma of the left shoulder after excision of the primary 1 year ago (Breslow 3.4 mm). The sentinel lymph node biopsy revealed microscopic tumor spread. PET/CT was performed for staging. **A:** Maximum intensity projection (MIP) fluorodeoxyglucose (FDG) PET scan demonstrated a focal lesion in the lower abdomen on the left. Transaxial PET section (**B**), corresponding CT section (**C**), and corresponding PET/CT section (**D**) showed focal FDG accumulation in the colon descendens. A metastasis or a second cancer could not been ruled out. Histologically a colon polyp was proven.

staging. It has been shown that FDG accumulation in nodal metastases is dependent on nodal tumor involvement of greater than 50% or capsular infiltration and by the size of the metastasis. In a study by Crippa et al. (38), FDG PET detected 100% of metastases 10 mm and larger, 83% of metastases 6 to 10 mm, but only 23% of metastases 5 mm or smaller. Steinert et al. (39) demonstrated the importance of image acquisition and processing to lesion detectability in a study comparing whole-body PET with planar gamma camera coincidence imaging. The sensitivities were 89% and 18%, respectively. Detection of lesions smaller than 22 mm in diameter showed a reduced sensitivity by coincidence imaging. Therefore, only dedicated PET scanners can be recommended for whole-body staging of malignant melanoma as the goal is to detect both large and small tumor foci.

EFFECTIVENESS OF WHOLE-BODY FLUORODEOXYGLUCOSE PET

Patients with stage I melanoma (Breslow tumor thickness less than 1 mm) are cured by surgery. Since most malignant melanomas develop in the cutis, these lesions are simply visible by clinical examination and amenable to diagnostic biopsy. In addition, the

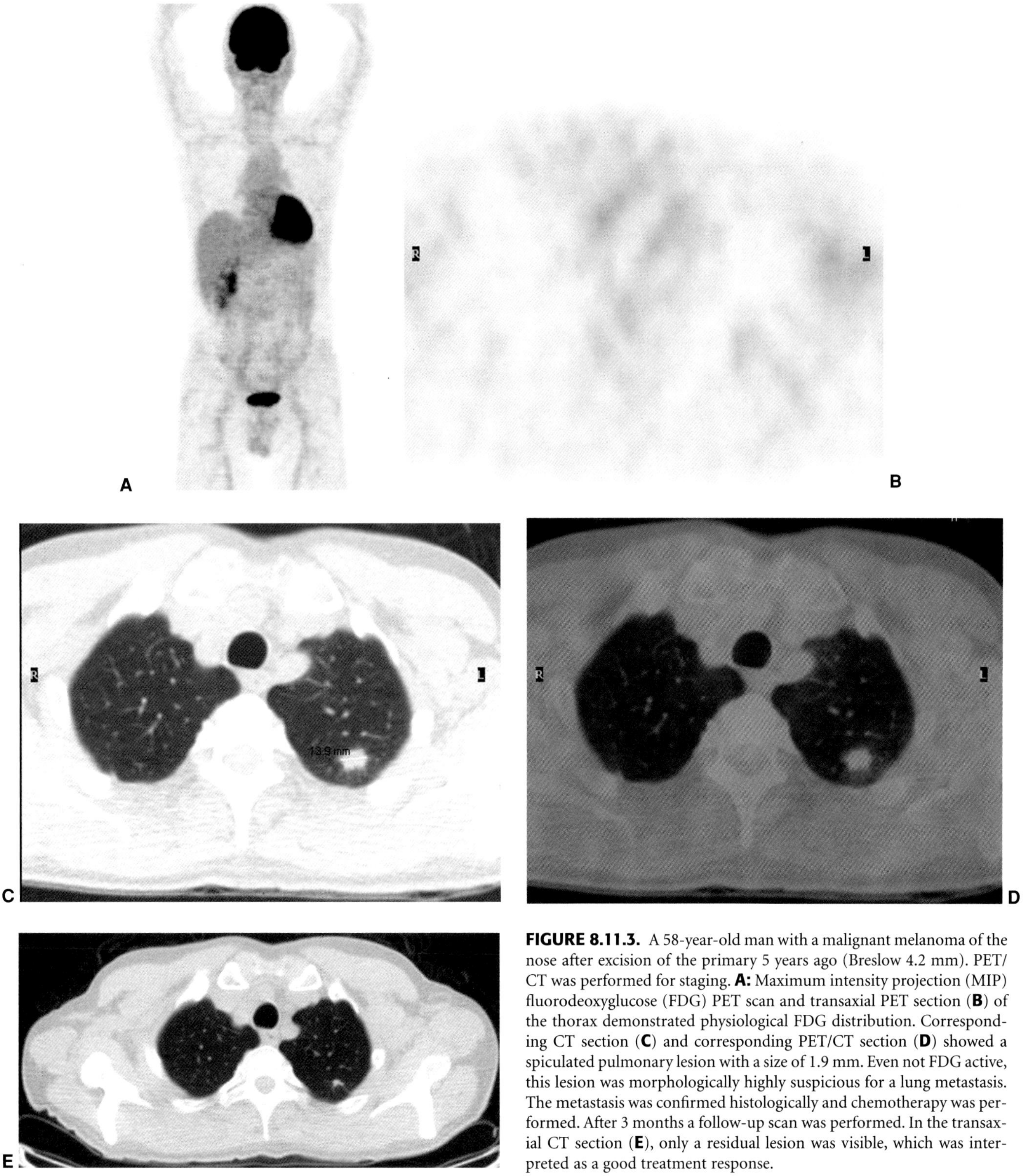

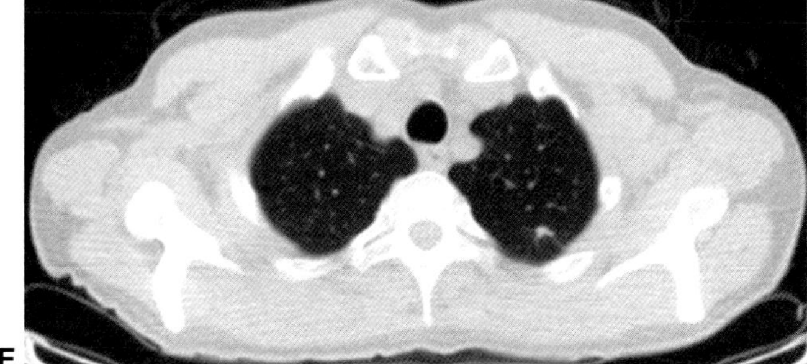

FIGURE 8.11.3. A 58-year-old man with a malignant melanoma of the nose after excision of the primary 5 years ago (Breslow 4.2 mm). PET/CT was performed for staging. **A:** Maximum intensity projection (MIP) fluorodeoxyglucose (FDG) PET scan and transaxial PET section (**B**) of the thorax demonstrated physiological FDG distribution. Corresponding CT section (**C**) and corresponding PET/CT section (**D**) showed a spiculated pulmonary lesion with a size of 1.9 mm. Even not FDG active, this lesion was morphologically highly suspicious for a lung metastasis. The metastasis was confirmed histologically and chemotherapy was performed. After 3 months a follow-up scan was performed. In the transaxial CT section (**E**), only a residual lesion was visible, which was interpreted as a good treatment response.

size of most primary melanomas is far below the spatial resolution of PET and PET/CT imaging. The likelihood of metastases is so small that staging with radiographic or PET and PET/CT imaging is not effective.

In patients with melanoma with a Breslow thickness from 1 to 4 mm, sentinel lymph node scintigraphy and biopsy is the most effective examination for staging at baseline (4). Dedicated PET scanners have a spatial resolution of 5 to 6 mm. Therefore, PET and PET/CT imaging are not useful to determine subclinical microscopic tumor spread to lymph nodes (40–45). The risk for distant metastases is also low in this patient group.

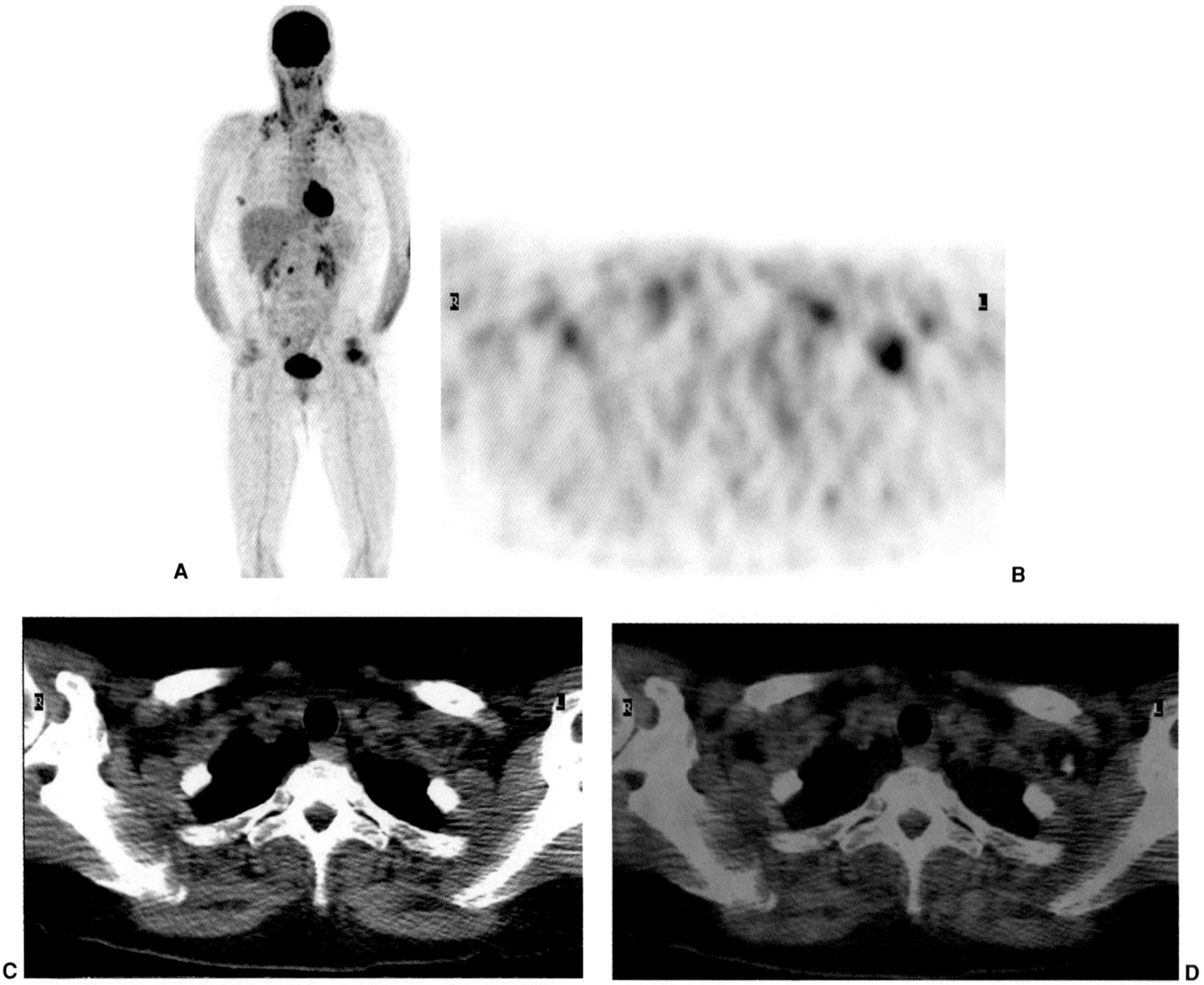

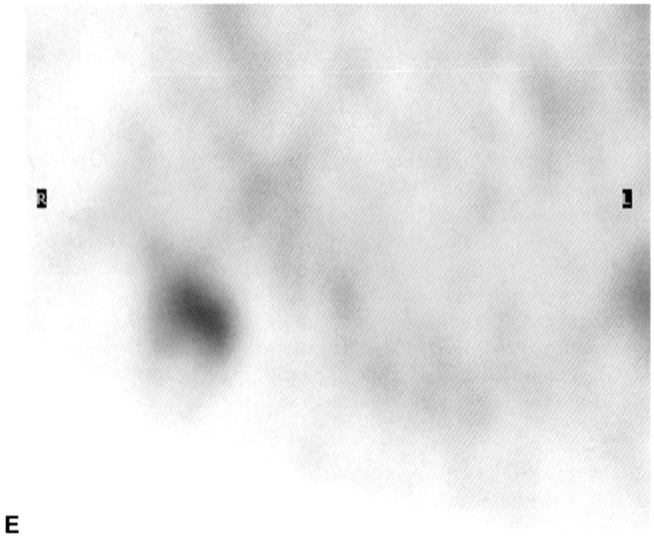

FIGURE 8.11.4. A 37-year-old woman with a malignant melanoma of unknown origin. A satellite metastasis in the right elbow was resected 2 years ago. There was a suspicion of a metastasis in the right lower thoracic wall. PET/CT was performed for staging to rule out further metastases. **A:** Maximum intensity projection (MIP) fluorodeoxyglucose (FDG) PET scan demonstrated symmetrical FDG uptake in the region of the shoulders and paravertebrally, in the right thoracic wall, in the lumbar spine, and in the right pelvis above the bladder. Transaxial PET section (**B**), corresponding CT section (**C**), and corresponding PET/CT section (**D**) of the upper thorax clearly showed FDG accumulation in the brown fat, which is a known physiological finding. Transaxial PET section (**E**), corresponding CT section (**F**), and corresponding PET/CT section (**G**) of the lower thorax demonstrated an FDG active soft tissue metastasis in the thoracic wall. (*continued*)

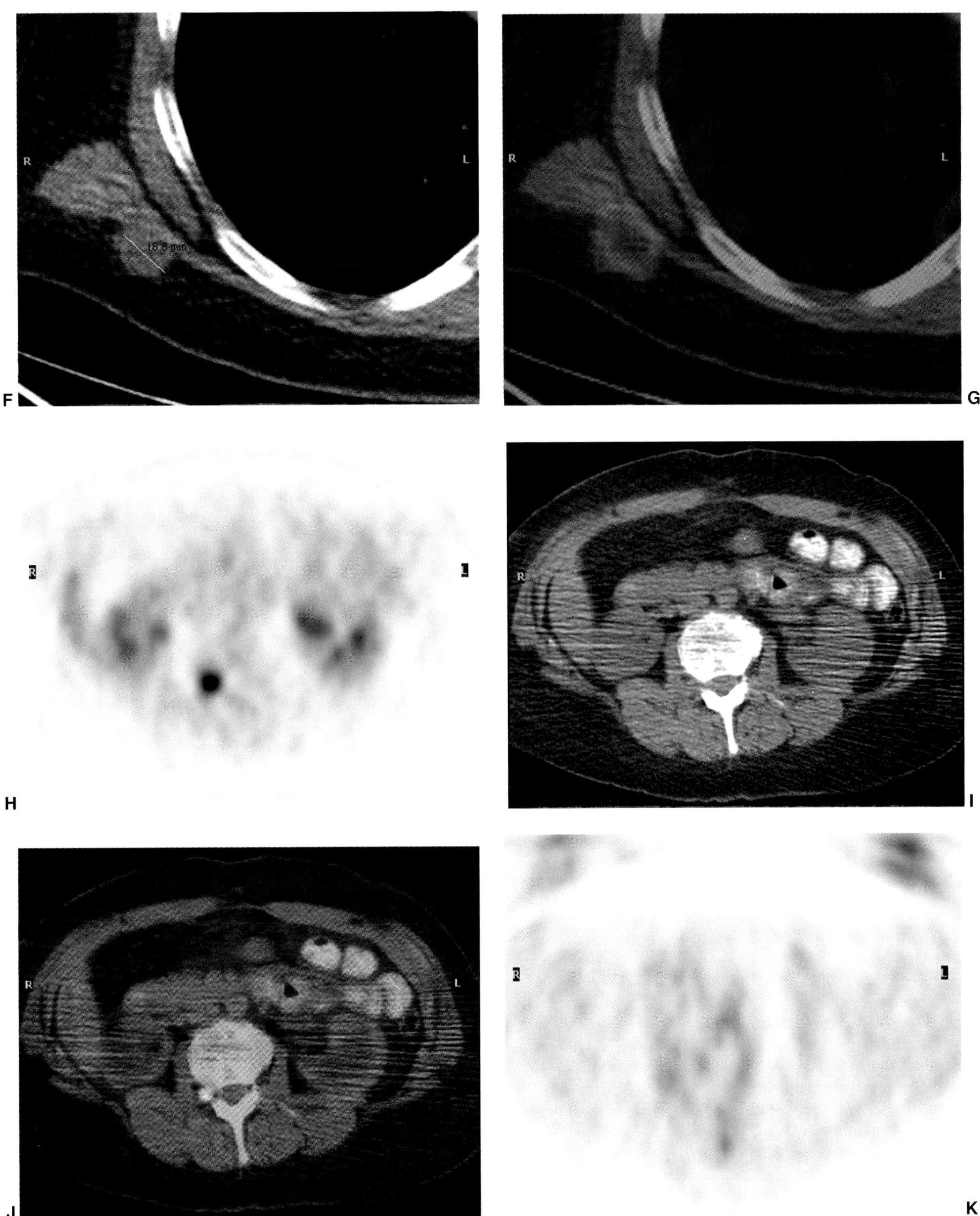

FIGURE 8.11.4. (*Continued*) In addition, transaxial PET section (**H**), corresponding CT section (**I**), and corresponding PET/CT section (**J**) of the lower abdomen showed an FDG active lesion in the right foramen of L2. (*continued*)

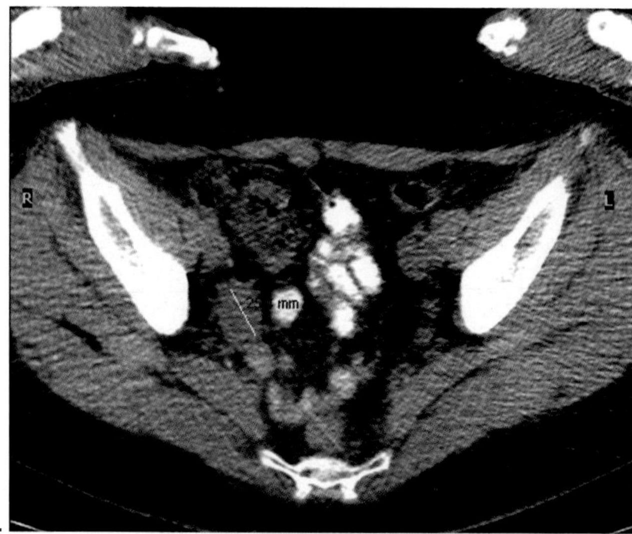

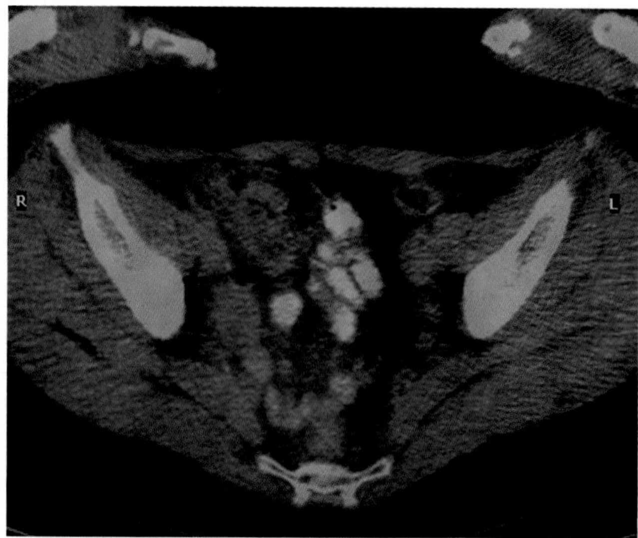

FIGURE 8.11.4. (*Continued*) Transaxial PET section (**K**), corresponding CT section (**L**), and corresponding PET/CT section (**M**) of the pelvis showed a slightly increased FDG activity in the right ovary, which was interpreted as physiologic finding of the menstrual circle. Both metastases in the thoracic wall and in the lumbar were resected.

Patients with a melanoma Breslow thickness higher than 4 mm or with known nodal metastases have a high risk of over 30% to develop distant metastases. The early detection of metastases is crucial for the optimal management of these patients. Several studies have demonstrated that whole-body FDG PET imaging is an accurate method for staging, in the follow-up of high-risk patients, and in the restaging of patients with known distant metastases to evaluate for tumor response. Surgical excision of metastases is recommended if only one or a few sites of disease is apparent (46). Therefore, the number and the location of metastases should be exactly defined. Today, whole-body integrated PET/CT imaging is the best single examination to identify and to localize the metastases.

In several studies the cost-effectiveness of whole-body FDG PET in patients with melanoma has been studied. Von Schulthess et al. (47) reviewed treatment records of 100 patients with newly diagnosed high-risk malignant melanoma. In patients with known metastatic disease, all metastases had been removed. Two staging procedures were defined. In the first, conventional staging consisted of physical examination, chest x-ray, and ultrasound of lymph nodes and the abdomen. Any suspicious lesion after conventional staging resulted in additional CT scans and histopathologic correlation. In the second procedure, staging with whole-body PET included inspection of the skin. Suspicious lesions were confirmed by biopsy or another imaging modality. The review found 172 staging protocols that could be analyzed for cost comparison. The total cost of conventional staging for the population was approximately $170,000, compared to approximately $173,000 for PET, thus only around 2% more. Among the 72 patients with metastatic disease, conventional staging costs were $145,000, while PET staging costs were $130,000. In this subset, the PET protocol cost approximately 11% less than conventional staging.

Gambhir et al. (48) compared the cost-effectiveness of the imaging strategies using conventional staging alone, including body CT and brain MRI, versus conventional staging with whole-body FDG PET. Sixty patients with suspected recurrence from malignant melanoma were included in this study. The study also predicted survival, using measures of life expectancy based on the literature, as well as savings due to changes in patient management resulting from the use of PET. The incremental cost-effectiveness ratio of the FDG PET strategy, compared with the conventional staging strategy, was $3,000 to $8,000 per year of life saved, a figure far below the standard of $50,000 per year of life saved used by U.S. health economists to characterize a cost-effective intervention.

In another study the impact of FDG PET on patient stage and management has been evaluated from the referring physician's perspective (49). Referring physicians indicated that whole-body FDG PET changed the clinical stage in 29% of patients. Twenty percent of patients were up-staged and 10% of patients were down-staged. The PET findings resulted in intermodality management changes in 29% of patients. Intramodality management change occurred in 18% of patients. This survey-based study of referring physicians demonstrated that FDG PET has a major impact on the management of patients with melanoma.

In the author's experience, PET changes the treatment in 20% of patients with high-risk melanoma. Other groups reported an even higher influence of FDG PET on the diagnostic and therapeutic management of patients. In one study, PET resulted in a change in surgical management in 16 of 45 patients (36%). Changes in management can include cancellation of surgery to remove "limited" stage melanoma when more extensive melanoma is actually present. The addition of FDG PET to the diagnostic algorithm resulted in a savings-to-cost ratio of 2:1 because of the avoidance of unnecessary procedures (50). In a study in patients with recurrent melanoma, PET results changed the clinical management of 36% of patients in comparison to conventional staging (30). Although the use of PET and PET/CT to follow the treatments of patients with melanoma is not yet widely supported in the literature, in part because of the limited number of effective therapies, an increasing use of PET with FDG is being seen in the monitoring of treatment response.

SUMMARY

Whole-body FDG PET is a very effective imaging modality to screen for metastases in patients with malignant melanoma and a high risk for metastases (Breslow thickness of more than 4 mm or already known metastases). The preselection of patients ensures high effectiveness of PET imaging and PET/CT imaging. The advantage of PET and PET/CT, particularly in melanoma with its unpredictable spread of metastases, is that the whole body can be easily examined. Limitations of FDG PET in the detection of lung metastases and brain metastases have been recognized. Recently it has been shown that integrated PET/CT is superior to conventional CT in lesion detection. Dedicated interpretation of the CT part of integrated PET/CT imaging improves the early detection of lung metastases. Due to the clear advantages of integrated PET/CT, it is not surprising that worldwide many conventional PET scanners are being replaced by combined PET/CT devices. Whole body FDG PET and PET/CT have a major impact on the management of patients with melanoma.

Surgical resection is the treatment of choice for regional lymph node metastases or a single distant metastasis. Whole-body FDG PET or PET/CT should be used to exclude unsuspected occult metastases in patients in whom surgery is planned. If multiple metastases are present, patients are referred to chemo- and/or immunotherapy. In extended metastatic disease, only palliative therapy is indicated. Whole-body FDG PET and PET/CT also play an important role in the evaluation of patients treated with recombinant interferon α and is only indicated in disease-free patients after resection of a high-risk cutaneous melanoma. PET and PET/CT are also helpful in following response to treatment. Assessment of the efficacy of treatments with PET is also becoming more frequent as the therapeutic options for systemic metastatic disease continue to grow.

REFERENCES

1. Jemal A, Tiwari RC, Murray T, et al. Cancer statistics, 2004. *CA Cancer J Clin* 2004;54:8–29.
2. Balch CM, Murad TM, Soong S-J, et al. A multifactorial analysis of melanoma: prognostic histopathological features comparing Clark's and Breslow's staging methods. *Ann Surg* 1978;188:732–742.
3. Balch CM, Sober AJ, Soong S-J, et al. The new melanoma staging system. *Semin Cutan Med Surg* 2004;22:42–51.
4. Hafner J, Schmid MH, Kempf W, et al. Baseline staging in cutaneous malignant melanoma. *Br J Dermatol* 2004;150:677–686.
5. Buzaid AD, Sandler AB, Mani S, et al. Role of computed tomography in the staging of primary melanoma. *J Clin Oncol* 2001;19:2674–2678.
6. Kalff V, Hicks RJ, Ware RE, et al. Evaluation of high-risk melanoma: comparison of [18F]FDG PET and high-dose 67Ga SPET. *Eur J Nucl Med* 2002;29:506–515.
7. Böni R, Huch-Böni R, Steinert HC, et al. Antimelanoma monoclonal antibody 225.28S immunoscintigraphy in metastatic melanoma. *Dermatology* 1995;191:119–123.
8. Hoefnagel CA, Rankin EM, Valdes Olmos RA, et al. Sensitivity versus specificity in melanoma using iodine-123 iodobenzamide and indium-111 pentetreotide. *Eur J Nucl Med* 1994;21:587–588.
9. Alonso O, Martinez M, Mut F, et al. Detection of recurrent malignant melanoma with 99mTc-MIBI scintigraphy. *Melanoma Res* 1998;8:355.
10. Steinert HC, Böni R, Huch-Böni R, et al. Jod-123-methyltyrosin-szintigraphie beim malignen melanom. *Nuklearmedizin* 1997;36:36–41.
11. Schreckenberger M, Kadalie C, Enk A, et al. First results of ^{18}F-fluoroethyl-tyrosine PET for imaging of metastatic malignant melanoma. *J Nucl Med* 2001; 42[Suppl]:30P.
12. Steinert HC, Huch-Böni R, Böni R, et al. Dopamin-D2-Rezeptorszintigraphie mit Jod-123-Jodbenzofuran beim malignen Melanom. *Nuklearmedizin* 1995;34:146–150.
13. Mishima Y, Imahori Y, Honda C, et al. *In vivo* diagnosis of human malignant melanoma with PET using specific melanoma seeking fluorine-18-DOPA analogue. *J Neurooncol* 1997;33:163–169.
14. Böni R, Bläuenstein P, Dummer R, et al. Non-invasive assessment of tumour cell proliferation with positron emission tomography and ^{76}Br-bromodeoxyuridine. *Melanoma Res* 1999;9:569–573.
15. Vogg AT, Glatting G, Möller P, et al. ^{18}F5-fluoro-2'-desoxyuridine as PET-tracer for imaging of solid malignomas. *J Nucl Med* 2001;42 [Suppl]:30P.
16. Wahl RL, Hutchins GD, Buchsbaum DJ, et al. 18F-2-deoxy-2-fluoro-D-glucose uptake into human tumour xenografts. *Cancer* 1991;67: 1544–1550.
17. Gritters LS, Francis IR, Zasadny KR, et al. Initial assessment of positron emission tomography using 2-fluorine-18-fluoro-2-deoxy-D-glucose in the imaging of malignant melanoma. *J Nucl Med* 1993;34: 1420–1427.
18. Steinert HC, Huch-Böni RA, Buck A, et al. Malignant melanoma: staging with whole-body positron emission tomography and 2-[F-18]-fluoro-2-deoxy-D-glucose. *Radiology* 1995;195:705–709.
19. Rinne D, Baum RP, Hör G, et al. Primary staging and follow-up of high risk melanoma patients with whole-body ^{18}F-fluorodeoxyglucose positron emission tomography. *Cancer* 1998;82:1664–1671.
20. Damian DL, Fulham MJ, Thompson E, et al. Positron emission tomography in the detection and management of metastatic melanoma. *Melanoma Res* 1996;6:325–329.
21. Holder WD Jr, White RL Jr, Zuger JH, et al. Effectiveness of positron emission tomography for the detection of melanoma metastases. *Ann Surg* 1998;227:764–769.
22. Hsueh EC, Gupta RK, Glass EC, et al. Positron emission tomography plus serum TA90 immune complex assay for detection of occult metastatic melanoma. *J Am Coll Surg* 1998;187:191–197.
23. Paquet P, Henry F, BelhocineT, et al. An appraisal of 18-fluorodeoxyglucose positron emission tomography for melanoma staging. *Dermatology* 2000;200:167–169.
24. Tyler DS, Onaitis M, Kherani A, et al. Positron emission tomography scanning in malignant melanoma. Clinical utility in patients with stage III disease. *Cancer* 2000;89:1019–1025.
25. Eigtved A, Andersson AP, Dahlstrom K, et al. Use of fluorine-18 fluorodeoxyglucose positron emission tomography in the detection of silent metastases from malignant melanoma. *Eur J Nucl Med* 2000;27: 70–75.
26. Reinhardt MJ, Joe AY, Huber A, et al. Diagnostic performance of whole body dual modality ^{18}F-FDG PET/CT imaging for N- and M-staging of malignant melanoma: experience with 250 consecutive patients. *J Clin Oncol* 2006;24:1178–1187.
27. Dummer R, Panizzon R, Bloch PH, et al. Updated Swiss guidelines fort he treatment and follow-up of cutaneous melanoma. *Dermatology* 2005;210:39–44.
28. Steinert HC, von Schulthess GK, Reuland P, et al. A meta-analysis of the literature for staging of malignant melanoma with whole-body FDG PET. *J Nucl Med* 2001;42[Suppl]:307P.
29. Gambhir SS, Czernin J, Schwimmer J, et al. A tabulated summary of the FDG PET literature. Oncologic applications: melanoma. *J Nucl Med* 2001;42[Suppl 1]:13S–15S.
30. Mijnhout GS, Hoekstra OS, van Tulder MW, et al. Systematic review of the diagnostic accuracy of ^{18}F-fluorodeoxyglucose positron emission tomography in melanoma patients. *Cancer* 2001;91:1530–1542.
31. Stas M, Stroobants S, Dupont P, et al. 18-FDG PET scan in the staging of recurrent melanoma: additional value and therapeutic impact. *Melanoma Res* 2002;12:479–490.
32. Fuster D, Chiang S, Johnson G, et al. Is ^{18}F-FDG PET more accurate than standard diagnostic procedures in the detection of suspected recurrent melanoma? *J Nucl Med* 2004;45:1323–1327.

33. Strauss LG. Fluorine-18 deoxyglucose and false-positive results: a major problem in the diagnostics of oncological patients. *Eur J Nucl Med* 1996;23:1409–1415.
34. Shreve PD, Anzai Y, Wahl RL. Pitfalls in oncologic diagnosis with FDG PET imaging: physiologic and benign variants. *Radiographics* 1999;19: 61–77.
35. Steinert HC, Bode B, Boeni R, et al. Malignant melanoma: Non-malignant "hot spots" in whole-body FDG PET with radiologic pathologic correlation. *Radiology* 2000;217[Suppl]:359.
36. Nguyen AT, Akhurst T, Larson SM, et al. PET scanning with FDG in patients with melanoma: benefits and limitations. *Clin Positron Imaging* 1999;2:93–98.
37. Strobel K, Dummer R, Husarik DB, et al. High-risk melanoma: accuracy of FDG PET/CT with added CT morphologic information for detection of metastases. *Radiology* 2007;244:566–574.
38. Crippa F, Leutner M, Belli F, et al. Which kinds of lymph node metastases can FDG PET detect? A clinical study in melanoma. *J Nucl Med* 2000;41:1491–1494.
39. Steinert HC, Voellmy DR, Trachsel C, et al. Planar coincidence scintigraphy and PET in staging malignant melanoma. *J Nucl Med* 1998;39: 1892–1897.
40. Acland KM, Healy C, Calonje E, et al. Comparison of positron emission tomography scanning and sentinel node biopsy in the detection of micrometastases of primary cutaneous malignant melanoma. *J Clin Oncol* 2001;19:2674–2678.
41. Belhocine T, Pierard G, de Labrassinne M, et al. Staging of regional nodes in AJCC stage I and II melanoma: ^{18}FDG PET imaging versus sentinel node detection. *Oncologist* 2002;7:271–278.
42. Wagner JD. PET detection of melanoma metastases in lymph nodes. *J Nucl Med* 2003;44:486.
43. Fink AM, Holle-Robatsch S, Herzog N, et al. Positron emission tomography is not useful in detecting metastasis in the sentinel lymph node in patients with primary malignant melanoma stage I and II. *Melanoma Res* 2004;14:141–145.
44. Wagner JD, Schauwecker DS, Davidson D, et al. Inefficacy of F-18 fluorodeoxy-D-glucose-positron emission tomography scans for initial evaluation in early-stage cutaneous melanoma. *Cancer* 2005:104:570–579.
45. Wagner JD, Schauwecker DS, Davidson D, et al. FDG-PET sensitivity for melanoma lymph node metastases is dependent on tumor volume. *J Surg Oncol* 2001;77:237–242.
46. Finkelstein SE, Carrasquillo JA, Hoffmann JM, et al. A prospective analysis of positron emission tomography and conventional imaging for detection of stage IV metastatic melanoma in patients undergoing metastasectomy. *Ann Surg Oncol* 2004;11:731–738.
47. Von Schulthess GK, Steinert HC, Dummer R, et al. Cost effectiveness of whole-body FDG imaging in non–small cell lung cancer and malignant melanoma. *Acad Radiol* 1998;5[Suppl 2]:S300–S302.
48. Gambhir SS, Hoh CK, Essner R, et al. A decision analysis model for the role of whole body FDG PET in the management of patients with recurrent melanoma. *J Nucl Med* 1998;39[Suppl]:94P.
49. Wong C, Silverman DH, Seltzre M, et al. The impact of 2-deoxy-2[18F]fluoro-D-glucose whole body positron emission tomography for managing patients with melanoma: the referring physician's perspective. *Mol Imag Biol* 2002;4:185–190.
50. Valk PE, Pounds TR, Tesar RD, et al. Cost-effectiveness of PET imaging in clinical oncology. *Nucl Med Biol* 1996;23:737–743.

CHAPTER

8.12 PET in Breast Cancers

FARROKH DEHDASHTI

Breast cancer is the most common malignancy in women, accounting for approximately 26% of all female cancers. It is estimated that in the year 2008 that there will have been nearly 182,460 new cases of breast cancer and approximately 40,480 breast cancer-related deaths in the United States (1). Despite progress in early diagnosis and treatment, breast cancer remains a significant health problem. An increase in availability and advances in imaging techniques have the potential to improve the management of breast cancer. The past decade has witnessed the emergence of functionally based methods, such as positron emission tomography (PET), which have added new dimensions to the radiological evaluation of breast cancer.

Currently the role of imaging is not limited to the early detection of breast cancer, but it also involves staging and restaging, assessment of tumor behavior and prognosis, and monitoring response to therapy. This chapter focuses on the current and potential clinical applications of PET and PET combined with computed tomography (CT), as well as their limitations, and discusses how PET can help resolve some of the shortcomings of conventional imaging modalities in the management of patients with breast cancer.

Although a variety of biological and functional characteristics of breast cancer, such as blood flow and receptor status, can be studied with PET, the clinical applications are mainly focused on the assessment of glucose metabolism using 2-fluorine-18-fluoro-2-deoxy-D-glucose (FDG). This focus is related to tracer availability as well as the superior performance of FDG in tumor evaluation and characterization relevant to clinical management of cancer patients, and the fact that PET assessment of some of the biological features of breast cancer, such as tumor blood flow, do not appear to be clinically relevant based on present data.

Clinical and preclinical studies have shown increased FDG accumulation in breast cancer. Several specific tumor characteristics have been demonstrated to determine the degree of glucose metabolism. In human breast cancer, marked overexpression of the *GLUT1* glucose transporter has been reported, and this is certainly an important factor contributing to the increased glucose accumulation within this cancer (2). Additionally, FDG uptake in breast cancer has been attributed to several other factors such as microvessel density, hexokinase activity, number of tumor cells/volume, proliferation rate (also reflected in necrosis), number of lymphocytes (not macrophages), and HIF1α for up-regulating GLUT1 (3,4).

The phosphorylation step may determine the uptake of FDG in breast cancer (5). *In vitro* studies of rat mammary tumors (RMT) and human breast cancer cells (*MCF7* and *HTB771P3*) have demonstrated an inverse relationship between extracellular glucose levels and tumor FDG uptake (6,7). It also has been shown that in breast cancer cell line (*MCF7*), abrogation of p53 is associated with specific changes in glucose metabolism (8).

IMAGING PROTOCOL AND IMAGE ANALYSIS

FDG PET imaging protocols differ from institution to institution; however, there are several important issues that should be considered for successful clinical FDG PET imaging of patients with breast cancer. In this group of patients, FDG should be administered intravenously in the arm opposite a suspected breast lesion or via a foot vein to avoid increased FDG uptake in normal axillary lymph nodes as a result of extravasation of FDG at the injection site. Patients should have been fasting for at least 4 hours prior to FDG injection and exercise should be avoided in the day prior to the PET scan.

Determination of blood glucose levels before FDG injection is recommended to identify patients with possible fasting hyperglycemia (7). *In vitro* studies of rodent and human mammary carcinoma cells in culture and *in vivo* studies in rodent tumors have demonstrated that acute hyperglycemia markedly impairs tumor FDG uptake (7). A significant decrease in tumor FDG uptake has been reported in the insulin-induced hypoglycemic state. Typically, patients are studied in the supine position; however, primary breast cancer may be visualized more clearly with the patient in the prone position using a scintimammography positioning pad, which provides less motion-related artifact and better separation of deep breast structures from the myocardium and liver and may decrease scatter from FDG uptake in these organs compared with that in the supine position (9).

It has been reported that the tumor-to-nontumor uptake ratio improves by obtaining delayed PET images 3 hours after administration of FDG (10). Kumar et al. (11) reported that over time (average time interval of approximately 38 minutes between two scans), FDG uptake increased in breast cancer, whereas FDG uptake decreased in inflammatory lesions and normal breast tissues. They found that a percentage change of +3.75 or more in standard uptake value (SUV) over time is highly sensitive and specific in differentiating inflammatory lesions from malignant lesions. However, it is yet to be proven whether prone imaging or delayed imaging improves lesion characterization or detection sensitivity.

FDG PET imaging is performed with or without attenuation correction. No significant difference has been demonstrated in lesion detectability of attenuation-corrected or noncorrected images (10). Currently, as PET/CT replaces PET alone, fewer studies are performed without attenuation correction. It is recommended that both attenuation-corrected and noncorrected images be evaluated, as some breast lesions may be better seen on noncorrected images.

Although clinical oncologic FDG PET images are most often interpreted qualitatively, semiquantitative measurements offer more objective criteria for differentiating benign from malignant lesions and monitoring response to therapy. The most commonly utilized semiquantitative method is the SUV, also known as the differential uptake ratio or the differential absorption ratio. SUV is an index of glucose metabolism based on tissue uptake of FDG normalized to body weight (or lean body mass or body surface area) and injected dose (12,13). In the fasting state body fat has a much lower uptake of FDG than other tissues, so the SUVs of many tissues show a strong positive correlation with weight and may be overestimated in obese patients. This may be important when FDG PET studies performed before and after cancer treatment are compared to assess response to therapy, as SUVs may not be comparable if the patient loses a significant amount of weight between the two PET studies. It has been shown that SUV normalized to lean body mass or body surface area instead of total body weight is a more accurate estimate that will be less affected by changes in body weight (12,13).

Overall, in patients undergoing cancer therapy, efforts should be made to perform the studies in a similar fashion. Probably the most common source of variability in SUV determination is related to the duration of the uptake phase, as the SUV for most tumors continues to increase slowly over time, and no methods to correct for this variable are available.

The Patlak graphical approach also has been used in a limited fashion for quantitative evaluation of the FDG metabolic rate in breast lesions. This graphical approach provides an estimate of the net FDG phosphorylation rate constant (mL/min/g); this value is proportional to the glucose utilization rate based on the assumptions that the flow of tracer is unidirectional into the cellular compartment and follows first-order kinetics, and that it occurs only in an irreversible manner if the tracer is metabolized so that the metabolites are also irreversibly trapped (14). Although this type of analysis may provide a more reliable estimate of regional glucose metabolism, it is time consuming and technically demanding and therefore is not recommended for routine clinical studies of cancer patients who are often too ill to tolerate the lengthy imaging required.

A recent study demonstrated similar diagnostic accuracy for visual and semiquantitative (SUV and Patlak, respectively) analysis in differentiating benign from malignant breast lesions (15). The average SUV normalized to body weight and blood glucose and corrected for partial volume averaging had the highest diagnostic accuracy, exceeding that achieved with either the Patlak method or both average and maximum SUV uncorrected for blood glucose level and partial volume averaging (15).

Physiologic accumulation of FDG in normal breast tissue is variable, reflecting the amount of proliferative glandular breast tissue present. FDG uptake in normal breast is typically mild and diffuse with focally increased uptake in the areolar complexes. However, FDG uptake is more prominent in premenopausal women with abundant proliferative glandular breast tissue and in postmenopausal women undergoing hormone replacement therapy.

In a recent study of 96 patients with documented unilateral breast cancer, menstrual status or age was shown to have no effect on the degree of FDG uptake in the normal breast (16). Intense FDG uptake has been reported in lactating breasts, but not in postpartum breasts of women who are not breastfeeding. FDG is detected in minimal concentration in breast milk despite intense uptake in the breast itself. Therefore, radiation exposure to an infant is mainly due to close contact with the mother's breast rather than to ingestion of radioactive milk. Interruption of breastfeeding for approximately 8 hours should be sufficient to keep the infant's exposure below 500 mrem. However, radiation dose to the lactating breast can be substantial if breastfeeding is not terminated, and careful consideration must be given as to the diagnostic information available from the PET versus the increased radiation dose to the patient in such cases.

DETECTION OF BREAST CANCER

In randomized clinical trials, screening mammography has resulted in a reduction of breast cancer mortality by about 25% to 45% in women over the age of 40 (17). Recent significant progress in mammographic technique, such as computer-aided lesion detection, as well as the appropriate use of supplementary imaging techniques, such as ultrasonography and magnetic resonance imaging (MRI), have played an important role in the early detection of breast cancer.

Currently, the diagnosis of breast cancer is based on breast self-examination, physical examination by trained personnel, mammography supplemented as necessary by ultrasonography and MRI, and histological examination of identified breast lesions. Breast examination has low specificity and is not very sensitive for detection of small lesions, but is useful for detection of palpable breast masses. Mammography has a relatively high sensitivity, ranging from 54% to 81% depending on age, breast density, and menopausal status (18). The use of computer-aided lesion detection with mammography has resulted in an increase in the rate of cancer detection (19). Although mammography has a higher sensitivity for detecting breast cancer in fatty breasts, it is of limited value in several situations, such as detection of malignancy in dense breasts or postsurgical breasts (e.g., after breast augmentation, lumpectomy, or breast-conserving therapy for breast cancer), early detection of tumor recurrence after surgery, and monitoring response to therapy (20,21).

Mammography has a low positive-predictive value (10% to 35%) for nonpalpable cancers, and the frequency of positive biopsy findings after abnormal mammography ranges from 10% to 50% (22–24). Because of the low specificity of mammography, the majority of breast lesions are subjected to biopsy. Although the commonly employed fine-needle aspiration and stereotactic core biopsy are less invasive than excisional biopsies, they suffer from sampling errors.

Recently, MRI of the breast has attracted significant attention and, although the initial results in assessing mammographically difficult-to-examine breasts are very promising, its clinical role for general population screening has not yet been established. Currently, MRI is recommended for screening women at high risk for developing breast cancer. A recent review of the literature has shown that MRI mammography is a valuable adjunct to conventional imaging in the preoperative local staging of invasive breast cancer, in particular in the assessment of tumor extent, including detection of multifocal, multicentric, and bilateral disease (25).

PET imaging of the breast offers physiological information complementary to that achieved from conventional imaging techniques and, therefore, can be used to better characterize disease. However, PET has important limitations such as high cost, significant radiation exposure, and limited resolution, suggesting that the clinical use of PET should be reserved for a selected subset of women with breast cancer.

FDG uptake is considerably higher in malignant tumors than in normal tissues. Several studies have demonstrated that FDG PET has high sensitivity (64% to 96%) and specificity (80% to 100%) for detection of primary breast cancer and for differentiating breast cancer from benign lesions (26–37). In a study of 144 patients with breast masses, visual qualitative analysis of parametric (SUV normalized) FDG PET images was assessed. FDG PET images were evaluated using conventional image reading (CIR), in which only focal areas of markedly increased FDG accumulation were considered to represent malignancy, and sensitive image reading (SIR), in which those with diffuse or focal areas of moderately increased FDG accumulation were also considered to represent malignancy. Breast cancer was identified with a sensitivity of 64% and 80% using CIR and SIR, respectively. However, the increased sensitivity using SIR resulted in a significant decrease in specificity (94% to 75%) (32).

Avril et al. (32) also demonstrated that the diagnostic accuracy of FDG PET is dependent on tumor size. None of four stage pT1a tumors (less than 0.5 cm) and only one of eight stage pT1b tumors (greater than 0.5 to 1.0 cm) were classified as malignant lesions by FDG PET. However, FDG PET had high sensitivity (81% and 92% using CIR and SIR, respectively) for detection of pT2 breast cancers (greater than 2.0 to 5.0 cm).

False-positive results have been reported in infectious and inflammatory lesions, including hemorrhagic inflammation after biopsy or surgery, due to accumulation of FDG in inflammatory cells (38,39). However, these conditions often can be easily recognized clinically. False-negative results are not limited to small lesions (typically less than 1 cm in diameter), but also are reported in slowly growing or well-differentiated tumors (such as tubular carcinomas, ductal carcinoma *in situ*, and lobular carcinomas) (27,32) (Fig. 8.12.1). The sensitivity of FDG PET for detection of breast cancer is also

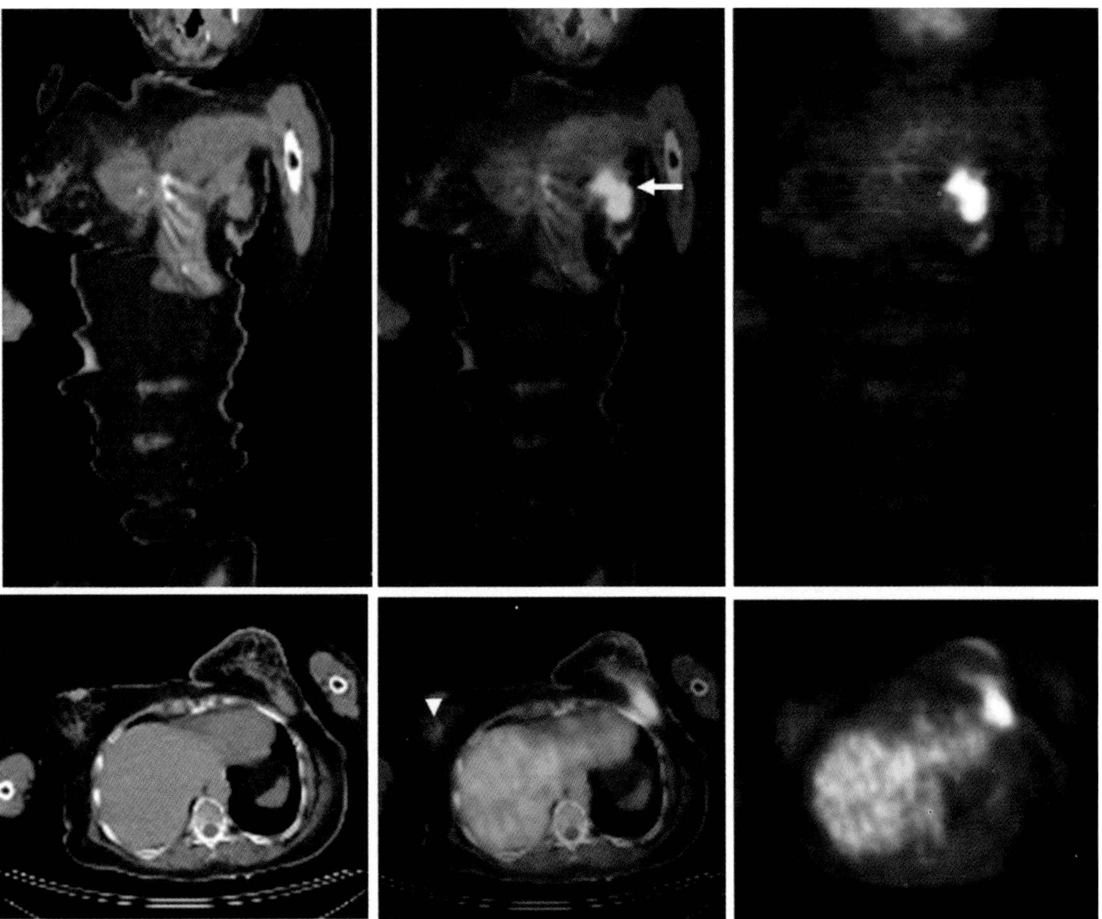

FIGURE 8.12.1. Breast cancer detection. Coronal (**top**) and transaxial (**bottom**) CT (**left**), PET/CT fusion (**middle**), and PET (**right**) images demonstrate intense fluorodeoxyglucose uptake within the left breast cancer (*arrow*) and mild fluorodeoxyglucose uptake within the small (0.8 cm) right breast cancer (*arrowhead*).

dependent on the degree of uptake within the lesion in comparison to uptake in the surrounding tissue (5). It may be difficult to identify lesions with mild to moderate intensity against a background of diffusely increased activity, which is often seen in women with an abundance of proliferative glandular breast tissue (particularly young women). Therefore, FDG PET is not suitable for breast cancer screening due to its limited sensitivity for detection of small lesions, technical complexity, availability, and high cost, at least with currently available whole-body PET scanners.

Recent technical advances that led to development of dedicated scanners specific for breast imaging may improve detection of small primary breast cancers by PET. One such device, a high-resolution PET scanner using mild breast compression (positron emission mammography [PEM]), consists of two moving detector heads, mounted on compression paddles, which perform volumetric acquisitions of the immobilized breast (40). PEM can be used as a stand-alone device or mounted on a stereotactic x-ray platform. In a recent study, Berg et al. (41) reported that PEM has sensitivity, specificity, positive-predictive value, negative-predictive value, and accuracy of 91%, 93%, 95%, 88%, 92%, respectively. When interpreted with mammographic and clinical findings PEM depicted 91% (10 of 11) ductal carcinoma *in situ* and 89% (33 of 37) invasive cancers. PEM was positive in one of two T1a tumors, four of six T1b tumors, and seven of seven T1c tumors. These scanners have the capability to coregister PET images and x-ray mammographic images.

The superior ability of PEM to depict early cancers compared to the whole-body PET scanners is likely a result of several factors, the capability to coregister PET images, better spatial resolution (1.5 mm FWHM vs. 4 mm), higher counting efficiency (leading to higher signal-to-noise ratios), and the use of modern iterative reconstruction techniques (42,43). The potential applications of this technique include evaluating mammographically difficult-to-examine breasts (i.e., radiodense breasts, postsurgical breasts), detecting an occult primary breast cancer in a patient with known axillary metastatic disease, and assessing the local extent of breast cancer (i.e., detecting multicentric or multifocal disease) (41) (Fig. 8.12.2). There may ultimately be a role for PEM as a supplemental screening tool considering the added functional information provided by this technique.

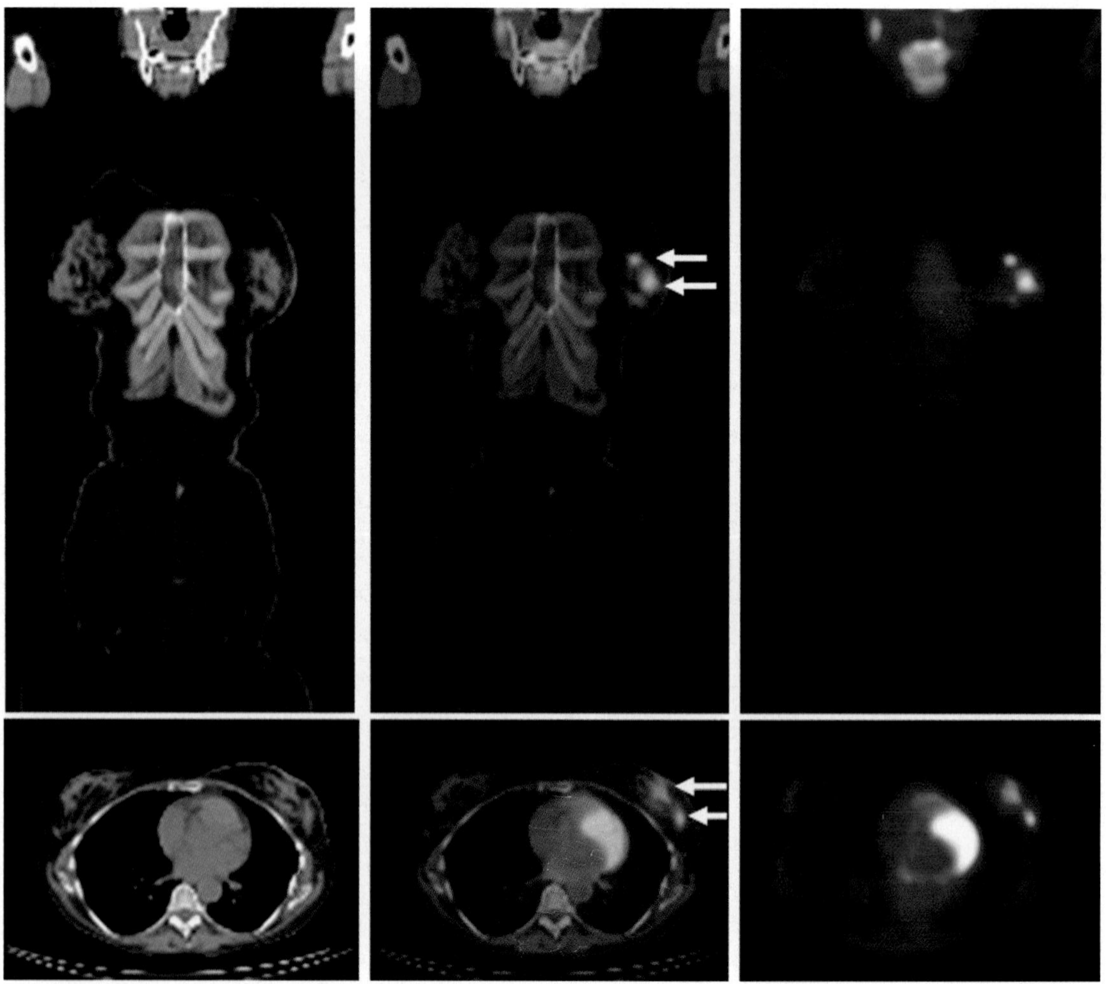

FIGURE 8.12.2. Multifocal primary breast cancer. Coronal (**top**) and transaxial (**bottom**) CT (**left**), PET/CT fusion (**middle**), and PET (**right**) images demonstrate foci of increased fluorodeoxyglucose uptake in a patient with multifocal breast cancer (*arrows*).

In untreated primary breast cancer, FDG uptake has been correlated with known prognostic factors by several investigators. This prognostic information provided by FDG PET may offer insight about the expected behavior of the tumor and guide the aggressiveness of the therapy. Strong positive correlations were found between FDG uptake (SUV) and several tumor characteristics, including histologic grade, cell proliferation indices, histologic type (with greater uptake in ductal cancers by comparison with lobular cancers), microvessel density, and number of tumor cells/volume (3,29,44–47).

No significant correlation has been reported between tumor FDG uptake and other known prognostic factors such as steroid-receptor levels (quantitative estrogen receptor [ER] and progesterone receptor [PR] concentrations], c-*erb* B2 expression, tumor size, presence of inflammatory cells, expression of *GLUT1*, percentage of necrotic, fibrotic, and cystic components, and the status of the axillary lymph nodes.

It has been shown that patient outcome may be predicted based on the degree of tumor FDG uptake (34,44,46–48). In one study, patients with a tumor differential absorption ratio SUV 3.0 or greater had a significantly worse overall survival ($P < .0005$) and disease-free survival ($P < .0001$) than those with tumor SUV less than 3.0 (45). In a multivariate analysis of known prognostic factors including tumor histologic grade, tumor size, number of positive lymph nodes, microvessel density, number of positive lymph nodes, and tumor FDG uptake assessed by SUV, FDG uptake was an independent predictor of disease-free survival ($P = .0377$). Similarly, Mankoff et al. (49) demonstrated that high tumor metabolic rate, as measured by FDG, relative to blood flow, as measured by [^{15}O]-water, predicted poorer survival in patients with locally advanced breast cancer. The degree of FDG uptake within the primary tumor, as measured by peak SUV (SUV_{max}), has been shown to be predictive of survival. Inoue et al. (50) demonstrated that 5-year disease-free survival is less (75% vs. 95%) in patients with high FDG uptake than those with low FDG uptake (mean ± standard deviation 5.87 ± 3.12 vs. 4.02 ± 2.89; $P = .011$). In addition, the combination of high SUV_{max} and PET-positive axillary lymph node status was shown to be a highly significant risk factor being independent of the clinical T and N stages; patients with high SUV_{max} and PET-positive lymph node status showed a significantly ($P < .001$) poorer prognosis than the remaining patients (5-year disease-free survival of 44.4% vs. 96.8%).

These studies demonstrate that tumor FDG uptake provides relevant and unique information about tumor biology, which predicts tumor behavior and prognosis preoperatively before histopathological examination of the breast cancer. These data may assist in the selection of the most appropriate therapy for an individual patient.

LYMPH NODE STAGING

The most common site of regional metastasis of breast cancer is the axillary lymph nodes. The status of the axillary lymph nodes is the single most important prognostic variable in the staging of early breast cancer and significantly influences the selection of treatment. Patients with histologically negative axillary nodes have significantly better survival rates than do patients with positive nodes, and survival among patients with positive nodes depends on the number of involved nodes (51,52). The 10-year survival rate in patients with histologically negative axillary nodes ranges from 65% to 80% versus 38% to 63% in those with involvement of one to three nodes and 13% to 27% in those with more than three positive axillary nodes (51). The likelihood of axillary nodal involvement is directly related to the size of the primary tumor at diagnosis (51).

Approximately 50% of patients with breast cancer evident on physical examination have histologic evidence of axillary nodal involvement (51). Clinical evaluation in predicting axillary nodal disease is inadequate, and, therefore, lymph node dissection (either conventional or more often limited with the use of sentinel node localization) is routinely performed to assess axillary nodal status. Currently the status of axillary lymph nodes is used to define patients in need of receiving axillary lymph node radiotherapy and also to determine the type and aggressiveness of adjuvant chemotherapy and hormonal therapy (53,54). Whether axillary nodal dissection also has therapeutic benefit for regional control of breast cancer remains controversial.

Currently, conventional or limited axillary nodal dissection, guided by lymphatic mapping using the sentinel lymph node technique, represents the standard of care in patients with invasive breast cancer. However, this procedure carries with it a relatively high cost and substantial morbidity. A noninvasive test that could reliably evaluate the status and extent of nodal involvement would be of great interest in the management of patients with breast cancer.

Accurate preoperative staging becomes even more important when one considers the increasing number of patients who are placed on neoadjuvant therapy prior to surgical removal of the primary tumor or lymph nodes. The surgical approach, including the role of sentinel node biopsy and delivery of radiation therapy after neoadjuvant therapy, in patients with breast cancer is evolving. Ongoing clinical trials will likely help to define which patients will benefit from neoadjuvant therapy and to determine the optimal multidisciplinary approach to the management of breast cancer.

If systemic neoadjuvant therapy prior to determination of the status of the axillary lymph nodes becomes routine, the histopathologic information about the number of involved axillary lymph nodes and the size of the primary tumor will no longer be available, and other methods will have to be identified to provide similar prognostic information. To address some of the limitations of such an approach, more recently the trend has been to assess the status of axillary lymph nodes prior to neoadjuvant therapy using the sentinel lymph node (SLN) technique or fine-needle aspiration with ultrasound or MRI guidance.

In preclinical studies of several types of tumors, Wahl et al. (55) demonstrated that FDG uptake in lymph nodes involved by metastatic tumor is greater than that in the normal lymph nodes. Although early studies suggested that FDG PET had the potential to be useful in noninvasive evaluation of locoregional nodal groups in patients with breast cancer and might reduce the number of patients requiring nodal sampling/dissection, more recent studies have been less encouraging (26–29,35–37,44,48,56–71). The reported sensitivities have ranged from 20% to 100% and specificities from 66% to 100% for detection of axillary nodal metastasis. False-negative results with PET occur chiefly in patients with small deposits of tumors (typically less than 1 cm). The results of studies with 20 patients or more are listed in Table 8.12.1.

Based on the current data, a positive FDG PET may alleviate the need for a complete axillary nodal dissection because of its high specificity; however, a negative FDG PET does not preclude axillary nodal sampling or dissection given the high false-negative

TABLE 8.12.1 Fluorodeoxyglucose PET Results for Detection of Axillary Lymph Node Metastases

Authors (year/ref.)	No. of patients	Analysis	% Sensitivity	% Specificity
Adler et al. (1993/29)[a]	20	Qualitative	90	100
Avril et al. (1996/35)[a]	51	Qualitative	79	96
T1 primary	18	Qualitative	33	100
>T1 primary	23	Qualitative	94	100
Utech et al. (1996/36)[a]	124	Qualitative	100	75
Crippa et al. (1997/48)[a]	66	Qualitative	84	85
Adler et al. (1997/58)[a]	20	Qualitative	95	66
Smith et al. (1998/59)[a]	50	Qualitative	90	97
Rostom et al. (1999/60)[a]	74	Qualitative	86	100
Schirrmeister et al. (2001/37)[b]	85	Qualitative	79	92
Greco et al. (2001/61)	167	Qualitative	94	86
Guller et al. (2002/62)	31	Qualitative	43	94
Barranger et al. (2003/63)	32	Qualitative	20	100
Wahl et al. (2004/64)	308	Qualitative	61	83
		Semiquant[c]	25	99
Zornoza et al. (2004/65)	200		84	98
van der Hoeven et al. (2002/66)	70	Qualitative	25	97
Lovrics et al. (2004/67)	98	Qualitative	40	97
Fehr et al. (2004/68)	24	Qualitative	20	93
Kumar et al. (2005/11)	80	Qualitative	44	95
Chung et al. (2006/70)	51	Semiquant[d]	64	89
Gil-Rendo et al. (2006/71)	275	Qualitative	84	98

[a]Attenuation corrected images.
[b]Without attenuation correction.
[c]Semiquantitative analysis using standard uptake value $(SUV)_{lean} \geq 2$.
[d]Semiquantitative analysis using SUV ≥ 2.

rate. The PET detection of axillary nodal metastases is directly related to the size of the primary tumor and the number of lymph nodes involved. Avril et al. (35) demonstrated sensitivity and specificity of 94% and 100%, respectively, in patients with primary tumors greater than 2 cm in diameter and 33% and 100%, respectively, in patients with tumors less than 2 cm. Further, PET identified one of four patients with a single lymph node metastasis, four of six with two to five lymph node metastases, and all ten patients with more than five lymph node metastases. Schirrmeister et al. (37) demonstrated that FDG PET is superior to clinical evaluation for predicting axillary nodal involvement; the sensitivity and specificity were 79% and 92%, respectively, for FDG PET and 41% and 96%, respectively, for clinical evaluation of lymph nodes.

Because of the limited resolution of PET, it is unlikely that this technique can detect small tumor deposits or determine accurately the number and pathological features of involved axillary nodes or extranodal spread. Thus, PET cannot replace axillary lymph nodal sampling, and treatment decisions should not be solely based on FDG PET results.

Axillary lymph node dissection is an important part of the surgical treatment of breast cancer. Axillary nodal dissection based on lymphatic mapping using SLN technique is an alternative to conventional complete axillary node dissection. The combined use of blue dye and lymphoscintigraphy gives the best SLN identification rate. SLN biopsy combined with immunohistochemical staining for cytokeratin to identify microscopic tumor foci accurately detects metastatic disease in lymph nodes and, thus, negative results identify patients who do not require complete axillary dissection. Several studies have compared FDG PET with histological results from SLN mapping and demonstrated low sensitivity, but high specificity of FDG PET for detection of axillary metastatic disease in early breast cancer (62,66,68,69,71–73) (Table 8.12.2). The high specificity may indicate that a complete axillary dissection without the need for SLN mapping should be performed in patients with positive PET.

MRI using ultrasmall superparamagnetic iron oxide (USPIO) particles has shown promise in noninvasive detection of metastatic disease in lymph nodes (74). The clinical use of this contrast agent is still under evaluation in clinical trials. The most widely utilized studied agent is ferumoxtran-10; the particles of this agent, at 20 to 30 nm, are too large to be filtered at the glomerulus. Twenty-four hours after injection almost all injected USPIO particles are phagocytized by macrophages and monocytes, which leads to a decrease in the signal intensity in normal or reactive lymph nodes because of the T2 shortening effects of the agent, whereas metastatic deposits in nodes, which replace the macrophages, will not undergo signal intensity changes when using T2-weighted sequences (74). USPIO-enhanced MRI has been used for staging axillary lymph nodes in patients with breast cancer.

TABLE 8.12.2 Fluorodeoxyglucose PET Results for Detection of Axillary Lymph Node Metastases Compared with Pathologic Results of Sentinel Node Lymph Node Biopsy

Authors (year/ref.)	No. of Patients	% Sensitivity	% Specificity
Yang et al. (2001/72)	18	50	100
Kelemen et al. (2002/73)	15	20	90
Guller et al. (2002/62)	31	43	94
van der Hoeven et al. (2002/66)	70	25	97
Fehr et al. (2004/68)	24	20	93
Lovrics et al. (2004/67)	72	27	96
Kumar et al. (2005/11)	80	44	95
Gil-Rendo et al. (2006/71)	125	79	98

Michel et al. (75) demonstrated that USPIO-enhanced MRI was true positive in 9, true negative in 7, false positive in zero, and false negative in 2 of 18 patients studied. In one preliminary study, USPIO-enhanced MRI has been compared with FDG PET for detection of axillary lymph node metastasis in ten patients with breast cancer who were scheduled for surgery and axillary node resection (76). Five patients had positive nodes at surgery and five had negative nodes. USPIO-enhanced MRI was false positive in one and FDG-PET was false negative in one. More studies are needed to define the role of USPIO-enhanced MRI in cancer imaging, and at the time this chapter was prepared, such agents were not yet approved by the Food and Drug Administration in the United States.

In addition to detection of axillary nodal involvement, FDG PET has the potential to detect involvement of other nodal groups, including the internal mammary and supraclavicular nodes. Involvement of the internal mammary nodes in the absence of axillary nodal involvement is uncommon (approximately 10%), and the prognosis of such patients does not differ significantly from that of patients with metastasis only to the axillary nodes (51). However, a poorer prognosis has been reported when both nodal groups are involved.

Because detection of internal mammary nodal metastasis is difficult with currently utilized staging methods and sampling is not routinely performed at surgery, the status of these lymph nodes has been largely ignored. However, with the use of the sentinel node technique (which can demonstrate that the primary route of drainage of the tumor is to the internal mammary nodes) and the increasing use of postsurgical adjuvant radiation therapy, the status of this nodal group has become important. It has been shown that FDG PET may have a role in noninvasive evaluation of internal mammary lymph nodes in patient with locally advanced breast cancer. In a retrospective study of 28 women with locally advanced breast cancer who underwent FDG PET before neoadjuvant chemotherapy, abnormal FDG uptake in the internal mammary nodes was seen in 25% of the patients (77). Increased FDG uptake in the internal mammary lymph nodes was associated with large size of the primary tumor ($P = .03$) and with inflammatory disease ($P = .04$). Involvement of internal mammary lymph nodes on FDG PET predicted the pattern of failure; 67% of patients with positive PET had a pattern of failure consistent with spread from internal mammary lymph node metastasis versus 16% in those with FDG-negative internal mammary nodes.

Knowledge of the status of ipsilateral supraclavicular lymph nodes is also important for effective treatment of these nodes. Currently, the ipsilateral supraclavicular lymph nodes are considered N3 rather than M1, and patients with involvement of these lymph nodes are treated with curative rather than palliative intent (78). There is evidence that prognosis improves with definitive therapy in patients with involvement of ipsilateral supraclavicular lymph nodes (78). SLN mapping is a very useful tool in delineating drainage to these lymph nodes. The status of supraclavicular lymph nodes can be determined by biopsy/minimally invasive surgery once drainage to these lymph nodes is documented. The role of PET in noninvasive staging of these nodal groups is not known, and prospective trials are needed.

DISTANT METASTATIC DISEASE

The presence of distant metastases is an important prognostic factor in patients with breast cancer and has a significant influence on determining therapy. Because breast cancer can metastasize to many organs (bone, liver, lung, brain, etc.), several radiological imaging studies such as bone scintigraphy, CT, MRI, and chest radiography are used to detect distant metastases at the time of primary diagnosis and during follow-up after therapy. Obviously, it is preferable to use a single imaging modality instead of several to detect the presence and extent of disease. Whole-body PET imaging has a major role in documenting the systemic extent of malignant disease as it can detect not only the primary tumor and nodal metastases, but also skeletal and visceral metastases in a single study. Several clinical studies have shown that FDG PET is more sensitive than other currently utilized noninvasive techniques for demonstrating the true extent of metastatic disease (6,35,57) and will quite often reveal unsuspected metastatic disease (Figs. 8.12.3 and 8.12.4) (2,27,35).

In patients with early breast cancer, the use of conventional imaging has been associated with a very low yield in detection of metastatic disease; thus, the routine use of imaging modalities in the management of early primary breast cancer has been questioned. A recent study by Port et al. (79) in 80 patients with operable breast cancer who were considered high risk for harboring metastatic disease (patients with T3 lesions and/or clinically positive N1/N2), demonstrated that the rate of false-positive results was greater with conventional imaging (CT or bone scintigraphy) than FDG PET (17% vs. 5%). The findings on the conventional imaging

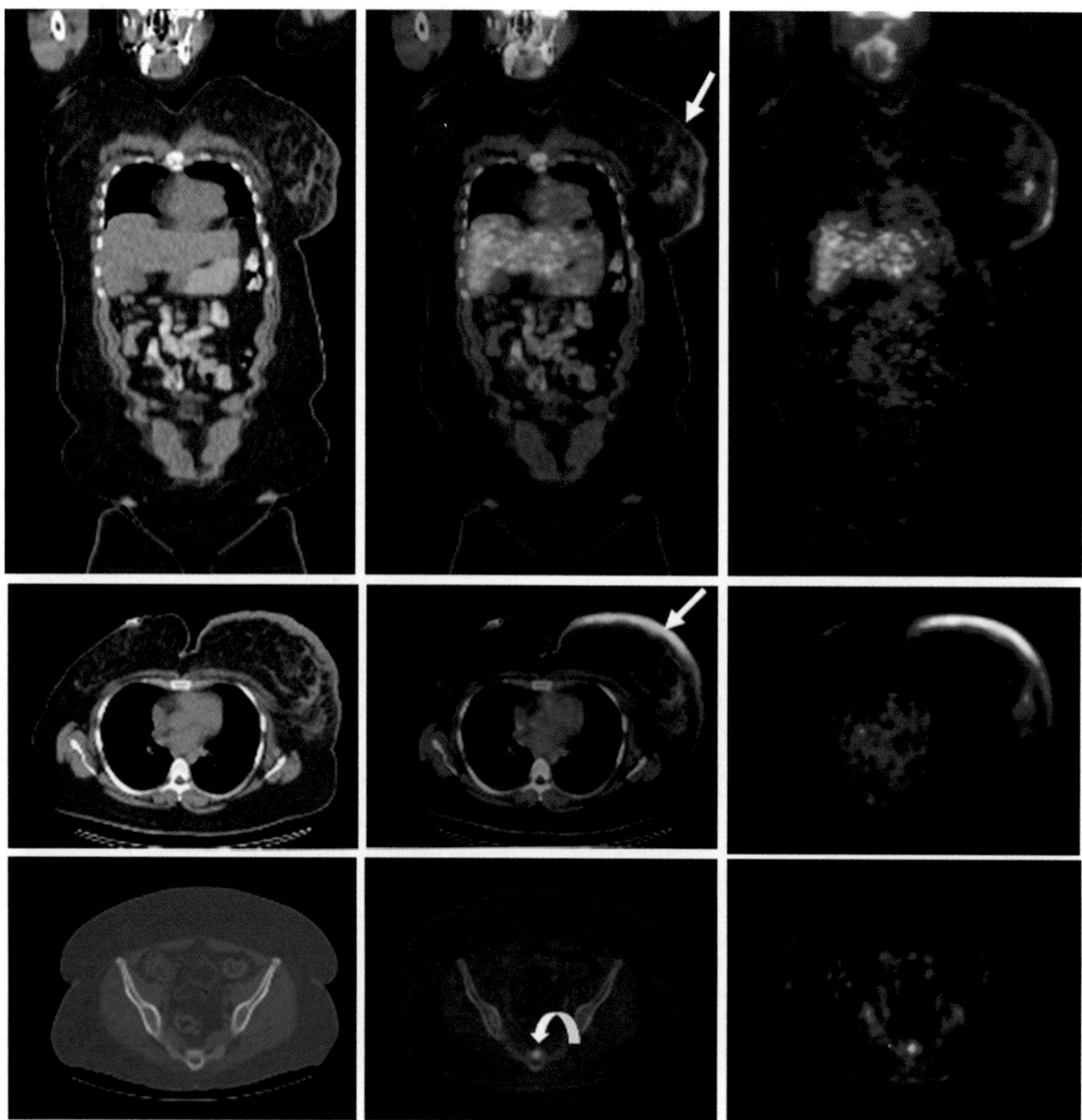

FIGURE 8.12.3. Metastatic breast cancer. Coronal (**top**) and transaxial (**middle, bottom**) CT (**left**), PET/CT fusion (**middle**), and PET (**right**) images demonstrate intense fluorodeoxyglucose uptake within the left inflammatory breast cancer involving the entire breast and overlying skin (*arrows*). A focal area of increased uptake is seen in the sacrum (*curved arrow*) without a corresponding osseous abnormality on the bone window of the CT scan, consistent with unsuspected liver metastasis.

generated additional tests and biopsies that eventually had negative results. In addition, eight patients (10%) had metastatic disease detected by both conventional imaging and PET; however, four (5%) other patients had additional metastatic disease seen only on PET that altered management. Avril et al. (35) studied 41 patients with breast cancer and reported that FDG PET demonstrated unsuspected distant metastatic disease in 12 of these patients (29%), with a resultant alteration in their management.

Breast cancer commonly metastasizes to bone. Overall, 8% of patients with breast cancer will develop an osseous metastasis; the frequency is nearly 70% among patients with advanced disease (80). The presence of osseous metastases alters both the management and prognosis. The median survival of patients with metastatic disease confined to the skeleton is 24 months and the 5-year survival rate is 20% (80). The presence of osseous metastatic disease also increases the morbidity and the cost of treatment. The role of bone scintigraphy and FDG PET for detection of bone metastases is not clearly defined. FDG PET has the advantage of demonstrating osseous and nonosseous metastatic sites, and its uptake within the bone is assumed to represent metabolic activity of the tumor cells.

Bone scintigraphy is limited to evaluation of osseous disease, and its uptake is assumed to represent local blood flow and osteoblastic response to bone destruction by tumor cells rather than the tumor itself. Thus, bone scintigraphy is not very specific. It is sensitive for detection of advanced osseous lesions, but is somewhat limited in evaluation of osteolytic metastatic foci or detection of early osseous involvement.

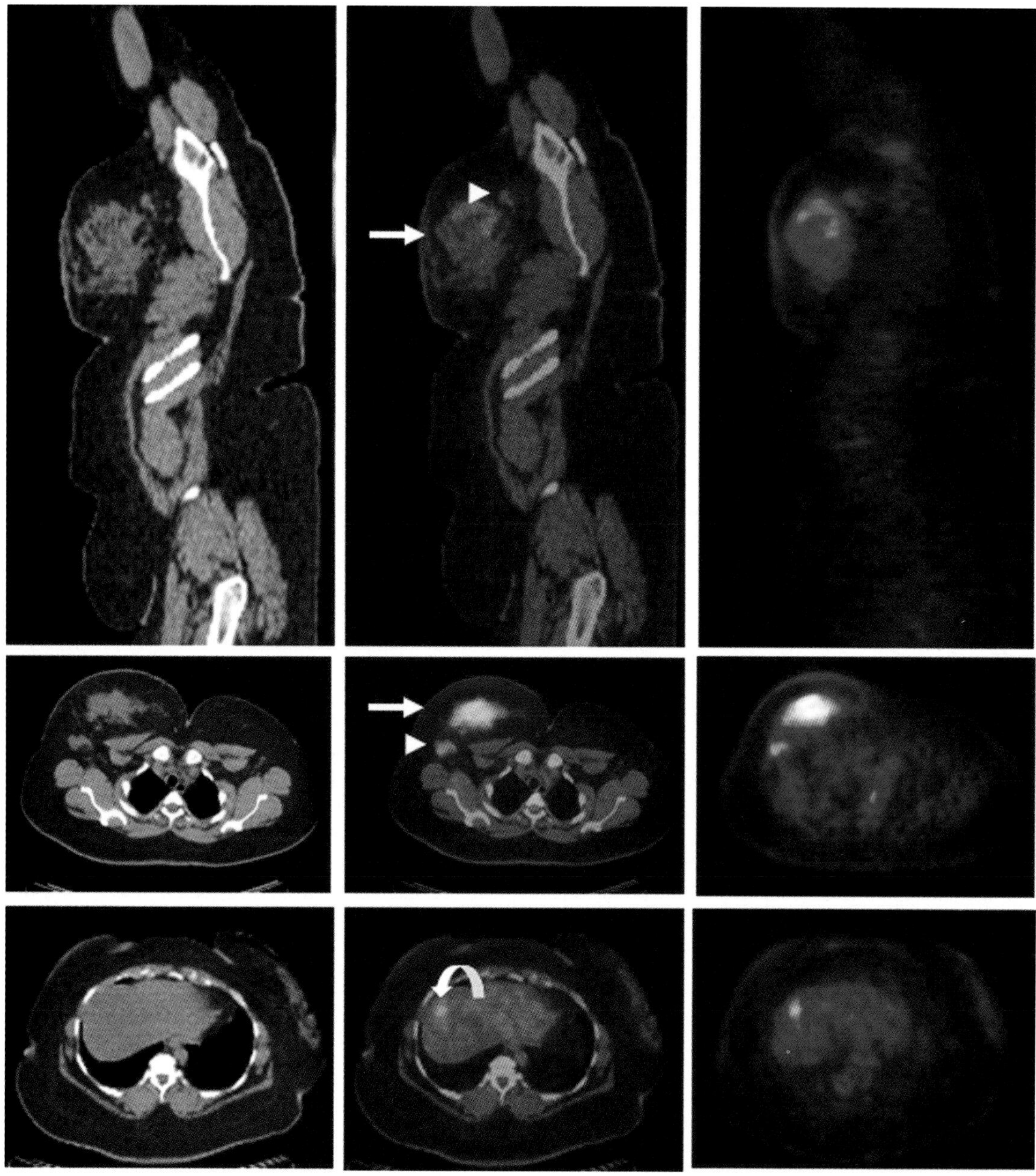

FIGURE 8.12.4. Metastatic breast cancer. Coronal (**top**) and transaxial (**middle, bottom**) CT (**left**), PET/CT fusion (**middle**), and PET (**right**) images demonstrate intense fluorodeoxyglucose uptake within the right breast cancer (*arrows*) and right axillary lymph node (*arrowheads*). A focal area of increased uptake is seen in the liver (*curved arrow*), consistent with unsuspected liver metastasis; CT became positive 10 months later.

Several studies have compared PET with bone scintigraphy (81–86). Many studies have shown that FDG PET detected more osseous metastatic lesions but fewer osteoblastic lesions than bone scintigraphy. Cook et al. (81) compared technetium-99m methylene diphosphonate (^{99m}Tc-MDP) bone scintigraphy with semiquantitative FDG PET in 23 patients with documented osseous metastatic breast cancer. They demonstrated that overall, FDG PET detected more osseous lesions than bone scintigraphy (mean of 14.1 vs. 7.8 lesions). This was most notable among the patients with osteolytic metastases (which were associated with a poor prognosis). Conversely, in patients with osteoblastic lesions, FDG PET detected significantly fewer lesions than bone scintigraphy (P <.05). Patients with a more aggressive breast cancer who tend to develop osteolytic metastatic lesions may benefit from earlier detection of osseous metastatic disease by FDG PET.

Kao et al. (82) studied 24 patients with suspected or proven osseous metastatic breast cancer. A total of 89 lesions were found by bone scintigraphy and/or FDG PET; there were concordant results in 59 lesions and discordant results in 39 lesions (bone scintigraphy+/FDG− in 31 lesions and bone scintigraphy–/FDG+ in 8 lesions). All 8 discordant lesions with bone scintigraphy−/FDG+ and 11 of 31 discordant lesions with scintigraphy+/FDG− were confirmed to be metastatic sites; the remaining 20 discordant lesions were benign.

Abe et al. (83) also demonstrated that FDG PET was superior to bone scintigraphy for detection of osteolytic (92% vs. 73%) metastasis, but inferior in detecting osteoblastic lesions (74% vs. 95%). Similarly, Nakai et al. (84) demonstrated that for detection of osteoblastic, osteolytic, and mixed lesions, PET had sensitivities of 56%, 100%, and 95%, respectively, while bone scintigraphy had sensitivities of 100%, 70%, and 84%, respectively.

Several studies have shown PET is superior to bone scintigraphy in its specificity. Yang et al. (85) evaluated 48 patients with breast cancer. A total of 127 bone lesions including 105 metastatic and 22 benign osseous lesions were found by either FDG PET or bone scintigraphy. FDG PET accurately detected 100 metastatic and 20 benign osseous lesions, while bone scintigraphy correctly detected 98 osseous metastatic and two benign lesions. The diagnostic sensitivity and accuracy of FDG PET were 95% and 94%, respectively, versus 93% and 79%, respectively, for bone scintigraphy. Thus, FDG PET shows a similar sensitivity and a better accuracy than bone scintigraphy for detecting osseous metastases in patients with breast cancer.

Ohta et al. (86) also demonstrated that the sensitivity, specificity, and accuracy were 78%, 98%, and 94%, respectively, for FDG PET and 78%, 81%, and 80%, respectively, for bone scintigraphy. Considering the differences in the mechanisms of uptake of FDG and conventional bone-seeking tracers, these two imaging techniques are likely complementary. One advantage of PET over bone scintigraphy is that PET can more readily assess the response to therapy, as changes due to successful therapy occur more rapidly with PET imaging in comparison to bone scintigraphy.

PET with fluoride-18 (^{18}F) has been used to assess osseous metastatic disease in breast cancer. The bone uptake of ^{18}F is approximately twofold higher than that of ^{99m}Tc-MDP, and its blood clearance is faster, resulting in a higher bone-to-background ratio (87–90). Schirrmeister et al. (91) compared ^{18}F PET with conventional bone scintigraphy in 34 patients with breast cancer. In 17 patients, ^{18}F PET detected 64 lesions, whereas bone scintigraphy detected 29 lesions in 11 of these patients. The results of ^{18}F PET altered clinical management in four patients (12%). On a lesion-by-lesion basis, the area under the receiver operating characteristic (ROC) curve was 0.99 for ^{18}F PET and 0.74 for bone scintigraphy ($P < .05$). On a patient-by-patient basis, the area under the ROC curve was 1.00 for ^{18}F PET and 0.82 for bone scintigraphy ($P < .05$). Not surprisingly, because of the greater sensitivity of ^{18}F PET, the number of benign lesions detected by ^{18}F PET was higher than that detected by conventional bone scintigraphy, leading to a higher number of false-positive studies.

With the improved image contrast and greater spatial resolution of PET, ^{18}F PET should allow for earlier detection of osseous metastases and more accurate definition of the extent of metastatic disease than is possible with conventional bone scintigraphy. Even-Sapir et al. (92) have shown that ^{18}F PET/CT was both sensitive and specific for the detection of lytic and sclerotic malignant lesions in 44 patients with various malignant diseases; 10 of these patients had breast cancer. [^{18}F]-fluoride-18 PET/CT accurately differentiated malignant from benign bone lesions. In a lesion-based analysis, the sensitivity of PET alone was 72% when inconclusive lesions were considered false negative and 90% when inconclusive lesions were considered true positive. PET/CT had an overall sensitivity (99% vs. 90%; $P < .05$) and specificity (97% vs. 72%; $P < .001$) significantly higher than that of PET alone. In a patient-based analysis, the sensitivity of PET and PET/CT was 88% and 100%, respectively ($P < .05$), and the specificity was 56% and 88%, respectively (not statistically significant).

For most lesions, the anatomic data provided by the low-dose CT of the PET/CT study obviates the performance of a full-dose diagnostic CT for correlation purposes. The use of PET/CT resulted in reduction of the false-positive rate by determining the morphology of the scintigraphic lesions on the CT data of the PET/CT. Even-Sapir et al. (93) confirmed these findings in a recent study in patients with high-risk prostate cancer. This added value of ^{18}F PET/CT may improve the clinical management of oncologic patients. However, more studies are needed before the role of this tracer is determined in evaluation of oncologic patients, although it appears to be a more than adequate substitute for the ^{99m}TC diphosphonate bone scan.

MONITORING RESPONSE TO THERAPY

An important role of FDG PET in breast cancer is predicting the response of the tumor to therapy, as well as assessing the effectiveness of therapy. PET has the ability to quantify tracer distribution *in vivo*. This capability, coupled with the observation that changes in tumor metabolism occur shortly after initiation of therapy before any change in tumor size, makes PET well suited for predicting and monitoring response to therapy. Conventional imaging modalities are limited in assessing response to therapy, and often a delay of several weeks after completion of therapy is required before the effectiveness of the treatment can be assessed. The ability to predict response to therapy before therapy has begun or shortly after institution of therapy, so that alternative treatments could be substituted in nonresponding patients, would be very desirable. In addition, the morbidity and costs associated with ineffective treatment could be avoided.

The use of neoadjuvant chemotherapy in the treatment of primary breast cancer is well established. A significant correlation has been noted between primary tumor response to neoadjuvant therapy and outcome; patients with marked response to neoadjuvant therapy have a better disease-free survival than those who fail to respond (94). Systemic neoadjuvant therapy is typically used in the treatment of patients with large or locally advanced breast cancer to reduce the size of the primary tumor in order to permit breast conservation surgery and to treat occult systemic disease.

Approximately one fourth of patients do not respond to therapy, and it is important to identify nonresponders early during therapy so that unsuccessful treatment can be discontinued and alternative treatment initiated. Conventional methods such as physical examination, mammography, and sonography are suboptimal in accurate assessment of response to therapy. A limited number of studies are available that have shown a potential role for MRI in monitoring response to neoadjuvant therapy in patients with breast cancer (95,96). Larger prospective studies are needed to define the role of MRI in the management of patients with breast cancer.

FDG PET has been used effectively to monitor neoadjuvant therapy in breast cancer. Histological response could be predicted during therapy with FDG PET (Fig. 8.12.5). Typically, a significant decline in the FDG uptake occurs early in the course of chemotherapy in responders, whereas no change or a slight increase occurs in those who do not respond to treatment. In a prospective study,

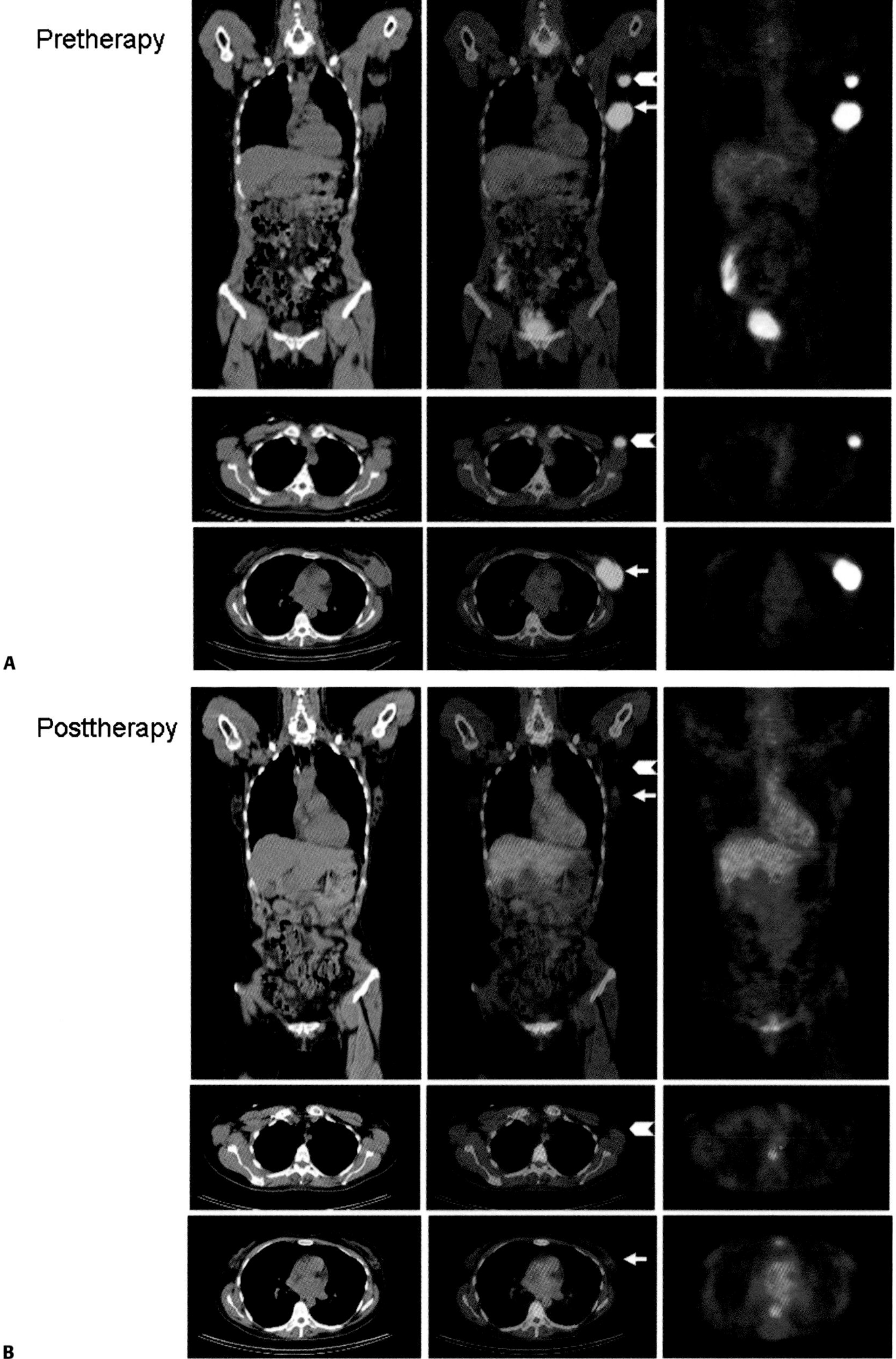

FIGURE 8.12.5. Response to therapy. **A:** Coronal (**top**) and transaxial (**middle**, **bottom**) CT (**left**), PET/CT fusion (**middle**), and PET (**right**) images demonstrate intense fluorodeoxyglucose uptake within the left breast cancer (*arrows*) and left axillary lymph node (*arrowheads*) in a patient with locally advanced breast cancer. **B:** Coronal (**top**) and transaxial (**middle**, **bottom**) CT (**left**), PET/CT fusion (**middle**), and PET (**right**) images performed after four cycles of neoadjuvant therapy demonstrate normalization of fluorodeoxyglucose uptake and resolution of the soft tissue masses, consistent with marked response to therapy. In addition, there is mild diffusely increased fluorodeoxyglucose accumulation in the bone marrow secondary to recent treatment with granulocyte colony-stimulating factor. Mastectomy revealed no residual tumor.

Wahl et al. (97) demonstrated an early and significant decrease in tumor glucose metabolism (both semiquantitatively and quantitatively) 8 days after institution of effective chemohormonotherapy in eight patients with locally advanced breast carcinoma; the reduction in tumor metabolism antedated changes in tumor size. No significant decline in tumor FDG uptake was noted in three nonresponders. Similar results have been reported by others in patients with advanced breast cancer (98,99).

In another study to assess the value of FDG PET in predicting response to therapy, Schelling et al. (100) studied 22 patients undergoing chemotherapy for locally advanced breast cancer. They compared semiquantitative tumor FDG uptake following the first (16 patients) and second (all 22 patients) courses of neoadjuvant chemotherapy with the histopathological response after completion of therapy. After the first course of therapy, all responders (defined as pathologic complete response or minimal residual disease) were identified using a decline in tumor SUV to a level below 55% of baseline (100% [3 of 3] sensitivity and 85% [11 of 13] specificity). After the second course of therapy using the same threshold, all but one of the responders were identified (91% [5 of 6] sensitivity and 94% [15 of 16] specificity).

In a study of 30 patients with advanced breast cancer, Smith et al. (101) compared histopathological response with semiquantitative and quantitative tumor FDG uptake before and after institution of chemotherapy (after the first, second, and fifth doses of therapy), as well as after the last dose of chemotherapy. After the first pulse of chemotherapy, FDG PET predicted complete pathological response with a sensitivity of 90% and specificity of 74% using a decline in tumor SUV to a level below 20% of baseline.

Kim et al. (102) showed in 50 patients with noninflammatory large or locally advanced breast cancer that using a 79% reduction in FDG uptake after completion of therapy as the cutoff value, pathologic responders can be differentiated from nonresponders with a sensitivity of 85% and specificity of 83%. McDermott et al. (103) studied 96 patients with large or locally advanced breast cancer before the first and second cycles, at the midpoint, and at completion of neoadjuvant therapy. They found that the best discrimination was achieved for the mean SUV at the midpoint of therapy, which identified 77% of low-responding tumors (no response to up to 90% reduction in cellularity) and 100% of high-responding tumors (more than 90% reduction in cellularity to no residual tumor) and had an ROC area of 0.93. They also found that FDG PET is ineffective for tumors with low image contrast (tumor-to-background ratio less than 5) on pretherapy PET.

Rousseau et al. (104) studied 64 patients with stage II and III breast cancer with FDG PET at baseline and after the first, second, third, and sixth courses of neoadjuvant chemotherapy. Patients underwent surgical resection after six courses of neoadjuvant chemotherapy. Histopathologic analysis revealed gross residual disease in 28 patients (nonresponders) and minimal residual disease in 36 patients (responders). FDG uptake, as measured by SUV, decreased markedly in 94% (34 of 36) of responders and did not vary much in nonresponders. When using 60% reduction in SUV as the cutoff value, the sensitivity, specificity, and negative predictive value of FDG PET were 61%, 96%, and 68% after one course of chemotherapy, 89%, 95%, and 85% after two courses, and 88%, 73%, and 83% after three courses, respectively. In these patients, ultrasound and mammography also were used to assess changes in tumor size with therapy. Conventional modalities (ultrasound and mammography) did not predict histologic response; the sensitivity, specificity, positive predictive value, and negative predictive value after six courses of chemotherapy were 64%, 43%, 53%, and 55% with ultrasound, and 31%, 56%, 42%, and 45% with mammography, respectively. The investigators concluded that pathologic response to neoadjuvant chemotherapy can be predicted accurately by FDG PET after two courses of chemotherapy.

In the neoadjuvant setting, changes in tumor blood flow, as measured by PET with [^{15}O]-water, have been evaluated. One of the factors that can have an important impact on the responsiveness of tumor to therapy is adequate blood flow to and within the tumor; tumors with low blood perfusion may respond poorly to therapy. Tseng et al. (105) evaluated 35 patients with locally advanced breast cancer with FDG PET and [^{15}O]-water PET before and 2 months after neoadjuvant chemotherapy. The investigators demonstrated that a low metabolism-to-blood-flow ratio prior to initiation of therapy was an independent predictor of complete pathologic response to therapy. In addition, after therapy, responders had a greater decline in tumor blood flow in comparison with nonresponders. The investigators also reported that the posttherapy blood flow measurement was the only statistically significant variable associated with improved survival. Although the results are encouraging and this technique allows for evaluation of a tumor feature other than glucose utilization rate, [^{15}O]-water has a very short half-life and is not available in centers without a cyclotron. Furthermore, quantitative analysis of blood flow with [^{15}O]-water is not yet fully standardized.

Distant metastases indicate incurable disease, and systemic treatments are given for palliative rather than curative purposes. Approximately 25% to 30% of patients with negative axillary lymph nodes and greater than two thirds of those with axillary node metastasis will have recurrent and/or metastatic disease and eventually die from advanced disease (106). The goals of therapy are to improve survival and quality of life; thus, it is important to identify nonresponders early in the course of therapy to prevent the morbidity associated with ineffective therapy. Several studies have shown that FDG PET is a useful tool in this group of patients and improves patient care by identifying nonresponders early in the course of therapy.

Minn and Soini (107) studied ten patients with breast cancer before and after therapy (chemotherapy alone in seven patients and in combination with radiotherapy in three), utilizing qualitative planar FDG imaging. They demonstrated that an increase in FDG uptake in breast cancer over time was associated with tumor progression. Schwarz et al. (108) studied 11 patients (26 metastatic lesions) with metastatic breast cancer with serial FDG PET to predict response after the first and second cycles of chemotherapy. The differences in changes in FDG uptake, as measured by SUV, between responding and nonresponding lesions were statistically significant after the first and second cycles. Visual analysis of FDG PET images correctly predicted the response in all patients as early as after the first cycle of chemotherapy. As assessed by FDG PET, the overall survival in nonresponders was shorter than that in responders (8.8 months vs. 19.2 months).

Assessment of response to therapy in osseous metastatic disease is difficult with conventional imaging, bone scintigraphy, plain radiography, CT, or MRI, as changes indicative of response to therapy occur slowly. In addition, the issue of scintigraphic "flare reaction" that often occurs early in the course of therapy on bone scans may mistakenly lead to discontinuation of therapy. Stafford et al. (109) used serial FDG PET in patients with breast cancer being treated for osseous metastatic disease. They found that changes in FDG uptake with therapy correlate well with the overall clinical assessment of response. The percentage of change in FDG uptake with therapy showed a strong correlation with the percentage of change in tumor marker values.

The role of high-dose chemotherapy followed by autologous stem cell transplantation is still controversial, and it may only be beneficial in selected patients with metastatic breast cancer (110). Considering the high toxicity of this therapy in comparison to standard therapy, it is even more important to identify patients who may not benefit from such therapy. Cachin et al. (111) demonstrated that a single FDG PET performed after completion of high-dose chemotherapy can strongly stratify for survival in patients with metastatic breast cancer. They studied 47 patients with metastatic breast cancer undergoing high-dose chemotherapy with autologous stem cell transplantation. Responsiveness to therapy was assessed by conventional imaging (ultrasonography, mammography, and bone scintigraphy, as clinically indicated, and CT in all patients) and FDG PET after the last cycle of high-dose chemotherapy. Complete responses were observed in 16 patients (37%) with conventional imaging and 34 patients (72%) with FDG PET. The FDG PET result was the most powerful and independent predictor of survival; patients with a negative posttreatment FDG PET had a longer median survival than patients with a positive FDG PET (24 months vs. 10 months; $P < .001$). By multivariate analysis the relative risk (RR) of death was higher in patients with positive FDG PET (RR, 5.3), prior anthracycline treatment (RR, 3.3), or with visceral metastasis (RR, 2.4). Thus, a single FDG PET performed after completion of high-dose chemotherapy can strongly stratify for survival.

With the increasing use of hematopoietic cytokines such as granulocyte colony-stimulating factor (G-CSF) and granulocyte-macrophage colony-stimulating factor (GM-CSF) in conjunction with chemotherapy for breast cancer, it is important to be familiar with the effect of such therapy on FDG uptake in the bone marrow. In a recent study, Sugawara et al. (112) studied the effects of G-CSF and GM-CSF on the biodistribution of FDG in rats and 11 patients with breast cancer. In rats, bone marrow activity was significantly higher in the group pretreated with G-CSF and GM-CSF compared to the control group ($P < .05$); however, the biodistribution in other normal tissues was comparable in both groups. In patients with breast cancer, chemotherapy alone did not result in increased FDG uptake in bone marrow; however, bone marrow uptake increased after treatment with G-CSF. The SUV_{lean} (SUV corrected for lean body mass) of the bone marrow was 1.56 ± 0.23 at baseline, 3.13 ± 1.40 after one cycle ($P < .01$), 2.22 ± 0.85 after two cycles ($P < .05$), and 2.14 ± 0.79 after three cycles of therapy ($P < .5$). The dose of G-CSF and the duration of treatment were correlated with the extent of increase in FDG uptake in the bone marrow. After completion of treatment with G-CSF, FDG uptake in the bone marrow declined, but was higher than the baseline level for up to 4 weeks following completion of therapy.

Markedly increased FDG uptake in the spleen was also noted after treatment with G-CSF, likely due to extramedullary hematopoiesis in the spleen (113). A uniform increase in bone marrow or splenic activity should be interpreted with caution; a history of recent therapy with cytokines would be helpful in making the distinction between diffuse metastatic disease and the drug effect. If possible, FDG PET should be delayed for a few weeks following completion of treatment with G-CSF or other hematopoietic cytokines as marked activity in bone marrow may interfere with accurate assessment of response to therapy.

RECURRENT DISEASE

Early detection and accurate restaging of recurrent breast cancer is important in selection of the most appropriate mode of therapy and in identifying patients with limited disease amenable to curative therapy. Conventional imaging modalities are limited in differentiating posttherapy changes from recurrent tumor, especially in a region of prior surgery and/or radiation therapy. Several studies have shown that FDG PET is a useful adjunct to the conventional imaging in evaluating patients with suspected locoregional or distant recurrent disease (Figs. 8.12.6 and 8.12.7).

Moon et al. (114) studied 57 patients with a clinical suspicion of recurrent breast cancer after initial therapy (surgery with or without adjuvant chemotherapy or radiotherapy). They reported that nonattenuation corrected whole-body FDG PET has sensitivity, specificity, positive- and negative-predictive values of 93%, 79%, 82%, and 92%, respectively, for detection of recurrent breast cancer.

Bender et al. (115) studied 75 patients with suspected recurrent breast cancer and demonstrated that FDG PET is a useful adjunct to MRI and/or CT in the detection of recurrent disease involving lymph nodes and visceral organs. For lymph node involvement, the sensitivity and specificity were 97% and 91%, respectively, for FDG PET and 74% and 95%, respectively, for CT and/or MRI. For detection of recurrent disease in visceral organs, the sensitivity was 96% for FDG PET and 57% for CT and/or MRI. FDG PET was shown to be a useful adjunct in detection of recurrent disease in 23 patients with stages II and III breast cancer who were symptomatic (an abnormal mammogram, a palpable mass at the surgical site, and/or symptoms suggestive of local recurrence and/or distant disease) (116). Overall sensitivity, specificity, accuracy, positive- and negative-predictive values of FDG PET were 81%, 100%, 87%, 100%, and 50%, respectively. FDG PET detected two recurrences that were missed by conventional imaging. Similar results have been reported by others (117).

In the follow-up of patients treated for breast cancer, elevation of serum tumor markers, such as cancer antigen 15-3 (CA15-3) and carcinoembryonic antigen (CEA), is often indicative of recurrent disease. However, tumor markers lack specificity and increased levels are not always consistent with cancer recurrence, nor do they indicate the site of involvement and whether the disease is limited or widespread. This is particularly difficult for the treating physicians when the patient is asymptomatic and conventional imaging is negative or equivocal. Several studies have evaluated the use of PET in this clinical stetting. Liu et al. (118) demonstrated that FDG PET had a sensitivity of 96% and accuracy of 90% in 30 patients with previously treated breast cancer who had asymptomatically elevated tumor markers and negative or equivocal imaging studies.

Lonneux et al. (119) studied 39 patients who had been treated (surgery with or without adjuvant chemotherapy or radiotherapy) for breast cancer; 34 of these patients had asymptomatically increased tumor markers and 5 had clinical findings suspicious for recurrent tumor. Thirty-three patients had recurrent disease at 39 sites, and the remaining 6 patients had no evidence of tumor recurrence after a mean follow-up of 18 months (range 12 to 24 months). FDG PET detected disease in 31 of 33 patients with disease recurrence (37 of 39 sites); conventional imaging was positive in only 6 of these patients.

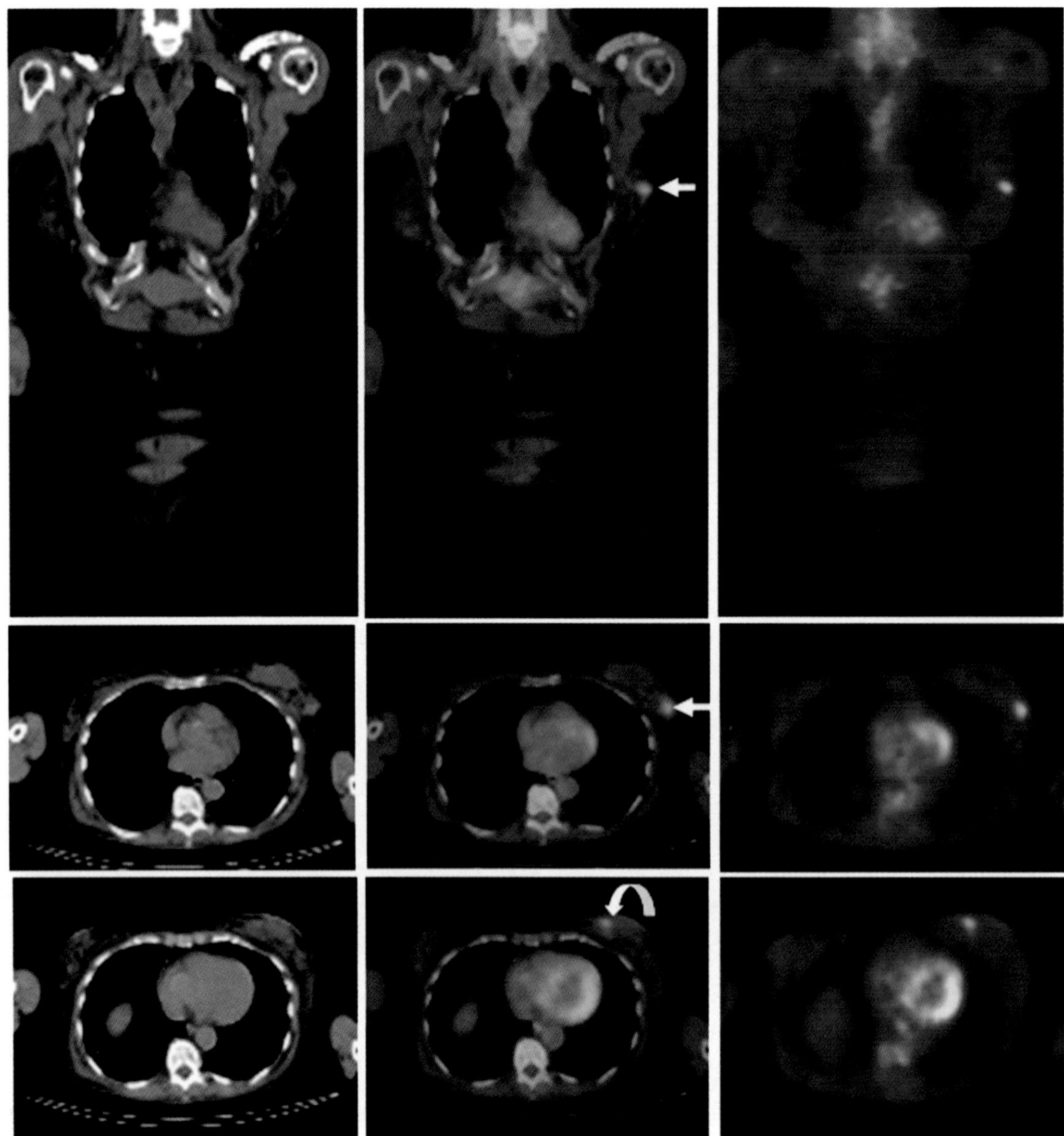

FIGURE 8.12.6. Recurrent breast cancer. Coronal (**top**) and transaxial (**middle, bottom**) CT (**left**), PET/CT fusion (**middle**), and PET (**right**) images demonstrate intense fluorodeoxyglucose uptake within the known local recurrence laterally (*arrows*) in a patient previously treated with neoadjuvant chemotherapy and lumpectomy. There is an unsuspected additional focal area of increased uptake within the breast medially (*curved arrow*), consistent with more multifocal local recurrence.

Therefore, FDG PET had 94% (31 of 33) sensitivity and 50% (3 of 6) specificity. FDG PET is a useful adjunct to conventional imaging in evaluation of patients with asymptomatic elevation of tumor markers. However, its low specificity indicates that histological or radiological confirmation is required when a change in management is intended based on the positive results of PET imaging.

In 2006 the American Society of Clinical Oncology (ASCO) announced its guidelines on breast cancer follow-up and management in the adjuvant setting (120). Based on the published literature through March 2006, ASCO concluded that there is evidence to support regular history, physical examination, and mammography as the cornerstone of appropriate breast cancer follow-up, at defined intervals, in this group of patients. The use of complete blood cell counts, chemistry panels, bone scans, chest radiographs, liver ultrasounds, CT, FDG PET, MRI, or tumor markers (carcinoembryonic antigen, CA15-3, and CA27.29) is not recommended for routine breast cancer follow-up in an otherwise asymptomatic patient with no specific findings on clinical examination.

Locoregional recurrence occurs in 7% to 30% of patients with breast cancer. Clinical detection of locoregional recurrence is limited because the signs and symptoms of locoregional recurrence often cannot be reliably distinguished from side effects of therapy. Conventional imaging techniques also are limited in differentiating posttherapeutic changes from tumor recurrence.

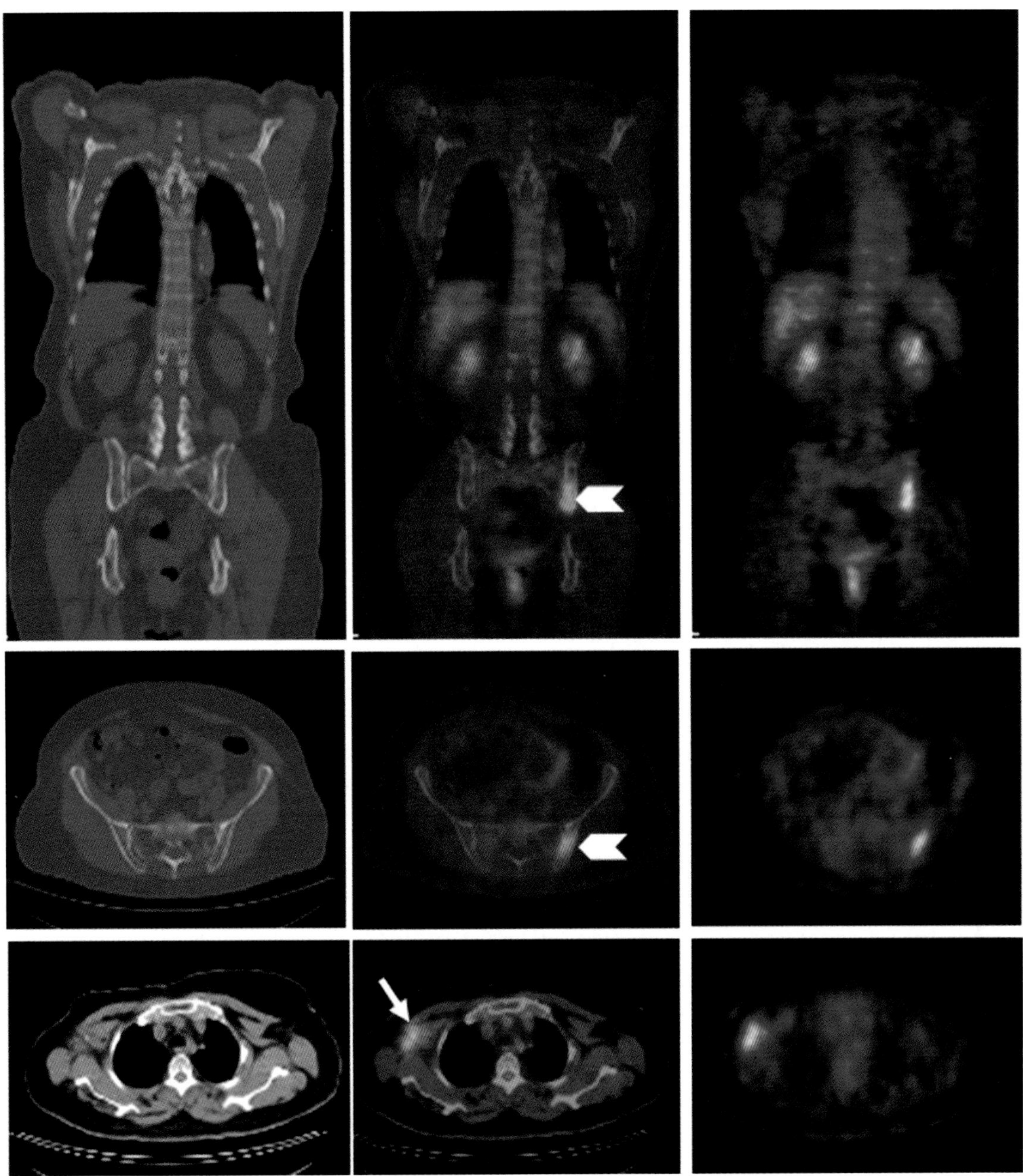

FIGURE 8.12.7. Recurrent breast cancer. Coronal (**top**) and transaxial (**middle, bottom**) CT (**left**), PET/CT fusion (**middle**), and PET (**right**) images demonstrate intense fluorodeoxyglucose uptake within the known local recurrence in the right axilla (*arrow*) in a patient previously treated with lumpectomy. There is an additional unsuspected focal area of increased uptake within the left iliac bone (*curved arrow*), without a corresponding osseous abnormality on the bone window of the CT scan, consistent with an osseous metastasis.

Hathaway et al. (121) compared FDG PET with MRI in evaluating the axillary and brachial plexus in ten patients with suspected locoregional recurrence. MRI correctly detected disease in five and was indeterminate in four of nine patients with disease recurrence, while FDG PET detected locoregional recurrence in all nine patients as well as additional unsuspected disease in six of these nine patients (distant metastatic disease in five and local breast recurrence in one). Both FDG PET and MRI were negative in the single patient without disease recurrence.

Bender et al. (115) demonstrated that MRI and/or CT were superior to FDG PET in the detection of local recurrence. FDG PET was negative in four patients with 7 to 10 mm lesions; therefore, the sensitivity and specificity of FDG PET were 80% and 96%, respectively, versus 93% and 98%, respectively, for CT and/or MRI.

Ahmad et al. (122) studied 19 patients with signs and symptoms suspicious for recurrence in the region of the brachial plexus; all but two of these patients had received local radiation therapy in the past. Fourteen patients had disease recurrence and four did not have recurrence. FDG PET was positive in all 14 patients with locoregional recurrence; CT was positive in three and negative in six of these patients who underwent CT. FDG PET was normal in four patients without disease recurrence; two of these patients underwent CT and MRI, which also were negative for disease recurrence. The remaining patient did not have locoregional disease, but had positive FDG PET findings for distant metastases in the sternum.

In one study, Eubank et al. (123) demonstrated that FDG PET contributes significantly to define the extent of disease and decide on treatment of patients with advanced breast cancer. The investigators retrospectively studied 125 patients with recurrent/metastatic disease. FDG PET was compared with conventional imaging performed before FDG PET. By comparison with conventional imaging, the extent of disease was changed by FDG PET in 84 (67%) patients. The results of FDG PET altered the therapeutic plan in 40 (32%) patients, directly helped to support the therapeutic plan in 34 (27%), and did not change the plan devised before FDG PET in the remaining 51 (41%). FDG PET altered therapy most frequently in the patients suspected of having locoregional recurrence and in those being evaluated for restaging after completion of therapy. The FDG PET results were confirmed in 61 (49%) of the patients by histopathology (n = 23) or follow-up imaging (n = 38; mean follow-up interval, 21.3 months). In this subset of patients, these studies demonstrate that FDG PET is reliable for assessment of recurrence/residual disease at distant and local sites and is a very useful adjunct to the conventional imaging modalities.

Recently, a meta-analysis of the literature regarding the utility of FDG PET in recurrent and metastatic disease was published (124). Patient-based analysis of 16 studies (n = 808 patients) demonstrated that FDG PET has a median sensitivity of 92.7% and median specificity of 81.6% for detection of metastatic or recurrent disease. The pooled sensitivity was 90% (95% confidence interval [CI], 86.8 to 93.2), and the pooled false-positive rate was 11% (95% CI, 7.8 to 14.6), after the exclusion of outliers. The maximum joint sensitivity and specificity was 88% (95% CI, 86.0 to 90.6). Lesion-based analysis of 8 studies (n = 1013 lesions) demonstrated that FDG PET has a median sensitivity of 91.7% and median specificity of 88.9% for detection of metastatic or recurrent disease. The pooled sensitivity was 85% (95% CI, 81.6 to 88.1), and the pooled false-positive rate was 6.9% (95% CI, 4.9 to 9.4), after the exclusion of outliers. The maximum joint sensitivity and specificity was 91% (95% CI, 87.1 to 94.4). These results further confirm that FDG PET is a valuable tool for detecting breast cancer recurrence and metastases.

RECEPTOR IMAGING

The majority of breast cancers are dependent on estrogen, progesterone, or both for their growth. The stimulatory effect is mediated through nuclear ERs and PRs. Therefore, these receptors have been targeted by hormonal agents in an effort to control tumor growth. Drugs based on both hormone antagonists and hormone agonists have been successfully used in treatment of breast cancer. It has long been known that the ER (and PR) status of the tumor is an important prognostic factor in breast cancer (125,126); hormone-dependent tumors, as indicated by increases in the ER and PR content of the tumor, are less aggressive than ER (and/or PR) negative tumors. Because of the importance of these receptors, *in vitro* assays of tissue obtained at biopsy or surgery are routinely used to estimate the ER and PR content of breast cancer. The most commonly used methods include ligand-binding assays, immunohistochemical analysis, and enzyme immunoassay. These assays have a number of shortcomings, most notably that they provide limited information about the functional status of the receptors and the responsiveness of tumor to hormonal therapy; only 55% to 60% of patients with ER-positive (ER+) disease respond to hormonal therapy (versus less than 10% of patients with ER-negative [ER–] disease) (125,127).

ER status is important not only in predicting the likelihood of response to first-line hormonal therapy, but also in predicting responsiveness to second-line and subsequent hormonal therapy. However, in recurrent or metastatic breast cancer, the ER status of the lesions may not always be the same as that of the original primary tumor; approximately 20% of ER+ primary breast cancers have ER– metastases (125). Indeed, the receptor status of recurrent or metastatic disease may be more predictive of response to hormonal therapy. Because some of these metastatic lesions are not amenable to biopsy, their receptor status cannot be easily determined. A method that can reliably determine both the quantity and the functional status of tumor ERs in individual lesions would be of critical importance in identifying patients who have less aggressive disease and would benefit from hormonal therapy.

Estrogen Receptor Imaging

Several decades ago, it was recognized that the presence of tumor receptors provides a mechanism for selective uptake of radiolabeled hormones as tumor imaging agents. The unique feature of PET, namely its ability to precisely quantify tracer distribution *in vivo*, has rendered it a very desirable method for evaluating receptors. The steroid receptor systems in breast cancer, and particularly the ER, have attracted the interest of numerous investigators. Efforts to identify a radioligand with high affinity and selectivity for the ER and with properties suitable for imaging have been ongoing for over two decades. Several steroidal and nonsteroidal estrogens labeled with bromine-77, bromine-75, iodine-123, and ^{18}F have been synthesized (128). One of the most promising positron-emitting radiolabeled estrogen analogues identified is 16-[^{18}F]-fluoro-17-estradiol (FES). This radioligand has high specific activity, high selective ER binding *in vitro*, and high affinity for ER+ target tissues (e.g., uterus and mammary tumors) in animal models (129–132).

Because of its favorable characteristics, FES has been most extensively studied in patients with breast cancer. FES PET has been successfully used to image ER+ breast cancers and to accurately determine the ER status of these tumors. An excellent correlation has been demonstrated between tumor FES uptake, measured on PET images (expressed as the percentage of injected dose per milliliter), and the ER concentration of the tumor determined by conventional quantitative ligand binding assays of the primary breast cancer ($r = 0.96$; $P < .001$) (133).

In patients with known metastatic breast cancer, FES PET also has been shown to be highly sensitive (93%) for detection of ER+ metastatic foci (134). FES accumulation within metastatic lesions decreased following institution of tamoxifen therapy, presumably related to the nonavailability of ERs to interact with FES because the receptors were occupied by tamoxifen and its bioactive metabolites. This confirmed that the tumor uptake of FES is a receptor-mediated process and suggests that FES may be useful for evaluating the availability of functional ERs in breast cancer and predicting the likelihood of response to hormonal therapy.

In patients (n = 43) with untreated advanced breast cancer, tumor uptake of FES was compared with *in vitro* ER levels and tumor uptake of FDG in order to determine the relationship between FDG uptake and ER status of breast cancer (34). Although ER– tumors are expected to be more aggressive than ER+ tumors, no significant relationship between FDG uptake and either the ER status or FES uptake was seen in this study. The study demonstrated a good correlation between the results of FES PET and *in vitro* ER assays and revealed that *in vitro* ER assays and/or FES PET provide unique information about tumor ER status that cannot be obtained indirectly from FDG PET. The overall rate of agreement between the results of *in vitro* ER assays and the results of FES PET was 88% in this study. This level of agreement is similar to that observed between replicate *in vitro* assays (with disagreements explained by such factors as interlaboratory variability, interassay variability, and specimen variability).

It is known that independent of the stage of disease, survival of women with ER+ disease is superior to that of women with ER– disease. Similar results were found in another study; the median survival of patients with FES– disease was relatively short at 21.6 months, while the median survival of FES+ patients had not yet been achieved in FES+ patients at a median follow-up interval of 22 months (135). In the same study, tumor heterogeneity and ER concordance between primary and metastatic lesions in individual patients also has been addressed with FES PET. Fifty individual metastatic lesions in 17 patients were evaluated with FES PET; concordance among multiple lesions within a patient was observed in 76% of patients (134). This level of concordance is comparable to that identified by *in vitro* ER determinations, when multiple sites have been biopsied.

Hormone receptor status of breast cancer directs systemic therapy; patients with hormone-sensitive (ER+ and/or PR+) advanced breast cancer are candidates for hormonal therapy. However, the inability to distinguish ER+, endocrine-therapy-resistant breast cancer from ER+, endocrine-therapy-sensitive disease leads to considerable over- or undertreatment. A known side effect of hormonal therapy is the so-called hormonal "flare" reaction, characterized by increased pain at sites of osseous metastatic disease, pain and erythema in soft tissue lesions, hypercalcemia, and apparent disease progression on bone scintigraphy that typically occurs within 7 to 10 days following institution of hormonal treatment in 5% to 20% of patients (136). Clinically, it is sometimes difficult to distinguish a flare reaction from disease progression. The clinical flare reaction has been shown to be predictive of response to hormonal therapy in 80% of patients (136–138) and is presumed to represent an initial agonist effect of the drug on the tumor before its antagonist effect supervenes (137).

Preclinical studies in immature female rats have shown that both tamoxifen and estrogen cause prompt increases in FDG accumulation in estrogen-responsive normal tissue (uterus) (139); presumably, both estrogen and tamoxifen initially stimulate cell proliferation and glucose metabolism and, thus, cause increased FDG uptake. These observations suggested that augmentation of tumor FDG uptake ("metabolic flare") early during a course of tamoxifen treatment would be indicative of an agonist effect of the drug on functional ERs and therefore predictive of a good response to therapy.

If "metabolic flare" can be detected early during the course of tamoxifen treatment, responders can be distinguished from nonresponders. In a recent prospective study of 11 patients with ER+ advanced breast cancer, this hypothesis was tested. The presence of metabolic flare, indicated by an increase in quantitative (SUV) tumor FDG uptake 7 to 10 days after tamoxifen therapy over pretherapy values, discriminated patients who subsequently responded to tamoxifen therapy from those who did not respond (Fig. 8.12.8) (140). Additionally, the pretherapy FES uptake in the tumor and the magnitude of ER blockade by tamoxifen, as measured by a decrease in quantitative tumor FES uptake after tamoxifen therapy, were superior to *in vitro* ER and PR assays in predicting response to tamoxifen therapy. These results recently have been confirmed in a larger series of patients (n = 40) with ER+ advanced breast cancer (141). A multivariate logistic regression analysis of the results demonstrated that the baseline FES uptake and the percentage of change in FDG uptake were the best predictors of response to tamoxifen therapy. In this study, it was demonstrated that the positive-predictive value for response to tamoxifen of a metabolic flare (if an increase in tumor FDG uptake of 10% or more was arbitrarily selected as the cutoff criterion) was 91% and the negative-predictive value was 94%. The corresponding positive- and negative-predictive values for the baseline FES uptake (with a cutoff SUV of 2.0) were 79% and 88%, respectively. Thus, both serial FDG and baseline FES can be useful adjuncts to *in vitro* assays to help further identify patients who are likely to respond from those who are unlikely to respond to hormonal therapy. It must be realized, however, that 10% variances in SUV can be due to intrinsic measurement methodology issues, so applying this threshold clinically may be problematic and warrants further study.

In a recent study, Linden et al. (142) also demonstrated that FES PET was superior to *in vitro* ER measurements in predicting response to both tamoxifen and aromatase inhibitors. The investigators studied 46 patients with ER+ primary or recurrent breast cancer with FES PET prior to initiation of hormonal therapy. They demonstrated that quantitative FES uptake at baseline is predictive of response to hormonal therapy in patients whose tumors do not over express *HER2/neu*. Treatment selection using quantitative FES PET in their patient population would have increased the rate of response from 23% to 34% overall, and from 29% to 46% in the subset of patients lacking *HER2/neu* overexpression. Thus, the baseline FES alone was superior to ER and PR status determined *in vitro* in predicting response to hormonal therapy. These studies demonstrated that PET provides unique information about tumor response at the biochemical level before or early during therapy that could be used to guide therapy.

Recently, several new hormonal therapeutic agents have been approved for treatment of hormone-sensitive breast cancer. These agents have different mechanisms of action than that of tamoxifen and, unlike tamoxifen, lack estrogenic effect. These agents include the aromatase inhibitors that prevent production of estrogen in the adrenal glands and fulvestrant that destroys estrogen receptors in breast cancer cells. Thus, in order to detect metabolic flare as the predictor of response to these new hormonal agents, the author has hypothesized that development of a "metabolic flare" in response to a challenge pulse of estradiol will be predictive of response to any type of therapy that either targets or is mediated via functional estrogen receptors. This is based on the hormonal challenge test, an old concept used in the management of breast cancer (34).

Researchers have investigated whether the "metabolic flare" in response to a challenge pulse of estradiol can predict the likelihood of response to aromatase inhibitors and fulvestrant prior to initiation of treatment, since these drugs are now more widely used than

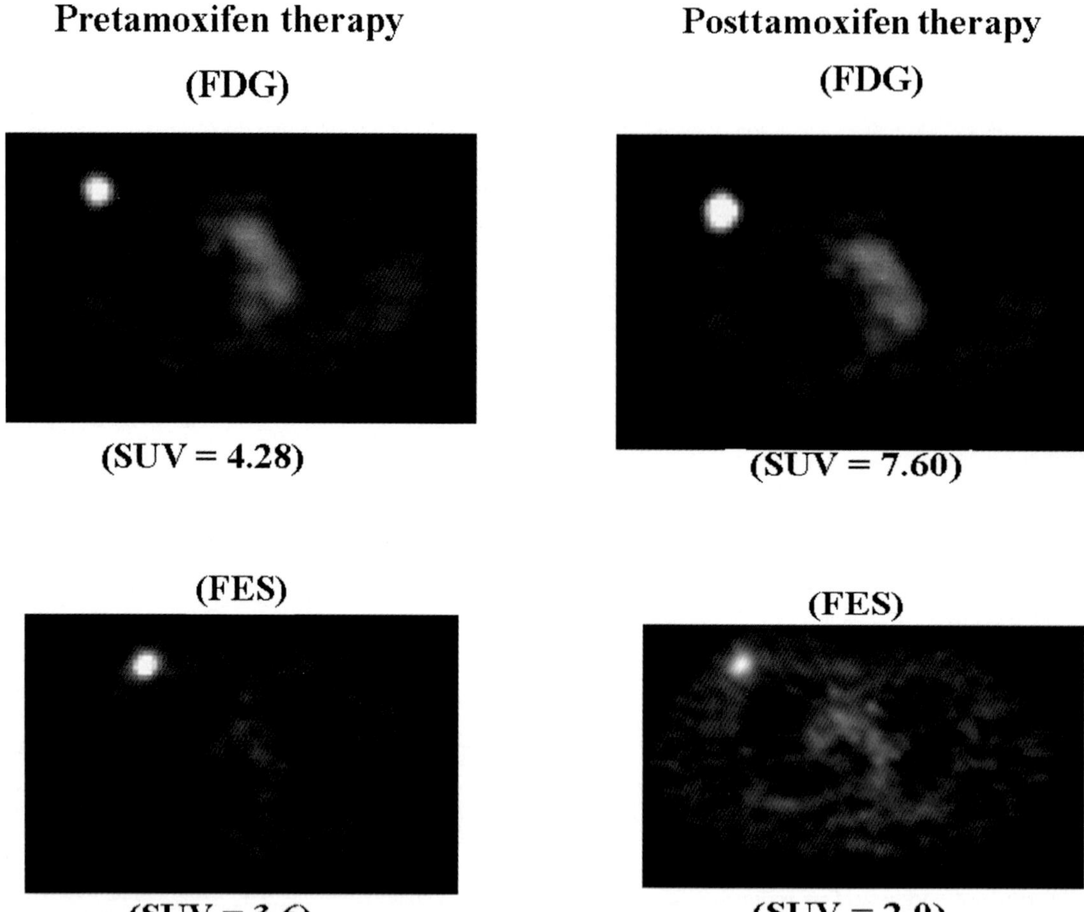

FIGURE 8.12.8. Metabolic flare. Anterior fluorodeoxyglucose (FDG) PET (**upper**) and 16-fluorine-18-fluoro-17-estradiol (FES) PET (**lower**) images before (**left**) and after (**right**) tamoxifen therapy. On the pretreatment images, there is intense FDG and FES uptake in the right primary breast cancer. After 1 week of tamoxifen therapy, there is an increase in the tumor FDG uptake (reflected by an increase in the maximum standard uptake value [SUV] of the tumor) and a concomitant decrease in FES uptake.

tamoxifen for treating advanced breast cancer (45,46). An ability to prospectively distinguish patients with hormone-sensitive disease who can safely forgo treatment with chemotherapy from patients with hormone-resistance disease who will not benefit from hormonal therapy would be a major advance in breast cancer management. The results confirm that metabolic flare in response to a challenge pulse of estradiol is predictive of response to therapy, and a negative baseline FES is highly predictive of lack of response to hormonal therapy in patients with advanced or recurrent breast cancer (143).

Progesterone Receptor Imaging

Although PR status is considered a weaker prognostic factor than ER status (125), the combination of ER and PR expression is a stronger predictor of response to hormone therapy than either alone (125,126,144,145). The presence of PR in a tumor is presumed to indicate a functionally intact estrogen-response mechanism, because PR is induced by estrogen stimulation. However, more recent data suggest an alternative explanation. Although many studies show that loss of PR predicts relative resistance to the antiestrogen tamoxifen, PR loss may not indicate resistance to aromatase inhibition (146). This may be related to crosstalk between ER and PR and growth factor receptor pathways such as *HER2*. Thus, the status of PR may help clinicians decide between initial use of an aromatase inhibitor or tamoxifen in the individual patient.

Reliable determination of PR status is extremely important. Efforts to develop radiolabeled ligands for PRs have been less successful than those for ER imaging. Several radiolabeled progesterone analogues have been developed (147,148); 21-[^{18}F]-fluoro-16-ethyl-19-norprogesterone (FENP) is one such compound that has been developed for imaging by PET. Although FENP had favorable *in vitro* and *in vivo* characteristics in preclinical testing, imaging results with this compound in patients with breast cancer were disappointing due to the low target-to-background uptake ratio, poor correlation of tumor uptake with PR content of the tumor, and high nonspecific uptake (147,149–151).

The search for a more suitable progesterone-based imaging compound continues and currently, several new ^{18}F radioligands are being developed, such as 21-[^{18}F]-fluoro-16α,17α [(*R*)-1'-α-furylmethylidene)dioxy]-19-norpregn-4-ene-3,20-dione (FFNP) is a new progestin-based PET radioligand with better imaging characteristics than FENP and is now proposed for evaluation in patients with breast cancer.

Imaging with Radiolabeled Antiestrogens

[^{18}F]-fluorotamoxifen, an analogue of tamoxifen, has been developed as a tracer to assess the tumor ER status and responsiveness to tamoxifen therapy (152,153). Limited clinical studies of [^{18}F]-fluorotamoxifen in patients with breast cancer have demonstrated that this compound has low specific binding to ERs and high nonspecific binding in other tissues (153).

OTHER RADIOPHARMACEUTICALS

Protein Metabolism

In a pilot study, L-[methyl-^{11}C] methionine (MET) has been used to evaluate amino acid metabolism and protein metabolism in breast cancer (154). Although tumor uptake of MET correlated with the S-phase fraction of the tumor measured by flow cytometry and response to systemic or radiotherapy, only lesions greater than 3 cm were identified. This, as well as the 20-minute half-life of carbon-11, has significantly limited the use of MET PET in the clinical or research setting.

In a preliminary study, PET with L-[1-^{11}C]-tyrosine (TYR) has been studied in patients with primary breast cancer. TYR has the potential to be useful in differentiating benign from malignant lesions, as high TYR uptake was noted in malignant tumors, while benign lesions had no uptake (30). More recently, breast cancer has been imaged with [^{18}F]-fluorothymidine (FLT). Smyczek-Gargya et al. (155) demonstrated that FLT PET can successfully image primary breast cancer. In patients with locally advanced and metastatic breast cancer, the retention of FLT correlated well with the Ki-67 labeling index from tumor biopsies and, thus, revealed information about the cellular proliferation of breast cancer (156).

More recently, FLT PET was used to monitor response to systemic therapy in 14 patients with breast cancer. Pio et al. (157) demonstrated that FLT PET obtained 2 weeks after the end of the first course of systemic therapy was useful for predicting long-term efficacy of therapy in these patients. Studies with larger numbers of patients are needed to confirm these results in patients with advanced breast cancer undergoing various systemic therapeutic regimens.

CONCLUSION

The past decade has witnessed a striking increase in interest in clinical and investigational use of PET in breast cancer. The unique functional information provided by PET has been shown to be of significant value for the evaluation of patients with breast cancer. PET is being increasingly used to resolve clinical questions that are not satisfactorily addressed by conventional imaging methods.

The current literature suggests that PET not only can improve breast cancer detection, staging, and management, but also can provide prognostic information. The functional information provided by PET has the potential to be useful in resolving some of the shortcomings of the conventional imaging methods in the evaluation of patients with breast cancer (e.g., patients with difficult-to-examine breasts). FDG PET has been shown to be limited in staging of regional lymph nodes.

There is increasing evidence that FDG PET is the preferred method to assess the extent of distant metastatic disease and is especially useful in patients with high clinical suspicion of disease who have normal conventional imaging studies. Similarly, FDG PET has been shown to be a useful adjunct to conventional imaging methods in evaluation of recurrent disease.

FDG PET has shown promise in assessing early response to chemotherapy and/or hormonal therapy. Significant progress has also been made in the development and testing of receptor imaging ligands, particularly ER-based ligands that provide unique information about the biology and behavior of breast cancer, leading to more effective treatment of this cancer.

REFERENCES

1. Jemal A, Siegel R, Ward E, et al. Cancer statistics, 2008. *CA Cancer J Clin* 2008;58:71–96.
2. Brown RS, Wahl RL. Overexpression of Glut-1 glucose transporter in human breast cancer. An immunohistochemical study. *Cancer* 1993; 72:2979–2985.
3. Bos R, van Der Hoeven JJ, van Der Wall E, et al. Biologic correlates of (18)fluorodeoxyglucose uptake in human breast cancer measured by positron emission tomography. *J Clin Oncol* 2002;20:379–387.
4. Brown RS, Leung JY, Fisher SJ, et al. Intratumoral distribution of tritiated fluorodeoxyglucose in breast carcinoma: I. Are inflammatory cells important? *J Nucl Med* 1995;36:1854–1861.
5. Torizuka T, Zasadny KR, Recker B, et al. Untreated primary lung and breast cancers: correlation between F-18 FDG kinetic rate constants and findings of *in vitro* studies. *Radiology* 1998;207:767–774.
6. Wahl RL, Cody RL, Hutchins GD, et al. Primary and metastatic breast carcinoma: initial clinical evaluation with PET with the radiolabeled glucose analogue 2-[F-18]-fluoro-2-deoxy-D-glucose. *Radiology* 1991;179:765–770.
7. Wahl RL, Henry CA, Ethier SP. Serum glucose: effects on tumor and normal tissue accumulation of 2-[F-18]-fluoro-2-deoxy-D-glucose in rodents with mammary carcinoma. *Radiology* 1992;183:643–647.
8. Smith TA, Sharma RI, Thompson AM, et al. Tumor ^{18}F-FDG incorporation is enhanced by attenuation of p53 function in breast cancer cells *in vitro*. *J Nucl Med* 2006;47:1525–1530.
9. Yutani K, Tatsumi M, Uehara T, et al. Effect of patients' being prone during FDG PET for the diagnosis of breast cancer. *AJR Am J Roentgenol* 1999;173:1337–1339.
10. Boerner AR, Weckesser M, Herzog H, et al. Optimal scan time for fluorine-18 fluorodeoxyglucose positron emission tomography in breast cancer. *Eur J Nucl Med* 1999;26:226–230.
11. Kumar R, Loving VA, Chauhan A, et al. Potential of dual-time-point imaging to improve breast cancer diagnosis with (18)F-FDG PET. *J Nucl Med* 2005;46:1819–1824.
12. Zasadny KR, Wahl RL. Standardized uptake values of normal tissues at PET with 2-[fluorine-18]-fluoro-2-deoxy-D-glucose: variations with body weight and a method for correction. *Radiology* 1993;189: 847–850.
13. Sugawara Y, Zasadny KR, Neuhoff AW, et al. Reevaluation of the standardized uptake value for FDG: variations with body weight and methods for correction. *Radiology* 1999;213:521–525.
14. Patlak CS, Blasberg RG. Graphical evaluation of blood-to-brain transfer constants from multiple-time uptake data. Generalizations. *J Cereb Blood Flow Metab* 1985;5:584–590.
15. Avril N, Bense S, Ziegler SI, et al. Breast imaging with fluorine-18-FDG PET: quantitative image analysis. *J Nucl Med* 1997;38:1186–1191.
16. Kumar R, Chauhan A, Zhuang H, et al. Standardized uptake values of normal breast tissue with 2-deoxy-2-[F-18]fluoro-D-glucose positron emission tomography: variations with age, breast density, and menopausal status. *Mol Imaging Biol* 2006;8:355–362.

17. Feig SA. Role and evaluation of mammography and other imaging methods for breast cancer detection, diagnosis, and staging. *Semin Nucl Med* 1999;29:3–15.
18. Whitman GJ. The role of mammography in breast cancer prevention. *Curr Opin Oncol* 1999;11:414–418.
19. Dean JC, Ilvento CC. Improved cancer detection using computer-aided detection with diagnostic and screening mammography: prospective study of 104 cancers. *AJR Am J Roentgenol* 2006;187:20–28.
20. Sickles EA. Mammographic features of early breast cancer. *AJR Am J Roentgenol* 1984;143:461–464.
21. Moskowitz M. The predictive value of certain mammographic signs in screening for breast cancer. *Cancer* 1983;51:1007–1011.
22. Kopans DB. The positive predictive value of mammography. *AJR Am J Roentgenol* 1992;158:521–526.
23. Franceschi D, Crowe J, Zollinger R, et al. Biopsy of the breast for mammographically detected lesions. *Surg Gynecol Obstet* 1990;171:449–455.
24. Skinner MA, Swain M, Simmons R, et al. Nonpalpable breast lesions at biopsy. A detailed analysis of radiographic features. *Ann Surg* 1988;208:203–208.
25. Van Goethem M, Tjalma W, Schelfout K, et al. Magnetic resonance imaging in breast cancer. *Eur J Surg Oncol* 2006;32:901–910.
26. Tse NY, Hoh CK, Hawkins RA, et al. The application of positron emission tomographic imaging with fluorodeoxyglucose to the evaluation of breast disease. *Ann Surg* 1992;216:27–34.
27. Nieweg OE, Kim EE, Wong WH, et al. Positron emission tomography with fluorine-18-deoxyglucose in the detection and staging of breast cancer. *Cancer* 1993;71:3920–3925.
28. Scheidhauer K, Scharl A, Pietrzyk U, et al. Qualitative [18F]FDG positron emission tomography in primary breast cancer: clinical relevance and practicability. *Eur J Nucl Med* 1996;23:618–623.
29. Adler LP, Crowe JP, al-Kaisi NK, et al. Evaluation of breast masses and axillary lymph nodes with [F-18] 2-deoxy-2-fluoro-D-glucose PET. *Radiology* 1993;187:743–750.
30. Kole AC, Nieweg OE, Pruim J, et al. Standardized uptake value and quantification of metabolism for breast cancer imaging with FDG and L-[1-11C]tyrosine PET. *J Nucl Med* 1997;38:692–696.
31. Palmedo H, Bender H, Grunwald F, et al. Comparison of fluorine-18 fluorodeoxyglucose positron emission tomography and technetium-99m methoxyisobutylisonitrile scintimammography in the detection of breast tumours. *Eur J Nucl Med* 1997;24:1138–1145.
32. Avril N, Rose CA, Schelling M, et al. Breast imaging with positron emission tomography and fluorine-18 fluorodeoxyglucose: use and limitations. *J Clin Oncol* 2000;18:3495–3502.
33. Noh DY, Yun IJ, Kim JS, et al. Diagnostic value of positron emission tomography for detecting breast cancer. *World J Surg* 1998;22:223–227; discussion 227–228.
34. Dehdashti F, Mortimer JE, Siegel BA, et al. Positron tomographic assessment of estrogen receptors in breast cancer: comparison with FDG-PET and in vitro receptor assays. *J Nucl Med* 1995;36:1766–1774.
35. Avril N, Dose J, Janicke F, et al. Assessment of axillary lymph node involvement in breast cancer patients with positron emission tomography using radiolabeled 2-(fluorine-18)-fluoro-2-deoxy-D-glucose. *J Natl Cancer Inst* 1996;88:1204–1209.
36. Utech CI, Young CS, Winter PF. Prospective evaluation of fluorine-18 fluorodeoxyglucose positron emission tomography in breast cancer for staging of the axilla related to surgery and immunocytochemistry. *Eur J Nucl Med* 1996;23:1588–1593.
37. Schirrmeister H, Kuhn T, Guhlmann A, et al. Fluorine-18 2-deoxy-2-fluoro-D-glucose PET in the preoperative staging of breast cancer: comparison with the standard staging procedures. *Eur J Nucl Med* 2001;28:351–358.
38. Avril N, Dose J, Janicke F, et al. Metabolic characterization of breast tumors with positron emission tomography using F-18 fluorodeoxyglucose. *J Clin Oncol* 1996;14:1848–1857.
39. Bakheet SM, Powe J, Kandil A, et al. F-18 FDG uptake in breast infection and inflammation. *Clin Nucl Med* 2000;25:100–103.
40. Weinberg I, Beylin D, Yarnall S, et al. Application of a PET device with 1.5 mm FWHM intrinsic spatial resolution to breast cancer imaging. In: *Proceedings of the 2004 IEEE International Symposium on Biomedical Imaging: 2004, from Nano to Macro, Arlington, VA, April 15–18, 2004*. New York: IEEE, 2004:1396–1399.
41. Berg WA, Weinberg IN, Narayanan D, et al. High-resolution fluorodeoxyglucose positron emission tomography with compression ("positron emission mammography") is highly accurate in depicting primary breast cancer. *Breast J* 2006;12:309–323.
42. Murthy K, Aznar M, Bergman AM, et al. Positron emission mammographic instrument: initial results. *Radiology* 2000;215:280–285.
43. Bergman AM, Thompson CJ, Murthy K, et al. Technique to obtain positron emission mammography images in registration with x-ray mammograms. *Med Phys* 1998;25:2119–2129.
44. Crippa F, Seregni E, Agresti R, et al. Association between [18F]fluorodeoxyglucose uptake and postoperative histopathology, hormone receptor status, thymidine labelling index and p53 in primary breast cancer: a preliminary observation. *Eur J Nucl Med* 1998;25:1429–1434.
45. Oshida M, Uno K, Suzuki M, et al. Predicting the prognoses of breast carcinoma patients with positron emission tomography using 2-deoxy-2-fluoro[18F]-D-glucose. *Cancer* 1998;82:2227–2234.
46. Avril N, Menzel M, Dose J, et al. Glucose metabolism of breast cancer assessed by 18F-FDG PET: histologic and immunohistochemical tissue analysis. *J Nucl Med* 2001;42:9–16.
47. Buck A, Schirrmeister H, Kuhn T, et al. FDG uptake in breast cancer: correlation with biological and clinical prognostic parameters. *Eur J Nucl Med Mol Imaging* 2002;29:1317–1323.
48. Crippa F, Agresti R, Donne VD, et al. The contribution of positron emission tomography (PET) with ^{18}F-fluorodeoxyglucose (FDG) in the preoperative detection of axillary metastases of breast cancer: the experience of the National Cancer Institute of Milan. *Tumori* 1997;83:542–543.
49. Mankoff DA, Dunnwald LK, Gralow JR, et al. Blood flow and metabolism in locally advanced breast cancer: relationship to response to therapy. *J Nucl Med* 2002;43:500–509.
50. Inoue T, Yutani K, Taguchi T, et al. Preoperative evaluation of prognosis in breast cancer patients by [(18)F]2-deoxy-2-fluoro-D-glucose-positron emission tomography. *J Cancer Res Clin Oncol* 2004;130:273–278.
51. Hellman S, Harris JR. Natural history of breast cancer. In: Harris JR, Lippman ME, Marrow M, et al., eds. *Diseases of the breast*, 2nd ed. Philadelphia: Lippincott Williams & Wilkins, 2000:407–423.
52. Singletary SE, Allred C, Ashley P, et al. Revision of the American Joint Committee on Cancer staging system for breast cancer. *J Clin Oncol* 2002;20:3628–3636.
53. Goldhirsch A, Glick JH, Gelber RD, et al. Meeting highlights: International Consensus Panel on the Treatment of Primary Breast Cancer. Seventh International Conference on Adjuvant Therapy of Primary Breast Cancer. *J Clin Oncol* 2001;19:3817–3827.
54. Recht A, Edge SB, Solin LJ, et al. Postmastectomy radiotherapy: clinical practice guidelines of the American Society of Clinical Oncology. *J Clin Oncol* 2001;19:1539–1569.
55. Wahl RL, Kaminski MS, Ethier SP, et al. The potential of 2-deoxy-2[18F]fluoro-D-glucose (FDG) for the detection of tumor involvement in lymph nodes. *J Nucl Med* 1990;31:1831–1835.
56. Wahl RL, Cody RL, August D. Initial evaluation of FDG-PET for staging of the axilla in newly diagnosed breast cancer patients. *J Nucl Med* 1991;32:981.
57. Hoh CK, Hawkins RA, Glaspy JA, et al. Cancer detection with whole-body PET using 2-[18F]fluoro-2-deoxy-D-glucose. *J Comput Assist Tomogr* 1993;17:582–589.
58. Adler LP, Faulhaber PF, Schnur KC, et al. Axillary lymph node metastases: screening with [F-18]2-deoxy-2-fluoro-D-glucose (FDG) PET. *Radiology* 1997;203:323–327.
59. Smith IC, Ogston KN, Whitford P, et al. Staging of the axilla in breast cancer: accurate in vivo assessment using positron emission tomogra-

phy with 2-(fluorine-18)-fluoro-2-deoxy-D-glucose. *Ann Surg* 1998;228:220–227.
60. Rostom AY, Powe J, Kandil A, et al. Positron emission tomography in breast cancer: a clinicopathological correlation of results. *Br J Radiol* 1999;72:1064–1068.
61. Greco M, Crippa F, Agresti R, et al. Axillary lymph node staging in breast cancer by 2-fluoro-2-deoxy-D-glucose-positron emission tomography: clinical evaluation and alternative management. *J Natl Cancer Inst* 2001;93:630–635.
62. Guller U, Nitzsche EU, Schirp U, et al. Selective axillary surgery in breast cancer patients based on positron emission tomography with ^{18}F-fluoro-2-deoxy-D-glucose: not yet! *Breast Cancer Res Treat* 2002;71:171–173.
63. Barranger E, Grahek D, Antoine M, et al. Evaluation of fluorodeoxyglucose positron emission tomography in the detection of axillary lymph node metastases in patients with early-stage breast cancer. *Ann Surg Oncol* 2003;10:622–627.
64. Wahl RL, Siegel BA, Coleman RE, et al. Prospective multicenter study of axillary nodal staging by positron emission tomography in breast cancer: a report of the staging breast cancer with PET Study Group. *J Clin Oncol* 2004;22:277–285.
65. Zornoza G, Garcia-Velloso MJ, Sola J, et al. ^{18}F-FDG PET complemented with sentinel lymph node biopsy in the detection of axillary involvement in breast cancer. *Eur J Surg Oncol* 2004;30:15–19.
66. van der Hoeven JJ, Hoekstra OS, Comans EF, et al. Determinants of diagnostic performance of [F-18]fluorodeoxyglucose positron emission tomography for axillary staging in breast cancer. *Ann Surg* 2002;236:619–624.
67. Lovrics PJ, Chen V, Coates G, et al. A prospective evaluation of positron emission tomography scanning, sentinel lymph node biopsy, and standard axillary dissection for axillary staging in patients with early stage breast cancer. *Ann Surg Oncol* 2004;11:846–853.
68. Fehr MK, Hornung R, Varga Z, et al. Axillary staging using positron emission tomography in breast cancer patients qualifying for sentinel lymph node biopsy. *Breast J* 2004;10:89–93.
69. Kumar R, Zhuang H, Schnall M, et al. FDG PET positive lymph nodes are highly predictive of metastasis in breast cancer. *Nucl Med Commun* 2006;27:231–236.
70. Chung A, Liou D, Karlan S, et al. Preoperative FDG-PET for axillary metastases in patients with breast cancer. *Arch Surg* 2006;141:783–788; discussion 788–789.
71. Gil-Rendo A, Zornoza G, Garcia-Velloso MJ, et al. Fluorodeoxyglucose positron emission tomography with sentinel lymph node biopsy for evaluation of axillary involvement in breast cancer. *Br J Surg* 2006;93:707–712.
72. Yang JH, Nam SJ, Lee TS, et al. Comparison of intraoperative frozen section analysis of sentinel node with preoperative positron emission tomography in the diagnosis of axillary lymph node status in breast cancer patients. *Jpn J Clin Oncol* 2001;31:1–6.
73. Kelemen PR, Lowe V, Phillips N. Positron emission tomography and sentinel lymph node dissection in breast cancer. *Clin Breast Cancer* 2002;3:73–77.
74. Weissleder R, Elizondo G, Wittenberg J, et al. Ultrasmall superparamagnetic iron oxide: an intravenous contrast agent for assessing lymph nodes with MR imaging. *Radiology* 1990;175:494–498.
75. Michel SC, Keller TM, Frohlich JM, et al. Preoperative breast cancer staging: MR imaging of the axilla with ultrasmall superparamagnetic iron oxide enhancement. *Radiology* 2002;225:527–536.
76. Stadnik TW, Everaert H, Makkat S, et al. Breast imaging. Preoperative breast cancer staging: comparison of USPIO-enhanced MR imaging and ^{18}F-fluorodeoxyglucose (FDG) positron emission tomography (PET) imaging for axillary lymph node staging-initial findings. *Eur Radiol* 2006;16:2153–2160.
77. Bellon JR, Livingston RB, Eubank WB, et al. Evaluation of the internal mammary lymph nodes by FDG-PET in locally advanced breast cancer (LABC). *Am J Clin Oncol* 2004;27:407–410.
78. Singletary SE, Greene FL. Revision of breast cancer staging: the 6th edition of the TNM classification. *Semin Surg Oncol* 2003;21:53–59.
79. Port ER, Yeung H, Gonen M, et al. ^{18}F-2-fluoro-2-deoxy-D-glucose positron emission tomography scanning affects surgical management in selected patients with high-risk, operable breast carcinoma. *Ann Surg Oncol* 2006;13:677–684.
80. Coleman RE, Rubens RD. The clinical course of bone metastases from breast cancer. *Br J Cancer* 1987;55:61–66.
81. Cook GJ, Houston S, Rubens R, et al. Detection of bone metastases in breast cancer by 18FDG PET: differing metabolic activity in osteoblastic and osteolytic lesions. *J Clin Oncol* 1998;16:3375–3379.
82. Kao CH, Hsieh JF, Tsai SC, et al. Comparison and discrepancy of ^{18}F-2-deoxyglucose positron emission tomography and Tc-99m MDP bone scan to detect bone metastases. *Anticancer Res* 2000;20:2189–2192.
83. Abe K, Sasaki M, Kuwabara Y, et al. Comparison of ^{18}FDG-PET with 99mTc-HMDP scintigraphy for the detection of bone metastases in patients with breast cancer. *Ann Nucl Med* 2005;19:573–579.
84. Nakai T, Okuyama C, Kubota T, et al. Pitfalls of FDG-PET for the diagnosis of osteoblastic bone metastases in patients with breast cancer. *Eur J Nucl Med Mol Imaging* 2005;32:1253–1258.
85. Yang SN, Liang JA, Lin FJ, et al. Comparing whole body (18)F-2-deoxyglucose positron emission tomography and technetium-99m methylene diphosphonate bone scan to detect bone metastases in patients with breast cancer. *J Cancer Res Clin Oncol* 2002;128:325–328.
86. Ohta M, Tokuda Y, Suzuki Y, et al. Whole body PET for the evaluation of bony metastases in patients with breast cancer: comparison with 99Tcm-MDP bone scintigraphy. *Nucl Med Commun* 2001;22:875–879.
87. Krishnamurthy GT, Thomas PB, Tubis M, et al. Comparison of 99mTc-polyphosphate and 18F. I. Kinetics. *J Nucl Med* 1974;15:832–836.
88. Hawkins RA, Choi Y, Huang SC, et al. Evaluation of the skeletal kinetics of fluorine-18-fluoride ion with PET. *J Nucl Med* 1992;33:633–642.
89. Hoh CK, Hawkins RA, Dlabom M. Whole body skeletal imaging with [F-18] fluoride ion with PET. *J Comput Assist Tomogr* 1992;17:34–41.
90. Schiepers C, Nuyts J, Bormans G, et al. Fluoride kinetics of the axial skeleton measured in vivo with fluorine-18-fluoride PET. *J Nucl Med* 1997;38:1970–1976.
91. Schirrmeister H, Guhlmann A, Kotzerke J, et al. Early detection and accurate description of extent of metastatic bone disease in breast cancer with fluoride ion and positron emission tomography. *J Clin Oncol* 1999;17:2381–2389.
92. Even-Sapir E, Metser U, Flusser G, et al. Assessment of malignant skeletal disease: initial experience with ^{18}F-fluoride PET/CT and comparison between ^{18}F-fluoride PET and ^{18}F-fluoride PET/CT. *J Nucl Med* 2004;45:272–278.
93. Even-Sapir E, Metser U, Mishani E, et al. The detection of bone metastases in patients with high-risk prostate cancer: 99mTc-MDP planar bone scintigraphy, single- and multi-field-of-view SPECT, ^{18}F-fluoride PET, and ^{18}F-fluoride PET/CT. *J Nucl Med* 2006;47:287–297.
94. Beresford M, Padhani AR, Goh V, et al. Imaging breast cancer response during neoadjuvant systemic therapy. *Expert Rev Anticancer Ther* 2005;5:893–905.
95. Londero V, Bazzocchi M, Del Frate C, et al. Locally advanced breast cancer: comparison of mammography, sonography and MR imaging in evaluation of residual disease in women receiving neoadjuvant chemotherapy. *Eur Radiol* 2004;14:1371–1379.
96. Wasser K, Klein SK, Fink C, et al. Evaluation of neoadjuvant chemotherapeutic response of breast cancer using dynamic MRI with high temporal resolution. *Eur Radiol* 2003;13:80–87.
97. Wahl RL, Zasadny K, Helvie M, et al. Metabolic monitoring of breast cancer chemohormonotherapy using positron emission tomography: initial evaluation. *J Clin Oncol* 1993;11:2101–2111.
98. Flanagan FL, Dehdashti F, Siegel BA. PET in breast cancer. *Semin Nucl Med* 1998;28:290–302.
99. Bassa P, Kim EE, Inoue T, et al. Evaluation of preoperative chemotherapy using PET with fluorine-18-fluorodeoxyglucose in breast cancer. *J Nucl Med* 1996;37:931–938.

100. Schelling M, Avril N, Nahrig J, et al. Positron emission tomography using [(18)F]Fluorodeoxyglucose for monitoring primary chemotherapy in breast cancer. *J Clin Oncol* 2000;18:1689–1695.
101. Smith IC, Welch AE, Hutcheon AW, et al. Positron emission tomography using [(18)F]-fluorodeoxy-D-glucose to predict the pathologic response of breast cancer to primary chemotherapy. *J Clin Oncol* 2000;18:1676–1688.
102. Kim SJ, Kim SK, Lee ES, et al. Predictive value of [18F]FDG PET for pathological response of breast cancer to neo-adjuvant chemotherapy. *Ann Oncol* 2004;15:1352–1357.
103. McDermott GM, Welch A, Staff RT, et al. Monitoring primary breast cancer throughout chemotherapy using FDG-PET. *Breast Cancer Res Treat* 2007;102:75–84.
104. Rousseau C, Devillers A, Sagan C, et al. Monitoring of early response to neoadjuvant chemotherapy in stage II and III breast cancer by [18F]fluorodeoxyglucose positron emission tomography. *J Clin Oncol* 2006;24:5366–5372.
105. Tseng J, Dunnwald LK, Schubert EK, et al. ^{18}F-FDG kinetics in locally advanced breast cancer: correlation with tumor blood flow and changes in response to neoadjuvant chemotherapy. *J Nucl Med* 2004;45:1829–1837.
106. Savio G, Laudani A, Leonardi V, et al. Treatment of metastatic breast cancer with vinorelbine and docetaxel. *Am J Clin Oncol* 2006;29:276–280.
107. Minn H, Soini I. [18F]fluorodeoxyglucose scintigraphy in diagnosis and follow up of treatment in advanced breast cancer. *Eur J Nucl Med* 1989;15:61–66.
108. Schwarz D, Bader M, Jenicke L, et al. Early prediction of response to chemotherapy in metastatic breast cancer using sequential ^{18}F-FDG PET. *J Nucl Med* 2005;46:1144–1150.
109. Stafford SE, Gralow JR, Schubert EK, et al. Use of serial FDG PET to measure the response of bone-dominant breast cancer to therapy. *Acad Radiol* 2002;9:913–921.
110. Tartarone A, Romano G, Galasso R, et al. Should we continue to study high-dose chemotherapy in metastatic breast cancer patients? A critical review of the published data. *Bone Marrow Transplant* 2003;31:525–530.
111. Cachin F, Prince HM, Hogg A, et al. Powerful prognostic stratification by [18F]fluorodeoxyglucose positron emission tomography in patients with metastatic breast cancer treated with high-dose chemotherapy. *J Clin Oncol* 2006;24:3026–3031.
112. Sugawara Y, Fisher SJ, Zasadny KR, et al. Preclinical and clinical studies of bone marrow uptake of fluorine-18-fluorodeoxyglucose with or without granulocyte colony-stimulating factor during chemotherapy. *J Clin Oncol* 1998;16:173–180.
113. Abdel-Dayem HM, Rosen G, El-Zeftawy H, et al. Fluorine-18 fluorodeoxyglucose splenic uptake from extramedullary hematopoiesis after granulocyte colony-stimulating factor stimulation. *Clin Nucl Med* 1999;24:319–322.
114. Moon DH, Maddahi J, Silverman DH, et al. Accuracy of whole-body fluorine-18-FDG PET for the detection of recurrent or metastatic breast carcinoma. *J Nucl Med* 1998;39:431–435.
115. Bender H, Kirst J, Palmedo H, et al. Value of 18-fluoro-deoxyglucose positron emission tomography in the staging of recurrent breast carcinoma. *Anticancer Res* 1997;17:1687–1692.
116. Wolfort RM, Li BD, Johnson LW, et al. The role of whole-body fluorine-18-FDG positron emission tomography in the detection of recurrence in symptomatic patients with stages II and III breast cancer. *World J Surg* 2006;30:1422–1427.
117. Landheer ML, Steffens MG, Klinkenbijl JH, et al. Value of fluorodeoxyglucose positron emission tomography in women with breast cancer. *Br J Surg* 2005;92:1363–1367.
118. Liu CS, Shen YY, Lin CC, et al. Clinical impact of [(18)F]FDG-PET in patients with suspected recurrent breast cancer based on asymptomatically elevated tumor marker serum levels: a preliminary report. *Jpn J Clin Oncol* 2002;32:244–247.
119. Lonneux M, Borbath II, Berliere M, et al. The place of whole-body PET FDG for the diagnosis of distant recurrence of breast cancer. *Clin Positron Imaging* 2000;3:45–49.
120. Khatcheressian JL, Wolff AC, Smith TJ, et al. American Society of Clinical Oncology 2006 update of the breast cancer follow-up and management guidelines in the adjuvant setting. *J Clin Oncol* 2006;24:5091–5097.
121. Hathaway PB, Mankoff DA, Maravilla KR, et al. Value of combined FDG PET and MR imaging in the evaluation of suspected recurrent local-regional breast cancer: preliminary experience. *Radiology* 1999;210:807–814.
122. Ahmad A, Barrington S, Maisey M, et al. Use of positron emission tomography in evaluation of brachial plexopathy in breast cancer patients. *Br J Cancer* 1999;79:478–482.
123. Eubank WB, Mankoff D, Bhattacharya M, et al. Impact of FDG PET on defining the extent of disease and on the treatment of patients with recurrent or metastatic breast cancer. *AJR Am J Roentgenol* 2004;183:479–486.
124. Isasi CR, Moadel RM, Blaufox MD. A meta-analysis of FDG-PET for the evaluation of breast cancer recurrence and metastases. *Breast Cancer Res Treat* 2005;90:105–112.
125. Elledge RM, Fuqua SAW. Estrogen and progesterone receptors In: Harris JR, Lippman ME, Marrow M, et al., eds. 2nd ed. *Diseases of the breast.* Philadelphia: Lippincott Williams & Wilkins, 2000:471–488.
126. Vollenweider-Zerargui L, Barrelet L, Wong Y, et al. The predictive value of estrogen and progesterone receptors' concentrations on the clinical behavior of breast cancer in women. Clinical correlation on 547 patients. *Cancer* 1986;57:1171–1180.
127. Ravdin PM, Green S, Dorr TM, et al. Prognostic significance of progesterone receptor levels in estrogen receptor-positive patients with metastatic breast cancer treated with tamoxifen: results of a prospective Southwest Oncology Group study. *J Clin Oncol* 1992;10:1284–1291.
128. Katzenellenbogen JA. Designing steroid receptor-based radiotracers to image breast and prostate tumors. *J Nucl Med* 1995;36:8S–13S.
129. Kiesewetter DO, Kilbourn MR, Landvatter SW, et al. Preparation of four fluorine-18-labeled estrogens and their selective uptakes in target tissues of immature rats. *J Nucl Med* 1984;25:1212–1221.
130. Mathias CJ, Welch MJ, Katzenellenbogen JA, et al. Characterization of the uptake of 16 alpha-([18F]fluoro)-17 beta-estradiol in DMBA-induced mammary tumors. *Int J Rad Appl Instrum B* 1987;14:15–25.
131. Brodack JW, Kilbourn MR, Welch MJ, et al. Application of robotics to radiopharmaceutical preparation: controlled synthesis of fluorine-18-16-alpha-fluoroestradiol-17 beta. *J Nucl Med* 1986;27:714–721.
132. Brodack JW, Kilbourn MR, Welch MJ, et al. NCA 16 alpha-[18F]fluoroestradiol-17 beta: the effect of reaction vessel on fluorine-18 resolubilization, product yield, and effective specific activity. *Int J Rad Appl Instrum A* 1986;37:217–221.
133. Mintun MA, Welch MJ, Siegel BA, et al. Breast cancer: PET imaging of estrogen receptors. *Radiology* 1988;169:45–48.
134. McGuire AH, Dehdashti F, Siegel BA, et al. Positron tomographic assessment of 16 alpha-[18F]-fluoro-17-beta-estradiol uptake in metastatic breast carcinoma. *J Nucl Med* 1991;32:1526–1531.
135. Mortimer JE, Dehdashti F, Siegel BA, et al. Positron emission tomography with 2-[18F]fluoro-2-deoxy-D-glucose and 16alpha-[18F]fluoro-17beta-estradiol in breast cancer: correlation with estrogen receptor status and response to systemic therapy. *Clin Cancer Res* 1996;2:933–939.
136. Plotkin D, Lechner JJ, Jung WE, et al. Tamoxifen flare in advanced breast cancer. *JAMA* 1978;240:2644–2646.
137. Legha SS. Tamoxifen in the treatment of breast cancer. *Ann Intern Med* 1988;109:219–228.
138. Vogel CL, Schoenfelder J, Shemano I, et al. Worsening bone scan in the evaluation of antitumor response during hormonal therapy of breast cancer. *J Clin Oncol* 1995;13:1123–1128.
139. Welch M, Bonasera TJ, Sherman E. [F18]fluorodeoxyglucose (FDG) and 16a[F-18]fluoroestradiol-17b (FES) uptake in estrogen-receptor (ER)-rich tissues following tamoxifen treatment: a preclinical study. *J Nucl Med* 1995;36:39.

140. Dehdashti F, Flanagan FL, Mortimer JE, et al. Positron emission tomographic assessment of "metabolic flare" to predict response of metastatic breast cancer to antiestrogen therapy. *Eur J Nucl Med* 1999;26:51–56.
141. Mortimer JE, Dehdashti F, Siegel BA, et al. Metabolic flare: indicator of hormone responsiveness in advanced breast cancer. *J Clin Oncol* 2001;19:2797–2803.
142. Linden HM, Stekhova SA, Link JM, et al. Quantitative fluoroestradiol positron emission tomography imaging predicts response to endocrine treatment in breast cancer. *J Clin Oncol* 2006;24:2793–2799.
143. Dehdashti F, Mortimer JE, Trinkaus K, et al. PET-based estradiol challenge as a predictive biomaker of response to endocrine therapy in women with estrogen-receptor-positive breast cancer. *Breast Cancer Res Treat* 2008 [Epub ahead of print]
144. Sledge GW Jr, McGuire WL. Steroid hormone receptors in human breast cancer. *Adv Cancer Res* 1983;38:61–75.
145. Clark GM. Prognostic and predictive factors. In: Harris JR, Lippman ME, Marrow M, et al., eds. *Diseases of the breast*. Philadelphia: Lippincott Williams & Wilkins, 2000:489–514.
146. Osborne CK, Schiff R, Arpino G, et al. Endocrine responsiveness: understanding how progesterone receptor can be used to select endocrine therapy. *Breast* 2005;14:458–465.
147. Pomper MG, Katzenellenbogen JA, Welch MJ, et al. 21-[18F]fluoro-16 alpha-ethyl-19-norprogesterone: synthesis and target tissue selective uptake of a progestin receptor based radiotracer for positron emission tomography. *J Med Chem* 1988;31:1360–1363.
148. Pomper MG, Pinney KG, Carlson KE, et al. Target tissue uptake selectivity of three fluorine-substituted progestins: potential imaging agents for receptor-positive breast tumors. *Int J Rad Appl Instrum B* 1990;17:309–319.
149. Katzenellenbogen JA, Welch MJ, Dehdashti F. The development of estrogen and progestin radiopharmaceuticals for imaging breast cancer. *Anticancer Res* 1997;17:1573–1576.
150. Verhagen A, Studeny M, Luurtsema G, et al. Metabolism of a [18F]fluorine labeled progestin (21-[18F]fluoro-16 alpha-ethyl-19-norprogesterone) in humans: a clue for future investigations. *Nucl Med Biol* 1994;21:941–952.
151. Dehdashti F, McGuire AH, Van Brocklin HF, et al. Assessment of 21-[18F]fluoro-16 alpha-ethyl-19-norprogesterone as a positron-emitting radiopharmaceutical for the detection of progestin receptors in human breast carcinomas. *J Nucl Med* 1991;32:1532–1537.
152. Yang D, Kuang LR, Cherif A, et al. Synthesis of [18F]fluoroalanine and [18F]fluorotamoxifen for imaging breast tumors. *J Drug Target* 1993;1:259–267.
153. Yang DJ, Li C, Kuang LR, et al. Imaging, biodistribution and therapy potential of halogenated tamoxifen analogues. *Life Sci* 1994;55:53–67.
154. Leskinen-Kallio S, Nagren K, Lehikoinen P, et al. Uptake of ^{11}C-methionine in breast cancer studied by PET. An association with the size of S-phase fraction. *Br J Cancer* 1991;64:1121–1124.
155. Smyczek-Gargya B, Fersis N, Dittmann H, et al. PET with [18F]fluorothymidine for imaging of primary breast cancer: a pilot study. *Eur J Nucl Med Mol Imaging* 2004;31:720–724.
156. Kenny LM, Vigushin DM, Al-Nahhas A, et al. Quantification of cellular proliferation in tumor and normal tissues of patients with breast cancer by [18F]fluorothymidine-positron emission tomography imaging: evaluation of analytical methods. *Cancer Res* 2005;65:10104–10112.
157. Pio BS, Park CK, Pietras R, et al. Usefulness of 3′-[F-18]fluoro-3'-deoxythymidine with positron emission tomography in predicting breast cancer response to therapy. *Mol Imaging Biol* 2006;8:36–42.

CHAPTER

8.13 Esophagus

WOLFGANG A. WEBER AND RICHARD L. WAHL

PRIMARY TUMOR DETECTION
LOCOREGIONAL NODAL DETECTION
SYSTEMIC METASTASES
DETECTION OF RECURRENT DISEASE
ASSESSING RESPONSE TO THERAPY
PET/CT IMAGING
RADIATION TREATMENT PLANNING
MANAGEMENT CHANGES AND COST-EFFECTIVENESS
REIMBURSEMENT
OTHER TRACERS FOR PET IN ESOPHAGEAL CANCER
SUMMARY

Esophageal carcinoma is considered the eighth most common cancer worldwide with nearly 400,000 new cases diagnosed annually. However, incidence rates of esophageal cancer vary greatly from one region to another. Incidence rates are highest in Asia and southern and eastern Africa. In these areas the incidence of esophageal cancer has been reported to be as high as 100 per 100,000 (1). In the United States, esophageal carcinoma is a relatively uncommon cancer, with an estimated incidence rate of 5.4 per 100,000 corresponding to 16,470 new cases in 2006 (12,970 men and 3,500 women) (2). The cancer is extremely lethal and has an estimated death rate of 14,280 patients per year in the United States, with 11,250 men and 3,030 women dying. This high mortality rate is consistent with a very low 5-year survival after diagnosis, which is only about 16% for all stages of the disease. Although the 5-year survival is still poor, it has improved slightly, but significantly ($P<.05$) from 5% in 1975 to 1977 to 16% in 1996 to 2003, presumably due to improved diagnosis and treatment (2).

Most esophageal cancers diagnosed worldwide are of squamous cell histology. However, in the Western world, there has been a substantial increase in the incidence and prevalence of adenocarcinoma of the esophagus, particularly those arising at the esophagogastric junction (3). In the United States, the incidence of adenocarcinoma of the esophagus has increased about fourfold between 1973 to 1982 and 1993 to 2002 (3). Most, if not all, adenocarcinomas of the distal esophagus arise from areas with specialized intestinal metaplasia, which develop as a consequence of chronic gastroesophageal (GE) reflux. In some patients, it can be difficult to determine if tumors at the GE junction arose from the esophagus or the stomach itself. A substantial focus on the prevention of GE reflux disease, including prevention and treatment of Barrett's esophagus, is an ongoing attempt to reduce the increase of adenocarcinoma of the esophagus in the Western world. When gastric carcinomas occur in the fundus, they can be difficult or impossible to distinguish from esophageal adenocarcinomas.

The most common sites of metastatic disease are the locoregional lymph nodes immediately adjoining the esophagus and the upper abdominal lymph nodes. Tumors in the lower esophagus and GE junction may metastasize to mesenteric nodes. Tumors of the upper esophagus commonly metastasize to the cervical nodes, as well as the liver, lungs, and other organs including bone.

Decisions concerning primary therapy of esophageal cancer are based on knowledge of the tumor stage. Staging for esophageal carcinoma is commonly tabulated using the American Joint Committee on Cancers Tumor, Node, Metastasis (TNM) system (Tables 8.13.1 and 8.13.2). Depending on tumor stage, current potentially curative treatment options for esophageal and gastric cancer range from endoscopic mucosal resection to preoperative chemoradiotherapy followed by esophagectomy (4). Most of these therapeutic approaches are associated with substantial morbidity and mortality as well as a long-term compromise in the quality of life. Accurate pretherapeutic staging by imaging techniques is therefore crucial in order to select the appropriate form of therapy. Generally the first step in this process is to distinguish between patients with locoregional and systemic disease. For patients presenting with hematogenous metastases or distant lymph node metastases (M1), no curative treatment is available and local tumor therapy is only applied for palliation of symptoms.

In patients with locoregional disease, assessment of local tumor infiltration (T stage) and regional lymph node involvement (N stage) is necessary in order to decide whether a complete tumor resection (R0) is feasible (5). Local tumor infiltration (T stage) is also frequently used as a criterion to use multimodality therapy instead of primary surgery. Although patients with T1 and T2 tumors are generally treated by primary resection and lymph node dissection, patients with T3 and T4 tumors are frequently offered preoperative chemo- or chemoradiotherapy in order to improve the rate of curative resections and potentially overall survival (6). When the primary tumor is limited to the mucosa or submucosa (T1), limited surgical resections may provide the same chance for cure as standard surgical procedures. As the frequency of lymph node metastases is very low in tumors limited to the mucosa, patients with these early cancers may even be cured by endoscopic mucosal resection (7).

Survival is dependent on stage and is much better for localized than locoregional or disseminated esophageal cancers. For patients with stage I esophageal cancer 5-year survival rates of 80% have been reported after surgical resection (8,9). Various methods have been used to stage esophageal cancer, including endoscopic ultrasound (EUS), computed tomography (CT), and more recently positron emission tomography (PET) imaging, particularly using fluorine-18 (^{18}F) fluorodeoxyglucose (FDG).

TABLE 8.13.1 Tumor, Node, Metastasis Staging System for Esophageal Cancer

PRIMARY TUMOR (T)	
Tis	Carcinoma *in situ*
T1	Tumor invades lamina propria or submucosa
T2	Tumor invades muscularis propria
T3	Tumor invades adventitia
T4	Tumor invades adjacent structures
REGIONAL LYMPH NODES (N)	
N0	No regional lymph node metastasis
N1	Regional lymph node metastasis
DISTANT METASTASIS (M)	
M0	No distant metastasis
M1	Distant metastasis (including metastasis in nonregional lymph nodes)[a]
	Tumors of the lower thoracic esophagus
M1a	Metastasis in celiac lymph nodes
M1b	Other distant metastasis
	Tumors of the midthoracic esophagus
M1a	Not applicable
M1b	Nonregional lymph nodes or other distant metastasis
	Tumors of the upper thoracic esophagus
M1a	Metastasis in cervical lymph nodes
M1b	Other distant metastasis

[a]regional lymph nodes: Cervical esophageal tumor: scalene, internal jugular, upper cervical, periesophageal, supraclavicular, cervical not otherwise specified. Intrathoracic esophageal tumor: tracheobronchial, superior mediastinal, peritracheal, carinal, hilar, periesophageal, perigastric, paracardial, mediastinal not otherwise specified.

(From American Joint Committee on Cancer: *AJCC cancer staging manual*, 6th ed. New York, NY: Springer, 2002, with permission.)

Imaging techniques are also used to evaluate tumor response to chemo- and chemoradiotherapy. Tumor response to preoperative therapy is a very strong prognostic factor in esophageal cancer (8). Multiple studies have demonstrated that patients with a substantial reduction in the number of viable tumor cells are characterized by a relatively favorable prognosis (5-year survival greater than 50%), even if they presented with locally advanced disease at diagnosis (8,10). Noninvasive assessment of tumor response thus provides important prognostic information and can be used to guide further patient management.

TABLE 8.13.2 American Joint Committee on Cancer Stage Groupings

Stage	T	N	M
0	Tis	N0	M0
I	T1	N0	M0
IIA	T2	N0	M0
	T3	N0	M0
IIB	T1	N1	M0
	T2	N1	M0
III	T3	N1	M0
	T4	Any N	M0
IV	Any T	Any N	M1
IVA	Any T	Any N	M1a
IVB	Any T	Any N	M1b

(From American Joint Committee on Cancer: *AJCC cancer staging manual*, 6th ed. New York, NY: Springer, 2002, with permission.)

PRIMARY TUMOR DETECTION

Nearly all localized primary esophageal carcinomas are detected first by clinical symptoms of dysphagia or in the context of endoscopy performed as part of an evaluation of the upper gastrointestinal (GI) tract for GE reflux—or in sequential management of patients with Barrett's esophagus. PET has not been used as a primary screening method for esophageal carcinoma. The precursor lesion to many cases of adenocarcinoma of the esophagus is Barrett's esophagus. It usually has a low total volume that would not be expected to be detected using whole-body PET imaging devices, although on rare occasions it can be (11). Similarly, some inflammations of the distal esophagus can have mildly increased FDG uptake (11). Several studies have shown that the vast majority of primary esophageal cancers that are first diagnosed by other methods are detectable by [^{18}F]-FDG PET, with sensitivities in the 90% to 100% range for T2 to T4 tumors (12–16). When PET results have been reported to be falsely negative in esophageal cancers, this was usually due to small tumor volume, such as in stage T1 primary lesions. Furthermore, some adenocarcinomas of the gastric cardia demonstrate only low FDG uptake and can be falsely negative on FDG PET even at advanced tumor stages. This is likely related to their growth pattern and mucin production (17).

Diagnostic challenges in esophageal cancer include determining whether there is abnormal or physiologic uptake at the GE junction. There may be some uptake in this location normally, so detecting small esophageal cancers can be problematic as they can be lost in the normal spectrum of mild FDG uptake in the distal esophagus. For these reasons, it is probable that early low-volume esophageal cancer can be much more easily detected by direct visualization using an endoscope or by careful barium studies than by PET.

LOCOREGIONAL NODAL DETECTION

The detection of nodal metastases with PET is dependent on the volume of tumor in the metastasis, the intensity of tracer uptake in the lesion, the background tracer activity (as well as the injected dose of radiotracer and the performance and resolution of the scanner), and the interpretation criteria. CT detects nodal metastases based on their size, and what constitutes a "positive or negative" node by CT differs with different observers. The larger the node, the more likely it is to represent a node involved by cancer, although the optimal cutoff size for "positive or negative" nodes is not clear in esophageal cancer.

Both PET and CT can fail to detect small metastases of esophageal cancer to locoregional lymph nodes. Lesions smaller than 5 mm are not usually detected on PET with FDG, which is consistent with other detection challenges encountered with current FDG PET technology. To achieve high sensitivity with CT, small lymph nodes must be called positive. For example, 5-mm and larger nodes may be called abnormal in some CT studies, whereas others may choose a 10-mm cutoff. The smaller the cutoff for node size, the more likely cancer will be detected, but at the price of a lower specificity. This results in a considerable range in the sensitivity and specificity of PET for assessing tumor involvement in regional lymph nodes and an even greater range in accuracy of CT (Table 8.13.3).

In general PET is not exceptionally sensitive, but it has a high specificity for the detection of locoregional lymph node metastases (typical sensitivities of 30% to 80%, but with specificities of 80% to 90%). A meta-analysis published in 2004 evaluating data from 421 patients reported a pooled sensitivity and specificity of FDG PET of 51% and 84%, respectively. Table 8.13.3 provides an overview of the largest studies used in the meta-analysis as well as of more recently published studies (18). By contrast, reported CT sensitivity/specificity pairs range from (31% to 86% to 87% to 14%), meaning CT can be either very insensitive or reasonably specific (although not as specific as PET) or very sensitive and extremely nonspecific. When directly compared, in several studies PET was an equivalent or more accurate method for nodal staging than CT (Table 8.13.3).

EUS has been reported to be more sensitive (70% to 80%) than either PET or CT for staging regional nodes and it is reasonably specific (70% to 80%) (15,19,20). EUS is also valuable for assessing tumor size and depth of invasion. According to a systematic review including a total of 2,508 patients, the diagnostic accuracy of EUS for differentiation of stages T1 and T2 from stages T3 and T4 was 91% (21). There are no data showing that PET or CT is accurate in evaluating the primary tumor stage of esophageal cancers. Neither can resolve the individual layers of the esophageal wall that form the basis of the T-staging system. A disadvantage of EUS is its operator dependency. Furthermore, EUS may be technically impossible if the tumor causes a stenosis that cannot be passed by the endoscope (21). There is some interest in using minimally invasive surgical techniques for staging esophageal cancer. Specifically, sentinel node dissection is currently being evaluated as a minimally invasive technique to improve lymph node staging (22).

SYSTEMIC METASTASES

In almost all studies to date, PET has been more accurate than other conventional diagnostic methods in detecting organ metastases or nonregional lymph node metastases (Table 8.13.4). Nonregional lymph node metastases are considered as M1 disease in esophageal cancer (Table 18.3.1). A recent meta-analysis reported a pooled sensitivity of FDG PET for detection of M1 disease of 67% at a speci-

TABLE 8.13.3 Diagnostic Accuracy of Fluorodeoxyglucose- PET and CT for Detection of Locoregional Lymph Node Metastases (N stage)

					FDG PET		CT	
Authors (ref.)	Year	No. of Patients	Histology (adeno/squamous/other)	Prevalence (%)	Sensitivity (%)	Specificity (%)	Sensitivity (%)	Specificity (%)
Block et al. (13)	1997	58	34/22/2	51	58	87	71	79
Choi et al. (49)	2000	48	0/48/0	58	81	88	41	100
Flamen et al. (15)	2000	74	53/21/0	55	28	90	55	82
Meltzer et al.(16)	2000	47	37/10/0	74	41	83	87	14
Yoon et al. (50)	2003	81	0/81/0	48	64	69	31	86
Kneist et al. (51)	2003	58	31/27/0	44–59[a]	6–42[a]	94–100[a]	67–73[a]	73–80[a]
Heeren et al. (52)	2004	71	62/12/0	66	55	71	44	90
Kato et al. (53)	2005	149[a,b]	7/134/8	52	55	90	48	79
Yuan et al. (35)	2006	45[c,d]	0/45/0	21	82 94[c]	87 92[c]	ND	ND

FDG, fluorodeoxyglucose; ND, not determined.

[a]Thoracic, cervical, thoracic, celiac, and abdominal lymph nodes were analyzed separately.

[b]Lymph node status evaluable in 81 patients.

[c]Analysis based on lymph node regions, not patients.

[d]FDG PET/CT.

TABLE 8.13.4 Diagnostic Accuracy of Fluorodeoxyglucose PET for Detection of Distant Metastases (M stage)

					FDG PET		CT	
Authors (ref.)	Year	No. of Patients	Histology (adeno/ squamous/ other)	Prevalence (%)	Sensitivity (%)	Specificity (%)	Sensitivity (%)	Specificity (%)
Block et al. (13)	1997	58	34/22/2	36	65	97	20	ND
Flamen et al. (15)	2000	74	53/21/0	46	74	90	41	83
Meltzer et al. (16)	2000	47	37/10/0	22	70	92	57	66
Rasanen et al. (54)	2003	42	0/42/0	36	47	89	33	96
Kneist et al. (55)	2004	81[a]	40/41/0	74	38	89	63	11
Heeren et al. (52)	2004	74	62/12/0	36	78	98	37	87
Bar-Shalom et al. (34)	2005	32[b]	25/7/0	68	100	54	ND	ND
					100[c]	69[c]		

FDG, fluorodeoxyglucose; ND, not determined.
[a]Analysis based on histopathologic analysis of 31 lesions in 28 patients.
[b]Analysis based on 41 studies in 32 patients.
[c]FDG PET/CT.

ficity of 97% (18). In studies comparing PET and CT the sensitivity and specificity of CT have been consistently lower than of PET (Table 8.13.4). An example of metastatic esophageal cancer is shown in Fig. 8.13.1.

Although PET is the most effective single imaging method for detecting distant metastases from esophageal carcinoma, other imaging modalities are superior to PET in specific body regions. For example, very small (a few millimeters) lung metastases are detected better by CT than by PET (23,24). It is also probable that brain metastases are less well seen with FDG PET than with CT or MRI, as is the case in lung cancer imaging (25).

The relative performance of PET versus bone scans in the detection of bone metastases is only reported to a limited extent. In one study FDG PET was shown to be more sensitive than bone scans for detection of bony metastases (26). The higher sensitivity was due to correct visualization of lytic metastases that were false negative on bone scans. Based on the available data, PET is recommended as an initial staging procedure for esophageal cancer.

DETECTION OF RECURRENT DISEASE

Detection of recurrent esophageal cancer has been evaluated by Flamen et al. (27) who evaluated 33 patients with 40 recurrent sites. PET was not as reliable in characterizing anastomotic recurrences as conventional diagnostic methods (CDMs), which included EUS and EUS-directed biopsy. PET tended to have false-positive results in patients with benign strictures after dilation, although PET was very sensitive (sensitivity, specificity, and accuracy of 100%, 57%, and 74% for PET, respectively, vs. 100%, 93%, and 96%, respectively, for CDMs). PET was very reliable for detecting systemic metastases, with sensitivity, specificity, and accuracy for PET being 94%, 82%, and 87%, respectively, compared with 81%, 82%, and 81%, respectively, for CDMs (P = not significant). Although the accuracy rates in these patients were comparable, PET provided additional information in about 27% of patients (27). The high sensitivity of PET for detection of recurrent esophageal cancer was confirmed in a recent study by Kato et al. (23). In this study the sensitivity, specificity, and accuracy of FDG PET for detection of recurrent esophageal cancer were 96%, 68%, and 82%, respectively. PET had a higher sensitivity for detection of bony metastases than CT, but it was less sensitive for detection of pulmonary metastases. Thus PET appears to add incremental value to CDMs for detection of recurrent esophageal cancer but in this setting is not clearly proven superior to CDMs. Based on available data, it seems the combination of CDMs and PET would be the most rational approach to detect recurrent disease. In practice, the combination of PET using FDG and a diagnostic quality CT scan (as part of PET/CT) can serve as a highly accurate method of following esophageal carcinoma after therapy.

ASSESSING RESPONSE TO THERAPY

Preoperative chemotherapy and chemoradiotherapy for locally advanced esophageal cancer have been investigated since the late 1970s. However, their role in patient management still remains controversial. Randomized trials comparing preoperative chemo- or chemoradiotherapy followed by surgical resection to surgical treatment alone have yielded conflicting results (28). Nevertheless, it has been a very consistent observation that histopathologic response to chemotherapy is one of the most important factors determining patient prognosis. Median survival of patients with histopathologically responding and nonresponding cancers has been shown to differ by a factor of 3 to 4 (8,10). However, this beneficial effect appears to be outweighed by the poor prognosis of patients with nonresponding tumors. Many investigators have emphasized the need for a noninvasive diagnostic test that allows the assessment, or even the prediction, of the histopathologic response to preoperative therapy. Since chemoradiotherapy results in complete tumor regression in up to 40% of the treated patients (28), it has been suggested that it might be feasible to eliminate the need for surgery if it were possible to determine with imaging that there was no residual tumor present—or at least predict this with high certainty.

Based on encouraging data in other tumor types, such as breast cancer (29), the use of FDG PET to monitor tumor response in esophageal cancer has been addressed in several studies. Table 8.13.5

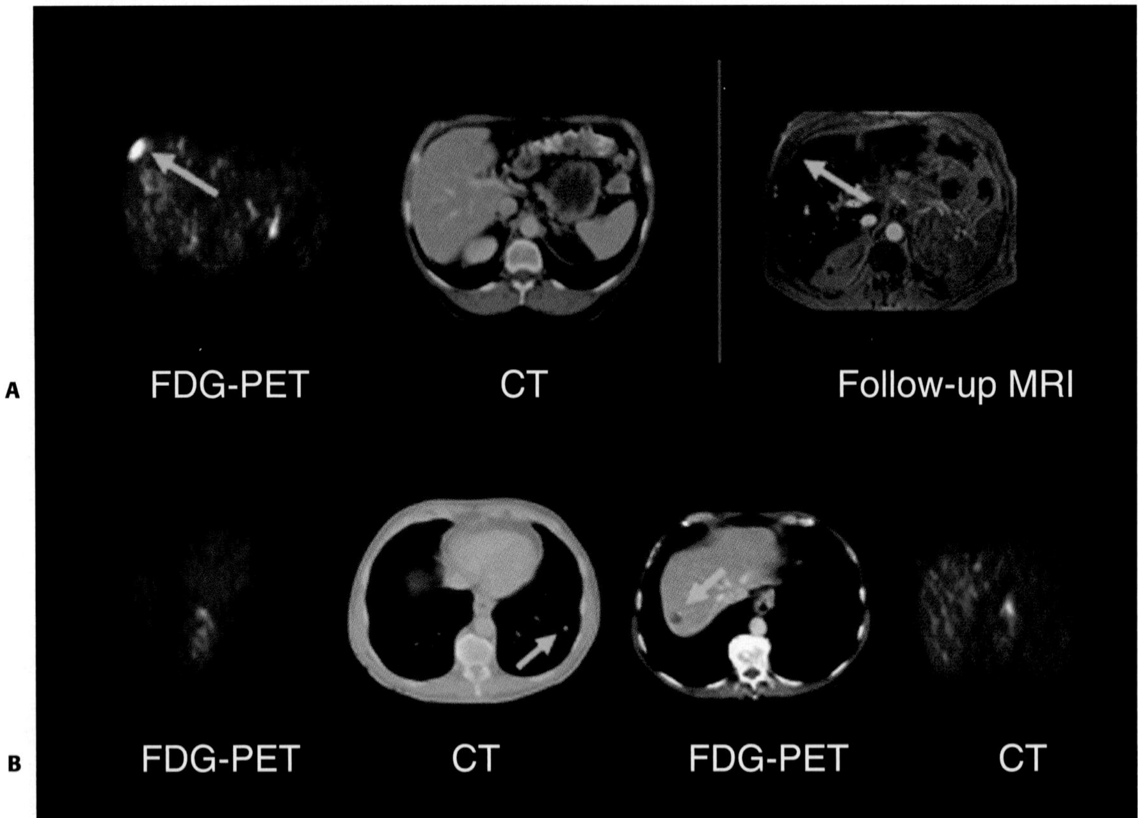

FIGURE 8.13.1. Staging of esophageal cancer by fluorodeoxyglucose (FDG) PET and CT. **A:** Bony metastasis of esophageal cancer. A right-sided rib lesion demonstrates intense FDG uptake without a corresponding abnormality on CT. Four months later a magnetic resonance image confirmed the presence of a metastatic lesion. **B:** A patient with esophageal cancer and a right-sided pulmonary nodule as well as a hypodense liver lesion. Both are suspicious for metastatic disease on CT, but are negative on FDG PET. Further diagnostic work-up and clinical follow-up revealed a granuloma and a liver hemangioma.

gives an overview of studies using FDG PET to assess tumor response after completion of preoperative chemoradiotherapy. In all of these studies, FDG PET was a sensitive test to detect tumor response (i.e., the absence or marked reduction of the number of viable tumor cells). The specificity for assessment of tumor response was relatively low and quite variable (26% to 88%). The variability of the reported specificities is likely related to the fact that different studies used different definitions for a histopathologic response as shown in Table 8.13.5. Although some studies defined histopathologic response by complete absence of viable tumor cells, other used "less than 10% viable tumor" cells or "microscopic residual disease" as criteria. Different criteria were also applied for the evaluation of the FDG PET scans (Table 8.13.5). The lower than perfect accuracy for assessment of tumor response reflects the inability of FDG PET to detect small amounts of residual tumor tissue. Almost all tumors with 10% or less viable tumor cells and a significant fraction of tumors with 10% to 50% viable cells are negative on FDG PET (30). Thus, a negative PET scan after completion of therapy does not rule out residual tumor tissue, and surgery cannot be avoided in these patients. On the other hand, a positive PET scan after chemoradiotherapy appears to be a relatively specific marker for macroscopic residual tumor tissue and is associated with a poor prognosis (Table 8.13.5).

Ideally, PET should be performed before and then again soon after treatment is started in an effort to determine longer-term response, as this would allow treatment adjustments. Several studies have now suggested that changes in tumor FDG uptake during preoperative chemo- or chemoradiotherapy predict histopathologic response and patient survival (Table 8.13.6). In the first of these studies, PET scans before and at 14 days after the start of a platinum-based chemotherapy regime for treatment of esophageal carcinoma were performed in 40 patients. Response was assessed after 3 months of therapy by EUS and histology (31). Responding tumors had a decrease in tracer uptake of 54% ± 17%, whereas nonresponding tumors showed only a minimal decline in tracer uptake of 15% ± 21%. A cutoff value of a 35% decline was about 95% effective in identifying tumors that did not respond histopathologically to preoperative therapy. The patients with a larger decline in FDG uptake also had significantly longer times to tumor progression and/or recurrence than those patients with only minimal drops in tracer uptake with treatment.

In a follow-up study the 35% threshold value for differentiation of responding and nonresponding tumors was prospectively validated in an independent group of 65 patients (32). In this study histopathologic response was predicted by FDG PET 14 days after the start of chemotherapy with a sensitivity and specificity of 82%

TABLE 8.13.5 Assessment of Tumor Response and Patient Survival after Completion of Therapy

			Response Assessment				Patient Survival (mo)		
Authors (ref.)	Year	No. of Patients	PET Criterion	Gold Standard	Sensitivity (%)	Specificity (%)	PET Responder	PET Nonresponder	*P* Value
Brucher et al. (56)	2001	27	ΔSUV >52%	<10% viable tumor cells	100	55	22	7	.001
Flamen et al. (57)	2002	36	Visual	Down-staging	82	71	16	6	.005
Downey et al. (58)	2003	17	ΔSUV >60%	ND	ND	ND	>50	30	.08
Swisher et al. (59)	2004	84	SUV <4	0% viable tumor cells	95	26	>24	15	.01
Wieder et al. (60)	2004	38	ΔSUV > 52%	<10% viable tumor cells	89	57	ND	ND	ND
Cerfolio et al. (61)	2005	48	Visual	0% viable tumor cells	87	88	ND	ND	ND
Duong et al. (62)	2006	53	Visual	ND	ND	ND	>30	9	<.001
Levine et al. (63)	2006	31	ΔSUV >40%	Microscopic residual disease	92	52	ND	ND	ND

ND, not determined; SUV, standard uptake value.

TABLE 8.13.6 Prediction of Tumor Response Early in the Course of Therapy

			Response Prediction				Patient Survival (mo)		
Authors (ref.)	Year	No. of Patients	PET Criterion	Gold Standard	Sensitivity (%)	Specificity (%)	PET Responder	PET Nonresponder	*P* value
Weber et al. (31)[a]	2001	40	ΔSUV >35%	<10% viable tumor cells	89	75	>50	19	.04
Wieder et al. (60)[b]	2004	38	ΔSUV >30%	<10% viable tumor cells	93	88	>30	18	.01
Ótt et al. (32)[a]	2006	65	ΔSUV >35%	<10% viable tumor cells	82	78	>50	18	.01
Westerterp et al. (64)[c]	2005	26	ΔSUV >31%	<10% viable tumor cells	75	75	ND	ND	ND

SUV, standard uptake value; ND, not determined.
[a]Preoperative chemotherapy.
[b]Preoperative chemoradiotherapy
[c]Preoperative chemoradiotherapy plus hyperthermia.

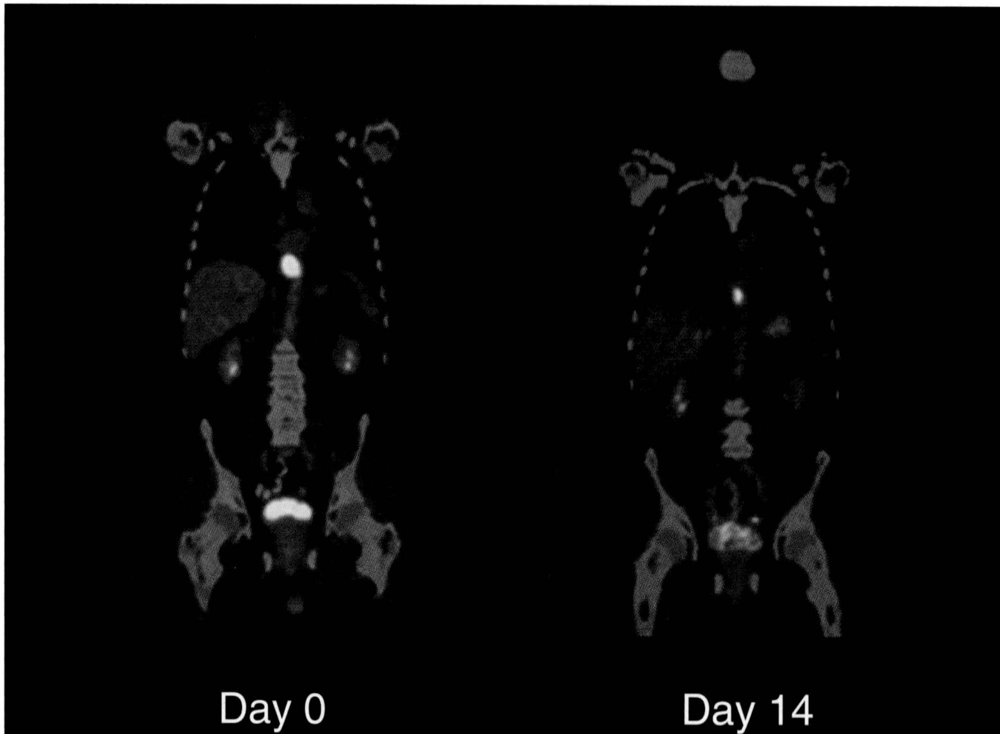

FIGURE 8.13.2. Early assessment of tumor response by fluorodeoxyglucose (FDG) PET/CT in a patient with locally advanced distal esophageal cancer. The tumor demonstrates intense FDG uptake prior to therapy (day 0). The FDG uptake decreases markedly on day 14 of the first chemotherapy cycle. Quantitatively tumor FDG uptake decreased from a standard uptake value of 9.2 to 4.2.

and 78%, respectively. A metabolic response in FDG PET (decrease of tumor FDG uptake by more than 35%) was also predictive for patient survival. Median overall survival of metabolic responders was more than 50 months, while it was only 18 months for metabolic nonresponders.

Based on these data it seems feasible to use early metabolic changes to individualize preoperative chemotherapy of esophageal cancer. The Metabolic response evalUatioN for individulization of neoadjuvant Chemotherapy in esOphageal and esophgogastric adeNocarcinoma (MUNICON) trial (33) has evaluated such a concept in 111 patients with locally advanced adenocarcinomas of the distal esophagus or cardia. FDG PET was performed prior to therapy and after a 2-week course of cisplatin-based chemotherapy. If tumor FDG uptake had decreased by more than 35% at the time of the second PET scan, patients received the full 3-month course of chemotherapy. Otherwise, the patients underwent immediate tumor resection. This study prospectively confirmed that FDG PET allows selection of patients with a high probability of a histopathological response (33). An example of a responding tumor is shown in Fig. 8.13.2.

PET/CT IMAGING

Only few studies on imaging of esophageal cancer with PET/CT have been published so far (34–36). Bar-Shalom et al. (34) compared the staging accuracy of PET and PET/CT in 32 patients with esophageal cancer. PET/CT provided better specificity and accuracy than PET for detecting sites of esophageal cancer (81% and 90% vs. 59% and 83%, respectively; $P < .01$). PET/CT image fusion was of special value for interpretation of cervical and abdominopelvic sites, for disease assessment in locoregional lymph nodes before surgery, and in regions of postoperative anatomical distortion.

Yuan et al. (35) studied 45 patients with esophageal squamous cell carcinoma prior to surgical resection. They compared the accuracy of PET/CT for detection of locoregional lymph node metastases with side-by-side review of PET and CT images. They found that PET/CT provided a remarkably high sensitivity and specificity (94% and 92%, respectively) for detection of lymph node metastases. This represented a significant improvement when compared to side-by-side review of PET and CT studies (sensitivity 82% and 87%, respectively).

RADIATION TREATMENT PLANNING

A number of studies have suggested that FDG PET may have a significant impact on radiation treatment planning in patients with esophageal cancer (37–41). PET/CT imaging has greatly facilitated integration of FDG PET in radiation treatment planning because misregistration of PET and CT scans, due to differences in patient positioning, are minimized. FDG PET can change radiation treatment fields by detection of lymph node metastases and better delineation of the longitudinal extent of the primary tumor, particularly in the region of the esophagogastric junction (39). In one study FDG-avid disease was found outside of the gross target volume defined by CT in 11 of 18 patients (69%). In five patients this would have resulted in excluding metabolically active tissue from the radiation treatment fields.

Although these data are encouraging, standardized algorithms for definition of tumor extension on FDG PET are lacking, and there are no detailed studies comparing tumor extension on FDG PET with histology. It is not clear how well FDG PET delineates the infiltrative growth of esophageal cancer. Further studies with histologic correlation are also necessary in order to determine the ability of FDG PET to differentiate between tumor infiltration and physiologic FDG uptake at the gastroesophageal junction or inflammatory changes surrounding the tumor. There have been no direct randomized comparative studies comparing radiation therapy planning with and without PET imaging in the plans.

MANAGEMENT CHANGES AND COST-EFFECTIVENESS

A comprehensive review of the PET literature in esophageal cancer, including abstracts, suggested that PET changed management in 14% to 20% of patients (42). This often involved finding disseminated metastatic disease not detected by other methods but can also include clarifying that a "positive" abnormality on CT is in fact not "positive" on FDG PET and thus not likely to represent a metastasis. A recent study of 68 patients found that FDG PET changed management in one third of the patients. Tumor stage as assessed by FDG PET was highly significantly correlated with patient survival, whereas tumor stage based on CT was not (43).

The cost-effectiveness of FDG PET was studied by decision-tree analysis (44) in 2002. Six staging strategies based on CT, EUS, and FDG PET as well as combinations of these modalities were investigated. Combined use of FDG PET and EUS was found to be the most effective strategy for staging of esophageal cancer. The cost-effectiveness ratio of this strategy was $60,544 per quality-adjusted life-year. However, the assumed costs of FDG PET in this analysis were high ($2,391 per scan) and the cost-effectiveness ratio of the PET-based staging strategy will improve with decreasing PET costs. Since average reimbursement for PET from Medicare is now much lower, the dollars/quality-adjusted life-year now falls at less than $50,000, a figure generally considered to be societally acceptable in the United States.

REIMBURSEMENT

FDG PET is currently approved by Medicare in the United States for diagnosis, staging, and restaging of esophageal cancer (45). Treatment monitoring with FDG PET is covered if the patient's referring physician and the provider submit data to a clinical registry (National Oncologic PET Registry) to assess the impact of PET on cancer patient management. Many insurers now cover PET in the assessment of treatment response as well.

OTHER TRACERS FOR PET IN ESOPHAGEAL CANCER

PET has been used most extensively with FDG as a tracer in patients with esophageal cancer and the results have been very good. Only modest work has been performed with other PET tracers. Carbon-11 (^{11}C)-choline and FDG PET were compared for accuracy in 33 patients with biopsy-proven esophageal carcinoma (46). [^{11}C]-choline PET was more effective than FDG PET and CT in detecting very small metastases localized in the mediastinum. It was ineffective, however, in detecting metastases localized in the upper abdomen because of the normal uptake of [^{11}C]-choline in the liver. These data were based on a small number of patients, but the authors believed PET with both tracers might be the most accurate approach for diagnosing esophageal carcinoma (46). A follow-up study evaluated 18 patients with esophageal carcinoma with both tracers. On a lesion basis, FDG PET detected 10 of 12 nonregional metastases (83% sensitivity), whereas [^{11}C]-choline PET detected 5 of 12 (42% sensitivity). Standard uptake values (SUV) were significantly higher for FDG (6.6 ± 3.5 vs. 5.5 ± 2.5 for [^{11}C]-choline; P = .04). The authors concluded [^{11}C]-choline PET was able to visualize esophageal carcinoma and its metastases but appeared to be inferior to FDG PET (47).

Esophageal cancer has also been studied with fluorine-18 (^{18}F)-fluorothymidine (FLT). In a pilot study including 10 patients with biopsy-proven cancer of the esophagus or esophagogastric junction tumors FDG uptake was significantly higher than FLT uptake (SUV 6.0 vs. 3.4). Two primary tumors and one metastatic lymph node were false negative on FLT PET. In contrast to other tumor types, there was no correlation between the degree of FLT uptake and tumor cell proliferation as assessed by Ki-67 labeling (47). This may be related to the fact that the studied tumors demonstrated only a relatively narrow range of Ki-67 labeling (57% to 85%). These preliminary data suggest only a limited role of FLT PET for detection and staging of esophageal cancer. Animal studies have indicated that FLT PET may be a useful technique to monitor response of esophageal cancer to radiotherapy (48). However, no clinical trials evaluating treatment monitoring with FLT PET in esophageal cancer have been published so far. Treatment monitoring does require disease detection first, so if FLT does result in frequent false-negative studies prior to treatment, its role in treatment monitoring may be restricted to those tumors that are strongly FLT avid—and then only if it provides superior predictive ability to FDG.

SUMMARY

PET with FDG is an accurate method for noninvasive detection of primary esophageal cancer, but endoscopy and EUS are more reliable methods for characterizing the size and local invasiveness of the untreated primary tumor. FDG PET is generally more specific than CT and is somewhat superior to CT in accuracy, but it can fail to detect small nodal metastases in many instances, especially those near the esophagus. EUS in skilled hands may be superior to PET for assessing locoregional periesophageal metastases to lymph nodes. FDG PET is superior to other imaging methods for detecting systemic metastatic disease. Data to date on assessment of response to treatment suggest PET provides an early and quite accurate readout of the efficacy of therapy. PET is incapable of detecting residual microscopic disease at the conclusion of treatment due to resolution limitations. Where directly compared, PET/CT has proven to be somewhat more accurate than PET alone. Tracers other than FDG, although of interest, have not demonstrated superiority to FDG in imaging this tumor.

REFERENCES

1. Parkin DM. International variation. *Oncogene* 2004;23(38):6329–6340.
2. Jemal A, Siegel R, Ward E, et al. Cancer statistics, 2006. *CA Cancer J Clin* 2006;56(2):106–130.
3. Holmes RS, Vaughan TL. Epidemiology and pathogenesis of esophageal cancer. *Semin Radiat Oncol* 2007;17(1):2–9.
4. Lerut T, Coosemans W, Decker G, et al. Cancer of the esophagus and gastro-esophageal junction: potentially curative therapies. *Surg Oncol* 2001;10(3):113–122.

5. Stein HJ, Brucher BL, Sendler A, et al. Esophageal cancer: patient evaluation and pre-treatment staging. *Surg Oncol* 2001;10(3):103–111.
6. Urschel JD, Vasan H. A meta-analysis of randomized controlled trials that compared neoadjuvant chemoradiation and surgery to surgery alone for resectable esophageal cancer. *Am J Surg* 2003;185(6):538–543.
7. Soetikno R, Kaltenbach T, Yeh R, et al. Endoscopic mucosal resection for early cancers of the upper gastrointestinal tract. *J Clin Oncol* 2005;23(20):4490–4498.
8. Swisher SG, Hofstetter W, Wu TT, et al. Proposed revision of the esophageal cancer staging system to accommodate pathologic response (pP) following preoperative chemoradiation (CRT). *Ann Surg* 2005;241(5):810–817; discussion 817–820.
9. Stein HJ, Feith M, Bruecher BL, et al. Early esophageal cancer: pattern of lymphatic spread and prognostic factors for long-term survival after surgical resection. *Ann Surg* 2005;242(4):566–573; discussion 573–575.
10. Berger AC, Farma J, Scott WJ, et al. Complete response to neoadjuvant chemoradiotherapy in esophageal carcinoma is associated with significantly improved survival. *J Clin Oncol* 2005;23(19):4330–4337.
11. Bakheet SM, Amin T, Alia AG, et al. F-18 FDG uptake in benign esophageal disease. *Clin Nucl Med* 1999;24(12):995–997.
12. Fukunaga T, Enomoto K, Okazumi S, et al. [Analysis of glucose metabolism in patients with esophageal cancer by PET: estimation of hexokinase activity in the tumor and usefulness for clinical assessment using ^{18}F-fluorodeoxyglucose]. *Nippon Geka Gakkai Zasshi* 1994;95(5): 317–325.
13. Block MI, Patterson GA, Sundaresan RS, et al. Improvement in staging of esophageal cancer with the addition of positron emission tomography. *Ann Thorac Surg* 1997;64(3):770–776; discussion 776–777.
14. Kole AC, Plukker JT, Nieweg OE, et al. Positron emission tomography for staging of oesophageal and gastroesophageal malignancy. *Br J Cancer* 1998;78(4):521–527.
15. Flamen P, Lerut A, Van Cutsem E, et al. Utility of positron emission tomography for the staging of patients with potentially operable esophageal carcinoma. *J Clin Oncol* 2000;18(18):3202–3210.
16. Meltzer CC, Luketich JD, Friedman D, et al. Whole-body FDG positron emission tomographic imaging for staging esophageal cancer comparison with computed tomography. *Clin Nucl Med* 2000;25(11):882–887.
17. Ott K, Weber WA, Fink U, et al. Fluorodeoxyglucose-positron emission tomography in adenocarcinomas of the distal esophagus and cardia. *World J Surg* 2003;27(9):1035–1039.
18. van Westreenen HL, Westerterp M, Bossuyt PM, et al. Systematic review of the staging performance of ^{18}F-fluorodeoxyglucose positron emission tomography in esophageal cancer. *J Clin Oncol* 2004;22(18): 3805–3812.
19. Kienle P, Buhl K, Kuntz C, et al. Prospective comparison of endoscopy, endosonography and computed tomography for staging of tumours of the oesophagus and gastric cardia. *Digestion* 2002;66(4):230–236.
20. Wu LF, Wang BZ, Feng JL, et al. Preoperative TN staging of esophageal cancer: comparison of miniprobe ultrasonography, spiral CT and MRI. *World J Gastroenterol* 2003;9(2):219–224.
21. Kelly S, Harris KM, Berry E, et al. A systematic review of the staging performance of endoscopic ultrasound in gastro-oesophageal carcinoma. *Gut* 2001;49(4):534–539.
22. Udagawa H. Sentinel node concept in esophageal surgery: an elegant strategy. *Ann Thorac Cardiovasc Surg* 2005;11(1):1–3.
23. Kato H, Miyazaki T, Nakajima M, et al. Value of positron emission tomography in the diagnosis of recurrent oesophageal carcinoma. *Br J Surg* 2004;91(8):1004–1009.
24. Stahl A, Stollfuss J, Ott K, et al. FDG PET and CT in locally advanced adenocarcinomas of the distal oesophagus. Clinical relevance of a discordant PET finding. *Nuklearmedizin* 2005;44(6):249–255; quiz N55–56.
25. Posther KE, McCall LM, Harpole DH Jr, et al. Yield of brain ^{18}F-FDG PET in evaluating patients with potentially operable non–small cell lung cancer. *J Nucl Med* 2006;47(10):1607–1611.
26. Kato H, Miyazaki T, Nakajima M, et al. Comparison between whole-body positron emission tomography and bone scintigraphy in evaluating bony metastases of esophageal carcinomas. *Anticancer Res* 2005;25(6C):4439–4444.
27. Flamen P, Lerut A, Van Cutsem E, et al. The utility of positron emission tomography for the diagnosis and staging of recurrent esophageal cancer. *J Thorac Cardiovasc Surg* 2000;120(6):1085–1092.
28. Schneider BJ, Urba SG. Preoperative chemoradiation for the treatment of locoregional esophageal cancer: the standard of care? *Semin Radiat Oncol* 2007;17(1):45–52.
29. Wahl RL, Zasadny K, Helvie M, et al. Metabolic monitoring of breast cancer chemohormonotherapy using positron emission tomography: initial evaluation. *J Clin Oncol* 1993;11(11):2101–2111.
30. Swisher SG, Erasmus J, Maish M, et al. 2-Fluoro-2-deoxy-D-glucose positron emission tomography imaging is predictive of pathologic response and survival after preoperative chemoradiation in patients with esophageal carcinoma. *Cancer* 2004;101(8):1776–1785.
31. Weber WA, Ott K, Becker K, et al. Prediction of response to preoperative chemotherapy in adenocarcinomas of the esophagogastric junction by metabolic imaging. *J Clin Oncol* 2001;19(12):3058–3065.
32. Ott K, Weber WA, Lordick F, et al. Metabolic imaging predicts response, survival, and recurrence in adenocarcinomas of the esophagogastric junction. *J Clin Oncol* 2006;24(29):4692–4698.
33. Lordick F, Ott K, Krause B. PET to assess early metabolic response and to guide treatment of adenocarcinoma of the oesophagogastric junction: the MUNICON phase II trial. *Lancet Oncol* 2007;8:797–805.
34. Bar-Shalom R, Guralnik L, Tsalic M, et al. The additional value of PET/CT over PET in FDG imaging of oesophageal cancer. *Eur J Nucl Med Mol Imaging* 2005;32(8):918–924.
35. Yuan S, Yu Y, Chao KS, et al. Additional value of PET/CT over PET in assessment of locoregional lymph nodes in thoracic esophageal squamous cell cancer. *J Nucl Med* 2006;47(8):1255–1259.
36. Jadvar H, Henderson RW, Conti PS. 2-deoxy-2-[F-18]fluoro-D-glucose-positron emission tomography/computed tomography imaging evaluation of esophageal cancer. *Mol Imaging Biol* 2006;8(3): 193–200.
37. Moureau-Zabotto L, Touboul E, Lerouge D, et al. Impact of CT and ^{18}F-deoxyglucose positron emission tomography image fusion for conformal radiotherapy in esophageal carcinoma. *Int J Radiat Oncol Biol Phys* 2005;63(2):340–345.
38. Konski A, Doss M, Milestone B, et al. The integration of 18-fluoro-deoxy-glucose positron emission tomography and endoscopic ultrasound in the treatment-planning process for esophageal carcinoma. *Int J Radiat Oncol Biol Phys* 2005;61(4):1123–1128.
39. Leong T, Everitt C, Yuen K, et al. A prospective study to evaluate the impact of FDG-PET on CT-based radiotherapy treatment planning for oesophageal cancer. *Radiother Oncol* 2006;78(3):254–261.
40. Gondi V, Bradley K, Mehta M, et al. Impact of hybrid fluorodeoxyglucose positron-emission tomography/computed tomography on radiotherapy planning in esophageal and non–small cell lung cancer. *Int J Radiat Oncol Biol Phys* 2007;67(1):187–195.
41. Hong TS, Crowley EM, Killoran J, et al. Considerations in treatment planning for esophageal cancer. *Semin Radiat Oncol* 2007;17(1):53–61.
42. Gambhir SS, Czernin J, Schwimmer J, et al. A tabulated summary of the FDG PET literature. *J Nucl Med* 2001;42[5 Suppl]:1S–93S.
43. Duong CP, Demitriou H, Weih L, et al. Significant clinical impact and prognostic stratification provided by FDG-PET in the staging of oesophageal cancer. *Eur J Nucl Med Mol Imaging* 2006;33(7): 759–769.
44. Wallace MB, Nietert PJ, Earle C, et al. An analysis of multiple staging management strategies for carcinoma of the esophagus: computed tomography, endoscopic ultrasound, positron emission tomography, and thoracoscopy/laparoscopy. *Ann Thorac Surg* 2002;74(4): 1026–1032.
45. Centers for Medicare and Medicaid Services. *Medicare national coverage determination manual.* 2006:chap. 1, Pt 4 (Secs. 200–310.1).
46. Kobori O, Kirihara Y, Kosaka N, et al. Positron emission tomography of esophageal carcinoma using (11)C-choline and (18)F-fluorodeoxyglucose: a novel method of preoperative lymph node staging. *Cancer* 1999;86(9):1638–1648.

47. Jager PL, Que TH, Vaalburg W, et al. Carbon-11 choline or FDG-PET for staging of oesophageal cancer? *Eur J Nucl Med* 2001;28(12): 1845–1849.
48. Apisarnthanarax S, Alauddin MM, Mourtada F, et al. Early detection of chemoradioresponse in esophageal carcinoma by 3′-deoxy-3′-3H-fluorothymidine using preclinical tumor models. *Clin Cancer Res* 2006;12(15):4590–4597.
49. Choi JY, Lee KH, Shim YM, et al. Improved detection of individual nodal involvement in squamous cell carcinoma of the esophagus by FDG PET. *J Nucl Med* 2000;41(5):808–815.
50. Yoon YC, Lee KS, Shim YM, et al. Metastasis to regional lymph nodes in patients with esophageal squamous cell carcinoma: CT versus FDG PET for presurgical detection prospective study. *Radiology* 2003;227(3): 764–770.
51. Kneist W, Schreckenberger M, Bartenstein P, et al. Positron emission tomography for staging esophageal cancer: does it lead to a different therapeutic approach? *World J Surg* 2003;27(10):1105–1112.
52. Heeren PA, Jager PL, Bongaerts F, et al. Detection of distant metastases in esophageal cancer with (18)F-FDG PET. *J Nucl Med* 2004;45(6): 980–987.
53. Kato H, Miyazaki T, Nakajima M, et al. The incremental effect of positron emission tomography on diagnostic accuracy in the initial staging of esophageal carcinoma. *Cancer* 2005;103(1):148–156.
54. Rasanen JV, Sihvo EIT, Knuuti MJ, et al. Prospective analysis of accuracy of positron emission tomography, computed tomography, and endoscopic ultrasonography in staging of adenocarcinoma of the esophagus and the esophagogastric junction. *Ann Surg Oncol* 2003;10(8):954–960.
55. Kneist W, Schreckenberger M, Bartenstein P, et al. Prospective evaluation of positron emission tomography in the preoperative staging of esophageal carcinoma. *Arch Surg* 2004;139(10):1043–1049.
56. Brucher BL, Weber W, Bauer M, et al. Neoadjuvant therapy of esophageal squamous cell carcinoma: response evaluation by positron emission tomography. *Ann Surg* 2001;233(3):300–309.
57. Flamen P, Van Cutsem E, Lerut A, et al. Positron emission tomography for assessment of the response to induction chemotherapy in locally advanced esophageal cancer. *Ann Oncol* 2002;13:361–368.
58. Downey RJ, Akhurst T, Ilson D, et al. Whole body ^{18}FDG-PET and the response of esophageal cancer to induction therapy: results of a prospective trial. *J Clin Oncol* 2003;21(3):428–432.
59. Swisher SG, Maish M, Erasmus JJ, et al. Utility of PET, CT, and EUS to identify pathologic responders in esophageal cancer. *Ann Thorac Surg* 2004;78(4):1152–1160; discussion 1152–1160.
60. Wieder HA, Brucher BL, Zimmermann F, et al. Time course of tumor metabolic activity during chemoradiotherapy of esophageal squamous cell carcinoma and response to treatment. *J Clin Oncol* 2004;22(5): 900–908.
61. Cerfolio RJ, Bryant AS, Ohja B, et al. The accuracy of endoscopic ultrasonography with fine-needle aspiration, integrated positron emission tomography with computed tomography, and computed tomography in restaging patients with esophageal cancer after neoadjuvant chemoradiotherapy. *J Thorac Cardiovasc Surg* 2005;129(6):1232–1241.
62. Duong CP, Hicks RJ, Weih L, et al. FDG-PET status following chemoradiotherapy provides high management impact and powerful prognostic stratification in oesophageal cancer. *Eur J Nucl Med Mol Imaging* 2006;33(7):770–778.
63. Levine EA, Farmer MR, Clark P, et al. Predictive value of 18-fluoro-deoxy-glucose-positron emission tomography (^{18}F-FDG-PET) in the identification of responders to chemoradiation therapy for the treatment of locally advanced esophageal cancer. *Ann Surg* 2006;243(4): 472–478.
64. Westerterp M, Omloo JM, Sloof GW, et al. Monitoring of response to pre-operative chemoradiation in combination with hyperthermia in oesophageal cancer by FDG-PET. *Int J Hyperther* 2006;22(2): 149–160.

CHAPTER

8.14 Applications for Fluorodeoxyglucose PET and PET/CT in the Evaluation of Patients with Colorectal Carcinoma

DOMINIQUE DELBEKE

Colorectal cancer is the third most common cause of cancer in men and women, and it affects 5% of the population in the United States and most Western countries. The American Cancer Society estimates that there are approximately 135,000 new cases of colorectal cancer per year in the United States, and approximately 57,000 patients per year die from this disease in the United States, representing 10% of all cancer deaths. Approximately 70% to 80% of patients are treated with curative intent, and the overall survival at 5 years after diagnosis is less than 60%.

SCREENING AND DIAGNOSIS OF COLORECTAL CARCINOMA

The diagnosis of colorectal carcinoma is based on colonoscopy and biopsy. The American Cancer Society recommends screening for colorectal cancer with yearly fecal occult blood test and flexible sigmoidoscopy every 5 years after the age of 50 for asymptomatic individuals (1). Colonoscopy evaluating the entire colon is a more comprehensive screening examination and has also been advocated in patients over 50. The role of virtual colonoscopy with multidetector computed tomography (CT) is still debated (2), but this screening technique will likely grow in prominence. Although fluorodeoxyglucose (FDG) positron emission tomography (PET) is not routinely used for screening or diagnostic purposes, it is not uncommon to incidentally detect colorectal carcinoma on whole-body studies performed for other indications.

Accurate interpretation of FDG PET images requires knowledge of the normal physiological distribution of FDG. Uptake in the gastrointestinal tract is variable from patient to patient. For example, FDG uptake along the esophagus is common, especially in the distal portion and at the gastroesophageal junction and in the presence of esophagitis. The wall of the stomach is usually faintly seen and can be used as an anatomical landmark, but occasionally the uptake can be relatively intense. There is FDG uptake in the cecum of many patients that may be related to abundant lymphoid tissue in the intestinal wall, among other factors. When marked activity is present in the bowel, evaluation for recurrence at the anastomotic site can be masked. Mild to moderate uptake is also usually seen at colostomy sites.

FDG uptake normally present in the gastrointestinal tract can occasionally be difficult to differentiate from a malignant lesion. Incidental colonic FDG uptake in 27 patients without colorectal carcinoma was correlated with colonoscopic and/or histopathologic findings (3). Diffuse uptake in eight patients was normal and associated with a normal colonoscopy. Segmental uptake was due to colitis in five of six patients. Focal uptake in seven patients was associated with benign adenomas. A study of 110 patients has demonstrated that precancerous adenomatous polyps can be detected incidentally on whole body images performed for other indications with a sensitivity of 24% (24 of 59). The positivity rate increased to 90% for lesions greater than 13 mm in size, and the false-positive rate was 5.5% (six of ten) (4).

Agress and Cooper (5) reviewed FDG PET studies of 1,750 patients referred for evaluation of known or suspected malignancies. They found 58 unexpected focal areas of FDG uptake that were unlikely to be related to the known primary in 53 (3.3%) patients. Forty-two lesions were pathologically confirmed and 30 of 42 (71%) were malignant or premalignant, including 18 colonic adenomas and 3 colon carcinomas. Similar data were published by Kamel et al. (6) on a review of 3,281 patients and Gutman et al. (7) on a review of 1,716 patients.

The clinical history, physical examination, pattern of uptake and correlation with anatomy are more helpful in avoiding false-positive interpretations than semiquantitative evaluation by the standard uptake value (SUV). The sensitivity of FDG PET is highly dependent on both the size of the lesion, reaching 72% sensitivity for lesions greater than 1 cm, and the degree of dysplasia reaching 89% for carcinomas, 76% for high-grade, and 36% for low-grade dysplasia (8). The sensitivity is more limited for flat premalignant lesions (9). Although PET is not recommended for detection or screening for precancerous or malignant colonic neoplasms, the identification of focal colon uptake should not be ignored. Fig. 8.14.1 illustrates incidental finding of colon carcinoma in a patient referred for FDG PET/CT follow-up of metastatic melanoma.

INITIAL STAGING OF COLORECTAL CANCER

The preoperative staging with imaging modalities is usually limited because most patients will benefit from colectomy to prevent intestinal obstruction and bleeding. The extent of the disease can be evaluated during surgery with excision of pericolonic and mesenteric lymph nodes along with peritoneal exploration. The performance of

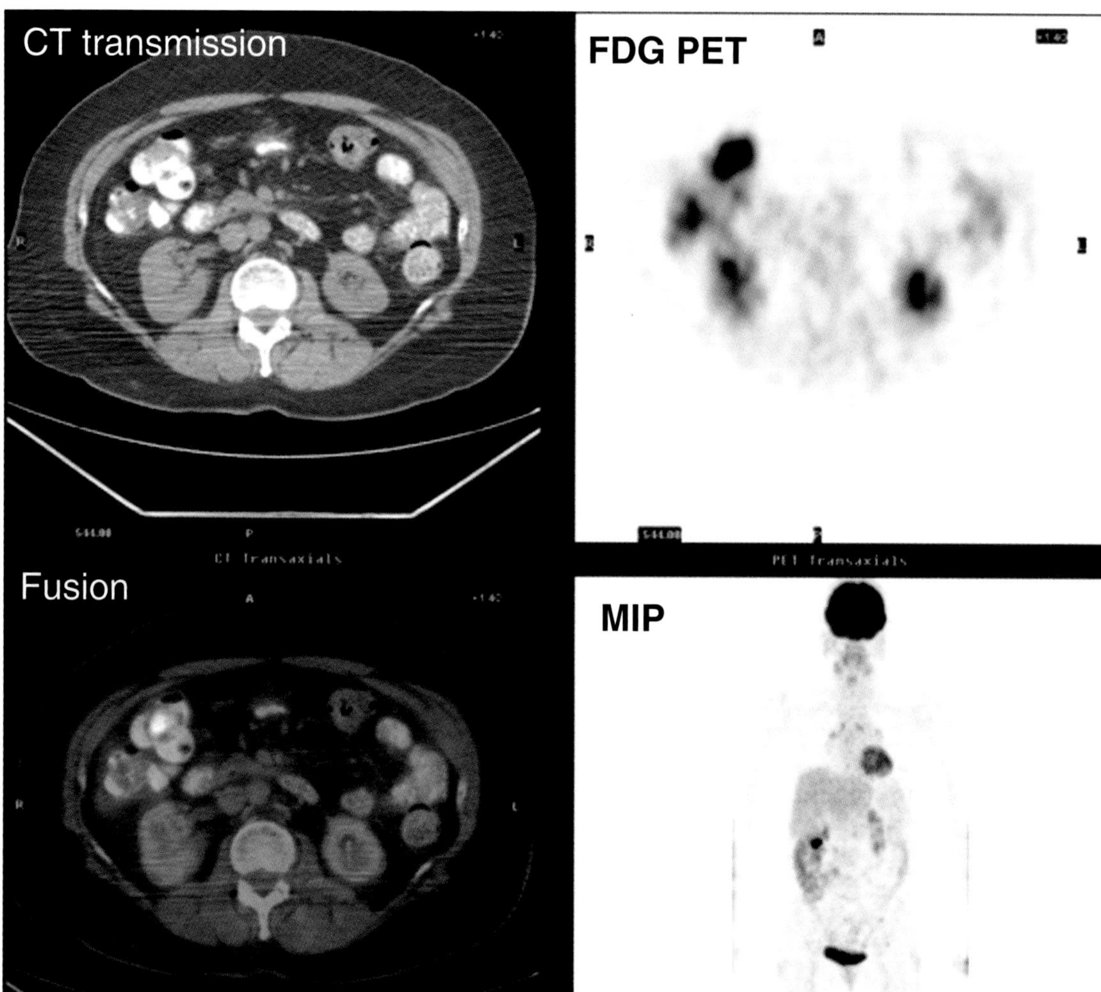

FIGURE 8.14.1. A 63-year-old woman with a history of recurrent melanoma 1 year earlier was referred for follow-up 1 year after treatment. Whole-body fluorodeoxyglucose (FDG) PET imaging was performed using an integrated PET/CT imaging system providing transmission CT images, FDG PET images, and fusion images. FDG PET maximum intensity projection (MIP) image demonstrates normal distribution of FDG with a focus of abnormal FDG uptake in the right upper quadrant just below the liver. The PET/CT transaxial slice through that area demonstrates that the FDG uptake corresponds with the wall of the colon and is worrisome for malignancy. Colonoscopy was performed for follow-up and revealed adenocarcinoma of the colon. Surgical resection revealed stage I disease.

FDG PET preoperatively may be helpful if the detection of distant metastases will cancel surgery in patients with increased surgical risk. It may also be helpful as a baseline evaluation prior to chemotherapy in patients with advanced stage disease. FDG PET imaging is a powerful tool for assessment of the response to therapy.

Three studies have been performed to evaluate the performance of FDG PET in the initial staging of colorectal cancer. Abdel-Nabi et al. (10) evaluated the usefulness of FDG PET for staging patients with known or suspected primary colorectal carcinomas. In 48 patients, FDG PET imaging identified all primary carcinomas. They found that both FDG and CT had a poor sensitivity of 29% for detecting local lymph node involvement. FDG PET was, however, superior to CT for detecting hepatic metastases, with sensitivity and specificity of 88% and 100%, respectively, compared to 38% and 97% for CT. These data were confirmed in the studies of Mukai et al. (11) and Kantorova et al. (12), which also reported that FDG PET changed the treatment modality in 8% of patients and the range of surgery in 13%. False-positive findings include abscesses, fistulas, diverticulitis, and occasionally adenomas. Although the sensitivity of FDG PET for the detection of a primary colon carcinoma may be high, its role in the preoperative staging is still debated except in high-risk patients for whom surgery can be avoided if metastases are identified, as illustrated in Fig. 8.14.2.

DETECTION OF RECURRENT OR METASTATIC COLORECTAL CARCINOMA

The 2005 recommendations from the American Society of Clinical Oncology for colorectal cancer surveillance are: (a) history and physical examination every 3 to 6 months for the first 3 years, every

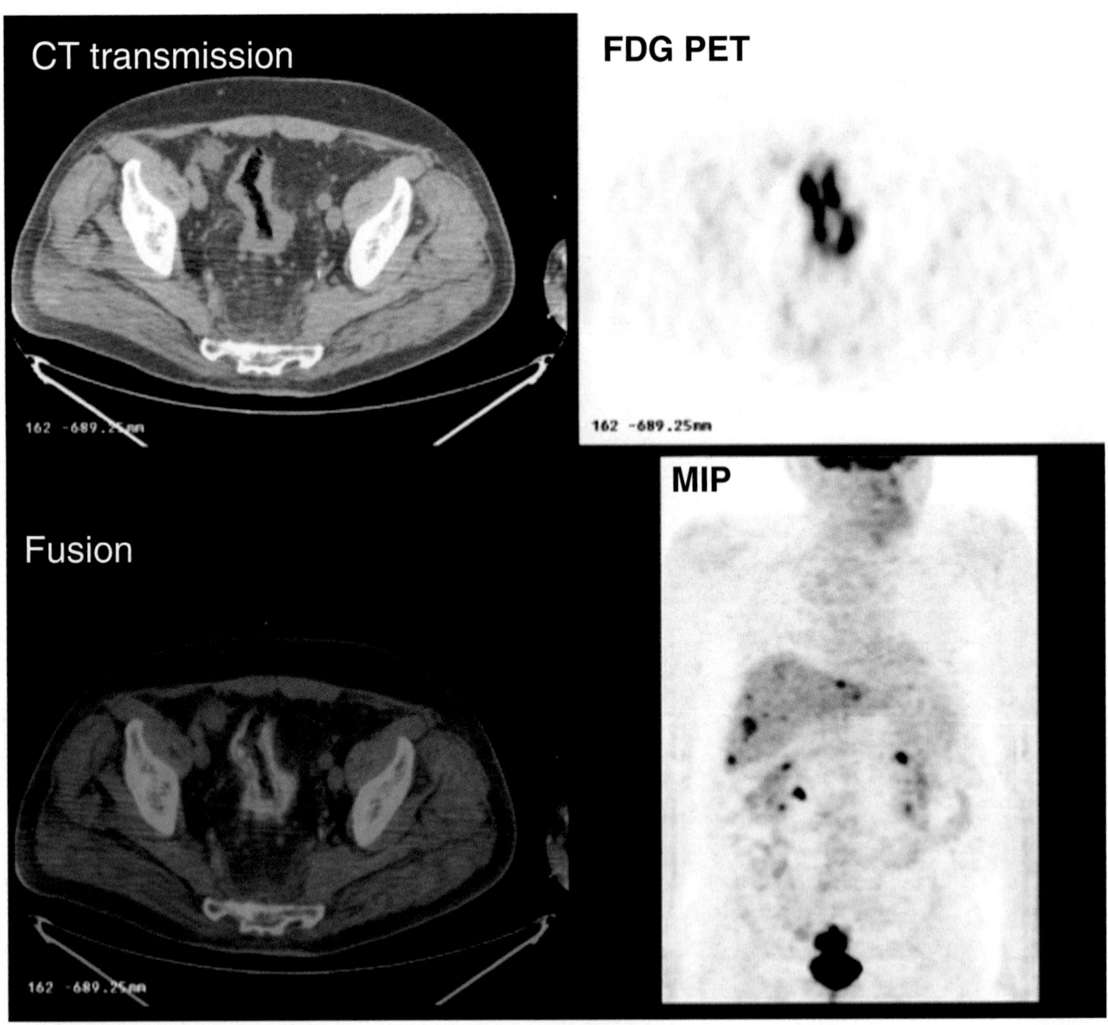

FIGURE 8.14.2. A 65-year-old man with recently diagnosed rectosigmoid carcinoma was referred for initial staging. Whole-body fluorodeoxyglucose (FDG) PET imaging was performed using an integrated PET/CT imaging system providing transmission CT images, FDG PET images, and fusion images. The FDG PET maximum intensity projection (MIP) image demonstrates focal FDG uptake above the bladder in the expected location of the primary tumor. In addition, multiple foci of FDG uptake are seen in the liver, indicating multiple hepatic metastases. Transaxial PET/CT slice through the lower pelvis demonstrated FDG uptake in a linear fashion corresponding to thickening of the wall of the sigmoid colon consistent with the primary carcinoma. In follow-up the patient was determined to have stage IV disease. He was a high-risk surgical candidate and elected to proceed with palliative chemotherapy.

6 months during years 4 and 5, and subsequently at the discretion of the physician, (b) carcinoembryonic antigen (CEA) serum levels every 3 months postoperatively for at least 3 years after diagnosis, (c) annual CT of the chest and abdomen for 3 years after primary therapy for patients who are at higher risk of recurrence and who could be candidates for curative-intent surgery; pelvic CT scan for rectal cancer surveillance, (d) colonoscopy at 3 years after operative treatment, and, if results are normal, every 5 years thereafter (13).

About 70% of the patients are resectable with curative intent but recurrence is noted in one third of these patients in the first 2 years after resection. Twenty-five percent of these patients have recurrence limited to one site and are potentially curable by surgical resection (14). For example, about 14,000 patients per year present with isolated liver metastases as their first recurrence, and about 20% of these patients die with metastases exclusively to the liver (15). Hepatic resection is the only curative therapy in these patients, but it is associated with a mortality of 2% to 7% and has the potential for significant morbidity (16). The poor prognosis of extrahepatic metastases is believed to be a contraindication to hepatic resection (17). Therefore, accurate noninvasive detection of inoperable disease with imaging modalities plays a pivotal role in selecting patients who would benefit from surgery.

Conventional Modalities for Detecting and Staging Recurrence

Elevated circulating levels of CEA occur in approximately two thirds of patients with colorectal carcinoma. Serial measurements of serum CEA levels are used to monitor these patients for recurrence and have a sensitivity of 59% and specificity of 84%. Imaging is necessary to localize the site of recurrence (18). Barium studies have been reported to detect local recurrence with an accuracy in the range of 80%, but are only 49% sensitive for overall recurrence; however, these are used relatively infrequently.

CT has been the conventional imaging modality used to localize recurrence with an accuracy of 25% to 73%, but it fails to demonstrate hepatic metastases in up to 7% of patients and underestimates the number of lobes involved in up to 33% of patients. In addition, metastases to the peritoneum, mesentery, and lymph nodes are commonly missed on CT, and the differentiation of postsurgical changes from local tumor recurrence is often equivocal (19–23). Among the patients with a negative CT, 50% will be found to have nonresectable lesions at the time of exploratory laparotomy. CT can also detect small lesions in the liver that are not due to malignancy resulting in false positives. CT portography (superior mesenteric arterial portography) is more sensitive (80% to 90%) than CT (70% to 80%) for detection of hepatic metastases, but has a considerable rate of false-positive findings, lowering the positive predictive value (24–27). In patients undergoing exploration for recurrent colorectal cancer, the presence of adhesions or the limitations of surgical exposure (transverse upper abdominal incision for liver resection) often preclude a detailed operative staging.

Detection and Staging Recurrent Colorectal Carcinoma with Fluorodeoxyglucose PET Imaging

A number of studies have demonstrated the role of FDG PET as a functional imaging modality for detecting recurrent or metastatic colorectal carcinoma (28–49). Overall, the sensitivity of FDG PET imaging is in the 90% range and the specificity greater than 70%, both superior to CT. A meta-analysis of 11 clinical reports and 577 patients determined that the sensitivity and specificity of FDG PET for detecting recurrent colorectal cancer were 97% and 76%, respectively (50). A comprehensive review of the PET literature (2,244 patients studied) has reported a weighted average for FDG PET sensitivity and specificity of 94% and 87%, respectively, compared to 79% and 73% for CT (51).

However, false-negative FDG PET findings have been reported with mucinous adenocarcinoma. Whiteford et al. (52) reported that the sensitivity of FDG PET imaging for detection of mucinous adenocarcinoma was 58% (n = 16), significantly lower than for nonmucinous adenocarcinoma at 92% (n = 93; $P = .005$). They suspect that the low sensitivity of FDG PET for detection of mucinous adenocarcinoma is due to the relative hypocellularity of these tumors. Similar findings (41% sensitivity) have been reported in a subsequent series of 22 patients (53).

Several studies have compared FDG PET and CT for differentiation of scar from local recurrence (29,30,33–35,39). CT was equivocal in most cases, and the accuracy of FDG PET imaging was greater than 90%. In the largest study (76 patients), the accuracy of FDG PET and CT were 95% and 65%, respectively (35).

Other studies have compared the accuracy of FDG PET and CT for detection of hepatic metastases (35,36,38,39,41). Overall, FDG PET was more accurate than CT. A meta-analysis performed to compare noninvasive imaging methods (ultrasound, CT, magnetic resonance imaging [MRI], and FDG PET) for the detection of hepatic metastases from colorectal, gastric, and esophageal cancers demonstrated that at an equivalent specificity of 85%, FDG PET had the highest sensitivity of 90% compared to 76% for MRI, 72% for CT, and 55% for ultrasound (54). A more recent meta-analysis confirmed these data (55). Vitola et al. (36) and Delbeke et al. (38) reported the comparison of FDG with CT and CT portography. CT portography, which is more invasive and more costly than FDG PET or CT alone, is regarded as the most effective means of determining resectability of hepatic metastasis by imaging. FDG PET had a higher accuracy (92%) than CT (78%) and CT portography (80%) for detection of hepatic metastases. Although the sensitivity of FDG PET (91%) was lower than that of CT portography (97%), the specificity of FDG PET was much higher, particularly at postsurgical sites.

Flanagan et al. (40) reported the use of FDG PET in 22 patients with unexplained elevation of serum CEA level after resection of colorectal carcinoma, and no abnormal findings on conventional work-up, including CT. Sensitivity and specificity of FDG PET for tumor recurrence were 100% and 71%, respectively. Valk et al. (41) reported sensitivity of 93% and specificity of 92% in a similar group of 18 patients. In both studies, PET correctly demonstrated tumor in two thirds of patients with rising CEA levels and negative CT scans.

Valk et al. (41) compared the sensitivity and specificity of FDG PET and CT for specific anatomic locations and found that FDG PET was more sensitive than CT in all locations except the lung, where the two modalities were equivalent. The largest difference between PET and CT was found in the abdomen, pelvis, and retroperitoneum, where over one third of PET-positive lesions were negative by CT. PET was also more specific than CT at all sites except the retroperitoneum, but the differences were smaller than the differences in sensitivity. Other investigators also found that FDG PET was especially useful for detecting retroperitoneal and pulmonary metastases (37,38). In addition, by the nature of being a whole-body technique, FDG PET imaging allowed identification of distant metastatic disease in the chest, abdomen, or pelvis which might not be in the field of view of routine CT staging examinations. Fig. 8.14.3 shows an example of a patient with residual/recurrent colon carcinoma for whom FDG PET/CT demonstrated both the local recurrence and distant metastases.

Impact of Fluorodeoxyglucose PET Imaging on Patient's Management

In a meta-analysis of the literature, FDG PET imaging changed the management in 29% of (102 of 349) patients (50). A comprehensive

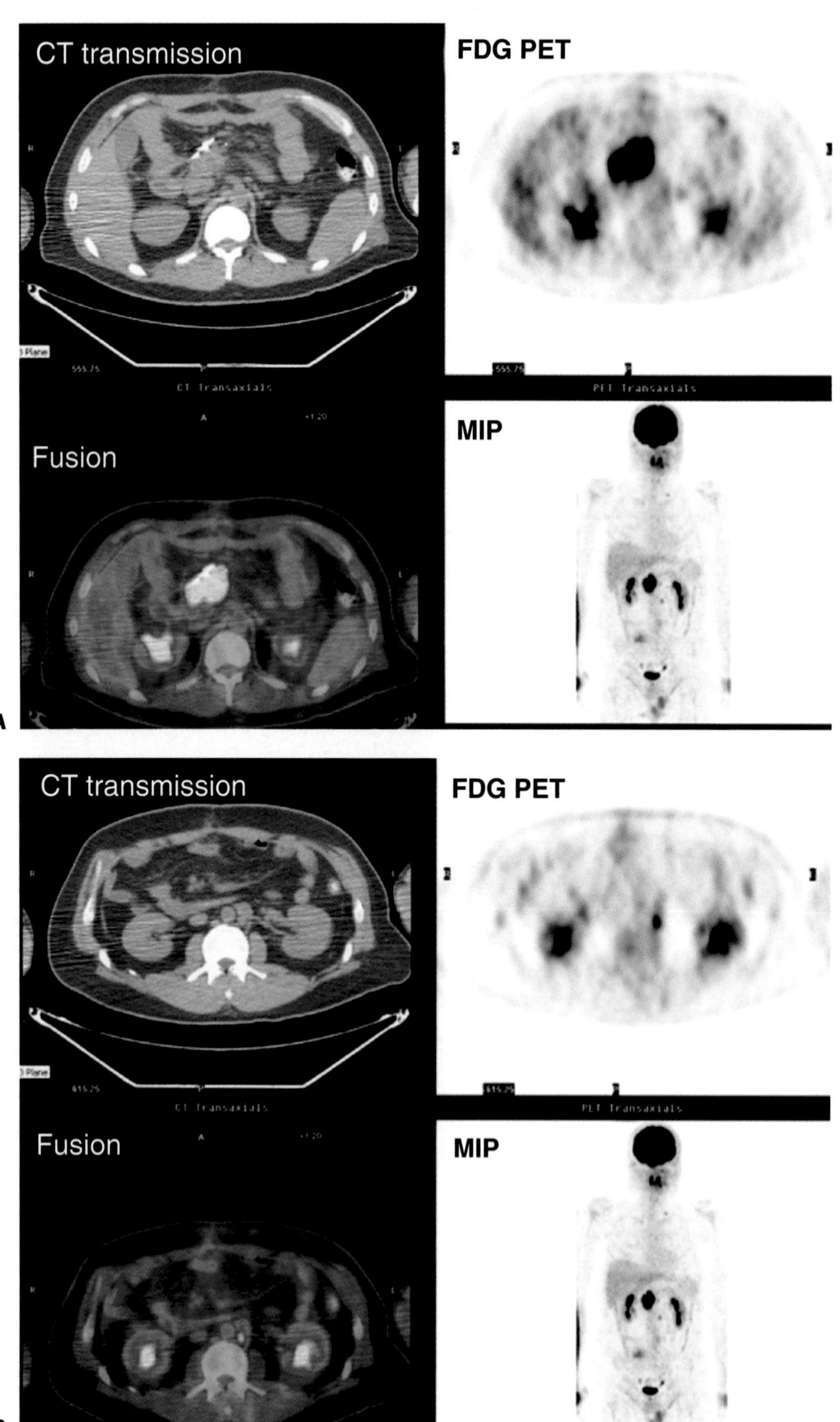

FIGURE 8.14.3. A 27-year-old man underwent an emergency exploratory laparotomy for abdominal pain 2 months earlier and a perforated adenocarcinoma of the transverse colon was found. He underwent a partial colectomy with colostomy but one margin of resection was positive. He was referred for staging prior to further therapy. Whole-body fluorodeoxyglucose (FDG) PET imaging was performed using an integrated PET/CT imaging system providing transmission CT images, FDG PET images, and fusion images. The FDG PET maximum intensity projection (MIP) image demonstrates a large area of focal FDG uptake in the midabdomen corresponding to the location of the primary tumor, indicating residual adenocarcinoma. In addition, at least two small foci of FDG uptake are seen projecting to the left of the lumbar spine and one focused in the left supraclavicular region. **A:** The transaxial slice through the midabdomen demonstrates that the foci of FDG uptake corresponds to the mass in the surgical bed at the root of the mesentery above the pancreatic head, consistent with residual adenocarcinoma. **B:** The PET/CT transaxial slice through the level of the mid-kidneys demonstrates that the focus of FDG uptake to the left of the spine corresponds to a small left retroperitoneal lymph node, indicating a metastasis. In follow-up, a CT angiogram revealed near total occlusion of the midsuperior mesenteric vein trunk as it courses through the tumor mass, and the residual/recurrent tumor was deemed unresectable. The presence of metastases also ruled out the possibility of resection in this patient. (*Continued*)

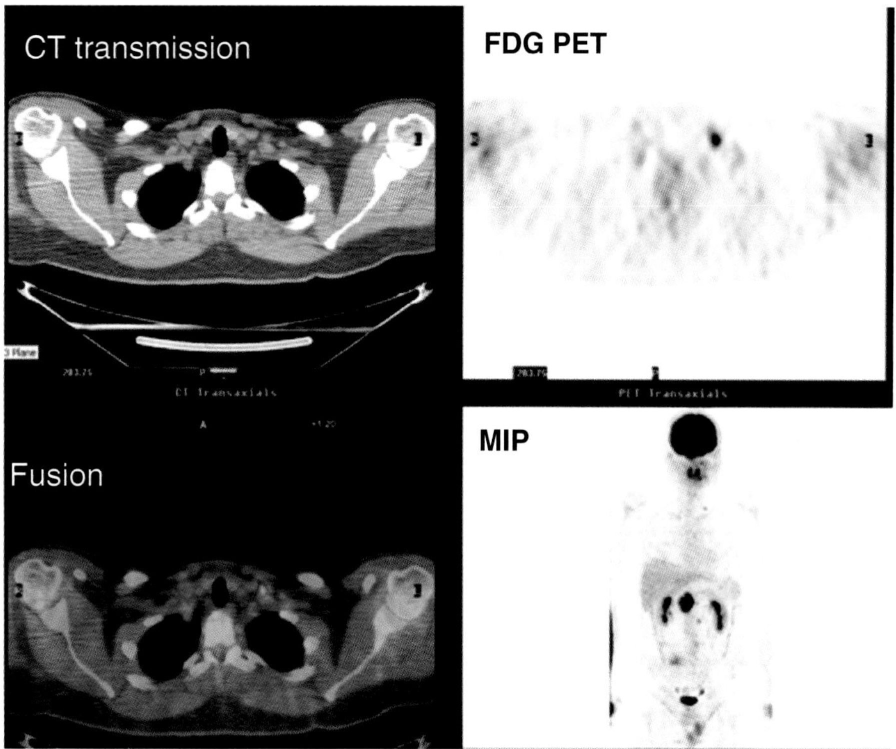

FIGURE 8.14.3. *Continued.* **C:** The transaxial slice through the upper chest demonstrates that the foci of FDG uptake corresponded to a small left supraclavicular lymph node, indicating a metastasis.

review of the PET literature has reported a weighted average change of management related to FDG PET findings in 32% of 915 patients (51).

The greater sensitivity of PET compared to CT in diagnosis and staging of recurrent tumor results from two factors: early detection of abnormal tumor metabolism, before changes have become apparent by anatomic imaging, and the whole-body nature of PET imaging, which permits diagnosis of tumor when it occurs in unusual and unexpected sites. FDG PET imaging allows detection of unsuspected metastases in 13% to 36% of patients and has a clinical impact in 14% to 65% (34,35,37–41,43,47–49,56,57). In the study of Delbeke et al. (38) surgical management was altered by PET in 28% of patients, in one-third by initiating surgery, and in two-thirds by avoiding surgery. In a survey-based study of 60 referring oncologists, surgeons, and generalists, FDG PET performed at initial staging had a major impact on the management of patients with colorectal cancer and contributed to a change in clinical stage in 42% (80% up-staged and 20% down-staged) and a change in the clinical management in over 60%. As a result of the PET findings, physicians avoided major surgery in 41% of patients for whom surgery was the intended treatment (58). In a recent prospective study of 51 patients evaluated for resection of hepatic metastases, clinical management decisions based on conventional diagnostic methods were changed in 20% of patients based on the findings on FDG PET imaging, especially by detecting unsuspected extrahepatic disease (57).

Although survival is not a typical end point for a diagnostic test, Strasberg et al. (56) have estimated the survival of patients who underwent FDG PET imaging in their preoperative evaluation for resection of hepatic metastases. The Kaplan-Meier test estimate of the overall survival at 3 years was 77% and the lower confidence limit was 60%. These percentages are higher than those in previously published series that ranged from 30% to 64%. In the patients undergoing FDG PET imaging prior to hepatic resection, the 3-year disease-free survival rate was 40%, again higher than that usually reported.

The same group of investigators recently reported the 5-year survival after resection of metastases from colorectal carcinoma (59). They established the 5-year survival of patients with conventional diagnostic imaging from the literature by pooling the data of 19 studies with a total of 6,090 patients. The 5-year survival rate was 30% and appeared not to have changed over time. These results were compared to their group of 100 patients with hepatic metastases, who were preoperatively staged for resection with curative intent with the addition of FDG PET imaging. The 5-year survival rate improved to 58%, indicating that they were able to define a subgroup after conventional imaging that has a better prognosis. The main contribution was in detecting occult disease, leading to a reduction of futile surgeries.

Fluorodeoxyglucose Imaging to Monitor Therapy of Colorectal Carcinoma

FDG PET is most helpful to monitor patients with advanced-stage colorectal carcinoma that is associated with a poor prognosis. Systemic chemotherapy with 5-fluorouracil has demonstrated effective palliation and improved survival (60), although response rates are only 10% to 20% in patients with advanced disease. In a study of 18 patients, Findlay et al. (61) reported that responders could be discriminated from nonresponders after 4 to 5 weeks of chemotherapy with 5-fluorouracil by measuring FDG uptake before and during therapy. More recently, newer chemotherapeutic agents, particularly irinotecan and oxaliplatin have been shown to improve survival in combination with 5-fluorouracil-based therapies.

Systemic chemotherapy with 5-fluorouracil in combination with radiotherapy has also been shown to improve survival. In these patients, radiation-induced inflammation and necrosis make it difficult to differentiate postradiation changes from residual tumor with ultrasound, CT, and MRI (62). A preliminary study on six patients demonstrated the FDG uptake decreased in the primary tumor during radiation therapy, whereas the tumor size did not change on CT. Another study of 44 patients demonstrated that FDG PET imaging can differentiate local recurrence from scarring after radiation therapy (63). However, increased FDG uptake immediately following radiation may be due to inflammatory changes and is not always associated with residual tumor. The time course of postirradiation FDG activity has not been studied systematically; it is, however, generally accepted that focal FDG activity present within 6 months after completion of radiation therapy likely represents tumor recurrence. A case-controlled study of 60 FDG PET studies performed 6 months following external beam radiation therapy for rectal cancer found a sensitivity of 84% and specificity of 88% for detection of local pelvic recurrence (64). In a study of 15 patients with locally advanced rectal carcinoma, Guillem et al. (65) demonstrated that FDG PET imaging performed before and 4 to 5 weeks after completion of preoperative radiation, and 5-fluorouracil-based chemotherapy had the potential to assess the pathological response. Subsequently, the same authors demonstrated that FDG PET imaging could predict long-term outcome after a median follow-up of 42 months (66). The mean percentage decrease in SUV_{max} was 69% for patients free from recurrence and 37% for patients with recurrence.

Hepatic metastases can be treated with regional therapy to the liver. A variety of procedures to administer regional therapy to hepatic metastases have been investigated, including chemotherapy administered through the hepatic artery using infusion pumps, selective chemoembolization, cryoablation and alcohol ablation, radiofrequency ablation, and yttrium-90 (^{90}Y) microsphere radioembolization (67–70). Regional therapy to the liver by chemoembolization can also be monitored with FDG PET imaging, as shown by Vitola et al. (71) and Torizuka et al. (72). FDG uptake decreases in responding lesions, and the presence of residual uptake in some lesions can help in guiding further regional therapy.

Radiofrequency ablation and ^{90}Y microsphere radioembolization are becoming the interventional techniques of choice for patients with unresectable hepatic metastases. Radiofrequency ablation is often indicated for patients with a limited number of hepatic metastases measuring less than 5 cm in size. It is usually performed percutaneously under ultrasound or CT guidance. The probe tip delivers current and energy that destroy the liver tissue as it reaches 55°C. Median survival has been shown to improve with radiofrequency ablation of colorectal hepatic metastases compared to historical data (73). CT and MRI have limitations for evaluation of residual tumor because of contrast enhancement at the periphery of the ablative necrosis for up to 3 months postradiofrequency ablation due to hyperemia and tissue regeneration (74).

Langenhoff et al. (75) have prospectively monitored 23 patients with liver metastases following radiofrequency ablation and cryoablation. Three weeks after therapy, 51 of 56 metastases became FDG negative, and there was no recurrence during 16 months' follow-up; whereas among the 5 of 56 lesions with persistent FDG uptake, 4 of 5 recurred. The single false-positive case was found to have an FDG-avid infection. Data in smaller series of patients support their findings (76,77). Donckier et al. (78) followed 17 patients with 28 hepatic metastases at 1 week and 1 month postradiofrequency ablation. FDG PET detected residual tumor in 4 of 28 lesions, although CT was negative. There was no recurrence in the 24 of 28 lesions negative with FDG PET after 11 months' follow-up. In another study, the sensitivity for detection of residual tumor was 65% for PET/CT and 45% for CT (79). However, other studies have reported FDG uptake in the inflammatory rim, making the interpretation difficult (79,80). Antoch et al. (81) studied minipigs who underwent radiofrequency ablation of nontumorous liver. There was no FDG uptake within 90 minutes after completion of the procedure and no tissue regeneration was seen on histology, but there was a rim of enhancement on morphological imaging. This suggests that FDG imaging should be performed immediately after the procedure.

Intra-arterial hepatic radioembolization with ^{90}Y microspheres is also an option for therapy of unresectable hepatic metastases and hepatocellular carcinoma. As most of the perfusion to the hepatic tumors comes from the hepatic artery, the labeled spheres administered intra-arterially and measuring approximately 30 μm in diameter are trapped in the capillaries. ^{90}Y has a half-life of 64 hours and emits β particles with an average range of 2.5 mm, maximizing tumor damage. Prior to the procedure, the vascular anatomy to the liver has to be assessed to avoid radioembolization in vessels perfusing other organs. Hepatopulmonary shunting can be evaluated on a separate, or the same, day with technetium-99m (^{99m}Tc) macroaggregated albumin scintigraphy, and a lung/liver shunt fraction greater than 20% is usually a contraindication to treatment to avoid radiation pneumonitis.

Wong et al. (82) have compared FDG PET imaging, CT, or MRI and serum levels of CEA to monitor the therapeutic response of hepatic metastases to ^{90}Y glass microspheres 3 months after therapy. They found a significant difference between the FDG PET changes and the changes on CT or MRI; the changes in FDG uptake correlated better with the changes in serum levels of CEA. This was confirmed in a subsequent study by the same investigators using quantitative analysis (83).

In summary, preliminary data suggest that FDG PET imaging may be able to effectively monitor the efficacy of regional therapy to hepatic metastases, but these data need to be confirmed in larger series of patients.

Cost Analysis

Including FDG PET in the evaluation of patients with recurrent colorectal carcinoma has been shown to be cost-effective in a study using clinical evaluation of effectiveness with modeling of costs and studies using decision-tree sensitivity analysis (41,84,85). In both types of studies, all cost calculations were based on Medicare reimbursement rates and a $1,800 cost for a PET scan. As Medicare reimbursement rates for PET have declined somewhat, the cost-benefit analyses would be expected to be even more favorable toward PET.

In a management algorithm where recurrence at more than one site was treated as nonresectable, Valk et al. (41) evaluated cost savings in 78 patients undergoing preoperative staging of recurrent colorectal carcinoma. This study was limited to preoperative patients and demonstrated potential savings of $3,003 per patient, resulting from diagnosis of nonresectable tumor by PET.

In 1997 Gambhir et al. (84) used a quantitative decision-tree model combined with sensitivity analysis to evaluate cost issues if all patients presenting with recurrent colorectal cancer undergo

FDG PET imaging. The conventional strategy for detection of recurrence and determination of resectability using CEA levels and CT was compared to the conventional strategy plus PET for all patients presenting with suspected recurrence. The assumptions included prevalence of resectable disease of 3%, sensitivity and specificity of 65% and 45%, respectively, for CT, and 90% and 85% for PET. The conventional strategy plus PET showed an incremental savings of $220 per patient without a loss of life expectancy.

Park et al. (85) used the decision-tree sensitivity analysis to evaluate the cost of adding FDG PET imaging in the evaluation of patients referred for suspected recurrence based on elevated CEA levels and candidates for hepatic resection. The CT plus PET strategy was higher in mean cost by $429 per patient, but resulted in an increase in the mean life expectancy of 9.5 days per patient. As PET prices have declined, more PET favorable cost analyses are expected.

Clinical Impact of Integrated PET/CT Imaging

Concurrent PET/CT imaging with an integrated system may be especially important in the abdomen and pelvis. PET images alone may be difficult to interpret owing to both the absence of anatomical landmarks (other than the kidneys and bladder), the presence of nonspecific uptake in the stomach, small bowel, and colon, and urinary excretion of FDG. Concurrent PET/CT imaging is helpful for differentiating focal retention of urine in the ureter, for example, versus an FDG-avid lymph node.

A study of 45 patients with colorectal cancer referred for FDG PET imaging using an integrated PET/CT system concluded that PET/CT imaging increases the accuracy of interpretation and certainty of location of the lesions (86). In this study performed at Johns Hopkins University, the frequency of equivocal and probable lesion characterization was reduced by 50% with PET/CT compared to PET alone, the number of definite lesion locations was increased by 25%, and the overall correct staging increased from 78% to 89% (86).

A study of 204 patients (34 with gastrointestinal tumors) performed at Rambam Medical Center using an integrated PET/CT system concluded that the diagnostic accuracy of PET is improved in approximately 50% of patients versus the use of PET alone (87). In that study, PET/CT fusion images improved characterization of equivocal lesions as definitely benign in 10% of sites and definitely malignant in 5% of sites. It precisely defined the anatomic location of malignant FDG uptake in 6% and led to retrospective lesion detection on PET or CT in 8%. The results of PET/CT images had an impact on the management of 14% (28 of 204) of patients, 7 of 28 patients with a change of management had colorectal cancer representing 20% (8 of 34) of patients with gastrointestinal tumors. The changes in management in the eight patients with colorectal cancer included guiding colonoscopy and biopsy for a local recurrence (n = 2), guiding biopsy to a metastatic supraclavicular lymph node (n = 1), guiding surgery to localized metastatic lymph nodes (n = 3), and referral to chemotherapy (n = 2). Similar conclusions were found in a study of 173 patients performed at Vanderbilt University, 24 of whom had colorectal carcinoma (88).

Selzner et al. (89) have compared contrast-enhanced CT and non–contrast-enhanced PET/CT in 76 patients referred for restaging prior to resection of hepatic metastases. For detection of hepatic metastases, contrast-enhanced CT and non–contrast-enhanced PET/CT had similar sensitivities of 95% and 91%, respectively. However, for evaluation of patients with a prior hepatic resection, the PET/CT had a superior specificity of 100% compared to 50% for contrast-enhanced CT. For local recurrence, PET/CT had a superior sensitivity of 93% compared to 53% for contrast-enhanced CT. A similar conclusion was reached for extrahepatic metastases with a sensitivity of 89% for PET/CT compared to 64% for contrast-enhanced CT. There was an impact of PET/CT on the management of 21% of patients. False-negative PET/CT studies were seen for small lesions (less than 5 mm) and in some patients who had undergone chemotherapy in the month prior to PET/CT.

CT transmission images have to be carefully reviewed for detection of malignant lesions that may not be FDG avid, such as mucinous tumors or renal cell carcinomas, for example, as well as other incidental findings relevant to a patient's care. An analysis of 250 patients demonstrated that these findings are uncommon (3% of patients) but could be important enough to warrant alterations in clinical management (90). Concurrent PET/CT fusion images have the potential to provide better maps than CT alone to modulate the field and dose of radiation therapy, including in patients with colorectal carcinoma (91,92).

LIMITATIONS OF FLUORODEOXYGLUCOSE IMAGING

Tumor detectability depends on both the size of the lesion and the degree of uptake, as well as surrounding background uptake and intrinsic resolution of the imaging system. False-negative lesions can be due to partial volume averaging, leading to underestimation of the uptake in small lesions (less than twice the resolution of the imaging system) or in necrotic, partly treated, or mucinous lesions, falsely classifying these lesions as benign instead of malignant.

False-positive findings are due to physiologic variations of FDG distribution and FDG avidity of inflammatory lesions. In view of the known high uptake of FDG by activated macrophages, neutrophils, fibroblasts, and granulation tissue, it is not surprising that inflamed tissue demonstrates FDG activity. Mild to moderate FDG activity seen early after radiation therapy along recent incisions, infected incisions, biopsy sites, drainage tubing and catheters, as well as colostomy sites can lead to errors in interpretation if the history is not known. Uptake after radiation therapy may persist for several months. Comparison with baseline FDG images and knowledge of the radiation port are helpful. Some inflammatory lesions, especially granulomatous ones, may be markedly FDG avid and can be mistaken for malignancies; this includes inflammatory bowel disease, tuberculosis, sarcoidosis, histoplasmosis, and aspergillosis, among others (93).

COST AND REIMBURSEMENT ISSUES

In July 2001, the Center for Medical Services (CMS) approved and implemented reimbursement by Medicare for six types of malignant tumors including colorectal carcinoma. This coverage is for diagnosis, staging, and restaging, but not monitoring therapy.

POTENTIAL NEW PET TRACERS FOR CLINICAL USE

Besides evaluation of glucose metabolism with FDG, PET can assess various other biologic parameters such as perfusion, accumulation/metabolism of other compounds, hypoxia, and receptor expression. Some of these radiopharmaceuticals are labeled with positron emitters that have a short half-life, such as oxygen-15 (T1/2 = 2 minutes), nitrogen-13 (T1/2 = 10 minutes), and carbon-11 (^{11}C) (T1/2 = 20 minutes). The short half-life of these radioisotopes prevents any timely distribution of the radiopharmaceuticals labeled with them, and, therefore, their use is restricted to institutions having a cyclotron and associated laboratories and personnel on-site. Some tracers labeled with fluorine-18 (^{18}F), such as [^{18}F]-fluoride and [^{18}F]-fluorothymidine (FLT), are being investigated for clinical use.

[^{18}F]-fluoride was first described as a skeletal imaging agent in the 1960s but then was replaced by the ^{99m}Tc-labeled diphosphonate radiopharmaceuticals (94). With the widespread applications of FDG PET in oncology, PET imaging systems are becoming more widely available, and there is a renewed interest in [^{18}F]-fluoride. Although the mechanism of uptake for [^{18}F]-fluoride is similar to that for other bone-imaging radiopharmaceuticals (95), the spatial resolution of the PET technology is superior to that of both planar and single-photon emission computed tomography imaging using the ^{99m}Tc radiopharmaceuticals. Because of the better spatial resolution and routine acquisition of tomographic images, [^{18}F]-fluoride PET imaging offers potential advantages over bone scintigraphy in detecting metastases. Although skeletal metastases are not common in colorectal cancer, [^{18}F]-fluoride may have a role in the future if skeletal metastases are suspected clinically.

The rate of DNA synthesis can be assessed using [^{11}C]-thymidine or FLT. Thymidine is a DNA precursor and allows direct assessment of tumor proliferation. Shields et al. (96) have developed and evaluated ^{18}F-FLT for clinical use because of its ^{18}F labeling. A report of 17 patients with colorectal cancer comparing FDG and FLT demonstrated all primary tumors were visualized with both tracers, but tumor FDG uptake was on average twofold higher as compared to FLT (97). Pulmonary and peritoneal metastases were visualized with both tracers, but the sensitivity of FLT for hepatic metastases was only 34% compared to 97% for FDG. This low sensitivity was due to the high physiologic hepatic background activity with FLT. Therefore, the authors concluded that it was unlikely that FLT would play an important role for evaluation of patients with colorectal carcinoma.

SUMMARY

Evaluation of patients with known or suspected recurrent colorectal carcinoma is now an accepted indication for FDG PET imaging. PET and CT are complementary and therefore, integrated PET/CT imaging should be performed where available. The most common indication is for diagnosis and staging of recurrence and for preoperative staging (node and metastasis) of known recurrence that is considered to be resectable. FDG PET/CT imaging is valuable for differentiation of posttreatment changes from recurrent tumor, differentiation of benign from malignant lesions (indeterminate lymph nodes and hepatic and pulmonary lesions), and evaluation of patients with rising tumor markers in the absence of a known source. Addition of FDG PET/CT to the evaluation of these patients reduces overall treatment costs by accurately identifying patients who will and will not benefit from surgical procedures.

Although initial staging at the time of diagnosis is often performed during colectomy, FDG PET/CT imaging is now commonly performed preoperatively. It is particularly useful if surgery can be avoided if FDG PET shows metastases. Screening for recurrence in patients at high risk has also been advocated. FDG PET imaging seems promising for monitoring patient response to a wide range of therapies, but larger studies are necessary.

The diagnostic implications of integrated PET/CT imaging include improved detection of lesions on both the CT and FDG PET images, better differentiation of physiologic from pathologic foci of metabolism, and better localization of the pathologic foci. This new powerful technology provides more accurate interpretation of both CT and FDG PET images and therefore more optimal patient care. PET/CT fusion images affect the clinical management by guiding further procedures (biopsy, surgery, radiation therapy), excluding the need for additional procedures, and changing both inter- and intramodality therapy.

REFERENCES

1. Smith RA, Cokkinides V, Eyre HJ. American Cancer Society Guidelines for the early detection of cancer, 2004. *CA Cancer J Clin* 2004;54:41–52.
2. Pickhardt PJ. Virtual colonoscopy: issues related to primary screening. *Eur Radiol* 2005;15[Suppl 4]:D133–D137.
3. Tatlidil R, Jadvar H, Bading JR, et al. Incidental colonic fluorodeoxyglucose uptake: correlation with colonoscopic and histopathologic findings. *Radiology* 2002;224(3):783–787.
4. Yasuda S, Fujii H, Nakahara T, et al. ^{18}F-FDG PET detection of colonic adenomas. *J Nucl Med* 2001;42:989–992.
5. Agress H, Cooper BZ. Detection of clinically unexpected malignant and premalignant tumors with whole-body FDG PET: histopathologic comparison. *Radiology* 2004;230(2):417–422.
6. Kamel EM, Thumshirn M, Truninger K, et al. Significance of incidental ^{18}F-FDG accumulations in the gastrointestinal tract in PET/CT: correlation with endoscopic and histopathological results. *J Nucl Med* 2004;45:1804–1810.
7. Gutman F, Alberini JL, Wartski M, et al. Incidental colonic focal lesions detected by FDG PET/CT. *Am J Roentgenol* 2005;185 (2):495–500.
8. Van Kouwen MC, Nagengast FM, Jansen JB, et al. 2-(18F)-fluoro-2-deoxy-D-glucose positron emission tomography detects clinical relevant adenomas of the colon: a prospective study. *J Clin Oncol* 2005;23(16):3713–3717.
9. Friedland S, Soetikno R, Carlisle M, et al. 18-Fluorodeoxyglucose positron emission tomography has limited sensitivity for colonic adenomas and early stage colon cancer. *Gastrointest Endosc* 2005;61(3): 305–400.
10. Abdel-Nabi H, Doerr RJ, Lamonica DM, et al. Staging of primary colorectal carcinomas with fluorine-18 fluorodeoxyglucose whole-body PET: correlation with histopathologic and CT findings. *Radiology* 1998;206:755–760.
11. Mukai M, Sadahiro S, Yasuda S, et al. Preoperative evaluation by whole-body ^{18}F-fluorodeoxyglucose positron emission tomography in patients with primary colorectal cancer. *Oncol Rep* 2000;7:85–87.
12. Kantorova I, Lipska L, Belohlavek O, et al. Routine ^{18}F-FDG PET preoperative staging of colorectal cancer: comparison with conventional staging and its impact on treatment decision making. *J Nucl Med* 2003;44:1784–1788.
13. Desch CE, Benson AB 3rd, Somerfield MR, et al. Colorectal cancer surveillance: 2005 update of an American Society of Clinical Oncology practice guideline. *J Clin Oncol* 2005;23(33):8512–8519.
14. August DA, Ottow RT, Sugarbaker PH. Clinical perspectives on human colorectal cancer metastases. *Cancer Metastases Rev* 1984;3:303–324.
15. Foster JH, Lundy J. Liver metastases. *Curr Probl Surg* 1981;18:158–202.
16. Holm A, Bradley E, Aldrete J. Hepatic resection of metastases from colorectal carcinoma: morality, morbidity and pattern of recurrence. *Ann Surg* 1989;209:428–434.
17. Hughes KS, Simon R, Songhorabodi S, et al. Resection of liver for colorectal carcinoma metastases: a multi-institutional study of indications for resection. *Surgery* 1988;103:278–288.
18. Moertel CG, Fleming TR, McDonald JS, et al. An evaluation of the carcinoembryonic antigen (CEA) test for monitoring patients with resected colon cancer. *JAMA* 1993;270:943–947.

19. Sugarbaker PH, Grianola FJ, Dwyer S, et al. A simplified plan for follow-up of patients with colon and rectal cancer supported by prospective studies of laboratory and radiologic test results. *Surgery* 1987;102: 79–87.
20. Steele G Jr, Bleday R, Mayer R, et al. A prospective evaluation of hepatic resection for colorectal carcinoma metastases to the liver: Gastrointestinal Tumor Study Group protocol 6584. *J Clin Oncol* 1991;9: 1105–1112.
21. Granfield CAJ, Charnsangaveg C, Dubrow RA, et al. Regional lymph node metastases in carcinoma of the left side of the colon and rectum: CT demonstration. *AJR Am J Roentgenol* 1992;159:757–761.
22. Charnsangavej C, Whitley NO. Metastases to the pancreas and peripancreatic lymph nodes from carcinoma of the right colon: CT findings in 12 patients. *AJR Am J Roentgenol* 1993;160:49–52.
23. McDaniel KP, Charnsangavej C, Dubrow R, et al. Pathways of nodal metastases in carcinoma of the cecum, ascending colon and transverse colon: CT demonstration. *AJR Am J Roentgenol* 1993;161:61–64.
24. Soyer P, Levesque M, Elias D, et al. Detection of liver metastases from colorectal cancer: comparison of intraoperative US and CT during arterial portography. *Radiology* 1992;183:541–544.
25. Nelson RC, Chezmar JL, Sugarbaker PH, et al. Hepatic tumors: comparison of CT during arterial portography, delayed CT and MR imaging for preoperative evaluation. *Radiology* 1989;172:27–34.
26. Small WC, Mehard WB, Langmo LS, et al. Preoperative determination of the resectability of hepatic tumors: efficacy of CT during arterial portography. *AJR Am J Roentgenol* 1993;161:319–322.
27. Peterson MS, Baron RL, Dodd GD 3rd, et al. Hepatic parenchymal perfusion detected with CTPA: imaging-pathologic correlation. *Radiology* 1992;183:149–155.
28. Yonekura Y, Benua RS, Brill AB, et al. Increased accumulation of 2-deoxy-2[^{18}F]fluoro-D-glucose in liver metastases from colon carcinoma. *J Nucl Med* 1982;23:1133–1137.
29. Strauss LG, Clorius JH, Schlag P, et al. Recurrence of colorectal tumors: PET evaluation. *Radiology* 1989;170:329–332.
30. Ito K, Kato T, Tadokoro M, et al. Recurrent rectal cancer and scar: differentiation with PET and MR imaging. *Radiology* 1992;182:549–552.
31. Kim EE, Chung SK, Haynie TP, et al. Differentiation of residual or recurrent tumors from post-treatment changes with F-18 FDG-PET. *Radiographics* 1992;12:269–279.
32. Gupta NC, Falk PM, Frank AL, et al. Pre-operative staging of colorectal carcinoma using positron emission tomography. *Nebr Med J* 1993; 78:30–35.
33. Falk PM, Gupta NC, Thorson AG, et al. Positron emission tomography for preoperative staging of colorectal carcinoma. *Dis Colon Rectum* 1994;37:153–156.
34. Beets G, Penninckx F, Schiepers C, et al. Clinical value of whole-body positron emission tomography with [18F]fluorodeoxyglucose in recurrent colorectal cancer. *Br J Surg* 1994;81:1666–1670.
35. Schiepers C, Penninckx F, De Vadder N, et al. Contribution of PET in the diagnosis of recurrent colorectal cancer: comparison with conventional imaging. *Eur J Surg Oncol* 1995;21:517–522.
36. Vitola JV, Delbeke D, Sandler MP, et al. Positron emission tomography to stage metastatic colorectal carcinoma to the liver. *Am J Surg* 1996;171:21–26.
37. Lai DT, Fulham M, Stephen MS, et al. The role of whole-body positron emission tomography with [18F]fluorodeoxyglucose in identifying operable colorectal cancer. *Arch Surg* 1996;131:703–707.
38. Delbeke D, Vitola J, Sandler MP, et al. Staging recurrent metastatic colorectal carcinoma with PET. *J Nucl Med* 1997;38:1196–1201.
39. Ogunbiyi OA, Flanagan FL, Dehdashti F, et al. Detection of recurrent and metastatic colorectal cancer: comparison of positron emission tomography and computed tomography. *Ann Surg Oncol* 1997;4: 613–620.
40. Flanagan FL, Dehdashti F, Ogunbiyi OA, et al. Utility of FDG PET for investigating unexplained plasma CEA elevation in patients with colorectal cancer. *Ann Surg* 1998;227(3):319–323.
41. Valk PE, Abella-Columna E, Haseman MK, et al. Whole-body PET imaging with F-18-fluorodeoxyglucose in management of recurrent colorectal cancer. *Arch Surg* 1999;134:503–511.
42. Ruhlmann J, Schomburg A, Bender H, et al. Fluorodeoxyglucose whole-body positron emission tomography in colorectal cancer patients studied in routine daily practice. *Dis Colon Rectum* 1997;40:1195–1204.
43. Flamen P, Stroobants S, Van Cutsem E, et al. Additional value of whole-body positron emission tomography with fluorine-18-2-fluoro-2-deoxy-D-glucose in recurrent colorectal cancer. *J Clin Oncol* 1999;17(3):894–901.
44. Akhurst T, Larson SM. Positron emission tomography imaging of colorectal cancer. *Semin Oncol* 1999;26(5):577–583.
45. Vogel SB, Drane WE, Ros PR, et al. Prediction of surgical resectability in patients with hepatic colorectal metastases. *Ann Surg* 1994;219:508–516.
46. Imbriaco M, Akhurst T, Hilton S, et al. Whole-body FDG-PET in patients with recurrent colorectal carcinoma. A comparative study with CT. *Clin Positron Imaging* 2000;3(3):107–114.
47. Imdahl A, Reinhardt MJ, Nitzsche EU, et al. Impact of ^{18}F-FDG-positron emission tomography for decision making in colorectal cancer recurrences. *Arch Surg* 2000;385(2):129–134.
48. Staib L, Schirrmeister H, Reske SN, et al. Is (18)F-fluorodeoxyglucose positron emission tomography in recurrent colorectal cancer a contribution to surgical decision making? *Am J Surg* 2000;180(1):1–5.
49. Kalff VV, Hicks R, Ware R. F-18 FDG PET for suspected or confirmed recurrence of colon cancer. A prospective study of impact and outcome. *Clin Pos Imaging* 2000;3:183.
50. Huebner RH, Park KC, Shepherd JE, et al. A meta-analysis of the literature for whole-body FDG PET detection of colorectal cancer. *J Nucl Med* 2000;41:1177–1189.
51. Gambhir SS, Czernin J, Schimmer J, et al. A tabulated review of the literature. *J Nucl Med* 2001;42[Suppl]:9S–12S.
52. Whiteford MH, Whiteford HM, Yee LF, et al. Usefulness of FDG-PET scan in the assessment of suspected metastatic or recurrent adenocarcinoma of the colon and rectum. *Dis Colon Rectum* 2000;43(6):759–767; discussion 767–770.
53. Berger KL, Nicholson SA, Dehadashti F, et al. FDG PET evaluation of mucinous neoplasms: correlation of FDG uptake with histopathologic features. *AJM Am J Roentgenol* 2000;174(4):1005–1008.
54. Kinkel K, Lu Y, Both M, et al. Detection of hepatic metastases from cancers of the gastrointestinal tract by using noninvasive imaging methods (US, CT, MRimaging, PET): a meta-analysis. *Radiology* 2002;224(3):748–756.
55. Bipat S, van Leeuwen MS, Comans EF, et al. Colorectal liver metastases: CT, MR imaging, and PET for diagnosis—meta analysis. *Radiology* 2005;237:123–131.
56. Strasberg SM, Dehdashti F, Siegel BA, et al. Survival of patients evaluated by FDG PET before hepatic resection for metastatic colorectal carcinoma: a prospective database study. *Ann Surg* 2001;233:320–321.
57. Ruers TJ, Langenhoff BS, Neeleman N, et al. Value of positron emission tomography with [F-18] fluorodeoxyglucose in patients with colorectal liver metastases: a prospective study. *J Clin Oncol* 2002;20 (2):388–395.
58. Meta J, Seltzer M, Schiepers C, et al. Impact of ^{18}F-FDG PET on managing patients with colorectal cancer: the referring physician's perspective. *J Nucl Med* 2001;42:586–590.
59. Fernandez FG, Drebin JA, Linehan DC, et al. Five-year survival after resection of hepatic metastases from colorectal cancer in patients screened by positron emission tomography with F-18 fluorodeoxyglucose (FDG-PET). *Ann Surg* 2004;240(3):438–447; discussion 447–450.
60. Venook A. Critical evaluation of current treatments in metastatic colorectal cancer. *Oncologist* 2005;10:250–261.
61. Findlay M, Young H, Cunningham D, et al. Noninvasive monitoring of tumor metabolism using fluorodeoxyglucose and positron emission tomography in colorectal cancer liver metastases: correlation with tumor response to fluorouracil. *J Clin Oncol* 1996;14:700–708.
62. Kahn H, Alexander A, Ratinic J, et al. Preoperative staging of irradiated rectal cancers using digital rectal examination, computed tomography,

endorectal ultrasound, and magnetic resonance imaging does not accurately predict T0, N0 pathology. *Dis Colon Rectum* 1997;40:140–144.
63. Haberkorn U, Strauss LG, Dimitrakopoulou A, et al. PET studies of fluorodeoxyglucose metabolism in patients with recurrent colorectal tumors receiving radiotherapy. *J Nucl Med* 1991;31:1485–1490.
64. Moore HG, Akhurst T, Larson SM, et al. A case controlled study of 18-fluorodeoxyglucose positron emission tomography in the detection of pelvic recurrence in previously irradiated rectal cancer patients. *J Am Coll Surg* 2003;197(1):22–28.
65. Guillem J, Calle J, Akhurst T, et al. Prospective assessment of primary rectal cancer response to preoperative radiation and chemotherapy using 18-fluorodeoxyglucose positron emission tomography. *Dis Colon Rectum* 2000;43:18–24.
66. Guillem JG, Moore HG, Akhurst T, et al. Sequential preoperative fluorodeoxyglucose-positron emission tomography assessment of response to preoperative chemoradiation: a means for determining long-term outcomes of rectal cancer. *J Am Coll Surg* 2004;199:1–7.
67. Liu LX, Zhang WH, Jiang HC. Current treatment for liver metastases from colorectal cancer. *World J Gastroenterol* 2003;9(2):193–200.
68. Ruers T, Bleichrodt RP. Treatment of liver metastases, an update on the possibilities and results. *Eur J Cancer* 2002;38(7):1023–1033.
69. Gray B, Van Hazel G, Hope M, et al. Randomized trial of Sir-spheres plus chemotherapy vs chemotherapy alone for treating patients with liver metastases from primary large bowel cancer. *Ann Oncol* 2001;12(12):1711–1720.
70. Nijsen JF, van het Schip AD, Hennink WE, et al. Advances in nuclear oncology: microspheres for internal radionuclide therapy of liver tumours. *Curr Med Chem* 2002;9(1):73–82.
71. Vitola JV, Delbeke D, Meranze SG, et al. Positron emission tomography with F-18-fluorodeoxyglucose to evaluate the results of hepatic chemoembolization. *Cancer* 1996;78:2216–2222.
72. Torizuka T, Tamaki N, Inokuma T, et al. Value of fluorine-18-FDG PET to monitor hepatocellular carcinoma after interventional therapy. *J Nucl Med* 1994;35(12):1965–1969.
73. Solbiati L, Livraghi T, Golberg SN, et al. Percutaneous radiofrequency ablation of hepatic metastases from colorectal cancer: long-term results in 117 patients. *Radiology* 2001;221:159–166.
74. Linamond P, Zimmerman P, Raman SS, et al. Interpretation of CT and MRI after radiofrequency ablation of hepatic malignancies. *AJR Am J Roentgenol* 2003;181:1635–1640.
75. Langenhoff BS, Oyen WJ, Jager GJ, et al. Efficacy of fluorine-18-deoxyglucose positron emission tomography in detecting tumor recurrence after local ablative therapy for liver metastases: a prospective study. *J Clin Oncol* 2002;20:4453–4458.
76. Anderson GS, Brinkmann F, Soulen MC, et al. FDG positron emission tomography in the surveillance of hepatic tumors treated with radiofrequency ablation. *Clin Nucl Med* 2003;28:192–197.
77. Ludwig V, Hopper OW, Martin WH, et al. FDG-PET surveillance of hepatic metastases from prostate cancer following radiofrequency ablation—case report. *Am Surg* 2003;69:593–598.
78. Donckier V, Van Laetham JL, Goldman S, et al. Fluorodeoxyglucose positron emission tomography as a tool for early recognition of incomplete tumor destruction after radiofrequency ablation for liver metastases. *J Surg Oncol* 2003;84:215–223.
79. Veit P, Antoch G, Stergar H, et al. Detection of residual tumor after radiofrequency ablation of liver metastasis with dual-modality PET/CT: initial results. *Eur Radiol* 2006;16:80–87.
80. Barker DW, Zagoria RJ, Morton KA, et al. Evaluation of liver metastases after radiofrequency ablation: utility of FDG PET and PET/CT. *AJR Am J Roentgenol* 2005;184:1096–1102.
81. Antoch G, Vogt FM, Veit P, et al. Assessment of liver tissue after radiofrequency ablation: findings with different imaging procedures. *J Nucl Med* 2005;46:520–525.
82. Wong CY, Salem R, Raman S, et al. Evaluating ^{90}Y-glass microsphere treatment response of unresectable colorectal liver metastases by [18F]FDG PET: a comparison with CT or MRI. *Eur J Nucl Med Mol Imaging* 2002;29:815–820.
83. Wong CY, Salem R, Qing F, et al. Metabolic response after intra-arterial ^{90}Y-glass microsphere treatment for colorectal metastases: comparison of quantitative and visual analyses by ^{18}F-FDG PET. *J Nucl Med* 2004;45:1892–1897.
84. Gambhir SS, Valk P, Shepherd J, et al. Cost effective analysis modeling of the role of FDG-PET in the management of patients with recurrent colorectal cancer. *J Nucl Med* 1997;38:90P.
85. Park KC, Schwimmer J, Sheperd JE, et al. Decision analysis for the cost-effective management of recurrent colorectal cancer. *Ann Surg* 2001;233:310–319.
86. Cohade C, Osman M, Leal J, et al. Direct comparison of FDG PET and PET-CT imaging in colorectal carcinoma. *J Nucl Med* 2003;44: 1797–1803.
87. Bar-Shalom R, Yefremov N, Guralnik L, et al. Clinical performance of PET/CT in the evaluation of cancer: additional value for diagnostic imaging and patient management. *J Nucl Med* 2003;44: 1200–1209.
88. Roman CD, Martin WH, Delbeke D. Incremental value of fusion imaging with integrated PET-CT in oncology. *Clin Nucl Med* 2005;30(5): 470–477.
89. Selzner M, Hany TF, Wildbrett P, et al. Does the novel PET/CT imaging modality impact on the treatment of patients with metastatic colorectal cancer of the liver? *Ann Surg* 2004;240:1027–1034.
90. Osman MM, Cohade C, Fishman E, et al. Clinically significant incidental findings on non-contrast CT portion of PET-CT studies: frequency in 250 patients. *J Nucl Med* 2005;46:1252–1355.
91. Dizendorf E, Ciernik IF, Baumert B, et al. Impact of integrated PET/CT scanning on external beam radiation treatment planning. *J Nucl Med* 2002;43:33P.
92. Ciernik IF, Dizendorf E, Baumert BG, et al. Radiation treatment planning with integrated positron emission and computed tomography (PET/CT): a feasibility study. *Int J Radiat Oncol Biol Phys* 2003;57(3): 853–863.
93. Kubota R, Yamada S, Kubota K, et al. Intratumoral distribution of fluorine-18-fluorodeoxyglucose *in vivo*: high accumulation in macrophages and granulocytes studied by microautoradiography. *J Nucl Med* 1992;33:1972–1980.
94. Blau M, Nagler W, Bender MA. A new isotope for bone scanning. *J Nucl Med* 1962;3:332–334.
95. Bang S, Baug CA. Topographical distribution of fluoride in iliac bone of a fluoride-treated osteoporotic patient. *J Bone Miner Res* 1990;5: S87–S89.
96. Shields AF, Grierson JR, Dohmen BM, et al. Imaging proliferation in vivo with [F-18]FLT and positron emission tomography. *Nat Med* 1998;4:1334–1336.
97. Francis DL, Visvikis D, Costa DC, et al. Potential impact of [(18)F]3′-deoxy-3′-fluorothymidine versus [(18)F]fluoro-2-deoxy-D-glucose in positron emission tomography for colorectal cancer. *Eur J Nucl Med Imaging* 2003;30(7):988–994.

CHAPTER

8.15 Pancreatic and Hepatobiliary Cancers

OLEG TEYTELBOYM, DOMINIQUE DELBEKE, AND RICHARD L. WAHL

PANCREATIC CARCINOMA

Pancreatic ductal adenocarcinoma is the most common type of pancreatic cancer, accounting for 5% of cancer related deaths in the United States (1). Pancreatic adenocarcinoma is characterized by diagnosis occurring when the disease is quite advanced, aggressive behavior with invasion into adjacent soft tissues, lymph nodal and hepatic metastasis, and a generally poor prognosis. Early diagnosis in a localized state and prompt and complete surgical resection offer the only opportunity for cure. The preoperative diagnosis, staging, and treatment of pancreatic adenocarcinoma remain challenging. Imaging of pancreatic carcinoma can be separated into several distinct tasks: (a) detecting the presence of a pancreatic mass, (b) lesion characterization, (c) image guidance for biopsy, (d) detection of unresectable disease, (e) detection of recurrent disease, and (f) monitoring therapy response.

Limitations of Conventional Imaging Modalities

Pancreatic cancer is most commonly initially detected by computed tomography (CT), presenting as a hypoenhancing mass (on intravenous [IV] contrast CT), causing obstruction of the common bile duct and or pancreatic duct. CT currently is the most common diagnostic imaging modality used in the preoperative diagnosis and staging of pancreatic cancer. Application of dual-phase CT protocols has been reported to demonstrate 97% sensitivity and 92% positive predictive value for pancreatic tumor detection, 75% sensitivity for hepatic metastasis, 54% sensitivity for nodal metastasis, with an overall 91% accuracy for determining nonresectability (2). Evolution of CT technology has significantly improved assessment of vascular involvement and invasion of adjacent organs. Recent studies have demonstrated negative predictive value of 100% for detection of vascular invasion and 87% negative predictive value for overall resectability (3). However, since many pancreatic cancers recur, including locally, the true definition of "resectability" probably shows somewhat limited good performance.

Unfortunately, interpretation of the CT scan is sometimes difficult in the setting of mass-forming pancreatitis or questionable findings such as enlargement of the pancreatic head without definite signs of malignancy or a discrete mass (4,5). Further, a variety of characteristics have been described to determine vascular invasion, which is on a continuum of certainty. The diagnosis of locoregional lymph node metastases is also difficult with CT because such nodes often are small. In addition, subcentimeter hepatic metastases cannot reliably be differentiated from cysts and hemangiomas (6).

The diagnostic performance of magnetic resonance imaging (MRI) remains similar to that of CT (7–10). Even with the latest technology improvements, MRI demonstrates sensitivity of 86% and specificity of 89% for detection of pancreatic tumors (11). Although MRI is probably superior to CT for evaluation of hepatic metastases, lower spatial resolution makes detection of small lymph nodes even more difficult.

Endoscopic ultrasonography (EUS) has a limited field of view but offers the possibility of tissue diagnosis with fine-needle aspiration (FNA) biopsy, with reported diagnostic yield of 68% and diagnostic accuracy of 74.4% (12). However, reported overall diagnostic rate, sensitivity, and negative predictive value of FNA biopsies guided using CT (97.7%, 94.9%, and 60%, respectively) are not significantly different from those guided using EUS (88.9%, 85%, and 57.1%, respectively) (13). Although both methods of biopsy offer definitive tissue diagnosis, there remains a substantial rate of inconclusive results. Biopsy accuracy is, of course, dependent on sampling the proper tissue, and false-negative biopsies can occur due to sampling errors.

The difficulty in making a preoperative diagnosis is associated with two types of adverse outcomes. First, less-aggressive surgeons may abort attempted resection due to a lack of tissue diagnosis. This is borne out by the significant rate of "reoperative" pancreaticoduodenectomy performed at major referral centers (14–16). A second type of adverse outcome, generated by failure to obtain a preoperative diagnosis, occurs when more aggressive surgeons inadvertently resect benign disease. This is particularly notable in those patients who present with suspected malignancy without an associated mass on CT scan. This has been reported to occur in up to 55% of patients in some series (17). Another adverse outcome can be aggressive surgical resection for "cure" of disease that is already systemically metastatic, if diagnostic testing is inadequately sensitive.

18-F Fluorodeoxyglucose PET in the Preoperative Diagnosis of Pancreatic Carcinoma

Metabolic imaging with fluorine-18 ([^{18}F])-fluorodeoxyglucose (FDG) positron emission tomography (PET) can be used to improve the accuracy of the preoperative diagnosis of pancreatic carcinoma by differentiating benign and malignant pancreatic masses (Fig. 8.15.1). Most malignancies, including pancreatic carcinoma, demonstrate increased glucose utilization due to an increased number of glucose transporter (GLUT) proteins and increased hexokinase and phosphofructokinase activity (18,19). There is evidence that the overexpression of GLUTs by malignant pancreatic cells contributes to the increased uptake of FDG by these neoplasms (20,21).

In 10 studies (22–31), the performance of FDG PET to differentiate benign from malignant lesions ranged from 85% to 100% for sensitivity, 67% to 99% for specificity, and 85% to 93% for accuracy. In most of these studies, the accuracy of FDG PET imaging was superior to that of CT. For example, in the study of Delbeke et al. (31), the sensitivity and specificity of FDG PET imaging was 92% and 85%, respectively, compared with 65% and 62%, respectively, for CT. In another study, 28% of patients had indeterminate or unrecognized pancreatic masses on CT clarified with FDG PET, while again demonstrating higher sensitivity and specificity than CT in correctly diagnosing pancreatic carcinoma (92% and 85% vs. 65% and 62%) (32). Additionally, this study showed that the sensitivity of CT imaging improves with the size of the lesion, but the sensitivity of FDG PET is not as dependent on lesion size (32). However, such findings are at variance with the principles of physics, and certainly at very small lesion sizes, both PET and CT would be expected to have diminished performance simply due to impaired signal detection. A recent review by Pakzad et al. (33) suggested that the overall detection sensitivity for PET at diagnosis varies between 90% and 95% and specificity from 82% to 100%, whereas for staging, sensitivity data vary from 61% to 100% and specificity data from 67% to 100% for PET.

Based on the then available data, the European Consensus Conference designated FDG PET as an established indication for differentiation of benign and malignant pancreatic masses (34). However, it is important to keep in mind that these studies do not reflect current clinical practice as PET/CT has rapidly replaced PET at most institutions. Further, uses in Europe are not uniform by country or provider.

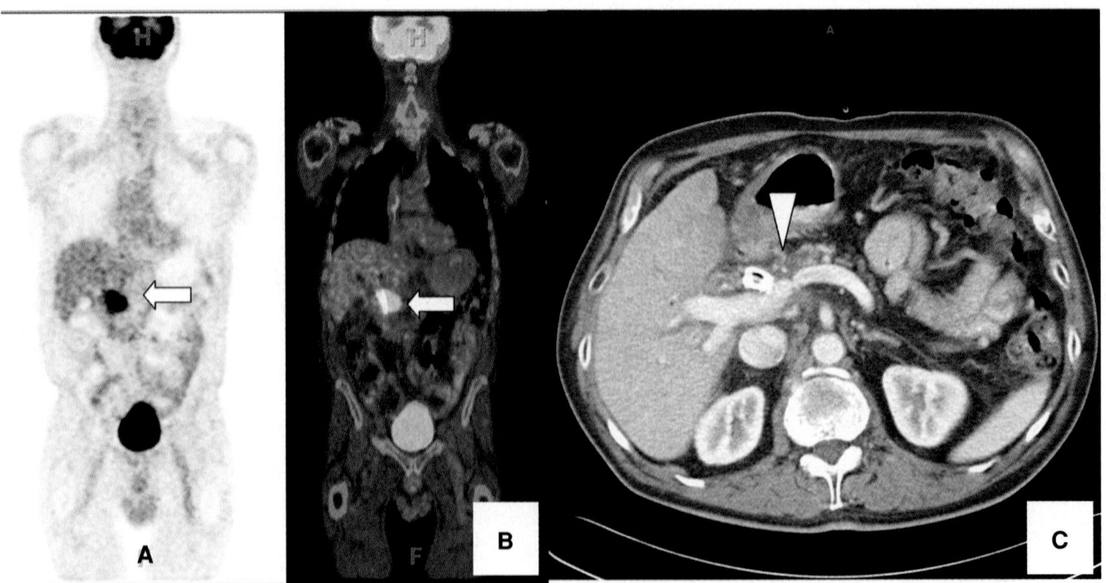

FIGURE 8.15.1. Locally advanced pancreatic adenocarcinoma. **A:** Coronal fluorodeoxyglucose (FDG) PET and (**B**) PET/CT fusion images demonstrate intensely FDG-avid tumor in the pancreatic head (*arrow*). **C:** Venous phase axial CT image demonstrates a hypodense tumor in the pancreatic head (*arrowhead*), narrowing the portal confluence.

There is evidence that the degree of FDG uptake has prognostic value. Nakata et al. (35) noted a correlation between standard uptake value (SUV) and survival in 14 patients with pancreatic adenocarcinoma. Patients with an SUV higher than 3.0 had a mean survival of 5 months, compared with 14 months in those with an SUV lower than 3.0. In a multivariate analysis of 52 patients with pancreatic carcinoma (36), the median survival of patients with an SUV higher than 6.1 was 5 months, compared with 9 months for patients with an SUV lower than 6.1.

Limitations of Fluorodeoxyglucose PET Imaging

As with any imaging modality, FDG PET has limitations in the evaluation of pancreatic cancer. The high incidence of glucose intolerance and diabetes exhibited by patients with pancreatic pathology represents a potential limitation of this modality in the diagnosis of pancreatic cancer. Elevated serum glucose levels result in decreased FDG uptake in tumors due to competitive inhibition; low SUVs with false-negative FDG PET scans have been noted in hyperglycemic patients. Several studies have reported a lower sensitivity in hyperglycemic compared with euglycemic patients (24,28,31). For example, in a study of 106 patients with a disease prevalence of 70% (28), FDG PET had a sensitivity of 98% in a subgroup of euglycemic patients versus 63% in hyperglycemic patients. This has led some investigators to suggest that the SUV be corrected according to serum glucose level (37–41). Although a study of 86 pancreatic lesions by Koyama et al. (41) demonstrated only modestly improved sensitivity and negative predictive value of serum glucose corrected SUV compared to uncorrected SUV (91% and 73% vs. 89% and 70%).

In the studies of Delbeke et al. (31) and Diederichs et al. (40), the presence of elevated serum glucose levels and/or diabetes mellitus may have contributed to false-negative interpretations; but correction of the SUV for serum glucose level has not significantly improved the sensitivity of FDG PET in the diagnosis of pancreatic carcinoma. The true impact of serum glucose levels on the accuracy of FDG PET in pancreatic cancer and other neoplasms remains somewhat controversial, although it is clear that elevated serum glucose levels can reduce tumor FDG uptake significantly.

False-negative study results may also occur when the tumor diameter is less than 1 cm (i.e., small ampullary carcinoma). Ampullary carcinomas arise from the ampulla of Vater and have a better prognosis than pancreatic carcinoma because they cause biliary obstruction and are diagnosed earlier in the course of the disease. The detection rate with FDG imaging is only 70% to 80%, probably because of their smaller size at the time of clinical presentation. In addition, such lesions can be located immediately adjoining bowel, which can be FDG avid, thus lowering tumor/background uptake ratios.

Both glucose and FDG are substrates for cellular mediators of inflammation. Some benign inflammatory lesions, including chronic and acute pancreatitis, can accumulate FDG and result in false-positive interpretations on PET images (24,27,42,43). However, Koyama et al. (41) reported significant differences in SUV of benign and malignant lesions by using an SUV cutoff of 2.1. Even better results were reported by Nakamoto et al. (44) in a study of 49 patients by obtaining an additional 2-hour delayed scan, showing diagnostic accuracy of 91.5% compared to 83% for standard protocol in differentiating malignant and benign lesions of the pancreas. Nakamoto et al. (44) also documented that SUVs of malignant lesions increase over time in comparison with those of benign pancreatic lesions after injection of FDG. Similar results were reported by Nitzsche et al. (45), who performed kinetic analysis of FDG uptake in normal patients and patients with acute pancreatitis, chronic pancreatitis, or pancreatic cancer. Recently, fairly high accuracy was observed in the differentiation of chronic pancreatitis from cancer. In 87% (67 of 77) of the patients with chronic pancreatitis, pancreatic FDG accumulation was absent. Six patients had significant accumulation of FDG, most likely due to active inflammation. In patients with pancreatic cancer, 24 of 26 patients had a positive PET scan. In practice, cancers are usually focal, while pancreatitis is usually diffuse. In some instances, it can be impossible to tell the two conditions apart, especially where there is, for example, mass-forming pancreatitis present.

FDG PET imaging is complementary to CT in the evaluation of patients with pancreatic masses or in whom the diagnosis of pancreatic carcinoma is suspected. In view of the probable decreased sensitivity seen in patients with hyperglycemia, the acquisition of PET images should be performed under controlled metabolic conditions and in the absence of acute inflammatory abdominal disease. If FDG PET findings are equivocal, measurement of FDG kinetics and or delayed images can be performed to differentiate between benign and malignant processes. In practice, parametric imaging is feasible only when dynamic image data are collected; thus, this can usually only be done prospectively. Close correlation with anatomic images is, of course, required for optimal imaging accuracy.

Fluorodeoxyglucose PET for Staging Pancreatic Carcinoma

Pancreatic adenocarcinoma is staged by the tumor, node, metastases (TNM) system (Tables 8.15.1 and 8.15.2). The resectability of a local tumor is determined by whether the tumor extends into major arterial structures and whether long segment involvement, or occlusion, of major venous structures is present (46). TNM classification has recently been updated to reflect advances in surgical technique permitting venous interposition grafts. Local extent of the tumor can only be evaluated with anatomic imaging modalities, which demonstrate the relationship between the tumor, adjacent organs, and vascular structures. Functional imaging modalities cannot replace anatomic imaging in the assessment of local tumor resectability. Even fusion imaging with FDG PET/CT may not significantly improve local staging given the limited intrinsic PET resolution, but this has not been fully resolved. PET can certainly help identify additional foci of disease that may help define resectability.

Sixty percent of patients presenting with pancreatic adenocarcinoma have advanced disease (47) (Figs. 8.15.2 and 8.15.3). Detection of nodal and peritoneal disease remains a challenge with all imaging modalities. FDG imaging is not consistently superior to helical CT for node staging but is more accurate than CT for metastases staging—but this area warrants further study with PET/CT. Reported FDG PET sensitivity and specificity for lymph node staging is 49% and 63%, respectively (40). In a study by Delbeke et al. (31), metastases were diagnosed both on CT and on PET in 10 of 21 patients with stage IV disease, but PET demonstrated hepatic metastases not identified or equivocal on CT and/or distant metastases unsuspected clinically in seven additional patients (33%). In four patients (19%), neither CT nor PET imaging showed evidence of metastases, but surgical exploration revealed carcinomatosis in three and a small liver metastasis in one patient.

TABLE 8.15.1 Tumor, Node, Metastases Classification for the Staging of Pancreatic Cancer

T (Tumor)	
TX	Primary tumor not assessed.
Tis	Carcinoma *in situ*
T1	Tumor is ≤2 cm in maximum diameter and confined to pancreas.
T2	Tumor is >2 cm and confined to pancreas
T3	Tumor extends beyond pancreas but does not involve celiac axis or superior mesenteric artery
T4	Primary tumor involves either celiac axis or superior mesenteric artery
N (Nodal involvement)	
NX	Regional lymph nodes not assessed
NO	No involvement of regional lymph nodes
N1	Involvement of regional lymph nodes
M (Metastases)	
MX	Distant metastasis cannot be assessed
MO	No distant metastases
M1	Distant metastasis present

(From Tamm EP, Silverman PM, Charnsangavej C, et al. Diagnosis, staging, and surveillance of pancreatic cancer. AJR Am J Roentgenol 2003;180:1311–1123, with permission.)

FDG PET is sensitive for detection of hepatic metastases, but false-positive findings have been reported in the livers of patients with dilated bile ducts and inflammatory granulomas (48). In a study by Diederichs et al. (40) FDG PET demonstrated sensitivity of 70% and a specificity of 95% for liver metastases, with sensitivity decreasing as lesion size decreased. A direct comparison of PET and MRI with hepatocyte iron contrast showed the MRI technique to be more sensitive, especially for small hepatic lesions, than was PET/CT. On a per patient basis, MRI and FDG PET were comparable in performance, with sensitivities of 96.6% and 93.3%, and accuracies of 97.1% and 85.3%, respectively. However, per-lesion analysis showed MRI to have a higher sensitivity than FDG PET at 81.4% and 67.0%, respectively. PET detected only about 40% of the lesions seen by MRI that were less than 1 cm in diameter. Although MRI liver specific contrast is not yet routinely available, these data do indicate that while PET is a sensitive tool for metastatic pancreatic cancer to the liver, the sensitivity is not as high as can probably ultimately be achieved with MRI given the superior resolution of MRI versus PET. In that study, PET did detect extrahepatic lesions missed by MRI, so the techniques are clearly complementary.

Impact of Fluorodeoxyglucose PET on the Management of Patients with Pancreatic Carcinoma

The rate at which FDG PET may lead to alterations in clinical management clearly depends on the specific therapeutic philosophy employed by the evaluating surgeon. In the study of Delbeke et al. (31), the surgeons advocated pancreaticoduodenectomy only for those patients with potentially curable pancreatic cancer. They also took an aggressive approach to resection, including *en bloc* retroperitoneal lymphadenectomy and selective resection of the superior mesenteric-portal vein confluence when necessary. Most patients with nonmalignant biliary strictures were managed without resection. In that series of 65 patients, the application of FDG PET imaging, in addition to CT, altered the surgical management in 41% of the patients, 27% by detecting CT-occult pancreatic carcinoma, and 14% by identifying unsuspected distant metastases, or by clarifying the benign nature of lesions equivocal on CT (31).

Fluorodeoxyglucose PET for Detection of Recurrent Pancreatic Carcinoma

FDG PET utility for monitoring of patients with pancreatic adenocarcinoma after surgical therapy, chemotherapy, and radiation has been confirmed in several studies (32,50,51) (Fig. 8.15.4). For example, Ruf et al. (50) evaluated 39 patients with subsequently

TABLE 8.15.2 Tumor, Node, Metastases Staging of Pancreatic Cancer

Stage	Description	TNM Levels	Comment
I	Resectable	T1–2 NO MO	No extrapancreatic disease No encasement of celiac axis or superior mesenteric artery
II	Typically resectable	T1–2 N1 MO T3 NO–1 MO	Regional lymph nodes may be involved No encasement of celiac axis or superior mesenteric artery May be extrapancreatic involvement
III	Unresectable	T4 NO–1 MO	Regional lymph nodes may be involved Encasement of celiac axis or superior mesenteric artery
IV	Unresectable	Any T any N M1	Liver, peritoneal, lung metastases

N, node; M, metastases; T, tumor.
(From Eriksson B, Orlefors H, Oberg K, et al. Developments in PET for the detection of endocrine tumours. Best Pract Res Clin Endocrinol Metab 2005;19:311–324, with permission.)

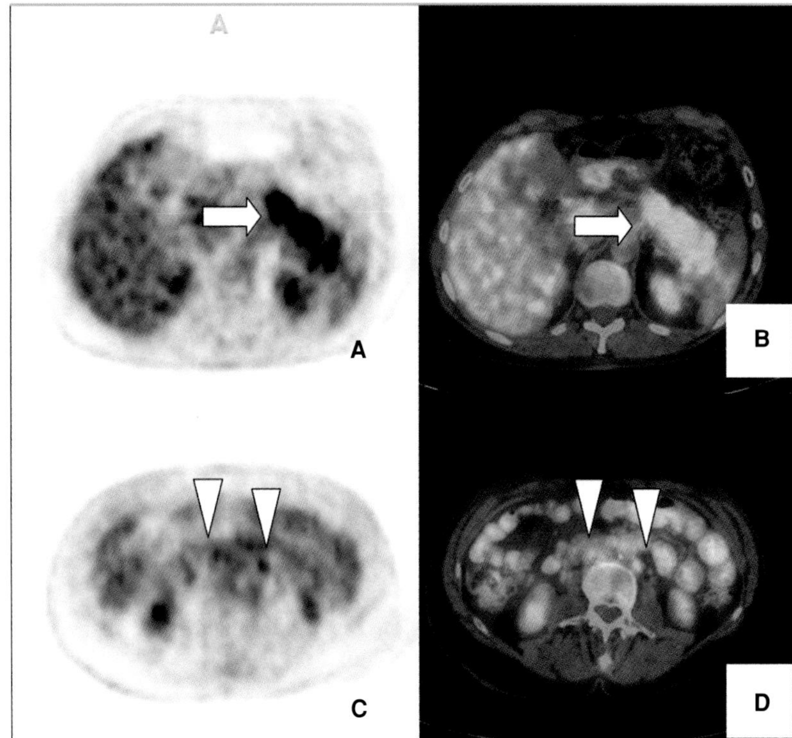

FIGURE 8.15.2. Pancreatic adenocarcinoma with lymph node metastasis at presentation. **A:** Axial fluorodeoxyglucose (FDG) PET and (**B**) PET/CT fusion images demonstrate intensely FDG-avid primary tumor in the pancreatic tail (*arrow*). **C:** Axial FDG PET and (**D**) PET/CT fusion images demonstrate smaller and somewhat lower-intensity, FDG-avid para-aortic lymph node metastasis (*arrowheads*).

confirmed recurrence after surgery, demonstrating that FDG PET reliably detected local and nonlocoregional recurrences, whereas CT-MRI was more sensitive for the detection of hepatic metastases. Of 25 patients with local recurrences on follow-up, initial imaging suggested relapse in 23 patients. Of these, FDG PET detected 96% (22 of 23) and CT-MRI 39% (9 of 23). Among 12 liver metastases, FDG PET detected 42% (5 of 12). CT-MRI detected 92% (11 of 12) correctly. Moreover, seven of nine abdominal lesions were malignant on follow-up, of which FDG PET detected seven of seven and CT-MRI detected none. Additionally, FDG PET detected extra-abdominal metastases in two patients.

Another study of 19 patients concluded that FDG PET added important incremental information in 50% of the patients, resulting in a change of therapeutic procedure (49). This included

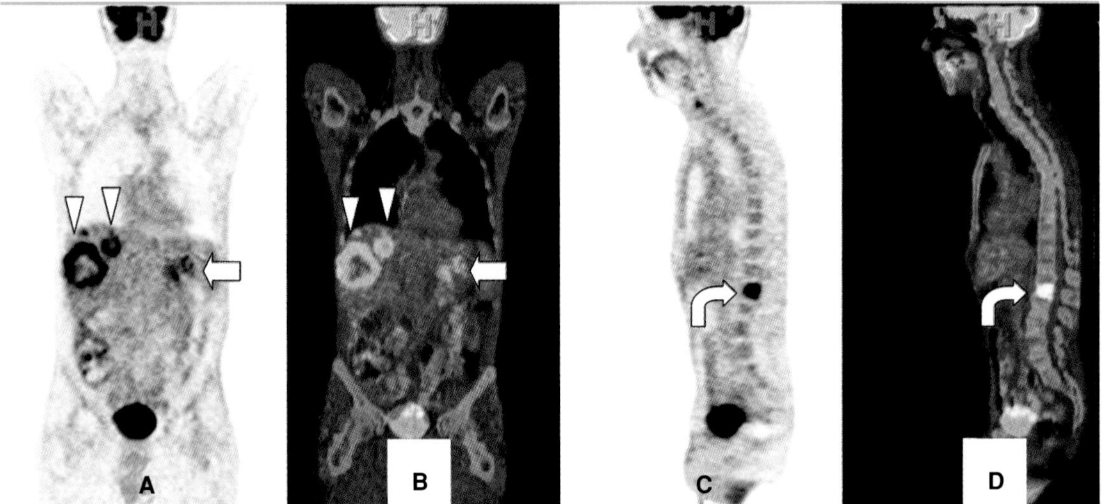

FIGURE 8.15.3. Pancreatic adenocarcinoma with distant metastasis at presentation. **A:** Coronal fluorodeoxyglucose (FDG) PET and (**B**) PET/CT fusion images demonstrate intensely FDG-avid primary tumor in the pancreatic tail (*arrow*) and hepatic metastasis. Central photopenia in these lesions is due to central necrosis. **C:** Sagittal FDG PET and (**D**) PET/CT fusion images demonstrate intensely FDG-avid vertebral body metastasis (*curved arrow*).

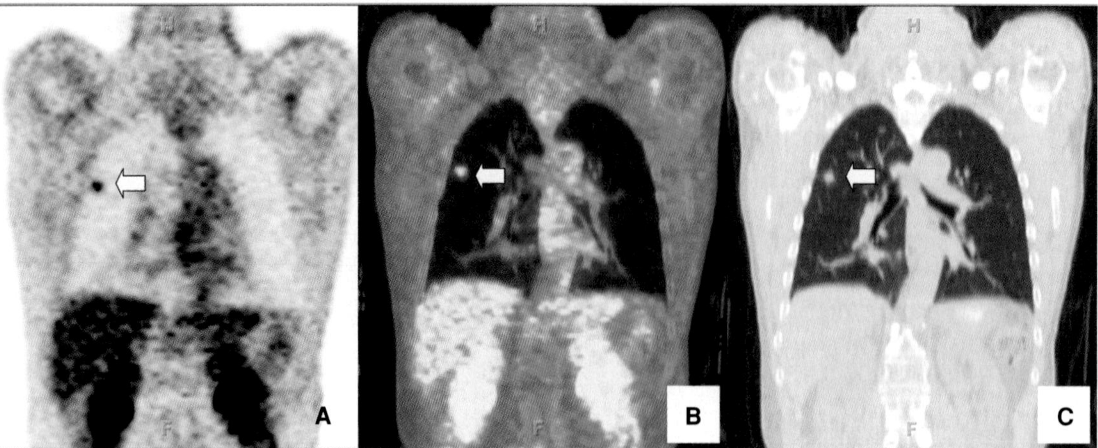

FIGURE 8.15.4. Pancreatic adenocarcinoma recurrence with lung metastasis in a patient after undergoing a Whipple procedure. **A:** Coronal fluorodeoxyglucose (FDG) PET, (**B**) PET/CT fusion, and (**C**) corresponding CT images demonstrate intensely FDG-avid lung nodule (*arrow*) consistent with metastatic disease.

patients with elevated serum tumor marker levels but no findings on anatomic imaging. Therefore, FDG PET may be particularly useful when (a) CT identifies an indistinct region of change in the bed of the resected pancreas that is difficult to differentiate from postoperative or postradiation fibrosis, (b) for the evaluation of new hepatic lesions that may be too small to biopsy, and (c) in patients with rising serum tumor marker levels and a negative conventional work-up. Given the poor prognosis of pancreatic cancer, it is not expected that large differences in patient outcome will result from such studies. However, it is probable that patients will benefit by giving the most appropriate treatment while eliminating treatments viewed as unlikely to be effective. The presentation of recurrent tumor may overlap substantially with that of pancreatic insufficiency or radiation enteritis, and accurate diagnosis is essential given the markedly different treatment approaches.

Fluorodeoxyglucose PET for Monitoring Therapy

In a study by Higashi et al. (51), FDG PET was useful in monitoring patients after intraoperative radiotherapy for unresectable pancreatic cancer, because the decrease in metabolism in pancreatic cancer could be detected earlier than the decrease in tumor size (Fig. 8.15.5).

A pilot study by Rose et al. (32), determined that FDG PET imaging might be useful for the assessment of tumor response to neoadjuvant therapy and the evaluation of suspected recurrent disease after resection. Nine patients underwent FDG PET imaging before and after neoadjuvant chemoradiation therapy. FDG PET successfully predicted histologic evidence of chemoradiation-induced tumor necrosis in the four patients who demonstrated at least a 50% reduction in tumor SUV after chemoradiation. Among these patients, none showed a measurable reduction in tumor diameter, as assessed by CT. This is consistent with past data that showed a more rapid drop in tumor glucose metabolism levels than the changes in tumor size. The four patients who had FDG PET evidence of tumor response went on to successful resection, all showing 20% to 80% tumor necrosis in the resected specimen. Three patients showed stable FDG uptake and two showed increasing FDG uptake indicative of tumor progression. Among the two patients with progressive disease demonstrated by FDG PET, one showed tumor progression on CT and the other demonstrated stable disease. Among the five patients who showed no response by FDG PET, the disease could be subsequently resected in only two, and only one patient who underwent resection showed evidence of chemoradiation-induced necrosis in the resected specimen.

Another pilot study suggests that the absence of FDG uptake at 1 month after chemotherapy is an indicator of improved survival versus patients in whom persistent uptake is present (52). Definitive conclusions regarding the role of FDG PET in assessing treatment response will obviously require evaluation in much larger populations of patients. However, given the poor track record of CT in assessing histologic response to neoadjuvant chemoradiation, the potential utility of FDG PET in this capacity deserves further investigation.

Fluorodeoxyglucose PET for Evaluation of Cystic Pancreatic Neoplasms

Evaluation of cystic pancreatic lesions has been a challenge for all imaging modalities. There is significant overlap between benign and malignant disease on both CT and MRI. FDG PET may be superior to CT in differentiating benign from malignant pancreatic cystic lesions. Sperti et al. (53) evaluated 56 patients with suspected cystic tumors, demonstrating FDG PET is more accurate than CT in identifying malignant pancreatic cystic lesions (Fig. 8.15.6). Sensitivity, specificity, and positive and negative predictive values for [^{18}F]-FDG PET and CT scanning in detecting malignant tumors were 94%, 97%, 94%, and 97% and 65%, 87%, 69%, and 85%, respectively.

A study of 39 patients with cystic pancreatic tumors by Tann et al. (54) compared CT, PET, and combined PET/CT images for determining whether cystic pancreatic tumors are malignant, demonstrating improved sensitivity of PET-CT in comparison to CT or PET only. Sensitivities of CT, PET, and combined PET/CT images were 67% to 71%, 57%, and 86%, respectively. Specificities of CT, PET, and combined PET/CT images were 87% to 90%, 65%, and 91%, respectively.

More studies are required to define the role of FDG PET in imaging of cystic pancreatic lesion; however, the available data indicate that FDG PET can play an important role with positive result

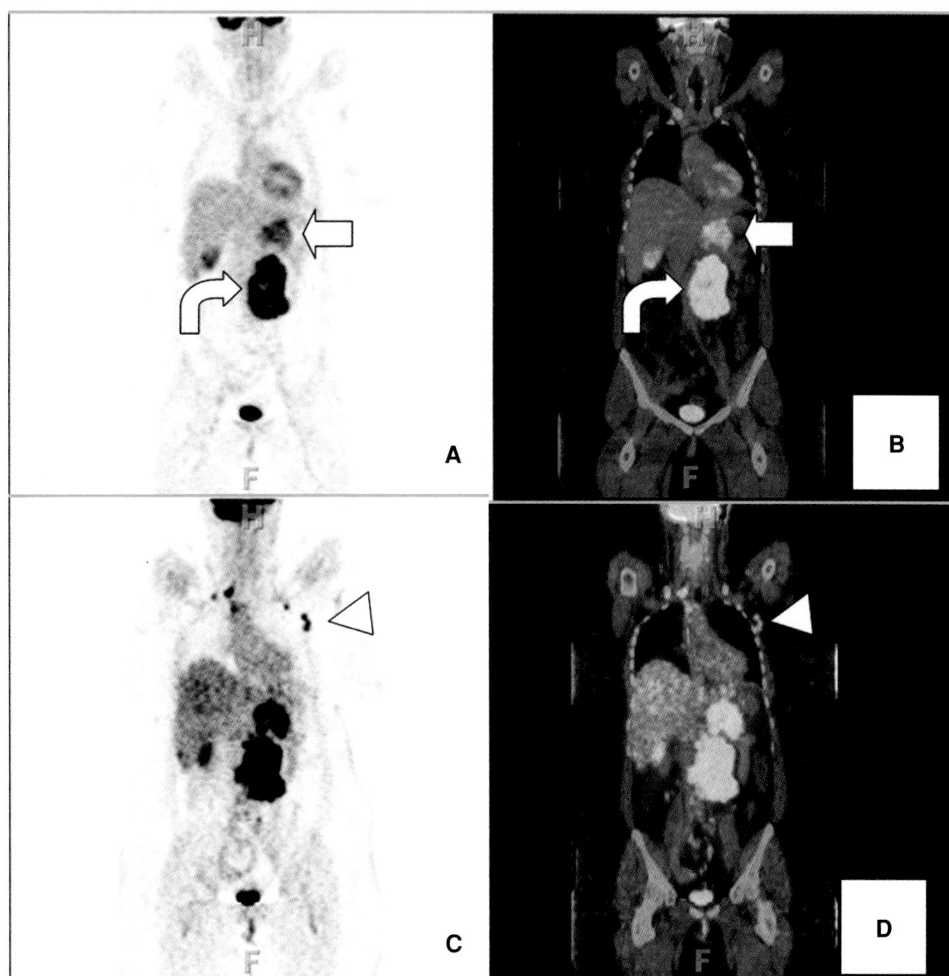

FIGURE 8.15.5. Pancreatic adenocarcinoma follow-up after chemotherapy. **A:** Coronal fluorodeoxyglucose (FDG) PET and (**B**) PET/CT fusion images demonstrate intensely FDG-avid pancreatic mass (*straight arrow*) and widespread metastatic disease (*curved arrow*). Six months later (**C**) coronal FDG PET and (**D**) PET/CT fusion images demonstrate disease progression, including the left axilla and other nodes (*arrowhead*).

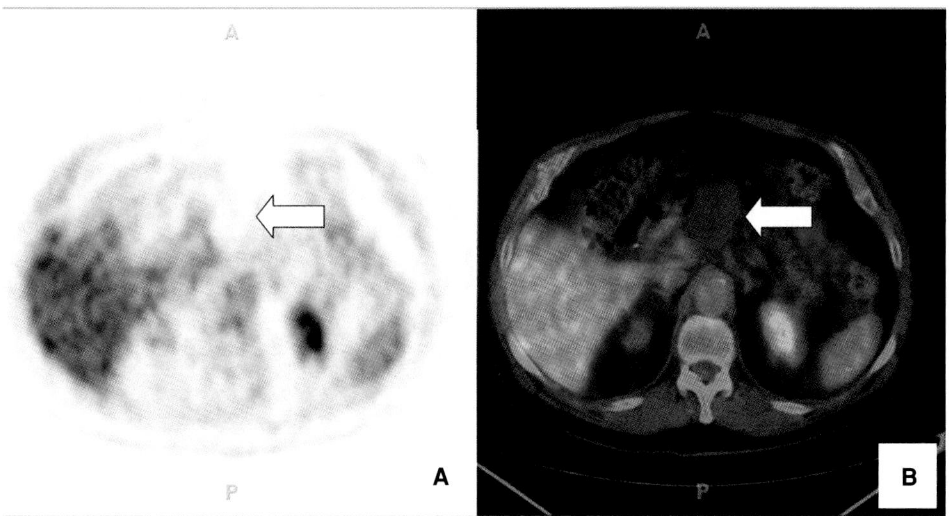

FIGURE 8.15.6. Pancreatic serous cystadenoma. **A:** Axial fluorodeoxyglucose (FDG) PET and (**B**) PET/CT fusion images demonstrate no FDG uptake in the cystic pancreatic lesion (*arrow*), suggesting benign etiology.

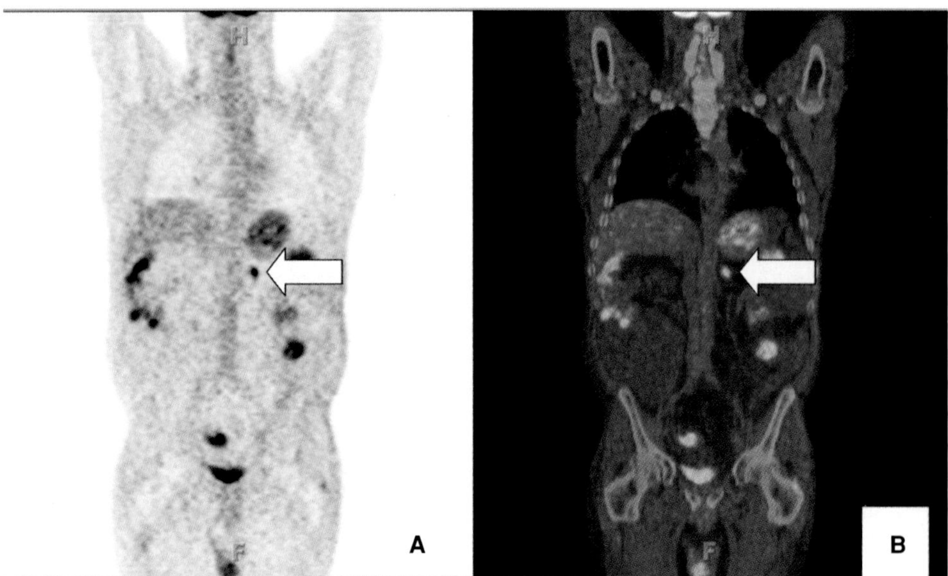

FIGURE 8.15.7. Recurrent fluorodeoxyglucose (FDG)-avid neuroendocrine neoplasm in para-aortic region (arrow). **A:** Coronal FDG PET and (**B**) PET/CT fusion images demonstrate intense FDG uptake in this lesion consistent with active tumor.

strongly suggesting malignancy. A negative result in a cystic pancreatic mass is suggestive of a benign lesion that may be treated more conservatively with follow-up, biopsy, or more limited resection in selected high-risk patients. An additional observation is that as CT techniques have improved, small cystic lesions appear more frequently using the 1.25 mm thickness slices than was the case with thicker slices. PET is expected to be challenged in evaluating very small pancreatic lesions due to resolution limitations.

Fluorodeoxyglucose PET for Evaluation of Endocrine Pancreatic Neoplasms

The endocrine tumors of the pancreas are composed of cells with a neuroendocrine phenotype. They can be classified as well-differentiated tumors, well-differentiated carcinomas, poorly differentiated carcinomas, functioning (insulinomas, gastrinomas, glucagonomas, etc.) and nonfunctioning tumors (55). Imaging of pancreatic endocrine tumors can be very challenging, since even tiny tumors can become symptomatic due to hormonal secretion. Furthermore, some of these tumors can be extrapancreatic, making detection even more difficult.

Gadolinium-enhanced MRI, CT, somatostatin receptor imaging with indium-111-pentetreotide, and endoscopic ultrasonography have all been reported to be useful for the detection and staging of pancreatic endocrine neoplasms (56–60). FDG PET does not improve detection of pancreatic neuroendocrine tumors compared to anatomic imaging, particularly if the tumor is small at presentation (Fig. 8.15.7). In a study by Nakamoto et al. (61), the sensitivity of FDG PET was 53%, whereas those of ultrasound, CT, and MRI were 53%, 50%, and 53%, respectively. In 9 of 19 tumors that were not detected by FDG PET, seven were small tumors, ranging from 1.5 to 8 mm in diameter, and were not identified by other imaging methods.

Endocrine tumors have the unique characteristics of taking up and decarboxylating amine precursors like L-DOPA (3,4 dihydroxy-L-phenylalanine) and 5-hydroxy-L-tryptophan, offering highly specific targets for PET tracers (62). In a study by Kauhanen et al. (63), seven of eight insulinomas were detected by [^{18}F]-DOPA PET, demonstrating superior performance to CT and MRI.

Several studies have also demonstrated promising results in diagnosing pancreatic endocrine tumors with carbon-11 ([^{11}C])-5-hydroxy-L-tryptopha, copper-64 ([^{64}Cu])-TETA-octreotide, and [^{11}C]-DOPA (64–66). Gallium-68-somatostatin receptor binding peptides also appear promising (67). Although more studies are required to further define the role of amine precursor PET tracers, patients with pancreatic endocrine tumors undetectable on anatomic imaging are likely to benefit from imaging with these PET tracers.

Summary: Pancreatic Cancer

FDG PET imaging appears to be a reasonably sensitive and specific adjunct to CT when applied to the preoperative diagnosis of pancreatic adenocarcinoma, particularly in patients with suspected pancreatic cancer in whom CT fails to identify a discrete tumor mass. PET/CT has also shown reasonable accuracy as a tool for characterizing pancreatic masses as malignant or benign. By providing preoperative documentation of pancreatic malignancy in these patients, laparotomy may be undertaken with a curative intent, and the risk of aborting resection due to diagnostic uncertainty is minimized. FDG PET imaging is also useful in detection of CT-occult metastatic disease, allowing nontherapeutic resection to be avoided altogether in this group of patients. Radiation therapy planning may also be possible using PET/CT methods. As is true with other neoplasms, FDG PET holds promise in the restaging of patients posttherapy. Rapid evolution of technology with widespread use of PET/CT will likely demonstrate increased diagnostic accuracy of fusion imaging compared to FDG PET or CT alone.

HEPATOBILIARY TUMORS

In the United States, metastases to the liver occur 20 times more often than primary hepatic carcinoma and are often multifocal. Although many tumors may metastasize to the liver, the most common primaries producing liver metastases are colorectal, gastric, pancreatic, lung, and breast carcinomas. Ninety percent of malignant primary liver tumors are epithelial in origin: hepatocellular carcinoma (HCC) and cholangiocarcinoma. Mesenchymal tumors such as angiosarcomas, epithelioid angioendothelioma, and primary lymphoma are relatively rare malignant tumors that can affect the liver.

Hepatocellular carcinoma is the most common primary hepatic tumor arising from malignant transformation of hepatocytes. It typically occurs in the setting of chronic liver disease due to viral hepatitis, alcohol, or in patients exposed to carcinogens. HCC is the fourth most common cause of cancer-related deaths in the world and is becoming increasingly common in the United States due to hepatitis C epidemic (68–70). Once cirrhosis is present, HCC develops in 1% to 4% of patients yearly (71). However, in North America, 42.6% of HCCs arose in noncirrhotic livers (72). HCC most frequently metastasizes to regional lymph nodes, lungs, and the skeleton. HCC is often associated with elevated serum levels of α-fetoprotein (AFP).

Cholangiocarcinomas account for approximately 30% of primary hepatic neoplasm (73,74). Adenocarcinoma is the most common histological subtype, arising from intra- or extrahepatic bile duct epithelium. About 20% of patients who develop cholangiocarcinomas have predisposing conditions, including sclerosing cholangitis, ulcerative colitis, Caroli disease, choledochal cyst, infestation by the fluke Clonorchis sinensis, cholelithiasis, or, rarely (and now, mainly historically) exposure to thorotrast (73–75).

Approximately 50% of cholangiocarcinomas occur in the liver and the other 50% are extrahepatic (73,74). These tumors are often unresectable at the time of diagnosis and have a poor prognosis. Intrahepatic cholangiocarcinomas can be further subdivided in two categories: the peripheral type arising from the interlobular biliary duct and the hilar type (Klatskin tumor) arising from the main hepatic duct or its bifurcation. In addition, they can develop in three morphologic types: infiltrating sclerosing lesions (most common), exophytic lesions, and polypoid intraluminal masses. Malignant tumors arising along the extrahepatic bile ducts are usually diagnosed early, because they cause biliary obstruction. Tumors arising near the hilum of the liver have a worse prognosis because of their direct extension into the liver and their unresectability. Distant metastases occur late in the disease and most often affect lungs.

Gallbladder carcinoma is the most common type of biliary cancer and is the fifth most common gastrointestinal malignancy, accounting for approximately 6,500 deaths per year in the United States (76). Adenocarcinoma is the most common histologic subtype, representing approximately 90% of the tumors. Gallbladder carcinoma is associated with porcelain gallbladder and chronic inflammation by gallstones (77). These tumors are insidious and usually unsuspected clinically until advanced disease is present. Gallbladder carcinoma is characterized by invasion into the liver and other adjacent tissues. The tumor can spread to regional lymph nodes and also frequently demonstrates intraperitoneal spread. Hematogenous metastases usually occur in advanced disease, most commonly involving lungs, liver, and bones.

Conventional Imaging Modalities for Evaluation of Hepatic Lesions

Ultrasound, dual phase contrast CT, and MRI are the standard modalities usually employed for hepatic imaging. The typical diagnostic issues include early detection of primary hepatic malignancies, differentiation from cirrhosis and other benign liver lesions, and evaluation of the response to therapy.

HCC screening has been recommended by an expert panel from the European Association for the Study of the Liver for cirrhotic patients (78). There are no randomized controlled clinical trials concerning survival benefit of HCC surveillance in patients with chronic liver disease. However, HCC screening with ultrasound and AFP serum levels in cirrhotic patients demonstrated survival benefit in retrospective or uncontrolled prospective studies (79–81). The sensitivity and specificity of AFP screening depends on the AFP threshold and the population risk of HCC. In a study by Trevisani et al. (82), the positive predictive value of an AFP level greater than 20 μg/L was only 21.5% at a 5% tumor prevalence in patients with viral hepatitis. AFP levels greater than 400 μg/L increases the positive predictive value to 60% to 97%, depending on the underlying population; however, it is generally considered diagnostic of HCC, especially when a liver mass is visualized at ultrasound or CT (82,83).

The sensitivity of ultrasound in the detection of HCC ranges from 35% to 84% (83–85). However, ultrasound is highly operator- and patient size dependent, likely accounting for the difference in sensitivity. CT is the conventional method used for assessing the liver at many institutions. Dual phase protocols with arterial and portal venous phase imaging take advantage of early arterial phase enhancement of most HCCs. In a literature review by Fung et al. (86), sensitivities of spiral CT for HCC nodules from nonexplant studies were 92% to 95% and the sensitivities from explant studies were just 53.8% to 71%, respectively.

MRI is also extensively used for hepatic imaging, permitting lesion characterization based on the enhancement pattern and intrinsic T1 and T2 signal properties. MRI may be slighter superior to CT, as in the review by Fung et al. (86), reporting sensitivities of 75% to 94% for HCC nodules from nonexplant studies and sensitivities of 53% to 77% from explant studies.

Diagnosis of HCC can be established noninvasively for patients with cirrhosis if a nodule with arterial hypervascularization is greater than 2 cm in diameter and AFP levels are greater than 400 μg/L (78,86). For the diagnosis of HCC not exceeding 2 cm diameter, biopsy of the nodule is recommended because the imaging techniques do not have sufficient accuracy to distinguish HCC from other benign or malignant conditions, and the AFP level is usually within normal values or is only slightly elevated (78,86).

Extrahepatic tumors are usually detected because of biliary ductal obstruction. Magnetic resonance cholangiopancreatography (MRCP) and endoscopic retrograde cholangiopancreatography (ERCP) are the two most commonly used techniques for evaluation of biliary obstruction. In a study by Park et al. (87), sensitivity, specificity, and accuracy of the two methods for differentiation of malignant from benign causes of biliary stricture were 81%, 70%, and 76%, respectively, for MRCP and 74%, 70%, and 72%, respectively, for ERCP.

Intrahepatic cholangiocarcinomas can be peripheral or central, producing variable amount of biliary obstruction. Peripheral tumors usually become symptomatic at more advanced stages of the disease. Detection of these tumors can be challenging with any imaging modality because of poor contrast enhancement on CT and MRI. Delayed contrast CT has been reported to improve tumor detection with reported sensitivity of 74% to 82% (88,89) and may be partially attributable to high fibrous content of these tumors.

Distinct patterns of enhancement have also been reported on MRI, exhibiting minimal or moderate initial rim enhancement followed by progressive and concentric filling with the contrast agent (90). MRI may also demonstrate intrahepatic bile duct dilatation or low T2 signals that are not commonly seen with metastatic disease.

Fluorodeoxyglucose PET in the Diagnosis of Hepatocellular Carcinoma

Differentiated hepatocytes normally have relatively high glucose-6-phosphatase activity, which allows dephosphorylation of intracellular FDG-6 phosphate to FDG and its egress from the liver. Although experimental studies have shown that glycogenesis decreases and glycolysis increases during carcinogenesis, the accumulation of FDG in HCC is variable, at least in part, due to varying degrees of activity of the enzyme glucose-6-phosphatase in these tumors (91,92). It has been postulated that FDG PET evaluation of liver tumors, particularly HCCs, will require dynamic imaging with blood sampling and kinetic analysis. Kinetic analysis is cumbersome to perform clinically and cannot be performed over the entire body, thus preventing staging. Studies using kinetic analysis have shown that the phosphorylation kinetic constant for glucose (k3) is elevated in the vast majority of HCCs. The dephosphorylation kinetic constant for FDG-6-phosphate to FDG (k4) is low in metastatic lesions and in cholangiocarcinomas, resulting in intratumoral accumulation of FDG. But k4 is similar to k3 for HCCs that do not accumulate FDG (93–95). Therefore, HCCs are hypermetabolic, but many do not accumulate FDG due to their inability to retain FDG intracellularly.

There are three patterns of uptake for HCC: FDG uptake higher than, equal to, or lower than liver background (55%, 30%, and 15%, respectively) (Fig. 8.15.8). FDG PET detects only 50% to 70% of HCCs but has a sensitivity of more than 90% for all other primaries (cholangiocarcinoma and sarcoma) and nearly all metastatic tumors to the liver, at least in their untreated state (96,97). Delayed imaging at 2 or 3 hours after FDG injection may increase FDG PET sensitivity (98,99). Lin et al. (98) reported 62.5% sensitivity for HCC detection on the 2- and 3-hour images compared to 56.3% on the 1-hour image. Imaging at 3 hours resulted in better tumor to background ratio than imaging at 2 hours, but did not increase the diagnostic sensitivity (98). Benign tumors, including focal nodular hyperplasia, adenoma, regenerating nodules, cysts, and hemangiomas typically demonstrate FDG uptake at the same level as normal liver. Abscesses or granulomatous inflammation will

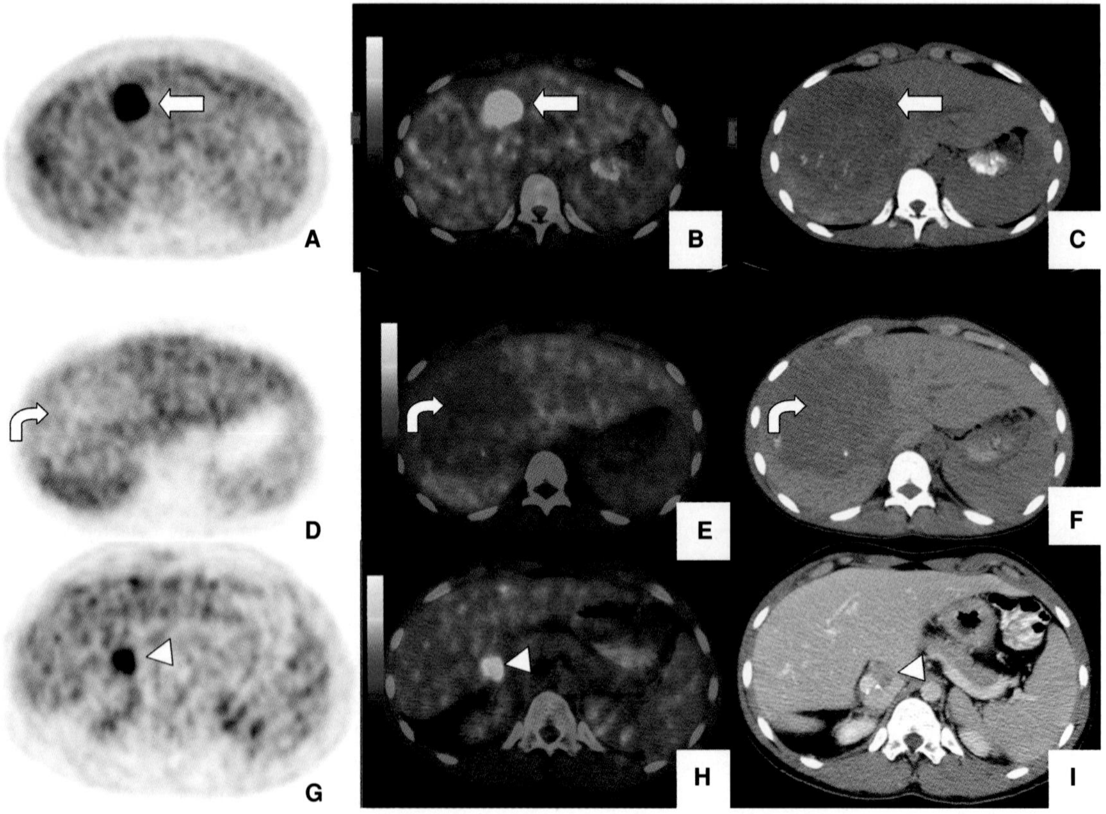

FIGURE 8.15.8. Hepatocellular carcinoma with increased fluorodeoxyglucose (FDG) uptake. **A:** Axial FDG PET, (**B**) PET/CT fusion, and (**C**) corresponding CT images demonstrate intensely FDG-avid focus of viable tumor (*arrow*) in periphery of the lesion that has been previously treated by chemoembolization. However, carbon-11-acetate (**D**) axial PET, (**E**) PET/CT fusion, and (**F**) corresponding CT images demonstrate no increased uptake by the viable tumor (*curved arrow*). On 6-month follow-up after subsequent resection, (**G**) axial FDG PET, (**H**) PET/CT fusion, and (**I**) corresponding intravenous contrast-enhanced CT images demonstrate intensely FDG-avid retroperitoneal lymph node (*arrowhead*), indicating recurrent disease.

commonly have higher levels of FDG uptake than normal liver. In addition, a positive correlation has been found between the degree of FDG uptake, including both the SUV and k3, and the grade of malignancy (94,95).

FDG imaging may have prognostic significance in the evaluation of patients with HCC. HCCs that accumulate FDG tend to be moderately to poorly differentiated and are associated with markedly elevated AFP levels (100,101). However, FDG PET has been reported to have only limited value for the differential diagnosis of focal liver lesions in patients with chronic hepatitis C virus infection because of the low sensitivity for the detection of HCC and the high prevalence of this tumor in that population of patients (102).

Fluorodeoxyglucose PET for Staging Hepatocellular Carcinoma

In patients with HCC that accumulate FDG, PET imaging is able to detect unsuspected regional and distant metastases, as with other tumors (103,104). In some cases, FDG PET is the only imaging modality that can demonstrate the tumor and its metastases. In a study by Sugiyama et al. (104), FDG PET had 83% sensitivity (24 of 29 metastases) for extrahepatic metastases larger than 1 cm in greatest diameter and 13% (1 of 8 metastases) for lesions less than or equal to 1 cm. PET revealed two bone metastases not depicted by bone scan and detected the nodal metastasis and intestinal metastases inconclusive on CT. No false-positive lesions were seen.

Fluorodeoxyglucose PET for Monitoring Therapy and Detection of Recurrent Hepatocellular Carcinoma

Surgical resection is often not possible for many patients with HCC because of advanced-stage tumors or underlying cirrhosis with impaired hepatic reserve. Nonsurgical treatment options include hepatic arterial chemoembolization, systemic chemotherapy, surgical cryoablation, ethanol ablation, radiofrequency ablation, and liver transplantation. In patients treated with hepatic arterial chemoembolization, FDG PET is more accurate than lipiodol retention on CT in predicting the presence of residual viable tumor. Due to the associated inflammatory response, it is recommended that FDG imaging be delayed for at least several weeks after ablative therapy. The presence of residual uptake in some lesions can help in guiding further regional therapy (105–107). However, dynamic MRI has become the standard of care for monitoring local response, with a reported 100% sensitivity and specificity, although these figures obviously may be diminished in smaller lesions, at least based on the physic principle for detectability (108).

FDG PET can be helpful in patients with treated HCC who have rising AFP levels and no detectable disease on anatomic imaging. In a study of 26 patients with previously treated HCC by Chen et al. (109), the sensitivity, specificity, and accuracy of FDG PET for detecting HCC recurrence was 73.3%, 100%, and 74.2%, respectively.

Carbon-11-Acetate and Dual-Tracer PET for Evaluation of Hepatocellular Carcinoma

There is growing evidence that [^{11}C]-acetate PET is complementary to FDG in the detection of primary HCC (Fig. 8.15.9) (110–112). Carbon-11-acetate is a metabolic substrate of β-oxidation, precursors of amino acid, fatty acid, and sterol, and is useful in evaluation for various malignancies (113). In a study by Ho et al. (110), HCC lesions nonapparent with [^{18}F]-FDG were detected by [^{11}C]-acetate, with none of the tumors missed by both tracers. The tracer uptake by the tumors was related to the tumor differentiation with preferential uptake of [^{11}C]-acetate by well-differentiated HCCs and FDG uptake by poorly differentiated tumors. Carbon-11-acetate was also highly specific for HCC, with no accumulation in cholangiocarcinoma or metastasis to the liver.

A follow-up study by Ho et al. (111) showed the value of dual-tracer PET/CT for evaluation of HCC metastasis, demonstrating 98% sensitivity, 86% specificity, and 96% accuracy in the detection of HCC metastasis on a per patient basis. The lesion-based and patient-based detection by both tracers was complementary, with 60% and 64% sensitivities by [^{11}C]-acetate, and 77% and 79% sensitivities by FDG. Since higher grade HCCs tend to be more FDG avid, metastasis were more likely to be detected with FDG. However, [^{11}C]-acetate was a better trace for detection of metastasis in patients previously treated for primary HCC and who had no evidence of local recurrence. Clinically significant changes in management were found in patients with true-positive metastasis, of whom 19% were affected by [^{11}C]-acetate PET alone (114). Carbon-11-choline–related compounds have also been used for detection of HCC, although the normal liver already has substantial choline accumulation.

Fluorodeoxyglucose PET for Evaluation of Biliary Tumors

There are multiple reports confirming utility of FDG PET in evaluation for cholangiocarcinoma with reported sensitivity of 61% to 90% (97,115–119) (Figs. 8.15.10 and 8.15.11). In a study by Anderson et al. (117), FDG PET was more helpful in patients with nodular cholangiocarcinomas (85% sensitivity) than in those with the infiltrating variety (18% sensitivity). Infiltrating cholangiocarcinoma may not have sufficient cellular density required to form a lesion that can be detected by PET, given 4 to 5 mm intrinsic resolution of modern PET cameras. False-positive findings can be seen in patients with biliary stents, probably related to inflammatory changes, as well as in patients with acute cholangitis (115,117).

In the study by Anderson et al. (117), FDG PET had 65% sensitivity for metastatic disease in patients with cholangiocarcinoma (11 of 17), resulting in significant change of management of these patients since the metastatic disease was unsuspected on other imaging modalities. PET imaging was falsely negative for metastatic disease in patients with carcinomatosis (three of three), which was subsequently discovered during surgery. All extra-abdominal metastases (six of six) were detected by FDG PET.

There is evidence that FDG PET imaging may be useful in the diagnosis and management of small cholangiocarcinomas in patients with primary sclerosing cholangitis (PSC) (115,116). Dynamic FDG PET appears superior to conventional imaging techniques for both detection and exclusion of cholangiocarcinoma in advanced PSC, and may be useful for screening for cholangiocarcinoma in the pretransplant evaluation of patients with PSC. In a study by Prytz et al. (116), dynamic FDG PET was performed in 24 consecutive patients with PSC within 2 weeks after listing for liver transplantation and with no evidence of malignancy on CT, MRI, or ultrasound. Three patients had cholangiocarcinomas that were correctly identified by PET. Dynamic FDG PET was negative in one patient with high-grade hilar duct dysplasia and was false positive in one patient with epithelioid granulomas in the liver.

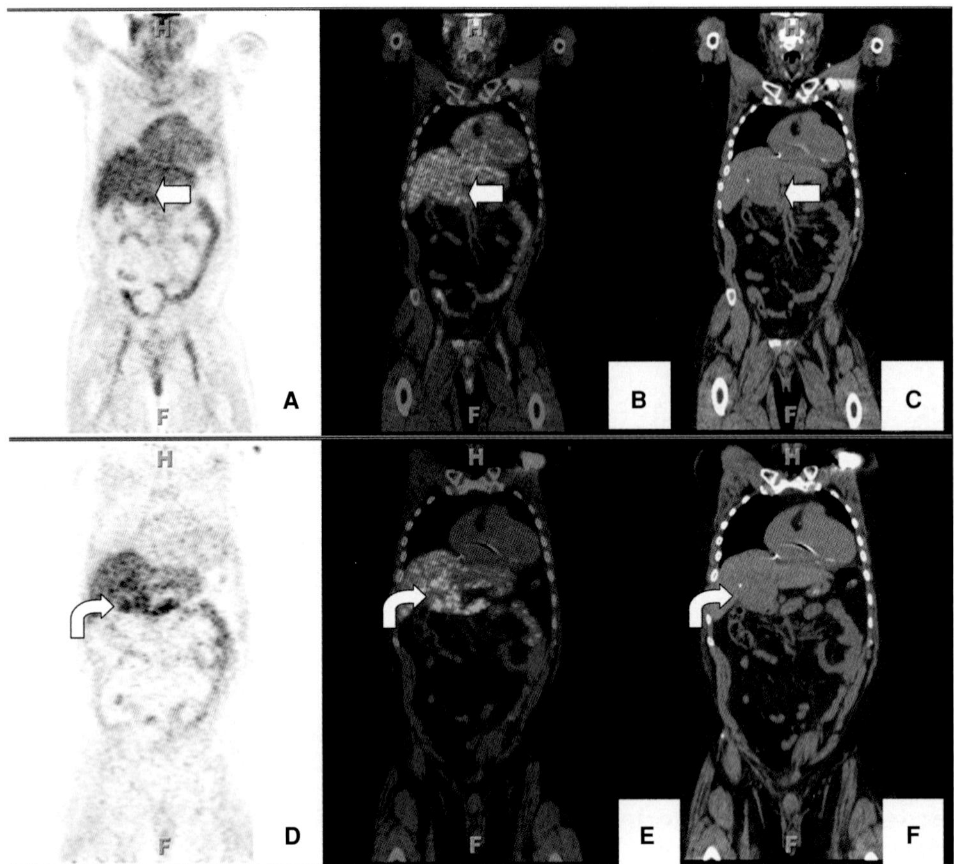

FIGURE 8.15.9. Hepatocellular carcinoma with increased carbon-11 (^{11}C)-acetate uptake. **A:** Axial fluorodeoxyglucose (FDG) PET, (**B**) PET/CT fusion, and (**C**) corresponding CT images demonstrate FDG uptake by the tumor (*arrow*) at the level of normal liver. However, ^{11}C-acetate (**D**) axial PET, (**E**) PET/CT fusion, and (**F**) corresponding CT images demonstrate moderately intense uptake by the tumor (*curved arrow*), compared to normal hepatic parenchyma. (Courtesy of Dr. Hubert Chuang, Johns Hopkins Hospital.)

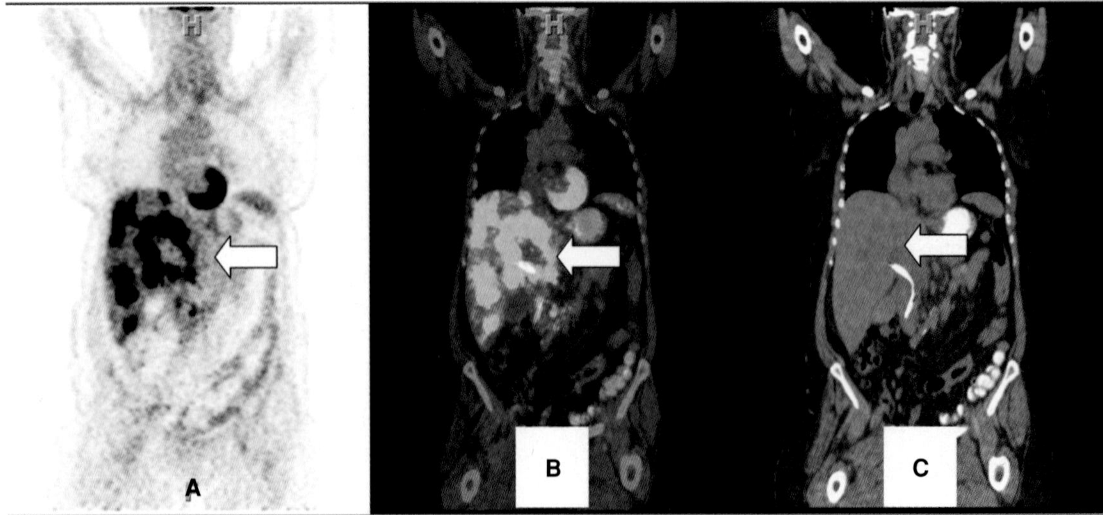

FIGURE 8.15.10. Cholangiocarcinoma with hepatic metastasis at presentation. **A:** Coronal fluorodeoxyglucose (FDG) PET, (**B**) PET/CT fusion, and (**C**) corresponding CT images demonstrate intensely FDG-avid primary tumor (*arrow*) and multiple hepatic metastases.

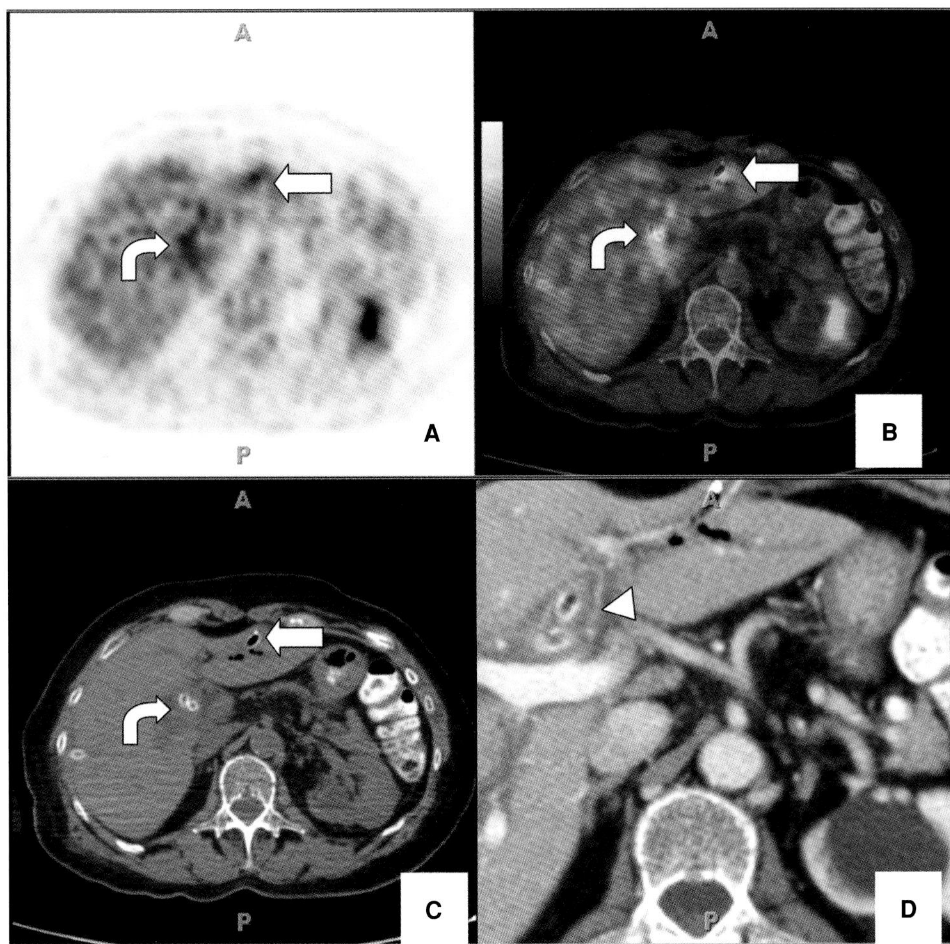

FIGURE 8.15.11. Cholangiocarcinoma and intense fluorodeoxyglucose (FDG) uptake around the biliary drainage catheter. **A:** Axial FDG PET, (**B**) PET/CT fusion, and (**C**) corresponding CT images demonstrate intense FDG uptake in the biliary hilum (*curved arrow*) due to the tumor or catheter-related inflammation. However, intense FDG uptake in the left hepatic lobe (*arrow*) is due to catheter-induced inflammation. **D:** Intravenous contrast-enhanced CT demonstrates hypoenhancing cholangiocarcinoma infiltrating along the biliary tree. In some instances, it can be very difficult to separate cholangiocarcinoma from stent/catheter-related inflammation.

FDG PET is not usually used for evaluation of primary gallbladder carcinoma since most patients are diagnosed incidentally after cholecystectomy (Fig. 8.15.12). Therefore, FDG PET is typically used for initial staging after cholecystectomy or restaging when recurrence is suspected. Occult gallbladder carcinoma found after laparoscopic cholecystectomy has been associated with reports of gallbladder carcinoma seeding of laparoscopic trochar sites (120,121). Increased FDG uptake has been demonstrated in gallbladder carcinoma (122) and has been helpful in identifying recurrence in the area of the incision when CT could not differentiate scar tissue from malignant recurrence (123). In the study by Anderson et al. (117), the overall sensitivity of FDG PET for residual gallbladder carcinoma was 78% and the specificity was 80%. The one false-positive result was seen in a patient after a recent cholecystectomy. The sensitivity for detecting metastatic gallbladder carcinoma was 56% due to an inability to detect carcinomatosis (117). Addition of delayed imaging may improve differentiating between malignant and benign lesions, with Nishiyama et al. (124) reporting a sensitivity increase from 82.6% to 95.7% and 100% for delayed imaging and combined early and delayed imaging, with SUV cutoffs of 4.5 (early) and 2.9 (delayed), and retention index of –8. However, the specificity decreased from 55.6% to 44.4% for delayed imaging and combined early and delayed imaging, respectively

Summary: Hepatobiliary Cancers

Nearly all secondary malignant hepatic tumors are FDG avid, and most benign processes accumulate FDG to the same level as normal hepatic parenchyma. Nearly all cholangiocarcinoma and cancers of the gallbladder are FDG avid as well. Approximately one third to one half of HCCs, particularly the low-grade tumors, do not accumulate FDG. However, higher grade tumors are more likely to metastasize, increasing the utility of FDG PET for staging or detecting tumor recurrence. There is growing evidence that [^{11}C]-acetate PET is complementary to FDG for evaluation of HCC, with preferential uptake in well-differentiated tumors. Dual-tracer PET/CT can have a significant impact on patient care by improving the accuracy of staging and detecting recurrent disease. Unfortunately,

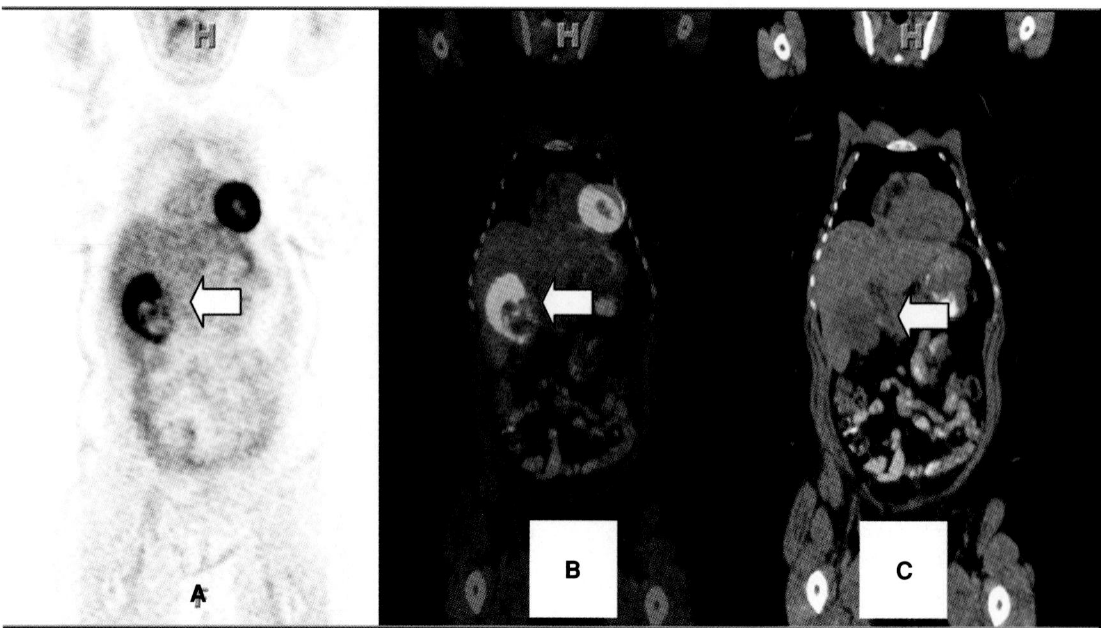

FIGURE 8.15.12. Gallbladder carcinoma. **A:** Coronal fluorodeoxyglucose (FDG) PET, (**B**) PET/CT fusion, and (**C**) corresponding CT images demonstrate FDG uptake by the tumor (*arrow*) that is invading the liver.

the 20-minute half-life of [^{11}C] is a major limitation to availability of this technique.

FDG PET may have an important role for evaluation of biliary malignancies by detecting unsuspected distant metastases. In addition, FDG PET imaging may be useful in the diagnosis and management of small cholangiocarcinomas in patients with primary sclerosing cholangitis. However, FDG PET has a high false-negative rate for infiltrating cholangiocarcinoma and for detection of low-volume peritoneal carcinomatosis. Inflammation along biliary stents, from acute cholangitis, or recent cholecystectomy can reduce specificity of FDG PET for residual or recurrent biliary neoplasm as well.

REFERENCES

1. American Cancer Society. *Cancer facts and figures 2007: year 2007 surveillance research from the American Cancer Society*. Bethesda, MD: American Cancer Society, 2007.
2. Diehl SJ, Lehman KJ, Sadick M, et al. Pancreatic cancer: value of dual-phase helical CT in assessing resectability. *Radiology* 1998;206:373–378.
3. Vargas R, Nino-Murcia M, Trueblood W, et al. MDCT in pancreatic adenocarcinoma: prediction of vascular invasion and resectability using a multiphasic technique with curved planar reformations. *AJR Am J Roentgenol* 2004;182:419–425.
4. Johnson PT, Outwater EK. Pancreatic carcinoma versus chronic pancreatitis: dynamic MR imaging. *Radiology* 1999;212(1):213–218.
5. Lammer J, Herlinger H, Zalaudek G, et al. Pseudotumorous pancreatitis. *Gastrointest Radiol* 1995;10:59–67.
6. Bluemke DA, Cameron IL, Hurban RH, et al. Potentially resectable pancreatic adenocarcinoma: spiral CT assessment with surgical and pathologic correlation. *Radiology* 1995;197:381–385.
7. Bluemke DA, Fishman EK. CT and MR evaluation of pancreatic cancer. *Surg Oncol Clin North Am* 1998;7:103–124.
8. Catalano C, Pavone P, Laghi A, et al. Pancreatic adenocarcinoma: combination of MR angiography and MR cholangiopancreatography for the diagnosis and assessment of resectability. *Eur Radiol* 1998;8: 428–434.
9. Irie H, Honda H, Kaneko K, et al. Comparison of helical CT and MR imaging in detecting and staging small pancreatic adenocarcinoma. *Abdom Imaging* 1997;22:429–433.
10. Trede M, Rumstadt B, Wendl, et al. Ultrafast magnetic resonance imaging improves the staging of pancreatic tumors. *Ann Surg* 1997;226: 393–405.
11. Birchard KR, Semelka RC, Hyslop WB, et al. Evaluation of pancreatic cancer by MRI. *AJR Am J Roentgenol* 2005;185:700–703.
12. Voss M, Hammel P, Molas G, et al. Value of endoscopic ultrasound guided fine needle aspiration biopsy in the diagnosis of solid pancreatic masses. *Gut* 2000;46:244–249.
13. Erturk SM, Mortele KJ, Tuncali K, et al. Fine-needle aspiration biopsy of solid pancreatic masses: comparison of CT and endoscopic sonography guidance. *AJR Am J Roentgenol* 2006;187(6):1531–1535.
14. McGuire GE, Pitt HA, Lillemoe KD, et al. Reoperative surgery for periampullary adenocarcinoma. *Arch Surg* 1991;126:1205–1212.
15. Tyler DS, Evans DB. Reoperative pancreaticoduodenectomy. *Ann Surg* 1994;219:211–221.
16. Robinson EK, Lee JE, Lowy AM, et al. Reoperative pancreaticoduodenectomy for periampullary carcinoma. *Am J Surg* 1996;172:432–438.
17. Thompson JS, Murayama KM, Edney JA, et al. Pancreaticoduodenectomy for suspected but unproven malignancy. *Am J Surg* 1994;169:571–575.
18. Flier JS, Mueckler MM, Usher P, et al. Elevated levels of glucose transport and transporter messenger RNA are induced by ras or src oncogenes. *Science* 1987;235:1492–1495.
19. Monakhov NK, Neistadt EL, Shavlovskil MM, et al. Physiochemical properties and isoenzyme composition of hexokinase from normal and malignant human tissues. *J Natl Cancer Inst* 1978;61:27–34.
20. Higashi T, Tamaki N, Honda T, et al. Expression of glucose transporters in human pancreatic tumors compared with increased F-18 FDG accumulation in PET study. *J Nucl Med* 1997;38:1337–1344.
21. Reske S, Grillenberger KG, Glatting G, et al. Overexpression of glucose transporter 1 and increased F-18 FDG uptake in pancreatic carcinoma. *J Nucl Med* 1997;38:1344–1348.
22. Bares R, Klever P, Hauptmann S, et al. F-18-fluorodeoxyglucose PET *in vivo* evaluation of pancreatic glucose metabolism for detection of pancreatic cancer. *Radiology* 1994;192:79–86.

23. Stollfuss JC, Glatting G, Friess H, et al. 2-(Fluorine-18)-fluoro-2-deoxy-D-glucose PET in detection of pancreatic cancer: value of quantitative image interpretation. *Radiology* 1995;195:339–344.
24. Inokuma T, Tamaki N, Torizuka T, et al. Evaluation of pancreatic tumors with positron emission tomography and F-18 fluorodeoxyglucose: comparison with CT and US. *Radiology* 1995;195:345–352.
25. Kato T, Fukatsu H, Ito K, et al. Fluorodeoxyglucose positron emission tomography in pancreatic cancer: an unsolved problem. *Eur J Nucl Med* 1995;22:32–39.
26. Friess H, Langhans J, Ebert M, et al. Diagnosis of pancreatic cancer by 2[F-18]-fluoro-2-deoxy-D-glucose positron emission tomography. *Gut* 1995;36:771–777.
27. Ho CL, Dehdashti F, Griffeth LK, et al. FDG PET evaluation of indeterminate pancreatic masses. *Comput Assisted Tomogr* 1996;20:363–369.
28. Zimny M, Bares R, Fass J, et al. Fluorine-18 fluorodeoxyglucose positron emission tomography in the differential diagnosis of pancreatic carcinoma: a report of 106 cases. *Eur J Nucl Med* 1997;24:678–682.
29. Keogan MT, Tyler D, Clark L, et al. Diagnosis of pancreatic carcinoma: role of FDG PET. *AJR Am J Roentgenol* 1998;171:1565–1570.
30. Imdahl SA, Nitzsche E, Krautmann F, et al. Evaluation of positron emission tomography with 2-[^{18}F]fluoro-2-deoxy-D-glucose for the differentiation of chronic pancreatitis and pancreatic cancer. *Br J Surg* 1999;86(2):194–199.
31. Delbeke D, Chapman WC, Pinson CW, et al. F-18 fluorodeoxyglucose imaging with positron emission tomography (FDG PET) has a significant impact on diagnosis and management of pancreatic ductal adenocarcinoma. *J Nucl Med* 1999;40:1784–1792.
32. Rose DM, Delbeke D, Beauchamp RD, et al. 18-Fluorodeoxyglucose-positron emission tomography (^{18}FDG-PET) in the management of patients with suspected pancreatic cancer. *Ann Surg* 1999;229: 729–738.
33. Pakzad F, Groves AM, Ell PJ. The role of positron emission tomography in the management of pancreatic cancer. *Sem Nucl Med* 2006; 36(3): 248–256.
34. Reske SN, Kotzerke J. FDG-PET for clinical use. Results of the 3rd German Interdisciplinary Consensus Conference, "Onko-PET III", 21 July and 19 September 2000. *Eur J Nucl Med* 2001;28:1707–1723.
35. Nakata B, Chung YS, Nishimura S, et al. ^{18}F-fluorodeoxyglucose positron emission tomography and the prognosis of patients with pancreatic carcinoma. *Cancer* 1997;79:695–699.
36. Zimny M, Fass J, Bares R, et al. Fluorodeoxyglucose positron emission tomography and the prognosis of pancreatic carcinoma. *Scand J Gastroenterol* 2000;35:883–888.
37. Wahl RL, Henry CA, Ethrer SP. Serum glucose: effects on tumor and normal tissue accumulation of 2-[F-18]-fluoro-2-deoxy-D-glucose in rodents with mammary carcinoma. *Radiology* 1992;183:643–647.
38. Lindholm P, Minn H, Leskinen-Kallio S, et al. Influence of the blood glucose concentration on FDG uptake in cancer—a PET study. *J Nucl Med* 1993;34:1–6.
39. Diederichs CG, Staib L, Glatting G, et al. FDG PET: elevated plasma glucose reduces both uptake and detection rate of pancreatic malignancies. *J Nucl Med* 1998;39:1030–1033.
40. Diederichs CG, Staib L, Vogel J, et al. Values and limitations of FDG PET with preoperative evaluations of patients with pancreatic masses. *Pancreas* 2000; 20:109–116.
41. Koyama K, Okamura T, Kawabe J, et al. Diagnostic usefulness of FDG PET for pancreatic mass lesions. *Ann Nucl Med* 2001;15(3): 217–224.
42. Zimny M, Buell U, Diederichs CG, et al. False positive FDG PET in patients with pancreatic masses: an issue of proper patient selection? *Eur J Nucl Med* 1998;25:1352.
43. Shreve PD. Focal fluorine-18-fluorodeoxyglucose accumulation in inflammatory pancreatic disease. *Eur J Nucl Med* 1998;25:259–264.
44. Nakamoto Y, Higashi T, Sakahara H, et al. Delayed (^{18})F-fluoro-2-deoxy-D-glucose positron emission tomography scan for differentiation between malignant and benign lesions in the pancreas. *Cancer* 2000;89:2547–2554.
45. Nitzsche EU, Hoegerle S, Mix M, et al. Non-invasive differentiation of pancreatic lesions: is analysis of FDG kinetics superior to semiquantitative uptake value analysis? *Eur J Nucl Med* 2002;29:237–242.
46. Tamm EP, Silverman PM, Charnsangavej C, et al. Diagnosis, staging, and surveillance of pancreatic cancer. *AJR Am J Roentgenol* 2003;180: 1311–1123.
47. Douglass HJ, Kim S, Meropol N. Neoplasms of the exocrine pancreas. In: Holland J, Frei EI, Bast RJ, et al., eds. *Cancer medicine*, 4th ed. Baltimore: Williams & Wilkins, 1997:1989–2018.
48. Frolich A, Diederichs CG, Staib L, et al. Detection of liver metastases from pancreatic cancer using FDG PET. *J Nucl Med* 1999;40:250–255.
49. Franke C, Klapdor R, Meyerhoff K, et al. 18-FDG positron emission tomography of the pancreas: diagnostic benefit in the follow-up of pancreatic carcinoma. *Anticancer Res* 1999;19:2437–2442.
50. Ruf J, Lopez Hänninen E, Oettle H, et al. Detection of recurrent pancreatic cancer: comparison of FDG-PET with CT/MRI. *Pancreatology* 2005;5(2–3):266–272.
51. Higashi T, Sakahara H, Torizuka T, et al. Evaluation of intraoperative radiation therapy for unresectable pancreatic cancer with FDG PET. *J Nucl Med* 1999;40:1424–1433.
52. Maisey NR, Webb A, Flux GD, et al. FDG PET in the prediction of survival of patients with cancer of the pancreas: a pilot study. *Br J Cancer* 2000;83:287–293.
53. Sperti C, Pasquali C, Chierichetti F, et al. Value of 18-fluorodeoxyglucose positron emission tomography in the management of patients with cystic tumors of the pancreas. *Ann Surg* 2001;234:675–680.
54. Tann M, Sandrasegaran K, Jennings SG, et al. Positron-emission tomography and computed tomography of cystic pancreatic masses. *Clin Radiol* 2007;62(8):745–751.
55. Klöppel G, Anlauf M. Pancreatic endocrine tumors. *Pathol Case Rev* 2006;11(6):256–267.
56. Horton KM, Hruban RH, Yeo C, et al. Multi-detector row CT of pancreatic islet cell tumors. *Radiographics* 2006;26:453–464.
57. Thoeni RF, Mueller-Lisse UG, Chan R, et al. Detection of small functional islet cell tumors in the pancreas: selection of MR imaging sequences for optimal sensitivity. *Radiology* 2000;214:483–490.
58. Gouya H, Vignaux O, Augui J, et al. CT, endoscopic sonography, and a combined protocol for preoperative evaluation of pancreatic insulinomas. *AJR Am J Roentgenol* 2003;181:987–992.
59. Ichikawa T, Peterson MS, Federle MP, et al. Islet cell tumor of the pancreas: biphasic CT versus MR imaging in tumor detection. *Radiology* 2000;216:163–171.
60. Lebtahi R, Le Cloirec J, Houzard C, et al. Detection of neuroendocrine tumors: 99mTc-P829 scintigraphy compared with ^{111}In-pentetreotide scintigraphy. *J Nucl Med* 2002;43:889–895.
61. Nakamoto Y, Higashi T, Sakahara H, et al. Evaluation of pancreatic islet cell tumors by fluorine-18 fluorodeoxyglucose positron emission tomography: comparison with other modalities. *Clin Nucl Med* 2000;25:115–119.
62. Eriksson B, Orlefors H, Oberg K, et al. Developments in PET for the detection of endocrine tumours. *Best Pract Res Clin Endocrinol Metab* 2005;19:311–324.
63. Kauhanen S, Seppanen M, Minn H, et al. Fluorine-18-L-dihydroxyphenylalanine (^{18}F-DOPA) positron emission tomography as a tool to localize an insulinoma or β-cell hyperplasia in adult patients. *J Clin Endocrinol Metab* 2007;92(4):1237–1244.
64. Ahlstrom H, Eriksson B, Bergstrom M, et al. Pancreatic neuroendocrine tumors: diagnosis with PET. *Radiology* 1995;195:333–337.
65. Eriksson B, Bergstrom M, Sundin A. The role of PET in localization of neuroendocrine and adrenocortical tumors. *Ann NY Acad Sci* 2002; 970:159–169.
66. Anderson CJ, Dehdashti F, Cutler PD. ^{64}Cu-TETA-octreotide as a PET imaging agent for patients with neuroendocrine tumors. *J Nucl Med* 2001;42:213–221.
67. Antunes P, Ginj M, Zhang H, et al. Are radiogallium-labelled DOTA-conjugated somatostatin analogues superior to those labelled with other radiometals? *Eur J Nucl Med Mol Imaging* 2007;34(7): 982–993.

68. Bosch FX, Ribes J, Borras J. Epidemiology of primary liver cancer. *Semin Liver Dis* 1999;19:271–285.
69. Russo MW, Wei JT, Thiny MT, et al. Digestive and liver disease statistics. *Gastroenterology* 2004;126:1448–1453.
70. El Serag HB, Davila JA, Petersen NJ, et al. The continuing increase in the incidence of hepatocellular carcinoma in the United States—an update. *Ann Intern Med* 2003;139:817–823.
71. Fattovich G, Giustina G, Degos F, et al. Morbidity and mortality in compensated cirrhosis C a retrospective follow-up study of 384 patients. *Gastroenterology* 1997;112:463–472.
72. Nzeako U, Goodman ZD, Ishak KG. Hepatocellular carcinoma in cirrhotic and noncirrhotic livers. A clinico-histopathologic study of 804 North American patients. *Am J Clin Pathol* 1996;105:65–75.
73. de Groen PC, Gores GJ, LaRusso NF, et al. Biliary tract cancers. *N Engl J Med* 1999;341(18):1368–1378.
74. Yalcin S. Diagnosis and management of cholangiocarcinomas: a comprehensive review. *Hepatogastroenterology* 2004;51(55):43–50.
75. Chalasani N, Baluyut A, Ismail A, et al. Cholangiocarcinoma in patients with primary sclerosing cholangitis: a multicenter case-control study. *Hepatology* 2000;31(1):7–11.
76. Donohue JH, Stewart AK, Menck HR. The National Cancer Data Base report on carcinoma of the gallbladder, 1989–1995. *Cancer* 1998;83(12): 2618–2628.
77. Vitetta L, Sali A, Little P, et al. Gallstones and gall bladder carcinoma. *Aust N Z J Surg* 2000;70(9):667–673.
78. Bruix J, Sherman M, Llovet JM, et al. Clinical management of hepatocellular carcinoma. Conclusions of the Barcelona 2000 EASL conference. *J Hepatol* 2001;35:421–430.
79. Lacrosse G, Sorokopud H, Berry G, et al. Sonographic screening for hepatocellular carcinoma in patients with chronic hepatitis or cirrhosis: an evaluation. *AJR Am J Roentgenol* 1998;171:433–435.
80. Colombo M, De Franchis R, Del Ninno E, et al. Hepatocellular carcinoma in Italian patients with cirrhosis. *N Engl J Med* 1991;325:675–680.
81. Cottone M, Turri M, Caltagirone M, et al. Screening for hepatocellular carcinoma in patients with Child's A cirrhosis: an 8-year prospective study by ultrasound and alphafetoprotein. *J Hepatol* 1994;21: 1029–1034.
82. Trevisani F, PE D'Intino PE, Morselli-Labate AM, et al. Serum alphafetoprotein for diagnosis of hepatocellular carcinoma in patients with chronic liver disease: influence of HBsAg and anti-HCV status. *J Hepatol* 2001;34:570–575.
83. Koteish A, Thuluvath PJ. Screening for hepatocellular carcinoma. *J Vasc Interv Radiol* 2002;13:9II.
84. Murakami T, Mochizuki K, Nakamura H. Imaging evaluation of the cirrhotic liver. *Semin Liver Dis* 2001;21:213–224.
85. Takayasu K, Moriyama N, Muramatsu Y, et al. The diagnosis of small hepatocellular carcinomas: efficacy of various imaging procedures in 100 patients. *AJR Am J Roentgenol* 1990;155:49–54.
86. Fung KT, Li FT, Raimondo ML, et al. Systematic review of radiological imaging for hepatocellular carcinoma in cirrhotic patients. *Br J Radiol* 2004;77(920):633–640.
87. Park MS, Kim TK, Kim KW, et al. Differentiation of extrahepatic bile duct cholangiocarcinoma from benign stricture: findings at MRCP versus ERCP. *Radiology* 2004;233(1):234–240.
88. Lacomis JM, Baron RL, Oliver JH 3rd, et al. Cholangiocarcinoma: delayed CT contrast enhancement patterns. *Radiology* 1997;203(1): 98–104.
89. Valls C, Guma A, Puig I, et al. Intrahepatic peripheral cholangiocarcinoma: CT evaluation. *Abdom Imaging* 2000;25:490–496.
90. Maetani Y, Itoh K, Watanabe C, et al. MR imaging of intrahepatic cholangiocarcinoma with pathologic correlation. *AJR Am J Roentgenol* 2001;176(6):1499–1507.
91. Weber G, Cantero A. Glucose-6-phosphatase activity in normal, precancerous, and neoplastic tissues. *Cancer Res* 1955;15:105–108.
92. Weber G, Morris HP. Comparative biochemistry of hepatomas, III: carbohydrate enzymes in liver tumors of different growth rates. *Cancer Res* 1963;23:987–994.
93. Messa C, Choi Y, Hoh CK, et al. Quantification of glucose utilization in liver metastases: parametric imaging of FDG uptake with PET. *J Comput Assisted Tomogr* 1992;16:684–689.
94. Okazumi S, Isono K, Enomoto D, et al. Evaluation of liver tumors using fluorine-18-fluorodeoxyglucose PET: characterization of tumor and assessment of effect of treatment. *J Nucl Med* 1992;33:333–339.
95. Torizuka T, Tamaki N, Inokuma T, et al. *In vivo* assessment of glucose metabolism in hepatocellular carcinoma with FDG PET. *J Nucl Med* 1995;36:1811–1817.
96. Khan MA, Combs CS, Brunt EM, et al. Positron emission tomography scanning in the evaluation of hepatocellular carcinoma. *J Hepatol* 2000;32:792–797.
97. Delbeke D, Martin WH, Sandler MP, et al. Evaluation of benign vs. malignant hepatic lesions with positron emission tomography. *Arch Surg* 1998;133:510–515.
98. Lin WY, Tsai SC, Hung GU. Value of delayed ^{18}F-FDG-PET imaging in the detection of hepatocellular carcinoma. *Nucl Med Commun* 2005;26(4):315–321.
99. Koyama K, Okamura T, Kawabe J, et al. The usefulness of ^{18}F-FDG PET images obtained 2 hours after intravenous injection in liver tumor. *Ann Nucl Med* 2002;16(3):169–176.
100. Iwata Y, Shiomi S, Sasaki N, et al. Clinical usefulness of positron emission tomography with fluorine-18-fluorodeoxyglucose in the diagnosis of liver tumors. *Ann Nucl Med* 2000;14:121–126.
101. Trojan J, Schroeder O, Raedle J, et al. Fluorine-18 FDG positron emission tomography for imaging of hepatocellular carcinoma. *Am J Gastroenterol* 1999;94:3314–3319.
102. Schroder O, Trojan J, Zeuzem S, et al. Limited value of fluorine-18-fluorodeoxyglucose PET for the differential diagnosis of focal liver lesions in patients with chronic hepatitis C virus infection. *Nuklearmedizin* 1998;37:279–285.
103. Rose AT, Rose DM, Pinson CW, et al. Hepatocellular carcinoma outcome based on indicated treatment strategy. *Am Surg* 1998;64: 1122–1135.
104. Sugiyama M, Sakahara H, Torizuka T, et al. ^{18}F-FDG PET in the detection of extrahepatic metastases from hepatocellular carcinoma. *J Gastroenterol* 2004;39(10):961–968.
105. Torizuka T, Tamaki N, Inokuma T, et al. Value of fluorine-18-FDG PET to monitor hepatocellular carcinoma after interventional therapy. *J Nucl Med* 1994;35:1965–1969.
106. Akuta K, Nishimura T, Jo S, et al. Monitoring liver tumor therapy with [^{18}F]FDG positron emission tomography. *J Comput Assisted Tomogr* 1990;14:370–374.
107. Vitola JV, Delbeke D, Meranze SG, et al. Positron emission tomography with F-18-fluorodeoxyglucose to evaluate the results of hepatic chemoembolization. *Cancer* 1996;78:2216–2222.
108. Kubota K, Hisa N, Nishikawa T, et al. Evaluation of hepatocellular carcinoma after treatment with transcatheter arterial chemoembolization: comparison of lipiodol-CT, power Doppler sonography, and dynamic MRI. *Abdom Imaging* 2001;26(2):184–190.
109. Chen YK, Hsieh DS, Liao CS, et al. Utility of FDG-PET for investigating unexplained serum AFP elevation in patients with suspected hepatocellular carcinoma recurrence. *Anticancer Res* 2005;25(6C): 4719–4725.
110. Ho CL, Yu SCH, Yeung DWC. ^{11}C-Acetate PET imaging in hepatocellular carcinoma and other liver masses. *J Nucl Med* 2003;44:213–221.
111. Ho CL, Chen S, Yeung DW, et al. Dual-tracer PET/CT imaging in evaluation of metastatic hepatocellular carcinoma. *J Nucl Med* 2007;48(6): 902–909.
112. Delbeke D, Pinson CW. ^{11}C-acetate: a new tracer for the evaluation of hepatocellular carcinoma. *J Nucl Med* 2003;44(2):222–223.
113. Liu RS. Clinical applications of C-11-acetate in oncology. *Clin Positron Imaging* 2000;3:185.
114. Lenzo NP, Anderson J, Campbell A, et al. Fluoromethylcholine PET in recurrent multifocal hepatoma. *Australas Radiol* 2007;51[Suppl]: B299–B302.

115. Keiding S, Hansen SB, Rasmussen HH, et al. Detection of cholangiocarcinoma in primary sclerosing cholangitis by positron emission tomography. *Hepatology* 1998;28:700–706.
116. Prytz H, Keiding S, Björnsson E, et al. Dynamic FDG-PET is useful for detection of cholangiocarcinoma in patients with PSC listed for liver transplantation. *Hepatology* 2007;44(6):1572–1580.
117. Anderson CD, Rice MH, Pinson CW, et al. Fluorodeoxyglucose PET imaging in the evaluation of gallbladder carcinoma and cholangiocarcinoma. *J Gastroint Surg* 2004;8(1):90–97.
118. Widjaja A, Mix H, Wagner S, et al. Positron emission tomography and cholangiocarcinoma in primary sclerosing cholangitis. *Z Gastroenterol* 1999;37:731–733.
119. Kluge R, Schmidt F, Caca K, et al. Positron emission tomography with $[(^{18})F]$fluoro-2-deoxy-D-glucose for diagnosis and staging of bile duct cancer. *Hepatology* 2001;33:1029–1035.
120. Drouart F, Delamarre J, Capron JP. Cutaneous seeding of gallbladder cancer after laparoscopic cholecystectomy. *N Engl J Med* 1991;325:1316.
121. Weiss SM, Wengert PA, Harkavy SE. Incisional recurrence of gallbladder cancer after laparoscopic cholecystectomy. *Gastrointest Endosc* 1994;40:244–246.
122. Hoh CK, Hawkins RA, Glaspy JA, et al. Cancer detection with whole-body PET using 2-$[^{18}F]$fluoro-2-deoxy-D-glucose. *J Comput Assisted Tomogr* 1993;17:582–589.
123. Lomis KD, Vitola JV, Delbeke D, et al. Recurrent gallbladder carcinoma at laparoscopy port sites diagnosed by PET scan: implications for primary and radical second operations. *Am Surg* 1997;63: 341–345.
124. Nishiyama Y, Yamamoto Y, Fukunaga K, et al. Dual-time-point ^{18}F-FDG PET for the evaluation of gallbladder carcinoma. *J Nucl Med* 2006;47(4):633–638.

CHAPTER

8.16 Cervical and Uterine Cancer

PERRY W. GRIGSBY

PATIENT PREPARATION AND IMAGING
CERVICAL CANCER
STAGING
PROGNOSIS
DIRECTING THERAPY
POSTTHERAPY MONITORING
ENDOMETRIAL CANCER

The initial diagnosis and staging of most gynecologic malignancies are commonly achieved by history and physical examination and by use of selected imaging studies. Accurate staging of gynecologic cancers is important both for selecting appropriate therapy and for prognosis. Most gynecologic cancers initially spread regionally and then through lymphatic channels before hematogenous dissemination to distant organs. With locally advanced disease, the status of pelvic and para-aortic lymph nodes is an important determinant of prognosis and guides treatment planning decisions. Computed tomography (CT) has been the most widely used imaging method for assessment of nodal involvement and detection of distant metastatic disease. Despite its high resolution and excellent depiction of anatomy, CT is limited by its inability to detect small-volume metastatic involvement in normal-sized lymph nodes and to determine whether enlarged nodes represent metastasis or reactive hyperplasia (which is particularly problematic in patients with large necrotic tumors with significant associated inflammation). Recognition of small peritoneal tumor deposits is also difficult on CT.

Positron emission tomography (PET) with the glucose analogue 2-fluorine-18-fluoro-2-deoxy-D-glucose (FDG) has become an established imaging tool for many cancers. The functional information about regional glucose metabolism provided by FDG PET provides for greater sensitivity and specificity in most cancer imaging applications by comparison with CT and other anatomic imaging methods. The role of PET in gynecological cancers is evolving, but the current literature suggests that PET is superior to conventional imaging modalities for evaluating patients with cervical cancer. The role of PET in other gynecological cancers is less well defined.

The development and rapid dissemination of integrated PET/CT scanners that allow functional and anatomical information to be obtained in a single examination represents an important advance in PET imaging technology, resulting in a synergistic improvement in the accuracy of interpretation of both PET and CT images (1). Accordingly, the performance of PET based on published studies performed with conventional PET scanners is now being re-evaluated in light of emerging PET/CT results (2).

PATIENT PREPARATION AND IMAGING

Patient preparation for PET imaging of gynecological tumors is similar to that for PET oncologic imaging. However, because of the potential for artifacts and interpretation errors related to intense FDG activity in urinary tract structures (e.g., streak artifacts, confusion of ureteral activity with lymph nodes), various interventions to minimize the amount of FDG in the urinary tract have been employed in different clinics. The current general use of iterative reconstruction algorithms instead of filtered back projection has eliminated most of the image artifacts related to intense urinary tract activity. Nevertheless, in some centers, urinary tract preparation is performed for evaluation of gynecologic cancers. Our procedure is to place a Foley catheter in the urinary bladder, administer intravenous fluids (1,000 to 1,500 mL of 0.9% or 0.45% saline solution to be infused during the course of the study), and intravenous administration of 20 mg furosemide before or after injection of FDG. The Foley catheter should be placed before injection of FDG to minimize radiation exposure to technical or nursing staff. Some investigators prefer the use of continuous bladder irrigation with a double-lumen catheter for the duration of the study.

For PET/CT, the administration of oral contrast agents is helpful for delineating bowel loops and makes image interpretation easier. There is no consensus regarding the need for administration of intravenous contrast agents. PET imaging is delayed for 1 hour after injection of FDG improves the sensitivity for detection of nodal metastasis in cervical cancer. Serum glucose levels are maintained at about 100 mg/dL, and studies are deferred if blood glucose concentration exceeds 200 mg/dL.

CERVICAL CANCER

Worldwide, cervical cancer is the second most common cause of cancer-related deaths in women. Although less common in the United States, cervical cancer is still expected to account for approximately 11,070 new cervical cancer diagnoses and 3,870 deaths in 2008 (3). Squamous cell carcinomas represent over 90% of cervical cancers and originate in the surface epithelium of the cervix; adenocarcinomas represent approximately 5% to 9% of cervical cancers and originate in the cervical glandular tissue. Adenosquamous carcinoma is relatively infrequent and represents about 2% to 5% of all cervical carcinomas. Rare cervical sarcomas and small cell carcinomas account for the remainder.

STAGING

Cervical cancer typically disseminates in a predictable fashion, with initial spread to local structures and regional lymphatics and later hematogenous spread to distant organs, such as bone, brain, liver, and lung. The pattern of nodal metastasis is also predictable: tumor spreads from the primary lesion sequentially to pelvic lymph nodes, para-aortic lymph nodes, and supraclavicular lymph nodes. Cervical cancer is staged clinically based on the Federation Internationale de Gynecologie et d'Obstetrique (FIGO) staging system. Involvement of pelvic or para-aortic lymph node does not alter the FIGO clinical stage of disease, but indicates a worse prognosis (4–7) and may have an important impact on therapy. Because of limitations of conventional radiological techniques for evaluating lymph nodes, surgical assessment of para-aortic nodes is considered the gold standard. However, exploratory laparotomy and nodal dissection has not had a demonstrable impact on survival. Moreover, because of the morbidity associated with surgical staging, this procedure is not widely used; thus, the search for an accurate noninvasive staging method is an ongoing process.

FDG PET appears to be well suited for imaging of cervical carcinoma. Most primary tumors, except for very small lesions, are readily seen on PET images and exhibit intense FDG uptake. In most series, primary squamous cell carcinoma and adenocarcinoma have similar FDG avidity. However, because of its relatively poor spatial resolution and inability to assess parametrial invasion or involvement of adjacent organs reliably, FDG PET is of limited value for staging of the primary tumor.

A number of studies have shown that FDG PET is superior to conventional imaging methods for detecting metastatic disease, particularly lymph node metastasis (8,9). Havrilesky et al. (10) recently reported a systematic review of the published literature up through 2003. They included only those studies involving 12 or more subjects who had PET performed with a dedicated scanner with specified resolution, and with clinical follow-up of 6 months or more or histopathology as the reference standards. In patients with newly diagnosed cervical cancer, the pooled sensitivity of PET was 79% (95% confidence interval [CI], 65% to 90%), and the pooled specificity was 99% (95% CI, 96% to 99%) for detection of pelvic lymph nodes metastasis (9,11–13). Two studies were identified that compared PET to magnetic resonance imaging (MRI) and CT (7,8). MRI had a pooled sensitivity of 72% (95% CI, 53% to 87%) and pooled specificity of 96% (95% CI, 92% to 98%), whereas CT had a pooled sensitivity of 47% (95% CI, 21% to 73%) (there were insufficient data to calculate a pooled specificity).

In four prospective studies in which histology after para-aortic lymphadenectomy was used as the reference standard, the pooled sensitivity of PET for the detection of para-aortic nodal metastasis was 84% (95% CI, 68% to 94%) and the pooled specificity was 95% (95% CI, 89% to 98%) (9,11,12,14). In three of these studies, the inclusion criteria for study entry included a negative CT or MRI of the abdomen (10,12,13). Thus, the accuracy of conventional imaging could not be calculated. Reinhardt et al. (9) did not require a negative abdominal imaging study prior to surgery. The sensitivity and specificity of MRI in the 12 patients who underwent aortic node sampling were 67% and 100%, respectively.

False-negative results for detection of nodal metastasis are chiefly related to the limited resolution of PET and, thus, its inability to detect microscopic disease and small macroscopic tumor deposits. In a recent study that evaluated the sensitivity of FDG PET by comparison with surgical lymphadenectomy in patients with early stage cervical cancer the mean size of tumor deposits was larger in PET-positive pelvic nodes (15.2 mm; range 2 to 35 mm) than in PET-negative nodes (7.3 mm; range 0.3 to 20 mm) (15). False-positive results are most likely related to uptake of FDG in hyperplastic nodes or misinterpretation of physiologic activity in bowel or the urinary tract as nodal metastasis. Sironi et al. (16) demonstrated similar findings in their prospective study of FDG PET/CT before radical hysterectomy.

Grigsby et al. (17) have shown that FDG PET is superior to CT and lymphangiography in showing unsuspected sites of metastasis in pelvic lymph nodes, extrapelvic lymph nodes, and visceral organs in patients with newly diagnosed advanced cervical cancer. FDG PET showed abnormalities consistent with metastasis more often than did CT in pelvic lymph nodes (67% vs. 20%) and in para-aortic lymph nodes (21% vs. 7%). PET also showed disease in supraclavicular lymph nodes in 8% (18). These initial results have been sustained in subsequent evaluations of data from a prospective registry that now includes over 400 patients (19).

The role of PET/CT in staging of cervical cancer needs to be determined. The literature currently contains limited data on the use of PET/CT in cervical cancer; however, it is expected that PET/CT image fusion will allow for easier distinction of pathologic and physiologic tracer uptake and, thus, improve the accuracy of image interpretation (20).

Based on the results in the literature to date, the U.S. Center for Medicare and Medicaid Services in January 2005 approved coverage for use of FDG PET in initial staging of patients with cervical cancer who have no evidence of extrapelvic metastatic disease on CT or MRI (21).

PROGNOSIS

Several prognostic factors have been identified for patients with carcinoma of the cervix. These include patient age, tumor histology, tumor stage, tumor size, lymph node metastasis, and tumor hypoxia (22,23). In a study of 101 patients with newly diagnosed cervical cancer, Grigsby et al. (18) demonstrated that the lymph node status determined by FDG PET is the most significant pretreatment independent predictor of progression-free and overall survival in patients with cervical cancer. The 2-year, disease-free survival was better predicted by PET evidence of lymph node involvement than by CT findings. Based on the imaging findings in the pelvic lymph nodes, the 2-year, disease-free survival was 84% for CT–/PET– patients, 64% for CT−/PET+ patients, and 48% for CT+/PET+ patients (P = .05). Based on the imaging findings in the para-aortic nodes, the 2-year, disease-free survival was 78% in CT–/PET– patients, 31% for CT−/PET+ patients, and 14% for CT+/PET+ patients ($P \leq .0001$). No patients with PET+ supraclavicular lymph nodes survived 2 years. The PET-determined status of the para-aortic nodes was the strongest predictor of survival in a multivariate logistic regression analysis. These results suggest an opportunity to cure patients with para-aortic nodal metastasis defined by PET, but were not otherwise detected by CT. A recent review of data from 256 patients in the author's registry found that the extent of lymph node involvement is inversely correlated with survival (19). It was also found that FDG PET demonstrated metastatic involvement in the left supraclavicular lymph nodes in 8% of this patient population (24). This finding had a positive predictive value of 100% and indicates a dismal prognosis, despite aggressive therapy. Similarly, it was found that the cause-specific survival for patients with FIGO stage IIIb carcinoma is highly dependent on the extent of lymph node metastasis demonstrated by whole-body FDG PET at initial presentation (25). The 3-year estimates of cause-specific survival were 73% for those with no lymph node metastasis, 58% for those with only pelvic lymph node metastasis, 29% for those with pelvic and para-aortic lymph node metastasis, and 0% for those with pelvic, para-aortic, and supraclavicular lymph node metastasis (P = .0005).

Extent of regional lymph node metastasis was also found by Unger et al. (26) to be a significant prognostic factor.

Miller and Grigsby (27) evaluated the usefulness of tumor volume measurement with FDG PET in 57 patients with cervical cancer. Tumor volume and lymph node status determined by PET and FIGO stage determined by clinical examination were predictive of progression-free survival; tumor volume and lymph node involvement by PET predicted overall survival (27). The avidity of FDG uptake in the primary cervical tumor is a predictor of survival outcome. Patient tumors that have a high maximum standardized uptake value (SUV_{max}) have a worse survival outcome than those with a low SUV_{max} (28).

In patients with cervical cancer, tumor hypoxia is an important prognostic factor indicating decreased overall and disease-free survival. Hypoxic tumors are resistant to radio- and chemotherapy. Various therapeutic strategies directed toward tumor hypoxia have been unsuccessful, in part because a clinically relevant tool for determining and monitoring tumor oxygenation has not been available. The only established method for assessing the oxygenation status of tumors *in vivo* used invasive oxygen electrodes. However, this method is not clinically practical because of its invasiveness, sampling errors, and the fact that it can only be used in readily accessible tumors. It has been demonstrated that the tracer, copper-60-labeled diacetyl-bis (N^4-methylthiosemicarbazone) (^{60}Cu-ATSM), accumulates avidly in hypoxic tissues but washes out rapidly from normoxic tissues. Dehdashti et al. (23) studied 27 patients with advanced cervical cancer and demonstrated an inverse relationship between tumor uptake of [^{60}Cu]-ATSM and response to therapy. In addition, progression-free and overall survival were significantly worse in patients with increased pretreatment primary tumor uptake of [^{60}Cu]-ATSM. In these same patients, we found no significant difference in tumor FDG uptake in subjects with hypoxic (ATSM-avid) tumors versus those with normoxic tumors. Thus, [^{60}Cu]-ATSM PET imaging of hypoxia provides prognostic information that cannot be derived from FDG PET, and this examination has the potential to be used to monitor hypoxic-directed therapy in patients with hypoxic cervical cancer.

DIRECTING THERAPY

The use of FDG PET in pretreatment clinical staging has had a significant impact on the therapeutic management of patients with cervic carcinoma. Patients with early stage cervical cancer often undergo a radical hysterectomy and lymph node dissection. Postoperative chemoradiation is administered only to those patients who are found to have positive lymph nodes or other high-risk factors. The pretreatment detection of lymph node metastasis can change management from planned surgery alone to chemoradiation alone, thus avoiding two forms of radical therapy. The standard treatment of advanced cervical carcinoma is radiotherapy with concurrent chemoradiation (29–31). Radiotherapy is directed at the pelvis to encompass primary disease as well as pelvic lymph nodes. The radiotherapy port is expanded to include the para-aortic lymph node region in patients who have evidence of para-aortic nodal disease. Patients who have evidence of disease beyond the para-aortic lymph nodes at the time of initial diagnosis have little chance of a cure and receive palliative therapy. Based on the findings in the study of Grigsby et al. (18), it is now routine to administer curative para-aortic irradiation to patients with CT-negative, FDG-positive para-aortic nodal disease, whereas no irradiation to this region would have been administered to such patients in the past before the use of PET to assess for para-aortic disease. Fourteen patients in that analysis had para-aortic disease that was not detected by CT, but detected by FDG PET. These patients had their radiation portals increased to include the para-aortic nodal region.

Radiotherapy treatment planning is routinely performed utilizing PET/CT simulation for all patients with cervical cancer. It has been demonstrated that with the use of CT the 40% isocontour of the SUV_{max} corresponded to tumor size (27) and validated with MRI (Fig. 8.16.1). Fig. 8.16.2 demonstrates that the metabolic tumor volume is contoured on the PET simulation images, and then the pelvic lymph node regions are contoured from the CT images of the PET/CT. The author currently uses PET/CT-guided intensity-modulated radiotherapy to deliver higher doses to para-aortic nodes that have FDG-avid disease by PET/CT (32,33). Fused PET/CT images are used to

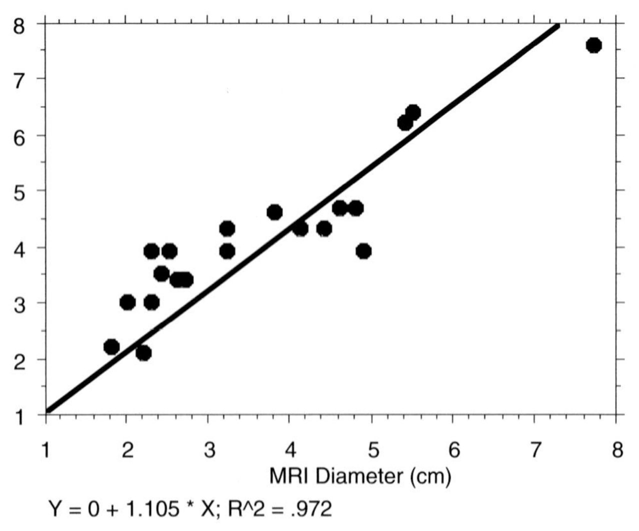

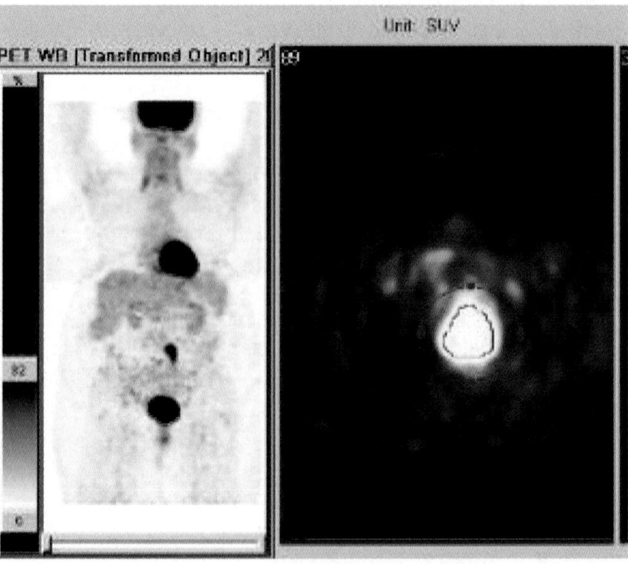

FIGURE 8.16.1. Definition of tumor volume for radiotherapy treatment planning. **A:** Magnetic resonance imaging correlation of tumor size and the 40% maximum standard uptake value isocountour. **B:** Forty percent isocountour defining the metabolic tumor volume (MTV) cervix.

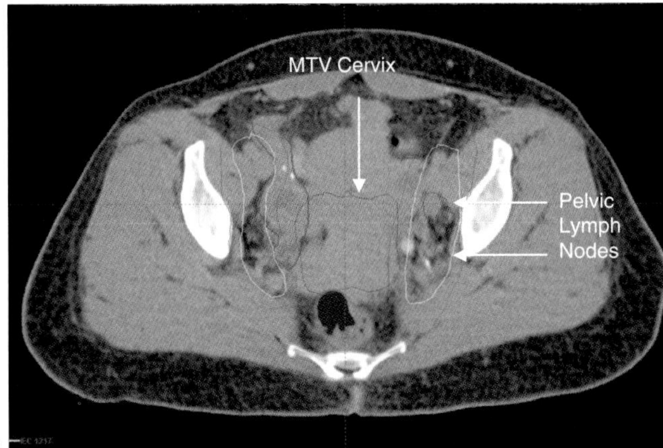

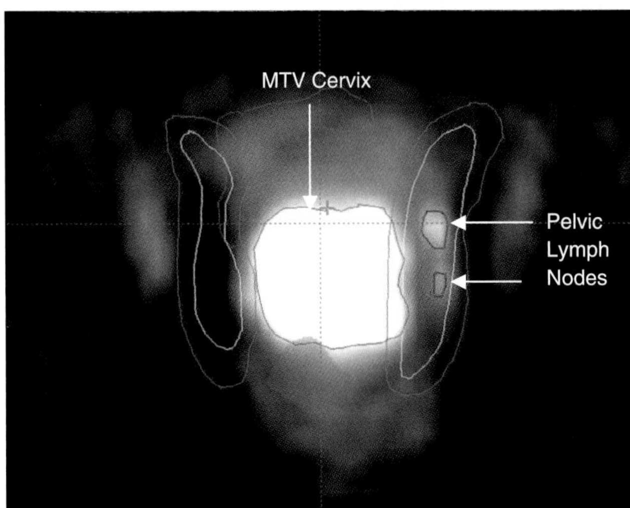

FIGURE 8.16.2. Cervical tumor volumes for radiotherapy planning. **A:** Pelvic lymph nodes and primary cervical tumor volumes contoured for radiotherapy treatment planning. **B:** FDG avid pelvic lymph nodes and primary cervix tumor (MTVCervix) are contoured on the PET image with contours then transferred to the CT image (A).

differentiate tumor from adjacent normal structures more reliably and thus allow for delivery of higher doses of radiation to the tumor while decreasing radiation dose to normal structures. Isodose distributions derived from PET/CT simulation and treatment planning are shown in Fig. 8.16.3.

FDG PET may also be useful in determining whether concurrent chemotherapy should be administered to patients with advanced-stage disease. A recent study from the Gynecologic Oncology Group (GOG 109) randomized patients with pathologically positive pelvic lymph nodes to either radiotherapy alone or to radiotherapy with concurrent and adjuvant cisplatin and 5-fluorouracil chemotherapy. The study demonstrated that there was both a superior disease-free and overall survival advantage when chemotherapy was added to radiation therapy (34). A subsequent report from this study demonstrated that there was no benefit to the use of concurrent chemotherapy in patients with only one positive lymph node (35). A similar finding was demonstrated by Grigsby et al. (36). In this retrospective analysis of 65 patients, there was no apparent clinical benefit to the use of concurrent chemotherapy with primary irradiation in patients who had no evidence of lymph node metastasis by FDG PET. Thus, FDG PET may be useful to select a subgroup of patients with locally advanced cervical cancer without lymph node metastasis who may not benefit from

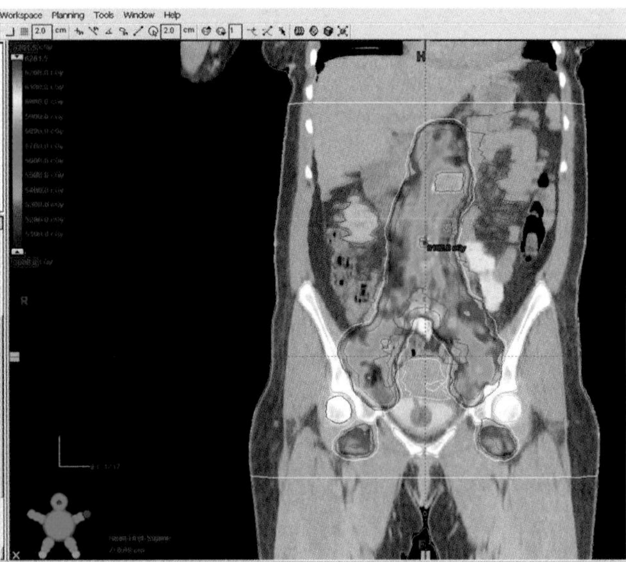

FIGURE 8.16.3. Radiotherapy isodose distributions using fluorodeoxyglucose PET/CT for radiotherapy target definitions. This patient had FDG avid pelvic and para-aortic lymph nodes treated with irradiation to 60 Gy (brown regions). The remainder of the clinical lymph node region received 50 Gy.

the administration of concurrent chemotherapy. Larger prospective studies need to be completed to confirm these results.

POSTTHERAPY MONITORING

Approximately 30% of cervical cancer patients with advanced stage disease will ultimately fail after definitive treatment (37). Clinical and radiological techniques have been used for early detection of recurrent disease. FDG PET has been shown to have a role in the posttreatment monitoring of patients with cervical cancer. In a large retrospective study by Ryu et al. (38), 249 women with previously treated cervical cancer without overt evidence of recurrence underwent FDG PET as part of their routine follow-up. Eighty patients (32%) were found to have abnormal FDG uptake; 28 (11%) had clinically or histologically confirmed recurrent disease. The sensitivity and specificity of FDG PET for detection of recurrent disease were 90% and 76%, respectively. The positive and negative predictive values were 35% and 98%, respectively. There was a high false-positive rate associated with FDG uptake in the pulmonary hila, lungs, neck, inguinal, and axillary regions. The majority of the recurrences were detected within 6 to 18 months after diagnosis. In another series by Unger et al. (39), FDG PET detected recurrences in 31% of asymptomatic patients and recurrences in 67% of symptomatic patients. In symptomatic patients, the sensitivity of FDG PET was 100%, the specificity was 86%, and the positive and negative predictive values were 93% and 100%, respectively. By comparison, in asymptomatic patients, the sensitivity of FDG PET was 80%, the specificity was 100%, and the positive and negative predictive values were 100% and 100%, respectively. In a study by Grigsby et al. (40), 152 patients previously treated with radiotherapy with or without concurrent chemotherapy who were free of FDG-avid sites on PET, obtained an average of 3 months posttherapy, had 5-year cause-specific and overall survival of 80% and 92%, respectively. Persistent abnormal uptake in the cervix or lymph nodes was found in 20 patients, and their cause-specific survival was 32%. New areas of increased FDG uptake in previously unirradiated regions

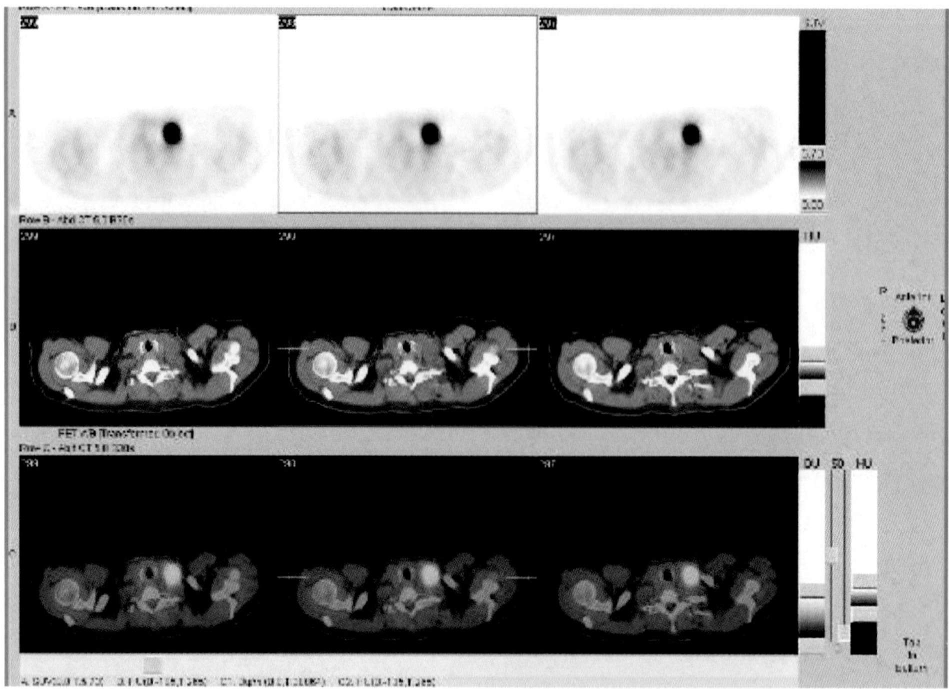

FIGURE 8.16.4. Metastatic cervical cancer in a left supraclavicular lymph node 3 months after completing chemoradiation.

were found in 18 patients, none of whom was alive at 5 years. Posttreatment PET abnormalities were found to be the most significant predictor of death from cervical cancer in this study. Together these results point to a significant impact of FDG PET findings on treatment strategy after primary therapy. Fig. 8.16.4 demonstrates abnormal FDG uptake in a left supraclavicular lymph node 3 months after completing chemoradiation.

Other groups have investigated the use of FDG PET in combination with other biomarkers, such as squamous cell carcinoma antigen (41). In a phase II study, 27 patients with previously treated cervical cancer underwent FDG PET for unexplained elevation of serum squamous cell carcinoma antigen levels found during follow-up evaluation. PET showed FDG-avid lesions in 17 of 18 patients with proven recurrent disease; 12 of these patients had distant recurrences only, 2 had local recurrences only, and 3 had both local and distant recurrences. Because of PET imaging, only 7 of the 18 patients with recurrent disease were treated with curative intent as compared to 16 of 30 patients treated with curative intent in the historical control group. PET imaging allowed better selection of patients for salvage therapy, which resulted in a trend toward increased overall survival compared with a historical control group. These promising results will need to be confirmed in further investigations to better define the role of FDG PET in combination with molecular biomarkers. Additionally, Yen et al. (42) reported on two prospective studies examining the role of FDG PET imaging in patients with biopsy confirmed relapse of disease or unexplained elevation of tumor marker serum levels with documented relapse after treatment. Fifty-five women were enrolled, 36 (66%) had treatment modifications because of the PET findings, and the remaining 19 were treated as originally planned. Of those patients whose plans were modified, 25% received salvage therapy with curative intent, but the modality or field of irradiation was changed, and 75% received only palliative treatment. Together these results demonstrate the usefulness of FDG PET for determining the intent and optimal scope of salvage therapy in patients with recurrent cervical cancer (43–46).

One way to overcome the limitation of PET to detect small lesions, at least in part, may be with the use of PET/CT scanners. PET/CT should improve disease detection by increasing radiological sensitivity and specificity. Fused PET/CT images clearly are helpful in localizing pathologic activity and differentiating this activity from physiologic radiotracer uptake.

In patients with cervical cancer, tumor hypoxia is an important prognostic factor indicating decreased overall and disease-free survival. The authors have shown that a new tracer, 60Cu-labeled diacetyl-bis(N4-methylthiosemicarbazone) (60Cu-ATSM), accumulates avidly in hypoxic tissues but washes out rapidly from normoxic tissues (Fig. 8.16.5). Increased 60Cu-ATSM uptake in cervical cancer results in decreased progression-free and overall survivals. 60Cu-ATSM-PET imaging appears to provide additional prognostic information and has the potential to be used to identify patients requiring more aggressive therapy due to their poor outcome.

ENDOMETRIAL CANCER

Endometrial cancer is the most common gynecologic cancer in the United States with an estimated 40,100 new endometrial cases and 7,470 deaths expected in 2008 (3). About 75% of endometrial cancers are adenocarcinoma that arises from the glands of the uterine lining. Endometrial cancer is a disease of postmenopausal women and is surgically staged and treated. There are no reports of the use of FDG PET for diagnosis of primary endometrial cancer. However, it might be expected that FDG PET would have limited accuracy for this purpose because increased uterine FDG uptake may occur with benign conditions, including uterine bleeding (e.g., menstruation, postpartum) and leiomyomata (47,48).

Surgical staging of endometrial cancer includes an exploratory laparotomy, total abdominal hysterectomy, bilateral salpingo-oophorec-

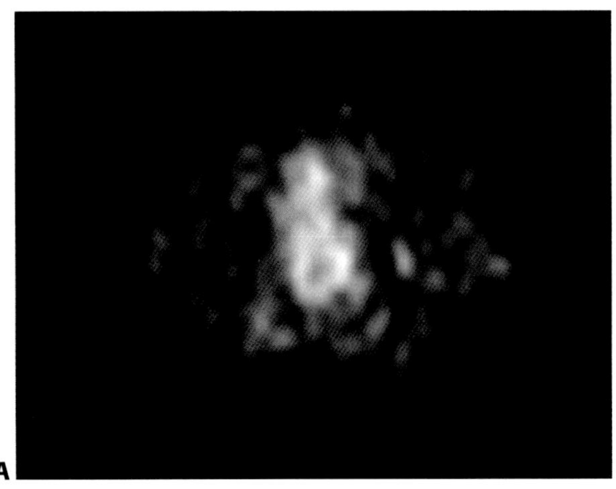

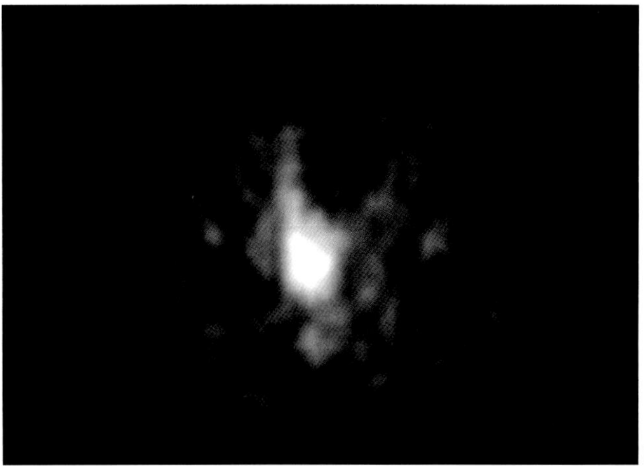

FIGURE 8.16.5. A: ^{60}Cu-ATSM PET showing hypoxia (T/M ratio 5.3). **B:** ^{60}Cu-ATSM PET showing normoxia (T/M ratio 2.1).

tomy, pelvic and para-aortic lymphadenectomy, and peritoneal cytology. The extent of lymph node sampling remains controversial (49). Conventional imaging methods, such as CT and MRI, have been unreliable in detecting pelvic and para-aortic lymph node metastasis (50,51). Grigsby et al. (52) conducted a prospective study evaluating the sensitivity and specificity of FDG PET imaging for detecting pelvic and para-aortic lymph node metastasis in patients undergoing surgical staging for newly diagnosed high-risk uterine corpus cancer. One of the 19 patients did not undergo lymphadenectomy because FDG PET was suspicious for nodal and pulmonary metastasis; disseminated disease was confirmed by percutaneous nodal biopsy. The primary tumor was seen on PET in 16 of 19 patients (84%). FDG PET was found to have 60% sensitivity and 98% specificity for detection of pelvic and para-aortic lymph node metastasis. Similar results were noted by Suzuki et al. (53). Because of its limited sensitivity, FDG PET should not replace lymphadenectomy in most patients, but it may be useful in guiding adjuvant therapy in patients who are poor surgical candidates.

Other groups have investigated the role of FDG PET in the postoperative or posttherapy setting (54,55). In a retrospective study by Belhocine et al. (55), 41 FDG PET studies were performed on 34 patients with previously treated endometrial cancer and compared with the results of clinical examination and conventional imaging procedures. They found the sensitivity, specificity, diagnostic accuracy, and positive and negative predictive values of FDG PET imaging for residual/recurrent disease to be 96%, 78%, 90%, 89%, and 91%, respectively. In 26 studies, FDG PET detected recurrent disease that was confirmed by histology (n = 7) or by clinical and radiological outcomes (n = 19). In 88% of these cases, FDG PET confirmed recurrence initially suspected based on the results of other studies. FDG PET was able to detect asymptomatic recurrences in the remaining 12% of patients. In 35% of cases, FDG PET significantly altered treatment decisions by detecting otherwise unsuspected distant metastasis.

Saga et al. (54) evaluated 21 postoperative patients with endometrial cancer (FIGO stages IA to IVA) who underwent 30 FDG PET examinations to evaluate for recurrence or to assess response to treatment. When evaluated in conjunction with anatomic information available from CT or MRI, FDG PET had a sensitivity of 100%, a specificity of 88%, and an accuracy of 93%. Additionally, FDG PET was able to detect unsuspected metastatic disease in 19% of patients and changed the management of seven patients (33%). FDG PET had a high negative predictive value for excluding recurrence, with no false-negative results after a minimal follow-up of 5 months.

Based on the current literature, FDG PET is more sensitive in the postoperative or posttherapy setting than in the preoperative setting in patients with endometrial cancer (56). This is likely because of the larger metastatic tumor burden present in the posttherapy setting versus the microscopic metastatic disease present at initial diagnosis. Larger prospective studies will be needed to confirm these results.

REFERENCES

1. Nakamoto Y, Saga T, Fujii S. Positron emission tomography application for gynecologic tumors. *Int J Gynecol Cancer* 2005;15(5):701–709.
2. Lin LL, Dehdashti F, Siegel B, et al. PET and PET-CT of tumors of the female genital tract. In: von Schulthess GK, ed. *Molecular anatomic imaging*. Philadelphia: Lippincott Williams & Wilkins, 2007:427–442.
3. Jemal A, Siegel R, Ward E, et al. Cancer statistics, 2008. *CA Cancer J Clin* 2008; 58(2): 71–96.
4. Heller PB, Malfetano PB, Bundy BN, et al. Clinical-pathologic study of stage IIB, III, and IVA carcinoma of the cervix: extended diagnostic evaluation for paraaortic node metastasis—a Gynecologic Oncology Group study. *Gynecol Oncol* 1990;38(3):425–430.
5. Delgado G, Bundy B, Zaino R, et al. Prospective surgical-pathological study of disease-free interval in patients with stage IB squamous cell carcinoma of the cervix: a Gynecologic Oncology Group study. *Gynecol Oncol* 1990;38:352–357.
6. Toita T, Nakano M, Higashi M, et al. Prognostic value of cervical size and pelvic lymph node status assessed by computed tomography for patients with uterine cervical cancer treated by radical radiation therapy. *Int J Radiat Oncol Biol Phys* 1995;33(4):843–849.
7. Sevin BU, Lu Y, Bloch DA, et al. Surgically defined prognostic parameters in patients with early cervical carcinoma. A multivariate survival tree analysis. *Cancer* 1996;78(7):1438–1446.
8. Belhocine T, Thille A, Fridman V, et al. Contribution of whole-body ^{18}FDG PET imaging in the management of cervical cancer. *Gynecol Oncol* 2002;87(1):90–97.
9. Reinhardt MJ, Ehritt-Braun C, Vogelgesang D, et al. Metastatic lymph nodes in patients with cervical cancer: detection with MR imaging and FDG PET. *Radiology* 2001;218:776–782.
10. Havrilesky LJ, Kulasingman SL, Matchar DB, et al. FDG-PET for management of cervical and ovarian cancer. *Gynecol Oncol* 2005;97(1): 183–191.
11. Rose PG, Adler LP, Rodriguez M, et al. Positron emission tomography for evaluating para-aortic nodal metastasis in locally advanced cervical cancer before surgical staging: a surgicopathologic study. *J Clin Oncol* 1999;17:41–45.

12. Yeh LS, Hung YC, Shen YY, et al. Detecting para-aortic lymph nodal metastasis by positron emission tomography of ^{18}F-fluorodeoxyglucose in advanced cervical cancer with negative magnetic resonance imaging findings. *Oncol Rep* 2002;9(6):1289–1292.
13. Sugawara Y, Eisbruch A, Kosuda S, et al. Evaluation of FDG PET in patients with cervical cancer. *J Nucl Med* 1999;40(7):1125–1131.
14. Lin WC, Hung YC, Yeh LS, et al. Usefulness of (18)F-fluorodeoxyglucose positron emission tomography to detect para-aortic lymph nodal metastasis in advanced cervical cancer with negative computed tomography findings. *Gynecol Oncol* 2003;89(1):73–76.
15. Wright JD, Dehdashti F, Herzog TJ, et al. Preoperative lymph node staging of early-stage cervical carcinoma by (18F)-fluoro-2-deoxy-D-glucose-positron emission tomography. *Cancer* 2005;104(11):2484–2491.
16. Sironi S, Buda A, Picchio M, et al. Lymph node metastasis in patients with clinical early-stage cervical cancer: detection with integrated FDG PET/CT. *Radiology* 2006;238(1):272–279.
17. Grigsby PW, Dehdashti F, Siegel BA. FDG-PET evaluation of carcinoma of the cervix. *Clin Positron Imaging* 1999;2(2):105–109.
18. Grigsby PW, Siegel BA, Dehdashti F. Lymph node staging by positron emission tomography in patients with carcinoma of the cervix. *J Clin Oncol* 2001;19(17):3745–3749.
19. Grigsby PW. 4th International Cervical Cancer Conference: update on PET and cervical cancer. *Gynecol Oncol* 2005;99:S173–S175.
20. Subhas N, Patel PV, Pannu HK, et al. Imaging of pelvic malignancies with in-line FDG PET-CT: case examples and common pitfalls of FDG PET. *Radiographics* 2005;25(4):1031–1043.
21. Carey PE, Coleman RE, Grigsby PW, et al. Medicare coverage of PET for cervical cancer. *J Am Coll Radiol* 2006;3:19–22.
22. Stehman F, Bundy B, DiSaia P, et al. Carcinoma of the cervix treated with irradiation therapy. I: a multivariate analysis of prognostic variables in the Gynecologic Oncology Group. *Cancer* 1991;67:2776–2785.
23. Dehdashti F, Grigsby PW, Mintun MA, et al. Assessing tumor hypoxia in cervical cancer by positron emission tomography with ^{60}Cu-ATSM: relationship to therapeutic response—a preliminary report. *Int J Radiat Oncol Biol Phys* 2003;55(5):1233–1238.
24. Tran BN, Grigsby PW, Dehdashti F, et al. Occult supraclavicular lymph node metastasis identified by FDG-PET in patients with carcinoma of the uterine cervix. *Gynecol Oncol* 2003;90(3):572–576.
25. Singh AK, Grigsby PW, Dehdashti F, et al. FDG-PET lymph node staging and survival of patients with FIGO stage IIIB cervical carcinoma. *Int J Radiat Oncol Biol Phys* 2003;56:489–493.
26. Unger JB, Lilien DL, Caldito G, et al. The prognostic value of pretreatment 2-(F)-fluoro-2-deoxy-d-glucose positron emission tomography scan in women with cervical cancer. *Int J Gynecol Cancer* 2007; .
27. Miller TR, Grigsby PW. Measurement of tumor volume by PET to evaluate prognosis in patients with advanced cervical cancer treated by radiation therapy. *Int J Radiat Oncol Biol Phys* 2002;53(2):353–359.
28. Xue F, Linn LL, Dehdashti F, et al. F-18 fluorodeoxyglucose uptake in primary cervical cancer as an indicator of prognosis after radiation therapy. *Gynecol Oncol* 2006;101(1):147–151.
29. Rose PG, Bundy BN, Watkins FB, et al. Concurrent cisplatin-based radiotherapy and chemotherapy for locally advanced cervical cancer. *N Engl J Med* 1999;340(15):1144–1153.
30. Morris M, Eifel PJ, Lu J, et al. Pelvic radiation with concurrent chemotherapy compared with pelvic and para-aortic radiation for high-risk cervical cancer. *N Engl J Med* 1999;340(15):1137–1143.
31. Keys HM, Bundy BN, Stehman FB, et al. Cisplatin, radiation, and adjuvant hysterectomy compared with radiation and adjuvant hysterectomy for bulky stage IB cervical carcinoma. *N Engl J Med* 1999;340(15):1154–1161.
32. Esthappan J, Mustic S, Malyapa RS, et al. Treatment planning guidelines regarding the use of CT/PET-guided IMRT for cervical carcinoma with positive para-aortic lymph nodes. *Int J Radiat Oncol Biol Phys* 2004;58(4):1289–1297.
33. Singh AK, Rader J, Dehdashti F, et al. Prospective trial of concurrent chemoradiation with IMRT to 60 Gy for positive para-aortic lymph nodes in carcinoma of the cervix. *Int J Radiat Oncol Biol Phys* 2006;66[3 Suppl]:S162.
34. Peters WA, Liu PY, Barrett RJ, et al. Concurrent chemotherapy and pelvic radiation therapy compared with pelvic radiation therapy alone as adjuvant therapy after radical surgery in high-risk early-stage cancer of the cervix. *J Clin Oncol* 2000;18(8):1606–1613.
35. Monk BJ, Wang J, Im S, et al. Rethinking the use of radiation and chemotherapy after radical hysterectomy: a clinical-pathologic analysis of a Gynecologic Oncology Group/Southwest Oncology Group/Radiation Therapy Oncology Group trial. *Gynecol Oncol* 2005;96(3):721–728.
36. Grigsby PW, Mutch DG, Rader J, et al. Lack of benefit of concurrent chemotherapy in patients with cervical cancer and negative lymph nodes by FDG-PET. *Int J Radiat Oncol Biol Phys* 2005;61(2):444–449.
37. DiSaia PJ, Creasman WT. *Clinical gynecologic oncology*, 6th ed. St. Louis: Saunders, 2001.
38. Ryu SY, Kim MH, Choi SC, et al. Detection of early recurrence with ^{18}F-FDG PET in patients with cervical cancer. *J Nucl Med* 2003;44(3):347–352.
39. Unger JB, Ivy JJ, Conner P, et al. Detection of recurrent cervical cancer by whole-body FDG PET scan in asymptomatic and symptomatic women. *Gynecol Oncol* 2004;94(1):212–216.
40. Grigsby PW, Siegel BA, Dehdashti F, et al. Posttherapy (^{18}F)fluorodeoxyglucose positron emission tomography in carcinoma of the cervix: response and outcome. *J Clin Oncol* 2004;22(11):2167–2171.
41. Chang TC, Law KS, Hong JH, et al. Positron emission tomography for unexplained elevation of serum squamous cell carcinoma antigen levels during follow-up for patients with cervical malignancies: a phase II study. *Cancer* 2004;101(1):164–171.
42. Yen T-C, See LC, Lai CH, et al. ^{18}F-FDG uptake in squamous cell carcinoma of the cervix is correlated with glucose transporter 1 expression. *J Nucl Med* 2004;45(1):22–29.
43. Chung HH, Kim SK, Kim TH, et al. Clinical impact of FDG-PET imaging in post-therapy surveillance of uterine cervical cancer: from diagnosis to prognosis. *Gynecol Oncol* 2006;103(1):165–170.
44. Lin CT, Yen TC, Chang TC, et al. Role of (18F)fluoro-2-deoxy-D-glucose positron emission tomography in re-recurrent cervical cancer. *Int J Gynecol Cancer* 2006;16(6):1994–2003.
45. Yen TC, Lai CH, Ma Sy, et al. Comparative benefits and limitations of (18)F-FDG PET and CT-MRI in documented or suspected recurrent cervical cancer. *Eur J Nucl Med Mol Imaging* 2006;33(12):1399–1407.
46. Sironi S, Picchio M, Landoni C, et al. Post-therapy surveillance of patients with uterine cancers: value of integrated FDG PET/CT in the detection of recurrence. *Eur J Nucl Med Mol Imaging* 2007;34(4):472–479.
47. Zhuang H, Yamamoto AJ, Sinha P, et al. Similar pelvic abnormalities on FDG-PET positron emission tomography of different origins. *Clin Nucl Med* 2001;26: 515–517.
48. Lee W-L, Liu RS, Yuan CC, et al. Relationship between gonadotropin-releasing hormone agonist and myoma cellular activity: preliminary findings on positron emission tomography. Fertil Steril 2001;75(3):638–639.
49. Aalders JG, Thomas G. Endometrial cancer—revisiting the importance of pelvic and para aortic lymph nodes. *Gynecol Oncol* 2007;104(1):222–231.
50. Connor JP, Andrews JI, Anderson B, et al. Computed tomography in endometrial carcinoma. *Obstet Gynecol* 2000;95(5):692–696.
51. Hricak H. Cancer of the uterus: the value of MRI pre- and post-irradiation. *Int J Radiat Oncol Biol Phys* 1991;21:1089–1094.
52. Grigsby P, Dehdashti F, Siegel BA. FDG-PET evaluation of recurrent endometrial carcinoma. In: Pecorelli S, Atlante G, Benedetti Panici P, et al., eds. *7th Biennial Meeting of the International Gynecologic Society*. Bologna, Italy: Monduzzi Editore, 1999.
53. Suzuki R, Miyagi E, Takahashi N, et al. Validity of positron emission tomography using fluoro-2-deoxyglucose for the preoperative evaluation of endometrial cancer. *Int J Gynecol Cancer* 2007; .
54. Saga T, Higashi T, Ishimori T, et al. Clinical value of FDG-PET in the follow up of post-operative patients with endometrial cancer. *Ann Nucl Med* 2003;17(3): 197–203.
55. Belhocine T, DeBarsy C, Hustinx R, et al. Usefulness of (18)F-FDG PET in the post-therapy surveillance of endometrial carcinoma. *Eur J Nucl Med Mol Imaging* 2002;29(9):1132–1139.
56. Belhocine T, Grigsby PW. FDG PET and PET-CT in uterine cancers [review]. *Cancer Ther* 2005;3:201–218.

CHAPTER

8.17 PET and PET/CT in Ovarian Cancer

HEDIEH ESLAMY, ROBERT BRISTOW, AND RICHARD L. WAHL

Ovarian cancer accounts for about 3% of all cancers among women and ranks second in frequency among gynecologic cancers in the United States, following cancer of the uterine corpus (1). However, in the United States, ovarian cancer has the highest mortality rate of all gynecologic cancers. An estimated 22,430 new cases of ovarian cancer and an estimated 15,280 deaths are expected in the United States in 2007 (1). This high mortality rate is in part related to the relatively advanced stage of disease in which ovarian cancer patients often present (1). Given the rather late state at which ovarian cancers are frequently diagnosed, it is clear why there is a considerable interest in developing earlier diagnostic methods for ovarian cancer.

At present, most ovarian cancers are judged as "sporadic." However, there are families at increased risk of ovarian cancer based on mutations in the *BRCA1* or *BRCA2* genes. It has been estimated that about 10% of ovarian cancers fall into this class of familial cancers. Relative risks of cancer of 20- to 45-fold over the general population have been described for carriers of these mutations. These same mutations are associated with markedly increased risks of breast cancer as well. Risk-reducing salpingo-oophorectomy has been applied in some of these women in an effort to reduce the probability of a new cancer developing (2).

Histologically, ovarian cancers are differentiated by the cell of origin: epithelial (90%), stromal, germ cell, or mixed the remainder. Ovarian cancer results in regional and distant spread through four main pathways:

1. Penetration of the ovarian capsule and direct invasion of contiguous organs or the pelvic peritoneum;
2. Spread via the lymphatic system to the pelvic and para-aortic lymph nodes;
3. Penetration of ovarian capsule and subsequent peritoneal spread;
4. Hematogenous spread (3,4).

The potential diagnostic tasks in ovarian cancer are several fold. First, accurate early diagnosis of ovarian cancer before it was clinically apparent as a pelvic mass or disseminated disease would be highly desirable. Second, characterization of an ovarian mass as malignant or benign, noninvasively, would be of great value. Once an ovarian mass was diagnosed as malignant, assessing the extent of disease would be very helpful as well (i.e., staging). After diagnosis and staging, predicting if a response would occur to a specific therapy or determining whether the disease is responding to treatment would also be very useful. Positron emission tomography (PET) has been evaluated in each of these settings to some extent, however, the role of PET must be considered in the context of other imaging and diagnostic approaches to ovarian cancer. PET has been most extensively evaluated in patients with known ovarian cancer, however.

BACKGROUND: PRIMARY DISEASE DETECTION

A robust method to screen for ovarian cancer has the potential to reduce mortality from this disease, much as has occurred with cervical cancer and the use of cytological staining. To date, a single modality screening method for ovarian cancer, using either the blood test for cancer antigen 125 (CA125) or transvaginal ultrasonography (TVS), has not provided the required accuracy necessary for reliable, cost-effective, early detection of this cancer. Multimodality screening using serum CA125 and pelvic or TVS appears to improve the median survival in the screened group (5–8). Currently there are at least two large ongoing trials for multimodal screening (CA125 and TVS) in ovarian cancer. The final assessment of the accuracy of such approaches will have to await the analysis of the complete cohort and longer follow-up to assess the impact on mortality (9,10). It is clear that such programs can identify patients with ovarian masses, which then need further work-up.

Most ovarian masses in premenopausal women are benign in etiology and functionally related to the menstrual cycle. When incidentally detected, these masses are typically followed for regression by physical examination or ultrasound. Those that do not regress have a great probability of malignancy. By contrast, ovarian masses in postmenopausal women are more commonly malignant in etiology and are far more concerning for cancer than masses in the premenopausal woman. Certainly, premenopausal women can develop ovarian cancer and a mass that does not resolve in such a patient is of considerable concern for cancer and requires further work-up.

Morphologic imaging may be used to characterize adnexal masses as benign or malignant and delineate regional or distant spread prior to surgery. In a recent meta-analysis, Liu et al. (11) compared ultrasound (US), computed tomography (CT), and magnetic resonance imaging (MRI) in differentiation of malignant from benign ovarian tumors. Sensitivity and specificity estimates of all imaging modalities were comparable: 89% (95% confidence interval [CI], 88% to 90%) for US, 85% (95% CI, 83% to 86%) for CT, and 89% (95% CI, 88% to 92%) for MRI ($P = .09$). Specificity estimates were also comparable: 95% CI, 83% to 85% for US, 76% to 92% for CT, and 84% to 88% for MRI ($P = .12$). The authors concluded that ultrasound techniques seem to be similar to CT and MRI in differentiation of malignant from benign ovarian tumors, and that ultrasound morphologic assessment still is the most important and common modality in the detection of ovarian cancer. However, since none of these imaging methods achieve total accuracy, persistent ovarian masses in postmenopausal women are commonly surgically excised to avoid delayed diagnosis of ovarian carcinoma.

Staging

Traditionally, ovarian cancer has been staged surgically. The TNM (Tumor, Node, Metastasis) and FIGO (Federation Internationale de Gynecologie et d'Obstetrique) staging systems classify ovarian cancers as:

Stage I: tumor limited to ovaries (one or both)
Stage II: tumor involves one or both ovaries with pelvic extension
Stage III: tumor involves one/both ovaries with microscopic/macroscopic peritoneal metastasis beyond the pelvis and/or regional lymph node metastasis
Stage IV: distant metastasis (excludes peritoneal metastasis) (12).

Essential elements of surgical staging of ovarian cancer include peritoneal cytology, intact tumor removal, complete abdominal exploration; removal of the remaining ovary, uterus, and fallopian tubes; infracolic omentectomy, pelvic, and para-aortic lymph node sampling; and multiple biopsies, including "blind biopsies" from areas at risk for spread (i.e., diaphragm, paracolic gutters, and pelvis). Prognosis is influenced by the diameter of the residual disease after primary cytoreductive surgery, with optimal and suboptimal debulking being defined as the largest diameter of a residual nodule as 1 cm or less or greater than 1 cm, respectively. Quite clearly, it is desirable to surgically reduce the tumor volume to the greatest extent feasible in such procedures (4).

Approximately 20% to 30% of patients with early stage disease (stage IA to IIA) and 50% to 75% of those with advanced disease (stage IIB to IV) who obtain a complete response following first-line chemotherapy will ultimately develop recurrent disease, which more frequently involves the pelvis and abdomen (13).

In a recent study preoperative CT and MRI were found to be reasonably accurate in the detection of inoperable tumor and in the prediction of suboptimal debulking (sensitivity, specificity, positive predictive value, and negative predictive value were 76%, 92%, 94%, and 96%, respectively). The two modalities were equally effective ($P = 1.0$) in the detection of inoperable tumor. This study suggests that imaging may help triage inoperable patients to a more appropriate neoadjuvant chemotherapy group (14). The 76% sensitivity indicates there are still major opportunities to improve imaging accuracy, especially for low tumor volume disease.

The standard of care for patients with ovarian carcinoma is primary cytoreductive surgery and adjuvant chemotherapy (the latter except in some stage IA and IB patients), typically intravenous paclitaxel and carboplatin. A number of phase III randomized trials in the United States have reported improved progression-free survival (PFS) and/or overall survival (OS) with the intraperitoneal (IP) administration of cisplatin. Hess et al. (15) identified six randomized trials of 1,716 ovarian cancer patients. The pooled hazard ratio (HR) for PFS of IP cisplatin as compared to intravenous treatment regimens reported was 0.792 (95% CI, 0.688 to 0.912; $P = .001$), and the pooled HR for OS was 0.799 (95% CI, 0.702 to 0.910; $P = .0007$), both favoring IP therapy to intravenous treatment. These findings strongly support the incorporation of an IP cisplatin regimen to improve survival in the front-line treatment of stage III, optimally debulked ovarian cancer.

Recently, a prospective trial by Armstrong et al. (16) showed in 415 patients enrolled that for the patients who could tolerate the rather toxic IP therapy approach, the median duration of PFS and OS were significantly prolonged in the IP therapy groups versus the intravenous PFS from 18.3 to 23.8 months and disease-free survival from 49.7 to 65.6 months ($P < .03$ and $< .05$, respectively).

In patients with advanced disease who are not candidates for primary cytoreductive surgery, neoadjuvant chemotherapy is commonly administered. Localized borderline histology tumors are sometimes not treated with chemotherapy.

Ovarian cancer primarily recurs in the peritoneal cavity and retroperitoneal lymph nodes. Patients are monitored for recurrence with periodic physical examinations, serum CA125 levels, and ultrasound examination. Additional imaging—CT, MRI, and fluorine 18-fluorodeoxyglucose ([^{18}F]-FDG) PET, or PET/CT—is performed when signs or symptoms suggestive of recurrence appear (4,13,17). However, both morphologic (CT and MRI) and functional imaging ([^{18}F]-FDG PET) are limited in their ability to detect small-volume (<5 to 10 mm) disease. Rising CA125 levels may precede the clinical detection of recurrence in 56% to 94% of the cases, with a median lead time of 3 to 5 months (13).

In the 1970s and 1980s, second-look surgery, defined as a comprehensive surgical exploration in an asymptomatic patient who has completed primary cytoreductive surgery and adjuvant chemotherapy, was widely used. Second-look surgery does not appear to have a role in the management of early stage ovarian cancer, and its role in the patients with advanced-stage disease is controversial (4).

The treatment options for recurrent ovarian cancer include salvage chemotherapy, experimental protocols, hormonal therapy, secondary cytoreductive surgery, palliative care, and hospice care. The choice of the chemotherapeutic regimen depends on whether the disease is platinum sensitive or platinum resistant. Patients with disease progression while receiving platinum-based therapy, patients who fail to achieve a complete clinical response, and those who relapse within 6 months of the end of chemotherapy are classified as platinum resistant (4,17).

Initiation of treatment in patients with biochemical relapse (CA125 greater than 35 U/mL or doubling of the posttreatment nadir level) and negative radiographic studies is a controversial topic, but is performed in some settings (4,17).

ROLE OF FLUORODEOXYGLUCOSE PET IN OVARIAN CANCER IMAGING

Ovarian cancers have been shown to be FDG avid in animal models, to express high levels of the glucose transporter *GLUT1*, and in human xenograft studies to have higher FDG uptake in areas of viable cancer than in normal tissues (including normal lymph nodes) in human xenograft studies. Pilot studies showing the feasibility of imaging ovarian cancer with PET were reported as early as 1991 (18–20). Nearly all PET imaging of ovarian cancer is currently performed with FDG as the radiotracer.

Much like other FDG-avid cancers, patients should be imaged in the fasting state to minimize insulin levels and the targeting of FDG to normal insulin-responsive tissues like skeletal muscle. The approach to imaging may vary slightly depending on the individual PET center but is generally rather consistent. In the authors' institution, patient preparation for ovarian cancer imaging is similar to that for oncologic imaging in general, with fasting for at least 4 hours (and ideally overnight), with no specific urinary tract preparation. The authors normally use dilute positive oral contrast to achieve definitive positive bowel visualization. In some centers, various interventions are utilized to decrease the amount of FDG in the urinary tract such as bladder catheterization, continuous bladder irrigation, and/or intravenous hydration (1,000 to 1,500 mL of 0.9% or 0.45% saline solution) followed by the intravenous administration of 20 to 40 mg of furosemide. Another way to deal with urinary tract activity can be use of an additional delayed image postvoiding if there is any confusion regarding the urinary tract radiotracer activity levels. Most centers now use iterative reconstruction methods as opposed to filtered back projection methods in order to image the pelvis, as these iterative imaging approaches appear less sensitive to imaging artifacts from the "hot" activity in the bladder or ureters. The proper time from tracer injection until imaging has to be long enough for the FDG to accumulate avidly into the tumors, but not so long that the radiotracer has decayed away substantially. Most imaging in ovarian cancer is started about 60 minutes posttracer injection, but longer delays of 90 minutes to 2 hours will commonly result in superior target/background uptake ratios but lower total counts in the images.

The potential role of [^{18}F]-FDG PET and/or PET/CT in ovarian carcinoma has been considered and/or investigated to varying extents in the following settings:

Screening: Detection of ovarian cancer in a woman at average or high risk of ovarian cancer through systematic use of PET imaging in large numbers of patients.

Diagnosis: Differentiation of benign from malignant masses in patients presenting with asymptomatic adnexal masses, diagnosed either by physical examination or by screening programs.

Staging: Preoperative staging of patients with known or suspected ovarian cancer.

Monitoring response to therapy: Evaluating response to neoadjuvant chemotherapy, adjuvant chemotherapy, standard chemotherapy, or radiotherapy.

Restaging: Evaluating ovarian tumor recurrence in patients with clinically suspected recurrence and/or treatment planning to accurately localize extent of disease.

Surveillance: Evaluating ovarian tumor recurrence in patients who are clinically disease free and not on specific therapies.

Prognosis: Determining prognosis at any of several times, including after cytoreductive surgery, adjuvant chemotherapy, or at presentation prior to any therapy.

DIAGNOSIS OF PRIMARY OVARIAN CANCER

Screening

There have been no systematic studies of FDG PET screening specifically for ovarian carcinoma detection. Radiation exposure with PET/CT is not minimal, and exposure of large numbers of patients to ionizing radiation in a screening program may result in a high population radiation burden. However, cancer screening of larger populations with FDG has been investigated by several groups, mainly in Asia (21). In addition, there are large numbers of patients with known or suspected cancers being imaged with PET for other reasons. Although a wide range of cancers have been detected in such programs, with a prevalence of 1% to 2%, ovarian cancer has not been detected with any substantive frequency. Given the radiation exposure from screening studies and the limited anecdotal data available, there is not an established role for PET screening in ovarian cancer. The use of PET/CT in screening for cancer is discussed in detail by Schöder et al. (22) in an excellent review. However, there is a not uncommon situation clinically in which there is increased radiotracer uptake in the ovary of an asymptomatic woman being imaged for other reasons using FDG PET.

Lerman et al. (23) detected increased ovarian FDG uptake in 21 of 119 premenopausal patients without known gynecologic malignancy. They concluded that increased ovarian uptake is associated with malignancy in postmenopausal patients but may be either functional or malignant in premenopausal patients. Typically in the premenopausal woman, such uptake is function in nature; however, such a finding requires additional follow-up imaging to ensure the lesion has resolved or is stable.

Kim et al. (24) correlated the finding of incidental FDG accumulation in the ovary with the menstrual history, concurrent morphologic imaging (MRI, CT, and ultrasound) and surgical or imaging (PET or CT) follow-up in 19 patients who did not have primary or metastatic ovarian malignancy. They concluded that the typical spherical or discoid FDG accumulation in the ovary during the luteal or ovulatory phase represents normal physiological uptake in ovarian follicles or corpus luteum.

A recent report from China had similar findings (25). Thus, if incidental ovarian uptake is identified in a younger woman, it is more likely benign than malignant, but must be followed closely as cancer can occur in younger women. In postmenopausal women such uptake is far more concerning for cancer.

PRIMARY OVARIAN CARCINOMA DIAGNOSIS

The literature regarding PET in ovarian carcinoma detection is somewhat variable and, at first inspection, somewhat confusing. The original literature was generated using PET only, while most recent studies have utilized PET/CT imaging. Given the complexities and variability of locations for the ovaries in the pelvis, it is not surprising that recent results with PET/CT have been generally more accurate than those with PET only.

The detection sensitivity using PET for ovarian cancer is likely dependent on the lesion histology as well as the lesion size. Small lesions, under 1 cm in size, are likely to be far less easily detected than larger lesions due to the resolution limitations of current PET systems. Similarly, mucinous tumors are less likely to be detected than more cellular tumors based on the experience in other mucinous tumors. In interpreting the results of PET imaging in ovarian carcinoma, it is critical to bear in mind the significant variability that may be present in the study populations included for imaging. Detection of microscopic disease is a task beyond the resolution of current PET systems. By contrast, the detection of macroscopic tumors before treatment-induced reductions in glucose metabolism occur is a much more realistic and feasible task for current imaging methodologies.

Ultrasound has been considered the modality of choice in the evaluation of patients with suspected adnexal masses, with MRI utilized in uncertain or problematic cases to further characterize masses as benign or malignant (26).

Hubner et al. (27) correlated the results of FDG PET and CT with pathology results in imaging ovarian masses. The calculated sensitivity, specificity, accuracy, positive predictive value, and negative predictive value were 83%, 80%, 82%, 86%, and 76%, respectively, for PET and 82%, 53%, 72%, 77%, and 62% for CT. However, when combining PET and CT results, the positive and negative predictive values would be 95% and 100%, respectively. This study was performed with an early generation PET-only system, not PET/CT. Further, filtered back projection was used for image reconstructions. This may have led to degradation of image quality due to streak artifacts, but the overall performance of the test remained encouraging.

Rieber et al. (28) prospectively compared the diagnostic performance of transvaginal ultrasound, PET, and MRI in 103 patients with suspicious adnexal findings on ultrasound, in whom subsequent histology revealed 12 malignant and 91 benign ovarian tumors. The calculated sensitivity, specificity, and accuracy were 58%, 78%, and 76%, respectively, for PET; 83%, 84%, and 83% for MRI; 92%, 59%, and 63% for ultrasound; and 92%, 84%, and 85% for all three modalities in consensus.

Kawahara et al. (29) prospectively compared MRI and FDG PET in 38 patients suspected of having ovarian cancer based on findings on physical examination and ultrasound. Histology revealed 23 malignant and 15 benign lesions. The calculated sensitivity, specificity, and accuracy were 78%, 87%, and 82%, respectively, for PET; 91%, 87%, and 92% for MRI; and 91%, 87%, 92% for the two modalities in consensus.

However, in a recent study combined PET/CT demonstrated a higher sensitivity and specificity of 100% and 92.5%, respectively ($P < .00005$) in diagnosing a malignant pelvic tumor in patients with a pelvic mass of unknown origin and elevated risk of malignancy based on a substantially elevated serum CA125, ultrasound examinations, and menopausal state (30). The authors suggested PET/CT was the image modality of choice when ultrasound showed a pelvic tumor and additional information prior to surgery was needed. It is worth noting that borderline tumors and benign tumors were lumped together into the benign group in this study, which may not be suitable for routine management.

Thus, the more recent results with PET/CT appear superior to those of PET alone, but it is improbable that 100% sensitivity will be reliably achieved with PET/CT in such masses. In other series, the presence of cystic tumors represented a particular challenge for detection of ovarian cancer as there was little viable tumor as a part of the whole mass.

The etiologies of false-positive and false-negative findings on FDG PET in patients with adnexal masses are summarized in Table 8.17.1 (27–29,31,32).

STAGING OF OVARIAN CANCER

Yoshida et al. (33) prospectively evaluated the incremental benefits of FDG PET over CT alone for the preoperative staging of 15 patients with suspected ovarian cancer on the basis of results of physical examination, sonography findings, and level of serum CA125. All patients underwent surgical staging within 2 weeks of the imaging examinations. The lesion-based sensitivity, specificity, accuracy, positive predictive value, and negative predictive value

TABLE 8.17.1 Etiologies of False-positive and False-negative Findings on Fluorodeoxyglucose PET in Patients With Adnexal Masses

Etiologies of Possible False-positive Findings on Fluorodeoxyglucose PET	Etiologies of False-negative Findings on Fluorodeoxyglucose PET
Endometrioma	Borderline tumors (mucinous and serous)
Dermoid cyst	Mucinous adenocarcinoma
Cystadenoma	Serous adenocarcinoma (well differentiated stage I)
Thecoma	Small tumors
Schwannoma (benign)	Hyperglycemia (potentially)
Follicular cyst	
Corpus luteum cyst	
Hydrosalpinx	
Adnexal abscess	
Cholesterol granuloma	

(From Hubner KF, McDonald TW, Niethammer JG, et al. Assessment of primary and metastatic ovarian cancer by positron emission tomography (PET) using 2-[F18]Deoxyglucose (2-[F18]FDG). *Gynecol Oncol* 1993;51:197–204; Rieber A, Nussla K, Stohr I, et al. Preoperative diagnosis of ovarian tumors with MR imnaging: comparison with transvaginal sonography, positron emission tomography, and histologic findings. *AJR Am J Roentgenol* 2001;177:123–129; Kawahara K, Yoshida Y, Kurokawa T, et al. Evaluation of positron emission tomography with tracer 18-fluorodeoxyglucose in addition ot magnetic resonance imaging in the diagnosis of ovarian cancer in selected women after ultrasonography. *J Comput Assist Tomogr* 2004;28:505–516; Fenchel S, Grab D, Nuessle K, et al. Asymptomatic adnexal masses: correlation of FDG PET and histopathologic findings. Radiology 2002;223:780–788; Schroder W, Zimny M, Rudlowski C, et al. The role of F18-fluorodeoxyglucose positron emission tomography (F18-FDG PET) in diagnosis of ovarian cancer. Int J Gynecol Cancer 1999;9:117–122.)

were 46%, 90%, 83%, 47%, and 90%, respectively, for CT; and 68%, 92%, 88%, 65%, and 93% for PET/CT. The authors did not report these values for FDG PET alone. The patient-based diagnostic accuracy was 53% for CT and 78% for CT with FDG PET. The authors concluded that the addition of FDG PET to CT increased accuracy in staging ovarian cancer.

Peritoneal carcinomatosis can present as either focal or uniform FDG uptake, corresponding to nodular and diffuse peritoneal disease, respectively, on FDG PET scans (34). Low-volume disease can fail to be detected on PET/CT.

MONITORING RESPONSE TO THERAPY

In a prospective study of 33 patients with advanced stage ovarian cancer (FIGO stage IIIC and IV) receiving neoadjuvant chemotherapy prior to cytoreductive surgery, FDG PET scans of the abdomen and pelvis were obtained before treatment and after the first and third cycles of chemotherapy (35). A significant correlation was observed between FDG PET metabolic response after the first and third cycles of chemotherapy and overall survival (Fig. 8.17.1). The authors concluded that FDG PET appears to be a promising tool for early prediction of response to chemotherapy. There is increased use of PET/CT in this setting, although the literature is clearly just evolving.

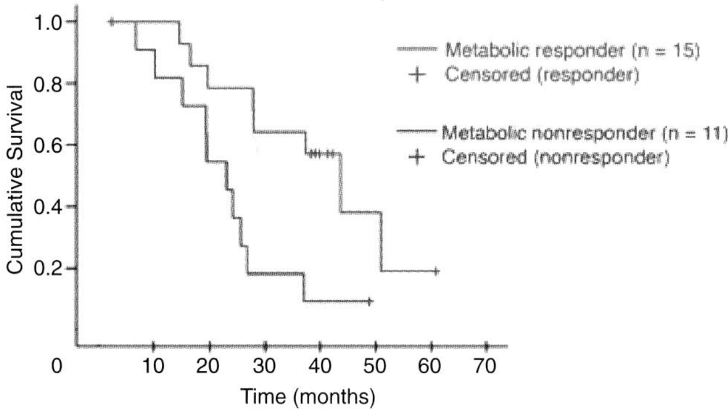

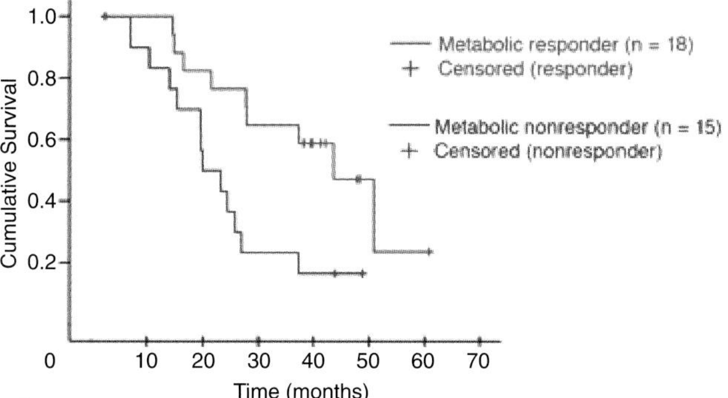

FIGURE 8.17.1. Survival in ovarian cancer patients following chemotherapy with two separate standard uptake value response criteria thresholds. A metabolic response was associated with longer survival. (From Avril N, Sassen S, Schmalfeldt B, et al. Prediction of response to neoadjuvant chemotherapy by sequential F-18-fluorodeoxyglucose positron emission tomography in patients with advanced-stage ovarian cancer. *J Clin Oncol* 2005;23:7445–7453, with permission.)

Restaging

Many authors have retrospectively or prospectively evaluated the diagnostic value of PET or PET/CT in patients with clinically suspected ovarian cancer recurrence (based on physical examination, serum tumor markers, morphologic imaging, or symptoms) and patients who are clinically disease free (i.e., restaging versus surveillance). As these two groups have potentially different pretest probabilities of a positive PET finding, they should be considered separately. Restaging is typically performed either in patients with suspected tumor recurrence or in patients with documented tumor recurrence on anatomical imaging to accurately localize extent of disease for treatment planning. The impact of restaging with functional imaging on patient management has also been studied. It should be noted that many of these studies have a small sample size and therefore lack statistical power, and that they also utilize different standards of reference and different imaging methodologies (PET vs. PET/CT vs. PET/CT with intravenous contrast). Some of these studies are summarized in Table 8.17.2 (36–46).

Bristow et al. (40) prospectively evaluated the utility of PET/CT in patient selection for secondary cytoreductive surgery. Their standard of reference was recurrent ovarian tumor measuring 1 cm or greater at the time of surgery, a size associated with an "optimal" debulking procedure. This size cutoff for macroscopic disease is somewhat different from other studies that also considered microscopic disease and macroscopic disease less than 1 cm in the calculation of sensitivity and specificity of PET. In this study, PET/CT had an estimated accuracy of 81.8% and sensitivity of 83.3% in detecting recurrent disease 1 cm or greater.

Bristow et al. (47) retrospectively evaluated 14 patients with rising serum CA125 levels and negative or equivocal conventional CT imaging 6 months or more after primary therapy who were identified as having recurrent disease limited to retroperitoneal lymph nodes by combined PET/CT and underwent surgical reassessment of targeted nodal basins. Eleven patients (78.6%) had recurrent ovarian cancer in retroperitoneal lymph nodes targeted by PET/CT. Of 143 nodes retrieved, 59 contained recurrent ovarian cancer (median nodal diameter, 2.5 cm; range, 0.8 to 5.2 cm). For all target nodal basins, the sensitivity, specificity, positive and negative predictive values, and accuracy for recurrent ovarian cancer in dissected lymph nodes were 40.7% (24/59), 94.0% (79/84), 82.8% (24/29), 69.3% (79/114), and 72.0% (103/143), respectively ($P < .001$). PET/CT failed to identify microscopic disease in 59.3% of pathologically positive nodes. The authors concluded that combined PET/CT demonstrates high positive predictive value in identifying recurrent ovarian cancer in retroperitoneal lymph nodes when conventional CT findings are negative or equivocal. The high incidence of occult disease within the target nodal basins suggests that regional lymphadenectomy may be necessary for complete secondary cytoreduction of recurrent disease. These findings in lymph nodes are very similar to those described in breast cancer where false-negative results in small tumor foci were not uncommon. In a small study from the same institution, Pannu et al. (48) showed a very low sensitivity of PET/CT for lesions less than 1 cm in diameter (13%), illustrating again the limitations of PET/CT in low-volume disease.

Sironi et al. (41) prospectively evaluated the accuracy of PET/CT for depicting persistent ovarian carcinoma after first-line treatment in 31 patients, with use of histologic findings as the reference standard. The overall lesion-based sensitivity, specificity, accuracy,

TABLE 8.17.2 Summary of Several Studies Assessing the Role of PET/CT in Restaging of Ovarian Cancer

Authors (ref.)	Modality	N	SN	SP
Yen et al. (36)	PET	24	91	92
Zimny et al. (37)	PET	58	94	75
Nakamoto et al. (38)	PET	12	80	50
Torizuka et al. (39)	PET	25	80	100
Bristow et al. (40)	PET/CT	22	81.8 (in detecting recurrent disease ≥1 cm)	83.3
Sironi et al. (41)	PET/CT	31	78	75
Takekuma et al. (42)	PET	29	84.6	100
Nanni et al. (43)	PET/CT	41	88.2	71.4 (acc 85.4)
Chung et al. (44)	PET/CT	77	93.3	96.9
Thrall et al. (45)	PET/CT	24	94	100
Sebastian et al. (46)	PET/CT	53	Acc 94%	–

N, number of cases; SN, sensitivity; SP, specificity.

positive predictive value, and negative predictive value of PET/CT were 78%, 75%, 77%, 89%, and 57%, respectively. All of the lesions missed on PET/CT were 0.5 cm or less in maximum diameter, again consistent with the limited ability of PET to detect microscopic disease.

Serum CA125 levels are often used to follow ovarian cancer patients and to suggest recurrence. Sheng et al. (49) reported the PET/CT findings on 26 patients with rising CA125 levels (doubling or greater in 2 months), with 14 of 17 greater than 35 kU/L typically with a negative CT scan. In nearly all patients, PET was able to detect recurrent tumor, although more foci appeared to be detected by PET in patients with higher CA125 levels. Thus, it is not uncommon to have a negative or equivocal CT scan and a positive PET scan if serum markers are elevated or elevating. Examples of PET/CT scans obtained in the setting of suspected recurrence with a rising CA125 level are shown in Figs. 8.17.2 and 8.17.3.

PET/CT was recently compared to CT in detecting ovarian carcinoma recurrence in 51 consecutive patients who underwent 53 restaging PET/CT scans (46). PET/CT accuracy exceeded CT for body 92% (49/53) versus 83% (44/53), chest 96% (51/53) versus 89% (47/53), and abdomen 91% (48/53) versus 79% (42/53). PET was more accurate than CT in the abdomen by receiver operating characteristic curve analysis (<0.01). Interobserver agreement was better for PET–CT than for CT alone. The authors concluded that PET/CT demonstrates greater accuracy and less interobserver variability than CT alone.

Surveillance

True prospective systematic surveillance studies have not been reported in ovarian cancer. Most of the studies have been retrospective in nature and were performed at varying points in the disease management algorithm. Thus, the precise role of PET/CT in surveillance remains in evolution. The study by Rose et al. (50) could possibly be viewed as restaging or as surveillance, as it involved an assessment after therapy was completed. These authors correlated FDG PET with findings on second-look laparotomy in 22 patients with advanced-stage ovarian cancer (n = 17) or peritoneal carcinoma (N = 5) who had achieved complete clinical remission and normal CA125 levels after six cycles of chemotherapy. Persistent disease was found in 13 of the 22 (59%) on second-look laparotomy: 1.5 cm macroscopic disease (n = 1), macroscopic disease less than 1 cm (n = 8), and microscopic disease (n = 4). PET only detected the 1.5 cm macroscopic disease and one of the sites with microscopic disease. It should be noted that this 10% sensitivity for all lesions is associated with a "100%" sensitivity for lesions greater than 1 cm in diameter, similar to that of Bristow et al (40). Thus, PET has consistently performed well for macroscopic disease, but fails in low tumor volume disease very commonly. The results of the studies by Rose et al. (50) Zimny et al. (37), and Nakamoto et al. (38) are summarized in Table 8.17.3.

In a retrospective chart review Thrall et al. (45) identified 59 FDG PET/CT scans with intravenous contrast (in 39 ovarian cancer patients) performed for restaging (47 scans), monitoring response to treatment (eight scans), or surveillance (four scans). Four patients were scanned in lieu of second-look laparoscopy, and all were negative with no recurrent disease detected during a follow-up period of 6 months.

Garcia-Velloso et al. (51) retrospectively evaluated the diagnostic yield of FDG PET for the diagnosis of recurrent ovarian cancer. Eighty FDG PET scans were performed on 55 patients owing to suspicion of relapse (restaging), and 45 FDG PET scans were performed on 31 patients who were clinically disease free (surveillance). In the patients who underwent imaging for surveillance the sensitivity, specificity, positive predictive value, negative predictive value, and accuracy were 55%, 88%, 78%, 71%, and 73%, respectively. Thus, PET can perform reasonably well in a surveillance setting, but more systematic study is essential to fully define the role of the method in this setting.

Prognosis

Kim et al. (52) retrospectively compared the prognostic value of FDG PET and second-look laparotomy in 55 patients with advanced ovarian cancer who had undergone cytoreductive surgery and adjuvant chemotherapy. Thirty patients underwent second-look laparotomy and 25 patients underwent FDG PET. Disease-free interval (40.5 +/– 11.6 months and 48.6 +/– 12.1 months,

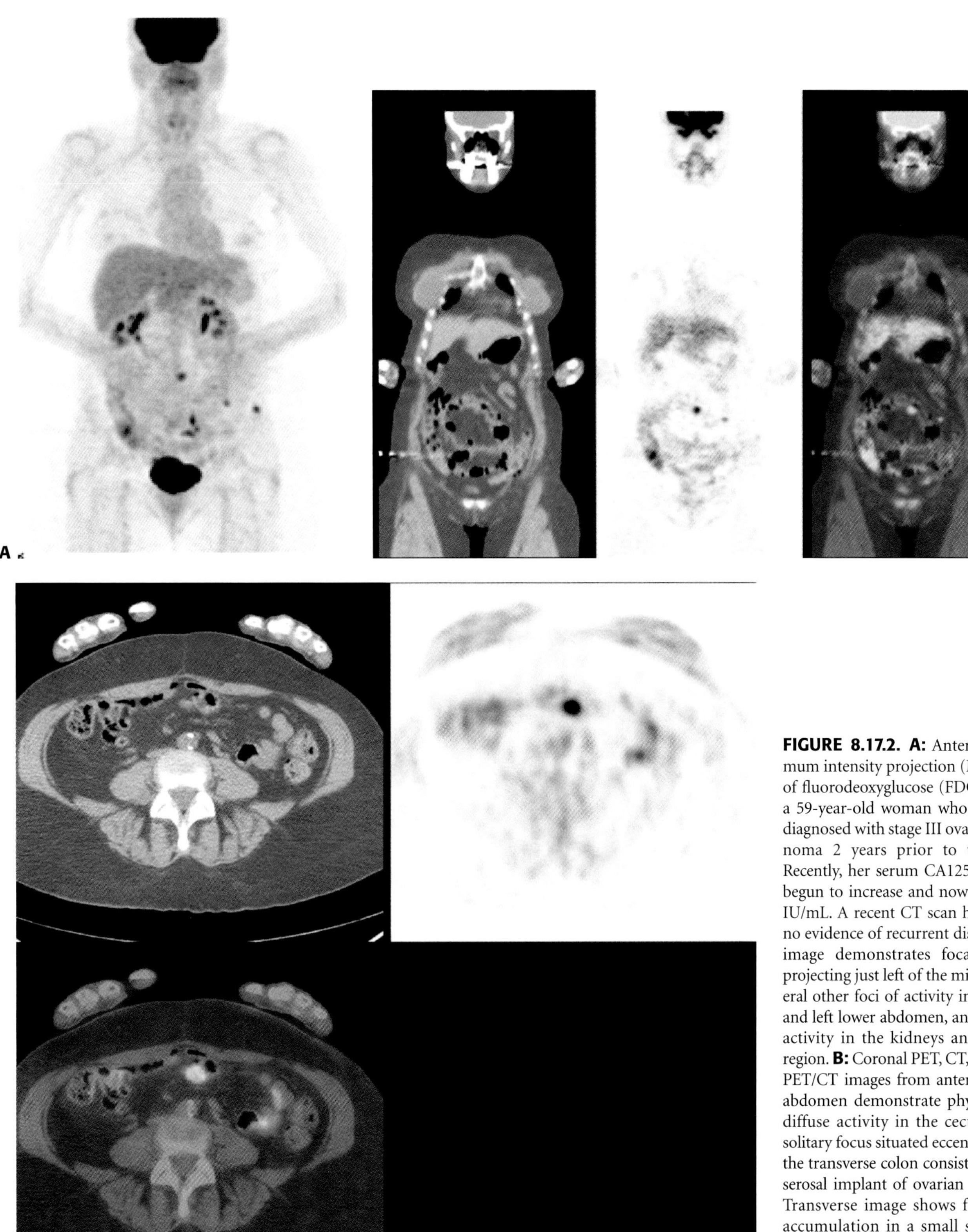

FIGURE 8.17.2. A: Anterior maximum intensity projection (MIP) view of fluorodeoxyglucose (FDG) scan in a 59-year-old woman who had been diagnosed with stage III ovarian carcinoma 2 years prior to this scan. Recently, her serum CA125 level had begun to increase and now was at 46 IU/mL. A recent CT scan had shown no evidence of recurrent disease. This image demonstrates focal activity projecting just left of the midline, several other foci of activity in the mid- and left lower abdomen, and excreted activity in the kidneys and bladder region. **B:** Coronal PET, CT, and fused PET/CT images from anterior in the abdomen demonstrate physiological diffuse activity in the cecum and a solitary focus situated eccentrically off the transverse colon consistent with a serosal implant of ovarian cancer. **C:** Transverse image shows focal FDG accumulation in a small soft tissue mass immediately adjoining the serosa of the transverse colon, representing a tumor implant situated on the bowel.

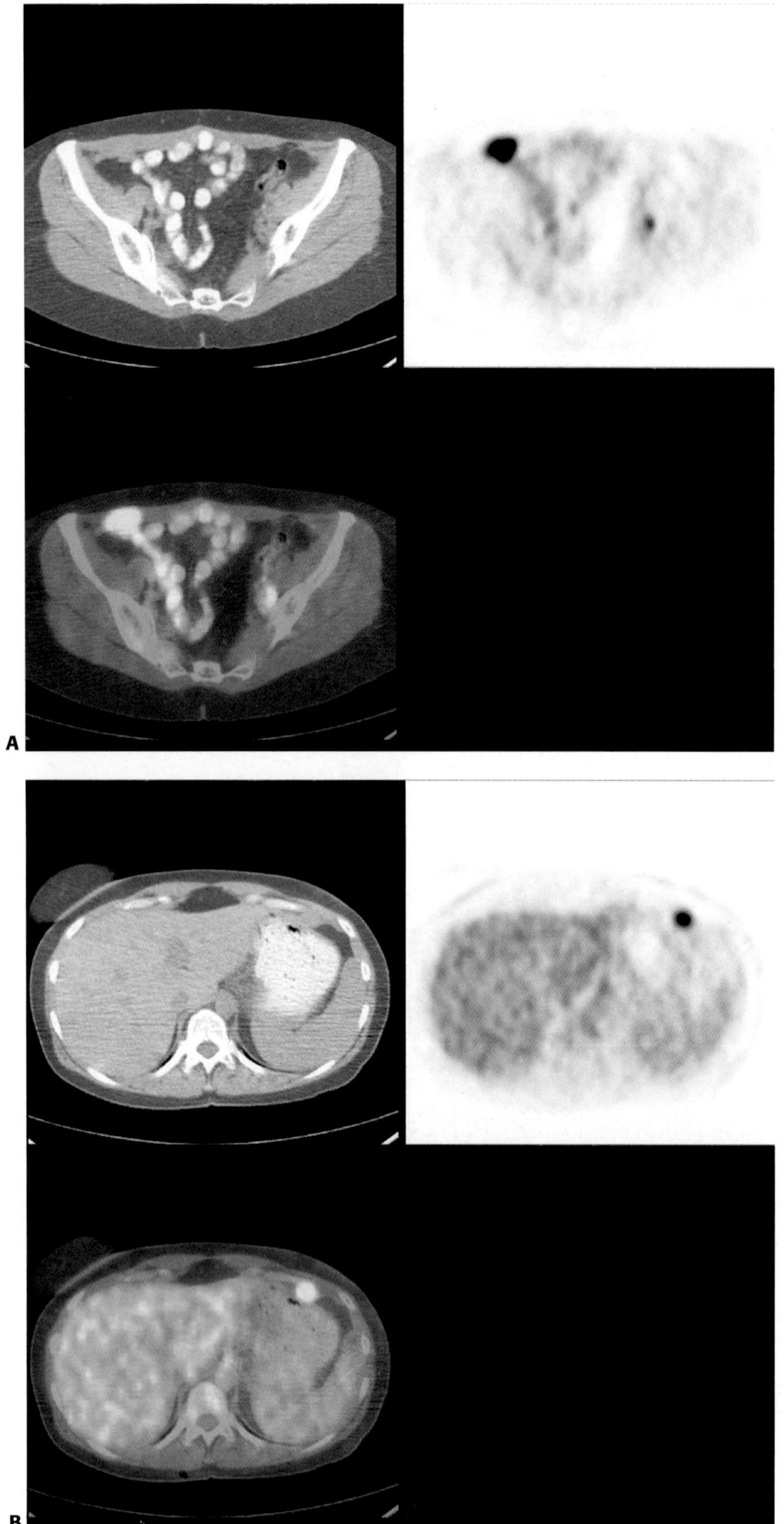

FIGURE 8.17.3. A 40-year-old woman with a history of stage 3C ovarian cancer diagnosed 5 years prior to this PET/CT. An outside CT demonstrated a 2-cm anterior abdominal mass. PET/CT was obtained to determine if there was any other tumor present. **A:** Transverse images demonstrate on PET and PET/CT an intense focus of tracer accumulation in the right anterior abdominal wall. In addition, there is focus of activity in a left internal iliac lymph node, both representing metastatic ovarian cancer. **B:** Transverse images in the upper abdomen demonstrate a nearly normal CT scan with a markedly abnormal PET, showing intense fluorodeoxyglucose (FDG) uptake in the peritoneal space just anterior to the stomach. Examination of the fused image clearly shows the uptake to be in a very subtle peritoneal implant. (*continued*)

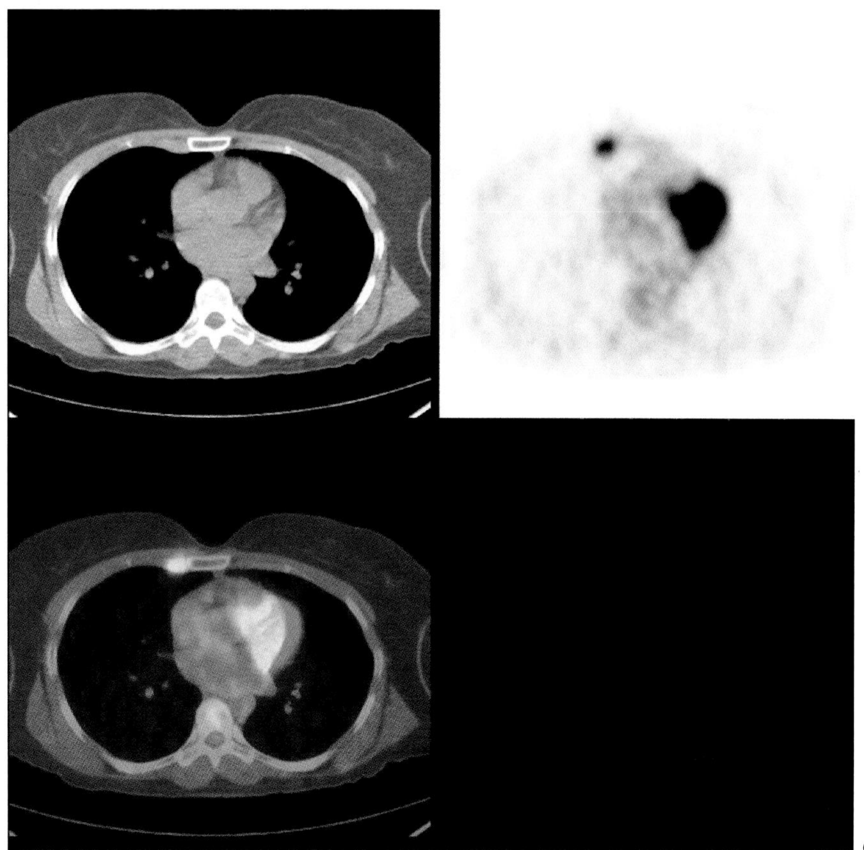

FIGURE 8.17.3. *Continued.* **C:** Transverse image of the thorax show intense FDG uptake in a right internal mammary node. The right internal mammary node is minimally enlarged. This represents an internal mammary lymph node metastasis. In addition, normal FDG uptake is identified in the heart.

respectively, in the PET and second-look laparotomy groups) and progression-free interval (28.8 +/− 12.7 months and 30.6 +/− 13.7 months, respectively, in the PET and second-look laparotomy groups) were similar in these two groups, and the authors concluded that FDG PET could be used as a substitute for second-look laparotomy in the follow-up of patients with ovarian cancer.

As discussed earlier, Avril et al. (35) has shown a better prognosis in patients who have a brisk decline in standard uptake value to chemotherapy than was seen in the nonresponding groups. Cho et al. (53) retrospectively assessed the correlation of PET positivity of tumor recurrence and vascularity, Ki-67, p53, and histologic grade in 19 patients with recurrent ovarian cancer prior to second-look surgery. FDG PET positivity revealed positive correlation with microvessel density and mitotic activity. Thus, it seems biologically reasonable to expect that declines in tumor metabolic activity would likely be linked to relevant biological changes.

Other PET Radiotracers

FDG has been the dominant tracer used in clinical studies of PET imaging in ovarian and other cancers. However, other tracers may have some advantages. Torizuka et al. (54) evaluated carbon-11 ([^{11}C])-choline in a small number of patients with ovarian cancer. They found that [^{11}C]-choline had less tracer uptake in the urine than that seen with FDG but had considerable normal gut uptake. Both FDG and [^{11}C]-choline failed to detect a tumor in a patient with a low tumor burden. At present, there has been too little experience with radiotracers other than FDG to draw firm conclusions regarding their value.

TABLE 8.17.3 Summary of Several Studies Assessing the Role of PET/CT in Surveillance of Ovarian Cancer

Authors (ref.)	N	SN	SP	Standard of Reference
Rose et al. (50)	22 (17 ovarian)	10	42	Second-look laparotomy
Zimny et al. (37)	48	65	86	Histology or median follow-up of 22 months
Nakamoto et al. (38)	12	67	89	Histopathology or at least 6 months of clinical follow-up

N, number of cases; SN, sensitivity; SP, specificity.

CHANGES IN MANAGEMENT BASED ON PET OR PET/CT

Simcock et al. (55) prospectively evaluated the impact of PET/CT in the management of recurrent epithelial ovarian cancer. PET/CT results showed a different from known (pre-PET/CT) disease distribution in 64% of scans; PET/CT showed less disease than known in 9% and more disease in 52% of scans. PET/CT resulted in a substantial management change in 58% of patients. The authors concluded that PET/CT modifies the assessment of the distribution of recurrent ovarian cancer, alters patient management in a substantial proportion of patients, and appears to offer prognostic information.

Another report examining management changes showed PET appeared to induce an intermodality change in management in 62.8% of patients with suspected recurrent ovarian carcinoma (56).

Mangili et al. (57) compared PET/CT to CT in 32 patients. Intermodality changes in management (i.e., use of a different treatment modality) after PET/CT examination were indicated in 14 of 32 (44%) patients in the chart review. The most common management change was from observation to chemotherapy.

Economic analyses of PET are limited, but in the setting of reducing the number of laparotomies for diagnosis, in one model, PET reduce the number of procedures from 70% to just 5%, with an estimated cost savings of $2,000 to $12,000 per case due to avoidance of many surgical procedures (58).

CONCLUSION

The use of PET/CT in ovarian carcinoma imaging continues to increase. There is not an established role for PET imaging in the screening for ovarian cancer. It is also not clear that ther performance of PET/CT is adequate to characterize ovarian masses as malignant or benign as some false negatives are seen in borderline tumors and those tumors with substantial cystic components, although recent results with PET/CT have been very encouraging. There appears to be sufficient data showing less than optimal sensitivity, so that an approach using FDG PET/CT to make the determination as to whether a mass requires surgery cannot be confidently recommended. Certainly in postmenopausal women it is clear that intense FDG uptake in an ovarian mass is highly concerning for ovarian cancer. Such a finding can be seen incidentally in a busy PET/CT practice due to the prevalence of ovarian cancer in the cancer population and warrants further investigation.

More data including careful prospective trials in adequate numbers of patients using state-of-the-art PET/CT will be required before PET/CT could be adopted as a tool to make triage decisions regarding ovarian masses.

A substantial amount of data now exist to show PET/CT to be consistently superior to CT alone in the detection of recurrent ovarian cancer for most histologies. Although prospective studies showing survival benefit in patients imaged with PET would be desirable, they are unlikely to be forthcoming, especially given the increasing clinical acceptance of PET/CT in patient management. Although many studies are retrospective, most have shown the limited ability of FDG PET and PET/CT to detect disease recurrence in those tumors less than 5 to 10 mm in maximum diameter.

The most established indication for PET/CT appears to be in patients with clinical suspicion of recurrent ovarian carcinoma based on rising CA125 levels (above 35 U/mL or doubling of the nadir achieved after primary treatment) and negative or equivocal morphological imaging findings. However, given the rapidly growing acceptance of PET/CT, it is increasingly common, despite a somewhat limited number of studies, to use PET/CT instead of CT alone in the imaging management of ovarian cancer, for treatment response assessment, as well as for follow-up. The roles of PET in ovarian cancer treatment response assessment are less well explored, but initial data are consistent with that of PET in other solid tumors (i.e., brisk declines in glycolysis are associated with better responses and prognosis). The role of PET in surveillance remains under evaluation, but it is increasingly applied if there are reasonable therapeutic alternatives for patients. It is anticipated this literature will continue to emerge over the coming years and that PET will assume an increasingly major role in the management of ovarian cancer patients.

REFERENCES

1. *Cancer facts and figures 2007*. Atlanta, GA: American Cancer Society. World Wide Web URL: http://www.cancer.org.
2. Kauff ND, Barakat RR. Risk-reducing salpingo-oophorectomy in patients with germline mutations in *BRCA1* or *BRCA2*. *J Clin Oncol* 2007;25:2921–2927.
3. Bhoola S, Hoskins W. Diagnosis and management of epithelial ovarian cancer. *Obstet Gynecol* 2006;107:1399–1410.
4. Sonoda Y, Spriggs D. Oncology: an evidence-based approach. In: Chang AE, Ganz PA, Hayes DF, eds. *Ovarian cancer*. New York: Springer, 2005:903–927.
5. Jacobs I, Stabile I, Bridges J, et al. Multimodal approach to screening for ovarian cancer. *Lancet* 1988;1:268–271.
6. Jacobs I, Davies AP, Bridges J, et al. Prevalence screening for ovarian cancer in postmenopausal women by CA125 measurement and ultrasonography. *BMJ* 1993;306:1030–1034.
7. Jacobs IJ, Skates SJ, MacDonald N, et al. Screening for ovarian cancer: a pilot randomised controlled trial. *Lancet* 1999;353:1207–1210.
8. Skates SJ, Menon U, MacDonald N, et al. Calculation of the risk of ovarian cancer from serial CA-125 values for preclinical detection in postmenopausal women. *J Clin Oncol* 2003;21[10 Suppl]:206–210.
9. Buys SS, Partridge E, Greene MH, et al. Ovarian cancer screening in the prostate, lung, colorectal and ovarian (PLCO) cancer screening trial: findings from the initial screen of a randomized trial. *Am J Obstet Gynecol* 2005;193:1630–1639.
10. Menon U, Skates SJ, Lewis S, et al. Prospective study using the risk of ovarian cancer algorithm to screen for ovarian cancer. *J Clin Oncol* 2005;23:7919–7926.
11. Liu J, Xu Y, Wang J. Ultrasonography, computed tomography and magnetic resonance imaging for diagnosis of ovarian carcinoma. *Eur J Radiol* 2007;62(3):328–334.
12. Greene FL, Compton CC, Fritz AG, et al., eds. *AJCC cancer staging atlas*. New York: Springer.
13. Gadducci A, Cosio S, Zola P, et al. Surveillance procedures for patients treated for epithelial ovarian cancer: a review of the literature. *Int J Gynecol Cancer* 2007;17(1):21–31.
14. Qayyum A, Coakley FV, Westphalen AC, et al. Role of CT and MR imaging in predicting optimal cytoreduction of newly diagnosed primary epithelial ovarian cancer. *Gynecol Oncol* 2005;96(2):301–306.
15. Hess LM, Benham-Hutchins M, Herzog TJ, et al. A meta-analysis of the efficacy of intraperitoneal cisplatin for the front-line treatment of ovarian cancer. *Int J Gynecol Cancer* 2007;17:561–570.
16. Armstrong DK, Bundy B, Wenzel L, et al. Intraperitoneal cisplatin and paclitaxel in ovarian cancer. *N Engl J Med* 2006;354(1):34–43.
17. See HT, Kavanaugh JJ. The MD Anderson manual of medical oncology. In: Kantarjian HM, Wolff RA, Koller CA, eds. *Ovarian cancer*. New York: McGraw-Hill, 2006:543–578.

18. Wahl RL, Hutchins GD, Buchsbaum DJ, et al. ^{18}F-2-deoxy-2-fluoro-D-glucose uptake into human tumor xenografts. Feasibility studies for cancer imaging with positron-emission tomography. *Cancer* 1991; 67(6):1544–1550.
19. Brown RS, Fisher SJ, Wahl RL. Autoradiographic evaluation of the intra-tumoral distribution of 2-deoxy-D-glucose and monoclonal antibodies in xenografts of human ovarian adenocarcinoma. *J Nucl Med* 1993;34(1):75–82.
20. Wahl RL, Hutchins GD, Roberts J. FDG-PET imaging of ovarian cancer: initial experience. *J Nucl Med* 1991;32:982.
21. Shen YY, Chen LK, Liao AC, et al. Application of PET and PET/CT imaging for cancer screening. *Anticancer Res* 2004;24(6):4103–4108.
22. Schöder H, Gönen M. Screening for cancer with PET and PET/CT: potential and limitations. *J Nucl Med* 2007;48[Suppl 1]:4S–18S.
23. Lerman H, Metser U, Grisaru D, et al. Normal and abnormal F18-FDG endometrial and ovarian uptake in pre- and postmenopausal patients: assessment by PET/CT. *J Nucl Med* 2004;45:266–271
24. Kim SK, Kang KW, Roh JW, et al. Incidental ovarian F18-FDG accumulation on PET: correlation with the menstrual cycle. *Eur J Nuc ed Mol Imaging* 2005;32:757–763.
25. Zhu ZH, Cheng WY, Cheng X, et al. [Characteristics of physiological uptake of uterus and ovaries on ^{18}F-fluorodeoxyglucose positron emission tomography]. *Zhongguo Yi Xue Ke Xue Yuan Xue Bao* 2007;29:124–129.
26. Togashi K. Ovarian cancer: the clinical role of US, CT, and MRI. *Eur Radiol* 2003;13:L87–L104.
27. Hubner KF, McDonald TW, Niethammer JG, et al. Assessment of primary and metastatic ovarian cancer by positron emission tomography (PET) using 2-[F18]Deoxyglucose (2-[F18]FDG). *Gynecol Oncol* 1993;51: 197–204.
28. Rieber A, Nussla K, Stohr I, et al. Preoperative diagnosis of ovarian tumors with MR imaging: comparison with transvaginal sonography, positron emission tomography, and histologic findings. *AJR Am J Roentgenol* 2001;177:123–129.
29. Kawahara K, Yoshida Y, Kurokawa T, et al. Evaluation of positron emission tomography with tracer 18-fluorodeoxyglucose in addition ot magnetic resonance imaging in the diagnosis of ovarian cancer in selected women after ultrasonography. *J Comput Assist Tomogr* 2004;28: 505–516.
30. Risum S, Hogdall C, Loft A, et al. The diagnostic value of PET/CT for primary ovarian cancer—a prospective study. *Gynecol Oncol* 2007;105: 145–149.
31. Fenchel S, Grab D, Nuessle K, et al. Asymptomatic adnexal masses: correlation of FDG PET and histopathologic findings. *Radiology* 2002;223: 780–788.
32. Schroder W, Zimny M, Rudlowski C, et al. The role of F18-fluorodeoxyglucose positron emission tomography (F18-FDG PET) in diagnosis of ovarian cancer. *Int J Gynecol Cancer* 1999;9:117–122.
33. Yoshida Y, Kurokawa T, Kawahara K, et al. Incremental benefits of FDG positron emission tomography over CT alone for the preoperative staging of ovarian cancer. *AJR Am J Roentgenol* 2004;182:227–233.
34. Turlakow A, Yeung HW, Salmon AS, et al. Peritoneal carcinomatosis: role of (^{18})F-FDG PET. *J Nucl Med* 2003;44(9):1407–1412.
35. Avril N, Sassen S, Schmalfeldt B, et al. Prediction of response to neoadjuvant chemotherapy by sequential F-18-fluorodeoxyglucose positron emission tomography in patients with advanced-stage ovarian cancer. *J Clin Oncol* 2005;23:7445–7453.
36. Yen RF, Sun SS, Shen YY, et al. Whole body positron emission tomography with ^{18}F-fluoro-2-deoxyglucose for the detection of recurrent ovarian cancer. *Anticancer Res* 2001;21:3691–3694.
37. Zimny M, Siggelkow W, Schroder W, et al. 2-[Fluorine-18]-fluoro-2-deoxy-D-glucose positron emission tomography in the diagnosis of recurrent ovarian cancer. *Gynecol Oncol* 2001;83:310–315.
38. Nakamoto Y, Saga T, Ishimori T, et al. Clinical value of positron emission tomography with FDG for recurrent ovarian cancer. *AJR Am J Roentgenol* 2001;176(6):1449-1454.
39. Torizuka T, Nobezawa S, Kanno T, et al. Ovarian cancer recurrence: role of whole-body positron emission tomography using 2-[fluorine-18]-fluoro-2-deoxy-D-glucose. *Eur J Nucl Med Mol Imaging* 2002;29: 797–803.
40. Bristow RE, del Carmen MG, Pannu HK, et al. Clinically occult recurrent ovarian cancer: patient selection for secondary cytoreductive surgery using combined PET/CT. *Gynecol Oncol* 2003;90:519–528.
41. Sironi S, Messa C, Mangili G, et al. Integrated FDG PET/CT in patients with persistent ovarian cancer: correlation with histologic findings. *Radiology* 2004;233:433–440.
42. Takekuma M, Maeda M, Ozawa T, et al. Positron emission tomography with ^{18}F-fluoro-2-deoxyglucose for the detection of recurrent ovarian cancer. *Int J Clin Oncol* 2005;10:177–181.
43. Nanni C, Rubello D, Farsad M, et al. (^{18})F-FDG PET/CT in the evaluation of recurrent ovarian cancer: a prospective study on forty-one patients. *Eur J Surg Oncol* 2005;31:792–797.
44. Chung HH, Kang WJ, Kim JW, et al. Role of [^{18}F]FDG PET/CT in the assessment of suspected recurrent ovarian cancer: correlation with clinical or histological findings. *Eur J Nucl Med Mol Imaging* 2007;34: 480–486.
45. Thrall MM, DeLoia JA, Gallion H, et al. Clinical use of combined positron emission tomography and computed tomography (FDG-PET/CT) in recurrent ovarian cancer. *Gynecol Oncol* 2007;105:17–22.
46. Sebastian S, Lee SI, Horowitz NS, et al. PET-CT vs. CT alone in ovarian cancer recurrence. *Abdom Imaging* 2008;33:112–118.
47. Bristow RE, Giuntoli RL 2nd, Pannu HK, et al. Combined PET/CT for detecting recurrent ovarian cancer limited to retroperitoneal lymph nodes. *Gynecol Oncol* 2005;99:294–300.
48. Pannu HK, Cohade C, Bristow RE, et al. PET-CT detection of abdominal recurrence of ovarian cancer: radiologic-surgical correlation. *Abdom Imaging* 2004;29:398–403.
49. Sheng XG, Zhang XL, Fu Z, et al. [Value of positron emission tomography-CT imaging combined with continual detection of CA125 in serum for diagnosis of early asymptomatic recurrence of epithelial ovarian carcinoma]. *Zhonghua Fu Chan Ke Za Zhi* 2007;42: 460–463.
50. Rose PG, Faulhaber P, Miraldi F, et al. Positive emission tomography for evaluating a complete clinical response in patients with ovarian or peritoneal carcinoma: correlation with second-look laparotomy. *Gynecol Oncol* 2001;82:17–21.
51. Garcia-Velloso MJ, Jurado M, Ceamanos C, et al. Diagnostic accuracy of FDG PET in the follow-up of platinum-sensitive epithelial ovarian carcinoma. *Eur J Nucl Med Mol Imaging* 2007;34(9):1396–1405.
52. Kim S, Chung JK, Kang SB, et al. [^{18}F]FDG PET as a substitute for second-look laparotomy in patients with advanced ovarian carcinoma. *Eur J Nucl Med Mol Imaging* 2004;31:196–201.
53. Cho SM, Park YG, Lee JM, et al. ^{18}F-fluorodeoxyglucose positron emission tomography in patients with recurrent ovarian cancer: in comparison with vascularity, Ki-67, p53, and histologic grade. *Eur Radiol* 2007;17:409–417.
54. Torizuka T, Kanno T, Futatsubashi M, et al. Imaging of gynecologic tumors: comparison of (^{11})C-choline PET with (^{18})F-FDG PET. *J Nucl Med* 2003;44:1051–1056.
55. Simcock B, Neesham D, Quinn M, et al. The impact of PET/CT in the management of recurrent ovarian cancer. *Gynecol Oncol* 2006;103:271–276.
56. Ruiz-Hernandez G, Delgado-Bolton RC, Fernandez-Perez C, et al. [Impact of positron emission tomography with FDG-PET in treatment of patients with suspected recurrent ovarian cancer]. *Rev Esp Med Nucl* 2005;24:113–126.
57. Mangili G, Picchio M, Sironi S, et al. Integrated PET/CT as a first-line re-staging modality in patients with suspected recurrence of ovarian cancer. *Eur J Nucl Med Mol Imaging* 2007;34:658–666.
58. Smith GT, Hubner KF, McDonald T, et al. Cost analysis of FDG PET for managing patients with ovarian cancer. *Clin Positron Imaging* 1999;2: 63–70.

CHAPTER

8.18 Genitourinary Malignancies

HEIKO SCHÖDER

GENERAL CONSIDERATIONS

Urologic malignancies account for approximately 25% of all new cancers in the United States (1). The clinical utility of positron emission tomography (PET) with various radiotracers has been studied to some extent for all of these tumors. The diagnostic yield is quite variable for the different malignancies, and the utility of a given radiotracer may depend on the clinical state of the malignancy in question. This chapter discusses some of the most important biochemical alterations in cancer as the basis for PET imaging in urologic tumors. Although most of these data come from experimental work in prostate cancer, much of this likely also applies to the other malignancies discussed in this chapter. In the second part of the chapter the clinical indications for PET imaging and the data of the more important PET studies are discussed in the appropriate clinical context.

Biochemical Alterations as the Basis for PET Imaging in Urologic Malignancies

Fluorodeoxyglucose

Fluorine-18 (^{18}F)-fluorodeoxyglucose (FDG), the agent used for 95% of all clinical PET examinations, traces glucose uptake and phosphorylation by hexokinase. Imaging with FDG takes advantage of the Warburg effect: aerobic glycolysis and an overall increase in glucose metabolism are metabolic characteristics of cancer cells as compared to normal tissue (2,3). The increased glucose metabolism in cancer is mediated through increased expression and activity of glucose transporters (GluT) in the cell surface membrane (4) and through characteristic changes in glycolytic enzyme expression and activity (5,6). Despite the presence of oxygen, glucose is largely metabolized to lactate (aerobic glycolysis). The alterations in glucose metabolism are early events in cancer development (7).

Recent experimental studies have clarified some of the mechanisms and the significance of increased glucose consumption in cancer. In the 1920s, Warburg et al. (2) originally proposed that the increased aerobic glycolysis in cancer cells was the consequence of defects in mitochondrial respiration. Although inhibition of mitochondrial respiration may indeed be one possible explanation (8), more recent theories have invoked alterations in signaling molecules and pathways as important mechanisms for aerobic glycolysis in cancer. One line of evidence has implicated an activation of the hypoxia inducible factor 1 (HIF-1), either as the consequence of intratumoral hypoxia or due to altered gene expression (9). Activation of HIF-1 causes overexpression of numerous proteins, including cell survival and proliferation factors, glucose transporters, and glycolytic enzymes (9). Interestingly, HIF-1 also induces the expression of pyruvate dehydrogenase (PDH) kinase 1, which inactivates PDH, the mitochondrial enzyme that converts pyruvate to acetyl-CoA (10), thereby inhibiting the citrate cycle and oxidative phosphorylation.

Another more recent line of evidence suggests that activation of the oncogene *Akt* and its gene product, the serine/threonine kinase Akt, may be sufficient to stimulate the switch to aerobic glycolysis (11). Activation of Akt is one of first steps in the PI3K/Akt signaling pathway, which promotes cell growth, survival, and resistance to apoptosis. Activation of Akt kinase in transformed cells stimulates glucose uptake (12) and consumption, and these cells are more susceptible to death than control cells after glucose withdrawal. Activation of the PI3K/Akt pathway causes activation of various other downstream kinases, including mammalian target of rapamycin (mTOR) (7,13). mTOR sensitizes nutrient availability within the cell and regulates cell growth and proliferation (14). In experimental studies, the pharmacologic inhibition of mTOR reverses the cancer-specific increases in glucose metabolism and inhibits the development of prostatic intraepithelial neoplasia (PIN) (7). mTOR may exert some of its effects through activation/stabilization of HIF-1 (15).

Because of the relationship between mTOR and glucose metabolism, PET imaging with FDG is under investigation for determining the treatment response to mTOR inhibitors in various malignancies, including prostate and renal cancers. Unfortunately, this process is not straightforward because mTOR also regulates Akt through both negative and positive feedback loops (16). This may explain the suboptimal clinical response rates with mTOR inhibitors in some cancers with known activation of the PI3K/Akt signaling pathway. It also highlights the potential limitations of "molecular targeted therapies." Inhibition of one molecule or pathway may slow down but not necessarily stop the progression of cancer, may only succeed in a subset of patients, or in some cases may even promote cancer progression (17).

Concerning urologic malignancies, the role of the PI3K/Akt pathway is particularly well documented in prostate cancer. Constitutive activation of this pathway is found in up to 50% of progressive prostate cancers (18) and correlates with a high Gleason score and pathological stage, a higher rate of biochemical recurrence, low response to hormonal manipulations, and progression to metastasis (19–22). The intensity of *Akt* expression and the number of *Akt* expressing cells increases from normal prostate tissue to benign prostatic hyperplasia then to prostate cancer (23).

In addition to *Akt*, *p53* is another frequently mutated gene in cancer. The *p53* deficient cancer cells produce similar amounts of adenosine triphosphate (ATP) as normal cells, but significantly higher levels of lactate, a measure of increased glycolysis. The reason is a lack of activation of the gene synthesis of cytochrome oxidase 2 (*SCO2*), an enzyme complex that is critical during oxidative phosphorylation. This inhibition of oxygen consumption may facilitate the survival of the cancer cell in an hypoxic environment (8). Interestingly, in other model systems, Akt attenuates mitochondrial p53 accumulation (24). This is just one example for many connecting points between various cancer pathways that may affect tumor metabolism and, hence, PET imaging. Indeed, decreased expression of p53 correlates with higher incorporation of FDG into tumor cells (25).

Aerobic glycolysis is not only characteristic for cancer cells, but is in fact mandatory for their continued growth and survival. Although it is possible experimentally to induce a switch from aerobic glycolysis to oxidative phosphorylation in some cancer cells by inhibition of lactate dehydrogenase (LDH), the growth of such cells is clearly inhibited (26). This proves that aerobic glycolysis is not just an epiphenomenon but is indeed necessary for growth and survival of the cancer cell. Among the postulated reasons for increased aerobic glycolysis in cancer is the fact that glycolysis can provide ATP faster that oxidative phosphorylation, and that the products of glycolysis are required for fatty acid synthesis and the maintenance of the nonessential amino acid pool during cell growth (27). In contrast to normal cells, which can switch from glucose consumption to fatty acid oxidation for generation of ATP depending on the substrate availability (28), *Akt*-expressing transformed cells are limited in their ability to do so (12). One of several possible mechanisms for suppressed β oxidation in cancer could be the Akt-dependent inhibition of CPT-1, the shuttle needed for transporting free fatty acids into the mitochondrion (12).

Before aerobic glycolysis can even start, transport across the cell membrane is the first rate-limiting step for sugar metabolism in cancer cells. Almost 20 years ago, experimental studies in fibroblasts showed that malignant transformation by *src* and *ras* oncogenes causes a rapid increase in glucose uptake and GluT-1 expression (29). This is a critical step in the survival of the cancer cell. Whereas normal mammalian cells depend on extracellular signals for maintaining cell surface transporters, growth, proliferation, and survival, cancer cells function autonomously. Despite a lack of external growth factors and survival stimuli, the constitutive expression of *Akt* in cancer cells can prevent apoptosis, in part by maintaining transporter molecules in the cell surface, such as GluT-1 and amino acid transporters.

Overexpression of glucose transporters (e.g., GluT-1, GluT-3, and GluT-12) has been documented in many malignancies (reviewed in Macheda et al. [4]), including urologic cancers. In prostate cancer, GluT-1 and GluT-12 are overexpressed (30,31), and GluT-1 is expressed to a higher degree in poorly differentiated prostate cancer cell lines, such as DU145 and PC3, than in hormone-responsive LNCaP cell line (31). In clinical prostate cancer specimens, the level of GluT-1 expression increases with advancing grade of malignancy (31).

Overexpression of GluT-1 also occurs in approximately 60% of bladder cancers, but not normal bladder tissue or benign papillomas (32). Among bladder cancers, invasive transitional cell carcinomas and tumors with a high nuclear grade exhibit a higher grade of Glut-1 protein expression than superficial bladder cancers and tumors with lower nuclear grade (32). In bladder cancer, the number of cancer cells with high GluT-1 expression shows an inverse relation with disease-specific and overall survival (33,34).

Increased glucose metabolism in cancer can also be a consequence of hypoxia (anaerobic glycolysis), which is a common feature in many malignancies and leads to overexpression of GluT proteins or alteration of GluT functional activity (34–36) and also causes overexpression of hexokinase II (37). Hypoxia is common in bladder cancer (34,38) and prostate cancer (39) and is a marker of poor prognosis. In bladder cancer, the severity of hypoxia correlates with the expression of GluT-1 (34). Of note, while hypoxia is associated with resistance to both radiation and chemotherapy, the inhibition of GluT in hypoxic cells can resensitize those cells to chemotherapeutic drugs and initiate their apoptosis (40), again highlighting the significance of glucose metabolism for the survival of the cancer cell.

For clinical PET imaging with FDG in urologic cancers, some organ-specific mechanisms need to be considered. Prostate cancer differs from other urologic malignancies because it is a hormone-dependent tumor. In the early stages of prostate cancer, FDG uptake may be regulated by the level of androgen stimulation and can be suppressed by androgen withdrawal (41,42). In logical extension of these experimental data, clinical observations suggest that the appearance of lesions with abnormal FDG uptake in patients on antiandrogen therapy indicates a transition to the castrate-resistant state (Fig. 8.18.1) and a worsening of the patient's prognosis. Moreover, in prostate cancer models, rapidly dividing DU145 prostate cancer cells depended on high levels of glucose, whereas relatively slow-growing LNCaP cells are much less dependent on glucose (43). These data may explain why prostate tumors with high Gleason scores are more likely to exhibit adequate FDG uptake than those with lower scores. They also explain why FDG may not be a good tracer for the diagnosis of primary prostate cancer but is a suitable agent for disease detection and treatment monitoring in patients with progressive castration-resistant metastatic disease.

Renal cancer shows a peculiar molecular abnormality that may have consequences for PET imaging with FDG. About 60% of sporadic renal cell carcinomas are clear cell carcinomas, showing a loss of the von Hippel-Lindau (*VHL*) tumor suppressor gene (44).

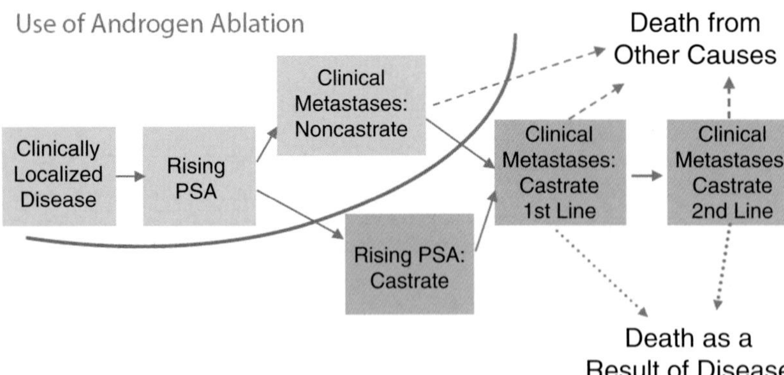

FIGURE 8.18.1. Model of prostate cancer states. Progressive prostate cancer can be characterized according to well-defined clinical states, which may require different therapies. Use of proper terminology is necessary when comparing the results of clinical and imaging studies in progressive prostate cancer. PSA, prostate-specific antigen. (Figure courtesy of Howard Scher, MD, at MSKCC. Reprinted with permission.)

Under normal conditions, VHL binds to the transcription factor HIF-1 and promotes its degradation. Loss of VHL causes HIF-1 accumulation (due to lack of breakdown), which then leads to overexpression of numerous proteins, including growth factors, glucose transporters, and glycolytic enzymes (9).

In experimental studies, HIF has been established as the key factor in promoting malignant transformation of kidney cells (45). HIF-dependent activation of glycolysis may be one reason for increased FDG uptake in a subset of renal cancers, which in fact occurs in a similar fraction (about 60%) of cases. HIF-1 expression in VHL deficient renal cancers is promoted by mTOR, one of the aforementioned signaling kinases (18). Consequently, the treatment with mTOR inhibitors suppresses the expression of HIF and the production of protein products of HIF target genes, such as GluT and glycolytic enzymes, which can be shown in cell cultures and imaging studies. Treatment with mTOR inhibitors (but not other chemotherapeutic drugs) causes a rapid and significant decrease in FDG uptake in VHL-deficient tumor xenografts. These preliminary experimental data provide some rationale for the use of FDG to identify VHL-deficient (i.e., HIF-dependent) renal cancers and monitor the response to novel anticancer drugs.

In summary, increased glucose uptake and metabolism, as well as some of the underlying molecular mechanism, are well documented in urologic malignancies. This highlights the significance of cancer imaging with FDG PET. Unfortunately, for clinical PET imaging of urologic malignancies, FDG has some limitations related to its physiologic excretion through the urinary tract. Moreover, FDG is not a suitable radiotracer for slow growing malignancies with low glucose metabolism (e.g., early prostate cancer) because the signal will be low and not detectable against background activity. In contrast, this tracer can provide clinically meaningful information in patients with more aggressive disease. This also includes a subset of patients with prostate-specific antigen (PSA) relapse and shorter doubling times, individuals with castrate-resistant metastatic prostate cancer, and patients with recurrent or metastatic renal, bladder, and testicular cancers.

In the interpretation of imaging studies, it should be recognized that aerobic glycolysis is a phenomenon of the cancer cell *per se* and may not involve the surrounding stroma that continues to rely on oxidative phosphorylation for the supply of energy (46). Accordingly, lactate released as the end product of aerobic glycolysis from cancer cells may be metabolized further by the surrounding stroma, enter the microcirculation (especially when local concentrations are high), or may cause normal cell death by collapse of the transmembrane proton gradient and a breakdown of the extracellular matrix (47). Because current PET scanners cannot distinguish between cancer and stromal cells, the signal obtained always reflects an admixture of metabolic events within a given tumor.

The image quality of FDG PET studies has markedly improved over the past 10 years so that some negative reports in the literature may be outdated. In particular, the routine use of iterative reconstruction algorithms and combined PET with computed tomography (CT) has led to a marked improvement in interpretation of PET studies in the abdomen and pelvis. Nevertheless, the unavoidable urinary excretion of FDG may sometimes interfere in the assessment of prostate, renal, or bladder cancer.

Acetate

Carbon-11 (^{11}C)-acetate is an established agent for tumor imaging. Good tumor-to-background ratios and little urinary excretion make it a suitable agent for imaging urologic malignancies. Acetate can also be labeled with ^{18}F, but methods for safe and efficient synthesis are still under investigation.

The biochemical rationale for cancer imaging with [^{11}C]-acetate is found in characteristic alterations in fatty acid metabolism, which are best documented in prostate cancer but may also apply in other malignancies. Under normal circumstances, exogenous acetate is activated to acetyl-CoA, which can enter various pathways, but predominantly the citrate cycle. In the prostate, normal glandular tissue in the central zone oxidizes citrate like many other mammalian tissues. In contrast, in the epithelial cells of the peripheral zone, the enzyme m-aconitase, responsible for conversion of citrate to isocitrate, is inhibited by high levels of zinc (48).

Testosterone stimulates the key enzyme pyruvate dehydrogenase in prostate tissue, which converts pyruvate to acetyl-CoA, the building block for citrate (49). High concentrations of citrate thus accumulate in the normal prostate and are thought to be essential for maintaining the pH and serve as an energy source for seminal fluid. This has been established in various *in vitro* studies as well as clinical studies using magnetic resonance (MR) spectroscopy (50,51).

In prostate cancer, inhibition of m-aconitase is no longer present and citrate levels decline. Conceivably, this would suggest increased acetate metabolism through the citrate cycle. However, *in vitro* studies tracing the metabolic fate of [^{14}C]-acetate in tumor cell lines (52) revealed that tumor cells incorporate ^{14}C activity mostly into phosphatidylcholine and neutral lipids, and this incorporation showed some correlation with growth activity. Only a small fraction of ^{14}C-acetate was converted into carbon dioxide and amino acids. This observation is in keeping with earlier studies, which had shown that endogenously synthesized fatty acids in cancer cells are predominantly esterified to phospholipids (which are building blocks for membranes), rather than to triglycerides as in normal tissues (53).

Several enzymes involved in fatty acid synthesis are up-regulated in prostate cancer, and the expression of the key enzyme fatty acid synthase (FAS) increases with increasing degree of malignancy (54). Overexpression of FAS has also been shown in bladder, lung, and endometrial cancers (55,56). FAS is a multifunctional enzyme that synthesizes palmitate from acetyl-CoA and malonyl-CoA. Under androgen stimulation, FAS expression is up-regulated in prostate cancer (57). Following androgen ablation, FAS expression initially decreases, but returns to higher levels after the transition from the androgen-responsive to the castrate-resistant state of the disease (58).

At least in prostate cancer, FAS expression appears to be regulated by the activity of the PI3K/Akt pathway. Studies have shown (a) a positive relationship between FAS and Akt expression (59), (b) an inverse relationship between PTEN and FAS expression (60), and (c) a reduction in FAS expression upon treatment with PI3K inhibitors (61). Signaling through the *HER2* (*ERBB2*)receptor, important in a subset of breast as well as prostate cancers, has also been associated with FAS expression. High FAS expression in breast cancer is associated with a poor prognosis (62).

Although increased FAS expression is important for the progression of cancer, the reverse is also true. In breast and prostate cancer cell lines the inhibition of FAS leads to accumulation of malonyl-CoA and apoptosis (63,64). In addition to FAS, the enzyme acetyl-CoA-carboxylase α may also be critical for prostate cancer progression (65). Importantly, the newly synthesized fatty acids in cancer cells are predominantly assembled in membrane lipid rafts (66), that is, membrane microdomains that are involved in signal transduction, intracellular trafficking, cell polarization, and migration (67).

Taken together, these data indicate that fatty acid synthesis is an important metabolic process in prostate cancer progression, that at least two enzymes are critical in this process, and that inhibition or silencing of these enzymes can induce apoptosis. Acetate incorporation in cancer is a consequence of the enhanced lipid synthesis. *In vitro*, acetate incorporation correlates with tritium thymidine incorporation into DNA, a measure of proliferation (52). Much work remains to be done to investigate whether labeled acetate accumulation in clinical cancer studies can indeed be linked to the specific alterations in fatty acid metabolism and critical enzymes as shown *in vitro* and described above.

Normal biodistribution of [^{11}C]-acetate involves intense acetate uptake in liver, spleen, and pancreas, and moderate uptake in the myocardium on early images. There is also a moderate uptake in the kidneys and varying degrees of renal excretion. Intestinal activity and uptake in skeletal muscle can vary in intensity. The effective dose equivalent is 6.2×10^{-3} mSv/MBq (68). Imaging with PET/CT is very valuable in distinguishing between bowel and urinary activity from tracer uptake in lymph nodes, bladder wall, or prostate (Table 8.18.1).

The potential pitfalls are that acetate not only accumulates in prostate and bladder cancer, but also in benign hyperplastic prostate tissue, in sites of focal prostatitis (in particular, when acute), and at sites of PIN, which may or may not progress to prostate cancer. In the prostate, acetate uptake may be age related and could be higher in individuals with normal prostate tissue who are less than 50 years of age than in normal prostate of older subjects (older than 50 years) or those with benign prostatic hyperplasia. The intensity of acetate uptake in the prostate was similar in older subjects with normal prostate (standard uptake value [SUV] 2.3 ± 0.7) and patients with proven prostate cancer (SUV 1.9 ± 0.6) (69). False positives can occur in inflammatory lymph nodes and inflammatory changes in the bladder wall.

Methionine

Amino acid uptake and protein synthesis are up-regulated in cancer. C-11-methionine is one of many possible tracers for measuring amino acid uptake in tumor cells (70). As shown in patients with castrate-resistant metastatic prostate cancer, methionine uptake in tumor occurs rapidly with a peak at about 10 minutes followed by plateau (71). Accordingly, PET imaging should start approximately 10 minutes after tracer injection. C-11-methionine undergoes rapid clearance from the blood pool, is primarily metabolized in liver and pancreas, and (in most cases) shows no significant renal excretion.

Normal biodistribution includes intense tracer uptake in the liver and pancreas and somewhat less intense uptake in spleen, kidneys, and intestines. The effective dose equivalent is 5×10^{-3} mSv/MBq (72).

Potential pitfalls include methionine uptake at sites of inflammation and misinterpretation of urinary or bowel activity as lymph node activity.

Choline

Radiolabeled choline is under investigation for imaging of prostate and bladder cancers. Studies with [^{14}C]-choline and investigations using MR spectroscopy have established that the majority (approximately 90%) of exogenous choline is converted to phosphocholine (73,74). Phosphorylation of choline to phosphocholine is the first step of choline metabolism. Increased levels of phosphocholine in tissues is a characteristic of the malignant phenotype (74). This is likely the result of overexpression of the enzyme choline kinase, which is a common feature in many malignancies, including prostate cancer (75,76). Moreover, in breast cancer cells, the suppression of choline kinase inhibits proliferation and induces redifferentiation (77). Carbon-14 incorporation into phosphocholine—an indirect assessment of choline kinase activity—is related to the proliferative activity in various cell lines (73), although this correlation is weaker than that seen with acetate incorporation.

For PET imaging, choline has been labeled with ^{11}C and ^{18}F. Although [^{11}C]-choline is an excellent agent for cancer imaging (78), the short 20-minute half-life of ^{11}C poses a logistical challenge in many institutions. The ^{18}F-labeled compounds include [^{18}F]-fluoro-ethyl-choline (FEC) (79) and [^{18}F]-fluoromethyl-dimethyl-2-hydroxyethylammonium (FCH) (80,81).

Clinically, all three labeled choline compounds show rapid clearance from blood pool and rapid uptake in prostate tissue (81–83), although peak uptake in prostate appears to occur at later time points with FEC than with FCH. Among the ^{18}F-labeled choline compounds, the cellular uptake and phosphorylation by

TABLE 8.18.1 PET Tracers for Imaging of Prostate Cancer

	[^{18}F]-FDG	[^{11}C]-methionine	[^{11}C]-choline	[^{18}F]-choline[a]	[^{11}C]-acetate	[^{18}F]-FDHT
Normal biodistribution	Myocardium, bowel, liver, spleen, kidney	Pancreas, liver, spleen, kidney, salivary glands	Lung, liver, kidney, adrenal	Renal cortex, liver, spleen, salivary glands	Lung, spleen, pancreas, liver, kidney (mild in bowel movement and bowel)	Liver, blood pool, small intestine (excretion)
Primary mode of excretion	Renal	Intestinal	Intestinal	Urinary	Intestinal	Intestinal
Urinary activity?	+++	+	+	++[b]	variable	++
Suitable for:						
Detection of primary PCA	–	–	(+)	(+)	–	–
Node and metastasis staging	–	?	+	+	+	–
PSA relapse						
Local recurrence	+	+(+)	+++	+++	+++	–
Distant metastases	+	++	+++	+++	+++	–
Prognostic value?	+	?	?	?	?	Likely
Therapy monitoring?	++	?	?	?	?	+
Typical activity in mCi (MBq)	296–555	370–740	370–925	185–370	555–925	296–555
Imaging start at minutes postinjection.	60	5–10	5–10	5–10[c]	5–10[c]	0 or 30
EDE in mSv/MBq	2×10^{-2}	5×10^{-3}[d]	5×10^{-3}	3.5×10^{-2}[e]	6.2×10^{-3}[a]	1.8×10^{-2}[f]

FDG, fluorodeoxyglucose; FDHT, 16–[^{18}F]-fluoro-5–dihydrotestosteron; PCA, prostate cancer; PSA, prostate-specific antigen; EDE, effective dose equivalent; ?, questionable or unclear; +, number of + signs indicates degree of usefulness; ++, +++, (+).

[a]From Seltzer MA, Jahan SA, Sparks R, et al. Radiation dose estimates in humans for (11) C-acetate whole-body PET. *J Nucl Med* 2004;45:1233–1236.

[b]Beginning at 5 minutes postinjection.

[c]Earlier dynamic images may be helpful in differentiating tumor from urinary and bowel activity.

[d]From Deloar HM, Fujiwara T, Nakamura T, et al. Estimation of internal absorbed dose of L-[methyl-11C]methionine using whole-body positron emission tomography. *Eur J Nucl Med* 1998;25:629–633.

[e]From DeGrado TR, Reiman RE, Price DT, Wang S, Coleman RE. Pharmacokinetics and radiation dosimetry of ^{18}F-fluorocholine. *J Nucl Med* 2002;43:92–96.

[f]From Zanzonico PB, Finn R, Pentlow KS, et al. PET-based radiation dosimetry in man of 18F-fluorodihydrotestosterone, a new radiotracer for imaging prostate cancer. *J Nucl Med* 2004;45:1966–1971.

choline kinase is very similar for FCH and natural choline, but is lower for FEC (80). In contrast to [^{11}C]-choline, which shows very little urinary excretion and whose activity concentration in the bladder is usually lower than in prostate cancer or metastases (84), excreted ^{18}F activity from both FCH and FEC appears in the bladder as early as 3 to 5 minutes postinjection. This may be related to incomplete tubular reabsorption of intact tracer or enhanced excretion of oxidized metabolites.

Excreted activity in the bladder may interfere with visualizing primary or recurrent prostate cancer. Similarly, excreted tracer in the ureter may be mistaken for uptake in nodal metastases or vice versa. Therefore, it may be helpful to start imaging of the pelvis as early as 1 minute postinjection (i.e., as soon as the majority of tracer has cleared from the blood pool). On dynamic images (e.g., 1-minute frames) true pathology will show early tracer accumulation, whereas excreted tracer in the ureters and bladder would not appear before 3 to 4 minutes after injection. Following these initial images of the lower pelvis, a PET scan of the torso, including a late image of the pelvis, is acquired. The use of combined PET/CT will aid in detecting abnormal tracer uptake in lymph nodes, in particular in smaller nodes along the course of the ureters, as well as in defining tracer accumulation in the bladder wall, prostate, or prostatic fossa after prostatectomy and distinguishing those from physiological bowel activity.

Normal biodistribution for all choline compounds includes intense uptake in liver and kidney parenchyma, and less prominent uptake in spleen, pancreas, and skeletal muscle. The effective dose equivalent is 5×10^{-3} mSv/MBq for [^{11}C]-choline, and 3.5×10^{-2} mSv/MBq for [^{18}F]-choline (85).

The potential pitfalls are that the intensity of choline uptake can be similar in prostate cancer, focal prostatitis, and benign prostate hyperplasia (84,86–89); SUVs as high as 5.0 were seen in benign prostatic hyperplasia. Other reasons for false-positive uptake outside of the prostate region include sarcoidosis (87), meningiomas (87), nonspecific inflammation and infection (87), and cystitis (90). Intense bowel activity can be observed with all choline compounds and can be a reason for false-positive findings (91). False-negative findings have been described for metastases in lymph nodes of less than 1 cm in size (90,91).

Imaging of the Androgen Receptor in Prostate Cancer

In the normal prostate gland, androgens mediate key physiological processes such as differentiation, secretory function, metabolism, morphology, proliferation, and survival. Androgen ablation results in prostate involution and the loss of epithelial cells via apoptosis. Animal experiments have suggested that the androgen receptor (AR) functions primarily to maintain the differentiated secretory function of prostate epithelial cells, and that the survival of these cells is regulated in large part by paracrine factors expressed and provided by the supporting AR-positive surrounding stromal cells (92).

Androgens, signaling through the AR, are also the primary regulators of prostate cancer cell growth and proliferation. Androgen withdrawal causes apoptosis in a proportion of cells, whereas those that survive will arrest in the G1 phase of the cell cycle (93). Clinical progression of prostate cancer may result from continued growth of cells that were primarily resistant to androgen ablation, or from regrowth of cells that arrest after a period of growth and undergo a series of genetic alterations that permit adaptation to a low-androgen environment (94).

Primary prostate cancer and early states of recurrent disease always respond to antiandrogen hormonal therapy. Therapeutically this is used for neoadjuvant therapy in combination with external-beam radiation therapy (EBRT) (95) and in the early state of metastatic disease (96). Historically, it was assumed that progressing prostate cancer eventually reaches a hormone-refractory state where further disease progression is androgen independent. Clinical and laboratory studies in the past 5 to 10 years have shown that this concept is not true. In fact, there is continued signaling through the AR in progressive prostate cancer despite castrate serum levels of testosterone, and this phenomenon continues into the late states of the disease (97–99). Intratumoral androgens are also found even in late stages of the disease.

Exactly why and how even advanced stages of the disease remain dependent on signaling through the AR is still under investigation. Recent experimental studies have shed some light into this. According to classic teaching, steroid hormones exert most of their effects by binding to specific nuclear receptors, which then act as transcription factors. For many years, such "genomic function" was also thought to be the main or only function of the androgen receptor: androgen binding to the AR → AR translocation to the nucleus → binding to androgen responsive elements on the DNA → stimulation of mRNA synthesis → protein synthesis.

It has been suggested that the progression from low-grade to high-grade prostate cancer and metastases is mediated by a selective down-regulation of those AR target genes that inhibit proliferation, induce differentiation, and mediate apoptosis, whereas target genes that promote the growth and survival of prostate cancer cells are still expressed (100). However, it is now clear that in addition to its genomic function the AR can also act directly as a cytoplasmic signaling molecule. For instance, signaling through the AR can stimulate the PI3K/Akt pathway through direct interaction of the AR with the p85α regulatory subunit of PI3K (101,102), thus protecting cells against apoptosis and promoting tumor proliferation.

In addition, stimulation of the AR by binding of its natural ligand dihydrotestosterone can cause direct activation of mTOR, which does not require activation of the PI3K/Akt or MAP (mitogen activated protein) kinase pathways (103). Evidence suggests that mTOR activation in this setting is responsible for the increased expression of multiple genes whose protein products are involved in enhancing the availability of nutrients in the cancer cell.

The various mechanisms explaining continued signaling through the AR in advanced prostate cancer include receptor activation by ligands other than testosterone (including AR antagonists), a lowering in the threshold for ligand necessary for the receptor activation, increased expression of steroid receptor coactivators, and many more (98,104). For instance, studies in mice have shown that signaling through the *Her2/Her3* receptor dimer stabilizes the AR and promotes its binding to target genes on the DNA (105). This is one example for how signaling through the AR does not necessarily require the presence of androgens for receptor activation. Other *in vivo* studies have demonstrated crosstalk between the AR and the epidermal growth factor receptor (EGFR) in prostate cancer cells. A functional AR appeared important in mediating the signaling through EGFR (106), again regardless of the presence or absence of androgens.

At the cellular level, a direct synergy between AR and Akt signaling can transform normal prostate epithelial cells and induce androgen insensitive carcinoma. Although these cells continue to proliferate despite androgen withdrawal, they do require an AR with maintained genomic and nongenomic function (see above). Akt seems to regulate the expression and stability of AR at multiple levels (107). Finally, hypoxia can also affect the function of the AR by stimulating the binding of the AR to the androgen-responsive element on the DNA and enhancing the activity of genes that are expressed under the control of the AR (108).

As mentioned before, the AR is expressed on both prostate epithelial as well as surrounding stromal cells. Most recent studies indicate that hormone-refractory prostate cancer is characterized by a stimulation of AR function on epithelial cells (thus promoting proliferation) and simultaneous blockage of AR function on surrounding stromal cells (thus blocking apoptosis-inducing paracrine signals from the stroma). This alteration in regional AR expression within prostate tissue appears to be a consequence of an activation of the PI3K/AKT pathway (and perhaps also the Erk/MAP kinase pathway) (109).

Because continued signaling through the AR occurs even in advanced prostate cancer and in fact promotes disease progression, pharmacologic studies are now under way to target the AR and cause its destruction or down-regulation. Experimental studies using HSP-90 inhibitors (110), RNA interference (111), or short hairpin RNA (112) have provided proof of concept in this regard. (HSP-90 is a "chaperone" protein needed for the stabilization and function of the androgen receptor.) It is therefore of increasing interest to develop a method to measure AR expression and activity. This should improve our understanding of prostate cancer biology and should be helpful in monitoring the response to drugs targeting this receptor. Potentially, such method could also identify candidates more likely to respond to certain classes of drugs or small molecules targeting the androgen receptor.

Verification of the AR expression in patients with metastatic prostate cancer would require repeated biopsies from multiple sites.

A noninvasive method for systemic and repeated study of AR expression and function would therefore be preferred. Several compounds were developed for this purpose (113), and the agent 16β-[^{18}F]-fluoro-5α-dihydrotestosteron (FDHT) is currently under clinical investigation for imaging and quantifying the androgen receptor expression in metastatic prostate cancer (114,115).

Larson et al. (114) studied the biodistribution and binding characteristics of FDHT. Among seven patients imaged with both FDG and FDHT, 46 of 59 lesions showed both FDG and FDHT uptake, and the remainder had FDG but not FDHT uptake. The normal biodistribution of this agent involves high uptake in liver with excretion through the hepatobiliary system, causing some bowel activity, uptake in kidneys with some excretion to bladder, and high blood pool activity in the heart and large arteries. The effective dose equivalent is 1.8×10^{-2} mSv/MBq, which is similar to FDG (116). FDHT is a suboptimal radiotracer because of its high lipophilicity, rapid metabolism, and the persistent high blood pool activity of breakdown products. Newer PET tracers for imaging the AR are therefore under development.

Tumor Proliferation

Fluorine-18-fluorothymidine (FLT) (117) is a promising proliferation marker for PET imaging studies, but there are currently no conclusive data on FLT imaging in patients with urologic cancers. In a mouse model using the CWR22 androgen-dependent xenograft, FLT uptake in tumor reached its plateau in 30 minutes and remained up to 60 minutes. Surgical castration or treatment with diethylstilbestrol caused a marked reduction of FLT uptake in the tumor (118). Because of high natural uptake in bone marrow, the agent may not be suitable for the imaging of osseous metastases. Whether FLT may be useful for treatment monitoring in metastatic renal or prostate cancer or for detecting viable cancer in residual nodal masses after chemotherapy for testicular cancer, remains to be seen, but concerns exist as to whether the degree of tumor targeting will be sufficient.

Summary and Recommendations

Imaging genitourinary cancers with PET poses several challenges. Although FDG is a useful tracer, it is clearly limited in several settings, and alternative tracers are necessary for optimum diagnosis. Given the rapid evolution of this field, the optimal diagnostic tracer is not yet fully clarified in several settings. Regardless, for each radiotracer employed, the interpreting physician needs to understand the normal biodistribution and normal variants in tracer accumulation. None of the available radiotracers is specific for cancer, and false-positive tracer uptake (in benign lesions or normal anatomic structures) can occur for many reasons. However, depending on the underlying disease, the location of a hypermetabolic lymph node might determine the probability for a metastasis. For instance, inguinal lymph nodes are an extremely unusual site for metastases from prostate or bladder cancer, whereas nonspecific enlargement and tracer uptake in inguinal nodes is a relatively common finding in many patients. It is helpful to establish a threshold for the intensity of tracer uptake that should be considered normal or abnormal in order to guarantee the reproducibility of study interpretation and standardize the reporting. Depending on the radiotracer, this could include a comparison to uptake in surrounding background, uptake in large blood vessels, or uptake in skeletal muscle. Measurements of the SUV may guide the interpretation in a given case, but they cannot be used categorically for differentiating between cancer versus normal tissue, inflammation or infection.

It is highly recommended that all studies be performed on a combined PET/CT machine. The fusion images are of great help in identifying excreted tracer in normal structures (including ureters, prostatic urethra, bowel, menstrual cycle–related activity in uterus and ovaries, and so forth) and distinguishing it from true pathology. A number of false-positive findings can thus be avoided (activity in bowel, ureter or bladder misinterpreted as lymph nodes or bladder tumor). In patients with extensive resections (e.g., cystoprostatectomy with neobladder or ileal conduit; pelvic exenteration), the interpreting physician needs to understand the technical details of the operation and establish close rapport with the referring surgeon or urologist. Knowledge of the surgical history, together with assessment of CT and fusion images, helps to prevent embarrassing reports and false-positive PET findings.

PROSTATE CANCER

Clinical Statement

In the United States, approximately 186,320 individuals will be diagnosed, and 28,660 are expected to die of prostate cancer in 2008 (1). Many primary lesions will be detected by screening. Indeed, over the past 20 years the incidence of clinically indolent as well as clinically relevant but potentially curable prostate cancers has increased significantly (119). The two main treatment modalities with curative intent for primary prostate cancer are radical prostatectomy and EBRT.

With prostatectomy, negative surgical margins are of critical importance (120). In patients with positive margins or other high-risk histological features (e.g., greater than or equal to pT3b, Gleason score 8 or more) or lymph node involvement, adjuvant irradiation or chemotherapy with mitoxantrone may be indicated; the latter is currently under study by the Southwest Oncology Group (SWOG). Among patients treated with EBRT, higher radiation doses are associated with better outcome (121). In patients with locally advanced prostate cancer, cure rates can be improved further with combined antiandrogen therapy and EBRT (122,123).

The goal for curative treatment in primary prostate cancer is an eradication of all sites of disease, which should be reflected clinically in undetectable PSA levels. The plasma half-time of PSA is about 3.15 days. Undetectable PSA levels are to be expected within 1 month after prostatectomy. In contrast, PSA levels decline more slowly after EBRT, and undetectable levels may not be reached for more than 1 year. This occurs because even with successful irradiation, irreversibly damaged and amitotic cancer cells may still survive and function for several months.

Progressive prostate cancer needs to be discussed according to clinical states (Fig. 8.18.1). Initially, about one third of patients treated with prostatectomy or EBRT will develop subclinical recurrence (also known as PSA relapse or biochemical recurrence). Among the many definitions for PSA relapse, an increase of PSA 0.4 ng/mL or greater followed by another increase best explains the development of distant metastasis among ten candidate definitions, after controlling for clinical variables and the use of secondary therapy. However, more sensitive definitions, such as PSA 0.2 or greater and rising, may be more appropriate to use when selecting patients for salvage radiotherapy (124).

Among patients with PSA relapse after prostatectomy, this state of the disease is reached within the first 2 years in about 50% and within the first 5 years in about 77% of cases (125). The majority of these individuals experience further disease progression. Without salvage therapy, 65% develop clinically apparent skeletal metastases (the most common site of metastatic disease from prostate cancer) within 10 years (125). Similar data are reported for the subset of patients who fail to achieve undetectable PSA levels after prostatectomy. The estimated rate for developing distant metastases is 32% at 3 years, 51% at 5 years, and 68% at 10 years (126). In general, patients with rapid PSA doubling time and higher initial Gleason score are more likely to develop metastases (125,126).

In a given patient, the likelihood for developing clinical metastasis after EBRT (127) and the likelihood for developing PSA relapse or clinical metastases after prostatectomy (128) can be estimated from nomograms. Among those with PSA relapse only, the likelihood for developing clinical metastases (129) as well as the time interval from study entry to clinical metastasis (130) can be estimated from histopathological features of the primary tumor and PSA doubling time.

Isolated local recurrence of prostate cancer may be amenable to salvage therapy with prostatectomy or irradiation. Among patients with proven or highly likely local recurrence, the results of salvage irradiation after failed prostatectomy depend on clinical and histopathological features. In a large multicenter study (131), the 4-year progression-free survival was 50% among patients with Gleason scores of 4 to 7, but it declined to 29% among those with Gleason score of 8 or more. In each of these two patient groups, the 4-year progression-free survival was significantly better when the PSA prior to salvage radiation therapy was below 2 ng/mL.

Positive surgical margins indicate a greater likelihood for local recurrence (rather than nodal or distant metastases) and were therefore positively correlated with outcome after salvage irradiation to the prostate bed. By comparison, among patients undergoing salvage prostatectomy for local recurrence after failed EBRT (132), the preoperative PSA level was the only significant pretreatment predictor of disease progression: PSA levels less than 4, 4 to 10, and greater than 10 ng/mL were associated with 5-year progression-free survivals of 86%, 55%, and 37%, respectively. Both studies show a common theme: regardless of the treatment modality, salvage therapy in patients with PSA relapse is more likely to succeed when performed early during this state of the disease.

With regard to medical treatment, recurrent prostate cancer, in general, initially responds well to hormonal therapy (inhibition of production of testosterone by luteinizing hormone-releasing hormone analogues or orchiectomy, treatment with antiandrogens, or a combination of these two approaches), but a durable response is rare. Further disease progression initially manifests itself as a continuous rise in PSA levels despite hormonal therapy. However, the natural history of disease progression among these patients is quite variable. For instance, the 2-year metastasis-free survival will be about 60%, 40%, or 80%, respectively, with a PSA doubling time of less than 6 months, 6 to 18 months, or greater than 18 months (133).

Established metastatic disease may still respond to hormonal manipulations, but overall, the median response time to antiandrogen therapy does not exceed 18 months. Nevertheless, patients with disease considered hormone refractory may still respond to secondary or tertiary hormonal manipulations. For instance, some patients treated with antiandrogens show clinical improvement when this therapy is discontinued (antiandrogen withdrawal syndrome). This is particularly well described for the drug flutamide. Moreover, other hormonal treatments (e.g., bicalutamide, glucocorticoids, or ketoconazole) may retain activity even in patients who have failed to respond to combined antiandrogen therapy and flutamide withdrawal (134). Because of this unpredictable and variable response, the term *hormone-independent* prostate cancer should no longer be used.

Metastatic disease most commonly occurs in the bones. About 60% to 80% of patients may present with bone metastases only, and almost all patients who die of prostate cancer have bone metastases. Once hormonal manipulations have failed, docetaxel is now the standard treatment for metastatic prostate cancer (135,136), with significant albeit relatively small survival and symptomatic benefits as compared to other regimens. There is likely a subset of patients with very aggressive prostate cancer who are bound to progress to the metastatic state despite optimal surgical and oncologic treatment.

Role of CT, Magnetic Resonance Imaging, and Bone Scan in Imaging Prostate Cancer

Histopathologically and on high-resolution imaging studies, such as endorectal MRI, the normal human prostate can be divided into central, transitional, and peripheral zones. The three zones are defined by their location in relationship to the urethra. Of note, most of the prostate tissue belongs to the peripheral zone, where about 70% of all cancers arise. In contrast, cancer occurs rarely in the central zone (1% to 5%), although it comprises approximately 25% of the glandular tissue. The transitional zone comprises 5% to 10% of glandular tissue and accounts for 20% of prostate cancers (137). Although these structures cannot be recognized on PET or CT, an understanding of the zonal prostate anatomy will help the nuclear medicine physician in establishing rapport with MR readers and urologists and is important as better resolution imaging of the prostate is developed.

CT is generally not helpful in detecting either primary prostate cancer or local recurrence. The sensitivity for lymph node staging in the primary setting is limited, with a sensitivity of 27% to 75% and a specificity of 66% to 100%. CT is still a standard test for the work-up of patients with PSA relapse, with the main goal to *rule out* obvious distant disease in lymph nodes and bones. The diagnostic yield is low as long as the PSA is less than 10 ng/mL, and even among individuals with PSA doubling time of less than 6 months, only about one fourth of CT scans will show disease (138). The sensitivity for detecting local recurrence is as low as 36% (139).

MRI with endorectal and pelvis-phased array coils has shown a high accuracy for determining organ-confined disease in individuals with primary prostate cancer (PCA) (140). In experienced hands, MR spectroscopy adds diagnostic value to MRI alone. Alterations in citrate and choline concentration in cancer form the basis for MR spectroscopy imaging of prostate cancer. Normal prostate shows high citrate concentrations, whereas prostate cancer shows high levels of choline and often diminished citrate and in particular an increased ratio of (choline plus creatine)/citrate (50).

It is now possible to actually quantify the absolute changes of these metabolites in prostate tissue (51): phosphocholine plus glycerophosphocholine (PC+GPC), total choline, lactate, and alanine concentrations are higher in prostate cancer than in healthy glandular and healthy stromal tissues, while citrate and polyamine concentrations are significantly higher in healthy glandular tissues than in healthy stromal and prostate cancer tissues. For clinical purposes and to guide patient management, MR spectroscopy data should be interpreted in conjunction with MRI findings (141). MRI can also detect local recurrence in many patients with PSA relapse but no palpable tumor in the prostatic fossa. Preliminary data suggest a very high sensitivity of 95% and specificity of 100% (142). Above all, MRI permits the simultaneous assessment of prostate bed, pelvic lymph nodes, and bones (early disease confined to bone marrow). Following EBRT, an MR spectroscopy imaging pattern of complete metabolic atrophy (essentially a flat line in the spectra) is a surrogate for successful therapy. However, false-positive MR spectroscopy findings are not uncommon after EBRT.

Among nuclear medicine methods, the bone scan is the most frequently used test. In the staging of primary prostate cancer, the diagnostic yield of the bone scan remains as low as 1% until the PSA level reaches 10 to 20 ng/mL. In patients with PSA relapse, a bone scan may be the most commonly ordered imaging test, although it will rarely show an abnormality when the PSA is less than 20 ng/mL (143,144). In a UCLA study, PSA doubling time (rather than a single PSA measurement alone) was a meaningful measure in identifying a subset of patients with more aggressive disease. Although only 11% of patients with PSA less than 10 ng/mL had a positive bone scan, this rate was 26% for those with PSA doubling time of less than 6 months as compared to 3% in individuals with PSA doubling time greater than 6 months (138).

Although most bone scans will be negative, it may sometimes be helpful to obtain this test to establish baseline conditions. Recently, a nomogram has been published that allows calculation of probability for a positive bone scan in patients with PSA relapse, based on clinical and laboratory parameters (145). In individuals with metastatic prostate cancer, the number of lesions on bone scans and an increasing spread to the peripheral skeleton correlate with prognosis.

Clinical Applications for PET According to Clinical State of Prostate Cancer

Different PET tracers may suit different states of primary or progressive prostate cancer. Most likely, there is no magic bullet imaging agent for all states of this disease. Even in patients with metastatic disease, metastases at different sites are biologically distinct (146). Clinical applications for PET are therefore discussed according to the clinical states model (Fig. 8.18.1).

Detection and Screening

There is no clear role for PET in detecting primary prostate cancer in nonselected healthy individuals or even those with elevated PSA. Focal radiotracer uptake in the prostate can be seen incidentally with FDG, acetate, or choline, suggesting focal prostatitis or prostate cancer. The finding should be pursued clinically, and, depending on the level of suspicion, a biopsy may be indicated (Fig. 8.18.2).

With choline, at least one focus of abnormal uptake can be identified in most patients with primary prostate cancer, although the sensitivity for individual cancer foci within the gland is only in

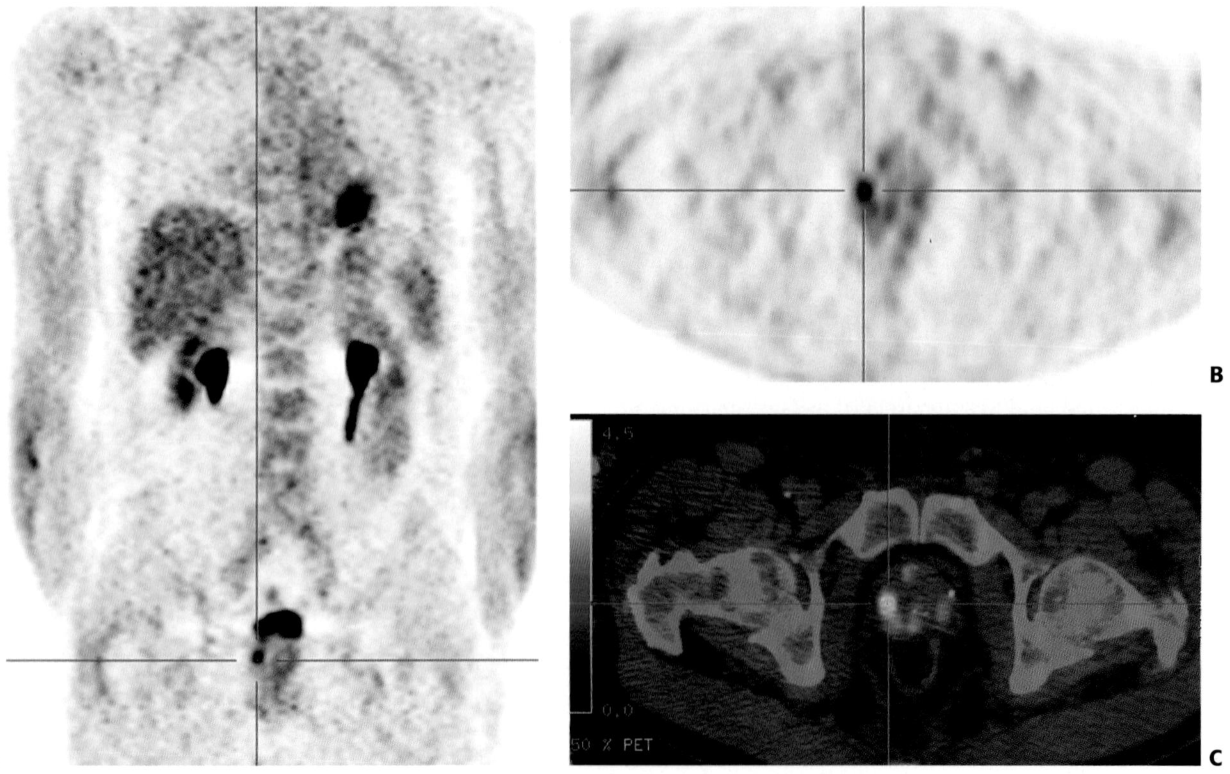

FIGURE 8.18.2. Incidental detection of prostate cancer on fluorodeoxyglucose (FDG) PET/CT. FDG PET **(A, B)** and PET/CT fusion **(C)** images in a 66-year-old man with newly diagnosed prostate cancer (two of seven cores, Gleason 6). Prostate-specific antigen was 7.23 ng/mL. The patient subsequently underwent external-beam radiation therapy. It is not proven that the intense FDG uptake precisely corresponded to the tumor.

the range of 60% to 80% (89,147). A possible indication for choline PET in the setting of primary disease might exist in guiding biopsies in patients with clinical suspicion but repeated negative transrectal-untrasonography–guided biopsies.

It is unclear if acetate or choline uptake in primary prostate cancer lesions can serve as an indicator of biologic aggressiveness. Acetate uptake does not correlate with PSA level or Gleason score (148,149). Similarly, choline uptake does not correlate with PSA levels, Gleason score, or the proliferation marker Ki-67 (84,147), but only with tumor stage (147), the latter likely reflecting poor count recovery in smaller tumors.

Primary Staging

The local extent of the disease (extracapsular extension, seminal vesicle invasion) cannot be assessed reliably with any PET tracer. FDG has insufficient accuracy for lymph node staging. Choline and acetate are under study for this purpose. In one study of 67 patients, choline PET had a sensitivity and specificity of 80% and 96%, respectively, as compared to 47% and 98% with CT or MRI (150). These promising but preliminary data need to be confirmed in larger groups of individuals. The clinical use of PET for lymph node staging, if any, will depend on the local surgical preference (i.e., whether the standard approach involves limited dissection or routine extended lymph node dissection). The role of sentinel lymph node mapping is also under investigation. In one small study, sentinel lymph node mapping showed a better sensitivity than [^{18}F]-choline PET (151).

Prostate-specific Antigen Relapse after Treatment with Curative Intent

The main purpose of imaging studies is to distinguish between local recurrence in and around the prostate bed and distant metastatic disease in lymph nodes, bones, or parenchymal organs. Although the probability for local versus distant recurrence can be estimated from clinical and pathological features (152,153), a rational treatment strategy will generally require the identification of disease sites on imaging studies or histopathology. The single exception to this rule might be the patient with PSA relapse in whom isolated local recurrence is very likely (although not necessarily proven by biopsy) based on clinical features and absence of distant disease on imaging studies. Local recurrence may be amenable to salvage prostatectomy or salvage irradiation. As pointed out before, local recurrence needs to be identified and treated early during PSA relapse in order to succeed (131,132). In contrast, distant disease generally requires systemic therapy, in the initial phase usually with antiandrogens.

There are three potential scenarios in which imaging tests can help in the management of patients with PSA relapse:

- *Show local recurrence early* (i.e., when PSA is less than 2 to 4 ng/mL). This may be elusive in many cases because of low volume disease.
- *Exclude distant disease* whenever local salvage therapy is planned (at whatever PSA level this may be).
- *Reveal distant (and/or local) disease* and determine the extent of disease. This information can then be used in treatment monitoring studies.

Local recurrence most commonly occurs at the perianastomotic or retrovesical regions. However, up to 30% of local recurrences may occur at other sites, such as retained seminal vesicles or at the lateral or anterior surgical margins. Transrectal ultrasonography and transrectal ultrasonography–guided biopsy are the most common diagnostic tests, but they may suffer from sampling error and a relatively high rate of false-negative findings. The likelihood for tumor detection may be higher if the PSA is greater than 4 ng/mL (154), and as many as 28% of patients with initial normal biopsies demonstrate recurrence on subsequent biopsies (154,155).

The true extent of recurrent disease may have been underestimated frequently in the past. In several studies, the success rates for salvage radiotherapy after prostatectomy ranged from 10% to 50%, suggesting that many patients already had occult distant metastases at the time of treatment and therefore did not benefit from salvage radiotherapy (131).

FDG PET can identify some sites of local recurrence or distant disease in patients with PSA relapse after prostatectomy (156). In a retrospective cohort study of 91 patients with a mean PSA of 4.3 ± 8.6 ng/mL, this test showed local recurrence and/or metastatic disease in 28 of the 91 patients (30%). The PSA was higher in patients with a positive as compared to those with a negative PET scan (9.5 ± 12.2 ng/mL vs. 2.1 ± 3.3 ng/mL). The probability for disease detection increased with higher PSA and PSA velocity. Of note, 52 of 60 patients without evidence for disease on PET underwent other concurrent imaging studies, and in 86% all of these tests were negative (156). This is in concordance with the clinical experience that a site of disease can often be missed in a large number of patients until the PSA reaches higher levels. Similarly, FDG PET was more likely to detect lymph node metastases in patients with PSA relapse when the PSA was greater than 4 ng/mL (157).

In comparison to FDG, the sensitivity for detecting sites of recurrent disease with acetate has been reported as 30% to 90% (158–161), and with [^{11}C]- or [^{18}F]-choline as 50% to 100% (162,163) (Figs. 8.18.3, 8.18.4, and 8.18.5). The reader is encouraged to interpret these data in the proper clinical context, in light of the chosen inclusion criteria and gold standard for verification of PET findings, and in conjunction with PSA values and kinetics. In some but not all studies with acetate or choline, the likelihood for disease detection increased with rising PSA levels. In one acetate study (158), the sensitivity was higher in patients with PSA greater than 3 ng/mL. In one small study with [^{11}C]-choline, local or systemic recurrence was identified in all cases with PSA greater than 2 ng/mL (161), whereas a larger study with [^{18}F]-choline (163) found a higher likelihood for disease detection among individuals with a PSA greater than 4 ng/mL and Gleason score greater than 8. Of note, 41 of the 52 patients (79%) with PSA less than 4 ng/mL had a negative PET scan. This later study included 100 patients with PSA relapse imaged with [^{18}F]-choline, the mean PSA was 38 ng/mL in patients with positive PET scan as compared to 2.1 ng/mL in those with negative PET scans (median PSA 9.6 and 0.98 ng/mL, respectively).

Few studies have directly compared FDG with other radiotracers, but there seems to be general agreement that imaging with acetate, methionine, or choline may be more sensitive than imaging with FDG in patients with PSA relapse (158,162). Overall, sites of disease can probably be identified in 30% of patients with FDG (156,162). The author believes that the eventual sensitivity with acetate or choline will be in the range of 50% to 70%. No difference in sensitivity was found in the only study comparing [^{11}C]-acetate with [^{11}C]-choline (164). A final assessment of the true clinical utility of PET in patients with PSA relapse (regardless of the specific tracer used) may require a prospective study, perhaps a

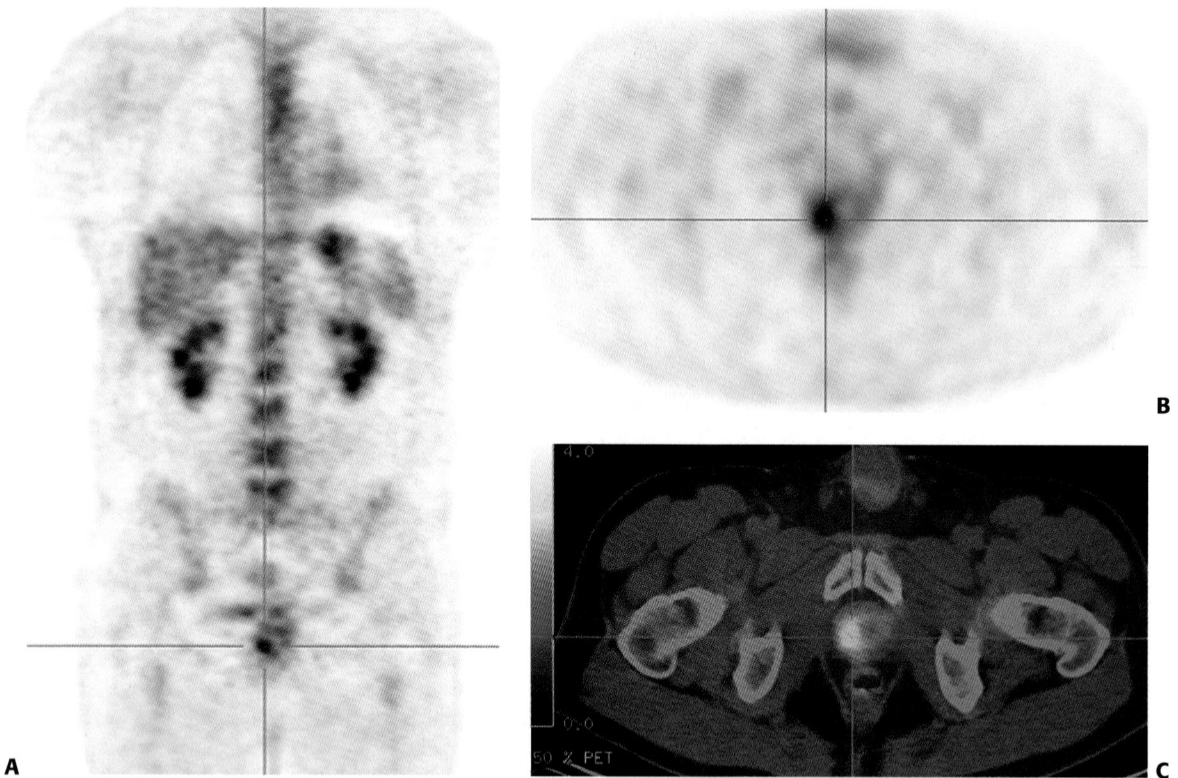

FIGURE 8.18.3. Local recurrence on fluorodeoxyglucose (FDG) PET/CT. FDG PET **(A, B)** and PET/CT fusion **(C)** images in a 57-year-old man with prostate-specific antigen relapse (PSA 2.86 ng/mL) approximately 4 years after external-beam radiation therapy to the prostate. Local recurrence was proven by biopsy and no other sites of disease were detected. He underwent salvage prostatectomy. The step section histology map showed cancer (Gleason 7) within the inked areas. There was extracapsular extension and invasion into the right seminal vesicle.

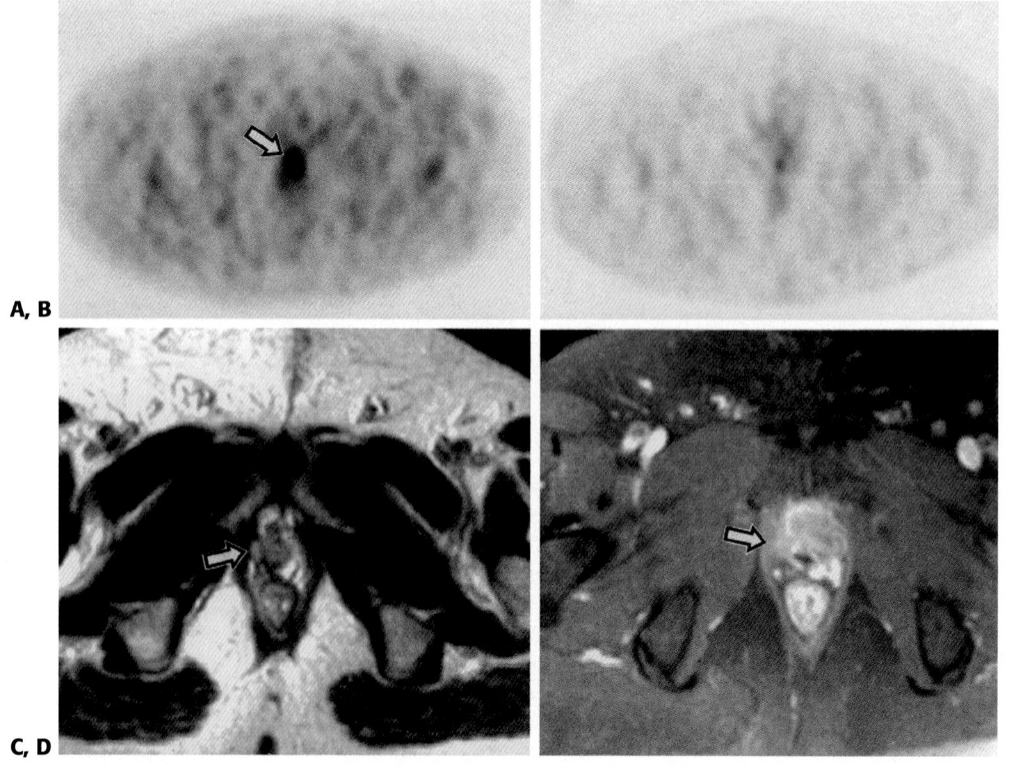

FIGURE 8.18.4. Local recurrence of prostate cancer seen with [^{11}C]-choline PET. Images of a man with prostate-specific antigen relapse (PSA 3.8 ng/mL) approximately 7 years after radical prostatectomy. Transaxial [^{11}C]-choline PET **(A)** shows abnormal tracer uptake in the prostate fossa (*arrow*), whereas FDG PET **(B)** is negative. Turbo spin-echo T2-weighted image **(C)** shows soft tissue with abnormal signal (*arrow*), and there is contrast enhancement after intravenous administration of gadolinium (*arrow*) on the spin-echo T1-weighted image with fat suppression **(D).** (From Picchio M, Messa C, Landoni C, et al. Value of [11C]choline-positron emission tomo-graphy for re-staging prostate cancer: a comparison with [18F]-fluorodeoxyglucose-positron emission tomography. *J Urol* 2003;169: 1337–1340, with permission.)

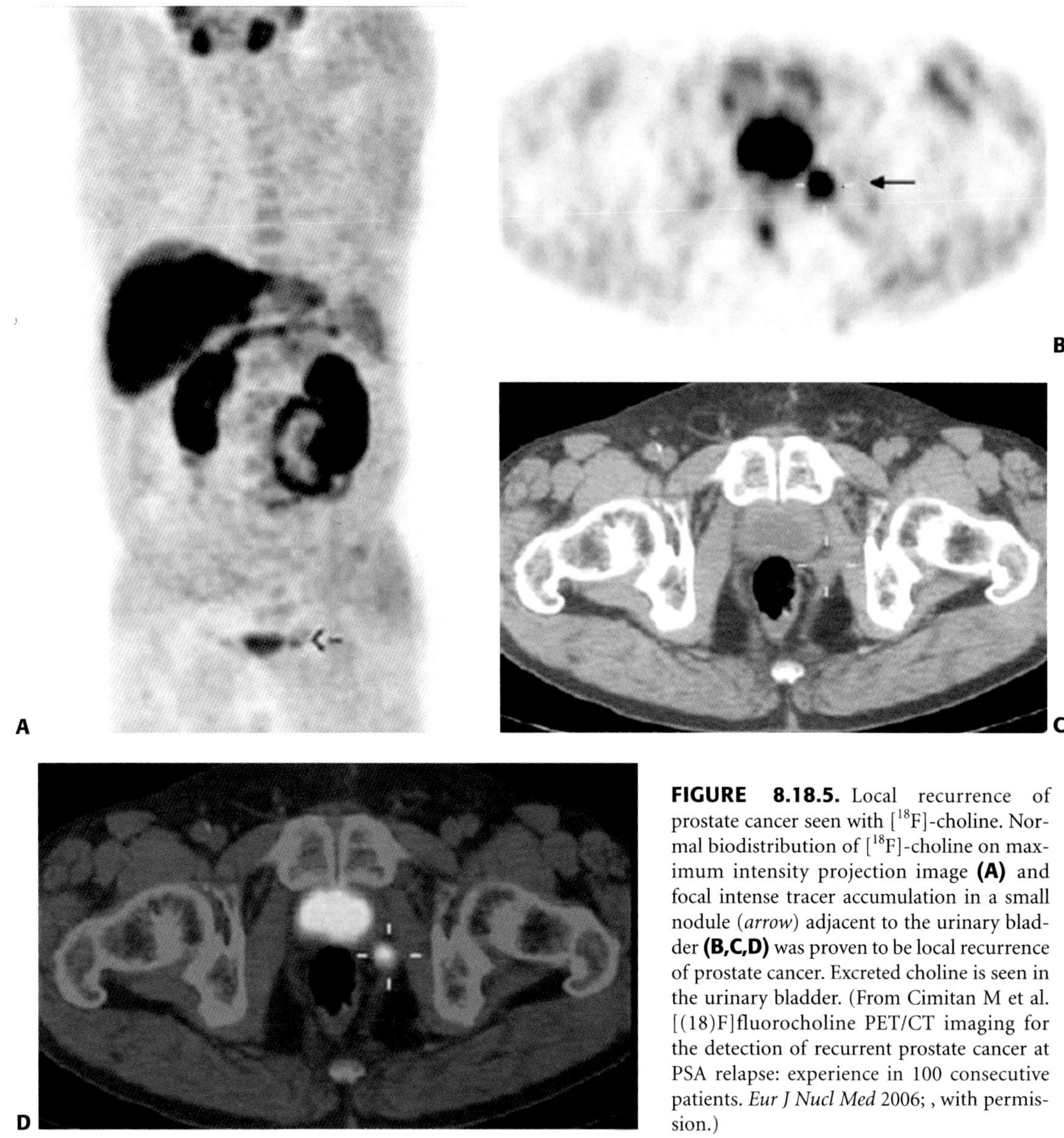

FIGURE 8.18.5. Local recurrence of prostate cancer seen with [^{18}F]-choline. Normal biodistribution of [^{18}F]-choline on maximum intensity projection image **(A)** and focal intense tracer accumulation in a small nodule (*arrow*) adjacent to the urinary bladder **(B,C,D)** was proven to be local recurrence of prostate cancer. Excreted choline is seen in the urinary bladder. (From Cimitan M et al. [(18)F]fluorocholine PET/CT imaging for the detection of recurrent prostate cancer at PSA relapse: experience in 100 consecutive patients. *Eur J Nucl Med* 2006; , with permission.)

multicenter study, with rigid inclusion criteria and routine use of combined PET/CT. It would be important to determine if PET could potentially replace a battery of other tests in the patient with PSA relapse and establish how the detection of disease sites on PET translates into changes in patient management and ultimate outcome.

Guiding Chemotherapy in Metastatic Disease

Changes in PSA and PSA doubling time under chemotherapy provide important prognostic information, but it would be desirable to have an imaging study that can actually show and quantify the response to chemotherapy in an individual patient.

Clinical evidence suggests an inverse relationship between the aggressiveness and its detectability on FDG PET (Fig. 8.18.6). In patients with metastatic prostate cancer, the response to chemotherapy can be monitored well with FDG PET, whereas this may not be possible on the bone scan (slow response, flare phenomenon) or CT (sclerotic bone lesions may appear stable, but this does not necessarily reflect the biologic activity of the disease). Indeed, FDG PET can show treatment effects that are usually described by a combination of PSA, bone scintigraphy, and soft tissue imaging (165). In experimental studies, a response to hormonal therapy could be monitored with FLT PET (118). Because of the intense uptake in normal bone marrow and the predominance of bone metastases, the clinical utility of FLT in metastatic prostate cancer appears doubtful.

Prognostic Value of PET

Imaging studies, in particular the bone scan, can provide prognostic information in patients with metastatic prostate cancer (166–168). In a study comparing bone scan and FDG PET in metastatic prostate cancer, nearly all lesions seen on bone scan

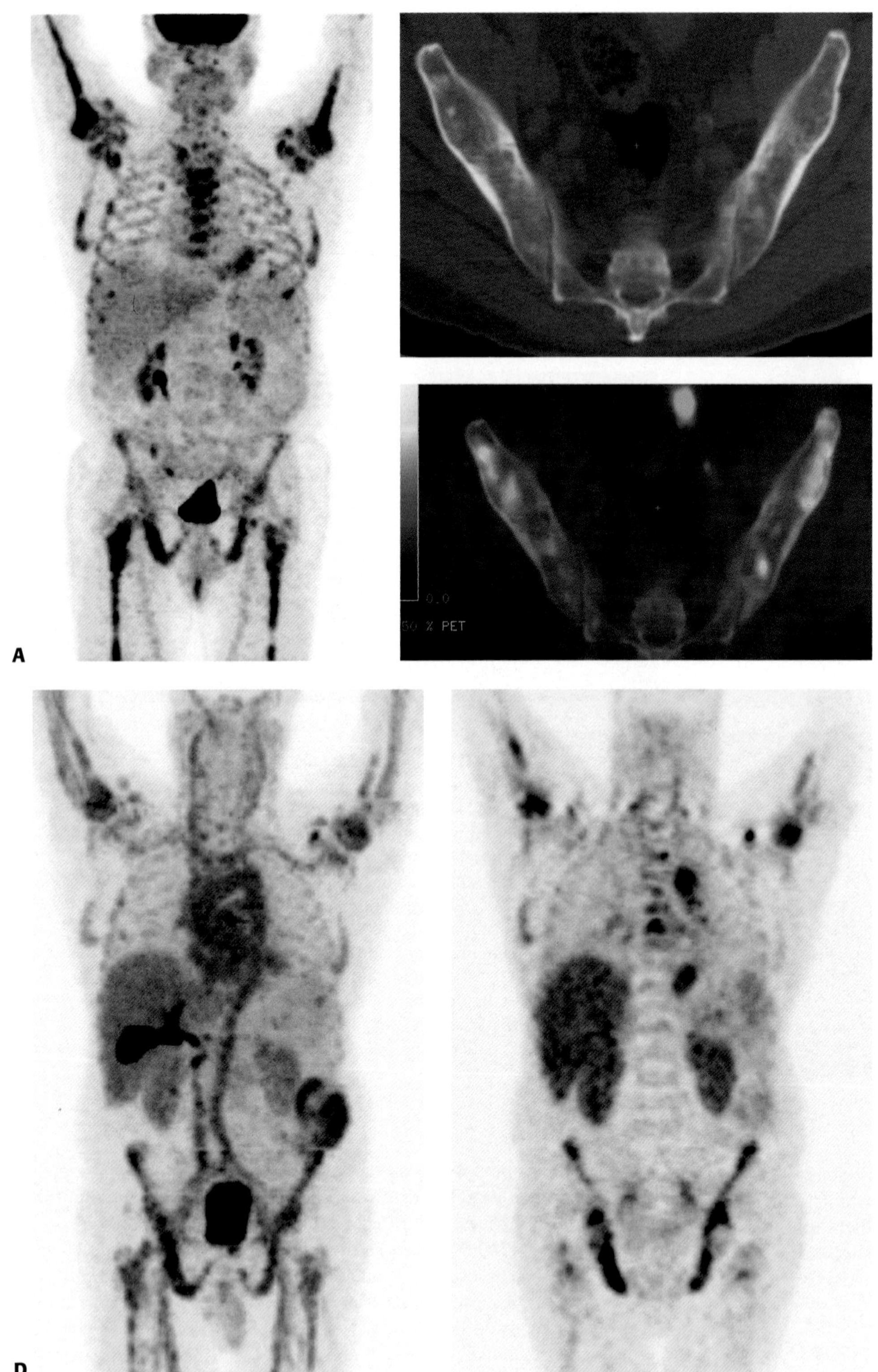

FIGURE 8.18.6. Widespread metastatic prostate cancer in bones seen with fluorodeoxyglucose (FDG) and 16β-[^{18}F]-fluoro-5α-dihydrotestosteron (FDHT) PET. A 66-year-old man with widespread metastatic prostate cancer. FDG maximum intensity projection (MIP) **(A)** image shows abnormal FDG uptake throughout the skeleton. Transaxial CT and PET/CT **(B,C)** fusion images demonstrate osteoblastic metastases with intense FDG uptake. MIP image of FDHT **(D)** shows normal blood pool activity, hepatobiliary clearance of tracer and intense, abnormal uptake in the skeleton. Uptake in bone metastases is better seen on coronal PET image **(E).** Prostate-specific antigen 885 ng/mL, castrate levels of testosterone at 4 ng/mL.

alone remained stable, whereas all lesions detected by FDG only progressed upon follow-up (169). This has recently been confirmed in a larger study of 51 patients (170). In the same population, an SUV greater than 6.0 at the site of most intense FDG uptake in the scan was associated with a median survival of 15 months, as compared to 28 months when the SUV was less than 6.0.

Imaging of the Androgen Receptor

FDHT is under study in patients with castrate-resistant metastatic prostate cancer (Fig. 8.18.6). The goal is to evaluate metabolic heterogeneity among metastatic lesions and to assess the potential clinical utility of this or similar agents in monitoring the response to molecular therapies targeting the androgen receptor. As proof of this principle, treatment with the AR blocker flutamide reduces FDHT uptake within 24 hours of therapy (115).

Summary of PET Indications

- No clear indication in screening or detection of primary prostate cancer when PSA is elevated.
- Possible indication in guiding biopsies when clinical suspicion and prior repeat biopsy is negative.
- No established role in primary staging; studies on nodal staging ongoing.
- PSA relapse may be a major indication: identify local or distant disease; acetate and choline likely more sensitive than FDG.
- Treatment monitoring of castrate-resistant metastatic disease with FDG.
- FDHT or similar compounds for study of tumor biology and possibly monitoring response to novel therapies targeting the androgen receptor.

RENAL CANCER

Clinical Statement

Renal cell cancer accounts for about 3% of all malignancies in the United States. About 54,390 cases are estimated for 2008 and about 13,000 people are expected to die (1). The vast majority of cases (about 75%) are conventional or clear cell carcinomas. About one quarter of patients present with locally advanced or metastatic disease and about one third of individuals who undergo resection will later develop some form of recurrence (171). The treatment traditionally has consisted of radical nephrectomy with resection of the kidney, Gerota fascia, ipsilateral adrenal gland, and local lymph nodes. Recent surgical advances include so-called nephron-sparing resections, in particular in patients with a single kidney, renal dysfunction, or bilateral involvement. Metastatic disease does not respond well to standard chemotherapy. Alternate treatments involve immunomodulation with interferon alfa or interleukin 2, and more recently various tyrosine kinase inhibitors (e.g., sunitinib, sorafenib), mTOR inhibitors, and antibodies against vascular endothelial growth factor, EGFR, and carbonic anhydrase IX (172). The role of FDG PET or other PET tracers in monitoring the response to these newer agents is under investigation.

Imaging of Renal Cancer

Diagnosis and Staging

Renal masses can be characterized reasonably well with dedicated thin-slice CT. Although a specific diagnosis may not be possible in all cases, renal masses can be divided into those that require further surgical exploration and those that require no further management or observation only. Diagnostic criteria include structural appearance and density, size, and contrast enhancement patterns. Overall, the sensitivity and specificity for the detection of renal cell carcinoma approaches 100% and 90%, respectively (173,174). The reported sensitivity for the detection of retroperitoneal lymph node metastases is as high as 95% (175), but using a nodal size of 1 cm or greater, false-positive findings can occur in 3% to 49% of cases (176).

Efforts to employ the traditional PET radiotracer FDG for the imaging of primary renal cancer have been hampered by physiologic tracer accumulation and excretion in the kidney. In general, it is not possible to reliably detect renal cell carcinoma or other renal malignancies on FDG PET. In exceptional cases, a large solid renal lesion may reveal mild to moderate FDG uptake (Figs. 8.18.7 and 8.18.8). In the largest study in patients with primary renal cell carcinoma, FDG PET had a sensitivity of 60% and specificity of 100% (177). False-positive uptake was reported in pheochromocytomas, angiomyolipomas, and pericytoma and large cell lymphoma. When using a combined PET/CT scanner, the CT features may help to define the nature of the lesion (e.g., negative density values in angiomyolipomas) better than would be possible with FDG. Little is known regarding the potential clinical utility of alternate PET radiotracers in renal cancer. One new experimental imaging agent for primary clear cell renal cell carcinoma is the antibody cG250, labeled with iodine-124 (^{124}I). The antibody is directed against carbonic anhydrase IX, which is consistently overexpressed in renal cell carcinoma. In preliminary studies conducted at the author's institution, PET imaging with [^{124}I]-cG250 could identify presence of clear cell cancer with sensitivity and specificity of greater than 90% (178). These findings will now be validated in a multicenter study. Other PET tracers with potential clinical application in renal cancer include the unnatural amino acid anti-1-amino-3-[^{18}F]-fluorocyclobutyl-1-carboxylic acid (FACBC).

The primary staging of renal cell carcinoma involves CT or MRI of the abdomen and pelvis and CT of the chest. Other imaging studies may be needed. PET with established radiotracers has not been shown to contribute meaningful information in the primary staging. The role of the newer PET agents for this purpose still needs to be studied. For instance, an agent with high specificity for clear cell carcinoma might be helpful in case of equivocal CT or MRI findings in lymph nodes or at distant sites.

Local Recurrence and Metastatic Disease

Recurrent or metastatic renal cancer can be identified with FDG PET in 65% to 80% of cases (177,179), but the intensity of FDG uptake in these lesions may be variable. Metastatic disease is rarely detected on PET when CT or MRI are negative (180). In the largest study to date, in which 172 soft tissue and bone lesions were assessed by CT, bone scan, and FDG PET, the sensitivity for PET was low at 67% (64% for soft tissue and 75% for bone lesions) (177). In this study, CT was superior for detecting soft tissue lesions, and the combination of CT and bone scan showed a better sensitivity in detecting osseous metastases. Nevertheless, it may be reasonable to include FDG PET imaging in the follow-up of high-risk patients when there is clinical suspicion for recurrence and metastasis and in particular when structural imaging studies are equivocal. FDG PET may affect patient management by characterizing anatomic lesions of unclear significance. Its role in monitoring the response of metastases to novel treatments with tyrosine kinase inhibitors or vascular endothelial growth factor antibodies is under investigation.

Summary of PET Indications

- No clear indication for FDG, choline, or acetate in primary lesion detection, renal mass characterization, or staging.
- Imaging with specific antibodies or artificial amino acids may prove helpful in assessment of renal masses and staging, but this requires much more study.
- PET with FDG may be helpful in suspected recurrence, especially when CT or MRI are equivocal.
- Role of FDG PET in monitoring response to tyrosine kinase inhibitors and mTOR inhibitors is under investigation.

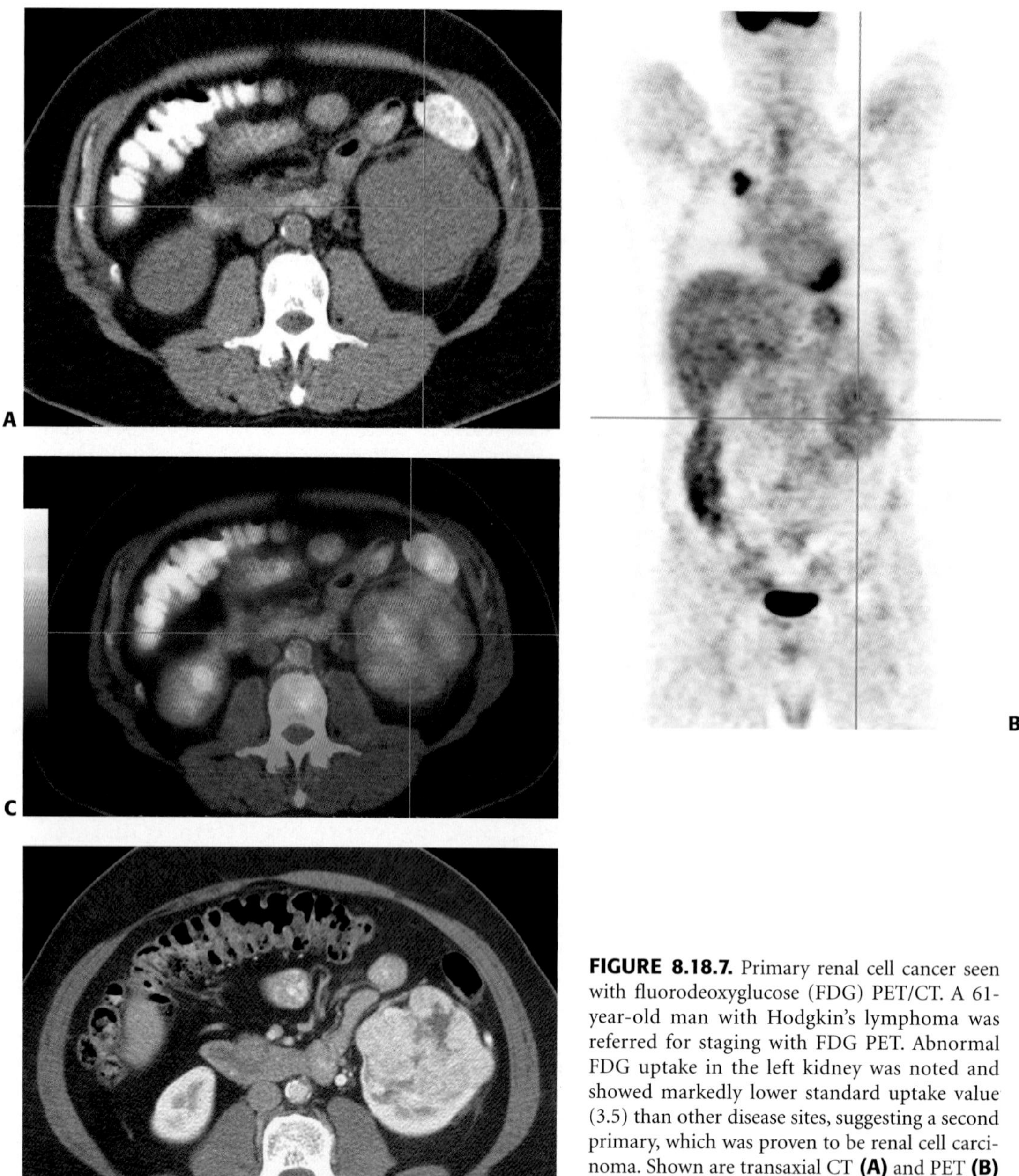

FIGURE 8.18.7. Primary renal cell cancer seen with fluorodeoxyglucose (FDG) PET/CT. A 61-year-old man with Hodgkin's lymphoma was referred for staging with FDG PET. Abnormal FDG uptake in the left kidney was noted and showed markedly lower standard uptake value (3.5) than other disease sites, suggesting a second primary, which was proven to be renal cell carcinoma. Shown are transaxial CT **(A)** and PET **(B)** as well as fusion **(C)** and CT with intravenous contrast **(D).** On the coronal FDG PET image, a lesion with higher FDG uptake in the right lung indicates a site of Hodgkin's lymphoma.

BLADDER CANCER

Clinical Statement

Transitional cell carcinoma of the urinary bladder is the second most common urologic malignancy behind prostate cancer. Sixty-eight thousand new cases are expected in 2008, with a male to female ratio of about 3:1, and about 14,000 are expected to die of this disease in 2008 (1). At the time of diagnosis, approximately 70% of tumors are superficial (without muscle invasion), and most of these tumors are low grade (181). However, they recur frequently and approximately 10% to 20% progress to muscle invasive or metastatic disease. Because of the frequent recurrence and need for surveillance, it is estimated that more than 600,000 patients in the United States are receiving active care for bladder cancer (182).

The standard management for superficial bladder cancer involves transurethral resection, "immuno-boost" therapy with BCG vaccine for all T1 and high-grade Ta lesions, and meticulous follow-up since most recurrences occur within the first 5 years (181). The role of intravesical chemotherapy is under investigation. In contrast, invasive bladder cancer is characterized by progressive local invasion, extension to adjacent organs, and the development of regional and distant metastases. Radical cystoprostatectomy in

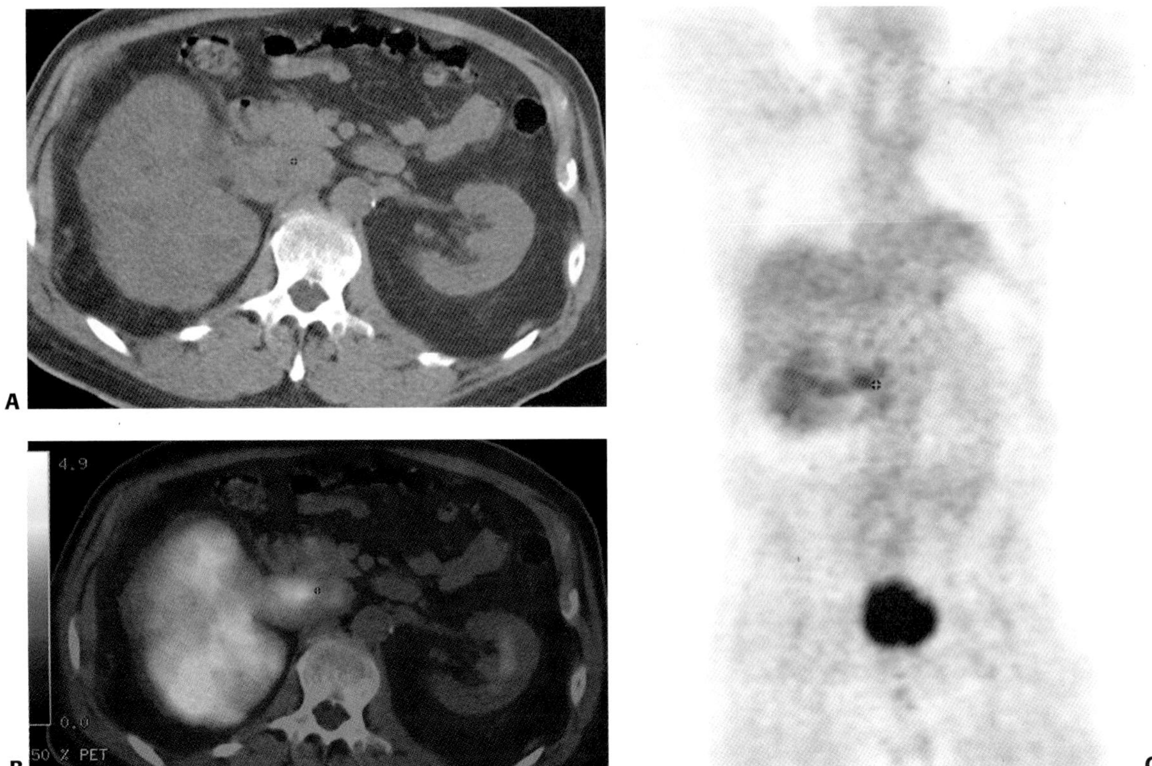

FIGURE 8.18.8. Advanced stage renal cell cancer seen with fluorodeoxyglucose (FDG) PET/CT. Locally advanced renal cell cancer in a 70-year-old man. There is diffuse enlargement of the right kidney on CT **(A).** Abnormal FDG uptake of moderate intensity extends from the right kidney into the right renal vein and inferior vena cava as seen on transaxial and coronal **(B,C)** PET images, indicating tumor thrombus.

male patients and anterior pelvic exenteration in female patients, coupled with *en bloc* pelvic lymphadenectomy, are the standard surgical approach to muscle invasive bladder carcinoma in the absence of metastatic disease (182).

The effectiveness of local therapy depends largely on the extent of primary tumor invasion and the presence of pelvic lymph node metastases. Organ-confined bladder cancer can be treated by surgery alone and may be curable in over 70% of patients (183–185). In comparison, the average relapse rate with local or distant disease may be as high as 66% in patients with lymph node metastases found at the time of cystectomy (183,186), and as a group, these individuals show a 5-year survival of only 20% to 25% (183–188). Local extravesical extension and lymph node involvement increase the probability for later metastatic disease (186). Nontransitional carcinoma of the bladder also confers a worse prognosis (189).

Accurate staging of bladder cancer is important to select the appropriate treatment strategy. Advances in surgical techniques for cystectomy and pelvic reconstruction have made it possible to tailor surgery to the specific needs of patients. Preoperative knowledge of local tumor extension would help in selecting appropriate patients for bladder-sparing surgery, nerve or vaginal-sparing procedures, or pelvic exenteration.

There is also an ongoing discussion regarding the appropriate anatomic extent of pelvic lymph node dissection in bladder cancer. It would be desirable to limit any unnecessary dissection in patients at low risk for metastases ("tailored approach"). However, the safety and potential benefits of such an approach are currently unproven. The main problem with this strategy lies in the inability of current imaging techniques to identify nodal disease with sufficient sensitivity. Approximately 20% to 25% of contemporary patients with bladder cancer treated with radical cystectomy will demonstrate pathologic evidence of regional lymph node involvement (183,186,188,190). In most cases this occurs without evidence for gross disease on presurgical imaging studies (186,188). The incidence for lymph node involvement increases with increasing tumor stage. Although pelvic lymph node dissection is primarily a staging procedure, it may also improve the disease-specific survival in some patients with limited nodal disease (188,191–194). The number of lymph nodes removed and the tumor volume in these nodes (lymph node density) are critical prognostic factors (194).

Some institutions advocate an extension of the standard pelvic lymph node dissection to just above the level of the aortic bifurcation to improve the staging accuracy. Surgical removal of all involved nodes carries an independent prognostic value (193). Patients with histologically proven nodal disease undergo systemic adjuvant chemotherapy (195). Of note, a subset of patients without evidence for metastasis by standard histopathological analysis may harbor subclinical micrometastases, which may also influence patient prognosis (196). Regardless of these important data, however, it remains true that a large number of patients do not harbor nodal metastases, and they are unnecessarily subjected to pelvic lymph node dissection. This suggests a need to improve the presurgical staging with newer imaging tests.

Imaging of Bladder Cancer

Primary Tumor Detection and Staging

The diagnosis of bladder cancer is based on cystoscopy and biopsy, and there is no proven role for PET imaging in this setting. The most important issue in the initial management of bladder cancer is to differentiate between superficial and muscle invasive tumors. None of the current imaging technologies can reliably and accurately assess the degree of muscle invasion. Among the structural imaging studies, CT has particular limitations. In a retrospective study of 85 patients the depth of invasion was correctly assessed in only one patient and extravesical tumor spread in four patients, likely because the invasion can be microscopic and below the resolution of these methods (190). MRI appears more accurate in demonstrating invasion into perivesical fat tissue or tumor extension into the ureter or adjacent soft tissue organs. However, even with modern techniques, overstaging is common, although superficial and muscle invasive tumors can be distinguished in 85% and organ-confined from non–organ-confined tumor in 82% of cases (197).

Among the available PET tracers, FDG is a suboptimal agent for the evaluation of primary bladder cancer. Because of urinary excretion it may be difficult to differentiate between excreted activity in the ureters and nodal activity, and lymph nodes adjacent to the bladder may not be distinguishable from excreted tracer in the bladder lumen. The use of delayed imaging, diuresis, fluid loading, and bladder catheterization can help with extravesicular disease detection, however. Although these shortcomings have been alleviated to some degree with the advent of clinical PET/CT machines and newer reconstruction algorithms (which reduce streak artifacts from high activity concentrations in the bladder), recent efforts with PET in bladder cancer staging have focused on alternate PET tracers, such as [^{11}C]- or [^{18}F]-choline or [^{11}C]-acetate (Figs. 8.18.9 and 8.18.10). However, at the time of this writing, fewer than 100 patients have been studied with these agents, the majority with [^{11}C]-choline (90,198,199).

On PET images, bladder cancer can show variable degrees of tracer uptake (regardless of the compound used). With FDG it is usually difficult to identify a lesion in the bladder wall because of excreted tracer in the bladder lumen. Even with an indwelling bladder catheter it may be impossible to empty the bladder completely; in addition, imaging of the bladder wall is generally easier when the organ is fluid filled. With methionine, tracer uptake in the bladder cancer is related to tumor stage (200). Only 78% of all bladder cancers could be visualized and PET did not improve the local staging of the disease. With [^{11}C]-choline, bladder primaries are well visualized, with mean SUV reported between 3.3 and 7.3 (90,198,199). Similarly, [^{11}C]-acetate also shows good uptake in most muscle invasive bladder primaries. With both agents, the normal bladder wall shows only very mild uptake. Premalignant lesions (carcinoma *in situ*, dysplasia) may be missed (90). Abundant urinary activity in the bladder may rarely interfere with tumor detection. False-positive uptake may be related to inflammatory changes in the bladder wall. Some PET studies have attempted to assess the presence of residual tumor tissue after transurethral resection, but with mixed results (198).

Lymph Node Staging and Distant Metastases

CT or MRI of the abdomen and pelvis are the standard tests in the evaluation for lymph node metastases. Their accuracy is limited. In a study of 85 patients with bladder cancer, CT identified lymph node metastases in only 4 of 21 cases; 17 CT studies were false negative, and 2 were false positive. The overall staging accuracy of CT was 55%, and 39% of cases were understaged (190). The introduction of multidetector row CT and new MR techniques could potentially improve the staging accuracy. In an initial study of 58 patients with bladder cancer, the new MR contrast agent ferumoxtran-10 showed a sensitivity and specificity of 95% for lymph node metastases, whereas the sensitivity was as low as 76% with nonenhanced MRI. Metastases sized 4 to 9 mm were found in 10 of 12 normal-sized (less than 10 mm) nodes analyzed with standard H/E staining (201).

With PET and FDG, sensitivities of 67% and specificities of 85% were reported in smaller studies (202). Data for other PET tracers are also limited. For instance, in one study with [^{11}C]-choline, 8 of 27 patients had lymph node metastases, and these were correctly detected in five patients with PET and in four patients with CT (198). PET did not identify metastatic nodes in three patients. The size of these false-negative nodes was 6 to 21 mm, and the size of the metastatic deposit within these nodes was 1 to 15 mm. Six lymph nodes were falsely classified as metastatic on CT, but none on PET. In another study of 18 patients with negative diagnostic CT, [^{11}C]-choline PET suspected nodal metastases in six individuals, and this was eventually confirmed in three (199). Data on the potential use of labeled amino acids or acetate are even more limited. Regardless of the tracer used, very small volume metastases are likely to be missed in lymph nodes due to resolution limitations of PET.

Distant metastases are rare in patients with primary bladder cancer, and the standard diagnostic work-up for primary bladder cancer is usually restricted to CT of the abdomen and pelvis and a radiograph of the chest. However, in one small study, combined PET/CT with [^{11}C]-choline detected unexpected widespread metastases in lymph nodes and bone in 2 of 18 patients whose diagnostic CT with intravenous contrast had been interpreted as negative. Planned cystectomy was therefore canceled. Small studies have shown good sensitivities for the detection of systemic metastatic prostate cancer with FDG. These preliminary data suggest that PET (with choline or one of the other PET tracers) may potentially be useful in patients with widely invasive bladder cancer and elevated risk for systemic disease. FDG PET is being used more commonly to detect metastatic bladder cancer under the Medicare registry.

Recurrent Disease

The risk of recurrence after radical cystectomy can be estimated by nomograms (203). Imaging studies can be applied according to the expected risk for recurrence during postsurgical surveillance. In contrast to the primary disease setting, FDG PET can be helpful in detecting recurrent or metastatic bladder cancer after radical cystectomy (Fig. 8.18.11). It is important for the nuclear medicine physician to be familiar with the surgical techniques used so that physiologic accumulation of excreted FDG (for instance in an ileal conduit) is not misinterpreted as disease recurrence. It is likely that other PET tracers, such as choline or acetate, will also find clinical application in patients with suspected recurrence or distant metastatic disease. The role of choline and acetate in recurrent bladder cancer is under investigation.

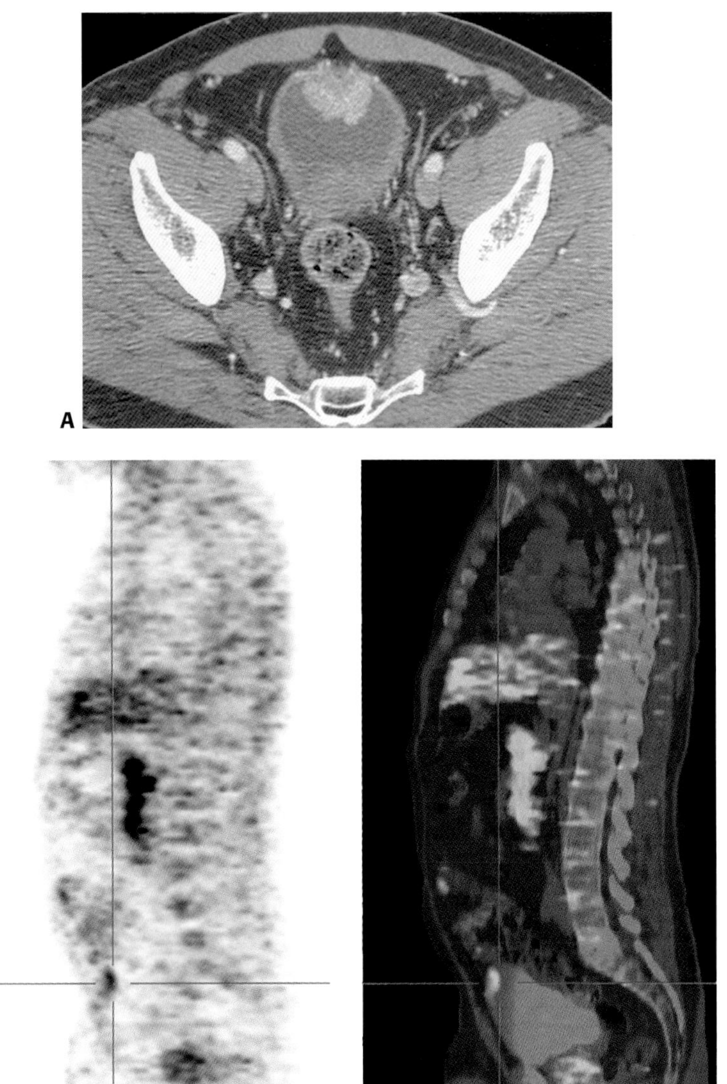

FIGURE 8.18.9. Bladder cancer seen with [^{11}C]-acetate PET/CT. Newly diagnosed bladder cancer in a 58-year-old man. CT with intravenous contrast shows exophytic tumor at the anterior wall of the urinary bladder **(A).** Sagittal [^{11}C]-acetate PET **(B)** and fusion **(C)** images demonstrate abnormal tracer uptake in the tumor. The fusion images also show intravenous contrast layering posterior in the bladder and increased acetate uptake inferior to the bladder (i.e., in the enlarged prostate), which showed nodular hyperplasia in the cystoprostatectomy specimen.

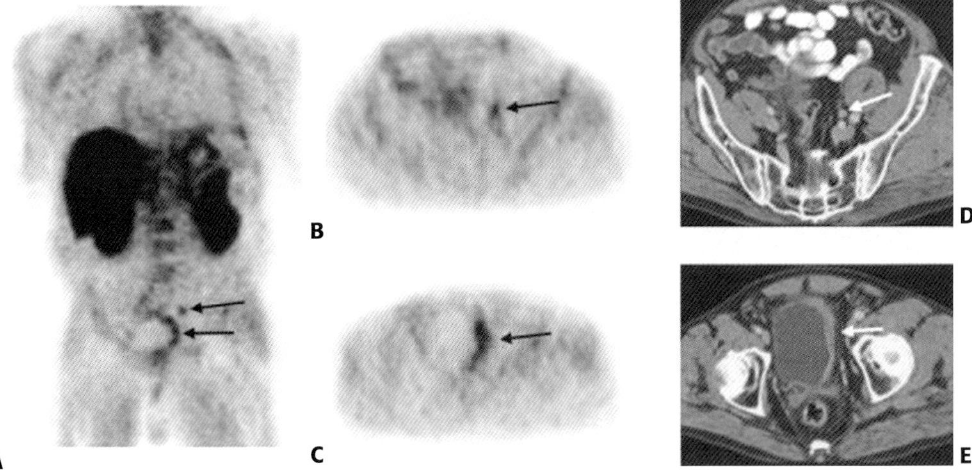

FIGURE 8.18.10. Metastatic bladder cancer seen with [^{11}C]-choline. Coronal and transaxial [^{11}C]-choline images show abnormal tracer uptake in the left lateral wall of the bladder and in a pelvic lymph nodes (**A–C**). Lymph node and bladder wall thickening are also seen on CT images (**D,E**; *arrows*). (From Picchio M, Treiber U, Beer AJ, et al. Value of ^{11}C-choline PET and contrast-enhanced CT for staging of bladder cancer: correlation with histopathologic findings. *J Nucl Med* 2006;47:938–944, with permission.)

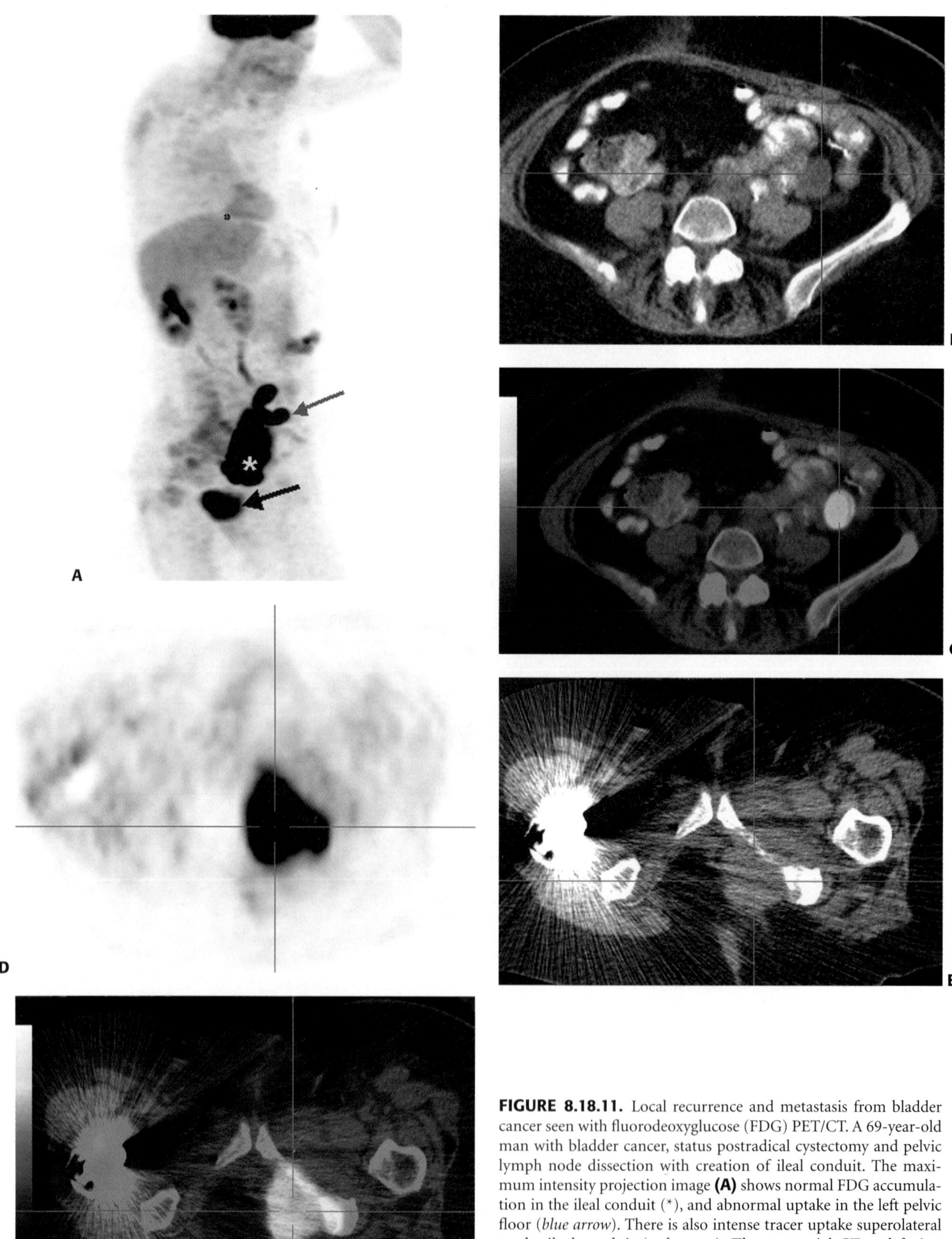

FIGURE 8.18.11. Local recurrence and metastasis from bladder cancer seen with fluorodeoxyglucose (FDG) PET/CT. A 69-year-old man with bladder cancer, status postradical cystectomy and pelvic lymph node dissection with creation of ileal conduit. The maximum intensity projection image **(A)** shows normal FDG accumulation in the ileal conduit (*), and abnormal uptake in the left pelvic floor (*blue arrow*). There is also intense tracer uptake superolateral to the ileal conduit (*red arrow*). The transaxial CT and fusion images prove that this is excreted tracer in the dilated left ureter **(B,C)**. A metastasis in the pelvic floor is seen on transaxial PET, CT, and fusion images **(D–F)**.

Summary of PET Indications

- No established indications for primary tumor detection.
- Investigative: choline and acetate for lymph node staging, staging of high-risk patients with widely muscle invasive disease.
- Probably useful: FDG for suspected recurrence (better results with combined PET/CT).

TESTICULAR CANCER

Clinical Statement

About 8,100 new testicular cancers will be diagnosed in the United States in 2008, and 380 individuals are expected to die of this disease (1). Thus, testicular cancer is relatively rare, but it is the most common malignancy in men aged 15 to 35 years. For practical purposes, testicular cancer is principally divided into two categories: seminoma and nonseminoma (includes choriocarcinoma, embryonal cell carcinoma, yolk sac tumor, teratocarcinoma, and, in more than 50% of cases, mixed histologies). The histology of the primary tumor determines the natural history of the disease: whereas 60% to 85% of all seminomas are clinically confined to the testis, 60% to 70% of nonseminomas present with demonstrable metastatic disease. Testicular cancer, in general, is considered a malignancy with a high cure rate even among patients with metastatic disease. Treatment strategies are based on the histology, extent of disease, and prognostic factors. Nowadays, cure rates of 95% to 99% are achievable for patients with early stage testicular cancer and 50% to 90% for patients with widely metastatic disease (204).

The primary treatment for all testicular neoplasms consists of radical orchiectomy. The need for additional treatment depends on the stage and histology of the disease. Among patients with seminoma, approximately 80% present with stage I (T1-4N0M0) disease. Without further adjuvant treatment, 15% to 20% of these individuals will subsequently relapse; nevertheless, the overall cure rate is 99% (204). Radiation therapy to para-aortic (and pelvic) lymph nodes has been the traditional approach. Because of concerns for long-term toxicity, studies are investigating the use of lower radiation doses (20 instead of 30 Gy) or use of chemotherapy instead of irradiation. In patients without demonstrable lymph node involvement and low risk (tumor size less than 4 cm and no invasion of rete testis), observation (surveillance) instead of adjuvant therapy may be an alternate approach when done as part of clinical studies. This might include the monitoring of tumor markers and, potentially, imaging with FDG PET/CT. In patients with advanced stage seminoma, adjuvant therapy includes irradiation and/or chemotherapy.

Patients with nonseminomatous germ cell tumor are subdivided into those with low- and high- or advanced-stage disease. Patients with low-stage nonseminomatous germ cell tumor may be candidates for surveillance, chemotherapy, or retroperitoneal lymph node dissection, depending on clinical stage, tumor markers, and tumor histology. Patients with advanced disease are further subcategorized into those with good, intermediate, and poor risk and undergo primary chemotherapy.

More than 50% of patients with testicular tumors present with metastatic disease. With the exception of choriocarcinoma, testicular cancer spreads in a predictable and stepwise fashion. Involvement of the epididymis or spermatic cord may lead to pelvic lymph node metastasis, whereas tumors confined to the testis itself usually spread to retroperitoneal nodes. Hematogenous metastases occur in lung, bone, and liver. Cisplatin-based combination chemotherapy, with or without resection of residual masses, remains the therapeutic mainstay for patients with metastatic disease. Because of the excellent treatment results achievable with this regimen, recent research efforts have mainly focused on reducing treatment-related toxicity while maintaining high cure rates. Testicular cancer is one of the few neoplasms associated with accurate serum markers: β-human chorionic gonadotropin and α-fetoprotein. These accurate tumor markers allow careful follow-up, with intervention early in the course of disease. This is also an area in which PET imaging could potentially contribute to patient management (see below).

Imaging of Testicular Cancer

Diagnosis and Staging

Ultrasonography has become the method of choice for imaging in diseases affecting the scrotum. High-resolution ultrasound, supplemented by color Doppler and pulsed Doppler, is now indispensable in the work-up of testicular masses. It is possible to distinguish between intra- and extratesticular lesions, as well as between cystic versus solid tumors (98% of which are malignant) (205).

FDG uptake in testicular cancer depends on the histology of the tumor: seminoma, choriocarcinoma, embryonal, and teratocarcinoma show varying degrees of FDG uptake, whereas mature teratoma has no or only very low FDG uptake that is similar to background activity. Although testicular cancer or metastatic disease from other primary tumors can occasionally be detected on FDG PET (206), very intense FDG uptake may also be observed in a normal testis, in particular among younger patients (i.e., the target population for testicular malignancies) (207).

CT and MRI of the abdomen and pelvis are the standard methods for lymph node staging. In the primary staging of nonseminomas, FDG PET could potentially be helpful in distinguishing between stage I (N0) versus IIA disease (N1 with less than 2 cm nodes); however, because of unproven benefit, this should only be done as part of prospective trials. In contrast, there is no clear indication for PET in the staging of seminomas.

Posttreatment Evaluation and Long-term Follow-up

The presence of residual disease after irradiation or chemotherapy is difficult to assess. Normalization of tumor marker levels after treatment is desirable but cannot be equated with the absence of residual disease. Between 10% and 20% of patients receiving combined systemic chemotherapy for bulky metastatic disease who subsequently undergo retroperitoneal lymph node dissection have viable tumor in the histologic specimen despite normal preoperative tumor marker levels (208). CT and MRI may show residual masses, but cannot determine the presence or absence of residual viable tumor tissue with certainty.

Among patients with seminoma, a residual retroperitoneal mass can be observed in 60% to 80% after combination chemotherapy. Most of these masses are stable or will eventually regress. Surgical resection is difficult but likely beneficial because the cure rate declines once disease becomes clinically manifest (209). Historically, size criteria have been used to determine the presence of residual viable tumor. In most institutions, patients with residual mass less than 3 cm in diameter will undergo observation only. Controversy exists in regard to management of residual masses greater than 3 cm, 25% to 55% of which will contain viable tumor. This

TABLE 8.18.2 Data of the Seminoma PET (SEMPET) Trial

56 PET scans in 51 patients with postchemo residual mass > 1 cm: Markers (human chorionic gonadotropin, lactate dehydrogenase) were negative. Visual analysis (location, shape, intensity of uptake). Standard of reference was histology of resected mass or clinical and imaging follow-up.

RESULTS

19 had mass >3cm: PET correct in all
37 had mass <3cm: PET correct in 35 of 37

	Sensitivity (%)	Specificity (%)	PPV (%)	NPV (%)
FDG PET	80	100	100	96
CT (< or >3 cm)	70	74	37	92

FDG, fluorodeoxyglucose; PPV, positive predictive value; NPV, negative predictive value.
(From De Santis M, Becherer A, Bokemeyer C, et al. 2-18fluoro-deoxy-D-glucose positron emission tomography is a reliable predictor for viable tumor in postchemotherapy seminoma: an update of the prospective multicentric SEMPET trial. *J Clin Oncol* 2004;22:1034–1039, with permission.)

implies that if size is used as the sole treatment criterion, 45% to 75% of patients will be overtreated with a technically demanding retroperitoneal lymph node dissection.

Tumor shrinkage on CT is an inconsistent sign (210). FDG PET has the potential to identify viable tumor tissue in a residual mass greater than 3 cm (210). In a multicenter study of 51 patients with seminoma and a residual mass greater than 1 cm following chemotherapy, FDG PET showed a high accuracy for the detection of residual disease (Table 8.18.2). Because of the high positive and negative predictive value, PET has the potential to replace standard retroperitoneal lymphadenectomy. However, until more data become available, this approach should probably be enacted only with patient consent and under close surveillance. Since seminomas are quite infrequent, the parallel to other tumors, such as lymphoma, is apparent, and it is reasonable to consider PET with FDG very seriously in the management of these patients.

In patients with nonseminoma and retroperitoneal lymph node metastases, one therapeutic approach involves induction chemotherapy, followed by assessment for residual viable tumor. The prognosis depends on the completeness of resection, histology of the residual mass, markers at the time of lymphadenectomy, and prior therapy burden. Histologic analysis of such residual masses shows necrosis in 50%, teratoma in 40%, and residual cancer in about 10% of cases (211). Retroperitoneal lymphadenectomy is considered the most rigorous diagnostic and therapeutic approach because models to predict residual disease have false-negative rates of 20% (212), and histological discordance between sites can be observed in 30% to 45% of cases. Of note, the size of the residual mass is an unreliable indicator for residual disease. In one study of 87 patients with a residual mass less than 2 cm, viable tumor was found in six individuals, and in five of these cases the residual mass was less than 1 cm in diameter (213).

In contrast to seminoma, FDG PET cannot provide all of the needed diagnostic information in residual masses in patients in the nonseminoma group. Among 45 patients with 85 residual masses from nonseminomatous germ cell tumor, the sensitivity and specificity for FDG PET were 59% and 92%, respectively, as compared to 55% and 86% for CT, and 42% and 100% for analysis of tumor markers only (214). The major limitation of FDG PET lies in its inability to differentiate between necrosis and mature teratoma (both show low FDG uptake). Although mature teratoma is *not* a malignant tumor, it can increase in size over time (growing teratoma syndrome) and thereby compromise vital organ functions. In addition, a malignant transformation to sarcoma or adenocarcinoma is well described, and chemotherapy or radiation therapy is ineffective. Therefore, surgical resection is necessary if there is growth of such masses.

FDG PET may provide prognostic information in patients with relapsed germ cell tumor (215). In a small study of 23 patients, 16 individuals had persistent abnormal FDG uptake at the end of standard chemotherapy, and 14 of these 16 developed early recurrence within 6 months despite additional high-dose chemotherapy. Clearly, intense FDG uptake in a mass would be highly suggestive of recurrent malignant tumor.

It is reasonable to integrate FDG PET in the long-term follow-up of high-risk patients with testicular cancer, in particular in patients with rising tumor markers and negative or equivocal CT findings. Whether the combined PET/CT should completely replace the current standard diagnostic CT for this purpose remains to be seen and will depend on costs, reimbursements, practicality, and the diagnostic yield of the combined test.

Summary of PET Indications

- Best validated indication: assess residual mass greater than 3 cm in seminoma.
- Possible indications (need more data): stage I versus IIA in primary staging (N0 vs. N1 less than 2 cm) and assessment of early response to high-dose chemotherapy.
- Already in clinical use despite lack of large study: rising tumor markers with or without negative or equivocal CT.
- Intense uptake in nonseminomatous germ cell tumor residual masses is most consistent with malignancy, however, low uptake can be seen in mature teratoma and scar.

REFERENCES

1. Jemal A, Siegel R, Ward E, et al. Cancer statistics, 2008. *CA Cancer J Clin* 2008;58:71–96.
2. Warburg O. *The metabolism of tumors*. New York: Richard R. Smith, 1931.

3. Gatenby RA, Gillies RJ. Why do cancers have high aerobic glycolysis? *Nat Rev Cancer* 2004;4:891–899.
4. Macheda ML, Rogers S, Best JD. Molecular and cellular regulation of glucose transporter (GLUT) proteins in cancer. *J Cell Physiol* 2005;202: 654–662.
5. Weber G. Enzymology of cancer cells (first of two parts). *N Engl J Med* 1977;296:486–492.
6. Weber G. Enzymology of cancer cells (second of two parts). *N Engl J Med* 1977;296:541–551.
7. Majumder PK, Febbo PG, Bikoff R, et al. mTOR inhibition reverses Akt-dependent prostate intraepithelial neoplasia through regulation of apoptotic and HIF-1-dependent pathways. *Nat Med* 2004;10: 594–601.
8. Matoba S, Kang JG, Patino WD, et al. p53 regulates mitochondrial respiration. *Science* 2006;312:1650–1653.
9. Semenza GL. Targeting HIF-1 for cancer therapy. *Nat Rev Cancer* 2003;3:721–732.
10. Kim JW, Tchernyshyov I, Semenza GL, et al. HIF-1-mediated expression of pyruvate dehydrogenase kinase: a metabolic switch required for cellular adaptation to hypoxia. *Cell Metab* 2006;3:177–185.
11. Elstrom RL, Bauer DE, Buzzai M, et al. Akt stimulates aerobic glycolysis in cancer cells. *Cancer Res* 2004;64:3892–3899.
12. Buzzai M, Bauer DE, Jones RG, et al. The glucose dependence of Akt-transformed cells can be reversed by pharmacologic activation of fatty acid beta-oxidation. *Oncogene* 2005;24:4165–4173.
13. Edinger AL, Thompson CB. Akt maintains cell size and survival by increasing mTOR-dependent nutrient uptake. *Mol Biol Cell* 2002;13: 2276–2288.
14. Bjornsti MA, Houghton PJ. The TOR pathway: a target for cancer therapy. *Nat Rev Cancer* 2004;4:335–348.
15. Zhong H, Chiles K, Feldser D, et al. Modulation of hypoxia-inducible factor 1alpha expression by the epidermal growth factor/phosphatidylinositol 3-kinase/PTEN/AKT/FRAP pathway in human prostate cancer cells: implications for tumor angiogenesis and therapeutics. *Cancer Res* 2000;60:1541–1545.
16. Sabatini DM. mTOR and cancer: insights into a complex relationship. *Nat Rev Cancer* 2006;6:729–734.
17. O'Reilly KE, Rojo F, She QB, et al. mTOR inhibition induces upstream receptor tyrosine kinase signaling and activates Akt. *Cancer Res* 2006; 66:1500–1508.
18. Thomas GV, Tran C, Mellinghoff IK, et al. Hypoxia-inducible factor determines sensitivity to inhibitors of mTOR in kidney cancer. *Nat Med* 2006;12:122–127.
19. McMenamin ME, Soung P, Perera S, et al. Loss of PTEN expression in paraffin-embedded primary prostate cancer correlates with high Gleason score and advanced stage. *Cancer Res* 1999;59:4291–4296.
20. Halvorsen OJ, Haukaas SA, Akslen LA. Combined loss of PTEN and p27 expression is associated with tumor cell proliferation by Ki-67 and increased risk of recurrent disease in localized prostate cancer. *Clin Cancer Res* 2003;9:1474–1479.
21. Ayala G, Thompson T, Yang G, et al. High levels of phosphorylated form of Akt-1 in prostate cancer and non-neoplastic prostate tissues are strong predictors of biochemical recurrence. *Clin Cancer Res* 2004; 10:6572–6578.
22. Edwards J, Krishna NS, Witton CJ, et al. Gene amplifications associated with the development of hormone-resistant prostate cancer. *Clin Cancer Res* 2003;9:5271–5281.
23. Liao Y, Grobholz R, Abel U, et al. Increase of AKT/PKB expression correlates with Gleason pattern in human prostate cancer. *Int J Cancer* 2003;107:676–680.
24. Yang X, Fraser M, Moll UM, et al. Akt-mediated cisplatin resistance in ovarian cancer: modulation of p53 action on caspase-dependent mitochondrial death pathway. *Cancer Res* 2006;66:3126–3136.
25. Smith TA, Sharma RI, Thompson AM, et al. Tumor ^{18}F-FDG incorporation is enhanced by attenuation of p53 function in breast cancer cells *in vitro*. *J Nucl Med* 2006;47:1525–1530.
26. Fantin VR, St-Pierre J, Leder P. Attenuation of LDH-a expression uncovers a link between glycolysis, mitochondrial physiology, and tumor maintenance. *Cancer Cell* 2006;9:425–434.
27. Bui T, Thompson CB. Cancer's sweet tooth. *Cancer Cell* 2006;9:419–420.
28. Frayn KN. The glucose-fatty acid cycle: a physiological perspective. *Biochem Soc Trans* 2003;31:1115–1119.
29. Birnbaum MJ, Haspel HC, Rosen OM. Transformation of rat fibroblasts by FSV rapidly increases glucose transporter gene transcription. *Science* 1987;235:1495–1498.
30. Chandler JD, Williams ED, Slavin JL, et al. Expression and localization of GLUT1 and GLUT12 in prostate carcinoma. *Cancer* 2003;97:2035–2042.
31. Effert P, Beniers AJ, Tamimi Y, et al. Expression of glucose transporter 1 (Glut-1) in cell lines and clinical specimens from human prostate adenocarcinoma. *Anticancer Res* 2004;24:3057–3063.
32. Chang S, Lee S, Lee C, et al. Expression of the human erythrocyte glucose transporter in transitional cell carcinoma of the bladder. *Urology* 2000;55:448–452.
33. Younes M, Juarez D, Lechago LV, et al. Glut 1 expression in transitional cell carcinoma of the urinary bladder is associated with poor patient survival. *Anticancer Res* 2001;21:575–578.
34. Hoskin PJ, Sibtain A, Daley FM, et al. GLUT1 and CAIX as intrinsic markers of hypoxia in bladder cancer: relationship with vascularity and proliferation as predictors of outcome of ARCON. *Br J Cancer* 2003;89:1290–1297.
35. Airley R, Loncaster J, Davidson S, et al. Glucose transporter GLUT-1 expression correlates with tumor hypoxia and predicts metastasis-free survival in advanced carcinoma of the cervix. *Clin Cancer Res* 2001;7:928–934.
36. Atkin GK, Daley FM, Bourne S, et al. The impact of surgically induced ischaemia on protein levels in patients undergoing rectal cancer surgery. *Br J Cancer* 2006;95:928–933.
37. Mathupala SP, Rempel A, Pedersen PL. Glucose catabolism in cancer cells: identification and characterization of a marked activation response of the type II hexokinase gene to hypoxic conditions. *J Biol Chem* 2001;276:43407–43412.
38. Wykoff CC, Beasley NJ, Watson PH, et al. Hypoxia-inducible expression of tumor-associated carbonic anhydrases. *Cancer Res* 2000;60:7075–7083.
39. Carnell DM, Smith RE, Daley FM, et al. An immunohistochemical assessment of hypoxia in prostate carcinoma using pimonidazole: implications for radioresistance. *Int J Radiat Oncol Biol Phys* 2006;65: 91–99.
40. Cao X, Fang L, Gibbs S, et al. Glucose uptake inhibitor sensitizes cancer cells to daunorubicin and overcomes drug resistance in hypoxia. *Cancer Chemother Pharmacol* 2006; .
41. Agus DB, Golde DW, Sgouros G, et al. Positron emission tomography of a human prostate cancer xenograft: association of changes in deoxyglucose accumulation with other measures of outcome following androgen withdrawal. *Cancer Res* 1998;58:3009–3014.
42. Jadvar H, Xiankui L, Shahinian A, et al. Glucose metabolism of human prostate cancer mouse xenografts. *Mol Imaging* 2005;4:91–97.
43. Singh G, Lakkis CL, Laucirica R, et al. Regulation of prostate cancer cell division by glucose. *J Cell Physiol* 1999;180:431–438.
44. Kim WY, Kaelin WG. Role of VHL gene mutation in human cancer. *J Clin Oncol* 2004;22:4991–5004.
45. Kondo K, Klco J, Nakamura E, et al. Inhibition of HIF is necessary for tumor suppression by the von Hippel-Lindau protein. *Cancer Cell* 2002;1:237–246.
46. Koukourakis MI, Giatromanolaki A, Harris AL, et al. Comparison of metabolic pathways between cancer cells and stromal cells in colorectal carcinomas: a metabolic survival role for tumor-associated stroma. *Cancer Res* 2006;66:632–637.
47. Gatenby RA, Gawlinski ET, Gmitro AF, et al. Acid-mediated tumor invasion: a multidisciplinary study. *Cancer Res* 2006;66:5216–5223.
48. Costello LC, Liu Y, Franklin RB, et al. Zinc inhibition of mitochondrial aconitase and its importance in citrate metabolism of prostate epithelial cells. *J Biol Chem* 1997;272:28875–28881.

49. Costello LC, Franklin RB. Testosterone regulates pyruvate dehydrogenase activity of prostate mitochondria. *Horm Metab Res* 1993;25:268–270.
50. Scheidler J, Hricak H, Vigneron DB, et al. Prostate cancer: localization with three-dimensional proton MR spectroscopic imaging—clinicopathologic study. *Radiology* 1999;213:473–480.
51. Swanson MG, Zektzer AS, Tabatabai ZL, et al. Quantitative analysis of prostate metabolites using 1H HR-MAS spectroscopy. *Magn Reson Med* 2006;55:1257–1264.
52. Yoshimoto M, Waki A, Yonekura Y, et al. Characterization of acetate metabolism in tumor cells in relation to cell proliferation: acetate metabolism in tumor cells. *Nucl Med Biol* 2001;28:117–122.
53. Kuhajda FP, Jenner K, Wood FD, et al. Fatty acid synthesis: a potential selective target for antineoplastic therapy. *Proc Natl Acad Sci U S A* 1994;91:6379–6383.
54. Swinnen JV, Roskams T, Joniau S, et al. Overexpression of fatty acid synthase is an early and common event in the development of prostate cancer. *Int J Cancer* 2002;98:19–22.
55. Visca P, Sebastiani V, Pizer ES, et al. Immunohistochemical expression and prognostic significance of FAS and GLUT1 in bladder carcinoma. *Anticancer Res* 2003;23:335–339.
56. Sebastiani V, Visca P, Botti C, et al. Fatty acid synthase is a marker of increased risk of recurrence in endometrial carcinoma. *Gynecol Oncol* 2004;92:101–105.
57. Swinnen JV, Ulrix W, Heyns W, et al. Coordinate regulation of lipogenic gene expression by androgens: evidence for a cascade mechanism involving sterol regulatory element binding proteins. *Proc Natl Acad Sci U S A* 1997;94:12975–12980.
58. Ettinger SL, Sobel R, Whitmore TG, et al. Dysregulation of sterol response element-binding proteins and downstream effectors in prostate cancer during progression to androgen independence. *Cancer Res* 2004;64:2212–2221.
59. Van de Sande T, Roskams T, Lerut E, et al. High-level expression of fatty acid synthase in human prostate cancer tissues is linked to activation and nuclear localization of Akt/PKB. *J Pathol* 2005;206:214–219.
60. Bandyopadhyay S, Pai SK, Watabe M, et al. FAS expression inversely correlates with PTEN level in prostate cancer and a PI 3-kinase inhibitor synergizes with FAS siRNA to induce apoptosis. *Oncogene* 2005;24:5389–5395.
61. Van de Sande T, De Schrijver E, Heyns W, et al. Role of the phosphatidylinositol 3'-kinase/PTEN/Akt kinase pathway in the overexpression of fatty acid synthase in LNCaP prostate cancer cells. *Cancer Res* 2002;62:642–646.
62. Zhang D, Tai LK, Wong LL, et al. Proteomic study reveals that proteins involved in metabolic and detoxification pathways are highly expressed in *HER-2/neu*-positive breast cancer. *Mol Cell Proteomics* 2005;4: 1686–1696.
63. Zhou W, Simpson PJ, McFadden JM, et al. Fatty acid synthase inhibition triggers apoptosis during S phase in human cancer cells. *Cancer Res* 2003;63:7330–7337.
64. Brusselmans K, Vrolix R, Verhoeven G, et al. Induction of cancer cell apoptosis by flavonoids is associated with their ability to inhibit fatty acid synthase activity. *J Biol Chem* 2005;280:5636–5645.
65. Brusselmans K, De Schrijver E, Verhoeven G, et al. RNA interference-mediated silencing of the acetyl-CoA-carboxylase-alpha gene induces growth inhibition and apoptosis of prostate cancer cells. *Cancer Res* 2005;65:6719–6725.
66. Swinnen JV, Van Veldhoven PP, Timmermans L, et al. Fatty acid synthase drives the synthesis of phospholipids partitioning into detergent-resistant membrane microdomains. *Biochem Biophys Res Commun* 2003;302:898–903.
67. Simons K, Toomre D. Lipid rafts and signal transduction. *Nat Rev Mol Cell Biol* 2000;1:31–39.
68. Seltzer MA, Jahan SA, Sparks R, et al. Radiation dose estimates in humans for (11)C-acetate whole-body PET. *J Nucl Med* 2004;45: 1233–1236.
69. Kato T, Tsukamoto E, Kuge Y, et al. Accumulation of [(11)C]acetate in normal prostate and benign prostatic hyperplasia: comparison with prostate cancer. *Eur J Nucl Med Mol Imaging* 2002;29:1492–1495.
70. Ishiwata K, Kubota K, Murakami M, et al. Re-evaluation of amino acid PET studies: can the protein synthesis rates in brain and tumor tissues be measured *in vivo*? *J Nucl Med* 1993;34:1936–1943.
71. Macapinlac HA, Humm JL, Akhurst T, et al. Differential metabolism and pharmacokinetics of L-[1-(11)C]-methionine and 2-[(18)F] fluoro-2-deoxy-D-glucose (FDG) in androgen independent prostate cancer. *Clin Positron Imaging* 1999;2:173–181.
72. Deloar HM, Fujiwara T, Nakamura T, et al. Estimation of internal absorbed dose of L-[methyl-11C]methionine using whole-body positron emission tomography. *Eur J Nucl Med* 1998;25:629–633.
73. Yoshimoto M, Waki A, Obata A, et al. Radiolabeled choline as a proliferation marker: comparison with radiolabeled acetate. *Nucl Med Biol* 2004;31:859–865.
74. Ackerstaff E, Pflug BR, Nelson JB, et al. Detection of increased choline compounds with proton nuclear magnetic resonance spectroscopy subsequent to malignant transformation of human prostatic epithelial cells. *Cancer Res* 2001;61:3599–3603.
75. Ramirez de Molina A, Rodriguez-Gonzalez A, Gutierrez R, et al. Overexpression of choline kinase is a frequent feature in human tumor-derived cell lines and in lung, prostate, and colorectal human cancers. *Biochem Biophys Res Commun* 2002;296:580–583.
76. Glunde K, Jie C, Bhujwalla ZM. Molecular causes of the aberrant choline phospholipid metabolism in breast cancer. *Cancer Res* 2004; 64:4270–4276.
77. Glunde K, Raman V, Mori N, et al. RNA interference-mediated choline kinase suppression in breast cancer cells induces differentiation and reduces proliferation. *Cancer Res* 2005;65:11034–11043.
78. Hara T, Kosaka N, Kishi H. PET imaging of prostate cancer using carbon-11-choline. *J Nucl Med* 1998;39:990–995.
79. Hara T, Kosaka N, Kishi H. Development of (18)F-fluoroethylcholine for cancer imaging with PET: synthesis, biochemistry, and prostate cancer imaging. *J Nucl Med* 2002;43:187–199.
80. DeGrado TR, Baldwin SW, Wang S, et al. Synthesis and evaluation of (18)F-labeled choline analogs as oncologic PET tracers. *J Nucl Med* 2001;42:1805–1814.
81. DeGrado TR, Coleman RE, Wang S, et al. Synthesis and evaluation of ^{18}F-labeled choline as an oncologic tracer for positron emission tomography: initial findings in prostate cancer. *Cancer Res* 2001;61:110–117.
82. Hara T. ^{18}F-fluorocholine: a new oncologic PET tracer. *J Nucl Med* 2001;42:1815–1817.
83. Roivainen A, Forsback S, Gronroos T, et al. Blood metabolism of [methyl-11C]choline; implications for in vivo imaging with positron emission tomography. *Eur J Nucl Med* 2000;27:25–32.
84. Sutinen E, Nurmi M, Roivainen A, et al. Kinetics of [(11)C]choline uptake in prostate cancer: a PET study [correction for study]. *Eur J Nucl Med Mol Imaging* 2004;31:317–324.
85. DeGrado TR, Reiman RE, Price DT, et al. Pharmacokinetics and radiation dosimetry of ^{18}F-fluorocholine. *J Nucl Med* 2002;43:92–96.
86. de Jong IJ, Pruim J, Elsinga PH, et al. Visualization of prostate cancer with ^{11}C-choline positron emission tomography. *Eur Urol* 2002;42: 18–23.
87. Schmid DT, John H, Zweifel R, et al. Fluorocholine PET/CT in patients with prostate cancer: initial experience. *Radiology* 2005;235:623–628.
88. Farsad M, Schiavina R, Castellucci P, et al. Detection and localization of prostate cancer: correlation of (11)C-choline PET/CT with histopathologic step-section analysis. *J Nucl Med* 2005;46:1642–1649.
89. Martorana G, Schiavina R, Corti B, et al. 11C-choline positron emission tomography/computerized tomography for tumor localization of primary prostate cancer in comparison with 12-core biopsy. *J Urol* 2006;176:954–960; discussion 960.
90. de Jong IJ, Pruim J, Elsinga PH, et al. Visualisation of bladder cancer using (11)C-choline PET: first clinical experience. *Eur J Nucl Med Mol Imaging* 2002;29:1283–1288.

91. Kotzerke J, Prang J, Neumaier B, et al. Experience with carbon-11 choline positron emission tomography in prostate carcinoma. *Eur J Nucl Med* 2000;27:1415–1419.
92. Kurita T, Wang YZ, Donjacour AA, et al. Paracrine regulation of apoptosis by steroid hormones in the male and female reproductive system. *Cell Death Differ* 2001;8:192–200.
93. Agus DB, Cordon-Cardo C, Fox W, et al. Prostate cancer cell cycle regulators: response to androgen withdrawal and development of androgen independence. *J Natl Cancer Inst* 1999;91:1869–1876.
94. Wang S, Gao J, Lei Q, et al. Prostate-specific deletion of the murine Pten tumor suppressor gene leads to metastatic prostate cancer. *Cancer Cell* 2003;4:209–221.
95. Roach M. Neoadjuvant hormonal therapy in men being treated with radiotherapy for localized prostate cancer. *Rev Urol* 2004;6[Suppl 8]:S24–S31.
96. Loblaw DA, Mendelson DS, Talcott JA, et al. American Society of Clinical Oncology recommendations for the initial hormonal management of androgen-sensitive metastatic, recurrent, or progressive prostate cancer. *J Clin Oncol* 2004;22:2927–2941.
97. Chen CD, Welsbie DS, Tran C, et al. Molecular determinants of resistance to antiandrogen therapy. *Nat Med* 2004;10:33–39.
98. Pienta KJ, Bradley D. Mechanisms underlying the development of androgen-independent prostate cancer. *Clin Cancer Res* 2006;12: 1665–1671.
99. Yoshida T, Kinoshita H, Segawa T, et al. Antiandrogen bicalutamide promotes tumor growth in a novel androgen-dependent prostate cancer xenograft model derived from a bicalutamide-treated patient. *Cancer Res* 2005;65:9611–9616.
100. Hendriksen PJ, Dits NF, Kokame K, et al. Evolution of the androgen receptor pathway during progression of prostate cancer. *Cancer Res* 2006;66:5012–5020.
101. Sun M, Yang L, Feldman RI, et al. Activation of phosphatidylinositol 3-kinase/Akt pathway by androgen through interaction of p85alpha, androgen receptor, and Src. *J Biol Chem* 2003;278:42992–43000.
102. Baron S, Manin M, Beaudoin C, et al. Androgen receptor mediates non-genomic activation of phosphatidylinositol 3-OH kinase in androgen-sensitive epithelial cells. *J Biol Chem* 2004;279:14579–14586.
103. Xu Y, Chen SY, Ross KN, et al. Androgens induce prostate cancer cell proliferation through mammalian target of rapamycin activation and post-transcriptional increases in cyclin D proteins. *Cancer Res* 2006; 66:7783–7792.
104. Isaacs JT, Isaacs WB. Androgen receptor outwits prostate cancer drugs. *Nat Med* 2004;10:26–27.
105. Mellinghoff IK, Vivanco I, Kwon A, et al. *HER2/neu* kinase-dependent modulation of androgen receptor function through effects on DNA binding and stability. *Cancer Cell* 2004;6:517–527.
106. Migliaccio A, Di Domenico M, Castoria G, et al. Steroid receptor regulation of epidermal growth factor signaling through Src in breast and prostate cancer cells: steroid antagonist action. *Cancer Res* 2005;65:10585–10593.
107. Xin L, Teitell MA, Lawson DA, et al. Progression of prostate cancer by synergy of AKT with genotropic and nongenotropic actions of the androgen receptor. *Proc Natl Acad Sci U S A* 2006;103:7789–7794.
108. Park SY, Kim YJ, Gao AC, et al. Hypoxia increases androgen receptor activity in prostate cancer cells. *Cancer Res* 2006;66:5121–5129.
109. Gao H, Ouyang X, Banach-Petrosky WA, et al. Combinatorial activities of Akt and B-Raf/Erk signaling in a mouse model of androgen-independent prostate cancer. *Proc Natl Acad Sci U S A* 2006;103: 14477–14482.
110. Solit DB, Zheng FF, Drobnjak M, et al. 17-Allylamino-17-demethoxygeldanamycin induces the degradation of androgen receptor and *HER-2/neu* and inhibits the growth of prostate cancer xenografts. *Clin Cancer Res* 2002;8:986–993.
111. Liao X, Tang S, Thrasher JB, et al. Small-interfering RNA-induced androgen receptor silencing leads to apoptotic cell death in prostate cancer. *Mol Cancer Ther* 2005;4:505–515.
112. Cheng H, Snoek R, Ghaidi F, et al. Short hairpin RNA knockdown of the androgen receptor attenuates ligand-independent activation and delays tumor progression. *Cancer Res* 2006;66:10613–10620.
113. Choe YS, Lidstrom PJ, Chi DY, et al. Synthesis of 11 beta-[18F]fluoro-5 alpha-dihydrotestosterone and 11 beta-[18F]fluoro-19-nor-5 alpha-dihydrotestosterone: preparation via halofluorination-reduction, receptor binding, and tissue distribution. *J Med Chem* 1995;38:816–825.
114. Larson SM, Morris M, Gunther I, et al. Tumor localization of 16beta-(18)F-fluoro-5alpha-dihydrotestosterone versus (18)F-FDG in patients with progressive, metastatic prostate cancer. *J Nucl Med* 2004;45:366–373.
115. Dehdashti F, Picus J, Michalski JM, et al. Positron tomographic assessment of androgen receptors in prostatic carcinoma. *Eur J Nucl Med Mol Imaging* 2005;32:344–350.
116. Zanzonico PB, Finn R, Pentlow KS, et al. PET-based radiation dosimetry in man of 18F-fluorodihydrotestosterone, a new radiotracer for imaging prostate cancer. *J Nucl Med* 2004;45:1966–1971.
117. Shields AF, Grierson JR, Dohmen BM, et al. Imaging proliferation *in vivo* with [F-18]FLT and positron emission tomography. *Nat Med* 1998;4:1334–1336.
118. Oyama N, Ponde DE, Dence C, et al. Monitoring of therapy in androgen-dependent prostate tumor model by measuring tumor proliferation. *J Nucl Med* 2004;45:519–525.
119. Cooperberg MR, Moul JW, Carroll PR. The changing face of prostate cancer. *J Clin Oncol* 2005;23:8146–8151.
120. Swindle P, Eastham JA, Ohori M, et al. Do margins matter? The prognostic significance of positive surgical margins in radical prostatectomy specimens. *J Urol* 2005;174:903–907.
121. Zietman AL, DeSilvio ML, Slater JD, et al. Comparison of conventional-dose vs high-dose conformal radiation therapy in clinically localized adenocarcinoma of the prostate: a randomized controlled trial. *JAMA* 2005;294:1233–1239.
122. Bolla M, Collette L, Blank L, et al. Long-term results with immediate androgen suppression and external irradiation in patients with locally advanced prostate cancer (an EORTC study): a phase III randomised trial. *Lancet* 2002;360:103–106.
123. D'Amico AV, Loffredo M, Renshaw AA, et al. Six-month androgen suppression plus radiation therapy compared with radiation therapy alone for men with prostate cancer and a rapidly increasing pretreatment prostate-specific antigen level. *J Clin Oncol* 2006;24:4190–4195.
124. Stephenson AJ, Kattan MW, Eastham JA, et al. Defining biochemical recurrence of prostate cancer after radical prostatectomy: a proposal for a standardized definition. *J Clin Oncol* 2006;24:3973–3978.
125. Pound CR, Partin AW, Eisenberger MA, et al. Natural history of progression after PSA elevation following radical prostatectomy. *JAMA* 1999;281:1591–1597.
126. Rogers CG, Khan MA, Craig Miller M, et al. Natural history of disease progression in patients who fail to achieve an undetectable prostate-specific antigen level after undergoing radical prostatectomy. *Cancer* 2004;101:2549–2556.
127. Kattan MW, Zelefsky MJ, Kupelian PA, et al. Pretreatment nomogram that predicts 5-year probability of metastasis following three-dimensional conformal radiation therapy for localized prostate cancer. *J Clin Oncol* 2003;21:4568–4571.
128. Stephenson AJ, Scardino PT, Eastham JA, et al. Postoperative nomogram predicting the 10-year probability of prostate cancer recurrence after radical prostatectomy. *J Clin Oncol* 2005;23:7005–7012.
129. Freedland SJ, Humphreys EB, Mangold LA, et al. Risk of prostate cancer-specific mortality following biochemical recurrence after radical prostatectomy. *JAMA* 2005;294:433–439.
130. Slovin SF, Wilton AS, Heller G, et al. Time to detectable metastatic disease in patients with rising prostate-specific antigen values following surgery or radiation therapy. *Clin Cancer Res* 2005;11:8669–8673.
131. Stephenson AJ, Shariat SF, Zelefsky MJ, et al. Salvage radiotherapy for recurrent prostate cancer after radical prostatectomy. *JAMA* 2004; 291:1325–1332.

132. Bianco FJ Jr, Scardino PT, Stephenson AJ, et al. Long-term oncologic results of salvage radical prostatectomy for locally recurrent prostate cancer after radiotherapy. *Int J Radiat Oncol Biol Phys* 2005;62: 448–453.
133. Smith MR, Kabbinavar F, Saad F, et al. Natural history of rising serum prostate-specific antigen in men with castrate nonmetastatic prostate cancer. *J Clin Oncol* 2005;23:2918–2925.
134. Small EJ, Vogelzang NJ. Second-line hormonal therapy for advanced prostate cancer: a shifting paradigm. *J Clin Oncol* 1997;15:382–388.
135. Petrylak DP, Tangen CM, Hussain MH, et al. Docetaxel and estramustine compared with mitoxantrone and prednisone for advanced refractory prostate cancer. *N Engl J Med* 2004;351:1513–1520.
136. Tannock IF, de Wit R, Berry WR, et al. Docetaxel plus prednisone or mitoxantrone plus prednisone for advanced prostate cancer. *N Engl J Med* 2004;351:1502–1512.
137. Che M, Grignon D. Pathology of prostate cancer. *Cancer Metastasis Rev* 2002;21:381–395.
138. Okotie OT, Aronson WJ, Wieder JA, et al. Predictors of metastatic disease in men with biochemical failure following radical prostatectomy. *J Urol* 2004;171:2260–2264.
139. Kramer S, Gorich J, Gottfried HW, et al. Sensitivity of computed tomography in detecting local recurrence of prostatic carcinoma following radical prostatectomy. *Br J Radiol* 1997;70:995–999.
140. Hricak H, Schoder H, Pucar D, et al. Advances in imaging in the postoperative patient with a rising prostate-specific antigen level. *Semin Oncol* 2003;30:616–634.
141. Hricak H. MR imaging and MR spectroscopic imaging in the pre-treatment evaluation of prostate cancer. *Br J Radiol* 2005;78(2): S103–S111.
142. Sella T, Schwartz LH, Swindle PW, et al. Suspected local recurrence after radical prostatectomy: endorectal coil MR imaging. *Radiology* 2004;231:379–385.
143. Cher ML, Bianco FJ Jr, Lam JS, et al. Limited role of radionuclide bone scintigraphy in patients with prostate specific antigen elevations after radical prostatectomy. *J Urol* 1998;160:1387–1391.
144. Kane CJ, Amling CL, Johnstone PA, et al. Limited value of bone scintigraphy and computed tomography in assessing biochemical failure after radical prostatectomy. *Urology* 2003;61:607–611.
145. Dotan ZA, Bianco FJ, Jr., Rabbani F, et al. Pattern of prostate-specific antigen (PSA) failure dictates the probability of a positive bone scan in patients with an increasing PSA after radical prostatectomy. *J Clin Oncol* 2005;23:1962–1968.
146. Shah RB, Mehra R, Chinnaiyan AM, et al. Androgen-independent prostate cancer is a heterogeneous group of diseases: lessons from a rapid autopsy program. *Cancer Res* 2004;64:9209–9216.
147. Reske SN, Blumstein NM, Neumaier B, et al. Imaging prostate cancer with ^{11}C-choline PET/CT. *J Nucl Med* 2006;47:1249–1254.
148. Oyama N, Akino H, Kanamaru H, et al. ^{11}C-acetate PET imaging of prostate cancer. *J Nucl Med* 2002;43:181–186.
149. Kotzerke J, Volkmer BG, Neumaier B, et al. Carbon-11 acetate positron emission tomography can detect local recurrence of prostate cancer. *Eur J Nucl Med Mol Imaging* 2002;29:1380–1384.
150. de Jong IJ, Pruim J, Elsinga PH, et al. Preoperative staging of pelvic lymph nodes in prostate cancer by (11)C-choline PET. *J Nucl Med* 2003;44:331–335.
151. Hacker A, Jeschke S, Leeb K, et al. Detection of pelvic lymph node metastases in patients with clinically localized prostate cancer: comparison of [18F]fluorocholine positron emission tomography-computerized tomography and laparoscopic radioisotope guided sentinel lymph node dissection. *J Urol* 2006;176:2014–2018; discussion 2018–2019.
152. Swindle PW, Kattan MW, Scardino PT. Markers and meaning of primary treatment failure. *Urol Clin North Am* 2003;30:377–401.
153. Kattan MW, Wheeler TM, Scardino PT. Postoperative nomogram for disease recurrence after radical prostatectomy for prostate cancer. *J Clin Oncol* 1999;17:1499–1507.
154. Leventis AK, Shariat SF, Slawin KM. Local recurrence after radical prostatectomy: correlation of US features with prostatic fossa biopsy findings. *Radiology* 2001;219:432–439.
155. Fowler JE Jr, Brooks J, Pandey P, et al. Variable histology of anastomotic biopsies with detectable prostate specific antigen after radical prostatectomy. *J Urol* 1995;153:1011–1014.
156. Schoder H, Herrmann K, Gonen M, et al. 2-[18F]fluoro-2-deoxyglucose positron emission tomography for the detection of disease in patients with prostate-specific antigen relapse after radical prostatectomy. *Clin Cancer Res* 2005;11:4761–4769.
157. Seltzer MA, Barbaric Z, Belldegrun A, et al. Comparison of helical computerized tomography, positron emission tomography and monoclonal antibody scans for evaluation of lymph node metastases in patients with prostate specific antigen relapse after treatment for localized prostate cancer. *J Urol* 1999;162:1322–1328.
158. Oyama N, Miller TR, Dehdashti F, et al. ^{11}C-acetate PET imaging of prostate cancer: detection of recurrent disease at PSA relapse. *J Nucl Med* 2003;44:549–555.
159. Wachter S, Tomek S, Kurtaran A, et al. ^{11}C-acetate positron emission tomography imaging and image fusion with computed tomography and magnetic resonance imaging in patients with recurrent prostate cancer. *J Clin Oncol* 2006;24:2513–2519.
160. Albrecht S, Buchegger F, Soloviev D, et al. (11)C-acetate PET in the early evaluation of prostate cancer recurrence. *Eur J Nucl Med Mol Im* 2007;34:185–196.
161. Sandblom G, Sorensen J, Lundin N, et al. Positron emission tomography with C11-acetate for tumor detection and localization in patients with prostate-specific antigen relapse after radical prostatectomy. *Urology* 2006;67:996–1000.
162. Picchio M, Messa C, Landoni C, et al. Value of [11C]choline-positron emission tomography for re-staging prostate cancer: a comparison with [18F]fluorodeoxyglucose-positron emission tomography. *J Urol* 2003;169:1337–1340.
163. Cimitan M, Bortolus R, Morassut S, et al. [(18)F]fluorocholine PET/CT imaging for the detection of recurrent prostate cancer at PSA relapse: experience in 100 consecutive patients. *Eur J Nucl Med Mol Im* 2006;33:1387–1398.
164. Kotzerke J, Volkmer BG, Glatting G, et al. Intraindividual comparison of [11C]acetate and [11C]choline PET for detection of metastases of prostate cancer. *Nuklearmedizin* 2003;42:25–30.
165. Morris MJ, Akhurst T, Larson SM, et al. Fluorodeoxyglucose positron emission tomography as an outcome measure for castrate metastatic prostate cancer treated with antimicrotubule chemotherapy. *Clin Cancer Res* 2005;11:3210–3216.
166. Soloway MS, Hardeman SW, Hickey D, et al. Stratification of patients with metastatic prostate cancer based on extent of disease on initial bone scan. *Cancer* 1988;61:195–202.
167. Sabbatini P, Larson SM, Kremer A, et al. Prognostic significance of extent of disease in bone in patients with androgen-independent prostate cancer. *J Clin Oncol* 1999;17:948–957.
168. Rigaud J, Tiguert R, Le Normand L, et al. Prognostic value of bone scan in patients with metastatic prostate cancer treated initially with androgen deprivation therapy. *J Urol* 2002;168:1423–1426.
169. Morris MJ, Akhurst T, Osman I, et al. Fluorinated deoxyglucose positron emission tomography imaging in progressive metastatic prostate cancer. *Urology* 2002;59:913–918.
170. Meirelles G, Ravizzini G, Schoder H, et al. Prognostic value of FDG PET in patients with bone metastases from castrate-resistant prostate cancer. *J Nucl Med* 2006;47:180(abst).
171. Cohen HT, McGovern FJ. Renal-cell carcinoma. *N Engl J Med* 2005; 353:2477–2490.
172. Motzer RJ, Bukowski RM. Targeted therapy for metastatic renal cell carcinoma. *J Clin Oncol* 2006;24:5601–5608.
173. Schreyer HH, Uggowitzer MM, Ruppert-Kohlmayr A. Helical CT of the urinary organs. *Eur Radiol* 2002;12:575–591.
174. Kopka L, Fischer U, Zoeller G, et al. Dual-phase helical CT of the kidney: value of the corticomedullary and nephrographic phase for evaluation of renal lesions and preoperative staging of renal cell carcinoma. *AJR Am J Roentgenol* 1997;169:1573–1578.
175. Hilton S. Imaging of renal cell carcinoma. *Semin Oncol* 2000;27:150–159.

176. Zagoria RJ, Bechtold RE, Dyer RB. Staging of renal adenocarcinoma: role of various imaging procedures. *AJR Am J Roentgenol* 1995;164:363–370.
177. Kang DE, White RL Jr, Zuger JH, et al. Clinical use of fluorodeoxyglucose F 18 positron emission tomography for detection of renal cell carcinoma. *J Urol* 2004;171:1806–1809.
178. Divgi CR, Pandit-Taskar N, Jungobluth A et al. Preoperative characterization of clear-cell renal cell carcinoma using iodine-124 labelled antibody chimeric G250 (124I–cG250) and PET in patients with renal masses: a phase I trial. *Lancet Oncol* 2007;8:304–310.
179. Safaei A, Figlin R, Hoh CK, et al. The usefulness of F-18 deoxyglucose whole-body positron emission tomography (PET) for re-staging of renal cell cancer. *Clin Nephrol* 2002;57:56–62.
180. Majhail NS, Urbain JL, Albani JM, et al. F-18 fluorodeoxyglucose positron emission tomography in the evaluation of distant metastases from renal cell carcinoma. *J Clin Oncol* 2003;21:3995–4000.
180. Jones JS, Campbell SC: Non-muscle invasive bladder cancer (Ta, T1, CIS). In: Wein AJ (ed): *Campbell-Walsh urology*. 9th ed, chapter 76. Saunders-Elsevier, Philadelphia 2007 http://www.mdconsult.com/das/book/body/98575437-3/0/1445/79.html?tocnode=54304745&fromURL=79.html.
181. Bajorin DF, Motzer RJ, Bosl GJ. Advances in urologic oncology: results progress from successful interdisciplinary research. *J Clin Oncol* 2006;24:5479–481.
182. Schoenberg MP, Gonzalogo ML: management of invasive and metastatic bladder cancer. In: Wein AJ (ed): *Campbell-Walsh urology*, 9th ed, chapter 77. Saunders-Elsevier, Philadelphia 2007 http://www.mdconsult.com/das/book/body/98575437-3/0/1445/80.html?tocnode=54304787&fromURL=80.html.
183. Stein JP, Lieskovsky G, Cote R, et al. Radical cystectomy in the treatment of invasive bladder cancer: long-term results in 1,054 patients. *J Clin Oncol* 2001;19:666–675.
184. Dalbagni G, Genega E, Hashibe M, et al. Cystectomy for bladder cancer: a contemporary series. *J Urol* 2001;165:1111–1116.
185. Ghoneim MA, el-Mekresh MM, el-Baz MA, et al. Radical cystectomy for carcinoma of the bladder: critical evaluation of the results in 1,026 cases. *J Urol* 1997;158:393–399.
186. Madersbacher S, Hochreiter W, Burkhard F, et al. Radical cystectomy for bladder cancer today—a homogeneous series without neoadjuvant therapy. *J Clin Oncol* 2003;21:690-696.
187. Frank I, Cheville JC, Blute ML, et al. Transitional cell carcinoma of the urinary bladder with regional lymph node involvement treated by cystectomy: clinicopathologic features associated with outcome. *Cancer* 2003;97:2425–2431.
188. Mills RD, Turner WH, Fleischmann A, et al. Pelvic lymph node metastases from bladder cancer: outcome in 83 patients after radical cystectomy and pelvic lymphadenectomy. *J Urol* 2001;166:19–23.
189. Rogers CG, Palapattu GS, Shariat SF, et al. Clinical outcomes following radical cystectomy for primary nontransitional cell carcinoma of the bladder compared to transitional cell carcinoma of the bladder. *J Urol* 2006;175:2048–2053; discussion 2053.
190. Paik ML, Scolieri MJ, Brown SL, et al. Limitations of computerized tomography in staging invasive bladder cancer before radical cystectomy. *J Urol* 2000;163:1693–1696.
191. Vieweg J, Gschwend JE, Herr HW, et al. Pelvic lymph node dissection can be curative in patients with node positive bladder cancer. *J Urol* 1999;161:449–454.
192. Konety BR, Joslyn SA, O'Donnell MA. Extent of pelvic lymphadenectomy and its impact on outcome in patients diagnosed with bladder cancer: analysis of data from the Surveillance, Epidemiology and End Results Program data base. *J Urol* 2003;169:946–950.
193. Honma I, Masumori N, Sato E, et al. Removal of more lymph nodes may provide better outcome, as well as more accurate pathologic findings, in patients with bladder cancer—analysis of role of pelvic lymph node dissection. *Urology* 2006;68:543–548.
194. Stein JP, Cai J, Groshen S, et al. Risk factors for patients with pelvic lymph node metastases following radical cystectomy with en bloc pelvic lymphadenectomy: concept of lymph node density. *J Urol* 2003;170:35–41.
195. Stein JP. Lymphadenectomy in bladder cancer: how high is "high enough"? *Urol Oncol* 2006;24:349–355.
196. Copp HL, Chin JL, Conaway M, et al. Prospective evaluation of the prognostic relevance of molecular staging for urothelial carcinoma. *Cancer* 2006;107:60–66.
197. Tekes A, Kamel I, Imam K, et al. Dynamic MRI of bladder cancer: evaluation of staging accuracy. *AJR Am J Roentgenol* 2005;184:121–127.
198. Picchio M, Treiber U, Beer AJ, et al. Value of ^{11}C-choline PET and contrast-enhanced CT for staging of bladder cancer: correlation with histopathologic findings. *J Nucl Med* 2006;47:938–944.
199. Gofrit ON, Mishani E, Orevi M, et al. Contribution of ^{11}C-choline positron emission tomography/computerized tomography to preoperative staging of advanced transitional cell carcinoma. *J Urol* 2006; 176:940–944; discussion 944.
200. Ahlstrom H, Malmstrom PU, Letocha H, et al. Positron emission tomography in the diagnosis and staging of urinary bladder cancer. *Acta Radiol* 1996;37:180–185.
201. Deserno WM, Harisinghani MG, Taupitz M, et al. Urinary bladder cancer: preoperative nodal staging with ferumoxtran-10-enhanced MR imaging. *Radiology* 2004;233:449–456.
202. Bachor R, Kotzerke J, Reske SN, et al. [Lymph node staging of bladder neck carcinoma with positron emission tomography]. *Urologe A* 1999;38:46–50.
203. Bochner BH, Kattan MW, Vora KC. Postoperative nomogram predicting risk of recurrence after radical cystectomy for bladder cancer. *J Clin Oncol* 2006;24:3967–3972.
204. Kollmannsberger C, Honecker F, Bokemeyer C. Treatment of germ cell tumors—update 2006. *Ann Oncol* 2006;17[Suppl 10]:X31–X35.
205. Lesnik G, Nickl S, Kuschnig P, et al. [Sonography of the scrotum]. *Rofo* 2006;178:165–179.
206. Weng LJ, Schoder H. Melanoma metastasis to the testis demonstrated with FDG PET/CT. *Clin Nucl Med* 2004;29:811–812.
207. Kosuda S, Fisher S, Kison PV, et al. Uptake of 2-deoxy-2-[18F]fluoro-D-glucose in the normal testis: retrospective PET study and animal experiment. *Ann Nucl Med* 1997;11:195–199.
208. Ritchie JP, Steele GS: Neoplasms of the testis. In: Wein AJ (ed): Campbell-Walsh urology, 9th ed, chapter 29. Saunders-Elsevier, Philadelphia 2007 http://www.mdconsult.com/das/book/body/98575437-3/0/1445/32.html?tocnode=54301601&fromURL=32.html#4-ul.0-B978-0-7216-0798-6.50031-5 2164.
209. Miller KD, Loehrer PJ, Gonin R, et al. Salvage chemotherapy with vinblastine, ifosfamide, and cisplatin in recurrent seminoma. *J Clin Oncol* 1997;15:1427–1431.
210. De Santis M, Becherer A, Bokemeyer C, et al. 2-18fluoro-deoxy-D-glucose positron emission tomography is a reliable predictor for viable tumor in postchemotherapy seminoma: an update of the prospective multicentric SEMPET trial. *J Clin Oncol* 2004;22:1034–1039.
211. Sheinfeld J. The role of adjunctive postchemotherapy surgery for nonseminomatous germ-cell tumors: current concepts and controversies. *Semin Urol Oncol* 2002;20:262–271.
212. Kuczyk M, Machtens S, Stief C, et al. Management of the postchemotherapy residual mass in patients with advanced stage non-seminomatous germ cell tumors (NSGCT). *Int J Cancer* 1999;83: 852–855.
213. Oldenburg J, Alfsen GC, Lien HH, et al. Postchemotherapy retroperitoneal surgery remains necessary in patients with nonseminomatous testicular cancer and minimal residual tumor masses. *J Clin Oncol* 2003;21:3310–3317.
214. Kollmannsberger C, Oechsle K, Dohmen BM, et al. Prospective comparison of [18F]fluorodeoxyglucose positron emission tomography with conventional assessment by computed tomography scans and serum tumor markers for the evaluation of residual masses in patients with nonseminomatous germ cell carcinoma. *Cancer* 2002;94: 2353–2362.
215. Bokemeyer C, Kollmannsberger C, Oechsle K, et al. Early prediction of treatment response to high-dose salvage chemotherapy in patients with relapsed germ cell cancer using [(18)F]FDG PET. *Br J Cancer* 2002;86:506–511.

CHAPTER

8.19 Sarcomas

JANET EARY

Sarcomas are thought of as relatively rare tumors, however, considering the entire group as a whole, they occur at a higher incidence than this term would suggest. The sarcomas are derived from mesenchymal tissue elements and as such are diagnosed in myriad clinical presentations. This complex group also has a wide variation in clinical outcomes, ranging from relatively indolent behavior that can be treated with surgical management to some of the most biologically aggressive and treatment resistant tumors that can be encountered in clinical practice. Commonly, the sarcomas are considered in two groups: the soft tissues sarcomas and the bone tumors. As with most descriptions of sarcomas, there are many exceptions to such classifications. Several soft tissue sarcomas can present as primary bone tumors, and there are notable presentations of bone tumors that arise in the soft tissues. Although positron emission tomography (PET) imaging in sarcomas presents challenges, it offers opportunities to make a significant contribution to patient care and to explore the utility of imaging in understanding tumor biological behavior.

SOFT TISSUE SARCOMAS

The classification schemes for sarcomas are designed to help assess tumor biologic behavior for treatment planning. They are largely based on histologic criteria that are described on the presumed tissue or origin for a given tumor. In large part, this scheme is successful at categorizing soft tissue sarcomas. Table 8.19.1 shows the most common soft tissue sarcomas classified on the basis of their tissue of origin. However, periodically the classification schemes for sarcoma undergo a certain amount of reconsideration, as this group contains clearly distinct tumors that have no known tissue of origin such as the alveolar soft sarcomas and the epithelioid subtypes. Currently, there is some thinking that although soft tissue sarcomas arise from mesenchymal tissues, their apparent differentiation is a result of local factors, and histologic appearance may not consistently reflect the tissue of origin.

Newer tissue analysis techniques such as immunocytochemistry, cytogenetics, and gene microarrays are suggesting that there is indeed overlap in tumor characteristics, some of which support the current classification schemes and some that do not. The histologic grade of the tumor, which may take into account all of these additional tissue analyses, is most commonly used for prediction of tumor biologic behavior or prognosis and treatment planning. The FNCLCC (Federation Nationale des Centre de Lutte Contre le Cancer) classification scheme for the assessment of the histologic grade of the tumor is most commonly used for the diagnosis of sarcoma (1). It assigns a point score for several tissue characteristics. Factors such as mitotic rate, cellularity, and differentiation are associated with high predictive values for patient outcome.

Soft tissue sarcomas have certain distributions of location within the body for the various tumor histologic subtypes. This factor in many ways also helps to account for differences in patient prognoses between the tumor subtypes and within the patient groups who seemingly display the same tumor subtype. As with tissue diagnosis in sarcomas, there are many exceptions to these descriptions, but their use assists in beginning the process of patient tumor assessment and treatment planning.

Most authorities agree that any given scheme for sarcoma classification and patient outcome prediction has weaknesses that are related to the complexities of these tumors. They often present as large heterogeneous masses that may be deep seated. Masses with a similar appearance on anatomic imaging may have widely differing biologic behavior. Because of this variety in presentation, there can be a significant error in diagnosis for soft tissue sarcomas. Errors in tumor grade that dictate the need for adjuvant therapy have the most consequences. Other errors in classification type and inclusion as sarcomas as opposed to other cancer histologies can also be significant for the purposes of treatment planning for optimal patient outcome and reduction in morbidity.

The trend toward core needle biopsy of these often very large tumors may be increasing these problems based on sampling error alone (2). Most often located for surgical convenience, these small biopsies may miss the most biologically aggressive area of the

TABLE 8.19.1 Soft Tissue Sarcoma Subtypes

Soft Tissue Sarcoma Subtypes
Leiomyosarcoma
Rhabdomyosarcoma
Subtypes
Alveolar (pediatric)
Embryonal (pediatric)
Pleomorphic (adult)
Fibrosarcoma
Malignant fibrous histiocytoma
Liposarcoma
Subtypes
Well differentiated
Myxoid
Round cell
Pleomorphic
De-differentiated
Malignant peripheral nerve sheath tumor
Malignant schwannoma
Angiosarcoma
Hemangiopericytoma
Lymphangiosarcoma
Other
Pleiomorphic sarcoma
Synovial sarcoma
Alveolar soft part sarcoma
Gastrointestinal stromal tumor

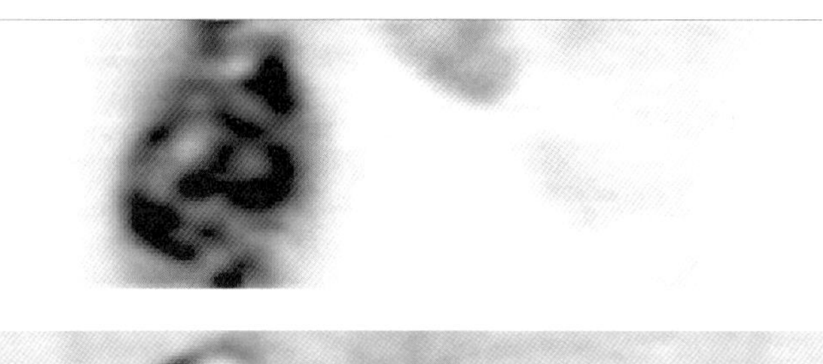

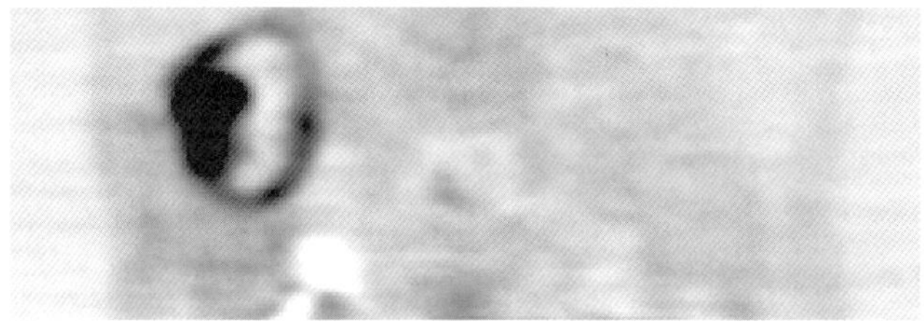

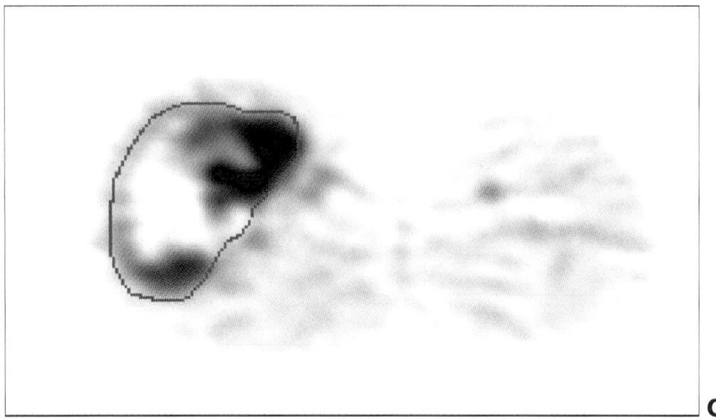

FIGURE 8.19.1. Examples of fluorodeoxyglucose PET images of soft tissue sarcomas where there is significant spatial heterogeneity in tumor uptake. These tumors are often high grade and expected to have relatively poor outcome. **A:** Shows a coronal image of a right thigh malignant fibrous histiocytoma grade III. At resection this tumor showed large areas of necrosis and fluid degeneration. **B:** A coronal image of a patient with a left pelvic high-grade pleomorphic sarcoma. Probable central necrosis is present. **C:** An axial image of a large thigh liposarcoma showing variable areas of differentiation.

tumor or an area of significant tumor necrosis. The presence of significant liquefactive necrosis is an important factor in the assessment of tumor grade; high-grade tumors are identified by the presence of necrosis. Most sarcoma treatment centers would agree that patients with large intermediate and high-grade tumors benefit from preoperative adjuvant treatment prior to resection. Radiation therapy also plays a role in situations where tumor resection margins are close or contaminated with infiltrating tumor. Fig. 8.19.1 shows fluorodeoxyglucose (FDG) PET images of soft tissue sarcomas with significant spatial heterogeneity in tracer uptake. It demonstrates the potential problem of sampling error for tumor assessment when core biopsy is used for diagnosis. This tumor has areas of low and high uptake as well as significant photopenic areas that likely correspond to tumor necrosis. This appearance indicates a high-grade tumor, with the expected aggressive behavior in the form of early local recurrence and metastases (3,4).

Fluorodeoxyglucose PET for Diagnosis of Soft Tissue Sarcomas

Work in PET imaging in soft tissue sarcomas has focused mainly on the problems in diagnosis and assessment of the biological aggressiveness of the tumor, as mentioned above in the discussion of histopathology. Many investigators have endeavored to evaluate the use of FDG PET for the diagnosis of sarcoma, with particular aims directed toward correlation of FDG uptake to describe tumor metabolism with tumor histologic grade. Their goal was to improve accuracy in diagnosis. Sarcomas have regional heterogeneity within the tumor mass, and some areas may be less well differentiated than others. These areas are reflected by a regional increase in FDG uptake, easily noted on a clinical scan. From experience with pathological diagnoses, it is known that the behavior of sarcomas is usually dictated by the most biologically aggressive component. Regional tumor areas with increased uptake have histologic correlates that have been used to support the use of FDG PET for tumor diagnosis and assessment of tumor grade.

Folpe et al. (4) found that an increased tumor standardized uptake value (SUV) was associated with increasing histopathological grade (grades I to III), tissue cellularity, mitotic activity, MIB labeling index, and p53 overexpression. These data suggest that FDG PET images can be used effectively to guide biopsy. Hain et al. (5) found that areas of the tumor with the highest SUV were the most malignant regions compared to the rest of the tumor. Benign tumors did not show significant FDG uptake.

There are numerous published reports from investigators exploring the use of FDG PET to grade sarcomas prior to treatment (6–14). Generally, FDG PET shows a significant ability to distinguish benign or low-grade from high-grade tumors. Lucas et al.

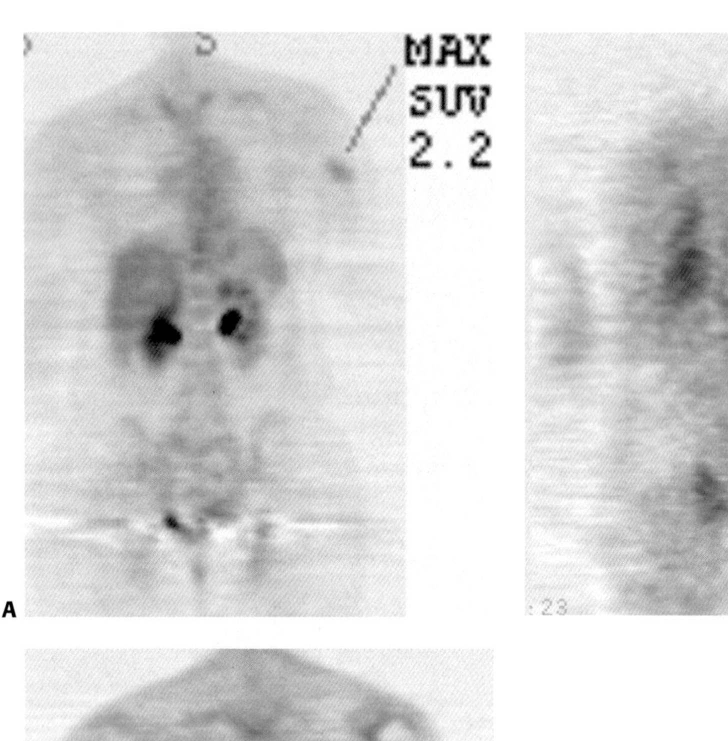

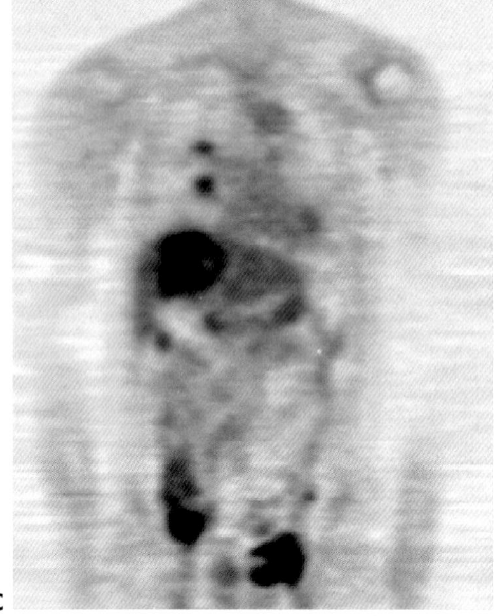

FIGURE 8.19.2. Some examples of fluorodeoxyglucose PET images of soft tissue sarcomas of various tumor grade and locations. **A:** A whole-torso image in a patient with an intermediate grade neurofibrosarcoma in the left shoulder region. The tumor SUV is relatively low, as is typical for this tumor histology. **B:** A large high-grade leiomyosarcoma in the left gluteal region. **C:** A coronal whole-body image of a patient with a pleomorphic sarcoma in the left pelvis that is widely metastatic.

(12), using a quantitative assessment, reported a 95% sensitivity and a 75% specificity for diagnosis. This result is similar to the work published in other studies. Figs. 8.19.2 and 8.19.3 show examples of soft tissue sarcomas.

Like most other efforts in sarcoma research, published reports are often hampered with low patient numbers and groups of patients with mixed histologic subtypes of tumor. With a number of published studies on the diagnosis of sarcoma in the literature over the past decade, several authors have performed meta-analyses to review the general pertinent findings from the group of studies. Ioannidis and Lau (15) performed a meta-analysis of 15 studies with 441 soft tissue lesions analyzed with receiver operator curves. The sensitivity for distinguishing benign from malignant tumors using visual techniques were 92% and 73%, respectively, and all intermediate- to high-grade tumors were identified visually. Tumors with SUV greater than 2.0 had a sensitivity of 87% and specificity of 79% for this same comparison. The quantitative FDG metabolic rate of 6.0 showed lower values for sensitivity (74%) and specificity (73%) for determination of tumor grade. The meta-analysis authors concluded that FDG PET is helpful in assessing soft tissue masses in recurrent and primary tumors, but performs less well in discriminating low-grade tumors from benign ones.

Franzius et al. (16) and Aoki et al. (17) both concluded that specific prospective studies in larger patient groups and groups with specific tumor histologies should be undertaken to further clarify this role of FDG PET in soft tissue sarcomas. Other meta-analyses of the available literature on the use of FDG PET in the management of patients with sarcoma showed that there is a significant ability of the technique to distinguish benign or low-grade from high-grade tumors.

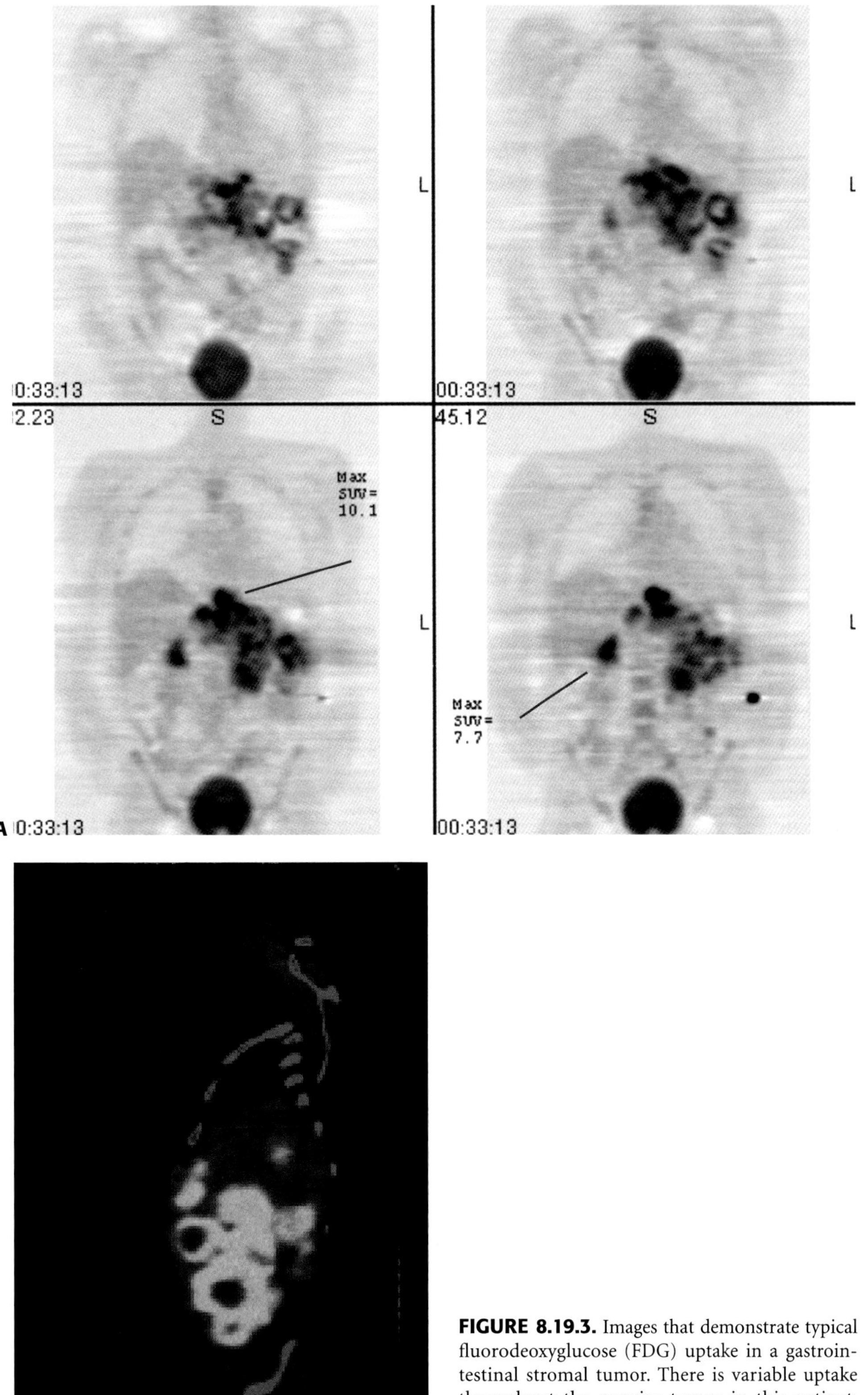

FIGURE 8.19.3. Images that demonstrate typical fluorodeoxyglucose (FDG) uptake in a gastrointestinal stromal tumor. There is variable uptake throughout the massive tumor in this patient. **A:** Several coronal views of the abdominal tumor. **B:** Shows a sagittal view of the patient with the FDG scan fused with the accompanying CT image. In this case, CT fusion with the PET emission scan was helpful in delineating the tumor involved structures.

The use of the FDG PET SUV is very helpful in tumor assessment, since, as a semiquantitative objective assessment, it can be used at baseline to describe the tumor metabolic activity, and in later evaluations, as a comparison for tumor progression or treatment effect. The use of the SUV for tumor assessment has met with controversy since the rapid rise in the use of FDG PET for cancer imaging. This is in large part due to valid criticisms that the tumor SUV data and conclusions from one patient series was often not comparable to those reported in another study. The source of this variability lies more in differences in the FDG PET scan procedures and techniques than with the variable itself as a valid biomarker for tumor biological behavior. Differences in patient preparation with respect to blood glucose levels, length of fast, other metabolic illnesses, FDG dose, length of FDG equilibration, the length of the scan acquisition, and method of attenuation correction are all factors that can influence the SUV determination. Recently, the U.S. National Cancer Institute Imaging Program convened a consensus panel to identify sources of irregularity in FDG PET parameters and procedures to begin establishment of its use as a valid biomarker for tumor response. The consensus opinion was published, and it presents a framework for conduct of FDG PET tumor imaging applications (18).

In sarcoma, the use of the tumor SUV maximum is recommended for reporting and understanding that the areas of highest FDG uptake correlate with tumor areas of increased cellularity and mitotic rate, and that these areas are the ones that have the most potential for aggressive behavior. It has long been known that the most biologically aggressive areas of tumor will control the overall behavior of the tumor, so the use of the FDG maximum uptake in a tumor has the advantage of describing the biological potential of the tumor most accurately.

The use of a global or average SUV for a sarcoma will often include large areas of necrosis, which, although important to identify, will interfere with the reporting of the most metabolically active areas. The technique of selecting the maximum SUV also has the advantage of being relatively independent from region of interest delineation and appears to have good reproducibility.

The use of combined PET/CT imaging has contributed to increasing the accuracy of tumor location in many cancers. There is not much literature to date on the improvement of FDG PET using emission scan images fused with CT for the diagnosis of sarcoma. A large patient group meta-analysis did not find an improvement in diagnostic sensitivity or specificity (15). In another report, magnetic resonance imaging (MRI) FDG PET image coregistration did not significantly add to regional tumor assessment for biopsy (5). With most other cancers, the use of PET/CT has only improved upon the results seen with PET alone. It is thus probable that once a larger experience is gained, that PET/CT will prove superior to PET alone in assessing sarcomas.

The addition of anatomic images to FDG PET for staging of patients with sarcoma does not yield an increase in specificity, but analysis of surgical margins and other anatomic features for surgical planning is facilitated by the use of PET and CT images that are coregistered. The anatomic precision and detail for combined functional imaging and anatomic assessment in the future are likely to be more effectively produced by the use of PET MRI coregistration techniques. There is early published literature in this area. Somer et al. (19) examined patients with soft tissue masses in the lower extremities or near the spine and used externally placed fiducials to assist with image coregistration. Although the variable spatial distortion in the MRI can make direct image overlay procedures difficult, groups are increasingly evaluating this technique.

Fluorodeoxyglucose PET for Staging Soft Tissue Sarcoma

Most soft tissues sarcomas present as masses in the extremities. In general, they tend to metastasize to the lungs, as the first site of metastases. In most cases, early metastases are small subcentimeter masses that are not conclusively detected with FDG PET. The concomitant use of a high-resolution CT scan of the chest for this purpose is a mandatory part of the patient staging work-up. Selected tumors metastasize to other sites such as lymph nodes, bones, and other soft tissues. The presence of these sites of metastases may be a clue to the tumor histologic subtype and grade.

A whole-body scan is required for a sarcoma staging study. Table 8.19.2 lists the soft tissue sarcomas that have unusual metastatic patterns or those where the primary and earliest metastasis is to the lungs. FDG PET has been shown to be a useful means for sarcoma restaging, similar to the way it is used for diagnosis. A whole-body scan with attention to areas of known metastases is required. The most effective time in the patient treatment sequence of events for an FDG PET restaging study is when a change in therapy is contemplated.

Fluorodeoxyglucose PET for Assessment of Response in Soft Tissue Sarcomas

FDG PET for the assessment of response of soft tissue sarcomas to treatment is an important area of active investigation. Standard anatomic imaging criteria for treatment response such as Response Evaluation Criteria in Solid Tumors (RECIST) in CT do not necessarily report sarcoma treatment responses (20,21). This is likely because sarcomas are derived from mesenchymal elements. Many tumors can contain populations of stromal or structural elements such as fibrous tissue, fat, and bone that do not decrease in volume in response to cytotoxic therapy.

However, FDG PET does identify treatment response in most cases (22). This determination assumes the use of careful criteria for definition of response. The images used to determine the response of sarcomas to treatment often show low levels of residual FDG uptake in the tumor. These tumors may certainly respond to treatment by loss of proliferating tumor cells, but there may also be fibrosis, granulation tissue formation, coagulative and liquefactive necrosis, hemorrhage, and serous fluid accumulation. Some of these processes, particularly scar and granulation tissue formation, are actively consuming energy and thus will accumulate FDG. A tumor residual SUV after treatment of 1.5 to 2.5 may appear on histologic examination as 100% nonviable in the resection specimen. These tissue repair processes, along with inflammation, are likely

TABLE 8.19.2 Soft Tissue Sarcoma Sites of Metastases

Most common for most histologic subtypes:
Lungs
Followed by
Bone.
Brain metastases
Epithelioid sarcomas
Synovial sarcomas
Lymph nodes

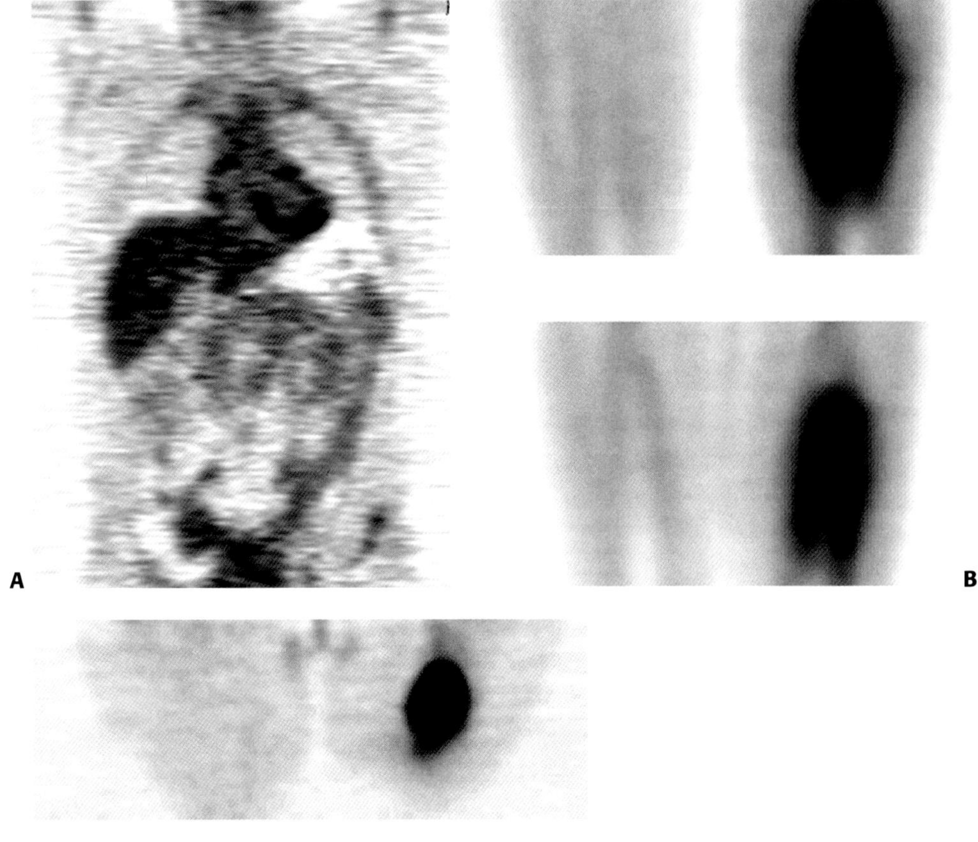

FIGURE 8.19.4. Tumor response to neoadjuvant chemotherapy is often demonstrated on fluorodeoxyglucose (FDG) PET. **A:** A whole-torso image of a patient with residual FDG uptake in a very large right lower abdomen liposarcoma. **B:** A single field of view coronal image of the legs before and after treatment. The patient had an intermediate-grade liposarcoma. **C:** Another single field of view example that compares a set of images acquired before treatment with those after treatment. The high-grade undifferentiated tumor in the gluteal region shows a nearly complete response. Residual FDG uptake is likely related to fibrosis and inflammation in the resolving tumor bed.

significant contributors to FDG uptake in a nonviable tumor or one that is still responding to treatment.

Fig. 8.19.4 shows several examples of soft tissue sarcomas that responded to treatment. The European Organisation for Research and Treatment of Cancer conference on tumor response to treatment guidelines state that at least a 25% decrease between pre- and posttreatment SUV be used to reliably indicate treatment response (23). Use of this system requires careful adherence to imaging time points after FDG injection, blood glucose levels, and image analysis. The neoadjuvant and adjuvant treatments are limited for this group of diseases. However, there are a number of new applications for molecularly targeted therapies that make accurate tumor response assessments particularly important for these patients who often have very poor responses, tolerate high levels of treatment related morbidity, and still expect poor outcomes. Consistency between imaging studies in a specific patient, and within the patient group, will increase confidence in the assessment of treatment response. This is particularly critical in patients where FDG PET is used as a biomarker for treatment response.

Fluorodeoxyglucose PET Imaging and Patient Outcome

It is possible to use FDG PET imaging in cancer to produce prognostic information about a patient's tumor. This is largely the goal of tumor grade assessment that is performed during histopathological diagnosis. The developing practice of prognosis by noninvasive imaging requires at least semiquantitative assessment of imaging data. Overall, in response assessment, response is associated with a more favorable patient outcome. These results have been found in sarcomas with FDG PET imaging protocols performed during treatment (24).

Eary et al. (25) found that the initial tumor SUV maximum was independently predictive of outcome compared to other clinical variables in a group of patients with both bone and soft tissue sarcomas. They later evaluated treatment response in a group of patients with high-grade extremity soft tissue sarcomas treated with neoadjuvant chemotherapy and evaluated the relationship of tumor FDG uptake and patient outcome (26). The results of two imaging variables were found to have prognostic information. These were the pretreatment tumor SUV maximum and the percentage decrease of the tumor SUV maximum after four cycles of neoadjuvant chemotherapy. Sarcomas with baseline SUV maximum greater than 6.0 and 40% or less decrease in tumor SUV maximum after treatment had a high rate of disease recurrence (90% at 4 years after starting treatment). The tumors with a better prognosis had greater than a 40% decrease in tumor SUV maximum.

The experience with FDG PET imaging of tumor response in gastrointestinal stromal tumors deserves special mention. These neoplasms have a mutation in the *KIT* gene, which promotes increased activation of tyrosine kinases (27,28). They can be successfully treated with imatinib mesylate (Gleevec), a tyrosine kinase inhibitor, and other tyrosine kinase inhibitors now being used as well. When gastrointestinal stromal tumor responses are observed as changes in size by anatomic imaging, they are often delayed because the early effect of this targeted therapy is a decrease in cellular metabolism, which eventually leads to cell death. Consequently, when the tumor metabolic responses are determined by FDG PET, decreases in tumor metabolism are highly predictive of patient outcome. In a major study, an FDG PET response was associated with a 92% progression-free survival compared to FDG PET nonresponders who had 12% survival over the same period of time (29). Most patients with complete responses showed these decreases in tumor uptake within 1 week after therapy. Others have reported this finding as well (30,31). They have also found that the use of PET/CT enabled improved tumor characterization (32).

MALIGNANT BONE TUMORS

Bone tumors are derived from bone and cartilage elements. On both imaging and histologic examination, they originate from the bone cortex, periosteum, marrow cavity, and joint surfaces (cartilage). Osteosarcomas have a peak incidence in the patients between 10 and 50 years of age and are located in the metaphysis (33). They are primarily aggressive tumors of the extremities, which often present with distant metastases. This stage implies a worse prognosis (34). In staging studies, 15% to 20% of patients present with pulmonary metastases (the most common site). Other metastatic sites include bone, lymph nodes, and brain. There are many subtypes of osteosarcomas. These are listed in Table 8.19.3. Osteosarcomas are classified according to the FNCLCC grading system for sarcomas (1) and are treated with neoadjuvant chemotherapy, which often consists of doxorubicin, cisplatin, and iphosphamide and high-dose methotrexate. Chemotherapy resistance can develop in patients with osteosarcoma, which results in a decreased disease-free interval. Overall 5-year survival using a combination chemotherapy and surgical approach is 60% to 80%. The low-grade osteosarcoma subtypes are treated with wide resection and recur in approximately 5% of cases.

TABLE 8.19.3 Osteosarcoma Histologic Subtypes

Chondroblastic
Fibroblastic
Osteoblastic
Parosteal
Telangiectatic (vascular)
Small cell
Periosteal
High-grade surface types
Secondary

Fluorodeoxyglucose PET for Diagnosis of Bone Tumor

The utility of FDG PET in bone tumor assessment at diagnosis has been described (14,35,37). Similar to findings in soft tissue sarcomas, several authors have found that the level of tumor metabolic activity assessed with FDG PET indicates tumor grade, and the distinction between benign and malignant tumors can be made. Generally, sarcomas have higher FDG uptake than benign bone tumors, as described by Schulte et al. (35), but active benign tumors cannot always be distinguished from malignant ones. Examples of active benign bone tumors include giant cell tumors and active cases of myositis ossificans. A tumor to background ratio greater than 3.0 in an FDG PET image was used to identify malignant tumors with a sensitivity of 93%, a specificity of 66.7%, and accuracy of 81.7% (35). Similar findings have been reported by other investigators (14). Analysis of these data suggests that FDG PET can be used in conjunction with standard clinical imaging to assess bone tumors for treatment planning. Fig. 8.19.5 shows examples of malignant bone tumors.

EWING'S TUMORS

Ewing's bone tumors, or Ewing's sarcoma family of tumors (ESFT), are aggressive tumors in young patients. Considered high-grade tumors arising from the neural crest precursors, they have a peak age incidence at 15 years. At histologic examination they are identified as having neuronal differentiation. The ESFT differ in several aspects from osteosarcomas and are listed in Table 8.19.4. Presenting with pain and a bone-based soft tissue mass, they may be present for several years before coming to clinical attention. They occur in all skeletal sites but most frequently in the extremities (53%) and pelvis (33). This group of tumors has been the subject of early studies on the relationship of cytogenetic abnormalities with tumor biologic aggressiveness. The presence of the EWS-FLI1 fusion protein implies a worse prognosis (38). There are no known risk factors for development of ESFT, but several links with a family history of other cancers have been described.

Fluorodeoxyglucose PET in Ewing's Sarcoma Family of Tumors

Patients with ESFT often present with distant bony metastases and "skip" lesions in an affected extremity, so a whole-body survey with FDG PET that includes the entire extremities is an important aspect

TABLE 8.19.4 The Ewing's Sarcoma Family of Tumors

Ewing's sarcoma of bone
Extraosseous Ewing's sarcoma
Askin tumor (chest wall primary tumor)
Peripheral primitive neuroectodermal tumor
Peripheral neuroepithelioma

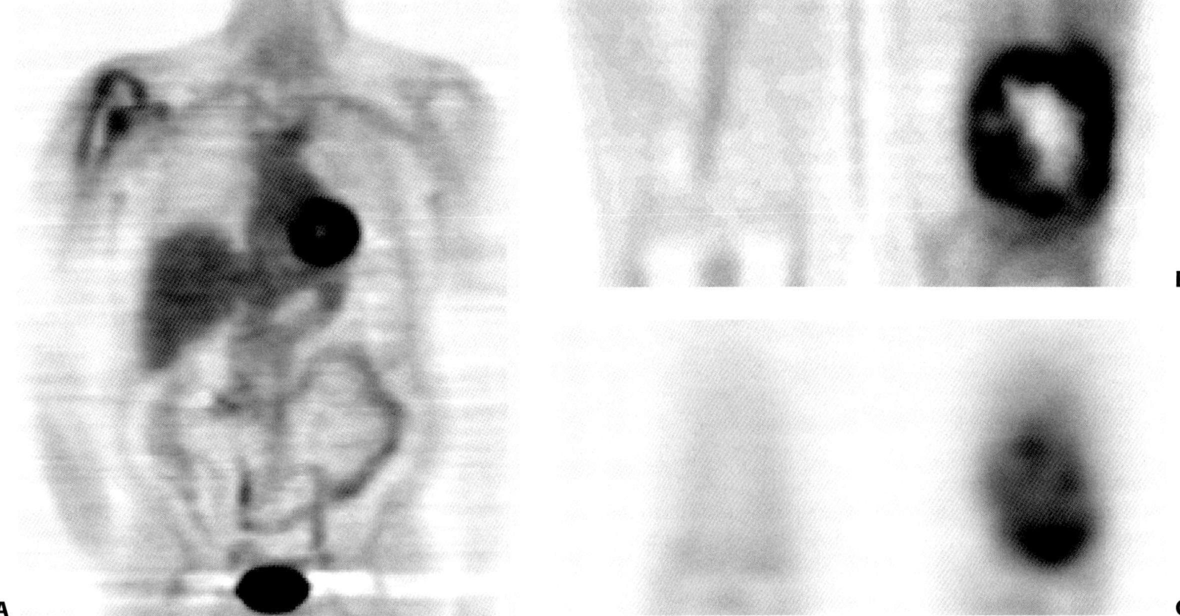

FIGURE 8.19.5. Bone tumors have variable appearances on fluorodeoxyglucose PET. **A:** A coronal whole-torso image of a patient with a Ewing's sarcoma in the right shoulder. **B:** An anterior coronal single field of view image of a patient with a leiomyosarcoma of bone in the left knee distal femur. **C:** A single field of view image of another patient with a chondroblastic osteosarcoma in the left distal femur.

of patient staging. Fifteen percent to 30% of patients have metastatic disease at diagnosis of the primary tumor. However, the most common site of metastasis is pulmonary (53%). In contrast to the osteosarcomas, the ESFT typically have a homogenous appearance on whole-body FDG PET. The tumor FDG SUV maximums are generally not as high as those for osteosarcoma, the average range being from 6.0 to 8.0. This is an interesting finding since these are very cellular high-grade tumors on microscopic appearance.

MALIGNANT CARTILAGE TUMORS

Malignant cartilage tumors (chondrosarcomas) present some of the greatest challenges in tumor assessment and treatment in the sarcoma group. They occur in older adults but are seen in most adult age groups. Table 8.19.5 lists the types of malignant cartilage tumors. The proximal humerus, proximal femur, pelvis in the obturator ring, and the medial wall of the acetabulum are the most common primary tumor sites. Chondrosarcomas have variable behavior and display low- to high-grade differentiation. This critical aspect of diagnosis may be difficult to distinguish with standard imaging and histological assessment.

High-grade chondrosarcomas are less common and have a poor prognosis with 50% survival at 5 years from diagnosis. However, most tumors present as low- to intermediate-grade types (75%), which have 5-year survival rates between 70% and 80%. Spine chondrosarcomas are a particularly high-risk form, where 75% of patients die of progressive disease. Secondary chondrosarcomas arise from pre-existing enchondromas and occur in similar sites as the primary tumors.

The clear cell and mesenchymal chondrosarcoma variants are rare tumors. The clear cell chondrosarcomas occur most frequently in the proximal femur (50%) and have low local recurrence and moderate overall survival (50% at 5 years) rates. The mesenchymal chondrosarcomas present as painful lytic tumors in the femur, ribs, pelvis, or face. They are biologically aggressive and have a 10% 5-year survival rate. Because of this aggressive behavior, they are treated with chemotherapy and wide resection for both local control and an attempt to reduce distant metastases.

TABLE 8.19.5 Chondrosarcomas

Central, primary, secondary
Peripheral
Mesenchymal
Clear cell

Fluorodeoxyglucose PET for Imaging Chondrosarcomas

In patients with chondrosarcomas, FDG PET can be helpful in assessment of biological aggressiveness. Although they usually have low metastatic potential, they are difficult to assess using conventional imaging techniques. The FDG PET scan can contribute to tumor assessment for treatment planning, since, as with other sarcomas, increased SUV maximum suggests higher grade behavior. High-grade tumors can be distinguished from low-grade and benign types easily with use of the tumor SUV. It is more difficult to separate benign cartilage tumors from low-grade chondrosarcomas using any of the standard FDG PET imaging criteria (39,40).

Recently it was found that a tumor SUV cutoff of 2.3 for grade II or III masses had a positive predictive value of 0.82 and a negative predictive value of 0.96 (41). In another study, a combination of tumor histologic grade with the tumor SUV maximum derived from FDG PET was used to identify patients at risk for tumor recurrence

(42). Local recurrences were rare in patients in this series who had tumor SUV maximums lower than 3.0 and diagnoses of intermediate- or low-grade tumor. Chondrosarcomas usually show homogenous FDG uptake with relatively low SUV compared to other tumor groups. This finding of low tissue metabolism may be a reason for the clinical observation that chondrosarcomas often do not exhibit response to chemo- and radiotherapy.

Assessment for Bone Tumor Response with Fluorodeoxyglucose PET

There is not a great amount of published literature on the identification of treatment response in bone sarcomas. Patients whose tumors display an FDG uptake decrease by 30% or more are likely to demonstrate good histologic response in the resected tumor specimen (43). In most cases, these responses were not observable on standard clinical imaging. The presence of large amounts of bone, cartilage, and other low metabolism tissue can result in little change in tumor size in response to successful treatment. In ESFT, Hawkins et al. (44) found that change in the SUV maximum in FDG tumor uptake compared to baseline was highly predictive of patient outcome. Tumor recurrence can also be detected with FDG PET, particularly when the level of metabolic activity in the primary tumor is known from previous baseline imaging studies. FDG PET is also useful in assessing patients with hardware present from a previous tumor resection, where there would be severe artifacts on conventional imaging studies. PET/CT combined scans will likely provide important information for delineation of involved structures when soft tissue tumor extension occurs, in response assessment after surgical resection, and after adjuvant radiotherapy treatment.

OTHER RADIOTRACERS FOR IMAGING SARCOMAS

Sarcomas often display a number of tissue characteristics that imply that they are under stress or have a biologic risk for aggressiveness. Various aspects of these tumors are the basis for investigation of PET radiotracers that are more specific for reporting on these processes than FDG. Some of the new radiopharmaceuticals that have been investigated for application to sarcomas and other cancer types using sarcomas as a model include fluorine-18 fluoromisonidazole (FMISO) to quantitate the levels of tissue hypoxia (45–47). Hypoxia is implied as a result or cause of increased unregulated tumor growth, neovascularization, and up-regulation of stress-reactive proteins. Preliminary work in sarcomas using FMISO has shown that they are often regionally hypoxic and that these areas of hypoxia do not necessarily relate to areas of increased tumor metabolism determined by FDG imaging (48). In the future, as new targeted therapies are tested for sarcomas, newer biologically specific PET radiopharmaceuticals will play an important role in quantitating clinically relevant responses. In this way, patients with sarcoma will benefit from the use of PET imaging data as validated biomarkers specific for their disease.

SUMMARY

Sarcomas represent a broad range of tumor types. Both soft tissue and bone sarcomas can be well imaged using FDG PET. As in other tumor types, higher levels of FDG uptake predict a more aggressive tumor type, although some overlap does occur. The use of PET can add complementary information to anatomic imaging. In assessing treatment response, rapid and substantial declines in FDG uptake with chemotherapy appear to be most predictive of a good outcome. Fusion with anatomic imaging is helpful, but in addition to PET/CT, software fusion of PET to MRI is promising. Although these tumors are reasonably infrequent, PET has a valuable and growing role in sarcoma management.

REFERENCES

1. Coindre JM, Terrier P, Guillou L, et al. Predictive value of grade for metastasis development in the main histologic types of adult soft tissue sarcomas: a study of 1240 patients from the French Federation of Cancer Centers Sarcoma Group. *Cancer* 2001;91:1914–1926.
2. Deyrup AT, Weiss SW. Grading of soft tissue sarcomas: the challenge of providing precise information in an imprecise world. *Histopathology* 2006;48(1):42–50.
3. O'Sullivan F, Roy S, Eary, J. A statistical measure of tissue heterogeneity with application to 3D PET sarcoma data. Biostatistics 2003;4(3):433–448.
4. Folpe AL, Lyles RH, Sprouse JT, et al. (F-18) fluorodeoxyglucose positron emission tomography as a predictor of pathologic grade and other prognostic variables in bone and soft tissue sarcoma. *Clin Cancer Res.* 2000;(4):1279–1287.
5. Hain SF, O'Foherty MJ, Bingham J, et al. Can FDG PET be used to successfully direct preoperative biopsy of soft tissue tumors? *Nucl Med Commun* 2003;24(11):1130–1143.
6. Adler LP, Blair HF, Makley JT, et al. Non-invasive grading of musculoskeletal tumors using PET. *J Nucl Med* 1990;32:1508–1512.
7. Griffeth LK, Dedashti F, McGuire AH, et al. PET evaluation of soft tissue masses with fluorine-18 fluoro-2-deoxy-glucose. *Radiology* 1992; 182:185–194.
8. Nieweg OE, Pruim J, van Ginkel RJ, et al. Fluorine-18-fluorodeoxyglucose PET imaging of soft-tissue sarcoma. *J Nucl Med* 1996;37(2):257–261.
9. Eary JF, Conrad EU, Bruckner JD, et al. Quantitative [F-18] fluorodeoxyglucose positron emission tomography in pretreatment and grading of sarcoma. *Clin Can Res* 1998;4(5):1215–1220.
10. Eary JF, Conrad EU. Positron emission tomography in grading soft tissue sarcomas. *Semin in Muskel Radiol* 1999;3(2):135–138.
11. Schwarzbach M, Willeke F, Dimitrakopoulou Strauss A, et al. Functional imaging and detection of local recurrence in soft tissue sarcomas by positron emission tomography. *Anticancer Res* 1999;19:1343–1349.
12. Lucas JD, O'Doherty MJ, Wong JCH, et al. Evaluation of fluorodeoxyglucose positron emission tomography in the management of soft-tissue sarcomas. *J Bone Joint Surg* 1998;80(3):441–447.
13. Wantanabe H, Shinozaki T. Yanagawa T, et al. Glucose metabolic analysis of musculoskeletal tumours using 18-fluorine-FDG PET as an aid to preoperative planning. *J Bone Joint Surg* 2000;82(5):760–767.
14. Feldman F, van Heertum R, Manos C. 18-FDG PET scanning of benign and malignant musculoskeletal lesions. *Skeletal Radiol* 2003;32:201–208.
15. Ioannidis JP, Lau J. ^{18}-F-FDG PET for the diagnosis and grading of soft-tissue sarcoma: a meta-analysis. *J Nucl Med* 2003;44(5):717–724.
16. Franzius C, Schulte M, Hillmann W, et al. Clinical value of position emission tomography (PET) in the diagnosis of bone and soft tissue tumors. 3rd Interdisciplinary Consensus Conference "PET in Oncology": results of the Bone and Soft Tissue Study Group. *Chirurg* 2001;72(9):1071–1077.
17. Aoki J, Endo K, Watanabe H, et al. FDG-PET for evaluating musculoskeletal tumors: a review. *J Orthop Sci* 2003;8:435–441.
18. Shankar LK, Hoffman JM, Bacharach S, et al. National Cancer Institute. Consensus recommendations for the use of 18F-FDG PET as an indicator of therapeutic response in patients in National Cancer Institute Trials. *J Nucl Med.* 2006;47(6):1059–1066.
19. Somer EJR, Marsden PK, Benatar NA, et al. PET-MR image fusion in soft tissue sarcoma: accuracy, reliability and practicality of interactive point-based and automated mutual information techniques. *Eur J Nucl Med* 2003;30:54–62.

20. Therasse P, Arbuck SG, Eisenhauer EA, et al. New guidelines to evaluate the response to treatment in solid tumors. *J Natl Cancer Inst* 2000;92: 205–216.
21. Ratain MJ, Eckhardt SG. Phase II studies of modern drugs directed against new target: if you are fazed, too, then resist RECIST. *J Clin Oncol* 2004;22(22):4442–4445.
22. Jones DN, McCowage GB, Sostman HD, et al. Monitoring of neoadjuvant therapy response of soft-tissue and musculoskeletal sarcoma using fluorine-18-FDG PET. *J Nucl Med* 1996;37(9):1438–1444.
23. Young H, Baum R, Cremerius U, et al. Measurement of clinical and subclinical tumour response using [F-18]-fluorodeoxyglucose and positron emission tomography: review and 1999 EORTC recommendations. *Eur J Cancer* 1999;35(13):1773–1782.
24. Weber W. Use of PET for monitoring cancer therapy and predicting outcome. *J Nucl Med* 2005;46:983–995.
25. Eary JF, O'Sullivan F, Powitan Y, et al. Sarcoma tumor FDG uptake measured by PET and patient outcome: a retrospective analysis. *Eur J Nucl Med* 2002;29(9):1149–1154.
26. Schuetze SM, Rubin BP, Vernon C, et al. Use of positron emission tomography in localized extremity soft tissue sarcoma treated with neoadjuvant chemotherapy. *Cancer* 2005;103(2):339–348.
27. Rubin BP, Schuetze SM, Eary JF, et al. Molecular targeting of platelet-derived growth factor B by imatinib mesylate in a patient with metastatic dermatofibrosarcoma protuberans. *J Clin Oncol* 2002;20(17): 3586–3591.
28. Singer S, Rubin BP, Lux MK, et al. *KIT* activation is a ubiquitous feature of gastrointestinal stromal tumors. *Cancer Res* 2001;61: 8118–8121.
29. Stroobants S, Goeminne J, Seegers M, et al. 18-FDG-positron emission tomography for the early prediction of response in advanced soft tissue sarcoma treated with imatinib mesylate (Glivec). *Eur J Cancer* 2003;39: 2012–2020:2003.
30. Jager PL, Gietema JA, van der Graaf WTA. Imatinib mesylate for the treatment of gastrointestinal stromal tumors:best monitored with FDG PET. *Nucl Med Commun* 2004;25:43308.
31. Schwarzbach MHM, Hinz U, Dimitrakopoulou-Strauss A, et al. Prognostic significance of preoperative [^{18}-F] fluorodeoxyglucose (FDG) positron emission tomography (PET) imaging in patients with resectable soft tissue sarcomas. *Ann Surg* 2005;241:286–294.
32. Goerres GW, Stupp R, Barghouth G, et al. The value of PET, CT and in-line PET/CT in patients with gastrointestinal stromal tumors: long-term outcome of treatment with imatinib mesylate. *Eur J Med Mol Imaging* 2005;32:153–162.
33. Pizzo PA. Management of pediatric cancer. *Hosp Pract* (Off Ed). 1986;21(3):111–8, 124–30. No abstract available.
34. Meyers PA, Gorlick R, Heller G, et al. Intensification of pre-operative chemotherapy for osteogenic sarcoma: results of the Memorial Sloan-Kettering protocol. *J Clinc Oncol* 1998;16(7):1020–1033.
35. Schulte M, Brecht-Krauss D, Heymer B, et al. Grading of tumors and tumorlike lesions of bone: evaluation by FDG PET. *J Nucl Med* 2000;41: 1695–1701.
36. Israel-Mardirosian N, Adler LP. Positron emission tomography of soft tissue sarcomas. *Curr Opin Oncol* 2003;15:327–330.
37. Conrad EU, Morgan HD, Vernon C, et al. Fluorodeoxyglucose position emission tomography scanning: basic principles and imaging of adult soft-tissue sarcomas. *J Bone Joint Surg Am* 2004; 86A[Suppl 2]:98–104.
38. de Alava E, Kawai A, Healey JH, et al. EWS-FLI1 fusion transcript structure is an independent determinant of prognosis in Ewing's sarcoma. *J Clin Oncol* 1998;16(4):1248–1255.
39. Eary JF, Conrad EU, Bruckner JD, et al. Quantitative [F-18] fluorodeoxyglucose positron emission tomography in pretreatment and grading of sarcoma. *Clin Can Res* 1998;4(5):1215–1220.
40. Aoki J, Watanabe H, Shinozaki A, et al. FDG-PET in differential diagnosis and grading of chondrosarcomas. *J Comput Asst Tomog* 1999;23(4): 603–608.
41. Lee FY, Yu J, Chang SS, et al. Diagnostic value and limitations of fluorine-18 fluorodeoxyglucose positron tomography for cartilaginous tumors of bone. *J Bone Joint Surg Am* 2004;86A(12):2677–2685.
42. Brenner W, Conrad EU, Eary JF. FDG PET imaging for grading and prediction of outcome in chondrosarcoma patients. *Eur J Nucl Med Mol Imaging* 2004;31(2):189–195.
43. Franzius C, Sciuk J, Brinkschmidt C, et al. Evaluation of chemotherapy in primary bone tumors with F-18 FDG positron emission tomography compared with histologically assessed tumor necrosis. *Clin Nucl Med* 2000;25(11):874–881.
44. Hawkins DS, Rajendran JG, Conrad EU, Bruckner JD, Eary JF. [F-18]Fluorodeoxyglucose positron emission tomography predicts outcome for Ewing's sarcoma family of tumors. *J Clin Oncol* 2005;23(34):8828–8834.
45. Moulder JE, Rockwell S. Tumor hypoxia: its impact on cancer therapy. *Cancer Metastasis Rev* 1987;5(4):313–341.
46. Rasey JS, Koh WJ, Evans ML, et al. Quantifying regional hypoxia in human tumors with positron emission tomography of [F-18]fluoromisonidazole: a pre-therapy study of 37 patients. *Int J Radiat Oncol Biol Phys* 1996;36:417–428.
47. Rajendran JG, Krohn KA. Imaging hypoxia and angiogenesis in tumors. *Radiol Clin North Am* 2005;43:169 187.
48. Rajendran JG, Wilson DC, Conrad EU, et al. [18-F]FMISO and [18-F] FDG PET imaging in soft tissue sarcomas: correlation of hypoxia, metabolism and VEGF expression. *Eur J Nucl Med Mol Imaging* 2003; 30(5):695–704.

CHAPTER

8.20 Gastrointestinal Stromal Tumors

ANNICK D. VAN DEN ABBEELE, ERTUK MEHMET, AND RICHARD J. TETRAULT

In 1983, Mazur and Clark (1) described gastrointestinal stromal tumors (GISTs) as a distinctive subgroup of gastrointestinal mesenchymal tumors not classified as neurogenic or smooth muscle-derived. Kindblom et al. (2) hypothesized that these tumors may originate from the interstitial cell of Cajal in the normal myenteric plexus, an intestinal pacemaker cell. This hypothesis was confirmed by Hirota et al. (3) in 2000, who demonstrated that neoplastic GIST cells show ultrastructural features and express cell markers typical of the normal interstitial cell of Cajal (4). Today, on the basis of pathological features, most gastrointestinal mesenchymal tumors previously designated as smooth muscle tumors, such as leiomyomas, leiomyoblastomas, and leiomyosarcomas, are classified as GISTs (4).

GIST is the most common mesenchymal neoplasm of the alimentary tract (5). Although it is a rare tumor and accounts for only approximately 3% of all gastrointestinal cancers, up to 20% of small bowel malignancies are GISTs (6). GISTs predominantly occur in the fifth to seventh decades of life, without any gender predilection (4). Primary GIST is solitary rather than multiple. GISTs arise throughout the whole length of the gastrointestinal tract, most commonly in the stomach (60% to 70%) followed by small bowel (20% to 25%) and rarely in the rectum, esophagus, colon, and appendix (7). The presentation symptoms are usually nonspecific and are typically related to mass effects dependent on the size and the location of the tumor (4). Small GISTs are usually detected incidentally at surgery, on radiographic imaging, or during endoscopy and are typically asymptomatic. In approximately half of the patients, bleeding may be the first manifestation of GIST (4). Another 20% of patients will present with abdominal discomfort that is typically associated with a large tumor size. Another clinical presentation is bowel obstruction or perforation. At first diagnosis, approximately 10% of patients have metastatic disease (7), but this incidence may be higher, with DeMatteo et al. (8) reporting metastatic disease found in nearly half of their patients. The liver is the most common site (65%) for metastatic disease, followed by the peritoneum (21%), mesentery and abdominal cavity, while metastases to lymph nodes, bone, and lung are rare. Most patients develop recurrent GISTs after an apparently complete surgical resection of the primary lesion, with the most common sites of recurrence being in the liver, peritoneum, or both (9).

GIST has a typical immunohistochemical profile that helps confirm the diagnosis. Approximately 95% of GISTs are positive for *KIT* (CD117), the c-*kit* receptor tyrosine kinase (10). In most GISTs, an activating mutation of c-*kit* leads to ligand-independent receptor dimerization and activation of *KIT* tyrosine kinase that promotes tumor survival and tumor growth (11). More than 80% of GISTs have an oncogenic mutation in the *KIT* tyrosine kinase (12), and most of the mutations occur in the juxtamembrane domain encoded by exon 11, but mutations may also occur in exons 9, 13, 17, or *PDGFRA* (platelet-derived growth factor receptor) (13–15). Approximately 10% to 15% of GISTs are negative for *KIT* and *PDGFRA* mutations. Interestingly, the kinase genotype has been shown to be predictive of response to imatinib therapy (13,16). The presence, as well as the location of mutations in *KIT* or *PDGFRA*, highly correlates with the clinical response to imatinib, the first tyrosine kinase inhibitor approved for the treatment of GIST (see below) (13,16). Patients who have an exon 11 mutation within their tumors show the best response to imatinib therapy, with an 85% response rate. There is also some suggestion that patients with exon 9 mutations may be more sensitive to sunitinib (17), the second drug approved for treatment of GIST (see below). Recent data even suggest that mutational screening might be useful in selecting the optimal dose of imatinib (16). It is too early to determine if mutational screening will become part of a standard diagnostic work-up for patients with GISTs. However, it is interesting to see how far the knowledge about GIST, as well as the molecular-targeted therapies used to treat it, have come in a relatively short period since the first trial was started in the summer of 2000.

GISTs are known to be both chemoresistant and insensitive to irradiation, and surgical resection is the initial therapy for patients with primary GIST who have no metastases and are considered resectable. Prior to 2002, the lack of therapeutic options in inoperable and metastatic disease resulted in a generally poor prognosis in patients with GISTs (18–20). Recent studies, however, have shown promising results and greatly improved survival when patients with GISTs were treated with a new line of therapy using a selective small molecule that inhibits tumor growth by competitive interaction at the adenosine triphosphate–binding site of the c-*kit* receptor (imatinib mesylate, STI571, Gleevec, Glivec; Novartis Pharmaceuticals, East Hanover, New Jersey).

Imatinib is an oral drug that inhibits several tyrosine kinases including *KIT* and *BCR-ABL* (20–24). The multidisciplinary team of Demetri et al. (20) participated in the first multicenter trial that tested imatinib in patients with unresectable and metastatic GISTs. The results of this trial showed a high incidence of durable responses with 85% of the patients still alive 76 weeks post-initiation of treatment. There was a close relationship between clinical outcome and the results seen on positron emission tomography (PET) using fluorine-18-fluoro-2-deoxy-D-glucose (FDG), or FDG PET, 1 month following initiation of imatinib, while objective response by computed tomography (CT) criteria (using the Southwest Oncologic Group [SWOG] criteria) were lagging weeks and months behind the response seen on FDG PET (25). Although no patient had achieved a complete response by standard anatomic criteria at that time point, clinical benefit was clearly observed even in patients with stable disease. It actually took a median of 3 months for patients to achieve partial response by SWOG criteria, while a marked decrease in glycolytic metabolism could be observed on FDG PET in all patients who responded to imatinib at 1 month, and even as early as 24 hours postinitiation of the drug (20,26).

Although most patients with advanced GISTs benefit from imatinib therapy, a small percentage of patients (less than 15%) may have primary resistance to the drug. Patients can also develop secondary resistance to the drug following a period of response to imatinib. This can occur months or years following continuous response to imatinib and is thought to be related to clonal differentiation within the tumor secondary to the acquisition of new mutations that confers resistance to the drug in this subpopulation of tumor cells (27).

In January 2006, the U.S. Food and Drug Administration approved a second line of molecular-targeted therapy (sunitinib malate, SU11428, Sutent; Pfizer, New York, New York) for the treatment of metastatic GISTs (28). This drug is an oral tyrosine kinase multitargeted inhibitor that inhibits *KIT* and platelet derived growth factor receptor *(PDGFR)*, as well as vascular endothelial growth factor receptor *(VEGFR)1-3*, *FLT-3*, and *RET*, adding a potential antiangiogenic effect. It is available to patients who are unresectable and have developed primary or secondary resistance to imatinib and who are progressing despite higher doses of imatinib (28). Here again, very few patients achieved objective anatomic response criteria by RECIST (Response Evaluation Criteria in Solid Tumors) (29), but clinical benefit was observed in the 58% of patients who showed stable disease as the best overall tumor response by standard RECIST criteria. This discrepancy between clinical benefit and standard anatomic response criteria has now been observed with more than one tyrosine kinase inhibitor.

GASTROINTESTINAL STROMAL TUMORS AND IMAGING STUDIES

Initial Evaluation

Although imaging studies play an important role in the management of patients with GISTs, there are no well-defined imaging examinations for the initial diagnosis of GISTs. Radiological investigations occasionally pick up incidental cases, but patients are typically referred for imaging to characterize an abdominal mass or to evaluate nonspecific abdominal symptoms, as discussed above, and CT and/or magnetic resonance imaging (MRI) are usually used in that context.

Ultrasonography, contrast-enhanced CT, and MRI are able to assess GISTs based on detailed morphological appearance, but CT is the modality of choice for characterizing and localizing an abdominal mass, as well as for the staging of biopsy-proven GISTs (4). Oral and intravenous contrast-enhanced cross-sectional imaging studies are strongly preferred over conventional planar radiography and barium studies in detecting and delineating both the primary disease and metastatic lesions.

CT may reliably localize GIST as well as determine tumor size and possibly reveal the presence of secondary metastatic localizations (e.g., hepatic metastases) (4). CT can also disclose an extraluminal mass originating from the digestive tract wall. The untreated tumor masses are usually dense and enhance following intravenous contrast administration. Large GISTs can be heterogeneous with areas of necrosis. Imaging features usually offer valuable information in distinguishing tumors of mesenchymal origin from lymphoma, where necrosis is less common, and from epithelial neoplasms of gastrointestinal tract.

FDG PET is also particularly useful for the staging of GISTs because the great majority of untreated GISTs show intense glycolytic activity resulting in significant FDG uptake within all tumor masses (Figs. 8.20.1, 8.20.2A, 8.20.3A). However, FDG PET has mainly been used in the clinic for patient follow-up (4) (see below). Some GISTs have been reported to be FDG negative, but these tumors represent a small percentage of all GISTs. A baseline FDG PET should always be obtained prior to treatment if one is considering using this modality to monitor response to therapy.

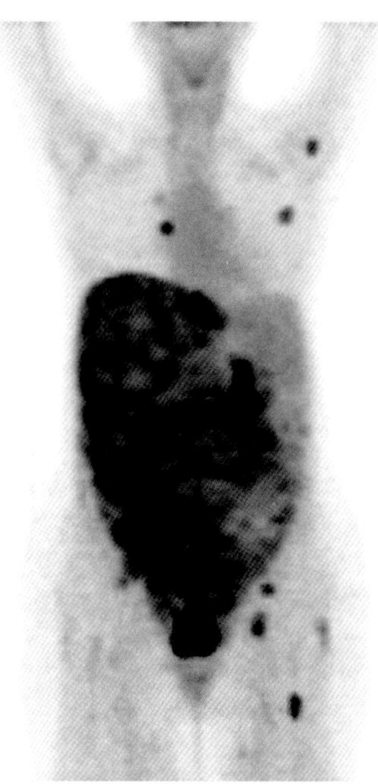

FIGURE 8.20.1. FDG PET in a patient with GIST with extensive metastatic involvement throughout the liver, the entire abdomen, and pelvis. The scan also demonstrates unsuspected skeletal/bone marrow metastases in the left humeral head, a right posterior rib, the pelvis, and the left femur, as well as unsuspected soft tissue involvement in the left breast and nodal involvement in the right internal mammary chain.

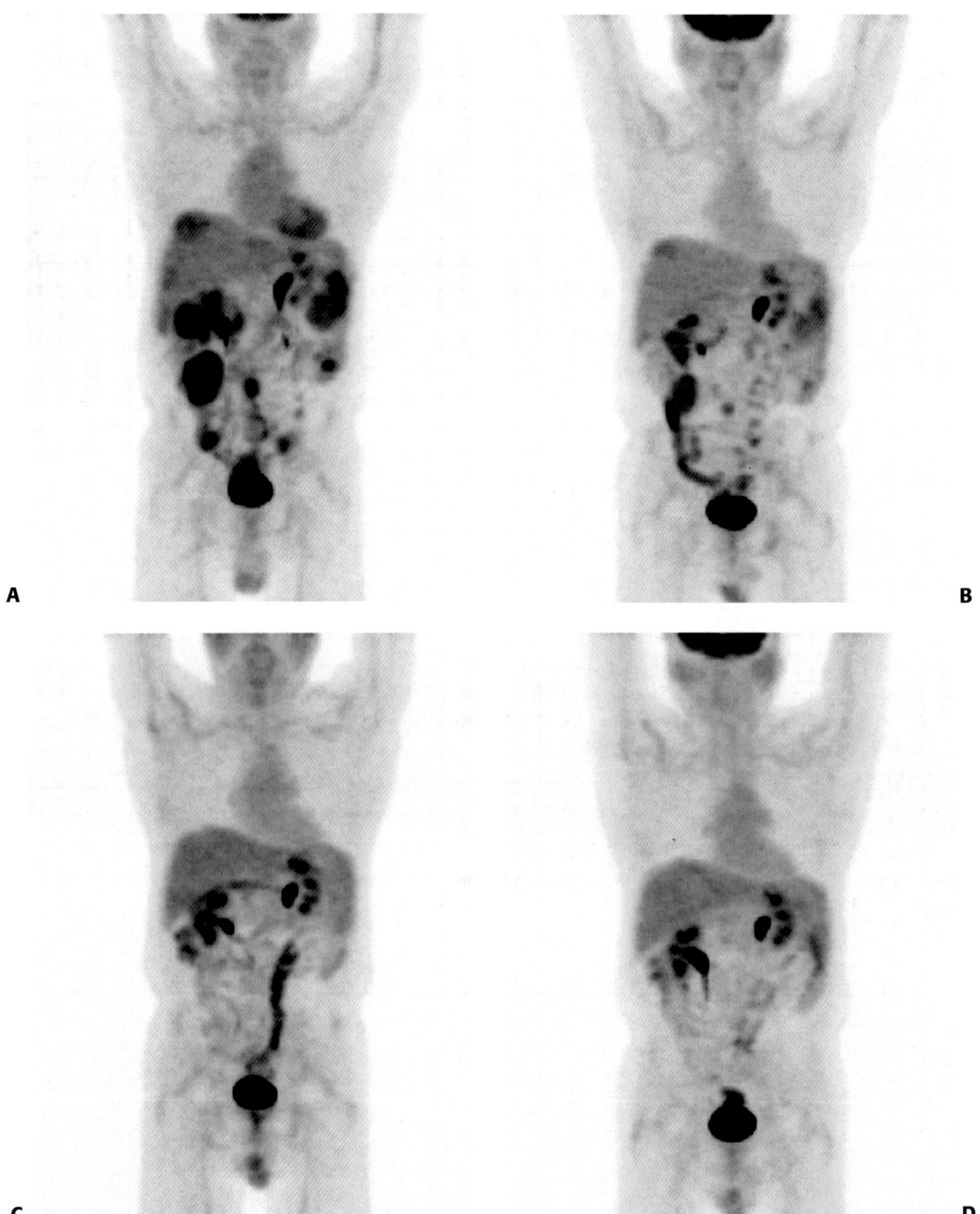

FIGURE 8.20.2. FDG PET in a patient with GIST metastatic to the liver, abdomen, and pelvis prior to and following initiation of imatinib therapy. **A:** Intense FDG uptake is seen in all tumor masses at baseline prior to imatinib therapy, reflecting intense glycolytic activity. **B:** A significant decrease in glycolytic activity can be seen in all tumor masses as early as 24 hours following a single dose (400 mg) of imatinib. **C:** Complete resolution of abnormal FDG uptake is seen in all tumor sites 1 month following initiation of treatment. **D:** Continuous response to imatinib is seen over time as shown in a follow-up scan performed 5.5 months following initiation of therapy. Physiologic FDG uptake is seen in the brain, the bowel, urinary collecting system in both kidneys, and the bladder in all images.

FDG PET also allows for semi-quantitative evaluation of metabolic activity within the tumor using the standardized uptake value (SUV) or maximum SUV (SUV_{max}) to characterize the glycolytic metabolism of the tumor and to evaluate response to therapy. Metabolic response criteria have been defined by the European Organisation for Research and Treatment of Cancer (EORTC) (30). These criteria are based on the magnitude of the decrease in SUV relative to baseline (hence the importance of obtaining a baseline study), and provide definitions for complete, partial, progressive, and stable metabolic disease. The prognostic value of

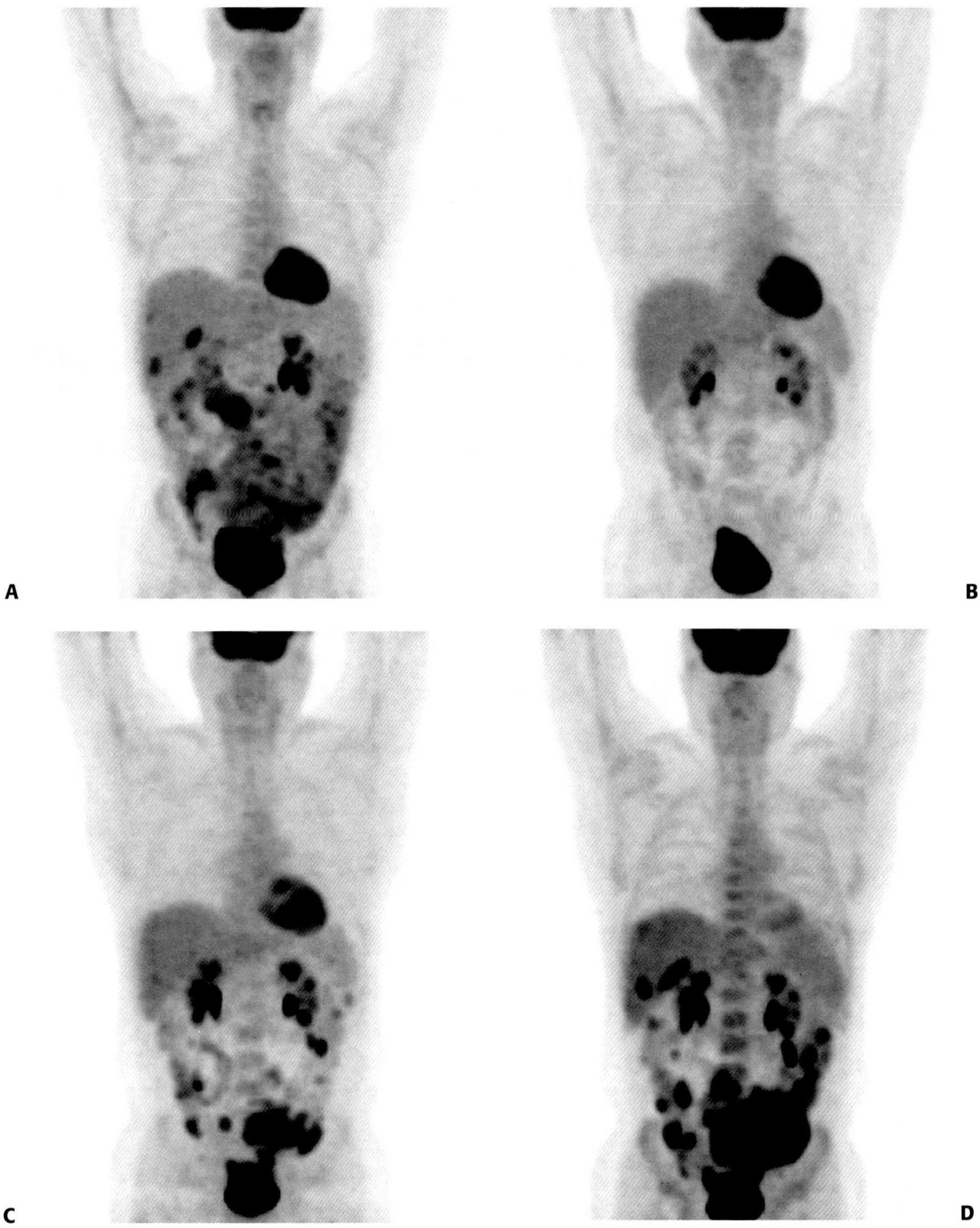

FIGURE 8.20.3. FDG PET in a patient with GIST metastatic to the liver, peritoneum, and pelvis. **A:** Baseline scan showing intense FDG uptake in all tumor sites including the liver, abdomen, peritoneal cavity, and pelvis prior to the initiation of imatinib. **B:** Complete resolution of abnormal FDG uptake is seen 1 month following initiation of imatinib in all tumor sites. Physiologic FDG uptake is seen in the brain, myocardium, urinary collecting system in both kidneys, and the bladder. **C:** Re-emergence of abnormal FDG uptake reflecting tumor progression due to secondary resistance is seen 18 months following initiation of therapy at sites that were originally involved prior to the start of imatinib including the liver, abdomen, peritoneal cavity, and pelvis. **D:** A "flare phenomenon" (i.e., a rebound in glycolytic activity) is seen in all tumor sites 3 weeks following cessation of imatinib therapy.

FDG PET has also been shown in various settings and in a variety of cancers (31–39).

In the past, attempts to predict potential malignant behavior of GISTs from its imaging features have been unsuccessful. Nevertheless, Kamiyama et al. (40) reported some promising results in this context. The malignant potential of GISTs is, however, difficult to diagnose before surgery, and the prognostic features should be based on tumor diameter and mitotic index (41), as these factors have been validated and serve as consensus criteria for the risk stratification of GISTs. In the study of Kamiyama et al. (40), ten patients diagnosed with gastric GISTs underwent FDG PET imaging before tumor resection. There was a significant correlation between the FDG uptake and both the Ki-67 index and the mitotic index, but the tumor diameter did not correlate with these indices, and the authors therefore concluded that FDG PET might be of value for predicting the malignant potential of gastric GISTs. However, tumor size and mitotic index remain the two most important prognostic features, as discussed above, and are needed to determine the malignant potential of GISTs (41). Metastases from GISTs are most often seen in the liver, omentum, and peritoneal cavity, and can be seen in soft tissues, but rarely in lung and pleura, and even more rarely in bone or lymph nodes.

Monitoring of Therapeutic Response and Patient Follow-up

In the past, the lack of nonsurgical therapeutic options for inoperable and metastatic disease caused a generally poor prognosis in patients with GISTs (42). As mentioned above, treatment with imatinib mesylate changed the management of GIST patients. The first report on the effect of imatinib in a solid tumor was published in a pilot study of a single Finnish patient with GIST that was metastatic to the liver (43). This patient was restaged 1 month after initiation of treatment with MRI and FDG PET. A marked decrease in gadolinium enhancement and in the density of the multiple hepatic metastases was seen on MRI. Complete resolution of the abnormal glycolytic activity seen prior to treatment was observed on FDG PET in all hepatic metastases.

To avoid unnecessary and costly treatment, the effect of imatinib on GISTs needs to be defined as soon as possible after the start of therapy. Early detection of tumor response ensures effective therapy, while a demonstrated lack of response to the drug identifies a group of patients who may benefit from alternative therapy.

As opposed to conventional cytotoxic chemotherapy, where a decrease in the size of a tumor mass often quite rapidly reflects response to therapy, reduction of viable tumor cells after therapy with tyrosine kinase inhibitors may not immediately result in a decrease in the tumor volume. In fact, in the case of imatinib and other molecular-targeted drugs, it may actually take weeks to months, even years, for tumors to shrink despite the fact that the patient is responding to treatment. Evaluation of objective tumor response through serial CT scanning using standard anatomic criteria such as World Health Organization (WHO) (44), SWOG (25), or RECIST (29) is therefore hampered by the fact that major volume changes tend to occur late (several weeks to months) after the start of imatinib treatment (26,45,46).

This observation was first reported in the original U.S. multicenter trial that tested imatinib in patients with metastatic GISTs (20,26,47). The imaging results in the first 25 patients entered into this trial at a single center (Dana-Farber Cancer Institute) were presented at the 2001 annual meeting of the American Society of Clinical Oncology (ASCO) (26). FDG PET was used in combination with diagnostic CT to evaluate response to imatinib. Response by FDG PET was assessed using the absolute value of SUV_{max} before and after therapy, as well as the percentage change in SUV_{max} relative to baseline. The SWOG criteria were used to assess response on CT. This report showed that the extent of disease was better defined by FDG PET compared with CT (Fig. 8.20.1) and that response to imatinib therapy could be seen on FDG PET as early as 24 hours after a single dose of the drug (Fig. 8.20.2B). It also demonstrated that 80% of patients had complete response by FDG PET 1 month after initiation of imatinib therapy (Figs. 8.20.2C and 8.20.3B) and that this early response was sustained over time (Fig. 8.20.2D). Conversely, as mentioned earlier, no patient showed complete response by anatomic criteria (SWOG) at that time point. The study concluded that "the functional information provided by FDG-PET may play an important role in the evaluation of therapies such as STI571 which target specific cell-signaling mechanisms," and that the roles of FDG PET and CT would need to be studied prospectively to determine their respective predictive values (26).

Further updates on this trial showed that based on these anatomic criteria, the overall response rate was only 38% (48), despite the fact that 85% of patients were still alive at 76 weeks (20,46). The imaging update on the first 64 patients enrolled at the same center by 2002 showed that the early results seen by FDG PET at 21 to 40 days were predictive of time-to-treatment failure, while CT measurements were not predictive of response at that time point (49). At 21 to 40 days, 79% of patients who showed decreases in SUV_{max} to 2.5 or less were still in remission 16 months after treatment initiation. The predictive value of FDG PET was also observed when the EORTC metabolic partial response criteria was used (i.e., a 25% decrease in SUV_{max} relative to baseline) (30). Interestingly, 52% of responders by FDG PET had not reached partial response by SWOG criteria (i.e., a 50% decrease in bidimensional tumor size on CT). These results were sustained over a longer follow-up of 35 months and still showed a more favorable outcome for patients who showed response by FDG PET at 1 month, while CT results at that time were not predictive of response (50). Holdsworth et al. (50) also showed that both PET and CT criteria could be optimized, and that the predictive value of CT could be significantly increased if absence of tumor growth was used as a criterion of response rather than a bidimensional decrease in tumor size as used in SWOG.

The early evidence of biologic response by FDG PET as well as the insensitivity of traditional tumor response criteria based on tumor size change, reported above, were both confirmed by subsequent studies in other centers (51,52). Stroobants et al. (51) studied 17 patients prior to and at 8 days, 28 days, and 8 weeks following imatinib. Eleven patients showed complete response by EORTC criteria and two had a partial response. FDG PET response preceded CT response by a median of 7 weeks (range 4 to 48 weeks). With a 12-month follow-up, response by FDG PET was associated with a longer progression-free survival compared with nonresponders (92% vs. 12%).

Choi et al. (52) studied 36 patients with metastatic GISTs using FDG PET and CT 2 months after initiation of imatinib and showed that a significant decrease in SUV_{max} was seen in 65% of patients. This correlated well with a subjective assessment of overall tumor response. However, 75% of patients had stable disease by RECIST criteria. The authors also reported that 70% of patients showing an FDG PET response also showed a decrease in tumor density on CT (53).

Heinicke et al. (54) studied 5 patients with GISTs and 1 patient with a *KIT*-positive small cell cancer undergoing imatinib mesylate therapy. The FDG PET scans were performed prior to and 1 week following the start of imatinib mesylate therapy. Metabolic responses were detected after only 1 week of therapy in all of the patients with GISTs (four partial responses and one complete response). The mean decrease of the SUV was 60% (range 43% to 77%). In contrast, the tumor of the non-GIST patient was metabolically stable. In this study, 4 of the 5 patients with GISTs achieved a partial response on CT after a mean duration of 23 weeks (range 6 to 48 weeks).

In the study of Jager et al. (55), 16 consecutive patients with unresectable or metastasized GISTs or another c-*kit* (CD117) positive mesenchymal tumor underwent FDG PET before and 1 week after the start of treatment with imatinib mesylate. The authors compared visual findings and SUV with the overall response to treatment, based on clinical and radiological response. They reported that FDG PET visualized all known and some unknown tumor locations. The separation by FDG PET after 1 week of treatment in "PET responders" (11 of 16 patients, mean SUV reduction 65%) versus "PET nonresponders" (5 of 16 patients, mean SUV increase 16%) appeared to match almost perfectly with overall treatment response and proved correct in 14 of 15 patients (prediction sensitivity 93%). FDG uptake changes after 1 week of treatment were of greater magnitude than tumor volume changes on CT at 8 weeks. Progression-free survival was significantly better in those patients with a PET response (P = .002). In this study, PET response predicted treatment outcome better than the radiological response.

The study of Gayed et al. (56) included 54 patients who underwent FDG PET and CT within 3 weeks before initiation of imatinib mesylate therapy. Forty-nine of these patients had repeat scans 2 months after therapy. The number of sites or organs containing lesions on FDG PET and CT scans were compared. Measurements of SUV_{max} on FDG PET and tumor size on CT were used for quantitative evaluation of early tumor response to therapy. A total of 122 and 114 sites and/or organs were involved on pre-therapy FDG PET and CT, respectively. The sensitivity and positive predictive values for CT were 93% and 100%, respectively, whereas these values for FDG PET were 86% and 98%. The differences between these values for CT and FDG PET were not statistically significant. Nevertheless, FDG PET predicted response to therapy earlier than CT in 22.5% of patients during a longer follow-up interval (4 to 16 months), whereas CT predicted lack of response to therapy earlier than FDG PET in 4.1%. The authors concluded that their findings suggest that FDG PET is superior to CT in predicting early response to therapy in patients with recurrent or metastatic GISTs.

Goerres et al. (57) studied the prognostic power of FDG PET, contrast enhanced CT, and FDG PET/CT in evaluating the therapeutic impact of imatinib mesylate in 34 patients with GISTs. In 28 patients, FDG PET/CT and contrast-enhanced CT were available after introduction of treatment with imatinib mesylate. Patients without FDG uptake after the start of treatment had a better prognosis than patients who showed residual activity. In comparison, contrast-enhanced CT criteria provided insufficient prognostic power. FDG PET/CT delineated active lesions better than did the combination of FDG PET and contrast-enhanced CT imaging. The authors concluded that both FDG PET and FDG PET/CT provided important prognostic information and that both have a significant impact on the clinical decision making in patients with GISTs.

Adding CT data to FDG PET increases the diagnostic accuracy by detecting additional lesions. Antoch et al. (58) examined 20 patients with histologically proven GISTs with FDG PET/CT imaging before and 1, 3, and 6 months after the start of imatinib therapy. Separate FDG PET and CT data sets, side-by-side FDG PET and CT data sets, and fused FDG PET/CT images were evaluated according to WHO, RECIST, and EORTC criteria for therapy response. Hounsfield units (HU) were assessed on CT images. The numbers of lesions detected in all patients were 135 with FDG PET, 249 with CT, 279 on side by-side evaluation, and 282 on fused FDG PET/CT images. Tumor response was correctly characterized in 95% of patients after 1 month and 100% after 3 and 6 months with FDG PET/CT. FDG PET and CT images viewed side by side were correct in 90% of patients at 1 month and 100% at 3 and 6 months. FDG PET accurately diagnosed tumor response in 85% of patients at 1 month and 100% at 3 and 6 months. CT was found to be accurate in 44% of patients at 1 month, 60% at 3 months, and 57% at 6 months. Hounsfield units were found to decrease by at least 25% in 12 of 14 responders after 1 month. The authors concluded that tumor response to imatinib should be assessed with a combination of morphologic and functional imaging. Image fusion with combined FDG PET/CT can provide additional information in individual cases when compared with side-by-side FDG PET and CT. In their study, Goerres et al. (57) reported that in comparison with FDG PET and contrast enhanced CT, FDG PET/CT delineated the lesions more precisely, allowing detailed surgical planning.

The observation that was originally made on MRI by Joensuu et al. (43) that GISTs responding to imatinib become hypodense and show a decrease in contrast enhancement on MRI has also been reported on CT, as mentioned above (52,53). This pattern of response is important to recognize because it may potentially lead to misinterpretation of progressive disease on CT when the patient is actually responding to the treatment. This situation is often seen in the context of hepatic metastases. After the initiation of treatment with imatinib, new hepatic lesions may be detected with a hypodense appearance. These lesions are most likely present prior to the start of imatinib, but, being isodense to the hepatic parenchyma they are difficult to characterize. In response to the treatment, these tumors become hypodense and can then be readily seen against the surrounding dense hepatic parenchyma. In the authors' experience, FDG PET can be of great help in resolving these types of ambiguous CT results. In the scenario described above, FDG PET will be negative, confirming that these patients are actually responding to the treatment. FDG PET can also be helpful when the findings on CT might suggest tumor growth, whether this increase in tumor size is actually the result of bleeding within the tumor mass or a result of other tumor swelling unrelated to progressive disease. In both of these cases, FDG PET will be negative confirming that the increase in size is not related to tumor progression.

It is clear that anatomic response assessment according to traditional criteria such as WHO, SWOG, or RECIST is not reflective of the true clinical benefit of tyrosine kinase inhibitors and that new anatomic methods are needed to monitor the effectiveness of molecular-targeted therapies such as imatinib. The newly proposed CT response criteria use either no growth in tumor size (50), or a combination of tumor density and size criteria (53) to assess the response of GIST patients to imatinib. As opposed to the standard SWOG or RECIST criteria, each of the new proposed methods show predictive values regarding time-to-treatment failure, as well as a close correlation with the results and predictive values demonstrated by FDG PET. These new criteria have each been validated in the center that produced them, and only in a patient population that was "naïve" to any treatment with tyrosine kinase inhibitors. These new criteria are not yet universally accepted, and they will need to be tested and validated outside of the specialized centers from which they originated. This should be done in a prospective multicenter setting and in different patient populations (including patients who have received prior tyrosine kinase inhibitors) before they can be considered as new anatomic guidelines for the evaluation of response to these drugs.

Patients who develop secondary resistance to imatinib generally show re-emergence of glycolytic activity within the site of the original tumor mass (Fig. 8.20.3A–C). FDG PET may therefore be useful during the surveillance of these patients to recognize clonal differentiation that leads to secondary resistance to imatinib. This re-emergence of glycolytic activity may or may not correlate with changes in the size of the mass as shown on CT. However, new patterns of recurrence have been defined on CT. One such pattern is a new intratumoral nodule arising from the wall of the mass ("nodule-within-a-mass") without a change in the overall size of the mass or an increase in the size of existing nodules (53,59–62).

Another interesting observation was made on FDG PET at the time of secondary resistance in patients receiving imatinib. As mentioned above, these patients showed increased FDG uptake at the tumor site (Fig. 8.20.3C). When this was first observed and disease recurrence was confirmed, these patients became eligible for enrollment in the trial that was then testing the second generation of tyrosine kinase inhibitors (sunitinib malate). Eligible patients were asked to stop imatinib prior to the start of the sunitinib therapy, and a repeat FDG PET was performed as the new baseline for the sunitinib trial. There was a significant rebound in glycolytic activity throughout the entire tumor mass in patients who underwent two FDG PET scans within 3 weeks or less between the end of imatinib therapy and prior to the initiation of sunitinib (Fig. 8.20.3D) (63). This "flare phenomenon" suggests that part of the mass is still responding to imatinib, and that cessation of the drug leads to reactivation of glycolytic metabolism in tumor cells that are still responding to imatinib, while the clonal differentiation that leads to secondary resistance and re-emergence of glycolytic activity probably affects another subpopulation of cells within that same tumor. This observation also suggests that compliance with the therapeutic regimen may be important to keep the tumor metabolism at bay, and that combination therapy with more than one tyrosine kinase inhibitor might need to be studied in the future.

CONCLUSION

Through the multidisciplinary collaborative efforts of many investigators, the GIST experience has resulted in the creation of several new paradigms that have helped to move new drugs along the experimental and regulatory pathways and to make these drugs available to the patients who need them. These new paradigms include the phenotypic and genotypic characterization of tumors, the design and testing of new molecular-targeting drugs, the monitoring of the response to these drugs, and the roles of anatomic and functional imaging in all of these steps.

Although contrast-enhanced CT has conventionally been the method of choice and will continue to play an important role in the management of patients with GISTs, it is also clear that FDG PET has been and continues to be instrumental to the success story of these drugs. The results of the first imatinib trial serve as the basis for the need to re-evaluate the traditional response assessment criteria when these types of drugs are used. Since most of the clinical PET studies done worldwide are now performed on combined hybrid PET/CT scanners (64,65), this gives us a unique opportunity to test and validate both new anatomic and functional response criteria in one setting (66). The use of PET/CT imaging with FDG or other PET tracers can potentially provide an *in vivo* pharmacodynamic assay of target hit, which can be a biomarker of response that is also predictive of outcome. This "one-stop shopping" concept may ultimately and cost-effectively shorten clinical trials and accelerate drug development. The lessons learned throughout the GIST experience are also helping to define the concept of personalized medicine and the design and implementation of new drugs and trials in other cancers including breast, lung, prostate, brain, and others.

ACKNOWLEDGMENTS

The authors thank Leonid Syrkin for his assistance with the figures, all the members of the nuclear medicine, radiology, and multidisciplinary teams for their expertise and dedication to our patients, and all the patients and their families who contributed so much of themselves for the benefit of all cancer patients.

REFERENCES

1. Mazur MT, Clark HB. Gastric stromal tumors. Reappraisal of histogenesis. *Am J Surg Pathol* 1983;7(6):507–519.
2. Kindblom LG, Remotti HE, Aldenborg F, et al. Gastrointestinal pacemaker cell tumor (GIPACT): gastrointestinal stromal tumors show phenotypic characteristics of the interstitial cells of Cajal. *Am J Pathol* 1998;152(5):1259–1269.
3. Hirota S, et al. Effects of loss-of-function and gain-of-function mutations of c-*kit* on the gastrointestinal tract. *J Gastroenterol* 2000;35[Suppl 12]:75–79.
4. Bucher P, Villiger P, Egger JF, et al Management of gastrointestinal stromal tumors: from diagnosis to treatment. *Swiss Med Wkly* 2004; 134(11–12):145–153.
5. Miettinen M, Lasota J. Gastrointestinal stromal tumors—definition, clinical, histological, immunohistochemical, and molecular genetic features and differential diagnosis. *Virchows Arch* 2001;438(1):1–12.
6. Blanchard DK, Budde J, Hatch GF 3rd, et al Tumors of the small intestine. *World J Surg* 2000;24(4):421–429.
7. Lau S, Tam K, Kam CK, et al. Imaging of gastrointestinal stromal tumor (GIST). *Clin Radiol* 2004;59(6):487–498.
8. DeMatteo RP, Lewis J, Leung D, et al. Two hundred gastrointestinal stromal tumors: recurrence patterns and prognostic factors for survival. *Ann Surg* 2000;231(1):51–58.
9. DeMatteo R. The GIST of targeted cancer therapy: a tumor (gastrointestinal stromal tumor), a mutated gene (c-*kit*), and a molecular inhibitor (STI571). *Ann Surg Oncol* 2002;9:831–839.
10. Fletcher CD, Berman JJ, Corless C, et al. Diagnosis of gastrointestinal stromal tumors: a consensus approach [comment]. *Hum Pathol* 2002; 33(5):459–465.
11. Lux ML, Rubin B, Biase TL, et al. *KIT* extracellular and kinase domain mutations in gastrointestinal stromal tumors. *Am J Pathol* 2000;156(3): 791–795.
12. Corless CL, Fletcher JA, Heinrich MC. Biology of gastrointestinal stromal tumors. *J Clin Oncol* 2004;22(18):3813–3825.
13. Heinrich MC, Corless CL, Demetri GC, et al. Kinase mutations and imatinib response in patients with metastatic gastrointestinal stromal tumor. *J Clin Oncol* 2003; 21(23):4342–4349.
14. Heinrich MC, Corless CL, Duensing A, et al. *PDGFRA* activating mutations in gastrointestinal stromal tumors. *Science* 2003;299(5607): 708–710.
15. Hirota S, Ohashi A, Nishida T, et al. Gain-of-function mutations of platelet-derived growth factor receptor alpha gene in gastrointestinal stromal tumors. *Gastroenterology* 2003;125(3):660–667.
16. Debiec-Rychter M, et al. *KIT* mutations and dose selection for imatinib in patients with advanced gastrointestinal stromal tumours. *Eur J Cancer* 2006;42(8):1093–1103.

17. Heinrich MC, Maki RG, Corless CL, et al. Sunitinib (SU) response in imatinib-resistant (IM-R) GIST correlates with *KIT* and *PDGFRA* mutation status. *Proc Am Assoc Clin Oncol* 2006;24:9502.
18. Strickland L, Letson GD, Muro-Cacho CA. Gastrointestinal stromal tumors. *Cancer Control* 2001;8(3):252–261.
19. Plaat BE, Hollema H, Molenaar WM, et al. Soft tissue leiomyosarcomas and malignant gastrointestinal stromal tumors: difference in clinical outcome and expression of multidrug resistance proteins. *J Clin Oncol* 2000;18(18):3211–3220.
20. Demetri GD, von Mehren M, Blanke CD, et al. Efficacy and safety of imatinib mesylate in advanced gastrointestinal stromal tumors [comment]. *N Engl J Med* 2002;347(7): 472–480.
21. Heinrich MC, Griffith DJ, Druker BJ, et al. Inhibition of c-*kit* receptor tyrosine kinase activity by STI571, a selective tyrosine kinase inhibitor. *Blood* 2000;96(3):925–932.
22. Tuveson DA, Willis NA, Jacks T, et al. STI571 inactivation of the gastrointestinal stromal tumor c-*KIT* oncoprotein: biological and clinical implications. *Oncogene* 2001;20(36):5054–5058.
23. Buchdunger E, Cioffi DL, Law N, et al. Abl protein-tyrosine kinase inhibitor STI571 inhibits in vitro signal transduction mediated by c-*kit* and platelet-derived growth factor receptors. *J Pharmacol Exp Ther* 2000;295(1): 139–145.
24. Perez EA, Livingstone AS, Franceschi D, et al. Current incidence and outcomes of gastrointestinal mesenchymal tumors including gastrointestinal stromal tumors. *J Am Coll Surg* 2006;202(4):623–629.
25. Green S, Weiss GR. Southwest Oncology Group standard response criteria, endpoint definitions and toxicity criteria. *Invest N Drugs* 1992; 10:239–253.
26. Van den Abbeele AD (for the GIST Collaborative PET Study Group Dana-Farber Cancer Institute, Boston, Massachusetts; OHSU, Portland, Oregon, Helsinki University Central Hospital, Turku University Central Hospital, Finland, Novartis Oncology). F18-FDG-PET provides early evidence of biological response to STI571 in patients with malignant gastrointestinal stromal tumors (GIST). *Proc Am Soc Clin Oncol* 2001; 20:362a.
27. Heinrich MC, Corless CL, Blanke CD, et al. Molecular correlates of imatinib resistance in gastrointestinal stromal tumors. *J Clin Oncol* 2006;24(29):4764–4774.
28. Demetri GD, van Oosterom AT, Garrett CR, et al. Efficacy and safety of sunitinib in patients with advanced gastrointestinal stromal tumour after failure of imatinib: a randomised controlled trial. *Lancet* 2006; 368(9544):1329–1338.
29. Therasse P, Arbuck SG, Eisenhauer EA, et al. New guidelines to evaluate the response to treatment in solid tumors. *J Natl Cancer Inst* 2000; 92:205–216.
30. Young H, Baum R, Cremerius U, et al. Measurement of clinical and subclinical tumor response using [18F]-fluorodeoxyglucose and positron emission tomography: review and 1999 EORTC recommendations. *Eur J Cancer* 1999;35:1773–1782.
31. Nguyen XC, Lee WW, Chung J-H, et al. FDG uptake, glucose transporter type 1, and Ki-67 expressions in non–small-cell lung cancer: correlations and prognostic values. *Eur J Radiol* 2007;62(2):214–219.
32. Lai CH, Yen T, Chang TC. Positron emission tomography imaging for gynecologic malignancy. *Curr Opin Obstet Gynecol* 2007;19:37–41.
33. Rademaker J. Hodgkin's and non-Hodgkin's lymphomas. *Radiol Clin North Am* 2007;45(1):69–83.
34. Blackstock AW, Farmer MR, Lovato J, et al. A prospective evaluation of the impact of 18-F-fluoro-deoxy-D-glucose positron emission tomography staging on survival for patients with locally advanced esophageal cancer. *Int J Radiat Oncol Biol Phys* 2006;64(2):455–460.
35. Weber WA, Ott K, Becker K, et al. Prediction of response to preoperative chemotherapy in adenocarcinomas of the esophagogastric junction by metabolic imaging. *J Clin Oncol* 2001;19:3058–3065.
36. Ott K, Fink U, Becker K, et al. Prediction of response to preoperative chemotherapy in gastric carcinoma by metabolic imaging: results of a prospective trial. *J Clin Oncol* 2003;21:4604–4610.
37. Hutchings M, Loft A, Hansen M, et al. FDG-PET after two cycles of chemotherapy predicts treatment failure and progression-free survival in Hodgkin lymphoma. *Blood* 2006;107(1):52–59.
38. Pottgen C, Levegrun S, Theegarten D, et al. Value of 18F-fluoro-2-deoxy-D-glucose-positron emission tomography/computed tomography in non–small-cell lung cancer for prediction of pathologic response and times to relapse after neoadjuvant chemoradiotherapy. *Clin Cancer Res* 2006;12(1):97–106.
39. Friedberg JW, Fischman A, Neuberg D, et al. FDG-PET is superior to gallium scintigraphy in staging and more sensitive in the follow-up of patients with *de novo* Hodgkin lymphoma: a blinded comparison. *Leukemia Lymphoma* 2004;45:85–92.
40. Kamiyama Y, Aihara R, Nakabayashi T, et al. 18F-fluorodeoxyglucose positron emission tomography: useful technique for predicting malignant potential of gastrointestinal stromal tumors. *World J Surg* 2005; 29(11):1429–1435.
41. Fletcher CD, Berman JJ, Corless C, et al. Diagnosis of gastrointestinal stromal tumors: a consensus approach. *Int J Surg Pathol* 2002;10(2): 81–89.
42. Rosenbaum SJ, Stergar H, Antoch G, et al. Staging and follow-up of gastrointestinal tumors with PET/CT. *Abdom Imaging* 2006;31(1): 25–35.
43. Joensuu H, Roberts PJ, Sarlomo-Rikala M, et al. Effect of the tyrosine kinase inhibitor ST1571 in a patient with a metastatic gastrointestinal stromal tumor. *N Engl J Med* 2001;344(14): 1052–1056.
44. Miller AB, Hoogstraten B, Staquet M, et al. Reporting results of cancer treatment. *Cancer Control* 1981;47:207–214.
45. Duffaud F, Blay YJ. Gastrointestinal stromal tumors: biology and treatment. *Oncology* 2003;65(3):187–197.
46. von Mehren M, Blanke C, Joensuu H, et al. High incidence of durable responses induced by imatinib mesylate (Gleevec) in patients with unresectable and metastatic gastrointestinal stromal tumors. *Proc Am Soc Clin Oncol* 2002;21:403a(abst 1608).
47. Van den Abbeele AD, Badawi RD. Use of positron emission tomography in oncology and its potential role to assess response to imatinib mesylate therapy in gastrointestinal stromal tumors (GISTs). *Eur J Cancer* 2002;38(5):S60–S65.
48. Dagher R, Cohen M, Williams G, et al. Approval summary: imatinib mesylate in the treatment of metastatic and/or unresectable malignant gastrointestinal stromal tumors. *Clin Cancer Res* 2002;8(10): 3034–3048.
49. Van den Abbeele AD, Badawi R, Cliché JP, et al. Response to imatinib mesylate therapy in patients with advanced gastrointestinal stromal tumors (GIST) is demonstrated by F-18-FDG-PET prior to anatomic imaging with CT. *Radiology* 2002;225:424P.
50. Holdsworth CH, Manola J, Badawi RD, et al. Use of computerized tomography (CT) as an early prognostic indicator of response to imatinib mesylate (IM) in patients with gastrointestinal stromal tumors (GIST). *Proc Am Soc Clin Oncol* 2004;22[Suppl 14]:3011.
51. Stroobants S, Goeminne J, Seegers M, et al. 18FDG-positron emission tomography for the early prediction of response in advanced soft tissue sarcoma treated with imatinib mesylate (Glivec). *Eur J Cancer* 2003; 39:2012–2020.
52. Choi H, Charnsangavej C, Macapinlac HA, et al. Correlation of computerized tomography (CT) and proton emission tomography (PET) in patients with metastatic GIST treated at a single institution with imatinib mesylate. *Proc Am Soc Clin Oncol* 2003;22:819.
53. Choi H, Charnsangavej C, de Castro Faria S, et al. CT evaluation of the response of gastrointestinal stromal tumors after imatinib mesylate treatment: a quantitative analysis correlated with FDG PET findings. *AJR Am J Roentgenol* 2004;183(6):1619–1628.
54. Heinicke T, Wardelmann E, Sauerbruch T, et al. Very early detection of response to imatinib mesylate for the treatment of gastrointestinal stromal tumours using 18fluoro-deoxyglucose-positron emission tomography. *Anticancer Res* 2005;25(6C):4591–4594.

55. Jager PL, Gietema JA, van der Graaf WT. Imatinib mesylate fro the treatment of gastrointestinal stromal tumours: best monitored with FDG PET. *Nucl Med Commun* 2004;25(5):433–438.
56. Gayed I, Vu T, Iyer R, et al. The role of ^{18}F-FDG PET in staging and early prediction of response to therapy of recurrent gastrointestinal stromal tumors. *J Nucl Med* 2004;45(1):17–21.
57. Goerres GW, Stupp R, Barghouth G, et al. The value of PET, CT and in-line PET/CT in patients with gastrointestinal stromal tumours: long-term outcome of treatment with imatinib mesylate. *Eur J Nucl Med Mol Imaging* 2005;32(2):153–62.
58. Antoch G, Kanja J, Bauer S, et al. Comparison of PET, CT, and dual-modality PET/CT imaging for monitoring of imatinib (ST1571) therapy in patients with gastrointestinal stromal tumors. *J Nucl Med* 2004; 45(3):357–365.
59. Shankar S, vanSonnenberg E., Desai J, et al. Gastrointestinal stromal tumor: new nodule-within-a-mass pattern of recurrence after partial response to imatinib mesylate. *Radiology* 2005;235:892–898.
60. Desai J, Shankar S, Heinrich MC, et al. Clonal evolution of resistance to imatinib (IM) in patients (pts) with gastrointestinal stromal tumor (GIST): molecular and radiologic evaluation of new lesions. *Clin Cancer Res* 2007;13(18):5398–5405.
61. Ryu M-H, Lee JL, Chang HM, et al. Patterns of progression in gastrointestinal stromal tumor treated with imatinib mesylate. *Jpn J Clin Oncol* 2006;36(1):17–24.
62. Hong X, Choi H, Loyer EM, et al. Gastrointestinal stromal tumor: role of CT in diagnosis and in response evaluation and surveillance after treatment with imatinib. *Radiographics* 2006;26(2): 481–495.
63. Van den Abbeele AD, Badawi R, Manola J, et al. Effects of cessation of imatinib mesylate (IM) therapy in patients (pts) with IM-refractory gastrointestinal stromal tumors (GIST) as visualized by FDG-PET scanning. *Proc Am Soc Clin Oncol* 2004;22:3012.
64. Beyer T, Townsend D, Brun T, et al. A combined PET/CT scanner for clinical oncology. *J Nucl Med* 2000;41:1369–1413.
65. Czernin J, Schelbert HR. Introduction. *J Nucl Med* 2007;48[1 Suppl]: 2S–3S.
66. Weber WA, Figlin R. Monitoring cancer treatment with PET/CT: does it make a difference? *J Nucl Med* 2007;48[1 Suppl]: 36S–44S.

CHAPTER

8.21 PET and PET/CT Imaging of Neuroendocrine Tumors

RICHARD P. BAUM AND VIKAS PRASAD

Neuroendocrine tumors (NET) are a heterogeneous group of neoplasms that are characterized by their endocrine metabolism and histology pattern. Several names such as carcinoid tumor, gastroenteropancreatic (GEP) tumor, islet cell tumor, neuroendocrine tumor, neuroendocrine carcinoma, and others have been suggested to cover the wide variety of tumor types belonging to NETs (1). The term *carcinoid* was first coined by Oberndorfer (2) in 1907 for endocrine tumors of the small intestine. Previously NETs have also been called APUD-oma (for *a*mine *p*recursor *u*ptake, and *d*ecarboxylation) and were suspected to have their origin from the neural crest, which was later found to be inappropriate because the peptide secreting cells of the tumors are not of the neuroectodermal unit (3).

The latest research has shown that pluripotent stem cells or differentiated neuroendocrine cells are responsible for the origin of different tumor subtypes (4). Apart from the diverse histological variants, the variable clinical manifestations, and the (frequently) slow growth, NETs present a unique challenge for the physicians to diagnose and treat these tumors at an early stage (5–7).

The various compounds produced by these tumors, along with their characteristic symptoms, although sometimes useful in the diagnosis of the disease, do not provide adequate information to allow a clinician to determine a treatment regime. The conventional imaging modalities like ultrasound, endoscopy, computed tomography (CT) scan, and magnetic resonance imaging (MRI), although very useful for detecting the site of the primary tumor, the number of lesions, and other anatomical parameters, do not give the functional status of the tumor, which is often essential for defining the prognosis (4).

The discovery of overexpression of receptors for peptide hormones in cancerous tissue in the mid-1980s led to the gradual upsurge in the role of nuclear medicine procedures in the diagnostic algorithms for NET (8). Since then, various radiopharmaceuticals targeting these tumor-related receptors, as well as various metabolic pathways peculiar to the neuroendocrine tumor cells, have been designed and used with great success (9).

INCIDENCE AND PATHOPHYSIOLOGY

The reported incidence of NET is low; however, because of the slow progression of many of these tumors, some patients may not get diagnosed during their lifetime. Traditionally, NETs are classified according to the site of origin (foregut, midgut, and hindgut), as tumors originating from the same site typically share functional properties, histochemistry, and secretory granules (3).

Based on histopathology, the World Health Organization (WHO) recently established a new classification system (10) (Table 8.21.1). Although NETs can occur at many sites in the body, the most common sites of origin are the GEP tract and the bronchus/lungs; other less common sites are the skin, the adrenal glands, the thyroid, and the genital tract (3). Neuroendocrine GEP tumors have been found to be derived from endodermal protodifferentiated stem cells (11) (Table 8.21.2). Approximately 70% of carcinoid tumors originating from gastrointestinal (GI) tissue are found in either the bronchus, jejuno-ileum, or colon/rectum (3).

HISTOLOGY

NETs consist of monotonous sheets of small, round cell nuclei and are characterized by their propensity for avidly staining with silver.

TABLE 8.21.1 World Health Organization Classification of Endocrine Tumors

Category
Well-differentiated endocrine tumor
Well-differentiated endocrine carcinoma
Poorly differentiated endocrine carcinoma
Mixed exocrine-endocrine tumor
Tumorlike lesion

Using immunohistochemical methods, typical markers of neuroendocrine tissues, like chromogranin, neuron-specific enolase (NSE), and synaptophysin can be detected. Electron microscopy reveals that these tumors possess numerous membrane-bound neurosecretory granules, which contain various hormones and biogenic amines (1).

CLINICAL MANIFESTATION

Based on clinical presentation, NETs can be broadly classified into functional and nonfunctional tumors. The functional tumors are characterized by the release of biogenic amines into the blood stream, which are responsible for producing characteristic clinical syndromes (3). The most common presenting symptoms of functional NETs are diarrhea, flushing, pain, asthma/wheezing, pellagra, and carcinoid heart disease like endocardial fibrosis (Hedinger syndrome). Approximately 33% to 50% of the NETs are nonfunctional. The symptoms present in this latter subset of patients with NET are largely related to the mass effect of the tumor, which varies by location. In many cases, these nonfunctional tumors are detected incidentally, often at a late stage when they have already metastasized.

The carcinoid tumors and tumors originating from the pancreas are mostly malignant in nature. Other than insulinomas, of which less than 10% are malignant, nearly all pancreatic NETs show malignant behavior. Among NETs of the GI tract, the highest incidence of metastases is found in jejuno-ileum tumors (58%), followed by lung/bronchus (6%) and rectum (4%). There are numerous factors determining the survival and the prognosis of patients; however, the presence of liver metastases is the single most important factor (6).

A correlation has been found between the size of the primary tumor and the chances of metastases in small intestinal carcinoids (3). Metastases to the liver occurred in 15% to 25% of tumors if the tumor diameter was less than 1 cm, in 58% to 80% if it was 1 to 2 cm, and greater than 75% if the tumor size was over 2 cm. These factors make it imperative to have a correct diagnostic algorithm before classifying a patient into a particular treatment regime (e.g., surgery, octreotide therapy, chemotherapy, or peptide receptor radionuclide therapy (PRRT).

TABLE 8.21.2 Origin of Gastroenteropancreatic Neuroendocrine Tumors

Derived from Protodifferentiated Adult Stem Cells	Tumor Type
Alpha cells	Gluganoma
Beta cells	Insulinoma
Delta cells	Somatostatinoma
EC cells	Enterochromaffin
G Cells	Gastrinoma
PP cells	PPoma

DIAGNOSIS

A detailed history and thorough clinical examination are essential and represent the first steps in the diagnostic algorithm for NET. The characteristic history of flushing and intractable diarrhea necessitates the measurement of urinary or plasma serotonin or its metabolites in the urine. Other NET markers like chromogranin A and NSE are also useful. These markers are generally elevated in carcinoid tumors. If a patient is suspected of having a gastrinoma (history of abdominal pain, diarrhea, and gastroesophageal reflex disease [GERD]), the fasting gastrin level should be measured. If the diagnosis of insulinoma is suspected (recurrent hypoglycemia), C-peptide and serum glucose levels are determined and an elevated insulin level should be demonstrated under fasting conditions. For pheochromocytoma, metanephrines, catecholamines, and their metabolites should be measured in blood and in the urine (3). In patients with severe watery diarrhea and hypokalemia (Verner Morrison syndrome), vasointestinal polypeptide (VIP) should be measured in serum. Cutaneous alterations (erythema necrolyticum migrans) are typical for glucagonoma syndrome and should lead to the measurement of glucagon in serum.

Imaging

After the determination of biochemical markers, the next step in the diagnostic algorithm is to localize the site of the primary tumor. A CT scan of the thorax should be performed if a thoracic origin of the tumor is suspected (12). The role of ultrasound in the diagnosis of NET depends largely on the site of disease. Ultrasound has a high diagnostic sensitivity for the detection of liver metastases. If a gastric or a pancreatic primary tumor is suspected, primarily endoscopic ultrasound (EUS) should be performed. For the assessment of the vascularity of a tumor, color Doppler and power Doppler ultrasound are useful as well as a contrast-enhanced CT scan. Very commonly CT scans from the neck through the pelvic floor are performed.

For preoperative staging, MRI and CT (primarily contrast-enhanced CT) are used for the localization of the primary tumor and metastases. These modalities are also useful in the follow-up of patients after primary surgery. The accurate measurement of tumor size and extent of spread can be evaluated using three-dimensional reconstruction. MRI is the method of choice for the study of cervical masses and is specifically useful in intracranial and intraspinal lesions as well as to evaluate for bone marrow involvement (12).

In spite of giving valuable anatomical information about the tumors, these morphologically oriented imaging methodologies are of limited use in the diagnosis of an unknown neuroendocrine primary tumor and in defining the prognosis of NETs. This is where nuclear medicine, with its armamentarium of radiopharmaceuticals, excels over morphological imaging. One other significant advantage of nuclear medicine imaging techniques is the ability to perform a whole-body scan in a single study.

Radionuclide Imaging of Neuroendocrine Tumors

Molecular imaging using diverse positron emission tomography (PET) radiopharmaceuticals has gained a special role in the diagnostic work-up of patients with NET only in the past decade, although radionuclide imaging with single photon tracers has been in use for the diagnosis of NET (e.g., using indium-labeled somatostatin analogues) for nearly 20 years (13,14).

PET Radiopharmaceuticals

To utilize the full potential of molecular imaging for tumor diagnosis, a metabolic pathway or a genuine molecular event (e.g., receptor binding of a peptide) that is specific for a certain kind of tumor or tissue/cells may be targeted. The wide range of biogenic amines and peptides secreted, and their receptor expression by NETs, has been extremely useful for the detection of these tumors. One of the radiopharmaceuticals, metaiodobenzylguanidine (MIBG), labeled with iodine-131 ([^{131}I]) (15) or with [^{123}I], utilizes the structural resemblance of MIBG to norepinephrine (NE). Just like NE, MIBG is taken up by an active amine uptake mechanism by the cell membrane of sympathomedullary tissue and also by the intracellular granules, which results in prolonged retention of the radiopharmaceutical in NETs.

Iodine-123 is the preferred radionuclide for labeling MIBG because of its better physical imaging characteristics and the ability to perform single-photon emission computed tomography (SPECT), whereas [^{131}I] MIBG can also be used for therapy. It is possible, however, that [^{124}I] MIBG may offer advantages over [^{123}I] MIBG in the coming years, but this requires further study.

Special care has to be taken to withdraw certain drugs (Table 8.21.3) that may interfere with the MIBG uptake (by interacting with vesicular monoamine transport mechanism) in order to avoid false-negative results (16–18). Despite the high specificity of [^{131}I] and [^{123}I]-labeled MIBG, the inherent drawback of gamma camera imaging (relatively low resolution and difficult to quantify) necessitated the development of radiopharmaceuticals based on positron-emitting radiotracers.

The list of PET tracers currently being employed for the imaging of NETs is growing rapidly (Table 8.21.4). In order to understand and compare the results of this wide range of PET radiopharmaceuticals, it is essential to first describe their respective molecular targets.

The molecular events/targets that are currently being utilized for PET-based radiopharmaceuticals are: (a) somatostatin receptor expression, (b) serotonin production pathway, (c) biogenic amine storage, (d) catecholamine transport, (e) glucose metabolism, (f) and other miscellaneous peptide receptor expression.

Pharmaceuticals Based on Somatostatin Receptor Expression of Neuroendocrine Tumors

Intact monoclonal antibodies and other smaller fragments of antibodies have been used extensively in nuclear medicine for both diagnosis and therapy. Although the U.S. Food and Drug Administration approval of yttrium-90 ([^{90}Y]) (e.g., Zevalin) and [^{131}I] (e.g., Bexxar)

TABLE 8.21.3 Drugs Interfering with Vesicular Monoamine Transporters, Potentially Leading to Wrong Interpretation of Iodine-123/131 Metaiodobenzylguanidine by Scintigraphy/SPECT

	Drugs		
Mechanism	Group/Use	Name	Suggested Withdrawal Period (in days)
Uptake-1 inhibition	Sympathomimetics	Cocaine, opiods	7–14
	Tricyclic antidepressants	Amitriptyline and its derivatives, imipramine and its derivatives, amoxapine, ioxapine, etc	7–21
	Antipsychotic/antiemetics	phenothiazines, thioxanthenes, butyrophenones	21–28
	Antihypertensive/cardiovascular	Labetalol, metoprolol	21
	Tetracyclic antidepressants	Maprotiline, mirtazapine	
Inhibition of granular uptake	Antihypertensive/cardiovascular	Reserpine	14
	Movement disorders	Tetrabenazine	
Competitive inhibition of granular uptake	Sympathomimetic	Norepinephrine	
	Antidepressant	Serotonin	14
	Antihypertensive	Guanethidine	
Depletion of storage granules	Antihypertensive/cardiovascular	Reserpine, guanethidine, labetalol, bethanidine, bretylium, debrisoquine	14–21
	Sympathomimetics	Phenylephrine, phenylpropanolamine, ephedrine, pseudoephedrine, amphetamine, dobutamine, dopamine, metaraminol	
Increased uptake and retention	Antihypertensives	Calcium channel blockers	14
		Angiotensin-converting enzyme inhibitors	14

TABLE 8.21.4 Different Radiopharmaceuticals Currently Employed for the Diagnosis of Neuroendocrine Tumors

Radiopharmaceutical		Radionuclide		Receptor/Metabolic Target		Imaging Protocol	
		Source	$T_{1/2}$		Dose (MBq)	Imaging Time Postinjection	Indication and Comments
PET	^{18}F-FDG	Cyclotron	110 min	Glycolytic pathway	340–740 (0.019mSv/ MBq)	60 min	Undifferentiated (small cell) NETs with a high proliferation rate. Not useful for highly differentiated NETs ("flip-flop" phenomenon when compared to Somatostatin Receptor [SMS-R] PET)
	^{68}Ga-DOTA-NOC	Generator	68.3 min	Somatostatin receptor (pan-somatostatin, high affinity for SSTR 2, 3, and 5)	100–150	60–90 min	All SSTR + VE NETs
	^{68}Ga-DOTA-TOC	Generator	68.3 min	Somatostatin receptor (high affinity for SSTR 2)	100–150	60–90 min	All SSTR + VE NETs
	^{11}C-5-HTP	Cyclotron	20.4 min	Serotonin production pathway	140–521	20 min	All serotonin-producing NETs
	^{11}C-DOPA	Cyclotron	20.4 min	Dopamine production pathway	–	–	Pheochromocytoma, paraganglioma, neuroblastoma. Difficult logistics (short half life), costly production.
	^{18}F-DOPA	Cyclotron	110 min	Dopamine production pathway	200–300 (2.7 mSv/ 100 MBq)	45–90 min	Pheochromocytoma, paraganglioma, neuroblastoma, glomus tumor
	^{18}F-FDA	Cyclotron	110 min	Catecholamine precursor	370–740	Immediately after injection	Pheochromocytoma, paraganglioma, neuroblastoma
	^{64}Cu-TETA-octretoide	Reactor/cyclotron	12.7 hr	Somatostatin receptor	111		All SSTR + VE NETs
	^{18}F-FP-Gluc-TOCA	Cyclotron	110 min	Somatostatin receptor	65–155	Immediately after injection (until 2 hr)	All SSTR + VE NETs
	^{11}C-ephidrine	Cylotron	20.4 min	Catecholamine transporter	–	–	Pheochromocytoma, neuroblastoma, study of sympathetic nervous system
	^{11}C-hydroxyeph-idrine	Cyclotron	20.4 min	Catecholamine transporter		Immediately after injection	Pheochromocytoma, neuroblastoma, study of sympathetic nervous system

Gamma camera	^{111}In-somatostatin analogues	Cyclotron	2.8 days	Somatostatin receptor	~220	4, 24, and 48 hr	All SSTR +VE NETs
	^{99m}Tc-HYNIC-TOC	Generator	6 hr	Somatostatin receptor	740–950	2 and 4 hr	All SSTR +VE NETs
	^{131}I-MIBG	Reactor	8 days	Catecholamine transporter	37–74 (specific activity ≥ 74 MBq/ mg)	24, 48, 72 hr (up to 120 hr)	Pheochromocytoma, neuroblastoma, paraganglioma
	^{123}I-MIBG	Cyclotron	159	Catecholamine transporter	370 (specific activity 300 MBq/mg)	4–6 hr and 24 hr	Pheochromocytoma, neuroblastoma, paraganglioma. SPECT possible
	^{99m}Tc DMSA(V)	Generator	140	Not clear, probably related to glucose-mediated acidosis in tumors/ structural similarity between DMSA(V) core and PO_4^{-3} which is avidly taken by tumors	740	2 hr	Medullary thyroid cancer

C, carbon, carbon-11-E/carbon-11-HED/fluorine-18-fluorodopamine PET scans; Cu, copper; DOPA, L-dihydroxyphenylalanine; DOTA-NOC, DOTA-1-Nal^3-octreotide; DOTA-TOC, DOTA-D-Phe1-Tyr3-octreotide; F, fluorine; FDA, fluorodopamine; Ga, gallium; 5-HTP, 5-hydroxytryptamine; HYNIC, ; I, iodine; In, indium; ^{99m}Tc, molybdenum-99-technetium; NET, neuroendocrine tumors; MIBG, metaiodobenzylguanidine; SPECT, single-photon emission computed tomography; SSTR, somatostatin receptors; TETA, ; VE, . (From Rufini V, Calcagni ML, Baum RP. Imaging of neuroendocrine tumors. *Semin Nucl Med* 2006;36:228–247; Win Z, Rahman L, Murrell J, et al. The possible role of ^{68}Ga-DOTATATE PET in malignant abdominal paraganglioma. *Eur J Nucl Med Mol Imaging* 2006;33:506; Horiuchi K, Saji H, Yokoyama A. Tc(V)-DMS tumor localization mechanism: a pH-sensitive Tc(V)-DMS-enhanced target/nontarget ratio by glucose-mediated acidosis. *Nucl Med Biol* 1998;25:549–555, with permission.)

labeled anti-CD20 antibodies for the treatment of B cell non-Hodgkin's lymphoma finally proved the success of radioimmunotherapy of hematological malignancies, the same is not true for imaging purposes because of the poor pharmacokinetics of whole monoclonal antibodies and the potential to generate an immune response. The discovery of overexpression of peptide receptors in various tumor cells in the 1980s opened a new chapter in the field of molecular imaging (8). Small peptides have better pharmacokinetic characteristics and no (or very low) antigenicity as compared to antibodies, making them nearly ideal ligands for receptor-based radionuclide imaging. Somatostatin, a cyclic peptide hormone, labeled with different radionuclides, is an example of such a peptide that has been used with high efficiency in the diagnosis of NETs.

There are two naturally occurring bioactive forms of somatostatin: somatostatin-14 and somatostatin-28. Somatostatin receptors are normally expressed in different organs, such as the pituitary gland, thyroid, pancreas, liver, in the spleen (activated lymphocytes), and GI tract in different quantities. The primary action of this peptide hormone is the inhibition of hormone secretion and modulation of neurotransmission and cell proliferation through specific membrane bound G-protein-coupled receptors (19). These somatostatin receptors (SSTR) have generated wide clinical interest as they are expressed on various tumor types (20).

Five different types of SSTR proteins have been cloned (SSTR 1 through 5). Recent studies revealed that SSTR 2 consists of two subtypes, SSTR 2a and SSTR 2b. Some of these receptors, especially SSTR 2, are overexpressed in NET, which forms the basis of peptide receptor imaging using radiolabeled somatostatin analogues (19). Of importance is also to understand the complex interaction between SSTR 2 and SSTR 5. Sharif et al. (21) have shown that the presence of SSTR 5 in the same cells modulates trafficking and cell surface regulation of SSTR 2a and cellular desensitization to the effects of the somatostatin (sometimes also known as somatotropin release-inhibiting factor). Prolonged treatment with Sandostatin LAR/s.c. (Novartis Oncology, East Hanover, New Jersey) may have some bearing on the imaging with radiolabeled somatostatin receptor ligands.

For defining the dosimetry of a radiopharmaceutical, and also for determining the potential cause of false-positive results, it is essential to know the expression of SSTR in normal and in nonmalignant tissues. Table 8.21.5 shows in detail the expression of SSTR

TABLE 8.21.5 Normal Organs/Tissues and Somatostatin Receptor Expression

Tissues	Somatostatin Receptor Subtypes (SSTR)
Vessels (veins and arteries) +	SSTR 1, 2, and 4
Endothelial cells +	SSTR 1
Nerve plexus (myenteric)	
Pancreatic islets	SSTR 1-3
Adrenal medulla	SSTR 3
Adrenal cortex	SSTR 1–3 & 5
Prostatic stroma	
Gastric mucosa	SSTR 1–5
Pituitary gland	SSTR 1–5
Colon mucosa	SSTR 5
Spleen	SSTR 2
Lymphocytes and monocytes	
Activated T cells	SSTR 5
Normal T cells (peripheral blood)	SSTR 1–5
Monocytes, macrophages, and dendritic cells	SSTR 2
Salivary glands	SSTR 2A, 2B, 3, & 5
Germinal center	SSTR 2
Fibroblasts	
Lymphoreticular tissues	SSTR 2, 3, & 5
Parathyroid	SSTR 1, 3, 4
Thymus	SSTR 1, 2A, & 3
Duodenum	SSTR 1–5
Ileum	SSTR 5
Bronchial glands	SSTR 1, 2B, 3–5
Cerebellum (Purkinje cells)	SSTR 5
Kidney	SSTR 1–5
Testes and ovary	SSTR 2a
Myocardium	SSTR 2a & 5
Bone marrow	SSTR 2a
Normal hepatocytes	No SSTR expression
Skeletal muscles	No SSTR expression
Trachea	No SSTR expression
Thyroid C cells	—

TABLE 8.21.6 Tumors with Proven Somatostatin Receptor Expression

Tumor Types	Receptor Subtypes
Gastroenteropancreatic neuroendocrine tumors	SSTR 1, SSTR 2, SSTR 5
Neuroblastoma	SSTR 2
Meningioma	SSTR 2
Breast carcinoma	SSTR 2
Medulloblastoma	SSTR 2
Lymphoma	SSTR 2, SSTR 5
Renal cell carcinoma	SSTR 2
Paraganglioma	SSTR 1, SSTR 2, SSTR 3
Small cell lung cancer	SSTR 2
Hepatoma	SSTR 2
Prostate carcinoma	SSTR 1
Sarcoma	SSTR 1, SSTR 2, SSTR 4
Inactive pituitary adenoma	SSTR 1, SSTR 2, SSTR 3, SSTR 5
Growth hormone-producing pituitary adenoma	SSTR 2, SSTR 3, SSTR 5
Gastric carcinomas	SSTR 1, SSTR 2, SSTR 5
Ependydomas	SSTR 1
Pheochromocytoma	SSTR 1, SSTR 2, SSTR 5
Non-small cell lung cancer	Not availabe
Pituitary adenoma	Not availabe
Medullary thyroid carcinoma	Not availabe
Merkel cell skin carcinoma	Not availabe
Ganglioma	Not availabe
Ganglioneuroblastoma	Not availabe

SSTR, somatostatin receptors.

in different normal tissues (22–28). Of particular importance is the expression of SSTR on activated lymphocytes, macrophages, and fibroblasts. Most of the tumors that have been studied with radiolabeled somatostatin analogues mainly express SSTR 2. However, recent results have shown that SSTR 1 and SSTR 3, 4, and 5 are also expressed on many tumors (Table 8.21.6) with varying percentages of expression (23).

SSTR 2 is expressed maximally (95%) in neuroendocrine tumors of midgut origin, followed by SSTR 1 (80%) and SSTR 5 (75%) (3). This observation has lead to the gradual modification of somatostatin analogue synthesis. Most of the currently used somatostatin radiopharmaceuticals (Table 8.21.7) are derivatives of octreotide, lanreotide, or vapreotide and show variable binding to SSTR (17,19,29,30).

TABLE 8.21.7 Affinity Profiles (IC50) of Somatostatin Receptor Subtypes for Different Somatostatin Analogues (the Smaller the Value, the Higher the Affinity)

Somatostatin Analogues	SSTR 1	SSTR 2	SSTR 3	SSTR 4	SSTR 5
Native somatostatin (SS28)	5.2	2.7	7.7	5.6	4.0
In-DTPA-octreotide	>10,000	22	182	>1,000	237
In-DOTA-[Tyr3]octreotide (DOTA-TOC)	>10,000	4.6	120	230	130
Y-DOTA-TOC	>10,000	11	389	>10,000	114
Ga-DOTA-TOC	>10,000	2.5	613	>1,000	73
DOTA-lanreotide (DOTA-LAN)	>10,000	26	771	>10,000	73
DOTA-[Tyr3]octreotate (DOTA-TATE)	>10,000	1.5	>1,000	453	547
In-DOTA[1-Nal3]octreotide (DOTA-NOC)	>10,000	2.9	8	227	11.2
Y-DOTA[1-Nal3]octreotide (DOTA-NOC)	>1,000	3.3	26	>1,000	10.4
In-DOTA-NOC-ATE	>10,000	2	13	160	4.3
In-DOTA-BOC-ATE [(DOTA, BzThi^3, Thr^8)-octreotide]	>1,000	1.4	5.5	135	3.9

Ga, gallium; In, indium; SSTR, somatostatin receptors; y, yttrium.

(Adapted from Antunes P, Ginj M, Zhang H, et al. Are radiogallium-labelled DOTA-conjugated somatostatin analogues superior to those labelled with other radiometals? *Eur J Nucl Med Mol Imaging* 2007; 34:982–993, with permission.)

The first radiolabeled somatostatin analogue to be approved for scintigraphy of NET was [^{111}In]-DTPA-D-Phe1-octreotide ([^{111}In]-pentetreotide; OctreoScan, Mallinckrodt, Inc, St. Louis, Missouri). Large clinical studies have shown that this radiopharmaceutical is well suited for the scintigraphic localization of primary and metastatic NETs (31,32). Molybdenum-99-technetium (^{99m}Tc)-labeled somatostatin analogues, such as ^{99m}Tc-depreotide (6-hydrazinonicotinic), ^{99m}Tc-vapreotide, ^{99m}Tc-P829, and ^{99m}Tc-EDDA-HYNIC-TOC, have also been used (32–37). Among these, only ^{99m}Tc-EDDA-HYNIC-TOC (or -TATE) has been shown in a larger patient population to be superior to [^{111}In]-pentetreotide for the detection of SSTR-positive tumors and metastases (33).

In an effort to find a somatostatin analogue with higher affinity for SSTR receptors, the next generation of somatostatin analogues (e.g., DOTA-TOC [DOTA-D-Phe1-Tyr3-octreotide]) (16) were developed and labeled with different radionuclides for imaging as well as for therapy (38–45). Replacement of the alcohol group at the C-terminus of the peptide by a carboxylic acid group resulted in the formation of DOTA-D-Phe^1-Tyr^3-Thr^8-octreotide (DOTA-TATE) and has been shown to have very high affinity for the SSTR 2 receptor, which even surpasses the binding affinity of natural somatostatin (29,46).

The binding affinity to other SSTR receptors is low (SSTR 5) or negligible (SSTR 3), and there is no significant affinity to SSTR 1 and SSTR 4 (19). Indium-111-DOTA-lanreotide (LAN; D-2-Nal-Cys-tyr-D-Trp-Lys-Val-Thr-NH2) has been postulated to be superior to [^{111}In]-DTPA-octreotide in the detection of neuroendocrine pancreatic carcinoma (47). However, the claim that [^{111}In]-DOTA-lanreotide targets SSTR 2 through 5 with higher affinity and SSTR 1 with lower affinity was not confirmed by Reubi et al. (29).

Next in the development of high-affinity somatostatin analogues was DOTA-NOC (DOTA-1-Nal^3-octreotide), which was the result of amino acid exchange at position 3 of octreotide (Fig. 8.21.1). This compound has improved affinity for SSTR 2 and higher affinity to SSTR 3 and SSTR 5 (19), resulting in coverage of a wider spectrum of SSTR (pansomatostatin analogue). It is expected to have a significant effect on staging, diagnosis, and therapy of NETs and various other somatostatin receptor–expressing tumors. All these somatostatin analogues labeled with various radionuclides have been used for scintigraphy or PET of SSTR positive tumors with variable success. Other somatostatin analogues, which are in the preclinical stage of development, are DOTA-NOC-ATE [(DOTA-1Nal^3,Thr^8)-octreotide] and DOTA-BOC-ATE [(DOTA, BzThi^3, Thr^8)-octreotide]. Also radiolabeled with [^{111}In], these "fourth-generation analogues" have been shown to have very high affinity for SSTR 2, SSTR 3, and SSTR 5 and intermediate high affinity to SSTR 4 (48).

SSTR antagonists, (NH(2)-CO-c(DCys-Phe-Tyr-DAgl(8)(Me,2-naphthoyl)-Lys-Thr-Phe-Cys)-OH (SST(3)-ODN-8) and (SST(2)-ANT) have also been labeled with [^{111}In], and their superiority over SSTR agonists (in murine models) for *in vivo* targeting of SSTR 2 and SSTR 3 rich tumors, as shown by the group of Ginj et al. (49) and Reubi et al. (50), has resulted in the shift in paradigm, and they are now being contemplated for use in tumor diagnosis. The intrinsic superior efficiency and resolution of PET imaging favors the use of PET-labeled SSTR binding agents if the kinetics of the PET tracer are similar to those of the single photon emitter. Thus, both PET and SPECT SSTR binding agents will likely be used in practice.

Pharmaceuticals Based on the Serotonin Production Pathway

Most of the clinical symptoms of a neuroendocrine tumor are due to the excessive production of serotonin. The name serotonin was coined by Maurice M. Robert in 1948 and literally means "a serum

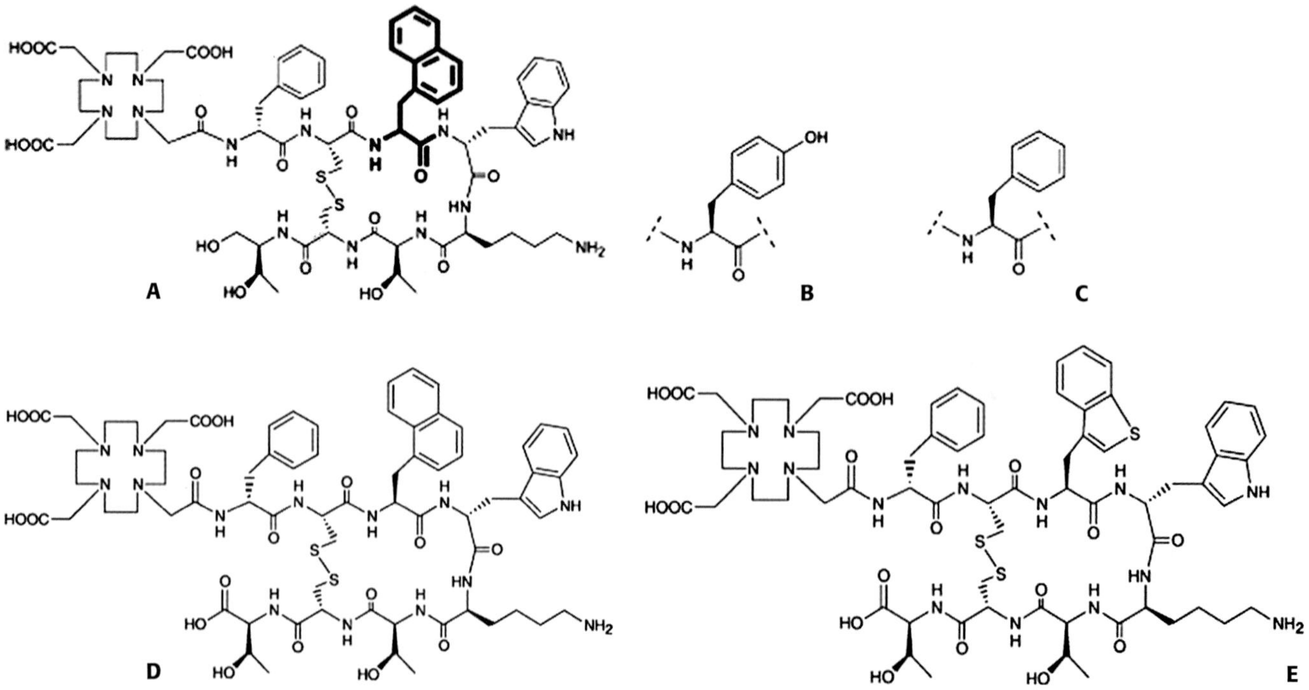

FIGURE 8.21.1. Chemical structure of different synthetic somatostatin analogues. **A:** DOTA-NOC (DOTA-1-Nal^3-octreotide). **B:** DOTA-TOC (DOTA-D-Phe1-Tyr3-octreotide). **C:** DOTA-OC (DOTA-octreotide). **D:** DOTA-NOC-ATE ([DOTA-1Nal^3, Thr^8]-octreotide). **E:** DOTA-BOC-ATE (DOTA, BzThi^3, Thr^8)-octreotide) For reference see text.

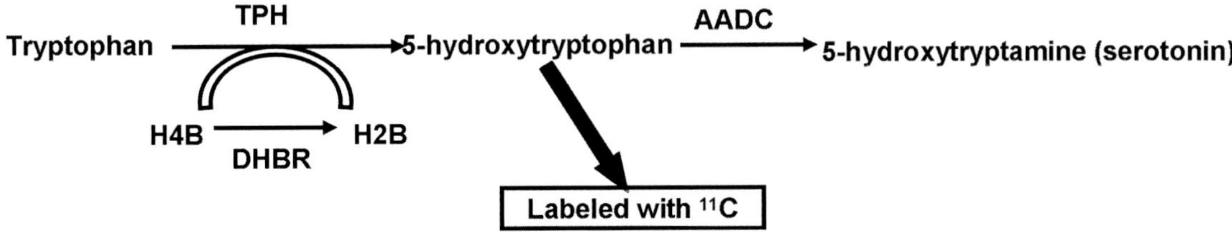

FIGURE 8.21.2. Serotonin production pathway. AADC, aromatic L-amino acid decarboxylase; DHPR, dihydropteridine reductase, H2B, dihydrobiopterin, H4B, tetrahydrobiopterin, TPH, tryptophan hydroxylase.

agent responsible for producing vasoconstriction." It was later identified as 5-hydroxytryptamine (HTP). The precursor for the production of 5-hydroxytryptamine is tryptophan (Fig. 8.21.2). One of the intermediates in the production pathway, HTP has been labeled successfully with carbon-11 ([^{11}C]) in a phase I clinical trial. After administration, the functionally active, serotonin-producing neuroendocrine tumor cells accumulate the radiopharmaceutical, leading to visualization on the PET images.

Pharmaceuticals Based on Biogenic Amine Production and Storage Mechanism

Neuroendocrine tumors are characterized by the production and storage of several biogenic amines. One radiopharmaceutical that has been designed based on this observation is [^{11}C]- or fluorine-18 ([^{18}F])-labeled L-dihydroxyphenylalanine (DOPA). The increase in the activity of L-DOPA decarboxylase is one of the hallmarks of NETs (51,52). The metabolic pathway leading to the production of dopamine by the decarboxylation reaction is shown in Fig. 8.21.3.

Pharmaceuticals Based on the Catecholamine Transport Pathway

The success achieved by MIBG encouraged scientists to develop PET radiopharmaceuticals based on the catecholamine transport mechanism. Pheochromocytoma, neuroblastoma and other chromaffin tumor tissues, due to their ability to produce epinephrine and norepinephrine, concentrate many synthetic amine precursors using catecholamine transporters. Carbon-11-epinephrine ([^{11}C]-E) and [^{11}C]-hydroxyepiphedrine (^{11}C-HED) are catecholamine analogues and [^{18}F]-fluorodopamine (^{18}F-FDA) is a catecholamine precursor, developed by the National Institutes of Health. Like [^{123}I]/[^{131}I]-MIBG, these radiopharmaceuticals may also be prone to interference by drugs (Table 8.21.3), acting on vesicular monoamine transporters and the norepinephrine transporter (16).

Pharmaceuticals Based on Increased Glucose Metabolism

The one molecule that has revolutionized the way nuclear medicine is being practiced these days is [^{18}F]-2-fluoro-2-deoxyglucose ([^{18}F]-FDG), the "molecule of the century," as it was termed by H. N. Wagner, Jr.). Its utilization for tumor imaging is based on the high glucose metabolism of many cancer cells for meeting their energy demand. Fluorine-18-FDG enters the glycolytic pathway like glucose in cytoplasm where it is phosphorylated by the enzyme hexokinase to [^{18}F]-FDG-6-phosphate; however, it is not significantly metabolized, resulting in further accumulation (trapping) inside the cancer cell.

Pharmaceuticals Based on Miscellaneous Other Peptides Produced by Neuroendocrine Tumors

The list of peptides that are secreted by NETs is growing steadily, and several of them have been used by nuclear medicine scientists for imaging purposes (Table 8.21.8).

One of the peptides that has been labeled with a positron emitter is bombesin (gallium-68 [^{68}Ga]-bombesin). Bombesin and its human counterpart, the gastrin-releasing peptide (GRP) receptors, are expressed mainly on undifferentiated prostate cancers, breast carcinomas, small cell lung cancer, as well as renal cell carcinomas and some neuroendocrine tumors. Initial results are encouraging both for diagnosis as well as for therapy (e.g., using lutetium-177-labeled AMBA (DO3A-CH2CO-G-4-aminobenzoyl-Q-W-A-G-H-L-MNH2) for the treatment of prostate cancer (53–59).

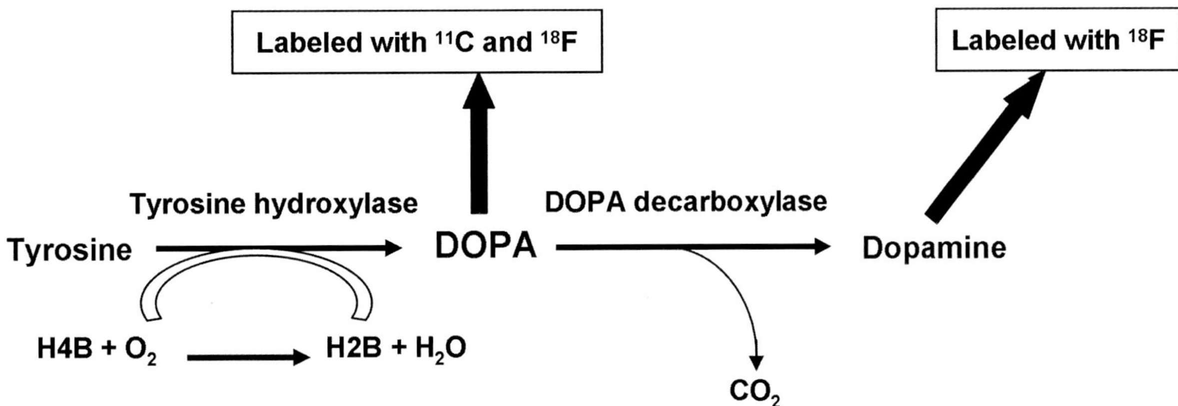

FIGURE 8.21.3. Dopamine production pathway. DOPA, dihydroxyphenylalanine; H2B, dihydrobiopterin; H4B, tetrahydrobiopterin.

TABLE 8.21.8 Peptides Targeted for Imaging and Therapy

Peptides	Radiolabeled Peptides	Receptor	Tumor-Expressing Receptors
Bombesin/GRP	^{99m}Tc-bombesin, ^{111}In-bombesin, ^{68}Ga-bombesin ^{177}Lu-AMBA (for therapy)	GRP-R	Prostate cancer, breast cancer, GIST, SCLC
CCK/gastrin	^{111}In-DTPA-minigastrin, ^{90}Y minigastrin (for therapy)	CCK-2	MTC, SCLC, GIST, insulinoma
GLP-1	^{123}I-GLP-1	GLP-1-R	Insulinoma, gastrinoma
Neuropeptide Y	^{99m}Tc-neuropeptide Y	NPY-R	Breast cancer, ovarian tumor, adrenal tumor
VIP	^{123}I-VIP, ^{99m}Tc-TP3654	VPAC1	Gastrointestinal, other epithelial cancer
Neurotensin	^{99m}Tc- neurotensin	NT-R1	Exocrine pancreatic cancer, Ewing sarcoma
Substance P	^{90}Y-DOTAGA-substance P (for therapy)	NK1	Glial tumors

AMBA, DO3A-CH2CO-G-4-aminobenzoyl-Q-W-A-G-H-L-MNH2; CCK, cholecystokinin; Ga, gallium; GLP, glucagon-like peptide, GIST, gastrointestinal stromal tumors; GRP-R, gastrin releasing peptide receptor; In, indium; Lu, lutetium; ^{99m}Tc, metastable state of technetium; MTC, medullary thyroid carcinomas; NK, neurokinin; SCLC, small cell lung cancer; VIP, vasoactive intestinal peptide; VPAC, VIP pituitary adenylate cyclase activating polypeptide; Y, yttrium.
(Modified from Rufini V, Calcagni ML, Baum RP. Imaging of neuroendocrine tumors. *Semin Nucl Med* 2006;36:228–247, with permission.)

VIP, a 28 amino acid peptide, initially isolated from porcine intestine, radiolabeled with either ^{99m}Tc or [^{123}I], has also been used for imaging of NETs. Two subtypes of VIP receptors (VIPAC1 and VIPAC2) have been described. VIP receptors, predominantly VIPAC1, are expressed in the majority of breast, prostate, lung, pancreas, colon, stomach, liver, and bladder carcinomas. Leiomyomas predominantly express VPAC2 receptors, whereas paragangliomas, glial tumors, neuroblastomas, pituitary adenomas, pheochromocytomas, and endometrial carcinomas most commonly express VPAC1 receptors. Although only a few results have been published, one potential clinical indication is the scintigraphic imaging of neuroendocrine GEP tumors, especially VIPomas (60–64).

Other peptides that have been used for receptor scintigraphy of NETs are cholecystokinin (CCK-B), gastrin, minigastrin, and others, and work is ongoing to find the best peptide for targeting various NE tumors (53,65–69).

Germanium-68/Gallium-68 Generator

The high cost associated with the establishment and maintenance of cyclotrons encouraged the development of generators for the production of positron emitters. The germanium-68 ([^{68}Ge]/gallium-68 ([^{68}Ga]) generator was first mentioned in 1961 (70), but due to the limited use of PET and the difficulties associated with the handling of later versions of the generator (71,72), it did not gain momentum until several decades later (73). Since the development of DOTA (a strong chelator for [^{68}Ga]), octreotide derivatives, mainly developed by Maecke et al. (9) and an industrially available [^{68}Ge]/[^{68}Ga] generator system constructed by the Rösch and Knapp (73), an increasing number of centers in Europe are using [^{68}Ga]- DOTA-somatostatin analogues for the diagnosis of NETs (with PET or PET/CT). A brief description of the generator is given here.

Gallium-68 ($t_{1/2}$= 68 min) is an excellent positron emitter with 89% positron emission and negligible gamma emission (1,077 keV) of 3.2 % only. The long half-life of the mother radionuclide [^{68}Ge] (270.8 days) means that the generator can be used for 9 months to 1 year depending on the demand of a particular center. Early generator systems used aluminum or zirconium oxide as the matrix and the eluted product of the generator, [^{68}Ga]-EDTA (ethylenediaminetetraacetic acid), was directly applied for tumor imaging with limited success. Subsequently, several different matrices have been used, but nowadays the most commonly used commercially available [^{68}Ge]/[^{68}Ga] generator is based on a TiO_2 phase containing as much as 1.85 GBq (50 mCi) of [^{68}Ge]. "Ionic" [^{68}Ga]$^{3+}$ is eluted in 0.1 N HCl (normal hydrochloric acid) solution with a [^{68}Ga] yield of more than 60% in 5 mL and [^{68}Ge] breakthrough not exceeding 5×10^{-3}%. However, prior to labeling, the eluate product undergoes several postprocessing steps (anion exchange, cation exchange, fractionation), because of the large volume, [^{68}Ge] breakthrough, high H^+ concentration, and impurities such as Zn(II), Ti(IV), and Fe(III). The most successful method of postprocessing is a cation exchange (73).

Zhernosekov et al. (74) have shown that processing on a cation exchanger in hydrochloric acid/acetone media represents an efficient strategy for the concentration and purification of generator-derived [^{68}Ga]-(III) eluates. The developed scheme guarantees high yields and safe preparation of injectable [^{68}Ga]-labeled radiopharmaceuticals for routine application and is easy to automate.

Labeling of DOTA-NOC, DOTA-TOC, and DOTA-TATE with Gallium-68

Various institutions use different labeling techniques (9,75–77) and a detailed discussion is beyond the scope of this chapter; therefore, only the [^{68}Ga]-labeling of DOTA-NOC, DOTA-TOC, and DOTA-TATE, as developed by Baum et al. (78) and first applied routinely in a large number of patients is discussed here.

Gallium-68 elute is first concentrated and purified using the microchromatography method as described by Rösch and Knapp (73). Following preconcentration and purification of the initial generator eluates, [^{68}Ga](III) is eluted with 400 μL 98% acetone/0.05 N HCl solution (2×10^{-5} mol HCl). This fraction is used directly for labeling of DOTA-octreotide derivatives such as DOTA-TOC, DOTA-NOC, or DOTA-TATE. In our clinical experience, using DOTA-NOC in over 1,500 patient studies, 1 GBq of [^{68}Ga] is put into a vial containing 30 to 50 μg of the peptide to produce [^{68}Ga] DOTA-NOC with a specific activity of 15 MBq/μg of peptide. Gallium-68 DOTA-NOC was purified and finally eluted using 0.5 mL ethanol into 4.5 mL of isotonic saline. Radiolabeling yields of greater than 95% were usually achieved within 15 minutes. Overall, 370 to 700 MBq of [^{68}Ga] DOTA-NOC were obtained within 20 minutes.

For DOTA-TOC, the processed eluate containing [^{68}Ga] (up to 700 MBq) is added to 4 to 4.5 mL of pure water in the reagent vial containing 7 to 14 nmol DOTA-TOC with the addition of Hepes buffer. Gallium-68-labeled DOTA-derivatized octreotide is purified from unreacted [^{68}Ga] species by reversed phase chromatography. The reaction mixture is then passed through a small C18 cartridge and after washing the cartridge with 5 mL water, the [^{68}Ga]-labeled peptide is recovered with 200 to 400 μL of pure ethanol. A radiolabeling yield of 88% at approximately 99°C is achieved within 10 minutes with specific activities of up to 450 MBq/μmol of peptide (76).

RADIONUCLIDE IMAGING METHODS

Rapid development in electronics, detector materials, and software has kept pace with the requirements of the present generation of molecular imaging agents. Nuclear medicine currently employs the following basic methods of imaging, which have their own merits and shortcomings: (a) planar imaging, (b) SPECT, (c) SPECT-CT, (d) PET, and (e) PET/CT.

Single-photon Emission Computed Tomography versus Planar Imaging

Planar imaging, being two-dimensional, has the major disadvantage of lacking the precise localization of the tumor site. SPECT has the advantage of three-dimensional reconstruction and thus assists in better localization. In addition, SPECT is more sensitive for the detection of deep-seated tumors.

Single-photon Emission Computed Tomography versus PET

One of the major disadvantages of SPECT imaging is that absolute quantification is not possible (or at least is very difficult), and reliable semiquantitative data are difficult to obtain. However, from a clinical point of view, it is essential to have quantitative (or semiquantitative) data apart from visual qualitative data for the proper follow-up of cancer patients under strict guidelines (like European Organisation for Research and Treatment of Cancer, Response Evaluation Criteria in Solid Tumors RECIST, WHO) and for better patient management. This is today routinely only possible through PET or PET/CT. The higher resolution of PET imaging also makes it much superior to SPECT. The only limiting factor with PET is the higher cost of the equipment, making SPECT the most commonly used imaging method in oncology in various countries (especially less developed/developing countries).

The maintenance of cyclotron units and the implementation of good manufacturing practice rules have made the running costs of a fully functional PET-cyclotron unit very high (and out of reach of many developing countries). This is where the in-house positron emitting radionuclide generators, because of their low cost and easy availability, play a very critical role in the further spread of this technology throughout the world.

PET vs. PET/CT and Single-photon Emission Computed Tomography versus Single-photon Emission Computed Tomography–CT

Because nuclear medicine imaging in general lacks detailed anatomical information, the addition of CT to PET or SPECT helps in the precise localization of lesions. The present generation of PET scanners used for oncologic imaging nearly all have an embedded CT in the gantry, which makes it possible to obtain contrast/noncontrast enhanced CT scans with excellent resolution. It is possible to obtain both the anatomical information and the functional information in one sitting. Indeed, PET/CT is already being heralded as the next generation molecular imaging methodology.

PET or PET/CT versus CT–Magnetic Resonance Imaging

The rapid advances in medical imaging have definitely increased the accuracy of diagnosis of diseases, but judicious use of these highly sophisticated imaging tools is necessary to prevent an economic burden on patients as well as to reduce the potential side effects of radiation or contrast materials. Both conventional and functional imaging tools play a critical role in the diagnosis of NET. CT alone or MRI cannot provide specific information regarding the functional status of the tumor. Since this is essential to know in most cases prior to starting any of the available therapies, the current medical consensus should be to use PET/CT (or SPECT-CT or SPECT when PET is not available) at all tumor stages, and add MRI or other specific imaging modalities only when needed (7).

CLINICAL INDICATIONS FOR PET/CT (AND PET) IN NEUROENDOCRINE TUMORS

Based on the personal experience Baum et al. (78) and a review of the literature, PET/CT (and to a certain degree also PET alone) can be used in NET for:

1. Diagnosis and staging
2. Follow-up of patients after surgery
3. Follow-up of patients after octreotide/interferon or chemotherapy
4. Choosing the appropriate therapeutic regime of PRRT
5. For predicting the response to PRRT
6. Defining the prognosis of patients (yet to be established).

CLINICAL STUDIES

Although NETs belong to a heterogeneous group of malignancies, many of them share common characteristics, making it easier to judge the clinical suitability of a radiopharmaceutical in different tumor subtypes. This section will present the gross summary of several studies that have been conducted in the diagnosis of NET up to now.

Role of the Nuclear Medicine Physician in the Management of Neuroendocrine Tumors

It is important to stress that most of the nuclear medicine studies have been performed on metastatic NETs, which remain the most common stage in which a patient is referred to a nuclear medicine physician. A surgeon's primary interest lies in the location, size, and resectability of the primary tumor (or of operable metastases). An oncologist, gastroenterologist, endocrinologist, as well as the nuclear medicine physician or the radiotherapist wants to have more detailed information regarding the total extent of the disease. This includes location of the primary (or multiple primaries), somatostatin receptor status (e.g., for use of octreotide therapy), exact location of the target (e.g., in the bone) for external beam radiotherapy, effectiveness of biotherapy or chemotherapy, and possibility of performing PRRT (e.g., density of SSTR receptor expression).

Taking into consideration the long protracted course of many NETs, these patients are frequently referred for serial studies. Since radiation exposure (and cost) is a concern especially in young patients, it is essential to ascertain the time gap between two serial studies based on the radiopharmaceutical being employed by a particular center. PET studies performed at too short an interval may not give adequate information to influence patient management and will only burden the patient with unnecessary radiation, thereby jeopardizing future studies. Similarly, PET studies performed at a much longer interval may expose the patient to protracted chemotherapy/PRRT with their inherent side effects.

It is also necessary for nuclear medicine physicians dealing with NETs to be aware of the ways and means to assess tumor response. As a guide, different criteria currently used in therapy monitoring (79) are mentioned in Table 8.21.9. Thus, the onus of performing these highly specialized molecular imaging techniques lies in the hands of the respective nuclear medicine physicians and nuclear radiologists (in strong collaboration with other specialities involved in the care of NET patients), necessitating the need for extensive training prior to being involved in the management of patients with NETs .

Gallium-68-DOTA-NOC/DOTA-TOC Receptor PET/CT

Gallium-68-DOTA-NOC/DOTA-TOC receptor PET/CT has been used in (78):

1. Neuroendocrine tumors, especially gastroenteropancreatic tumors Fig. 8.21.4, Fig. 8.21.12
2. Pheochromocytoma and paraganglioma Fig. 8.21.9
3. Thyroid cancer (medullary as well as papillary/follicular cancer) Fig. 8.21.11
4. Glomus tumors and meningioma Fig. 8.21.5 and Fig. 8.21.6
5. Neuroblastoma
6. Small cell lung cancer
7. Merkel cell tumors and other rare tumors expressing SMS receptors like aesthesioneuroblastoma, thymoma, hepatoblastoma, neuroendocrine prostate cancer
8. Nonmalignant conditions/diseases with aggressive behavior (e.g., retroperitoneal fibrosis, fibrocystoma).

Patient Preparation, Imaging, and Reporting

Before enrolling the patient for a somatostatin receptor PET/CT, it is essential to inform the patient about the application of "cold" octreotide therapy. To minimize receptor blockade, Sandostatin LAR injections must be stopped 4 to 6 weeks prior to the scan and subcutaneous treatment with octreotide should be stopped at least 2 days before.

Proper hydration of the patient is achieved by having the patient drink 500 mL of water just prior to the acquisition 1.5 L of water-equivalent oral contrast dispersion (e.g., Gastrografin, Bracco Diagnostics, Princeton, New Jersey) is given.

PET/CT acquisition starts at 60 minutes (30 to 180 minutes) after intravenous injection of 100 MBq (75 to 250 MBq) of the radiolabeled peptide (e.g., [^{68}Ga]-DOTA-NOC). In order to increase renal elimination (and to reduce the radiation exposure to the urinary bladder), furosemide is given at the time of injection of [^{68}Ga] DOTA-NOC. Before the PET acquisition, a low-dose, contrast-enhanced CT scan is performed based on the specification of the PET/CT scanner. For scientific purposes, and if the dynamic mode is available, it is advisable to perform a dynamic study as it gives more detailed and precise information about the kinetics of the radiopharmaceutical and allows absolute quantification. However, practically speaking, static delayed injections are usually diagnostically sufficient and offer quantitative information of considerable value.

Image analysis should always start with an examination of the maximum intensity projection images Fig. 8.21.4c to get an impression about the whole-body biodistribution of the radiopharmaceutical

TABLE 8.21.9 Criteria for Tumor Response to Treatment Based on Anatomical and Metabolic Tumor Imaging Methods

	CR	PR	PD	SD
EORTC (^{18}F-FDG PET)	No uptake of ^{18}F-FDG in the target lesion	Reduction in SUV 15%–25% after one cycle and >25% afterward	Increase in SUV >25%, visible increase in extent of tumor uptake by 20%, appearance of new ^{18}F-FDG uptake in metastatic lesions	Increase in SUV <25% or decrease in SUV <15%, no visible change in extent of tumor
WHO	Complete disappearance of all disease manifestations in two observations at an interval of at least 4 weeks	≥50% decrease in tumor size	>25% increase in tumor lesions and/or appearance of new foci of tumor	Increase or decrease in tumor size of <25%
RECIST	Disappearance of all tumor lesions	At least 30% decrease in the sum of longest diameter of tumor lesion	At least 20% increase in sum of the longest diameter of tumor lesion	Neither PR nor PD

CR, complete response; EORTC, European Organisation for Research and Treatment of Cancer; F, fluorine; PR, partial response; PD, progressive disease; RECIST, Response Evaluation Criteria in Solid Tumors; SD, stable disease; SUV, standard uptake value; WHO, World Health Organization.

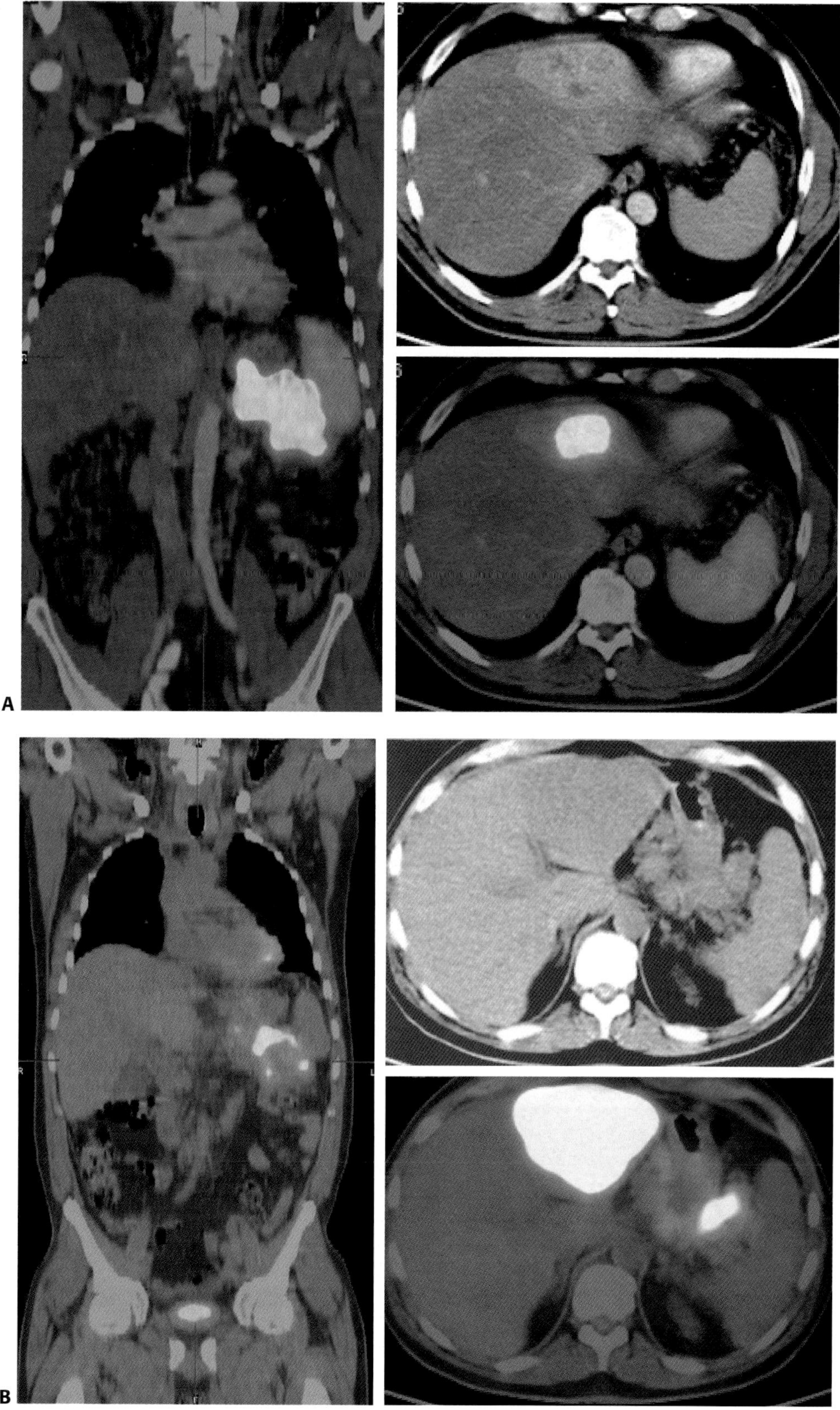

FIGURE 8.21.4. **A:** Extensive, inoperable neuroendocrine carcinoma of the stomach (gastrinoma) with liver metastases (shown is one in the left lobe), progressive after chemotherapy and octreotide/interferon treatment before PRRT. Receptor PET/CT (^{68}Ga DOTA-NOC) demonstrates intense somatostatin receptor expression of the primary tumor and the liver lesion. The patient was treated with three cycles of PRRT (^{90}Y and ^{177}Lu DOTA-TATE, total 12.7 GBq) and achieved a stable disease. **B:** Fifteen months after the last PRRT course, the patient developed severe paraneoplastic hypercalcemia with renal insufficiency. CT scan showed progression of the liver metastases, and ^{18}F-FDG PET/CT, which was unremarkable before, now revealed intense glucose hypermetabolism of the fast-growing metastases in the left liver lobe. (*continued*)

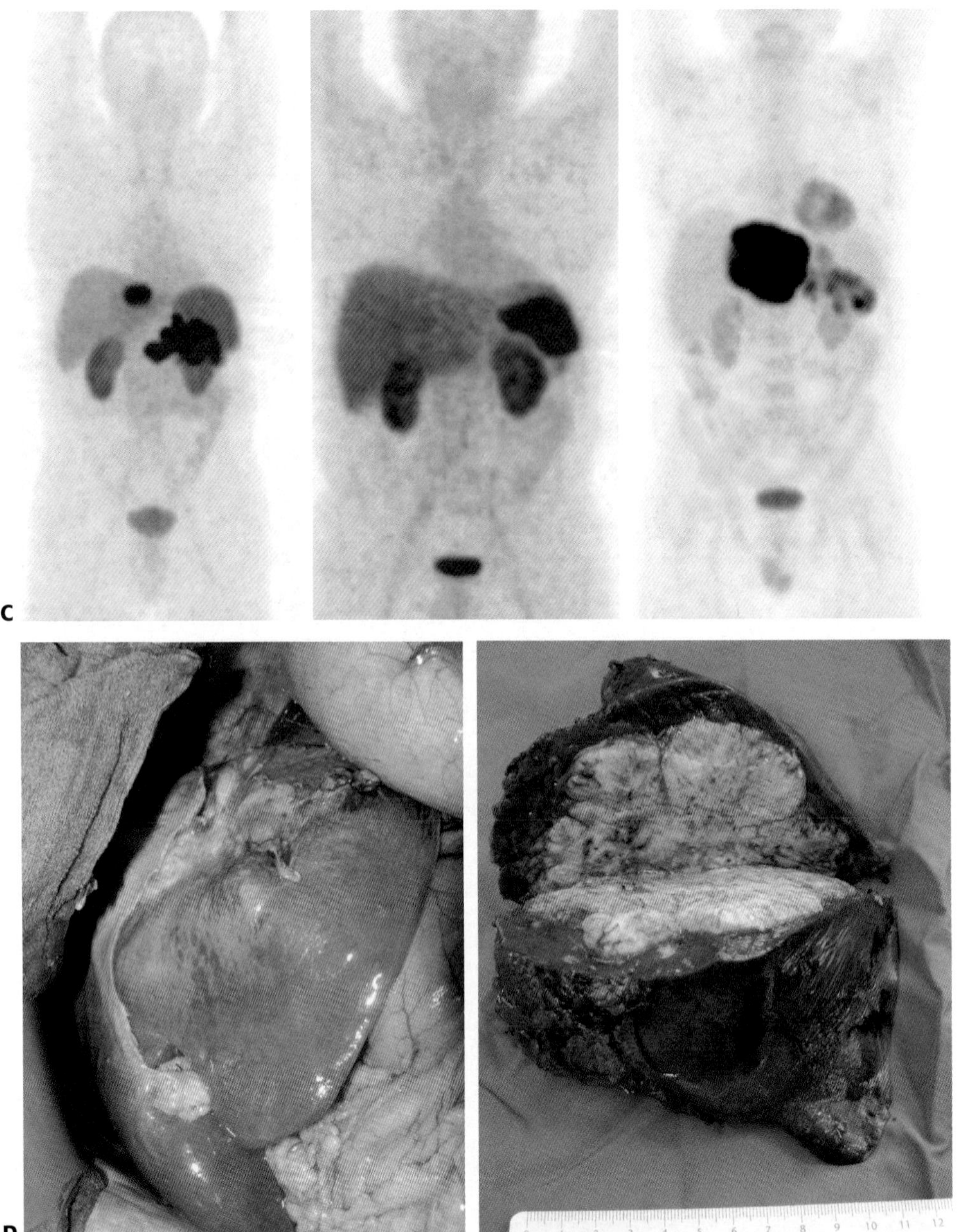

FIGURE 8.21.4. *Continued.* **C:** MIP images: ^{68}Ga DOTA-NOC receptor PET on the left before PRRT and after three cycles (**middle**), ^{18}F-FDG PET on the right. Dedifferentiation of the tumor is related to high FDG uptake and loss of somatostatin receptors (the "vanishing receptor sign"). **D:** Extended left hemihepatectomy resulted in immediate normalization of the calcium in serum and normalization of kidney function. DOTA-NOC, DOTA-1-Nal^{3}-octreotide; DOTA-TATE, DOTA-D-Phe^{1}-Tyr^{3}-Thr^{8}-octreotide; F, fluorine; Ga, gallium; MIP, maximum intensity projection; PRRT, peptide receptor radionuclide therapy. (Images courtesy of Merten Hommann, MD, Dept. of Surgery, Zentralklinik Bad Berka.)

and the relevant uptake in metastases; as a rule of thumb, all focal lesions with higher uptake than the liver are suspicious for malignancy. This is followed by detailed examination of the transverse slices and the PET/CT fusion images from head Fig. 8.21.7 to midthigh and the standard uptake value (SUV) measurement of each lesion and relevant normal organs (e.g., pituitary gland, thyroid, lung, liver, spleen, adrenals, gluteus muscle/background).

Normal Biodistribution and Pharmacokinetics of Gallium-68-DOTA-NOC and -DOTA-TOC

Analysis of the normal biodistribution in patients with metastasized NET in over 1,500 studies (80) showed [^{68}Ga]-DOTA- NOC is fairly uniformly distributed in brain, pituitary gland, thyroid, lungs, kidneys, normal liver, and gluteus muscle. The distribution in spleen, and to some extent in adrenals, is highly variable. Octreotide

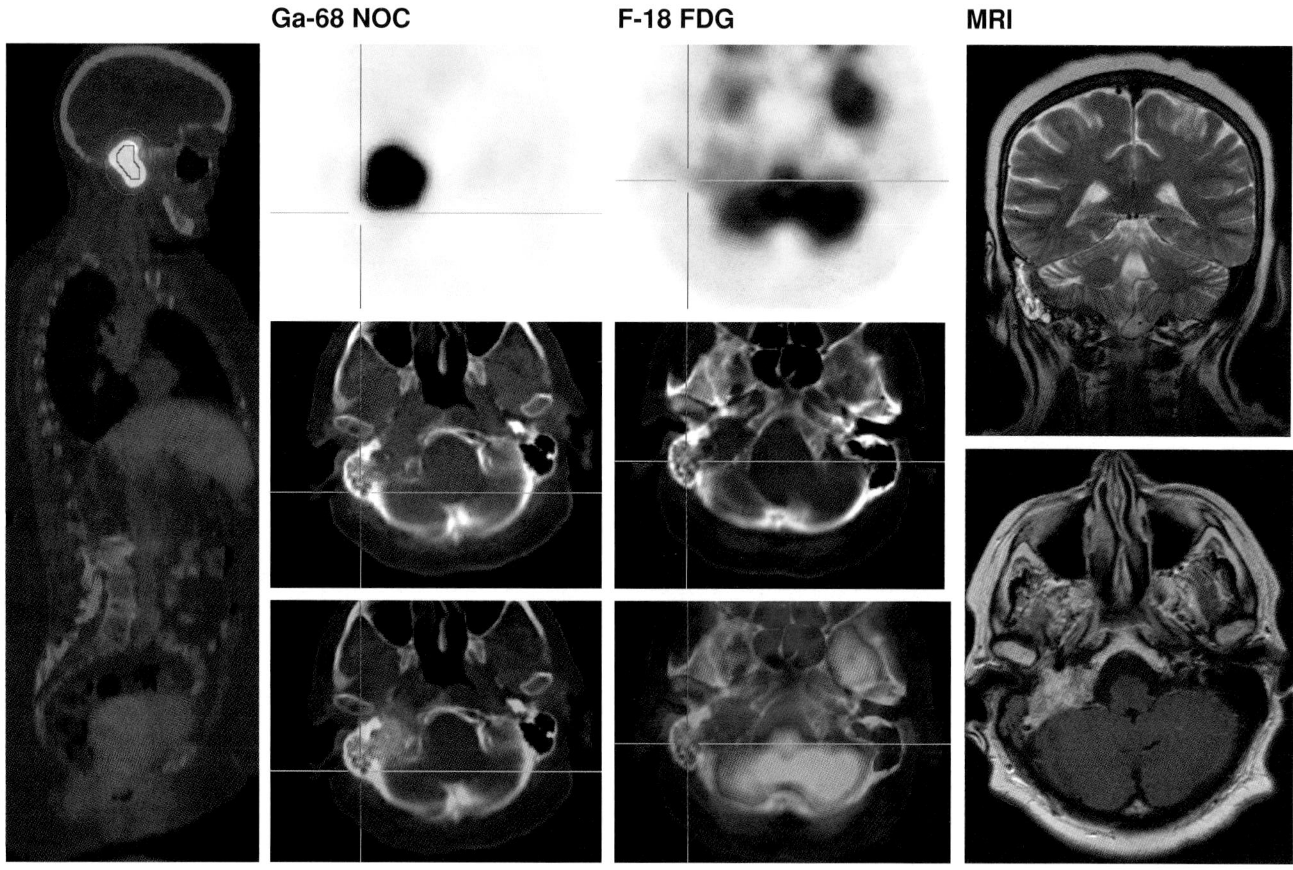

FIGURE 8.21.5. Gallium-68 DOTA-NOC receptor PET/CT shows very high (SUVmax 112) SSTR expression in a patient with an inoperable glomus tumor invading the base of the skull, as demonstrated by magnetic resonance imaging (**on the right**), whereas fluorine-18-FDG PET/CT does not reveal any glucose hypermetabolism (the "flip-flop sign"). The tumor was progressive even after external beam radiation with 60 Gy. After two courses of PRRT there was a remarkable tumor response with significant clinical improvement. DOTA-NOC, DOTA-1-Nal^3-octreotide; FDG, fluorodeoxyglucose; SSTR, somatostatin receptors; SUVmax, maximum standard uptake value.

given subcutaneously immediately before the study or as depot intramuscular (Sandostatin LAR) within 3 to 4 weeks prior to the study significantly reduces the uptake in spleen and normal liver (and also in tumor). This observation supports the true receptor-radioligand binding property (competitive binding) of [^{68}Ga]-DOTA-NOC.

In carcinoid heart disease (Hedinger syndrome), the [^{68}Ga]-DOTA-NOC uptake is significantly reduced because these patients are mostly on long-standing octreotide therapy to reduce the effect of serotonin on the endocardium. Chemotherapeutic drugs like gemcitabine, 5-fluorouracil, cisplatin, doxorubicin, and camptothecin, which are often used for the treatment of patients with pancreatic NETs, have been shown to reduce the expression of DOTA-LAN (synthetic somatostatin analogues) in pancreatic tumor cell lines (81). This observation may have some implication in the outcome of somatostatin receptor PET/CT studies.

The excretion of DOTA-NOC is primarily through the kidneys, making it the critical organ. Urinary bladder, spleen, and liver (in the order of appearance) also receive high radiation dose; however, overall [^{68}Ga]-DOTA-NOC delivers a radiation dose to the organs comparable to, and even lower than, other diagnostic analogues. This, in spite of the fact that DOTA-NOC covers the wider range of somatostatin receptors, makes it a very interesting and positive observation. Other organs having known physiologic SSTR expression, such as the pituitary glands, adrenals, and so forth, also show mild to moderate uptake (82).

The normal biodistribution of [^{68}Ga]-DOTA-TOC shows a similar uptake pattern in different organs. Hoffman et al. (75) have reported a biexponential decay of [^{68}Ga]-DOTA-TOC in arterialized venous blood and very fast renal clearance. It is also reported that the time to peak in 95% of tumors (also in the spleen) is achieved within 50 to 90 minutes. Koukouraki et al. (83) have observed that [^{68}Ga]-DOTA-TOC uptake in NETs is based on specific receptor binding and fractional blood volume. It is also important to remember that after receptor binding [^{68}Ga]-DOTA-NOC/DOTA-TOC is internalized into the tumor cells, and there is minimal washout of the radiopeptides from the tumor cells (84–86). A recent study by Cescato et al. (87), using immunocytochemical methods, has shown that [^{90}Y]-DOTA-TATE, [^{90}Y]-DOTA-NOC, and [^{177}Lu]-DOTA-BOC-ATE were more potent in internalizing SSTR 2 as compared to DTPA-OC (octreotide) and also this internalization was blocked by specific SSTR antagonists.

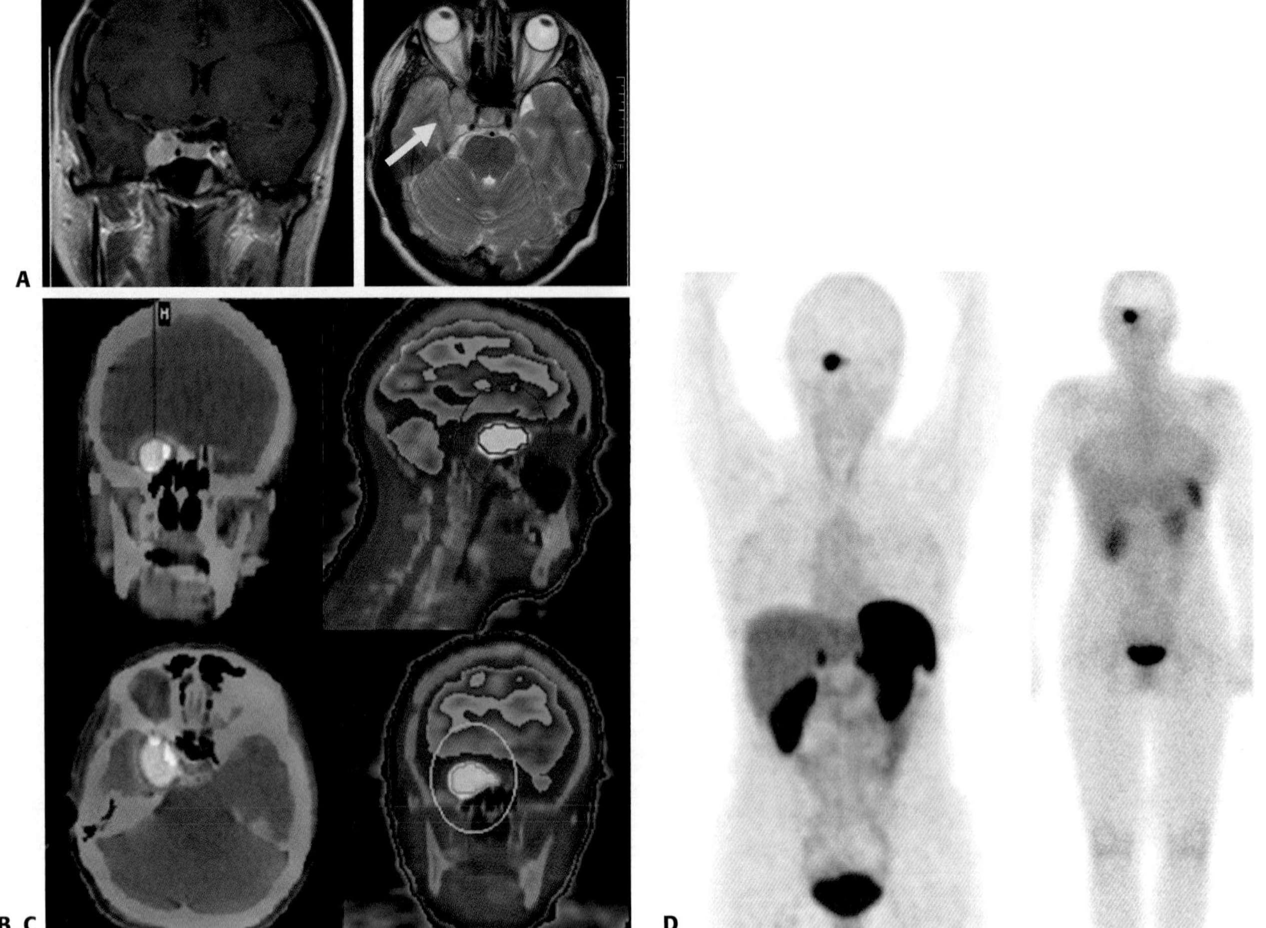

FIGURE 8.21.6. Meningioma (*arrow*) growing near the right optical nerve, causing nerve compression and loss of vision of the right eye (the patient, a computer worker, had inborn amblyopia of the left eye and was losing her sight). Gallium-68 DOTA-NOC PET/CT showed high SSTR expression of the meningioma. **A:** Coronal and transversal magnetic resonance images. **B:** Coronal and transversal PET/CT images. **C:** Coronal and transversal region of interest images (SUVmax 17.2). **D:** MIP gallium-68 DOTA-TATE PET/CT. **E:** Whole-body scan 3 hours after administration of 5.3 GBq lutetium-177 DOTA-TATE. SPECT dosimetry revealed a tumor dose of 27 Gy. Two years after a second PRRT course, her vision became nearly normal. DOTA-NOC, DOTA-1-Nal^3-octreotide; DOTA-TATE, DOTA-D-Phe^1-Tyr^3-Thr^8-octreotide; PRRT, peptide receptor radionuclide therapy; SPECT, single-photon emission computed tomography; SSTR, somatostatin receptors; SUVmax, maximum standard uptake value.

Clinical Results

Although somatostatin receptor scintigraphy has been validated as the most specific tool for the detection of NET and is used extensively for the follow-up of patients after receiving octreotide therapy, the few studies that have compared somatostatin-based PET radiopharmaceuticals and OctreoScan have found that PET was significantly more sensitive in detecting tumor lesions (Fig. 8.21.8). This may be attributed in part to the decreased sensitivity of gamma camera imaging as compared to PET. One of the advantages of [^{68}Ga]-DOTA-NOC/DOTA-TOC PET or PET/CT over [^{111}In]-octreotide scintigraphy is better visualization of bone lesions Fig. 8.21.9, which are difficult to detect on planar and SPECT images (88).

Buchmann et al (88), compared the diagnostic accuracy of [^{68}Ga]-DOTA-TOC PET and [^{111}In]-OctreoScan SPECT. The conclusion was that [^{68}Ga]-DOTA-TOC PET is superior to [^{111}In]-DTPA-TOC SPECT in the detection of NET manifestations in the lung and skeleton and similar for the detection of NET manifestations in the liver and brain. Gallium-68 DOTA-TOC PET was found to be advantageous in guiding the clinical management.

In a preliminary clinical study, Hofmann et al. (75) have shown that [^{68}Ga]-DOTA-TOC is superior to [^{111}In]-octreotide SPECT (CT was taken as the reference for comparison) in detecting upper abdominal metastases. Kowalski et al. (77) described that in comparison to the [^{111}In]-octreotide scan, [^{68}Ga]-DOTA-TOC PET appears superior, especially in detecting small tumors or tumors bearing only a low density of somatostatin receptors.

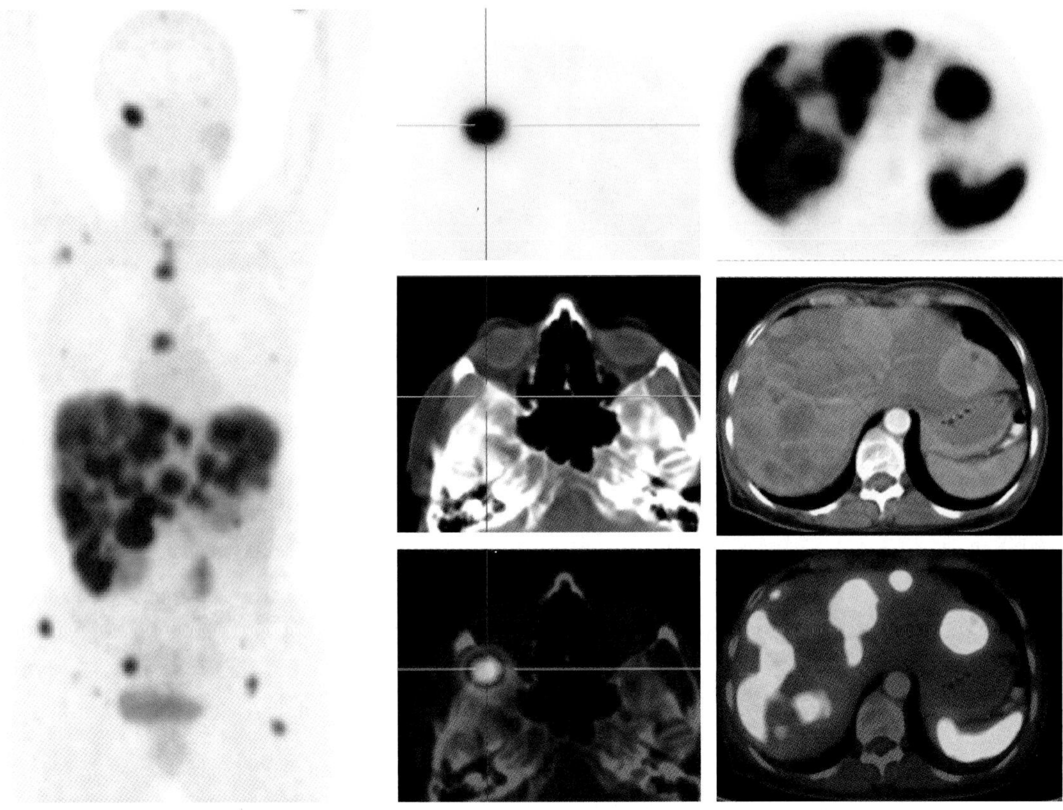

FIGURE 8.21.7. Retro-orbital metastasis of neuroendocrine carcinoma (CUP syndrome), localized in the os sphenoidale. Gallium-68 DOTA-NOC receptor PET/CT demonstrates also extensive liver and additional osseous metastases. DOTA-NOC, DOTA-1-Nal^3-octreotide.

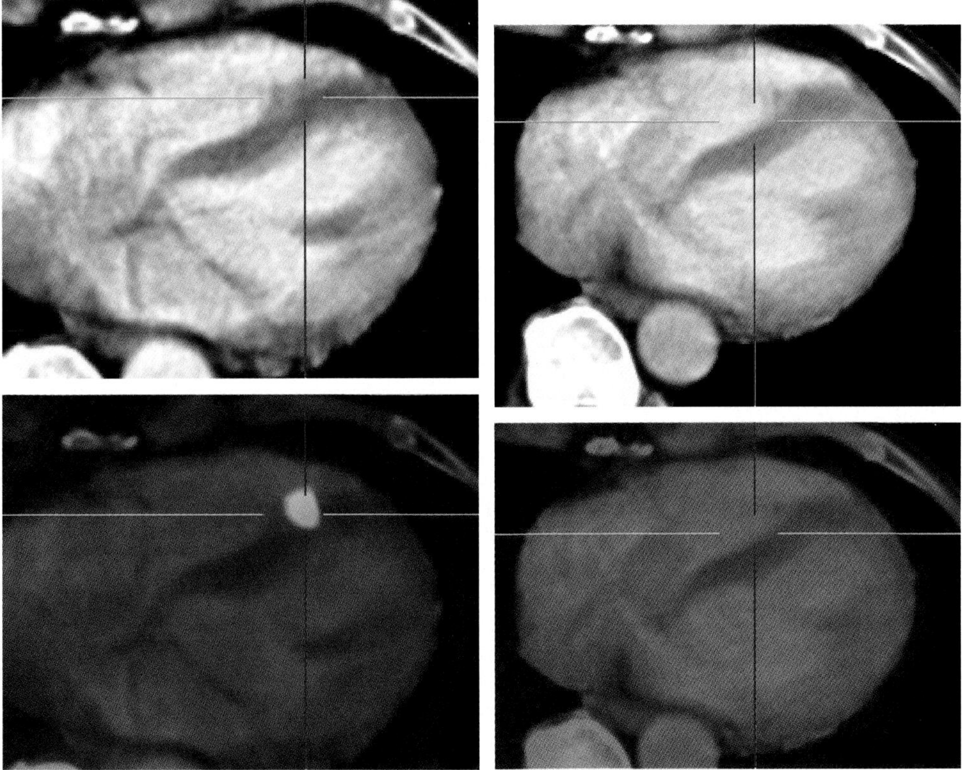

FIGURE 8.21.8. Cardiac metastasis of ileum carcinoid before (**left**) and after (**right**) PRRT. Gallium-68 DOTA-NOC PET/CT shows complete response after therapy. DOTA-NOC, DOTA-1-Nal^3-octreotide; PRRT, peptide receptor radionuclide therapy.

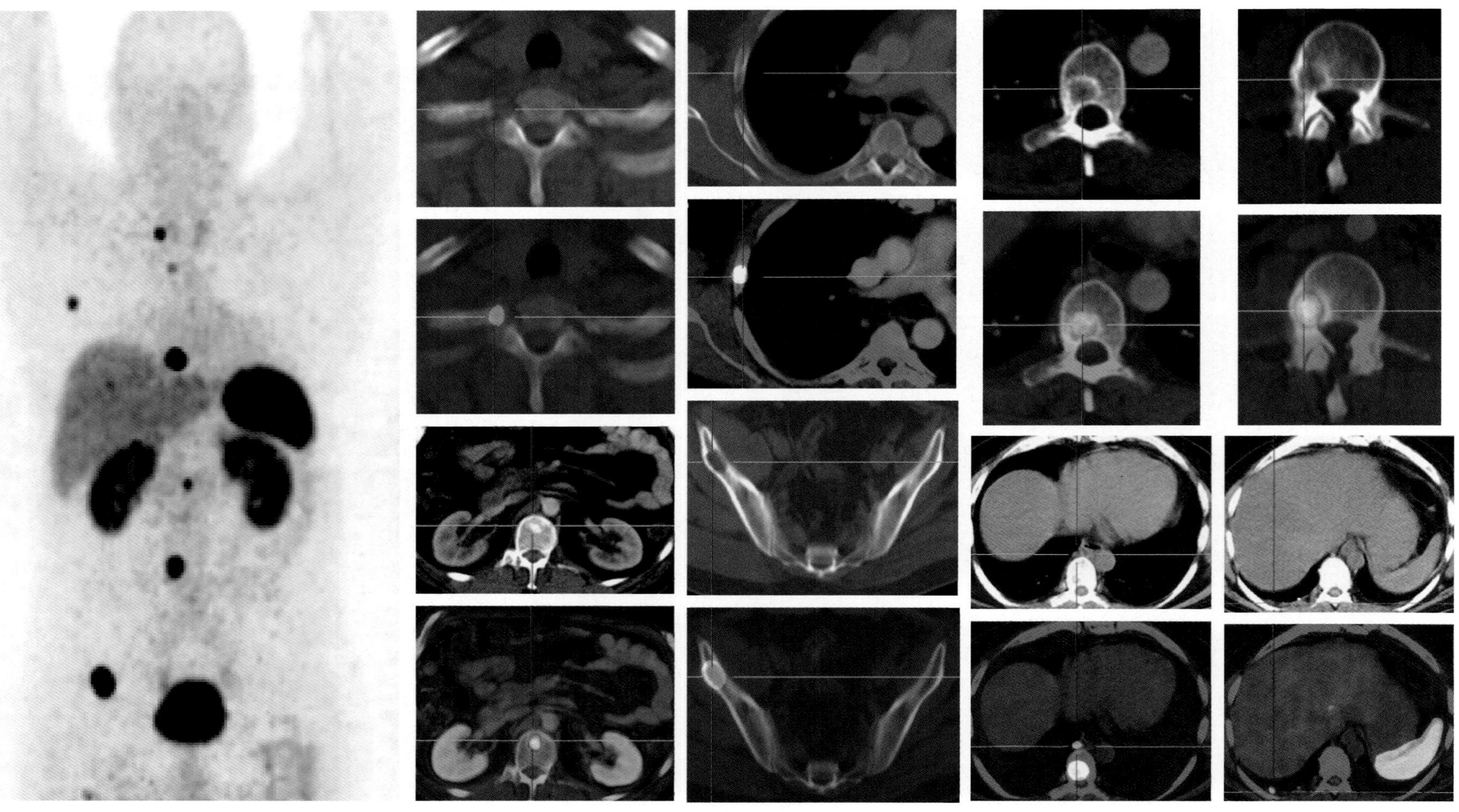

FIGURE 8.21.9. A 38-year-old patient with malignant pheochromocytoma/paraganglioma (mutation of the *SDHB* gene), diagnosed at age 25. Multiple bone metastases (e.g., in the ribs, thoracic and lumbar vertebrae, and in the iliac bone), mostly lytic, but also osteoblastic with very high SSTR expression (SUVmax 100 in Th 7). Gallium-68 DOTA-NOC PET/CT also detected pleural metastasis and prevertebral paraganglioma. DOTA-NOC, DOTA-1-Nal^3-octreotide; SSTR, somatostatin receptors; SUVmax, maximum standardized uptake value.

Apart from GEP tumors, [^{68}Ga]-DOTA-TOC PET has also been envisaged to have a potential role in small cell lung cancer, as this tumor is known to express somatostatin receptors (9). In an intraindividual study comparing the diagnostic efficacy of [^{68}Ga]-DOTA-NOC and [^{68}Ga]-DOTA-TATE, it was demonstrated for the first time that [^{68}Ga]-DOTA-NOC is superior to [^{68}Ga]-DOTA-TATE (90). In more than 1,500 receptor PET/CT studies performed in our hospital over the past 3 years, it was found that (a) [^{68}Ga]-DOTA-NOC PET was able to detect many lesions that could not be detected by CT Fig. 8.21.13, (b) [^{68}Ga]-DOTA-NOC PET is of significant value in monitoring patients with NETs Fig. 8.21.8 before and after PRRT (in over 350 patients treated with [^{90}Y]- or [^{177}Lu]-labeled DOTA-TATE in the authors' center), (c) PET/CT provides additional information about the tumor status as compared to the PET study alone Fig. 8.21.10, and (d) [^{68}Ga]-DOTA-NOC PET is a useful adjunct in deciding on the amount of

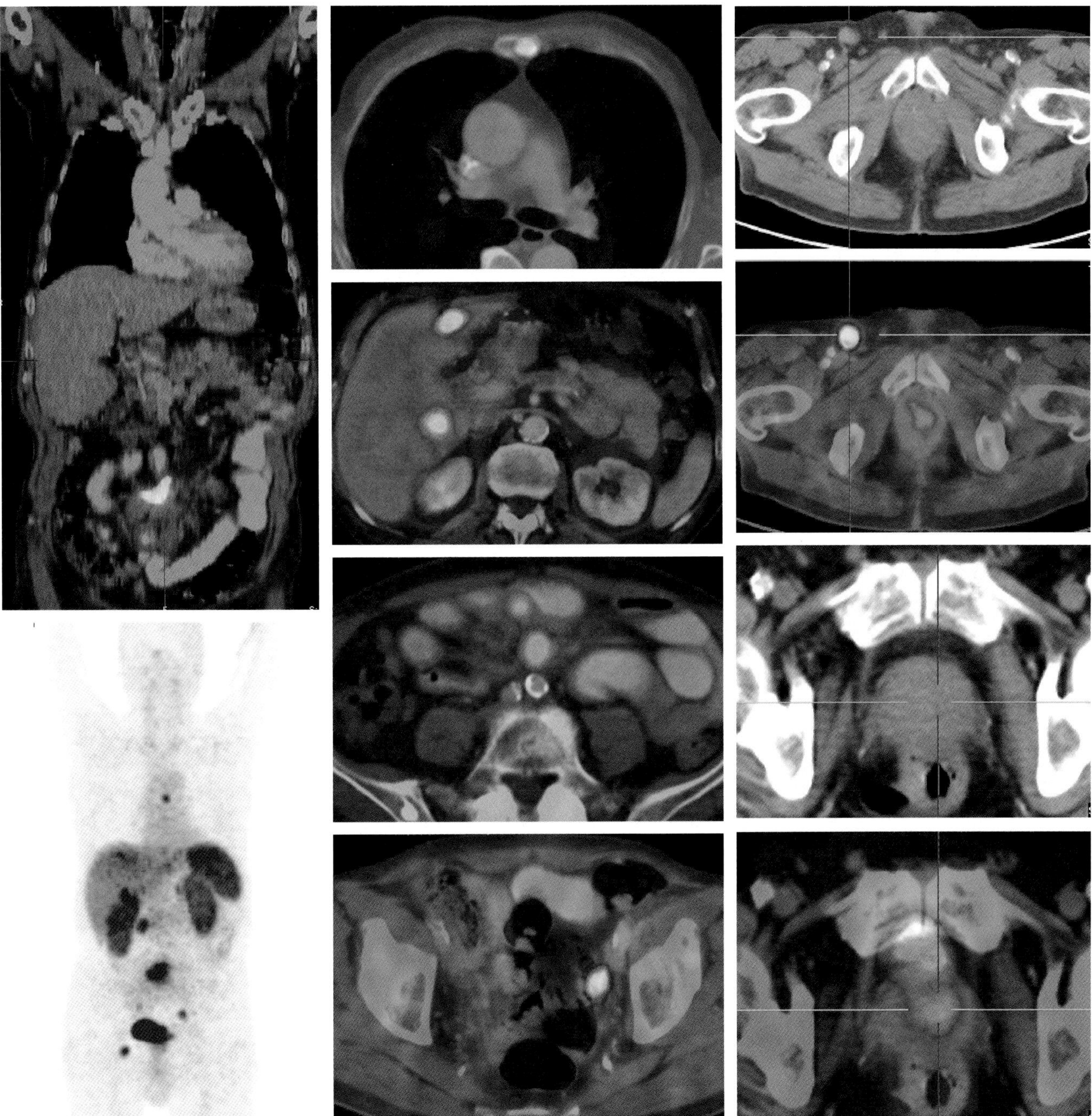

FIGURE 8.21.10. Neuroendocrine carcinoma of the small bowel with metastases in the sternum, liver, and in mesenteric lymph nodes as shown by gallium-68 DOTA-TATE PET/CT. In addition, a neuroendocrine prostate cancer was revealed (confirmed by biopsy) with iliac and inguinal lymph node metastases. DOTA-TATE, DOTA-D-Phe^{1}-Tyr^{3}-Thr^{8}-octreotide.

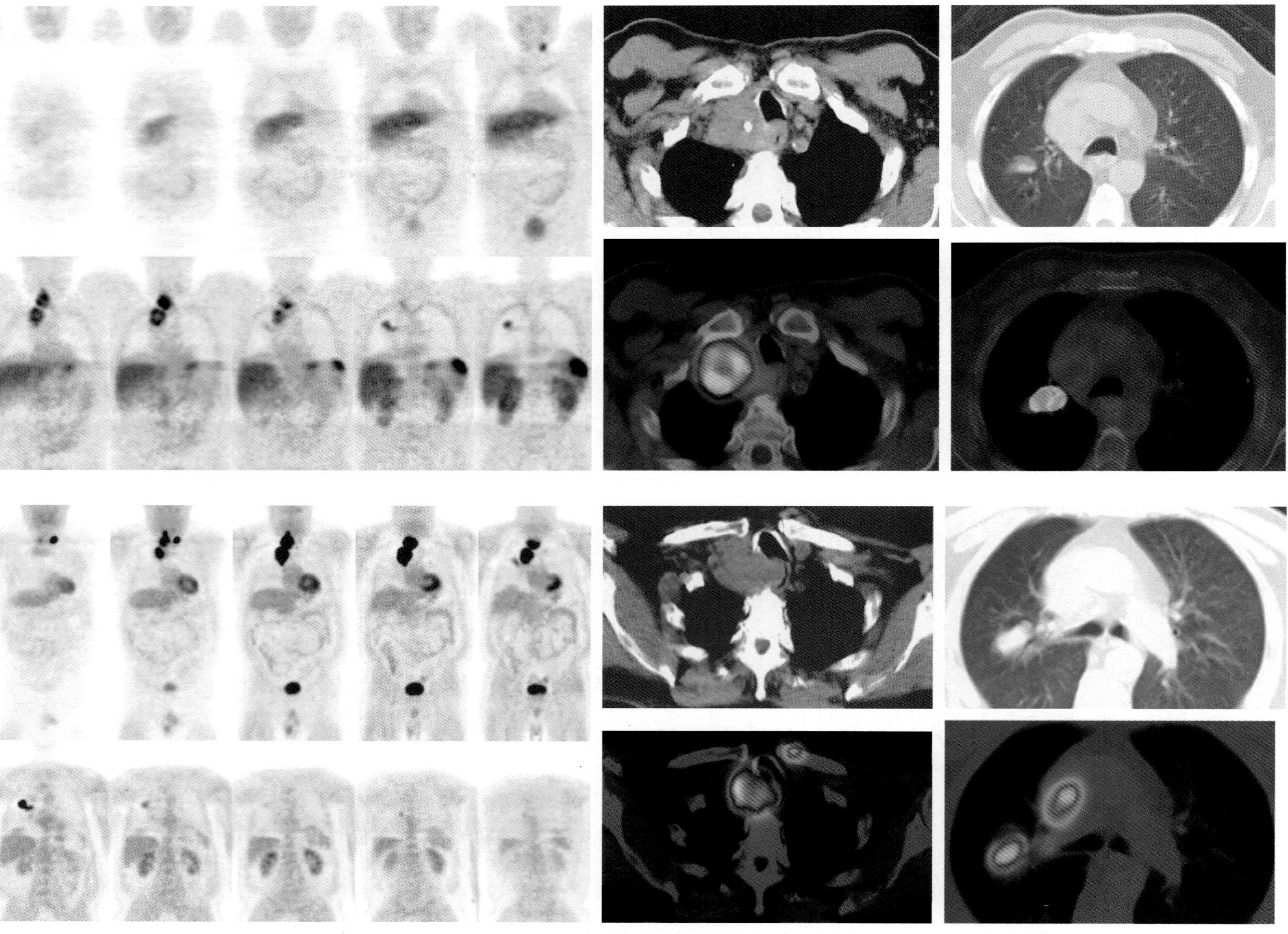

FIGURE 8.21.11. Thyroid cancer (mixed follicular and medullary carcinoma with human thyroglobulin and calcitonin production). Radioiodine negative metastases after radioiodine therapy with a cumulative administered activity of 37 GBq (1,000 mCi). Upper row (**A**): gallium-68 DOTA-TATE PET/CT (coronal slices and selected transversal slices) showing high SSTR expression (SUVmax 25). Lower row (**B**): fluorine-18 FDG PET/CT demonstrating very high metabolic activity in a paratracheal recurrence, infiltrating the trachea, and in multiple metastases in the mediastinum and in the lung. DOTA-TATE, DOTA-D-Phe^1-Tyr^3-Thr^8-octreotide; FDG, fluorodeoxyglucose; SUVmax, maximum standardized uptake value.

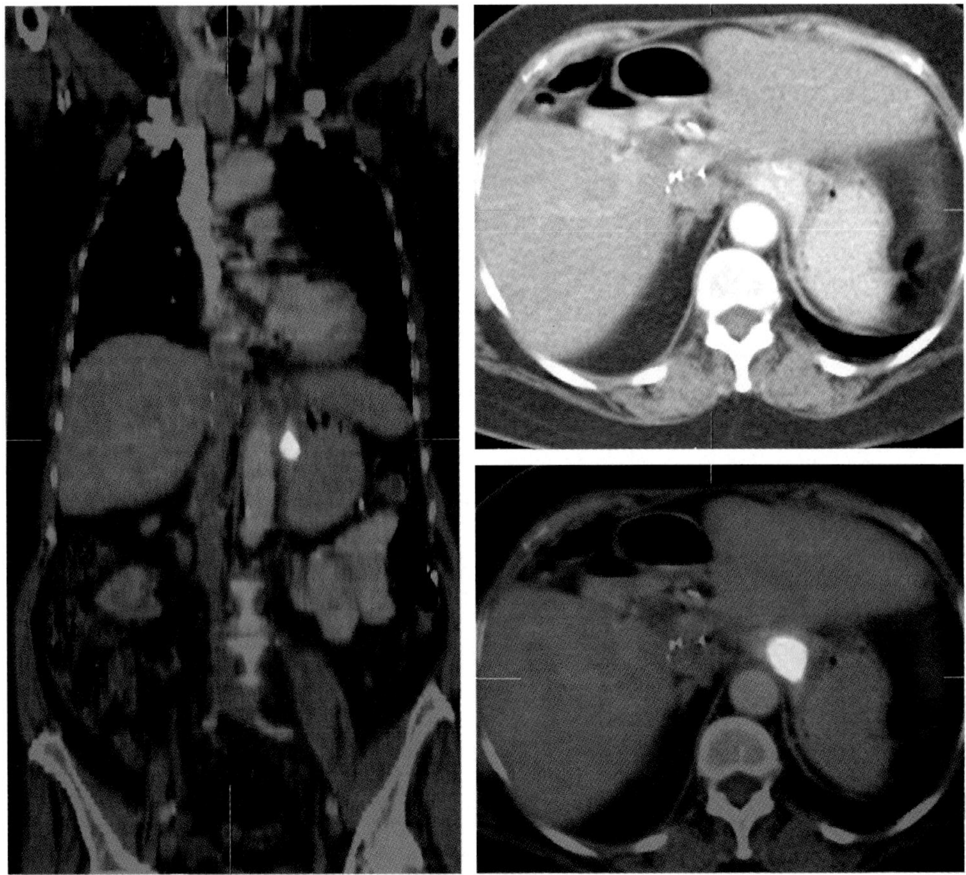

FIGURE 8.21.12. Gallium-68 DOTA-NOC PET/CT: local recurrence of pancreatic neuroendocrine tumors. DOTA-NOC, DOTA-1-Nal^3-octreotide.

radioactivity to be administered for PRRT (pretherapeutic dosimetry).

Care must be taken while reporting the scans of patients having documented vasculitis, sarcoidosis, Crohn disease, rheumatoid arthritis, and tuberculosis as activated lymphocytes (showing SSTR expression) may be present at the site of the pathology.

Fluorine-18- and Carbon-11-dihydroxyphenylalanine and Fluorine-18-fluorodopamine PET

The possible indications for use of [^{18}F]- and [^{11}C]-dihydroxyphenylalanine, and [^{18}F]-fluorodopamine PET include:

1. Neuroendocrine tumors, especially pancreatic tumors
2. Pheochromocytoma
3. Paraganglioma
4. Medullary thyroid cancer
5. Neuroblastoma

Imaging

The adult dose of [^{18}F]-DOPA is 200 to 300 MBq. PET acquisition is started 45 to 90 minutes postinjection.

Results

The first study that demonstrated the utility of [^{11}C]-DOPA in the detection of neuroendocrine pancreatic tumors was done by Ahlstrom et al. (91) in 1995. However, the high cost, short half-life, and limited availability of [^{11}C] has marred its development as a potential agent for NET imaging. Fluorine-18-DOPA performs better than OctreoScan scintigraphy in visualizing advanced NETs. The authors also proposed that [^{18}F]-DOPA performs better than CT in detection of bone lesions (92). However, in small cell lung cancer, [^{18}F]-DOPA was found to be significantly inferior to [^{18}F]-FDG PET (93). Recent studies have demonstrated an increased L-DOPA decarboxylase activity in 80% of NET, and it has been suggested that this parameter could be used as a marker of tumor activity (94). In recent years, preliminary studies have shown that [^{18}F]-DOPA is useful for the assessment of NET, performing better than conventional morphologic (ultrasound, CT, MRI) and nuclear medicine (somatostatin receptor scintigraphy [SRS]) procedures with reported sensitivities ranging from 65% to 100% (92,95–97). In 2001 Hoegerle et al. (95) reported that [^{18}F]-DOPA PET allowed the detection of a higher number of NET lesions in the GI tract as compared to SRS and [^{18}F]-FDG PET (respectively, true positive findings at primary sites: 7 vs. 4 vs. 2; nodes metastasis: 41 vs. 27 vs. 14). In a prospective single-center study, Koopmans et al. (96) compared [^{18}F]-DOPA PET results with SRS and CT in 53 patients with metastatic carcinoid tumor. The authors observed that[^{18}F]-DOPA PET detected more lesions, more positive regions, and more lesions per region that combined SRS and CT. In region-based analysis, sensitivity of [^{18}F]-DOPA PET was 95% (90–98) as compared to 66% (57–74) for SRS, 57% (48–66) for CT, and 79% (70–86) for combined CT and SRS (p = 0.0001, PET vs combined CT and SRS).

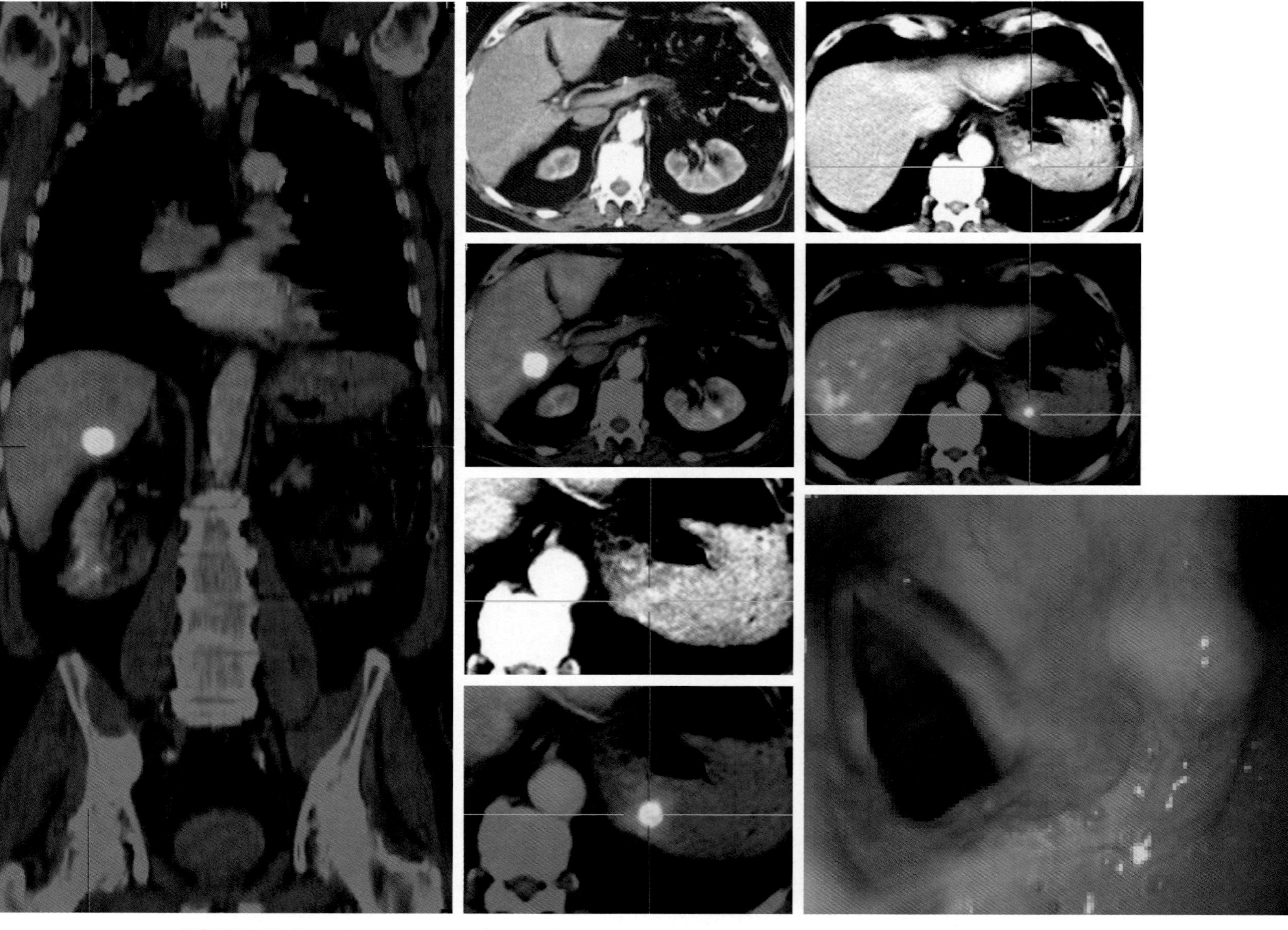

FIGURE 8.21.13. Patient presenting with rising chromogranin A level in serum (545 ng/mL, cutoff 100 ng/mL) after resection of a neuroendocrine carcinoma of the pancreatic tail, splenectomy, partial resection of the stomach and of the left colon flexure followed by extirpation of a liver metastasis (S4/5) 18 months after the primary tumor operation. A previous CT scan described a questionable liver lesion; octreotide scintigraphy, performed 1 month earlier, was described as normal. Gallium-68 DOTA-NOC PET/CT clearly shows a liver metastasis in the posterior segment of S5 (just in front of the kidney, which explains that the lesion was not detected on the OctreoScan image) and in addition a SSTR positive infiltration of the stomach wall, which was confirmed by endoscopy. DOTA-NOC, DOTA-1-Nal^3-octreotide; SSTR, somatostatin receptors. (Gastroscopy image courtesy of Dieter Hörsch, MD, Dept. of Internal Medicine, Zentralklinik Bad Berka.)

In patients with pheochromocytoma, both [^{18}F]-DOPA PET and MRI were found to have better sensitivity and specificity (100% each) than [^{131}I]-MIBG scanning (however, [^{131}I]-MIBG scintigraphy is not the current gold standard as [^{123}I]-MIBG SPECT is superior) (97). Fluorine-18-DOPA PET has also been found to be useful in the detection of congenital hyperinsulinism (the most common cause of persistent hypoglycemia in infants and children). In a recent study, Hardy et al. (99) have shown in 24 patients that [^{18}F]-DOPA PET has high sensitivity (96%) in detecting focal or diffuse congenital hyperinsulinism. The diagnostic accuracy of 100% for focal disease prompted the authors to suggest that [^{18}F]-DOPA PET should be considered prior to pancreatectomy for treatment of congenital hyperinsulinism in infants (Fig. 8.21.14).

In a preliminary study Ambrosini et al. (100) have shown that [^{18}F]-DOPA PET/CT has a promising role in GEP patients with negative or inconclusive findings at conventional radiological imaging and [^{111}In]-pentetreotide scintigraphy. The authors observed that the findings were helpful in biopsy guidance and played a major role in changing the management of those patients.

The potential limitation of [^{18}F]-DOPA PET is high physiologic uptake in the duodenum and pancreas, which might cause problems in localization of tumors in these regions. Apart from this, the nonspecific accumulation of [^{18}F]-DOPA in the intestine is a potential source of false-positive interpretation.

Carbon-11 5-hydroxytryptamine PET

In a study comparing 5-HTP PET with CT and somatostatin receptor scintigraphy in patients with carcinoid and endocrine pancreatic tumors, 5-HTP PET was found to be superior to CT and somatostatin receptor scintigraphy for tumor visualization. Many small, previously overlooked lesions were diagnosed by [^{11}C]-5-HTP PET (101,102).

Gluc-Lys Fluorine-18-FP-TOCA PET

The success of PET and PET/CT made scientists work towards using [^{18}F] as a radioligand for somatostatin analogues (103). Gluc-Lys ([^{18}F])-FP)-TOCA N^{α}-(1-deoxy-D-fructosyl)-N^{ε}-(2-[^{18}F] fluropropionyl-Lys^{0}-Tyr^{3}-octreotate PET, in a preliminary comparative study, was superior to [^{111}In]-DTPA-octreotide scan in the diagnosis of NETs. In the same study (based on literature survey) it was stressed that Gluc-Lys [^{18}F]-FP-TOCA PET is comparable with [^{68}Ga]-DOTA-TOC PET findings in NET (104).

Copper-64-TETA-octreotide PET

Copper-64 (half-life 12.7 hours; $\beta +$ 0.653 MeV [17.4%]; $\beta -$, 0.579 MeV [39%], 43.6% electron capture) has shown good potential as a positron-emitting radionuclide for PET imaging and radiotherapy (105–107). The possibility of performing dosimetry for PRRT based on [^{64}Cu] is one other possible advantage. In a preliminary study, [^{64}Cu]-TETA-octreotide (TETA, 14,8,11-tetraazacyclotetradecane-N,N9,N99,N999-tetraacetic acid) PET was found to have high sensitivity, favorable dosimetry, and pharmacokinetics (106).

Fluorine-18-fluorodeoxyglucose PET

Fluorine-18-fluorodeoxyglucose is useful for evaluating the early phases of tumor glucose utilization, which is often increased in tumor cells because of an accelerated rate of glycolysis. Fluorine-18-fluorodeoxyglucose PET is primarily used in tumors for the purpose

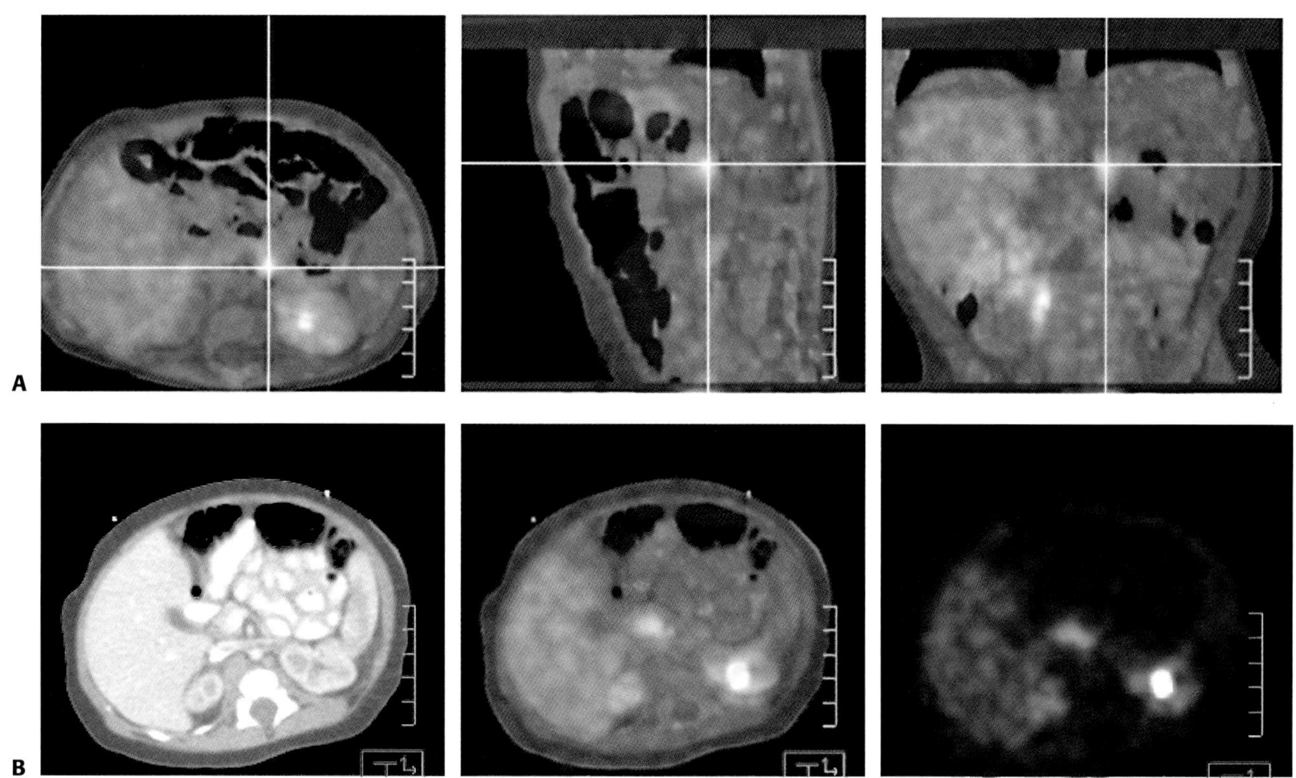

FIGURE 8.21.14. Diagnosis of focal (**A**) and diffuse (**B**) congenital hyperinsulinism by fluorine-18-fluorodopa PET. (Images courtesy of Abass Alavi, MD, University of Pennsylvania School of Medicine, Philadelphia, Pennsylvania.)

of diagnosis, staging, restaging, and evaluation of the response to treatment. The use of FDG PET in the diagnosis of NETs depends on the grade of differentiation and/or the aggressiveness of NETs (101,109–113).

In a study comparing [^{18}F]-FDG PET, [^{111}In]-pentetreotide somatostatin receptor scintigraphy (SS-R) and ^{99m}Tc(V)-DMSA scintigraphy (dual radionuclide technique, DNS equals SS-R plus ^{99m}Tc(V)-DMSA) in patients with GEP and medullary thyroid carcinoma, it was shown that FDG PET was more sensitive than SS-R in picking up less differentiated GEP tumors but was less sensitive in the detection of differentiated GEP tumors (109).

In patients with recurrent medullary thyroid carcinomas (MTC) and rapidly increasing carcinoembryonic antigen (CEA) levels, FDG PET was found to be superior to DNS (DNS, dual-radionuclide scintigraphy (SS-R and ^{99m}Tc(V)-DMSA) (109). Similar finding were observed in another study conducted on 16 patients with NETs (110). The [^{18}F]-FDG PET uptake in NETs was related to the aggressiveness and rapid tumor growth. It was also concluded that FDG PET contributes to better staging of advanced stages as compared to CT scans and SS-R (110). In a multicenter study, it was demonstrated that FDG PET is a useful method for the staging and follow-up of patients with MTC (the highest diagnostic accuracy as compared to other imaging modalities like CT scan, SS-R, ^{99m}Tc(V) DMSA, etc.) (114). For NETs in the pancreatic-duodenal region, FDG PET had the potential to change the treatment protocol in 17% of patients. FDG PET was best suited for patients suspected of having a malignant tumor or a pancreatic mass of more than 2 cm, or MEN1 cases with at least one visible lesion. FDG PET was not useful in duodenal tumors, benign insulinomas, and small, single pancreatic neuroendocrine lesions (115).

Carbon-11-epinephrine, Carbon-11-hydroxyepiphedrine PET

The indications for use of [^{11}C]-epinephrine, [^{11}C]-hydroxyepiphedrine PET are: (a) pheochromocytoma, (b) paraganglioma, (c) neuroblastoma, or (d) sympathetic nerve study.

Results

In eight patients with neuroblastoma, Shulkin et al. (116) have demonstrated that [^{11}C]-HED (hydroxyepiphedrine) PET has high sensitivity for neuroblastoma. The tumor uptake of [^{11}C]-HED was rapid, and most of the tumors were visualized within 5 minutes. Most of the tumor lesions visible on the [^{11}C]-HED PET were also localized by [^{123}I]-MIBG, provided they were within the field of view. In addition, the high uptake of [^{11}C]-HED in liver was found to be a hindrance for localization of tumor. In another study conducted by the same group, similar results were observed in ten patients with pheochromocytoma, suggesting a potential role of [^{11}C]-HED (117). However, high cost, short half-life, and limited availability of [^{11}C] have been obstacles for the wider clinical utilization of [^{11}C]-HED. Carbon-11-epinephrine is under evaluation as well, and has the potential as an agent for imaging neuroblastomas, although it suffers from the typical logistical challenges of the 20-minute half life of [^{11}C].

FUTURE PERSPECTIVES

Over the past decade, medical science has advanced tremendously, making it possible to unravel hitherto mysterious molecular events. The paramount importance of targeting small molecules for *in vivo* diagnostic purposes became clear when medical scientists were using intact monoclonal antibodies. The poor pharmacokinetics of these antibodies forced the development of smaller antibody fragments like minibodies, diabodies, and affibodies. Indeed, the use of [^{124}I]-labeled, genetically engineered anti-CEA minibodies and diabodies resulted in high contrast images (118). Intraoperative gamma probe detection of neuroendocrine tumors has been superior to scintigraphy and surgical palpation (119,120), offering the potential to shorten the operation time as well as minimizing the extent of surgical trauma.

PRRT is getting increasing acceptance among specialists dealing with NET patients. To individualize the patient's treatment, efforts are ongoing to deliver PRRT based on the results of pretherapeutic dosimetry, thereby also increasing its therapeutic index. New synthetic SSTR analogues, covering a wider range of SSTR subtypes ("pansomatostatin" analogues), and optimal radiometal-peptide combinations have been explored (90) (e.g., [^{68}Ga]-DOTA-TATE PET has already been shown to have a significant role in the detection of malignant paraganglioma) (121).

Looking at the present scenario, it can only be said that, just as FDG PET has revolutionized the care of patients with lymphoma, it will not be too long before receptor PET/CT imaging and peptide receptor radionuclide therapy will be well integrated into the routine management of patients with neuroendocrine tumors. An additional challenge in the United States, at present, is that the promising gallium-based generator systems and the various positron emitter "labelable" peptides are not yet approved by the U.S. Food and Drug Administration. Thus, the number of agents available in some locations for clinical practice is more limited than in other areas. In most areas, FDG and F-DOPA can be obtained, and these two agents can contribute significantly to the imaging of some NETs. The emerging availability of other PET-labeled NET imaging agents can only be viewed as an exciting enhancement to the field.

REFERENCES

1. Solcia E, Kloppel G, Sobin LH, et al. Histological typing of tumors. In World Health Organization, ed. *International histological classification of tumors.* Berlin, Heidelberg, New York: Springer, 2000.
2. Oberndorfer S. Karzinoidtumoren des Dünndarms. *Frankf Z Pathol* 1907;1:426–429.
3. Jensen RT. Endocrine tumors of the gastrointestinal tract and pancreas. In: Kasper DL, Fauci AS, Longo DL, et al., eds. *Harrison's principles of internal medicine.* New York: McGraw-Hill, 2005:2347–2358.
4. Li S, Beheshti M. The radionuclide molecular imaging and therapy of neuroendocrine tumors. *Curr Cancer Drug Targets* 2005;5:139–148.
5. Jensen RT. Carcinoid and pancreatic endocrine tumors:recent advances in molecular pathogenesis, localization, and treatment. *Curr Opin Oncol* 2000;12:368–377.
6. Kaltsas GA, Besser GM, Grossman AB. The diagnosis and medical management of advanced neuroendocrine tumors. *Endocr Rev* 2004;25: 458–511.
7. Baum RP, Hofmann M. Nuklearmedizinische Diagnostik neuroendokriner Tumoren. *Onkologe* 2004;10:598–610.
8. Reubi JC. Peptide receptors as molecular targets for cancer diagnosis and therapy. *Endocr Rev* 2003;24:389–427.
9. Maecke HR, Hofmann M, Haberkorn U. (68)Ga-labeled peptides in tumor imaging. *J Nucl Med* 2005;46[Suppl 1]:172S–178S.
10. Schmitt-Gräff A, Hezel B, Wiedenmann B. Pathologisch-diagnostische Aspekte neuroendokriner Tumoren des Gastrointestinaltrakts. *Onkologe* 2000;6:613–623.
11. Vinik AI, Woltering EA, O'Dorisio TM, et al. *Neuroendocrine tumors: a comprehensive guide to diagnosis and management.* Edmonton University of Alberta. Inter Science Institute, 2006.

12. Bombardieri E, Seregni E, Villano C, et al. Position of nuclear medicine techniques in the diagnostic work-up of neuroendocrine tumors. *Q J Nucl Med Mol Imaging* 2004;48:150–163.
13. Krenning EP, Bakker WH, Kooij PP, et al. Somatostatin receptor scintigraphy with indium-111-DTPA-D-Phe-1-octreotide in man: metabolism, dosimetry and comparison with iodine-123-Tyr-3-octreotide. *J Nucl Med* 1992;33:652–658.
14. Krenning EP, Bakker WH, Lamberts SW. [Receptor scintigraphy with somatostatin analog in oncology]. *Ned Tijdschr Geneeskd* 1990;134: 1077–1080.
15. Shapiro B, Copp JE, Sisson JC, et al. Iodine-131 metaiodobenzylguanidine for the locating of suspected pheochromocytoma: experience in 400 cases. *J Nucl Med* 1985;26:576–585.
16. Kolby L, Bernhardt P, Levin-Jakobsen AM, et al. Uptake of metaiodobenzylguanidine in neuroendocrine tumours is mediated by vesicular monoamine transporters. *Br J Cancer* 2003;89:1383–1388.
17. Rufini V, Calcagni ML, Baum RP. Imaging of neuroendocrine tumors. *Semin Nucl Med* 2006;36:228–247.
18. Troncone L, Rufini V. *MIBG in diagnosis of neuroendocrine tumors.* Edinburgh: Churchill Livingstone, 2004.
19. Wild D, Schmitt JS, Ginj M, et al. DOTA-NOC, a high-affinity ligand of somatostatin receptor subtypes 2, 3 and 5 for labelling with various radiometals. *Eur J Nucl Med Mol Imaging* 2003;30:1338–1347.
20. Reubi JC, Laissue JA. Multiple actions of somatostatin in neoplastic disease. *Trends Pharmacol Sci* 1995;16:110–115.
21. Sharif N, Gendron L, Wowchuk J, et al. Coexpression of somatostatin receptor subtype 5 affects internalization and trafficking of somatostatin receptor subtype 2. *Endocrinology* 2007;148:2095–2105.
22. Curtis SB, Hewitt J, Yakubovitz S, et al. Somatostatin receptor subtype expression and function in human vascular tissue. *Am J Physiol Heart Circ Physiol* 2000;278:H1815–H1822.
23. Reubi JC, Waser B, Schaer JC, et al. Somatostatin receptor SST1–SST5 expression in normal and neoplastic human tissues using receptor autoradiography with subtype-selective ligands. *Eur J Nucl Med* 2001; 28:836–846.
24. Taniyama Y, Suzuki T, Mikami Y, et al. Systemic distribution of somatostatin receptor subtypes in human: an immunohistochemical study. *Endocr J* 2005;52:605–611.
25. Unger N, Tourne H, Redmann A, et al. Immunohistochemical expression of somatostatin receptor subtypes in various normal human tissues. *Exp Clin Endocrinol Diabetes* 2005;113.
26. Ferone D, Pivonello R, Van Hagen PM, et al. Age-related decrease of somatostatin receptor number in the normal human thymus. *Am J Physiol Endocrinol Metab* 2000;279:E791–E798.
27. Dalm VA, van Hagen PM, van Koetsveld PM, et al. Expression of somatostatin, cortistatin, and somatostatin receptors in human monocytes, macrophages, and dendritic cells. *Am J Physiol Endocrinol Metab* 2003;285:E344–E353.
28. Neumann I, Mirzaei S, Birck R, et al. Expression of somatostatin receptors in inflammatory lesions and diagnostic value of somatostatin receptor scintigraphy in patients with ANCA-associated small vessel vasculitis. *Rheumatology* (Oxford) 2004;43:195–201.
29. Reubi JC, Schar JC, Waser B, et al. Affinity profiles for human somatostatin receptor subtypes SST1–SST5 of somatostatin radiotracers selected for scintigraphic and radiotherapeutic use. *Eur J Nucl Med* 2000;27:273–282.
30. Wild D, Macke HR, Waser B, et al. ^{68}Ga-DOTANOC: a first compound for PET imaging with high affinity for somatostatin receptor subtypes 2 and 5. *Eur J Nucl Med Mol Imaging* 2005;32:724.
31. Krenning EP, Kwekkeboom DJ, et al. Somatostatin receptor scintigraphy with [^{111}In-DTPA-D-Phe1]- and [^{123}I-Tyr3]-octreotide: the Rotterdam experience with more than 1000 patients. *Eur J Nucl Med* 1993;20: 716–731.
32. Lebtahi R, Le Cloirec J, Houzard C, et al. Detection of neuroendocrine tumors: ^{99m}Tc-P829 scintigraphy compared with ^{111}In-pentetreotide scintigraphy. *J Nucl Med* 2002;43:889–895.
33. Decristoforo C, Melendez-Alafort L, Sosabowski JK, et al. ^{99m}Tc-HYNIC-[Tyr3]-octreotide for imaging somatostatin-receptor-positive tumors: preclinical evaluation and comparison with ^{111}In-octreotide. *J Nucl Med* 2000;41:1114–1119.
34. Maina T, Nock B, Nikolopoulou A, et al. [^{99m}Tc]Demotate, a new ^{99m}Tc-based [Tyr3]octreotate analogue for the detection of somatostatin receptor-positive tumours: synthesis and preclinical results. *Eur J Nucl Med Mol Imaging* 2002;29:742–753.
35. Forrer F, Uusijarvi H, Storch D, et al. Treatment with ^{177}Lu-DOTATOC of patients with relapse of neuroendocrine tumors after treatment with ^{90}Y-DOTATOC. *J Nucl Med* 2005;46:1310–1316.
36. Virgolini I. *Peptide imaging.* Berlin, Heidelberg: Springer-Verlag, 2000.
37. Storch D, Behe M, Walter MA, et al. Evaluation of [^{99m}Tc/EDDA/HYNIC0]octreotide derivatives compared with [^{111}In-DOTA0,Tyr3, Thr8]octreotide and [^{111}In-DTPA0]octreotide: does tumor or pancreas uptake correlate with the rate of internalization? *J Nucl Med* 2005; 46:1561–1569.
38. Smith-Jones PM, Stolz B, Bruns C, et al. Gallium-67/gallium-68-[DFO]-octreotide—a potential radiopharmaceutical for PET imaging of somatostatin receptor-positive tumors: synthesis and radiolabeling in vitro and preliminary *in vivo* studies. *J Nucl Med* 1994;35:317–325.
39. de Jong M, Bakker WH, Krenning EP, et al. Yttrium-90 and indium-111 labelling, receptor binding and biodistribution of [DOTA0,d-Phe1, Tyr3]octreotide, a promising somatostatin analogue for radionuclide therapy. *Eur J Nucl Med* 1997;24:368–371.
40. Otte A, Herrmann R, Heppeler A, et al. Yttrium-90 DOTATOC: first clinical results. *Eur J Nucl Med* 1999;26:1439–1447.
41. Otte A, Mueller-Brand J, Dellas S, et al. Yttrium-90-labelled somatostatin-analogue for cancer treatment. *Lancet* 1998;351:417–418.
42. Paganelli G, Zoboli S, Cremonesi M, et al. Receptor-mediated radiotherapy with ^{90}Y-DOTA-D-Phe1-Tyr3-octreotide. *Eur J Nucl Med* 2001;28:426–434.
43. Stolz B, Weckbecker G, Smith-Jones PM, et al. The somatostatin receptor-targeted radiotherapeutic [^{90}Y-DOTA-DPhe1, Tyr3]octreotide (^{90}Y-SMT 487) eradicates experimental rat pancreatic CA20948 tumours. *Eur J Nucl Med* 1998;25:668–674.
44. Waldherr C, Pless M, Maecke HR, et al. Tumor response and clinical benefit in neuroendocrine tumors after 7.4 GBq (^{90})Y-DOTATOC. *J Nucl Med* 2002;43:610–616.
45. Heppeler A, Froidevaux S, Maecke HR. Radiometal-labelled macrocyclic chelator-derivatised somatostatin analogue with superb tumour-targeting properties and potential for receptor-mediated internal radiotherapy. *Chem Eur J* 1999;5:1016–1023.
46. Kwekkeboom DJ, Bakker WH, Kooij PP, et al. [^{177}Lu-DOTAOTyr3] octreotate: comparison with [^{111}In-DTPAo]octreotide in patients. *Eur J Nucl Med* 2001;28:1319–1325.
47. Raderer M, Pangerl T, Leimer M, et al. Expression of human somatostatin receptor subtype 3 in pancreatic cancer *in vitro* and *in vivo*. *J Natl Cancer Inst* 1998;90:1666–1668.
48. Ginj M, Chen J, Walter MA, et al. Preclinical evaluation of new and highly potent analogues of octreotide for predictive imaging and targeted radiotherapy. *Clin Cancer Res* 2005;11:1136–1145.
49. Ginj M, Zhang H, Waser B, et al. Radiolabeled somatostatin receptor antagonists are preferable to agonists for *in vivo* peptide receptor targeting of tumors. *Proc Natl Acad Sci U S A* 2006;103:16436–16441.
50. Reubi JC, Schaer JC, Wenger S, et al. SST3-selective potent peptidic somatostatin receptor antagonists. *Proc Natl Acad Sci U S A* 2000;97: 13973–13978.
51. Baylin SB, Abeloff MD, Goodwin G, et al. Activities of L-DOPA decarboxylase and diamine oxidase (histaminase) in human lung cancers and decarboxylase as a marker for small (oat) cell cancer in cell culture. *Cancer Res* 1980;40:1990–1994.
52. Gazdar AF, Helman LJ, Israel MA, et al. Expression of neuroendocrine cell markers L-DOPA decarboxylase, chromogranin A, and dense core granules in human tumors of endocrine and nonendocrine origin. *Cancer Res* 1988;48:4078–4082.

53. Breeman WA, De Jong M, Bernard BF, et al. Pre-clinical evaluation of [(^{111})In-DTPA-Pro(1), Tyr(4)]bombesin, a new radioligand for bombesin-receptor scintigraphy. *Int J Cancer* 1999;83:657–663.
54. Van de Wiele C, Dumont F, Vanden Broecke R, et al. Technetium-99m RP527, a GRP analogue for visualisation of GRP receptor-expressing malignancies: a feasibility study. *Eur J Nucl Med* 2000;27:1694–1699.
55. Hoffman TJ, Gali H, Smith CJ, et al. Novel series of ^{111}In-labeled bombesin analogs as potential radiopharmaceuticals for specific targeting of gastrin-releasing peptide receptors expressed on human prostate cancer cells. *J Nucl Med* 2003;44:823–831.
56. Scopinaro F, De Vincentis G, Varvarigou AD, et al. ^{99m}Tc-bombesin detects prostate cancer and invasion of pelvic lymph nodes. *Eur J Nucl Med Mol Imaging* 2003;30:1378–1382.
57. Nock B, Nikolopoulou A, Chiotellis E, et al. [^{99m}Tc]Demobesin 1, a novel potent bombesin analogue for GRP receptor-targeted tumour imaging. *Eur J Nucl Med Mol Imaging* 2003;30:247–258.
58. Reubi JC, Korner M, Waser B, et al. High expression of peptide receptors as a novel target in gastrointestinal stromal tumours. *Eur J Nucl Med Mol Imaging* 2004;31:803–810.
59. Schuhmacher J, Zhang H, Doll J, et al. GRP receptor-targeted PET of a rat pancreas carcinoma xenograft in nude mice with a ^{68}Ga-labeled bombesin(6-14) analog. *J Nucl Med* 2005;46:691–699.
60. Moody TW, Hill JM, Jensen RT. VIP as a trophic factor in the CNS and cancer cells. *Peptides* 2003;24:163–177.
61. Reubi JC, Waser B. Concomitant expression of several peptide receptors in neuroendocrine tumours: molecular basis for in vivo multireceptor tumour targeting. *Eur J Nucl Med Mol Imaging* 2003;30: 781–793.
62. Thakur ML, Marcus CS, Saeed S, et al. ^{99m}Tc-labeled vasoactive intestinal peptide analog for rapid localization of tumors in humans. *J Nucl Med* 2000;41:107–110.
63. Virgolini I, Kurtaran A, Raderer M, et al. Vasoactive intestinal peptide receptor scintigraphy. *J Nucl Med* 1995;36:1732–1739.
64. Virgolini I, Raderer M, Kurtaran A, et al. Vasoactive intestinal peptide-receptor imaging for the localization of intestinal adenocarcinomas and endocrine tumors. *N Engl J Med* 1994;331:1116–1121.
65. Behe M, Becker W, Gotthardt M, et al. Improved kinetic stability of DTPA-dGlu as compared with conventional monofunctional DTPA in chelating indium and yttrium: preclinical and initial clinical evaluation of radiometal labelled minigastrin derivatives. *Eur J Nucl Med Mol Imaging* 2003;30:1140–1146.
66. Behr TM, Behe M, Angerstein C, et al. Cholecystokinin-B/gastrin receptor binding peptides: preclinical development and evaluation of their diagnostic and therapeutic potential. *Clin Cancer Res* 1999;5: 3124s–3138s.
67. Behr TM, Jenner N, Radetzky S, et al. Targeting of cholecystokinin-B/gastrin receptors *in vivo*: preclinical and initial clinical evaluation of the diagnostic and therapeutic potential of radiolabelled gastrin. *Eur J Nucl Med* 1998;25:424–430.
68. Kwekkeboom DJ, Bakker WH, Kooij PP, et al. Cholecystokinin receptor imaging using an octapeptide DTPA-CCK analogue in patients with medullary thyroid carcinoma. *Eur J Nucl Med* 2000;27: 1312–1317.
69. Reubi JC, Waser B, Schaer JC, et al. Unsulfated DTPA- and DOTA-CCK analogs as specific high-affinity ligands for CCK-B receptor-expressing human and rat tissues *in vitro* and *in vivo*. *Eur J Nucl Med* 1998; 25:481–490.
70. Green MW, Tucker D. An improved gallium-68 cow. *Int J Appl Radiat Isot* 1961;12:62–63.
71. Schumacher J, Maier-Borst W. A new ^{68}Ge/^{68}Ga radioisotope generator system for production of ^{68}Ga in dilute HCl. *Int J Appl Radiat Isot* 1981;32:31–36.
72. Arino H, Skraba W, Kramer HH. A new ^{68}Ge/^{68}Ga radioisotope generator system. *Int J Appl Radiat Isot* 1978;29:117–120.
73. Rösch F, Knapp FFR. *Radionuclide generators.* Rotterdam: Kluwer Academic Publishers, 2003.
74. Zhernosekov KP, Filosofov DV, Baum RP, et al. Processing of generator-produced ^{68}Ga for medical application. *J Nucl Med* 2007;48: 1741–1748.
75. Hofmann M, Maecke H, Borner R, et al. Biokinetics and imaging with the somatostatin receptor PET radioligand (^{68})Ga-DOTATOC: preliminary data. *Eur J Nucl Med* 2001;28:1751–1757.
76. Meyer GJ, Macke H, Schuhmacher J, et al. ^{68}Ga-labelled DOTA-derivatised peptide ligands. *Eur J Nucl Med Mol Imaging* 2004;31: 1097–1104.
77. Kowalski J, Henze M, Schuhmacher J, et al. Evaluation of positron emission tomography imaging using [^{68}Ga]-DOTA-D Phe(1)-Tyr(3)-Octreotide in comparison to [^{111}In]-DTPAOC SPECT. First results in patients with neuroendocrine tumors. *Mol Imaging Biol* 2003;5: 42–48.
78. Baum RP, Schmücking M, Niesen A, et al. Receptor-PET/CT of neuroendocrine tumors using the gallium-68 labelled somatostatin analog DOTA-NOC: first clinical results. *Eur Radiol* 2005;15[Suppl 1]: C0409.
79. Baum RP, Prasad V. Monitoring treatment. In: Cook GJR, Maisey MN, Britton KE, et al., eds. *Clinical nuclear medicine.* London: Hodder Arnold, 2006:57–78.
80. Baum RP, Prasad V, Hommann M, et al. Receptor PET/CT imaging of neuroendocrine tumors. *Recent Res Cancer Res* 2008;170: 225–242.
81. Fueger BJ, Hamilton G, Raderer M, et al. Effects of chemotherapeutic agents on expression of somatostatin receptors in pancreatic tumor cells. *J Nucl Med* 2001;42:1856–1862.
82. Pettinato C, Sarnelli A, Di Donna M, et al. (^{68})Ga-DOTANOC: biodistribution and dosimetry in patients affected by neuroendocrine tumors. *Eur J Nucl Med Mol Imaging* 2008;35:72–79
83. Koukouraki S, Strauss LG, Georgoulias V, et al. Evaluation of the pharmacokinetics of (^{68})Ga-DOTATOC in patients with metastatic neuroendocrine tumours scheduled for (^{90})Y-DOTATOC therapy. *Eur J Nucl Med Mol Imaging* 2006;33:460–466.
84. Henze M, Schuhmacher J, Dimitrakopoulou-Strauss A, et al. Exceptional increase in somatostatin receptor expression in pancreatic neuroendocrine tumour, visualised with (^{68})Ga-DOTATOC PET. *Eur J Nucl Med Mol Imaging* 2004;31:466.
85. Henze M, Dimitrakopoulou-Strauss A, Milker-Zabel S, et al. Characterization of ^{68}Ga-DOTA-D-Phe1-Tyr3-octreotide kinetics in patients with meningiomas. *J Nucl Med* 2005;46:763–769.
86. Henze M, Schuhmacher J, Hipp P, et al. PET imaging of somatostatin receptors using [^{68}GA]DOTA-D-Phe1-Tyr3-octreotide: first results in patients with meningiomas. *J Nucl Med* 2001;42:1053–1056.
87. Cescato R, Schulz S, Waser B, et al. Internalization of SST2, SST3, and SST5 receptors: effects of somatostatin agonists and antagonists. *J Nucl Med* 2006;47:502–511.
88. Kwekkeboom DJ, Kho GS, Lamberts SW, et al. The value of octreotide scintigraphy in patients with lung cancer. *Eur J Nucl Med* 1994;21: 1106–1113.
89. Buchmann I, Henze M, Engelbrecht S, et al. Comparison of ^{68}Ga-DOTATOC PET and ^{111}In-DTPAOC (OctreoScan) SPECT in patients with neuroendocrine tumours. *Eur J Nucl Med Mol Imaging* 2007;34: 1617–1626.
90. Antunes P, Ginj M, Zhang H, et al. Are radiogallium-labelled DOTA-conjugated somatostatin analogues superior to those labelled with other radiometals? *Eur J Nucl Med Mol Imaging* 2007;34:982–993 .
91. Ahlstrom H, Eriksson B, Bergstrom M, et al. Pancreatic neuroendocrine tumors: diagnosis with PET. *Radiology* 1995;195:333–337.
92. Becherer A, Szabo M, Karanikas G, et al. Imaging of advanced neuroendocrine tumors with (^{18})F-FDOPA PET. *J Nucl Med* 2004;45: 1161–1167.
93. Jacob T, Grahek D, Younsi N, et al. Positron emission tomography with [(^{18})F]FDOPA and [(^{18})F]FDG in the imaging of small cell lung carcinoma: preliminary results. *Eur J Nucl Med Mol Imaging* 2003;30: 1266–1269.

94. Eldrup E, Clausen N, Scherling B, et al. Evaluation of plasma 3,4-dihydroxyphenylacetic acid (DOPAC) and plasma 3,4-dihydroxyphenylalanine (DOPA) as tumour markers in children with neuroblastoma. *Scand J Clin Lab Invest* 2001;61(6):479–490.
95. Hoegerle S, Altehoefer C, Ghanem N, et al. Whole-body ^{18}F DOPA PET for detection of gastrointestinal carcinoid tumors. *Radiology* 2001;220: 373–380.
96. Koopmans KP, de Vries EG, Kema IP, et al. Staging of carcinoid tumours with ^{18}F-DOPA PET: a prospective, diagnostic accuracy study. *Lancet Oncol* 2006;7:728–734.
97. Nanni C, Fanti S, Rubello D. ^{18}F-DOPA PET and PET/CT. *J Nucl Med* 2007;48:1577–1579.
98. Hoegerle S, Nitzsche E, Altehoefer C, et al. Pheochromocytomas: detection with ^{18}F DOPA whole body PET—initial results. *Radiology* 2002;222:507–512.
99. Hardy OT, Hernandez-Pampaloni M, Saffer JR, et al. Diagnosis and localization of focal congenital hyperinsulinism by ^{18}F-fluorodopa PET scan. *J Pediatr* 2007;150:140–145.
100. Ambrosini V, Tomassetti P, Rubello D, et al. Role of ^{18}F-DOPA PET/CT imaging in the management of patients with ^{111}In-pentetreotide negative GEP tumours. *Nucl Med Commun* 2007;28:473–477.
101. Eriksson B, Bergstrom M, Orlefors H, et al. Use of PET in neuroendocrine tumors. *In vivo* applications and *in vitro* studies. *Q J Nucl Med* 2000;44:68–76.
102. Orlefors H, Sundin A, Ahlstrom H, et al. Positron emission tomography with 5-hydroxytryprophan in neuroendocrine tumors. *J Clin Oncol* 1998;16:2534–2541.
103. Wester HJ, Schottelius M, Scheidhauer K, et al. PET imaging of somatostatin receptors: design, synthesis and preclinical evaluation of a novel ^{18}F-labelled, carbohydrated analogue of octreotide. *Eur J Nucl Med Mol Imaging* 2003;30:117–122.
104. Meisetschlager G, Poethko T, Stahl A, et al. Gluc-Lys([^{18}F]FP)-TOCA PET in patients with SSTR-positive tumors: biodistribution and diagnostic evaluation compared with [^{111}In]DTPA-octreotide. *J Nucl Med* 2006;47:566–573.
105. Sprague JE, Peng Y, Sun X, et al. Preparation and biological evaluation of copper-64-labeled tyr3-octreotate using a cross-bridged macrocyclic chelator. *Clin Cancer Res* 2004;10:8674–8682.
106. Anderson CJ, Dehdashti F, Cutler PD, et al. ^{64}Cu-TETA-octreotide as a PET imaging agent for patients with neuroendocrine tumors. *J Nucl Med* 2001;42:213–221.
107. Lewis JS, Lewis MR, Cutler PD, et al. Radiotherapy and dosimetry of ^{64}Cu-TETA-Tyr3-octreotate in a somatostatin receptor-positive, tumor-bearing rat model. *Clin Cancer Res* 1999;5:3608–3616.
108. Wang M, Caruano AL, Lewis MR, et al. Subcellular localization of radiolabeled somatostatin analogues: implications for targeted radiotherapy of cancer. *Cancer Res* 2003;63:6864–6869.
109. Adams S, Baum R, Rink T, et al. Limited value of fluorine-18 fluorodeoxyglucose positron emission tomography for the imaging of neuroendocrine tumours. *Eur J Nucl Med* 1998;25:79–83.
110. Pasquali C, Rubello D, Sperti C, et al. Neuroendocrine tumor imaging: can ^{18}F-fluorodeoxyglucose positron emission tomography detect tumors with poor prognosis and aggressive behavior? *World J Surg* 1998;22:588–592.
111. Scanga DR, Martin WH, Delbeke D. Value of FDG PET imaging in the management of patients with thyroid, neuroendocrine, and neural crest tumors. *Clin Nucl Med* 2004;29:86–90.
112. Sundin A, Eriksson B, Bergstrom M, et al. PET in the diagnosis of neuroendocrine tumors. *Ann N Y Acad Sci* 2004;1014:246–257.
113. Zhao DS, Valdivia AY, Li Y, et al. ^{18}F-fluorodeoxyglucose positron emission tomography in small-cell lung cancer. *Semin Nucl Med* 2002;32: 272–275.
114. Diehl M, Risse JH, Brandt-Mainz K, et al. Fluorine-18 fluorodeoxyglucose positron emission tomography in medullary thyroid cancer: results of a multicentre study. *Eur J Nucl Med* 2001;28: 1671–1676.
115. Pasquali C, Sperti C, Scappin S, et al. Role and indications of fluorodeoxyglucose positron emission tomography (FDG-PET) in neuroendocrine pancreaticoduodenal tumors. *J Pancreas* 2004;6[5 Suppl]: 528–529.
116. Shulkin BL, Wieland DM, Baro ME, et al. PET hydroxyephedrine imaging of neuroblastoma. *J Nucl Med* 1996;37:16–21.
117. Shulkin BL, Wieland DM, Schwaiger M, et al. PET scanning with hydroxyephedrine: an approach to the localization of pheochromocytoma. *J Nucl Med* 1992;33:1125–1131.
118. Sundaresan G, Yazaki PJ, Shively JE, et al. ^{124}I-labeled engineered anti-CEA minibodies and diabodies allow high-contrast, antigen-specific small-animal PET imaging of xenografts in athymic mice. *J Nucl Med* 2003;44:1962–1969.
119. Adams S, Baum RP. Intraoperative use of gamma-detecting probes to localize neuroendocrine tumors. *Q J Nucl Med* 2000;44: 59–67.
120. Adams S, Baum RP, Hertel A, et al. Intraoperative gamma probe detection of neuroendocrine tumors. *J Nucl Med* 1998;39:1155–1160.
121. Win Z, Rahman L, Murrell J, et al. The possible role of ^{68}Ga-DOTATATE PET in malignant abdominal paraganglioma. *Eur J Nucl Med Mol Imaging* 2006;33:506.

CHAPTER

8.22

Carcinoma of Unknown Primary: Including Paraneoplastic Neurological Syndromes

JENNIFER RODRIGUEZ-FERRER AND RICHARD L. WAHL

PARANEOPLASTIC NEUROLOGICAL SYNDROMES

Carcinoma of unknown primary (CUP) accounts for 3% to 5% of all new cancer diagnoses. It is the seventh most common malignancy and the fourth most common cause of cancer death in both males and females. The median age at presentation is 60, with CUP more frequent in men than in women. The prognosis of patients with CUP is generally poor. The median survival rate is approximately 3 to 11 months with less than 25% of patients surviving over 1 year. Survival rates differ among histological subgroups and are worse in those patients who present with widely disseminated disease (1–3).

CUP is defined as histologically confirmed metastatic cancer with no identifiable primary site after a complete history and physical examination (including a pelvic and rectal examination), complete blood count, biochemistry, urinalysis, occult fecal blood test, serum tumor markers, histopathology review of biopsy material with the use of immunohistochemistry, mammography in females, computed tomography (CT) of the chest, abdomen and pelvis, or any other relevant test. Until recently, 18-F-fluoro-2-deoxy-D-glucose (FDG) positron emission tomography (PET) was not one of these tests. There is some variability in the literature as to the intensity of the work-up for CUP, likely contributing to some variability in the rates of identification of the previously occult primary lesions by imaging tests like PET. In the majority of cases the primary site will never be found during the patient's lifetime using a work-up that does not include PET. Twenty percent of patients have no detectable primary tumor site even at postmortem studies. Conventional radiological imaging identifies about 20% to 27% of the primary tumors after intensive investigation. Most commonly, patients seek medical attention because of the recent enlargement of a superficial lymph node or present with visceral masses, bone lesions either symptomatic or detected at radiographic examinations for an unrelated indication. Possible explanations for the inability to detect the primary tumor include: (a) spontaneous regression (the primary is not detectable when metastasis becomes evident, not a common phenomenon but this process has been described in several tumors such as melanoma; approximately 5% of patients with malignant melanoma present without a identifiable primary site); (b) immune-modulated destruction of the primary cancer; or (c) the primary tumor's malignant phenotype and genotype favor metastatic ability over local tumor growth (1–3).

CUPs are categorized into four major subtypes by routine light microscopy criteria:

(a) adenocarcinomas, well to moderately differentiated 50% to 60%; (b) poorly differentiated adenocarcinomas or carcinomas 30% to 40%; (c) squamous cell carcinoma (SCC) 5% to 8%; and (d) undifferentiated neoplasms 2% to 5% (including lymphoma, sarcoma, melanoma, primitive neuroendocrine tumors, germ cell tumors, and embryonal tumors). Patients with poorly differentiated carcinomas and metastatic adenocarcinoma of unknown primary have the poorest prognosis, while metastatic SCC has a more favorable prognosis. CUP has an unpredictable metastatic pattern that differs from the pattern distribution seen in tumors with identifiable primary lesions. For example, patients eventually diagnosed with prostate cancer who present as CUP have a high incidence of metastases to nonosseous sites such as lung, liver, and brain. Bone metastases are less common than lung metastases in thyroid cancer presenting as CUP than in other presentations of thyroid cancer.

CUP falls into two major categories of anatomical presentation: those with metastatic involvement to lymph nodes or patients presenting with visceral tumor involvement. As discussed later, CUP can also present with neurological syndromes. The most common sites for involvement of metastatic disease are lymph nodes, liver, lung, or bone. Lymph nodes in the cervical and supraclavicular region are the most common metastatic sites for CUP. Histologically, these tumors are usually SCC, but occasionally may be adenocarcinoma, melanoma, or anaplastic tumors. If the metastatic lymph nodes are located in the upper and middle cervical levels, especially in the case of SCC, a primary tumor of the head and neck region is highly suspected. If the lower cervical lymph nodes are only involved, the primary tumor is often located below the clavicles. Also, cervical metastases of non-SCC at any level can be due to a primary tumor located outside the head and neck area, and most likely the primary is found in the lung, gastrointestinal, or urogenital system. Although axillary nodal involvement in a middle-aged women is highly suggestive of primary breast carcinoma, nonpalpable breast cancer presenting as axillary metastases is quite rare, accounting for less than 0.5% of all breast cancers (although since breast cancers are quite common, this presentation of CUP is not infrequent). Metastases to inguinal nodes more commonly originate from primary tumors of the anogenital area, where diffuse metastatic involvement of the peritoneum or retroperitoneal lymph nodes are most consistent with primary tumors of the ovary, peritoneum, prostate, or testis. Pulmonary and hepatic metastases may arise from any site, whereas the most common origin of bone metastases are thyroid, breast, and prostate cancers (1–3).

FDG PET has been used for the evaluation of patients with CUP, particularly in patients with isolated neck metastases, but very few data are available on its usefulness in extracervical metastases. The detection rates in the literature for FDG PET have ranged widely, from 8% to 57% (Table 8.22.1). This wide range is attributed to the different definitions used for CUP between studies, differing make up of the patient populations, differing techniques (e.g., PET vs. PET/CT), and likely differing reader thresholds for positivity. Overall, the PET detection rate of primary lesions is about 39% (4–20).

A close review of Table 8.22.1 illustrates that much of the literature with PET in CUP is for patients presenting with head and neck nodal metastases. The number of cases with non–head and neck SCC is rather low. In addition, it is worth noting that when PET is used, while true-positive results dominate, they often occur in less than half of the patients evaluated. Further, false-positive results are not uncommon in such patients. Indeed in at least one of the studies, the false-positive rate exceeded the true-positive rate, raising questions regarding the value of the scan. However, many of the earlier studies were performed with FDG PET and not PET/CT. Based on the results of PET/CT in other tumors, it is probable that specificity is superior with PET/CT rather than PET alone, and it is probable, although not proven, that diagnostic accuracy is superior in this setting with PET/CT. Thus, use of FDG PET in such cases must be accompanied by a realistic expectation that while a primary lesion may be found, this is by no means the rule and that false-positive results may be expected in some instances. Thus, even with PET/CT, the diagnosis of CUP is far from a fully solved matter.

CUP accounts for the presentation of 1% to 2% of patients with head and neck cancer. The diagnostic work-up of cervical nodal metastasis of an unknown primary includes physical examination, CT, and/or magnetic resonance imaging of the neck, fine-needle biopsy of the lymph node, and panendoscopy with blind and directed biopsies. Imaging of the chest and abdomen are usually performed for adenocarcinomas and undifferentiated cancers. Even after such extensive work-up the detection rate of the primary tumor is still less than 50%. If a head and neck primary is suspected but cannot be localized, the usual treatment includes neck dissection and tonsillectomy followed by radiotherapy of all areas of the neck that may harbor the primary tumor. Therefore, correct identification of the primary tumor results in a definitive treatment with curative intent. Further, the therapeutic procedure can be adapted according to treatment protocol for specific tumor and reduces the risk of complications of radiotherapy by decreasing the size of the radiation field and by reducing excessive surgery. Survival is also probably improved in patients when the primary tumor is identified, likely attributable to better regional treatment options in these patients.

False-negative FDG PET results can be obtained due to a very small primary tumor, because the primary was actually removed at the time of neck dissection, because of low metabolic activity due to necrotic or cystic tumor, or because of a nodal metastasis next to the primary tumor that may not be detectable as a separate hypermetabolic focus when both the primary and the nodal metastasis show intense FDG uptake, undetectably merging primary with the nodal metastasis.

FDG PET is a valuable tool in localizing a primary tumor in patients with metastases of unknown primary. FDG PET can also identify additional sites of metastases that can alter the patient's management, which probably improves survival time and at the same time can serve as a guide for biopsies (Figs. 8.22.1 and 8.22.2). FDG PET is also useful for treatment monitoring following a therapeutic intervention. Various reviews have proposed that FDG PET should be the first imaging procedure performed in the case of cervical metastases since it is unlikely that other imaging modalities will identify a primary tumor that cannot be detected by FDG PET. If the FDG PET is positive, biopsies can be obtained from the suspected area. As indicated earlier, false-positive results can also occur, so to achieve high sensitivity for PET an understanding of the possibility of false positives must be present. If the FDG PET is negative, panendoscopy with biopsy sampling can be performed. If FDG PET is performed in the head and neck cancer setting, it is the authors' recommendation that it be done with PET/CT, and it is the authors' expectation that the use of intravenous contrast may help in precisely locating foci of increased tracer uptake.

PARANEOPLASTIC NEUROLOGICAL SYNDROMES

Paraneoplastic neurological syndromes (PNS) are rare neurologic manifestations of nonneurological cancers as a result of the development of antibodies directed against tumors that cross-react with normal neuronal tissue, which leads to progressive neurological damage. These syndromes includes Lambert-Eaton myasthenic syndrome, stiff man (person) syndrome, encephalomyelitis, myasthenia gravis, cerebellar degeneration, limbic and/or brain stem encephalitis, neuromyotonia, opsoclonus, and sensory neuropathy. PNS affect 1% to 3% of all cancer patients and are characterized by rapidly progressive subacute neurological dysfunction (21).

Paraneoplastic cerebellar degeneration (PCD) is the most common paraneoplastic syndrome affecting the brain, and it is found most commonly in patients with small cell lung cancer (SCLC), adenocarcinoma of the ovary and breast, and Hodgkin's lymphoma. Neurologic symptoms begin with the acute onset of cerebellar dysfunction over the course of days to weeks and typically occur prior to primary tumor detection (22,23). As the disease progresses there may be pancerebellar symptoms including nystagmus, vertigo, diplopia, dysarthria, symmetrical truncal, and appendicular ataxia, leaving the patient in a severely disabled state. PCD is believed to be caused by immune-mediated damage to the nervous system, which has been supported by the presence of high titers of anti-Purkinje cell antibodies in the serum or cerebral spinal fluid that reacts specifically with cerebellar Purkinje cells. Antineuronal antibodies are found in approximately 60% of these patients. Pathologically, PCD is characterized by marked loss of Purkinje cells throughout the cerebellar cortex and may be accompanied by neuronal loss in the granular cell layer and deep cerebellar nuclei. The most frequent

TABLE 8.22.1 Unknown Primary Carcinomas Detected by Fluorodeoxyglucose PET

Study	No. of Patients	No. of Cervical Metastases	No. of Extracervical Metastases	TP	% of Tumor Detected by FDG-PET	FP	FN
Bohuslavizki et. al.	53	44 (7 undifferentiated ca, 28 SCC, 8 undecisive cytology or histology, 1 other)	9 (3 adenoca, 2 SCC, 1 undifferentiated ca, 3 undecisive cytology or histology)	20	37.8%	6	4
Regelink et. al.	50	50 (30 SCC, 18 large cell ca, 1 adenoca, 1 neuroendocrine ca)	0	16	32.0%	2	0
Aassar et. al.	17	17 (14 SCC, 3 adenoca)	0	9	53.0%	3	0
Greven et. al.	13	13 (SCC)	0	1	8.0%	6	2
Braams et. al.	13	13 (10 SCC, 1 adenoca, 1 plasmacytoma, 1 PTC)	0	4	30.0%	0	1
Lassen et. al.	20	11 (6 SCC, 4 adenoca, 1 poorly differentiated ca)	9 (7 adenoca, 2 poorly differentiated ca)	9	45.0%	4	2
Kole et. al.	29	16 (11 SCC, 3 adenoca, 1 plasmacytoma, 1 large cell ca)	13 (8 melanoma, 4 adenoca, 1 not specified)	7	24.0%	0	3
Lonneux et. al.	24	3 (2 SCC, 1 unknown)	21 (18 adenoca, 2 poorly differentiated ca, 1 unknown)	13	54.0%	5	0
Gutzeit et. al.	45	18^	27^	15	33.0%	3	2
Nanni et. al.*	21	4 (1 melanoma, 3 SCC)	17 (8 adenoca, 4 SCC, 1 poorly differentiated ca, 1 germ cell tumor, 3 others)	12	57.0%	1	0
Mantaka et. al.	25	15 (7 SCC, 3 adenoca, 2 small cell ca, 1 well differentiated ca, 1 differentiated papillary ca, 1 malignant tumor)	10 (2 adenoca, 2 poorly differentiated ca, 1 small cell ca, 1 well diferentiated ca, 1 undifferentiated ca, 2 dysplasia, 1 data not available)	12	48.0%	5	0
Pelosi et. al.*	68	18 (3 adenoca, 15 carcinoma)	50 (4 melanoma, 15 adenoca, 31 carcinoma)	24	35.3%	5	5
Paul et. al.*	14	14 (2 adenoca, 7 undifferentiated adenoca, 3 undifferentiated ca, 1 undifferentiated neuroendocrine tumor, 1 low-grade sarcoma)	0	7	50.0%	1	2

*FDG-PET/CT; ca = Carcinoma; ^Not specified (total of 25 adenoca, 15 SCC, 5 undifferential ca); SCC = Squamous Cell Carcinoma; PTC = Papillary Thyroid Carcinoma; TP = True Positive; FP = False Positive; FN = False Negative

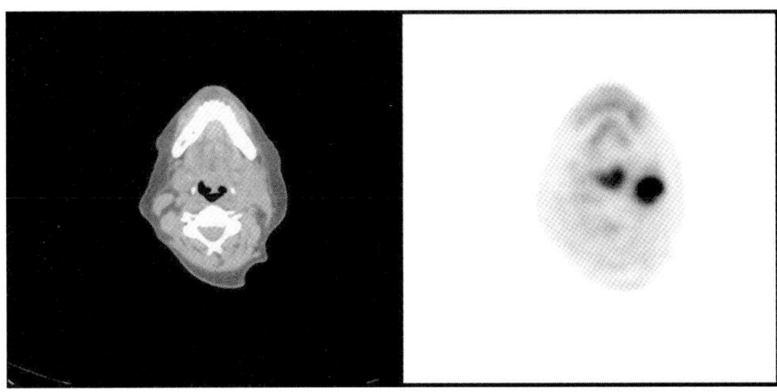

FIGURE 8.22.1. A 51-year-old man who presented with a left neck mass. Fine-needle aspiration was positive for squamous cell carcinoma. CT and magnetic resonance imaging of the neck only revealed left cervical adenopathy. Fluorodeoxyglucose (FDG) PET/CT performed for detection of primary tumor shows a small focus of intense FDG uptake in the left tonsillar region in addition to the intense FDG uptake in the left neck nodal mass. On the noncontrast CT scan no clear abnormality is seen in the region of the left palatine tonsil. Biopsy of the left palatine tonsil revealed squamous cell carcinoma.

antineuronal antibodies associated with PCD are anti-Hu, anti-Yo, anti-Tr, and anti-Ri (23). There is an association between these antibodies and specific tumors. Anti-Hu antibodies are usually associated with SCLC, anti-Yo antibodies have been associated with ovarian cancer and breast cancer, anti-Tr antibodies are specific for Hodgkin's lymphoma, and anti-Ri antibodies are associated with breast cancer. The onset of neurological symptoms and the presence of antineuronal antibodies in the serum or cerebrospinal fluid establishes the diagnosis of PCD and typically prompts an extensive diagnostic work-up for underlying tumor (24).

FDG PET has been shown to be useful in detecting unknown primary tumors and small metastatic lesions when conventional imaging studies are negative or inconclusive in this setting. For the clinicians it is important to recognized this syndrome, since early detection can lead to resection of the tumor before it has metastasized, and early treatment is likely the only chance to stabilized PCD before irreversible cerebellar damage has occurred. At times the primary malignancy is discovered up to 4 years after the initial onset of PCD. Mathew et al. (25) reported on a patient with anti-Yo associated PCD whose tumor was demonstrated 5 years after follow-up. In a study performed by Linke et al. (26) that includes 13 patients with antibody-positive PNS (8 anti-Hu; 4 anti-Yo; 1 anti-Tr), a new tumor or tumor recurrence was found in 10 of 13 patients (5 SCLC, 2 ovarian cancer, 1 neuroblastoma, 1 Hodgkin's lymphoma, 1 lymph node metastasis of adenocarcinoma). In that study, FDG PET was positive in nine of ten patients (90% sensitivity), compared with CT, which was positive in three of ten patients (30% sensitivity); and a 100% sensitivity was obtained with the combination of FDG PET with CT. Another study by Younes-Mhenni et al. (27) evaluated 20 patients with paraneoplastic antibodies (12 anti-Hu; 4 anti-Yo; 1 anti-Hu and anti-CV2; 1 anti-CV2, 1 anti-Ri; 1 anti-amphiphysin) in whom conventional imaging was negative or inconclusive, but FDG PET was positive for tumor in 18 of 20 patients. A histological diagnosis was made in 14 patients (8 SCLC, 2 breast adenocarcinoma, 2 lung adenocarcinoma, 1 axillary metastasis of ovarian carcinoma, 1 malignant thymoma). The sensitivity of FDG PET to detect tumor was reported to be 70% to 83% and the specificity 25%. In a retrospective study by Rees et al. (28), 43 unselected patients with suspect PNS were evaluated with FDG PET after having been investigated previously with conventional imaging. Of the 43 patients 16 had positive FDG PET scans. Histological diagnosis was confirmed in only seven patients, and CT imaging suggested malignancy in one patient. FDG PET detection rate of the malignancy was only 32% with a false-positive rate of approximately 10%. Only six patients with positive FDG PET scan had positive serum antineuronal antibodies, which could explain the results. Thus, it is clear that a significant fraction of patients with PNS will have positive PET scans, but not all. The PET scan is likely of greatest utility for identification of the primary tumor site when antineuronal antibodies are identified in the serum.

In summary, CUP can present in several ways, with overt metastatic disease to lymph nodes or elsewhere or with a paraneoplastic syndrome. Although the rate of PET scan positivity can vary greatly in these groups, it is increasingly clear that FDG PET should be considered and performed as part of the standard work-up of such tumors and syndromes suggesting occult tumors. It must also be recognized that false-negative results are common and that false-positive results are not uncommonly seen. Thus, histological confirmation of the PET findings is very important.

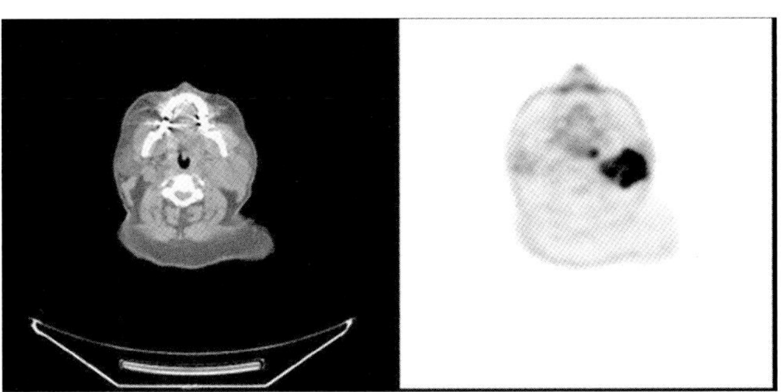

FIGURE 8.22.2. A 55-year-old woman with metastatic squamous cell carcinoma in a left neck mass. Panendoscopy with biopsies did not reveal the primary tumor. Fluorodeoxyglucose (FDG) PET/CT to evaluate for primary tumor shows asymmetric intense FDG uptake in the left base of tongue and intense FDG uptake in the patient's known left neck nodal mass. Subsequently, the patient underwent left neck dissection and direct laryngoscopy with biopsy of the left base of tongue. Pathology confirms squamous cell carcinoma of the left base of tongue.

REFERENCES

1. Pavlidis N, Briasoulis E, Hainsworth J, et al. Diagnostic and therapeutic management of cancer of unknown primary. *Eur J Cancer* 2003;39: 1990–2005.
2. Chorost M, Lee MC, Yeoh CB, et al. Unknown primary. *J Surg Oncol* 2004;87:191–203.
3. Abbruzzese JL, Abbruzzese MC, Lenzi R, et al. Analysis of a diagnostic strategy for patients with suspected tumors of unknown origin. *J Clin Oncol* 1995; 13:2094–2110.
4. Bohuslavizki KH, Klutmann S, Kroger S, et al. FDG PET detection of unknown primary tumors. *J Nucl Med* 2000;41:816–822.
5. Regelink G, Brouwer J, de Bree R, et al. Detection of unknown primary tumours and distant metastases in patients with cervical metastases: value of FDG-PET versus conventional modalities. *Eur J Nucl Med Mol Imaging* 2002;29:1024–1030.

6. OS AA, Fischbein NJ, Caputo GR, et al. Metastatic head and neck cancer: role and usefulness of FDG-PET in locating occult primary tumors. *Radiology* 1999;210:177–181.
7. Kole AC, Nieweg OE, Pruim J, et al. Detection of unknown occult primary tumors using positron emission tomography. *Cancer* 1998;82: 1160–1166.
8. Lassen U, Daugaard G, Eigtved A, et al. ^{18}F-FDG whole body positron emission tomography (PET) in patients with unknown primary tumours (UPT). *Eur J Cancer* 1999;35:1076–1082.
9. Braams JW, Pruim J, Kole AC, et al. Detection of unknown primary head and neck tumors by positron emission tomography. *Int J Oral Maxillofac Surg* 1997;26:112–115.
10. Greven KM, Keyes JW, Jr., Williams DW, et al. Occult primary tumors of the head and neck: lack of benefit from positron emission tomography imaging with 2-F18 fluoro-2-deoxy-D-glucose. *Cancer* 1999:86:114–118.
11. Lonneux M, Reffad A. Metastases from unknown primary tumor: PET-FDG as initial diagnostic procedure? *Clin Positron Imaging* 2000;3: 137–141.
12. Gutzeit A, Antoch G, Kuhl H, et al. Unknown primary tumors;dtection with dual-modality PET/CT: initial experience. *Radiology* 2005;234: 227–234.
13. Nanni C, Rubello D, Castellucci P, et al. Role of ^{18}F-FDG PET-CT imaging for the detection of an unknown primary tumour: preliminary results in 21 patients. *Eur J Nucl Mol Imaging* 2005;32:589–592.
14. Mantaka P, Baum RP, Hertel A, et al. PET with 2-[F-18]-fluoro-2-deoxy-D-glucose (FDG) in patients with cancer of unknown primary (CUP): influence on patients' diagnostic and therapeutic management. *Cancer Biother Radiopharm* 2003;18:47–58.
15. Pelosi E, Pennone M, Deandreis D, et al. Role of whole body positron emission tomography/computed tomography scan with ^{18}F-fluorodeoxyglucose in patients with biopsy proven tumor metastases from unknown primary site. *Q J Nucl Med Mol Imaging* 2006;50:15–22.
16. Paul SA, Stoeckli SJ, von Schulthess GK, et al. FDG PET/CT for the detection of the primary tumour in patients with cervical non-squamous cell carcinoma metastasis of an unknown primary. *Eur Arch Otorhinolaryngol* 2007;264(2): 189–195.
17. Seve P, Billotey C, Broussolle C, et al. The role of 2-deoxy-2-[F-18]fluoro-D-glucose positron emission tomography in disseminated carcinoma of unknown primary site. *Cancer* 2007;109(2):292–299.
18. Rades D, Kuhnel G, Wildfang I, et al. Localised disease in cancer of unknown primary (CUP): the value of positron emission tomography (PET) for individual therapeutic management. *Ann Oncol* 2001;12: 1605–1609.
19. Schoder H, Yeung HWD. Positron emission imaging of head and neck cancer, including thyroid carcinoma. *Sem Nucl Med* 2004;3:180–197.
20. Kresnik E, Mikosch P, Gallowitsch HJ, et al. Evaluation of the head and neck cancer with F-18 FDG PET: a comparison with MRI/CT. *Eur J Nucl Med* 2004;31: 590–595.
21. Posner JB. Paraneoplastic syndromes. Neurologic complications of systemic cancer. *Neurol Clin* 1991;9:919.
22. Lin JT, Lachmann E, Nagler W. Paraneoplastic cerebellar degeneration as the first manifestation of cancer. *J Womens Health Gend Based Med* 2001;10:495–502.
23. Shams'ili S, Grefkens J, de Leeuw B, et al. Paraneoplastic cerebellar degeneration associated with antineuronal antibodies: analysis of 50 patients. *Brain* 2003;126;1409–1418.
24. Frings M, Antoch G, Knorn P, et al. Strategies in detection of the primary tumour in anti-Yo associated paraneoplastic cerebellar degeneration. *J Neurol* 2005;252:197–201.
25. Mathew RM, Cohen AB, Galetta SL, et al. Paraneoplastic cerebellar degeneration: Yo-expressing tumor revealed after 5 year follow-up with FDG-PET. *J Neurol Sci* 2006;250:1–2.
26. Linke R, Schroeder M, Helmberger T, et al. Antibody-positive paraneoplastic neurologic syndromes. Value of CT and PET for tumor diagnosis. *Neurology* 2004;63:282–286.
27. Younes-Mhenni S, Janier MF, Cinotti L, et al. FDG-PET improves tumour detection in patients with paraneoplastic neurological syndromes. *Brain* 2004;124:2331–2338.
28. Rees JH, Hain SF, Johnson MR, et al. The role of [18F]fluoro-2-deoxyglucose-PET scanning in the diagnosis of paraneoplastic neurological disorders. *Brain* 2001;124:2223–2231.

CHAPTER

8.23 Pediatrics

HOSSEIN JADVAR, LEONARD P. CONNOLLY, FREDERIC H. FAHEY, AND BARRY L. SHULKIN

The use of positron emission tomography (PET) and the more recent hybrid PET with computed tomography (PET/CT) systems is rapidly expanding. The development and validation of applications for PET in pediatrics has proceeded more slowly than in adult medicine, but PET and PET/CT are becoming important in the diagnostic imaging evaluation of children with a variety of disorders, particularly cancer.

The initial slow proliferation of PET in pediatrics was partly because diseases to which PET has been most widely applied in adults are uncommon in pediatrics. Only about 2% of all cancers, for example, occur in patients <15 years of age. Experience has therefore been gained more slowly in pediatrics. Accrual of experience has been further slowed since there are few PET units in pediatric hospitals.

The labor-intensive nature of imaging sick children has limited the ability of adult-oriented PET centers, which are faced with a shortage of available imaging slots, to take on a substantial number of time-consuming, challenging pediatric cases. Despite these considerations, PET and PET/CT are emerging as important tools in pediatric nuclear medicine. This chapter will review the clinical applications of PET and PET/CT in pediatrics with an emphasis on the more common applications in epilepsy and oncology. General considerations in patient preparation and radiation dosimetry will also be discussed.

PATIENT PREPARATION

Preparation of children and parents for nuclear medicine imaging has been thoroughly reviewed elsewhere (1,2). As with any imaging study, gaining the trust and allaying the fears of both the patient and the parents are essential before attempting to image. Because parental attitudes and anxieties are readily conveyed to children, it is essential that the parents be well informed and cooperative if their child's trust is to be gained. Patient cooperation, once achieved, may be assisted by relatively simple methods. Sheets wrapped around the body, sandbags, and/or special holding devices are often sufficient for immobilization. Parents may accompany their child during the course of the study to provide emotional support. However, on occasion, an anxious parent may impair the performance of the study.

Sedation is indicated when, on the basis of careful consideration, it is anticipated that simpler approaches will be inadequate. Sedation protocols, particularly regarding the recommended medications and the level of sedation required for an imaging procedure, vary from institution to institution. Guidelines such as those advanced by the Society of Nuclear Medicine are useful in developing an institutional sedation program and a sedation formulary (3). Also important to consider is the potential effect of sedatives on fluorodeoxyglucose (FDG) distribution. Many sedatives may affect cerebral metabolism. When performing FDG PET of the brain, it is best if sedatives are not administered for 30 minutes after FDG administration because it is during this interval that the majority of cerebral FDG uptake occurs. Sedatives are not known to cause significant changes in tumoral metabolism and can be administered at any time relative to FDG administration for studies of tumors outside the central nervous system (4). It should be noted that the effects of sedation on FDG uptake in tumors have not been exhaustively studied, however, and it is suggested that a similar approach to brain PET imaging might be considered, with sedation starting after the FDG uptake has been substantial, such as after 30 minutes post tracer injection.

Other important technical issues specific for the performance of PET studies in pediatric patients (e.g., consent, intravenous access, bladder catheterization) have been reviewed (5,6). The recent introduction of PET/CT imaging systems also presents unique issues that will need to be addressed. Kaste (7) has reviewed the experience with implementing PET/CT at a tertiary pediatric hospital. Issues such as physical location of the PET/CT unit, the roles of CT and nuclear medicine technologists, and the methodology for study interpretation are discussed. Additional important considerations deliberated are the use of intravenous and sugar-free oral contrasts for the CT portion of the PET/CT examinations and the management of hyperglycemia. Procedure guidelines for tumor imaging with PET and PET/CT have been published (8,9).

TABLE 8.23.1 Radiation Dosimetry for Fluorodeoxyglucose

	1 Year	5 Years	10 Years	15 Years	Adult
Mass (kg)[a]	9.8	19.0	32.0	55.0	70.0
Administered activity (MBq)	54.5	105.6	177.8	305.6	389.0
Bladder	32.1	33.8	49.8	64.2	62.2
Brain	2.6	3.6	5.3	8.6	10.9
Heart	19.1	21.1	21.3	24.8	24.1
Kidneys	5.2	5.7	6.4	7.6	8.2
Red marrow	3.3	3.4	3.9	4.3	4.3
Effective dose (mSv)[b]	5.2	5.3	6.4	7.6	7.4

[a]Patient masses represent the 50% percentile for that age. (From ICRP Report 56, Age-dependent doses to members of the public from intake of radionuclides: Part 1, International Commission on Radiation Protection, 1989, p. 4, with permission.)

[b](From ICRP Report 80, Radiation dose to patients from radiopharmaceuticals, International Commission on Radiation Protection, 1998, pp. 49–110, with permission.)

RADIATION DOSIMETRY

Several factors affect the dosimetry of positron emitters relative to single photon imaging agents. On the one hand, the energy per photon is higher (511 keV as compared to 140 keV for technetium-99m [^{99m}Tc]), and there are two photons emitted per disintegration. This leads to higher energy per unit activity than with most single photon agents. However, the higher photon energy also leads to a smaller fraction of the photons being absorbed within the patient. Table 8.23.1 summarizes the dosimetry of FDG for selected organs as well as the effective dose in the pediatric population based on the administered activity of 5.55 kBq/kg (0.15 μCi/kg).

Since the administered activities are scaled by body weight, the doses are similar across the age range being slightly higher in adults. The effective dose is 5.1 and 7.4 mSv for the 1-year-old and the adult, respectively. The critical organ is the bladder wall with the dose being six to eight times higher than the effective dose (based on a 2-hour voiding; however, patients routinely void before image acquisition starts about 1-hour postinjection). Table 8.23.2 compares the effective dose from FDG to a number of commonly used, single photon imaging agents. From this table, it can be seen that the radiation absorbed dose to the patient from an FDG PET scan is very similar to the dose received from other nuclear medicine imaging procedures (10,11).

In many cases in pediatric imaging, the parents of the patient prefer to remain with the patient during the procedure. The exposure rate constants for fluorine-18 ([^{18}F]) and ^{99m}Tc are 0.0154 and 0.00195 mR/h per MBq at 1 m, respectively. The difference is primarily due to the higher photon energy for [^{18}F] as compared to ^{99m}Tc, and the fact that two photons are emitted per disintegration. It is also therefore prudent to consider the radiation exposure to the parent during these procedures. As shown in Table 8.23.1, pediatric patients receive a range of administered activities depending on patient size. Consider the following assumptions: the patient receives 260 MBq and is considered to be a point source with no self-absorption. The patient sits in a preparatory room for 60 minutes during uptake and then is imaged for 60 minutes. These assumptions are considered quite conservative; that is, these will probably lead to an overestimation of the radiation dose to the parent. Table 8.23.3 estimates the total exposure to the parent during both the uptake and imaging periods, provided the parent maintains the distance from the patient specified.

Even if the parent stayed within 1 m of the patient during the entire uptake and imaging periods, the exposure to the parent

TABLE 8.23.2 Effective Dose in Pediatrics for a Variety of Radiopharmaceuticals

Radiopharmaceutical	Maximum Administered Activity (MBq)[a]	1 Year	5 Years	10 Years	15 Years	Adult
FDG	389	5.2	5.3	6.4	7.6	7.4
^{67}Ga-citrate	222	19.9	19.9	20.3	22.7	22.2
^{99m}Tc HMPAO	740	5.1	5.4	5.8	6.4	6.9
^{99m}Tc MDP	740	2.8	2.8	3.7	4.1	4.2
^{99m}Tc SestaMIBI	740	4.7	4.6	5.4	5.8	5.8

FDG, fluorodeoxyglucose; ^{67}Ga, gallium citrate; ^{99m}TC, technetium-99m; HMPAO, hexamethylpropylene; MDP, methylene diphosphonate; MIBI, methoxyisobutylisonitrile.

The doses are reported in mSv.

[a]The maximum administered activity is that which would be administered to a 70-kg adult. The pediatric dose administered is scaled by the patient's weight as in Table 8.23.1 (From ICRP Report 80, Radiation dose to patients from radiopharmaceuticals, International Commission on Radiation Protection, 1998, pp. 49–110, ; ICRP Report 56, Age-dependent doses to members of the public from intake of radionuclides: Part 1, International Commission on Radiation Protection, 1989, p. 4, with permission.)

TABLE 8.23.3 Total Exposure to The Parent from a Patient Receiving 260 MBq of Fluorine-18 for a Fluorodeoxyglucose PET Study

Distance From Patient During Uptake Period (m)	Distance From Patient During Imaging Period (m)	Total Exposure to Parent (mR)
1	1	5.5
1	2	4.0
2	2	1.4
2	3	1.1

It is assumed that the parent stayed with the patient during a 60-minute uptake period and a 60-minute imaging period.

would be no more than 5.5 mR. Therefore, the parents can be allowed to stay with the patient during the procedure but are instructed to stay as far from the patient as they feel comfortable. Hybrid PET/CT scanners use the CT portion of the examination for attenuation correction. The dose to the patient from CT can vary greatly depending on the tube voltage and current and the size of the patient. Table 8.23.4 summarizes the dose to patients of various ages (based on a phantom study using phantoms of various sizes) as a function of tube voltage.

Smaller patients receive a substantially higher dose from the same CT acquisition parameters. For example, a 10-year-old will receive approximately twice the radiation dose of a medium-sized adult for the same CT acquisition parameters. An alternative to using CT for attenuation correction is to use rotating rod sources. Based on a phantom study using phantoms of different sizes, the dose to the patient is between 0.05 and 0.2 mGy for 15 minutes of scanning with a total activity in the rods of 370 MBq. Thus the dose to the patient from a CT scan used for attenuation correction is substantially higher than that associated with the rotating rods' sources. However, the CT scan provides anatomical correlation to the functional images, a feature that is not available using the rod sources and is considerably quicker, which can be of particular value for pediatric imaging.

Comparing the values in Tables 8.23.1 and 8.23.4, the dose to the patient from the CT portion of the scan can be equal to, if not higher than, the dose received from the radiopharmaceutical. The acquisition parameters for the CT portion of the scan should be tailored to the patient's size. For diagnostic CT, reduction of exposure by 30% to 50% relative to adult has been suggested (12). Reducing the milliamperes proportionately decreases the absorbed radiation dose without significant loss in the information provided. In addition, there is the potential to further reduce the tube voltage and current without adversely affecting the quality of the attenuation correction in those cases where precise anatomical correlation is less important.

PET IN PEDIATRIC NEUROLOGY

A discussion of brain PET imaging in all age groups is present in Chapter 9.1. In the following sections the PET imaging in neurologic applications is discussed.

Normal Brain Development

An understanding of the normal brain development and evolution of cerebral glucose utilization is important when FDG PET is considered as a diagnostic functional imaging study. Functional maturation proceeds phylogenetically. Glucose metabolism is initially high in the sensorimotor cortex, thalamus, brainstem, and cerebellar vermis. During the first 3 months of life, glucose metabolism gradually increases in the basal ganglia and in the parietal, temporal, calcarine, and cerebellar cortices. Maturation of the frontal cortex, which proceeds from lateral to medial, and the dorsolateral cortex occurs during the second 6 months of life. Cerebral FDG distribution in children after the age of 1 year resembles that of adults (Fig. 8.23.1) (13–15).

Epilepsy in Childhood

Epilepsy is a relatively common and potentially devastating neurologic condition during childhood. Its incidence in children and adolescents is between 40 and 100 per 100,000 (16). The 1990 National Institutes of Health Consensus Conference on Surgery for Epilepsy estimated that 10% to 20% of epilepsy cases prove medically

TABLE 8.23.4 Dose from CT at Different Ages

Kv(p)	Newborn	1 Year	5 Year	10 Year	Med Adult
80	7.0	5.7	4.5	3.8	1.5
100	13.5	11.3	9.0	7.9	3.5
120	21.4	18.2	14.9	12.9	6.0
140	30.1	25.8	21.8	18.9	9.0

Kv(p), kilovolt peak.
All doses are reported in mGy. All data were obtained at 130 mAs and a pitch of helical 1.5:1.

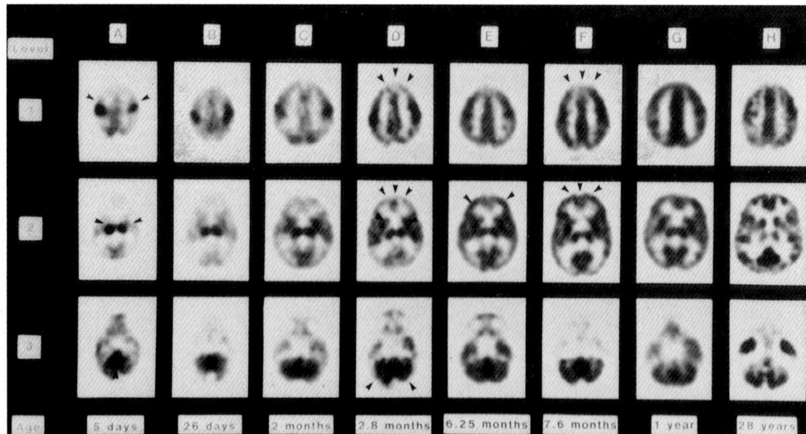

FIGURE 8.23.1. Normal brain maturation. PET scans showing ontogenic changes in local cerebral glucose metabolism of the normal human infant. **A:** In the 5-day-old, glucose metabolism is highest in the sensorimotor cortex, thalamus, cerebellar vermis (*arrows*), and brainstem (not shown). **B,C,D:** Glucose metabolism increases gradually in the parietal, temporal, and calcarine cortices, basal ganglia, and cerebellar cortex (*arrows*), especially during the second and third months. **E:** In the frontal cortex, glucose metabolism increases first in the lateral prefrontal regions by approximately 6 months. **F:** By about 8 months, glucose metabolism also increases in the medial aspects of the frontal cortex (*arrows*) as well as the dorsolateral occipital cortex. **G:** By 1 year, the glucose metabolic pattern resembles that of a normal adult, although metabolic rates are two- to threefold elevated in comparison to values expected in normal adults (**H**). (Photo kindly provided by Harry T. Chugani, MD. From Chugani HT. Positron emission tomography. In: Berg BO, ed. *Principles of child neurology*. New York: McGraw-Hill, 1996:113–128, with permission.)

intractable, and that 2,000 to 5,000 epilepsy patients per year can benefit from surgical resection of the seizure focus (17). Accurate preoperative localization of the epileptogenic region is an essential but difficult task that is best accomplished by finding a concordance between results obtained with clinical examination, electroencephalography (EEG), neuropsychological evaluation, and imaging studies. CT and magnetic resonance imaging (MRI) are used to detect anatomic lesions that may cause the seizures. However, structural lesions occur in a relatively small percentage of patients with epilepsy, and when such lesions are detected, they may not necessarily correspond to the epileptogenic region (18). Ictal or interictal single-photon emission tomography (SPECT) evaluation of regional cerebral blood flow (rCBF) with tracers such as ^{99m}Tc-hexamethylpropylene (^{99m}Tc-HMPAO) and ^{99m}Tc-ethylcysteinate dimer (^{99m}Tc-ECD) can localize the epileptogenic region in the presence or absence of structural abnormalities. The characteristic appearance of an epileptogenic region is relative zonal hyperperfusion on ictal SPECT and relative zonal hypoperfusion on interictal SPECT.

The sensitivity of ictal rCBF SPECT may approach 90%, while that of interictal SPECT is in the range of 50% (19). The utility of ictal SPECT is somewhat reduced by the difficulty in coordinating tracer administration with seizures. Noninvasive evaluation is often unsuccessful in precisely localizing an epileptogenic region. As a result, surgical placement of electrode grids on the brain surface or insertion of depth electrodes becomes necessary.

FDG PET has proven useful in preoperative localization of the epileptogenic region (Fig. 8.23.2) (20). FDG PET is generally performed following an interictal injection. Although metabolic alterations might be localized better ictally than interictally, the relatively short half-life of [^{18}F] limits the window of opportunity during which it can be administered ictally. Even when FDG can be administered at seizure onset, the approximately 30-minute brain uptake time of FDG means that the study may depict peri-ictal as well as ictal FDG distribution. Ictal FDG studies may also show areas of seizure propagation, which could be confused with the actual seizure focus. Despite these considerations, some favorable results have been reported employing ictal PET for patients with continuous or frequent seizures (21).

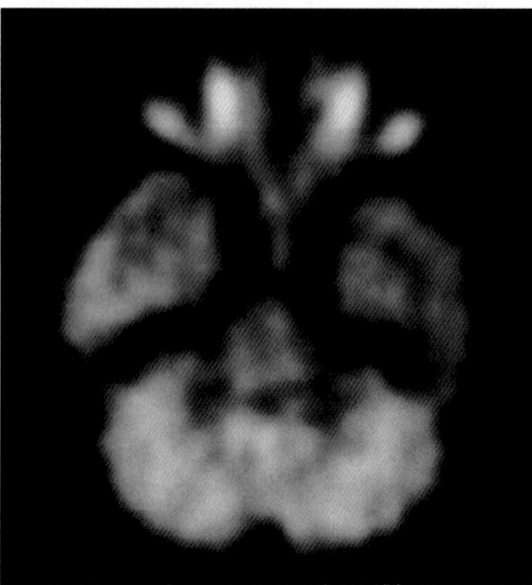

FIGURE 8.23.2. A transaxial fluorodeoxyglucose PET brain scan of a 14-year-old girl shows a hypometabolic epileptogenic left temporal lobe. (From Jadvar H, Connolly LP, Shulkin BL, et al. Positron-emission tomography in pediatrics. *Nucl Med Annu* 2000:53–83, with permission.)

For interictal PET, FDG should be administered in a setting such as a quiet room with dim lights where environmental stimuli are minimal during the 30 minutes following FDG administration. It is best to have the child remain awake with minimal parental interaction during this period. EEG monitoring is essential to identify seizure activity that might affect FDG distribution.

The sensitivity of interictal FDG PET approaches that of ictal rCBF SPECT in localizing the epileptogenic region, which is detected as regional hypometabolism (22). Importantly, the hypometabolism may predominantly affect cortex bordering the epileptogenic focus. Epileptic activity may originate in cortical areas bordering the hypometabolic regions rather than the hypometabolic region itself (23). A recent study also suggested that persistent or increased seizure frequency (one or more seizures per day) results in enlargement in the area of hypometabolic cortex on sequential PET scans. In contrast, patients whose seizure frequency decreases below daily seizures show a decrease in the size of the hypometabolic cortex on serial scans (24).

Incorporation of FDG PET into preoperative evaluation of patients with epilepsy reduces the need for intracranial EEG monitoring and the cost of preoperative evaluation (25,26). The best results have been obtained in temporal lobe epilepsy, for which metabolic abnormalities may be evident in as many as 90% of surgical candidates (25,27). Coregistered FDG PET and MRI in association with diffusion tensor imaging has also been recently shown to accurately localize the epileptogenic cortex in patients with tuberous sclerosis complex (28).

Extratemporal epileptogenic regions are more difficult to identify, but some success has been achieved in children with intractable frontal lobe epilepsy and normal CT or MRI studies (29). FDG PET has been reported as being of particular help in the evaluation of infantile spasms, a subtype of seizure disorder. This condition, which has an incidence of 2 to 6 per 10,000 live births, consists of a characteristic pattern of infantile myoclonic seizures and is frequently associated with profound developmental delay despite medical treatment (15,30). Prior to the availability of FDG PET, surgical intervention was attempted and successful in only isolated instances. Incorporation of FDG PET into the evaluation of children with infantile spasms has resulted in identification of a substantial number of children who have benefited from cortical resection. FDG PET has revealed marked focal cortical glucose hypometabolism associated with malformative or dysplastic lesions that are not evident on anatomic imaging. There is a marked decline in seizure frequency and in some patients reversal of developmental delay when a single metabolic abnormality that correlates with EEG findings is shown by FDG PET. Patients with bitemporal hypometabolism on FDG PET have a poor prognosis and typically are not candidates for resective surgery (31–34).

In addition to FDG, PET tracers that assess an altered abundance or function of receptors, enzymes, and neurotransmitters in epileptogenic regions have been applied to localizing the epileptogenic region. Among alterations that have been observed are relatively reduced uptake of carbon-11 ([^{11}C])-flumazenil, a central benzodiazepine receptor antagonist, and [^{11}C]-labeled (S)-[*N*-methyl] ketamine, which binds to the *N*-methyl-D-aspartate receptor-gated ion channel, and the amino acid methyl-L-tryptophan (35–41). Relative increases in uptake of [^{11}C]-carfentanil, a selective mu opiate receptor agonist, and [^{11}C]-deuterium-deprenyl, an irreversible inhibitor of monoamine oxidase type B, have also been described (42,43).

Other Neurologic Applications

PET with oxygen-15 ([^{15}O])-water has also been investigated in infants with intraventricular hemorrhage and hemorrhagic infarction and in infants with hypoxic ischemic encephalopathy (44,45). Cerebral blood flow was markedly reduced not only in the hemorrhagic areas but also in the remainder of the involved hemisphere, suggesting that neurologic deficits may be caused by ischemia rather than the presence of blood within the brain parenchyma or cerebral ventricles (44). In full-term infants with perinatal asphyxia, diminished blood flow to the parasagittal cortical regions suggested that injury to the brain in these infants was also ischemic in etiology (45).

PET has also been employed to study the pathophysiology of many other childhood brain disorders such as autism (46), attention deficit hyperactivity disorder (47,48), mental retardation and developmental disabilities (49), age-associated metabolic changes in deafness (50), schizophrenia (51), sickle cell encephalopathy (52), and anorexia and bulimia nervosa (53,54), Rasmussen syndrome (55), Krabbe disease (56), Sturge-Weber syndrome (57), and cognitive impairment in Duchenne muscular dystrophy (58). However, the exact role of PET in these clinical settings remains unclear. Further experience may result in an expanded role of PET in many childhood neurological disorders.

PET IN PEDIATRIC CARDIOLOGY

Currently, PET plays a relatively minor role in pediatric cardiology. Quinlivan et al. (59) have reviewed the cardiac applications of PET in children. PET with nitrogen-13 ([^{13}N])-ammonia has been employed to measure myocardial perfusion in infants after anatomic repair of congenital heart defects and after Norwood palliation for hypoplastic left heart syndrome (60). Infants with repaired heart disease had higher resting blood flow and less coronary flow reserve than previously reported for adults. Infants with Norwood palliation also had less perfusion and oxygen delivery to the systemic ventricle than the infants with repaired congenital heart lesion, explaining in part the less favorable outcome for patients with Norwood palliation. Evaluation of myocardial perfusion with [^{13}N]-ammonia PET in infants following a neonatal arterial switch operation has demonstrated that patients with myocardial perfusion defects may have a more complicated postoperative course (61). The higher resolution of PET versus SPECT may have advantages in pediatric cardiac imaging, but this requires further study in specialized centers.

A major application of PET in adult cardiology is the assessment of myocardial viability with FDG as a tracer for glucose metabolism. Rickers et al. (62) evaluated regional glucose metabolism and contractile function by gated FDG PET in seven infants and seven children after arterial switch operation and suspected myocardial infarction. Gated FDG PET was found to contribute pertinent information to guide additional therapy including high-risk revascularization procedures. Other reports have also provided evidence for the utility of PET in the assessment of myocardial perfusion and viability in infants and children with coronary abnormalities (63,64).

In another study of children with Kawasaki disease, PET with [^{13}N]-ammonia and FDG showed abnormalities in about 60% of patients during the acute and subacute stages and about 40% of patients in the convalescent stage of disease (65). PET was valuable in assessing the response to immunoglobulin therapy at differing doses and administration schedules. PET and ammonia may also reveal reduction of coronary flow reserve in children with Kawasaki disease and angiographically normal epicardial coronary arteries (66).

Beyond the more common assessment of myocardial perfusion and oxidative metabolism, PET has been used to study such fundamental functional abnormalities as mitochondrial dysfunction in children with hypertrophic or dilated cardiomyopathy (67). Dynamic PET with [^{11}C]-acetate demonstrated reduced myocardial Krebs cycle activity (i.e., decreased oxidative metabolism) in children with cardiomyopathy despite normal myocardial perfusion. The diminished oxidative metabolism was associated with compensatory increased glycolytic activity as demonstrated on FDG PET.

PET IN PEDIATRIC ONCOLOGY

The incidence of cancer is estimated to be 133.3 per million children in the United States (68). Although cancer is much less common in children than in adults, it is still an important cause of mortality in pediatrics. Approximately 10% of deaths during childhood are attributable to cancer, making it the leading cause of childhood death from disease (69).

Childhood cancers often differ from those encountered in adults. This is illustrated in Table 8.23.5, which delineates the estimated incidences of the more commonly encountered cancers in U.S. children. Of the adult cancers to which FDG PET has been most widely applied, only lymphomas and brain tumors occur with an appreciable incidence in children. However, the diagnostic utility of FDG PET and its impact on patient management have been reported for many pediatric cancers (70–81). In decreasing order of frequency, PET led to important changes in clinical management of lymphoma (32%), brain tumors (15%), and sarcomas (13%) (71).

PET/CT has also been shown to improve on PET alone by precise CT localization of metabolic abnormalities on PET and by metabolic characterization of abnormal and normal findings on CT, thereby increasing diagnostic confidence and reducing equivocal image interpretations (82–85). Before reviewing the applications of PET in pediatric oncology, it is important to consider potential causes of confusion on FDG PET that relate to physiologic FDG distribution in children. High FDG uptake by thymus, adenoids, tonsils, and skeletal growth centers (particularly the long bone physes) as well as the greater extent of hematopoietic marrow in the immature skeleton compared to the adult skeleton are important physiological variations in FDG distribution encountered in children (Figs. 8.23.3 and 8.23.4) (86–90). Specifically, the thymic FDG uptake appears to have a significant relationship with lymphocyte count and may be physiologically elevated after chemotherapy (Fig. 8.23.5) (91). Normal thymic uptake must be recognized to avoid confusion with mediastinal malignancy.

With the introduction of PET/CT imaging systems, it has been recognized that elevated FDG uptake in the normal brown adipose

TABLE 8.23.5 Cancer Incidence Rates Per Million Children Younger Than 15 Years in The United States as Derived from The Surveillance, Epidemiology, and End Results (SEER) Program

	Total[b]			Men		Women			Whites		Blacks		
Histology	No.	Rate	(%)	No.	Rate	No.	Rate	Male: Female	No.	Rate	No.	Rate	White: Black
All histologic types	10,555	133.3	(100)	5,711	140.9	4,844	125.1	1.13	8,756	139.5	1,064	108.3	1.29
Acute lymphoid leukemia	2,484	30.9	(23.2)	1,383	33.7	1,101	28.0	1.20	2,092	32.9	169	16.9	1.95
All central nervous system (CNS)	2,205	27.6	(20.7)	1,195	29.3	1,010	26.0	1.13	1,847	29.3	239	23.8	1.23
Astrocytomas and gliomas	1,329	16.8	(12.6)	692	17.1	637	16.2	1.06	1,130	17.9	144	14.3	1.25
Primitive neurectodermal	532	6.6	(5.0)	311	7.7	221	5.6	1.38	433	6.8	56	5.9	1.15
Other CNS	344	4.3	(3.2)	192	4.6	152	3.9	1.18	284	4.6	37	3.6	1.28
Neuroblastoma	754	9.7	(7.3)	389	9.8	365	9.6	1.02	632	10.2	78	7.8	1.31
Non-Hodgkin's lymphoma	666	8.4	(6.3)	484	12.0	182	4.6	2.61	578	9.1	53	5.4	1.69
Wilms tumor	638	8.1	(6.1)	287	6.9	351	8.9	0.78	520	8.3	94	9.4	0.88
Hodgkin's disease	511	6.6	(5.0)	295	7.4	216	5.6	1.32	451	7.3	46	4.7	1.55
Acute myeloid leukemia	454	5.6	(4.2)	224	5.5	230	6.0	0.92	358	5.8	47	4.8	1.21
Rhabdomyosarcoma	354	4.5	(3.4)	211	5.2	143	3.6	1.44	294	4.7	40	4.1	1.15
Retinoblastoma	306	3.9	(2.9)	144	3.6	162	4.2	0.86	234	3.9	44	4.5	0.87
Osteosarcoma	262	3.4	(2.6)	130	3.3	132	3.4	0.97	197	3.4	38	3.9	0.87
Ewing sarcoma	208	2.8	(2.1)	109	2.8	99	2.6	1.08	194	3.3	3	0.3	11.00
All other histologic types	1,713	21.8	(16.4)	860	21.4	853	22.6	0.95	1,359	21.3	213	22.7	0.94

[a]Rates are standardized to the 1980 SEER population and reported per million children per year.
[b]Includes all races and both sexes.
(From Gurney JG, Severson RK, Davis S, et al. Incidence of cancer in children in the United States. *Cancer* 1995;75:2186–2195, with permission.)

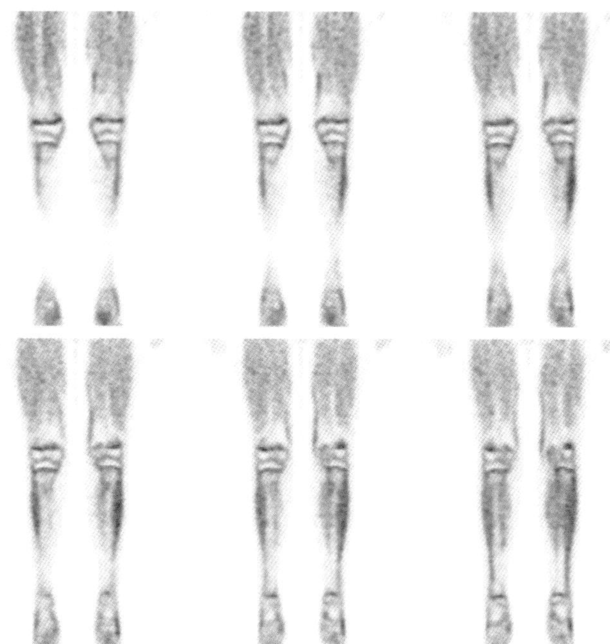

FIGURE 8.23.3. Coronal fluorodeoxyglucose PET images of the lower extremities of an 11-year-old boy with a history of Hodgkin's lymphoma, off therapy for 3 years, show high physiologic uptake in the growth plates bilaterally.

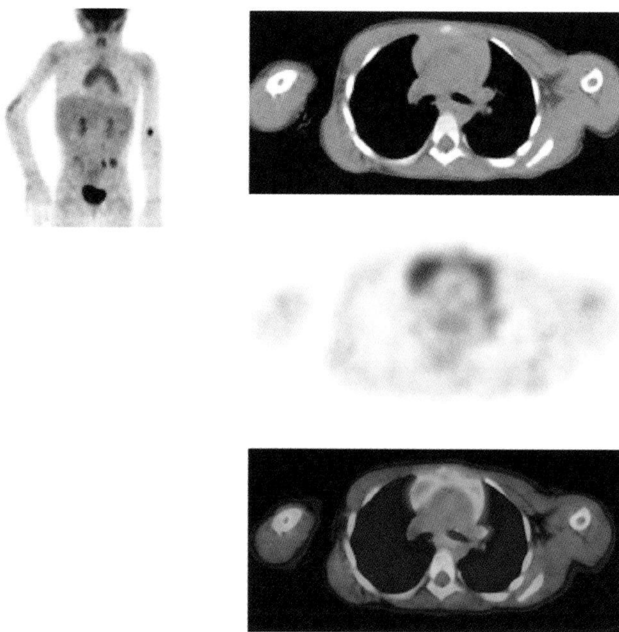

FIGURE 8.23.5. Thymic rebound. Fluorodeoxyglucose (FDG) PET/CT images of a 12-year-old boy treated for embryonal sarcoma of the liver (same patient as in Fig. 8.23.4) off therapy for 6 months. **Left panel:** An anterior maximal intensity projection image shows intense uptake in the upper chest in a configuration typical for thymus. **Right panel:** CT (**top**), FDG PET (**middle**), and fusion (**bottom**) images of the upper chest show increased uptake in the thymus, which appears prominent.

tissue may also be a source of false-positive finding (92–94). The common anatomic areas involved include the neck and shoulder region, axillae, mediastinum, and the paravertebral and perinephric regions. Neck brown fat hypermetabolism is seen significantly more in the pediatric population than in the adult population (15% vs. 2% respectively; $P < .01$) and appears to be stimulated by cold temperatures (92,93). Recent data have shown that brown fat metabolic activity may be suppressed pharmacologically (e.g., propranolol, fentanyl) (95,96) or even more simply by controlling environmental temperature in the hours before injection and during the uptake phase (97).

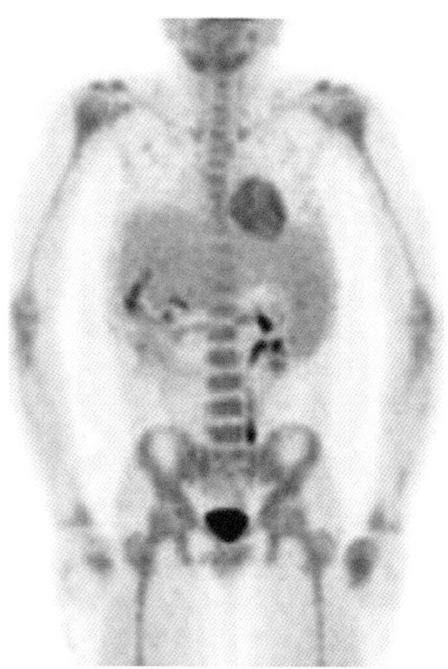

FIGURE 8.23.4. An anterior maximal intensity projection image of a 12-year-old boy undergoing therapy for embryonal sarcoma of the liver shows no discernible thymic uptake.

Other potential pitfalls, which also apply to imaging adults, include variable FDG uptake in the working skeletal muscles, the myocardium, the thyroid gland, and the gastrointestinal tract, as well as accumulation of FDG excreted into the renal pelves and bladder, and possible tracer accumulation in draining lymph nodes from extravasated tracer at the time of injection (98).

Diffuse high bone marrow and splenic FDG uptake following administration of hematopoietic stimulating factors, which is correlated with increasing white blood cell counts and decreasing hemoglobin levels, may also resemble disseminated metastatic disease (Fig. 8.23.6) (99–101). Elevated bone marrow FDG uptake has been observed in patients as long as 4 weeks following completion of treatment with granulocyte colony-stimulating factor (99). This observation is probably reflective of increased bone marrow glycolytic metabolism in response to hematopoietic growth factors. High FDG uptake may occasionally be seen in some benign lesions (e.g., adenoma, nonossifying fibroma, osteochondroma) (102–104).

Another important issue specific to PET imaging of pediatric patients is the choice of measurement parameter for the standardized uptake value (SUV), which is commonly used as a semiquantitative measure of FDG localization in a region of interest. The calculation of SUV based on body surface area appears to be a more

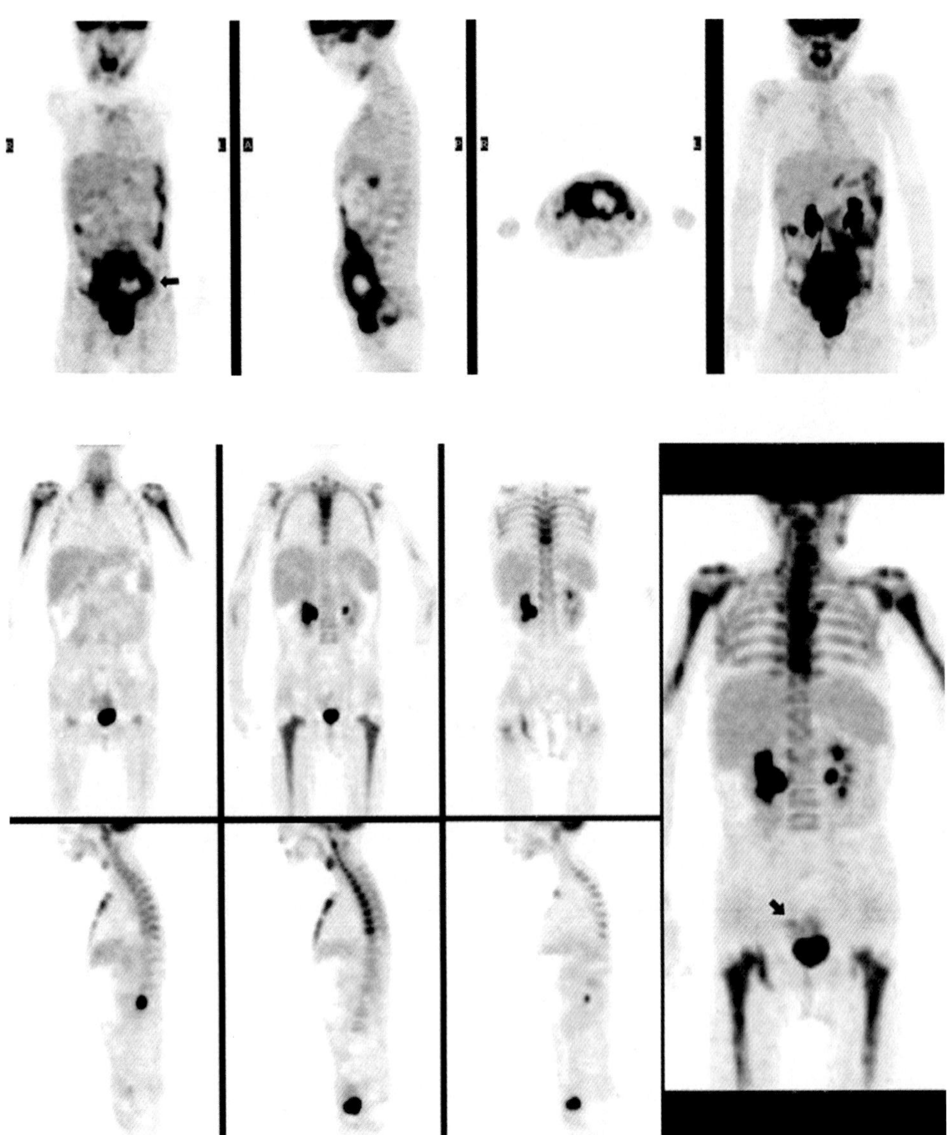

FIGURE 8.23.6. High fluorine-18 fluorodeoxyglucose uptake is seen in a large pelvic mass and at multiple sites within the abdomen of a 7-year-old girl with embryonal rhabdomyosarcoma and omental metastases (**top line:** coronal, sagittal, transverse, and maximal intensity projection images). The patient received chemotherapy and radiotherapy (2,250 cGy to the whole abdomen and a boost of 2,490 cGy to the pelvis). Three months after completing radiotherapy, a restaging PET scan (**middle line:** serial coronal views, serial sagittal views) was obtained while the patient was receiving 5 μg/kg of granulocyte colony-stimulating factor daily for chemotherapy-induced neutropenia. Low-grade uptake is seen in the mass (*arrow*, **far right lower panel:** maximal intensity projection image). Uptake is high throughout the hematopoietic marrow except the regions that had been included within the radiation port. (From Drubach LA, Dubois S, Frazier L, et al. Combined effects of granulocyte colony stimulating factor and radiation. *Clin Nucl Med* 2007:32:39–41, with permission.)

uniform parameter than that calculated based on body weight in pediatric patients (105).

Central Nervous System Tumors

Taken as a group, tumors of the central nervous system (CNS) are the most common nonhematologic tumors of childhood. They account for about 20% of all pediatric malignancies. The grouping includes many histologically diverse tumors of both neuroepithelial and nonneuroepithelial origin. The majority of pediatric brain tumors arise from neuroepithelial tissue. CNS tumors are subclassified histopathologically by cell type and graded for degree of malignancy using criteria that include mitotic activity, infiltration, and anaplasia (106,107).

To grasp the wide variety of pediatric CNS tumors, one need only consider the distribution of the most common tumors according to the major anatomic compartment involved. In the posterior fossa, medulloblastoma, cerebellar astrocytoma, ependymoma, and brainstem gliomas are most common. Tumors about the third ventricle include tumors that arise from suprasellar, pineal, and ventricular tissue. The most common neoplasms about the third ventricle are optic and hypothalamic gliomas, craniopharyngiomas, and germ cell tumors. Supratentorial tumors are most often astrocytomas, many of which are low grade (107).

MRI and CT are the principal imaging modalities used in staging and following children with CNS tumors. Their main limitation is the inability to distinguish viable recurrent or residual tumor from abnormalities resulting from surgery or radiation. SPECT with thallium-201 ([^{201}Tl]) and ^{99m}Tc-methoxyisobutylisonitrile (MIBI) have proven valuable for this determination in a number of pediatric brain tumors (108–111). The use of FDG PET in brain tumors has been widely reported in series that predominantly include adult patients for whom FDG PET has helped distinguish viable tumor from posttherapeutic changes (112–114). In general, high FDG uptake relative to adjacent brain indicates residual or recurrent tumor, whereas low or absent FDG uptake is observed in areas of necrosis. This distinction is most readily made with high-grade tumors that show high uptake of FDG at diagnosis. Even with

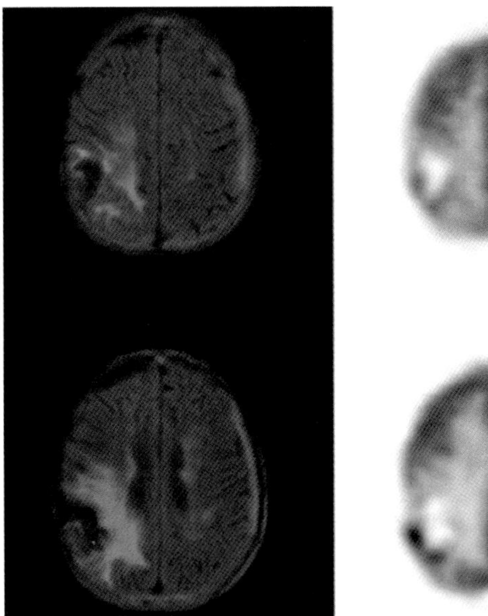

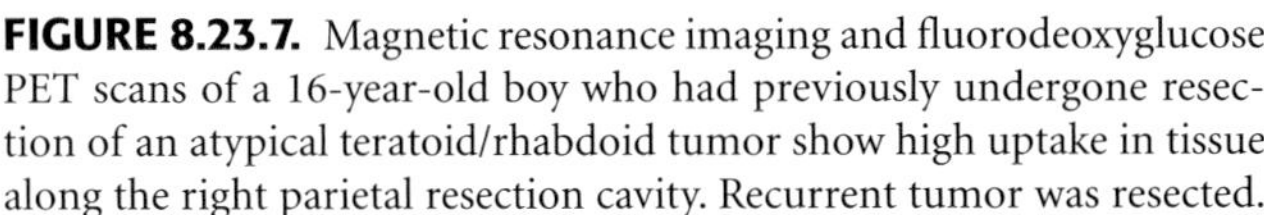

FIGURE 8.23.7. Magnetic resonance imaging and fluorodeoxyglucose PET scans of a 16-year-old boy who had previously undergone resection of an atypical teratoid/rhabdoid tumor show high uptake in tissue along the right parietal resection cavity. Recurrent tumor was resected.

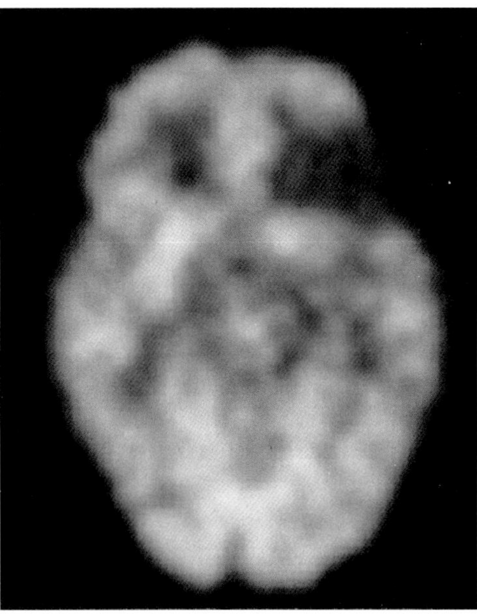

FIGURE 8.23.8. A transaxial fluorodeoxyglucose PET brain image from a 4-and-a-half-year-old boy with generalized tonic-clonic seizure demonstrates hypometabolism in the left frontal lobe. This area was resected and shown to be a low-grade glioma. (From Jadvar H, Connolly LP, Shulkin BL, et al. Positron-emission tomography in pediatrics. *Nucl Med Annu* 2000:53–83, with permission.)

high-grade tumors, the presence of microscopic tumor foci is not excluded by an FDG PET study that does not show increased uptake. This is particularly true after intensive radiation therapy, in which case FDG PET results may not accurately correlate with tumor progression (115). Furthermore, in the immediate posttherapy period, elevated FDG uptake may persist (116).

FDG PET has been applied to tumor grading and prognostic stratification. Higher-grade aggressive tumors typically have higher FDG uptake than do lower grade tumors (Figs. 8.23.7 and 8.23.8) (117,118). Among low-grade tumors, some show insufficient FDG uptake to be distinguished from adjacent brain and some appear hypometabolic. The development of hypermetabolism as evidenced by increased FDG uptake in a low-grade tumor that appeared hypometabolic at diagnosis indicates degeneration to a higher grade (119). The biological behavior of high-grade tumors may be reflected in their appearance on FDG PET. Shorter survival times have been reported for patients whose tumors show the highest degree of FDG uptake (120).

Data, although limited, suggest that FDG PET findings also correlate well with pathology and clinical outcome in children (121–125). A potential pediatric application of this entails a reported excellent correlation between FDG PET findings and clinical outcome in children affected by neurofibromatosis who have low-grade astrocytomas (126). In that series, high tumoral glucose metabolism shown by FDG PET was a more accurate predictor of tumor behavior than was histological analysis.

Combining FDG PET and MRI in the planning of stereotactic brain biopsies has been reported to improve the diagnostic yield in infiltrative, ill-defined lesions and to reduce sampling in high-risk function areas (127). The combined imaging also facilitates tumor resection planning (128). Another positron-emitting radiotracer that has been used to study pediatric brain tumors is $[^{11}C]$-L-methionine ($[^{11}C]$-MET), which localizes to only a minimal degree in normal brain. Uptake of this labeled amino acid reflects transport and to some extent transmethylation pathways that are present in some tumors. However, as with FDG, some low-grade gliomas may escape detection (129–131). $[^{11}C]$-MET PET has been reported to be useful in differentiating viable tumor from treatment-induced changes (129,132–134). It is worth noting, however, that $[^{11}C]$-MET is not tumor specific as it has been shown to accumulate in some nontumoral CNS diseases, probably as a result of blood–brain barrier disruption (135).

Both FDG PET and $[^{11}C]$-MET PET have been shown to be independent predictors of event-free survival (136,137). $[^{11}C]$-MET, because of the short 20-minute half-life of $[^{11}C]$, must be produced on-site for administration and is not commercially available. Potential uses of $[^{18}F]$-3′-deoxy-3′-fluorothymidine, $[^{11}C]$-methyl-L-tryptophan, and $[^{18}F]$-fluoroethyl-L-tyrosine in assessing brain tumors have recently been described (138–142).

Lymphoma

Lymphomas of non-Hodgkin's and Hodgkin's types account for between 10% and 15% of pediatric malignancies. Non-Hodgkin's lymphoma occurs throughout childhood. Lymphoblastic and small-cell tumors, including Burkitt lymphoma, are the most common histological types. The disease is usually widespread at diagnosis. Mediastinal and hilar involvement are common with lymphoblastic lymphoma. Burkitt lymphoma most often occurs in the abdomen. Hodgkin's lymphoma has a peak incidence during adolescence and accounts for about 6% of all childhood cancers (143). Nodular sclerosing and mixed cellularity are the most common histologic types. The disease is rarely widespread at diagnosis, and the majority of cases have intrathoracic nodal involvement (68,144).

Gallium-67 ([^{67}Ga])-citrate scintigraphy has proven useful in staging and monitoring therapeutic response of patients with non-Hodgkin's and Hodgkin's lymphomas (145–149). In numerous studies, which have included predominantly adult patient populations, FDG has been shown to accumulate in non-Hodgkin's and Hodgkin's lymphoma tissue (Fig. 8.23.9) (98,150–168). Similar to [^{67}Ga]-citrate, FDG uptake is generally greater in higher than in lower grade lymphomas (157,159). FDG PET has been shown to reveal sites of nodal and extranodal disease that are not detected by conventional staging methods, resulting in upstaging of disease (155–162,169). FDG PET, when performed at the time of initial evaluation, has also been shown to change disease stage and treatment in up to 10% to 23% of children with lymphoma (170–174). The much shorter half-life of FDG can result in favorable radiation dosimetry, as well, versus [^{67}Ga].

Identification of areas of intense FDG uptake within the bone marrow can be particularly useful in directing the site of biopsy or even eliminating the need for biopsy at staging (155,168). FDG PET is also useful for assessing residual soft tissue masses shown by CT after therapy. Absence of FDG uptake in a residual mass is predictive of remission while high uptake indicates residual or recurrent tumor (162,175). A negative FDG PET scan after completion of chemotherapy, however, does not exclude the presence of residual microscopic disease (176). FDG PET can predict clinical outcome with a higher accuracy than conventional imaging (91% vs. 66%, respectively; $P < .05$) in patients previously treated for Hodgkin lymphoma (177).

Levine et al. (178) reported on the frequency of false-positive studies with PET-only systems after completion of therapy. Scans were considered positive if the interpretation was most consistent with malignancy. Diagnostic validation was by pathologic evaluation, resolution on follow-up scan, or absence of disease progression over at least 1 year without intervention. A false-positive rate of 16% was observed with etiologies such as fibrosis, progressive transformation of germinal centers, abdominal wall hernia, appendicitis, thymus, and human immunodeficency virus (HIV)-associated lymphadenopathy.

Positive PET scans after treatment should be interpreted cautiously, and therapeutic decisions should not generally be made without histologic confirmation (179). Despite this however, the hybrid systems, which incorporate both structural and metabolic information, will provide a more accurate assessment (180). In fact, in a recent German study, it was demonstrated that a correlative imaging strategy that also incorporates FDG PET provides the most accurate imaging evaluation that improves diagnostic confidence and impacts therapeutic management (181). Another study from Israel that utilized PET/CT in 24 Hodgkin's and seven non-Hodgkin's lymphoma patients showed that PET/CT resulted in a stage change in 32% of patients (22% upstaged and 10% downstaged) (182). In general, however, it is suggested that a negative PET/CT during routine follow-up for lymphoma in children strongly suggests the absence of recurrence (high negative predictive value), but a positive finding should be interpreted with caution (less than perfect, although very good, positive predictive value) (183). The potential role of FDG PET in radiation treatment planning for pediatric oncology including lymphoma has also been described (184–186). It is possible that PET can help determine which lymphoma patients require radiation to residual masses after therapy, as well as the field of radiation, but the precise role of PET in planning radiation therapy in children continues to evolve. FDG PET has been compared to [^{11}C]-MET PET in a relatively small series of 14 patients with non-Hodgkin's lymphoma. [^{11}C]-MET PET provided superior tumor-to-background contrast, while FDG PET was superior in distinguishing between high- and low-grade lymphomas (153).

Neuroblastoma

Neuroblastoma is the most common extracranial solid malignant tumor in children. The mean age of patients at presentation is 20 to 30 months, and it is rare after the age of 5 years (144). The most common location of neuroblastoma is the adrenal gland. Other sites of origin include the paravertebral and presacral sympathetic chain, the organ of Zuckerkandl, posterior mediastinal sympathetic ganglia, and cervical sympathetic plexuses. Gross or microscopic calcification is often present in the tumor. Two related neural crest tumors, ganglioneuroma and ganglioneuroblastoma, have been described.

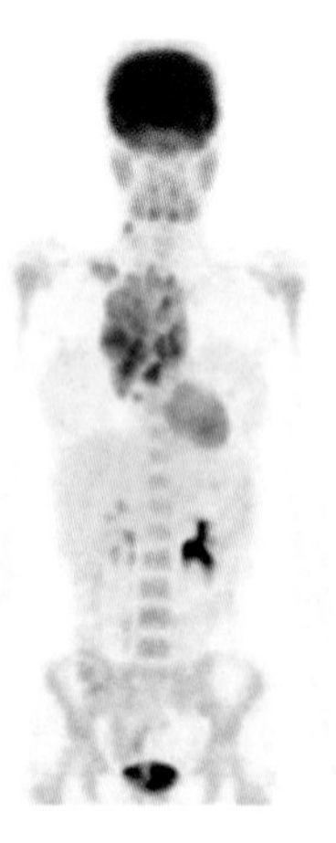

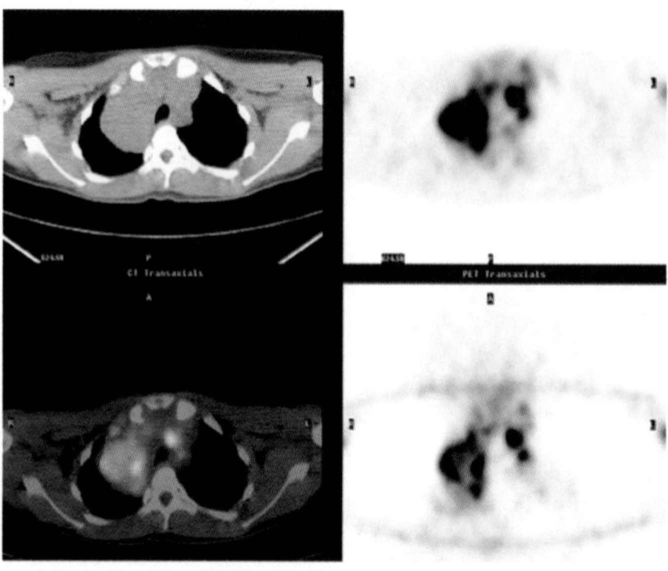

FIGURE 8.23.9. A 15-year-old girl with newly diagnosed Hodgkin's lymphoma. **Left panel:** Anterior maximal intensity projection image. **Upper panel left:** Computed tomography, fluorodeoxyglucose (FDG) PET (**upper panel right**), fusion (**lower panel left**), and FDG PET nonattenuation-corrected images show a large right- and left-sided mediastinal mass with irregular but markedly increased uptake.

Some neuroblastomas spontaneously regress or mature into ganglioneuroma, which is benign. However, the unpredictability and apparent infrequency of spontaneous regression and maturation and the consequences of delaying therapy require that treatment be instituted at diagnosis in most cases. Ganglioneuroblastoma is a malignant tumor that contains both undifferentiated neuroblasts and mature ganglion cells.

Disseminated disease is present at diagnosis in up to 70% of cases of neuroblastoma and most commonly involves cortical bone and bone marrow. Less frequently, there is involvement of liver, skin, or lung. A primary tumor is not detected in up to 10% of children with disseminated neuroblastoma (187). The primary tumor may also go undetected in patients who present with paraneoplastic syndromes such as infantile myoclonic encephalopathy. Surgical excision is the preferred treatment of localized neuroblastoma. When local disease is extensive, intensive preoperative chemotherapy may be utilized. When distant metastases are present, surgical removal is not likely to improve survival. The prognosis in these cases is poor but high-dose chemotherapy, total-body irradiation, and bone marrow reinfusion are beneficial for some children with this presentation.

Delineation of local disease extent is achieved with MRI, CT, and scintigraphic studies (188). These tests are also utilized in localizing the primary site in children who present with disseminated disease or with a paraneoplastic syndrome. Metaiodobenzylguanidine (MIBG) and indium-111 ([^{111}In])-pentetreotide scintigraphy have been employed in these settings with a sensitivity of >85% for detecting neuroblastoma. Uptake of MIBG, which is an analogue of guanethidine and norepinephrine, into neuroblastoma is by a neuronal sodium- and energy-dependent transport mechanism. The localization of [^{111}In]-pentetreotide in neuroblastoma reflects the presence of somatostatin type 2 receptors on some neuroblastoma cells (189). Bone scintigraphy has been most widely used for detection of skeletal involvement for staging. MIBG and, to a lesser extent, [^{111}In]-pentetreotide imaging have also been increasingly used for detecting skeletal involvement (190).

Patients with residual unresected primary tumors are periodically evaluated with MRI or CT. However, these studies cannot distinguish viable tumor from treatment-related scar or tumor that has matured into ganglioneuroma. Specificity in establishing residual viable tumor can be improved with MIBG or [^{111}In]-pentetreotide imaging when the primary tumor has been shown to accumulate one of these agents. These agents are also useful in assessing residual skeletal disease in patients with MIBG or [^{111}In]-pentetreotide-avid skeletal metastases. Bone scintigraphy, however, is unable to distinguish active disease from bony repair on the basis of tracer uptake.

Neuroblastomas are metabolically active tumors. Neuroblastomas and/or their metastases avidly concentrated FDG prior to chemotherapy or radiation therapy in 16 of 17 patients studied with FDG PET and MIBG imaging (190).Uptake after therapy was variable but tended to be lower. FDG and MIBG results were concordant in most instances (Fig. 8.23.10). However, there were occasions that one agent accumulated at a site of disease and the other did not. MIBG imaging was overall considered superior to FDG PET, particularly in delineation of residual disease. As the patients in this series had aggressive tumors and poor prognoses, the value of FDG PET for assessing therapeutic response could not be determined. An advantage of FDG PET is the initiation of imaging 30 to 60 minutes after FDG administration, while MIBG imaging is performed 1 or more days following tracer administration.

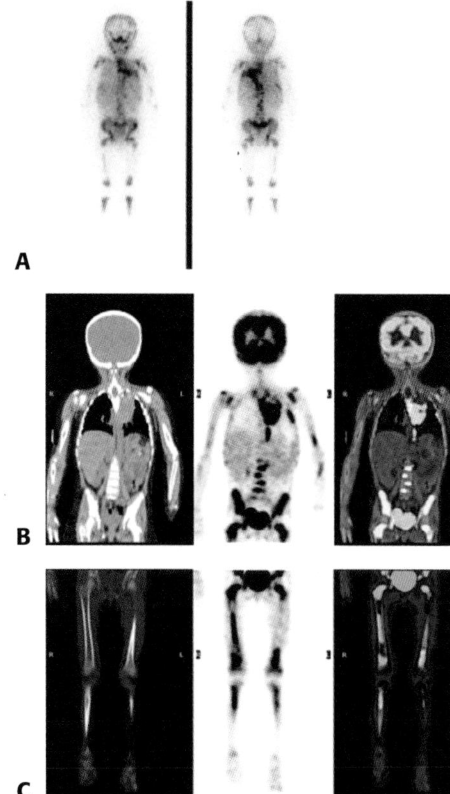

FIGURE 8.23.10. Images from of a 2-year-old girl with neuroblastoma at presentation. **A: Top panel.** Anterior (left) and posterior (right) planar views of a iodine-123-metaiodobenzylguanidine (MIBG) scan at 24 hours. There is extensive uptake of MIBG within the axial and much of the appendicular skeleton, and a left posterior upper thoracic mass. **B: Middle panel.** Selected coronal images of a fluorodeoxyglucose (FDG) PET scan (CT **left,** PET **middle,** fusion **right**) show the mediastinal mass and extensive irregular skeletal uptake. **C: Bottom panel.** Coronal images of the lower extremities (CT **left,** PET **middle,** fusion **right**) shows widespread abnormal osseous uptake. The distribution of abnormal uptake in the MIBG and FDG PET scans is similar.

FDG PET may be of limited value for the evaluation of the bone marrow involvement of neuroblastoma due to mild FDG accumulation by the normal bone marrow (191). Pitfalls resulting from physiologic FDG uptake in the bowel and the thymus are additional factors that may limit the role for FDG PET in neuroblastoma. It has been reported that once the primary tumor is resected, PET and bone marrow examination suffice for monitoring patients with neuroblastoma at high risk for progressive disease in soft tissue, bone, and bone marrow (188). Currently, however, the primary role of FDG PET in neuroblastoma is in the evaluation of known or suspected neuroblastomas that do not demonstrate MIBG uptake. Variable uptake of FDG in ganglioneuromas has also been noted. This suggests that FDG may not reliably differentiate between neuroblastomas and ganglioneuromas.

Carbon-11-hydroxyephedrine ([^{11}C]-HED), an analogue of norepinephrine, and [^{11}C]-epinephrine PET have also been used in evaluating neuroblastoma (Fig. 8.23.11). All seven neuroblastomas studied showed uptake of [^{11}C]-HED (192), and four of five neuroblastomas studied showed uptake of [^{11}C]-epinephrine (193). A

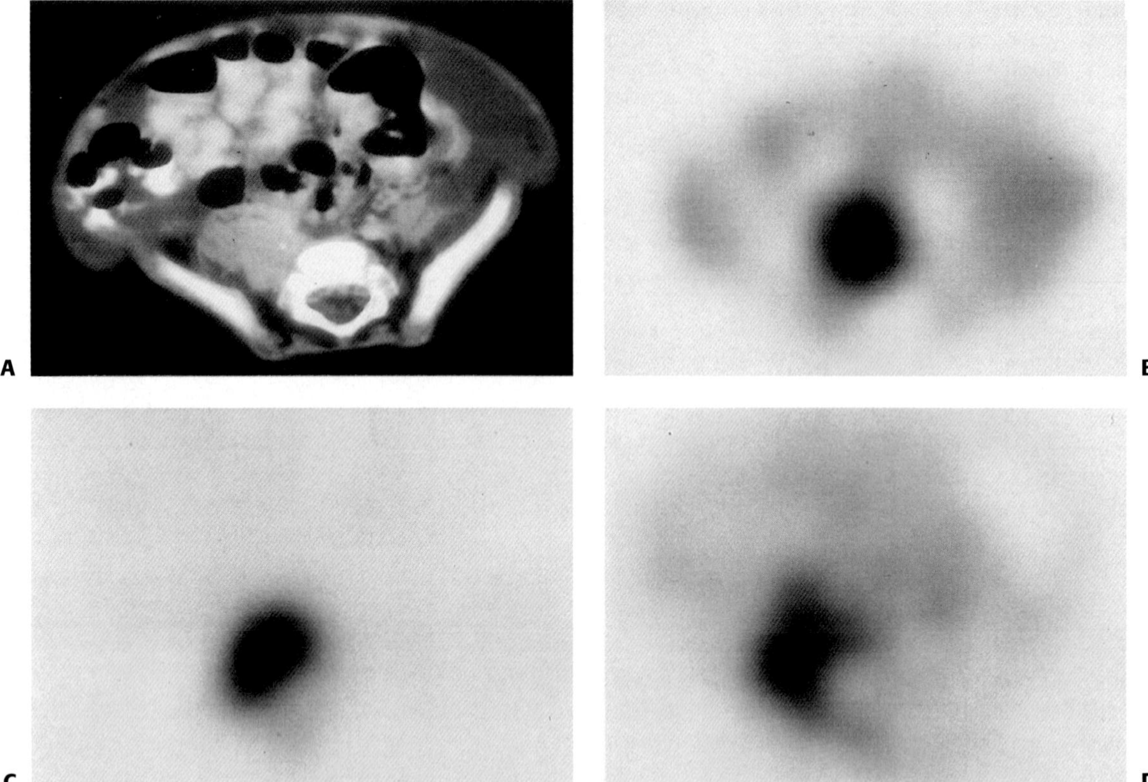

FIGURE 8.23.11. A: A CT scan of the pelvis of a 6-month-old boy following surgical debulking of abdominal-pelvic neuroblastoma: There is abnormal soft tissue with speckled calcification in the right posterior pelvis. **B:** Metaiodobenzylguanidine (MIBG) single-photon emission computed tomography (SPECT) scan at 24 hours shows uptake into the tumor. **C:** Hydroxyephedrine (HED) PET scan at 20 minutes following injection. There is excellent uptake within the neuroblastoma, and the image appears similar to the MIBG SPECT examination. **D:** Fluorodeoxyglucose (FDG) PET scan at 50 minutes. There is moderate accumulation of FDG within the mass relative to surrounding background. However, the tumor appears better delineated with the more specific adrenergic tumor imaging agent HED. (From Shulkin BL, Wieland DM, Baro ME, et al. PET hydroxyephedrine imaging of neuroblastoma. *J Nucl Med* 1996;37:16–21, with permission.)

recent study reported a higher sensitivity for [^{11}C]-HED PET/CT than that for iodine-123 ([^{123}I])-MIBG SPECT-CT (99% vs. 93%, respectively) (194). Uptake of these tracers is demonstrated within minutes after administration, which is an advantage over MIBG imaging. Limitations regarding cost and the need for on-site synthesis of short-lived [^{11}C] (half-life of 20 minutes) suggest that neither [^{11}C]-HED nor [^{11}C]-epinephrine PET is likely to replace MIBG imaging. These tracers may prove useful adjuncts in difficult cases where a primary tumor is difficult to identify with more readily available agents and to further the understanding of this disease. Compounds labeled with [^{18}F], such as fluoronorepinephrine, fluorometaraminol, and fluorodopamine, may also be useful tracers (195). PET using 4-[^{18}F]-fluoro-3-iodobenzylguanidine (196) and [^{124}I]-labeled MIBG (197) has also been described.

Wilms Tumor

Wilms tumor is the most common renal malignancy of childhood, predominantly seen in younger children and uncommonly encountered after the age of 5 years (47). Bilateral renal involvement occurs in about 5% of all cases and can be identified synchronously or metachronously (198). An asymptomatic abdominal mass is the typical mode of presentation. Nephrectomy with adjuvant chemotherapy is the treatment of choice. Radiation therapy is used in selected cases when resection is incomplete.

Scintigraphy has not played an important role in imaging of Wilms tumor. Radiography, ultrasonography, CT, and MRI are commonly employed in anatomic staging and detection of metastases, which predominantly involve lung, occasionally liver, and only rarely other sites. Anatomic imaging, however, is of limited value in the assessment for residual or recurrent tumor (198). Uptake of FDG by Wilms tumor (Fig. 8.23.12) has been described (199), but a role for FDG PET in Wilms tumor has not been established. Normal excretion of FDG through the kidney is a limiting factor. However, careful correlation with anatomic cross-sectional imaging allows distinction of tumor uptake from normal renal FDG excretion.

Bone Tumors

Osteosarcoma and Ewing sarcoma are the two primary bone malignancies of childhood; of the two, osteosarcoma is the more common and predominantly affects adolescents and young adults. A

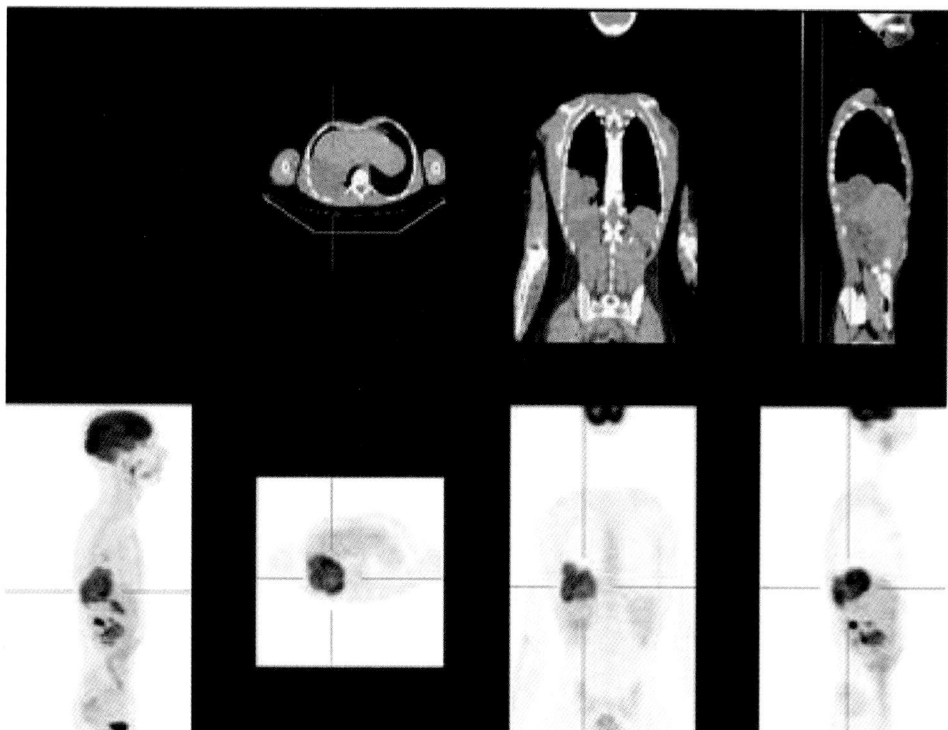

FIGURE 8.23.12. A 16-year-old boy with recurrent Wilms tumor. CT scan (**top panel**). PET scan (**bottom panel**—right lateral projection image on left). Markedly increased uptake of FDG (*cross bars*) is present within the right-sided mass seen on CT (*cross bars*).

second peak affects older adults, predominantly individuals with a history of prior radiation to bone or Paget disease. This tumor rarely affects children younger than 7 years of age. Osteosarcoma is typically a lesion of the long bones. The treatment of choice for osteosarcoma of an extremity is wide resection and limb-sparing surgery. Limb-sparing procedures entail the resection of tumor with a cuff of surrounding normal tissue at all margins, skeletal reconstruction, and muscle and soft tissue transfers. Employing current chemotherapeutic regimens pre- and postoperatively and imaging to define tumor extent and tumor viability preoperatively, limb-sparing procedures can be performed in 80% of patients with osteosarcoma (200).

Almost all cases of Ewing sarcoma occur between the ages of 5 and 30, with the highest incidence being in the second decade of life. In patients younger than 20 years, Ewing sarcoma most often affects the appendicular skeleton. Beyond that age, pelvic, rib, and vertebral lesions predominate. The tumor is believed to be of neuroectodermal origin and, along with the primitive neuroectodermal tumor, to be part of a spectrum of a single biologic entity (201). Ewing sarcoma is considered an undifferentiated variant and primitive neuroectodermal tumor a more differentiated peripheral neural tumor. Therapy for Ewing sarcoma involves multiagent chemotherapy for eradication of microscopic or overt metastatic disease and irradiation and/or surgery for control of the primary lesion. Because late recurrence is not uncommon, resection of the primary tumor is gaining favor for local disease control (202).

MRI is used to define the local extent of osteosarcoma and Ewing sarcoma in bone and soft tissue. However, signal abnormalities caused by peritumoral edema can result in an overestimation of tumor extension (203). Scintigraphy has been used primarily to detect skeletal metastases of these tumors at diagnosis and during follow-up. With osteosarcoma, skeletal scintigraphy occasionally demonstrates extraosseous metastases, most often pulmonary, due to osteoid production by the metastatic deposits.

Determination of preoperative chemotherapeutic response is important in planning limb-salvage surgery. Due to nonspecific appearance of viable tumor on MRI, variable results have been reported for assessing chemotherapeutic response (204–209). Scintigraphy with [^{201}Tl] has been shown to be useful for assessing therapeutic response in osteosarcoma (210–215) and perhaps Ewing sarcoma (211,212). A marked decrease in tumoral [^{201}Tl] uptake indicates a favorable response to chemotherapy. When tumoral [^{201}Tl] uptake does not decrease within weeks of chemotherapy, a therapeutic change may be needed. ^{99m}Tc-MIBI may also be useful in osteosarcoma but seemingly not with Ewing sarcoma (216,217).

The exact role of FDG PET in osteosarcoma and Ewing sarcoma has not yet been determined (Figs. 8.23.13 and 8.23.14). However, early experience suggests that in patients with Ewing sarcoma, FDG PET may play a role in assessing the extent of disease, in monitoring response to therapy, and in predicting long-term outcome after therapy (218–226). The posttherapy level of FDG uptake may underestimate the extent of tumor necrosis when compared to histological assessment probably due to some increase in the metabolic activity in response to therapy-induced inflammation and healing (227).

When compared to bone scintigraphy, FDG PET may be superior for detecting osseous metastases from Ewing sarcoma, but may be less sensitive for those from osteosarcoma (228). A second potential role is in assessing patients with suspected or known pulmonary metastasis, which is particularly common with osteosarcoma. In a recent retrospective study of 55 patients with bone tumors, PET detected metastases in 22% of patients, with 67% of these harboring disease outside the lung; 7% of patients were upstaged to stage IV with the most important alteration in treatment decisions being the substitution of irradiation *in lieu* of surgery for local control (229).

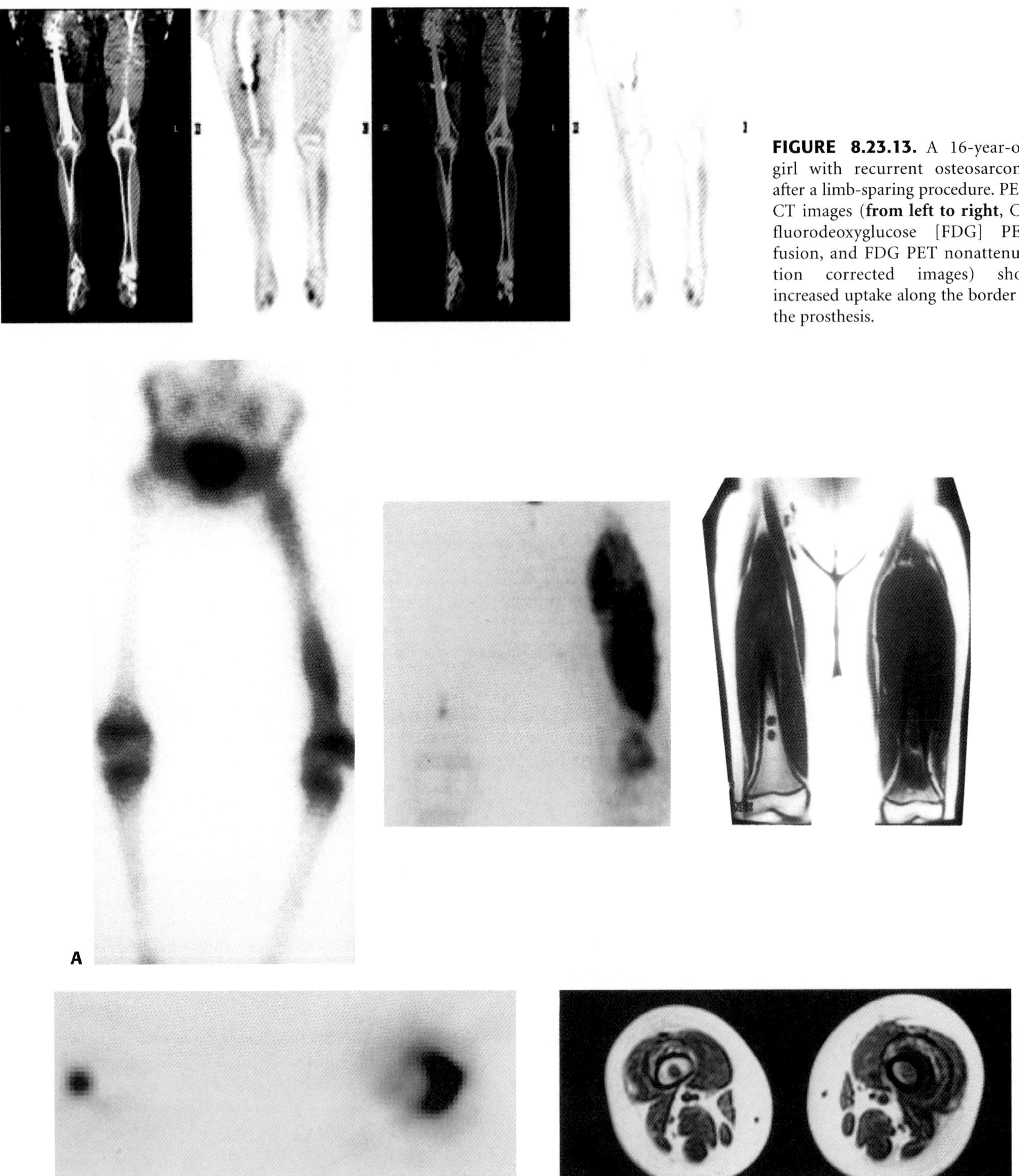

FIGURE 8.23.13. A 16-year-old girl with recurrent osteosarcoma after a limb-sparing procedure. PET/CT images (**from left to right**, CT, fluorodeoxyglucose [FDG] PET, fusion, and FDG PET nonattenuation corrected images) show increased uptake along the border of the prosthesis.

FIGURE 8.23.14. An 11-year-old girl complained of pain and swelling in the left thigh. Plain film radiographs showed findings suggestive of Ewing sarcoma, subsequently confirmed on biopsy. **A (left panel):** A bone scan obtained 2 hours following injection of technetium-99m methylene diphosphonate (^{99m}Tc-MDP). Abnormal accumulation of tracer is seen throughout the left femur. The right femur is unremarkable (**center panel**). The anterior projection image from the PET study shows intense, irregular uptake of fluorodeoxyglucose (FDG) within the soft tissues of the left thigh. Two small foci of activity are seen in the region of the distal right femur that are not present on the bone scan (**right panel**). The T1 weighted coronal magnetic resonance image shows a soft tissue mass in the left thigh, replacement of normal marrow of the left femur, and two focal lesions in the distal right femur. **B (left panel):** A transverse image from a PET scan at the level of the distal femurs. Intense uptake of FDG is present in the soft tissues surrounding the left femur and focally within the right femur (**right panel**). T1 weighted magnetic resonance image at same level shows the soft tissue mass surrounding the left femur, replacement of marrow of the left femur, and a lesion in the center of the right femur. (From Shulkin BL, Mitchell DS, Ungar DR, et al. Neoplasms in a pediatric population: 2-[F-18]-fluoro-2-deoxy-D-glucose PET studies. *Radiology* 1995;194:495–500, with permission.)

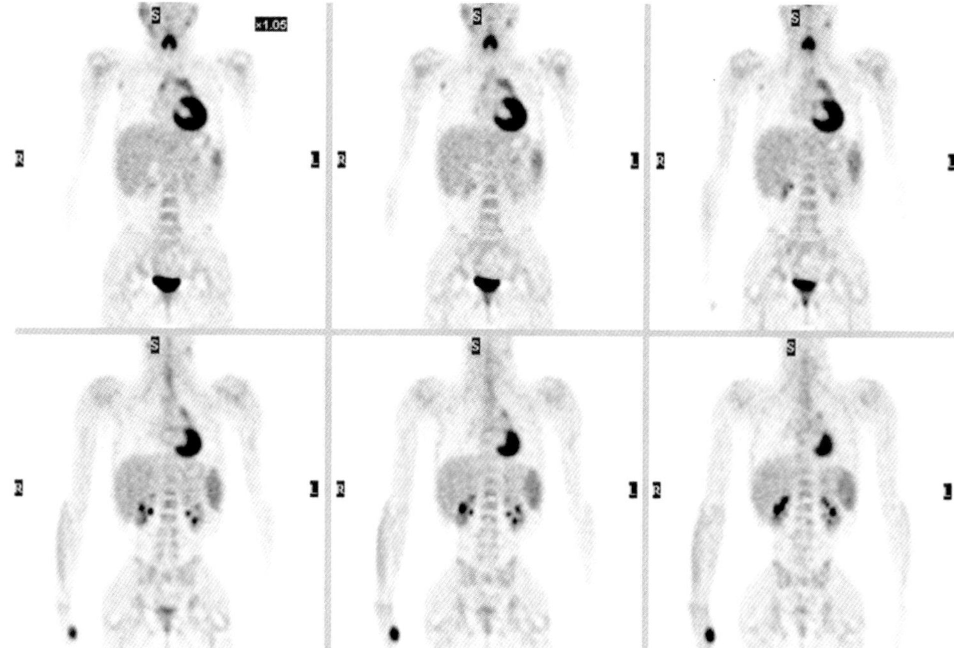

FIGURE 8.23.15. Coronal images of a 10-year-old girl show marked fluorine-18-fluorodeoxyglucose uptake by an alveolar rhabdomyosarcoma in the right hand and focal high uptake in the right axilla where metastatic nodal involvement was later confirmed by biopsy. High thymic uptake is also evident.

Soft Tissue Tumors

Rhabdomyosarcoma is the most common soft tissue malignancy of childhood. The peak incidence occurs between 3 and 6 years of age. Rhabdomyosarcomas can develop in any organ or tissue but, contrary to what the name implies, this tumor does not usually arise in muscle. The most common anatomic locations are the head, particularly the orbit and paranasal sinuses, the neck, and the genitourinary tract. CT or MRI is important for establishing the extent of local disease. Radiography and CT are used for detecting pulmonary metastases, and skeletal scintigraphy is employed for identifying osseous metastases. Radiation therapy and surgery are utilized for local disease control, and chemotherapy is employed for treatment of metastases.

Rhabdomyosarcomas show variable degrees of FDG accumulation. Cases showing the clinical utility of FDG PET have been described, but the exact role of FDG PET in rhabdomyosarcoma is yet to be determined (Fig. 8.23.15) (4,218,230,231). A recent study has shown that in patients with soft tissue sarcomas, the pretreatment tumor SUV_{max} (maximum) and change in SUV_{max} after neoadjuvant chemotherapy independently identified patients at high risk of tumor recurrence (232).

PET IN PEDIATRIC INFECTION AND INFLAMMATION

The diagnostic utility of PET is expanding to include infectious and inflammatory disorders of adult patients. There have also been reports on the use of PET in pediatric population in these clinical settings. Sturm et al. (233) evaluated how FDG PET can contribute to the management of pediatric liver transplantation candidates who present with fever of unknown origin. Nonhepatic origins of systemic infections may render the patient unsuitable for transplantation, whereas infections within the liver may require organ resection for a cure. This study included 11 children with biliary cirrhosis and fever of unknown origin during the waiting period for liver transplantation. In five children, true positive intrahepatic findings corresponded to bacterial cultures of the excised liver and/or anatomic or histologic signs of infection. These patients underwent transplantation after continuous antibiotic treatment. In the remaining six children, no abnormal hepatic findings were found. Transplantation in these patients was performed only after becoming afebrile. Standard imaging techniques were negative in all these children. The authors concluded that in children with biliary cirrhosis and fever of unknown origin on the waiting list for liver transplantation, FDG PET imaging might be useful for decisions on when to proceed with liver transplantation.

Loffler et al. (234) evaluated the diagnostic potential of FDG PET in 23 children with suspected inflammatory bowel disease. PET findings were compared to endoscopic, histologic, and abdominal ultrasound findings. FDG PET, endoscopy, and ultrasound demonstrated sensitivity and specificity of 98% and 68%, 90% and 75%, and 56% and 92%, respectively. The study concluded that because of its high sensitivity, FDG PET is an excellent noninvasive diagnostic tool for evaluating suspected inflammatory bowel disease in children. In a similar investigation from Canada, PET correctly identified active inflammatory disease in 80% of children with inflammatory bowel disease (81.5% with Crohn disease; 76.4% with ulcerative colitis) and correctly showed no evidence of inflammation in children with recurrent abdominal pain (235).

SUMMARY

FDG PET is being applied increasingly to study diseases of childhood, especially tumors. Because the tumors encountered are relatively rare, it will be difficult to perform well-designed, prospective clinical trials at single institutions. The recent merger of the CCG (Children's Cancer Group) and the POG (Pediatric Oncology Group) to form COG (Children's Oncology Group) brings an opportunity to examine the use of FDG PET in the management of childhood tumors in multi-institutional, cooperative efforts. It is expected that future data will show that FDG PET and PET/CT do contribute unique, valuable information for the care of childhood disorders.

REFERENCES

1. Gordon I. Issues surrounding preparation, information, and handling the child and parent in nuclear medicine. *J Nucl Med* 1998;39:490–494.
2. Treves ST. Introduction. In: Treves ST, ed. *Pediatric nuclear medicine*, 2nd ed. New York: Springer-Verlag, 1995:1–11.
3. Mandell GA, Cooper JA, Majd M, et al. Procedure guidelines for pediatric sedation in nuclear medicine. *J Nucl Med* 1997;38:1640–1643.
4. Shulkin BL. PET applications in pediatrics. *Q J Nucl Med* 1997;41: 281–291.
5. Borgwardt L, Larsen HJ, Pedersen K, et al. Practical use and implementation of PET in children in a hospital PET center. *Eur J Nucl Med Mol Imaging* 2003;30:1389–1397.
6. Roberts EG, Shulkin BL. Technical issues in performing PET studies in pediatric patients. *J Nucl Med Technol* 2004;32:5–9.
7. Kaste SC. Issues specific to implementing PET-CT for pediatric oncology: what we have learned along the way. *Pediatr Radiol* 2004; 34:205–213.
8. Delbeke D, Coleman RE, Guiberteau MJ, et al. Procedure guideline for tumor imaging with ^{18}F-FDG PET-CT 1.0. *J Nucl Med* 2006;47:885–895.
9. Schelbert H, Hoh CK, Royal HD, et al. Procedure guideline for tumor imaging using fluorine-18-FDG. *J Nucl Med* 1998;39:1302–1305.
10. Jones SC, Alavi A, Christman D, et al. The radiation dosimetry of 2-[^{18}F]fluoro-2-deoxy-D-glucose in man. *J Nucl Med* 1982;23:613–617.
11. Ruotsalainen U, Suhonen-Povli H, Eronen E, et al. Estimated radiation dose to the newborn in FDG-PET studies. *J Nucl Med* 1996;37: 387–393.
12. Brenner D, Elliston C, Hall E, et al. Estimated risks of radiation-induced fatal cancer from pediatric CT. *Am J Roentgenol* 2001;176: 289–296.
13. Chugani HT, Phelps ME. Maturational changes in cerebral function in infants determined by ^{18}FDG positron emission tomography. *Science* 1986;231:840–843.
14. Chugani HT, Phelps ME, Mazziotta JC. Positron emission tomography study of human brain functional development. *Ann Neurol* 1987;22:487–497.
15. Chugani HT. Positron emission tomography. In: Berg BO, ed. *Principles of child neurology*. New York: McGraw-Hill, 1996:113–128.
16. Hauser W. Epidemiology of epilepsy in children. *Neurosurg Clin North Am* 1995;6:419–428.
17. National Institutes of Health Consensus Development Conference Statement: surgery for epilepsy. *Epilepsia* 1990;31:806–812.
18. Kuzniecky R, Suggs S, Gaudier J, et al. Lateralization of epileptic foci by magnetic resonance imaging in temporal lobe epilepsy. *J Neuroimaging* 1991;1:163–167.
19. Treves ST, Connolly LP. Single photon emission computed tomography in pediatric epilepsy. *Neurosurg Clin North Am* 1995;6:473–480.
20. Snead OC III, Chen LS, Mitchell WG, et al. Usefulness of [^{18}F]fluorodeoxyglucose positron emission tomography in pediatric epilepsy surgery. *Pediatr Neurol* 1996;14:98–107.
21. Meltzer CC, Adelson PD, Brenner RP, et al. Planned ictal FDG PET imaging for localization of extratemporal epileptic foci. *Epilepsia* 2000;41(2):193–200.
22. Lee JJ, Kang WJ, Lee DS, et al. Diagnostic performance of ^{18}F-FDG PET and ictal ^{99m}Tc-HMPAO SPET in pediatric temporal lobe epilepsy: quantitative analysis by statistical mapping, statistical probabilistic anatomical map, and subtraction ictal SPET. *Seizure* 2005;14:213–220.
23. Juhasz C, Chugani DC, Muzik O, et al. Is epileptogenic cortex truly hypometabolic on interictal positron emission tomography? *Ann Neurol* 2000;48(1):88–96.
24. Benedek K, Juhasz C, Chugani DC, et al. Longitudinal changes in cortical glucose hypometabolism in children with intractable epilepsy. *J Child Neurol* 2006;21:26–31.
25. Cummings TJ, Chugani DC, Chugani HT. Positron emission tomography in pediatric epilepsy. *Neurosurg Clin North Am* 1995;6:465–472.
26. Ollenberger GP, Byrne AJ, Berlangieri SU, et al. Assessment of the role of FDG PET in the diagnosis and management of children with refractory epilepsy. *Eur J Nucl Med Mol Imaging* 2005;32:1311–1316.
27. Engel J Jr, Kuhl DE, Phelps ME. Patterns of human local cerebral glucose metabolism during epileptogenic seizures. *Science* 1982;218:64–66.
28. Chandra PS, Salamon N, Hunag J, et al. FDG PET/MRI coregistration and diffusion-tensor imaging distinguish epileptogenic tubers and cortex in patients with tuberous sclerosis complex: a preliminary report. *Epilepsia* 2006;47:1543–1549.
29. da Silva EA, Chugani DC, Muzik O, et al. Identification of frontal lobe epileptic foci in children using positron emission tomography. *Epilepsia* 1997;38:1198–1208.
30. Hrachovy R, Frost J. Infantile spasms. *Pediatr Clin North Am* 1989; 36:311–329.
31. Chugani HT, Shields WD, Shewmon DA, et al. Infantile spasms: I PET identifies focal cortical dysgenesis in cryptogenic cases for surgical treatment. *Ann Neurol* 1990;27:406–413.
32. Chuagni HT, Shewmon DA, Shields WD, et al. Surgery for intractable infantile spasms: neuroimaging perspectives. *Epilepsia* 1993;34:764–771.
33. Chugani HT, Da Silva E, Chugani DC. Infantile spasms: III prognostic implications of bitemporal hypometabolism on positron emission tomography. *Ann Neurol* 1996;39:643–649.
34. Chugani HT, Conti JR. Etiologic classification of infantile spasms in 140 cases: role of positron emission tomography. *J Child Neurol* 1996;11:44–48.
35. Savic I, Svanborg E, Thorell JO. Cortical benzodiazepine receptor changes are related to frequency of partial seizures: a positron emission tomography study. *Epilepsia* 1996;37:236–244.
36. Arnold S, Berthele A, Drzezga A, et al. Reduction of benzodiazepine receptor binding is related to the seizure onset zone in extratemporal focal cortical dysplasia. *Epilepsia* 2000;41(7):818–824.
37. Richardson MP, Koepp MJ, Brooks DJ, et al. ^{11}C-flumanezil PET in neocortical epilepsy. *Neurology* 1998;51:485–492.
38. Debets RM, Sadzot B, van Isselt JW, et al. Is ^{11}C-flumazenil PET superior to ^{18}FDG PET and ^{123}I-iomazenial SPECT in presurgical evaluation of temporal lobe epilepsy? *J Neurol Neurosurg Psychiatry* 1997;62:141–150.
39. Kumlien E, Hartvig P, Valind S, et al. NMDA-receptor activity visualized with (S)-[*N*-methyl-11-C]ketamine and positron emission tomography in patients with medial temporal epilepsy. *Epilepsia* 1999;40:30–37.
40. Kagawa K, Chugani DC, Asano E, et al. Epilepsy surgery outcome in children with tuberous sclerosis complex evaluated with alpha-[^{11}C]methyl-L-tryptophan positron emission tomography (PET). *J Child Neurol* 2005;20:429–438.
41. Sood S, Chugani HT. Functional neuroimaging in the preoperative evaluation of children with drug-resistant epilepsy. *Childs Nerv Syst* 2006;22:810–820.
42. Mayberg HS, Sadzot B, Meltzer CC, et al. Quantification of mu and non-mu opiate receptors in temporal lobe epilepsy using positron emission tomography. *Ann Neurol* 1991;30:3–11.
43. Kumlien E, Bergstrom M, Lilja A, et al. Positron emission tomography with [C-11]deuterium deprenyl in temporal lobe epilepsy. *Epilepsia* 1995;36:712–721.
44. Volpe JJ, Herscovitch P, Perlman JM, et al. Positron emission tomography in the newborn: extensive impairment of regional cerebral blood flow with intraventricular hemorrhage and hemorrhagic intracerebral involvement. *Pediatrics* 1983;72(5):589–601.
45. Volpe JJ, Herscovitch P, Perlman JM, et al. Positron emission tomography in the asphyxiated term newborn: parasagittal impairment of cerebral blood flow. *Ann Neurol* 1985;17(3):287–296.

46. Zilbovicius M, Boddaert N, Belin P, et al. Temporal lobe dysfunction in childhood autism: a PET study. *Am J Psychiatry* 2000;157(12):1988–1993.
47. Ernst M, Zametkin AJ, Matochik JA, et al. High midbrain [^{18}F]DOPA accumulation in children with attention deficit hyperactivity disorder. *Am J Psychiatry* 1999;156(8):1209–1215.
48. Volkow ND, Wang GJ, Newcorn J, et al. Brain dopamine transporter levels in treatment and drug naive adults with ADHD. *Neuroimage* 2007;34:1182–1190.
49. Sundaram SK, Chugani HT, Chugani DC. Positron emission tomography methods with potential for increased understanding of mental retardation and developmental disabilities. *Ment Retard Dev Disabil Res Rev* 2005;11:325–330.
50. Kang E, Lee DS, Kang H, et al. Age-associated changes of cerebral glucose metabolism activity in both male and female deaf children: parametric analysis using objective volume of interest and voxel-based mapping. *Neuroimage* 2004;22:1543–1553.
51. Jacobson LK, Hamburger SD, Van Horn JD, et al. Cerebral glucose metabolism in childhood onset schizophrenia. *Psychiatry Res* 1997;75 (3):131–144.
52. Reed W, Jagust W, Al-Mateen M, et al. Role of positron emission tomography in determining the extent of CNS ischemia in patients with sickle cell disease. *Am J Hematol* 1999;60(4):268–272.
53. Delvenne V, Lotstra F, Goldman S, et al. Brain hypometabolism of glucose in anorexia nervosa: a PET scan study. *Biol Psychiatry* 1995;37(3): 161–169.
54. Delvenne V, Goldman S, Simon Y, et al. Brain hypometabolism of glucose in bulimia nervosa. *Int J Eat Disord* 1997;21(4):313–320.
55. Lee JS, Juhasz C, Kaddurah AK, et al. Patterns of cerebral glucose metabolism in early and late stages Rasmussen's syndrome. *J Child Neurol* 2001;16:798–805.
56. Al-Essa MA, Bakheet SM, Patay ZJ, et al. Clinical and cerebral FDG PET scan in a patient with Krabbe's disease. *Pediatr Neurol* 2000;22: 44–47.
57. Lee JS, Asano E, Muzik O, et al. Sturge-Weber syndrome: correlation between clinical course and FDG PET findings. *Neurology* 2001;57: 189–195.
58. Lee JS, Pfund Z, Juhasz C, et al. Altered regional brain glucose metabolism in Duchenne muscular dystrophy: a PET study. *Muscle Nerve* 2002;26:506–512.
59. Quinlivan RM, Robinson RO, Maisey MN. Positron emission tomography in pediatric cardiology. *Arch Dis Child* 1998;79(6):520–522.
60. Donnelly JP, Raffel DM, Shulkin BL, et al. Resting coronary flow and coronary flow reserve in human infants after repair or palliation of congenital heart defects as measured by positron emission tomography. *J Thorac Cardiovasc Surg* 1998;115(1):103–110.
61. Yates RW, Marsden PK, Badawi RD, et al. Evaluation of myocardial perfusion using positron emission tomography in infants following a neonatal arterial switch operation. *Pediatr Cardiol* 2000;21(2): 111–118.
62. Rickers C, Sasse K, Buchert R, et al. Myocardial viability assessed by positron emission tomography in infants and children after the arterial switch operation and suspected infarction. *J Am Coll Cardiol* 2000;36(5):1676–1683.
63. Singh TP, Muzik O, Forbes TF, et al. Positron emission tomography myocardial perfusion imaging in children with suspected coronary abnormalities. *Pediatr Cardiol* 2003;24:138–144.
64. Hernandez-Pampaloni M, Allada V, Fishbein MC, et al. Myocardial perfusion and viability by positron emission tomography in infants and children with coronary abnormalities: correlation with echocardiography, coronary angiography, and histopathology. *J Am Coll Cardiol* 2003;41:618–626.
65. Hwang B, Liu RS, Chu LS, et al. Positron emission tomography for the assessment of myocardial viability in Kawasaki disease using different therapies. *Nucl Med Commun* 2000;21(7):631–636.
66. Huaser M, Bengel F, Kuehn A, et al. Myocardial blood flow and coronary flow reserve in children with "normal" epicardial coronary arteries after the onset of Kawasaki disease assessed by positron emission tomography. *Pediatr Cardiol* 2004;25:108–112.
67. Litvinova I, Litvinov M, Loeonteva I, et al. PET for diagnosis of mitochondrial cardiomyopathy in children. *Clin Positron Imaging* 2000;3(4):172.
68. Gurney JG, Severson RK, Davis S, et al. Incidence of cancer in children in the United States. *Cancer* 1995;75:2186–2195.
69. Robison L. General principles of the epidemiology of childhood cancer. In: Pizzo P, Poplack D, eds. *Principles and practice of pediatric oncology*. Philadelphia: Lippincott-Raven, 1997:1–10.
70. Franzius C, Schober O. Assessment of therapy response by FDG PET in pediatric patients. *Q J Nucl Med* 2003;47:41–45.
71. Wegner EA, Barrington SF, Kingston JE, et al. The impact of PET scanning on management of paediatric oncology patients. *Eur J Nucl Med Mol Imaging* 2005;32:23–30.
72. Shulkin BL. PET imaging in pediatric oncology. *Pediatr Radiol* 2004;34:199–204.
73. Pacak K, Ilias I, Chen CC, et al. The role of ^{18}F-fluorodeoxyglucose positron emission tomography and In-111-diethylenetriaminepentaacetate-D-Phe-pentetreotide scintigraphy in the localization of ectopic adrenocorticotropin-secreting tumors causing Cushing's syndrome. *J Clin Endocrinol Metab* 2004;89:2214–2221.
74. Figarola MS, McQuiston SA, Wilson F, et al. Recurrent hepatoblastoma with localization by PET-CT. *Pediatr Radiol* 2005;35:1254–1258.
75. Kinoshita H, Shimotake T, Furukawa T, et al. Mucoepidermal carcinoma of the lung detected by positron emission tomography in a 5-year-old girl. *J Pediatr Surg* 2005;40:E1–E3.
76. Philip I, Shun A, McCowage G, et al. Positron emission tomography in recurrent hepatoblastoma. *Pediatr Surg Int* 2005;21:341–345.
77. Franzius C, Juergens KU, Vomoor J. PET-CT with diagnostic CT in the evaluation of childhood sarcoma. *AJR Am J Roentgenol* 2005;184: 1293–1304.
78. Sasi OA, Sathiapalan R, Rifai A, et al. Colonic neuroendocrine carcinoma in a child. *Pediatr Radiol* 2005;35:339–343.
79. Buchler T, Cervinek L, Belohlavek O, et al. Langerhans cell histiocytosis with central nervous system involvement: follow up by FDG PET during treatment with cladribine. *Pediatr Blood Cancer* 2005;44:286–288.
80. Mackie GC, Shulkin BL, Ribeiro RC, et al. Use of [^{18}F]fluorodeoxyglucose positron emission tomography in evaluating locally recurrent and metastatic adrenocortical carcinoma. *J Clin Endocrinol Metab* 2006;91:2665–2671.
81. Mody RJ, Pohlen JA, Malde S, et al. FDG PET for the study of primary hepatic malignancies in children. *Pediatr Blood Cancer* 2006;47:51–55.
82. Bar-Sever Z, Keidar Z, Ben-Barak A, et al. The incremental value of ^{18}F-FDG PET-CT in pediatric malignancies. *Eur J Nucl Med Mol Imaging* 2007;34:630–637.
83. Nanni C, Rubello D, Castelluci P, et al. ^{18}F-FDG PET-CT fusion imaging in pediatric solid extracranial tumors. *Biomed Pharmacother* 2006;60:593–606.
84. Yeung HW, Schoder H, Smith A, et al. Clinical value of combined positron emission tomography/computed tomography imaging in the interpretation of 2-deoxy-2-[F-18]fluoro-D-glucose positron emission tomography studies in cancer patients. *Mol Imaging Biol* 2005;7:229–235.
85. Moon L, McHugh K. Advances in pediatric tumor imaging. *Arch Dis Child* 2005;90:608–611.
86. Patel PM, Alibazoglu H, Ali A, et al. Normal thymic uptake of FDG on PET imaging. *Clin Nucl Med* 1996;21:772–775.
87. Weinblatt ME, Zanzi I, Belakhlef A, et al. False positive FDG-PET imaging of the thymus of a child with Hodgkin's disease. *J Nucl Med* 1997;38:888–890.
88. Brink I, Reinhardt MJ, Hoegerle S, et al. Increased metabolic activity in the thymus gland studied with 18F-FDG PET: age dependency and frequency after chemotherapy. *J Nucl Med* 2001;42:591–595.
89. Ferdinand B, Gupta P, Kramer EL. Spectrum of thymic uptake at ^{18}F-FDG PET. *Radiographics* 2004;24:1611–1616.

90. Nakamoto Y, Tatsumi M, Hammoud D, et al. Normal FDG distribution patterns in the head and neck: PET-CT evaluation. *Radiology* 2005;234:879–885.
91. Kawano T, Suzuki A, Ishida A, et al. The clinical relevance of thymic fluorodeoxyglucose uptake in pediatric patients after chemotherapy. *Eur J Nucl Med Mol Imaging* 2004;31:831–836.
92. Yeung HW, Grewal RK, Gonen M, et al. Patterns of (^{18}F)-FDG uptake in adipose tissue and muscles: a potential source of false-positives for PET. *J Nucl Med* 2003;44:1789–1796.
93. Cohade C, Mourtzikos KA, Wahl RL. "USA-fat": prevalence is related to ambient outdoor temperature—evaluation with ^{18}F-FDG PET/CT. *J Nucl Med* 2003;44:1267–1270.
94. Truong MT, Erasmus JJ, Munden RF, et al. Focal FDG uptake in mediastinal brown fat mimicking malignancy: a potential pitfall resolved on PET-CT. *AJR Am J Roentgenol* 2004;183:1127–1132.
95. Tatsumi M, Engles JM, Ishimori T, et al. Intense (^{18})F-FDG uptake in brown fat can be reduced pharmacologically. *J Nucl Med* 2004;45: 1189–1193.
96. Gelfand MJ, O'Hara SM, Curtwright LA, et al. Pre-medication to block [(^{18})F]FDG uptake in the brown adipose tissue of pediatric and adolescent patients. *Pediatr Radiol* 2005;35:984–990.
97. Garcia CA, Van Nostrand D, Atkins F, et al. Reduction of brown fat 2-deoxy-2-[F-18]fluoro-D-glucose uptake by controlling environmental temperature prior to positron emission tomography scan. *Mol Imaging Biol* 2006;8:24–29.
98. Delbeke D. Oncological applications of FDG PET imaging: colorectal cancer, lymphoma, and melanoma. *J Nucl Med* 1999;40:591–603.
99. Sugawara Y, Fisher SJ, Zasadny KR, et al. Preclinical and clinical studies of bone marrow uptake of fluorine-1-fluorodeoxyglucose with or without granulocyte colony-stimulating factor during chemotherapy. *J Clin Oncol* 1998;16:173–180.
100. Hollinger EF, Alibazoglu H, Ali A, et al. Hematopoietic cytokine-mediated FDG uptake simulates the appearance of diffuse metastatic disease on whole-body PET imaging. *Clin Nucl Med* 1998;23:93–98.
101. Nunez R, Rini JN, Tronco GG, et al. Correlation of hematologic parameters with bone marrow and spleen uptake in FDG PET. *Rev Esp Med Nucl* 2005;24:107–112.
102. Goodin GS, Shulkin BL, Kaufman RA, et al. PET-CT characterization of fibroosseous defects in children: 18F-FDG uptake can mimic metastatic disease. *AJR Am J Roentgenol* 2006;187:1146.
103. Feldman F, Van Heertum R, Saxena C. ^{18}Fluorodeoxyglucose positron emission tomography evaluation of benign versus malignant osteochondromas: preliminary observation. *J Comput Assist Tomogr* 2006;30:858–864.
104. Iagaru A, Henderson R. PET-CT follow-up in nonossifying fibroma. *AJR Am J Roentgenol* 2006;187:830–832.
105. Yeung HW, Sanches A, Squire OD, et al. Standardized uptake value in pediatric patients: an investigation to determine the optimum measurement parameter. *Eur J Nucl Med Mol Imaging* 2002;29:61–66.
106. Kleihues P, Burger P, Scheithauer B. The new WHO classification of brain tumors. *Brain Pathol* 1993;3:255–268.
107. Robertson R, Ball WJ, Barnes P. Skull and brain. In: Kirks D, ed. *Practical pediatric imaging. Diagnostic radiology of infants and children.* Philadelphia: Lippincott-Raven, 1997:65–200.
108. Maria B, Drane WB, Quisling RJ, et al. Correlation between gadolinium-diethylenetriaminepentaacetic acid contrast enhancement and thallium-201 chloride uptake in pediatric brainstem glioma. *J Child Neurol* 1997;12:341–348.
109. O'Tuama L, Janicek M, Barnes P, et al. Tl-201/Tc-99m HMPAO SPECT imaging of treated childhood brain tumors. *Pediatr Neurol* 1991;7:249–257.
110. O'Tuama L, Treves ST, Larar G, et al. Tl-201 versus Tc-99m MIBI SPECT in evaluation of childhood brain tumors. *J Nucl Med* 1993;34: 1045–1051.
111. Rollins N, Lowry P, Shapiro K. Comparison of gadolinium-enhanced MR and thallium-201 single photon emission computed tomography in pediatric brain tumors. *Pediatr Neurosurg* 1995;22:8–14.
112. Valk PE, Budinger TF, Levin VA, et al. PET of malignant cerebral tumors after interstitial brachytherapy. Demonstration of metabolic activity and correlation with clinical outcome. *J Neurosurg* 1988;69: 830–838.
113. Di Chiro G, Oldfield E, Wright DC, et al. Cerebral necrosis after radiotherapy and/or intraarterial chemotherapy for brain tumors: PET and neuropathologic studies. *AJR Am J Roentgenol* 1988;150:189–197.
114. Glantz MJ, Hoffman JM, Coleman RE, et al. Identification of early recurrence of primary central nervous system tumors by [^{18}F]fluorodeoxyglucose positron emission tomograph. *Ann Neurol* 1991;29:347–355.
115. Janus T, Kim E, Tilbury R, et al. Use of [^{18}F]fluorodeoxyglucose positron emission tomography in patients with primary malignant brain tumors. *Ann Neurol* 1993;33:540–548.
116. Rozental JM, Levine RL, Nickles RJ. Changes in glucose uptake by malignant gliomas: preliminary study of prognostic significance. *J Neurooncology* 1991;10:75–83.
117. Schifter T, Hoffman JM, Hanson MW, et al. Serial FDG-PET studies in the prediction of survival in patients with primary brain tumors. *J Comput Assist Tomogr* 1993;17:509–561.
118. Borgwardt L, Hojgaard L, Carstensen H, et al. Increased fluorine-18 2-fluoro-2-deoxy D-glucose (FDG) uptake in childhood CNS tumors is correlated with malignancy grade: a study with FDG positron emission tomography/magnetic resonance imaging coregistration and image fusion. *J Clin Oncol* 2005;23:3030–3037.
119. Francavilla TL, Miletich RS, Di Chiro G, et al. Positron emission tomography in the detection of malignant degeneration of low-grade gliomas. *Neurosurgery* 1989;24:1–5.
120. Patronas NJ, Di Chiro G, Kufta C, et al. Prediction of survival in glioma patients by means of positron emission tomography. *J Neurosurg* 1985;62:816–822.
121. Molloy PT, Belasco J, Ngo K, et al. The role of FDG PET imaging in the clinical management of pediatric brain tumors. *J Nucl Med* 1999;40:129P(abst).
122. Holthof VA, Herholz K, Berthold F, et al. *In vivo* metabolism of childhood posterior fossa tumors and primitive neuroectodermal tumors before and after treatment. *Cancer* 1993;1394–1403.
123. Hoffman JM, Hanson MW, Friedman HS, et al. FDG-PET in pediatric posterior fossa brain tumors. *J Comput Assist Tomogr* 1992;16:62–68.
124. Gururangan S, Hwang E, Herndon JE, 2nd, et al. [^{18}F]fluorodeoyglucose positron emission tomography in patients with medulloblastoma. *Neurosurgery* 2004;55:1280–1288.
125. Wang SX, Boethus J, Ericson K. FDG-PET on irradiated brain tumor: ten years summary. *Acta Radiol* 2006;47:85–90.
126. Molloy PT, Defeo R, Hunter J, et al. Excellent correlation of FDG PET imaging with clinical outcome in patients with neurofibromatosis type I and low-grade astrocytomas. *J Nucl Med* 1999;40:129P(abst).
127. Pirotte B, Goldman S, Salzberg S, et al. Combined positron emission tomography and magnetic resonance imaging for the planning of stereotactic brain biopsies in children: experience in 9 cases. *Pediatr Neurosurg* 2003;38:146–155.
128. Pirotte B, Goldman S, Dewitte O, et al. Integrated positron emission tomography and magnetic resonance imaging-guided resection of brain tumors: a report of 103 consecutive procedures. *J Neurosurg* 2006;104:238–253.
129. O'Tuama LA, Phillips PC, Strauss LC, et al. Two-phase [^{11}C]-methionine PET in childhood brain tumors. *Pediatr Neurol* 1990;6:163–170.
130. Mosskin M, von Holst H, Bergstrom M, et al. Positron emission tomography with ^{11}C-methionine and computed tomography of intracranial tumors compared with histopathologic examination of multiple biopsies. *Acta Radiologica* 1987;28:673–681.
131. Torii K, Tsuyuguchi N, Kawabe J, et al. Correlation of amino-acid uptake using methionine PET and histological classification in various gliomas. *Ann Nucl Med* 2005;19:677–683.
132. Lilja A, Lundqvist H, Olsson Y, et al. Positron emission tomography and computed tomography in differential diagnosis between recurrent or residual glioma and treatment-induced brain lesion. *Acta Radiologica* 1989;38:121–128.

133. Pirotte B, Levivier M, Morelli D, et al. Positron emission tomography for the early postsurgical evaluation of pediatric brain tumors. *Childs Nerv Syst* 2005;21:294–300.
134. Ceyssens S, Van Laere K, de Groot T, et al. [^{11}C]methionine PET, histopathology, and survival in primary brain tumors and recurrence. *AJNR Am J Neurolradiol* 2006;27:1432–1437.
135. Mineura K, Sasajima T, Kowada M, et al. Indications for differential diagnosis of nontumor central nervous system diseases from tumors. A positron emission tomography study. *J Neuroimaging* 1997;7:8–15.
136. Utriainen M, Metsahonkala L, Salmi TT, et al. Metabolic characterization of childhood brain tumors: comparison of ^{18}F-fluorodeoxyglucose and ^{11}C-methionine positron emission tomography. *Cancer* 2002;95: 1376–1386.
137. Van Laere K, Ceyssens S, Van Calenbergh F, et al. Direct comparison of ^{18}F-FDG and ^{11}C-methionine PET in suspected recurrence of glioma: sensitivity, inter-observer variability and prognostic value. *Eur J Nucl Med Mol Imaging* 2005;32:39–51.
138. Choi SJ, Kim JS, Kim JH, et al. [^{18}F]3'-deoxy-3'-fluorothymidine PET for the diagnosis and grading of brain tumors. *Eur J Nucl Med Mol Imaging* 2005;32:653–659.
139. Juhasz C, Chugani DC, Muzik O, et al. *In vivo* uptake and metabolism of alpha-[^{11}C]methyl-L-tryptophan in human brain tumors. *J Cereb Blood Flow Metab* 2006;26:345–357.
140. Floeth FW, Pauleit D, Wittsack HJ, et al. Multimodal metabolic imaging of cerebral gliomas: positron emission tomography with [^{18}F]fluoroethyl-L-tyrosine and magnetic resonance spectroscopy. *J Neurosurg* 2005;102:318–327.
141. Pauleit D, Floeth F, Hamacher K, et al. O-(2-[^{18}F]fluoroethyl)-L-tyrosine PET combined with MRI improves the diagnostic assessment of cerebral gliomas. *Brain* 2005;128(Pt 3):678–687.
142. Weckesser M, Langen KJ, Rickert CH, et al. O-(2-[^{18}F]fluorethyl)-L-tyrosine PET in the clinical evaluation of primary brain tumors. *Eur J Nucl Med Mol Imaging* 2005;32:422–429.
143. Kaste SC, Howard SC, McCarville EB, et al. ^{18}F-FDG-avid sites mimicking active disease in pediatric Hodgkin's. *Pediatr Radiol* 2005;35:141–154.
144. Cohen MD. *Imaging of children with cancer*. St. Louis: Mosby Yearbook, 1992.
145. Nadel HR, Rossleigh MA. Tumor imaging. In: Treves ST, ed. *Pediatric nuclear medicine*, 2nd ed. New York: Springer-Verlag, 1995:496–527.
146. Rossleigh MA, Murray IPC, Mackey DWJ. Pediatric solid tumors: evaluation by gallium-67 SPECT studies. *J Nucl Med* 1990;31: 161–172.
147. Howman-Giles R, Stevens M, Bergin M. Role of gallium-67 in management of pediatric solid tumors. *Aust Paediatr J* 1982;18:120–125.
148. Yang SL, Alderson PO, Kaizer HA, et al. Serial Ga-67 citrate imaging in children with neoplastic disease: concise communication. *J Nucl Med* 1979;20:210–214.
149. Sty JR, Kun LE, Starshak RJ. Pediatric applications in nuclear oncology. *Semin Nucl Med* 1985;15:171–200.
150. Barrington SF, Carr R. Staging of Burkitt's lymphoma and response to treatment monitored by PET scanning. *Clin Oncol* 1995;7:334–335.
151. Bangerter M, Moog F, Buchmann I, et al. Whole-body 2-[^{18}F]-fluoro-2-deoxy-D-glucose positron emission tomography (FDG PET) for accurate staging of Hodgkin's disease. *Ann Oncol* 1998;9:1117–1122.
152. Jerusalem G, Warland V, Najjar F, et al. Whole-body ^{18}F-FDG PET for the evaluation of patients with Hodgkin's disease and non-Hodgkin's lymphoma. *Nucl Med Commun* 1999;20:13–20.
153. Leskinen-Kallio S, Ruotsalainen U, Nagren K, et al. Uptake of carbon-11-methionine and fluorodeoxyglucose in non-Hodgkin's lymphoma: a PET study. *J Nucl Med* 1991;32:1211–1218.
154. Moog F, Bangerter M, Kotzerke J, et al. ^{18}-F-fluorodeoxyglucose positron emission tomography as a new approach to detect lymphomatous bone marrow. *J Clin Oncol* 1998;16:603–609.
155. Moog F, Bangerter M, Diederichs CG, et al. Extranodal malignant lymphoma: detection with FDG PET versus CT. *Radiology* 1998;206: 475–481.
156. Moog F, Bangerter M, Diederichs CG, et al. Lymphoma: role of whole-body 2-deoxy-2-[F-18]fluoro-D-glucose (FDG) PET in nodal staging. *Radiology* 1997;203:795–800.
157. Okada J, Yoshikawa K, Imazeki K, et al. The use of FDG-PET in the detection and management of malignant lymphoma: correlation of uptake with prognosis. *J Nucl Med* 1991;32:686–691.
158. Okada J, Yoshikawa K, Itami M, et al. Positron emission tomography using fluorine-18-fluorodeoxyglucose in malignant lymphoma: a comparison with proliferative activity. *J Nucl Med* 1992;33:325–329.
159. Rodriguez M, Rehn S, Ahlstrom H, et al. Predicting malignancy grade with PET in non-Hodgkin's lymphoma. *J Nucl Med* 1995;36:1790–1796.
160. Paul R. Comparison of fluorine-18-2-fluorodeoxyglucose and gallium-67 citrate imaging for detection of lymphoma. *J Nucl Med* 1987;28:288–292.
161. Newman JS, Francis IR, Kaminski MS, et al. Imaging of lymphoma with PET with 2-[F-18]-fluoro-2-deoxy-D-glucose: correlation with CT. *Radiology* 1994;190:111–116.
162. de Wit M, Bumann D, Beyer W, et al. Whole-body positron emission tomography (PET) for diagnosis of residual mass in patients with lymphoma. *Ann Oncol* 1997;8[Suppl 1]:57–60.
163. Cremerius U, Fabry U, Neuerburg J, et al. Positron emission tomography with ^{18}F-FDG to detect residual disease after therapy for malignant lymphoma. *Nucl Med Commun* 1998;19:1055–1063.
164. Hoh CK, Glaspy J, Rosen P, et al. Whole-body FDG PET imaging for staging of Hodgkin's disease and lymphoma. *J Nucl Med* 1997;38: 343–348.
165. Romer W, Hanauske AR, Ziegler S, et al. Positron emission tomography in non-Hodgkin's lymphoma: assessment of chemotherapy with fluorodeoxyglucose. *Blood* 1998;91:4464–4471.
166. Stumpe KD, Urbinelli M, Steinert HC, et al. Whole-body positron emission tomography using fluorodeoxyglucose for staging of lymphoma: effectiveness and comparison with computed tomography. *Eur J Nucl Med* 1998;25:721–728.
167. Lapela M, Leskinen S, Minn HR, et al. Increased glucose metabolism in untreated non-Hodgkin's lymphoma: a study with positron emission tomography and fluorine-18-fluorodeoxyglucose. *Blood* 1995;86: 3522–3527.
168. Carr R, Barrington SF, Madam B, et al. Detection of lymphoma in bone marrow by whole-body positron emission tomography. *Blood* 1998;91:3340–3346.
169. Hudson MM, Krasin MJ, Kaste SC. PET imaging in pediatric Hodgkin's lymphoma. *Pediatr Radiol* 2004;34:190–198.
170. Montravers F, McNamara D, Landman-Parker J, et al. [(^{18})F]FDG in childhood lymphoma: clinical utility and impact on management. *Eur J Nucl Med Mol Imaging* 2002;29:1155–1165.
171. Depas G, De Barsy C, Jerusalem G, et al. ^{18}F-FDG PET in children with lymphomas. *Eur J Nucl Med Mol Imaging* 2005;32:31–38.
172. Amthauer H, Furth C, Denecke T, et al. FDG-PET in 10 children with non-Hodgkin's lymphoma: initial experience in staging and follow-up. *Klin Pediatr* 2005;217:327–333.
173. Hernandez-Pampaloni M, Takalkar A, Yu JQ, et al. F-18 FDG-PET imaging and correlation with CT in staging and follow-up of pediatric lymphomas. *Pediatr Radiol* 2006;36:524–531.
174. Kabickova E, Sumerauer D, Cumlivska E, et al. Comparison of (^{18})F-FDG-PET and standard procedures for the pretreatment staging of children and adolescents with Hodgkin's disease. *Eur J Nucl Med Mol Imaging* 2006;33:1025–1031.
175. Keresztes K, Lengyel Z, Devenyi K, et al. Mediastinal bulky tumor in Hodgkin's disease and prognostic value of positron emission tomography in the evaluation of post treatment residual masses. *Acta Haematol* 2004;112:194–199.
176. Lavely WC, Delbeke D, Greer JP, et al. FDG PET in the follow-up of management of patients with newly diagnosed Hodgkin and non-Hodgkin lymphoma after first-line chemotherapy. *Int J Radiat Oncol Biol Phys* 2003;57:307–315.
177. Filmont JE, Yap CS, Ko F, et al. Conventional imaging and 2-deoxy-2-[^{18}F]fluoro-D-glucose positron emission tomography for predicting

the clinical outcome of patients with previously treated Hodgkin's disease. *Mol Imaging Biol* 2004;6:47–54.

178. Levine JM, Weiner M, Kelly KM. Routine use of PET scans after completion of therapy in pediatric Hodgkin disease results in a high false positive rate. *J Pediatr Hematol Oncol* 2006;28:711–714.
179. Meany HJ, Gidvani VK, Minniti CP. Utility of PET scans to predict disease relapse in pediatric patients with Hodgkin lymphoma. *Pediatr Blood Cancer* 2007;48:399–402.
180. Tatsumi M, Cohade C, Nakamoto Y, et al. Direct comparison of FDG PET and CT findings in patients with lymphoma: initial experience. *Radiology* 2005;237:1038–1045.
181. Furth C, Denecke T, Steffen I, et al. Correlative imaging strategies implementing CT, MR, and PET for staging of childhood Hodgkin disease. *J Pediatr Hematol Oncol* 2006;28:501–512.
182. Miller E, Metser U, Avrahami G, et al. Role of ^{18}F-FDG PET/CT in staging and follow-up of lymphoma in pediatric and young adult patients. *J Comput Assist Tomogr* 2006;30:689–694.
183. Rhodes MM, Delbeke D, Whitlock JA, et al. Utility of FDG PET-CT in follow-up of children treated for Hodgkin and non-Hodgkin lymphoma. *J Pediatr Hematol Oncol* 2006;28:300–306.
184. Swift P. Novel techniques in the delivery of radiation in pediatric oncology. *Pediatr Clin North Am* 2002;49:1107–1129.
185. Korholz D, Kluge R, Wickmann L, et al. Importance of F18-fluorodeoxy-D-2-glucose positron emission tomography (FDG-PET) for staging and therapy control of Hodgkin's lymphoma in childhood and adolescence—consequences for the GPOH-HD 2003 protocol. *Onkologie* 2003;26:489–493.
186. Krasin MJ, Hudson MM, Kaste SC. Positron emission tomography in pediatric radiation oncology: integration in the treatment-planning process. *Pediatr Radiol* 2004;34:214–221.
187. Bousvaros A, Kirks DR, Grossman H. Imaging of neuroblastoma: an overview. *Pediatr Radiol* 1986;16:89–106.
188. Kushner BH, Yeung HW, Larson SM, et al. Extending positron emission tomography scan utility to high-risk neuroblastoma: fluorine-18 fluorodeoxyglucose positron emission tomography as sole imaging modality in follow-up of patients. *J Clin Oncol* 2001;19:3397–3405.
189. Briganti V, Sestini R, Orlando C, et al. Imaging of somatostatin receptors by indium-111-pentetreotide correlates with quantitative determination of somatostatin receptor type 2 gene expression in neuroblastoma tumor. *Clin Cancer Res* 1997;3:2385–2391.
190. Shulkin BL, Shapiro B, Hutchinson RJ. ^{131}I-MIBG and bone scintigraphy for the detection of neuroblastoma. Presented at the Fifth Biennial Congress of the South African Society of Nuclear Medicine, Capetown, South Africa, September, 1992. *South African Med J* 1993;83:53.
191. Shulkin BL, Hutchinson RJ, Castle VP, et al. Neuroblastoma: positron emission tomography with 2-[fluorine-18]-fluoro-2-deoxy-D-glucose compared with metaiodobenzylguanidine scintigraphy. *Radiology* 1996;199:743–750.
192. Shulkin BL, Wieland DM, Baro ME, et al. PET hydroxyephedrine imaging of neuroblastoma. *J Nucl Med* 1996;37:16–21.
193. Shulkin BL, Wieland DM, Castle VP, et al. Carbon-11 epinephrine PET imaging of neuroblastoma. *J Nucl Med* 1999;40:129P(abst).
194. Franzius C, Hermann K, Weckesser M, et al. Whole-body PET-CT with ^{11}C-meta-hydroxyephedrine in tumors of the sympathetic system: feasibility study and comparison with ^{123}I-MIBG SPECT-CT. *J Nucl Med* 2006;47:1635–1642.
195. Brink I, Schaefer O, Walz, et al. Fluorine-18 DOPA PET imaging of paraganglioma syndrome. *Clin Nucl Med* 2006;31:39–41.
196. Vaidyanathan G, Affleck DJ, Zalutsky MR. Validation of 4-[fluorine-18]fluoro-3-iodobenzylguanidine as a positron-emitting analog of MIBG. *J Nucl Med* 1995;36:644–650.
197. Ott RJ, Tait D, Flower MA, et al. Treatment planning for ^{131}I-mIBG radiotherapy of neural crest tumors using ^{124}I-mIBG positron emission tomography. *Br J Radiol* 1992;65:787–791.
198. Barnewolt CE, Paltiel HJ, Lebowitz RL, et al. Genitourinary system. In: Kirks DR, ed. *Practical pediatric imaging. Diagnostic radiology of infants and children*, 3rd ed. Philadelphia: Lippincott-Raven, 1997:1009–1170.
199. Shulkin BL, Chang E, Strouse PJ, et al. PET FDG studies of Wilms tumors. *J Pediatr Hematol Oncol* 1997;19:334–338.
200. McDonald DJ. Limb salvage surgery for sarcomas of the extremities. *AJR Am J Roentgenol* 1994;163:509–513.
201. Triche TJ. Pathology of pediatric malignancies. In: Pizzo PA, Poplack DG, eds. *Principles and practice of pediatric oncology*, 2nd ed. Philadelphia: Lippincott, 1993:115–152.
202. O'Connor MI, Pritchard DJ. Ewing's sarcoma. Prognostic factors, disease control, and the reemerging role of surgical treatment. *Clin Orthop* 1991;262:78–87.
203. Jaramillo D, Laor T, Gebhardt M. Pediatric musculoskeletal neoplasms. Evaluation with MR imaging. *MRI Clin North Am* 1996;4:1–22.
204. Frouge C, Vanel D, Coffre C, et al. The role of magnetic resonance imaging in the evaluation of Ewing sarcoma—a report of 27 cases. *Skeletal Radiol* 1988;17:387–392.
205. MacVicar AD, Olliff JFC, Pringle J, et al. Ewing sarcoma: MR imaging of chemotherapy-induced changes with histologic correlation. *Radiology* 1992;184:859–864.
206. Lemmi MA, Fletcher BD, Marina NMm et al. Use of MR imaging to assess results of chemotherapy for Ewing sarcoma. *AJR Am J Roentgenol* 1990;155:343–346.
207. Erlemann R, Sciuk J, Bosse A, et al. Response of osteosarcoma and Ewing sarcoma to preoperative chemotherapy: assessment with dynamic and static MR imaging and skeletal scintigraphy. *Radiology* 1990;175:791–796.
208. Holscher HC, Bloem JL, Vanel D, et al. Osteosarcoma: chemotherapy-induced changes at MR imaging. *Radiology* 1992;182:839–844.
209. Lawrence JA, Babyn PS, Chan HS, et al. Extremity osteosarcoma in childhood: prognostic value of radiologic imaging. *Radiology* 1993;189:43–47.
210. Connolly LP, Laor T, Jaramillo D, et al. Prediction of chemotherapeutic response of osteosarcoma with quantitative thallium-201 scintigraphy and magnetic resonance imaging. *Radiology* 1996;201:349(abst).
211. Lin J, Leung WT. Quantitative evaluation of thallium-201 uptake in predicting chemotherapeutic response of osteosarcoma. *Eur J Nucl Med* 1995;22:553–555.
212. Menendez LR, Fideler BM, Mirra J. Thallium-201 scanning for the evaluation of osteosarcoma and soft tissue sarcoma. *J Bone Joint Surg* 1993;75:526–531.
213. Ramanna L, Waxman A, Binney G, et al. Thallium-201 scintigraphy in bone sarcoma: comparison with gallium-67 and technetium-99m MDP in the evaluation of chemotherapeutic response. *J Nucl Med* 1990;31:567–572.
214. Rosen G, Loren GJ, Brien EW, et al. Serial thallium-201 scintigraphy in osteosarcoma. Correlation with tumor necrosis after preoperative chemotherapy. *Clin Orthop* 1993;293:302–306.
215. Ohtomo K, Terui S, Yokoyama R, et al. Thallium-201 scintigraphy to assess effect of chemotherapy to osteosarcoma. *J Nucl Med* 1996;37:1444–1448.
216. Bar-Sever Z, Connolly LP, Treves ST, et al. Technetium-99m MIBI in the evaluation of children with Ewing's sarcoma. *J Nucl Med* 1997;38:13P(abst).
217. Caner B, Kitapel M, Unlu M, et al. Technetium-99m-MIBI uptake in benign and malignant bone lesions: a comparative study with technetium-99m-MDP. *J Nucl Med* 1992;33:319–324.
218. Lenzo NP, Shulkin B, Castle VP, et al. FDG PET in childhood soft tissue sarcoma. *J Nucl Med* 2000;41[5 Suppl]:96P(abst).
219. Abdel-Dayem HM. The role of nuclear medicine in primary bone and soft tissue tumors. *Semin Nucl Med* 1997;27:355–363.
220. Shulkin BL, Mitchell DS, Ungar DR, et al. Neoplasms in a pediatric population: 2-[F-18]-fluoro-2-deoxy-D-glucose PET studies. *Radiology* 1995;194:495–500.

221. Jadvar H, Connolly LP, Shulkin BL, et al. Positron-emission tomography in pediatrics. *Nucl Med Annu* 2000:53–83.
222. Franzius C, Sciuk J, Brinkschmidt C, et al. Evaluation of chemotherapy response in primary bone tumors with F-18 FDG positron emission tomography compared with histologically assessed tumor necrosis. *Clin Nucl Med* 2000;25:874–881.
223. Hawkins DS, Rajendran JG, Conrad EU 3rd, et al. Evaluation of chemotherapy response in pediatric bone sarcomas by [F-18]-fluorodeoxy-D-glucose positron emission tomography. *Cancer* 2002; 94:3277–3284.
224. Jadvar H, Alavi A, Mavi A, et al. PET in pediatric diseases. *Radiol Clin North Am* 2005;43:135–152.
225. Hawkins DS, Schuetze SM, Butrynski JE, et al. [^{18}F]fluorodeoxyglucose positron emission tomography predicts outcome for Ewing sarcoma family of tumors. *J Clin Oncol* 2005;23:8828–8834.
226. Gyorke T, Zajic T, Lange A, et al. Impact of FDG PET for staging of Ewing sarcomas and primitive neuroectodermal tumors. *Nucl Med Commun* 2006;27:17–24.
227. Huang TL, Liu RS, Chen TH, et al. Comparison between F-18-FDG positron emission tomography and histology for the assessment of tumor necrosis rates in primary osteosarcoma. *J Chin Med Assoc* 2006;69:372–376.
228. Franzius C, Sciuk J, Daldrup-Link HE, et al. FDG-PET for detection of osseous metastases from malignant primary bone tumors: comparison with bone scintigraphy. *Eur J Nucl Med* 2000;27:1305–1311.
229. Kneisl JS, Patt JC, Johnson JC, et al. Is PET useful in detecting occult nonpulmonary metastases in pediatric bone sarcomas? *Clin Orthop Relat Res* 2006;450:101–104.
230. Ben Arush MW, Bar Shalom R, Potovsky S, et al. Assessing the use of FDG-PET in the detection of regional and metastatic nodes in alveolar rhabdomyosarcoma of extremities. *J Pediatr Hematol Oncol* 2006;28:440–445.
231. Peng F, Rabkin G, Muzik O. Use of 2-deoxy-[F-18]-fluoro-D-glucose positron emission tomography to monitor therapeutic response by rhabdomyosarcoma in children: report of a retrospective case. *Clin Nucl Med* 2006;31:394–397.
232. Schuetze SM, Rubin BP, Vernon C, et al. Use of positron emission tomography in localized extremity soft tissue sarcoma treated with neoadjuvant chemotherapy. *Cancer* 2005;103:339–348.
233. Sturm E, Rings EH, Scholvinck EH, et al. Fluorodeoxyglucose positron emission tomography contributes to management of pediatric liver transplantation candidates with fever of unknown origin. *Liver Transpl* 2006;12:1698–1704.
234. Loffler M, Weckesser M, Franzius C, et al. High diagnostic value of ^{18}F-FDG-PET in pediatric patients with chronic inflammatory patients with chronic inflammatory bowel disease. *Ann N Y Acad Sci* 2006;1072:379–385.
235. Lemberg DA, Issenman RM, Cawdron R, et al. Positron emission tomography in the investigation of pediatric inflammatory bowel disease. *Inflamm Bowel Dis* 2005;11:733–738.

CHAPTER

8.24 Hypoxia Imaging

MORAND PIERT

DEFINITION OF HYPOXIA

A continued source of molecular oxygen is essential for cellular respiration and energy supply. Hypoxia is defined as a metabolic state in which the concentration of oxygen is below physiological levels (normoxia) but above the complete lack of oxygen (anoxia). Even under physiologic conditions, tissue oxygenation levels may vary considerably between different tissues and may display a marked heterogeneity even in tissues that are considered well perfused (1). Hypoxia should be differentiated from ischemia, the latter describing a lack of blood flow to a particular organ or tissue. Although ischemia can be caused by prolonged severe tissue hypoxia and by anoxia, these terms are clearly not interchangeable.

CELLULAR REGULATION OF OXYGEN HOMEOSTASIS

The transcription factor hypoxia-inducible factor 1 (HIF-1) is a key regulator of hypoxia-induced gene expressions. Since the discovery of the HIF-1 system by Semenza and Wang (2), HIF-1 has been of particular interest for cancer biologists. HIF-1 is a heterodimeric protein that is composed of two polypeptides, the HIF-1α and HIF-1β subunits (3,4). With the completion of the human genome project, two additional HIF α members, the closely related HIF-2α (5,6) and more distantly related HIF-3α (7), were identified, although their function is less well defined.

The phosphatidylinositol 3-kinase (PI3K) and ERK mitogen-activated protein kinase (MAPK) pathways regulate the HIF-1α protein synthesis (8). HIF-1 activity is regulated at the posttranscriptional level by protein degradation of HIF α subunits (9). Under normoxic cellular conditions, HIF-1α is targeted by the oxygen-dependent prolyl hydroxylase to undergo ubiquitylation by E3 ubiquitin-protein ligases. These ligases contain the von Hippel-Lindau (VHL) protein.

Ubiquitylated HIF-1α is rapidly degraded by the proteasome (8). By contrast, under hypoxic cellular conditions, the prolyl hydroxylation is inactive and the HIF α members are not complexed with VHL and remain available in the cell. As a result, HIF-1β binds to the HIF-1α subunit, leading to the transcriptional activation of multiple genes responsible for cellular proliferation and cell survival, apoptosis, oxygen and nutrient delivery (angiogenesis), and anaerobic energy metabolism (glucose metabolism), all of which are involved in the basic biology of cancer (10,11). Chronic tumor cell hypoxia increases genomic instability and heterogeneity and selects for tumor cells that survive severe microenvironmental stresses (12).

The regulation of HIF-1 signaling is a rather complex process. Suppression of HIF-1α degradation has not only been observed as a result of intracellular oxygen depletion but also due to environmental stresses like extracellular acidosis (13). Most importantly, growth factors like insulin-like growth factor receptor, epidermal growth factor receptor, human epidermal growth factor receptor 2, and others can also stimulate HIF-1 signaling (14), indicating that the regulation of the HIF-1 oxygen sensing system is more complex than previously appreciated.

HYPOXIA IN CARDIOVASCULAR DISEASE

The oxidative phosphorylation of adenosine diphosphate to adenosine triphosphate is the main source of energy needed to provide sustained contractility of the heart muscle. Because of that, ischemic conditions (thus inadequate oxygen supply) are likely to cause hypoxia of variable degrees. However, under certain pathophysiological conditions such as infections, hypoxia may occur in the heart muscle even if perfusion is well maintained. One important consequence of coronary artery disease, left ventricular dysfunction, can result from acute myocardial ischemia or myocardial infarction. In addition, transient postischemic "stunned" myocardium and chronic but potentially reversible ischemic "hibernating" myocardium are also associated with left ventricular dysfunctions. It has been shown that hibernating myocardium is characterized by an up-regulation of genes and corresponding proteins involved in anti-apoptosis, cell growth, angiogenesis, and cytoprotection, including the activation of the HIF-1 cascade (15). Since hibernating myocardium can be significantly improved by successful revascularization, the identification of this condition is of great clinical importance.

Currently, accessible noninvasive imaging approaches for the detection of myocardial ischemia are based on the recognition of flow impairment or the identification of a mismatch between flow and regional myocardial metabolism. All existing approaches are indirect methods assessing regional myocardial ischemia and are affected by sympathetic activation and substrate availability. The direct visualization of myocardial tissue hypoxia has great potential. It has been speculated that the assessment of tissue oxygenation using hypoxia tracers may potentially be the best indicator of the balance between blood flow and oxygen consumption (16). Consequently, hypoxia tracers have been suggested to identify dysfunctional chronically ischemic but viable hibernating myocardium.

HYPOXIA IN ONCOLOGY

Tumor hypoxia is a common, if not characteristic, feature of malignant tumors. It is related but not exclusively determined by a less ordered, often chaotic, and leaky vasculature. The structure and function of the tumor microcirculation is often disturbed and results in a deterioration of the diffusion geometry. Tumor-associated anemia further aggravates tumor tissue hypoxia. The existence of tumor hypoxia had long been suspected by histological observation of necrosis and disordered vasculature and was confirmed in animals and humans by microelectrode and bioreductive drug measurements. Tumor hypoxia has the well-known effect of decreasing the sensitivity of hypoxic cells to ionizing radiation. It has also been identified as a major adverse prognostic factor for tumor progression and for resistance to anticancer treatment (17–19).

Clinically relevant tumor tissue hypoxia is generally considered to be present at an oxygen partial pressure in tissue (tpO_2) of less than 8 to 10 mm Hg (12,20), while severely hypoxic tissue usually displays tpO_2 values below 3 to 5 mm Hg. Tumor tissue hypoxia plays an important role in radiation treatment because the extent of DNA damage following exposure to indirectly ionizing radiation is largely dependent on oxygen. Severely hypoxic cells require two to three times higher radiation dose compared to well-oxygenated cells to produce an equivalent amount of cell kill following indirectly ionizing radiation or low linear energy transfer radiation (17). The difference in radiosensitivity between hypoxic and normoxic cells has been called oxygen enhancement ratio. Oxygen is believed to prolong the lifetime of the short-lived free radicals produced by the interaction of x-rays and cellular water. In the absence of intracellular oxygen, free radicals formed by ionizing radiation are able to recombine without causing the expected cellular damage (21). Besides causing radioresistance, tumor hypoxia interferes with many chemotherapy regimes that require sufficient amounts of intracellular oxygen for the desired cytotoxic activities (22). The inefficient microvasculature of hypoxic tumors hampers sufficient drug delivery (17). Sustained hypoxia may also reduce tumor sensitivity by indirect mechanisms that include proteomic and genomic changes, the secretion of hypoxic stress proteins, and the loss of apoptotic potential (23–25). Fig. 8.24.1 summarizes the current knowledge of mechanisms for hypoxia-related treatment resistance and their deleterious effects on tumor aggressiveness and metastatic potential.

CHALLENGES OF HYPOXIA MEASUREMENTS

Many approaches to measure tissue hypoxia have been proposed. Most of the clinical experience has been obtained with polarographic oxygen-electrode systems. Although the measurements are quantitative, the results were generally reported as the fractional percentage of measurements below a certain cutoff tpO_2 value. Due to the heterogeneous distribution of tpO_2 values, results were generally reported as the "hypoxic tumor fraction," which was found to be a more robust parameter derived from such polarographic methods when compared to the average tpO_2 in tissue.

In the past decade, a large body of evidence was derived from oxygen electrode measurements. Studies have subsequently shown that pretreatment oxygenation can predict outcome of treatment in several solid tumors including head and neck cancer (26,27), lung

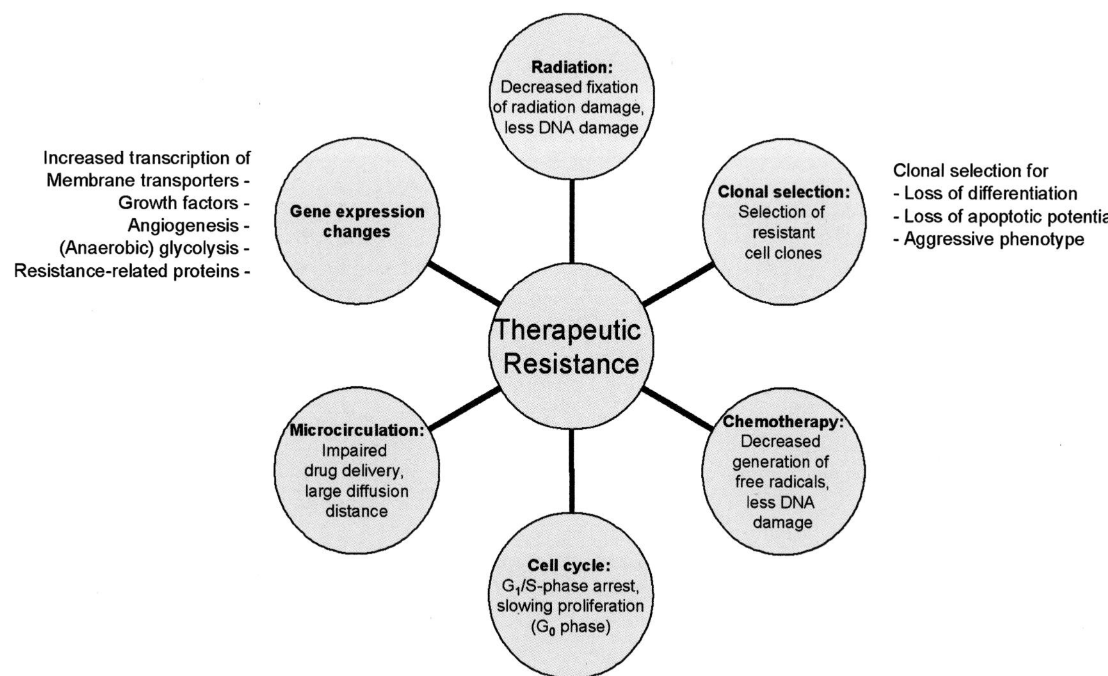

FIGURE 8.24.1. Selected mechanisms for hypoxia-related treatment resistance.

cancer, cervical cancer (18), and sarcomas (28). However, oxygen electrode measurements are rarely used routinely in human malignancies, mainly because they are invasive, limited to readily accessible tumor sites, and technically demanding (29). The exact localization of the probe's tip within the tumor volume is difficult, and oxygen electrode systems are unable to determine the tumor's oxygenation distribution on a truly regional basis, which is a necessary precondition for individually adapted therapeutic approaches. A noninvasive identification and quantification of regional tumor tissue hypoxia is, therefore, nearly a necessity for effective treatment selection, individual treatment planning, and treatment monitoring in oncology.

PET RADIOPHARMACEUTICALS FOR HYPOXIA IMAGING AND PRECLINICAL TESTING

Nitroimidazole Compounds

The discovery of azomycin (2-nitroimidazole) (30) and its synthesis in 1965 (31) started decades of research in hypoxic cell radiosensitization and was the basis for the development of a whole group of nitroimidazole tracers for single-photon emission computed tomography and positron emission tomography (PET) imaging. Chapman (32) suggested that nitroimidazoles should be useful for imaging of oxygen-deprived cells due to their radiosensitization capabilities and potential covalent binding to hypoxic cells. Intracellular accumulation is related to radical formation following reduction by ubiquitous nitroreductases. Under hypoxic conditions, reduction of these molecules involves a series of one electron steps (33). Products of this reduction are believed to covalently bind to intracellular macromolecules such as DNA, RNA, and proteins, which prevents back-diffusion across the cell membrane, causing the hypoxia-dependent accumulation of compound metabolites. Conversely under well-oxygenated conditions, the nitro radical anion of these compounds are reoxidized, facilitating back-diffusion and contributing to clearance of radioactivity from tissue (34). However, even under hypoxic conditions, some diffusible compounds are formed indicating complex biokinetics.

Fluorine-18 labeled fluoromisonidazole (1-(2-nitroimidazolyl)-2-hydroxy-3-fluoropropane) ([^{18}F]-FMISO) was the first nitroimidazole PET tracer described and synthesized by Jerabek et al. (35) and Grierson et al. (36). The evaluation of this tracer was first performed using [^{3}H]-FMISO, demonstrating that the FMISO uptake was dependent on the cellular oxygenation in rat myocytes (37) and tumor cell spheroids (38). Studies performed in several rodent tumor models using [^{3}H]-FMISO revealed tumor-to-blood ratios suitable for *in vivo* imaging (39,40). The hypoxia-specific uptake mechanism of [^{18}F]-FMISO was validated in an occlusion model and demonstrated tracer accumulation at radiobiologically relevant tpO_2 levels (41,42). The radiopharmaceutical [^{18}F]-FMISO is stable and robust and is currently the single most commonly used hypoxia PET tracer (43). However, its biokinetics suffer from relatively high lipophilicity (octanol/water partition coefficient of log $P = 2.6$), which results in protracted *in vivo* accumulation in hypoxic tissues and slow plasma clearance, resulting in relatively low target-to-background ratios. Imaging with nitroimidazole compounds is, therefore, generally performed at later time points (2 to 4 hours postinjection) when sufficient amounts of radioactivity have been cleared from plasma and normoxic tissues.

Several other nitroimidazole compounds have subsequently been labeled with positron emitters. [^{18}F]-fluoroetanidazole ([^{18}F]-FETA) and [^{18}F]-fluoroerythronitroimidazole ([^{18}F]-FETNIM) were evaluated as hypoxia markers in animal models (44,45) and the latter also in humans (46,47). Tumor-to-background ratios did not indicate significant advantages over [^{18}F]-FMISO for either tracer (45,48). Newer nitroimidazole tracers, 2-(2-nitroimidazol-1-yl)-N-(3,3,3-[^{18}F]-trifluoropropyl)acetamide ([^{18}F]-EF3), and [^{18}F]-EF5 ([^{18}F]-2-(2-nitro-1[H]-imidazol-1-yl)-N-(2,2,3,3,3-pentafluoropropyl)-acetamide) have undergone successful preclinical testing (49,50), but a direct comparison with [^{18}F]-FMISO or human data are yet not available. The iodine-124 labeled iodoazomycin galactoside ([^{124}I]-IAZG) shows promise as a tumor hypoxia marker in preclinical testing (51). Because of its long physical half-life, the compound allows for imaging at very late time points (24 to 48 hours). In fact, tumor-to-background ratios were generally higher (factor 1.5 to 2) as compared to [^{18}F]-FMISO at 3 hours postinjection. Very late time point imaging, however, may be compromised by deiodination as well as potential loss of initially bound radioactivity from hypoxic tissues.

Recently, [^{18}F]-fluoro-azomycin arabinoside ([^{18}F]-FAZA) had been evaluated in several rodent tumor models. Like the iodinated parent compound, iodoazomycin arabinoside (IAZA) (52), it displayed rapid clearance from the blood and nontarget tissues, yielding more favorable tumor-to-background ratios 3 hours postinjection as compared to [^{18}F]-FMISO (factor 1.9 to 2.2) (53). [^{18}F]-FAZA displays a lower octanol/water partition coefficient (log $P = 1.1$), indicating the potential for both rapid diffusion through tissue and faster renal excretion (54). Moreover, the arabinosyl-N1-α-glycosidic bond displays enhanced *in vivo* stability against enzymatic cleavage. The first clinical results in 11 head and neck cancer patients have been encouraging (55).

Copper Complexes

The development of newer radiopharmaceuticals involving copper isotopes has been pursued due to the relatively simple chemistry as well as an array of radiopharmaceuticals that are suitable for both imaging and radiotherapy of cancer. Several copper isotopes ([^{60}Cu], [^{61}Cu], [^{62}Cu], and [^{64}Cu]) with different physical half-lives (between 0.4 and 12.7 hours) are positron emitters and are applicable for PET imaging.

Cu-diacetyl-bis(N^4-methylthiosemicarbazone) (Cu-ATSM) is a Cu-labeled dithiosemicarbazone that has been shown to be selectively retained in hypoxic tissues. Cu-ATSM can be rapidly and quantitatively produced in high yields. The uptake mechanism is less well understood than that of the nitroimidazoles. Cu-ATSM retention is dependent on the inherent redox properties of the complex and uses reduction as the major trapping mechanism. It was proposed that the selectivity of Cu-ATSM for hypoxic tissue is due in part to its redox potential of -293 mV, which enables more Cu-ATSM to be reduced in hypoxic cells compared to normoxic cells (56). A similar compound Cu-pyruvaldehyde-bis(N^4-methylthiosemicarbazone) (Cu-PTSM) has been developed as a blood flow tracer for PET imaging in animals and humans (57).

Cu-ATSM was shown to have an oxygenation-dependent retention mechanism in an isolated perfused rat heart model that varied the oxygen concentration in the perfusate (58). In subsequent experiments in canine models, the Cu-ATSM retention was found to be independent of blood flow, allowing the delineation of hypoxia in clinically relevant acute coronary syndromes and for demand-induced ischemia (59). In solid tumor models, the Cu-ATSM uptake was found to correlate with the tpO_2, which further strengthened the role of Cu-ATSM as an *in vivo* hypoxia marker (60). These studies involving oxygen electrode measurements, PET imaging, and autoradiography were the basis for subsequent testing of this compound in human cancers.

In comparison to [^{18}F]-FMISO, Cu-ATSM exhibits higher uptake ratios between hypoxic and normoxic tissues (61). A particular advantage is the rapid kinetics of Cu-ATSM, which allows the identification of hypoxic tissue within 10 to 15 minutes postinjection using quantitative and semiquantitative approaches (62). This hypoxia marker is an attractive alternative to nitroimidazole-based compounds. More recent studies of the Cu-ATSM kinetics in experimental tumors have uncovered more differentiated uptake kinetics. O'Donoghue et al. (63) investigated Cu-ATSM in comparison with [^{18}F]-FMISO, using oxygen electrode measurements and immunofluorescence microscopy with pimonidazole. The 24-hour postinjection Cu-ATSM uptake correlated well with the [^{18}F]-FMISO uptake as assessed by autoradiography as well as with oxygen electrode measurements and pimonidazole stains. However, early Cu-ATSM imaging did not correlate with direct tissue assays nor with [^{18}F]-FMISO imaging, indicating more complex kinetics than previously thought. Yuan et al. (64) found intertumoral differences in the hypoxia selectivity of Cu-ATSM that challenged the use of Cu-ATSM as a universal PET hypoxia marker.

Newer semicarbazone complexes are currently being investigated. McQuade et al. (65) identified Cu-64-diacetyl.bis(N4-ethylthiosemicarbazone) (Cu-ATSE) as being most promising with improved hypoxia selectivity and most suitable *in vivo* properties for hypoxia imaging compared to Cu-ATSM. Cu-ATSM has also been used to study ischemic heart disease in experimental settings. The principal advantage of hypoxia imaging in ischemic heart disease compared to the current approach of separate stress and rest imaging would be the potential necessity of only one imaging study. Fujibayashi et al. (58) used Cu-ATSM to visualize hypoxic rat heart tissue in a model of an acute occluded left anterior descending coronary artery. Their results indicated that Cu-ATSM would be useful for the detection of hypoxia within minutes after tracer injection. Using canine models of hypoxic myocardium, Lewis et al. (59) reported on Cu-ATSM PET for the delineation of ischemic and hypoxic myocardium. Using protocols of clinically relevant acute coronary syndromes and demand-induced ischemia, they demonstrated that Cu-ATSM was able to delineate hypoxic myocardium.

Although the direct visualization of hypoxic myocardium has great potential, it likely faces limitations in the clinical environment where the immediate availability of imaging is a requirement. Several pathophysiological circumstances such as myocardial infarction, reperfusion following successful therapeutic intervention, hibernation, and stunning may complicate the interpretation of hypoxia imaging. Further clinical studies are required to fully assess the potential of this promising imaging approach.

APPLICATIONS OF HYPOXIA IMAGING IN ONCOLOGY

Since tumor tissue hypoxia is associated with poor response to treatment, the identification of tumor hypoxia holds great potential for a pretreatment prediction of the therapeutic outcome. Recent studies have demonstrated this potential by identifying hypoxia as an adverse prognostic factor for radiation treatment in several types of cancer.

Dehdashti et al. (62) investigated a small group of patients with cervical cancers and found that the tumor uptake of Cu-ATSM was inversely related to progression-free survival and overall survival. An arbitrarily selected tumor-to-muscle ratio discriminated tumors likely to develop recurrence. In a second study involving 14 patients with non–small cell lung cancer, low pretreatment tumor uptake of Cu-ATSM was predictive for response to therapy, while FDG PET imaging results were not correlated with outcome measures (66).

Rajendran et al. (67) investigated the changes in [^{18}F]-FMISO and fluorine-18-fluoro-2-deoxy-D-glucose ([^{18}F]-FDG) uptake over the time course of neoadjuvant chemotherapy in a small group of patients with soft tissue sarcomas. Most tumors showed evidence of reduced uptake of both FMISO and FDG following chemotherapy. However, there was a discrepancy between intratumoral [^{18}F]-FDG and [^{18}F]-FMISO uptake, indicating that regional hypoxia and glucose metabolism do not necessarily correlate. Similarly, they did not find any relationship between the hypoxic volume and vascular endothelial growth factor expression as an indicator for tumor angiogenesis.

In a study involving 40 patients with advanced head and neck ($n = 26$) or non–small cell lung cancer ($n = 14$), Eschmann et al. (68) investigated the predictive value of [^{18}F]-FMISO prior to radiotherapy with curative intent. All patients with a FMISO tumor-to-muscle ratio greater than 2.0 in non–small cell lung cancer and greater than 1.6 in head and neck cancer presented with tumor recurrence, further supporting the negative predictive value of significant hypoxia prior to radiation treatment. Fig. 8.24.2 shows the [^{18}F]-FDG and [^{18}F]-FMISO uptake of a large squamous cell cancer of the right lung and displays partial discordance between glucose consumption and tissue hypoxia. Hypoxic but viable cells up-regulate glycolysis to maintain cellular energy production because adenosine triphosphate can be produced from glucose without requiring molecular oxygen. In acute hypoxia, glycolysis can be increased as much as twofold, which was found to be associated with increased expression or modified forms of glucose transporters (GLUT1 and GLUT3) and increased levels and mitochondrial redistribution of hexokinase (69). Thus, hypoxia significantly contributes to the [^{18}F]-FDG uptake, but [^{18}F]-FDG is not generally considered a surrogate marker of tissue hypoxia as its uptake is dependent on a wide variety of factors.

One potential way to overcome resistance to radiation treatment would be to maximize the radiation dose to the hypoxic subfraction of malignancies. Intensity-modulated radiation therapy (IMRT) allows selective targeting of tumor and improved sparing of normal surrounding tissues. In a feasibility study, Chao et al. (70) proposed hypoxia-guided IMRT using Cu-ATSM and investigated in a single case of head and neck cancer the ability to deliver a higher dose of radiation to the hypoxic tumor subvolume. The plan delivered 80 Gy to the ATSM-avid tumor subvolume, while the remainder of the tumor received 70 Gy in 35 fractions without increasing the recommended doses to nearby critical organs (salivary glands).

Fig. 8.24.3 displays the simulation of hypoxia-directed IMRT using [^{18}F]-FAZA in a patient with untreated floor of the mouth squamous cell cancer. Tumor tissue hypoxia was arbitrarily defined as a tumor-to-muscle ratio of 1.5 or above. Treatment simulation resulted in a moderate increase of the radiation dose to the "hypoxic" subvolume, while the remainder of the tumor volume received 95% of the typically prescribed dose. As expected, hypoxia

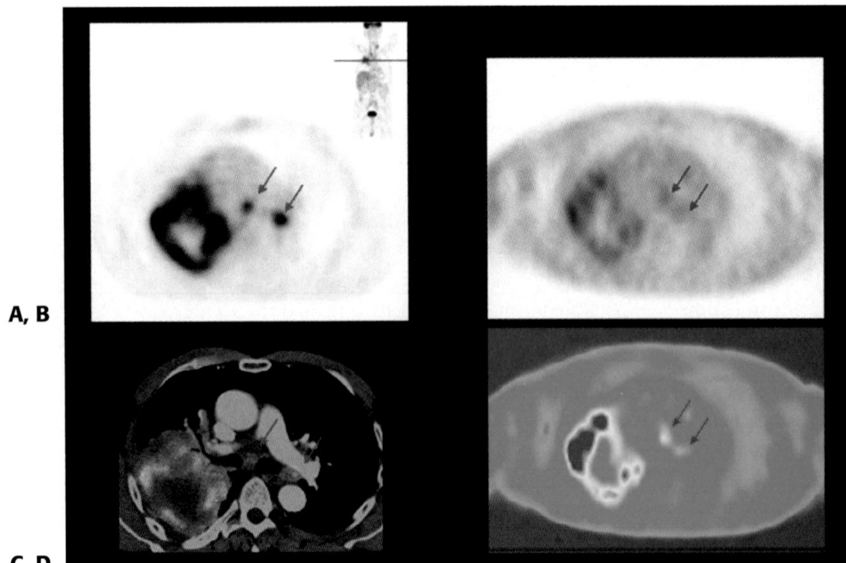

FIGURE 8.24.2. Transaxial images of a primary squamous cell cancer of the right upper lobe of the lung. **A:** 2-fluorine-18-fluoro-2-deoxy-D-glucose PET and **(B)** PET/CT fusion images obtained on a Siemens Biograph 16 (Malvern, Pennsylvania) high resolution scanner displaying a large tumor mass with central necrosis and inhomogeneous hypermetabolism in the periphery as well as two hypermetabolic mediastinal lymph node metastases (*red arrows*). **C,D:** Fluorine-18 labeled fluoromisonidazole (1-(2-nitroimidazolyl)-2-hydroxy-3-fluoropropane) ([^{18}F]-FMISO) PET images of the mass obtained from a GE Healthcare Advance (Uppsala, Sweden) PET scanner. The maximum [^{18}F]-FMISO uptake is at the lateral and anterior aspect of the tumor mass, while the remainder of the primary tumor, and especially the lymph node metastases, do not show significant [^{18}F]-FMISO uptake, indicating that glucose metabolism and hypoxia are not necessarily correlated. (Courtesy of M. Eschmann, PET Center Tuebingen, Germany.)

tracers such as Cu-ATSM and [^{18}F]-FAZA display heterogeneous uptake in tumor tissues. This raises concerns regarding the stability of the hypoxic signal as it may change during the time course of radiation treatment. If IMRT is used to enhance the radiation dose to the hypoxic subvolume, such behavior might necessitate in-treatment changes to the radiation plan. Although the general concept of hypoxia-guided IMRT may be appealing, it remains to be established whether a moderate increase in the delivered radiation dose to the hypoxic tumor volume improves local control or overall outcome after radiation treatment.

Although tumor hypoxia is a negative prognostic factor, it also constitutes a major difference between tumor and normal tissues. It, therefore, represents an opportunity for therapeutic exploitation. Bioreductive drugs or hypoxia-selective cytotoxins such as tirapazamine (TPZ) are inactive prodrugs that are favorably activated by reductive enzymes only in the hypoxic environment of tumors (71,72). Upon activation, they release toxic metabolites that can cause cell damage and death by various mechanisms. Beck et al. (73) investigated the effect of radiation, TPZ, and combined radiochemotherapy on murine breast cancers and compared the results with the pretreatment [^{18}F]-FAZA uptake. Radiochemotherapy involving TPZ displayed a synergistic effect in hypoxic, but not in well-oxygenated tumors.

Hicks at al. (74) investigated the effect of radiochemotherapy with TPZ in a small group of patients with advanced head and neck cancers that had been found to be positive on [^{18}F]-FMISO PET imaging. These investigators have also compared the [^{18}F]-FMISO and [^{18}F]-FAZA uptake in a series of patients with head and neck cancer (personal communication). Fig. 8.24.4 shows the superior tumor to background ratio that can be obtained with [^{18}F]-FAZA.

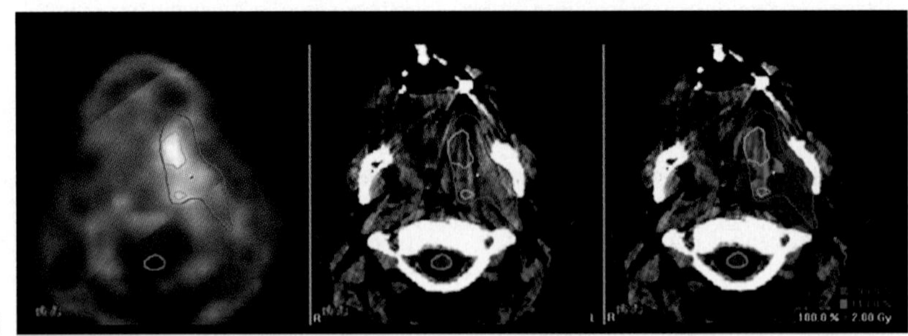

FIGURE 8.24.3. Transaxial realigned images of a left-sided floor of the mouth squamous cell cancer prior to primary radiochemotherapy. **A:** PET image obtained 2 hours after injection of 10.8 mCi of [^{18}F]fluoro-azomycin arabinoside displaying inhomogeneous tracer distribution. Individual regions of interest (ROI, *orange lines*) are defined in tumor areas exceeding an arbitrary threshold of 1.5 above muscle activity. **B:** The radiation planning CT loaded into the planning software with ROIs defining the gross tumor volume (GTV, *pink line*) as well as the "hypoxic" subvolume (*orange lines*) of the primary tumor. **C:** Treatment planning using IMRT (intensity-modulated radiation therapy) resulted in an increase of the radiation dose to the "hypoxic" subvolume to 113% of the typically prescribed single dose of 2 Gy. The remainder of the tumor volume received 95% of the prescribed dose, keeping the total radiation dose to the tumor tissue unchanged while reducing the radiation dose to the normal tissue. (Courtesy of A. L. Grosu [radiation oncology] and M. Souvatzoglou [nuclear medicine], Technical University of Munich, Germany.)

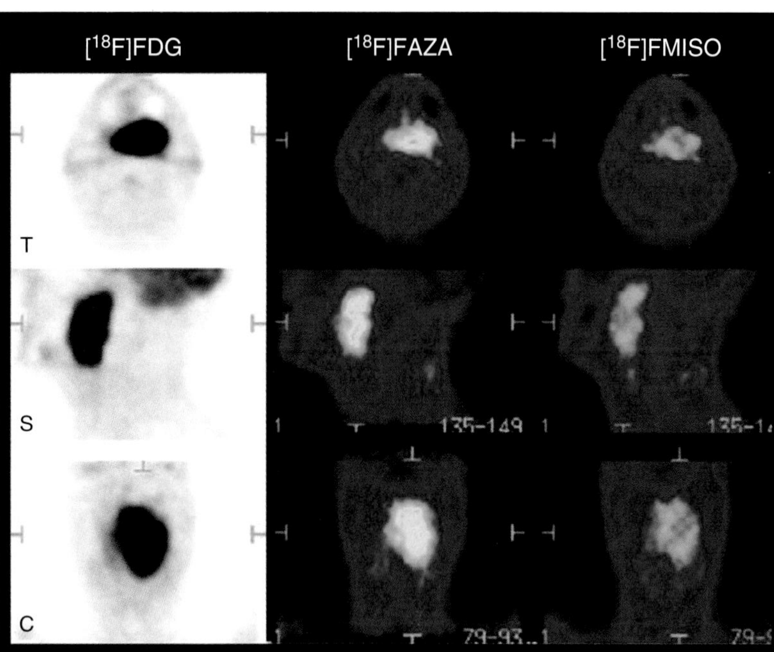

FIGURE 8.24.4. Transaxial (T), sagittal (S), and coronal (C) images of an oropharyngeal squamous cell cancer at primary diagnosis. 2-fluorine-18-fluoro-2-deoxy-D-glucose ([^{18}F]-FDG) PET shows an extensive hypermetabolic mass in comparison with hypoxia imaging performed with [^{18}F]-fluoro-azomycin arabinoside ([^{18}F]-FAZA) and [^{18}F]-fluoromisonidazole ([^{18}F]-FMISO). [^{18}F]-FAZA results in more favorable tumor-to-background image contrast compared to [^{18}F]-FMISO. [^{18}F]-FDG and [^{18}F]-FAZA PET imaging were performed within 24 hours, while the [^{18}F]-FMISO scan was performed 7 days after the [^{18}F]-FAZA scan. Hypoxia scans were started 2 hours postinjection of 5.8 mCi [^{18}F]-FAZA and 6.6 mCi [^{18}F]-FMISO using three-dimensional imaging. This image indicates the two hypoxia agents are not equivalent to each other. (Courtesy of R. Hicks, Melbourne, Australia.)

Evidence of the early resolution of [^{18}F]-FMISO abnormalities during treatment, associated with excellent locoregional control in this patient cohort, supports further investigation of hypoxia-targeting agents in advanced head and neck cancer. Based on these results, hypoxia imaging should be further investigated regarding the capability of guiding targeted chemotherapy using hypoxia-selective cytotoxins.

In summary, hypoxia imaging using PET can be recommended for further preclinical and clinical testing to identify tumor hypoxia in order to improve therapeutic strategies to either specifically target the hypoxic subvolume of tumors (via IMRT) or by taking advantage of the intratumoral lack of oxygen to apply hypoxia-directed chemotherapies. The optimal agent for hypoxia imaging remains under study, but this area of research is one with great potential for altering patient therapies.

REFERENCES

1. Vanderkooi JM, Erecinska M, Silver IA. Oxygen in mammalian tissue: methods of measurement and affinities of various reactions. *Am J Physiol* 1991;260:C1131–1150.
2. Semenza GL, Wang GL. A nuclear factor induced by hypoxia via *de novo* protein synthesis binds to the human erythropoietin gene enhancer at a site required for transcriptional activation. *Mol Cell Biol* 1992; 12:5447–5454.
3. Wang GL, Semenza GL. Characterization of hypoxia-inducible factor 1 and regulation of DNA binding activity by hypoxia. *J Biol Chem* 1993; 268:21513–21518.
4. Wang GL, Semenza GL. Purification and characterization of hypoxia-inducible factor 1. *J Biol Chem* 1995;270:1230–1237.
5. Tian H, McKnight SL, Russell DW. Endothelial PAS domain protein 1 (EPAS1), a transcription factor selectively expressed in endothelial cells. *Genes Dev* 1997;11:72–82.
6. Ema M, Taya S, Yokotani N, et al. A novel bHLH-PAS factor with close sequence similarity to hypoxia-inducible factor 1alpha regulates the VEGF expression and is potentially involved in lung and vascular development. *Proc Natl Acad Sci U S A* 1997;94:4273–4278.
7. Makino Y, Cao R, Svensson K, et al. Inhibitory PAS domain protein is a negative regulator of hypoxia-inducible gene expression. *Nature* 2001;414: 550–554.
8. Semenza GL. Targeting HIF-1 for cancer therapy. *Nat Rev Cancer* 2003; 3:721–732.
9. Kaelin WG. Proline hydroxylation and gene expression. *Annu Rev Biochem* 2005;74:115–128.
10. Semenza GL. Hypoxia-inducible factor 1 and the molecular physiology of oxygen homeostasis. *J Lab Clin Med* 1998;131:207–214.
11. Carmeliet P, Jain RK. Angiogenesis in cancer and other diseases. *Nature* 2000;407:249–257.
12. Hockel M, Vaupel P. Biological consequences of tumor hypoxia. *Semin Oncol* 2001;28:36–41.
13. Mekhail K, Khacho M, Gunaratnam L, et al. Oxygen sensing by H+: implications for HIF and hypoxic cell memory. *Cell Cycle* 2004;3: 1027–1029.
14. Semenza GL. HIF-1 and tumor progression: pathophysiology and therapeutics. *Trends Mol Med* 2002;8:S62–S67.
15. Depre C, Kim SJ, John AS, et al. Program of cell survival underlying human and experimental hibernating myocardium. *Circ Res* 2004;95: 433–440.
16. Sinusas AJ. The potential for myocardial imaging with hypoxia markers. *Semin Nucl Med* 1999;29:330–338.
17. Teicher BA. Angiogenesis and cancer metastases: therapeutic approaches. *Crit Rev Oncol Hematol* 1995;20:9–39.
18. Hockel M, Schlenger K, Aral B, et al. Association between tumor hypoxia and malignant progression in advanced cancer of the uterine cervix. *Cancer Res* 1996;56:4509–4515.
19. Brizel DM, Dodge RK, Clough RW, et al. Oxygenation of head and neck cancer: changes during radiotherapy and impact on treatment outcome. *Radiother Oncol* 1999;53:113–117.
20. Vaupel P, Thews O, Hoeckel M. Treatment resistance of solid tumors: role of hypoxia and anemia. *Med Oncol* 2001;18:243–259.
21. Holland, F. *Cancer Med* 2003;6. http://www.ncbi.nlm.nih.gov/books/bv.fcgi?rid=cmed6.chapter.9197.
22. Harrison L, Blackwell K. Hypoxia and anemia: factors in decreased sensitivity to radiation therapy and chemotherapy? *Oncologist* 2004;9 [Suppl 5]:31–40.

23. Greijer AE, de Jong MC, Scheffer GL, et al. Hypoxia-induced acidification causes mitoxantrone resistance not mediated by drug transporters in human breast cancer cells. *Cell Oncol* 2005;27:43–49.
24. Sakata K, Kwok TT, Murphy BJ, et al. Hypoxia-induced drug resistance: comparison to P-glycoprotein-associated drug resistance. *Br J Cancer* 1991;64:809–814.
25. Makin G, Hickman JA. Apoptosis and cancer chemotherapy. *Cell Tissue Res* 2000;301:143–152.
26. Stadler P, Becker A, Feldmann HJ, et al. Influence of the hypoxic subvolume on the survival of patients with head and neck cancer. *Int J Radiat Oncol Biol Phys* 1999;44:749–754.
27. Lartigau E, Lusinchi A, Weeger P, et al. Variations in tumour oxygen tension (pO2) during accelerated radiotherapy of head and neck carcinoma. *Eur J Cancer* 1998;34:856–861.
28. Nordsmark M, Alsner J, Keller J, et al. Hypoxia in human soft tissue sarcomas: adverse impact on survival and no association with p53 mutations. *Br J Cancer* 2001;84:1070–1075.
29. Raleigh JA, Dewhirst MW, Thrall DE. Measuring tumor hypoxia. *Semin Radiat Oncol* 1996;6:37–45.
30. Maeda K, Osato T, Umezawa H. A new antibiotic, azomycin. *J Antibiot (Tokyo)* 1953;6:182.
31. Lancini GC, Lazzari E. The synthesis of azomycin (2-nitroimidazole). *Experientia* 1965;21:83.
32. Chapman JD. Hypoxic sensitizers—implications for radiation therapy. *N Engl J Med* 1979;301:1429–1432.
33. McClelland RA. Molecular interactions and biological effects of the products of reduction of nitroimidazoles. In: Adams GE, Breccia A, Fiedlen EN, et al., eds. *NATO advanced research workshop on selective activation of drugs by redox processes.* New York: Plenum Press, 1990:125–136.
34. Machulla H-J. *Imaging of hypoxia: tracer developments.* Dordrecht, Boston: Kluwer Academic, 1999.
35. Jerabek PA, Patrick TB, Kilbourn MR, et al. Synthesis and biodistribution of ^{18}F-labeled fluoronitroimidazoles: potential *in vivo* markers of hypoxic tissue. *Int J Rad Appl Instrum [A]* 1986;37:599–605.
36. Grierson JR, Link JM, Mathis CA, et al. A radiosynthesis of fluorine-18 fluoromisonidazole. *J Nucl Med* 1989;30:343–350.
37. Martin GV, Cerqueira MD, Caldwell JH, et al. Fluoromisonidazole. A metabolic marker of myocyte hypoxia. *Circ Res* 1990;67:240–244.
38. Casciari JJ, Rasey JS. Determination of the radiobiologically hypoxic fraction in multicellular spheroids from data on the uptake of [^{3}H]fluoromisonidazole. *Radiat Res* 1995;141:28–36.
39. Rasey JS, Grunbaum Z, Magee S, et al. Characterization of radiolabeled fluoromisonidazole as a probe for hypoxic cells. *Radiat Res* 1987;111: 292–304.
40. Rasey JS, Koh WJ, Grierson JR, et al. Radiolabelled fluoromisonidazole as an imaging agent for tumor hypoxia. *Int J Radiat Oncol Biol Phys* 1989;17:985–991.
41. Piert M, Machulla H, Becker G, et al. Introducing fluorine-18 fluoromisonidazole positron emission tomography for the localisation and quantification of pig liver hypoxia. *Eur J Nucl Med* 1999;26:95–109.
42. Piert M, Machulla HJ, Becker G, et al. Dependency of the [^{18}F]fluoromisonidazole uptake on oxygen delivery and tissue oxygenation in the porcine liver. *Nucl Med Biol* 2000;27:693–700.
43. Silverman DH, Hoh CK, Seltzer MA, et al. Evaluating tumor biology and oncological disease with positron-emission tomography. *Semin Radiat Oncol* 1998;8:183–196.
44. Yang DJ, Wallace S, Cherif A, et al. Development of F-18-labeled fluoroerythronitroimidazole as a PET agent for imaging tumor hypoxia. *Radiology* 1995;194:795–800.
45. Rasey JS, Hofstrand PD, Chin LK, et al. Characterization of [^{18}F]fluoroetanidazole, a new radiopharmaceutical for detecting tumor hypoxia. *J Nucl Med* 1999;40:1072–1079.
46. Lehtio K, Oikonen V, Gronroos T, et al. Imaging of blood flow and hypoxia in head and neck cancer: initial evaluation with [^{15}O]H_2O and [^{18}F]fluoroerythronitroimidazole PET. *J Nucl Med* 2001;42: 1643–1652.
47. Lehtio K, Eskola O, Viljanen T, et al. Imaging perfusion and hypoxia with PET to predict radiotherapy response in head-and-neck cancer. *Int J Radiat Oncol Biol Phys* 2004;59:971–982.
48. Gronroos T, Bentzen L, Marjamaki P, et al. Comparison of the biodistribution of two hypoxia markers [^{18}F]FETNIM and [^{18}F]FMISO in an experimental mammary carcinoma. *Eur J Nucl Med Mol Imaging* 2004;31:513–520.
49. Mahy P, De Bast M, Leveque PH, et al. Preclinical validation of the hypoxia tracer 2-(2-nitroimidazol-1-yl)- N-(3,3,3-[(18)F]trifluoropropyl)acetamide [(^{18})F]EF3. *Eur J Nucl Med Mol Imaging* 2004;31: 1263–1272.
50. Ziemer LS, Evans SM, Kachur AV, et al. Noninvasive imaging of tumor hypoxia in rats using the 2-nitroimidazole ^{18}F-EF5. *Eur J Nucl Med Mol Imaging* 2003;30:259–266.
51. Zanzonico P, O'Donoghue J, Chapman JD, et al. Iodine-124-labeled iodo-azomycin-galactoside imaging of tumor hypoxia in mice with serial microPET scanning. *Eur J Nucl Med Mol Imaging* 2004;31:117–128.
52. Mannan RH, Somayaji VV, Lee J, et al. Radioiodinated 1-(5-iodo-5-deoxy-beta-D-arabinofuranosyl)-2-nitroimidazole (iodoazomycin arabinoside: IAZA): a novel marker of tissue hypoxia. *J Nucl Med* 1991;32: 1764–1770.
53. Piert M, Machulla H-J, Picchio M, et al. Hypoxia-specific tumor imaging with ^{18}F-fluoroazomycin arabinoside. *J Nucl Med* 2005;46:106–113.
54. Kumar P, Stypinski D, Xia H, et al. Fluoroazomycin arabinoside (FAZA): synthesis, ^{2}H and ^{3}H-labelling and preliminary biological evaluation of a novel 2-nitroimidazole marker of tissue hypoxia. *J Label Comp Radiopharm* 1999;42:3–16.
55. Souvatzoglou M, Grosu A, Roeper B, et al. Tumour hypoxia imaging with [^{18}F]FAZA PET in head and neck cancer patients: a pilot study. *Eur J Nucl Med* 2007;34:1566–1575.
56. Dearling JL, Lewis JS, Mullen GE, et al. Copper bis(thiosemicarbazone) complexes as hypoxia imaging agents: structure-activity relationships. *J Biol Inorg Chem* 2002;7:249–259.
57. Green MA, Mathias CJ, Welch MJ, et al. Copper-62-labeled pyruvaldehyde bis(N4-methylthiosemicarbazonato)copper(II): synthesis and evaluation as a positron emission tomography tracer for cerebral and myocardial perfusion. *J Nucl Med* 1990;31:1989–1996.
58. Fujibayashi Y, Cutler CS, Anderson CJ, et al. Comparative studies of Cu-64-ATSM and C-11-acetate in an acute myocardial infarction model: *ex vivo* imaging of hypoxia in rats. *Nucl Med Biol* 1999;26:117–121.
59. Lewis JS, Herrero P, Sharp TL, et al. Delineation of hypoxia in canine myocardium using PET and copper(II)-diacetyl-bis(N(4)-methylthiosemicarbazone). *J Nucl Med* 2002;43:1557–1569.
60. Lewis JS, Sharp TL, Laforest R, et al. Tumor uptake of copper-diacetyl-bis (N4-methylthiosemicarbazone): effect of changes in tissue oxygenation. *J Nucl Med* 2001;42:655–661.
61. Lewis JS, McCarthy DW, McCarthy TJ, et al. Evaluation of 64-Cu-ATSM *in vitro* and *in vivo* in a hypoxic tumor model. *J Nucl Med* 1999;40: 177–183.
62. Dehdashti F, Grigsby PW, Mintun MA, et al. Assessing tumor hypoxia in cervical cancer by positron emission tomography with ^{60}Cu-ATSM: relationship to therapeutic response—a preliminary report. *Int J Radiat Oncol Biol Phys* 2003;55:1233–1238.
63. O'Donoghue JA, Zanzonico P, Pugachev A, et al. Assessment of regional tumor hypoxia using ^{18}F-fluoromisonidazole and 64-Cu(II)-diacetyl-bis (N4-methylthiosemicarbazone) positron emission tomography: comparative study featuring microPET imaging, pO2 probe measurement, autoradiography, and fluorescent microscopy in the R3327-AT and FaDu rat tumor models. *Int J Radiat Oncol Biol Phys* 2005;61: 1493–1502.
64. Yuan H, Schroeder T, Bowsher JE, et al. Intertumoral differences in hypoxia selectivity of the PET imaging agent 64-Cu(II)-diacetyl-bis (N4-methylthiosemicarbazone). *J Nucl Med* 2006;47:989–998.
65. McQuade P, Miao Y, Yoo J, et al. Imaging of melanoma using 64-Cu-and 86Y-DOTA-ReCCMSH(Arg11), a cyclized peptide analogue of alpha-MSH. *J Med Chem* 2005;48:2985–2992.

66. Dehdashti F, Mintun MA, Lewis JS, et al. *In vivo* assessment of tumor hypoxia in lung cancer with ^{60}Cu-ATSM. *Eur J Nucl Med Mol Imaging* 2003;30:844–850.
67. Rajendran JG, Wilson DC, Conrad EU, et al. [(^{18})F]FMISO and [(^{18})F]FDG PET imaging in soft tissue sarcomas: correlation of hypoxia, metabolism and VEGF expression. *Eur J Nucl Med Mol Imaging* 2003;30:695–704.
68. Eschmann SM, Paulsen F, Reimold M, et al. Prognostic impact of hypoxia imaging with ^{18}F-misonidazole PET in non–small cell lung cancer and head and neck cancer before radiotherapy. *J Nucl Med* 2005; 46:253–260.
69. Burgman P, Odonoghue JA, Humm JL, et al. Hypoxia-induced increase in FDG uptake in MCF7 cells. *J Nucl Med* 2001;42:170–175.
70. Chao KS, Bosch WR, Mutic S, et al. A novel approach to overcome hypoxic tumor resistance: Cu-ATSM-guided intensity-modulated radiation therapy. *Int J Radiat Oncol Biol Phys* 2001;49:1171–1182.
71. Stratford IJ, Workman P. Bioreductive drugs into the next millennium. *Anticancer Drug Des* 1998;13:519–528.
72. Denny WA. Prodrug strategies in cancer therapy. *Eur J Med Chem* 2001; 36:577–595.
73. Beck R, Röper B, Carlsen JM, et al. Pretreatment [^{18}F]FAZA PET predicts success of hypoxia-directed radiochemotherapy using tirapazamine. *J Nucl Med* 2007;48:973–9800.
74. Hicks RJ, Rischin D, Fisher R, et al. Utility of FMISO PET in advanced head and neck cancer treated with chemoradiation incorporating a hypoxia-targeting chemotherapy agent. *Eur J Nucl Med Mol Imaging* 2005;32:1384–1391.

CHAPTER

8.25

Newer Tracers for Cancer Imaging

RODNEY J. HICKS

Although positron emission tomography (PET) has been recognized to have unique capabilities for the evaluation of neurological and cardiac diseases, the recent growth in clinical PET has been largely driven by its multiple roles in oncology. This clinical growth has been based almost exclusively on a single tracer, fluorine-18-fluoro-2-deoxy-D-glucose (FDG). As detailed elsewhere in this book, FDG performs admirably in a wide range of malignancies. However, despite its excellent diagnostic performance, it has recognized limitations. Broadly, these relate to the nonspecificity of glucose metabolic changes for cancer, lack of contrast between physiological and pathological uptake, and low FDG avidity of some cancer types, which limit to varying extent the accuracy of FDG PET in some cancers.

Although pattern recognition, knowledge of typical locations and routes of spread of metastases, and clinical judgment based on all historical and clinical data play important roles in differentiating inflammatory from malignant processes (1), biopsy may be necessary to characterize FDG PET abnormalities definitively. Even when cancer is known to be present, high uptake in adjacent tissues due to physiological processes can reduce lesion contrast and thereby impair the sensitivity of FDG PET for the detection of disease. This is particularly evident in the brain where high glucose use by the normal cerebral cortex can mask the presence of brain tumors (2). Similarly, high background normal organ FDG accumulation can also adversely affect test performance in the liver, bowel, stomach, kidneys, genitourinary system, and in areas of brown fat distribution.

Low FDG avidity can also occur with certain tumors, including some adenocarcinomas of the lung, breast, and prostate, reducing contrast and thereby reducing sensitivity. Despite these considerations, the diagnostic accuracy of FDG in cancer is so good in most clinical situations (3) that there is little incentive to develop new oncologic tracers. These new tracers would first have to match FDG and then be demonstrated to improve on this already high sensitivity and specificity, particularly if proposed to be a replacement for FDG as the workhorse agent for cancer imaging. However, the new tracers in development have the potential to combat the limitations of FDG and establish new applications for PET. More probably, such agents will fill important gaps where FDG's performance is substantially deficient.

In an era when molecular profiling is identifying specific and mechanistically important genomic and proteomic alterations in diseased cells, a logical progression of PET tracer development is to go beyond the probing of basic substrate metabolism, which is simply an indicator of the extent of viable tumor cells. The trend is toward evaluation of more specific features of cancer biology including proliferation and receptor expression (4). Many conventional nuclear medicine procedures are now performed in the oncology setting that could be replaced with PET tracers and provide superior spatial resolution and contrast, greater convenience, and lower radiation burden.

MOST SUITABLE RADIONUCLIDE FOR NEW CANCER IMAGING TRACERS

One of the great theoretical strengths of PET is the availability of a wide range of cyclotron and generator produced radionuclides with varying physical and chemical characteristics (5). Of these, carbon-11 ([^{11}C]), has the greatest flexibility for labeling biological compounds, and it does not perturb the biological behavior of the chemical. However, the short physical half-life of this radionuclide poses significant logistical problems in the clinical setting. Carbon-11 requires rapid synthesis and quality assurance processes to allow administration of adequate quantities for human imaging. It also significantly constrains the number of patients that can be imaged from each synthetic run, thereby increasing the cost per unit dose. Also important is whether the short half-life of [^{11}C] is best suited to the kinetics of the biological process that is to be addressed. Slower biological processes may not be appropriate for [^{11}C] imaging.

Fluorine-18 ([^{18}F]), on the other hand, has an adequate half-life to allow both synthesis and distribution of PET radiotracers, even to sites remote from a cyclotron, but is also sufficiently short to allow relatively low radiation dosimetry. The half-life of 109 minutes is well matched to many physiological processes. Medical cyclotrons involved in the production of FDG routinely produce [^{18}F]-fluoride, and increasing experience with fluorination chemistry enables an ever-wider range of PET tracers to be produced. The low positron energy of [^{18}F] provides high-quality images with modern

PET scanners. Based on these factors, the authors, and others, have focused on evaluating fluorinated PET tracers in oncology applications.

Generator-produced radionuclides such as gallium-68 may also have a role for facilities remote from a cyclotron (5), particularly for receptor imaging through chelation to peptides (6). Other long-lived radionuclides may have particular advantages in tracing biological processes with slow kinetics. An example of this is the use of iodine-124 to evaluate the localization of monoclonal antibodies in tumors (7).

SUBSTRATE METABOLITES THAT ADDRESS RECOGNIZED LIMITATIONS OF FLUORODEOXYGLUCOSE

PET metabolic imaging has traditionally focused on tracers of cellular substrate metabolism, especially FDG in oncology. Extending this paradigm, multiple radiolabeled amino acids suitable for PET imaging have been developed (8). Up-regulation of amino acid transport and enhanced protein synthesis is a hallmark of cancer. Amino acids are taken up much less avidly in inflammatory lesions, or by the brain, compared to FDG.

PET imaging of amino acid analogues has been seen as a means to address the limitations of FDG with respect to both specificity for cancer and for sensitivity of lesion detection in the brain where high background uptake can mask tumoral radiotracer accumulation. Carbon-11-L-methionine has been shown to have a sensitivity similar to FDG for detection of various nonbrain cancers, including head and neck and lung cancers. Its specificity is somewhat higher due to a reduced tendency to accumulate in inflammatory lesions. Carbon-11-L-methionine is one of the few radiopharmaceuticals to compete favorably with FDG in terms of diagnostic accuracy in cancer (9). It is also significantly more sensitive than FDG PET for brain tumors including glioma (10). It is clearly superior to FDG when lesions have lower or similar uptake of FDG compared to normal brain (2).

Unfortunately, as discussed above, the short physical half-life of [^{11}C] makes this an impractical tracer for routine clinical applications. Consequently, there has been a global effort to develop fluorinated amino acids for oncology imaging. One of the most promising of these is [^{18}F]-fluoroethyl-L-tyrosine (FET), which was developed as an alternative cancer-imaging agent (11) and was shown to have similar characteristics to [^{11}C]-L-methionine in comparative studies (12). However, FET has the practical advantages of using [^{18}F] as the imaging radionuclide. Since this agent demonstrates very low uptake in the normal brain and relatively high uptake in brain tumors (12,13), it provides a more sensitive detection of disease and better characterization of the extent of tumor involvement than does FDG (Fig. 8.25.1).

Although the specificity of FET for ring-enhancing lesions of the brain is superior to that of FDG, it remains imperfect and necessitates biopsy of positive lesions (14). The experience with this agent suggests reasonable uptake in squamous cell carcinomas of the head and neck (15), but the sensitivity for other extra-cranial malignancies has been disappointing (16) (Fig. 8.25.2).

Other fluorinated amino acids are also currently in development (17–19). Unless the sensitivity of these tracers can be demonstrated to be comparable to FDG, the higher specificity may not be an advantage since it may falsely reassure clinicians that a negative result in patients with a positive FDG PET scan is indicative of inflammation rather than malignancy. It may also be advantageous to have radiolabeled amino acids for patients who have poor glucose control and for low-grade brain tumors. Thus, there may be a niche for such agents, even if they do not generally replace FDG in

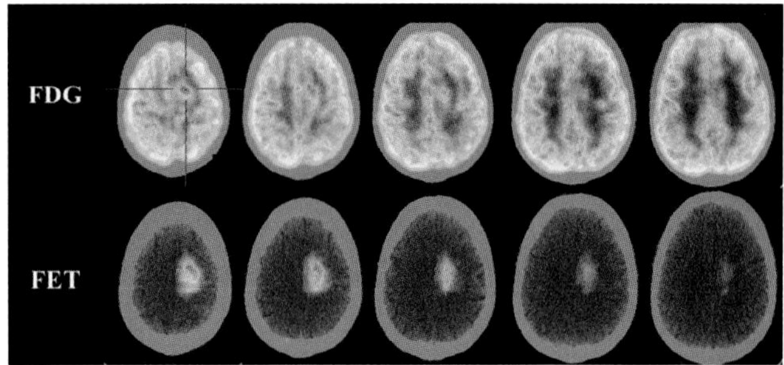

FIGURE 8.25.1. A comparison of fluorodeoxyglucose (FDG) (**upper row**) and fluorine-18-fluoroethyl-L-tyrosine (FET) (**lower row**) uptake in a glioblastoma multiforme demonstrates much higher contrast between tumor and normal brain tissue with FET despite a lower measured standard uptake value. This enables greater sensitivity for detection of tumor and particularly for defining the extent of tumor for surgical and radiotherapy planning.

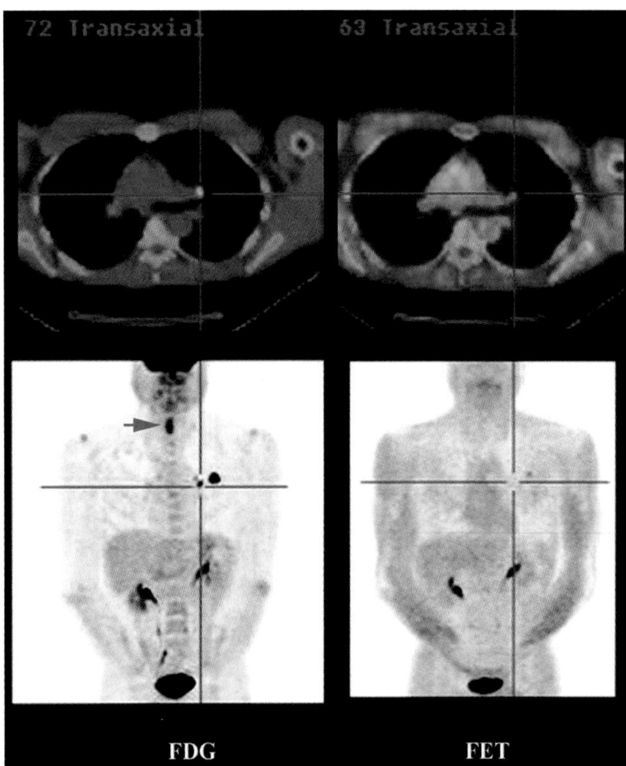

FIGURE 8.25.2. A comparison of fused PET/CT images (upper row) of fluorodeoxyglucose (FDG) and fluorine-18-fluoroethyl-L-tyrosine (FET) uptake in a primary squamous cell carcinoma of the lung demonstrates substantially higher contrast with FDG and, therefore, despite theoretically higher specificity for malignancy, the lower sensitivity of FET decreases confidence in the veracity of a negative result. Prominent FDG uptake at the site of recent laser surgery in the larynx (*arrow*) demonstrates no significant FET uptake (lower row), consistent with the lower uptake of FET than of FDG in regions of inflammation.

all applications. Recently, nonmetabolizable amino acid tracers have been fluorinated and applied to human imaging, an area of considerable interest and promise.

Increased sterol synthesis is another potential cancer-imaging target based on substrate metabolism. Tumor tissues have a requirement for increased synthesis of phosphatidylcholine, an important constituent of cell membranes. Increased rates of transmembrane transport and subsequent phosphorylation of choline by the enzyme choline kinase in tumors have been demonstrated.

Carbon-11-choline (20) has been used to successfully image a variety of tumors, including prostate cancer, brain tumors, esophageal cancer, and lung cancer, but because of the short half-life of [^{11}C] (20 minutes), fluorinated analogues are potentially more suitable for clinical studies. Fluorine-18 fluoromethyl-dimethyl-2-hydroxyethyl-ammonium or fluorocholine (FCH) is one such tracer. Preliminary studies suggested that FCH might be more sensitive than FDG for detection of nodal and bone metastases in prostate cancer (21). Subsequent studies in staging and restaging of patients with prostate cancer are continuing to define the potential clinical role of this tracer (22–27). The authors' experience suggests that FCH is more sensitive than FDG PET for detecting sites of relapse in patients with rising prostate-specific antigen levels (Fig. 8.25.3). High uptake in the liver and kidneys is a limitation of this tracer in detecting primary or secondary lesions in these organs. This is not a major limitation for prostate cancer, which seldom spreads to these organs, but it is for breast cancer, which commonly does (Fig. 8.25.4). A discussion of the use of [^{11}C] and [^{18}F]-choline analogues in genitourinary cancer imaging, especially prostate cancer, is present in Chapter 8.18 of this book.

Since FDG avidity of breast cancer is variable, FCH may have a role when there is a strong clinical suspicion of recurrence but a negative or equivocal FDG PET study. Despite the high uptake of FCH in the liver, preliminary results suggest that FCH may also be a useful imaging agent for hepatocellular carcinoma (28), which has variable FDG avidity. As with amino acid analogues, FCH is not taken up significantly in the normal brain, and preliminary studies suggest that this agent might also be useful for brain tumor imaging (29).

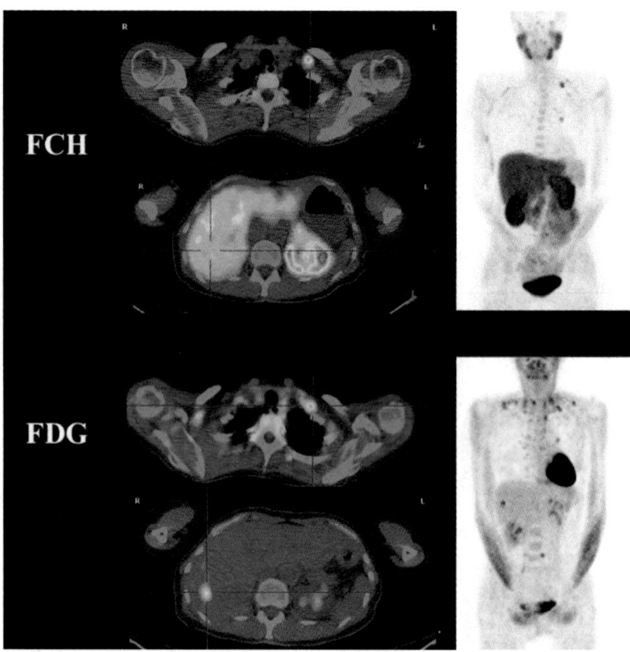

FIGURE 8.25.4. Breast cancers can show variable fluorodeoxyglucose (FDG) avidity but are generally well visualized on FDG PET. Physiological brown fat can be problematic for identifying axillary and supraclavicular nodal involvement. In this patient, the lack of [^{18}F]-fluorocholine (FCH) uptake in brown fat made identification of a left supraclavicular nodal metastasis much easier (top right) than on the corresponding FDG image (top left). However, high uptake of FCH in the liver decreased contrast and therefore detectability of a hepatic metastasis (bottom left).

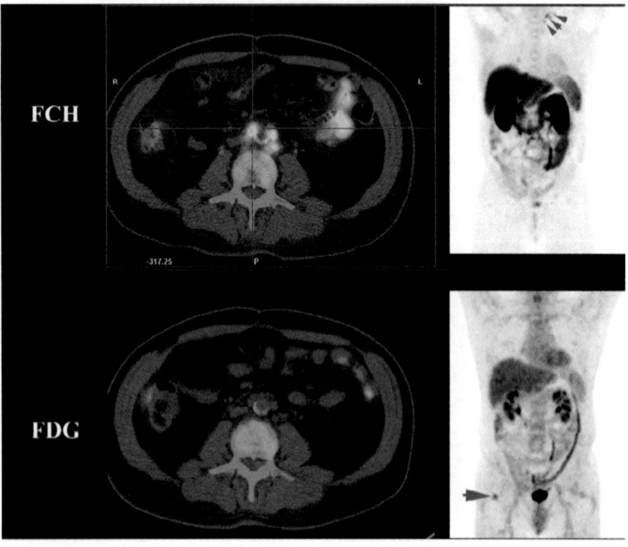

FIGURE 8.25.3. Low fluorodeoxyglucose (FDG) avidity is a recognized feature of some adenocarcinomas, particularly prostate cancer. In this patient with rising prostate-specific antigen levels, [^{18}F]-fluorocholine (FCH) PET (top left) demonstrated extensive uptake in nonenlarged para-aortic and left supraclavicular lymph nodes (*small arrows* on maximum intensity projection [MIP] image) (top right) that were negative on FDG PET (bottom left). A positive right inguinal node on FDG PET (*large arrow, bottom right*) was negative on FCH PET, consistent with a reactive node.

[^{11}C]-acetate is another substrate metabolite that has been used for cancer imaging (30–33), with potential application in urological malignancies. A fluorinated analogue of this compound, [^{18}F]-fluoroacetate has also been shown to have uptake in prostate cancer (34). These agents are also discussed in Chapter 8.18 as related to genitourinary cancer imaging.

Because most normal cells have some degree of versatility in their substrate metabolism, all the above tracers are, to some extent, nonspecific for cancer and measure processes that are well downstream from the key genetic mechanisms responsible for cancer. An appropriate objective of PET tracer development has been to design and validate tracers that are more specific and enhance the rapidly advancing knowledge regarding the molecular biology of cancer cells.

EVALUATION OF BIOLOGICAL PROCESSES MORE SPECIFIC TO CANCER

The discovery of oncogenes initially led to an overly simplistic view that cancer was caused by mutations in key individual genes. It is now apparent that there are many genes that are involved in the development, survival, progression, and metastases of cancer cells (35). This diversity of genomic abnormality and the interaction between tumor cells and host stromal cells accounts for the variability in the clinical behavior of cancers that by standard histopathological appearances may appear to be the same. Increasingly, advances in molecular profiling are beginning to provide information regarding the natural history of cancers of any given histology. For example, microarray analyses of breast cancer are providing prognostic insights and have the potential to suggest new treatment approaches (36).

Although metastasis is clearly an adverse event in the natural history of any individual cancer, there are many patients with metastatic disease who may still be able to have a relatively long survival. Other patients presenting with relatively small primaries and no evidence of metastatic disease may rapidly succumb to their diseases. The prototypical examples of this are carcinoma of the breast and prostate. For both malignancies, metastatic bone disease may be an indolent process that is well controlled by relatively innocuous therapies including hormone manipulation and bisphosphonates. In other, generally younger, individuals, the progress from diagnosis of an apparently localized primary to death may be rapid and inexorable despite aggressive therapies including toxic chemotherapeutic combinations.

Although standard pathological parameters like mitotic rate, cellular differentiation, and hormone receptor expression provide useful prognostic information, it is likely in the future that molecular profiling techniques, such a gene microarrays and serum proteomics, will provide a much more robust prediction of the cancers that will be "bad players." Inter- and intralesional heterogeneity related to genomic instability and microenvironmental factors will often limit the ability to extrapolate from a tiny pathological sample obtained at one point during the evolution of a cancer to a reliable prediction of its progress at later time points in individual patients. The ability to assay presumptive biological targets *in vivo* and on a whole-body basis is likely to provide unique complementary information. This is the intellectual rationale underpinning the current concept of molecular imaging and its application to molecular medicine.

Several of the key genes involved in cancer transformation lead to unrestrained proliferation. This is one of the hallmarks of cancer and therefore is a target of several anticancer therapeutics. The cellular uptake of thymidine provides evaluation of DNA synthesis, which is essential for up-regulated cellular proliferation. DNA synthesis is regulated by thymidine kinase 1 (TK-1) activity. This enzyme increases more than tenfold during the DNA synthetic (S) phase of the cell cycle. Radiolabeled thymidine analogues that are substrates for TK-1 show significant potential as PET imaging agents for this important process.

There has been a strong motivation to develop PET tracers of DNA synthesis. Initial studies with [^{11}C]-thymidine encouraged development of related fluorinated compounds, however, [^{11}C] agents are quite limited by their half-lives to centers with or (near) cyclotrons. Of these, the most promising currently is [^{18}F]-fluorothymidine (FLT). Although this compound is not incorporated into DNA, a theoretical advantage in relation to potential mutagenic risk, it is a substrate for TK-1 that undergoes phosphorylation and is trapped in cells. Its accumulation has been shown to closely correlate with tumor proliferation in a variety of situations (37–40). As with amino acid analogues, the lack of significant FLT uptake in the brain has encouraged evaluation of its role for brain tumor imaging, and the results have been encouraging (Fig. 8.25.5), particularly with respect to grading of primary brain lesions (41).

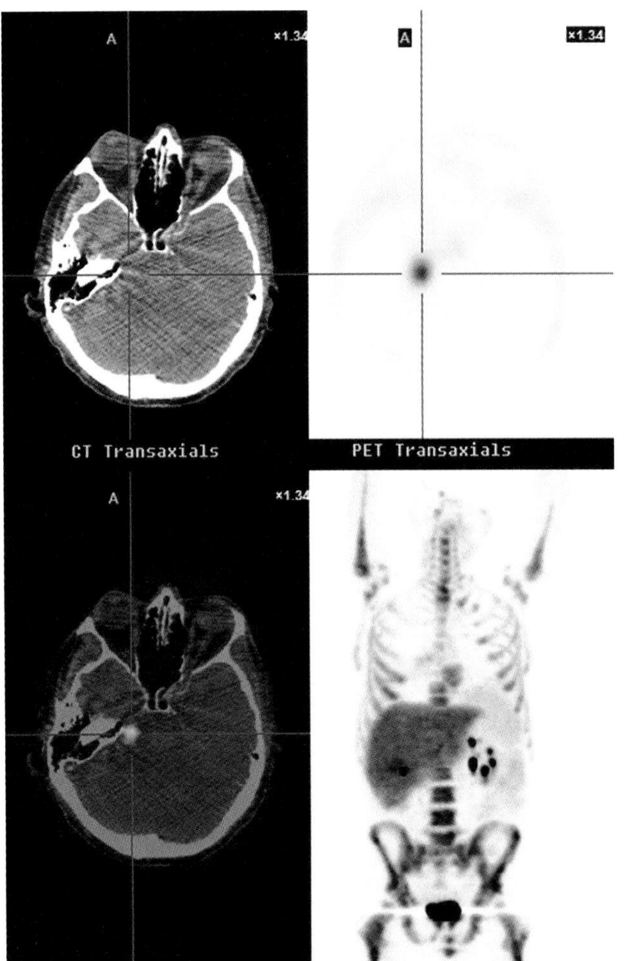

FIGURE 8.25.5. [^{18}F]-fluorothymidine (FLT) is a useful tracer of cellular proliferation. There is normal visualization of proliferating hematopoietic marrow and of crypt cells in the small bowel. Uptake in the liver in humans reflects the metabolism of this tracer. Physiologic uptake in these sites can mask metastases (bottom right). However, the lack of uptake in the brain facilitates detection of brain metastases. In this patient with non–small lung cancer treated with radiotherapy, FLT PET demonstrates reduced bone marrow activity in the sternum and thoracic spine, consistent with the prior radiation portal. The persisting uptake in the primary tumor indicates recurrent local disease. FLT PET also led to incidental detection of several previously unknown brain metastases, including a subcentimeter cerebellar metastasis. (Corresponding CT, top left, PET, top right, and fused PET/CT, bottom left).

A somewhat lower sensitivity in whole-body tumor imaging may limit the theoretical advantages of higher specificity (42), as does the relatively high uptake of FLT in bone, liver, and bone marrow, important sites of metastatic involvement. It has been noted that active germinal centers in reactive lymph nodes draining areas of inflammation can be positive on FLT scanning, limiting the specificity of nodal uptake in cases of cancer that also have an associated infective or inflammatory process. Nevertheless, the authors believe that this agent will have a major role in the assessment of therapeutic response, particularly for therapies that have a primarily tumoristatic rather than tumoricidal activity.

As tumors grow, they require formation of new blood vessels to maintain an adequate oxygen supply. Generally, this requires formation of new vessels in a process known as neovascularization. In many tumors this process is not adequate to provide the nutrient needs of the tumor cells, which leads to hypoxia and eventually to necrosis. Hypoxia is also known to be associated with a proliferation block, limiting the ability of tracers such as FLT to identify these cancer cell populations. Hypoxia within tumors is associated with a poor prognosis in a variety of cancer types and is a major factor implicated in resistance to radiation and cytotoxic drugs (43).

A number of therapeutic strategies to target or exploit hypoxia have been developed and include the hypoxic cytotoxin tirapazamine (44), and radiation dose painting (45,46), resulting in a need to accurately identify hypoxia within tumors.

Extensive efforts have been made to develop PET tracers to enable the noninvasive imaging of hypoxia. [^{18}F]-fluoromisonidazole (FMISO) is the most extensively studied agent in human cancers (44,47–51). FMISO is, however, a relatively lipophilic compound and demonstrates relatively low uptake in hypoxic tissue relative to normal tissue. This is due to its slow clearance from normal tissues. This necessitates delayed scanning and the consequential reduction in statistical image quality or the administration of a high dose of radioactivity. This has led to the development of other hypoxic probes that have more favorable imaging properties. Fluorine-18-fluoro-azomycin arabinoside (FAZA) is one such agent (52,53).

Preliminary results have been obtained at the authors' institution with the use of FAZA to image hypoxia within head and neck squamous cell carcinomas (Fig. 8.25.6). The authors have also used FAZA in lung cancer, cervical cancer, and sarcoma. These early results suggest that FAZA is likely to be a superior agent, compared to FMISO, for imaging hypoxia due to more rapid clearance of background soft tissues but similar tumoral uptake and thus to higher tumor to background contrast. This should provide more reproducible definition of hypoxic subvolumes and greater diagnostic confidence, but further studies to validate its ability to provide important prognostic stratification are required. Other fluorinated hypoxia tracers have also been developed are being evaluated clinically (54–56), as well as copper-labeled agents such as Cu-ATSM [Cu-diacetyl-bis(N^4-methylthiosemicarbazone)] (see Chapter 8.16).

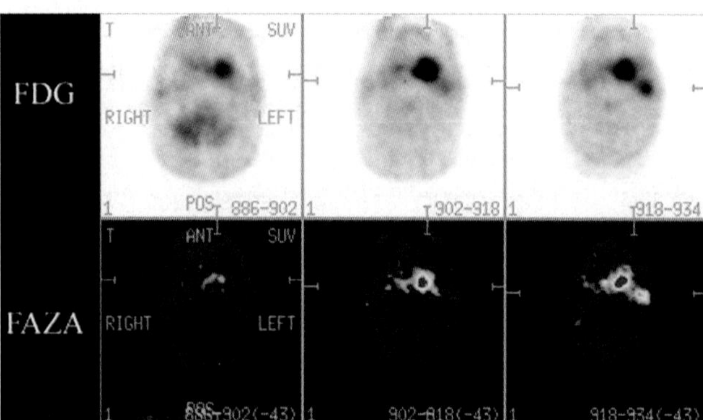

FIGURE 8.25.6. Noninvasive imaging of hypoxia may have both prognostic and therapeutic planning implications. High contrast between normal tissues and tumor is an advantage in localizing sites of disease. The new hypoxia agent fluorine-18-fluoro-azomycin arabinoside (FAZA) has more rapid soft tissue clearance than [^{18}F]-fluoromisonidazole (FMISO), and this generally leads to a higher tumor to background contrast. Comparison of fluorodeoxyglucose (FDG) PET (top row) and FAZA (bottom row) distributions can potentially identify hypoxic subvolumes for dose painting using highly conformal radiotherapy. Unlike FMISO, FAZA is not appreciably concentrated in the brain.

FUTURE DIRECTIONS

Proliferation and hypoxia are generic biological processes that are more common in cancer cell populations than in normal cells, but there are many other potential biological targets for cancer imaging. The list of these is long and increasing and is beyond the scope of this discussion. It is, however, likely that new targeted cancer therapeutics will become available and demonstrate the presence of a target expression in an individual lesion and its modulation by the targeting therapy. This will provide an increasingly important role in proof-of-mechanism studies and possibly in personalized treatment selection and dosing (57).

The favorable imaging characteristics and ready availability of [^{18}F] make it likely that there will be an increasing focus on fluorinated tracers, but a wide range of both cyclotron and generator-produced isotopes will also become relevant for cancer imaging. These include yttrium-86, gallium-68, and iodine-124.

These tracers lend themselves to form complexes with biological macromolecules, such as peptides (6) and antibodies. The availability of long-lived positron emitting radionuclides offers opportunities for translational research in the labeling of larger molecular species, including monoclonal antibodies, which can have slow accumulation in tissues (7,58).

IMPACT OF NEW PET TRACERS ON THE PRACTICE OF ONCOLOGICAL NUCLEAR MEDICINE

FDG PET has already had a significant impact on the use of traditional oncological tracers such as gallium-67-citrate in lymphoma and melanoma, thallium-201 in sarcoma, and technetium-99m (^{99m}Tc)-sestamibi in breast cancer. New tracers provide new applications for which no equivalent single-photon emission computed tomography tracer is available and will potentially also replace existing tracers. One such example is the replacement of indium-111-octreotide for the localization of neuroendocrine malignancy by gallium-68-DOTATOC ([DOTA0,Tyr3]octreotide) (6) and iodine-131 and iodine-123 for thyroid cancer staging by iodine-124 (59). In absolute terms, bone scanning remains one of the most commonly performed nuclear medicine tests for oncological staging. A long experience with [^{18}F]-fluoride as a bone tracer dates back to the time of rectilinear scanners. This tracer fell out of favor, not because of its performance as a tracer of bone metabolism, but because of suboptimal imaging characteristics with the gamma camera and, perhaps more importantly, due to the availability of ^{99m}Tc-based radiotracers for bone metastases (60,61). Recent experience suggests that [^{18}F]-fluoride bone scanning with modern combined PET and computed tomography (CT) scanners will result in superior characterization of bone lesions with both higher sensitivity and specificity than conventional bone scanning (27).

CONCLUSION

The development of new PET tracers for oncology is littered with failures, in part because of the great success of the existing yardstick, FDG. Nevertheless, there are still many opportunities for new tracers to complement existing diagnostic methods and potentially to supplant them in some situations. The focus of such development is to identify areas of clinical need that are not currently met by FDG and to be responsive to evolving information regarding cancer diagnosis and management that will provide more personalized management and thereby deliver better health outcomes. Several PET tracers already show such promise.

REFERENCES

1. Wang G, Lau EW, Shakher R, et al. How do oncologists deal with incidental abnormalities on whole-body fluorine-18 fluorodeoxyglucose PET/CT? *Cancer* 2007;109:117–124.
2. Chung JK, Kim YK, Kim SK, et al. Usefulness of ^{11}C-methionine PET in the evaluation of brain lesions that are hypo- or isometabolic on ^{18}F-FDG PET. *Eur J Nucl Med Mol Imaging* 2002;29:176–182.
3. Gambhir SS, Czernin J, Schwimmer J, et al. A tabulated summary of the FDG PET literature. *J Nucl Med* 2001;42:1S–93S.
4. Phelps ME. PET: the merging of biology and imaging into molecular imaging. *J Nucl Med* 2000;41:661–681.
5. Saha GB, MacIntyre WJ, Go RT. Cyclotrons and positron emission tomography radiopharmaceuticals for clinical imaging. *Semin Nucl Med* 1992;22:150–161.
6. Hofmann M, Maecke H, Borner R, et al. Biokinetics and imaging with the somatostatin receptor PET radioligand (68)Ga-DOTATOC: preliminary data. *Eur J Nucl Med* 2001;28:1751–1757.
7. Pagani M, Stone-Elander S, Larsson SA. Alternative positron emission tomography with non-conventional positron emitters: effects of their physical properties on image quality and potential clinical applications. *Eur J Nucl Med* 1997;24:1301–1327.
8. Jager PL, Vaalburg W, Pruim J, et al. Radiolabeled amino acids: basic aspects and clinical applications in oncology. *J Nucl Med* 2001;42: 432–445.
9. Kubota K, Matsuzawa T, Ito M, et al. Lung tumor imaging by positron emission tomography using C-11 L-methionine. *J Nucl Med* 1985;26: 37–42.
10. Van Laere K, Ceyssens S, Van Calenbergh F, et al. Direct comparison of ^{18}F-FDG and ^{11}C-methionine PET in suspected recurrence of glioma: sensitivity, inter-observer variability and prognostic value. *Eur J Nucl Med Mol Imaging* 2005;32:39–51.
11. Wester HJ, Herz M, Weber W, et al. Synthesis and radiopharmacology of O-(2-[^{18}F]fluoroethyl)-L-tyrosine for tumor imaging. *J Nucl Med* 1999;40:205–212.
12. Weber WA, Wester HJ, Grosu AL, et al. O-(2-[^{18}F]fluoroethyl)-L-tyrosine and L-[methyl-11C]methionine uptake in brain tumours: initial results of a comparative study. *Eur J Nucl Med* 2000;27:542–549.
13. Popperl G, Gotz C, Rachinger W, et al. Value of O-(2-[^{18}F]fluoroethyl)-L-tyrosine PET for the diagnosis of recurrent glioma. *Eur J Nucl Med Mol Imaging* 2004;31:1464–1470.
14. Floeth FW, Pauleit D, Sabel M, et al. ^{18}F-FET PET differentiation of ring-enhancing brain lesions. *J Nucl Med* 2006;47:776–782.
15. Langen KJ, Hamacher K, Weckesser M, et al. O-(2-[^{18}F]fluoroethyl)-L-tyrosine: uptake mechanisms and clinical applications. *Nucl Med Biol* 2006;33:287–294.
16. Pauleit D, Stoffels G, Schaden W, et al. PET with O-(2-^{18}F-fluoroethyl)-L-tyrosine in peripheral tumors: first clinical results. *J Nucl Med* 2005;46:411–416.
17. Imahori Y, Ueda S, Ohmori Y, et al. Fluorine-18-labeled fluoroboronophenylalanine PET in patients with glioma. *J Nucl Med* 1998;39:325–333.
18. Tang G, Wang M, Tang X, et al. Synthesis and evaluation of O-(3-[^{18}F]fluoropropyl)-L-tyrosine as an oncologic PET tracer. *Nucl Med Biol* 2003;30:733–739.
19. Chen W, Silverman DH, Delaloye S, et al. ^{18}F-FDOPA PET imaging of brain tumors: comparison study with ^{18}F-FDG PET and evaluation of diagnostic accuracy. *J Nucl Med* 2006;47:904–911.
20. Hara T, Inagaki K, Kosaka N, et al. Sensitive detection of mediastinal lymph node metastasis of lung cancer with ^{11}C-choline PET. *J Nucl Med* 2000;41:1507–1513.
21. DeGrado TR, Coleman RE, Wang S, et al. Synthesis and evaluation of ^{18}F-labeled choline as an oncologic tracer for positron emission tomography: initial findings in prostate cancer. *Cancer Res* 2001;61:110–117.
22. Price DT, Coleman RE, Liao RP, et al. Comparison of [^{18}F]fluorocholine and [^{18}F]fluorodeoxyglucose for positron emission tomography of androgen dependent and androgen independent prostate cancer. *J Urol* 2002;168:273–280.
23. Kwee SA, Coel MN, Lim J, et al. Prostate cancer localization with 18-fluorine fluorocholine positron emission tomography. *J Urol* 2005;173:252–255.
24. Schmid DT, John H, Zweifel R, et al. Fluorocholine PET/CT in patients with prostate cancer: initial experience. *Radiology* 2005;235:623–628.
25. Cimitan M, Bortolus R, Morassut S, et al. [(^{18})F]fluorocholine PET/CT imaging for the detection of recurrent prostate cancer at PSA relapse: experience in 100 consecutive patients. *Eur J Nucl Med Mol Imaging* 2006;33:1387–1398.
26. Heinisch M, Dirisamer A, Loidl W, et al. Positron emission tomography/computed tomography with F-18-fluorocholine for restaging of prostate cancer patients: meaningful at PSA $<$ 5 ng/mL? *Mol Imaging Biol* 2006;8:43–48.
27. Langsteger W, Heinisch M, Fogelman I. The role of fluorodeoxyglucose, ^{18}F-dihydroxyphenylalanine, ^{18}F-choline, and ^{18}F-fluoride in bone imaging with emphasis on prostate and breast. *Semin Nucl Med* 2006;36:73–92.
28. Talbot JN, Gutman F, Fartoux L, et al. PET/CT in patients with hepatocellular carcinoma using [(^{18})F]fluorocholine: preliminary comparison with [(^{18})F]FDG PET/CT. *Eur J Nucl Med Mol Imaging* 2006;33:1285–1299.
29. Wong TZ, van der Westhuizen GJ, Coleman RE. Positron emission tomography imaging of brain tumors. *Neuroimaging Clin North Am* 2002;12:615–626.
30. Shreve P, Chiao PC, Humes HD, et al. Carbon-11-acetate PET imaging in renal disease. *J Nucl Med* 1995;36:1595–1601.
31. Kotzerke J, Volkmer BG, Neumaier B, et al. Carbon-11 acetate positron emission tomography can detect local recurrence of prostate cancer. *Eur J Nucl Med Mol Imaging* 2002;29:1380–1384.
32. Oyama N, Akino H, Kanamaru H, et al. ^{11}C-acetate PET imaging of prostate cancer. *J Nucl Med* 2002;43:181–186.
33. Fricke E, Machtens S, Hofmann M, et al. Positron emission tomography with ^{11}C-acetate and ^{18}F-FDG in prostate cancer patients. *Eur J Nucl Med Mol Imaging* 2003;30:607–611.
34. Matthies A, Ezziddin S, Ulrich EM, et al. Imaging of prostate cancer metastases with ^{18}F-fluoroacetate using PET/CT. *Eur J Nucl Med Mol Imaging* 2004;31:797.
35. Hanahan D, Weinberg RA. The hallmarks of cancer. *Cell* 2000;100: 57–70.
36. Glinsky GV, Higashiyama T, Glinskii AB. Classification of human breast cancer using gene expression profiling as a component of the survival predictor algorithm. *Clin Cancer Res* 2004;10:2272–2283.
37. Shields AF, Grierson JR, Dohmen BM, et al. Imaging proliferation in vivo with [F-18]FLT and positron emission tomography. *Nat Med* 1998;4:1334–1336.
38. Mier W, Haberkorn U, Eisenhut M. [^{18}F]FLT; portrait of a proliferation marker. *Eur J Nucl Med Mol Imaging* 2002;29:165–169.
39. Vesselle H, Grierson J, Muzi M, et al. *In vivo* validation of 3'deoxy-3'-[(^{18})F]fluorothymidine ([(^{18})F]FLT) as a proliferation imaging tracer in humans: correlation of [(^{18})F]FLT uptake by positron emission tomography with Ki-67 immunohistochemistry and flow cytometry in human lung tumors. *Clin Cancer Res* 2002;8:3315–3323.
40. Buck AK, Halter G, Schirrmeister H, et al. Imaging proliferation in lung tumors with PET: ^{18}F-FLT versus ^{18}F-FDG. *J Nucl Med* 2003;44:1426–1431.
41. Chen W, Cloughesy T, Kamdar N, et al. Imaging proliferation in brain tumors with ^{18}F-FLT PET: comparison with ^{18}F-FDG. *J Nucl Med* 2005;46:945–952.

42. van Westreenen HL, Cobben DC, Jager PL, et al. Comparison of ^{18}F-FLT PET and ^{18}F-FDG PET in esophageal cancer. *J Nucl Med* 2005;46: 400–404.
43. Evans SM, Koch CJ. Prognostic significance of tumor oxygenation in humans. *Cancer Lett* 2003;195:1–16.
44. Rischin D, Hicks RJ, Fisher R, et al. Prognostic significance of [^{18}F]-misonidazole positron emission tomography-detected tumor hypoxia in patients with advanced head and neck cancer randomly assigned to chemoradiation with or without tirapazamine: a substudy of Trans-Tasman Radiation Oncology Group Study 98.02. *J Clin Oncol* 2006;24: 2098–2104.
45. Grosu AL, Piert M, Weber WA, et al. Positron emission tomography for radiation treatment planning. *Strahlenther Onkol* 2005;181:483–499.
46. Gregoire V, Haustermans K, Geets X, et al. PET-based treatment planning in radiotherapy: a new standard? *J Nucl Med* 2007;48[Suppl 1]:68S–77S.
47. Koh WJ, Rasey JS, Evans ML, et al. Imaging of hypoxia in human tumors with [F-18]fluoromisonidazole. *Int J Radiat Oncol Biol Phys* 1992;22:199–212.
48. Rasey JS, Koh WJ, Evans ML, et al. Quantifying regional hypoxia in human tumors with positron emission tomography of [^{18}F]fluoromisonidazole: a pretherapy study of 37 patients. *Int J Radiat Oncol Biol Phys* 1996;36:417–428.
49. Eschmann SM, Paulsen F, Reimold M, et al. Prognostic impact of hypoxia imaging with ^{18}F-misonidazole PET in non–small cell lung cancer and head and neck cancer before radiotherapy. *J Nucl Med* 2005;46:253–260.
50. Hicks RJ, Rischin D, Fisher R, et al. Utility of FMISO PET in advanced head and neck cancer treated with chemoradiation incorporating a hypoxia-targeting chemotherapy agent. *Eur J Nucl Med Mol Imaging* 2005;32:1384–1391.
51. Rajendran JG, Schwartz DL, O'Sullivan J, et al. Tumor hypoxia imaging with [F-18] fluoromisonidazole positron emission tomography in head and neck cancer. *Clin Cancer Res* 2006;12:5435–5441.
52. Sorger D, Patt M, Kumar P, et al. [^{18}F]fluoroazomycinarabinofuranoside (^{18}FAZA) and [^{18}F]Fluoromisonidazole (^{18}FMISO): a comparative study of their selective uptake in hypoxic cells and PET imaging in experimental rat tumors. *Nucl Med Biol* 2003;30:317–326.
53. Piert M, Machulla HJ, Picchio M, et al. Hypoxia-specific tumor imaging with ^{18}F-fluoroazomycin arabinoside. *J Nucl Med* 2005;46:106–113.
54. Rasey JS, Hofstrand PD, Chin LK, et al. Characterization of [^{18}F]fluoroetanidazole, a new radiopharmaceutical for detecting tumor hypoxia. *J Nucl Med* 1999;40:1072–1079.
55. Lehtio K, Oikonen V, Nyman S, et al. Quantifying tumour hypoxia with fluorine-18 fluoroerythronitroimidazole ([^{18}F]FETNIM) and PET using the tumour to plasma ratio. *Eur J Nucl Med Mol Imaging* 2003;30:101–108.
56. Mahy P, De Bast M, Leveque PH, et al. Preclinical validation of the hypoxia tracer 2-(2-nitroimidazol-1-yl)-N-(3,3,3-[(^{18})F]trifluoropropyl) acetamide, [(^{18})F]EF3. *Eur J Nucl Med Mol Imaging* 2004;31:1263–1272.
57. Haubner R, Wester HJ, Reuning U, et al. Radiolabeled alpha(v)beta3 integrin antagonists: a new class of tracers for tumor targeting. *J Nucl Med* 1999;40:1061–1071.
58. Pentlow KS, Graham MC, Lambrecht RM, et al. Quantitative imaging of I-124 using positron emission tomography with applications to radioimmunodiagnosis and radioimmunotherapy. *Med Phys* 1991;18: 357–366.
59. Eschmann SM, Reischl G, Bilger K, et al. Evaluation of dosimetry of radioiodine therapy in benign and malignant thyroid disorders by means of iodine-124 and PET. *Eur J Nucl Med Mol Imaging* 2002;29: 760–767.
60. Krishnamurthy GT, Walsh C, Winston MA, et al. Comparison of fluorine-18 bone studies obtained with rectilinear scanner and scintillation camera equipped with high-energy diverging-hole collimator. *Radiology* 1972;103:365–369.
61. Rosenfield N, Treves S. Osseous and extraosseous uptake of fluorine-18 and technetium-99m polyphosphate in children with neuroblastoma. *Radiology* 1974;111:127–133.

CHAPTER

9.1 Movement Disorders, Stroke, and Epilepsy

NICOLAAS I. BOHNEN

Anatomic imaging, such as computed tomography (CT) and magnetic resonance imaging (MRI), has revolutionized the diagnosis and management of the neurological patient. However, a brain lesion may be present functionally rather than associated with a macroscopic structural abnormality detectable by noninvasive anatomical imaging. For example, anatomical imaging in early idiopathic Parkinson disease may not reveal disease-specific changes, while positron emission tomography (PET) has clearly demonstrated the dopaminergic system abnormalities in this disorder.

PET is a molecular imaging technique that uses radiolabeled molecules to image molecular interactions of biological processes *in vivo*. Low doses of positron emitting radiotracers are being used for the radiolabeling of molecules or drugs that have binding sites in the brain, such as receptors, follow regional cerebral blood flow, or are metabolized by cerebral enzymes. PET can be used to perform neurochemical and functional brain imaging studies of cerebral blood flow or glucose metabolism.

Neurochemical imaging studies allow assessment of the regional distribution and quantitative measurement of neurotransmitters, enzymes, or receptors in the living brain. Neurochemical imaging studies are mainly performed for research purposes.

Functional brain imaging studies can measure regional cerebral blood flow or glucose metabolism. These studies may be performed in the resting state or following a specific intervention (e.g., a mental task, sensory stimulus or motor task) to "activate" specific regions in the brain.

Imaging of resting glucose metabolism and/or blood flow in the brain represent the major clinical applications of PET in neurology and will be mainly discussed in this chapter. The recent introduction of PET/CT into clinical practice may have limited utility when evaluating small lesions that are better visualized on MRI but offers the advantage of increased spatial accuracy when evaluating normal metabolic variants or artifacts due to partial volume effects. In addition, the intrinsically registered nature of the CT images from PET/CT can be helpful in both lesion localization as well as attenuation correction specific for the patient. PET studies of specific neurochemical markers, in particular dopamine, will also be discussed when clinically useful or promising. The precise correlation of anatomic findings with PET through image fusion is often useful and is facilitated through PET/CT fusion imaging as well as software fusion of PET with MRI images.

GENERAL PRINCIPLES OF CEREBRAL BLOOD FLOW AND METABOLIC IMAGING: FUNCTIONAL COUPLING AND PHYSIOLOGICAL CORRELATES

The energy metabolism of the adult human brain depends almost completely on the oxidation of glucose (1). Because the brain is unable to store either oxygen or glucose, it is thought that regional cerebral blood flow (rCBF) is continuously regulated to supply these substrates locally. The functional coupling of rCBF and local cerebral glucose metabolism has been established in a wide range of experiments using autoradiographic techniques in animals as well as double-tracer techniques in humans. Increased function of the central neurons results in increased neuronal metabolism and, as a consequence, increased concentration of metabolic end products (H^+, K^+, adenosine) results in increased rCBF (2).

A model has been proposed where neurogenic stimuli via perivascular nerve endings may act as rapid initiators responsible for moment-to-moment dynamic adjustment of rCBF to the metabolic demands (2). Functional activation of the brain (e.g., motor or visual activity) is accompanied by increases in rCBF and glucose consumption but only minimal increases in oxygen consumption (3,4). Therefore, large changes in blood flow are required to support small changes in the oxygen metabolic rate during neuronal stimulation (5). Increased oxygen consumption may result from a combined effect of increased blood flow and increased oxygen diffusion capacity in the region of brain activation (6). Factors other than local requirements in oxygen also underlie the increase in rCBF associated with physiological activation (7).

Oxygen-15 radiolabeled water ($H_2[^{15}O]$) is the most commonly used PET tracer for the measurement of rCBF. CBF can also be assessed by the inhalation of Oxygen-15 labeled carbon dioxide ($C[^{15}O_2]$). The very short half-life of oxygen-15 [^{15}O] (123 seconds) allows repeated and rapid rCBF assessments in the same individual. Fluorine-18 [^{18}F]-fluorodeoxyglucose (FDG) is a PET tracer used for the study of regional cerebral glucose metabolism. The majority of glucose in the brain is needed for maintenance of membrane potentials and restoration of ion gradients. The linking between synaptic activity and glucose utilization is a central physiological principle of brain function that has provided the basis for FDG brain PET imaging (8). Although the FDG PET signal represents neuronal and more specifically synaptic activity (9), glutamate-mediated uptake of the radioligand into astrocytes also appears to be a major mechanism (10). The basic mechanism involves glutamate-stimulated aerobic glycolysis: the sodium-coupled reuptake of glutamate by astrocytes and the ensuing activation of the sodium-potassium-adenosine triphosphatase (Na-K-ATPase) triggers glucose uptake and processing via glycolysis, resulting in the release of lactate from astrocytes. Lactate can then contribute to the activity-dependent fueling of the neuronal energy demands associated with synaptic transmission.

An operational model, the *astrocyte-neuron lactate shuttle*, is supported experimentally by a large body of evidence, which provides a molecular and cellular basis for interpreting data obtained from functional brain imaging studies (8). In addition, this neuron-glia metabolic coupling undergoes plastic adaptations in parallel with adaptive mechanisms that characterize synaptic plasticity (8).

READING BRAIN PET IMAGES: NORMAL VARIANTS, AGING, AND OTHER FACTORS THAT MAY AFFECT BLOOD FLOW OR GLUCOSE METABOLISM

The spatial resolution of the PET camera determines the extent of the partial volume effect that causes the edges of small brain structures to blur one another due to averaging of radioactivity. Therefore, the size of the imaged structure determines the recovery of counts by the camera from that structure (11). A structure must have dimensions greater than twice the resolution of the PET camera at full width half maximum in order to recover 100% of true tissue activity from that structure.

Partial volume effects may give a blurred or smoothed scan appearance of small brain structures, atrophied gyri, and smaller brain volumes, such as the inferior orbitofrontal and inferior temporal regions. Conversely, a cerebral sulcus, where two gray matter gyri face each other closely, may show relatively higher activity when a scanner does not have sufficient spatial resolution to resolve the two gyri (12). For instance, the pre- and postcentral gyri opposed at the central sulcus may form a single focus of relatively high activity (12). Similarly, the adjacent areas of the insular cortex and the superior temporal gyral cortex generate sufficiently similar FDG activity so that they may appear as one lateral mass at certain levels of scanning (13). Higher resolution PET cameras can help in this regard and are available in some centers.

It should be noted that a normal individual's brain is not completely symmetric. For example, the sylvian fissure in right-handed individuals is longer and more horizontal in the left hemisphere. Normal irregularity of gyral convolutions may give a heterogeneous scan appearance. Therefore, a commonly observed rule of visual PET analysis is the requirement that an area of apparent functional alteration of a brain structure should be seen on at least several adjacent slices in order to be deemed significant (13). Further, direct correlation with an anatomic imaging study is often required to recognize normal structural variability.

Studies of left-to-right hemispheric asymmetries in normal subjects are limited and have not been conclusive. An rCBF PET study reported slightly higher mean right hemispheric flow compared to left-sided values (14). An rCBF single-photon computed emission tomography (SPECT) study demonstrated consistent hemispheric asymmetry (right side greater than left side) in the cuneus, occipital cortex, occipital pole, middle temporal gyrus, and posterior middle frontal gyrus in 83% to 100% of individuals (15).

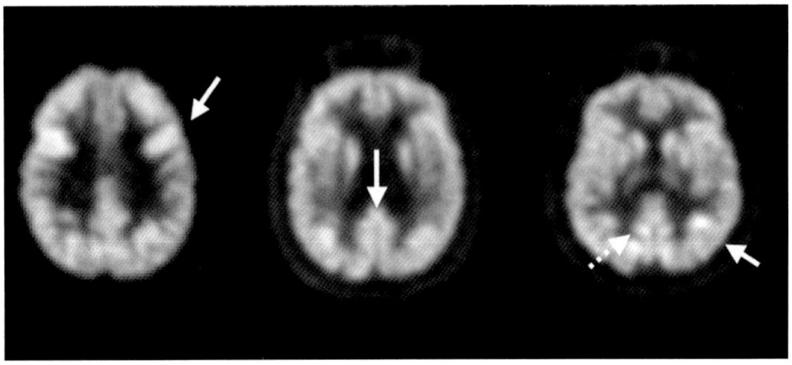

A, B C

FIGURE 9.1.1. PET images showing normal glucose metabolic variants in healthy volunteers. Examples of more prominent uptake in the frontal eye fields (**A**), posterior cingulate cortex (**B**), and an area of more intense uptake in the posterior parietal lobe (**C**) are shown by arrows. The angular gyrus is demonstrated by the dashed arrow in image C.

FDG PET studies have indicated that hemispheric asymmetries may depend on whether subjects are studied with open versus closed eyes or ears that are covered (16). For example, studies performed on subjects with eyes closed and ears covered demonstrated greater left than right hemispheric glucose metabolism. Subjects studied with closed eyes and ears also had a progressive overall decrease in glucose metabolism, reflecting general sensory deprivation (16). Decreased tracer uptake in the visual cortex is typical as well in patients whose eyes are covered.

Normal Variants

There are several normal variants that should be recognized when interpreting cerebral metabolic or blood flow PET scans. Some normal brain regions have focally more prominent metabolic or flow activity. These include the frontal eye fields (which can be asymmetric), posterior cingulate cortex and adjacent angular gyrus, Wernicke's region, the visual cortex (when subjects are injected with the eyes open), and an area of more intense uptake in the posterior parietal lobe (Fig. 9.1.1) (17,18).

The frontal eye fields have an approximate dimension of about 1 cm and are located a few centimeters anterior to the primary motor cortex (17). Wernicke's region is defined as an area of moderately intense activity measuring a few centimeters in size and is located in the posterior-superior temporal lobe. The posterior cingulate cortex is situated superior and anterior to the occipital cortex. An area of focally intense activity in the posterior parietal region is seen in about 50% of the normal population and appears mostly symmetric (Table 9.1.1) (17,18). Basal ganglia to cortex ratios are greater than unity, indicating relatively higher activity in the basal ganglia compared to the average cortex (17). Some brain regions, like the very anterior aspect of the frontal poles, may have less prominent or decreased tracer uptake (17).

TABLE 9.1.1 Frequency of Prominent Normal Fluorodeoxyglucose Brain PET Variants in the General Population

	Right (%)	Left (%)
Frontal eye field	84	77
Wernicke's area	80	85
Posterior parietal lobe	58	46

(From Loessner A, Alavi A, Lewandrowski KU, et al. Regional cerebral function determined by FDG-PET in healthy volunteers: normal patterns and changes with age. *J Nucl Med* 1995;36:11411149, with permission.)

Normal Aging: From Infancy to Adulthood

CBF PET studies in children have shown lower flow values in neonates compared to older children (19). The rCBF will reach adult values during adolescence (19). No major difference in rCBF has been observed between the basal ganglia and cortical gray matter in children with the exception of more prominent occipital flow.

FDG metabolic studies in infants and children have shown that infants less than 5 weeks old have highest metabolic activity in the sensorimotor cortex, thalamus, brainstem, and cerebellar vermis. By 3 months, metabolic activity increases in parietal, temporal, and occipital cortices, basal ganglia, and cerebellar cortex (20). Frontal and dorsolateral occipital cortical regions display a maturational rise in glucose metabolic activity by approximately 6 to 8 months.

Absolute values of glucose metabolic rate for various gray matter regions are low at birth (13 to 25 μmol/min/100 g), and rapidly rise to reach adult values (19 to 33 μmol/min/100 g) by 2 years. Glucose metabolic rate continues to rise until, by 3 to 4 years, reaching values of 49 to 65 μmol/min/100 g in most regions (20). These high rates are maintained until approximately 9 years, when they begin to decline, and reach adult rates again by the latter part of the second decade. The highest increases over adult values have been noted in cerebral cortical structures. Lesser increases have been found to be present in the basal ganglia and cerebellum. This time course of metabolic change matches the process describing initial overproduction and subsequent elimination of excessive neurons, synapses, and dendritic spines known to occur in the developing brain.

An FDG PET study of infants during the first 6 months of life reported glucose metabolic rates for various cortical brain regions and the basal ganglia to be low at birth (from 4 to 16 μmol/min/100 g) (21). In infants 2 months of age and younger rates were highest in the sensorimotor cortex, thalamus, and brainstem. By 5 months, rates had increased in the frontal, parietal, temporal, occipital, and cerebellar cortical regions. In general, the whole brain glucose metabolic activity correlated with postconceptional age, reflecting the functional maturation of these brain regions (21).

A statistical brain mapping study of metabolic aging from 6 to 38 years found greatest age-associated changes in the thalamus and anterior cingulate cortex (22). These findings were explained by relative increase of synaptic activities in the thalamus, possibly as a consequence of improved corticothalamic connections. Knowledge of the changing metabolic patterns during normal brain development is a necessary prelude to the study of abnormal brain development.

Normal Aging: From Adulthood to the Elderly

Postmortem studies have shown relatively stable neuronal numbers but loss in cell size and a decreased number of glial cells with advancing age (23). However, it remains a matter of controversy as to whether cerebral perfusion declines with healthy aging. $H_2[^{15}O]$ rCBF PET studies have shown a negative correlation between age and rCBF in the mesial frontal cortex, involving the anterior cingulate region (24). Age-related flow decreases have also been reported for the cingulate, parahippocampal, superior temporal, medial frontal, and posterior parietal cortices bilaterally, and in the left insular and left posterior prefrontal cortices (25). It should be realized that the affected areas represent limbic or neocortical association areas and, therefore, bias from possible preclinical dementia cannot be excluded.

It has been suggested that lack of partial volume correction for the dilution effect of age-related cerebral volume loss on PET measurements may be another reason for the observed age-related decline. For example, one study found a significant difference in mean cortical CBF between young/midlife (age range, 19 to 46 years; mean $\pm$ standard deviation [SD], 56 $\pm$ 10 mL/100 mL/min) and elderly (age range, 60 to 76 years; mean $\pm$ SD, 49 $\pm$ 2.6 mL/100 mL/min) subgroups before correcting for partial-volume effects (26). However, this group difference resolved after partial-volume correction (young/midlife: mean $\pm$ SD, 62$\pm$ 10 mL/100 mL/min; elderly: mean $\pm$ SD, 61 $\pm$ 4.8 mL/100 mL/min).

FDG PET imaging studies have shown decreased cortical metabolism with normal aging, particularly in the frontal lobes (17). Temporal, parietal, and occipital lobe metabolism varied considerably among subjects within the same age group as well as over decades (17). Basal ganglia, hippocampal area, thalami, cerebellum, posterior cingulate gyrus, and visual cortex remained metabolically unchanged with advancing age (17). An FDG PET study found bilateral medial prefrontal, including anterior cingulate cortices, and dorsolateral prefrontal reductions with normal aging (27). Brain scans of the aging and atrophied brain will demonstrate widened cerebral sulci, increased separation of the caudate nuclei and thalami, as well as widening of the anterior fissure. However, a Japanese study found that age-associated metabolic reductions that were present in bilateral perisylvian and medial frontal regions largely resolved after correction for partial volume effects (28).

Factors that May Affect Resting Cerebral Blood Flow or Glucose Metabolic Studies

A number of other factors need to be considered when interpreting brain PET images. Metabolism or blood flow activity will be most prominent in gray matter when compared to white matter (about four times higher). It should be emphasized that brain glucose metabolic or blood flow PET images are functional in nature. For example, if a patient is moving or talking around the time of injection, increased activity in specific brain regions like the basal ganglia, motor cortex, or language centers may be present. Subjects studied with eyes open will have increased metabolic activity in the visual cortex when compared to a baseline with the eyes closed (16). An FDG PET study found that passive audiovisual stimulation (watching a movie) led to significant glucose metabolic increases in visual and auditory cortical areas but significant decreases in frontal areas in normal volunteers (29).

Metabolic factors, such as hyperglycemia, may impair cortical FDG uptake (30). Therefore, knowledge of the clinical or behavioral state of the patient at the time of the injection and study is critical for proper image interpretation. As with any nuclear medicine study, better image quality will depend on improved count statistics. Since PET images are an average of radioactivity over a certain period of time, FDG acquisitions taken over 10 to 30 minutes will lead to better image quality compared to short-lasting (1 to 2 minutes) $H_2[^{15}O]$ CBF studies.

Drugs are also known to induce cerebral blood flow or glucose metabolic changes. For example, diazepam sedation has been found to reduce cerebral glucose metabolism globally by about 20% (31). A study by Wang et al. (32) found that lorazepam significantly decreased whole-brain metabolism over 10%. However, regional effects of lorazepam were largest in the thalamus and occipital cortex (about 20% reduction). An FDG PET study of propofol sedation in children found significant hypometabolism in the medial parieto-occipital cortex bilaterally, including the lingual gyrus, cuneus, and middle occipital gyrus (33). The bilateral parieto-occipital hypometabolism is likely to be a sedation-specific effect and should be taken into account when evaluating cerebral FDG PET scans in sedated patients.

Antiepileptic drugs have also been found to reduce glucose metabolism and rCBF. Studies of valproate have shown global FDG (9% to 10%) and global CBF (about 15%) reductions with greatest regional reductions in the thalamus (34). Phenytoin has been found to cause an average reduction of cerebral glucose metabolism by 13% (35). Cerebellar metabolism may also be reduced by phenytoin, although the effect of the drug is probably less than that due to early onset of uncontrolled epilepsy (Fig. 9.1.2) (36,37).

Lamotrigine may cause regional cerebral hypometabolism in the bilateral thalami, basal ganglia, and multiple regions of the cerebral cortex (38). Studies of the barbiturate phenobarbital and cerebral glucose metabolism have shown very prominent global reductions of about 37% (39). Neuroleptic drugs can cause differential regional metabolic effects. For example, haloperidol caused cerebellar and putaminal glucose metabolic increases, while significant reductions were evident in the frontal, occipital, and anterior cingulate cortex in normal volunteers (40).

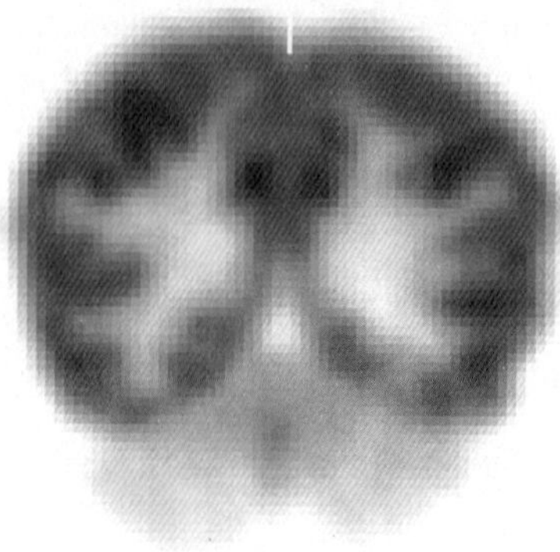

FIGURE 9.1.2. A fluorodeoxyglucose PET image of a patient with epilepsy showing bilateral cerebellar hypometabolism. Cerebellar hypometabolism may be caused by phenytoin therapy, although the effect of the drug is probably less than that due to early onset of uncontrolled epilepsy.

Diaschisis: Remote Functional Effects of Focal Brain Lesions

The functional nature of PET images may reveal metabolic or blood flow changes as a result of focal disturbance in another remote but functionally connected brain region. This phenomenon of remote effect is called diaschisis and was originally recognized by Von Monakow (41) in 1914 (42). Diaschisis in the cerebellum was first described by Baron and Marchal (43) in a patient whose PET study showed cerebellar hypoperfusion contralateral to a supratentorial stroke. Remote metabolic depression is characterized by coupled reductions in perfusion and metabolism in brain structures remote from, but connected with, the area damaged by a structural lesion. This effect has been explained as depressed synaptic activity as a result of disconnection (either direct or transneural) (44). Thus, remote effects allow mapping of the disruption in distributed networks as a result of a focal brain lesion.

Diaschisis may also occur as subcorticocortical effects. Subcorticocortical effects may lead to clinical symptoms, like subcortical aphasia due to thalamic or thalamocapsular stroke. Right-sided subcortical lesions may present with left hemineglect (subcortical neglect) (43). Small thalamic infarcts may induce metabolic depression of the ipsilateral cortical mantle (thalamocortical diaschisis) (45). Striatal and thalamic hypometabolism ipsilateral to corticosubcortical stroke is a frequent finding.

Thalamic hypometabolism may develop a few days after a stroke and presumably represents retrograde degeneration of damaged thalamocortical neurons, whereas striatal hypometabolism probably reflects loss of glutamatergic input from the cortex (43). Crossed cerebrocerebellar diaschisis may occur as early as 3 hours after stroke, is closely related to the volume of supratentorial hypoperfusion, and might be reversible (46). Persistence of diaschisis after stroke is strongly associated with outcome (46).

SPECT studies performed as ictal studies during seizure activity have demonstrated a pattern called *reverse crossed cerebrocerebellar diaschisis* where a supratentorial ictal seizure focus of hyperperfusion is associated with contralateral cerebellar hyperperfusion (Fig. 9.1.3) (47). This phenomenon also can be detected with PET.

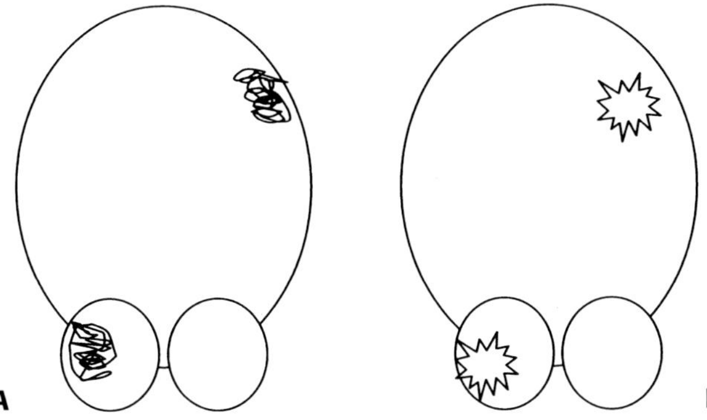

FIGURE 9.1.3. A: A diagrammatic representation of crossed cerebrocerebellar diaschisis showing cerebellar hypoperfusion contralateral to a supratentorial structural lesion. **B:** Reverse crossed cerebrocerebellar diaschisis can be observed during ictal seizure activity where a supratentorial ictal focus of hyperperfusion is associated with contralateral cerebellar hyperperfusion.

MOVEMENT DISORDERS

PET imaging of cerebral blood flow, metabolic pathways, or neurotransmission systems has contributed to researchers' understanding of the pathophysiology of movement disorders. PET measurements of dopaminergic pathways in the brain have confirmed the importance of dopamine and the basal ganglia in the pathophysiology of movement disorders, such as Parkinson disease. Brain activation studies can be performed using CBF or FDG PET. These studies compare regional brain activity during specific motor or mental tasks compared to control conditions. Activation studies have shown that the basal ganglia are activated whenever movements are performed, planned, or imagined (48). These studies support the existence of functionally independent distributed basal ganglia frontal loops. The caudate–prefrontal loop appears to mediate novel sequence learning, problem solving, and movement selection, while the putamen–premotor loop may facilitate automatic sequential patterns of limb movement and implicit acquisition of motor skills (48). Patients with movement disorders may have abnormal blood flow or metabolism in the basal ganglia (Table 9.1.2).

Cortical changes may represent primary cortical abnormalities or deafferentation effects because of subcortical abnormalities. Patients with movement disorders who also develop dementia typically will show more widespread cortical metabolic or blood flow changes. Table 9.1.3 provides a summary of the major subcortical and cortical glucose metabolic changes in neurodegenerative movement disorders.

Parkinson Disease

Parkinson disease is a clinical syndrome consisting of a variable combination of symptoms of tremor, rigidity, postural imbalance, and bradykinesia (49,50). Although Parkinson disease accounts for most patients who have parkinsonian symptoms, parkinsonism can be seen with neurodegenerative disorders other than Parkinson disease, such as progressive supranuclear palsy (PSP) or multiple system atrophy (MSA) (49). Idiopathic Parkinson disease distinguishes itself from other parkinsonian syndromes by marked left–right asymmetry in symptom severity and good symptomatic response to levodopa therapy (49,50). The additional presence of certain clinical findings may raise the clinical suspicion for an atypical parkinsonian syndrome, such as prominent autonomic dysfunction, cerebellar symptoms, or abnormal eye movements (49).

TABLE 9.1.2 Examples of Disorders or Conditions with Altered Glucose Metabolism of the Basal Ganglia

Increased fluorodeoxyglucose (FDG) metabolic activity basal ganglia	Early Parkinson disease Hepatocerebral degeneration Neuroleptic drug effects HIV infection
Decreased FDG metabolic activity basal ganglia	Atypical parkinsonism, such as progressive supranuclear palsy, multiple system atrophy or corticobasal degeneration Wilson disease

TABLE 9.1.3 Main Regional Subcortical and Cortical Glucose Metabolic Changes in Neurodegenerative Movement Disorders

	PD (early)	PD Dementia	Huntington	PSP	MSA	CBD
Caudate nucleus		↓	↓↓	↓	↓	↓[a]
Putamen	↑[a]	normal/↓	↓	↓	↓	↓[a]
Thalamus				↓		↓[a]
Cortex	↓ (occipital)	↓↓ (esp. temporoparietal, precuneus, occipital)	↓ (with dementia)	↓ (esp. frontal)		↓ (fronto-parietal)
Midbrain				↓↓		
Pons					↓↓	
Cerebellum					↓↓	

PD, Parkinson disease; PSP, progressive supranuclear palsy; MSA, multiple system atrophy; CBD, (15) corticobasal degeneration.
[a]Contralateral to (most) involved body side.

The clinical features of Parkinson disease to a large degree result from loss of nigrostriatal nerve terminals in the striatum secondary to the degeneration of dopamine-producing pigmented neurons in the substantia nigra in the brainstem (51,52). The greater the neuronal loss in the substantia nigra, the lower the concentration of dopamine in the striatum, and the more severe the parkinsonian symptoms. It should be noted that the cellular component of nigrostriatal nerve terminals within the striatum is far less than the number of intrinsic striatal interneurons and projection neurons. Therefore, resting glucose metabolic studies primarily reflect the synaptic activity of interneurons and only to a lesser extent afferent projection neurons.

Resting glucose metabolic and cerebral blood flow studies of patients with early Parkinson disease have shown increased striatal activity contralateral to the clinically most affected body side, which may represent a compensatory mechanism of intrinsic striatal cells (53,54). However, striatal glucose metabolism may decrease with advancing disease (55,56). FDG PET studies have also been used to predict levodopa response in parkinsonian patients. A study found that relatively increased FDG activity in the striatum contralateral to the clinically most affected body side was associated with a good levodopa response. In contrast, relatively decreased striatal FDG uptake was associated with poor levodopa responsiveness (57).

Parkinsonian or Lewy Body Dementia

Alzheimer disease is the most common type of dementia. The second most common form of degenerative dementia in most clinical series is parkinsonian or Lewy body dementia (58). An arbitrary but generally accepted distinction has been made in current international consensus diagnostic criteria between patients presenting with parkinsonism prior to the onset of dementia (Parkinson disease dementia) and developing parkinsonism and dementia concurrently (dementia with Lewy bodies) (59–61). These duration-based criteria would diagnose patients with Parkinson disease who subsequently develop dementia more than 1 year after their initial Parkinson disease motor symptoms as Parkinson disease dementia. Patients meeting the 1-year rule between the onset of dementia and parkinsonism would be diagnosed as dementia with Lewy bodies (60).

Although there are relative differences in temporal manifestation and relative severity of clinical symptoms between these clinically defined subgroups of parkinsonian dementia, the underlying neuropathological findings are more similar than dissimilar and suggest these subgroups should be grouped together (62). Parkinsonian dementia is characterized neuropathologically by neuronal losses and Lewy body inclusions in midbrain dopaminergic nuclei (as in Parkinson disease), but involving limbic and neocortical regions as well (58,60).

Cortical neuropathologic changes in Alzheimer disease are heterogeneous topographically but are not randomly distributed. It has been demonstrated that primary somatosensory and motor cortical regions are relatively spared, while association cortices are more severely involved (63). In the Alzheimer brain, FDG PET imaging reveals characteristic hypometabolism in neocortical structures, especially in posterior cingulate/precuneus, parietal, temporal, and to a lesser and more variable degree in frontal association cortices, the same locations where coexisting cortical neuronal degeneration is also found in postmortem studies (64,65). Parietotemporal hypometabolism can also be seen with parkinsonian or Lewy body dementias.

Vander Borght et al. (56) compared metabolic differences between Alzheimer disease and parkinsonian dementia matched for severity of dementia and found similar glucose metabolic reductions globally and regionally, involving the lateral parietal, lateral temporal, lateral frontal association cortices, and posterior cingulate gyrus when compared to controls. However, patients with parkinsonian dementia had greater metabolic reductions in the primary visual cortex and relatively preserved metabolism in the medial temporal lobe.

Decreased occipital metabolism has also been observed in nondemented patients with Parkinson disease (66). Patients with Alzheimer disease showed only mild reductions in the visual cortex but relatively more pronounced reduction in the medial temporal lobe. Metabolic reduction in the posterior cingulate cortex and precuneus demonstrated in Alzheimer disease has also been found in parkinsonian dementia (56) (Table 9.1.4).

TABLE 9.1.4 Metabolic Differences Between Alzheimer Disease and Parkinsonian Dementia

	Alzheimer Disease	Parkinsonian Dementia
Lateral parietal cortex	↓	↓
Lateral temporal cortex	↓	↓
Lateral frontal cortex	↓	↓
Posterior cingulate cortex	↓	↓
Medial temporal cortex	↓	"sparing"
Visual cortex	"sparing"	↓

There are similar glucose metabolic reductions globally and regionally involving the lateral parietal, lateral temporal, lateral frontal association cortices, and posterior cingulate gyrus when compared to controls. However, patients with parkinsonian dementia have greater metabolic reductions in the primary visual cortex and relatively preserved metabolism in the medial temporal lobe. In contrast, patients with Alzheimer disease showed only mild reductions in the visual cortex but relatively more pronounced hypometabolism in the medial temporal lobe.
(From Vander Borght T, Minoshima S, Giordani B, et al. Cerebral metabolic differences in Parkinson's and Alzheimer's disease matched for dementia severity. *J Nucl Med* 1997;38:797–802, with permission.)

Progressive Supranuclear Palsy

PSP or Steele-Richardson-Olszewski syndrome is an atypical parkinsonian syndrome characterized by severe gait and balance disturbances, abnormal eye movements (especially vertical supranuclear gaze palsy), and pseudobulbar palsy. More advanced disease is often associated with a frontal lobe type of dementia. Pathological changes consist of neurofibrillary tangle formation and neuronal loss in the superior colliculi, brainstem nuclei, periaqueductal gray matter, and basal ganglia (67).

PET studies of patients with progressive supranuclear palsy have shown reduced glucose metabolism in the caudate nucleus, putamen, thalamus, pons, and cerebral cortex, but not in the cerebellum (68). There are significant metabolic reductions in most regions throughout the cerebral cortex but are more prominent in the frontal lobe (Fig. 9.1.4) (69). Although frontal metabolism decreases with increasing disease duration, relative frontal hypometabolism has been found to already be present in the early stages of the disease (70).

Statistical brain mapping studies have demonstrated decreased glucose metabolism in the anterior cingulate, adjacent supplementary motor area, precentral cortex, middle prefrontal cortex, midbrain tegmentum, globus pallidus, and ventrolateral and dorsomedial nuclei of the thalamus (71,72). Clinical parkinsonian motor scores have been reported to correlate with caudate and thalamic glucose metabolic values (70). These data highlight predominant metabolic impairment in subcorticocortical connections in PSP.

Corticobasal Degeneration

Corticobasal degeneration is an atypical parkinsonian syndrome characterized clinically by marked asymmetric limb rigidity with apraxia. Patients may also exhibit alien limb phenomenon, cortical sensory loss, and myoclonus. Cognitive functions are relatively well preserved in most patients. Neuropathological findings consist of swollen, achromatic, tau-staining Pick bodies that may be present in the inferior parietal, posterior frontal, and superior temporal lobes, dentate nucleus, and substantia nigra (73). FDG PET studies have shown significantly reduced cerebral glucose metabolism in the hemisphere contralateral to the clinically most affected side. This reduction can occur in the dorsolateral frontal, medial frontal, inferior parietal, sensorimotor, and lateral temporal cortex as well as in the corpus striatum and the thalamus in patients with corticobasal degeneration (74–76).

Statistical brain mapping analysis of patients with corticobasal degeneration have confirmed the asymmetric glucose metabolic impairment in the putamen, thalamus, precentral, lateral premotor and supplementary motor areas, dorsolateral prefrontal cortex, and parietal cortex (77). A Japanese study found the most prominent loss in the parietal lobe in patients with corticobasal degeneration

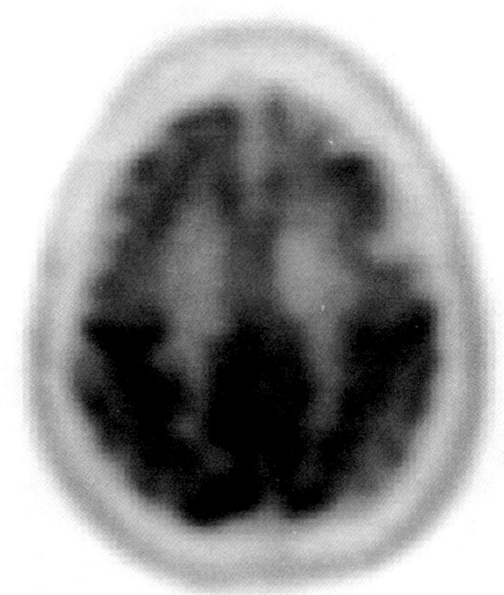

FIGURE 9.1.4. A fluorodeoxyglucose PET image of patient with progressive supranuclear palsy showing prominent frontal hypometabolism.

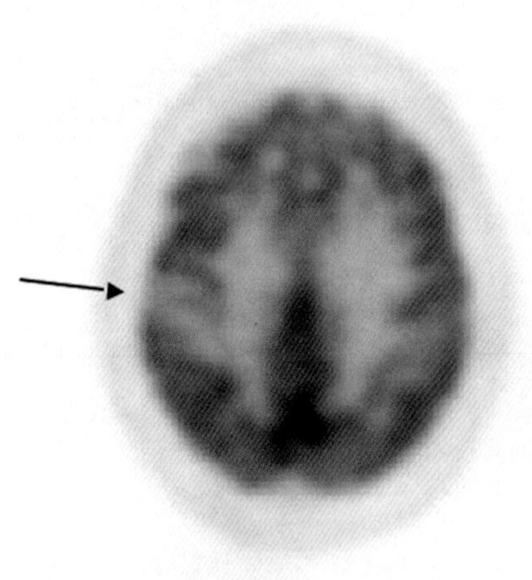

FIGURE 9.1.5. A fluorodeoxyglucose PET image of patient with corticobasal degeneration showing regionally prominent asymmetric (**right**) parietal hypometabolism.

(78). These results confirm the marked asymmetric cerebral involvement, particularly in the parietal cortex and thalamus, in patients with corticobasal degeneration (Fig. 9.1.5) (72,78–80).

Multiple System Atrophy

MSA is an atypical parkinsonian syndrome covering a clinical spectrum of parkinsonism in variable combination with symptoms of cerebellar ataxia or dysautonomia. This group of disorders includes Shy-Drager syndrome (MSA of the dysautonomia type), olivopontocerebellar atrophy (MSA of the cerebellar type), and striatonigral degeneration, which resembles Parkinson disease but does not respond to dopaminergic drugs. The pathology of MSA is distinct from Parkinson disease and consists of neuronal loss in the substantia nigra, striatum, cerebellum, brainstem, and spinal cord with argyrophilic and glial inclusions (81).

An FDG PET study found reduced caudate, putaminal, cerebellar, brainstem, and frontal and temporal cortical glucose metabolism in patients with MSA compared to normal controls (82). A voxel-based analysis of glucose metabolism found significant hypometabolism in the putamen, pons, and cerebellum in patients with MSA (83).

Reductions of cerebellar and brainstem glucose metabolism have been reported to be most prominent in patients with olivopontocerebellar atrophy (84). Although cerebellar and brainstem glucose metabolism correlated with the severity of MRI-measured atrophy, some patients who had no MR evidence of tissue atrophy still showed decreased glucose metabolism in these regions (85). Patients with the striatonigral degeneration subtype had relatively preserved brainstem and cerebellar glucose metabolic rates (85).

Essential Tremor

Essential tremor represents a variable combination of postural and kinetic tremor. It most commonly affects the hands, but also occurs in the head, voice, face, trunk, and lower extremities (86). Postmortem studies have found evidence of cerebellar degeneration; Lewy body deposition in the brainstem including the locus ceruleus has been found in a subset of subjects (87,88). A PET study found significant glucose hypermetabolism of the medulla and thalami, but not of the cerebellar cortex in patients with essential tremor during resting conditions (89). CBF PET studies using [^{15}O]-water in patients with essential tremor demonstrated abnormally increased bilateral cerebellar, red nuclear, and thalamic blood flow during tremor (90–93). Therefore, the cerebellum and thalamus appear to play important roles as part of a cerebral circuitry that is abnormally activated during tremor.

Huntington Disease and Choreiform Movement Disorders

Huntington disease is an autosomal dominant neurodegenerative disorder with complete penetrance (94). The gene for Huntington disease, containing an amplified number of cytosine-adenine-guanine (CAG) trinucleotide repeats, is located on the short arm of chromosome 4 (95). Chorea is the most commonly recognized involuntary movement abnormality in adult patients with Huntington disease, but the presence of psychiatric symptoms and dementia may vary (96). Pathologically, Huntington disease is characterized by marked neuronal loss and atrophy in the caudate nucleus and putamen (97,98). Glucose metabolic PET studies in Huntington disease have demonstrated decreased glucose utilization in the caudate nucleus and putamen even before striatal atrophy is apparent on brain CT or MRI scans (99–101). Metabolic covariance analysis of FDG PET data of patients with Huntington disease not only demonstrated caudate and putaminal hypometabolism, but there were reductions in mediotemporal metabolism as well as relative metabolic increases in the occipital cortex (102).

Chorea as a hyperkinetic movement disorder can also be seen with other disorders, such as dentatorubropallidoluysian atrophy, neuroacanthocytosis, or Sydenham chorea. Striatal, especially caudate, glucose hypometabolism has been demonstrated in dentatorubropallidoluysian atrophy and neuroacanthocytosis. This is similar to Huntington disease but striatal glucose metabolism has been found to be increased in a patient with Sydenham chorea and in a patient with antiphospholipid antibody syndrome and chorea (103–107). Patients with hyperglycemia-induced unilateral basal ganglion lesions with and without hemichorea may have reduced ipsilateral glucose metabolism (108).

Dopaminergic Neurochemical Imaging: Diagnosis of Parkinson Disease

The basal ganglia and the neurotransmitter dopamine have been key targets for research exploring the pathophysiology underlying movement disorders. Dopaminergic neurons from the substantia nigra project as nigrostriatal nerve terminals to the striatum where they have synaptic connections with striatal interneurons or projection neurons. Presynaptic nigrostriatal dopaminergic activity can be imaged using PET radiotracers like [^{18}F]-fluorodopa (FDOPA) or dopamine transporter protein ligands, such as the cocaine analogue [^{11}C]-WIN35428 (Fig. 9.1.6) (109–111). Postsynaptic dopamine D_2 receptor binding can be imaged using the PET tracer [^{11}C]-raclopride (112).

PET studies using presynaptic dopaminergic tracers have objectively demonstrated nigrostriatal nerve terminal loss in Parkinson disease even at a very early or preclinical stage of the disease (113).

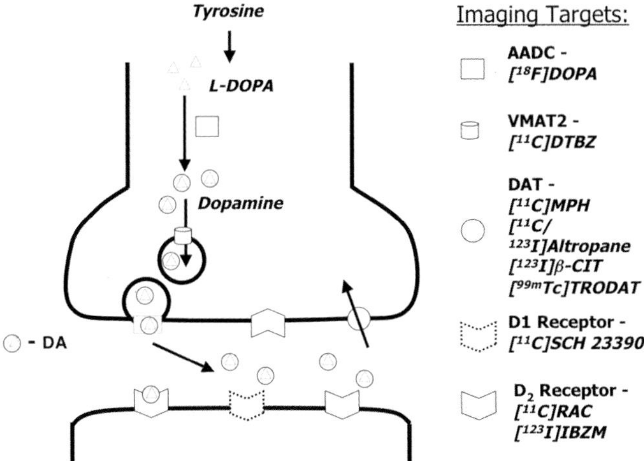

FIGURE 9.1.6. A schematic overview of the nigrostriatal dopamine nerve terminal and a postsynaptic dopamine neuron. Dopamine metabolism (DOPA decarboxylase enzyme activity), vesicular monoamine transporter type 2 (VMAT2), synaptic membrane dopamine transporter, and postsynaptic dopamine receptor type 1 and 2 activity can be studied by PET neurochemical imaging.

Reductions are more severe in the posterior putamen (when compared to the anterior putamen and caudate nucleus) and contralateral to the clinically most affected body side (Fig. 9.1.7) (114,115).

Putaminal FDOPA uptake is also correlated with clinical measures of disease severity, particularly bradykinesia (54,116–118). Therefore, these techniques can provide neurochemical markers to follow progression of disease or evaluate the effects of therapeutic or neurorestorative interventions. For example, fiber outgrowth from transplanted embryonic dopamine neurons, as indicated by an increase in putaminal FDOPA uptake, was detected in patients with severe Parkinson disease (119).

Pre- and Postsynaptic Dopaminergic Neurochemical Imaging: Atypical Parkinsonian Disorders

Nigrostriatal denervation is not specific for Parkinson disease. Presynaptic dopaminergic denervation has also been demonstrated in patients with multiple system atrophy, PSP, corticobasal degeneration, or spinocerebellar atrophy (120–122). Imaging of nigrostriatal dopaminergic system in PSP reveals consistent reductions, with relative regional differences in the intrastriatal pattern of denervation in comparison to Parkinson disease (121,123–127). For example, Ilgin et al. (128) found that striatal dopamine transporter reductions were more pronounced in the posterior putamen in patients with Parkinson disease, while patients with PSP had a relatively uniform degree of involvement of the caudate and putamen.

In addition to presynaptic changes in the nigrostriatal neurons, striatal dopamine receptors are altered in Parkinson disease. For instance, in early idiopathic Parkinson disease uptake of [^{11}C]-raclopride, which is a selective dopamine D_2 receptor ligand, increases in the striatum contralateral to the predominant parkinsonian symptoms compared to the uptake in the ipsilateral striatum (129). This up-regulation may disappear 3 to 5 years later (130). A combined FDG and D_2 receptor PET study found a positive correlation between striatal glucose metabolic activity and receptor expression in Parkinson disease (131).

Studies of the postsynaptic D_2 status have demonstrated normal or increased D_2 receptor density in early Parkinson disease and decreased receptor density in patients with advanced Parkinson disease or atypical parkinsonism, such as multiple system atrophy and progressive supranuclear palsy. Therefore, combined pre- and postsynaptic dopaminergic imaging may distinguish early idiopathic Parkinson disease from atypical parkinsonian disorders (Table 9.1.5). However, combined pre- and postsynaptic dopaminergic imaging may not be able to distinguish atypical parkinsonian disorders from each other or from advanced idiopathic Parkinson disease.

Dopaminergic PET studies should not be used as a substitute for the clinical diagnosis of Parkinson disease. However, neurochemical and functional activation studies may play an important clinical role in the selection of patients with abnormal movements who may benefit from electrical deep brain stimulation. Dopaminergic studies may have a limited clinical role in the diagnosis of patients with symptoms suggestive of Parkinson diseases yet do not respond to typical anti-Parkinson drugs. There is some interest in using dopaminergic PET tracers to aid in the differential diagnosis of essential tremor from early Parkinson disease.

Dopaminergic Neurochemical Imaging: Differential Diagnosis of Parkinsonian or Lewy Body Dementia from Alzheimer Disease

Nigrostriatal dopamine neurons are involved in virtually all patients with parkinsonian dementia, and imaging research studies have demonstrated reduced presynaptic nigrostriatal markers (132,133). Striatal dopaminergic markers are, conversely, normal in Alzheimer disease, and therefore presynaptic dopaminergic imaging can be used for the differential diagnosis between parkinsonian dementia and Alzheimer disease. A subset of patients with parkinsonian dementia present clinically with Parkinson disease, followed later by cognitive decline. These demented subjects have subtle differences from

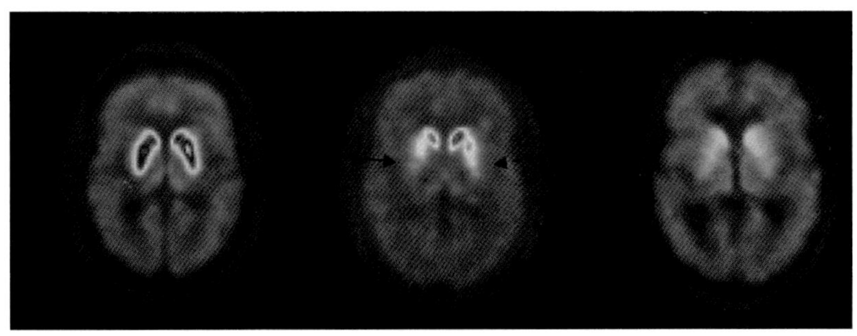

FIGURE 9.1.7. Carbon-11(+) dihydroletrabenazine (DTBZ) PET images of a normal person (**left**), patient with Parkinson disease (**middle**), and parkinsonian dementia (**right**). There is prominent predominant posterior putaminal (*arrow*) and asymmetric (*dashed arrow*) dopaminergic denervation in the patient with Parkinson disease. The patient with parkinsonian dementia has more diffuse and bilateral striatal dopaminergic denervation involving both the putamen and caudate nucleus.

TABLE 9.1.5 Pre- and Postsynaptic Dopaminergic Activity in Idiopathic Parkinson Disease and Atypical Parkinsonian Disorders

	Presynaptic Dopaminergic Nigrostriatal Activity	Postsynaptic Striatal Dopamine Receptor Activity
Early idiopathic Parkinson disease	↓ (esp. posterior putamen)	↑ (up-regulation)
Advanced Parkinson disease	↓	normal or ↓
Atypical parkinsonism (e.g., progressive supranuclear palsy or multiple system atrophy)	↓	↓

Parkinson disease in their nigrostriatal dopamine imaging patterns, with relatively symmetrical and diffuse reduction in presynaptic markers in comparison with the side-to-side and putamen-to-caudate nucleus heterogeneity typical of Parkinson disease (Fig. 9.1.7).

STROKE

Current management of patients with acute stroke is centered on CT and MRI. CT has traditionally played a prominent role by detecting the presence of hemorrhage. However, gradient recalled echo MR may be as accurate as CT for the detection of acute hemorrhage and is also more accurate than CT for the detection of chronic intracerebral hemorrhage (134). MR blood oxygen level-dependent functional imaging is now playing a key role in the very early diagnosis of ischemic stroke (135,136). Multitracer PET imaging has allowed major new insights into the pathophysiology of stroke in humans (137–139). Determinations of CBF, cerebral blood volume (CBV), and cerebral metabolic rate of oxygen ($CMRO_2$) permit the discrimination of various compensatory mechanisms in occlusive vascular disease. For example, compensatory changes in the CBF/CBV ratio (indicating a perfusion reserve) and increases in the oxygen extraction fraction (OEF, a marker of metabolic reserve), may prevent ischemic tissue damage during graded flow decreases (138). It has been possible to document the compensatory responses of the brain to reductions in perfusion pressure using PET and to directly relate these responses to prognosis (139).

Measurement of Cerebral Oxygen Metabolism, Cerebral Blood Volume, and Oxygen Extraction Fraction Using PET

PET measurements of rCBF, cerebral blood volume, oxygen extraction, oxygen and glucose consumption permit a detailed investigation of the pathophysiology of stroke (140). The short-lived PET tracer [^{15}O] (half-life of 123 seconds) was first used to study CBF and cerebral oxygen utilization in man by Ter-Pogossian et al. (141,142). Jones et al. (143) described a noninvasive inhalational method, using steady state kinetics, to measure the distribution of CBF and OEF in the human brain. The continuous inhalation of either molecular [^{15}O] or C^{15}[O_2] produces complementary images in that they relate to regional oxygen uptake and blood flow, offering a direct insight to the regional demand-to-supply relationships within the brain (144).

The method of quantitative measurement of rCBF and $CMRO_2$ has been described in detail by Frackowiak et al. (145). OEF reflects the arterial-venous oxygen difference divided by the arterial oxygen content. Reliable OEF estimates can be obtained by combining dynamic C[^{15}O] and [$^{15}O_2$] scans (146). An expression for OEF can be obtained by dividing the cerebral activity obtained during [^{15}O] inhalation by that obtained during C^{15}[O_2] inhalation with some additional computations (145). The $CMRO_2$ can be derived from the relationship (145):

$$CMRO_2 = CBF \times OEF \times \text{Total blood oxygen count (from arterial blood sample)}.$$

Using these methods Frackowiak et al. found normal values of $CMRO_2$ of 1.81 ± 0.22 mL O_2/100 mL/min in mean white matter and 5.88 ± 0.57 mL O_2/100 mL/min in temporal gray matter. Corresponding values for CBF were 21.4 ± 1.9 mL /100 mL/min in mean white matter and 65.3 ± 7.0 mL /100 mL/min in mean temporal lobe gray matter (145).

Methods other than the steady-state inhalation method have been developed to measure CBF and $CMRO_2$, such as the autoradiographic CBF method using intravenous H_2[^{15}O] and newer dynamic methods (147). Cerebral blood volume can be measured by inhalation of C[^{15}O] (148). Quantitative imaging of the OEF has been shown to be of invaluable help in the assessment of the pattern of CBF-$CMRO_2$ coupling (149). Ideally, glucose utilization should be measured simultaneously with $CMRO_2$ in order to provide an accurate assessment of regional energy metabolism. Glucose utilization and oxygen use may become uncoupled in acute stroke and this uncoupling may go in two opposite directions, either aerobic glycolysis with relatively increased glucose consumption, or use of substrates for oxidation other than glucose (149). Table 9.1.6

TABLE 9.1.6 Different Pathophysiological Conditions in Stroke

Condition	CBF	$CMRO_2$	OEF
Ischemia	low	low	very high
Oligemia	moderately low	normal	high
Luxury perfusion	low/normal/high	low	low

CBF, cerebral blood flow; $CMRO_2$, cerebral metabolic rate of oxygen; OEF, oxygen extraction fraction.
(From Baron JC, Frackowiak RS, Herholz K, et al. Use of PET methods for measurement of cerebral energy metabolism and hemodynamics in cerebrovascular disease. *J Cereb Blood Flow Metab* 1989;9:723–742, with permission.)

TABLE 9.1.7 Ischemic Thresholds and Regional Cerebral Blood Flow in Human and Nonhuman Primates

CBF Threshold	Clinical Correlates
20 cc/100 g/min	EEG and evoked cortical potential abnormalities appear, paralysis seen in awake monkeys
15 cc/100 g/min	EEG and evoked cortical potentials are lost
12 cc/100 g/min	Flow values at this level in excess of 120 minutes produce infarction in animals
6 cc/100 g/min	Massive loss of intracellular potassium

CBF, cerebral blood flow; EEG, electroencephalogram.
(From Morawetz RB, Crowell RH, DeGirolami U, et al. Regional cerebral blood flow thresholds during cerebral ischemia. *Fed Proc* 1979;38: 2493–2494, with permission.)

summarizes different pathophysiological conditions in stroke (from Baron et al. [149]).

Acute Ischemic Stroke

Brain tissue infarction may follow a critical reduction in rCBF and may lead to neurological deficits. The more severe the drop in perfusion the higher the chance of irreversible brain tissue damage (150). The development of methods of determining rCBF has made possible the determination of thresholds for the appearance of cerebral ischemia (Table 9.1.7). These thresholds vary depending on the method used for assessing cerebral ischemia. The presence of low attenuation changes on CT in acute stroke has been found to correlate with severe hypoperfusion (less than 12 mL/100 g/min) on CBF PET (151). It should be noted that not only the level of residual CBF but also the duration of ischemia will determine the presence of irreversible infarction.

A prerequisite for the successful treatment of acute ischemic stroke is the existence of viable tissue that is morphologically intact but functionally impaired due to flow decreases below a certain threshold. The ischemic penumbra is defined as tissue with flow falling within the thresholds for maintenance of function and of morphologic integrity (152). Early in the course of acute ischemia, CBF and $CMRO_2$ levels falling below certain thresholds may lead to irreversible tissue damage, while preservation of $CMRO_2$ with decreased flow resulting in increased OEF ("misery" perfusion) still suggests viable tissue ("penumbra") (153).

Identification of viable or penumbra tissue is the key target for interventional therapy in acute ischemic stroke. Rapid restoration of blood flow to the penumbra even in the presence of a fixed deficit at the center of the stroke may improve stroke outcome. Identification of penumbra tissue can be achieved by multitracer PET (138). It should be noted that MR-defined mismatch between diffusion-weighted and perfusion-weighted imaging does not reliably detect elevated OEF and overestimates the penumbra defined by PET (154). Diffusion-weighted imaging lesions on MR showed impaired tissue integrity (low $CMRO_2$ and low OEF); mismatch areas were viable (normal $CMRO_2$) but showed largely varying OEF (154). Therefore, the MR-defined diffusion-perfusion mismatch overestimates the volume of penumbra and therefore the tissue at risk.

Subacute Changes in Ischemic Stroke

In subacute states of cerebral ischemia reduced blood flow can be compensated by increased blood volume and, when perfusion reserve is exhausted, OEF may increase up to 48 hours after the onset of stroke (138). This condition, also called misery perfusion, implies that blood flow is inadequate relative to the energy metabolic tissue demand for oxygen (138). Penumbra tissue can be seen as a stable rim of tissue surrounding the core of infarction but may also change in time as a dynamic phenomenon, involving new adjacent tissue compartments while others are becoming permanently necrotic (138). Studies identifying penumbra tissue could be of value in the development of effective therapeutic strategies even in the subacute stage of stroke (138).

Some patients may have postischemic reactive hyperemia that occurs within hours or days after stroke onset. This phenomenon is called luxury perfusion and is seen in the periphery of an ischemic stroke. Unlike misery perfusion, luxury perfusion is seen as increased CBF and a low OER (138,149). Luxury perfusion may reflect recanalization of an occluded artery (149).

Chronic Arterial Occlusive Disease and Hemodynamic Reserve

Hemodynamic factors may play an important role in the pathogenesis of ischemic stroke in patients with cerebrovascular disease (155). Patients with arterial occlusive disease are protected against ischemic episodes to a certain extent by compensatory mechanisms, which may help to prevent ischemia when perfusion pressure drops (138). Severe atherosclerotic disease of the carotid and vertebral arteries may lead to reduced perfusion pressure (156). This may cause hemodynamic impairment of the distal cerebral circulation. It should be noted that CBF studies alone do not adequately assess cerebral hemodynamic status as CBF may be maintained by autoregulatory vasodilation and even low CBF values may not correlate with perfusion pressures (155).

Functional imaging techniques can be used to assess two basic categories of hemodynamic impairment. The first category reflects a state of autoregulatory vasodilation secondary to reduced perfusion pressure that can be assessed by the measurement of either increased cerebral blood volume or an impaired CBF response to a vasodilatory stimulus. The second category is defined on the basis of OEF measurements (increased OEF) (155).

Compensatory regional vasodilation may manifest itself as a focal increase in CBV in the supply territory of the occluded artery (138,157). Here, the ratio of CBF to CBV has been used as an indicator of local perfusion pressure or perfusion reserve (normal: 10) (138). The lower the value, the lower the flow velocity (138). When the perfusion pressure is exhausted (i.e., at maximal vasodilatation), any further decrease in arterial input pressure will produce a proportional decrease in both CBF and the CBF/CBV ratio (138). In this type of hemodynamic decompensation, the brain will exploit oxygen carriage reserve to prevent energy failure and loss of function, as evidenced by an increase in OEF (156,157).

The relative importance of hemodynamic factors in the pathogenesis of stroke in patients with carotid arterial occlusive disease was investigated in the St. Louis Carotid Occlusion Study (158,159).

This study demonstrated that increased cerebral OEF detected by PET scanning predicted future stroke in patients with symptomatic carotid occlusion. The study demonstrated that ipsilateral increased OEF measured by PET is a powerful independent risk factor for subsequent stroke in patients with symptomatic complete carotid artery occlusion. The ipsilateral ischemic stroke rate at 2 years was shown to be 5.3% in 42 patients with normal OEF and 26.5% in 39 patients with increased OEF. In patients in whom hemispheric symptoms developed within 120 days, the 2-year ipsilateral stroke rates were 12% in 27 patients with normal OEF and 50% in 18 patients with increased OEF (159). Previous PET studies have demonstrated that anastomosis of the superficial temporal artery to a middle cerebral artery cortical branch can restore OEF to normal. Consequently, a trial of extracranial-to-intracranial arterial bypass for this group of patients is being conducted in St. Louis (159,160).

It should be noted that correlation between different methods to assess impaired blood flow response to a vasodilatory stimulus with each other and with methods that assess OEF is quite variable (155). Vasodilatory hemodynamic stress testing relies on paired blood flow measurements with the initial measurement obtained at rest and the second measurement obtained following a cerebral vasodilatory stimulus (155). A comparison of the reststress perfusion may provide an estimate of cerebrovascular reserve. Acetazolamide or inhaling carbon dioxide have been used as vasodilatory stimuli (155). Acetazolamide is a carbonic anhydrase inhibitor that increases the carbon dioxide in the brain. Each vasodilator stimulus will result in a significant increase in CBF in normal persons. If the CBF response is muted or absent, pre-existing autoregulatory cerebral vasodilatation due to reduced cerebral perfusion pressure is inferred (155). The blood flow responses to vasodilator stress have been categorized into several grades of hemodynamic impairment: (a) reduced augmentation (relative to the contralateral hemisphere or normal controls); (b) absent augmentation (same as baseline); and (c) paradoxical reduction in rCBF ("steal" phenomenon) (155). Although commonly applied, it should be noted that there is a lack of well-controlled prognostic studies on the use of these vasodilator rest-stress techniques in patients with cerebrovascular disease (155,161). However, a recent study measuring OEF reactivity with acetazolamide found preliminary evidence that positive OEF reactivity may identify hemodynamic compromise despite normal baseline OEF (162). Abnormal OEF reactivity may also be associated with subcortical white matter infarcts (162).

Hemorrhagic Stroke

The importance of ischemia as a secondary mechanism of brain injury has been addressed in subarachnoid hemorrhage and intracranial hematoma (139). Multitracer PET studies of patients with subarachnoid hemorrhage but without vasospasm have shown a significant reduction in global $CMRO_2$ with no significant change in global OEF, suggesting a primary reduction in $CMRO_2$ in the absence of vasospasm (163). However, subarachnoid hemorrhage complicated by vasospasm has been found to be associated with significantly increased regional OEF with unchanged $CMRO_2$, indicative of cerebral ischemia without infarction (163). PET studies of patients with intracerebral intraparenchymal hemorrhage have shown reduced CBF surrounding the primary bleeding site (164). PET demonstrated that hematomas exert a primary depression of metabolism rather than inducing ischemia in the surrounding tissue. It also documented the integrity of autoregulation and provided clinically useful information regarding the safety of blood pressure reduction after intracranial hematoma (139).

Estimation of Prognosis After Stroke

Functional recovery after focal brain lesions is dependent on the adaptive plasticity of the cerebral cortex and of the nonaffected elements of the functional network (165). Therefore, the degree of functional recovery after a stroke is related to the location and size of the lesion, the presence of remaining neurons in the neighborhood of the lesion, and the presence of compensatory mechanisms in functionally connected networks (138). Rather than a complete substitution of function, the main mechanism underlying recovery of motor abilities involves enhanced activity in pre-existing networks, including the disconnected motor cortex in subcortical stroke and the infarct rim after cortical stroke (166). Although the regional cerebral metabolic rate of glucose in early ischemia is often not coupled to flow or $CMRO_2$ and might even be increased, regional cerebral glucose metabolism is the best indicator of permanent impairment of tissue function (138). A normal FDG PET or the presence of a mild metabolic abnormality has been strongly associated with good clinical outcome or complete reversal of the neurological dysfunction (167). In contrast, patients with poor clinical outcomes had more severe glucose metabolic deficits (167).

The presence of early luxury perfusion in the context of little or no metabolic alteration may also indicate a favorable prognosis (168). A study comparing early and delayed PET studies in patients with stroke found that in hyperperfused regions, the acute-stage perfusion, blood volume, and oxygen consumption were significantly increased, and the OEF was significantly reduced, while all these variables had significantly returned toward normality in the chronic-stage PET study. The ultimately infarcted area did not exhibit significant hyperperfusion in the acute stage (168). These data indicate that early reperfusion into metabolically active tissue is beneficial.

Clinical Applicability of Multitracer PET in the Management of Patients with Stroke

In the field of cerebrovascular disease, PET has served as a specialized research tool at a few centers to help elucidate the pathophysiology of stroke. PET studies are time-consuming, expensive, and require extensive facilities and technical support. Although PET has not been demonstrated to be necessary for making patient care decisions (139), knowledge gained from PET regarding acute ischemic stroke and chronic oligemia from arterial occlusive disease is growing more important with the increasing availability of CT and MR perfusion techniques.

New Emerging Clinical Applications of PET in Stroke: Neuronal and Hypoxia Imaging

New tracers, such as receptor ligands or hypoxia markers, may further improve the identification of penumbra tissue in the future (152,169). Clinical application of such techniques may permit the extension of the critical time period for inclusion of patients for aggressive stroke management strategies. CBF and FDG PET studies of patients with stroke may not only show the local effects caused by the primary stroke lesion but also demonstrate remote effects because of diaschisis. Central benzodiazepine receptor ligands, such as [^{11}C]-flumazenil, are markers of neuronal integrity and therefore may be useful in the differentiation of functionally and morphologically damaged tissue in stroke. [^{11}C]-flumazenil PET imaging has the potential to depict damaged brain tissue by directly assessing neuronal loss. A study demonstrated the feasibility of [^{11}C]-flumazenil PET imaging in distinguishing between irreversibly damaged and viable penumbra tissue early after acute stroke (170). In subacute and chronic states after stroke, functional impairment without morphologic lesions on CT could be attributed to silent infarctions characterized by significant reduction of benzodiazepine binding (171).

[^{18}F]-fluoromisonidazole (FMISO) is a PET hypoxia marker that has been validated to map the penumbra in acute stroke (172,173). A rat study demonstrated elevated FMISO uptake in the stroke area only in the early phase of arterial occlusion, but not after early reperfusion nor when tissue necrosis has developed (174). FMISO PET may be able to identify true penumbral tissue that would be amenable to rescue interventions even beyond 12 to 24 hours after stroke onset (173).

EPILEPSY

Epileptic syndromes are classified as generalized and partial types of seizures. Primary generalized epilepsy is associated with diffuse and bilateral epileptiform discharges on electroencephalogram (EEG) without evidence of focal brain lesions. In contrast, partial epilepsy is thought to arise from a focal gray matter lesion. Partial-onset seizures may remain partial or may secondarily generalize. Medically refractory epilepsy is defined by seizure syndromes that are not effectively controlled by antiepileptic drugs.

The management of medically refractory partial epilepsy has been revolutionized by neurosurgical techniques aimed at the resection of the epileptogenic brain focus. Therefore, precise seizure localization is the prime goal of presurgical work-up. EEG monitoring and structural brain imaging using MRI are part of the standard work-up of patients with epilepsy undergoing presurgical evaluation. FDG PET can provide additional localizing information in patients with nonlocalizing surface ictal EEG and can reduce the number of patients requiring intracranial EEG studies (175). Even when intracranial EEG is required, FDG PET can be helpful in guiding placement of subdural grids or depth electrodes prior to surgical ablative therapy. PET imaging should always be performed before intracranial EEG as prior depth electrode insertion can cause small hypometabolic regions that may lead to false-positive PET interpretations (176).

Regional Glucose Hypometabolism as Interictal Expression of Epileptogenic Foci

Unlike patients with primary generalized epilepsy who have no interictal abnormalities on CBF or FDG PET studies (177), interictal FDG PET studies can identify epileptogenic foci in patients with partial epilepsy on the basis of regional cortical glucose hypometabolism (178). It should be noted that FDG PET may show more widespread hypometabolism than suspected on the basis of the scalp-recorded EEG (175). The pathophysiology of interictal cortical hypometabolism in partial epilepsy is poorly understood. Areas of interictal hypometabolism in epileptogenic cortex appear to be partially uncoupled from blood flow with metabolic reductions being greater relative to flow (179).

Although there are significant correlations between hippocampal volume and inferior mesial and lateral temporal lobe cerebral metabolic rates in patients with temporal lobe epilepsy (180), studies have failed to find a significant correlation between cortical metabolism on preoperative FDG PET imaging and neuronal density of resected hippocampi (181). Therefore, hippocampal neuronal loss cannot fully account for the regional interictal hypometabolism of temporal lobe epilepsy. It is possible that synaptic mechanisms rather than cell loss may contribute to the observed hypometabolism (182). Children with a new onset of seizures are less likely to have hypometabolism (177). A longer duration of temporal lobe epilepsy is associated with greater hippocampal hypometabolism, suggesting that epilepsy is a progressive disease (183). Hypometabolism may reflect the effects of persistent epilepsy on the brain (184).

Regional Glucose Hypometabolism in Temporal Lobe Epilepsy

Mesial temporal lobe epilepsy is the most common type of partial epilepsy and is commonly associated with hippocampal sclerosis. FDG PET has high sensitivity in detecting temporal hypometabolic foci and can be visualized as a region of reduced metabolism, which when compared to the normal temporal lobe may show a significant asymmetry in FDG uptake (185). The severity of glucose hypometabolism correlates with the amount of interictal delta activity on EEG (186). It should be noted that false lateralization is rare but may occur. For example, unrecognized epileptic activity can make the contralateral temporal lobe appear spuriously depressed (176). Normal right-to-left asymmetry between temporal lobes should not be interpreted as pathological hypometabolism.

Although FDG PET images can be analyzed visually, additional information can be obtained by semiquantitative analysis, such as left-to-right asymmetry indices. Semiquantitative analysis using the asymmetry index is generally considered significant when a difference of 15% or greater exists between the affected and contralateral sides (187). Quantitative asymmetry indices should reduce potential error due to misinterpreting these normal left-to-right variations (188). Registration programs can be used to align structural MRI and PET for more precise anatomic localization of the hypometabolic area.

Although regional hypometabolism is typically present in the temporal lobe ipsilateral to EEG seizure onset, other brain regions may also show patterns of glucose hypometabolism (Fig. 9.1.8). For example, an FDG PET study of patients with temporal lobe epilepsy demonstrated hypometabolic regions ipsilateral to seizure onset that included lateral temporal (in 78% of patients), mesial temporal (70%), thalamic (63%), basal ganglia (41%), frontal (30%), parietal (26%), and occipital (4%) regions (189).

The prevalence of thalamic hypometabolism suggests a pathophysiologic role for the thalamus in initiation or propagation of temporal lobe seizures (189). Cerebellar hypometabolism may be ipsilateral, contralateral, or bilateral, depending on the distribution and spread of ictal activity and possible effects of phenytoin therapy (Fig. 9.1.2) (36,176). Bilateral cerebellar hypometabolism, which is often present, cannot be fully explained by the effects of phenytoin (36).

Unilateral temporal hypometabolism predicts good surgical outcome from temporal lobectomy. The greater the metabolic asymmetry the greater the chance of becoming seizure free (176). Bilateral temporal hypometabolism may represent a relative

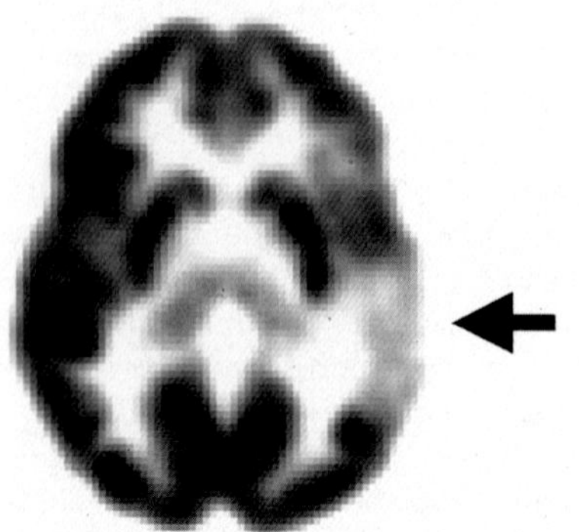

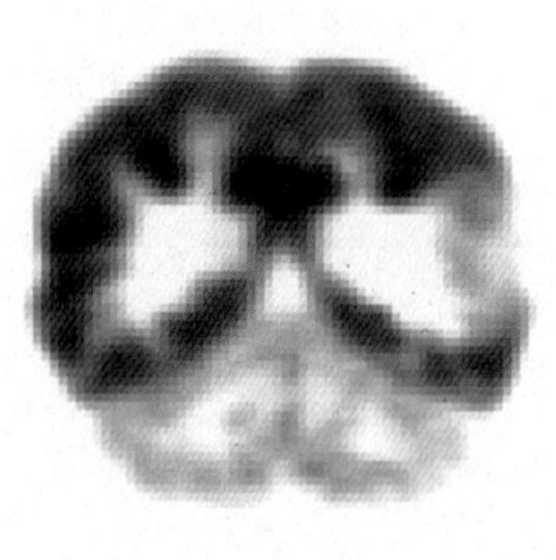

FIGURE 9.1.8. An interictal fluorodeoxyglucose PET study of a patient with a left lateral and posterior temporal seizure focus. There is an extensive area of hypometabolism (*arrow*) in addition to bilateral thalamic and cerebellar hypometabolic changes.

contraindication for surgery (176). Similarly, thalamic asymmetry on FDG PET is a strong predictor of surgical outcome; hypometabolism in the thalamus contralateral to the presumed EEG focus almost invariably predicts poor surgical outcome (190). Extratemporal cortical hypometabolism outside the seizure focus, in particular hypometabolism in the contralateral cerebral cortex, may also be associated with a poorer postoperative seizure outcome in temporal lobe epilepsy and may represent underlying pathology that is potentially epileptogenic (191). Preoperative extratemporal hypometabolism of the inferior frontal lobe and thalamus in temporal lobe epilepsy may be partially reversible after ipsilateral temporal lobe resection (192).

FDG PET is most useful for those patients with temporal lobe epilepsy who have equivocal or no structural MRI abnormalities to provide the necessary lateralization information (180,193). Although most patients with temporal lobe epilepsy will have the finding of hippocampal sclerosis on a high resolution MRI, a significant minority of patients with electroclinically well-lateralized temporal lobe seizures have no evidence of sclerosis on MRI (194). A recent study from Australia found that patients with MRI-negative temporal lobe epilepsy had interictal glucose hypometabolism that primarily involved the lateral neocortical rather than the mesiotemporal structures (195). Statistical parametric mapping analysis may help to distinguish lateral from mesial temporal lobe epilepsy (196).

Extratemporal Epilepsy

FDG PET may not be as valuable in the evaluation of patients with extratemporal seizures, such as frontal lobe epilepsy, because of limited sensitivity (188,197). Areas of hypometabolism in extratemporal lobe epilepsy have been found to be focal, regional, or hemispheric (Fig. 9.1.9) (198).

Large zones of extrafrontal, particularly temporal, hypometabolism are commonly observed ipsilateral to frontal hypometabolism in frontal lobe epilepsies (13). Recent data show that observer-independent automatic statistical brain mapping techniques may increase the usefulness of FDG PET in patients with extratemporal lobe epilepsy (199). For example, a study using an automated brain mapping method found significantly higher sensitivity in detecting the epileptogenic focus (67%) than visual analysis (19% to 38%) in patients with extratemporal epilepsy (200).

Hypometabolic regions in partial epilepsies of neocortical origin have usually been associated with structural imaging abnormalities (197). Therefore, PET data should always be interpreted in the context of high-quality anatomical MRI, providing a structural-functional correlation. Interictal hypometabolism may be uncommon in the absence of a colocalized structural imaging abnormality in frontal lobe epilepsy (13). Interictal FDG PET studies will have limited usefulness in the presence of multiple hypometabolic regions in patients with multifocal brain syndromes, such as in children with tuberous sclerosis. Such children with multifocal lesions represent a special challenge during presurgical evaluation. The goal of functional imaging in these cases is to identify the epileptogenic lesions and differentiate them from nonepileptogenic ones. In this context, ictal rCBF SPECT may have useful clinical applications but may be technically challenging when seizures are short, as is particularly common in frontal lobe epilepsy and in children who have infantile spasms that are associated with multifocal cortical dysplasia (201).

Glucose Metabolic PET Studies of Children with Infantile Spasms

Infantile spasms (West syndrome) are age-specific epileptic phenomena with many underlying etiologies. An infantile spasm is an epileptic syndrome that begins in early infancy where children have tonic

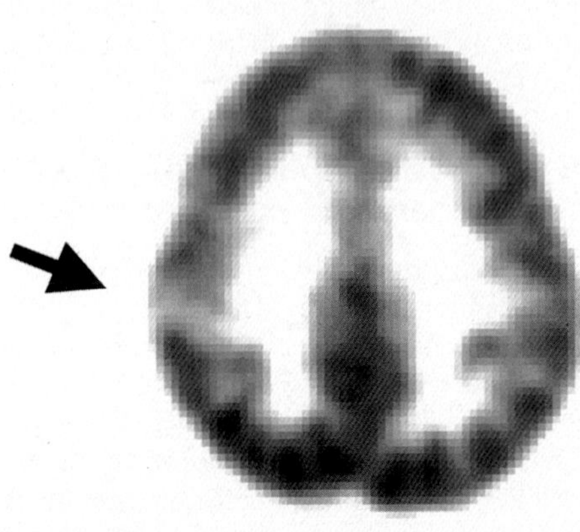

FIGURE 9.1.9. An interictal fluorodeoxyglucose PET study of patient with partial epilepsy shows a focus of right parietal hypometabolism (*arrow*).

and myoclonic seizures, arrhythmia on EEG, and developmental arrest. When the comprehensive evaluation, including MRI scan, fails to reveal the cause of the spasms and the seizures are refractory to medical treatment, a PET scan of glucose metabolism should be performed without further delay (202). Glucose metabolism PET studies in children with intractable cryptogenic infantile spasms have shown unifocal and, more commonly, multifocal cortical areas of hypometabolism interictally (203). Most infants who are diagnosed with "cryptogenic" spasms have, in fact, focal or multifocal cortical regions of decreased (or even occasionally increased) glucose metabolic activity on PET that are often consistent with areas of cortical dysplasia missed by MRI (204,205). When a single region of abnormal glucose hypometabolism is apparent on PET and is congruent with the EEG findings and the seizures are intractable, surgical removal of the PET focus results in seizure control and in complete or partial reversal of the associated developmental delay (201). When the pattern of glucose hypometabolism is generalized and symmetric, a lesional cause is not likely and neurogenetic or neurometabolic disorders should be considered when further evaluating the child (201).

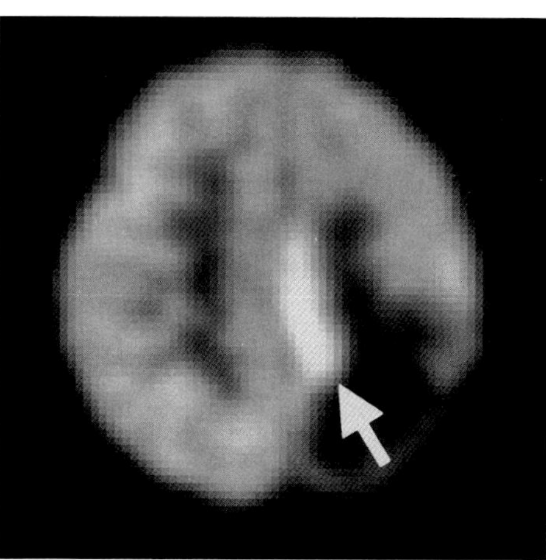

FIGURE 9.1.10. Five-year-old child suffered a left parieto-occipital stroke caused by left thalamic and intraventricular hemorrhage and subsequently the onset of seizures. An ictal fluorodeoxyglucose PET study demonstrates metabolic activation of the left posterior cinguloparietal cortex (*arrow*) adjacent to the stroke lesion.

Glucose Metabolic PET Studies in Lennox-Gastaut Syndrome

Lennox-Gastaut syndrome is a childhood epileptic encephalopathy characterized by an electroclinical triad of 1.0 to 2.5 Hz spike-wave pattern on EEG, intellectual impairment, and multiple types of epileptic seizures. Although the etiology is cryptogenic in about a fourth of all patients, symptomatic cases are due to diverse cerebral conditions, which are usually bilateral, diffuse, or multifocal, and involve cerebral gray matter (206). FDG PET studies have shown that Lennox-Gastaut syndrome can be classified into four predominant subtypes, each with a distinct metabolic pattern: normal, unilateral focal hypometabolism, unilateral diffuse hypometabolism, and bilateral diffuse hypometabolism (207). Patients who have the unilateral focal or unilateral diffuse patterns may be considered for cortical resection (201). Correlation of FDG PET and EEG studies in the Lennox-Gastaut syndrome suggest that an EEG pattern of 1.0 to 2.5 Hz spike-wave activity (slow spike-wave pattern) is an interictal phenomenon (208).

Interictal $H_2[^{15}O]$ Cerebral Blood Flow PET Studies

It should be noted that interictal $H_2[^{15}O]$ CBF PET studies when compared to FDG PET studies have reduced sensitivity in localizing epileptogenic zones and sometimes may even be false lateralizing (209). Furthermore, CBF PET scans are noisier compared to FDG PET, which may increase partial volume effects and make detection of a hypoperfused area more difficult. Therefore, interictal CBF PET studies are unreliable markers for epileptic foci and should not be used in the presurgical evaluation of patients with epilepsy (179).

Ictal PET

Although logistically challenging, FDG PET can also be used for ictal studies in patients who have frequent seizures (Fig. 9.1.10) (210,211). Chugani et al. (210) identified three ictal glucose metabolic patterns in children based on the degree and type of subcortical involvement. Nine children had type I: asymmetric glucose metabolism of the striatum and thalamus. Of these, the seven oldest children showed unilateral cortical hypermetabolism (always including frontal cortex) and crossed cerebellar hypermetabolism. Two infants (aged less than 1 year) had a similar ictal PET pattern but no cerebellar asymmetry, presumably owing to immaturity of corticopontocerebellar projections. Five children had type II: symmetric metabolic abnormalities of striatum and thalamus. This pattern was accompanied by hippocampal or insular cortex hypermetabolism, diffuse neocortical hypometabolism, and absence of any cerebellar abnormality. Four children had type III: hypermetabolism restricted to the cerebral cortex.

FDG PET may be less accurate for ictal compared to interictal glucose metabolic measurements since seizures may alter the "lumped constant," which describes the relationship between FDG and its physiologic substrate glucose (176). Furthermore, a typical seizure is much shorter than the average 30-minute FDG uptake period. Therefore, an "ictal" scan may include interictal, ictal, and postictal metabolic changes with combinations of hypermetabolic and hypometabolic regions (176). $H_2[^{15}O]$ PET imaging has been used to study quantitative alterations in rCBF accompanying seizures induced by pentylenetetrazol (212). Patients with generalized tonic-clonic seizures demonstrated asymmetric flow increases. One patient with a complex partial seizure demonstrated 70% to 80% increases in bitemporal flow. Thalamic flow increased during both complex partial and generalized seizures, indicating the importance of this subcortical structure during ictal activation (212).

Mapping of Cognitive or Language Functions

Changes in the functional activity of the brain (e.g., motor activity, language, or cognitive tasks) are accompanied by increases in rCBF and can be mapped to specific brain regions (3,4). Language-based PET activation studies have shown good correlation with the Wada language lateralization test (213). More detailed cortical mapping can be performed to better delineate the motor cortex from the epileptogenic zone. Cortical mapping using PET activation studies have shown comparable results to electrical stimulation mapping of the cortex using subdural electrodes (214).

Emerging Clinical Applications of Benzodiazepine Neuroreceptor and Serotonin Synthesis Imaging in Epilepsy

The inhibitory neurotransmitter γ-aminobutyric acid (GABA) has anticonvulsant properties. Benzodiazepine receptor ligands, such as [^{11}C]-flumazenil (FMZ), have been used to study the regional cerebral distribution of benzodiazepine receptor binding sites that are related to $GABA_A$ receptors. The high density of $GABA_A$ receptors in the normal hippocampus accounts for the high sensitivity of FMZ PET to detect even mild decreases in binding that are consistent with hippocampal sclerosis in temporal lobe epilepsy. FMZ PET, where available, provides a useful alternative to FDG PET in the evaluation of patients with epilepsy.

A regional decrease in benzodiazepine receptor binding has been associated with the presence of a possible epileptogenic focus. Unilaterally decreased temporal FMZ binding can also help to lateralize the epileptic focus in patients who have temporal lobe epilepsy that is associated with bilateral temporal hypometabolism on FDG PET (201). When compared to FDG studies, FMZ PET studies have been reported to demonstrate less extensive cortical involvement. For example, a study comparing FDG and FMZ PET imaging in patients with temporal lobe epilepsy found a wide range of mesial temporal, lateral temporal, and thalamic glucose hypometabolism ipsilateral to ictal EEG changes as well as extratemporal hypometabolism. In contrast, each patient demonstrated decreased benzodiazepine receptor binding in the ipsilateral anterior mesial temporal region, without neocortical changes.

Interictal metabolic dysfunction can be variable and usually is extensive in temporal lobe epilepsy, whereas decreased central benzodiazepine receptor density appears to be more restricted to the mesial temporal areas (215). Similar benzodiazepine receptor findings have been reported for patients with extratemporal lobe seizures caused by focal cortical dysplasia (216). Unlike the more widespread glucose hypometabolic patterns, benzodiazepine receptor changes may reflect localized neuronal loss that is more specific to the epileptogenic zone (215). Therefore, FMZ imaging may be useful in the presurgical evaluation of patients with epilepsy. However, focal increases of benzodiazepine receptor binding have also been reported in the temporal lobe as well as extratemporal sites in patients with temporal lobe epilepsy when statistical brain mapping analysis is performed (217). This may lead to false-localizing information when attention is only paid to areas of decreased uptake.

A potential clinical application of FMZ PET is the detection of periventricular increases of FMZ binding, indicating the presence of heterotopic neurons in patients with temporal lobe epilepsy (218). The presence of such increases correlates with a poorer outcome.

Another promising direction in the development of PET for epilepsy is to target serotonergic neurotransmission. A novel tracer, α-[^{11}C]-methyl-L-tryptophan (AMT), which accumulates in epileptic foci in the interictal state, can be a useful approach to identify epileptogenic sites in children with multifocal brain lesions (201,219). FMISO PET helps to differentiate between epileptogenic and nonepileptogenic lesions in a patient with multifocal lesions. Because fluoromisonidazole accumulates in the vicinity of the seizure focus, PET scanning of this radiotracer reveals an increased signal in the interictal state compared to FDG and FMZ, which both reveal decreased uptake (202). This radiotracer may also be useful in identifying nonresected epileptic cortex in young patients with a previously failed neocortical epilepsy surgery (220).

CONCLUSION

PET is a method for quantitative and qualitative imaging of regional physiological and biochemical parameters. With the tomographic principle of the PET scanner the quantitative distribution of the administered isotope can be determined in the brain, and images can be provided as well as dynamic information on blood flow, metabolism, and neuroreceptor function. Glucose metabolic and blood flow studies have been used for the study of patients with brain disorders, such as epilepsy, tumor, stroke, or dementia. New techniques for quantitative image processing and statistical brain mapping analysis using normative databases will aid the clinical utility of brain PET. Measurement of receptors or neurotransmitter metabolism is a unique ability of PET that has not achieved its full potential in the study of patients with neurological disorders. PET has the ability to visualize and quantify key pathophysiological processes underlying specific brain disorders and may serve as a tool not only for diagnosis but also for the assessment of effects of therapeutic interventions.

FDG PET imaging can identify specific topographic patterns that can aid the clinical differential diagnosis of the major atypical parkinsonian movement disorders (i.e., corticobasal degeneration, multiple system atrophy, and progressive supranuclear palsy). Parkinsonian dementia can be distinguished from Alzheimer disease on the basis of occipital hypometabolism. Neurochemical dopaminergic imaging can identify nigrostriatal denervation seen in Parkinson disease and may serve as a diagnostic or outcome biomarker in this disorder. Other parkinsonian neurodegenerations, including progressive supranuclear palsy and multiple system atrophy, also involve nigrostriatal dopaminergic projection losses but are characterized by additional degeneration within the striatum and other subcortical nuclei.

Multitracer PET imaging permits the accurate and quantitative assessment of regional hemodynamics and metabolism in stroke that may guide therapeutic decisions and predict the severity of permanent deficits. However, PET studies are time consuming, expensive, and require extensive facilities and technical support. Although PET has not been demonstrated to be necessary for making patient care decisions in stroke patients, knowledge gained from PET regarding acute ischemic stroke and chronic oligemia from arterial occlusive disease is growing more important with the increasing availability of CT and MR perfusion techniques. A new potential clinical role for PET in stroke may be the application of new hypoxia PET tracers, such as FMISO, that identify true penumbral tissue that would be amenable to rescue interventions even beyond 12 to 24 hours after the onset of stroke.

Although the primary imaging modality in the management of epilepsy is MRI, FDG and benzodiazepine receptor PET imaging often provide complementary information and, in patients with normal or nonlocalizing MRI, may provide unique localizing information. AMT PET has the potential to differentiate between epileptogenic and nonepileptogenic lesions in a patient with multifocal lesions, such as in a child with tuberous sclerosis.

REFERENCES

1. Siesjo BK. *Brain energy metabolism*. New York: Wiley, 1978.
2. Sandor P. Nervous control of the cerebrovascular system: doubts and facts. *Neurochem Int* 1999;35:237–259.
3. Raichle ME. Circulatory and metabolic correlates of brain function in normal humans. In: Mountcastle VB, Plum F, eds. *Handbook of physiology. The nervous system*. Bethesda: American Physiological Society, 1987: vol V, 643–674.
4. Raichle ME. The metabolic requirements of functional activity in the brain. In: Vranic M, Efendie S, Hollenberg CH, eds. *Fuel homeostasis and the nervous system*. New York: Plenum Press, 1991:1–4.
5. Buxton RB, Frank LR. A model for the coupling between cerebral blood flow and oxygen metabolism during neural stimulation. *J Cereb Blood Flow Metab* 1997;17:64–72.
6. Vafaee MS, Gjedde A. Model of blood–brain transfer of oxygen explains nonlinear flow-metabolism coupling during stimulation of visual cortex. *J Cereb Blood Flow Metab* 2000;20:747–754.
7. Mintun MA, Lundstrom BN, Snyder AZ, et al. Blood flow and oxygen delivery to human brain during functional activity: theoretical modeling and experimental data. *Proc Natl Acad Sci U S A* 2001;98: 6859–6864.
8. Magistretti PJ. Neuron-glia metabolic coupling and plasticity. *J Exp Biol* 2006;209:2304–2311.
9. Jueptner M, Weiller C. Review: does measurement of regional cerebral blood flow reflect synaptic activity? Implications for PET and fMRI. *Neurimage* 1995;2:148–156.
10. Magistretti PJ, Pellerin L. Cellular mechanisms of brain energy metabolism and their relevance to functional brain imaging. *Philos Trans R Soc Lond B Biol Sci* 1999;354:1155–1163.
11. Hoffman EJ, Huang SC, Phelps ME. Quantitation in positron emission computed tomography: 1. Effect of object size. *J Comput Assist Tomogr* 1979;3:299–308.
12. Minoshima S, Koeppe RA, Frey KA, et al. Stereotactic PET atlas of the human brain: aid for visual interpretation of functional brain images. *J Nucl Med* 1994;35:949–954.
13. Henry TR, Mazziotta JC, Engel JJ. The functional anatomy of frontal lobe epilepsy studied with PET. *Adv Neurol* 1992;57:449–463.
14. Perlmutter JS, Powers WJ, Herscovitch P, et al. Regional asymmetries of cerebral blood flow, blood volume, and oxygen utilization and extraction in normal subjects. *J Cereb Blood Flow Metab* 1987; 7:64–67.
15. Lobaugh NJ, Caldwell CB, Black SE, et al. Three brain SPECT region-of-interest templates in elderly people: normative values, hemispheric asymmetries, and a comparison of single- and multihead cameras. *J Nucl Med* 2000;41:45–56.
16. Mazziotta JC, Phelps ME, Carson RE, et al. Tomographic mapping of human cerebral metabolism: sensory deprivation. *Ann Neurol* 1982; 12:435–444.
17. Loessner A, Alavi A, Lewandrowski KU, et al. Regional cerebral function determined by FDG-PET in healthy volunteers: normal patterns and changes with age. *J Nucl Med* 1995;36:1141–1149.
18. Ivancevic V, Alavi A, Souder E, et al. Regional cerebral glucose metabolism in healthy volunteers determined by fluorodeoxyglucose positron emission tomography: appearance and variance in the transaxial, coronal, and sagittal planes. *Clin Nucl Med* 2000;25:596–602.
19. Takahashi T, Shirane R, Sato S, et al. Developmental changes of cerebral blood flow and oxygen metabolism in children. *Am J Neuroradiol* 1999;20:917–922.
20. Chugani HT, Phelps ME, Mazziotta JC. Positron emission tomography study of human brain functional development. *Ann Neurol* 1987;22: 487–497.
21. Kinnala A, Suhonen-Polvi H, Aarimaa T, et al. Cerebral metabolic rate for glucose during the first six months of life: an FDG positron emission tomography study. *Arch Dis Child Fetal Neonatal Ed* 1996;74: F153–157.
22. Van Bogaert P, Wikler D, Damhaut P, et al. Regional changes in glucose metabolism during brain development from the age of 6 years. *Neuroimage* 1998;8:62–68.
23. Terry RD, DeTeresa R, Hansen LA. Neocortical cell counts in normal human adult aging. *Ann Neurol* 1987;21:530–539.
24. Schultz SK, O'Leary DS, Boles Ponto LL, et al. Age-related changes in regional cerebral blood flow among young to mid-life adults. *Neuroreport* 1999;10:2493–2496.
25. Martin AJ, Friston KJ, Colebatch JG, et al. Decreases in regional cerebral blood flow with normal aging. *J Cereb Blood Flow Metab* 1991; 11:684–689.
26. Meltzer CC, Cantwell MN, Greer PJ, et al. Does cerebral blood flow decline in healthy aging? A PET study with partial-volume correction. *J Nucl Med* 2000;41:1842–1848.
27. Garraux G, Salmon E, Degueldre C, et al. Comparison of impaired subcortico-frontal metabolic networks in normal aging, subcortico-frontal dementia, and cortical frontal dementia. *Neuroimage* 1999;10: 149–162.
28. Yanase D, Matsunari I, Yajima K, et al. Brain FDG PET study of normal aging in Japanese: effect of atrophy correction. *Eur J Nucl Med Mol Imaging* 2005;32:794–805.
29. Pietrini P, Alexander GE, Furey ML, et al. Cerebral metabolic response to passive audiovisual stimulation in patients with Alzheimer's disease and healthy volunteers assessed by PET. *J Nucl Med* 2000;41:575–583.
30. Ishizu K, Nishizawa S, Yonekura Y, et al. Effects of hyperglycemia on FDG uptake in human brain and glioma. *J Nucl Med* 1994;35:1104–1109.
31. Foster NL, VanDerSpek AF, Aldrich MS, et al. The effect of diazepam sedation on cerebral glucose metabolism in Alzheimer's disease as measured using positron emission tomography. *J Cereb Blood Flow Metab* 1987;7:415–420.
32. Wang GJ, Volkow ND, Overall J, et al. Reproducibility of regional brain metabolic responses to lorazepam. *J Nucl Med* 1996;37:1609–1613.
33. Juengling FD, Kassubek J, Martens-Le Bouar H, et al. Cerebral regional hypometabolism caused by propofol-induced sedation in children with severe myoclonic epilepsy: a study using fluorodeoxyglucose positron emission tomography and statistical parametric mapping. *Neurosci Lett* 2002;335:79–82.
34. Gaillard WD, Zeffiro T, Fazilat S, et al. Effect of valproate on cerebral metabolism and blood flow: an ^{18}F-2-deoxyglucose and ^{15}O water positron emission tomography study. *Epilepsia* 1996;37:515–521.
35. Theodore WH, Bairamian D, Newmark ME, et al. Effect of phenytoin on human cerebral glucose metabolism. *J Cereb Blood Flow Metab* 1986;6:315–320.
36. Theodore WH, Fishbein D, Dietz M, et al. Complex partial seizures: cerebellar metabolism. *Epilepsia* 1987;28:319–323.
37. Seitz RJ, Piel S, Arnold S, et al. Cerebellar hypometabolism in focal epilepsy is related to age of onset and drug intoxication. *Epilepsia* 1996;37:1194–1199.
38. Joo EY, Tae WS, Hong SB. Regional effects of lamotrigine on cerebral glucose metabolism in idiopathic generalized epilepsy. *Arch Neurol* 2006;63:1282–1286.
39. Theodore WH. Antiepileptic drugs and cerebral glucose metabolism. *Epilepsia* 1988;29[Suppl 2]:S48–S55.
40. Bartlett EJ, Brodie JD, Simkowitz P, et al. Effects of haloperidol challenge on regional cerebral glucose utilization in normal human subjects. *Am J Psychiatry* 1994;151:681–686.
41. Von Monakow C. *Die Lokalisation im Grosshirn und der Abbau der Funktion durch Kortikale Herde.* Weisbaden, J. F. Bergman, 1914.
42. Meyer JS, Obara K, Muramatsu K. Diaschisis. *Neurol Res* 1993;15: 362–366.
43. Baron JC, Marchal G. Functional imaging in vascular disorders. In: Mazziotta JC, Toga AW, Frackowiak RSJ, eds. *Brain mapping: the disorders*. New York: Academic Press, 2000:299–316.
44. Baron JC, Bonsser MG, Comar D, et al. Crossed cerebellar diaschisis in human supratentorial brain infarction. *Trans Am Neurol Assoc* 1980;105:459–461.
45. Baron JC, D'Antona R, Pantano P, et al. Effects of thalamic stroke on energy metabolism of the cerebral cortex. A positron tomography study in man. *Brain* 1986;109:1243–1259.

46. Sobesky J, Thiel A, Ghaemi M, et al. Crossed cerebellar diaschisis in acute human stroke: a PET study of serial changes and response to supratentorial reperfusion. *J Cereb Blood Flow Metab* 2005;25: 1685–1691.
47. Park CH, Kim SM, Streletz LJ, et al. Reverse crossed cerebellar diaschisis in partial complex seizures related to herpes simplex encephalitis. *Clin Nucl Med* 1992;17:732–735.
48. Brooks DJ. Imaging basal ganglia function. *J Anat* 2000;196:543–554.
49. Quinn N. Parkinsonism-recognition and differential diagnosis. *BMJ* 1995;310:447–452.
50. Gelb DJ, Oliver E, Gilman S. Diagnostic criteria for Parkinson disease. *Arch Neurol* 1999;56:33–39.
51. Hughes AJ. Clinicopathological aspects of Parkinson's disease. *Eur Neurol* 1997;38[Suppl 2]:13–20.
52. Hughes AJ, Daniel SE, Blankson S, et al. A clinicopathologic study of 100 cases of Parkinson's disease. *Arch Neurol* 1993;50:140–148.
53. Wolfson LI, Leenders KL, Brown LL, et al. Alterations of regional cerebral blood flow and oxygen metabolism in Parkinson's disease. *Neurology* 1985;35:1399–1405.
54. Antonini A, Vontobel P, Psylla M, et al. Complementary positron emission tomographic studies of the striatal dopaminergic system in Parkinson's disease. *Arch Neurol* 1995;52:1183–1190.
55. Eidelberg D, Moeller JR, Dhawan V, et al. The metabolic topography of parkinsonism. *J Cereb Blood Flow Metab* 1994;14:783–801.
56. Vander Borght T, Minoshima S, Giordani B, et al. Cerebral metabolic differences in Parkinson's and Alzheimer's disease matched for dementia severity. *J Nucl Med* 1997;38:797–802.
57. Dethy S, Van Blercom N, Damhaut P, et al. Asymmetry of basal ganglia glucose metabolism and dopa responsiveness in parkinsonism. *Mov Disord* 1998;13:275–280.
58. Zaccai J, McCracken C, Brayne C. A systematic review of prevalence and incidence studies of dementia with Lewy bodies. *Age Ageing* 2005; 34:561–566.
59. McKeith IG, Galasko D, Kosaka K, et al. Consensus guideline for the clinical and pathological diagnosis of dementia with Lewy bodies (LBD): report of the Consortium on DLB International Workshop. *Neurology* 1996;47:1113–1124.
60. McKeith IG, Dickson DW, Lowe J, et al. Diagnosis and management of dementia with Lewy bodies: third report of the DLB Consortium. *Neurology* 2005;65:1863–1872.
61. Emre M. Dementia associated with Parkinson's disease. *Lancet Neurol* 2003;2:229–237.
62. Ballard C, Ziabreva I, Perry R, et al. Differences in neuropathologic characteristics across the Lewy body dementia spectrum. *Neurology* 2006;67:1931–1934.
63. Braak H, Braak E. Staging of Alzheimer's disease-related neurofibrillary changes. *Neurobiol Aging* 1995;16:271–284.
64. Friedland RP, Brun A, Budinger TF. Pathological and positron emission tomographic correlations in Alzheimer's disease. *Lancet* 1985;8422:228.
65. Mielke R, Schroder R, Fink GR, et al. Regional cerebral glucose metabolism and postmortem pathology in Alzheimer's disease. *Acta Neuropathol* 1996;91:174–179.
66. Bohnen NI, Minoshima S, Giordani B, et al. Motor correlates of occipital glucose hypometabolism in Parkinson's disease without dementia. *Neurology* 1999;52:541–546.
67. Steele JC, Richardson JC, Olszewski J. Progressive supranuclear palsy: a heterogeneous degeneration involving the brainstem, basal ganglia, and cerebellum, with vertical gaze and pseudobulbar palsy. *Arch Neurol* 1964;10:333–359.
68. Foster NL, Gilman S, Berent S, et al. Cerebral hypometabolism in progressive supranuclear palsy studied with positron emission tomography. *Ann Neurol* 1988;24:399–406.
69. D'Antona R, Baron JC, Samson Y, et al. Subcortical dementia. Frontal cortex hypometabolism detected by positron tomography in patients with progressive supranuclear palsy. *Brain* 1985;108:785–799.
70. Blin J, Baron JC, Dubois B, et al. Positron emission tomography study in progressive supranuclear palsy. Brain hypometabolic pattern and clinicometabolic correlations. *Arch Neurol* 1990;47:747–752.
71. Salmon E, Van der Linden MV, Franck G. Anterior cingulate and motor network metabolic impairment in progressive supranuclear palsy. *Neuroimage* 1997;5:173–178.
72. Juh R, Pae CU, Kim TS, et al. Cerebral glucose metabolism in corticobasal degeneration comparison with progressive supranuclear palsy using statistical mapping analysis. *Neurosci Lett* 2005;383:22–27.
73. Feany MB, Ksiezak-Reding H, Liu WK, et al. Epitope expression and hyperphosphorylation of tau protein in corticobasal degeneration: differentiation from progressive supranuclear palsy. *Acta Neuropathol (Berl)* 1995;90:37–43.
74. Eidelberg D, Dhawan V, Moeller JR, et al. The metabolic landscape of cortico-basal ganglionic degeneration: regional asymmetries studied with positron emission tomography. *J Neurol Neurosurg Psychiatry* 1991;54:856–862.
75. Nagahama Y, Fukuyama H, Turjanski N, et al. Cerebral glucose metabolism in corticobasal degeneration: comparison with progressive supranuclear palsy and normal controls. *Mov Disord* 1997;12:691–696.
76. Coulier IM, de Vries JJ, Leenders KL. Is FDG-PET a useful tool in clinical practice for diagnosing corticobasal ganglionic degeneration? *Mov Disord* 2003;18:1175–1178.
77. Garraux G, Salmon E, Peigneux P, et al. Voxel-based distribution of metabolic impairment in corticobasal degeneration. *Mov Disord* 2000;15:894–904.
78. Hosaka K, Ishii K, Sakamoto S, et al. Voxel-based comparison of regional cerebral glucose metabolism between PSP and corticobasal degeneration. *J Neurol Sci* 2002;199:67–71.
79. Blin J, Vidailhet MJ, Pillon B, et al. Corticobasal degeneration: decreased and asymmetrical glucose consumption as studied with PET. *Mov Disord* 1992;7:348–354.
80. Lutte I, Laterre C, Bodart JM, et al. Contribution of PET studies in diagnosis of corticobasal degeneration. *Eur Neurol* 2000;44:12–21.
81. Papp MI, Lantos PL. The distribution of oligodendroglial inclusions in multiple system atrophy and its relevance to clinical symptomatology. *Brain* 1994;117:235–243.
82. Otsuka M, Kuwabara Y, Ichiya Y, et al. Differentiating between multiple system atrophy and Parkinson's disease by positron emission tomography with ^{18}F-dopa and ^{18}F-FDG. *Ann Nucl Med* 1997;11: 251–257.
83. Juh R, Pae CU, Lee CU, et al. Voxel based comparison of glucose metabolism in the differential diagnosis of the multiple system atrophy using statistical parametric mapping. *Neurosci Res* 2005;52:211–219.
84. Gilman S, Koeppe RA, Junck L, et al. Patterns of cerebral glucose metabolism detected with positron emission tomography differ in multiple system atrophy and olivopontocerebellar atrophy. *Ann Neurol* 1994;36:166–175.
85. Otsuka M, Ichiya Y, Kuwabara Y, et al. Glucose metabolism in the cortical and subcortical brain structures in multiple system atrophy and Parkinson's disease: a positron emission tomographic study. *J Neurol Sci* 1996;144:77–83.
86. Gerstenbrand F, Klingler D, Pfeiffer B. Der essentialle Tremor. Phänomenologie und Epidemiologie. *Nervenarzt* 1983;43:46–53.
87. Louis ED, Vonsattel JP, Honig LS, et al. Essential tremor associated with pathologic changes in the cerebellum. *Arch Neurol* 2006;63:1189–1193.
88. Louis ED, Vonsattel JP, Honig LS, et al. Neuropathologic findings in essential tremor. *Neurology* 2006;66:1756–1759.
89. Hallett M, Dubinsky RM. Glucose metabolism in the brain of patients with essential tremor. *J Neurol Sci* 1993;114:45–48.
90. Colebatch JG, Findley LJ, Frackowiak RS, et al. Preliminary report: activation of the cerebellum in essential tremor. *Lancet* 1990;336: 1028–1030.
91. Jenkins IH, Bain PG, Colebatch JG, et al. A positron emission tomography study of essential tremor: evidence for overactivity of cerebellar connections. *Ann Neurol* 1993;34:82–90.
92. Wills AJ, Jenkins IH, Thompson PD, et al. Red nuclear and cerebellar but no olivary activation associated with essential tremor: a positron emission tomographic study. *Ann Neurol* 1994;36:636–642.
93. Wills AJ, Jenkins IH, Thompson PD, et al. A positron emission tomography study of cerebral activation associated with essential and writing tremor. *Arch Neurol* 1995;52:299–305.

94. Albin RL, Tagle DA. Genetics and molecular biology of Huntington's disease. *Trends Neurosci* 1995;18:11–14.
95. Huntington's Disease Collaborative Research Group. A novel gene containing a trinucleotide repeat that is expanded and unstable on Huntington's disease chromosomes. *Cell* 1993;72:971–983.
96. Vonsattel J-P, DiFiglia M. Huntington's disease. *J Neuropathol Exp Neurol* 1998;57:369–384.
97. Bernheimer H, Birkmayer W, Hornykiewicz O, et al. Brain dopamine and the syndromes of Parkinson and Huntington. Clinical, morphological and neurochemical correlations. *J Neurol Sci* 1973;20:415–455.
98. Vonsattel J-P, Meyers R, Stevens T, et al. Neuropathological classification of Huntington's disease. *J Neuropathol Exp Neurol* 1985;44:559–577.
99. Kuhl DE, Phelps ME, Markham CH, et al. Cerebral metabolism and atrophy in Huntington's disease determined by [18]FDG and computed tomographic scan. *Ann Neurol* 1982;12:425–434.
100. Kuhl DE, Metter EJ, Riege WH, et al. Patterns of cerebral glucose utilization in Parkinson's disease and Huntington's disease. *Ann Neurol* 1984;15[Suppl]:S119–S125.
101. Maziotta JH, Phelps ME, Pahl JJ, et al. Reduced cerebral glucose metabolism in asymptomatic subjects at risk for Huntington's disease. *N Engl J Med* 1987;316:357–362.
102. Feigin A, Leenders KL, Moeller JR, et al. Metabolic network abnormalities in early Huntington's disease: an [(18)F]FDG PET study. *J Nucl Med* 2001;42:1591–1595.
103. Hosokawa S, Ichiya Y, Kuwabara Y, et al. Positron emission tomography in cases of chorea with different underlying diseases. *J Neurol Neurosurg Psychiatry* 1987;50:1284–1287.
104. Dubinsky RM, Hallett M, Levey R, et al. Regional brain glucose metabolism in neuroacanthocytosis. *Neurology* 1989;39:1253–1255.
105. Weindl A, Kuwert T, Leenders KL, et al. Increased striatal glucose consumption in Sydenham's chorea. *Mov Disord* 1993;8:437–444.
106. Bohlega S, Riley W, Powe J, et al. Neuroacanthocytosis and aprebetalipoproteinemia. *Neurology* 1998;50:1912–1914.
107. Sunden-Cullberg J, Tedroff J, Aquilonius SM. Reversible chorea in primary antiphospholipid syndrome. *Mov Disord* 1998;13:147–149.
108. Hsu JL, Wang HC, Hsu WC. Hyperglycemia-induced unilateral basal ganglion lesions with and without hemichorea. A PET study. *J Neurol* 2004;251:1486–1490.
109. Garnett ES, Firnau G, Chan PKH, et al. [^{18}F]fluoro-dopa, an analogue of dopa, and its use in direct measurement of storage, degeneration, and turnover of intracerebral dopamine. *Proc Natl Acad Sci U S A* 1978;75:464–467.
110. Garnett ES, Firnau G, Nahmias C. Dopamine visualized in the basal ganglia of living man. *Nature* 1983;305:137–138.
111. Frost JJ, Rosier AJ, Reich SG, et al. Positron emission tomographic imaging of the dopamine transporter with ^{11}C-WIN35428 reveals marked declines in mild Parkinson's disease. *Ann Neurol* 1993;34:423–431.
112. Antonini A, Schwarz J, Oertel WH, et al. [^{11}C]raclopride and positron emission tomography in previously untreated patients with Parkinson's disease: influence of L-dopa and lisuride therapy on striatal dopamine D_2-receptors. *Neurology* 1994;44:1325–1329.
113. Brooks D. The early diagnosis of Parkinson's disease. *Ann Neurol* 1998;44[Suppl 1]:S10–S18.
114. Frey KA, Koeppe RA, Kilbourn MR, et al. Presynaptic monoaminergic vesicles in Parkinson's disease and normal aging. *Ann Neurol* 1996;40:873–884.
115. Bohnen NI, Albin RL, Koeppe RA, et al. Positron emission tomography of monoaminergic vesicular binding in aging and Parkinson disease. *J Cereb Blood Flow Metab* 2006;26:1198–1212.
116. Eidelberg D, Moeller JR, Dhawan V, et al. The metabolic anatomy of Parkinson's disease: complementary [^{18}F]fluorodeoxyglucose and [^{18}F]fluorodopa positron emission tomographic studies. *Mov Dis* 1990;5:203–213.
117. Morrish PK, Sawle GV, Brooks DJ. An [^{18}F]dopa-PET and clinical study of the rate of progression in Parkinson's disease. *Brain* 1996;119:585–591.
118. Vingerhoets FJG, Schulzer M, Calne DB, et al. Which clinical sign of Parkinson's disease best reflects the nigrostriatal lesion? *Ann Neurol* 1997;41:58–64.
119. Freed CR, Greene PE, Breeze RE, et al. Transplantation of embryonic dopamine neurons for severe Parkinson's disease. *N Engl J Med* 2001;344:710–719.
120. Brooks DJ, Ibanez V, Sawle GV, et al. Striatal D_2 receptor status in patients with Parkinson's disease, striatonigral degeneration, and progressive supranuclear palsy, measured with ^{11}C-raclopride and positron emission tomography. *Ann Neurol* 1992;31:184–192.
121. Gilman S, Frey KA, Koeppe RA, et al. Decreased striatal monoaminergic terminals in olivopontocerebellar atrophy and multiple system atrophy demonstrated with positron emission tomography. *Ann Neurol* 1996;40:885–892.
122. Pirker W, Asenbaum S, Bencsits G, et al. [^{123}I]beta-CIT SPECT in multiple system atrophy, progressive supranuclear palsy, and corticobasal degeneration. *Mov Disord* 2000;15:1158–1167.
123. Sawle GV, Brooks DJ, Marsden CD, et al. Corticobasal degeneration. A unique pattern of regional cortical oxygen hypometabolism and striatal fluorodopa uptake demonstrated by positron emission tomography. *Brain* 1991;114(Pt 1B):541–556.
124. Rinne JO, Burn DJ, Mathias CJ, et al. Positron emission tomography studies on the dopaminergic system and striatal opioid binding in the olivopontocerebellar atrophy variant of multiple system atrophy. *Ann Neurol* 1995;37:568–573.
125. Antonini A, Leenders KL, Vontobel P, et al. Complementary PET studies of striatal neuronal function in the differential diagnosis between multiple system atrophy and Parkinson's disease. *Brain* 1997;120(Pt 12):2187–2195.
126. Gilman S, Koeppe RA, Junck L, et al. Decreased striatal monoaminergic terminals in multiple system atrophy detected with positron emission tomography. *Ann Neurol* 1999;45:769–777.
127. Laureys S, Salmon E, Garraux G, et al. Fluorodopa uptake and glucose metabolism in early stages of corticobasal degeneration. *J Neurol* 1999;246:1151–1158.
128. Ilgin N, Zubieta J, Reich SG, et al. PET imaging of the dopamine transporter in progressive supranuclear palsy and Parkinson's disease. *Neurology* 1999;52:1221–1226.
129. Rinne UK, Laihinen A, Rinne JO, et al. Positron emission tomography demonstrates dopamine D_2 receptor supersensitivity in the striatum of patients with early Parkinson's disease. *Mov Disord* 1990;5:55–59.
130. Antonini A, Schwarz J, Oertel WH, et al. Long-term changes of striatal dopamine D_2 receptors in patients with Parkinson's disease: a study with positron emission tomography and [[11C]]raclopride. *Mov Disord* 1997;12:33–38.
131. Nakagawa M, Kuwabara Y, Taniwaki T, et al. PET evaluation of the relationship between D_2 receptor binding and glucose metabolism in patients with parkinsonism. *Ann Nucl Med* 2005;19:267–275.
132. Walker Z, Costa DC, Walker RW, et al. Striatal dopamine transporter in dementia with Lewy bodies and Parkinson disease: a comparison. *Neurology* 2004;62:1568–1572.
133. Koeppe RA, Gilman S, Joshi A, et al. ^{11}C-DTBZ and ^{18}F-FDG PET measures in differentiating dementias. *J Nucl Med* 2005;46:936–944.
134. Kidwell CS, Chalela JA, Saver JL, et al. Comparison of MRI and CT for detection of acute intracerebral hemorrhage. *JAMA* 2004;292:1823–1830.
135. Baird AE, Warach S. Imaging developing brain infarction. *Curr Opin Neurol* 1999;12:65–71.
136. Albers GW, Thijs VN, Wechsler L, et al. Magnetic resonance imaging profiles predict clinical response to early reperfusion: the diffusion and perfusion imaging evaluation for understanding stroke evolution (DEFUSE) study. *Ann Neurol* 2006;60:508–517.
137. Powers WJ. Hemodynamics and metabolism in ischemic cerebrovascular disease. *Neurol Clin* 1992;10:31–48.
138. Heiss WD, Herholz K. Assessment of pathophysiology of stroke by positron emission tomography. *Eur J Nucl Med* 1994;21:455–465.
139. Powers WJ, Zazulia AR. The use of positron emission tomography in cerebrovascular disease. *Neuroimaging Clin North Am* 2003;13:741–758.
140. Powers WJ, Raichle ME. Positron emission tomography and its application to the study of cerebrovascular disease in man. *Stroke* 1985;16:361–376.

141. Ter-Pogossian MM, Eichling JO, Davis DO, et al. The determination of regional cerebral blood flow by means of water labeled with radioactive oxygen-15. *Radiology* 1969;93:31–40.
142. Ter-Pogossian MM, Eichling JO, Davis DO, et al. The measure *in vivo* of regional cerebral oxygen utilization by means of oxyhemoglobin labeled with radioactive oxygen-15. *J Clin Invest* 1970;49:381–391.
143. Jones T, Chesler DA, Ter-Pogossian MM. The continuous inhalation of oxygen-15 for assessing regional oxygen extraction in the brain of man. *Br J Radiol* 1976;49:339–343.
144. Lenzi GL, Jones T, McKenzie CG, et al. Study of regional cerebral metabolism and blood flow relationships in man using the method of continuously inhaling oxygen-15 and oxygen-15 labelled carbon dioxide. *J Neurol Neurosurg Psychiatry* 1978;41:1–10.
145. Frackowiak RS, Lenzi GL, Jones T, et al. Quantitative measurement of regional cerebral blood flow and oxygen metabolism in man using ^{15}O and positron emission tomography: theory, procedure, and normal values. *J Comput Assist Tomogr* 1980;4:727–736.
146. Lammertsma AA, Frackowiak RSJ, Hoffman JM, et al. Simultaneous measurement of regional cerebral blood flow and oxygen metabolism: a feasibility study. *J Cereb Blood Flow Metab* 1987;7[Suppl 1]:S587.
147. Herscovitch P, Markham J, Raichle ME. Brain blood flow measured with intravenous $H2^{15}O$. I. Theory and error analysis. *J Nucl Med* 1983;24:782–789.
148. Grubb RLJ, Raichle ME, Higgins CS, et al. Measurement of regional cerebral blood volume by emission tomography. *Ann Neurol* 1978;4:322–328.
149. Baron JC, Frackowiak RS, Herholz K, et al. Use of PET methods for measurement of cerebral energy metabolism and hemodynamics in cerebrovascular disease. *J Cereb Blood Flow Metab* 1989;9:723–742.
150. Jones TH, Morawetz RB, Crowell RM, et al. Thresholds of focal cerebral ischemia in awake monkeys. *J Neurosurg* 1981;54:773–782.
151. Sobesky J, von Kummer R, Frackowiak M, et al. Early ischemic edema on cerebral computed tomography: its relation to diffusion changes and hypoperfusion within 6 h after human ischemic stroke. A comparison of CT, MRI and PET. *Cerebrovasc Dis* 2006;21:336–339.
152. Heiss WD. Ischemic penumbra: evidence from functional imaging in man. *J Cereb Blood Flow Metab* 2000;20:1276–1293.
153. Heiss WD, Graf R, Grond M, et al. Quantitative neuroimaging for the evaluation of the effect of stroke treatment. *Cerebrovasc Dis* 1998;8[Suppl 2]:23–29.
154. Sobesky J, Zaro Weber O, et al. Does the mismatch match the penumbra? Magnetic resonance imaging and positron emission tomography in early ischemic stroke. *Stroke* 2005;36:980–985.
155. Derdeyn CP, Grubb RLJ, Powers WJ. Cerebral hemodynamic impairment: methods of measurement and association with stroke risk. *Neurology* 1999;53:251–259.
156. Powers WJ, Press GA, Grubb RLJ, et al. The effect of hemodynamically significant carotid artery disease on the hemodynamic status of the cerebral circulation. *Ann Intern Med* 1987;106:27–34.
157. Gibbs JM, Wise RJ, Leenders KL, et al. Evaluation of cerebral perfusion reserve in patients with carotid-artery occlusion. *Lancet* 1984;I:310–314.
158. Grubb RLJ, Derdeyn CP, Fritsch SM, et al. Importance of hemodynamic factors in the prognosis of symptomatic carotid occlusion. *JAMA* 1998;280:1055–1060.
159. Grubb RL Jr, Powers WJ, Derdeyn CP, et al. The carotid occlusion surgery study. *Neurosurg Focus* 2003;14:e9.
160. Derdeyn CP, Grubb RL Jr, Powers WJ. Indications for cerebral revascularization for patients with atherosclerotic carotid occlusion. *Skull Base* 2005;15:7–14.
161. Derdeyn CP. Is the acetazolamide test valid for quantitative assessment of maximal cerebral autoregulatory vasodilation? *Stroke* 2000;31:2271–2272.
162. Nemoto EM, Yonas H, Pindzola RR, et al. PET OEF reactivity for hemodynamic compromise in occlusive vascular disease. *J Neuroimaging* 2007;17:54–60.
163. Carpenter DA, Grubb RLJ, Tempel LW, et al. Cerebral oxygen metabolism after aneurysmal subarachnoid hemorrhage. *J Cereb Blood Flow Metab* 1991;11:837–844.
164. Videen TO, Dunford-Shore JE, Diringer MN, et al. Correction for partial volume effects in regional blood flow measurements adjacent to hematomas in humans with intracerebral hemorrhage: implementation and validation. *J Comput Assist Tomogr* 1999;23:248–256.
165. Ward NS. Plasticity and the functional reorganization of the human brain. *Int J Psychophysiol* 2005;58:158–161.
166. Calautti C, Baron JC. Functional neuroimaging studies of motor recovery after stroke in adults: a review. *Stroke* 2003;34:1553–1566.
167. Kushner M, Reivich M, Fieschi C, et al. Metabolic and clinical correlates of acute ischemic infarction. *Neurology* 1987;37:1103–1110.
168. Marchal G, Furlan M, Beaudouin V, et al. Early spontaneous hyperperfusion after stroke. A marker of favourable tissue outcome? *Brain* 1996;119:409–419.
169. Kuroda S, Shiga T, Houkin K, et al. Cerebral oxygen metabolism and neuronal integrity in patients with impaired vasoreactivity attributable to occlusive carotid artery disease. *Stroke* 2006;37:393–398.
170. Heiss WD, Kracht L, Grond M, et al. Early [^{11}C]flumazenil/H_2O positron emission tomography predicts irreversible ischemic cortical damage in stroke patients receiving acute thrombolytic therapy. *Stroke* 2000;31:366–369.
171. Nakagawara J, Sperling B, Lassen NA. Incomplete brain infarction of reperfused cortex may be quantitated with iomazenil. *Stroke* 1997;28:124–132.
172. Markus R, Donnan G, Kazui S, et al. Penumbral topography in human stroke: methodology and validation of the "Penumbragram." *Neuroimage* 2004;21:1252–1259.
173. Markus R, Reutens DC, Kazui S, et al. Hypoxic tissue in ischaemic stroke: persistence and clinical consequences of spontaneous survival. *Brain* 2004;127:1427–1436.
174. Takasawa M, Beech JS, Fryer TD, et al. Imaging of brain hypoxia in permanent and temporary middle cerebral artery occlusion in the rat using (18)F-fluoromisonidazole and positron emission tomography: a pilot study. *J Cereb Blood Flow Metab* 2007;23:679–689.
175. Theodore WH, Newmark ME, Sato S, et al. [^{18}F]fluorodeoxyglucose positron emission tomography in refractory complex partial seizures. *Ann Neurol* 1983;14:429–437.
176. Theodore WH. Positron emission tomography in the evaluation of seizure disorders. *Neurosci News* 1998;1:18–22.
177. Theodore WH. Cerebral blood flow and glucose metabolism in human epilepsy. In: *Advances in neurology*. Philadelphia: Lippincott Williams & Wilkins, 1999: vol 79, 873–881.
178. Kuhl DE, Engel J, Phelps ME, et al. Epileptic patterns of local cerebral metabolism and perfusion in humans determined by emission computed tomography of ^{18}FDG and $^{13}NH3$. *Ann Neurol* 1980;8:348–360.
179. Gaillard WD, Fazilat S, White S, et al. Interictal metabolism and blood flow are uncoupled in temporal lobe cortex of patients with complex partial epilepsy. *Neurology* 1995;45:1841–1847.
180. Gaillard WD, Bhatia S, Bookheimer SY, et al. FDG-PET and volumetric MRI in the evaluation of patients with partial epilepsy. *Neurology* 1995;45:123–126.
181. Henry TR, Babb TL, Engel J Jr, et al. Hippocampal neuronal loss and regional hypometabolism in temporal lobe epilepsy. *Ann Neurol* 1994;36:925–927.
182. Hajek M, Wieser HG, Khan N, et al. Preoperative and postoperative glucose consumption in mesiobasal and lateral temporal lobe epilepsy. *Neurology* 1994;44:2125–2132.
183. Theodore WH, Kelley K, Toczek MT, et al. Epilepsy duration, febrile seizures, and cerebral glucose metabolism. *Epilepsia* 2004;45:276–279.
184. Gaillard WD, Kopylev L, Weinstein S, et al. Low incidence of abnormal (18)FDG-PET in children with new-onset partial epilepsy: a prospective study. *Neurology* 2002;58:717–722.
185. Henry TR, Van Heertum RL. Positron emission tomography and single photon emission computed tomography in epilepsy care. *Semin Nucl Med* 2003;33:88–104.

186. Erbayat Altay E, Fessler AJ, Gallagher M, et al. Correlation of severity of FDG-PET hypometabolism and interictal regional delta slowing in temporal lobe epilepsy. *Epilepsia* 2005;46:573–576.
187. Delbeke D, Lawrence SK, Abou-Khalil BW, et al. Postsurgical outcome of patients with uncontrolled complex partial seizures and temporal lobe hypometabolism on ^{18}FDG-positron emission tomography. *Invest Radiol* 1996;31:261–266.
188. Theodore WH, Sato S, Kufta CV, et al. FDG-positron emission tomography and invasive EEG: seizure focus detection and surgical outcome. *Epilepsia* 1997;38:81–86.
189. Henry TR, Mazziotta JC, Engel J. Interictal metabolic anatomy of mesial temporal lobe epilepsy. *Arch Neurol* 1993;50:582–589.
190. Newberg AB, Alavi A, Berlin J, et al. Ipsilateral and contralateral thalamic hypometabolism as a predictor of outcome after temporal lobectomy for seizures. *J Nucl Med* 2000;41:1964–1968.
191. Choi JY, Kim SJ, Hong SB, et al. Extratemporal hypometabolism on FDG PET in temporal lobe epilepsy as a predictor of seizure outcome after temporal lobectomy. *Eur J Nucl Med Mol Imaging* 2003;30: 581–587.
192. Spanaki MV, Kopylev L, DeCarli C, et al. Postoperative changes in cerebral metabolism in temporal lobe epilepsy. *Arch Neurol* 2000;57: 1447–1452.
193. Lamusuo S, Jutila L, Ylinen A, et al. [^{18}F]FDG-PET reveals temporal hypometabolism in patients with temporal lobe epilepsy even when quantitative MRI and histopathological analysis show only mild hippocampal damage. *Arch Neurol* 2001;58:933–939.
194. Carne RP, O'Brien TJ, Kilpatrick CJ, et al. MRI-negative PET-positive temporal lobe epilepsy: a distinct surgically remediable syndrome. *Brain* 2004;127:2276–2285.
195. Carne RP, Cook MJ, Macgregor LR, et al. "Magnetic resonance imaging negative positron emission tomography positive" temporal lobe epilepsy: FDG-PET pattern differs from mesial temporal lobe epilepsy. *Mol Imaging Biol* 2007;9:32–42.
196. Kim YK, Lee DS, Lee SK, et al. Differential features of metabolic abnormalities between medial and lateral temporal lobe epilepsy: quantitative analysis of (18)F-FDG PET using SPM. *J Nucl Med* 2003;44:1006–1012.
197. Henry TR, Sutherling WW, Engel J, et al. Interictal cerebral metabolism in partial epilepsies of neocortical origin. *Epilepsy Res* 1991;10:174–182.
198. Swartz BE, Halgren E, Delgado-Escueta AV, et al. Neuroimaging in patients with seizures of probable frontal lobe origin. *Epilepsia* 1989; 30:547–558.
199. Knowlton RC, Lawn ND, Mountz JM, et al. Ictal SPECT analysis in epilepsy: subtraction and statistical parametric mapping techniques. *Neurology* 2004;63:10–15.
200. Drzezga A, Arnold S, Minoshima S, et al. ^{18}F-FDG PET studies in patients with extratemporal and temporal epilepsy: evaluation of an observer-independent analysis. *J Nucl Med* 1999;40:737–746.
201. Juhasz C, Chugani HT. Imaging the epileptic brain with positron emission tomography. *Neuroimag Clin North Am* 2003;13:705–716.
202. Sood S, Chugani HT. Functional neuroimaging in the preoperative evaluation of children with drug-resistant epilepsy. *Childs Nerv Syst* 2006;22:810–820.
203. Chugani HT, Conti JR. Etiologic classification of infantile spasms in 140 cases: role of positron emission tomography. *J Child Neurol* 1996;11:44–48.
204. Chugani HT, Shields WD, Shewmon DA, et al. Infantile spasms: I. PET identifies focal cortical dysgenesis in cryptogenic cases for surgical treatment. *Ann Neurol* 1990;27:406–413.
205. Chugani HT, Shewmon DA, Shields WD, et al. Surgery for intractable infantile spasms: neuroimaging perspectives. *Epilepsia* 1993;34:764–771.
206. Markand ON. Lennox-Gastaut syndrome (childhood epileptic encephalopathy). *J Clin Neurophysiol* 2003;20:426–441.
207. Chugani HT, Mazziotta JC, Engel JJ, et al. The Lennox-Gastaut syndrome: metabolic subtypes determined by 2-deoxy-2[^{18}F]fluoro-D-glucose positron emission tomography. *Ann Neurol* 1987;21:4–13.
208. Chugani HT, Chugani DC. Basic mechanisms of childhood epilepsies: studies with positron emission tomography. *Adv Neurol* 1999;79: 883–891.
209. Leiderman DB, Balish M, Sato S, et al. Comparison of PET measurements of cerebral blood flow and glucose metabolism for the localization of human epileptic foci. *Epilepsy Res* 1992;13:153–157.
210. Chugani HT, Rintahaka PJ, Shewmon DA. Ictal patterns of cerebral glucose utilization in children with epilepsy. *Epilepsia* 1994;35: 813–822.
211. Meltzer CC, Adelson PD, Brenner RP, et al. Planned ictal FDG PET imaging for localization of extratemporal epileptic foci. *Epilepsia* 2000;41:193–200.
212. Theodore WH, Balish M, Leiderman D, et al. Effect of seizures on cerebral blood flow measured with $^{15}O-H_2O$ and positron emission tomography. *Epilepsia* 1996;37:796–802.
213. Hunter KE, Blaxton TA, Bookheimer SY, et al. ^{15}O water positron emission tomography in language localization: a study comparing positron emission tomography visual and computerized region of interest analysis with the Wada test. *Ann Neurol* 1999;45:662–665.
214. Bookheimer SY, Zeffiro TA, Blaxton T, et al. A direct comparison of PET activation and electrocortical stimulation mapping for language localization. *Neurology* 1997;48:1056–1065.
215. Henry TR, Frey KA, Sackellares JC, et al. *In vivo* cerebral metabolism and central benzodiazepine-receptor binding in temporal lobe epilepsy. *Neurology* 1993;43:1998–2006.
216. Arnold S, Berthele A, Drzezga A, et al. Reduction of benzodiazepine receptor binding is related to the seizure onset zone in extratemporal focal cortical dysplasia. *Epilepsia* 2000;41:818–824.
217. Koepp MJ, Hammers A, Labbe C, et al. ^{11}C-flumazenil PET in patients with refractory temporal lobe epilepsy and normal MRI. *Neurology* 2000;54:332–339.
218. Hammers A, Koepp MJ, Brooks DJ, et al. Periventricular white matter flumazenil binding and postoperative outcome in hippocampal sclerosis. *Epilepsia* 2005;46:944–948.
219. Juhasz C, Chugani DC, Muzik O, et al. Alpha-methyl-L-tryptophan PET detects epileptogenic cortex in children with intractable epilepsy. *Neurology* 2003;60:960–968.
220. Juhasz C, Chugani DC, Padhye UN, et al. Evaluation with alpha-[^{11}C]methyl-L-tryptophan positron emission tomography for reoperation after failed epilepsy surgery. *Epilepsia* 2004;45:124–130.
221. Morawetz RB, Crowell RH, DeGirolami U, et al. Regional cerebral blood flow thresholds during cerebral ischemia. *Fed Proc* 1979;38:2493–2494.

CHAPTER

9.2 Fluorodeoxyglucose PET Imaging of Dementia: Principles and Clinical Applications

SATOSHI MINOSHIMA, TAKAHIRO SASAKI, AND ERIC PETRIE

In many countries, life spans have lengthened considerably in the past several decades. The incidence of dementia increases with age, and imaging to detect dementia is of increasing importance for both clinical and research applications (1). Although exact prevalence figures vary across studies, it is estimated that more than 10% of persons over the age of 70 may suffer from dementia, the most common type, in most populations, being Alzheimer's disease (2).

Applications of positron emission tomography (PET) to imaging of dementia date back to the early stages of PET research developments in the late 1970s and early 1980s. In contrast to common clinical beliefs of the time that global reductions in cerebral perfusion and metabolic activity would be evident in dementia, early PET imaging demonstrated distinct patterns of regional heterogeneity in both hypoperfusion and hypometabolism (3). In 2004, more than 20 years after the initial application of PET imaging to dementia, and after considerable experience with fluorine-18-fluorodeoxyglucose (FDG) PET technology, the U.S. Center for Medicare and Medicaid Services announced their final decision to reimburse for FDG PET imaging for the differentiation of Alzheimer's disease and frontotemporal dementia. This approval has ignited renewed clinical and industrial interests in PET imaging of dementia in parallel to continuing efforts to refine research applications of these imaging modalities.

IMAGING IN THE CLINICAL WORK-UP OF DEMENTING DISORDERS

Dementia is defined as the development of multiple cognitive deficits manifested by (a) memory impairment, and (b) at least one of the following cognitive disturbances—aphasia, apraxia, agnosia, and declines in executive functioning (4). It is important to recognize that memory loss alone does not define dementia. Also, other cognitive disturbances can be prominent clinical features in certain dementing disorders. Dementia patients often manifest associated features such as impaired visuospatial functioning; poor judgment and insight; personality changes; anxiety, mood, and sleep disturbances; delusions and hallucinations; fluctuations in attention; and parkinsonian motor signs. Some of these features can give clues as to the type of dementing disorder present. These diverse symptoms also imply that dementing disorders may alter neural activity in widespread brain regions, the effects of which are often reflected on PET imaging.

Dementia can be manifested in many medical disorders, some of which are common differential diagnoses in PET imaging practice. Table 9.2.1 describes examples of dementing disorders. In the category of neurodegenerative diseases, Alzheimer's disease is the most common form, likely followed by dementia with Lewy bodies.

TABLE 9.2.1 Examples of Dementing Disorders

NEURODEGENERATIVE DISEASES
- Alzheimer's disease
- Dementia with Lewy bodies
- Frontotemporal dementia (including Pick disease)
- Parkinson's disease
- Huntington disease

ACQUIRED CEREBRAL DISORDERS
- Vascular dementia (micro- and macrovascular)
- Brain tumors (frontal lobe)
- Head trauma
- Multiple sclerosis
- Hydrocephalus
- Transmittable encephalopathies (e.g., Creutzfeldt-Jakob's disease)

OTHER MEDICAL CONDITIONS
- Metabolic disorder (e.g., chronic drug intoxication, alcoholism)
- Malnutrition (e.g., vitamin B_{12} deficiency),
- Infections (e.g., human immunodeficiency virus, neurosyphilis, tuberculosis, cryptococcosis)
- Depression

Vascular dementia includes both microvascular and macrovascular diseases, but classical multi-infarct dementia is now less commonly seen in imaging practice, in part due to improved control of risk factors for vascular diseases. Other medical conditions, such as metabolic disorders and infections, are typically diagnosed during a standard medical work-up but occasionally are part of the imaging differential diagnosis.

Clinical work-up of dementia patients involves medical, neurological, and laboratory examinations. Table 9.2.2 describes an example of the typical diagnostic work-up. The goals of the diagnostic work-up are to (a) confirm the presence of dementia; (b) identify the potential cause of dementia; and (c) establish a differential diagnosis for treatment decision making. It is important to note that the diagnosis of Alzheimer's disease and other neurodegenerative diseases is made only after the exclusion of other detectable causes of dementia. Structural imaging (computed tomography [CT] and magnetic resonance imaging [MRI]) is suggested as a part of the work-up. However, the use of structural imaging is primarily to exclude other causes of dementia, such as brain tumor and vascular disease. In contrast, diagnostic applications of PET and single-photon emission computed tomography (SPECT) imaging are primarily designed to identify "positive" markers, such as characteristic changes in cerebral perfusion or glucose metabolism. Thus, the goal of PET and SPECT imaging in the dementia work-up is to identify diagnostic *biomarkers* of the underlying neurodegenerative disease processes, similar to other biomarkers such as cerebrospinal fluid levels of pathologic β amyloid (i.e., $A\beta_{1-42}$) and tau protein (5).

TABLE 9.2.2 Clinical Work-up for Dementia

- Interview with patient/family member
- Physical examination
- Neurological examination
- Mini-Mental status examination (MMSE)
- Assessment for functional status
- Laboratory tests (e.g., complete blood cell count, thyroid, B_{12})
- Neuropsychological examination
- Neuroimaging (computed tomography or magnetic resonance imaging)
- Electroencephalogram, lumbar puncture (when required)
- Genetic test (e.g., apolipoprotein E) not clinically accepted

BRAIN PET AND SINGLE-PHOTON EMISSION COMPUTED TOMOGRAPHY IMAGING FOR DEMENTIA DIAGNOSIS

In the current radiology/nuclear medicine practice, both PET and SPECT imaging can be applied to the diagnostic work-up of dementias. As described previously, the current Medicare reimbursement for FDG PET is limited to the differential diagnosis of suspected Alzheimer's disease versus frontotemporal dementia. However, a large amount of research evidence suggests that FDG PET may also be capable of differentiating other dementing disorders. SPECT imaging can also be applied more generally in the dementia work-up, but the diagnostic accuracy of brain perfusion SPECT may not be as high as FDG PET imaging (6) presumably due to a combination of limited spatial resolution, sensitivity, and the nature of the perfusion tracers typically used in clinical SPECT imaging. For SPECT perfusion imaging, both technetium-99m (^{99m}Tc) ethyl cysteinate dimer (ECD) and ^{99m}Tc HMPAO (hexamethylpropyleneamine oxime) are available in the United States. In Japan, iodine-123 ([^{123}I]) IMP (N-isopropyl-p-iodoamphetamine) is also available for routine clinical applications. These "perfusion" tracers accumulate in the brain proportional to regional blood flow. Since regional neuronal activity and blood flow are tightly coupled, decreased neuronal activity due to neurodegenerative processes can be detected indirectly by SPECT imaging of secondary changes in blood flow. In contrast, FDG PET directly detects changes in regional neuronal activity as reflected in rates of neuronal glucose metabolism (Table 9.2.3).

TABLE 9.2.3 Radiotracers: Brain PET and Single-photon Emission Computed Tomography for Clinical Dementia Work-up

BRAIN PERFUSION SPECT
- [^{99m}Tc]-ECD, [^{99m}Tc]-HMPAO, [^{123}I]-IMP
- Regional brain uptake determined by:
- (1) Blood flow
- (2) Neuronal (synaptic) activity (coupled to blood flow)

BRAIN FDG PET
- [^{18}F]-2-fluoro-2-deoxy-D-glucose (FDG)
- Regional brain uptake determined by
- Neuronal (synaptic) activity

SPECT, single-photon emission computed tomography; [^{99m}Tc], technetium-99m; ECD, ethyl cysteinate dimer; HMPAO, hexamethylpropyleneamine oxime; [^{123}I]-IMP, iodine-123 N-isopropyl-p-iodoamphetamine.

Brain PET Tracer: [^{18}F]-2-fluoro-2-deoxy-D-glucose

The brain uses glucose as a major energy source but does not have substantial glucose storage capacity. Therefore, it requires a continuous supply of glucose from plasma to maintain its functions. If neurons in a certain part of the brain are not functioning normally, the change can be sensitively reflected by the amount of glucose utilization. If a glucose analogue is labeled with a positron emitting radionuclide and injected intravenously, areas of hypofunctioning neurons can be depicted as areas of decreased tracer uptake.

Sokoloff et al. (7) originally developed the glucose analogue, 2-deoxyglucose, for the study of regional brain function. Deoxyglucose is transported from plasma to brain cells through the neuronal membrane glucose transporter. Deoxyglucose is then phosphorylated by hexokinase to form deoxyglucose-6-phosphate (deoxy-G6P). However, deoxy-G6P cannot be further metabolized by enzymes in the glycolytic pathway and therefore accumulates within neurons. When deoxyglucose is labeled with a positron emitter such as [^{18}F] (8), PET imaging can detect this activity from outside the brain in three dimensions.

Despite more than a decade of research and clinical use of FDG in brain imaging, the exact microscopic locus of glucose consumption in neurons is still a matter of investigation. Sokoloff et al. demonstrated, in dorsal root ganglion neurons, that glucose consumption at synapses increased in proportion to neuronal activity, while glucose consumption in cell bodies was stable. To the degree that this model applies to the central nervous system, FDG uptake observed by PET imaging would be expected to preferentially reflect synaptic activity, possibly coupled with surrounding astrocyte uptake (9). This would be consistent with the sensitivity of FDG PET imaging in detecting regional reductions in cortical glucose uptake and metabolism in the early stages of Alzheimer's disease (10,11), as dysfunction and loss of synapses have been shown to be very early pathological processes in this disorder (12,13). This also implies that the degeneration of cortical projection neurons known to occur in Alzheimer's disease could result in spatial discordance between structural imaging measures of neuron loss and cortical atrophy and FDG PET imaging measures of synaptic loss and cortical hypometabolism. This illustrates the importance of understanding major pathways of neuronal connectivity in the brain for correctly interpreting the interrelationship between regional hypometabolism and atrophy (an example of the more general phenomenon of diaschisis, which is more commonly encountered in the interpretation of imaging findings in stroke).

PET VERSUS PET/CT

Combined PET/CT technology is replacing dedicated PET scanners in many clinical operations. Significant advantages of PET/CT for oncologic work-up are outlined elsewhere in this book. Although dedicated PET scanners can provide sufficient information for dementia work-up, the use of PET/CT has certain additional advantages. The use of CT for attenuation correction will reduce overall scanning time. This is a clear benefit for imaging elderly and demented patients who may have difficulty remaining still during prolonged scans. Simultaneous noncontrast CT also allows screening for gross anatomic abnormalities, such as tumors or subdural hematomas, which could potentially cause dementia. PET/CT scanners that use newer generation PET components can also provide better image quality that may potentially contribute to better diagnostic accuracy. Because head motion between CT and PET scans can be substantial in dementia patients, even with reduced scanning times, application of quality control measures prior to image reconstruction is critical.

Brain Fluorodeoxyglucose PET Imaging Protocols

A protocol for brain FDG PET imaging shares many procedural steps with oncologic FDG PET imaging. However, there are specific precautions that need to be taken for brain imaging. As an FDG PET scan is capable of detecting very subtle metabolic changes associated with dementing disorders, alterations in brain activity produced by environmental stimuli during the tracer uptake phase following intravenous injection of FDG can introduce artifactual metabolic alterations on brain PET images. The most noticeable changes occur in the primary sensory cortices. For example, if patients are exposed to light or visual stimulation, metabolic activity in the visual cortex increases. If auditory stimulation is given during the uptake phase, metabolic activity in the primary auditory cortex increases. This is similar to the muscle uptake occasionally seen in whole-body PET imaging when patients contract their muscles after FDG injection. To reduce metabolic variations due to external stimuli, a patient should be kept in a dimly lit room with low ambient noise levels both before and after FDG injection. An intravenous injection line should be established at least 10 minutes before FDG injection, so that brain activation due to intravenous line placement can subside prior to imaging. The patient should be instructed not to speak, read, listen to music, or watch television in the injection room. At many institutions, and recommended in several protocols, FDG injection is typically performed with the patient's eyes open. It is important to minimize interaction with the patient during at least the first 20 minutes after FDG injection, during the period of maximal brain tracer uptake. With respect to tracer dosing, 300 to 600 MBq (typically 370 MBq) and 125 to 250 MBq (typically 150 MBq) of FDG are recommended for two-dimensional and three-dimensional image acquisition protocols, respectively (14).

The patient should fast for at least 4 to 6 hours prior to FDG PET imaging. It is desirable if the patient can avoid caffeine, alcohol, and other substances or drugs that may affect brain chemistry and function. If plasma glucose levels are more than 160 to 200 mg/dL, many institutions recommend rescheduling the study, since a high plasma glucose level will degrade image quality as a result of competitive inhibition of neuronal FDG uptake by high levels of endogenous, unlabeled, plasma glucose.

Image acquisition can be started after allowing at least 20 minutes of tracer uptake following the intravenous injection of FDG. A brain FDG PET emission scan is typically acquired in three-dimensional data acquisition mode for 5 to 20 minutes. As mentioned previously, a shorter scanning time is desirable for elderly and dementia patients. Images can be reconstructed by either filtered back-projection or iterative image reconstruction methods.

Fluorodeoxyglucose PET Image Interpretation

Many neurodegenerative diseases are known to affect certain parts of the brain both pathologically and metabolically. The differential diagnosis of dementia on FDG PET relies on identification of these characteristic patterns of altered cerebral metabolic activity.

FIGURE 9.2.1. Effects of different color scales on brain PET image interpretation—Alzheimer disease. The right four images represent white background with different lower cutoff thresholds. Different color scales give different impressions for the degree of hypometabolism. Color scales tend to be more sensitive for subtle changes than black and white scales. Applying different color scales and cutoff thresholds when interpreting PET images on a workstation can confirm consistency of the findings.

Owing to widespread availability of high-speed computer workstations, interpretation of FDG PET images is typically performed on a computer monitor using image display software. In this setting, image features such as the color scale and the intensity/contrast can be changed interactively by the interpreter. This helps the interpreter identify subtle metabolic changes and confirm the consistency of findings across different display modes (Fig. 9.2.1). Image interpretation based solely on printed films is not a desirable method of image interpretation. Also, it is often helpful to view all images in a multislice display, instead of scrolling through single slices, to better understand the overall distribution of hypometabolism in the brain. In addition to transverse images, reformatted sagittal and coronal images provide better structural definition in certain structures, such as temporal lobe, subcortical structures, and midline structures. Coronal images are also useful for comparison of metabolic asymmetry when the head position is tilted. To achieve consistent structural identification, it is desirable to reslice reconstructed images parallel to the line passing through anterior and posterior commissures (AC-PC line). The AC-PC line defines the standard stereotactic coordinate system for human brains (15) and allows consistent localization of cortical and subcortical structures. Since the anterior and posterior commissures cannot be appreciated on brain PET images, the AC-PC line can be approximated by a line passing through anterior and posterior poles of the brain (Fig. 9.2.2).

Structures that provide diagnostic clues for dementing disorders include frontal, parietal, temporal, and occipital association cortices; posterior and anterior cingulate cortices; primary sensorimotor and visual cortices; thalamus; striatum; pons; and cerebellum. These structures need to be identified on PET images to allow identification of regional metabolic alterations (Table 9.2.4). Modern PET and PET/CT scanners have sufficient spatial resolution to depict cortical gyri and subcortical structures (Fig. 9.2.3). However, the resolution is typically not sufficient to resolve individual gyri facing each other at a sulcus. As a result, in a normal brain, FDG uptake often appears accentuated at the sulcus. In contrast, if there is atrophy present and a sulcus is widened, the two gyri facing the sulcus can be seen separately.

In normal subjects, brain FDG uptake is greatest in the primary visual cortex, especially if the eyes are open during the uptake period. Other primary cortices, such as sensorimotor and primary auditory cortex, also show relatively high uptake. The posterior cingulate cortex often shows very high uptake as well, almost equivalent to that of the primary visual cortex (11). Within the association cortices, the frontal lobe should have general FDG uptake comparable to or greater than that of parietal or temporal association cortices (hyperfrontality). This hyperfrontality can be lost in many conditions. In the aging brain, FDG uptake in the frontal lobe, in particular the medial frontal cortex, tends to decrease more than other parts of the brain (16). This decrease is often associated with

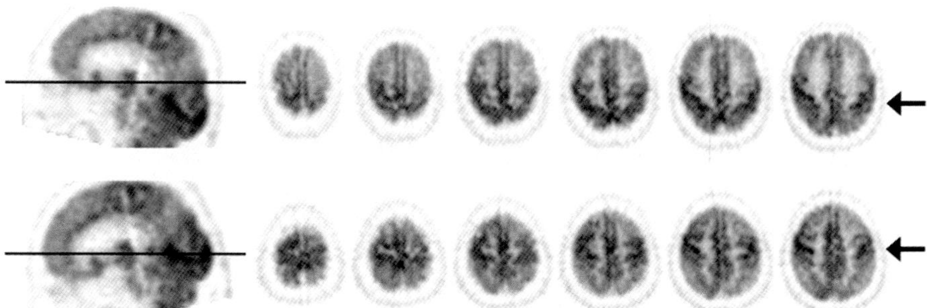

FIGURE 9.2.2. Effects of slice orientation on brain PET image interpretation—Alzheimer disease. Top row (**A**): transverse slices when images are obtained when the neck is extended. Bottom row (**B**): transverse slices when images are realigned parallel to the line passing through the anterior and posterior commissures (AC-PC). Arrows indicate locations of the primary sensorimotor cortex. In (**A**), relatively preserved fluorodeoxyglucose (FDG) uptake in the primary sensorimotor cortex is localized posteriorly in the superior part of the brain and creates an impression that FDG uptake in the parietal association cortex would be relatively preserved in contrast to decreased frontal uptake. In (**B**), the primary sensorimotor cortex is localized in between frontal and parietal lobes in the stereotactic orientation. FDG uptake in frontal and parietal association cortices is clearly diminished in comparison to that of the primary sensorimotor cortex, a diagnostic feature of Alzheimer disease.

TABLE 9.2.4 Structures Identification on PET Images for Dementia Diagnosis

CORTICAL STRUCTURES
Frontal association cortex
Parietal association cortex
Temporal association cortex
Occipital association cortex
Posterior and anterior cingulate cortices
Primary visual cortex, primary sensorimotor cortex
Watershed areas (anterior-middle, middle-posterior cerebral arteries)
SUBCORTICAL STRUCTURES
Caudate
Putamen
Thalamus
Cerebellum
Brainstem

a widened interhemispheric fissure in the medial frontal lobe that can be appreciated on PET images. Decreases in glucose metabolism may also extend to the lateral frontal cortex and anterior perisylvian regions in advanced age populations (Fig. 9.2.4).

Quantification, Pixel Normalization, and Statistical Mapping of Fluorodeoxyglucose PET Images

Using FDG PET imaging data, absolute regional glucose metabolic rates can be quantified by mathematical tracer kinetic modeling. The tracer kinetic modeling typically requires a plasma input function of tracer concentration, which can be measured by arterial sampling, arterialized venous sampling (warming of the arm to increase arterial-venous shunting), or image-based region of interest analysis of arterial activity on dynamic PET images. Early PET investigations with absolute glucose metabolic quantification demonstrated global metabolic reductions in Alzheimer's disease as well as other types of dementias in addition to focally and differentially accentuated hypometabolism (17,18). Due to the requirement for arterial input function measurement, absolute quantification of glucose metabolism by FDG PET is not practical in many clinical settings. Clinical interpretation of FDG PET imaging for dementia is therefore typically based on the *relative* distribution of FDG uptake in the brain. (In this chapter, the terms *FDG uptake* and *glucose metabolism* are used interchangeably for convenience.)

Despite administration of a similar dose of FDG, the level of FDG uptake in the brain can vary significantly and is influenced by several factors, including endogenous plasma glucose levels and the distribution of FDG within the body. The standard uptake value, which is often used for semiquantitative analysis in oncologic image interpretation, is not commonly used for brain PET image interpretation due to limited quantitative accuracy. Instead, pixel values of FDG PET images can be normalized to FDG uptake in a reference region that is known not to be, or at least is expected not to be, significantly affected by the disease processes under study (i.e., brain pixel values/averaged pixel values within the reference region). Traditionally, the thalamus and the cerebellum have been used for this purpose in Alzheimer's disease. Minoshima et al. (19) previously compared normalized FDG uptake by different reference regions, including thalamus, cerebellum, primary sensorimotor cortex, whole brain, and pons, in comparison to absolute glucose metabolic rates measured using an arterial input function in the same Alzheimer's disease subjects and found that pixel normalization using the pons produced the most accurate and precise estimates of absolute glucose metabolism. It is important to note that normalization

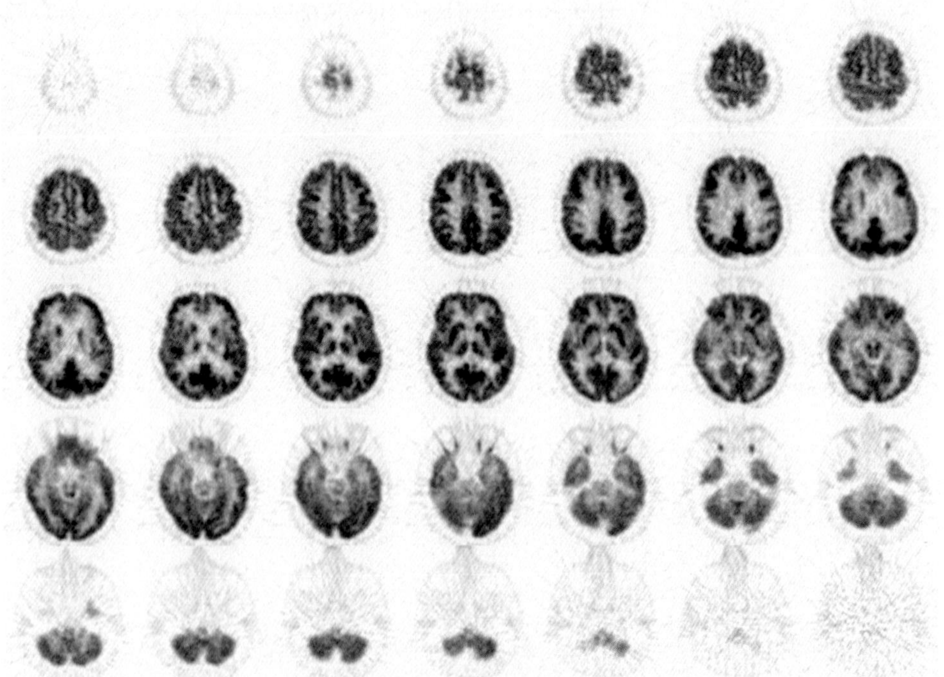

FIGURE 9.2.3. Normal fluorodeoxyglucose PET images. Cortical and subcortical structures are clearly depicted by the current generation of a PET scanner.

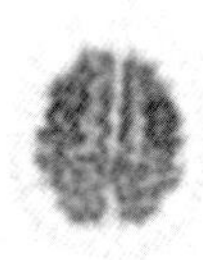
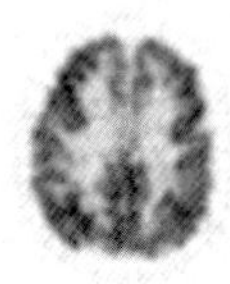
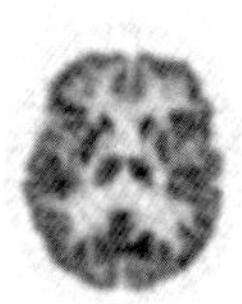
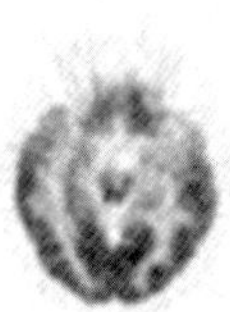
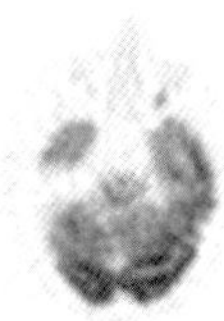
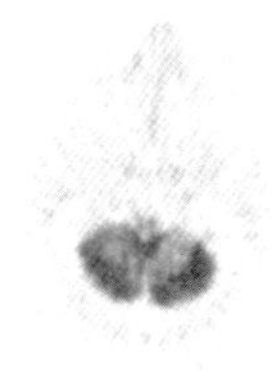

FIGURE 9.2.4. Normal fluorodeoxyglucose (FDG) PET images obtained in an elderly subject. Mildly decreased FDG uptake and widened interhemispheric fissure in the medial frontal lobe are common for an elderly subject.

by averaged whole-brain activity, as is often used in brain mapping analyses, can underestimate the degree and extent of hypometabolism in dementias as these disorders often affect relatively large areas of the brain and the averaged whole-brain activity is therefore affected by the disease processes. Also, particularly when global normalization is used, artifactual *relatively* increased regional FDG uptake may be observed. A caution should be exercised not to interpret this finding as *increased* regional glucose metabolism, as it often represents regionally less severe hypometabolism.

Owing to significant advancements in PET brain activation studies and mapping technology developed in late 1980s and early 1990s (20–24), modern interpretations of brain PET images are often performed statistically in the standard stereotactic coordinate system (15). In these analyses, brain PET images are resliced to match with the standard coordinate system, and individual differences in regional brain shape are minimized by computer algorithms that perform nonlinear warping. Once brain image data sets are standardized, image sets from different subjects can be compared on a pixel-by-pixel basis for various statistical assessments. To objectively and quantitatively estimate regional metabolic changes in dementias, we developed a brain mapping method in which individual brain PET data sets can be compared to a normative data set (often called a normal database) that is created from scans of multiple normal control subjects (25). For each pixel, a Z score, defined as [(individual pixel value minus normal control mean)/normal control standard deviation], can be calculated and displayed for image interpretation (Fig. 9.2.5). In this analysis, areas of hypometabolism can be detected as higher Z scores. This significantly improves the diagnostic accuracy of Alzheimer's disease using brain PET images (26). The concept of this image analysis is similar to that used in cardiac image interpretation (bull's eye). Statistical brain mapping analyses of FDG PET and perfusion SPECT are now used extensively for research investigations of dementia (16,27–32), and similar brain mapping software is now commercially available for routine clinical applications.

RADIOTRACERS OTHER THAN FLUORODEOXYGLUCOSE FOR DEMENTIA PET AND SINGLE-PHOTON EMISSION COMPUTED TOMOGRAPHY IMAGING

Numerous radiotracers have been developed and used for PET and SPECT investigations of dementing disorders. These include tracers for assessment of (a) oxygen metabolism ([^{15}O]-O_2); (b) blood flow ([^{15}O]-water, ^{123}I-IMP, ^{99m}Tc-HMPAO, ^{99m}Tc-ECD); (c) cholinergic system (carbon-11 [^{11}C]-scopolamine, [^{11}C]-TRB, [^{11}C]-NMPB, [^{123}I]-IBVM, [^{123}I]-QNB, [^{11}C]-PMP, [^{11}C]-BMP); (d) dopaminergic system ([^{18}F]-dopa, [^{11}C]-nomifensine, [^{11}C]-raclopride, [^{11}C]-DTBZ, [^{123}I]-IBZP, [^{123}I]-IBF, [^{123}I]-IBZM; (d) serotonergic system ([^{18}F]-setoperone); (e) central and peripheral benzodiazepine receptors ([^{11}C]-FMZ, [^{123}I]-IMZ, [^{11}C]-PK11195); and (f) amyloid ([^{11}C]-PIB, [^{18}F]-FDDNP, [^{11}C]-SB-13) (abbreviations found in MEDLINE). Significant efforts have been directed toward imaging of the cholinergic system in Alzheimer's disease (33–42) owing to the cholinergic hypothesis (43) and the widespread availability of cholinergic treatments for Alzheimer's disease. Beyond traditional perfusion, metabolic, and neurotransmitter receptor imaging, recent PET investigations have also been directed at characterizing immune activity in Alzheimer's brain using [^{11}C]-PK11195 and amyloid deposition using tracers such as [^{11}C]-PIB, [^{18}F]-FDDNP, and [^{11}C]-SB-13. Some of these tracers are described elsewhere in this book.

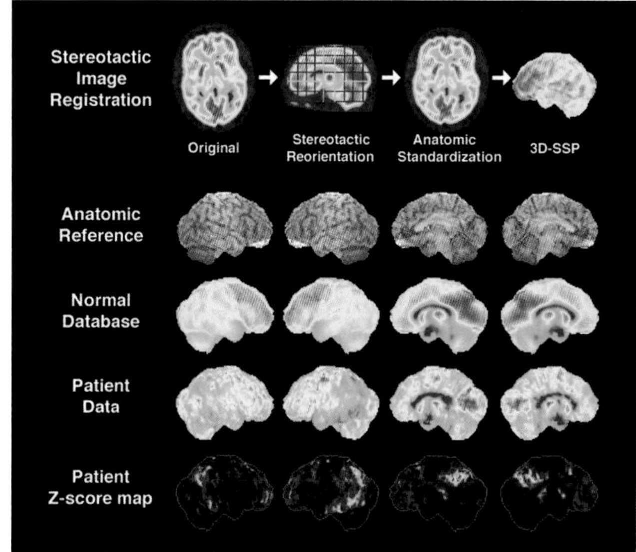

FIGURE 9.2.5. Statistical mapping of brain PET images for image interpretation. Original images are first standardized in the stereotactic coordinate system (stereotactic reorientation parallel to the anterior and posterior line and anatomic standardization to minimize individual anatomic variances), and gray matter activity is extracted into three dimensions (3D-stereotatic surface projections [3D-SSP]) (25). Data from multiple normal subjects constitute normal database (mean and standard deviation for each pixel). When patient data in question are processed in the same way, each pixel value of the patient data is compared to the mean value of the normal database relative to the standard deviation and generates a Z score to indicate the degree of deviation from the normal mean. This forms Z-score maps indicating areas of decreased FDG uptake in the patient in comparison to the normal database. Z-score maps significantly improve diagnostic accuracy of brain FDG PET for dementia (26).

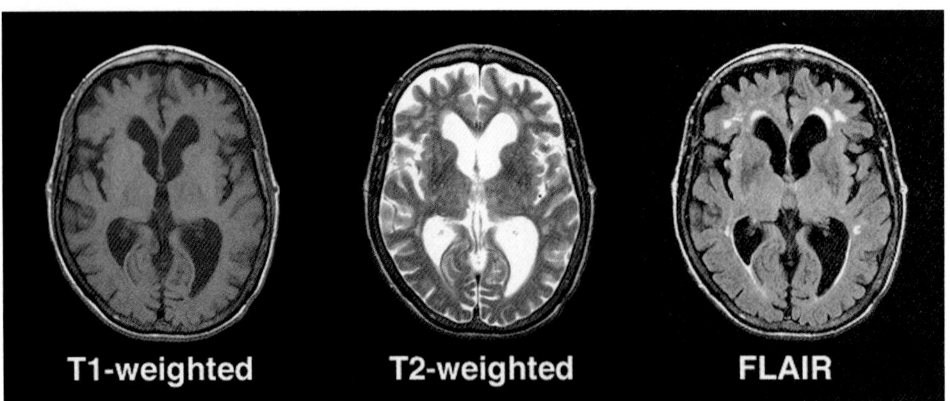

FIGURE 9.2.6. Magnetic resonance imaging for routine clinical evaluation. T1-weighted (**left**), T2-weighted (**middle**), and fluid-attenuated inversion recovery (FLAIR) (**right**) images are routinely obtained for dementia work-up.

MAGNETIC RESONANCE IMAGING FOR ROUTINE DEMENTIA EVALUATION

Structural imaging is often employed to exclude disorders such as stroke, frontal lobe tumor, and subdural hematoma in dementia patients. The cost-effectiveness of CT and MRI in dementia care has been debated. For clinical interpretation of FDG PET images, comparison with MRI is often useful for the evaluation of white matter changes, such as microvascular disease, which can affect cortical metabolic activity. For a typical dementia work-up, a noncontrast MRI can be obtained with pulse sequences including T1-weighted images, T2-weighted images, and fluid-attenuated inversion recovery (FLAIR) images (Fig. 9.2.6). T2-weighted and FLAIR images are useful for the evaluation of white matter abnormalities that cannot be appreciated by FDG PET imaging. T2-weighted images can also be used to evaluate a large vessel *flow void*. T1-weighted images provide detailed information regarding anatomy. It is important to note that neurodegenerative diseases can coexist with vascular disease (*mixed* dementia) (44). These patients can present with clinical symptoms that are not typical for each condition and are diagnostically challenging. Documentation of ischemic changes on MRI and neurodegenerative features on FDG PET help to establish the diagnosis of mixed dementia.

Significant efforts have been made in the field of MRI research to generate markers of neurodegenerative diseases. In addition to traditional hippocampal volume measurements, structural measurement can now be done for cortical gray matter using voxel-based analysis. Quantitative MR perfusion imaging has also been used for dementia evaluation. In addition, diffusion tensor imaging has been used to evaluate white matter tract abnormalities in Alzheimer's disease. Spectroscopic analysis of neurodegenerative disorders is another example. More recently, the feasibility of imaging amyloid in animals using fluorine-19-labeled tracer (45) as well as without tracer (46) have both been demonstrated. Although a detailed review of these technologies is outside the scope of this chapter, they may significantly enhance *in vivo* investigations and represent possible future advances in clinical approaches to imaging of dementing disorders.

METABOLIC PATTERNS OF MAJOR DEMENTING DISORDERS

One goal of FDG PET evaluation is to differentiate dementias with treatment options (e.g., symptomatic treatments for Alzheimer's disease, dementia with Lewy bodies, treatment and risk management for cerebrovascular disease) from nontreatable dementias. Different dementing disorders are often associated with unique metabolic features (47). In the clinical setting, a systematic approach to image interpretation contributes to diagnostic accuracy. An example of a systematic image interpretation is shown in Fig. 9.2.7. Major neurodegenerative disorders are described below.

Alzheimer's Disease

Alzheimer's disease is considered to be the most common cause of dementia. The disease was first described by Dr. Alzheimer's in 1906 (48). Clinical diagnostic criteria for *probable* Alzheimer's disease defined by National Institute of Neurological and Communicative Disorders and Stroke/Alzheimer's Disease and Related Disorders Association (NINCDS-ADRDA) (49) include: (a) dementia established by clinical examination and neuropsychological tests (e.g., Mini-Mental State Examination); (b) deficits in two or more areas of cognition; (c) progressive worsening of memory and other cognitive functions; (d) no disturbance of consciousness; (e) onset between ages 40 and 90, most often after age 65; and (f) absence of systemic disorders or other brain diseases that in and of themselves could account for the progressive deficits in memory

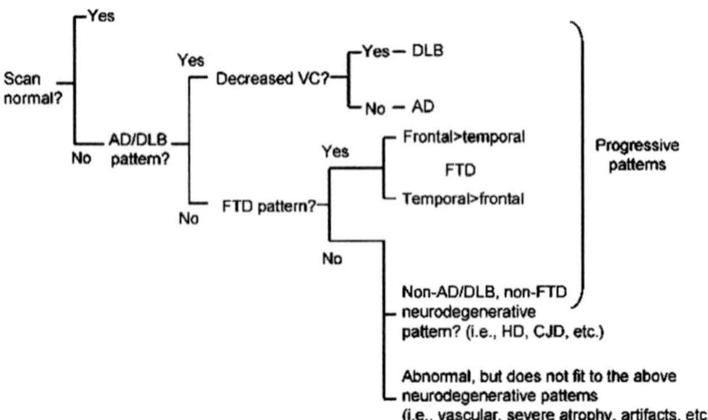

FIGURE 9.2.7. An example of a systematic interpretation of fluorodeoxyglucose PET images. The interpretation starts with a question if the scan is normal, then evaluate Alzheimer changes, frontotemporal changes, and then atypical changes. AD, Alzheimer disease; DLB, dementia with Lewy bodies; VC, visual cortex; FTD, frontotemporal dementia; HD, Huntington's disease; CJD, Creutzfeldt-Jakob's disease.

and cognition. Confirmatory neuropathologic changes include senile plaques containing $A\beta_{1-42}$ fibrils and neurofibrillary tangles made up of hyperphosphorylated tau isoforms. Several causative gene abnormalities (e.g., mutations in amyloid precursor protein [APP], presenilin-1 [PS-1], presenilin-2 [PS-2]) as well as genes that carry risk factors for earlier age of onset (e.g., apolipoprotein E [APOE] genotype) have been identified, but common genetic abnormalities for the majority of sporadic cases are yet to be elucidated. Mechanisms of amyloid deposition have been extensively investigated, and the involvement of APP processing by γ-secretase and other enzymes has been unveiled. There have been numerous publications to date concerning both research and clinical applications of PET imaging in Alzheimer's disease, and the role of PET imaging agents for amyloid is discussed in Chapter 9.1 in this book.

Metabolic features of Alzheimer's disease seen on FDG PET images vary depending on the stage of the disease. In mild dementia, FDG uptake in the parietotemporal association cortices as well as posterior cingulate cortex and precuneus is typically decreased. FDG uptake in the frontal association cortex varies, but mild reductions may be present in patients with mild dementia. In contrast, FDG uptake in the primary sensorimotor cortex, primary visual cortex, thalamus, putamen, pons, and cerebellum is relatively preserved (Fig. 9.2.8). It is important to note that this contrast between areas relatively *affected* and areas relatively *preserved* gives a diagnostic clue to Alzheimer's disease. If FDG uptake is decreased in areas supposed to be relatively preserved in Alzheimer's disease, despite the presence of parietotemporal hypometabolism, these findings might indicate either non-Alzheimer's disease or coexisting diseases such as ischemic vascular changes. When the disease progresses, FDG uptake in all of the association cortices, including frontal lobe, decreases. However, FDG uptake in primary cortices and subcortical structures remains relatively preserved, even in advanced disease (Fig. 9.2.9).

Positive and negative predictive values of the aforementioned FDG PET findings are influenced by the pretest probability of the disease. Risk factors for Alzheimer's disease include advanced age; gender (women greater than men); family history; previous head trauma; and APOE ε4 allele status (50). The association with APOE ε4 allele status has prompted consideration of combining information on genetic risk factors and PET findings to improve the diagnostic accuracy of Alzheimer's disease (51).

In a meta-analysis, the diagnostic accuracy of FDG PET, based on *DSM-III-R* or NINCDS-ADRDA clinical diagnostic criteria for Alzheimer's disease, was approximately 80% sensitivity and 70% specificity (averaged over data from three class I articles) (52–54), although these values varied somewhat depending on clinical settings, physician expertise, and patient populations. In contrast, the FDG PET diagnostic accuracy for Alzheimer's disease in comparison to autopsy results was approximately 90% sensitivity and 76% specificity (averaged over two class II articles) (47,55). These data demonstrate that the accuracy of an FDG PET diagnosis of Alzheimer's disease is comparable to, or even better than, that of a clinical diagnosis. In addition, FDG PET can produce objective diagnostic imaging findings in a single laboratory visit without necessitating a follow-up office visit to confirm progression of cognitive decline.

There are certain "normal variants" of the classic pattern of regional metabolic hypometabolism associated with Alzheimer's disease. Alzheimer's findings are commonly described as *bilateral*, but a certain degree of hemispheric asymmetry is also common. In some cases, only one hemisphere shows substantial abnormalities, and abnormalities in the other hemisphere could be subtle (Fig. 9.2.10). The FDG PET diagnosis for Alzheimer's disease should be based on confirmation of areas typically *affected* and *preserved* in each hemisphere as described above. Metabolic asymmetry often correlates with clinical symptoms (i.e., more prominent visuospatial dysfunction with right hemisphere dominant hypometabolism, more prominent language problem with left hemispheric hypometabolism (56).

Minoshima et al. (57,58) previously described significant hypometabolism in the posterior cingulate cortex and precuneus in Alzheimer's disease. Hypometabolism in the posterior cingulate cortex is difficult to appreciate on transverse slices and it is best visualized by sagittal slices or by the use of statistical mapping techniques. However, some fraction of patients may not demonstrate

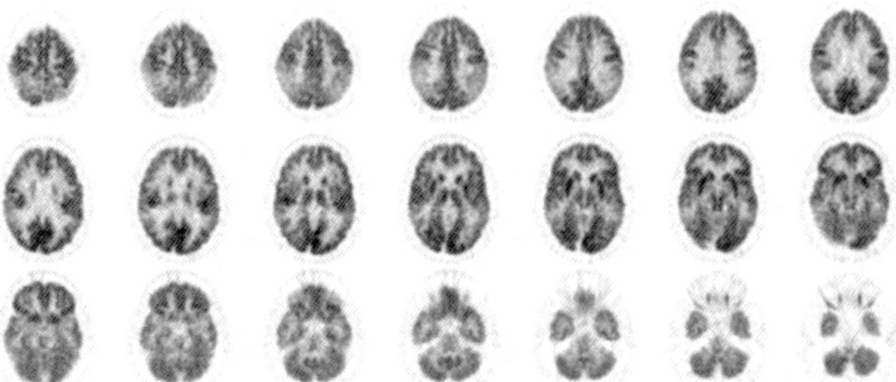

FIGURE 9.2.8. Mild Alzheimer disease. Mild metabolic reductions involving parietotemporal association cortices bilaterally. Fluorodeoxyglucose uptake in the primary sensorimotor cortex (**top row**), primary visual cortex (**middle row**), striatum and thalamus (**middle row**), and cerebellum (**bottom row**) is relatively preserved. Statistical mapping (see Fig. 9.2.17) shows additional metabolic reductions in the posterior cingulate cortex and precuneus. A contrast between areas affected and areas preserved (selective vulnerability) is the diagnostic feature of Alzheimer disease. Both hemispheres are often affected, but asymmetry is also common (Fig. 9.2.10).

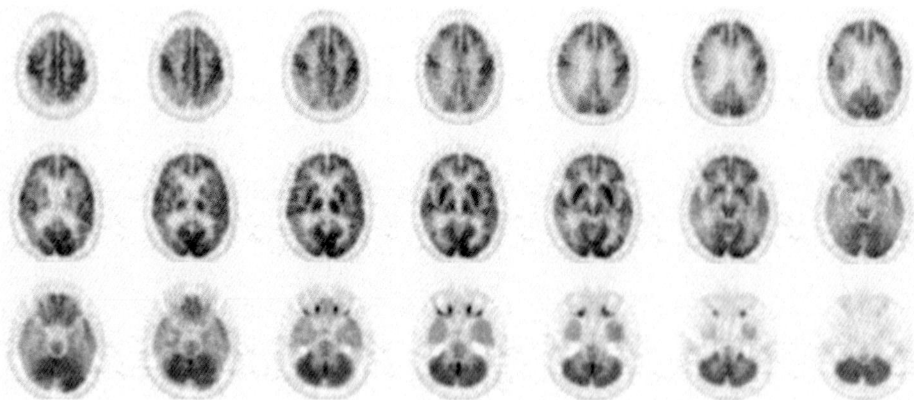

FIGURE 9.2.9. Severe Alzheimer disease. Fluorodeoxyglucose (FDG) uptake in the parietotemporal as well as frontal association cortices is severely decreased (the right hemisphere more severe than the left). Even at this late stage of the disease, FDG uptake in the primary sensorimotor and visual cortices, striatum, thalamus, and cerebellum is relatively preserved.

significant abnormalities in the posterior cingulate cortex (59). Early onset patients (younger than 65 years old) are known to demonstrate more marked metabolic abnormalities compared to late onset patients (60). This translates to clinical implications that, if a suspected dementia patient with age below 65 years old does not show convincing metabolic abnormalities, this patient probably does not have Alzheimer's disease. Mixed dementia is also common and can have somewhat atypical metabolic features, such as decreased and asymmetric FDG uptake in subcortical structures. If FDG PET images show major metabolic findings of Alzheimer's disease, such as parietotemporal hypometabolism, but also asymmetric reduction in FDG uptake in subcortical structures (e.g., thalamus, cerebellum) and/or watershed areas, coexisting micro- or macrovascular disease becomes a consideration. Crossed-cerebellar diaschisis associated with abnormalities in the contralateral hemisphere is commonly seen in stroke and other pathologic conditions, but is not prominently seen in Alzheimer's disease. The presence of apparent crossed-cerebellar diaschisis should raise the possibility of non-Alzheimer's changes or coexisting non-Alzheimer's pathology.

Mild Cognitive Impairment

Progressive neurodegenerative processes, particularly Alzheimer's disease, have been shown to have a long prodromal phase. Significant neuronal loss has occurred by the time clinical symptoms of dementia become evident. Currently, no therapies are available that directly target the underlying neurodegenerative processes in this disorder. Several classes of drugs, such as HMG-CoA reductase inhibitors (statins), nonsteroidal anti-inflammatory drugs, hormone replacement therapy in women, and antioxidants (e.g., vitamin E and vitamin C) have shown promise for preventing or delaying the onset of Alzheimer's disease *in vivo* or in epidemiological studies, but have not proven effective when tested in controlled clinical trials. A possible explanation for these discordant findings is that these agents act to prevent or delay the underlying neurodegenerative processes in Alzheimer's disease but are unable to reverse neuronal damage once it has occurred and therefore are not effective in the treatment of the disease once it has progressed to the point of clinical signs and symptoms. This being the case, the identification of patients still in the early, presymptomatic, stage of the disease would facilitate efforts at disease modification or prevention.

To help identify patients with early stage dementia who may derive greater benefit from treatment, the concept of *mild cognitive impairment* (MCI) has been developed (61,62). MCI patients are identified based on diagnostic criteria including (a) complaint of memory impairment; (b) normal activities of daily living; (c) normal general cognitive function; (d) abnormal memory function for age, and (e) absence of dementia. In some studies, approximately 10% to 15% of MCI patients convert to Alzheimer's disease every year. Subsequent research has identified other subgroups of MCI patients who present with cognitive deficits in domains other than, or in addition to, short-term memory (e.g., language, visuospatial skills, executive function [planning, sequencing, abstract reasoning]) and determined that multiple etiologic factors other than, or

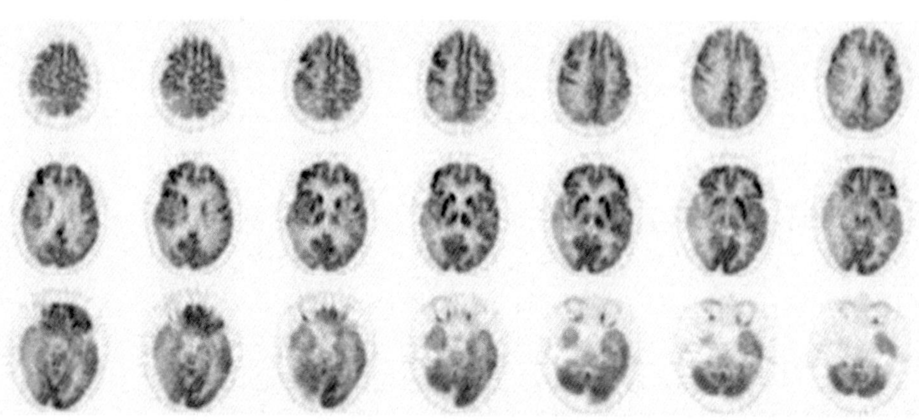

FIGURE 9.2.10. Alzheimer disease. Hemispheric asymmetry. Right parietotemporal cortices show decreased fluorodeoxyglucose (FDG) uptake. FDG uptake in the right primary sensorimotor cortex is relatively preserved (**top row**). The patient's head was tilted in the scanner, which would give impressions of asymmetric striatal and thalamic uptake.

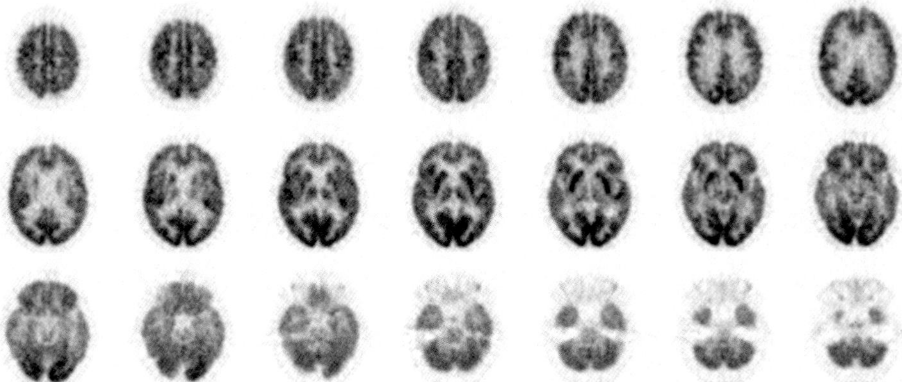

FIGURE 9.2.11. Very early Alzheimer disease identified in a patient with mild cognitive impairment (MCI). Very mild metabolic reductions in the left lateral parietal association cortex (**top row**), but it may not be difficult to appreciate such changes by visual inspection. Mildly accentuated fluorodeoxyglucose uptake in the region of the primary sensorimotor cortex bilaterally (**top row**) is often a sign of mild metabolic reductions in adjacent association cortices. Statistical mapping of this patient (Fig. 9.2.17) clearly demonstrates mild metabolic reductions in the parietotemporal association cortices, frontal association cortices, and posterior cingulate cortex and precuneus, bilaterally (the left hemisphere more severe than the right), but relative preservation of primary sensorimotor and visual cortices, findings consistent with very mild Alzheimer disease.

in addition to, incipient Alzheimer's disease may be present (i.e., degenerative, vascular, metabolic, traumatic, psychiatric disorders) (63,64).

Metabolic features of MCI are, for the most part, consistent with those seen in Alzheimer's disease, but of milder degree (11). Metabolic reduction in the posterior cingulate cortex is a relatively consistent finding. Identification of Alzheimer-type metabolic changes in MCI patients is highly predictive of subsequent cognitive decline and development of frank dementia (31). In a clinical setting, however, mild metabolic changes associated with very early Alzheimer's disease in MCI patients may not be easily identified on FDG PET images (Fig. 9.2.11). However, application of statistical mapping techniques can clearly improve diagnostic accuracy of FDG PET imaging in these circumstances (see Fig. 9.2.17) (26). Another approach is to combine imaging findings and other biomarkers such as risk genotypes to improve diagnostic accuracy (51). Combination of multiple diagnostic biomarkers is one of the directions of current research in Alzheimer's disease.

The extreme sensitivity of FDG PET in detecting very early changes in dementia is further demonstrated by findings of subtle Alzheimer's changes in cognitively normal middle-aged APOE $\varepsilon4$ homozygotes (65) and in normal elderly subjects who later developed cognitive decline (66). It remains to be determined just how early in the course of Alzheimer's disease altered glucose metabolic activity can be demonstrated and whether this occurs earlier or later than detectable changes in other Alzheimer's disease biomarkers, such as amyloid PET tracer uptake or alterations in cerebral spinal fluid β-amyloid and tau levels.

Frontotemporal Dementia

In contrast to Alzheimer's disease, frontotemporal dementia is more common among younger patients (onset under 65 years of age), and more prevalent in men (67). In the United States, the first government approval for dementia work-up by FDG PET was the differential diagnosis of Alzheimer's disease versus frontotemporal dementia. It is important to note that the pathological and clinical characterization and classification of frontotemporal dementia is an evolving field of research. A spectrum of neurodegenerative disorders that affects predominantly frontal and temporal lobes is included in the category of frontotemporal dementia. Mutations of the tau gene on chromosome 17 cause some forms of familial frontotemporal dementia (68). Mutations in progranulin genes have recently been associated with other familial forms of frontotemporal dementia (69). Other cases of frontotemporal dementia are associated with amyotrophic lateral sclerosis (70,71). Both the clinical presentations and pathologic features of frontotemporal dementia are similarly heterogeneous (72) and also do not necessarily show one-to-one correspondence (Table 9.2.5).

TABLE 9.2.5 Heterogeneity of Frontotemporal Dementia

PATHOLOGY
Classic Pick's disease (PiD)
Corticobasal degeneration (CBD)
Progressive supranuclear palsy (PSP)
Frontotemporal lobar degeneration with motor neuron disease or motor neuron disease-type inclusions (FTLD-MND/MNI)
Neurofibrillary tangle dementia (NFTD)
Dementia lacking distinctive histopathologic features (DLDH)
CLINICAL PRESENTATIONS
Frontal lobe dementia
Primary progressive aphasia
Corticobasal degeneration syndrome
Progressive supranuclear palsy
Amyotrophic lateral sclerosis

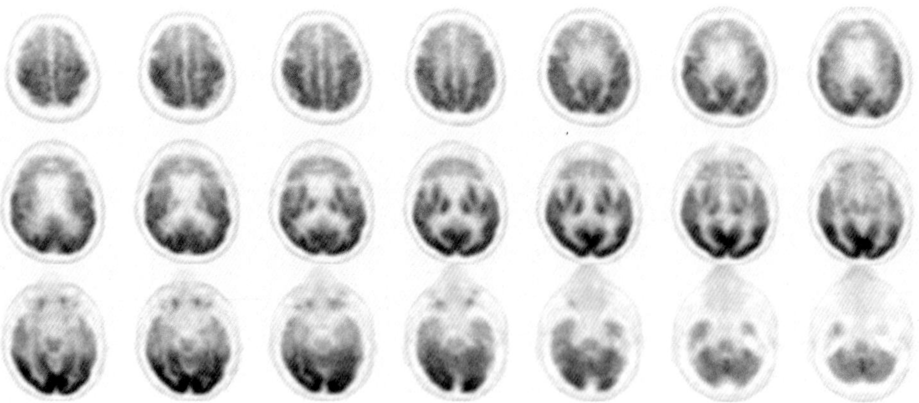

FIGURE 9.2.12. Frontotemporal dementia. Classical case of frontal lobar hypometabolism (bilateral). Additional metabolic reductions are seen in the anterior temporal lobe and caudate. Fluorodeoxyglucose uptake in the primary sensorimotor cortex and occipital cortex is relatively preserved.

Reflecting the pathologic and clinical heterogeneities of frontotemporal dementia, the metabolic features of these disorders are also variable. Classical *lobar* hypometabolism affecting predominantly frontal lobe may be seen in Pick's disease (Fig. 9.2.12). Although frontal and temporal lobes are often involved bilaterally, hypometabolism can be significantly asymmetric (Fig. 9.2.13). In addition to the frontal hypometabolism, the caudate nucleus and anterior temporal lobe often show hypometabolism. Similar to Alzheimer's disease, FDG uptake in the primary sensorimotor cortex (as well as other primary cortices such as primary visual cortex) is relatively preserved. When the disease progresses, areas of hypometabolism extend to the parietal and temporal association cortices (73). This progressive pattern is an important contrast to that of Alzheimer's disease in which parietotemporal association cortices are initially involved, and the frontal association cortex is affected in more severe cases. These metabolic features provide differential diagnostic clues for Alzheimer's disease versus frontotemporal dementia. However, other types of frontotemporal dementia demonstrate more variable metabolic features. Progressive supranuclear palsy shows milder superior frontal hypometabolism as well as subcortical hypometabolism (74–76) (Fig. 9.2.14). Frontotemporal dementia resulting from mutations of the tau gene on chromosome 17 can show more temporal lobe-dominant metabolic reductions with milder frontal hypometabolism (Fig. 9.2.15). It is sometimes difficult to distinguish temporal-dominant hypometabolism in frontotemporal dementia from those seen in Alzheimer's disease. Other biomarkers such as amyloid PET imaging may be helpful to better differentiate these conditions.

Many other medical and psychiatric conditions are known to affect metabolic activity in the frontal lobe (Table 9.2.6). Among these, vascular disease, alcoholism, and depression can be seen relatively frequently in patients referred for imaging studies. Correlation with medical history as well as structural MRI becomes essential for accurate differential diagnosis especially when FDG PET findings are somewhat atypical.

Dementia with Lewy Bodies and Parkinson's Disease with Dementia

A pathologic hallmark for Parkinson's disease is the presence of Lewy bodies in the brainstem (77) (Fig. 9.2.16). In the 1970s, demented patients were described who had numerous cortical Lewy bodies (78). Owing to the development of antiubiquitin immunocytochemistry (79,80), cortical Lewy bodies were subsequently described in larger numbers of patients presenting with dementia. After decades of debate and various proposals for taxonomy, a consensus of pathologic and clinical diagnostic criteria for dementia with Lewy bodies were established in 1996 (81). Dementia with Lewy bodies is now considered to be the second most common cause of dementia (81,82), following Alzheimer's disease, and

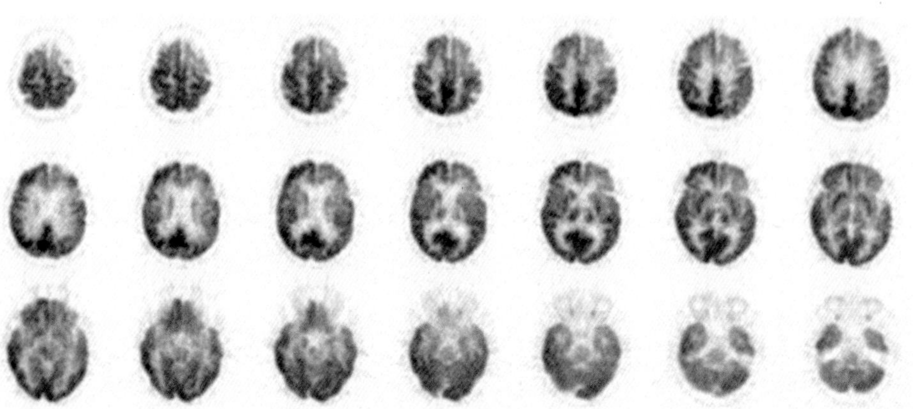

FIGURE 9.2.13. Frontotemporal dementia. Hemispheric asymmetry. The left frontal lobe, caudate, and anterior temporal lobe are more severely involved than the right hemisphere. These asymmetric findings are seen often in frontotemporal dementia as well as in Alzheimer disease. Fluorodeoxyglucose uptake in the primary sensorimotor cortex is relatively preserved in both hemispheres.

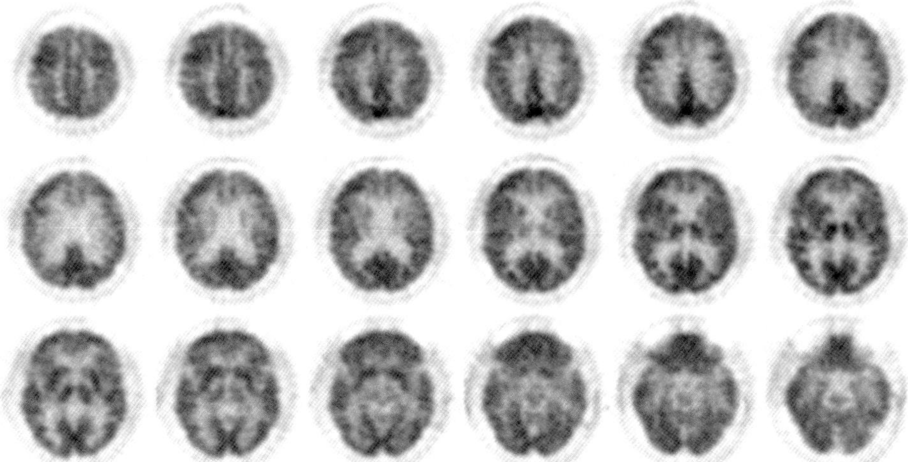

FIGURE 9.2.14. Progressive supranuclear palsy. Mild metabolic reductions are seen in the superior frontal cortex (more prominent in the medial frontal cortex), the left hemisphere more severely involved than the right (**top row**). Mild metabolic reduction is also seen in the left caudate (**middle row**).

followed by vascular dementia and frontotemporal dementia. Three distinctive clinical features are (a) spontaneous motor features of parkinsonism occurring early in the course of the disease; (b) marked fluctuations in cognitive function; and (c) persistent well-formed visual hallucinations. However, these symptoms are not necessarily consistent among patients, and clinical diagnosis remains challenging. Patients with dementia with Lewy bodies are sensitive to the side effects of neuroleptics, and adverse events can be severe and fatal (83), requiring careful selection of agent and dosage. Also, response to cholinesterase treatment can be more favorable in comparison to Alzheimer's disease (81). Because of these therapeutic implications, differential diagnosis of Alzheimer's disease versus dementia with Lewy bodies is critical.

Albin et al. (84) reported the first FDG PET findings of autopsy-proven cases of dementia with Lewy bodies, which was followed by a larger number of autopsy confirmed cases of both dementia with Lewy bodies and Alzheimer's disease (55). Dementia with Lewy bodies showed metabolic changes nearly identical to Alzheimer's disease in the cerebral cortex, but additional significant hypometabolism was observed in the occipital lobe, including the primary visual cortex (which is typically relatively preserved in Alzheimer's disease). Such occipital hypometabolism was seen in dementia with Lewy bodies with and without coexisting Alzheimer's changes. When using occipital hypometabolism as a marker of dementia with Lewy bodies, the sensitivity and specificity to distinguish dementia with Lewy bodies from Alzheimer's disease were 90% and 80%, respectively (autopsy-confirmed cases). These findings have been confirmed by other investigators (85,86) and are now considered to be a supportive feature of dementia with Lewy bodies in the most recent consensus diagnostic criteria (87). It is interesting to note that, despite the diagnostic value of the occipital hypometabolism in dementia with Lewy bodies, Lewy bodies are not prominent in the occipital lobe at autopsy. The pathophysiological mechanisms of occipital hypometabolism in dementia with Lewy bodies have yet to be elucidated.

More than half of Parkinson's disease patients eventually develop dementia. Many of these patients exhibit cortical Lewy bodies identical to dementia with Lewy bodies. Despite differences in the temporal sequences of symptoms (motor symptoms first in Parkinson's disease with dementia, dementia first in dementia with Lewy bodies), both diseases share similar pathological findings—abnormal neuronal α-synuclein inclusions forming Lewy bodies (88). Treatment responses to cholinesterase inhibitors are also similar in the two disorders (89). Reflecting close similarities between Parkinson's disease with dementia and dementia with Lewy bodies, FDG PET findings are also similar in these two disorders. Parkinson's disease with dementia is characterized by hypometabolism in the parietotemporal association cortices and additional hypometabolism in the occipital cortex including the primary visual cortex (30). When compared to Alzheimer's disease, metabolic reductions in the medial temporal cortex are relatively mild.

Imaging biomarkers other than FDG PET for dementia with Lewy bodies have been investigated. Consistent with the fact that dementia with Lewy bodies and Parkinson's disease with dementia

FIGURE 9.2.15. Frontotemporal dementia. Temporal-dominant hypometabolism. Fluorodeoxyglucose uptake is decreased in the anterior temporal lobe bilaterally. Additional metabolic reductions are seen in the medial frontal cortex bilaterally and caudate nucleus.

TABLE 9.2.6 Differential Diagnosis for Frontal Hypometabolism

Advanced aging
Frontotemporal dementia
Ischemia (microvascular, macrovascular)
Depression
Alcoholism
Schizophrenia
Brain trauma
Substance exposure
Others

exhibit neuropathological overlap with Parkinson's disease, PET and SPECT imaging of dopamine systems demonstrate decreased dopaminergic markers in all three of these conditions (87,90,91). In contrast, Alzheimer's disease is associated with only mild decrease in dopaminergic markers. Decreased dopamine uptake in the striatum is considered to be a *suggestive* feature of dementia with Lewy bodies in the current consensus diagnostic criteria (87). More recently, loss of cardiac sympathetic innervation in dementia with Lewy bodies was found using metaiodobenzylguanidine SPECT imaging (92,93). Decreased metaiodobenzylguanidine uptake in the heart can help distinguish dementia with Lewy bodies from Alzheimer's disease (94–96). Expanded commercial availability of these imaging biomarkers will likely further improve the ability to differentiate dementia with Lewy bodies, Alzheimer's disease, and related disorders in clinical settings.

HEALTH EFFECTS AND COST-BENEFIT CONSIDERATION OF FLUORODEOXYGLUCOSE PET IN DEMENTIA WORK-UP

Despite the government approval of reimbursement for FDG PET concerning differential diagnosis of Alzheimer's versus frontotemporal dementia in the United States, there is limited evidence concerning the cost effectiveness of FDG PET diagnosis in dementia care in comparison to that without PET diagnosis. Due to logistic difficulties in obtaining such evidence (i.e., the time required for final [pathologic] diagnostic confirmation; limited outcome variables; limited funding to conduct large-scale, prospective studies), attempts have been made to utilize statistical models to estimate the effectiveness of PET imaging in the diagnosis of dementia (the Agency for Healthcare Research and Quality, Contract No. 290-97-0014, Task Order 7, December 14, 2001). This analysis evaluated costs per life-years saved and quality-adjusted life years resulting from instituting cholinesterase inhibitor treatment in three clinical scenarios (mild to moderate dementia, mild cognitive impairment, and subjects at risk for dementia) with treatment based on presence or absence of PET imaging findings and concluded that "treatment without testing" in all three groups was the best outcome. However, the conclusions of this analysis have been criticized on several grounds, including limited outcome measures and limited input data for patients with mild cognitive impairment and subjects at risk for dementia, and there are still ongoing efforts to generate more evidence to assess the size of health effects in a prospectively designed research protocol. One example is a Center for Medicare and Medicaid Services supported study of FDG PET in the diagnosis of questionable dementia.

Cost-benefit considerations become an important factor in the implementation and widespread use of FDG PET imaging for dementia work-up. The literature evidence concerning cost of dementia care with and without FDG PET imaging is also limited. One study estimated that the use of FDG PET could result in greater numbers of patients being accurately diagnosed for the same level of financial expenditure over a wide range of tested values for PET diagnostic accuracy, costs of PET imaging, and long-term care costs, as well as varying degrees of use of structural neuroimaging (97). Another study argued that the use of functional imaging studies for the diagnosis of Alzheimer's disease is not cost effective in light of the effectiveness of currently available treatments (98). Given the impending implementation of new, potentially disease-modifying treatments (i.e., γ-secretase inhibitors, β-amyloid antibodies) and improving imaging technologies such as amyloid PET imaging, further cost-benefit analyses of PET imaging for

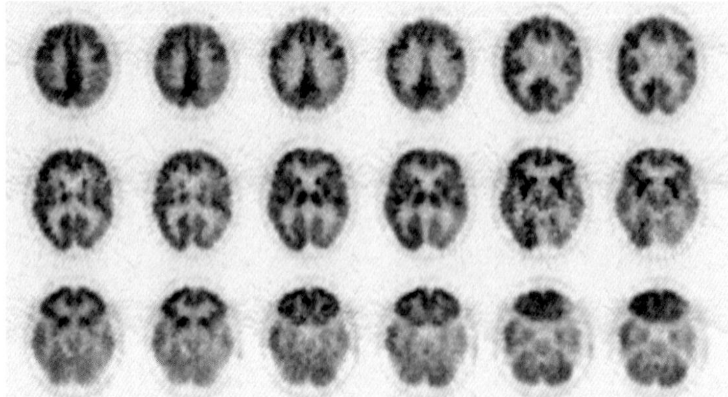

FIGURE 9.2.16. Dementia with Lewy bodies. Hypometabolism in the parietotemporal association cortices (the left hemisphere more severe than the right) similar to Alzheimer disease is seen. When compared to Alzheimer disease (Fig. 9.2.8), fluorodeoxyglucose (FDG) uptake in the primary visual cortex and occipital cortex is decreased, metabolic features of dementia with Lewy bodies. Typically, FDG uptake in the primary visual cortex is comparable to that of the thalamus. This case clearly shows metabolic reductions in the visual cortex in comparison to those in the thalamus (**middle row**).

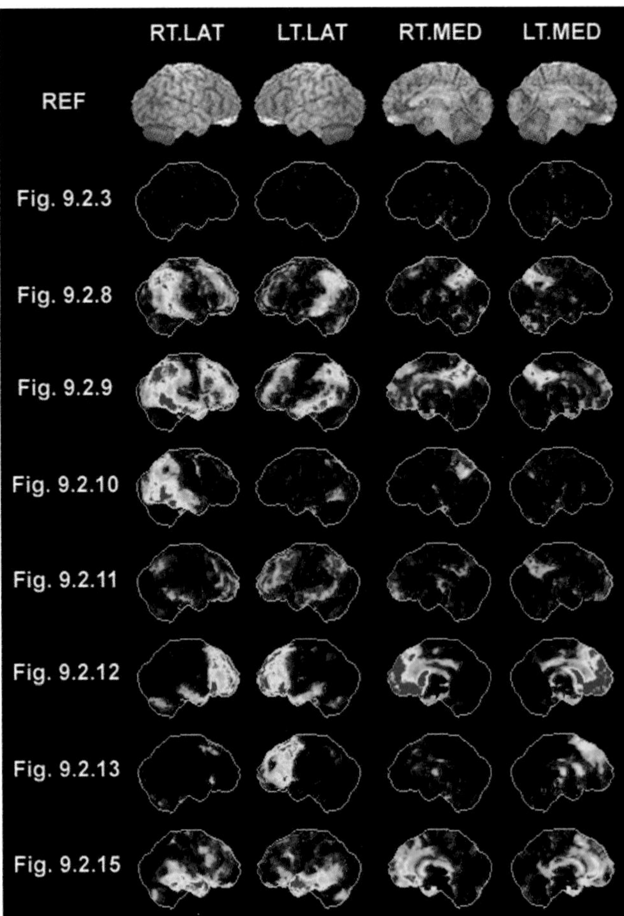

FIGURE 9.2.17. Sample Z-score maps of fluorodeoxyglucose PET images presented in this chapter. Anatomic reference images at the top (REF). Right lateral (RT.LAT), left lateral (LT.LAT), right medial (RT.MED), and left medial (LT.MED) hemispheres are demonstrated in 3D-SSP format. Color images represent Z scores that indicate the degree of regional hypometabolism relative to the normal database. Normal (Fig. 9.2.3); mild Alzheimer disease (Fig. 9.2.8); severe Alzheimer's disease (Fig. 9.2.9); asymmetric Alzheimer disease (Fig. 9.2.10); mild cognitive impairment (very mild Alzheimer disease) (Fig. 9.2.11); frontotemporal dementia (frontal lobar hypometabolism) (Fig. 9.2.12); asymmetric frontotemporal dementia (Fig. 9.2.13); and frontotemporal dementia, temporal dominant (Fig. 9.2.15).

Alzheimer's disease and other dementing illnesses are likely to be initiated to allow informed and cost-effective diagnostic and treatment decisions in clinical settings.

SUMMARY

In this chapter PET imaging of dementia, with a particular emphasis on FDG PET, has been reviewed. The clinical work-up of dementia, common fluorodeoxyglucose PET imaging protocols, principles of image interpretation, metabolic features of major neurodegenerative disorders, and cost-benefit relationships have been summarized. Extensive research and clinical applications of FDG PET in dementia have been published by numerous investigators. Given the increasing availability of PET imaging in routine clinical settings and ongoing developments of imaging technology, PET imaging can be expected to improve the diagnosis and management of patients with dementia in the future.

ACKNOWLEDGMENTS

The authors thank Yoshimi Anzai, MD, and Donna Cross, PhD, for their expert input. Data presented in this article are in part supported by NIH/NINDS RO1-NS045254.

REFERENCES

1. Kukull WA, Higdon R, Bowen JD, et al. Dementia and Alzheimer disease incidence: a prospective cohort study. *Arch Neurol* 2002;59:1737–1746.
2. Bachman DL, Wolf PA, Linn R, et al. Prevalence of dementia and probable senile dementia of the Alzheimer type in the Framingham Study. *Neurology* 1992;42:115–119.
3. Frackowiak RS, Pozzilli C, Legg NJ, et al. Regional cerebral oxygen supply and utilization in dementia. A clinical and physiological study with oxygen-15 and positron tomography. *Brain* 1981;104:753–778.
4. *Diagnostic and statistical manual of mental disorders* (DSM-IV). Washington, DC: American Psychiatric Association, 1994.
5. Fagan AM, Csernansky CA, Morris JC, et al. The search for antecedent biomarkers of Alzheimer's disease. *J Alzheimers Dis* 2005;8:347–358.
6. Ishii K, Minoshima S. PET is better than perfusion SPECT for early diagnosis of Alzheimer's disease. *Eur J Nucl Med Mol Imaging* 2005;32:1463–1465.
7. Sokoloff L, Reivich M, Kennedy C, et al. The [14C]deoxyglucose method for the measurement of local cerebral glucose utilization: theory, procedure, and normal values in the conscious and anesthetized albino rat. *J Neurochem* 1977;28:897–916.
8. Reivich M, Kuhl D, Wolf A, et al. Measurement of local cerebral glucose metabolism in man with ^{18}F-2-fluoro-2-deoxy-d-glucose. *Acta Neurol Scand Suppl* 1977;64:190–191.
9. Magistretti PJ, Pellerin L. Cellular bases of brain energy metabolism and their relevance to functional brain imaging: evidence for a prominent role of astrocytes. *Cerebral Cortex* 1996;6:50–61.
10. Reiman EM, Caselli RJ, Yun LS, et al. Preclinical evidence of Alzheimer's disease in persons homozygous for the epsilon 4 allele for apolipoprotein E. *N Engl J Med* 1996;334:752–758.
11. Minoshima S, Giordani B, Berent S, et al. Metabolic reduction in the posterior cingulate cortex in very early Alzheimer's disease. *Ann Neurol* 1997;42:85–94.
12. Masliah E, Mallory M, Hansen L, et al. Synaptic and neuritic alterations during the progression of Alzheimer's disease. *Neurosci Lett* 1994;174:67–72.
13. Masliah E, Terry RD, Alford M, et al. Cortical and subcortical patterns of synaptophysinlike immunoreactivity in Alzheimer's disease. *Am J Pathol* 1991;138:235–246.
14. Bartenstein P, Asenbaum S, Catafau A, et al. European Association of Nuclear Medicine procedure guidelines for brain imaging using [(^{18})F]FDG. *Eur J Nucl Med Mol Imaging* 2002;29:BP43–48.
15. Talairach J, Tournoux P. *Co-planar stereotaxic atlas of the human brain.* New York: Thieme, 1988.
16. Petit-Taboue MC, Landeau B, Desson JF, et al. Effects of healthy aging on the regional cerebral metabolic rate of glucose assessed with statistical parametric mapping. *Neuroimage* 1998;7:176–184.
17. Benson DF, Kuhl DE, Hawkins RA, et al. The fluorodeoxyglucose ^{18}F scan in Alzheimer's disease and multi-infarct dementia. *Arch Neurol* 1983;40:711–714.
18. Kuhl DE, Metter EJ, Riege WH. Patterns of local cerebral glucose utilization determined in Parkinson's disease by the [^{18}F]fluorodeoxyglucose method. *Ann Neurol* 1984;15:419–424.

19. Minoshima S, Frey KA, Foster NL, et al. Preserved pontine glucose metabolism in Alzheimer disease: a reference region for functional brain image (PET) analysis. *J Comput Assist Tomogr* 1995;19: 541–547.
20. Fox PT, Perlmutter JS, Raichle ME. A stereotactic method of anatomical localization for positron emission tomography. *J Comput Assist Tomogr* 1985;9:141–153.
21. Friston KJ, Passingham RE, Nutt JG, et al. Localisation in PET images: direct fitting of the intercommissural (AC-PC) line. *J Cereb Blood Flow Metab* 1989;9:690–695.
22. Minoshima S, Koeppe RA, Mintun MA, et al. Automated detection of the intercommissural line for stereotactic localization of functional brain images. *J Nucl Med* 1993;34:322–329.
23. Woods RP. Modeling for intergroup comparisons of imaging data. *Neuroimage* 1996;4:S84–S94.
24. Friston KJ, Frith CD, Liddle PF, et al. The relationship between global and local changes in PET scans. *J Cereb Blood Flow Metab* 1990;10: 458–466.
25. Minoshima S, Frey KA, Koeppe RA, et al. A diagnostic approach in Alzheimer's disease using three-dimensional stereotactic surface projections of fluorine-18-FDG PET. *J Nucl Med* 1995;36:1238–1248.
26. Burdette JH, Minoshima S, Vander Borght T, et al. Alzheimer disease: improved visual interpretation of PET images by using three-dimensional stereotaxic surface projections. *Radiology* 1996;198:837–843.
27. Ishii K, Sasaki M, Yamaji S, et al. Demonstration of decreased posterior cingulate perfusion in mild Alzheimer's disease by means of $H_2{}^{15}O$ positron emission tomography. *Eur J Nucl Med* 1997;24:670–673.
28. Signorini M, Paulesu E, Friston K, et al. Rapid assessment of regional cerebral metabolic abnormalities in single subjects with quantitative and nonquantitative [^{18}F]FDG PET: a clinical validation of statistical parametric mapping. *Neuroimage* 1999;9:63–80.
29. Bartenstein P, Minoshima S, Hirsch C, et al. Quantitative assessment of cerebral blood flow in patients with Alzheimer's disease by SPECT. *J Nucl Med* 1997;38:1095–1101.
30. Vander Borght T, Minoshima S, Giordani B, et al. Cerebral metabolic differences in Parkinson's and Alzheimer's diseases matched for dementia severity. *J Nucl Med* 1997;38:797–802.
31. Drzezga A, Lautenschlager N, Siebner H, et al. Cerebral metabolic changes accompanying conversion of mild cognitive impairment into Alzheimer's disease: a PET follow-up study. *Eur J Nucl Med Mol Imaging* 2003;30:1104–1113.
32. Nobili F, Koulibaly M, Vitali P, et al. Brain perfusion follow-up in Alzheimer's patients during treatment with acetylcholinesterase inhibitors. *J Nucl Med* 2002;43:983–990.
33. Holman BL, Gibson RE, Hill TC, et al. Muscarinic acetylcholine receptors in Alzheimer's disease. *In vivo* imaging with iodine 123-labeled 3-quinuclidinyl-4-iodobenzilate and emission tomography. *JAMA* 1985;254:3063–3066.
34. Weinberger DR, Mann U, Gibson RE, et al. Cerebral muscarinic receptors in primary degenerative dementia as evaluated by SPECT with iodine-123-labeled QNB. *Adv Neurol* 1990;51:147–150.
35. Kuhl DE, Koeppe RA, Fessler JA, et al. *In vivo* mapping of cholinergic neurons in the human brain using SPECT and IBVM. *J Nucl Med* 1994;35:405–410.
36. Kuhl DE, Minoshima S, Fessler JA, et al. *In vivo* mapping of cholinergic terminals in normal aging, Alzheimer's disease, and Parkinson's disease. *Ann Neurol* 1996;40:399–410.
37. Kuhl DE, Koeppe RA, Minoshima S, et al. *In vivo* mapping of cerebral acetylcholinesterase activity in aging and Alzheimer's disease. *Neurology* 1999;52:691–699.
38. Kuhl DE, Minoshima S, Frey KA, et al. Limited donepezil inhibition of acetylcholinesterase measured with positron emission tomography in living Alzheimer cerebral cortex. *Ann Neurol* 2000;48:391–395.
39. Kuhl DE, Koeppe RA, Snyder SE, et al. *In vivo* butyrylcholinesterase activity is not increased in Alzheimer's disease synapses. *Ann Neurol* 2006;59:13–20.
40. Namba H, Irie T, Fukushi K, et al. *In vivo* measurement of acetylcholinesterase activity in the brain with a radioactive acetylcholine analog. *Brain Res* 1994;667:278–282.
41. Irie T, Fukushi K, Namba H, et al. Brain acetylcholinesterase activity: validation of a PET tracer in a rat model of Alzheimer's disease. *J Nucl Med* 1996;37:649–655.
42. Iyo M, Namba H, Fukushi K, et al. Measurement of acetylcholinesterase by positron emission tomography in the brains of healthy controls and patients with Alzheimer's disease. *Lancet* 1997;349:1805–1809.
43. Bartus RT, Dean RLd, Beer B, et al. The cholinergic hypothesis of geriatric memory dysfunction. *Science* 1982;217:408–414.
44. Rockwood K, Macknight C, Wentzel C, et al. The diagnosis of "mixed" dementia in the Consortium for the Investigation of Vascular Impairment of Cognition (CIVIC). *Ann N Y Acad Sci* 2000;903:522–528.
45. Higuchi M, Iwata N, Matsuba Y, et al. ^{19}F and ^{1}H MRI detection of amyloid beta plaques *in vivo*. *Nat Neurosci* 2005;8:527–533.
46. Jack CR Jr, Garwood M, Wengenack TM, et al. *In vivo* visualization of Alzheimer's amyloid plaques by magnetic resonance imaging in transgenic mice without a contrast agent. *Magn Reson Med* 2004;52:1263–1271.
47. Silverman DH, Small GW, Chang CY, et al. Positron emission tomography in evaluation of dementia: regional brain metabolism and long-term outcome. *JAMA* 2001;286:2120–2127.
48. Alzheimer A. Uber einen eigenartigen schweren Erkrankungsprozeb der Hirnrinde. Neurologisches Centralblatt. *Neurologisches Centralblatt* 1906;23:1129–1136.
49. Tierney MC, Fisher RH, Lewis AJ, et al. The NINCDS-ADRDA Work Group criteria for the clinical diagnosis of probable Alzheimer's disease: a clinicopathologic study of 57 cases. *Neurology* 1988;38:359–364.
50. Corder EH, Saunders AM, Strittmatter WJ, et al. Gene dose of apolipoprotein E type 4 allele and the risk of Alzheimer's disease in late onset families. *Science* 1993;261:921–923.
51. Drzezga A, Grimmer T, Riemenschneider M, et al. Prediction of individual clinical outcome in MCI by means of genetic assessment and (^{18})F-FDG PET. *J Nucl Med* 2005;46:1625–1632.
52. Holmes C, Cairns N, Lantos P, et al. Validity of current clinical criteria for Alzheimer's disease, vascular dementia and dementia with Lewy bodies. *Br J Psychiatry* 1999;174:45–50.
53. Jobst KA, Barnetson LP, Shepstone BJ. Accurate prediction of histologically confirmed Alzheimer's disease and the differential diagnosis of dementia: the use of NINCDS-ADRDA and *DSM-III-R* criteria, SPECT, x-ray CT, and APO E4 in medial temporal lobe dementias. Oxford Project to Investigate Memory and Aging. *Int Psychogeriatr* 1998;10:271–302.
54. Lim A, Tsuang D, Kukull W, et al. Clinico-neuropathological correlation of Alzheimer's disease in a community-based case series. *J Am Geriatr Soc* 1999;47:564–569.
55. Minoshima S, Foster NL, Sima AA, et al. Alzheimer's disease versus dementia with Lewy bodies: cerebral metabolic distinction with autopsy confirmation. *Ann Neurol* 2001;50:358–365.
56. Foster NL, Chase TN, Fedio P, et al. Alzheimer's disease: focal cortical changes shown by positron emission tomography. *Neurology* 1983;33: 961–965.
57. Minoshima S, Foster NL, Kuhl DE. Posterior cingulate cortex in Alzheimer's disease. *Lancet* 1994;344:895.
58. Minoshima S, Foster NL, Frey KA, et al. Metabolic differences in Alzheimer's disease with and without cortical Lewy bodies as revealed by PET. *J Cereb Blood Flow Metab* 1997;17:S437.
59. Bonte FJ, Harris TS, Roney CA, et al. Differential diagnosis between Alzheimer's and frontotemporal disease by the posterior cingulate sign. *J Nucl Med* 2004;45:771–774.
60. Ichimiya A, Herholz K, Mielke R, et al. Difference of regional cerebral metabolic pattern between presenile and senile dementia of the Alzheimer type: a factor analytic study. *J Neurol Sci* 1994;123:11–17.
61. Petersen RC. Normal aging, mild cognitive impairment, and early Alzheimer's disease. *Neurologist* 1995;1:326–344.
62. Petersen RC, Smith GE, Waring SC, et al. Aging, memory, and mild cognitive impairment. *Int Psychogeriatr* 1997;9:65–69.

63. Petersen RC, Doody R, Kurz A, et al. Current concepts in mild cognitive impairment. *Arch Neurol* 2001;58:1985–1992.
64. Petersen RC, Stevens JC, Ganguli M, et al. Practice parameter: early detection of dementia: mild cognitive impairment (an evidence-based review). Report of the Quality Standards Subcommittee of the American Academy of Neurology. *Neurology* 2001;56:1133–1142.
65. Reiman EM, Caselli RJ, Yun LS, et al. Preclinical evidence of Alzheimer's disease in persons homozygous for the epsilon 4 allele for apolipoprotein E. *N Engl J Med* 1996;334:752–758.
66. de Leon MJ, Convit A, Wolf OT, et al. Prediction of cognitive decline in normal elderly subjects with 2-[(^{18})F]fluoro-2-deoxy-D-glucose/poitron-emission tomography (FDG/PET). *Proc Natl Acad Sci U S A* 2001;98:10966–10971.
67. Ratnavalli E, Brayne C, Dawson K, et al. The prevalence of frontotemporal dementia. *Neurology* 2002;58:1615–1621.
68. Poorkaj P, Bird TD, Wijsman E, et al. Tau is a candidate gene for chromosome 17 frontotemporal dementia. *Ann Neurol* 1998;43:815–825.
69. Baker M, Mackenzie IR, Pickering-Brown SM, et al. Mutations in progranulin cause tau-negative frontotemporal dementia linked to chromosome 17. *Nature* 2006;442:916–919.
70. Lomen-Hoerth C, Anderson T, Miller B. The overlap of amyotrophic lateral sclerosis and frontotemporal dementia. *Neurology* 2002;59:1077–1079.
71. Ringholz GM, Greene SR. The relationship between amyotrophic lateral sclerosis and frontotemporal dementia. *Curr Neurol Neurosci Rep* 2006;6:387–392.
72. Mott RT, Dickson DW, Trojanowski JQ, et al. Neuropathologic, biochemical, and molecular characterization of the frontotemporal dementias. *J Neuropathol Exp Neurol* 2005;64:420–428.
73. Diehl-Schmid J, Grimmer T, Drzezga A, et al. Decline of cerebral glucose metabolism in frontotemporal dementia: a longitudinal ^{18}F-FDG-PET-study. *Neurobiol Aging* 2007;28:42–50.
74. Foster NL, Gilman S, Berent S, et al. Progressive subcortical gliosis and progressive supranuclear palsy can have similar clinical and PET abnormalities. *J Neurol Neurosurg Psychiatry* 1992;55:707–713.
75. Karbe H, Grond M, Huber M, et al. Subcortical damage and cortical dysfunction in progressive supranuclear palsy demonstrated by positron emission tomography. *J Neurol* 1992;239:98–102.
76. Foster NL, Minoshima S, Johanns J, et al. PET measures of benzodiazepine receptors in progressive supranuclear palsy. *Neurology* 2000;54:1768–1773.
77. Lewy FH. Zur pathologischen Anatomie der Paralysis agitans. *Dtsch Z Nervenheilk* 1913;50:50–55.
78. Kosaka K. Lewy bodies in cerebral cortex, report of three cases. *Acta Neuropathol (Berl)* 1978;42:127–134.
79. Kuzuhara S, Mori H, Izumiyama N, et al. Lewy bodies are ubiquitinated. A light and electron microscopic immunocytochemical study. *Acta Neuropathol (Berl)* 1988;75:345–353.
80. Lennox G, Lowe J, Morrell K, et al. Anti-ubiquitin immunocytochemistry is more sensitive than conventional techniques in the detection of diffuse Lewy body disease. *J Neurol Neurosurg Psychiatry* 1989;52:67–71.
81. McKeith LG, Galasko D, Kosaka K, et al. Consensus guidelines for the clinical and pathologic diagnosis of dementia with Lewy bodies (DLB): report of the consortium on DLB international workshop. *Neurology* 1996;47:1113–1124.
82. Barker WW, Luis CA, Kashuba A, et al. Relative frequencies of Alzheimer disease, Lewy body, vascular and frontotemporal dementia, and hippocampal sclerosis in the State of Florida Brain Bank. *Alzheimer Dis Assoc Disord* 2002;16:203–212.
83. McKeith I, Fairbairn A, Perry R, et al. Neuroleptic sensitivity in patients with senile dementia of Lewy body type. *BMJ* 1992;305:673–678.
84. Albin RL, Minoshima S, D'Amato CJ, et al. Fluoro-deoxyglucose positron emission tomography in diffuse Lewy body disease. *Neurology* 1996;47:462–466.
85. Ishii K, Imamura T, Sasaki M, et al. Regional cerebral glucose metabolism in dementia with Lewy bodies and Alzheimer's disease. *Neurology* 1998;51:125–130.
86. Okamura N, Arai H, Higuchi M, et al. [^{18}F]FDG-PET study in dementia with Lewy bodies and Alzheimer's disease. *Prog Neuropsychopharmacol Biol Psychiatry* 2001;25:447–456.
87. McKeith IG, Dickson DW, Lowe J, et al. Diagnosis and management of dementia with Lewy bodies: third report of the DLB Consortium. *Neurology* 2005;65:1863–1872.
88. Lippa CF, Duda JE, Grossman M, et al. DLB and PDD boundary issues: diagnosis, treatment, molecular pathology, and biomarkers. *Neurology* 2007;68:812–819.
89. Thomas AJ, Burn DJ, Rowan EN, et al. A comparison of the efficacy of donepezil in Parkinson's disease with dementia and dementia with Lewy bodies. *Int J Geriatr Psychiatry* 2005;20:938–944.
90. Hu XS, Okamura N, Arai H, et al. ^{18}F-fluorodopa PET study of striatal dopamine uptake in the diagnosis of dementia with Lewy bodies. *Neurology* 2000;55:1575–1577.
91. Walker Z, Costa DC, Janssen AG, et al. Dementia with Lewy bodies: a study of post-synaptic dopaminergic receptors with iodine-123 iodobenzamide single-photon emission tomography. *Eur J Nucl Med* 1997;24:609–614.
92. Yoshita M, Taki J, Yamada M. A clinical role for [(^{123})I]MIBG myocardial scintigraphy in the distinction between dementia of the Alzheimer's-type and dementia with Lewy bodies. *J Neurol Neurosurg Psychiatry* 2001;71:583–588.
93. Watanabe H, Ieda T, Katayama T, et al. Cardiac (^{123})I-meta-iodobenzylguanidine (MIBG) uptake in dementia with Lewy bodies: comparison with Alzheimer's disease. *J Neurol Neurosurg Psychiatry* 2001;70:781–783.
94. Hanyu H, Shimizu S, Hirao K, et al. Comparative value of brain perfusion SPECT and [(^{123})I]MIBG myocardial scintigraphy in distinguishing between dementia with Lewy bodies and Alzheimer's disease. *Eur J Nucl Med Mol Imaging* 2006;33:248–253.
95. Jindahra P, Vejjajiva A, Witoonpanich R, et al. Differentiation of dementia with Lewy bodies, Alzheimer's disease and vascular dementia by cardiac ^{131}I-meta-iodobenzylguanidine (MIBG) uptake (preliminary report). *J Med Assoc Thai* 2004;87:1176–1181.
96. Kitagawa Y. Usefulness of [^{123}I] MIBG myocardial scintigraphy for differential diagnosis of Alzheimer's disease and dementia with Lewy bodies. *Intern Med* 2003;42:917–918.
97. Silverman DH, Gambhir SS, Huang HW, et al. Evaluating early dementia with and without assessment of regional cerebral metabolism by PET: a comparison of predicted costs and benefits. *J Nucl Med* 2002;43:253–266.
98. McMahon PM, Araki SS, Neumann PJ, et al. Cost-effectiveness of functional imaging tests in the diagnosis of Alzheimer disease. *Radiology* 2000;217:58–68.

CHAPTER 10

Psychiatric Disorders

MARC LARUELLE AND ANISSA ABI-DARGHAM

SCHIZOPHRENIA
- Dopamine Transmission
- Serotonin Transmission
- Gamma-aminobutyric Acid Secretion Transmission
- Antipsychotic Drug Occupancy Studies

AFFECTIVE DISORDERS
- Major Depressive Disorder
- Bipolar Disorder

ANXIETY DISORDERS
- Generalized Anxiety Disorder
- Panic Disorder
- Social Phobia
- Obsessive-Compulsive Disorder
- Posttraumatic Stress Disorder

PERSONALITY DISORDERS

CONDUCT DISORDER

SUBSTANCE ABUSE
- Cocaine
- Methamphetamine
- Ecstasy
- Heroin
- Nicotine
- Alcohol

CONCLUSION

Psychiatric conditions were once qualified as "functional" illnesses, that is, disorders in which no major abnormalities of brain integrity such as tumors, inflammation, or infection could be detected by neuropathological examination. Indeed, following a century of postmortem studies, only subtle abnormalities have been found at autopsy in brains of patients who suffered from major psychiatric illnesses, and few of these have been consistently replicated. These observations led to the impression that these illnesses were due to *functional* rather than *structural* brain abnormalities. Computed tomography (CT) and magnetic resonance imaging (MRI) studies have consistently observed abnormalities in brain regional volumes in many of these conditions, but these abnormalities remain for the most part within the limits of normal variability. None of them is pathognomonic or diagnostic. Therefore, the advent of molecular imaging with positron emission tomography (PET) and single-photon emission computed tomography (SPECT) held enormous promises for the field of psychiatry because, for the first time, living brain functions were directly accessible to clinical investigation.

Using PET and SPECT, a large body of studies has documented that psychiatric disorders are associated with regional alterations in flow and metabolism under both resting and activation conditions. In this regard, PET and SPECT have played a major role in unraveling alterations in brain function associated with these conditions. Today these techniques have largely been replaced by functional MRI (fMRI), which offers clear advantages in terms of spatial and temporal resolution, not to mention the lack of radiation exposure. Therefore, it is foreseeable that the role of PET and SPECT studies of flow and, to some extent, metabolism in psychiatry research may be greatly reduced in the future.

On the other hand, the ability of nuclear medicine techniques to image specific biomolecules is unmatched by any other method currently available to clinical investigators. Studies of receptors, transporters, enzymes, and other processes such as transmitter release clearly constitute the uniqueness of PET for current and future psychiatric research. These techniques have already yielded a number of fundamental observations. So far none of these findings has led to clinical applications useful in the diagnosis or treatment of these disorders in individual patients. However, it is anticipated that such applications may surface from this line of research in the near future.

The aim of this chapter is to describe the major findings stemming from this line of research and their implications for our understanding of the pathophysiology and treatment of major psychiatric illnesses. For the reasons discussed above, the chapter will focus on imaging studies of specific biomolecules as opposed to the study of flow and metabolism. Nonetheless, important flow and metabolism studies will be discussed, particularly when molecular imaging studies provide clues to the pathophysiology underlying their observations. The chapter will include both PET and SPECT studies, as it would not be feasible to provide a comprehensive review of this field without describing the important contributions of SPECT.

Technical considerations critical to the discussion of the findings will be included when appropriate, but, for an overview of the technical background of these studies, the reader is referred to Chapters 1–3, and 5 in this book. In line with the clinical orientation of this chapter, the studies will be reviewed by disorder (schizophrenia, mood, anxiety, personality, conduct, and substance abuse disorders) rather than by transmitter system.

The main neurotransmitter systems that have been studied with PET or SPECT in relation to psychiatric disorders and their treatment include dopamine (DA), serotonin (5-HT), γ-aminobutyric acid (GABA), and opiate systems. Radiotracers most frequently used include those for the DA $D_{2/3}$ receptor: carbon-11 [^{11}C]-*N*-methylspiperone, [^{11}C]-raclopride, iodine-123 [^{123}I]-IBZM (benzamide derivative (*S*)-3-[^{123}I]-iodo-*N*-[(1-ethyl-2-pyrrolidinyl)])-methyl-2-hydroxy-6-methoxybenzamide), [^{123}I]-epidipride, fluorine-18 [^{18}F]-fallypride, [^{11}C]-FLB457, [^{11}C]-PHNO (11)C](+)-PHNO ([(11)C](+)-4-propyl-3,4,4a,5,6,10b-hexahydro-2H-naphtho[1,2-b][1,4]oxazin-9-ol; D_1 receptors: [^{11}C]-SCH23390, [^{11}C]-NNC112; DA transporters: [^{11}C]-cocaine, [^{11}C]-methylphenidate, [^{123}I]-*β*-CIT (^{123}I-labeled 2-β-carbomethoxy-3-β-(4-iodophenyl)-tropane),

[^{11}C]/[^{18}F]-CFT (2-β-carbomethoxy-3-β-(4-fluorophenyl) tropane), technetium-99m [^{99m}Tc]-TRODAT-1; dopa decarboxylase: [^{18}F]/[^{11}C]-DOPA; monoamine oxydase: [^{11}C]-deprenyl and [^{11}C]-clorgyline; 5-HT_2 receptors: [^{18}F]-altanserin, [^{18}F]-setoperone, [^{11}C]-MDL100907; 5-HT_{1A} receptors: [^{11}C]-WAY100635; 5-HT transporters: [^{123}I]-β-CIT, [^{11}C]-McN5652, [^{11}C]-DASB; benzodiazepine receptors: [^{123}I]-iomazenil, [^{11}C]-flumazenil; and mu opiate receptors: [^{11}C]-carfentanil, [^{18}F]-cyclofoxy.

SCHIZOPHRENIA

Dopamine Transmission

The classical DA hypothesis, formulated over 40 years ago, proposed that schizophrenia is associated with hyperactivity of dopaminergic neurotransmission (1,2). This hypothesis was essentially based on the observation that all effective antipsychotic drugs provided at least some degree of D_2 receptor blockade (3,4), an observation that is still true today. As D_2 receptor blockade is most effective against positive symptoms (delusions and hallucinations), the DA hyperactivity model appeared to be most relevant to the pathophysiology of these symptoms. This idea was further supported by the fact that sustained exposure to DA agonists such as amphetamine can induce a psychotic state characterized by some features of schizophrenic positive symptomatology (emergence of paranoid delusions and hallucinations in the context of a clear sensorium) (5,6). These pharmacological effects suggest, but do not establish, a dysregulation of DA systems in schizophrenia.

On the other hand, negative and cognitive symptoms are generally resistant to treatment by antipsychotic drugs. Functional brain imaging studies have suggested that these symptoms are associated with prefrontal cortex (PFC) dysfunction (7). Studies in nonhuman primates have demonstrated that deficits in DA transmission in the PFC produce cognitive impairments reminiscent of those observed in schizophrenic patients (8), suggesting that a deficit in DA transmission in the PFC may be implicated in the cognitive impairments associated with schizophrenia (9,10).

Thus, a contemporary view of the role of DA in schizophrenia is that subcortical mesolimbic DA projections may be hyperactive (resulting in positive symptoms) and that the mesocortical DA projections to the PFC may be hypoactive (resulting in negative symptoms and cognitive impairment). Furthermore, these two abnormalities may be related, as the cortical DA system generally exerts an inhibitory action on subcortical DA systems (11,12). The advent in the early 1980s of techniques based on PET and SPECT to measure indices of DA activity in the living human brain opened the possibility of direct investigation of these hypotheses.

Subcortical Dopamine Transmission

Studies of striatal DA transmission in schizophrenia examined both postsynaptic (D_2 receptors and D_1 receptors) and presynaptic ([DOPA] decarboxylase activity, stimulant-induced DA release, baseline DA release, and dopamine transporter [DAT]) functions.

Striatal Dopamine Receptors

Striatal D_2 receptor density in schizophrenia has been extensively studied with PET and SPECT imaging (unless specified otherwise, the term D_2 receptor is used in this chapter to designate both D_2 and D_3 receptors). A meta-analysis (13) of these studies identified 17 studies comparing D_2 receptor parameters in patients with schizophrenia (included a total of 245 patients, 112 neuroleptic naive, and 133 neuroleptic free), and controls (n = 231), matched for age and sex (14–30). Radiotracers included butyrophenones ([^{11}C]-*N*-methyl-spiperone, [^{11}C]-NMSP, n = 4 studies, and bromine-76 [^{76}Br]-bromospiperone, n = 3 studies), benzamides ([^{11}C]-raclopride, n = 3 studies, and [^{123}I]-IBZM, n = 5 studies) or the ergot derivative [^{76}Br]-lisuride, n = 2 studies). Only 2 of 17 studies detected a significant elevation of D_2 receptor density parameters. However, meta-analysis revealed a small (12%) but significant elevation of striatal D_2 receptors in patients with schizophrenia. No clinical correlates of increased D_2 receptor binding parameters have been reliably identified. Studies performed with butyrophenones (n = 7) show an effect size of 0.96 ± 1.05, significantly larger than the effect size observed with other ligands (benzamides and lisuride, n = 10; 0.20 ± 0.26; P = .04). This difference has been attributed to differences in vulnerability of the binding of these tracers, to competition by endogenous DA, and to elevation of endogenous DA in schizophrenia (31,32). Interestingly, a recent study in unaffected monozygotic twins of patients with schizophrenia suggested that a modest elevation of D_2 receptors in the caudate might be associated with genetic vulnerability to schizophrenia (33).

Regarding striatal D_1 receptors, several imaging studies have confirmed the results of postmortem studies of unaltered levels of these receptors in the striatum of patients with schizophrenia (20,34,35).

Several lines of evidence suggest that D_3 receptors might play an important role in the pathophysiology and treatment of schizophrenia (36). An increase in the concentration of D_3 receptors has been reported in postmortem brains of patients with schizophrenia (37). In addition to their role in schizophrenia, D_3 receptors are also believed to play an important role in drug addiction (38). Until recently, imaging D3 receptor was not feasible: PET radiotracers commonly used to study D_2 and D_3 receptors exhibit similar affinities for both receptors and the concentration of D_3 receptors in the human striatum is lower than that of D_2 receptors. The recent discovery that [^{11}C]-PHNO is a D_3 preferring imaging agent might open a window to the *in vivo* study of this important target (39).

Striatal DOPA Decarboxylase Activity

Several studies have reported rates of activity of DOPA decarboxylase in patients with schizophrenia, using [^{18}F]-DOPA (40–45) or [^{11}C]-DOPA (46). The majority of these studies reported increased accumulation of DOPA in the striatum of patients with schizophrenia, and the combined analysis yielded a significant effect size (P = .01) (13). Together, these studies provide the strongest evidence for the existence of a dysregulation of DA function in the striatum of untreated patients with schizophrenia. In addition, several of these studies reported that high DOPA accumulation was more pronounced in psychotic paranoid patients, while low accumulation was observed in patients with negative or depressive symptoms and catatonia. Although the relationship between DOPA decarboxylase and the rate of DA synthesis is unclear (DOPA decarboxylase is not the rate-limiting step of DA synthesis), these observations are compatible with higher DA synthesis activity of DA neurons in schizophrenia, at least in subjects experiencing psychotic symptoms.

Striatal Amphetamine-induced Dopamine Release

D_2 receptor imaging, combined with pharmacological manipulation of DA release, enables more direct evaluation of DA presynaptic activity. Numerous groups have demonstrated that an acute increase in synaptic DA concentration is associated with decreased *in vivo* binding of benzamide radioligands, such as [^{11}C]-raclopride, [^{18}F]-fallypride, or [^{123}I]-IBZM. These interactions have been demonstrated in rodents, nonhuman primates, and humans, using a variety of methods to increase synaptic DA (for review of this abundant literature, see Laruelle [47]). It has also been consistently observed that the *in vivo* binding of spiperone and other butyrophenones is not as affected by acute fluctuations in endogenous DA levels, as is the binding of benzamides (47).

The decrease in [^{11}C]-raclopride and [^{123}I]-IBZM *in vivo* binding following acute amphetamine challenge has been well validated as a measure of the change in D_2 receptor stimulation by DA due to amphetamine-induced DA release. Manipulations that are known to inhibit amphetamine-induced DA release, such as pretreatment with the DA synthesis inhibitor α-methyl-para-tyrosine (αMPT) or with the DAT blocker GR12909, also inhibit the amphetamine-induced decrease in [^{123}I]-IBZM or [^{11}C]-raclopride binding (48,49). The effect of methamphetamine on [^{11}C]-raclopride *in vivo* binding is also significantly blunted in patients with Parkinson disease (50). Combined microdialysis and imaging experiments in primates demonstrated that the magnitude of the decrease in ligand binding was correlated with the magnitude of the increase in extracellular DA induced by the challenge (26,49), suggesting that this noninvasive technique provides an appropriate measure of the changes in synaptic DA levels.

Three of three studies demonstrated that the amphetamine-induced decrease in [^{11}C]-raclopride or [^{123}I]-IBZM binding was elevated in untreated patients with schizophrenia compared to well-matched controls (24,26,27). A significant relationship was observed between the magnitude of DA release and the transient induction or deterioration of positive symptoms. The increased amphetamine-induced DA release was observed in both first episode/drug-naive patients and patients previously treated with antipsychotic drugs (51). Patients who were experiencing an episode of illness exacerbation (or a first episode of illness) at the time of the scan showed elevated amphetamine-induced DA release, while patients in remission showed DA release values not different from controls (51), suggesting that the dysregulation of the DA system revealed by this challenge might represent a state rather than a trait factor. This exaggerated response of the DA system to amphetamine exposure did not appear to be a nonspecific effect of stress, as elevated anxiety before the experiment was not associated with a larger amphetamine effect. Furthermore, nonpsychotic subjects with unipolar depression, who reported levels of anxiety similar to the schizophrenic patients at the time of the scan, showed normal amphetamine-induced displacement of [^{123}I]-IBZM (52).

These findings were generally interpreted as reflecting a larger DA release following amphetamine in the schizophrenic group. Another interpretation of these observations would be that schizophrenia is associated with increased affinity of D_2 receptors for DA. Over the past few years, several D_2 receptor radiolabeled agonists such as [^{11}C]-NPA ([^{11}C]N-propyl-norapomorphine) and [^{11}C]-PHNO have been successfully developed, and studies using these agents in patients with schizophrenia are needed to solve this issue (39,53–57).

Striatal Baseline Dopamine Activity

A limitation of the amphetamine challenge of imaging studies is that they measure changes in synaptic DA transmission following a nonphysiological challenge (i.e., amphetamine) and do not provide any information about synaptic DA levels at baseline (i.e., in the unchallenged state). Several laboratories have reported that, in rodents, acute depletion of synaptic DA is associated with an acute increase in the *in vivo* binding of [^{11}C]-raclopride or [^{123}I]-IBZM to D_2 receptors (for review, see Laruelle [47]). The increased binding was observed *in vivo* but not *in vitro*, indicating that it was not due to receptor up-regulation (58), but to removal of endogenous DA and unmasking of D_2 receptors previously occupied by DA. The acute DA depletion technique was developed in humans using αMPT, to assess the degree of occupancy of D_2 receptors by DA (58–61). Using this technique, higher occupancy of D_2 receptors by DA was reported in patients with schizophrenia experiencing an episode of illness exacerbation, compared to healthy controls (28). Again, assuming normal affinity of D_2 receptors for DA, the data are consistent with higher DA synaptic levels in patients with schizophrenia. Increased D_2 receptor stimulation by DA at intake, as measured with the αMPT paradigm, was predictive of rapid clinical response to antipsychotic drugs (28). This finding illustrates the potential of molecular imaging to predict treatment response (Fig. 10.1).

Striatal Dopamine Transporters

The data reviewed above are consistent with higher DA output in the striatum of patients with schizophrenia, which could be explained by increased density of DA terminals. Since striatal DAT are exclusively localized on DA terminals, this question was investigated by measuring binding of [^{123}I]-β-CIT (62) or [^{18}F]-CFT (63) in patients with schizophrenia. Both studies reported no differences in DAT binding between patients and controls. In addition, Laruelle et al. (62) reported no association between amphetamine-induced DA release and DAT density. Thus, the increased presynaptic output

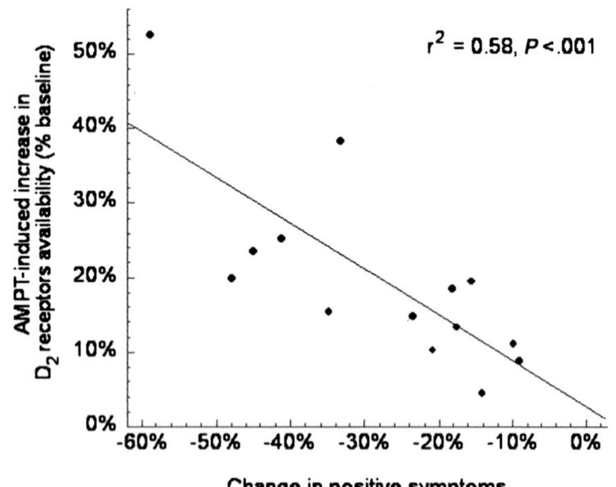

FIGURE 10.1. Imaging dopamine transmission and prediction of therapeutic response in schizophrenia. Relationship between dopamine synaptic levels at intake, as estimated by the α-methyl-para-tyrosine (αMPT) effect on [^{123}I]-IBZM binding potential (BP), and the decrease in positive symptoms measured after 6 weeks of antipsychotic treatments. Patients with high DA synaptic levels showed a larger decrease in positive symptoms following treatment than patients with DA levels similar to controls (effect of αMPT on [^{123}I]-IBZM BP in control subjects was 9% ± 7%). (From Abi-Dargham A, Rodenhiser J, Printz D, et al. Increased baseline occupancy of D2 receptors by dopamine in schizophrenia. *Proc Natl Acad Sci U S A* 2000;97(14):8104–8109, with permission.)

suggested by the studies reviewed above does not appear to be due to higher terminal density, an observation consistent with postmortem studies that failed to identify alteration in striatal DAT binding in schizophrenia (for references, see Laruelle et al. [62]).

Taken together, studies of striatal DA transmission in schizophrenia have provided support for the time-honored DA hypothesis of schizophrenia. As animal data suggest, the antipsychotic effect of D_2 receptor antagonism is mediated by blockade of D_2 receptors in the mesolimbic as opposed to the nigrostriatal DA system (64–66), and future studies will focus on studying striatal subsystems. Recent progress in PET instrumentation has provided the resolution necessary to differentiate the signal from ventral (i.e., limbic) and dorsal (i.e., motor) regions of the anterior striatum (67–69).

Extrastriatal D_2 Receptors

The development of radiotracers suitable for imaging extrastriatal D_2 receptors such as [^{11}C]-FLB497 (70) and [^{18}F]-fallypride (71) enabled the study of D_2 receptor transmission in extrastriatal areas. Lower D_2 receptor density has been described in untreated schizophrenia in the thalamus in three studies (72–74), as well as in the midbrain (75), in temporal cortex (76), and cingulated cortex (77). Additional studies are needed to replicate and extend these findings and explore their pathophysiological basis and significance.

Prefrontal Dopamine Transmission

The majority of DA receptors in the PFC are of the D_1 subtype (78,79). Cortical D_1 receptors have been studied in schizophrenia using [^{11}C]-SCH23390 (80) and [^{11}C]-NNC112 (81,82). In humans, [^{11}C]-NNC112 provides higher specific to nonspecific ratios compared to [^{11}C]-SCH23390 (82,83), a property that is important for quantification of cortical D_1 receptors. It should be noted that both ligands display only moderate *in vivo* selectivity for D_1 relative to 5-HT$_{2A}$ receptors, and that 20% to 30% of cortical binding of both radiotracers correspond to binding to 5-HT$_{2A}$ receptors (84,85).

PET studies with [^{11}C]-SCH23390 reported decreased (20) or unchanged (86) prefrontal D_1 receptor availability in untreated patients with schizophrenia. In contrast, a study using [^{11}C]-NNC112 reported increased D_1 receptor availability in the dorsolateral PFC (DLPFC) of patients with schizophrenia (35). Interestingly, increased [^{11}C]-NNC112 binding was associated with poor performance on the *n-back* test of working memory (35). The reason for the discrepancy in the results obtained with [^{11}C]-SCH23390 and [^{11}C]-NNC112 remains to be elucidated, but it is interesting to note that the binding of both radiotracers is differentially affected by endogenous DA competition and receptor trafficking (47). For example, chronic DA depletion in rodents is associated with decreased and increased *in vivo* binding of [^{11}C]-SCH23390 and [^{11}C]-NNC112, respectively (87). Thus, the contradictory observations of decreased [^{11}C]-SCH23390 binding (20) and increased [^{11}C]-NNC112 binding (35) observed in the PFC in patients with schizophrenia might in fact mean that both represent consequences of a sustained deficit in prefrontal DA function. Much work remains to be done to validate this hypothesis. This point illustrates that the *in vivo* binding of radiotracers is affected by several factors that are not present in the typical *in vitro* situation, such as the impact of receptor trafficking on ligand affinity (47). This situation represents both a challenge, because the interpretation of the results is less straightforward, and an opportunity, because more information can be gained on the functions of the living neurons.

Serotonin Transmission

Abnormalities of 5-HT transporters (SERT), 5-HT$_{2A}$ receptors, and, more consistently, 5-HT$_{1A}$ receptors have been described in postmortem studies in schizophrenia (see references in Abi-Dargham and Krystal [88]). However, these postmortem results were generally not confirmed by molecular imaging studies.

The concentration of SERT in the midbrain measured by [^{123}I]-β-CIT is unaltered in patients with schizophrenia (62). This observation was confirmed and extended to thalamus and striatum using the more selective radiotracer [^{11}C]-DASB (89). Yet, SERT imaging agents currently available are not valid to study SERT in areas of relatively low SERT density, such as the PFC, where SERT has been reported to be reduced in three of four postmortem studies in schizophrenia (88).

Decreased 5-HT$_{2A}$ receptors have been reported in the PFC in four of eight postmortem studies (see references in Abi-Dargham and Krystal [88]). Three PET studies in drug-naive or drug-free patients with schizophrenia reported normal cortical 5-HT$_{2A}$ receptor binding (90–92), while one study reported a significant decrease in PFC 5-HT$_{2A}$ binding in a small group ($n = 6$) of drug-naive schizophrenic patients (93).

The most consistent abnormality of 5-HT parameters reported in postmortem studies in schizophrenia is an increase in the density of 5-HT$_{1A}$ receptors in the PFC, reported in seven of eight studies (88). Several groups evaluated the binding of this receptor *in vivo* with PET and [^{11}C]-WAY100907 in schizophrenia and reported inconsistent results. One study reported increased 5-HT$_{1A}$ binding in the temporal lobe of patients with schizophrenia (94), another study reports decreased binding in the amygdala (95), and a third study failed to detect any changes in regional 5-HT$_{1A}$ availability (96). These inconsistencies indicate that the alterations of 5-HT$_{1A}$ receptors demonstrated in postmortem studies in schizophrenia could not be reliably detected with PET and might not be related to the pathophysiology of the illness.

Gamma-aminobutyric Acid Secretion Transmission

A robust body of findings suggests a deficiency of GABAergic function in the PFC in schizophrenia (for reviews, see Lewis [97] and Benes [98]). *In vivo* evaluation of GABAergic systems in schizophrenia has so far been limited to evaluation of benzodiazepine receptor densities with SPECT and [^{123}I]-iomazenil, and three of three studies comparing patients with schizophrenia and controls reported no significant regional differences (99–101). Although significant correlations between symptom clusters and regional benzodiazepine densities have been observed in some studies, these relationships have not been replicated. Thus, taken together, these studies are consistent with an absence of marked abnormalities of benzodiazepine receptor concentration in the cortex and patients with schizophrenia. Alterations of GABAergic systems in schizophrenia might not involve benzodiazepine receptors (102), or be restricted to certain cortical layers or classes of GABAergic cells that are beyond the resolution of current radionuclide-based imaging techniques.

Antipsychotic Drug Occupancy Studies

Perhaps the most widespread use of neuroreceptor imaging in schizophrenia over the past two decades has been the assessment of receptor occupancy achieved by typical and atypical antipsychotic drugs, a topic that has been reviewed elsewhere (103,104). The main focus has been on D_2 receptor occupancy, but 5-HT_{2A} and D_1 receptors have also been studied. Studies have repeatedly confirmed the existence of a threshold of occupancy of striatal D_2 receptors (about 80%) above which extrapyramidal side effects (EPS) are likely to occur (105). In general, studies have failed to observe a relationship between the degree of D_2 receptor occupancy and clinical response (106,107). However, most studies were performed at doses achieving more than 50% occupancy. Two studies performed with low doses of relatively selective D_2 receptor antagonists (haloperidol and raclopride) suggested that 50% to 60% occupancy was required to observe a rapid clinical response (108,109). Clozapine, at clinically therapeutic doses, has been found to achieve only 40% to 60% D_2 receptor occupancy (105,107,110), which, in conjunction with its anticholinergic properties, may account for its low risk for EPS. Occupancy of 5-HT_{2A} receptors by "5-HT_{2A}/D_2 balanced antagonists" such as risperidone does not confer protection against EPS, since the threshold of D_2 receptor occupancy associated with EPS is not markedly different between these drugs and drugs devoid of 5-HT_{2A} antagonism (111–114). Studies with quetiapine suggest that, at least with this agent, transient high occupancy of D_2 receptors might be sufficient to elicit a clinical response (115,116).

An interesting question relates to putative differences in the degree of occupancy achieved by antipsychotic drugs in striatal and extrastriatal areas. Pilowsky et al. (117) initially reported lower occupancy of striatal D_2 receptors compared to temporal cortex D_2 receptors in seven patients treated with the atypical antipsychotic drug clozapine, using the high affinity SPECT ligand [^{123}I]-epidipride. In contrast, typical antipsychotics were reported to achieve similar occupancy in striatal and extrastriatal areas, as measured with [^{11}C]-FLB457 (118) or [^{123}I]-epidipride (119). It should be noted, however, that these very high affinity ligands do not allow accurate determination of D_2 receptor availability in the striatum (120). Conversely, [^{18}F]-fallypride enables accurate determination of D_2 receptor availability in both striatal and extrastriatal areas (121). Occupancy studies using [^{18}F]-fallypride confirmed that clozapine and quetiapine, but not olanzepine or haloperidol, achieved higher D_2 receptor occupancy in temporal compared to striatal regions (122–124). Occupancy studies performed with [^{76}Br]-FLB457 also reported higher occupancies in cortex compared to striatum for a number of antipsychotic drugs, including typical antipsychotic drugs (125). Conversely, a study combining [^{11}C]-FLB457 imaging for extrastriatal D_2 receptor receptors and [^{11}C]-raclopride imaging for striatal D_2 receptors suggested similar occupancy of D_2 receptors in both regions for both typical and atypical antipsychotic drugs (126). Thus, at this point in time, there is a strong suggestion that many, if not most, antipsychotic drugs achieve higher occupancies in temporal cortex compared to striatum, although this phenomenon has not been universally observed. Factors underlying this difference remain to be elucidated.

Finally, it is important to point out that the most robust preclinical evidence relative to the site of therapeutic effect of antipsychotic drugs points toward the ventral striatum (65,127), while the imaging studies reviewed above contrasted striatal versus mesotemporal D_2 receptor binding. Furthermore, D_2 receptor occupancy levels in striatum have been shown to be more predictive of therapeutic response than in temporal cortex (128). Thus, the observation that, in a restricted dose range, D_2 receptor occupancy by antipsychotic drugs is higher in temporal cortex than in striatum does not necessarily imply that the temporal cortex is the therapeutic site of actions of these agents.

Another unresolved question is the discrepancy in the value of D_2 receptor occupancy obtained with [^{11}C]-raclopride versus [^{11}C]-NMSP. The haloperidol plasma concentration associated with 50% inhibition of [^{11}C]-NMSP binding (3 to 5 mg/mL) (129) is ten times higher than that associated with 50% inhibition of [^{11}C]-raclopride binding (0.32 ng/mL) (130). Quetiapine, at a dose of 750 mg, decreased [^{11}C]-raclopride specific binding by 51%, but failed to affect [^{11}C]-NMSP specific binding (131). These observations contribute to the debate regarding differences between benzamide and butyrophenone binding to D_2 receptors.

AFFECTIVE DISORDERS

Numerous abnormalities of regional cerebral blood flow (rCBF) and metabolism (rCMRglu) have been demonstrated in affective disorders using SPECT and PET. These studies have implicated anatomical circuits involving subregions of prefrontal cortex, striatum, amygdala, and hippocampus in the pathophysiology of these disorders (132,133). From a neurochemical perspective, abnormalities in several neurotransmitter systems may be relevant to the pathophysiology of depression. The 5-HT system has been the most extensively implicated, in part because of the antidepressant effect of medications that inhibit the synaptic reuptake of serotonin, as well as a wealth of postmortem, preclinical, and clinical data suggesting that reduced serotonergic function may be associated with depression (134). The recent availability of suitable PET radioligands for 5-HT_{2A} receptors, 5-HT_{1A} receptors, and SERT has allowed the *in vivo* investigation of their putative abnormalities in depression. In addition, a number of studies have evaluated potential alterations in DA systems in major depression.

This relatively recent literature is characterized by conflicting and inconsistent results, presumably related to the heterogeneity of major depression and to the relatively low number of subjects included in most studies. Effects of the clinical presentation (unipolar versus bipolar), clinical status (in episode versus in recovery), and medications have not yet been fully explored. Nonetheless, these studies have suggested that depression might be associated with lower SERT availability in the midbrain and lower 5-HT_{1A} receptor availability in various limbic and cortical regions. No consistent pattern of alterations has yet emerged from the study of DA parameters in depression.

Major Depressive Disorder

Serotonin (5-HT) Transmission

5-HT_2 Receptors

The earliest PET study of 5-HT_2 receptors and depressive symptoms used [^{11}C]-*N*-methyl-spiperone to investigate binding in patients with poststroke depression and reported increased binding (135). Yet, it is not clear how this finding can be generalized to more common clinical presentations of depression. Another early study using 2-[^{123}I]-ketanserin and SPECT reported increased and asymmetrical cortical uptake of the tracer in depressed patients when compared to controls (136). However, 2-[^{123}I]-ketanserin has significant limitations due to high nonspecific binding.

Since then, several PET studies have used newer 5-HT_2 PET radiotracers, [^{18}F]-setoperone (137) and [^{18}F]-altanserin (138), to investigate cortical 5-HT$_{2A}$ receptor binding in drug-free depressed patients. Biver et al. (139), using [^{18}F]-altanserin, reported reduced tracer uptake in a region of the right hemisphere including the orbitofrontal cortex and the anterior insular cortex. Two studies investigated midlife depression using [^{18}F]-setoperone and concluded that there is no major change or asymmetry in 5-HT$_{2A}$ receptors (140,141). In both studies the great majority of patients had been free of antidepressant medication for over 6 months. One study supported these negative findings and reported no significant alteration in 5-HT$_{2A}$ receptor binding in an untreated group of patients with late-life depression without cognitive impairment (142). Conversely, decreased 5-HT$_{2A}$ receptor binding was reported in the hippocampus of subjects suffering from late-life depression (143). Finally, the largest study to date (144) found a widespread reduction in 5-HT$_{2A}$ receptor binding potential (BP) and concluded that brain 5-HT$_{2A}$ receptors are decreased in patients with major depression. However, 40% of the patients in this study had been drug free for only 2 weeks before scanning. This factor may be significant as the majority of antidepressants down-regulate 5-HT$_{2A}$ receptors (141,145,146).

In summary, three studies reported no significant alteration in 5-HT$_{2A}$ receptor binding in major depression, and three studies found reduced 5-HT$_{2A}$ receptors. Differences between studies might stem from methodological issues, illness heterogeneity, and medication effects. None of the recent studies confirmed the earlier findings of increased binding (135,136). Similarly, the increase in 5-HT$_{2A}$ receptors found in some, but not all, postmortem studies of suicide depressed victims (for review see Mann [147]) has not been confirmed by *in vivo* investigations. Therefore, there is currently no strong evidence supporting the hypothesis that depression *per se* is associated with marked alterations of 5-HT$_{2A}$ receptor density.

5-HT$_{1A}$ Receptors

Two lines of evidence have implicated the 5-HT$_{1A}$ receptors in depression. The first is the finding that depressed patients have blunted neuroendocrine responses to 5-HT$_{1A}$ receptor agonists *in vivo*, and the second is the dense distribution of these receptors in the hippocampus. Recent theories have implicated interactions between stress, corticosteroids, growth factors, and hippocampal 5-HT$_{1A}$ receptors in depression (148–150). Postmortem studies of 5-HT$_{1A}$ receptors in suicide and depression have been inconsistent, showing increased, decreased, and unchanged 5-HT$_{1A}$ receptors levels in various regions (151–155). These discrepancies may reflect the possible confounding effects of suicidality, antemortem medications, differences between radioligands, and differences in the regulation of 5-HT$_{1A}$ receptors by corticosteroids and local levels of 5-HT in different brain regions. The results of *in vivo* PET imaging of 5-HT$_{1A}$ receptors in depressed patients are therefore of interest.

Several PET studies have investigated 5-HT$_{1A}$ receptors in unmedicated depressed subjects using [^{11}C]-WAY100635. The first study (156) found modest (approximately 10%) but significant widespread reductions in 5-HT$_{1A}$ receptor availability in cortical regions including medial temporal cortex (hippocampus and amygdala) in men with major depression. The same group reported a similar finding in patients with a history of major depression who were scanned after clinical recovery (157). Drevets et al. (148) reported comparable findings: reductions in the medial temporal cortex (27%) and raphe (41%). This group of subjects included both unipolar and bipolar depressed patients. The finding of lower raphe 5-HT$_{1A}$ receptor availability in depression was confirmed in a group of subjects with late-life depression (158). However, a study carried out in a large sample of subjects with major depressive disorder reported the opposite finding, an increase in 5-HT$_{1A}$ receptor availability in untreated subjects with major depression and no changes in treated patients (159). Higher baseline 5-HT$_{1A}$ receptor availability was associated with poorer response to antidepressant treatment (160).

Additional studies are warranted to further clarify the association between altered 5-HT$_{1A}$ receptor expression and depression. Since a major depressive episode is associated with hyperactivity of the hypothalamic-pituitary-adrenal axis, and increased cortisol levels might be associated with 5-HT$_{1A}$ receptor down-regulation (161–164), reduced 5-HT$_{1A}$ receptor availability might be secondary to the neuroendocrine dysregulation associated with depression. However, a direct test of this hypothesis found that a single dose of hydrocortisone failed to affect 5-HT$_{1A}$ receptor availability in recovered depressed patients (165).

Serotonin Transporter

Reductions in SERT levels in depressed patients have been reported in numerous postmortem studies (for review, see Mann [147]). The first ligand used to image SERT *in vivo* was the SPECT radiotracer [^{123}I]-β-CIT. β-CIT binds to both DAT and SERT with comparable affinity (Ki 1.4 and 2.4 nM for DAT and SERT, respectively) (166,167). The lack of DAT versus SERT selectivity is not a problem for measuring DAT in the striatum, as the density of SERT in striatum is much lower than that of DAT (167). However, in the midbrain, this proportion is reversed, and the β-CIT midbrain uptake mostly corresponds to SERT binding (168,169). Studies in nonhuman primates and humans have shown that, in the midbrain, [^{123}I]-β-CIT is selectively displaced by administration of selective serotonin reuptake inhibitors (SSRIs), but not by DAT selective drugs (168,170). [^{123}I]-β-CIT has been extensively used in clinical studies both for striatal DAT (62,171–176) and midbrain SERT evaluation (62,177–179).

In depression, findings from three SPECT studies using [^{123}I]-β-CIT were in agreement with postmortem results. A reduction in SERT binding was found in the midbrain in patients with unipolar depression (177) and in patients with atypical or melancholic depression (180), and in thalamus-hypothalamus in depressed patients with seasonal affective disorder (181).

The development of more selective SERT radiotracers was required to investigate SERT density in other regions of the brain. The first selective PET radiotracer available to measure SERT in humans was [^{11}C]-McN5652 (182). The usefulness of [^{11}C]-McN5652 as a PET tracer for SERT was validated in primates (183) and humans (184–186). However, [^{11}C]-McN5652 has many limitations, which include high nonspecific binding, low signal to noise ratio, and slow clearance from the brain, restricting the use of this ligand to regions with relatively high SERT densities, such as midbrain, thalamus, and striatum (185).

Using [^{11}C]-McN5652, one study found increased SERT availability in thalamus and unchanged SERT availability in midbrain in patients with major depression (187). In contrast, a [^{11}C]-McN5652 study including a larger number of subjects with major depression found reduced SERT availability in midbrain (188). A study conducted in patients with bipolar disorder with [^{11}C]-McN5652 reported lower SERT availability in midbrain, thalamus, and striatal regions (189).

Compounds from the phenylamine class have emerged as the most useful PET and SPECT SERT imaging agents to date. [^{123}I]-ADAM (2-((2-dimethylamino)methyl)phenyl)thio)-5-iodophenylamine and [^{11}C]-ADAM (190–193) were the first imaging agents reported from this class and are highly selective SERT SPECT and PET imaging agents. Studies conducted with [^{123}I]-ADAM in depression reported decreased (194) or unchanged (195) midbrain SERT availability.

Another compound in this series, [^{11}C]-DASB, was found to provide good imaging qualities for SERT quantification (196–198) and to be superior to [^{11}C]-McN5652 in humans (199) (Fig. 10.2). Using [^{11}C]-DASB, one study reported no changes in regional SERT availability in patients with major depressive episodes (200).

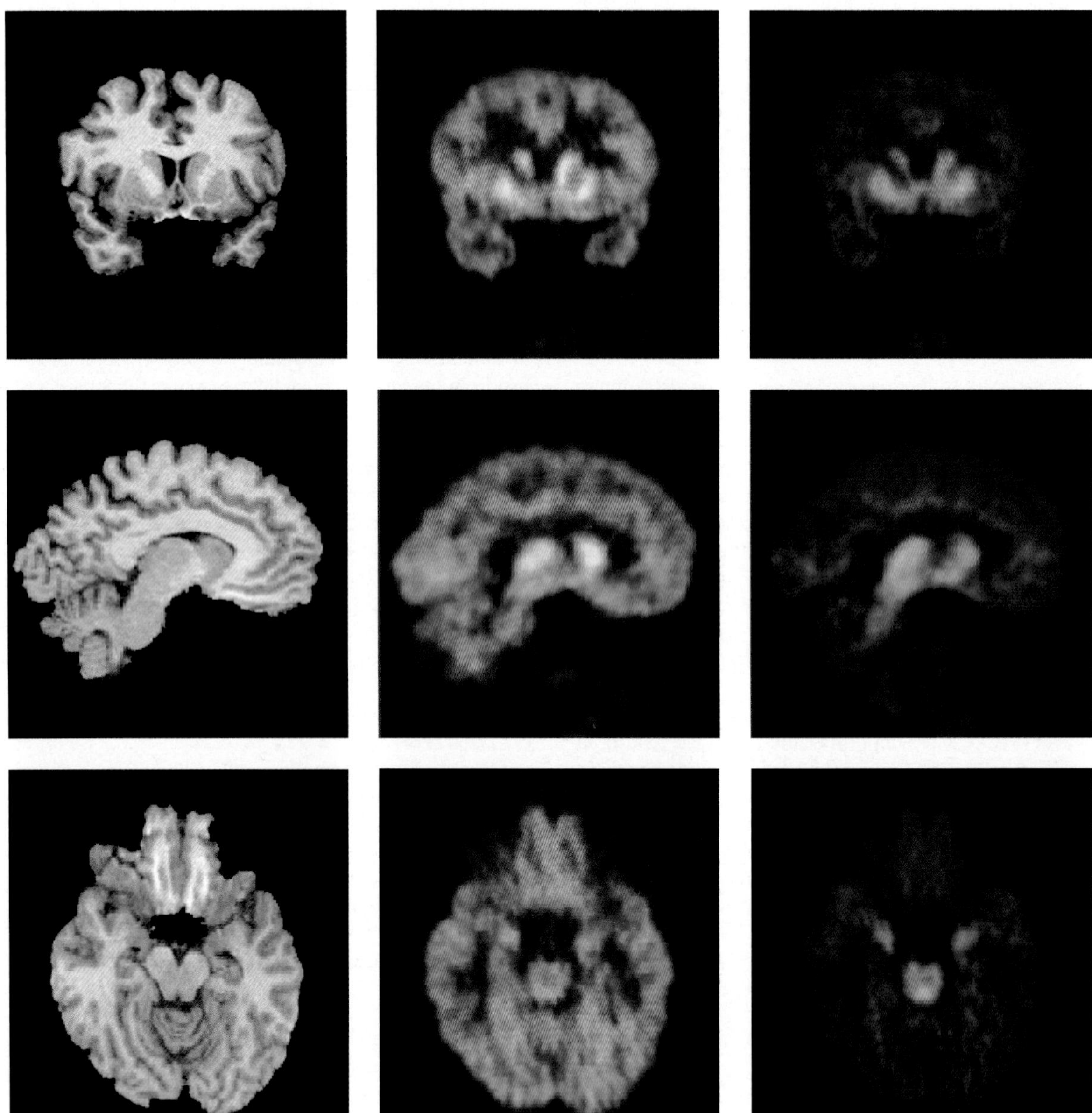

FIGURE 10.2. PET imaging of serotonin transporters (SERT): from [^{11}C]-McN5652 to [^{11}C]-DASB. Magnetic resonance imaging **(left)** and coregistered PET images acquired from 40 to 90 minutes following injection of 599 MBq [^{11}C]-McN5652 **(center)** and 659 MBq [^{11}C]-DASB **(right)** in the same subject (33-year-old healthy man volunteer). Activity was normalized to the injected dose and color coded using an identical scale. **Upper row:** Coronal plane, illustrating the ventrodorsal gradient of SERT in the striatum. **Middle row:** Sagittal plane close to the midline, showing accumulation of activity in the thalamus and caudate. This image also illustrates the low level of activity in the cerebellum, and the small difference in uptake between the cerebellum and neocortical regions. **Lower row:** Transaxial plane at the level of the midbrain. There is very high activity concentrated in the dorsal raphe on the [^{11}C]-DASB scan, just ventral to the fourth ventricle. The concentration of activity in the amygdala is also noticeable on the [^{11}C]-DASB image. The improvements in signal to noise achieved with [^{11}C]-DASB compared to [^{11}C]-McN5652 are readily noticeable on these images, which illustrates the critical contribution of radiotracer development for psychiatry research. (From Frankle WG, Huang Y, Hwang DR, et al. Comparative evaluation of serotonin transporter radioligands ^{11}C-DASB and ^{11}C-McN 5652 in healthy humans. *J Nucl Med* 2004;45(4):682–694 with permission.)

Together, studies of SERT availability suggest that depression might be associated with lower SERT availability in the midbrain, although this finding has not been reported in all studies. One should note that even the best SERT radiotracer reported to date, [^{11}C]-DASB, is inadequate to measure SERT in regions with relatively low SERT density, such as the frontal cortex. Novel SERT imaging agents with higher signal-to-noise characteristics are actively being developed to fill this gap (see for example Huang et al. [201]).

Dopamine Transmission

The critical role of DA in brain reward systems, the reports of low cerebrospinal fluid homovanillic acid levels in depressed patients, the association of major depression with Parkinson disease, and the enhancement of dopaminergic activity by several antidepressant treatments suggest that a deficiency of dopaminergic function might be associated with major depression (for review see Kapur and Mann [202]) (203–205). Five studies compared striatal D_2 receptor availability with [^{123}I]-IBZM and SPECT in patients with major depression and control subjects. Two of five studies reported higher [^{123}I]-IBZM specific binding in the striatum of depressed subjects compared to controls (206,207), whereas three studies reported no changes (52,208,209). Using [^{11}C]-raclopride and PET, one study reported elevated D_2 receptor availability in putamen in patients with depression with motor retardation (210). Amphetamine-induced DA release was also assessed in patients with major depression and found to be unchanged (52).

Two studies examined [^{123}I]-β-CIT striatal binding to DAT in patients with major depression and yielded conflicting results: one study reported normal levels of striatal DAT in patients with major depression (177), while the other reported increased DAT levels (211). One study reported decreased DAT density in depression using [^{11}C]-RTI32 (212). SPECT studies conducted with [^{99m}Tc]-TRODAT1 also reported conflicting results, with studies reporting increased (213) or unchanged (214) striatal [^{99m}Tc]-TRODAT1 uptake in patients with major depression.

Finally, [^{18}F]-DOPA uptake in the left caudate was observed to be significantly lower in depressed patients with psychomotor retardation than in depressed patients with high impulsivity and in comparison subjects (215). Thus, major depression *per se* does not appear to be consistently associated with alteration of the dopaminergic parameters at the level of the whole striatum. However, DA might play a role in the neurobiology underlying some clinical features of depression, such as psychomotor retardation.

Antidepressant Drugs Occupancy Studies

SSRIs are the most widely prescribed drugs for the treatment of depression, and molecular imaging studies reported on the degree of SERT occupancy by these drugs during treatment with them (reviewed in Meyer [216]).

Pirker et al. (170) compared [^{123}I]-β-CIT midbrain specific binding to SERT in depressed patients treated with 20 to 60 mg/d of citalopram for a minimum of 1 week and a group of control subjects. The reduction in [^{123}I]-β-CIT binding in the midbrain of the citalopram-treated patients was reported to be approximately 50% of controls. The [^{123}I]-β-CIT midbrain signal was also used to measure occupancy of SERT during venlafaxine extended release treatment (75 mg/d for 4 days followed by 150 mg/d for 5 days) and was found to be 55% (217).

Meyer et al. (218), using [^{11}C]-DASB, reported 77% SERT occupancy during treatment with 20 mg/d of citalopram. Kent et al. (219), using [^{11}C]-McN5652 and Meyer et al. (218), using [^{11}C]-DASB, reported near complete (greater than 80%) occupancy of SERT by paroxetine at therapeutic doses (20 to 40 mg/kg). High SERT occupancies (80% range) were also reported following therapeutic doses of fluvoxamine and clomipramine with [^{11}C]-McN5652 (220) and fluoxetine, sertraline, and venlafaxine with [^{11}C]-DASB (221,222). Thus, high SERT occupancies are achieved following administration of these drugs at therapeutic doses. The higher occupancy measured with [^{11}C]-McN5652 and [^{11}C]-DASB compared to [^{123}I]-β-CIT might reflect the contamination of the midbrain [^{123}I]-β-CIT signal by DAT from the nigra.

High SERT occupancy levels observed with SSRIs during the treatment of depression contrasts with DAT occupancy levels reported during antidepressant treatment with the DAT inhibitor bupropion, which are moderate in the range of 20% to 30% (214,223,224). Thus, these data suggest that effective antidepressant effects require lower DAT occupancy than SERT occupancy, although the contribution of norepinephrine transporter (NET) blockade to the mechanism of action of bupropion remains to be measured *in vivo*.

It has been suggested that the time lag (typically 1 to 2 weeks) in the onset of therapeutic effect of several classes of antidepressant medication may be related to the need for down-regulation of 5-HT_{1A} somatodendritic autoreceptors in the raphe before a net increase in forebrain 5-HT neurotransmission can occur (225). Because of this phenomenon, several groups have investigated whether the concomitant use of pindolol (antagonist at 5-HT_{1A} receptor and β-adrenoceptor) with an SSRI antidepressant might accelerate the onset of an improvement in mood. The results of clinical trials were inconsistent (for reviews, see Martinez et al. [226] and Artigas et al. [227]). Most clinical studies have used a dose of 7.5 mg daily of pindolol. Several PET centers have recently conducted human occupancy studies of pindolol at the postsynaptic and somatodendritic 5-HT_{1A} receptor (228–230) (Fig. 10.3). The consensus from these studies is that the dose used in clinical studies was too low to provide appropriate and reliable blockade of 5-HT_{1A} receptors, and that this factor might explain the limited success of this strategy in previous clinical trials. These studies provide another illustration of the potential of PET neuroreceptor imaging to facilitate drug development.

Bipolar Disorder

In comparison to major depressive disorder, only limited radioligand PET studies have been reported in patients with bipolar disorders. As discussed above, it may be significant that the findings of reduced 5-HT_{1A} receptor binding in the medial temporal cortex and raphe of depressed patients (148) was largely accounted for by the subjects with bipolar disorder and those with unipolar depression who had relatives with bipolar disorder.

Because of the relationship between mania and psychosis, a number of PET studies have investigated the DA system in bipolar disorders. D_1 receptor binding in the frontal cortex was reported to be decreased in a study of ten symptomatically heterogeneous, drug-free bipolar patients (231). Increases in D_2-like (i.e., D_2, D_3, and D_4) receptor density in the striatum were found in seven psychotic patients with bipolar disorder when compared to seven nonpsychotic patients with bipolar disorder and 24 control subjects. The authors concluded that an increase in D_2-like receptors is associated with the state of psychosis rather than with a diagnosis of bipolar disorder (232). As part of the same studies, Gjedde and Wong (233) also reported findings consistent with an elevated concentration of synaptic DA in bipolar patients with psychosis, but

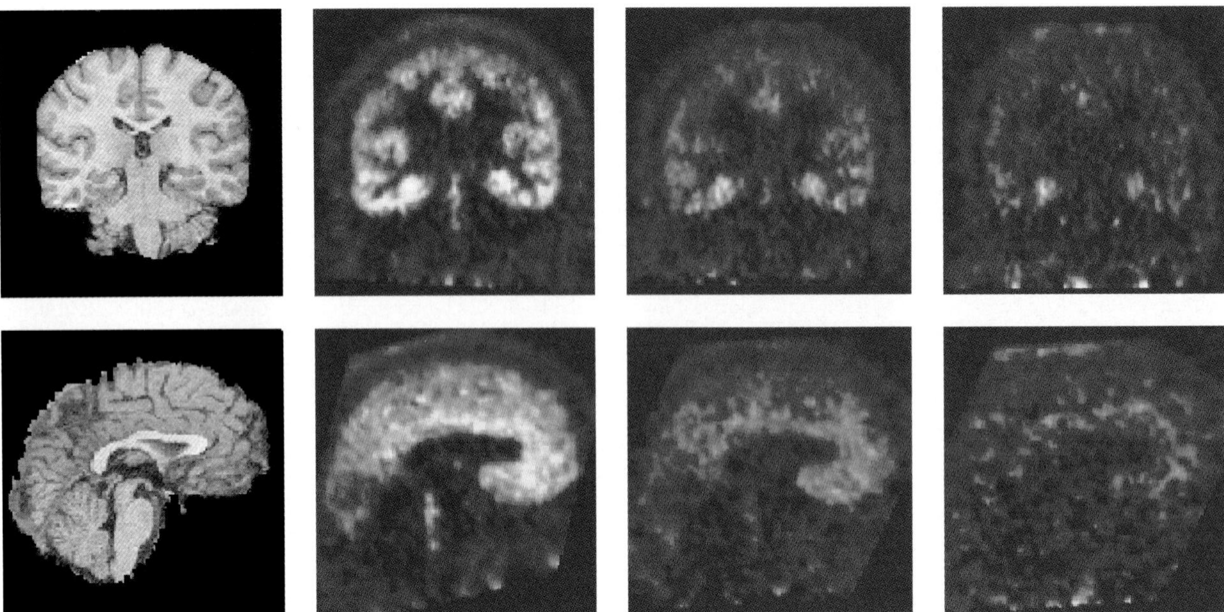

FIGURE 10.3. Contribution of PET to psychopharmacology. Coronal **(top row)** and sagittal **(bottom row)** MRI and coregistered PET images following injection of [^{11}C]-WAY100635 in a 29-year-old man under baseline conditions, and following administration of the 5-HT$_{1A}$ partial agonist pindolol 7.5 mg and 30 mg. The PET image is the sum of five frames of 10 minutes collected between 30 and 80 minutes. Activity was corrected for the injected dose and color coded using the same scale across the three scans. At each dose, pindolol administration is associated with a decrease in specific binding of the radiotracer to 5-HT$_{1A}$ receptors. This study revealed that the dose of pindolol used in clinical trials of augmentation of selective serotonin reuptake inhibitor therapeutic action in depression (7.5 mg every day) induced only low and variable occupancy of 5-HT$_{1A}$ receptors. This factor presumably accounts for the inconsistent results of these clinical studies. (From Martinez D, Hwang D, Mawlawi O, et al. Differential occupancy of somatodendritic and postsynaptic 5-HT$_{1A}$ receptors by pindolol. A dose-occupancy study with [^{11}C]-WAY100635 and positron emission tomography in humans. *Neuropsychopharmacology* 2001;24(3):209–229, with permission.)

not in nonpsychotic bipolar patients. On the other hand, amphetamine-induced DA release was reported to be normal in euthymic patients with bipolar disorders (234).

In conclusion, few investigations have been reported using PET molecular imaging techniques in patients with bipolar disorders, and the findings reported so far might be related to clinical states (depression, mania with psychosis) rather than to the bipolar condition *per se.*

ANXIETY DISORDERS

A number of PET studies have investigated rCBF changes associated with induced anxiety in healthy volunteers (235–240). Although there is considerable variability in the findings, a number of paralimbic-cortical regions have been consistently implicated including medial prefrontal cortex, anterior cingulate cortex, orbital prefrontal cortex, anterior temporal cortex, parahippocampal gyrus, and the claustrum-insular-amygdala region. In contrast to this abundant functional literature, anxiety disorders have been less studied with PET molecular imaging techniques.

Generalized Anxiety Disorder

As benzodiazepines (BDZ) are the prototypical anxiolytic drugs, evaluation of potential abnormalities in the BDZ receptor distribution is of interest in anxiety disorders. An initial study in generalized anxiety disorder (GAD) with [^{123}I]-NNC13-8241 reported reduced binding in the left temporal pole in ten drug-naive female patients with GAD compared with age- and sex-matched healthy controls (241). However, this has not been confirmed in a PET study using [^{11}C]-flumazenil, which found no differences in drug-free patients (242).

Panic Disorder

Two studies using [^{123}I]-iomazenil SPECT reported decreased uptake in the lateral temporal region (243) and increased binding in the right orbitofrontal cortex in benzodiazepine-naive patients (244). A third [^{123}I]-iomazenil SPECT study, using a more quantitative measurement of regional binding potential, reported decreased binding in left hippocampus and precuneus in patients with panic disorder relative to controls. Interestingly, patients who had a panic attack at the time of the scan had a relative decrease in binding in prefrontal cortex, suggesting that benzodiazepine function in prefrontal cortex may be involved in changes in state-related panic (245). In a fully quantitative PET study using [^{11}C]-flumazenil in medication-free patients, Malizia et al. (246) found a global reduction in BDZ binding throughout the brain in patients with panic disorder compared to controls. The largest regional decreases were in the right orbitofrontal cortex and right insula. Thus, there is relatively consistent evidence that panic disorder might be associated with alterations in the GABAergic system, the primary "endogenous" anxiolytic system. Nevertheless, the anatomical localization of these changes and their relationship with illness states remain to be clarified. A recent study identified a reduction in 5-HT_{1A} receptor availability in cingulate cortex and raphe nuclei in patients with panic disorder, an intriguing observation given the implication of 5-HT_{1A} receptors in anxiety in preclinical models (247).

Social Phobia

Neurobiological mechanisms underlying social phobia (social anxiety disorder), including neuroimaging findings, have been reviewed recently (248–250). One SPECT study using [^{123}I]-β-CIT to label DAT in the striatum reported that densities were markedly lower in patients with social phobia than in age- and gender-matched controls (251). Another study using [^{123}I]-IBZM reported a significant decrease in D_2 receptor binding potential in patients with social phobia compared to controls (252). Together, these studies suggest that the DA system might play a role in the pathophysiology of this illness. A recent study using [^{11}C]-McN5652 failed to find marked alterations in SERT in patients with social phobia (219). A deficit in 5-HT_{1A} receptors availability in several brain regions, including the amygdala, has recently been reported in patients with social anxiety (253). Together with the findings in panic disorder described above, these studies support the involvement of this transmission system in anxiety. Interestingly, a negative relationship was reported in healthy subjects between 5-HT_{1A} receptor availability and trait anxiety (254).

Obsessive-Compulsive Disorder

Obsessive-compulsive disorder (OCD) has been extensively studied with SPECT and PET metabolism studies. These studies have generated remarkably consistent results (i.e. increased metabolism in orbitofrontal cortex and striatum in symptomatic patients, which normalizes with successful treatment) (255–261). These findings have implicated abnormalities in the prefrontal cortex-basal ganglia-thalamic circuits, which originate from the orbitofrontal cortex, in the pathophysiology of OCD and the related neuropsychiatric disorder Gilles de la Tourette syndrome. Lower pretreatment metabolism in the orbitofrontal cortex has been found to predict greater improvement in patients on SSRI medication (259), however, different treatment modalities may have different predictive levels of pretreatment metabolism (261).

Abnormalities of serotonergic neurotransmission in OCD have been hypothesized on the basis of the therapeutic efficacy of medications that selectively increase synaptic 5-HT levels (including SSRIs and clomipramine) in nondepressed OCD patients and the high level of comorbid depression in OCD. Measurements of SERT in OCD subjects yielded conflicting results, with one study reporting elevated midbrain SERT availability with SPECT and [^{123}I]-β-CIT (262), one study reporting no alteration of regional SERT densities using PET and [^{11}C]-McN5652 (263), and two studies reporting low SERT midbrain binding with SPECT [^{123}I]-β-CIT (264,265). All studies included a relatively low number of subjects, which might account for the discrepant results. An increase in 5-HT_{2A} receptor availability in the caudate nuclei has been reported with PET and [^{18}F]-altanserin, which is interesting given the involvement of this structure in the pathophysiology of this condition (266).

Posttraumatic Stress Disorder

The results of functional neuroimaging and other studies in posttraumatic stress disorder (PTSD) have recently been reviewed in depth (267,268). It has been hypothesized that symptoms of PTSD are mediated by a dysfunction of the anterior cingulate, with a failure to inhibit amygdala activation and/or an intrinsic lower threshold of amygdalar response to fearful stimuli. The model further proposes that hippocampal atrophy is a result of the chronic hyperarousal symptoms mediated by amygdalar activation (267). One neuroreceptor imaging study has been reported in this population showing lower [^{123}I]-iomazenil binding in the prefrontal cortex of PTSD patients compared to similar normal subjects, suggesting that this condition is associated, like panic disorder and perhaps general anxiety disorder, with low BDZ receptor levels (269).

PERSONALITY DISORDERS

Personality disorders (PD) are characterized by stable patterns of maladaptive behavior. Some, such as paranoid, schizoid, schizotypal, avoidant, and obsessive-compulsive PD, have stable patterns of behavior reminiscent of their corresponding clinical disorders but do not reach a sufficient severity and their response to medication is generally poor. It therefore might be expected that some personality disorders could be associated with neurobiological abnormalities similar to, but less marked than, the disorders described in this chapter. Functional imaging studies have now begun to address the issue of how neurochemical brain functions may be associated with normal and pathological personality traits.

A number of studies have investigated differences within the normal range of personality traits or temperaments in healthy subjects. Most receptor PET studies have so far investigated dopaminergic neurotransmission. Studies using [^{11}C]-raclopride report that the traits of depression and personal detachment are related to low D_2 receptor density in the striatum (270,271). However, the relationship is not evident on all measures of detachment (271,272). Detachment was also found to be associated with low DAT binding in the putamen (273). These findings are also interesting in view of the association between social phobia and low DAT and D_2 receptors (251,252), and it has been argued that these neurobiological findings might underlie a commonality between detachment and social phobia (274).

Beyond the DA system, a significant negative correlation has been reported between cortical 5-HT_{1A} binding potential and trait anxiety (255). Zhuang et al. (275) report that this is consistent both with animal models that have shown higher anxiety in mice lacking 5-HT_{1A} receptors and clinical trials demonstrating anxiolytic properties of partial 5-HT_{1A} agonists.

Abnormalities of serotonergic neurotransmission are implicated in the pathophysiology of impulsive-aggressive behaviors, and PET studies have contributed to this body of evidence. 18-F Fluorodeoxyglucose (FDG) studies of the effects of fenfluramine-stimulated serotonin release report a significantly blunted response in areas of prefrontal cortex associated with regulation of impulsive behavior in patients with impulsive-aggressive personality difficulties (276,277). Serotonin synthesis and SERT availability have both been shown to be low in cortical areas in patients with borderline PD (278,279). This limited set of data is consistent with the hypothesis that impulsive and aggressive behaviors are associated with low cortical serotonin function.

CONDUCT DISORDER

Interesting findings have been reported in the study of attention deficit hyperactivity disorder (ADHD), a condition treated with psychostimulants. In a preliminary study of six adult subjects with ADHD, Dougherty et al. (280) observed a large increase in DAT availability (70%) compared to controls. This finding was replicated in a larger samples of adults with ADHD by Dresel et al. (281), using [^{99m}Tc]-TRODAT-1, by Larisch et al. (282), using [^{123}I]-FP-CIT, and by Spencer et al. (283), using [^{18}F]-altropane. In these subsequent studies, the magnitude of DAT elevation was considerably lower than in the original study. Elevated DAT availability was also replicated in children with ADHD (284). On the other hand, this findings has not been replicated in several studies carried out by other groups (285–287) using [^{123}I]-β-CIT SPECT, [^{11}C]-PE2I PET, and [^{11}C]-cocaine PET, respectively. Here again, the heterogeneity of this condition might account for the discrepant results.

The DAT blocker methylphenidate is the treatment of choice of ADHD, and oral therapeutic doses induce a significant decrease in [^{11}C]-raclopride binding (288), presumably due to increased synaptic DA levels. This method might provide a tool to monitor the biological effectiveness (increased synaptic DA) of the treatment and be useful in the evaluation of nonresponders.

SUBSTANCE ABUSE

Molecular imaging investigations yielded important information about the mode of action of addictive substances and neurochemical abnormalities associated with addictions. Given the central role of DA in mediating the rewarding effects of drugs of abuse (for reviews, see Wise and Romprè [289]) (290–294), it is not surprising that many imaging studies focused on this transmitter system. In general, studies demonstrated that acute administration of addictive drugs is associated with increased DA transmission in the limbic striatum, and that the pleasurable effects of these drugs is associated with the magnitude of DA system stimulation. In patients suffering from addiction, studies demonstrated deficits of both pre- and postsynaptic DA function, a finding not readily predicted from animal data.

Cocaine

Cocaine abuse has been extensively studied using molecular imaging techniques. Most of the work has focused on changes in striatal DA that occur with chronic cocaine use. The studies have generated a remarkably consistent set of data and illustrate admirably the ability of molecular imaging to unravel neurochemical abnormalities in the human brain associated with pathological conditions.

D_2 Receptors

A reduction in striatal DA D_2 receptors has been demonstrated by Volkow et al. (295–298) using both [^{18}F]-*N*-methylspiroperidol and [^{11}C]-raclopride, a finding that has been independently replicated (299). Volkow et al. (296) also noted that this decrease in striatal D_2 receptor availability correlated with years of use. This deficit appear to be long lasting in a group of subjects rescanned after 3 months of inpatient rehabilitation (296). PET studies also revealed reduction in striatal D_2 receptor availability in heroin abuse (300), methamphetamine abuse (301), and alcoholism (302–304), suggesting that decreased striatal D_2 receptor availability might be a general feature of the addicted brain (Fig. 10.4).

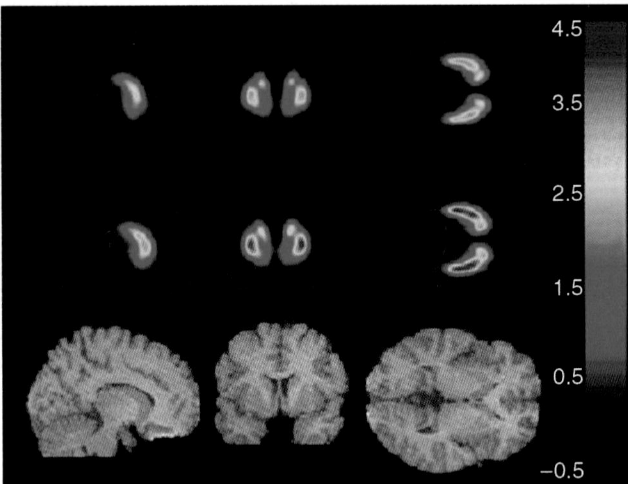

FIGURE 10.4. D_2 receptors and addiction. Comparison of D_2 receptor availability measured during bolus plus constant infusion of [^{11}C]-raclopride between recently detoxified alcoholic subjects (n = 15, **top row**) and matched healthy controls (n = 15, **middle row**). For each subject, a binding potential (BP) map was created on magnetic resonance coregistered PET data according to the formula BP (voxel) = activity (voxel)/mean cerebellum value − 1. Maps were then normalized into a common template space (Statistical Parametric Mapping [SPM] software environment) to facilitate averaging across subjects. The bottom row is the MRI of one subject normalized into the template space to show anatomic location of D_2 receptor maps. Alcoholism was associated with significant reduction in D_2 receptor availability compared to control subjects. Comparable findings were reported by other groups in alcoholic subjects, as well as in subjects suffering from other addictions, such as cocaine and heroin (see text). (From Volkow ND, Wang GJ, Fowler JS, et al. Decreases in dopamine receptors but not in dopamine transporters in alcoholics. *J Nucl Med* 1996;37:33P, with permission.)

The results of these studies raise the question of whether a decrease in D_2 receptors is the result of years of drug abuse or represents a neurochemical risk factor for developing substance abuse. Two observations suggested that low D_2 receptor availability might constitute a risk factor for the development of addiction. First, studies in healthy subjects suggested that low striatal D_2 receptor availability was predictive of a pleasurable experience following administration of the psychostimulant methylphenidate (305,306). Second, studies in nonhuman primates demonstrated that low striatal D_2 receptor availability was predictive of an increased propensity to self-administer cocaine (307). It should be noted, however, that low D_2 receptor availability is not predictive of a pleasurable experience following amphetamine use in healthy subjects (68,308,309) as it is in cocaine abusers (299). Thus, while the association between low striatal D_2 receptor availability and a history of chronic cocaine abuse is well established, the direction of causality in this relationship remains to be clarified.

Stimulant-induced Dopamine Release

As described above, PET and SPECT studies can been used to measure changes in subcortical DA transmission in the human brain following psychostimulant administration (for review see Laruelle [47]). In healthy subjects, a number of independent studies have shown that the percentage decrease in radioligand binding (i.e., the increase in DA release) is positively correlated with the pleasurable subjective effects induced by psychostimulant administration (69,308–312). This observation is consistent with the preclinical body of evidence indicating that DA transmission in the ventral striatum mediates the reinforcing effects of drugs of abuse (313,314). PET studies showed a greater decrease in [^{11}C]-raclopride binding in the ventral versus dorsal striatum in healthy controls in response to an amphetamine challenge (69,299) and in response to a monetary reward (315). Collectively, these studies suggest that a strong DA response would correlate with increased reward value, and might mediate the reinforcing effects of drugs of abuse and therefore constitute a risk factor toward the development of addiction.

However, cocaine abusers have been shown to have a blunted DA response to psychostimulants. A study of Volkow et al. (298) used [^{11}C]-raclopride to measure the change in D_2 receptor availability before and after an intravenous dose of 0.5 mg/kg methylphenidate in healthy controls and cocaine abusers who had been abstinent for 3 to 6 weeks. The authors reported a 9% decrease in [^{11}C]-raclopride binding in the cocaine abusers compared to a 21% decrease in healthy controls. Malison et al. (316) performed a similar study in abstinent cocaine abusers and controls using [^{123}I]-IBZM and an amphetamine challenge (0.3 mg/kg intravenous) and reported a 1% change in binding in the cocaine abusers compared to a 10% decrease in controls. Similarly, Martinez et al. (299) showed that the effect of amphetamine (0.3 mg/kg intravenous) on [^{11}C]-raclopride binding is markedly blunted in cocaine abusers in all striatal subregions. In the ventral striatum, this response was completely blunted. Furthermore, blunted dopamine transmission in the ventral striatum and anterior caudate was predictive of the choice for cocaine over money, suggesting that this deficit might confer vulnerability to relapse (299).

Dihydroxyphenylalanine (DOPA) Decarboxylase

The findings above of blunted presynaptic DA function in cocaine abusers are supported by the study of Wu et al. (317) showing a reduction in the rate of uptake of [^{18}F]-6-FDOPA in abstinent cocaine abusers.

Dopamine Transporter

Imaging studies of DAT in cocaine abusers have been published, and this body of work has failed to provide a clear picture of the status of DAT in cocaine abusers. Using [^{11}C]-cocaine, no changes in DAT were observed in detoxified (greater than 1 month) cocaine abusers (297). In contrast, Malison et al. (176) showed a significant up-regulation of DA transporters, measured with SPECT and [^{123}I]-β-CIT, in the striatum of recently detoxified (less than 96 hours) cocaine abusers. Such up-regulation was not observed following prolonged abstinence.

Dopamine Transporter Occupancy by Cocaine

Studies of DAT occupancy by cocaine have generated valuable information. Volkow et al. (318) reported that a DAT occupancy of about 50% or more is needed to produce the subjective effects of cocaine. These data suggest that any treatment approach to cocaine abuse in which the transporter is blocked would need to produce somewhere between 60% and 90% occupancy of the transporters. This issue was addressed in an occupancy study of mazindol, a nonselective catecholamine reuptake inhibitor (319). This study showed that the clinical dosage generally used produced only a modest occupancy of 16% to 23%, and would therefore not be expected to have sufficient efficacy to block the reinforcing effects of cocaine.

Although the magnitude of DAT blockade is important for the experience of the rewarding effect, the kinetic of occupancy is an important feature of the addictive process (320,321). Thus, cocaine exhibits very rapid association and dissociation from DAT and is highly addictive. The reinforcing effects of methylphenidate are stronger after intravenous compared to oral administration, due to faster access to DAT after intravenous administration. Antidepressants like bupropion or radafaxine are associated with moderated and sustained DAT occupancy due to slow peripheral clearance and are devoid of abuse liability (322).

Cue-induced Cocaine Craving

Two studies showed that cue-induced cocaine craving is associated with an acute decrease in [^{11}C]-raclopride availability, presumably related to acute changes in synaptic DA (323,324). Interestingly, craving intensity is associated with DA release in the dorsal rather than the ventral striatum, suggesting the involvement of this region in the habituation process associated with craving and addiction.

Serotonin Transporter (SERT)

Jacobsen et al. (325) reported increased SERT availability in the diencephalon and midbrain (17% and 32%, respectively) using [^{123}I]-β-CIT (325), suggesting that chronic cocaine abuse affects the serotonin system as well.

Mu Opiate Receptors

Zubieta et al. (326) reported an increase in mu opioid receptor availability using [^{11}C]-carfentanil in the caudate, thalamus, cingulate, and frontal and temporal cortices. This finding is of particular interest given the interaction between the dopaminergic and opioid systems in the direct and indirect pathways of the striatum (327,328).

Overall, the studies in cocaine abuse demonstrate a clear and pronounced dysregulation of the DA system in this disorder. The findings of decreased [^{18}F]-DOPA accumulation, decreased amphetamine- and methylphenidate-induced DA release, and decreased D_2 receptor density suggest a functional deficit in D_2 receptor transmission at the level of the whole striatum in this population. This alteration in DA transmission might contribute to the addictive process and the relapse risk.

Methamphetamine

Two imaging studies in methamphetamine abusers have demonstrated a significant decrease in DAT using PET (329,330). The authors also found that the decrease in DAT availability correlated with years of abuse and with impairment in motor and memory tasks. Both studies are in agreement with a postmortem report of reduced DA transporter density in the striata of chronic methamphetamine abusers, as well as decreases in DA and tyrosine hydroxylase (331). Evidence from studies in Parkinson disease support the hypothesis that the reduction in DAT availability reflects a loss of DA neurons, which is detectable with functional imaging (332–334). Based on this interpretation, these studies raise the issue of whether this decrease is reversible, or whether methamphetamine abuse results in neurotoxicity to the dopaminergic neurons. PET and postmortem studies in nonhuman primates have shown that methamphetamine exposure results in decreased DAT and other markers of dopaminergic transmission, suggesting a frank loss of dopaminergic neurons (335,336). However, one study suggested that this reduction might be reversible after prolonged abstinence (337). Overall, the PET data demonstrate that methamphetamine abuse in humans results in a reduction in the DAT and raise concerns about the DA neurotoxicity associated with this addiction.

Ecstasy

It has been known for over 25 years that methylenedioxymethamphetamine (MDMA, Ecstasy) is a potent and selective brain 5-HT neurotoxin in animals (for a review see Ricaurte et al. [338]). Rats treated with MDMA developed long-lasting decreases in brain 5-HT, without evidence for long-term effects on other brain monoaminergic systems (339–343). MDMA produces dose-related reductions in the levels of 5-HT and 5-hydroxyindoleacetic acid (5-HIAA, the major metabolite of 5-HT) (339,341–343), SERT density (342), and tryptophan hydroxylase (TPH), the rate-limiting enzyme in the 5-HT synthetic pathway (341,344).

PET and SPECT were used to evaluate the potential neurotoxic effects of MDMA on SERT density in human MDMA users. This literature has generated controversial results, mostly due to significant technical limitations of the early studies (for review see Lyvers [345] and Cowan [346]).

The first study was carried out in the United States. McCann et al. (347) measured SERT availability in 14 subjects who had abused MDMA on at least 25 occasions using both active and inactive enantiomer of [^{11}C]-McN5652. The difference between the distribution volume (DV) of the active and inactive enantiomers was used as an estimate of the specific DV. The authors used the natural logarithm of the DV as an outcome measure, a transformation that is not standard in the PET literature. MDMA users showed a significantly lower ln(DV) values than controls in all regions, a finding interpreted as evidence of significant decrease in SERT availability in MDMA users compared to controls. However, calculating the reverse transform of reported ln(DV) values yields DV values that are about ten times the range for the control group compared to control values reported by other groups (185,186), suggesting that this early report was associated with significant technical problems.

Two subsequent studies imaged MDMA abusers with the SPECT radioligand [^{123}I]-β-CIT (348,349). The first [^{123}I]-β-CIT study, carried out in the United Kingdom (348), reported a significant decrease in [^{123}I]-β-CIT uptake in posterior neocortical regions. Yet, the suitability of [^{123}I]-β-CIT to quantify SERT in cortical regions has not been firmly established (168,350,351). No differences were noted in the caudate and putamen (which is consistent with unaffected striatal DAT density), in the thalamus (a region where the binding of [^{123}I]-β-CIT mostly reflects binding to SERT), or in the midbrain (mostly if not exclusively SERT).

The second [^{123}I]-β-CIT study, carried out in the Netherlands (352), reported a significant decrease in specific binding in all regions (midbrain, thalamus, frontal, temporal, occipital, and parietal cortex) in heavy female users. No differences were found in any regions in male heavy users, in male or female light users, or in male and female ex-users. In other terms, this study suggested that alterations in SERT densities in MDMA users was only detected in females, but not in males, and was reversible upon abstinence.

The fourth study came from Germany (353), and was, by far, the best study published at the time: the number of subjects engaged in this study was higher than in previous studies, a control group of subjects using drugs other than MDMA was included, and the authors assessed SERT availability using [^{11}C]-McN5652 and well-validated analytical methods. This study reported results essentially similar to the study from the Netherlands (352): SERT availability in current MDMA users was significantly reduced in most regions compared with all other groups. Reduction was more pronounced in female than in male subjects. No significant difference in SERT availability was observed between former MDMA users and the drug-naive and polydrug comparison subjects.

More recently, the Baltimore group reported the results of a second study (354), that addressed most of the methodological limitations of their first study(347). The authors used both [^{11}C]-McN5652 and [^{11}C]-DASB to measure SERT availability in MDMA users and controls. Using both ligands, SERT reductions were found in MDMA users in several cortical and subcortical areas. As previously described (352,353), data suggested that SERT availability recovered with time.

In conclusion, the evidence to date suggests that a reduction in SERT availability is detectable in current and recently abstinent MDMA users, that this observation might be more frequent in female compared to male users, and that this alteration normalizes upon sustained abstinence. The mechanism underlying this observation (reversible neurotoxicity, functional down-regulation, residual occupancy of SERT by MDMA) remains to be clarified.

Heroin

Two groups measured opioid receptor occupancy in heroin-dependent subjects undergoing treatment. Kling et al. (355) reported on heroin-dependent subjects maintained on methadone using [^{18}F]-cyclofoxy, a mu and kappa opioid antagonist (356). A decrease in receptor availability of 19% to 32% was seen in methadone-treated subjects compared to healthy volunteers. Zubieta et al. (357) reported on the occupancy of buprenorphine, a partial mu agonist soon to be approved as an alternative to methadone. Subjects were given 2 mg and 16 mg sublingual doses, and scanned using the radioligand [^{11}C]-carfentanil, which is selective for the mu opioid receptor (358). The 2-mg dose resulted in 36% to 50% occupancy and the 16-mg dose resulted in 79% to 95% occupancy of the mu receptors across brain regions. Behavioral pharmacology studies show that doses of 8 to 16 mg of buprenorphine are needed to reduce heroin self-administration (359,360). Therefore, the study of Zubieta et al. suggests that a higher occupancy of the mu receptor than that reported by Kling et al. may be necessary for a therapeutic effect.

Zubieta et al. (357) reported marked increases in mu receptor availability in detoxified heroin-dependent subjects compared to healthy controls. However, this study included only three heroin-dependent subjects. Lastly, reductions in D_2 receptor availability of 18% in the putamen and 13% in the caudate were reported in the opiate-dependent subjects compared to healthy controls (300). This study is of particular interest given the reduction in D_2 receptor availability associated with other addictions, as described above.

Nicotine

Relative to the impact of smoking on public health, relatively few molecular imaging studies have been carried out to understand the impact of smoking on brain chemistry. Molecular imaging of nicotinic receptors demonstrated that typical cigarette smoking results in rapid and sustained near saturation of the $\alpha 2$-$\beta 4$ nicotinic receptors measured with 2-[^{18}F]-85380 (361). One SPECT study in nonhuman primates suggested that this was associated with significant and prolonged up-regulation of these receptors (362).

Several studies evaluated the effect of nicotine on striatal DA release, as measured with the [^{11}C]-raclopride binding reduction method. In rhesus monkeys, intravenous nicotine doses ranging from 0.01 to 0.06 mg/kg caused a significant albeit small reduction (5%) in [^{11}C]-raclopride availability (363). In humans, a first study (364) failed to detect a significant effect of cigarette smoking in regular smokers on striatal [^{11}C]-raclopride binding, but detected a relationship between the hedonic response to nicotine and decreased [^{11}C]-raclopride binding. Another study in nicotine-dependent subjects demonstrated a 30% reduction in [^{11}C]-raclopride binding in the ventral striatum following one cigarette (365). The magnitude of this effect was surprising, as it exceeded the magnitude of the [^{11}C]-raclopride reduction observed in the same region following 0.3 mg/kg intravenous amphetamine (15% to 20%) (69,311). In a subsequent study with a larger group of subjects, this group reported a much lower decrease in [^{11}C]-raclopride striatal binding following cigarette smoking (8%) (366). Finally, Montgomery et al. (367) failed to detect changes in [^{11}C]-raclopride binding in regular smokers following intranasal nicotine administration, while relationships were reported between positive subjective effects of the drug and decreased [^{11}C]-raclopride binding in striatal subregions. Together, these studies demonstrated that nicotine exposure in human smokers is associated with an increase in synaptic DA, and that this effect is generally of lower magnitude than the one observed with psychostimulants (for review see Laruelle [47]) and close to the detection limit associated with this imaging method. As previously described for stimulants (69,308, 309,311,312), the subjective effects of the drugs are associated with the extent of DA release.

Fowler et al. (368–371) investigated levels of monoamine oxidase (MAO) A and B in smokers, and showed marked and global decreases in both enzymes. MAO A and B exist in neurons and glial cells and both enzymes degrade DA. MAO B activity was measured using [^{11}C]-L-deprenyl (372). Smokers were found to have a 42% decrease in global MAO B activity compared to controls (368,371). Interestingly, a study of former smokers showed that levels of MAO B activity returned to baseline after smoking cessation (370). In a later study, this same group demonstrated a decrease in MAO A activity in the brains of cigarette smokers using [^{11}C]-clorgyline (369). In this study smokers had an average reduction of 28% in MAO A activity across brain regions, with a 22% decrease in the basal ganglia (369). Decreased activities of MAO A and B are expected to be associated with increased DA availability.

Salokongas et al. (373) used [^{18}F]-fluorodopa to measure presynaptic DA and reported higher uptake in the striatum in smokers, a finding which could be explained by an increase in DOPA decarboxylase activity or a decrease in MAO activity. A study by Dagher et al. (374) reported a reduction in D_1 receptor availability using [^{11}C]-SCH23390 in the striatum. Lastly, Staley et al. (375) investigated DAT and SERT density in the striatum and midbrain, respectively, in smokers and healthy controls using [^{123}I]-β-CIT. No difference was seen in DAT availability between these groups, but there was a trend level increase in [^{123}I]-β-CIT binding in the midbrain.

Overall, these findings are consistent with the hypothesis of alterations of DA system in cigarette smokers, but much work remains to be done to better understand the potential role of this dysregulation in the maintenance of nicotine addiction.

Alcohol

The DA system has been the most investigated neurochemical system using SPECT and PET in alcohol research, due to the wealth of preclinical data suggesting a role for DA in the reward system and clinical data suggesting alterations in DA function in alcoholic patients.

Acute effects of alcohol on DA release in humans have been studied with the [^{11}C]-raclopride reporting method. Similar to results reported with nicotine, alcohol administration in humans is not associated with major changes in [^{11}C]-raclopride binding, but the pleasurable effects of the drugs are associated with reduction in [^{11}C]-raclopride binding (376).

A number of well-controlled and independent studies have consistently demonstrated a reduction in D_2 receptor availability in recently detoxified alcoholics (302,304,377,378), an alteration that does not appear to be reversible following sustained abstinence (379). The majority of preclinical data do not indicate that chronic alcohol exposure affects D_2 receptor density (380–384), but conflicting results have been published suggesting that the effects of chronic alcohol use on DA receptors might vary according to the dose and duration of exposure (385–388). Such differences in duration of exposure, as well as interspecies differences in the response of D_2 receptors to alcohol, may undermine the relevance of rodent studies in answering the question of whether decreased D_2 receptor BP measured with PET in chronic alcoholics is a risk factor for, or an effect of, chronic alcohol intake. Another important question is whether the alterations in D_2 receptor density in recently detoxified alcoholics are transient or permanent (i.e., if this abnormality persists with a prolonged period of abstinence). Interestingly, recent data suggest that low D_2 receptor availability might be associated with high relapse risk (389). Studies reporting DAT measurements in chronic alcoholics have failed to detect consistent alterations of DAT binding in alcoholism (179,377,390–392).

Alcoholism is also associated with reduced amphetamine-induced DA release in the ventral striatum (304). Together with the evidence of reduced D_2 receptor availability, these findings suggest that alcoholism, like cocaine and maybe other addictions, is associated with a significant decrease in DA transmission at D_2 receptors. Interestingly, a recent study (393) in nonalcoholic offspring from families with a positive history of alcohol dependence failed to detect alteration of DA transmission (D_2 receptor availability and amphetamine-induced DA release) compared to nonalcoholic subjects without a family history of alcohol dependence. Therefore, one might conclude that these alterations are a consequence rather than a risk factor of alcoholism. However, it could also be argued that a normal DA transmission in these subjects might provide protective effects, counterbalancing other genetically mediated risks. Short of a long-term prospective study, the status of these DA alterations as risk factors or consequences of addiction is likely to remain unsolved.

Finally, PET imaging has contributed to the study of alterations in brain GABAergic function related to alcoholism. A blunted metabolic response to lorazepam in the thalamus, basal ganglia, and orbitofrontal cortex has been described in alcoholic subjects (394) and in the cerebellum of subjects at risk for alcoholism (395). Initial *in vivo* studies of BDZ receptor density failed to demonstrate abnormalities in [^{11}C]-flumazenil binding in limited samples of patients (396–398). However, a larger study reported a significant decrease in [^{11}C]-flumazenil V_T in the medial frontal lobes and cingulate gyrus in nine alcoholic subjects, and a decrease in the same regions as well as the cerebellum in eight alcoholic subjects with alcoholic cerebellar degeneration (399). Another study, using SPECT and [^{123}I]-iomazenil, found lower receptor levels in patients compared to controls in the frontal, anterior cingulate, and cerebellar cortices (400). These alterations have also been reported by a third group (401). Taken together, these studies suggest that alcoholism might be associated with a decrease in the BDZ/$GABA_A$ receptor complex in some brain regions such as the frontal cortex, the cingulate cortex, the hippocampus, and the cerebellum. However, the studies do not all agree on which regions are implicated. The heterogeneity of the alcoholic patients, including the presence of neurological impairment in some, might have contributed to the discrepancies between studies in the regions involved.

CONCLUSION

This chapter has reviewed key findings from PET and SPECT molecular imaging studies that have contributed to our understanding of the pathophysiology and treatment of psychiatric disorders. Since 1986, the year of publication of the seminal paper of Wong et al. (14), this field has undergone a major expansion. So far, it is clear that these techniques have already provided unique insights into the neurochemical imbalances underlying some of these conditions and the pharmacological mechanisms involved in their treatment. It is foreseeable that this contribution will continue to expand in the near future.

Psychiatric conditions are generally characterized by clinical heterogeneity. It is likely that a number of illnesses with different etiologies and neurobiological mechanisms are currently subsumed under the same name by our diagnostic classifications. Despite this, a number of findings have been remarkably consistent and replicated across studies, suggesting that the clinical commonality underlying these diagnostic syndromes might be associated with unique and perhaps specific final common pathophysiological pathways. Furthermore, the examination of the biological processes involved in clinical conditions with nuclear medicine techniques also provides an opportunity for redefining illnesses (402).

For example, one study reported that elevated DA synaptic levels in acute schizophrenia were predictive of rapid symptomatic response to antipsychotic (i.e., antidopaminergic) treatment (28). A subgroup of patients showed no detectable abnormality of striatal DA function despite frank psychotic symptoms and failed to respond to treatment. It is possible that, in these patients, the psychotic state is not driven by excess DA activity, and that the antidopaminergic treatment fails because the problem being treated does not exist in these patients. This result has led to the concept of dopaminergic- versus nondopaminergic-driven psychotic states in schizophrenia (28). This biological, rather than clinical, classification might prove to be useful in evaluation of nondopaminergic antipsychotic pharmacological strategies.

Another example is the constellation of conditions that have been reliably shown to be associated with low D_2 receptor availability in the striatum. This finding has been associated with a personality trait (detachment), anxiety disorder (social phobia), and addiction to a variety of substances, including cocaine, heroin, alcohol, and even food. These conditions are not similar but are frequently overlapping or comorbid. Therefore, imaging studies might reveal common biological processes across conditions that were hitherto unsuspected, and might help to delineate psychopathological features more directly related to altered biological brain functions than these current diagnostic classifications.

Despite these successes, a substantial number of studies yielded discordant results, and it is important to examine potential sources of discrepancies. An important drawback of this literature is the generally low number of subjects included in studies (typically less than 20 per group). In conditions characterized by marked heterogeneity, such as major depressive disorders, this factor is bound to yield divergent results across studies. Small samples are obviously due to the cost of these investigations, but also, in some instances, to the difficulty in recruiting appropriate clinical subjects (such as drug-free patients with schizophrenia). Another source of discrepancy is the variety of technical approaches to data acquisition and analysis. For example, analytical methods range from "empirical" or "semiquantitative" methods (typically a region of interest to a region of reference ratio measured at one time point) to model-based methods using an arterial input function. The limitations associated with empirical analytical methods are discussed in other chapters of this book and might account for artifactual results, especially when the effect size of the between-group difference and the number of subjects are small (403).

In addressing these limitations it will be important to increase the availability of these techniques beyond a few academic centers, to promote multicenter studies in well-characterized populations, and to standardize analytical methods. Until recently, SPECT was the only widely available technique, and SPECT studies have so far provided a substantial contribution to this field. With the current increase in PET camera availability, the development of [^{18}F]-based molecular imaging probes will provide unique opportunities for further dissemination of these techniques.

The greatest challenge facing this field is to develop molecular imaging probes suitable for imaging neurochemical processes beyond those currently available. Basically, four transmitter systems (DA, 5-HT, GABA, and opiates) dominate the psychiatric PET and SPECT molecular imaging literature. These systems are clearly involved in a very critical way in the mechanisms of action of psychiatric medications and drugs of abuse. However, a large number of other critical transmitter systems have not been investigated. Radiotracers suitable for studying transmitter systems as important as the glutamatergic or adrenergic systems in the brain are only emerging. The ability to image brain chemistry beyond neurotransmission itself and to examine growth factors or intracellular signaling pathways is still in its infancy. A sustained collaboration between industry and academic institutions will be required to expand the study of brain biomolecular processes beyond the current, and still relatively limited, arsenal.

In conclusion, the chapter has reviewed seminal findings obtained with PET and SPECT molecular imaging of psychiatric conditions. These techniques do not yet play a major role in the diagnosis and treatment of these disorders, and at present remain essentially research tools. However, the results produced by this field so far suggest that PET will significantly contribute to unraveling the biological bases of these conditions and might play an increasing role in their clinical management. Moreover, it is foreseeable that PET will become more and more involved in the development of new psychiatric medications. Expanding the availability of

PET and the current radiopharmaceutical portfolio will be critical for these predictions to become reality.

REFERENCES

1. Rossum V. The significance of dopamine receptor blockade for the mechanism of action of neuroleptic drugs. *Arch Int Pharmacodyn Ther* 1966;160:492–494.
2. Carlsson A, Lindqvist M. Effect of chlorpromazine or haloperidol on formation of 3-methoxytyramine and normetanephrine in mouse brain. *Acta Pharmacol Toxicol* 1963;20:140–144.
3. Seeman P, Lee T. Antipsychotic drugs: direct correlation between clinical potency and presynaptic action on dopamine neurons. *Science* 1975;188:1217–1219.
4. Creese I, Burt DR, Snyder SH. Dopamine receptor binding predicts clinical and pharmacological potencies of antischizophrenic drugs. *Science* 1976;19:481–483.
5. Connell PH. *Amphetamine psychosis*. London: Chapman and Hill, 1958.
6. Angrist BM, Gershon S. The phenomenology of experimentally induced amphetamine psychosis—preliminary observation. *Biol Psychiatry* 1970;2:95–107.
7. Weinberger DR, Berman KF. Prefrontal function in schizophrenia: confounds and controversies. *Philos Trans R Soc Lond B Biol Sci* 1996;351(1346):1495–1503.
8. Goldman-Rakic PS, Selemon LD. Functional and anatomical aspects of prefrontal pathology in schizophrenia. *Schizophrenia Bull* 1997;23: 437–458.
9. Weinberger DR. Implications of the normal brain development for the pathogenesis of schizophrenia. *Arch Gen Psychiatry* 1987;44: 660–669.
10. Knable MB, Weinberger DR. Dopamine, the prefrontal cortex and schizophrenia. *J Psychopharmacol* 1997;11(2):123–131.
11. Deutch AY. Prefrontal cortical dopamine systems and the elaboration of functional corticostriatal circuits: implications for schizophrenia and Parkinson's disease. *J Neural Transm Gen Sect* 1993;91(2–3): 197–221.
12. Wilkinson LS. The nature of interactions involving prefrontal and striatal dopamine systems. *J Psychopharmacol* 1997;11(2):143–150.
13. Weinberger DR, Laruelle M. Neurochemical and neuropharmacological imaging in schizophrenia. In: Davis KL, Charney DS, Coyle JT, et al., eds. *Neuropharmacology: The fifth generation of progress*. Philadelphia: Lippincott Williams & Wilkins, 2001:883–885.
14. Wong DF, Wagner HN, Tune LE, et al: Positron emission tomography reveals elevated D_2 dopamine receptors in drug-naive schizophrenics. *Science* 1986;234:1558–1563.
15. Crawley JC, Owens DG, Crow TJ, et al. Dopamine D_2 receptors in schizophrenia studied *in vivo*. *Lancet* 1986;2(8500):224–225.
16. Blin J, Baron JC, Cambon H, et al. Striatal dopamine D_2 receptors in tardive dyskinesia: PET study. *J Neurol Neurosurg Psychiatry* 1989; 52(11):1248–1252.
17. Martinot J-L, Peron-Magnan P, Huret J-D, et al. Striatal D_2 dopaminergic receptors assessed with positron emission tomography and 76-Br-bromospiperone in untreated patients. *Am J Psychiatry* 1990;147: 346–350.
18. Tune LE, Wong DF, Pearlson G, et al. Dopamine D_2 receptor density estimates in schizophrenia: a positron emission tomography study with ^{11}C-N-methylspiperone. *Psychiatry Res* 1993;49(3):219–237.
19. Nordstrom AL, Farde L, Eriksson L, et al. No elevated D_2 dopamine receptors in neuroleptic-naive schizophrenic patients revealed by positron emission tomography and [^{11}C]N-methylspiperone [comments]. *Psychiatry Res* 1995;61(2):67–83.
20. Okubo Y, Suhara T, Suzuki K, et al. Decreased prefrontal dopamine D_1 receptors in schizophrenia revealed by PET. *Nature* 1997;385(6617): 634–636.
21. Farde L, Wiesel F, Stone-Elander S, et al. D_2 dopamine receptors in neuroleptic-naive schizophrenic patients. A positron emission tomography study with [^{11}C]raclopride. *Arch Gen Psychiatry* 1990;47: 213–219.
22. Hietala J, Syvälahti E, Vuorio K, et al. Striatal D_2 receptor characteristics in neuroleptic-naive schizophrenic patients studied with positron emission tomography. *Arch Gen Psychiatry* 1994;51:116–123.
23. Pilowsky LS, Costa DC, Ell PJ, et al. D_2 dopamine receptor binding in the basal ganglia of antipsychotic-free schizophrenic patients. An I-123-IBZM single photon emission computerized tomography study. *Br J Psychiatry* 1994;164:16–26.
24. Laruelle M, Abi-Dargham A, van Dyck CH, et al. Single photon emission computerized tomography imaging of amphetamine-induced dopamine release in drug free schizophrenic subjects. *Proc Natl Acad Sci U S A* 1996;93:9235–9240.
25. Knable MB, Egan MF, Heinz A, et al. Altered dopaminergic function and negative symptoms in drug-free patients with schizophrenia. [^{123}I]-iodobenzamide SPECT study. *Br J Psychiatry* 1997;171: 574–577.
26. Breier A, Su TP, Saunders R, et al. Schizophrenia is associated with elevated amphetamine-induced synaptic dopamine concentrations: evidence from a novel positron emission tomography method. *Proc Natl Acad Sci U S A* 1997;94(6):2569–2574.
27. Abi-Dargham A, Gil R, Krystal J, et al. Increased striatal dopamine transmission in schizophrenia: confirmation in a second cohort. *Am J Psychiatry* 1998;155:761–767.
28. Abi-Dargham A, Rodenhiser J, Printz D, et al. Increased baseline occupancy of D_2 receptors by dopamine in schizophrenia. *Proc Natl Acad Sci U S A* 2000;97(14):8104–8109.
29. Martinot JL, Paillère-Martinot ML, Loc'h C, et al. The estimated density of D_2 striatal receptors in schizophrenia. A study with positron emission tomography and ^{76}Br-bromolisuride. *Br J Psychiatry* 1991; 158:346–350.
30. Martinot JL, Paillère-Martinot ML, Loch'H C, et al. Central D_2 receptors and negative symptoms of schizophrenia. *Br J Pharmacol* 1994; 164:27–34.
31. Seeman P, Guan H-C, Niznik HB. Endogenous dopamine lowers the dopamine D_2 receptor density as measured by [^{3}H]raclopride: implications for positron emission tomography of the human brain. *Synapse* 1989;3:96–97.
32. Seeman P. Brain dopamine receptors in schizophrenia: PET problems. *Arch Gen Psychiatry* 1988;45:598–660.
33. Hirvonen J, van Erp TG, Huttunen J, et al. Increased caudate dopamine D_2 receptor availability as a genetic marker for schizophrenia. *Arch Gen Psychiatry* 2005;62(4):371–378.
34. Karlsson P, Farde L, Halldin C, et al. D_1-dopamine receptors in schizophrenia examined by PET. *Schizophrenia Res* 1997;24:179.
35. Abi-Dargham A, Gil R, Mawlawi O, et al. Selective alteration in D_1 receptors in schizophrenia: a PET *in vivo* study. *J Nucl Med* 2001; 42:17P.
36. Sokoloff P, Diaz J, Le Foll B, et al. The dopamine D_3 receptor: a therapeutic target for the treatment of neuropsychiatric disorders. *CNS Neurol Disord Drug Targets* 2006;5(1):25–43.
37. Gurevich EV, Bordelon Y, Shapiro RM, et al. Mesolimbic dopamine D_3 receptors and use of antipsychotics in patients with schizophrenia. A postmortem study. *Arch Gen Psychiatry* 1997;54(3):225–232.
38. Pilla M, Perachon S, Sautel F, et al. Selective inhibition of cocaine-seeking behaviour by a partial dopamine D_3 receptor agonist [comments] [published erratum appears in *Nature* 1999;401(6751):403]. *Nature* 1999;400(6742):371–375.
39. Narendran R, Slifstein M, Guillin O, et al. Dopamine ($D_2/_3$) receptor agonist positron emission tomography radiotracer [^{11}C]-(+)-PHNO is a D_3 receptor preferring agonist *in vivo*. *Synapse* 2006;60(7): 485–495.
40. Reith J, Benkelfat C, Sherwin A, et al. Elevated dopa decarboxylase activity in living brain of patients with psychosis. *Proc Natl Acad Sci U S A* 1994;91:11651–11654.

41. Hietala J, Syvalahti E, Vuorio K, et al. Presynaptic dopamine function in striatum of neuroleptic-naive schizophrenic patients. *Lancet* 1995;346(8983):1130–1131.
42. Dao-Castellana MH, Paillere-Martinot ML, Hantraye P, et al. Presynaptic dopaminergic function in the striatum of schizophrenic patients. *Schizophrenia Res* 1997;23(2):167–174.
43. Hietala J, Syvalahti E, Vilkman H, et al. Depressive symptoms and presynaptic dopamine function in neuroleptic-naive schizophrenia. *Schizophrenia Res* 1999;35(1):41–50.
44. Meyer-Lindenberg A, Miletich RS, Kohn PD, et al. Reduced prefrontal activity predicts exaggerated striatal dopaminergic function in schizophrenia. *Nat Neurosci* 2002;5(3):267–271.
45. McGowan S, Lawrence AD, Sales T, et al. Presynaptic dopaminergic dysfunction in schizophrenia: a positron emission tomographic [^{18}F]fluorodopa study. *Arch Gen Psychiatry* 2004;61(2):134–142.
46. Lindstrom LH, Gefvert O, Hagberg G, et al. Increased dopamine synthesis rate in medial prefrontal cortex and striatum in schizophrenia indicated by L-(beta-^{11}C) DOPA and PET. *Biol Psychiatry* 1999;46(5): 681–688.
47. Laruelle M. Imaging synaptic neurotransmission with *in vivo* binding competition techniques: a critical review. *J Cereb Blood Flow Metab* 2000;20(3):423–451.
48. Villemagne VL, Wong DF, Yokoi F, et al. GBR12909 attenuates amphetamine-induced striatal dopamine release as measured by [(^{11})C] raclopride continuous infusion PET scans. *Synapse* 1999;33(4): 268–273.
49. Laruelle M, Iyer RN, Al-Tikriti MS, et al. Microdialysis and SPECT measurements of amphetamine-induced dopamine release in nonhuman primates. *Synapse* 1997;25:1–14.
50. Piccini P, Pavese N, Brooks DJ. Endogenous dopamine release after pharmacological challenges in Parkinson's disease. *Ann Neurol* 2003;53(5):647–653.
51. Laruelle M, Abi-Dargham A, Gil R, et al. Increased dopamine transmission in schizophrenia: relationship to illness phases. *Biol Psychiatry* 1999;46(1):56–72.
52. Parsey RV, Oquendo MA, Zea-Ponce Y, et al. Dopamine D(2) receptor availability and amphetamine-induced dopamine release in unipolar depression. *Biol Psychiatry* 2001;50(5):313–322.
53. Hwang D, Kegeles LS, Laruelle M. (-)-N-[(^{11})C]propyl-norapomorphine: a positron-labeled dopamine agonist for PET imaging of D(2) receptors. *Nucl Med Biol* 2000;27(6):533–539.
54. Narendran R, Hwang DR, Slifstein M, et al. *In vivo* vulnerability to competition by endogenous dopamine: comparison of the D_2 receptor agonist radiotracer (-)-N-[^{11}C]propyl-norapomorphine ([^{11}C]NPA) with the D_2 receptor antagonist radiotracer [^{11}C]-raclopride. *Synapse* 2004;52(3):188–208.
55. Willeit M, Ginovart N, Kapur S, et al. High-affinity states of human brain dopamine $D_2/_3$ receptors imaged by the agonist [^{11}C]-(+)-PHNO. *Biol Psychiatry* 2006;59(5):389–394.
56. Ginovart N, Willeit M, Rusjan P, et al. Positron emission tomography quantification of [^{11}C]-(+)-PHNO binding in the human brain. *J Cereb Blood Flow Metab* 2007;27(4):857–871.
57. Seneca N, Finnema SJ, Farde L, et al. Effect of amphetamine on dopamine D_2 receptor binding in nonhuman primate brain: a comparison of the agonist radioligand [^{11}C]MNPA and antagonist [^{11}C]raclopride. *Synapse* 2006;59(5):260–269.
58. Laruelle M, DSouza CD, Baldwin RM, et al. Imaging D_2 receptor occupancy by endogenous dopamine in humans. *Neuropsychopharmacology* 1997;17(3):162–174.
59. Fujita M, Verhoeff NP, Varrone A, et al. Imaging extrastriatal dopamine D(2) receptor occupancy by endogenous dopamine in healthy humans. *Eur J Pharmacol* 2000;387(2):179–188.
60. Verhoeff NP, Christensen BK, Hussey D, et al. Effects of catecholamine depletion on D(2) receptor binding, mood, and attentiveness in humans: a replication study. *Pharmacol Biochem Behav* 2003;74(2): 425–432.
61. Verhoeff NP, Hussey D, Lee M, et al. Dopamine depletion results in increased neostriatal D(2), but not D(1), receptor binding in humans. *Mol Psychiatry* 2002;7(3):233, 322–328.
62. Laruelle M, Abi-Dargham A, van Dyck C, et al. Dopamine and serotonin transporters in patients with schizophrenia: an imaging study with [^{123}I]beta-CIT. *Biol Psychiatry* 2000;47(5):371–379.
63. Laakso A, Vilkman H, Alakare B, et al. Striatal dopamine transporter binding in neuroleptic-naive patients with schizophrenia studied with positron emission tomography. *Am J Psychiatry* 2000;157(2):269–271.
64. Robertson G, Fibiger H. Neuroleptics increase C-fos expression in the forebrain: contrasting effects of haloperidol and clozapine. *Neuroscience* 1992;46:315–328.
65. Robertson GS, Matsumura H, Fibiger HC. Induction patterns of Fos-like immunoreactivity in the forebrain as predictors of atypical antipsychotic activity. *J Pharmacol Exp Ther* 1994;271(2):1058–1066.
66. Deutch A, Moghadam B, Innis R, et al. Mechanisms of action of atypical antipsychotic drugs. Implication for novel therapeutic strategies for schizophrenia. *Schizophrenia Res* 1991;4:121–156.
67. Mawlawi O, Martinez D, Slifstein M, et al. Imaging human mesolimbic dopamine transmission with positron emission tomography: I. Accuracy and precision of D_2 receptor parameter measurements in ventral striatum. *J Cereb Blood Flow Metab* 2001;21(9):1034–1057.
68. Martinez D, Slifstein M, Broft A, et al. Imaging human mesolimbic dopamine transmission with positron emission tomography. Part II: amphetamine-induced dopamine release in the functional subdivisions of the striatum. *J Cereb Blood Flow Metab* 2003;23(3):285–300.
69. Drevets WC, Gautier C, Price JC, et al. Amphetamine-induced dopamine release in human ventral striatum correlates with euphoria. *Biol Psychiatry* 2001;49(2):81–96.
70. Halldin C, Farde L, Hogberg T, et al. Carbon-11-FLB 457: a radioligand for extrastriatal D_2 dopamine receptors. *J Nucl Med* 1995;36(7): 1275–1281.
71. Mukherjee J, Yang ZY, Das MK, et al. Fluorinated benzamide neuroleptics—III. Development of (S)-N-[(1-allyl- 2-pyrrolidinyl) methyl]-5-(3-[^{18}F]fluoropropyl)-2, 3-dimethoxybenzamide as an improved dopamine D_2 receptor tracer. *Nucl Med Biol* 1995;22(3): 283–296.
72. Talvik M, Nordstrom AL, Olsson H, et al. Decreased thalamic D_2/D_3 receptor binding in drug-naive patients with schizophrenia: a PET study with [^{11}C]FLB 457. *Int J Neuropsychopharmacol* 2003;6(4): 361–370.
73. Talvik M, Nordstrom AL, Okubo Y, et al. Dopamine D_2 receptor binding in drug-naive patients with schizophrenia examined with raclopride-C^{11} and positron emission tomography. *Psychiatry Res* 2006; 148(2–3):165–173.
74. Yasuno F, Suhara T, Okubo Y, et al. Low dopamine D(2) receptor binding in subregions of the thalamus in schizophrenia. *Am J Psychiatry* 2004;161(6):1016–1022.
75. Tuppurainen H, Kuikka JT, Laakso MP, et al. Midbrain dopamine $D_2/_3$ receptor binding in schizophrenia. *Eur Arch Psychiatry Clin Neurosci* 2006;256(6):382–387.
76. Tuppurainen H, Kuikka J, Viinamaki H, et al. Extrastriatal dopamine $D_2/_3$ receptor density and distribution in drug-naive schizophrenic patients. *Mol Psychiatry* 2003;8(4):453–455.
77. Suhara T, Okubo Y, Yasuno F, et al. Decreased dopamine D_2 receptor binding in the anterior cingulate cortex in schizophrenia. *Arch Gen Psychiatry* 2002;59(1):25–30.
78. De Keyser J, Ebinger G, Vauquelin G. Evidence for a widespread dopaminergic innervation of the human cerebral neocortex. *Neurosci Lett* 1989;104:281–285.
79. Hall H, Sedvall G, Magnusson O, et al. Distribution of D_1- and D_2-dopamine receptors, and dopamine and its metabolites in the human brain. *Neuropsychopharmacology* 1994;11:245–256.
80. Halldin C, Stone-Elander S, Farde L, et al. Preparation of ^{11}C-labelled SCH 23390 for the in vivo study of dopamine D_1 receptors using positron emission tomography. *Appl Radiat Isot* 1986;37:1039–1043.

81. Andersen PH, Gronvald FC, Hohlweg R, et al. NNC-112, NNC-687 and NNC-756, new selective and highly potent dopamine D_1 receptor antagonists. *Eur J Pharmacol* 1992;219(1):45–52.
82. Halldin C, Foged C, Chou YH, et al. Carbon-11-NNC 112: a radioligand for PET examination of striatal and neocortical D_1-dopamine receptors. *J Nucl Med* 1998;39(12):2061–2068.
83. Abi-Dargham A, Simpson N, Kegeles L, et al. PET studies of binding competition between endogenous dopamine and the D_1 radiotracer [^{11}C]NNC 756. *Synapse* 1999;32(2):93–109.
84. Ekelund J, Slifstein M, Narendran R, et al. *In vivo* DA D(1) receptor selectivity of NNC 112 and SCH 23390. *Mol Imaging Biol* 2007;9(3): 117–125.
85. Slifstein M, Kegeles LS, Gonzales R, et al. [(^{11})C]NNC 112 selectivity for dopamine D(1) and serotonin 5-HT(2A) receptors: a PET study in healthy human subjects. *J Cereb Blood Flow Metab* 2007;27(10): 1733–1741.
86. Karlsson P, Farde L, Halldin C, et al. PET study of D(1) dopamine receptor binding in neuroleptic-naive patients with schizophrenia. *Am J Psychiatry* 2002;159(5):761–767.
87. Guo N, Hwang DR, Lo ES, et al. Dopamine depletion and *in vivo* binding of PET D_1 receptor radioligands: implications for imaging studies in schizophrenia. *Neuropsychopharmacology* 2003;28(9): 1703–1711.
88. Abi-Dargham A, Krystal J. Serotonin receptors as target of antipsychotic medications. In: Lidow MS, ed. *Neurotransmitter receptors in actions of antipsychotic medications*. Boca Raton, FL: CRC Press, 2000:79–107.
89. Frankle WG, Narendran R, Huang Y, et al. Serotonin transporter availability in patients with schizophrenia: a positron emission tomography imaging study with [^{11}C]DASB. *Biol Psychiatry* 2005;57(12): 1510–1516.
90. Lewis R, Kapur S, Jones C, et al. Serotonin 5-HT_2 receptors in schizophrenia: a PET study using [^{18}F]setoperone in neuroleptic-naive patients and normal subjects. *Am J Psychiatry* 1999;156(1):72–78.
91. Trichard C, Paillere-Martinot ML, Attar-Levy D, et al. No serotonin 5-HT_{2A} receptor density abnormality in the cortex of schizophrenic patients studied with PET. *Schizophr Res* 1998;31(1):13–17.
92. Okubo Y, Suhara T, Suzuki K, et al. Serotonin 5-HT_2 receptors in schizophrenic patients studied by positron emission tomography. *Life Sci* 2000;66(25):2455–2464.
93. Ngan ET, Yatham LN, Ruth TJ, et al. Decreased serotonin 2A receptor densities in neuroleptic-naive patients with schizophrenia: a PET study using [(^{18})F]setoperone. *Am J Psychiatry* 2000;157(6):1016–1018.
94. Tauscher J, Kapur S, Verhoeff NP, et al. Brain serotonin 5-HT(1A) receptor binding in schizophrenia measured by positron emission tomography and [^{11}C]WAY-100635. *Arch Gen Psychiatry* 2002;59(6): 514–520.
95. Yasuno F, Suhara T, Ichimiya T, et al. Decreased 5-HT_{1A} receptor binding in amygdala of schizophrenia. *Biol Psychiatry* 2004;55(5): 439–444.
96. Frankle WG, Lombardo I, Kegeles LS, et al. Serotonin 1A receptor availability in patients with schizophrenia and schizo-affective disorder: a positron emission tomography imaging study with [^{11}C]WAY 100635. *Psychopharmacology (Berl)* 2006;189(2):155–164.
97. Lewis DA. GABAergic local circuit neurons and prefrontal cortical dysfunction in schizophrenia. *Brain Res Rev* 2000;31(2–3):270–276.
98. Benes FM. Emerging principles of altered neural circuitry in schizophrenia. *Brain Res Rev* 2000;31(2–3):251–269.
99. Busatto GF, Pilowsky LS, Costa DC, et al. Correlation between reduced *in vivo* benzodiazepine receptor binding and severity of psychotic symptoms in schizophrenia. *Am J Psychiatry* 1997;154(1):56–63.
100. Verhoeff NP, Soares JC, D'Souza CD, et al. [^{123}I]Iomazenil SPECT benzodiazepine receptor imaging in schizophrenia. *Psychiatry Res* 1999;91(3):163–173.
101. Abi-Dargham A, Laruelle M, Krystal J, et al. No evidence of altered *in vivo* benzodiazepine receptor binding in schizophrenia. *Neuropsychopharmacology* 1999;20(6):650–661.
102. Benes FM, Wickramasinghe R, Vincent SL, et al. Uncoupling of GABA(A) and benzodiazepine receptor binding activity in the hippocampal formation of schizophrenic brain. *Brain Res* 1997;755(1): 121–129.
103. Kapur S, Zipursky RB, Remington G. Clinical and theoretical implications of 5-HT_2 and D_2 receptor occupancy of clozapine, risperidone, and olanzapine in schizophrenia. *Am J Psychiatry* 1999;156(2): 286–293.
104. Nyberg S, Nilsson U, Okubo Y, et al. Implications of brain imaging for the management of schizophrenia. *Int Clin Psychopharmacol* 1998;13[Suppl 3]:S15–S20.
105. Farde L, Nordström AL, Wiesel FA, et al. Positron emission tomography analysis of central D_1 and D_2 dopamine receptor occupancy in patients treated with classical neuroleptics and clozapine. *Arch Gen Psychiatry* 1992;49:538–544.
106. Wolkin A, Barouche F, Wolf AP, et al. Dopamine blockade and clinical response: evidence for two biological subgroups of schizophrenia. *Am J Psychiatry* 1989;146(7):905–908.
107. Pilowsky LS, Costa DC, Ell PJ, et al. Clozapine, single photon emission tomography, and the D_2 dopamine receptor blockade hypothesis of schizophrenia. *Lancet* 1992;340:199–202.
108. Nordstrom AL, Farde L, Wiesel FA, et al. Central D_2-dopamine receptor occupancy in relation to antipsychotic drug effects: a double-blind PET study of schizophrenic patients. *Biol Psychiatry* 1993;33(4): 227–235.
109. Kapur S, Zipursky R, Jones C, et al. Relationship between dopamine D(2) occupancy, clinical response, and side effects: a double-blind PET study of first-episode schizophrenia. *Am J Psychiatry* 2000;157(4): 514–520.
110. Nordstrom AL, Farde L, Nyberg S, et al. D_1, D_2, and 5-HT_2 receptor occupancy in relation to clozapine serum concentration: a PET study of schizophrenic patients. *Am J Psychiatry* 1995;152(10):1444–1449.
111. Nyberg S, Farde L, Eriksson L, et al. 5-HT_2 and D_2 dopamine receptor occupancy in the living human brain. A PET study with risperidone. *Psychopharmacology* 1993;110:265–272.
112. Kapur S, Remington G, Zipursky RB, et al. The D_2 dopamine receptor occupancy of risperidone and its relationship to extrapyramidal symptoms: a PET study. *Life Sci* 1995;57(10):L103–L107.
113. Knable MB, Heinz A, Raedler T, et al. Extrapyramidal side effects with risperidone and haloperidol at comparable D_2 receptor occupancy levels. *Psychiat Res Neuroimaging* 1997;75(2):91–101.
114. Kapur S, Zipursky RB, Remington G, et al. 5-HT_2 and D_2 receptor occupancy of olanzapine in schizophrenia: a PET investigation. *Am J Psychiatry* 1998;155(7):921–928.
115. Gefvert O, Bergstrom M, Langstrom B, et al. Time course of central nervous dopamine-D_2 and 5-HT_2 receptor blockade and plasma drug concentrations after discontinuation of quetiapine (Seroquel) in patients with schizophrenia. *Psychopharmacology (Berl)* 1998;135(2):119–126.
116. Kapur S, Zipursky R, Jones C, et al. A positron emission tomography study of quetiapine in schizophrenia: a preliminary finding of an antipsychotic effect with only transiently high dopamine D_2 receptor occupancy. *Arch Gen Psychiatry* 2000;57(6):553–559.
117. Pilowsky LS, Mulligan RS, Acton PD, et al. Limbic selectivity of clozapine. *Lancet* 1997;350(9076):490–491.
118. Farde L, Suhara T, Nyberg S, et al. A PET study of [C-11]FLB 457 binding to extrastriatal D-2-dopamine receptors in healthy subjects and antipsychotic drug-treated patients. *Psychopharmacology* 1997;133(4): 396–404.
119. Bigliani V, Mulligan RS, Acton PD, et al. *In vivo* occupancy of striatal and temporal cortical D_2/D_3 dopamine receptors by typical antipsychotic drugs. [^{123}I]epidepride single photon emission tomography (SPET) study. *Br J Psychiatry* 1999;175:231–238.
120. Olsson H, Farde L. Potentials and pitfalls using high affinity radioligands in PET and SPET determinations on regional drug induced D_2 receptor occupancy—a simulation study based on experimental data. *Neuroimage* 2001;14(4):936–945.

121. Abi-Dargham A, Hwang DR, Huang Y, et a l. Reliable quantification of both striatal and extrastriatal D_2 receptors in humans with [^{18}F]fallypride. *J Nucl Med* 2000;41:139P.
122. Kessler RM, Ansari MS, Riccardi P, et al. Occupancy of striatal and extrastriatal dopamine D_2 receptors by clozapine and quetiapine. *Neuropsychopharmacology* 2006;31(9):1991–2001.
123. Grunder G, Landvogt C, Vernaleken I, et al. The striatal and extrastriatal D_2/D_3 receptor-binding profile of clozapine in patients with schizophrenia. *Neuropsychopharmacology* 2006;31(5):1027–1035.
124. Kessler RM, Ansari MS, Riccardi P, et al. Occupancy of striatal and extrastriatal dopamine D_2/D_3 receptors by olanzapine and haloperidol. *Neuropsychopharmacology* 2005;30(12):2283–2289.
125. Xiberas X, Martinot JL, Mallet L, et al. Extrastriatal and striatal D(2) dopamine receptor blockade with haloperidol or new antipsychotic drugs in patients with schizophrenia. *Br J Psychiatry* 2001;179: 503–508.
126. Talvik M, Nordstrom AL, Nyberg S, et al. No support for regional selectivity in clozapine-treated patients: a PET study with [(^{11})C]raclopride and [(^{11})C]FLB 457. *Am J Psychiatry* 2001;158(6): 926–930.
127. Deutch AY, Lee MC, Iadarola MJ. Regionally specific effects of atypical antipsychotic drugs on striatal fos expression: the nucleus accumbens shell as a locus of antipsychotic action. *Mol Cell Neurosci* 1992;3:332–341.
128. Agid O, Mamo D, Ginovart N, et al. Striatal vs extrastriatal dopamine D(2) receptors in antipsychotic response—a double-blind PET study in schizophrenia. *Neuropsychopharmacology* 2007;32(6):1209–1215.
129. Wolkin A, Brodie JD, Barouche F, et al. Dopamine receptor occupancy and plasma haloperidol levels. *Arch Gen Psychiatry* 1989;46(5):482–484.
130. Fitzgerald PB, Kapur S, Remington G, et al. Predicting haloperidol occupancy of central dopamine D_2 receptors from plasma levels. *Psychopharmacology (Berl)* 2000;149(1):1–5.
131. Hagberg G, Gefvert O, Bergstrom M, et al. N-[^{11}C]methylspiperone PET, in contrast to [^{11}C]raclopride, fails to detect D_2 receptor occupancy by an atypical neuroleptic. *Psychiatry Res* 1998;82(3):147–160.
132. Drevets WC. Neuroimaging studies of mood disorders. *Biol Psychiatry* 2000;48:813–829.
133. Mayberg HS, Liotti M, Brannan SK, et al. Reciprocal limbic-cortical function and negative mood: converging PET findings in depression and normal sadness. *Am J Psychiatry* 1999;156(5):675–682.
134. Blier P, de Montigny C, Chaput Y. A role for the serotonin system in the mechanism of action of antidepressant treatments: preclinical evidence. *J Clin Psychiatry* 1990;51[Suppl]:14–20; discussion 21.
135. Mayberg H, Robinson R, Wong D, et al. PET imaging of cortical S2 serotonin receptors after stroke: lateralized changes and relationship to depression. *Am J Psychiatry* 1988;145(8):937–943.
136. D'haenen H, Bossuyt A, Mertens J, et al. SPECT imaging of serotonin 2 receptors in depression. *Psychiatry Res Neuroimaging* 1992; 45(4): 227-237
137. Blin J, Pappata S, Kijosawa M, et al. [^{18}F]setoperone: a new high-affinity ligand for positron emission tomography study of the serotonin-2 receptors in baboon brain *in vivo*. *Eur J Pharmacol* 1988;147:73–82.
138. Lemaire C, Cantineau R, Guillaume M, et al. Fluorine-18-altanserin: a radioligand for the study of serotonin receptors with PET: radiolabeling and *in vivo* biologic behavior in rats. *J Nucl Med* 1991;32(12): 2266–2272.
139. Biver F, Wikler D, Lotstra F, et al. Serotonin 5-HT_2 receptor imaging in major depression: focal changes in orbito-insular cortex. *Br J Psychiatry* 1997;171:444–448.
140. Meyer JH, Kapur S, Houle S, et al. Prefrontal cortex 5-HT_2 receptors in depression: an [^{18}F]setoperone PET imaging study. *Am J Psychiatry* 1999;156(7):1029–1034.
141. Attar-Levy D, Martinot J-L, Blin J, et al. The cortical serotonin 2 receptors studied with positron-emission tomography and [^{18}F]-setoperone during depressive illness and antidepressant treatment with clomipramine. *Biol Psychiatry* 1999;45(2):180–186.
142. Meltzer CC, Price JC, Mathis CA, et al. PET imaging of serotonin type 2A receptors in late-life neuropsychiatric disorders. *Am J Psychiatry* 1999;156(12):1871–1878.
143. Sheline YI, Mintun MA, Barch DM, et al. Decreased hippocampal 5-HT(2A) receptor binding in older depressed patients using [^{18}F]altanserin positron emission tomography. *Neuropsychopharmacology* 2004;29(12):2235–2241.
144. Yatham LN, Liddle PF, Shiah I-S, et al. Brain serotonin 2 receptors in major depression: a positron emission tomography study. *Arch Gen Psychiatry* 2000;57(9):850–858.
145. Meyer JH, Kapur S, Eisfeld B, et al. The effect of paroxetine on 5-HT_{2A} receptors in depression: an [^{18}F]setoperone PET imaging study. *Am J Psychiatry* 2001;158(1):78–85.
146. Yatham LN, Liddle PF, Dennie J, et al. Decrease in brain serotonin 2 receptor binding in patients with major depression following desipramine treatment: a positron emission tomography study with fluorine-18-labeled setoperone. *Arch Gen Psychiatry* 1999;56(8): 705–711.
147. Mann JJ. Role of the serotonergic system in the pathogenesis of major depression and suicidal behavior. *Neuropsychopharmacology* 1999; 21[2 Suppl]:99S–105S.
148. Drevets WC, Frank E, Price JC, et al. PET imaging of serotonin 1A receptor binding in depression. *Biol Psychiatry* 1999;46(10):1375–1387.
149. Fujita M, Charney DS, Innis RB. Imaging serotonergic neurotransmission in depression: hippocampal pathophysiology may mirror global brain alterations. *Biol Psychiatry* 2000;48(8):801–812.
150. Duman RS, Heninger GR, Nestler EJ. A molecular and cellular theory of depression. *Arch Gen Psychiatry* 1997;54(7):597–606.
151. Lowther S, DePaermentier F, Cheetham SC, et al. 5-HT_{1A} receptor binding sites in post-mortem brain samples from depressed suicides and controls. *J Affective Disord* 1997;42(2–3):199–207.
152. Dillon KA, Gross-Isseroff R, Israeli M, et al. Autoradiographic analysis of serotonin 5-HT_{1A} receptor binding in the human brain postmortem: effects of age and alcohol. *Brain Res* 1991;554(1–2):56–64.
153. Matsubara S, Arora RC, Meltzer HY. Serotonergic measures in suicide brain: 5-HT_{1A} binding sites in frontal cortex of suicide victims. *J Neural Transm Gen Sect* 1991;85(3):181–194.
154. Arranz B, Eriksson A, Mellerup E, et al. Brain 5-HT_{1A}, 5-HT_{1D}, and 5-HT_2 receptors in suicide victims. *Biol Psychiatry* 1994;35(7):457–463.
155. Arango V, Underwood MD, Gubbi AV, et al. Localized alterations in pre- and postsynaptic serotonin binding sites in the ventrolateral prefrontal cortex of suicide victims. *Brain Res* 1995;688(1–2):121–133.
156. Sargent PA, Kjaer KH, Bench CJ, et al. Brain serotonin (1A) receptor binding measured by positron emission tomography with [^{11}C]WAY-100635: effects of depression and antidepressant treatment. *Arch Gen Psychiatry* 2000;57(2):174–180.
157. Bhagwagar Z, Rabiner EA, Sargent PA, et al. Persistent reduction in brain serotonin 1A receptor binding in recovered depressed men measured by positron emission tomography with [^{11}C]WAY-100635. *Mol Psychiatry* 2004;9(4):386–392.
158. Meltzer CC, Price JC, Mathis CA, et al. Serotonin 1A receptor binding and treatment response in late-life depression. *Neuropsychopharmacology* 2004;29(12):2258–2265.
159. Parsey RV, Oquendo MA, Ogden RT, et al. Altered serotonin 1A binding in major depression: a [carbonyl-C-^{11}]WAY100635 positron emission tomography study. *Biol Psychiatry* 2006;59(2):106–113.
160. Parsey RV, Olvet DM, Oquendo MA, et al. Higher 5-HT_{1A} receptor binding potential during a major depressive episode predicts poor treatment response: preliminary data from a naturalistic study. *Neuropsychopharmacology* 2006;31(8):1745–1749.
161. Porter RJ, McAllister-Williams RH, Jones S, et al. Effects of dexamethasone on neuroendocrine and psychological responses to L-tryptophan infusion. *Psychopharmacology (Berl)* 1999;143(1):64–71.
162. Lopez JF, Liberzon I, Vazquez DM, et al. Serotonin 1A receptor messenger RNA regulation in the hippocampus after acute stress. *Biol Psychiatry* 1999;45(7):934–937.

163. Lopez JF, Vazquez DM, Chalmers DT, et al. Regulation of 5-HT receptors and the hypothalamic-pituitary-adrenal axis. Implications for the neurobiology of suicide. *Ann N Y Acad Sci* 1997;836:106–134.
164. Chaouloff F. Regulation of 5-HT receptors by corticosteroids: where do we stand? *Fundam Clin Pharmacol* 1995;9(3):219–233.
165. Bhagwagar Z, Montgomery AJ, Grasby PM, et al. Lack of effect of a single dose of hydrocortisone on serotonin (1A) receptors in recovered depressed patients measured by positron emission tomography with [^{11}C]WAY-100635. *Biol Psychiatry* 2003;54(9):890–895.
166. Wang S, Gao Y, Laruelle M, et al. Enantioselectivity of cocaine recognition sites: binding of (1S)- and (1R)-2 beta-carbomethoxy-3 beta-(4-iodophenyl)tropane (beta-CIT) to monoamine transporters. *J Med Chem* 1993;36(13):1914–1917.
167. Laruelle M, Giddings SS, Zea-Ponce Y, et al. Methyl 3 beta-(4-[125I]iodophenyl)tropane-2 beta-carboxylate *in vitro* binding to dopamine and serotonin transporters under "physiological" conditions. *J Neurochem* 1994;62(3):978–986.
168. Laruelle M, Baldwin RM, Malison RT, et al. SPECT imaging of dopamine and serotonin transporters with [^{123}I]beta-CIT: pharmacological characterization of brain uptake in nonhuman primates. *Synapse* 1993;13(4):295–309.
169. Brücke T, Kornhuber J, Angelberger P, et al. SPECT imaging of dopamine and serotonin transporters with [^{123}I]b-CIT. Binding kinetics in the human brain. *J Neural Transm Gen Sect* 1993;94(2): 137–146.
170. Pirker W, Asenbaum S, Kasper S, et al. Beta-CIT SPECT demonstrates blockade of 5HT-uptake sites by citalopram in the human brain *in vivo*. *J Neural Transm Gen Sect* 1995;100(3):247–256.
171. Seibyl JP, Marek KL, Quinlan D, et al. Decreased single-photon emission computed tomographic [^{123}I]beta-CIT striatal uptake correlates with symptom severity in Parkinson's disease. *Ann Neurol* 1995; 38(4):589–598.
172. Marek KL, Seibyl JP, Zoghbi SS, et al. [^{123}I] beta-CIT/SPECT imaging demonstrates bilateral loss of dopamine transporters in hemi-Parkinson's disease. *Neurology* 1996;46(1):231–237.
173. Eising EG, Muller TT, Zander C, et al. SPECT-evaluation of the monoamine uptake site ligand [I-^{123}](1R)-2-beta-carbomethoxy-3-beta-(4-iodophenyl)-tropane ([I-^{123}]beta-CIT) in untreated patients with suspicion of Parkinson disease. *J Invest Med* 1997;45(8): 448–452.
174. Seibyl JP, Marek K, Sheff K, et al. Iodine-123-beta-CIT and iodine-123-FPCIT SPECT measurement of dopamine transporters in healthy subjects and Parkinson's patients. *J Nucl Med* 1998;39(9): 1500–1508.
175. Muller U, Wachter T, Barthel H, et al. Striatal [^{123}I]beta-CIT SPECT and prefrontal cognitive functions in Parkinson's disease. *J Neural Transm* 2000;107(3):303–319.
176. Malison RT, Best SE, van Dyck CH, et al. Elevated striatal dopamine transporters during acute cocaine abstinence as measured by [^{123}I] beta-CIT SPECT. *Am J Psychiatry* 1998;155(6):832–834.
177. Malison RT, Price LH, Berman R, et al. Reduced brain serotonin transporter availability in major depression as measured by [^{123}I]-2 beta-carbomethoxy-3 beta-(4-iodophenyl)tropane and single photon emission computed tomography. *Biol Psychiatry* 1998;44(11): 1090–1098.
178. Heinz A, Ragan P, Jones DW, et al. Reduced central serotonin transporters in alcoholism. *Am J Psychiatry* 1998;155(11):1544–1549.
179. Heinz A, Knable MB, Wolf SS, et al. Tourette's syndrome: [I-^{123}]beta-CIT SPECT correlates of vocal tic severity. *Neurology* 1998;51(4): 1069–1074.
180. Lehto S, Tolmunen T, Joensuu M, et al. Midbrain binding of [^{123}I]nor-beta-CIT in atypical depression. *Prog Neuropsychopharmacol Biol Psychiatry* 2006;30(7):1251–1255.
181. Willeit M, Praschak-Rieder N, Neumeister A, et al. [^{123}I]-beta-CIT SPECT imaging shows reduced brain serotonin transporter availability in drug-free depressed patients with seasonal affective disorder. *Biol Psychiatry* 2000;47(6):482–489.
182. Suehiro M, Scheffel U, Ravert HT, et al. [^{11}C](+)McN5652 as a radiotracer for imaging serotonin uptake sites with PET. *Life Sci* 1993; 53(11):883–892.
183. Szabo Z, Scheffel U, Suehiro M, et al. Positron emission tomography of 5-HT transporter sites in the baboon brain with [^{11}C]McN5652. *J Cereb Blood Flow Metab* 1995;15(5):798–805.
184. Szabo Z, Scheffel U, Mathews WB, et al. Kinetic analysis of [^{11}C]McN5652: a serotonin transporter radioligand. *J Cereb Blood Flow Metab* 1999;19(9):967–981.
185. Parsey RV, Kegeles LS, Hwang DR, et al. *In vivo* quantification of brain serotonin transporters in humans using [^{11}C]McN 5652. *J Nucl Med* 2000;41(9):1465–1477.
186. Buck A, Gucker PM, Schonbachler RD, et al. Evaluation of serotonergic transporters using PET and [^{11}C](+)McN-5652: assessment of methods. *J Cereb Blood Flow Metab* 2000;20(2):253–262.
187. Ichimiya T, Suhara T, Sudo Y, et al. Serotonin transporter binding in patients with mood disorders: a PET study with [^{11}C](+)McN5652. *Biol Psychiatry* 2002;51(9):715–722.
188. Parsey RV, Hastings RS, Oquendo MA, et al. Lower serotonin transporter binding potential in the human brain during major depressive episodes. *Am J Psychiatry* 2006;163(1):52–58.
189. Oquendo MA, Hastings RS, Huang YY, et al. Brain serotonin transporter binding in depressed patients with bipolar disorder using positron emission tomography. *Arch Gen Psychiatry* 2007;64(2): 201–208.
190. Oya S, Choi SR, Hou C, et al. 2-((2-((dimethylamino)methyl)phenyl) thio)-5-iodophenylamine (ADAM): an improved serotonin transporter ligand. *Nucl Med Biol* 2000;27(3):249–254.
191. Vercouillie J, Tarkiainen J, Halldin C, et al. Precursor synthesis and radiolabeling of [^{11}C]ADAM: a potent radioligand for the serotonin transporter exploration by PET. *J Labelled Cpd Radiopharm* 2001; 44:113–120.
192. Sacher J, Asenbaum S, Klein N, et a l. Binding kinetics of ^{123}I[ADAM] in healthy controls: a selective SERT radioligand. *Int J Neuropsychopharmacol* 2007;10(2):211–218.
193. Catafau AM, Perez V, Penengo MM, et al. SPECT of serotonin transporters using ^{123}I-ADAM: optimal imaging time after bolus injection and long-term test-retest in healthy volunteers. *J Nucl Med* 2005;46(8):1301–1309.
194. Newberg AB, Amsterdam JD, Wintering N, et al. ^{123}I-ADAM binding to serotonin transporters in patients with major depression and healthy controls: a preliminary study. *J Nucl Med* 2005;46(6):973–977.
195. Herold N, Uebelhack K, Franke L, et al. Imaging of serotonin transporters and its blockade by citalopram in patients with major depression using a novel SPECT ligand [^{123}I]-ADAM. *J Neural Transm* 2006;113(5):659–670.
196. Wilson AA, Ginovart N, Schmidt M, et al. Novel radiotracers for imaging the serotonin transporter by positron emission tomography: synthesis, radiosynthesis, and *in vitro* and *ex vivo* evaluation of (^{11})C-labeled 2-(phenylthio)araalkylamines. *J Med Chem* 2000;43(16):3103–3110.
197. Houle S, Ginovart N, Hussey D, et al. Imaging the serotonin transporter with positron emission tomography: initial human studies with [^{11}C]DAPP and [^{11}C]DASB. *Eur J Nucl Med* 2000;27(11): 1719–1722.
198. Frankle WG, Slifstein M, Gunn RN, et al. Estimation of serotonin transporter parameters with ^{11}C-DASB in healthy humans: reproducibility and comparison of methods. *J Nucl Med* 2006;47(5):815–826.
199. Frankle WG, Huang Y, Hwang DR, et al. Comparative evaluation of serotonin transporter radioligands ^{11}C-DASB and ^{11}C-McN 5652 in healthy humans. *J Nucl Med* 2004;45(4):682–694.
200. Meyer JH, Houle S, Sagrati S, et al. Brain serotonin transporter binding potential measured with carbon 11-labeled DASB positron emission tomography: effects of major depressive episodes and severity of dysfunctional attitudes. *Arch Gen Psychiatry* 2004;61(12): 1271–1279.
201. Huang Y, Hwang DR, Narendran R, et al. Comparative evaluation in nonhuman primates of five PET radiotracers for imaging the serotonin

transporters: [^{11}C]McN 5652, [^{11}C]ADAM, [^{11}C]DASB, [^{11}C]DAPA, and [^{11}C]AFM. *J Cereb Blood Flow Metab* 2002;22(11):1377–1398.

202. Kapur S, Mann JJ. Role of the dopaminergic system in depression. *Biol Psychiatry* 1992;32(1):1–17.
203. Brown AS, Gershon S. Dopamine and depression. *J Neural Transm Gen Sect* 1993;91(2–3):75–109.
204. Diehl DJ, Gershon S.The role of dopamine in mood disorders. *Compr Psychiatry* 1992;33(2):115–120.
205. Willner P, Muscat R, Papp M. Chronic mild stress-induced anhedonia: a realistic animal model of depression. *Neurosci Biobehav Rev* 1992;16(4):525–534.
206. D'Haenen HA, Bossuyt A. Dopamine D_2 receptors in depression measured with single photon emission computed tomography. *Biol Psychiatry* 1994;35(2):128–132.
207. Shah PJ, Ogilvie AD, Goodwin GM, et al. Clinical and psychometric correlates of dopamine D_2 binding in depression. *Psychol Med* 1997;27(6):1247–1256.
208. Ebert D, Feistel H, Loew T, et al. Dopamine and depression—striatal dopamine D_2 receptor SPECT before and after antidepressant therapy. *Psychopharmacology (Berl)* 1996;126(1):91–94.
209. Klimke A, Larisch R, Janz A, et al. Dopamine D_2 receptor binding before and after treatment of major depression measured by [^{123}I]IBZM SPECT. *Psychiatry Res* 1999;90(2):91–101.
210. Meyer JH, McNeely HE, Sagrati S, et al. Elevated putamen D(2) receptor binding potential in major depression with motor retardation: an [^{11}C]raclopride positron emission tomography study. *Am J Psychiatry* 2006;163(9):1594–1602.
211. Laasonen-Balk T, Kuikka J, Viinamaki H, et al. Striatal dopamine transporter density in major depression. *Psychopharmacology (Berl)* 1999;144(3):282–285.
212. Meyer JH, Kruger S, Wilson AA, et al. Lower dopamine transporter binding potential in striatum during depression. *Neuroreport* 2001; 12(18):4121–4125,
213. Brunswick DJ, Amsterdam JD, Mozley PD, et al. Greater availability of brain dopamine transporters in major depression shown by [^{99m}Tc] TRODAT-1 SPECT imaging. *Am J Psychiatry* 2003;160(10): 1836–1841.
214. Argyelan M, Szabo Z, Kanyo B, et al. Dopamine transporter availability in medication free and in bupropion treated depression: a 99mTc-TRODAT-1 SPECT study. *J Affect Disord* 2005;89(1–3):115–123.
215. Martinot M, Bragulat V, Artiges E, et al. Decreased presynaptic dopamine function in the left caudate of depressed patients with affective flattening and psychomotor retardation. *Am J Psychiatry* 2001;158(2):314–316.
216. Meyer JH. Imaging the serotonin transporter during major depressive disorder and antidepressant treatment. *J Psychiatry Neurosci* 2007; 32(2):86–102.
217. Shang Y, Gibbs MA, Marek GJ, et al. Displacement of serotonin and dopamine transporters by venlafaxine extended release capsule at steady state: a [^{123}I]2beta-carbomethoxy-3beta-(4-iodophenyl)-tropane single photon emission computed tomography imaging study. *J Clin Psychopharmacol* 2007;27(1):71–75.
218. Meyer JH, Wilson AA, Ginovart N, et al. Occupancy of serotonin transporters by paroxetine and citalopram during treatment of depression: a [(^{11})C]DASB PET imaging study. *Am J Psychiatry* 2001;158(11):1843–1849.
219. Kent JM, Coplan JD, Lombardo I, et al. Imaging the serotonin transporter in social phobia with (+)[C-^{11}]McN5652. *J Nucl Med* 2000;41: 200P.
220. Suhara T, Takano A, Sudo Y, et al. High levels of serotonin transporter occupancy with low-dose clomipramine in comparative occupancy study with fluvoxamine using positron emission tomography. *Arch Gen Psychiatry* 2003;60(4):386–391.
221. Meyer JH, Wilson AA, Sagrati S, et al. Serotonin transporter occupancy of five selective serotonin reuptake inhibitors at different doses: an [^{11}C]DASB positron emission tomography study. *Am J Psychiatry* 2004;161(5):826–835.
222. Parsey RV, Kent JM, Oquendo MA, et al. Acute occupancy of brain serotonin transporter by sertraline as measured by [^{11}C]DASB and positron emission tomography. *Biol Psychiatry* 2006;59(9):821–828.
223. Meyer JH, Goulding VS, Wilson AA, et al. Bupropion occupancy of the dopamine transporter is low during clinical treatment. *Psychopharmacology (Berl)* 2002;163(1):102–105.
224. Learned-Coughlin SM, Bergstrom M, Savitcheva I, et al. *In vivo* activity of bupropion at the human dopamine transporter as measured by positron emission tomography. *Biol Psychiatry* 2003;54(8):800–805.
225. Blier P, de Montigny C. Possible serotonergic mechanisms underlying the antidepressant and anti-obsessive-compulsive disorder responses. *Biol Psychiatry* 1998;44(5):313–323.
226. Martinez D, Broft A, Laruelle M. Pindolol augmentation of antidepressant treatment: recent contributions from brain imaging studies. *Biol Psychiatry* 2000;48(8):844–853.
227. Artigas F, Celada P, Laruelle M, et al. How does pindolol improve antidepressant action? *Trends Pharmacol Sci* 2001;22(5):224–228.
228. Martinez D, Hwang D, Mawlawi O, et al. Differential occupancy of somatodendritic and postsynaptic 5HT(1A) receptors by pindolol. A dose-occupancy study with [^{11}C]WAY 100635 and positron emission tomography in humans. *Neuropsychopharmacology* 2001;24(3):209–229.
229. Andree B, Thorberg SO, Halldin C, et al. Pindolol binding to 5-HT_{1A} receptors in the human brain confirmed with positron emission tomography. *Psychopharmacology* 1999;144(3):303–305.
230. Rabiner EA, Gunn RN, Castro ME, et al. Beta-blocker binding to human 5-HT(1A) receptors *in vivo* and *in vitro*: implications for antidepressant therapy. *Neuropsychopharmacology* 2000;23(3):285–293.
231. Suhara T, Nakayama K, Inoue O, et al. D_1 dopamine receptor binding in mood disorders measured by positron emission tomography. *Psychopharmacology* 1992;106(1):14–18.
232. Wong WF, Pearlson GD, Tune LE, et al. Quantification of neuroreceptors in the living human brain: IV. Effect of aging and elevations of D_2-like receptors in schizophrenia and bipolar illness. *J Cereb Blood Flow Metab* 1997;17(3):331–342.
233. Gjedde A, Wong DF. Quantification of neuroreceptors in living human brain. V. Endogenous neurotransmitter inhibition of haloperidol binding in psychosis. *J Cereb Blood Flow Metab* 2001;21(8):982–994.
234. Anand A, Verhoeff P, Seneca N, et al. Brain SPECT imaging of amphetamine-induced dopamine release in euthymic bipolar disorder patients. *Am J Psychiatry* 2000;157(7):1108–1114.
235. Benkelfat C, Bradwejn J, Meyer E, et al. Functional neuroanatomy of CCK4-induced anxiety in normal healthy volunteers [comments]. *Am J Psychiatry* 1995;152(8):1180–1184.
236. Javanmard M, Shlik J, Kennedy SH, et al. Neuroanatomic correlates of CCK-4-induced panic attacks in healthy humans: a comparison of two time points. *Biol Psychiatry* 1999;45(7):872–882.
237. Chua P, Krams M, Toni I, et al. A functional anatomy of anticipatory anxiety. *Neuroimage* 1999;9(6 Pt 1):563–571.
238. Simpson JR Jr, Drevets WC, Snyder AZ, et al. Emotion-induced changes in human medial prefrontal cortex: II. During anticipatory anxiety. *Proc Natl Acad Sci U S A* 2001;98(2):688–693.
239. Kimbrell TA, George MS, Parekh PI, et al. Regional brain activity during transient self-induced anxiety and anger in healthy adults. *Biol Psychiatry* 1999;46(4):454–465.
240. Liotti M, Mayberg HS, Brannan SK, et al. Differential limbic–cortical correlates of sadness and anxiety in healthy subjects: implications for affective disorders. *Biol Psychiatry* 2000;48(1):30–42.
241. Tiihonen J, Kuikka J, Rasanen P, et al. Cerebral benzodiazepine receptor binding and distribution in generalized anxiety disorder: a fractal analysis. *Mol Psychiatry* 1997;2(6):463–471.
242. Abadie P, Boulenger JP, Benali K, et al. Relationships between trait and state anxiety and the central benzodiazepine receptor: a PET study. *Eur J Neurosci* 1999;11(4):1470–1478.
243. Kaschka W, Feistel H, Ebert D. Reduced benzodiazepine receptor binding in panic disorders measured by iomazenil SPECT. *J Psychiatr Res* 1995;29(5):427–434.

244. Brandt CA, Meller J, Keweloh L, et al. Increased benzodiazepine receptor density in the prefrontal cortex in patients with panic disorder. *J Neural Transm (Budapest)* 1998;105(10–12):1325–1333.
245. Bremner JD, Innis RB, White T, et al. SPECT [I-[123]]iomazenil measurement of the benzodiazepine receptor in panic disorder. *Biol Psychiatry* 2000;47(2):96–106.
246. Malizia AL, Cunningham VJ, Bell CJ, et al. Decreased brain GABA(A)-benzodiazepine receptor binding in panic disorder: preliminary results from a quantitative PET study. *Arch Gen Psychiatry* 1998; 55(8):715–720.
247. Neumeister A, Bain E, Nugent AC, et al. Reduced serotonin type 1A receptor binding in panic disorder. *J Neurosci* 2004;24(3):589–591.
248. Dewar KM, Stravynski A. The quest for biological correlates of social phobia: an interim assessment. *Acta Psychiatr Scand* 2001;103(4): 244–251.
249. Bell CJ, Malizia AL, Nutt DJ. The neurobiology of social phobia [review]. *Eur Arch Psychiatry Clin Neurosci* 1999;249[Suppl 1]: S11–S18.
250. Nutt DJ, Bell CJ, Malizia AL. Brain mechanisms of social anxiety disorder [review]. *J Clin Psychiatry* 1998;59[Suppl 17]:4–11.
251. Tiihonen J, Kuikka J, Bergstrom K, et al. Dopamine reuptake site densities in patients with social phobia. *Am J Psychiatry* 1997;154(2): 239–242.
252. Schneier FR, Liebowitz MR, Abi-Dargham A, et al. Low dopamine D(2) receptor binding potential in social phobia. *Am J Psychiatry* 2000;157(3):457–459.
253. Lanzenberger RR, Mitterhauser M, Spindelegger C, et al. Reduced serotonin-1A receptor binding in social anxiety disorder. *Biol Psychiatry* 2007;61(9):1081–1089.
254. Tauscher J, Bagby RM, Javanmard M, et al. Inverse relationship between serotonin 5-HT(1A) receptor binding and anxiety: a [([11])C]WAY-100635 PET investigation in healthy volunteers. *Am J Psychiatry* 2001;158(8):1326–1328.
255. Perani D, Colombo C, Bressi S, et al. [^{18}F]FDG PET study in obsessive-compulsive disorder. A clinical/metabolic correlation study after treatment. *Br J Psychiatry* 1995;166(2):244–250.
256. Biver F, Goldman S, Francois A, et al. Changes in metabolism of cerebral glucose after stereotactic leukotomy for refractory obsessive-compulsive disorder: a case report. *J Neurol Neurosurg Psychiatry* 1995;58(4):502–505.
257. Rauch SL, Savage CR, Alpert NM, et al. Probing striatal function in obsessive-compulsive disorder: a PET study of implicit sequence learning. *J Neuropsychiatry Clin Neurosci* 1997;9(4):568–573.
258. Mallet L, Mazoyer B, Martinot JL. Functional connectivity in depressive, obsessive-compulsive, and schizophrenic disorders: an explorative correlational analysis of regional cerebral metabolism. *Psychiatry Res* 1998;82(2):83–93.
259. Saxena S, Brody AL, Maidment KM, et al. Localized orbitofrontal and subcortical metabolic changes and predictors of response to paroxetine treatment in obsessive-compulsive disorder. *Neuropsychopharmacology* 1999;21(6):683–693.
260. Baxter LR Jr. Positron emission tomography studies of cerebral glucose metabolism in obsessive compulsive disorder [review]. *J Clin Psychiatry* 1994;55[Suppl]:54–59.
261. Brody AL, Saxena S, Schwartz JM, et al. FDG-PET predictors of response to behavioral therapy and pharmacotherapy in obsessive compulsive disorder. *Psychiatry Res* 1998;84(1):1–6.
262. Pogarell O, Hamann C, Popperl G, et al. Elevated brain serotonin transporter availability in patients with obsessive-compulsive disorder. *Biol Psychiatry* 2003;54(12):1406–1413.
263. Simpson HB, Lombardo I, Slifstein M, et al. Serotonin transporters in obsessive-compulsive disorder: a positron emission tomography study with [([11])C]McN 5652. *Biol Psychiatry* 2003;54(12):1414–1421.
264. Hasselbalch SG, Hansen ES, Jakobsen TB, et al. Reduced midbrain-pons serotonin transporter binding in patients with obsessive-compulsive disorder. *Acta Psychiatr Scand* 2007;115(5):388–394.
265. Hesse S, Muller U, Lincke T, et al. Serotonin and dopamine transporter imaging in patients with obsessive-compulsive disorder. *Psychiatry Res* 2005;140(1):63–72.
266. Adams KH, Hansen ES, Pinborg LH, et al. Patients with obsessive-compulsive disorder have increased 5-HT_{2A} receptor binding in the caudate nuclei. *Int J Neuropsychopharmacol* 2005;8(3):391–401.
267. Villarreal G, King CY. Brain imaging in posttraumatic stress disorder. *Sem Clin Neuropsychiatry* 2001;6(2):131–145.
268. Bremner JD. Alterations in brain structure and function associated with post-traumatic stress disorder. *Sem Clin Neuropsychiatry* 1999; 4(4):249–255.
269. Bremner JD, Innis RB, Southwick SM, et al. Decreased benzodiazepine receptor binding in prefrontal cortex in combat-related posttraumatic stress disorder. *Am J Psychiatry* 2000;157(7):1120–1126.
270. Farde L, Gustavsson JP, Jonsson E. D_2 dopamine receptors and personality traits. *Nature* 1997;385(6617):590.
271. Breier A, Kestler L, Adler C, et al. Dopamine D_2 receptor density and personal detachment in healthy subjects. *Am J Psychiatry* 1998; 155(10):1440–1442.
272. Kestler LP, Malhotra AK, Finch C, et al. The relation between dopamine D_2 receptor density and personality: preliminary evidence from the NEO Personality Inventory-Revised. *Neuropsychiatry Neuropsychol Behav Neurol* 2000;13(1):48–52.
273. Laakso A, Vilkman H, Kajander J, et al. Prediction of detached personality in healthy subjects by low dopamine transporter binding. *Am J Psychiatry* 2000;157(2):290–292.
274. Schneier FR, Liebowitz MR, Laruelle M. Detachment and generalized social phobia. *Am J Psychiatry* 2001;158(2):327.
275. Zhuang X, Gross C, Santarelli L, et al. Altered emotional states in knockout mice lacking 5-HT_{1A} or 5-HT_{1B} receptors. *Neuropsychopharmacology* 1999;21[2 Suppl]:52S–60S.
276. Soloff PH, Meltzer CC, Greer PJ, et al. A fenfluramine-activated FDG-PET study of borderline personality disorder. *Biol Psychiatry* 2000; 47(6):540–547.
277. Siever LJ, Buchsbaum MS, New AS, et al. d,l-Fenfluramine response in impulsive personality disorder assessed with [^{18}F]fluorodeoxyglucose positron emission tomography. *Neuropsychopharmacology* 1999;20(5): 413–423.
278. Leyton M, Okazawa H, Diksic M, et al. Brain regional [alpha]-[^{11}C]methyl-L-tryptophan trapping in impulsive subjects with borderline personality disorder. *Am J Psychiatry* 2001;158(5): 775–782.
279. Frankle WG, Lombardo I, New AS, et al. Brain serotonin transporter distribution in subjects with impulsive aggressivity: a positron emission study with [^{11}C]McN 5652. *Am J Psychiatry* 2005;162(5):915–923.
280. Dougherty DD, Bonab AA, Spencer TJ, et al. Dopamine transporter density in patients with attention deficit hyperactivity disorder. *Lancet* 1999;354(9196):2132–2133.
281. Dresel S, Krause J, Krause KH, et al. Attention deficit hyperactivity disorder: binding of [99mTc]TRODAT-1 to the dopamine transporter before and after methylphenidate treatment. *Eur J Nucl Med* 2000;27(10):1518–1524.
282. Larisch R, Sitte W, Antke C, et al. Striatal dopamine transporter density in drug naive patients with attention-deficit/hyperactivity disorder. *Nucl Med Commun* 2006;27(3):267–270.
283. Spencer TJ, Biederman J, Madras BK, et al. Further evidence of dopamine transporter dysregulation in ADHD: a controlled PET imaging study using altropane. *Biol Psychiatry* 2007;62(9):1059–1061.
284. Cheon KA, Ryu YH, Kim YK, et al. Dopamine transporter density in the basal ganglia assessed with [^{123}I]IPT SPET in children with attention deficit hyperactivity disorder. *Eur J Nucl Med Mol Imaging* 2003;30(2):306–311.
285. Jucaite A, Fernell E, Halldin C, et al. Reduced midbrain dopamine transporter binding in male adolescents with attention-deficit/hyperactivity disorder: association between striatal dopamine markers and motor hyperactivity. *Biol Psychiatry* 2005;57(3):229–238.

286. van Dyck CH, Quinlan DM, Cretella LM, et al. Unaltered dopamine transporter availability in adult attention deficit hyperactivity disorder. *Am J Psychiatry* 2002;159(2):309–312.
287. Volkow ND, Wang GJ, Newcorn J, et al. Brain dopamine transporter levels in treatment and drug naive adults with ADHD. *Neuroimage* 2007;34(3):1182–1190.
288. Volkow ND, Wang GJ, Fowler JS, et al. Therapeutic doses of oral methylphenidate significantly increase extracellular dopamine in the human brain. *J Neurosci* 2001;21(2):RC121.
289. Wise R, Romprè P. Brain dopamine and reward. *Ann Rev Psychol* 1989;40:191–225.
290. Kuhar MJ, Ritz MC, Boja JW. The dopamine hypothesis of the reinforcing properties of cocaine. *Trends Neurosci* 1991;14(7):299–302.
291. Di Chiara G. The role of dopamine in drug abuse viewed from the perspective of its role in motivation. *Drug Alcohol Depend* 1995;38(2): 95–137.
292. Nestler EJ, Berhow MT, Brodkin ES. Molecular mechanisms of drug addiction: adaptations in signal transduction pathways. *Mol Psychiatry* 1996;1(3):190–199.
293. Self DW, Nestler EJ. Molecular mechanisms of drug reinforcement and addiction. *Annu Rev Neurosci* 1995;18:463–495.
294. Koob GF. Drugs of abuse: anatomy, pharmacology and function of reward pathways. *Trends Pharmacol Sci* 1992;13(5):177–184.
295. Volkow ND, Fowler JS, Wolf AP, et al. Effects of chronic cocaine abuse on postsynaptic dopamine receptors. *Am J Psychiatry* 1990;147(6):719–724.
296. Volkow ND, Fowler JS, Wang GJ, et al. Decreased dopamine D_2 receptor availability is associated with reduced frontal metabolism in cocaine abusers. *Synapse* 1993;14(2):169–177.
297. Volkow ND, Wang GJ, Fowler JS, et al. Cocaine uptake is decreased in the brain of detoxified cocaine abusers. *Neuropsychopharmacology* 1996;14(3):159–168.
298. Volkow ND, Wang GJ, Fowler JS, et al. Decreased striatal dopaminergic responsiveness in detoxified cocaine-dependent subjects. *Nature* 1997;386:830–833.
299. Martinez D, Broft A, Foltin RW, et al. Cocaine dependence and D_2 receptor availability in the functional subdivisions of the striatum: relationship with cocaine-seeking behavior. *Neuropsychopharmacology* 2004;29(6):1190–1202.
300. Wang GJ, Volkow ND, Fowler JS, et al. Dopamine D_2 receptor availability in opiate-dependent subjects before and after naloxone-precipitated withdrawal. *Neuropsychopharmacology* 1997;16(2):174–182.
301. Volkow ND, Chang L, Wang GJ, et al. Low level of brain dopamine D_2 receptors in methamphetamine abusers: association with metabolism in the orbitofrontal cortex. *Am J Psychiatry* 2001;158(12): 2015–2021.
302. Hietala J, West C, Syvälahti E, et al. Striatal D_2 dopamine receptor binding characteristics *in vivo* in patients with alcohol dependence. *Psychopharmacology* 1994;116:285–290.
303. Volkow ND, Wang GJ, Fowler JS, et al. Decreases in dopamine receptors but not in dopamine transporters in alcoholics. *J Nucl Med* 1996;37:33P.
304. Martinez D, Gil R, Slifstein M, et al. Alcohol dependence is associated with blunted dopamine transmission in the ventral striatum. *Biol Psychiatry* 2005;58(10):779–786.
305. Volkow ND, Wang GJ, Fowler JS, et al. Prediction of reinforcing responses to psychostimulants in humans by brain dopamine D_2 receptor levels. *Am J Psychiatry* 1999;156(9):1440–1443.
306. Volkow ND, Wang GJ, Fowler JS, et al. Brain DA D_2 receptors predict reinforcing effects of stimulants in humans: replication study. *Synapse* 2002;46(2):79–82.
307. Morgan D, Grant KA, Gage HD, et al. Social dominance in monkeys: dopamine D_2 receptors and cocaine self-administration. *Nat Neurosci* 2002;5(2):169–174.
308. Laruelle M, Abi-Dargham A, van Dyck CH, et al. SPECT imaging of striatal dopamine release after amphetamine challenge. *J Nucl Med* 1995;36:1182–1190.
309. Abi-Dargham A, Kegeles LS, Martinez D, et al. Dopamine mediation of positive reinforcing effects of amphetamine in stimulant naive healthy volunteers: results from a large cohort. *Eur Neuropsychopharmacol* 2003;13(6):459–468.
310. Volkow ND, Wang GJ, Fowler JS, et al. Reinforcing effects of psychostimulants in humans are associated with increases in brain dopamine and occupancy of D_2 receptors. *J Pharmacol Exp Ther* 1999;291(1): 409–415.
311. Martinez D, Mawlawi O, Simpson N, et al. Comparison of amphetamine-induced endogenous dopamine release in striatal substructures in humans using PET. *Soc Neurosci Abst* 2000;26:1327.
312. Oswald LM, Wong DF, McCaul M, et al. Relationships among ventral striatal dopamine release, cortisol secretion, and subjective responses to amphetamine. *Neuropsychopharmacology* 2005; 30(4):821–832.
313. Di Chiara G, Imperato A. Drugs abused by humans preferentially increase synaptic dopamine concentrations in the mesolimbic system of freely moving rats. *Proc Natl Acad Sci U S A* 1988;85(14): 5274–5278.
314. Le Moal M, Simon H. Mesocorticolimbic dopamine network: functional and regulatory role. *Physiol Rev* 1991;71:155–234.
315. Koepp MJ, Gunn RN, Lawrence AD, et al. Evidence for striatal dopamine release during a video game. *Nature* 1998;393(6682):266–268.
316. Malison RT, Mechanic KY, Klummp H, et al. Reduced amphetamine-stimulated dopamine release in cocaine addicts as measured by [^{123}I]IBZM SPECT. *J Nucl Med* 1999;40(5 (Suppl):110P.
317. Wu JC, Bell K, Najafi A, et al. Decreasing striatal 6-FDOPA uptake with increasing duration of cocaine withdrawal. *Neuropsychopharmacology* 1997;17(6):402–409.
318. Volkow ND, Wang GJ, Fischman MW, et al. Relationship between subjective effects of cocaine and dopamine transporter occupancy. *Nature* 1997;386(6627):827–830.
319. Malison RT, McCance E, Carpenter LL, et al. [^{123}I]beta-CIT SPECT imaging of dopamine transporter availability after mazindol administration in human cocaine addicts. *Psychopharmacology (Berl)* 1998;137(4):321–325.
320. Volkow N, Wang G, Fischman M, et al. Relationship between subjective effects of cocaine and dopamine transporter occupancy. *Nature* 1997;386:827–830.
321. Volkow ND, Ding YS, Fowler JS, et al. Is methylphenidate like cocaine? Studies on their pharmacokinetics and distribution in the human brain. *Arch Gen Psychiatry* 1995;52(6):456–463.
322. Volkow ND, Wang GJ, Fowler JS, et al. The slow and long-lasting blockade of dopamine transporters in human brain induced by the new antidepressant drug radafaxine predict poor reinforcing effects. *Biol Psychiatry* 2005;57(6):640–646.
323. Wong DF, Kuwabara H, Schretlen DJ, et al. Increased occupancy of dopamine receptors in human striatum during cue-elicited cocaine craving. *Neuropsychopharmacology* 2006;31(12):2716–2727.
324. Volkow ND, Wang GJ, Telang F, et al. Cocaine cues and dopamine in dorsal striatum: mechanism of craving in cocaine addiction. *J Neurosci* 2006;26(24):6583–6588.
325. Jacobsen LK, Staley JK, Malison RT, et al. Elevated central serotonin transporter binding availability in acutely abstinent cocaine-dependent patients. *Am J Psychiatry* 2000;157(7):1134–1140.
326. Zubieta JK, Gorelick DA, Stauffer R, et al. Increased mu opioid receptor binding detected by PET in cocaine-dependent men is associated with cocaine craving. *Nat Med* 1996;2(11):1225–1259.
327. Hurd YL, Herkenham M. Molecular alterations in the neostriatum of human cocaine addicts. *Synapse* 1993;13(4):357–369.
328. Steiner H, Gerfen CR. Role of dynorphin and enkephalin in the regulation of striatal output pathways and behavior. *Exp Brain Res* 1998;123(1–2):60–76.
329. McCann UD, Wong DF, Yokoi F, et al. Reduced striatal dopamine transporter density in abstinent methamphetamine and methcathinone users: evidence from positron emission tomography studies with [^{11}C]WIN-35428. *J Neurosci* 1998;18(20):8417–8422.

330. Volkow ND, Wang G, Fowler JS, et al. Therapeutic doses of oral methylphenidate significantly increase extracellular dopamine in the human brain. *J Neurosci* 2001;21(2):RC121.
331. Wilson JM, Kalasinsky KS, Levey AI, et al. Striatal dopamine nerve terminal markers in human, chronic methamphetamine users. *Nat Med* 1996;2(6):699–703.
332. Wilson JM, Levey AI, Rajput A, et al. Differential changes in neurochemical markers of striatal dopamine nerve terminals in idiopathic Parkinson's disease. *Neurology* 1996;47(3):718–726.
333. Seibyl JP, Marek K, Sheff K, et al. Test/retest reproducibility of iodine-123-betaCIT SPECT brain measurement of dopamine transporters in Parkinson's patients. *J Nucl Med* 1997;38(9):1453–1459.
334. Guttman M, Burkholder J, Kish SJ, et al. [^{11}C]RTI-32 PET studies of the dopamine transporter in early dopa-naive Parkinson's disease: implications for the symptomatic threshold. *Neurology* 1997;48(6): 1578–1583.
335. Villemagne V, Yuan J, Wong DF, et al. Brain dopamine neurotoxicity in baboons treated with doses of methamphetamine comparable to those recreationally abused by humans: evidence from [^{11}C]WIN-35,428 positron emission tomography studies and direct *in vitro* determinations. *J Neurosci* 1998;18(1):419–427.
336. Melega WP, Lacan G, Harvey DC, et al. Dizocilpine and reduced body temperature do not prevent methamphetamine- induced neurotoxicity in the vervet monkey: [^{11}C]WIN 35,428—positron emission tomography studies. *Neurosci Lett* 1998;258(1):17–20.
337. Harvey DC, Lacan G, Tanious SP, et al. Recovery from methamphetamine induced long-term nigrostriatal dopaminergic deficits without substantia nigra cell loss. *Brain Res* 2000;871(2):259–270.
338. Ricaurte GA, Yuan J, McCann UD. (+/−)3,4-Methylenedioxymethamphetamine ("Ecstasy")-induced serotonin neurotoxicity: studies in animals. *Neuropsychobiology* 2000;42(1):5–10.
339. Schmidt CJ, Wu L, Lovenberg W. Methylenedioxymethamphetamine: a potentially neurotoxic amphetamine analogue. *Eur J Pharmacol* 1986;124(1–2):175–178.
340. Ricaurte G, Bryan G, Strauss L, et al. Hallucinogenic amphetamine selectively destroys brain serotonin nerve terminals. *Science* 1985; 229(4717):986–988.
341. Stone DM, Stahl DC, Hanson GR, et al. The effects of 3,4-methylenedioxymethamphetamine (MDMA) and 3,4-methylenedioxyamphetamine (MDA) on monoaminergic systems in the rat brain. *Eur J Pharmacol* 1986;128(1–2):41–48.
342. Commins DL, Vosmer G, Virus RM, et al. Biochemical and histological evidence that methylenedioxymethylamphetamine (MDMA) is toxic to neurons in the rat brain. *J Pharmacol Exp Ther* 1987;241(1): 338–345.
343. Schmidt CJ. Neurotoxicity of the psychedelic amphetamine, methylenedioxymethamphetamine. *J Pharmacol Exp Ther* 1987;240(1):1–7.
344. Schmidt CJ, Taylor VL. Depression of rat brain tryptophan hydroxylase activity following the acute administration of methylenedioxymethamphetamine. *Biochem Pharmacol* 1987;36(23):4095–4102.
345. Lyvers M. Recreational ecstasy use and the neurotoxic potential of MDMA: current status of the controversy and methodological issues. *Drug Alcohol Rev* 2006;25(3):269–276.
346. Cowan RL. Neuroimaging research in human MDMA users: a review. *Psychopharmacology (Berl)* 2007;189(4):539–556.
347. McCann UD, Szabo Z, Scheffel U, et al. Positron emission tomographic evidence of toxic effect of MDMA ("Ecstasy") on brain serotonin neurons in human beings. *Lancet* 1998;352(9138): 1433–1437.
348. Semple DM, Ebmeier KP, Glabus MF, et al. Reduced *in vivo* binding to serotonin transporter in the cerebral cortex of MDMA ('Ecstasy') users. *Br J Psychiatry* 1999;175:63–69.
349. Reneman L, Lavalaye J, Schmand B, et al. Cortical serotonin transporter density and verbal memory in individuals who stopped using 3,4-methylenedioxymethamphetamine (MDMA or "Ecstasy"): preliminary findings. *Arch Gen Psychiatry* 2001;58(10):901–906.
350. Heinz A, Jones DW. Serotonin transporters in ecstasy users. *Br J Psychiatry* 2000;176:193–195.
351. Laruelle M, Wallace E, Seibyl JP, et al. Graphical, kinetic, and equilibrium analyses of *in vivo* [^{123}I] beta-CIT binding to dopamine transporters in healthy human subjects. *J Cereb Blood Flow Metab* 1994;14(6):982–994.
352. Reneman L, Booij J, de Bruin K, et al. Effects of dose, sex, and long-term abstention from use on toxic effects of MDMA (Ecstasy) on brain serotonin neurons. *Lancet* 2001;358(9296):1864–1869.
353. Buchert R, Thomasius R, Wilke F, et al. A voxel-based PET investigation of the long-term effects of "Ecstasy" consumption on brain serotonin transporters. *Am J Psychiatry* 2004;161(7):1181–1189.
354. McCann UD, Szabo Z, Seckin E, et al. Quantitative PET studies of the serotonin transporter in MDMA users and controls using [^{11}C]McN5652 and [^{11}C]DASB. *Neuropsychopharmacology* 2005;30(9): 1741–1750.
355. Kling MA, Carson RE, Borg L, et al. Opioid receptor imaging with positron emission tomography and [(^{18})F]cyclofoxy in long-term, methadone-treated former heroin addicts. *J Pharmacol Exp Ther* 2000;295(3):1070–1076.
356. Carson RE, Channing MA, Blasberg RG, et al. Comparison of bolus and infusion methods for receptor quantitation: application to [^{18}F]cyclofoxy and positron emission tomography. *J Cereb Blood Flow Metab* 1993;13(1):24–42.
357. Zubieta J, Greenwald MK, Lombardi U, et al. Buprenorphine-induced changes in mu-opioid receptor availability in male heroin-dependent volunteers: a preliminary study. *Neuropsychopharmacology* 2000;23(3): 326–334.
358. Frost JJ, Douglass KH, Mayberg HS, et al. Multicompartmental analysis of [^{11}C]-carfentanil binding to opiate receptors in humans measured by positron emission tomography. *J Cereb Blood Flow Metab* 1989;9(3):398–409.
359. Mello NK, Mendelson JH, Kuehnle JC. Buprenorphine effects on human heroin self-administration: an operant analysis. *J Pharmacol Exp Ther* 1982;223(1):30–39.
360. Comer SD, Collins ED, Fischman MW. Buprenorphine sublingual tablets: effects on IV heroin self-administration by humans. *Psychopharmacology (Berl)* 2001;154(1):28–37.
361. Brody AL, Mandelkern MA, London ED, et al. Cigarette smoking saturates brain alpha 4 beta 2 nicotinic acetylcholine receptors. *Arch Gen Psychiatry* 2006;63(8):907–915.
362. Kassiou M, Eberl S, Meikle SR, et al. *In vivo* imaging of nicotinic receptor upregulation following chronic (−)-nicotine treatment in baboon using SPECT. *Nucl Med Biol* 2001;28(2):165–175.
363. Marenco S, Carson RE, Berman KF, et al. Nicotine-induced dopamine release in primates measured with [^{11}C]raclopride PET. *Neuropsychopharmacology* 2004;29(2):259–268.
364. Barrett SP, Boileau I, Okker J, et al. The hedonic response to cigarette smoking is proportional to dopamine release in the human striatum as measured by positron emission tomography and [^{11}C]raclopride. *Synapse* 2004;54(2):65–71.
365. Brody AL, Olmstead RE, London ED, et al. Smoking-induced ventral striatum dopamine release. *Am J Psychiatry* 2004;161(7): 1211–1218.
366. Brody AL, Mandelkern MA, Olmstead RE, et al. Gene variants of brain dopamine pathways and smoking-induced dopamine release in the ventral caudate/nucleus accumbens. *Arch Gen Psychiatry* 2006;63(7): 808–816.
367. Montgomery AJ, Lingford-Hughes AR, et al. The effect of nicotine on striatal dopamine release in man: a [(^{11})C]raclopride PET study. *Synapse* 2007;61(8):637–645.
368. Fowler JS, Volkow ND, Wang GJ, et al. Inhibition of monoamine oxidase B in the brains of smokers. *Nature* 1996;379(6567):733–736.
369. Fowler JS, Volkow ND, Wang GJ, et al. Brain monoamine oxidase A inhibition in cigarette smokers. *Proc Natl Acad Sci U S A* 1996;93(24): 14065–14069.

370. Fowler JS, Volkow ND, Wang GJ, et al. Neuropharmacological actions of cigarette smoke: brain monoamine oxidase B (MAO B) inhibition. *J Addict Dis* 1998;17(1):23–34.
371. Fowler JS, Wang GJ, Volkow ND, et al. Maintenance of brain monoamine oxidase B inhibition in smokers after overnight cigarette abstinence. *Am J Psychiatry* 2000;157(11):1864–1866.
372. Logan J, Fowler JS, Volkow ND, et al. Reproducibility of repeated measures of deuterium substituted [^{11}C]L-deprenyl ([^{11}C]L-deprenyl-D2) binding in the human brain. *Nucl Med Biol* 2000;27(1):43–49.
373. Salokangas RK, Vilkman H, Ilonen T, et al. High levels of dopamine activity in the basal ganglia of cigarette smokers. *Am J Psychiatry* 2000;157(4):632–634.
374. Dagher A, Bleicher C, Aston JA, et al. Reduced dopamine D_1 receptor binding in the ventral striatum of cigarette smokers. *Synapse* 2001; 42(1):48–53.
375. Staley JK, Krishnan-Sarin S, Zoghbi S, et al. Sex differences in [^{123}I]beta-CIT SPECT measures of dopamine and serotonin transporter availability in healthy smokers and nonsmokers. *Synapse* 2001;41(4):275–284.
376. Yoder KK, Constantinescu CC, Kareken DA, et al. Heterogeneous effects of alcohol on dopamine release in the striatum: a PET study. *Alcohol Clin Exp Res* 2007;31(6):965–973.
377. Volkow ND, Wang GJ, Fowler JS, et al. Decreases in dopamine receptors but not in dopamine transporters in alcoholics. *Alcohol Clin Exp Res* 1996;20(9):1594–1598.
378. Heinz A, Siessmeier T, Wrase J, et al. Correlation between dopamine D_2 receptors in the ventral striatum and central processing of alcohol cues and craving. *Am J Psychiatry* 2004;161(10):1783–1789.
379. Volkow ND, Wang GJ, Maynard L, et al. Effects of alcohol detoxification on dopamine D_2 receptors in alcoholics: a preliminary study. *Psychiatry Res* 2002;116(3):163–172.
380. Tabakoff B, Hoffman P. Development of functional dependence on ethanol in dopaminergic systems. *J Pharmacol Exp Ther* 1979;208: 216–222.
381. Muller P, Britton R, Seman P. The effects of long term ethanol on brain receptors for dopamine, acetylcholine, serotonin and noradrenaline. *Eur J Pharmacol* 1980;65:31–37.
382. Rabin RA, Wolfe BB, Dibner MD, et al. Effects of ethanol administration and withdrawal on neurotransmitter receptor systems in C57 mice. *J Pharmacol Exp Ther* 1983;213:491–496.
383. Fuchs V, Coper H, Rommelspacher H. The effects of ethanol and haloperidol on dopamine receptors (D_2) density. *Neuropharmacology* 1987;26:1231–1233.
384. Hietala J, Salonen I, Lappalainen J, et al. Ethanol administration does not alter dopamine D_1 and D_2 receptor characteristic in rat brain. *Neurosci Lett* 1990;108:289–294.
385. Lai H, Carino MA, Hrita A. Effects of ethanol on central dopamine function. *Life Sci* 1980;27:299–304.
386. Hruska RE. Effects of ethanol administration on striatal D_1 and D_2 receptors. *J Neurochem* 1988;50:1929–1933.
387. Lucchi L, Moresco RM, Govoni S, et al. Effect of chronic ethanol treatment on dopamine receptor subtypes in rat striatum. *Brain Res* 1988;449(1–2):347–351.
388. Hamdi A, Prasad C. Bidirectional changes in striatal D_2-dopamine receptor density during chronic ethanol intake. *Alcohol* 1993;93: 203–206.
389. Heinz A, Siessmeier T, Wrase J, et al. Correlation of alcohol craving with striatal dopamine synthesis capacity and $D_2/_3$ receptor availability: a combined [^{18}F]DOPA and [^{18}F]DMFP PET study in detoxified alcoholic patients. *Am J Psychiatry* 2005;162(8):1515–1520.
390. Tiihonen J, Kuikka J, Bergström K, et al. Altered striatal dopamine reuptake site densities in habitually violent and non-violent alcoholics. *Nat Med* 1995;1:654–657.
391. Laine TP, Ahonen A, Rasanen P, et al. Dopamine transporter availability and depressive symptoms during alcohol withdrawal. *Psychiatry Res* 1999;90(3):153–157.
392. Laine TP, Ahonen A, Torniainen P, et al. Dopamine transporters increase in human brain after alcohol withdrawal. *Mol Psychiatry* 1999;4(2):189–91, 104–105.
393. Munro CA, McCaul ME, Oswald LM, et al. Striatal dopamine release and family history of alcoholism. *Alcohol Clin Exp Res* 2006;30(7): 1143–1151.
394. Volkow ND, Wang GJ, Hitzemann R, et al. Decreased cerebral response to inhibitory neurotransmission in alcoholics. *Am J Psychiatry* 1993;150(3):417–422.
395. Volkow ND, Wang GJ, Begleiter H, et al. Regional brain metabolic response to lorazepam in subjects at risk for alcoholism. *Alcohol Clin Exp Res* 1995;19(2):510–516.
396. Pauli S, Liljequist S, Farde L, et al. PET analysis of alcohol interaction with the brain disposition of [^{11}C]flumazenil. *Psychopharmacology* 1992;107:180–185.
397. Litton J-E, Neiman J, Pauli S, et al. PET analysis of [^{11}C]flumazenil binding to benzodiazepine receptors in chronic alcohol-dependent men and healthy controls. *Psychiatry Res Neuroimaging* 1992;50: 1–13.
398. Farde L, Pauli S, Litton JE, et al. PET-determination of benzodiazepine receptor binding in studies on alcoholism. *EXS* 1994;71:143–153.
399. Gilman S, Koeppe RA, Adams K, et al. Positron emission tomographic studies of cerebral benzodiazepine-receptor binding in chronic alchoholics. *Ann Neurol* 1996;40:163–171.
400. Abi-Dargham A, Krystal JH, Anjilvel S, et al. Alterations of benzodiazepine receptors in type II alcoholic subjects measured with SPECT and [^{123}I]iomazenil. *Am J Psychiatry* 1998;155(11):1550–1555.
401. Lingford-Hughes AR, Acton PD, Gacinovic S, et al. Reduced levels of GABA-benzodiazepine receptor in alcohol dependency in the absence of grey matter atrophy. *Br J Psychiatry* 1998;173:116–122.
402. Wagner HW Jr. Highlights 2001 lecture. *J Nucl Med* 2001;42: 12N–30N.
403. Laruelle M. The role of model-based methods in the development of single scan techniques. *Nucl Med Biol* 2000;27(7):637–642.

Evaluation of Myocardial Perfusion

KEIICHIRO YOSHINAGA, NAGARA TAMAKI, TERRENCE D. RUDDY, ROBERT A. deKEMP, AND ROB S. B. BEANLANDS

Coronary artery disease (CAD) continues to be a major cause of death not only in modern industrialized society but also in developing countries. Techniques for evaluating myocardial blood flow (MBF) plays an important role in the identification of patients with CAD and determination of their prognosis. Patients at high risk for subsequent cardiac events can be treated with aggressive interventional therapy and low-risk patients managed medically. Measurement of regional myocardial perfusion permits measurement of coronary flow reserve and the evaluation of the physiologic significance of coronary lesions and adequacy of collateral supply. These MBF measurements are often essential for characterizing the functional significance of CAD and are complementary to coronary angiography. As well, positron emission tomography (PET) measurements of MBF reserve and endothelial function are useful for the serial evaluation of patients with the goals of determining the response to therapy and progression of disease. In the past the clinical use of cardiac PET has been limited by the cost of the technology, but the development of less expensive PET cameras and the increased use of PET for other indications have resulted in wider clinical application of cardiac PET as well. Furthermore, PET is uniquely suited to be a quantitative research tool for studies evaluating myocardial perfusion *in vivo* in man.

PET has become accepted as the most accurate technique for the measurement of regional MBF. Tissue perfusion in milliliters per minute per gram of weight can be measured *in vivo* by relating myocardial tracer kinetics to arterial tracer input. The accuracy of these noninvasive measurements requires (a) a radiotracer with retention or clearance kinetics related to MBF during normal and pathophysiologic states, (b) accurate measurement of the arterial blood and myocardial activity of the radiotracer with adequate temporal resolution to define the tracer kinetics, and (c) established

TABLE 11.1.1 PET Myocardial Blood Flow Tracers

Pharmaceutical	Radioisotopes	Half-life	Positron Energy (MeV)
Rubidium	Rb-82	76 sec	3.15
Water	O-15	110 sec	1.72
Potassium	K-38	7.6 min	2.7
PTSM	Cu-62	9.8 min	2.94
Ammonia	N-13	10 min	1.19
Acetate	C-11	20 min	0.96
Butanol			
FBnTP	F-18	110 min	0.63

PTSM, pyruvaldehyde bis (N^4-methylthiosemicarbazone); FBnTP, fluorobenzyl triphenyl phosphonium.

methods of modeling of the tracer kinetics to permit calculation of regional flow measurements. Current PET technology has spatial resolution of 4 to 6 mm and accurate attenuation correction, permitting measurement of myocardial radiotracer concentration at frequent time intervals. Integration of PET instrumentation with a computed tomography (CT) scanner (PET/CT) can provide the means for accurate attenuation correction of myocardial perfusion imaging (MPI) and coronary arteries anatomical information in a single setting. Suitable kinetic modeling has been developed for several PET flow tracers and makes the accurate measurement of tissue blood flow possible (1–7).

MYOCARDIAL BLOOD FLOW TRACERS

The commonly used PET blood flow tracers can be divided into (a) inert freely diffusible tracers such as oxygen-15 ([^{15}O])-labeled water and (b) physiologically retained tracers such as nitrogen-13 ([^{13}N])-ammonia and rubidium-82 ([^{82}Rb]). The commonly used PET MBF tracers are listed in Table 11.1.1 in order of increasing half-life.

Diffusible tracers such as [^{15}O]-labeled water diffuse freely across membranes, resulting in a distribution of tracer between vascular and extravascular space related to the partition coefficient. This partition coefficient for [^{15}O]-labeled water is stable over a wide range of flow rates such that uptake of [^{15}O]-labeled water is not diffusion limited. Conversely, the extraction fraction of physiologically retained radiotracers decreases with increasing blood flow and results in underestimation of MBF based on the measurement of tissue uptake. These physiologic properties are incorporated into the kinetic models for determination of MBF.

Nitrogen-13-Ammonia

[^{13}N]-ammonia is the most commonly used myocardial perfusion tracer in PET centers with an on-site cyclotron. Nitrogen-13 is produced with a cyclotron and a water target via the [^{16}O] (p,α) [^{13}N] nuclear reaction to yield the radionuclide. Ammonium ions can be converted readily with reducing agents.

Following intravenous administration of [^{13}N]-ammonia, [^{13}N]-ammonia crosses capillary and cell membranes via passive diffusion and is retained in myocardial tissue by the incorporation of the label into the amino acid pool as glutamine. The synthesis of glutamine is the rate-limiting process of tissue retention of [^{13}N]-ammonia. Nitrogen-13-ammonia in blood is in an equilibrium state with ionic [^{13}N]-ammonium (8,9). The first pass extraction fraction is nearly 100%, since [^{13}N]-ammonia diffuses freely across membranes (9). In myocardium, [^{13}N]-ammonia is either incorporated into synthesis of [^{13}N]-glutamine or back-diffuses into the vascular space (10). The net extraction fraction is approximately 80% in the resting flow range, but decreases with higher flow rates.

The image quality achieved with [^{13}N]-ammonia is considered to be the best among all of the PET perfusion tracers due to the relatively long physical half-life, relatively high extraction fraction, low background, and low positron energy (Fig. 11.1.1).

Rubidium-82

[^{82}Rb] is produced from a strontium-82/rubidium-82 generator that can be eluted every 10 minutes (11). [^{82}Rb] is a widely used PET perfusion tracer in centers without immediate access to an on-site cyclotron (7,12). The half-life of the parent isotope is 25.5 days and results in a generator life of about 4 to 6 weeks. Not needing a cyclotron is a major advantage of this radiotracer. Although the commercial generator is expensive, a high volume of cardiac studies significantly reduces the cost of radiotracer per examination. The short physical half-life of 76 seconds makes [^{82}Rb] suitable for repeated and sequential perfusion studies (Fig. 11.1.2). As well, the short half-life necessitates rapid image acquisition shortly after tracer administration. The relatively high positron energy of [^{82}Rb] of 3.15 MeV is associated with a positron range averaging 7.5 mm and results in lower spatial resolution than seen with [^{13}N]-ammonia with a positron range of 2.5 mm.

[^{82}Rb] is an analogue of potassium and has similar biological activity to thallium-201 [^{201}Tl] (13,14). [^{82}Rb] is rapidly extracted from the blood and concentrated by the myocardium. In animal models, the first-pass extraction fraction is 50% to 60% at rest and decreases to 25% to 30% at peak flow (13,15,16). In addition, the extraction fraction may remain reduced in myocardium recovering from transient ischemia (17). This radiotracer is retained in the myocardium and equilibrates in the potassium pool. Thus, cell membrane disruption may cause rapid tissue loss of radioactivity, and [^{82}Rb] kinetics can be used as a marker of tissue viability (18).

A small and mobile generator infusion system is used for eluting [^{82}Rb] every 10 to 15 minutes with low radiation exposure to personnel or patient (11). Quantitative assessment of MBF and flow reserve is quite feasible and clinically practical with this generator as compared to cyclotron-produced compounds (19–23).

Copper-62 PTSM

Copper-62 ([^{62}Cu]) pyruvaldehyde bis (N^4-methylthiosemicarbazone) (PTSM) is another generator-produced PET perfusion tracer and is produced from zinc-62 ([^{62}Zn])/copper-62 generator (24,25). [^{62}Cu] PTSM is quite suitable for serial measurement of MBF since the physical half-life of 9.7 minutes is short (26). Unfortunately, the relatively short half-life of 9.2 hours of the parent, [^{62}Zn], results in the need for a fresh generator on a daily basis.

Following intravenous administration of [^{62}Cu] PTSM, the radiotracer clears rapidly from blood with high tracer uptake in the myocardium. The uncharged lipophilic copper PTSM rapidly diffuses across cell membranes. Within the cell, the [^{62}Cu] PTSM is

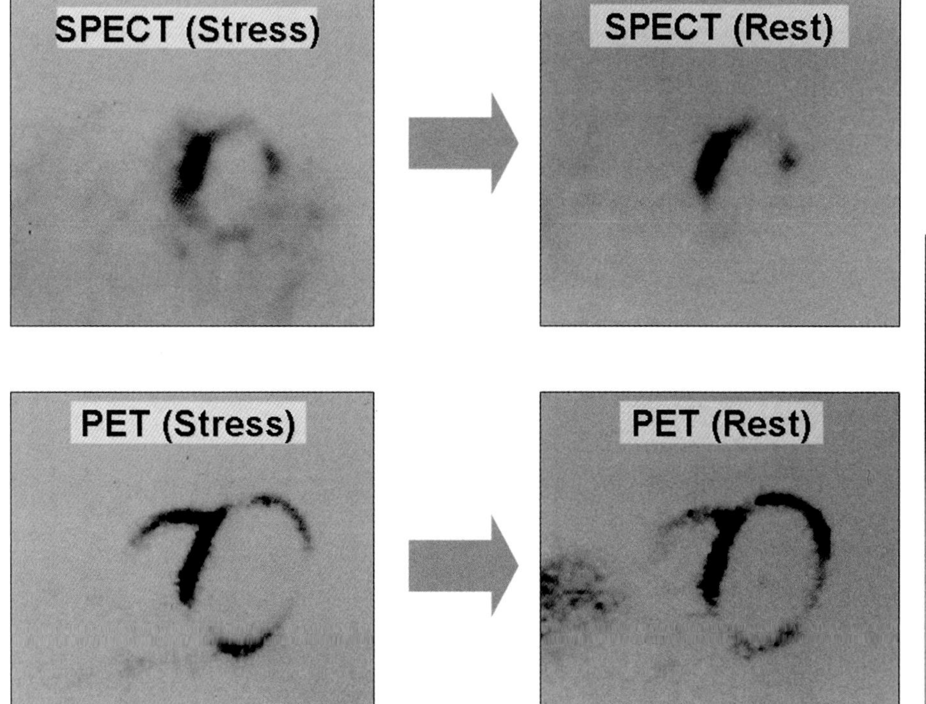

FIGURE 11.1. Transverse stress (**left**) and rest (**right**) myocardial perfusion images using nitrogen-13-ammonia PET (**bottom**) and thallium-201 single-photon emission computed tomography (SPECT) (**top**) acquired in a patient with an inferior wall myocardial infarction. The perfusion defect in the posterolateral region is well demonstrated by both studies, but the stress-induced perfusion abnormality is more clearly seen in the PET perfusion study.

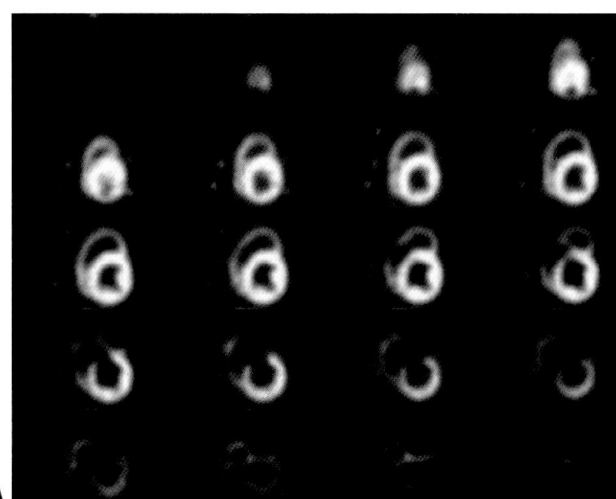

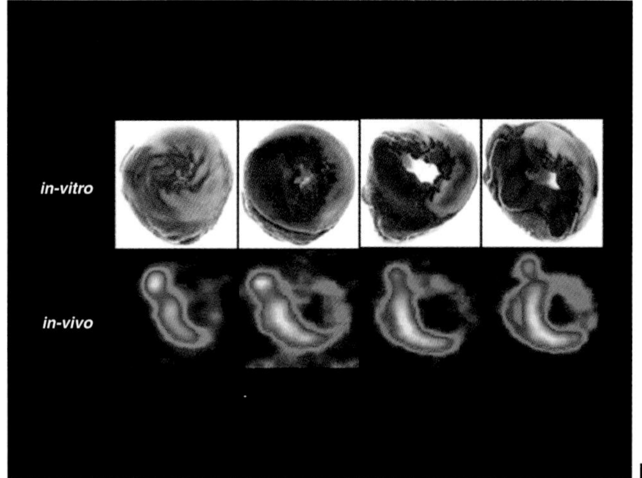

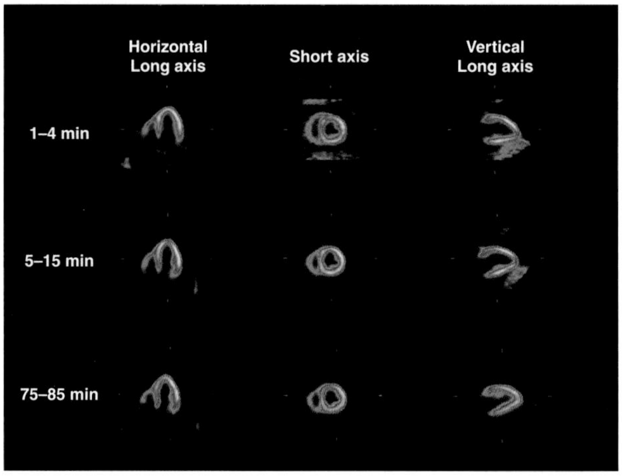

FIGURE 11.2. **A:** Fluorine-18 ([^{18}F])-labeled myocardial perfusion agents: [^{18}F]-fluorobenzyl triphenyl phosphonium (FBnTp) axial PET images of dog myocardium. Images represent [^{18}F]-FBnTp activity over 30 to 60 minutes after administration. Apex (**upper left corner**); base (**lower right corner**). (From Madar I, Ravert HT, Du Y, et al. Characterization of uptake of the new PET imaging compound ^{18}F-fluorobenzyl triphenyl phosphonium in dog myocardium. *J Nucl Med* 2006;47:1359–1366, with permission.) **B:** Reconstructed single-photon emission computed tomography (SPECT) images of RP-1012-18 in nonhuman primates at 1 to 4, 5 to 15, and 75 to 85 minutes (min) following intravenous injection of the agent. Excellent image quality is noted early and late following injection. (From Bristol-Myers Squibb Medical Imaging, with permission.) **C:** Comparison of *in vivo* and *in vitro* myocardial slices. In the rat model RP-1012-18 was injected after brief coronary artery ligation and reperfusion. The extent of infracted myocardium on *in vitro* histologically stained slices correlated very well with areas of perfusion defect. (From Bristol-Myers Squibb Medical Imaging, with permission.)

susceptible to reductive decomposition by reaction with ubiquitous intracellular enzymes. As a result, an effectively irreversible deposition of ionic copper is seen in the cells.

[^{62}Cu] PTSM is a promising tracer for the evaluation of myocardial and cerebral perfusion. High-quality myocardial perfusion images can be obtained shortly after tracer administration in the animal as well as human studies (26,27). Five percent to 10% of the injected dose of copper PTSM remains in the circulation due to binding to red blood cells. Therefore, the quantitative measurement of regional MBF using the microsphere model requires correction of the arterial blood time activity curve for blood pool binding (28). A significant reduction of extraction fraction is observed in the high flow range and requires correction to express data as absolute MBF (28).

In myocardial perfusion images acquired at rest and during pharmacological stress, myocardial contrast is high, although liver uptake interfered with the evaluation of the inferior wall (26,29).

Oxygen-15-Water

[^{15}O]-labeled water was one of the first radiopharmaceuticals developed for PET use and is considered the gold standard for quantification of myocardial perfusion. [^{15}O]-labeled water is usually obtained from [^{15}O]-oxygen gas combined with hydrogen gas. The [^{15}O] gas is produced either by [^{14}N] (d,n) [^{15}O] reaction or [^{15}N] (p,n) [^{15}O] method. Since the physical half-life of [^{15}O] is only 2 minutes, an in-house cyclotron is required to use [^{15}O]-labeled water.

One of the major advantages of [^{15}O]-labeled water is feasibility for quantitative assessment of MBF.

Carbon-11-Butanol

Radiolabeled aliphatic alcohols have been evaluated in the search for better blood flow tracers. Butanol seems to be a nearly optimal flow tracer since it has a better partition coefficient than [^{15}O]-labeled water. Carbon-11 ([^{11}C])-butanol can be produced with a simple synthesis with a high yield (30,31). However, this tracer has been mainly used for cerebral perfusion studies and not yet well evaluated for measurement of MBF.

Fluorine-18 Fluorobenzyl Triphenyl Phosphonium

Fluorine-18 ([^{18}F])-labeled compounds have relatively long physical half-life (110 minutes) and can be delivered to PET centers without an on-cite cyclotron in the same manner as [^{18}F]-fluorodeoxyglucose (FDG). Among [^{18}F]-labeled radio tracers, [^{18}F]-fluorobenzyl triphenyl phosphonium ([^{18}F]-FBnTP) represents a promising tracer. [^{18}F]-FBnTP is rapidly accumulated to myocardium and has a long retention time. Thus, [^{18}F]-FBnTP yielded high quality images in preliminary canine studies (32). This early results are encouraging (Fig. 11.1.2A). In healthy dogs, FBnTP accumulates rapidly in the myocardium (time to plateau <60 seconds) and distributes uniformly throughout the myocardium (6% to 8% coefficient of variance). In dogs with coronary stenosis, FBnTP flow defect contrast was 2.7 times greater than tetrofosmin *ex vivo*. A near identical qualitative and quantitative estimate of stenosis severity was obtained by early, short (5 to 15 minutes) and delayed, prolonged (30 to 60 minutes) [^{18}F]-FBnTP PET scans. Although animal results are promising, this tracer needs further investigation in human studies. An additional PET tracer, labeled with [^{18}F], has recently been reported, RP-1012-18. This agent is a structural analogue of pyridaben, a known mitochondrial complex 1 (MC-1) inhibitor (Figs. 11.1.2B, 11.1.2C).

CLINICAL INDICATION AND IMAGING PROTOCOLS

Clinical Indication

Current clinical guidelines (33) and a joint position statement (34) address patients with intermediate likelihood of CAD when the patient has had a nondiagnostic or equivocal single-photon emission computed tomography (SPECT) myocardial perfusion imaging (MPI) or other noninvasive imaging tests. For such patients, indications for PET MPI for diagnosis and detection of ischemia are considered class I (level of evidence B). In general, patients who are unable to exercise or have left bundle branch block (LBBB) or ventricular pacing rhythm may also benefit from PET MPI for diagnosis and detection of ischemia (class IIa; Class I [level of evidence B]) (Fig. 11.1.3) (33,34).

Imaging Protocol

Patient Preparation

Patients should be instructed to fast for 6 hours or more, to abstain from caffeine-containing products (i.e., coffee, tea, chocolate, and cola) at least 12 hours, and to avoid theophylline-containing medications for 48 hours prior to adenosine/adenosine triphosphate

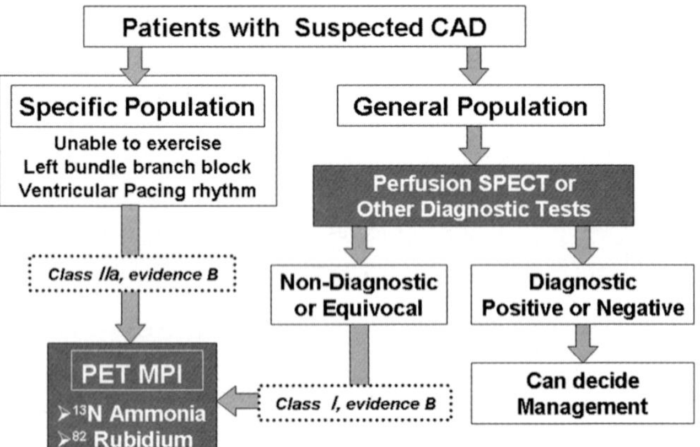

FIGURE 11.1.3. Indications of PET myocardial perfusion imaging for diagnosis of coronary artery disease based on American College of Cardiology/American Heart Association/American Society of Nuclear Cardiology guidelines. CAD, coronary artery disease; MPI, myocardial perfusion imaging; SPECT, single-photon emission computed tomography. (From Klocke FJ, Baird MG, Lorell BH, et al. ACC/AHA/ASNC guidelines for the clinical use of cardiac radionuclide imaging—executive summary: a report of the American College of Cardiology/American Heart Association Task Force on Practice Guidelines (ACC/AHA/ASNC Committee to Revise the 1995 Guidelines for the Clinical Use of Cardiac Radionuclide Imaging). *J Am Coll Cardiol* 2003;42:1318–1333, with permission.)

(ATP)/dipyridamole pharmacological stress tests (35). Patients who would have dobutamine stress tests should stop β-blockers 48 hours before the tests if the goal is diagnosis of CAD and if it is clinically safe to do so.

Stress Protocol

Vasodilator Pharmacological Stress

Adenosine, ATP, and dipyridamole stress are the established clinical stress methods for myocardial perfusion PET imaging. These vasodilator agents block transport of adenosine into the cells and/or increase extra cellular levels of adenosine, which causes coronary vasodilatation by interacting with the adenosine A_2 receptors in the cell membrane. Activation of A_2 receptors dilates coronary vasculatures via the production of adenylate cyclase and cyclic adenosine monophosphate stimulation of potassium channels, which results decreased intracellular calcium uptake. These agents increase MBF and permit measurement of MBF reserve. Adenosine and dipyridamole increase MBF by three- to fivefold in normal coronary territories without increasing oxygen demand. In contrast, myocardial regions supplied by diseased coronary arteries already have dilated coronary arterioles at rest in order to maintain resting blood supply. Thus, the hyperemic response is attenuated and coronary flow reserve is reduced (5).

Dipyridamole (0.56 mg/kg) is infused intravenously over 4 minutes. The radiotracer should be injected 3 to 5 minutes after the completion of dipyridamole infusion (Fig. 11.1.4). Adenosine should be administered as a continuous infusion (140 μg/kg/min) over a 6-minute period, and the radiotracer should be injected at the 3-minute mark of the 6-minute infusion period (36).

Dobutamine Stress

Dobutamine stress is a feasible alternative in the situation when adenosine, ATP, or dipyridamole is contraindicated because of severe reactive airway disease or caffeine intake (36). However, dobutamine perfusion imaging has not been as extensively studied as vasodilator stress agents. Dobutamine increases regional MBF based on physiologic principles of coronary flow reserve. Flow increases to meet increasing demand. However, this response is attenuated during high-dose dobutamine administration (20 to 40 μg/kg/min) in segments supplied by diseased vessels.

In practice, dobutamine can start 5 to 10 μg/kg/min, and dobutamine dose can be increased 5 μg/kg/min at 3-minute intervals up to a maximum dose of 40 μg/kg/min to achieve >85% of target heart rate (0.85 × [220 – age]).

Exercise Stress

An exercise stress test can evaluate the imbalance of oxygen demand and blood supply and thus provides physiological information as well as functional capacity. Although exercise stress is considered to be a physiological stress and is widely applied for SPECT myocardial perfusion imaging, in general pharmacological stress is preferred in PET imaging because imaging starts shortly after tracer administration and pharmacological stress can better avoid body movements during image acquisitions. However, [^{13}N]-ammonia can be used in conjunction with treadmill or upright bicycle exercise test. The tracer is administrated at peak exercise and exercise should be continued for an additional 30 to 60 seconds after tracer injection. The patient is then repositioned in the PET camera to start the acquisition within 4 to 6 minutes (37–39). Accurate repositioning is important to minimize artifact due to incorrect attenuation correction. A bicycle ergometer can be attached to the PET bed, which makes this approach more feasible in terms of attenuation correction (39), although patient body position may shift during the supine exercise. Exercise stress is also available for the [^{82}Rb] imaging (35,40). Using treadmill exercise, patients should continue their peak exercise 1.0 to 1.5 minutes after [^{82}Rb] intravenous

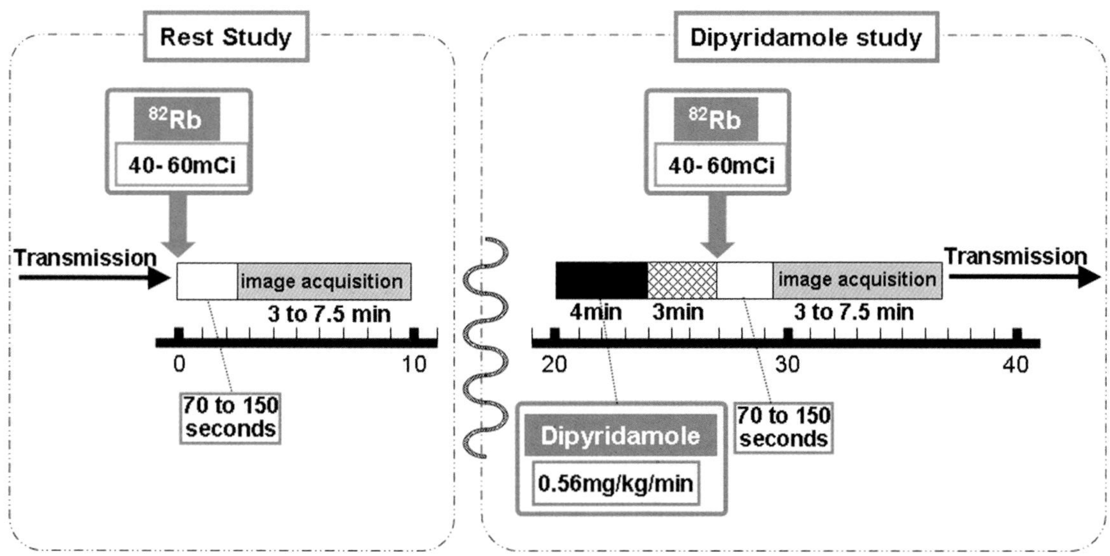

FIGURE 11.1.4. Imaging protocol of dipyridamole stress rubidium-82 ([^{82}Rb]) PET myocardial perfusion imaging.

administration. The patient is then repositioned in the PET scanner and the image acquisition should begin approximately 3 minutes after tracer injection (35,40).

Image Acquisition and Processing

Nitrogen-13-Ammonia

For relative perfusion imaging, [^{13}N]-ammonia is injected as a bolus of 10 to 20 mCi (370 to 740 MBq) and static images are acquired 1.5 to 3 minutes after tracer administration for an imaging time of 5 to 15 minutes (35).

For quantitative measurement of MBF, serial dynamic PET imaging begins simultaneously with tracer administration. From the dynamic images, time activity curves are generated for the myocardium and the blood pool. Global and regional MBF can be measured with use of compartmental tracer kinetic modeling fit to myocardial activity data and corrected for the arterial input function. Previously, the arterial input function was measured by sequential arterial blood sampling. However, blood pool time activity data obtained from left ventricular cavity provides an accurate measurement without the use of arterial cannulation and makes acquisitions more feasible and easier for the patient.

Rubidium-82

A large amount of tracer can be administered to the patient because of the short physical half-life of [^{82}Rb]. Forty to 60 mCi (1,480 to 2,220 MBq) of [^{82}Rb] can be injected as a bolus of 30 seconds or less followed by serial dynamic acquisition using a PET camera with a high-count rate and high sensitivity with a short acquisition time (35). After a 70- to 150-second completion of tracer injection, a 3- to 7.5-minute image acquisition is initiated (35,41). Alternatively, the newer generation of PET cameras can acquire data in three-dimensional modes and without septa, resulting in higher sensitivity and the need for smaller doses of [^{82}Rb] (19).

For quantitative assessment of regional MBF, a two-compartment model has been used, which includes activity in the vascular space and within the tissue compartment (42). Following bolus injection of the tracer, predominantly unidirectional transport is assumed from the vascular space into the tissue space. In the canine model, regional MBF can be accurately estimated using [^{82}Rb] (43). A simplified approach using a summed late image corrected for the input function, similar to that described for [^{13}N]-ammonia, has also been used. This approach allows reasonable quantification for perfusion that may be easier to apply in the clinical setting (Fig. 11.1.5) (19,21,22).

Semiquantitative Image Interpretation

Myocardial perfusion defects are usually identified by visual analysis of the reconstructed slices. Such perfusion defects should be characterized by their location as they relate to a specific coronary artery, their extent, and the defect severity. Defects noted during stress imaging whose severity and extent improve at rest are typically categorized as reversible, which indicates myocardial ischemia (Fig. 11.1.6). On the other hand, defects that are fixed in extent and severity at both stress and rest are categorized as myocardial injury or infarction. Perfusion defect description, including extent, severity, reversibility, location, and specific coronary territories, should be reported routinely (44). Moreover, cardiac event risk over 2 to 3 years may be addressed in the report based on the following risk stratifications guidelines that recommend semiquantitative analysis: normal perfusion = 0, mild = 1, moderate = 2, severe = 3, and absent uptake = 4, using a 17-segment model (Figs. 11.1.7A, 11.1.B) (34,45). Using this approach, the summed perfusion defect score can be calculated and is useful for cardiac risk stratification (34,46). A number of previous SPECT data have confirmed the critical cutoff for abnormal scan is summed stress score >4 in a 20-segment model (34). Berman et al. (47) confirmed this cutoff value can apply for the currently recommended 17-segment model in SPECT perfusion studies. Yoshinaga et al. (41) also reported that abnormal cutoff value of SSS 4 or greater can apply to [^{82}Rb] PET studies with the 17-segment model.

Common Artifacts with Nitrogen-13-Ammonia and Rubidium-82

[^{13}N]-ammonia studies in normal volunteers have shown a slight heterogeneity of regional tracer retention (Fig. 1.11.1) (29). [^{13}N]-ammonia retention was decreased by 10% in the lateral wall of the left ventricle as compared to the septum. The underlying mechanism of

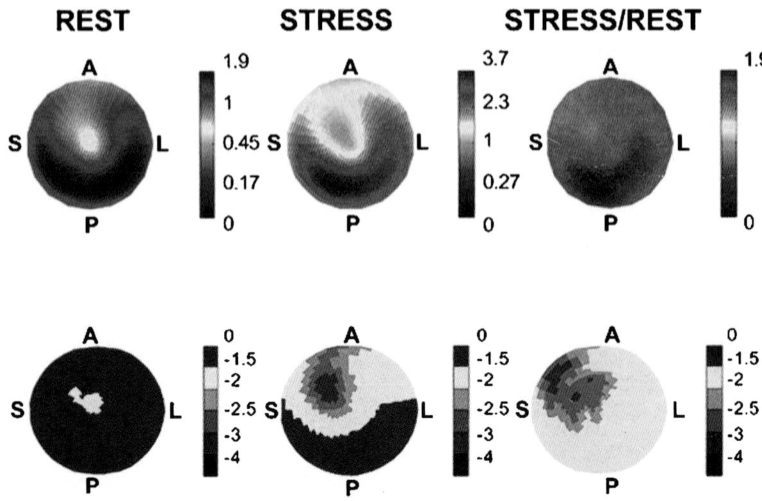

FIGURE 11.1.5. Rest and stress rubidium-82 ([^{82}Rb] uptake plus stress/rest (flow reserve) polar maps in a patient with anomalous left coronary artery arising from the pulmonary artery. **Upper panel:** Calculated flows (mL/min/g) are on the right of the color bar. **Lower panel:** Each increment represents a degree of standard deviation (SD) below the mean of a normal population (<5% likelihood of coronary artery disease). The blue segments represent sectors greater than 2 SD below the mean of a normal population. Note that the stress and stress/rest maps indicate impaired stress flow and flow reserve in the vascular bed of the left anterior descending (LAD). (From Beauchesne L. *Can J Cardiol* 2006; 22(12):1069–1070, with permission.)

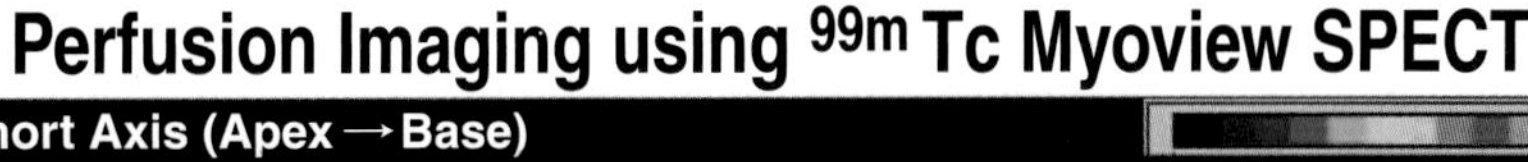

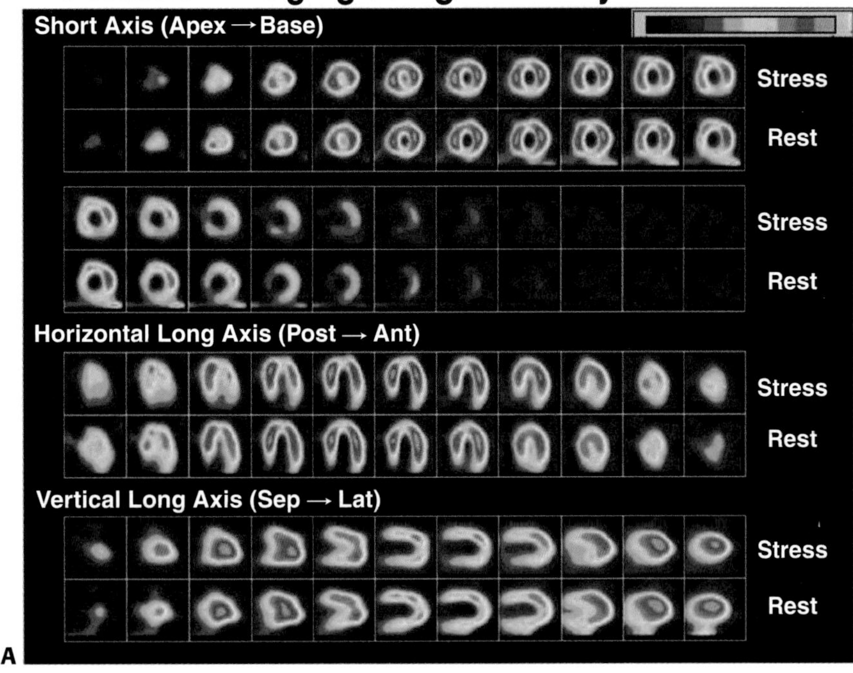

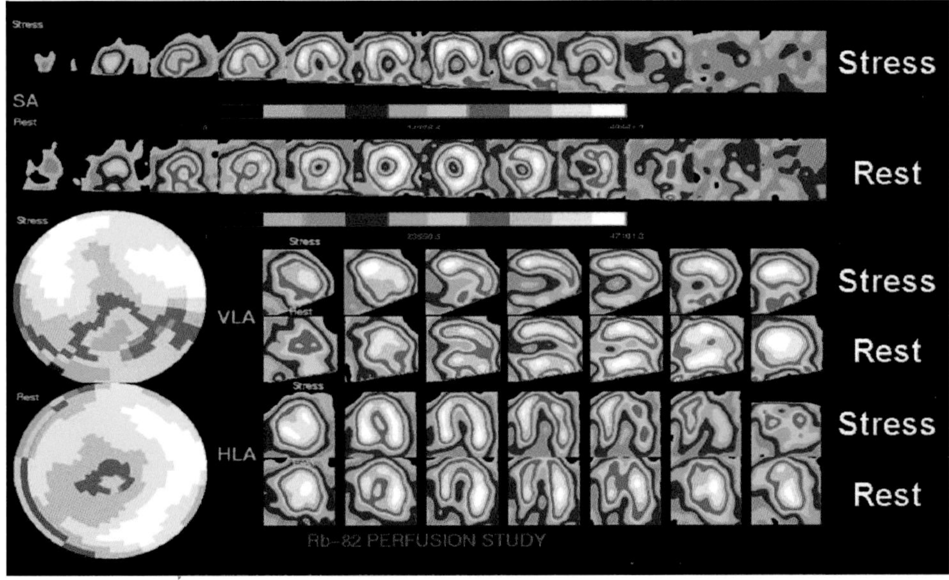

FIGURE 11.1.6. Representative images from a 44-year-old obese man who had exertional and atypical chest pain and positive exercise stress test. **A:** The technetium-99m (^{99m}Tc) tetrofosmin single-photon emission computed tomography (SPECT) images show a predominately fixed perfusion defect in the inferior wall. **B:** Rubidium-82 ([^{82}Rb]) PET images show reversible perfusion defect in inferior indicating severe myocardial ischemia right coronary artery territory.

this phenomenon is poorly understood. However, this mild heterogeneity has to be appreciated when interpreting [^{13}N]-ammonia perfusion images. Changes in the metabolic and hemodynamic environment within physiologic ranges do not significantly alter the retention of [^{13}N]-ammonia (9,10). Other factors to consider with [^{13}N]-ammonia imaging include excess liver activity, which can interfere with evaluation of the inferior wall, and excess lung activity in patients with pulmonary disease or congestion.

[^{82}Rb] images sometimes have excessive bowel radioactivity, which can make it difficult to interpret the inferior region. This excessive tracer accumulation is similarly observed using [^{201}Tl] SPECT. This may be resolved by water intake. In clinical practice at

Seventeen-segment nomenclature

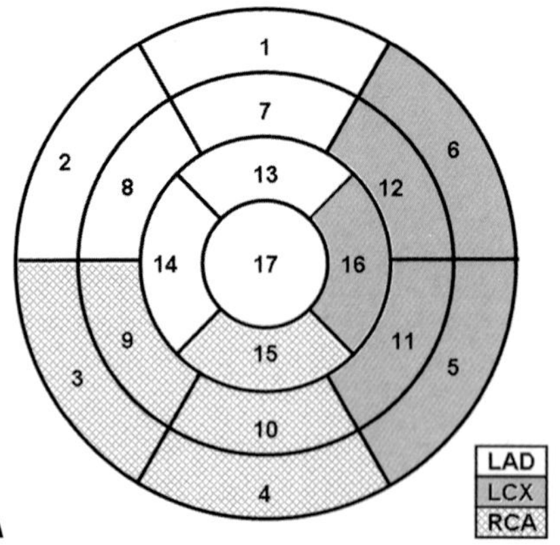

1	basal anterior
2	basal anteroseptal
3	basal inferoseptal
4	basal inferior
5	basal inferolateral
6	basal anterolateral
7	mid anterior
8	mid anteroseptal
9	mid inferoseptal
10	mid inferior
11	mid inferolateral
12	mid anterolateral
13	apical anterior
14	apical septal
15	apical inferior
16	apical lateral
17	apex

A

Semiquantitative Scoring System

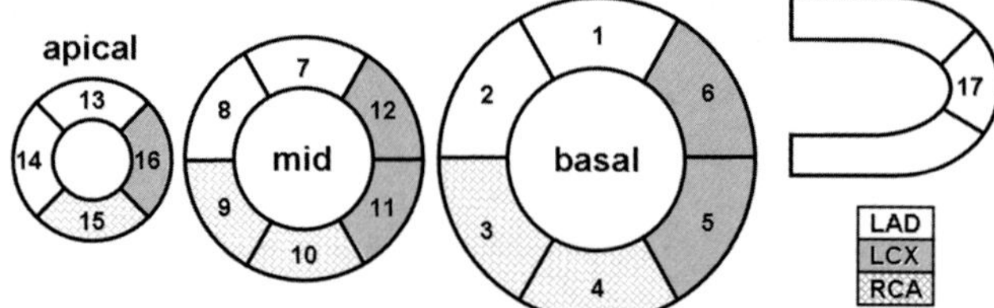

Five-point scoring system
0 = normal
1 = mildly reduced
2 = moderately reduced
3 = severely reduced
4 = absent uptake

SSS = Sum of segment score at stress
SRS = Sum of segment score at rest
SDS = Differences between stress & rest

B

FIGURE 11.1.7. Seventeen-segment nomenclature recommended by American College of Cardiology/American Heart Association/American Society of Nuclear Cardiology guidelines. LAD, left anterior descending; LCX, left circumflex; RCA, right coronary artery. (From Machac J, Bacharach SL, Bateman TM, et al. Positron emission tomography myocardial perfusion and glucose metabolism imaging. *J Nucl Cardiol* 2006;13:e121–151; American Society of Nuclear Cardiology. Imaging guidelines for nuclear cardiology procedures, part 2. *J Nucl Cardiol* 1999;6:G47–G84, with permission.)

the authors' facility, when a patient has strong bowel activity at rest imaging, the patient would have a cup of water and the resting study would be repeated.

Assessment of Absolute Myocardial Blood Flow

Absolute measurement of physiological or biochemical function are obtained by tracer kinetics. A parametric physical model uses the time course of radioactivity of the arterial blood input function *Ca*(*t*), which usually can measure blood radio activity in the left ventricle (LV) cavity, and myocardial response function *Cm*(*t*) to estimate a quantitative rate constant (48,49). A simple net retention model can be used to calculate absolute MBF directly from short dynamic sequential images. The net retention equals the measured radio tracer concentration at time *T* divided by the integral of the blood input function curve to that time (50) or an earlier time point. The net retention reflects the effects of both MBF and cellular radiotracer extraction. This approach is mainly used for [^{13}N]-tritium and [^{82}Rb] blood flow quantification (22).

Compartment models have been developed for MBF quantification. The compartments represent tissue volumes that include physical factors (arterial blood and intracellular fluid) or biochemical factors (tracer compound and labeled metabolite). A mathematical model is constructed with parameters such as a flux of radioactivity between the compartments. The compartment model approach is mainly applied for [^{13}N]-tritium and [^{15}O]-water blood flow quantification (51,52).

Nitrogen-13-Ammonia Blood Flow Quantification

The most common approach assumes a three-compartment model with the compartments being the vascular, extravascular, and metabolic spaces (51). The first pass extraction is assumed to be 100%. K_1 representing the transport of the tracer from the vascular space into the extravascular space is an estimate of MBF. These PET measurements have been well validated with microsphere measurements in experimental preparations confirming that regional MBF can be quantitatively measured over a wide blood flow range with [^{13}N]-ammonia and this three compartmental approach (53–55). A number of simplified approaches have been used to quantify regional MBF with [^{13}N]-ammonia. The simplest method is the microsphere model, which requires one static scan and arterial input function and correction for the net extraction fraction (50,56,57). However, the quantitative value is quite variable depending on the time of measurement after tracer administration. To minimize this effect, Patlak graphic analysis of the early uptake phase has recently been applied for the quantitative estimate of MBF (58,59).

Oxygen-15-Water Myocardial Blood Flow Quantification

Since water is freely diffusible in the myocardium without dependence on metabolism, the biological behavior of [^{15}O]-labeled water can be modeled with a simple one-compartment model as originally described by Bergmann et al. (60) and Kety (61). Rapid sequential image acquisition is needed after tracer administration. Because of the short physical half-life, a large amount of activity is administrated that requires a high count rate and high sensitivity PET camera for quantification of radioactivity concentration after dead time correction.

Tomographic visualization of the [^{15}O]-labeled water perfusion images requires correction of blood pool activity. A separate scan is acquired after inhalation of [^{15}O]-carbon monoxide, which labels erythrocytes and delineates the vascular blood pool. High contrast myocardial perfusion images can be obtained after subtraction of the blood pool images from the [^{15}O]-water images (Fig. 11.1.8) (60,62). Principal component analysis has been used to define the blood and myocardial signals, without the need for an additional blood pool scan. Patient motion between the two scans can introduce significant error into the subtraction images. The kinetic model used in the determination of MBF accounts for partial volume and blood-to-tissue spillover effects.

Iida et al. (52) proposed a mathematical model to correct the input function for the tissue-to-blood spillover (63) and partial volume effect (64). This model permits estimation of the perfusable

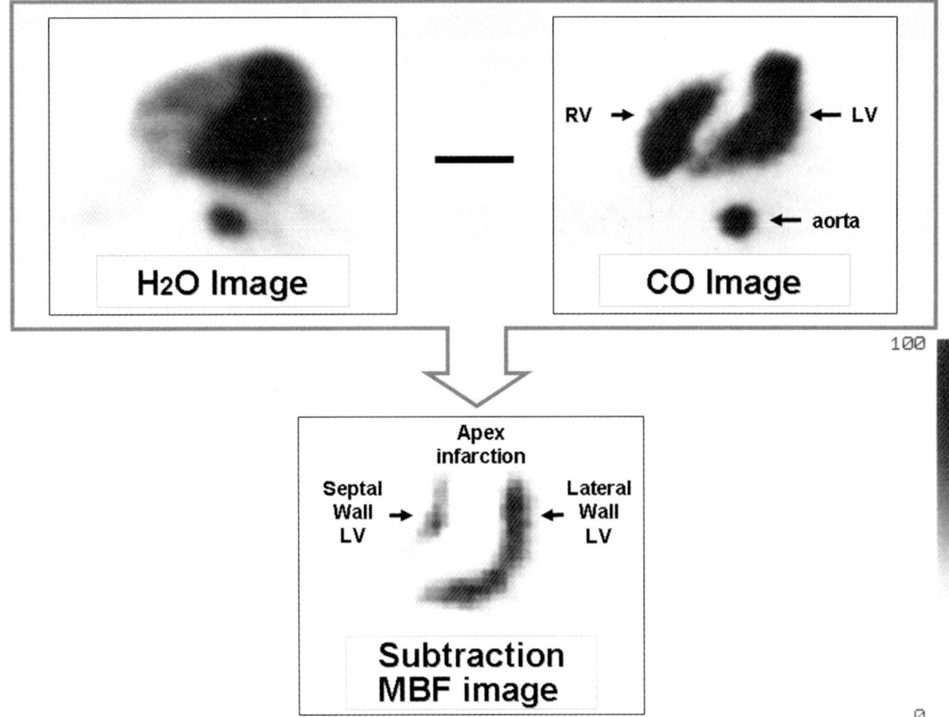

FIGURE 11.1.8. Oxygen-15 ([^{15}O])-labeled water perfusion transverse slice (**H_2O Image**) demonstrates myocardial and blood pool activity. A corresponding [^{15}O]-carbon monoxide image (**CO Image**) delineates the vascular blood pool and is acquired after inhalation of [^{15}O]-carbon monoxide and subsequent labeling of erythrocytes. The myocardial perfusion image (**Subtraction MBF Image**) is obtained after subtraction of the blood pool image from the [^{15}O]-water image.

tissue fraction defined as the water perfusable tissue divided by total extravascular anatomical tissue. This parameter is independent of the size of the region of interest and may discriminate water perfusable viable tissue from nonperfusable infarcted tissue, assuming that irreversibly damaged tissue cannot exchange water rapidly (65,66).

Manual positioning of regional myocardial regions of interest takes a long time and depends on the operator because [^{15}O]-water uptake is not easily visualized as it is not retained in the myocardium. Katoh et al. (67) developed an automatic algorithm to calculate regional MBF using semiautomatic regions of interests setting algorithm and uniform input function. This approach could facilitate quantitative blood flow analysis using [^{15}O]-labeled water PET in a clinical setting.

Hyperemic Myocardial Blood Flow and Coronary Flow Reserve

Hyperemic MBF represents microcirculatory vascular function, including both vascular smooth muscle and endothelial function. Vasodilatation is induced through both these mechanisms (68). Coronary flow reserve (CFR) is a ratio of near maximal MBF during pharmacologically induced hyperemia to MBF at rest. Thus, CFR represents coronary vascular function (5). The CFR measured by PET accurately reflects regional MBF as measured by intracoronary Doppler flow guide wire (69,70) and has good reproducibility using [^{13}N]-ammonia or [^{15}O]-water PET (71,72). Normal CFR measured using PET is 3.0 to 5.0 either by [^{13}N]-ammonia, [^{15}O]-water, or [^{82}Rb] (Table 11.1.2). Dobutamine stress may have less increase in MBF: a 2.4-fold increase at peak dobutamine dose (40 μg/kg/min) (73). Adding atropine to the maximum dose of dobutamine can increase MBF comparable to dipyridamole stress (74).

Visual interpretation of relative tracer uptake both in PET and SPECT MPI is the standard approach for image interpretations. However, blood flow quantification seems to be more sensitive than the conventional approach (Fig. 11.1.9). Parkash et al. (20) evaluated the clinical importance of coronary flow reserve over conventional visual analysis in patients with three-vessel CAD using [^{82}Rb] PET. The perfusion defect sizes were larger using quantification comparison with conventional relative uptake evaluation (69% $\pm$ 24% vs. 44% $\pm$ 18%; P = .008). Moreover, Yoshinaga et al. (75) compared the clinical value of MBF quantification and coronary flow reserve using [^{15}O]-water PET with relative perfusion estimation using technetium-99m (^{99m}Tc) SPECT MPI. Segments with coronary stenosis without a perfusion abnormality observed by ^{99m}Tc SPECT MPI had reduced coronary flow reserve compared with remote segments (2.22 $\pm$ 0.87 vs. 2.92 $\pm$ 1.21; P <.02). These data indicate MBF quantification can add valuable information to conventional approaches. However, further investigations in a large study population are needed to fully understand the clinical utility and added value of this approach.

Endothelial Function

Coronary endothelial cells protect the coronary artery as mechanical barrier and through production of vasoactive factors, anticoagulant factors, and anti-inflammatory factors. Endothelial dysfunction is the earliest abnormality in the development of coronary atherosclerosis.

Coronary angiography or Doppler flow measurements during intracoronary administration of acetylcholine are the standard approaches for measurement of coronary endothelial function. Blood flow response is well correlated between intracoronary administration of acetylcholine and cold pressor test. The cold pressor test is also available for perfusion PET studies. It is now possible to define early stages of coronary atherosclerosis that

TABLE 11.1.2 Normal Values in Baseline Myocardial Blood Flow and Coronary Flow Reserve in Normal Subjects

Authors (ref.)	Tracer	Stress Agent	No. of Subjects	Age (Years)	MBF at Rest	MBF at Hyperemia	CFR
Camici et al. (169)	$^{13}NH_3$	Dipy	12	51 ± 8	1.0 ± 0.2	2.7 ± 0.2	2.9 ± 1.0
Chan et al. (170)	$^{13}NH_3$	ADO	20	35 ± 16	1.1 ± 0.2	4.4 ± 0.9	4.4 ± 1.5
Chan et al. (170)	$^{13}NH_3$	Dipy	20	35 ± 16	1.1 ± 0.2	4.3 ± 1.3	4.3 ± 1.9
Czernin et al. (109)	$^{13}NH_3$	Dipy	22	64 ± 9	0.9 ± 0.3	2.7 ± 0.6	3.0 ± 0.7
Beanlands et al. (100)	$^{13}NH_3$	ADO	5	27 ± 4	0.62 ± 0.09	2.51 ± 0.27	4.1 ± 0.7
Beanlands et al. (100)	$^{13}NH_3$	ADO	7	53 ± 6	0.68 ± 0.15	2.58 ± 0.68	3.7 ± 0.4
Laine et al. (143)	$H_2{}^{15}O$	Dipy	19	35 ± 3	0.8 ± 0.2	3.8 ± 1.4	4.9 ± 2.5
Kaufmann et al. (118)	$H_2{}^{15}O$	ADO	61	45 ± 7	0.8 ± 0.1	3.6 ± 1.0	4.2 ± 1.2
Yoshinaga et al. (75)	$H_2{}^{15}O$	ATP	11	57 ± 12	0.9 ± 0.1	3.6 ± 1.2	3.8 ± 1.2
Furuyama et al. (162)	$H_2{}^{15}O$	ATP	12	26 ± 3	0.79 ± 0.1	3.8 ± 1.0	4.9 ± 1.3
Lin et al. (171)	^{82}Rb	Dipy	11	44	1.15 ± 0.46	2.50 ± 0.54	—
Wassenaar et al. (172)	^{82}Rb	Dipy	15	34 ± 6	0.95 ± 0.35	3.0 ± 0.70	3.2 ± 0.8
Lortie et al. (173)	^{82}Rb	Dipy	14	31 ± 7	0.69 ± 0.14	2.83 ± 0.81	4.25 ± 1.37
Total	Weighted Mean		Total 229	42.4	0.89	3.43	3.83
	Mean			41.3	0.88	3.26	3.97

ADO, adenosine; ATP, adenosine triphosphate; CFR, coronary flow reserve; Dipy, dipyridamole; H, hydrogen; MBF, myocardial blood flow; N, nitrogen; O, oxygen; Rb, rubidium.

(Adapted from Yoshinaga K, Chow BJ, deKemp RA, et al. Application of cardiac molecular imaging using positron emission tomography in evaluation of drug and therapeutics for cardiovascular disorders. *Curr Pharm Des* 2005;11:903–932, with permission.)

demonstrate endothelial dysfunction and vascular smooth muscle dysfunction measured as impaired coronary flow reserve or using cold pressor test or pharmacological vasodilator stress using adenosine or dipyridamole. MBF usually increases 30% to 60% of resting flow in normal volunteers (Table 11.1.3). PET MBF measurements during cold pressor test show high repeatability in both normal and smokers ($r = 0.81$; $P < .0001$) (76).

ADVANCED IMAGING SYSTEMS

Integrated PET/CT

PET/CT has become widely accepted for whole-body oncology imaging because of supplemental anatomical information over metabolic information alone (77). In recent years, PET/CT also has been applied for cardiac imaging (6).

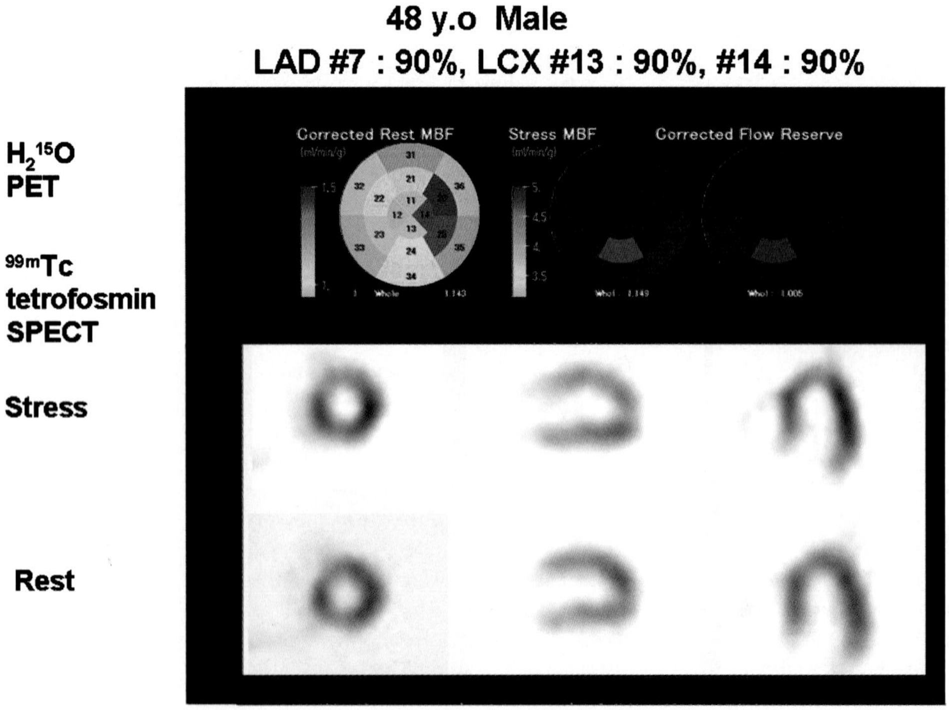

FIGURE 11.1.9. A comparison of myocardial perfusion images obtained using technetium-99m (^{99m}Tc) tetrofosmin single-photon emission computed tomography (SPECT) and oxygen-15 ([^{15}O])-water PET. Representative images from a 48-year-old man who had two-vessel coronary artery disease in left anterior descending and left circumflex arteries. The ^{99m}Tc tetrofosmin SPECT images show reversible perfusion defect in the anterior wall, while the [^{15}O]-water PET myocardial blood flow data show reduced hyperemic blood flow not only in the left anterior descending but also left circumflex territories. These abnormalities are also seen as reduced coronary flow reserve. LAD, left anterior descending; LCX, left circumflex.

TABLE 11.1.3 Mean Left Ventricle Myocardial Blood Flow Response During Cold Pressor Test in Normal Subjects

Authors (ref.)	Tracer	No. of Subjects	Age (Years)	MBF at Rest	MBF at CPT	% Change of MBF from Rest (%)
Campisi et al. (134)	$^{13}NH_3$	17	49 ± 9	0.68 ± 0.2	0.91 ± 0.18	—
Bottcher et al. (160)	$^{13}NH_3$	15	24 ± 5	0.66 ± 0.14	0.84 ± 0.25	—
Campisi et al. (174)	$^{13}NH_3$	12	22 ± 4	0.66 ± 0.14	1.03 ± 0.27	59 ± 36
Prior et al. (175)	$^{13}NH_3$	50	42 ± 13	0.64 ± 0.12	0.87 ± 0.15	39 ± 18
Furuyama et al. (162)	$H_2{}^{15}O$	12	26 ± 3	0.82 ± 0.15	1.12 ± 0.27	54 ± 26
Siegrist et al. (76)	$H_2{}^{15}O$	10	27 ± 3	0.91 ± 0.15	1.26 ± 0.07	42 ± 26
Total		116				
Weighted						
Mean			35.7	0.69	0.95	49.4
Mean			31.7	0.72	1.01	48.5

CPT, cold pressor test; H, hydrogen; MB, myocardial blood flow; N, nitrogen; O, oxygen.
(Adapted from Yoshinaga K, Chow BJ, deKemp RA, et al. Application of cardiac molecular imaging using positron emission tomography in evaluation of drug and therapeutics for cardiovascular disorders. *Curr Pharm Des* 2005;11:903–932, with permission.)

One of the advantages of cardiac PET over SPECT imaging is its better spatial resolution using attenuation correction. A germanium-68 ([^{68}Ge]) source is commonly used for the attenuation correction for the PET myocardial perfusion imaging. However, it requires a long acquisition time because of its low photon flux. One of the fundamental differences between PET/CT and conventional PET is the use of CT images for PET attenuation correction (78). Short acquisition time and lower x-ray energies of CT attenuation correction may raise concerns about the accuracy of CT-based attenuation correction. Kinahan et al. (78) reported in their phantom study that converting the CT attenuation map from an effective CT photon energy of 70 keV was comparable to the PET photon energy of 511 keV. Koepfli et al. (79) compared [^{68}Ge] and CT attenuation correction for the assessment of MBF. CT-based attenuation correction provided comparable MBF data to the conventional [^{68}Ge] attenuation correction. Thus, low-dose CT scan–based attenuation correction can provide advantages for cardiac PET/CT imaging. However, further validation studies are warranted.

PET/CT with CT angiography (CTA) can also be expected to provide coronary artery anatomy stenosis information in conjunction with the physiological perfusion data in an integrated single study (Fig. 11.1.10). Although CTA is an accurate diagnostic test,

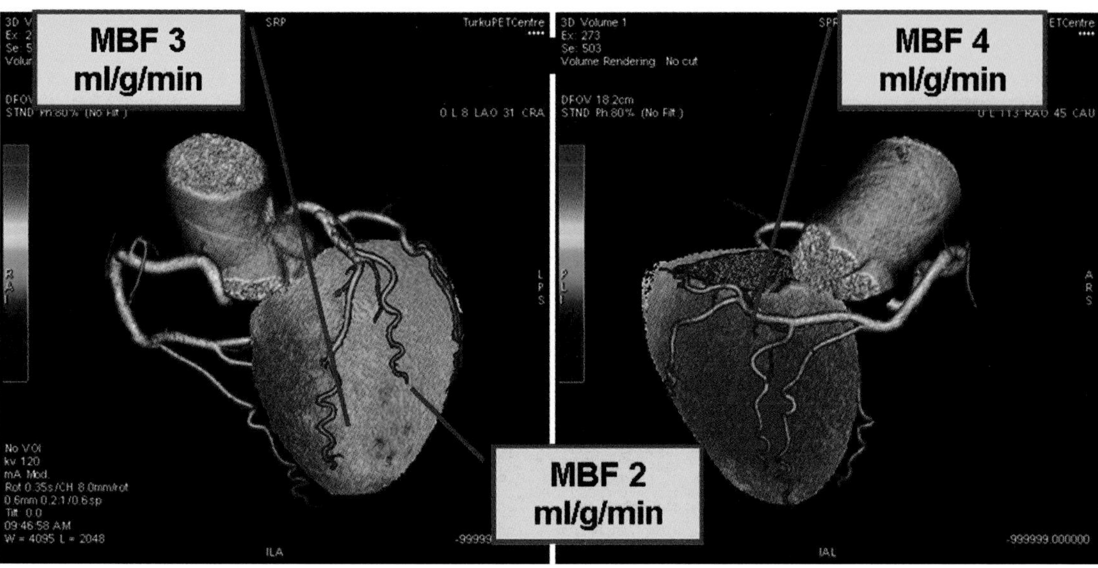

FIGURE 11.1.10. PET/CT imaging of myocardial perfusion demonstrating reduced myocardial flood flow. CTA, CT angiography; MBF, myocardial blood flow. (Courtesy of professor Juhani Knuuti and the Turku PET Center, Turku, Finland.)

especially in excluding the presence of coronary stenosis, the ability of CTA to accurately assess the degree of luminal narrowing is modest (80). Thus, myocardial perfusion imaging would be required after the CTA for considering coronary angiography and/or revascularization. Integrated approach to the diagnosis of CAD can improve sensitivity of myocardial perfusion imaging and CTA (81). Indeed, preliminary data by Di Carli et al. (82) showed 51% of patients suspected of CAD with normal [^{82}Rb] PET had some degree of coronary atherosclerosis. Namdar et al. (83) evaluated the diagnostic accuracy of PET/CT based on the diagnosis made by conventional approach such as [^{13}N]-tritium PET and coronary angiography in 25 patients with CAD. The sensitivity and specificity of this PET/CT approach were 90% and 98%, and positive and negative predictive values were 82% and 99%, respectively. Integrated anatomic and physiological information may facilitate decision making for coronary revascularization.

CLINICAL APPLICATIONS

Diagnosis in Coronary Artery Disease

Standard visual perfusion imaging assessment is based on defining regional uptake reduction relative to the maximum uptake in the heart. These so-called defects represent functionally significant CAD. This approach is applied for both PET and SPECT MPI.

Recently, the Canadian Cardiovascular Society conducted a systematic literature review for [^{82}Rb] and [^{13}N]-ammonia PET MPI in CAD diagnosis. The mean sensitivity and specificity of PET MPI were 89% and 89%, respectively, with ranges from 83% to 100% and 73% to 100% in 14 studies including a total 1,460 patients (Table 11.1.4) (33).

The diagnostic accuracy for detecting CAD with PET stress perfusion imaging has been compared to results with conventional SPECT stress perfusion imaging in the same patient population (Table 11.1.5). The first report from Tamaki et al. (84) showed similar high diagnostic accuracy for both techniques, although the image quality of the PET perfusion images was superior with better delineation of stress-induced ischemia than observed with [^{201}Tl] SPECT (Fig. 11.1.1). The other two studies, which compared [^{82}Rb] PET with [^{201}Tl] SPECT, included a greater number of patients with suspected CAD and reported higher sensitivity and specificity of PET perfusion imaging (85,86). In addition, the localization of CAD was more accurate with PET than SPECT (86). These early investigations compared PET MPI with [^{201}Tl] SPECT MPI. Today, ^{99m}Tc SPECT MPI has largely replaced [^{201}Tl] SPECT in many North American jurisdictions because ^{99m}Tc SPECT MPI has better image quality than [^{201}Tl] due to its higher photon energy. Important data from Bateman et al. (87) evaluated the diagnostic accuracy of electrocardiography (ECG)-gated [^{82}Rb] PET MPI versus ECG gated ^{99m}Tc-sestamibi SPECT in 112 MPI studies. Using a 50% threshold of coronary artery stenosis, the diagnostic accuracy was higher in PET than SPECT (P = .002). Overall, the accuracy for detection of CAD from pooled data was greater for PET versus SPECT with greater sensitivity of 90% versus 84%, specificity of 91% versus 74%, and diagnostic accuracy of 91% versus 82% (Table 11.1.5). MacIntyre et al. (88) studied the clinical outcome of patients with a false-negative [^{210}Tl] SPECT but true-positive [^{82}Rb] PET and observed that the majority were recommended for revascularization procedures.

Myocardial perfusion imaging using PET has several advantages over the conventional single-photon perfusion imaging. First, the higher sensitivity of the PET camera provides more photons from the myocardium and higher quality myocardial images. Second, accurate correction of photon attenuation can be performed with PET. This reduces attenuation artifact and makes accurate quantitative analysis of myocardial perfusion a possibility. In the future, SPECT perfusion imaging with new attenuation correction methods may also provide higher specificity and accuracy for detection of CAD. Third, the commonly used perfusion tracers, such as [^{13}N]-ammonia and generator-produced agent [^{82}Rb] have relatively high extraction fractions, which may permit detection of mild degrees of ischemia. These advantages of PET may be particularly important for the comparison of perfusion imaging with PET versus SPECT using ^{99m}Tc perfusion agents, which have a lower extraction fraction than [^{201}Tl]. Fourth, although stress perfusion abnormalities can be identified with conventional SPECT in the majority cases, the interpretation of PET perfusion images is less equivocal, possibly due to the better quality images.

Prognosis in Coronary Artery Disease

Defining prognosis in patients with suspected or known CAD is important in clinical care. Previous SPECT MPI studies have shown good prognostic value, and patients with normal stress perfusion imaging have a low hard cardiac event rate (<1% year) (34). In an early report using [^{82}Rb], PET perfusion imaging results were independent predictors of cardiac death and total cardiac events. The results of PET perfusion imaging yielded incremental prognostic information in comparison with clinical and angiographic findings alone (89). Chow et al. (90) reported a very low hard cardiac event rate (0.09%/year) in a group of patients with [^{82}Rb] PET MPI clinically reported as normal. Yoshinaga et al. (41) reported that normal PET MPI had a low hard cardiac event rate of 0.4%/year, and that a PET perfusion defect was a significant predictor for hard cardiac events including cardiac death and nonfatal myocardial infarction (Fig. 11.1.11A; Table 11.1.6). Importantly, [^{82}Rb] PET also seems to have prognostic value in patients whose diagnosis remains uncertain after SPECT MPI and obese patients (Fig. 11.1.11B). This study indicates PET MPI has prognostic value and may be useful in this important population. This incremental prognostic value is most likely due to the additional value of assessment of the physiological severity of abnormalities of myocardial perfusion and perfusion reserve by stress perfusion PET, similar to results observed with SPECT stress perfusion imaging.

Cost-effectiveness

The higher cost of PET studies with more expensive technology compared to echocardiography or SPECT raises questions about the cost-effectiveness of PET perfusion imaging. Patterson et al. (91) used a straightforward mathematical model based on Bayes theorem to compare the cost-effectiveness and utility of four diagnostic strategies using exercise ECG, stress SPECT MPI, stress PET MPI, and coronary angiography for the diagnosis of CAD. The risk, cost, and diagnostic accuracy of each test was calculated based on literature data and fitted using a management algorithm for each diagnostic strategy. PET stress MPI had the lowest cost per effect or cost per utility unit in patients with a pretest probability of less than 70%, whereas coronary angiography had the lowest cost per effect

TABLE 11.1.4 PET Coronary Artery Disease Diagnosis

Authors (ref.)	Year	Number	Stress	Tracer	Reference	Sensitivity			Specificity		
					CAG	Positive Test	Patients with CAD	%	Negative Test	Patients without CAD	%
Schelbert et al. (176)	1982	45	dipyridamole	$^{13}NH_3$	>50%	31	32	97	13	13	100
Tamaki et al. (38)	1985	25	exercise	$^{13}NH_3$	N/R	18	19	95	6	6	100
Yonekura et al. (177)	1987	50	exercise	$^{13}NH_3$	>75%	37	38	97	12	12	100
Tamaki et al. (84)	1988	51	exercise	$^{13}NH_3$	>50%	47	48	98	3	3	100
Gould et al. (178)[a]	1986	50	dipyridamole	$^{82}Rb/^{13}NH_3$	QCA SFR <3	21	22	95	9	9	100
Demer et al. (96)[a]	1989	193	dipyridamole	$^{82}Rb/^{13}NH_3$	QCA SFR<4	126	152	83	39	41	95
Go et al. (85)	1990	202	dipyridamole	^{82}Rb	>50%	142	152	93	39	50	78
Stewart et al. (86)	1991	81	dipyridamole	^{82}Rb	QCA >50%[b]	50[c]	60	84	18[c]	21	88
Marwick et al. (179)	1992	74	dipyridamole	^{82}Rb	>50%	63	70	90	4	4	100
Grover-McKay et al. (180)	1992	31	dipyridamole	^{82}Rb	>50%	16	16	100	11	15	73
Laubenbacher et al. (181)	1993	34	dipyridamole/ adenosine	$^{13}NH_3$	QCA >50%[b]	14	16	88	15	18	83
Bateman et al. (87)[d]	2006	112	dipyridamole	^{82}Rb	>50%[b]	64	74	86	38	38	100
Williams et al. (12)[e]	1994	287	dipyridamole	^{82}Rb	>67%	88	101	87	99	112	88
Simone et al. (182)[e]	1992	225	dipyridamole	^{82}Rb	>67%	—[e]	—[e]	83	—[e]	—[e]	91
Totals											
Weighted mean		1,460				696	778	89	297	333	89
Weighted mean excluding R/S						544	603	90	160	183	87
Nonweighted											
Mean								91			91

CAD, coronary artery disease; CAG, coronary angiography; H, hydrogen; N, nitrogen; N/R not reported; QCA, quantitative coronary angiography; Rb, rubidium; R/S, retrospective; SFR, stenosis flow reserve based on QCA data.

[a] Study reported that 50 patients in Gould et al. 1986 were included. Thus Gould et al. not included in mean calculations.

[b] Other cutoffs reported; >50% noted here.

[c] Derived from reported sensitivity and specificity.

[d] Electronic database, matched cohort design; values derived from reported population, sensitivity, and specificity.

[e] Retrospective study; MPI influenced CAG decision; mixed patient and region method for sensitivity/specificity; patients with disease could not be easily determined in one study.

(From Beanlands R, Chow BJ, Dick A, et al. CCS/CAR/CANM/CNCS/CanSCMR joint position statement on advanced non-invasive cardiac imaging using positron emission tomography, magnetic resonance imaging and multi-detector computed tomographic angiography in the diagnosis and evaluation of ischemic heart disease—abbreviated report. *Can J Cardiol* 2007;23:107–119; with permission.)

TABLE 11.1.5 Detection of Coronary Artery Disease with PET Versus Single-Photon Emission Computed Tomographic Imaging

				Sensitivity (%)		Specificity (%)		Accuracy (%)	
Authors (ref.)	Year	No. of Patients	Tracer	PET	SPECT	PET	SPECT	PET	SPECT
Bateman et al. (87)	2006	112	^{82}Rb vs. ^{99m}Tc	86	81	100[a]	66	91[a]	76
Stewart et al. (86)	1991	81	^{82}Rb vs. ^{201}Tl	84	84	88[a]	53	85	79
Go et al. (85)	1990	202	^{82}Rb vs. ^{201}Tl	93[a]	76	78	76	90[a]	77
Tamaki et al. (84)	1988	51	$^{13}NH_3$ vs. ^{201}T	98	96	100	100	98	96
Total		446		90	84	91	74	91	82

H, hydrogen; N, nitrogen; Rb, rubidium; SPECT, single-photon emission computed tomographic imaging; ^{99m}Tc, technetium-99m; Tl, thallium.
[a]$P < .05$ vs. SPECT.

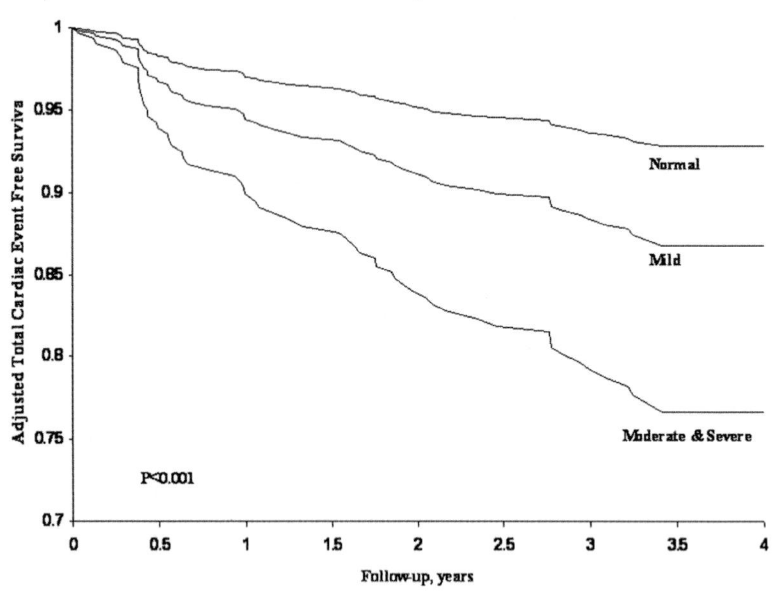

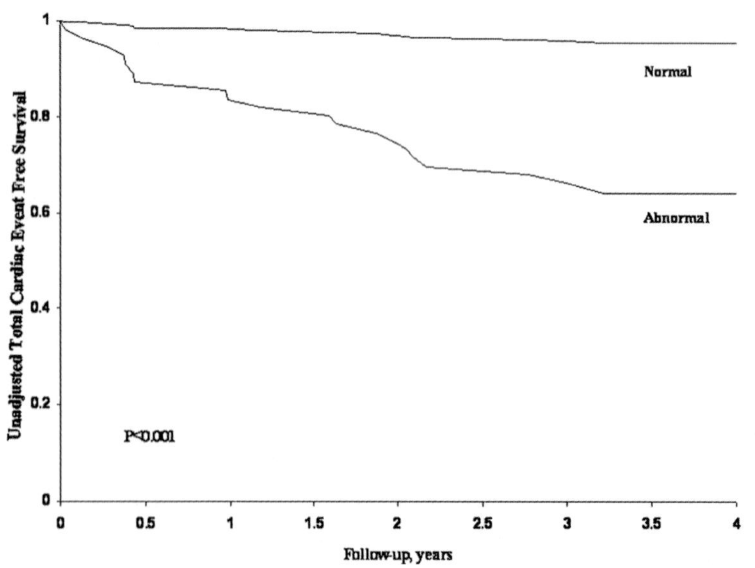

FIGURE 11.1.11. **A:** Risk-adjusted survival, free from any (total) cardiac events, as a function of summed stress score. **B:** Unadjusted survival free from any (total) cardiac events as a function of normal and abnormal summed stress score on PET myocardial perfusion imaging (MPI) in patients with obesity (body mass index ≥30 kg/m^2). (From Yoshinaga K, Chow BJ, Williams K, et al. What is the prognostic value of myocardial perfusion imaging using rubidium-82 positron emission tomography? *J Am Coll Cardiol* 2006;48:1029–1039, with permission.)

TABLE 11.1.6 PET Coronary Artery Disease Prognosis

Authors (ref.)	Year	No. of Patients	Stress	Tracer	Outcomes	Follow-up Time (Years)	Normal Scan–Annual Event Rate (%/yr)		Abnormal scan–annual Event Rate (%/yr)	
							Hard Events	Total Events	Hard Events	Total Events
Yoshinaga et al. (46)	2005	367	dipyridamole	^{82}Rb	death, MI, Rev, Hosp	3.1	0.4	1.7	mild: 2.3 mod/sev: 7.0	mild: 12.9 mod/sev: 13.2
Chow e al. (90)	2005	629	dipyridamole	^{82}Rb	death, MI, Rev, CAG	2.3	0.09	0.98	ECG +ve Normal MP: 0.6	ECG +ve Normal MP: 1.9
Marwick et al. (89)	1997	581	dipyridamole	^{82}Rb	death, MI, Rev, UAP	3.4	0.9	4	4	7
Marwick et al. (183)	1995	Prediction of perioperative and late cardiac events before vascular surgery								
MacIntrye et al. (88)	1993	Outcomes in patients with false negative thallium-201 SPECT								

CAG, coronary angiography; ECG, electrocardiogram; Hosp, hospitalized; MI, myocardial infarction; MP, myocardial perfusion; Rb, rubidium; Rev, revascularization; UAP, unstable angina

(From Beanlands R, Chow BJ, Dick A, et al. CCS/CAR/CANM/CNCS/CanSCMR joint position statement on advanced non-invasive cardiac imaging using positron emission tomography, magnetic resonance imaging and multi-detector computed tomographic angiography in the diagnosis and evaluation of ischemic heart disease—abbreviated report. *Can J Cardiol* 2007;23:107–119, with permission.)

in patients with a pretest probability of more than 70%. The relative savings of PET perfusion imaging was related to the high specificity. Using the PET strategy may reduce unnecessary coronary angiography. Furthermore, a high fraction of stress treadmill tests had undetermined results and may lead to greater number of unnecessary coronary angiograms. PET perfusion imaging appears to be the method of choice for detection of CAD in centers with access to both PET and SPECT. However, improved specificity for detecting CAD may be possible with SPECT imaging due to the recent development of attenuation correction and the addition of functional assessment with gated acquisitions.

In a decision-analysis study including a comprehensive literature review, Maddahi and Gambhir (92) showed that exercise ECG, followed by PET or SPECT if the stress was positive, was the most cost-effective approach for patients with low pretest likelihood of disease. For intermediate-risk patients, performing PET or SPECT first was the most cost-effective approach; while in high-risk patients direct angiography was best first test (similar to Patterson et al. [91]). Thus PET appears in some, but not all studies, to be a cost-effective approach for patients with intermediate pretest likelihood of CAD.

Assessment of Myocardial Blood Flow Reserve in Coronary Artery Disease

Quantitative measurements of MBF reserve with PET MPI provide a noninvasive means to determine the functional severity of coronary stenosis. Although coronary angiography defines stenosis severity on the basis of morphologic alterations, the measurement of MBF or flow reserve represents a more physiological evaluation of cellular perfusion as the net result of antegrade epicardial coronary flow and collateral circulation. Gould et al. (93,94) described the value of MBF reserve as a measure of the functional severity of CAD. Although MBF at rest remains normal during the progression of coronary lesions until there is a 80% to 85% diameter stenosis, coronary flow reserve begins to decrease at 40% to 50% diameter stenosis (95). In contrast to coronary flow measurement by invasive Doppler flow wire, PET provides three-dimensional information about MBF and flow reserve and facilitates easy assessment of the extent of perfusion abnormalities.

Demer et al. (96) first reported a significant relationship between the severity of relative perfusion abnormalities on PET perfusion images and coronary flow reserve measurements from quantitative coronary angiography. Uren et al. (97) showed a relationship between coronary artery stenosis on angiography and coronary flow reserve data obtained by [^{15}O]-labeled water PET perfusion studies. A similar relationship was also described with [^{13}N]-ammonia PET perfusion data (98,99). Despite a significant correlation between the severity of coronary stenosis and coronary flow reserve in these studies, there was considerable scatter between the two parameters. A quantitative measurement of coronary stenosis may possibly provide closer correlation. On the other hand, there seems to be inherent differences between the anatomical stenosis on angiography and functional coronary flow reserve on PET, such as accounting for collateral flow. In a study of patients with single vessel disease, coronary flow and flow reserve were significantly decreased in the remote areas supplied with no significant stenosis in patients compared to normal subjects. Quantitative measurement of MBF by PET may be a more sensitive method than coronary angiography to detect altered coronary flow dynamics in patients with CAD (100). Conversely, quantitative measurements of MBF with PET may provide high sensitivity but low specificity for detecting significant CAD (when coronary stenosis was used as a gold standard in the study of high-risk CAD). Since myocardial flow reserve reflects the functional status of tissue flow, this parameter may be discordant with the anatomical stenosis of major coronary arteries (101).

A number of other factors, such as collateral circulation (102,103) and endothelial modulation of vascular smooth muscle tone (104,105), may play major roles to determine the coronary flow reserve measured by PET study. Atherosclerosis may introduce potential variability in the behavior of both the epicardial coronary vessels and the coronary resistance vessels. A coronary stenosis in a patient may not produce a fixed degree of anatomic narrowing of the epicardial artery, and the resistance vessels may not undergo maximal vasodilatation in the response to pharmacologic vasodilators. Thus, interpretation of coronary flow reserve may require consideration of dynamic characteristics of both epicardial coronary artery and resistance vessels.

Altered MBF and flow reserve may be much more extensive than angiographic documentation of regional CAD. Accordingly, PET has been used to detect the early stages of vascular alterations and to monitor response to therapy. Van Tosh et al. (106) reported regions of abnormal flow reserve with [^{82}Rb] PET imaging and dipyridamole stress in the areas of restenosis after angioplasty. In addition, PET perfusion imaging has been used to delineate the efficacy of interventional therapies (21,107,108). Thus, PET can be used to objectively identify the patients who would benefit and recover their functional flow reserve.

Coronary Flow Reserve in Relation to Coronary Risk Factors and Evaluation of Therapies

A number of risk factors associated with atherosclerosis may cause a reduction of coronary flow reserve despite angiographically normal coronary arteries. PET has been extensively used to investigate the relationship of coronary flow reserve and such risk factors for CAD, including hypercholesterolemia, diabetes, smoking, and hypertension.

Coronary flow reserve is a complex physiological parameter influenced by many factors other than coronary artery stenosis. For example, coronary flow reserve may slightly decrease with age mainly due to increased workload at rest rather than abnormal vasodilator capacity (109,110). PET perfusion studies have demonstrated reduction of flow reserve in many cardiac disorders without evidence of CAD. About 10% to 30% of patients with chest pain who undergo cardiac catheterization are found to have angiographic normal coronary arteries. However, PET perfusion studies indicated about 40% to 50% of those patients showed high flow at rest and impaired flow reserve in response to dipyridamole (111,112).

Hyperlipidemia and Lipid Lowering Therapy

Dayanikli et al. (113) first described a linear relationship between coronary flow measurement and serum cholesterol levels in asymptomatic patients with high risk for developing CAD. Yokoyama et al. (114,115) confirmed these results by describing reduction of coronary flow reserve in asymptomatic patients with familial hypercholesterolemia. A significant inverse correlation was demonstrated between total cholesterol and coronary flow reserve in individual patients. Pitkanen et al. (116,117) showed a significant reduction of coronary flow reserve in patients less than 40 years of age with familial hypercholesterolemia in comparison to an age-matched control population. The baseline MBF was similar between the two groups, but the flow at maximal vasodilatation was 29% lower in patients with hypercholesterolemia than the healthy control subjects. As well, reduction of coronary flow reserve was related to lipid phenotype (116). Kaufmann et al. (118) showed a reduction of coronary flow reserve in patients with hypercholesterolemia and demonstrated that low-density lipoprotein cholesterol, but not total cholesterol, correlated inversely with coronary flow reserve in these patients. Mellwig et al. (119) showed the acute improvement of coronary vasodilatation capacity by single low-density lipoprotein (LDL) apheresis.

A number of large clinical trials have shown that lipid lowering therapy using statins (hydroxymethyl glutaryl-coenzyme A. [HMG-CoA] reductase inhibitors), reduces cardiovascular events in both primary and secondary preventions. The clinical benefits of statin therapy are considered to be mediated by the stabilization of atherosclerotic plaques and the improvement in endothelial function. Gould et al. (120) showed that short-term cholesterol lowering therapy decreased the size and severity of PET perfusion abnormalities in patients with CAD. Guethlin et al. (121) evaluated the coronary flow reserve before, at 3 months, and 6 months after initiation of therapy with fluvastatin. All patients showed significant reduction of cholesterol, LDL, and triglycerides early after therapy. Coronary flow reserve did not increase with 3 months of therapy but increased only after 6 months of therapy. These findings are in agreement with the evaluation of endothelial function with quantitative coronary angiography and acetylcholine injection (122). Similar improvement in coronary flow reserve has been reported after cholesterol-lowering treatment using simvastatin (123–125).

Lifestyle Modification Including Exercise Training

Czernin et al. (126) evaluated the effect of short-term cardiovascular conditioning such as combination of exercise training and low-fat diet on MBF and flow reserve in middle-aged volunteers. MBF reserve increased in association with an improvement in exercise capacity and serum lipid profiles. Yoshinaga et al. (23) evaluated the effect of exercise training effect on regional MBF in patients with stable CAD. The exercise training increased hyperemic MBF in diseased segments compared to sedentary lifestyle group (percentage of increase in MBF: 12.5% ± 22.1% vs. 2.6% ± 16.3%; $P = .02$). These data may indicate favorable evidence to support the effect of exercise training on MBF to ischemic myocardium.

Diabetes Mellitus

Diabetes mellitus and impaired glucose tolerance are well-established risk factors for coronary atherosclerosis and increase cardiovascular event risk. Alteration of coronary flow reserve has also been demonstrated in patients with diabetes. Yokoyama et al. (127,128) showed a significant reduction of coronary flow reserve in noninsulin-dependent diabetes compared to age-matched control subjects. The coronary flow reserve values were comparable between the diet and medication therapy groups. Coronary flow reserve was inversely correlated with average hemoglobin A_{1c} and hyperglycemia for 5 years but not lipid fractions or insulin resistance. Di Carli et al. (129) confirmed the reduction of coronary flow reserve in diabetic patients and also showed a decreased myocardial flow response to cold pressor in diabetics with sympathetic nerve dysfunction over those without dysfunction. These results are consistent with previous reports showing a reduction of angiographic coronary vasodilator capacity in human diabetes (130,131).

Acute administration of insulin has been shown to improve regional MBF and hyperemic blood flow in ischemic myocardium in patients with type 2 diabetes and CAD (132). These data suggest that insulin improves endothelial function and increases the threshold of ischemia in this population.

Prior et al. (133) evaluated endothelial dysfunction in patients with insulin resistance, impaired glucose tolerance, and diabetes mellitus. The magnitude of this endothelial dysfunction is associated with severity of insulin resistance.

Cigarette Smoking

Cigarette smoke may alter the vascular endothelium via oxidative stress. Czernin et al. (126) evaluated the acute effect of smoking on myocardial vasculature reactivity to vasodilator stimulation. Short-term smoking markedly reduced coronary flow reserve from 3.4 ± 0.8 at baseline to 2.3 ± 0.3 after smoking in smokers. On the other hand, MBF and flow reserve were similar in young, long-term smokers and age-matched healthy nonsmokers. Campisi et al. (134) demonstrated an altered response of MBF during a cold pressor test, despite normal coronary flow reserve in long-term smokers. This suggests long-term smokers have endothelial dysfunction. Furthermore, even in young smokers, coronary endothelial function may already be blunted (135). On the other hand, Morita et al. (136) reported relatively short-term (1-month) smoking cessation restored coronary endothelial function, and this effect was retained 6 months after smoking cessation in young smokers. These results support the reports of endothelial dysfunction in brachial and coronary arteries in long-term smokers and even passive smokers (137–139).

Antioxidants Therapy for Smokers

Since coronary dysfunction may be partly caused by increased oxidative stress, a number of trials have attempted to improve coronary vasomotor tone by use of antioxidants such as vitamin C and L-arginine. Kaufmann et al. (68) demonstrated that acute administration of vitamin C restored coronary microcirculatory responsiveness and coronary flow reserve in smokers, suggesting that the altered coronary circulation in smokers may be partly accounted for by increased oxidative stress. Acute administration of L-arginine also restored blunted MBF response to cold pressor test in long-term smokers (140).

Hypertension and Antihypertensive Therapy

Arterial hypertension often causes reduced coronary flow reserve. Hypertension with and without left ventricular hypertrophy reduces coronary flow reserve by altering the coronary vasculature and resistance (141,142). Laine et al. (143) demonstrated a reduced coronary flow reserve in young patients with borderline hypertension with no clinical signs of angina or left ventricular hypertrophy. Since resting MBF was unchanged, this reduction of coronary flow reserve may be dependent on impaired maximal vasodilator capacity. Gistri et al. (144) reported improvement in the altered flow reserve after verapamil treatment of hypertension, indicating reversible reduction of coronary flow reserve in these patients. Short-term intravenous angiotensin-converting inhibitors administration improves hyperemic blood flow and flow reserve in ischemic segments (145). Akinboboye et al. (146) compared the long-term treatment effects with angiotensin-converting inhibitors and angiotensin receptor blockers in patients with hypertension and left ventricular hypertrophy. Angiotensin-converting inhibitors improved hyperemic MBF and coronary flow reserve but angiotensin receptor blockers did not.

Endothelial Dysfunction in Patients Who Have Coronary Risk Factors

Coronary endothelial dysfunction is one of the earliest abnormalities to be seen in the development of CAD. Endothelial dysfunction is considered to be associated with future cardiac events. Schindler et al. (147) evaluated the prognostic value of MBF response during a cold pressor test using PET MPI. The blunted blood flow response was associated with cardiovascular events (log-rank test, $P = .033$) and tended to be an independent cardiovascular event risk factor. Altered endothelial function was associated with systemic microinflammation such as elevated C-reactive protein in patients who had coronary risk factors without overt coronary stenosis (148).

PET PERFUSION IMAGING IN NONATHEROSCLEROTIC HEART DISEASE

Hypertrophic and Dilated Cardiomyopathy

In patients with hypertrophic cardiomyopathy, Camici et al. (149) showed decreased coronary flow reserve with dipyridamole stress not only in the hypertrophic septal wall but also in lateral free wall, suggesting that reductions in coronary flow reserve was not a consequence of hypertrophy. They also described subendocardial hypoperfusion following dipyridamole administration (150). Altered coronary microvascular function is strongly associated with poor outcomes including death, progression of functional class, and ventricular arrhythmias in patients with hypertrophic cardiomyopathy (151).

In patients with dilated cardiomyopathy, Parodi et al. (152) reported global reduction of coronary flow reserve with dipyridamole infusion. This coronary flow reduction is seen in the subclinical stage of cardiomyopathy and may be due to a microvascular abnormality in these patients. Neglia et al. (153) reported lower resting flow with decreased flow reserve in patients with dilated cardiomyopathy without overt heart failure.

Valvular Heart Disease

Aortic stenosis with left ventricular hypertrophy is accompanied by coronary microcirculatory dysfunction. Rajappan et al. (154) observed that the subendocardial coronary flow reserve was lower than subepicardial coronary flow reserve (1.43 ± 0.33 vs. 1.78 ± 0.35; $P = .01$) in patients with aortic stenosis and normal coronary arteries. There were logarithmic relationships between hemodynamic load of the left ventricle and either subendocardial or epicardial coronary flow reserve. Coronary flow reserve improved after valve replacement, and the change in coronary flow reserve was correlated with an increase in aortic valve area and diastolic perfusion time during hyperemia postdipyridamole (155). As expected, left ventricular hypertrophy causes a greater degree of microcirculatory dysfunction in the subendocardium, which may be associated with left ventricular hemodynamics and diastolic perfusion time. This approach clarified the mechanism of angina in patients with aortic stenosis, which is difficult to detect by other standard diagnostic methods. Preliminary work also suggests that alterations in flow may help distinguish true low-flow, low-gradient aortic stenosis from pseudoaortic stenosis in patients with severe ventricular dysfunction (156).

Heart Transplant

In patients with cardiac transplantation, Rechavia et al. (157) demonstrated higher resting MBF with reduction of coronary flow reserve. Chan et al. (158) described a decrease in hyperemic flow with an increase in resting flow in excess of cardiac work in patients with transplant rejection. During a follow-up study after successful treatment, patients with transplant rejection had significant improvement, suggesting the role and possible importance of serial noninvasive flow measurements by PET.

Cardiac allograft vasculopathy is a diffuse and obliterate form of arteriosclerosis, which is a chief determinant of long-term outcomes after cardiac transplantation. Kofoed et al. (159) reported hyperemic MBF was lower in patients who had cardiac transplant than control and was inversely related to maximal intimal thickness. This finding suggests the potential use of PET using blood flow measurements to identify noninvasively patients at risk for allograft vasculopathy.

Syndrome X

Syndrome X is defined as a heart disease associated with chest pain with ischemic ECG changes but normal coronary arteries. Camici et al. (111) first reported the reduction of coronary flow reserve in 30% of patients with syndrome X with no correlation of alteration of coronary blood flow with ECG or other signs of ischemia. Bottcher et al. (160) found preserved microcirculatory endothelial function but markedly attenuated hyperemic flow in these patients. Conversely, Rosen et al. (161) studied 29 patients with syndrome X and 20 age-matched normal controls and found no differences of coronary flow reserve after correction of rate pressure product.

Myocardial Perfusion Imaging in Pediatrics

Muzik et al. (162) found reduced hyperemic flow and coronary flow reserve but normal resting blood flow in patients with a history of Kawasaki disease and normal epicardial coronary arteries. This reduction of coronary flow reserve may be the result of inflammation of the coronary arteries. Furuyama et al. (163) also reported reduced coronary flow reserve in regressed aneurysmal regions compared to controls (3.53 ± 0.95 vs. 4.60 ± 1.14; $P < .05$).

Impaired flow reserve has been observed in an anomalous origin of the left coronary artery (164) (Fig. 11.1.5). Coronary flow reserve has also been assessed in long-term survivors of repair of this rare congenital disorder. There is association with poor LV function due to inadequate coronary flow resulting in myocardial infarction or ischemic cardiomyopathy. After surgical repair to establish blood flow to the left coronary arteries from the aorta, dramatic improvement in LV function is seen. However, PET perfusion imaging has shown reduced coronary flow reserve in these patients after the repair, which may contribute to impaired exercise performance by limited cardiac output reserve (165).

Singh et al. (166) studied the coronary flow reserve in long-term survivors with transposition of the great arteries after the atrial switch operation (Mustard operation). Coronary flow reserve was reduced in these patients compared to healthy control subjects, suggesting possible systemic ventricular dysfunction in these patients. Hauser et al. (167) compared MBF and flow reserve in the patients who received the atrial switch operation to patients with pulmonary autograft aortic valve replacement (Ross operation). Patients with the atrial switch operation had stress-induced perfusion defects with attenuated coronary flow reserve. Although the long-term prognosis remains unclear in these patients after surgery of the congenital heart disease, PET may provide important information of myocardial perfusion and flow reserve and may predict cardiac dysfunction.

ASSESSMENT OF NEW THERAPIES

The recent development of new treatments for improving impaired myocardial perfusion have created the need for noninvasive and quantitative measurements of MBF using PET to confirm the improvement with these therapies. One of the most exciting areas is gene therapy for neovascularization in severe CAD.

A number of studies have been focused on imaging of reporter gene expression (168,184). In addition, to the imaging of genotype expression, the actual improvement on myocardial perfusion have been well demonstrated by SPECT imaging (185). Bengel et al. (186) successfully imaged gene expression in a pig study and showed mild increase in rest regional MBF in reporter gene injection sites compared with remote regions (0.99 ± 0.23 vs. 0.85 ± 0.26 mL/min^{-1}/g^{-1}; $P = .045$) using [^{13}N] ammonia PET. This may represent adenovirus-induced inflammatory reaction (186).

Cardiac Stem Cell Therapy

Cell transplantation represents a novel therapeutic approach for the treatment of acute myocardial infarction and end-stage heart disease for human. Initial studies have focused on assessment of cell tracking and cell survival. Thus, these early studies have been performed by FDG PET or SPECT MPI (187). Stem cells labeled with FDG may allow short-term tracking. (187). Further investigations evaluating transplanted cell survival and improved cell function are needed.

Cardiac Resynchronization Therapy

Cardiac resynchronization therapy simultaneously stimulates both ventricles and can optimize contractile synchrony. Knaapen et al. (188) reported cardiac resynchronization therapy changed inhomogeneous rest blood flow distribution to homogeneous distribution, which was evaluated as septal-to-lateral MBF ratio (0.77 ± 0.27 to 0.97 ± 0.34; $P = .049$), and improved blunted hyperemic global MBF (1.91 ± 1.03 to 2.66 ± 1.66 mL/min^{-1}/g^{-1}; $P = .013$) in patients with dilated cardiomyopathy accompanied with wide QRS complex. Reduced wall stress and increased diastolic perfusion time may improve the global hyperemic MBF.

SUMMARY

PET myocardial perfusion imaging provides accurate evaluation of regional MBF at rest and during stress. The role of PET myocardial perfusion imaging is now well established for diagnosis of CAD. Recent data have shown prognostic value of PET myocardial perfusion imaging in patients with suspected CAD. In the past, widespread clinical use has been limited by the cost of the technology and access to the radiotracers. However, clinical use is increasing as the expense of PET instrumentation decreases, and both cyclotrons and generator-produced radiotracers become more widely available. This trend is expected to continue.

PET perfusion imaging is the most validated noninvasive method for quantification of absolute MBF and flow reserve. PET imaging also has been applied for endothelial function measurements capable of defining early stage coronary arteriosclerosis. The ability of PET to quantify absolute perfusion provides a new dimension in addition to the traditional applications of standard perfusion imaging. Recent developments of integrated PET/CT now provide a new means for attenuation correction but also the capability to evaluate coronary function and anatomy together. More studies are needed to determine whether this hybrid approach will help optimize clinical decision making for therapy selection and whether this will improve patient outcomes. PET remains an ideal research tool for the study of the pathophysiology of CAD and other cardiac diseases. PET is also well suited for the evaluation of treatment acutely and longitudinally and will be very useful in the future as new therapies continue to develop.

ACKNOWLEDGMENTS

The authors thank Dr. Osamu Manabe and Sherri Nipius for their help in preparing this chapter.

REFERENCES

1. Bergmann SR. Cardiac positron emission tomography. *Semin Nucl Med* 1998;28:320–340.
2. Schelbert HR. Current status and prospects of new radionuclides and radiopharmaceuticals for cardiovascular nuclear medicine. *Semin Nucl Med* 1987;17:145–181.
3. Schwaiger M, Ziegler S, Bengel F. Assessment of myocardial blood flow with positron emission tomography. In: Pohost G, O'Rourke RA, Berman DS, eds. *Radionuclide-based methods/nuclear cardiology*. Philadelphia: Lippincott Williams & Wilkins, 2000:195–212.
4. Tamaki N. PET perfusion tracer. In: Taillefer R, Tamaki N, eds. *New radiotracers in cardiac imaging: principles and applications*. Stanford, CT: Appleton & Lange, 1999:213–227.
5. Camici PG. Positron emission tomography and myocardial imaging. *Heart* 2000;83:475–480.
6. Schwaiger M, Ziegler S, Nekolla SG. PET/CT: challenge for nuclear cardiology. *J Nucl Med* 2005;46:1664–178.
7. Yoshinaga K, Chow BJ, deKemp RA, et al. Application of cardiac molecular imaging using positron emission tomography in evaluation of drug and therapeutics for cardiovascular disorders. *Curr Pharm Des* 2005;11:903–932.
8. Schelbert HR, Phelps ME, Hoffman EJ, et al. Regional myocardial perfusion assessed with N-13 labeled ammonia and positron emission computerized axial tomography. *Am J Cardiol* 1979;43:209–218.
9. Schelbert HR, Phelps ME, Huang SC, et al. N-13 ammonia as an indicator of myocardial blood flow. *Circulation* 1981;63:1259–1272.

10. Krivokapich J, Huang SC, Phelps ME, et al. Dependence of $^{13}NH_3$ myocardial extraction and clearance on flow and metabolism. *Am J Physiol* 1982;242:H536–H542.
11. Alvarez-Diez TM, deKemp R, Beanlands R, et al. Manufacture of strontium-82/rubidium-82 generators and quality control of rubidium-82 chloride for myocardial perfusion imaging in patients using positron emission tomography. *Appl Radiat Isot* 1999;50:1015–1023.
12. Williams BR, Mullani NA, Jansen DE, et al. A retrospective study of the diagnostic accuracy of a community hospital-based PET center for the detection of coronary artery disease using rubidium-82. *J Nucl Med* 1994;35:1586–1592.
13. Mullani NA, Gould KL. First-pass measurements of regional blood flow with external detectors. *J Nucl Med* 1983;24:577–581.
14. Nishiyama H, Sodd VJ, Adolph RJ, et al. Intercomparison of myocardial imaging agents: ^{201}Ti, ^{129}Cs, ^{43}K, and ^{81}Rb. *J Nucl Med* 1976;17: 880–889.
15. Mullani NA, Goldstein RA, Gould KL, et al. Myocardial perfusion with rubidium-82. I. Measurement of extraction fraction and flow with external detectors. *J Nucl Med* 1983;24:898–906.
16. Ziegler WH, Goresky CA. Kinetics of rubidium uptake in the working dog heart. *Circ Res* 1971;29:208–220.
17. Wilson RA, Shea M, Landsheere CD, et al. Rubidium-82 myocardial uptake and extraction after transient ischemia: PET characteristics. *J Comput Assist Tomogr* 1987;11:60–66.
18. Gould KL, Yoshida K, Hess MJ, et al. Myocardial metabolism of fluorodeoxyglucose compared to cell membrane integrity for the potassium analogue rubidium-82 for assessing infarct size in man by PET. *J Nucl Med* 1991;32:1–9.
19. deKemp RA, Ruddy TD, Hewitt T, et al. Detection of serial changes in absolute myocardial perfusion with ^{82}Rb PET. *J Nucl Med* 2000;41: 1426–1435.
20. Parkash R, deKemp RA, Ruddy TD, et al. Potential utility of rubidium 82 PET quantification in patients with 3-vessel coronary artery disease. *J Nucl Cardiol* 2004;11:440–449.
21. Scott NS, Le May MR, de Kemp R, et al. Evaluation of myocardial perfusion using rubidium-82 positron emission tomography after myocardial infarction in patients receiving primary stent implantation or thrombolytic therapy. *Am J Cardiol* 2001;88:886–889.
22. Yoshida K, Mullani N, Gould KL. Coronary flow and flow reserve by PET simplified for clinical applications using rubidium-82 or nitrogen-13-ammonia. *J Nucl Med* 1996;37:1701–1712.
23. Yoshinaga K, Beanlands RS, Dekemp RA, et al. Effect of exercise training on myocardial blood flow in patients with stable coronary artery disease. *Am Heart J* 2006;151:1324.
24. Green MA, Mathias CJ, Welch MJ, et al. Copper-62-labeled pyruvaldehyde bis(N4-methylthiosemicarbazonato)copper(II): synthesis and evaluation as a positron emission tomography tracer for cerebral and myocardial perfusion. *J Nucl Med* 1990;31:1989–1996.
25. Shelton ME, Green MA, Mathias CJ, et al. Assessment of regional myocardial and renal blood flow with copper-PTSM and positron emission tomography. *Circulation* 1990;82:990–997.
26. Beanlands RS, Muzik O, Mintun M, et al. The kinetics of copper-62-PTSM in the normal human heart. *J Nucl Med* 1992;33:684–690.
27. Wallhaus TR, Lacy J, Whang J, et al. Human biodistribution and dosimetry of the PET perfusion agent copper-62-PTSM. *J Nucl Med* 1998;39:1958–1964.
28. Mathias CJ, Bergmann SR, Green MA. Development and validation of a solvent extraction technique for determination of Cu-PTSM in blood. *Nucl Med Biol* 1993;20:343–349.
29. Beanlands RS, Muzik O, Hutchins GD, et al.. Heterogeneity of regional nitrogen 13-labeled ammonia tracer distribution in the normal human heart: comparison with rubidium 82 and copper 62-labeled PTSM. *J Nucl Cardiol* 1994;1:225–235.
30. Herscovitch P, Raichle ME, Kilbourn MR, et al. Positron emission tomographic measurement of cerebral blood flow and permeability-surface area product of water using [^{15}O]water and [^{11}C]butanol. *J Cereb Blood Flow Metab* 1987;7:527–542.
31. Kabalka GW, Lambrecht RM, Sajjad M, et al. Synthesis of ^{15}O-labeled butanol via organoborane chemistry. *Int J Appl Radiat Isot* 1985;36: 853–855.
32. Madar I, Ravert HT, Du Y, et al. Characterization of uptake of the new PET imaging compound ^{18}F-fluorobenzyl triphenyl phosphonium in dog myocardium. *J Nucl Med* 2006;47:1359–1366.
33. Beanlands R, Chow BJ, Dick A, et al. CCS/CAR/CANM/CNCS/CanSCMR joint position statement on advanced non-invasive cardiac imaging using positron emission tomography, magnetic resonance imaging and multi-detector computed tomographic angiography in the diagnosis and evaluation of ischemic heart disease—abbreviated report. *Can J Cardiol* 2007;23:107–119.
34. Klocke FJ, Baird MG, Lorell BH, et al. ACC/AHA/ASNC guidelines for the clinical use of cardiac radionuclide imaging—executive summary: a report of the American College of Cardiology/American Heart Association Task Force on Practice Guidelines (ACC/AHA/ASNC Committee to Revise the 1995 Guidelines for the Clinical Use of Cardiac Radionuclide Imaging). *J Am Coll Cardiol* 2003;42:1318–1333.
35. Machac J, Bacharach SL, Bateman TM, et al. Positron emission tomography myocardial perfusion and glucose metabolism imaging. *J Nucl Cardiol* 2006;13:e121–151.
36. American Society of Nuclear Cardiology. Imaging guidelines for nuclear cardiology procedures, part 2. *J Nucl Cardiol* 1999;6:G47–G84.
37. Chow BJ, Beanlands RS, Lee A, et al. Treadmill exercise produces larger perfusion defects than dipyridamole stress N-13 ammonia positron emission tomography. *J Am Coll Cardiol* 2006;47:411–416.
38. Tamaki N, Yonekura Y, Senda M, et al. Myocardial positron computed tomography with ^{13}N-ammonia at rest and during exercise. *Eur J Nucl Med* 1985;11:246–251.
39. Wyss CA, Koepfli P, Mikolajczyk K, et al. Bicycle exercise stress in PET for assessment of coronary flow reserve: repeatability and comparison with adenosine stress. *J Nucl Med* 2003;44:146–154.
40. Chow BJ, Ananthasubramaniam K, deKemp RA, et al. Comparison of treadmill exercise versus dipyridamole stress with myocardial perfusion imaging using rubidium-82 positron emission tomography. *J Am Coll Cardiol* 2005;45:1227–1234.
41. Yoshinaga K, Chow BJ, Williams K, et al. What is the prognostic value of myocardial perfusion imaging using rubidium-82 positron emission tomography? *J Am Coll Cardiol* 2006;48:1029–1039.
42. Herrero P, Markham J, Shelton ME, et al. Implementation and evaluation of a two-compartment model for quantification of myocardial perfusion with rubidium-82 and positron emission tomography. *Circ Res* 1992;70:496–507.
43. Herrero P, Markham J, Shelton ME, et al. Noninvasive quantification of regional myocardial perfusion with rubidium-82 and positron emission tomography. Exploration of a mathematical model. *Circulation* 1990;82:1377–1386.
44. Hendel RC, Wackers FJ, Berman DS, et al. American Society of Nuclear Cardiology consensus statement: reporting of radionuclide myocardial perfusion imaging studies. *J Nucl Cardiol* 2003;10:705–708.
45. Schelbert HR, Beanlands R, Bengel F, et al. PET myocardial perfusion and glucose metabolism imaging: part 2—guidelines for interpretation and reporting. *J Nucl Cardiol* 2003;10:557–571.
46. Yoshinaga K, Chow BJ, deKemp RA, et al. Prognostic value of rubidium-82 perfusion positron emission tomography in patients referred after SPECT imaging. *J Nucl Cardiol* 2005;12:S43.
47. Berman DS, Abidov A, Kang X, et al. Prognostic validation of a 17-segment score derived from a 20-segment score for myocardial perfusion SPECT interpretation. *J Nucl Cardiol* 2004;11:414–423.
48. Iida H, Rhodes CG, de Silva R, et al. Use of the left ventricular time-activity curve as a noninvasive input function in dynamic oxygen-15-water positron emission tomography. *J Nucl Med* 1992;33:1669–1677.

49. Weinberg IN, Huang SC, Hoffman EJ, et al. Validation of PET-acquired input functions for cardiac studies. *J Nucl Med* 1988;29:241–247.
50. Nienaber CA, Ratib O, Gambhir SS, et al. A quantitative index of regional blood flow in canine myocardium derived noninvasively with N-13 ammonia and dynamic positron emission tomography. *J Am Coll Cardiol* 1991;17:260–269.
51. Hutchins GD, Schwaiger M, Rosenspire KC, et al. Noninvasive quantification of regional blood flow in the human heart using N-13 ammonia and dynamic positron emission tomographic imaging. *J Am Coll Cardiol* 1990;15:1032–1042.
52. Iida H, Kanno I, Takahashi A, et al. Measurement of absolute myocardial blood flow with $H_2{}^{15}O$ and dynamic positron-emission tomography. Strategy for quantification in relation to the partial-volume effect. *Circulation* 1988;78:104–115.
53. Bol A, Melin JA, Vanoverschelde JL, et al. Direct comparison of [^{13}N]ammonia and [^{15}O]water estimates of perfusion with quantification of regional myocardial blood flow by microspheres. *Circulation* 1993;87:512–525.
54. Kuhle WG, Porenta G, Huang SC, et al. Quantification of regional myocardial blood flow using ^{13}N-ammonia and reoriented dynamic positron emission tomographic imaging. *Circulation* 1992;86:1004–1017.
55. Muzik O, Beanlands RS, Hutchins GD, et al. Validation of nitrogen-13-ammonia tracer kinetic model for quantification of myocardial blood flow using PET. *J Nucl Med* 1993;34:83–91.
56. Bellina CR, Parodi O, Camici P, et al. Simultaneous in vitro and in vivo validation of nitrogen 13 ammonia for the assessment of regional myocardial blood flow. *J Nucl Med* 1990;31:1335–1343.
57. Shah A, Schelbert HR, Schwaiger M, et al. Measurement of regional myocardial blood flow with N-13 ammonia and positron-emission tomography in intact dogs. *J Am Coll Cardiol* 1985;5:92–100.
58. Choi Y, Huang SC, Hawkins RA, et al. A simplified method for quantification of myocardial blood flow using nitrogen-13-ammonia and dynamic PET. *J Nucl Med* 1993;34:488–497.
59. Tadamura E, Tamaki N, Yonekura Y, et al. Assessment of coronary vasodilator reserve by N-13 ammonia PET using the microsphere method and Patlak plot analysis. *Ann Nucl Med* 1995;9:109–118.
60. Bergmann SR, Fox KA, Rand AL, et al. Quantification of regional myocardial blood flow in vivo with $H_2{}^{15}O$. *Circulation* 1984;70:724–733.
61. Kety SS. The theory and applications of the exchange of inert gas at the lungs and tissues. *Pharmacol Rev* 1951;3:1–41.
62. Walsh MN, Bergmann SR, Steele RL, et al. Delineation of impaired regional myocardial perfusion by positron emission tomography with $H_2(^{15})O$. *Circulation* 1988;78:612–620.
63. Henze E, Huang SC, Ratib O, et al. Measurements of regional tissue and blood-pool radiotracer concentrations from serial tomographic images of the heart. *J Nucl Med* 1983;24:987–996.
64. Hoffman EJ, Huang SC, Phelps ME. Quantitation in positron emission computed tomography: 1. Effect of object size. *J Comput Assist Tomogr* 1979;3:299–308.
65. Iida H, Rhodes CG, de Silva R, et al. Myocardial tissue fraction—correction for partial volume effects and measure of tissue viability. *J Nucl Med* 1991;32:2169–2175.
66. Yamamoto Y, de Silva R, Rhodes CG, et al. A new strategy for the assessment of viable myocardium and regional myocardial blood flow using ^{15}O-water and dynamic positron emission tomography. *Circulation* 1992;86:167–178.
67. Katoh C, Morita K, Shiga T, et al. Improvement of algorithm for quantification of regional myocardial blood flow using ^{15}O-water with PET. *J Nucl Med* 2004;45:1908–1916.
68. Kaufmann PA, Gnecchi-Ruscone T, di Terlizzi M, et al. Coronary heart disease in smokers: vitamin C restores coronary microcirculatory function. *Circulation* 2000;102:1233–1238.
69. De Bruyne B, Baudhuin T, Melin JA, et al. Coronary flow reserve calculated from pressure measurements in humans. Validation with positron emission tomography. *Circulation* 1994;89:1013–1022.
70. Merlet P, Mazoyer B, Hittinger L, et al. Assessment of coronary reserve in man: comparison between positron emission tomography with oxygen-15-labeled water and intracoronary Doppler technique. *J Nucl Med* 1993;34:1899–1904.
71. Kaufmann PA, Gnecchi-Ruscone T, Yap JT, et al. Assessment of the reproducibility of baseline and hyperemic myocardial blood flow measurements with ^{15}O-labeled water and PET. *J Nucl Med* 1999;40:1848–1856.
72. Nagamachi S, Czernin J, Kim AS, et al. Reproducibility of measurements of regional resting and hyperemic myocardial blood flow assessed with PET. *J Nucl Med* 1996;37:1626–1631.
73. Krivokapich J, Czernin J, Schelbert HR. Dobutamine positron emission tomography: absolute quantitation of rest and dobutamine myocardial blood flow and correlation with cardiac work and percent diameter stenosis in patients with and without coronary artery disease. *J Am Coll Cardiol* 1996;28:565–572.
74. Tadamura E, Iida H, Matsumoto K, et al. Comparison of myocardial blood flow during dobutamine-atropine infusion with that after dipyridamole administration in normal men. *J Am Coll Cardiol* 2001;37:130–136.
75. Yoshinaga K, Katoh C, Noriyasu K, et al. Reduction of coronary flow reserve in areas with and without ischemia on stress perfusion imaging in patients with coronary artery disease: a study using oxygen 15-labeled water PET. *J Nucl Cardiol* 2003;10:275–283.
76. Siegrist PT, Gaemperli O, Koepfli P, et al. Repeatability of cold pressor test-induced flow increase assessed with $H_{(2)}(^{15})O$ and PET. *J Nucl Med* 2006;47:1420–1426.
77. Lardinois D, Weder W, Hany TF, et al. Staging of non-small-cell lung cancer with integrated positron-emission tomography and computed tomography. *N Engl J Med* 2003;348:2500–2507.
78. Kinahan PE, Townsend DW, Beyer T, et al. Attenuation correction for a combined 3D PET/CT scanner. *Med Phys* 1998;25:2046–2053.
79. Koepfli P, Hany TF, Wyss CA, et al. CT attenuation correction for myocardial perfusion quantification using a PET/CT hybrid scanner. *J Nucl Med* 2004;45:537–542.
80. Hacker M, Jakobs T, Matthiesen F, et al. Comparison of spiral multidetector CT angiography and myocardial perfusion imaging in the noninvasive detection of functionally relevant coronary artery lesions: first clinical experiences. *J Nucl Med* 2005;46:1294–1300.
81. Di Carli MF, Dorbala S, Hachamovitch R. Integrated cardiac PET-CT for the diagnosis and management of CAD. *J Nucl Cardiol* 2006; 13:139–144.
82. Di Carli M, Dorbala S, Limaye A, et al. Clinical value of hybrid PET/CT cardiac imaging: complementary roles of multi-detector CT coronary angiography and stress PET perfusion imaging. *J Am Coll Cardiol* 2006;47[Suppl]:115A.
83. Namdar M, Hany TF, Koepfli P, et al. Integrated PET/CT for the assessment of coronary artery disease: a feasibility study. *J Nucl Med* 2005;46:930–935.
84. Tamaki N, Yonekura Y, Senda M, et al. Value and limitation of stress thallium-201 single photon emission computed tomography: comparison with nitrogen-13 ammonia positron tomography. *J Nucl Med* 1988;29:1181–1188.
85. Go RT, Marwick TH, MacIntyre WJ, et al. A prospective comparison of rubidium-82 PET and thallium-201 SPECT myocardial perfusion imaging utilizing a single dipyridamole stress in the diagnosis of coronary artery disease. *J Nucl Med* 1990;31:1899–1905.
86. Stewart RE, Schwaiger M, Molina E, et al. Comparison of rubidium-82 positron emission tomography and thallium-201 SPECT imaging for detection of coronary artery disease. *Am J Cardiol* 1991;67: 1303–1310.
87. Bateman TM, Heller GV, McGhie AI, et al. Diagnostic accuracy of rest/stress ECG-gated Rb-82 myocardial perfusion PET: comparison with ECG-gated Tc-99m sestamibi SPECT. *J Nucl Cardiol* 2006;13: 24–33.

88. MacIntyre WJ, Go RT, King JL, et al. Clinical outcome of cardiac patients with negative thallium-201 SPECT and positive rubidium-82 PET myocardial perfusion imaging. *J Nucl Med* 1993;34:400–404.
89. Marwick TH, Shan K, Patel S, et al. Incremental value of rubidium-82 positron emission tomography for prognostic assessment of known or suspected coronary artery disease. *Am J Cardiol* 1997;80:865–870.
90. Chow BJ, Wong JW, Yoshinaga K, et al. Prognostic significance of dipyridamole-induced ST depression in patients with normal ^{82}Rb PET myocardial perfusion imaging. *J Nucl Med* 2005;46:1095–1101.
91. Patterson RE, Eisner RL, Horowitz SF. Comparison of cost-effectiveness and utility of exercise ECG, single photon emission computed tomography, positron emission tomography, and coronary angiography for diagnosis of coronary artery disease. *Circulation* 1995;91:54–65.
92. Maddahi J, Gambhir SS. Cost-effective selection of patients for coronary angiography. *J Nucl Cardiol* 1997;4:S141–S151.
93. Gould KL, Kirkeeide RL, Buchi M. Coronary flow reserve as a physiologic measure of stenosis severity. *J Am Coll Cardiol* 1990;15:459–474.
94. Gould KL, Lipscomb K, Hamilton GW. Physiologic basis for assessing critical coronary stenosis. Instantaneous flow response and regional distribution during coronary hyperemia as measures of coronary flow reserve. *Am J Cardiol* 1974;33:87–94.
95. Gould KL. Quantification of coronary artery stenosis *in vivo*. *Circ Res* 1985;57:341–353.
96. Demer LL, Gould KL, Goldstein RA, et al. Assessment of coronary artery disease severity by positron emission tomography. Comparison with quantitative arteriography in 193 patients. *Circulation* 1989;79:825–835.
97. Uren NG, Melin JA, De Bruyne B, et al. Relation between myocardial blood flow and the severity of coronary-artery stenosis. *N Engl J Med* 1994;330:1782–1788.
98. Beanlands R, Melon P, Muzik O, et al. N-13 ammonia PET identifies reduced perfusion reserve in angiographically normal regions of patients with CAD. *Circulation* 1992;86[Suppl I]:I-184(abst).
99. Di Carli M, Czernin J, Hoh CK, et al. Relation among stenosis severity, myocardial blood flow, and flow reserve in patients with coronary artery disease. *Circulation* 1995;91:1944–1951.
100. Beanlands RS, Muzik O, Melon P, et al. Noninvasive quantification of regional myocardial flow reserve in patients with coronary atherosclerosis using nitrogen-13 ammonia positron emission tomography. Determination of extent of altered vascular reactivity. *J Am Coll Cardiol* 1995;26:1465–1475.
101. Wilson RF, Marcus ML, White CW. Prediction of the physiologic significance of coronary arterial lesions by quantitative lesion geometry in patients with limited coronary artery disease. *Circulation* 1987;75:723–732.
102. Demer LL, Gould KL, Goldstein RA, et al. Noninvasive assessment of coronary collaterals in man by PET perfusion imaging. *J Nucl Med* 1990;31:259–270.
103. Holmvang G, Fry S, Skopicki HA, et al. Relation between coronary "steal" and contractile function at rest in collateral-dependent myocardium of humans with ischemic heart disease. *Circulation* 1999;99:2510–2516.
104. Maseri A, Crea F, Cianflone D. Myocardial ischemia caused by distal coronary vasoconstriction. *Am J Cardiol* 1992;70:1602–1605.
105. Zeiher AM, Drexler H, Wollschlager H, et al. Endothelial dysfunction of the coronary microvasculature is associated with coronary blood flow regulation in patients with early atherosclerosis. *Circulation* 1991;84:1984–1992.
106. Van Tosh A, Garza D, Roberti R, et al. Serial myocardial perfusion imaging with dipyridamole and rubidium-82 to assess restenosis after angioplasty. *J Nucl Med* 1995;36:1553–1560.
107. Stewart RE, Miller DD, Bowers TR, et al. PET perfusion and vasodilator function after angioplasty for acute myocardial infarction. *J Nucl Med* 1997;38:770–777.
108. Walsh MN, Geltman EM, Steele RL, et al. Augmented myocardial perfusion reserve after coronary angioplasty quantified by positron emission tomography with $H_2(^{15})O$. *J Am Coll Cardiol* 1990;15:119–127.
109. Czernin J, Muller P, Chan S, et al. Influence of age and hemodynamics on myocardial blood flow and flow reserve. *Circulation* 1993;88:62–69.
110. Uren NG, Camici PG, Melin JA, et al. Effect of aging on myocardial perfusion reserve. *J Nucl Med* 1995;36:2032–2036.
111. Camici PG, Gistri R, Lorenzoni R, et al. Coronary reserve and exercise ECG in patients with chest pain and normal coronary angiograms. *Circulation* 1992;86:179–186.
112. Geltman EM, Henes CG, Senneff MJ, et al. Increased myocardial perfusion at rest and diminished perfusion reserve in patients with angina and angiographically normal coronary arteries. *J Am Coll Cardiol* 1990;16:586–595.
113. Dayanikli F, Grambow D, Muzik O, et al. Early detection of abnormal coronary flow reserve in asymptomatic men at high risk for coronary artery disease using positron emission tomography. *Circulation* 1994;90:808–817.
114. Yokoyama I, Murakami T, Ohtake T, et al. Reduced coronary flow reserve in familial hypercholesterolemia. *J Nucl Med* 1996;37:1937–1942.
115. Yokoyama I, Ohtake T, Momomura S, et al. Reduced coronary flow reserve in hypercholesterolemic patients without overt coronary stenosis. *Circulation* 1996;94:3232–3238.
116. Pitkanen OP, Nuutila P, Raitakari OT, et al. Coronary flow reserve in young men with familial combined hyperlipidemia. *Circulation* 1999;99:1678–1684.
117. Pitkanen OP, Raitakari OT, Niinikoski H, et al. Coronary flow reserve is impaired in young men with familial hypercholesterolemia. *J Am Coll Cardiol* 1996;28:1705–1711.
118. Kaufmann PA, Gnecchi-Ruscone T, Schafers KP, et al. Low density lipoprotein cholesterol and coronary microvascular dysfunction in hypercholesterolemia. *J Am Coll Cardiol* 2000;36:103–109.
119. Mellwig KP, Baller D, Gleichmann U, et al. Improvement of coronary vasodilatation capacity through single LDL apheresis. *Atherosclerosis* 1998;139:173–178.
120. Gould KL, Martucci JP, Goldberg DI, et al. Short-term cholesterol lowering decreases size and severity of perfusion abnormalities by positron emission tomography after dipyridamole in patients with coronary artery disease. A potential noninvasive marker of healing coronary endothelium. *Circulation* 1994;89:1530–1538.
121. Guethlin M, Kasel AM, Coppenrath K, et al. Delayed response of myocardial flow reserve to lipid-lowering therapy with fluvastatin. *Circulation* 1999;99:475–481.
122. Huggins GS, Pasternak RC, Alpert NM, et al. Effects of short-term treatment of hyperlipidemia on coronary vasodilator function and myocardial perfusion in regions having substantial impairment of baseline dilator reverse. *Circulation* 1998;98:1291–1296.
123. Baller D, Notohamiprodjo G, Gleichmann U, et al. Improvement in coronary flow reserve determined by positron emission tomography after 6 months of cholesterol-lowering therapy in patients with early stages of coronary atherosclerosis. *Circulation* 1999;99:2871–2875.
124. Treasure CB, Klein JL, Weintraub WS, et al. Beneficial effects of cholesterol-lowering therapy on the coronary endothelium in patients with coronary artery disease. *N Engl J Med* 1995;332:481–487.
125. Yokoyama I, Momomura S, Ohtake T, et al. Improvement of impaired myocardial vasodilatation due to diffuse coronary atherosclerosis in hypercholesterolemics after lipid-lowering therapy. *Circulation* 1999;100:117–122.
126. Czernin J, Sun K, Brunken R, et al. Effect of acute and long-term smoking on myocardial blood flow and flow reserve. *Circulation* 1995;91:2891–2897.
127. Yokoyama I, Momomura S, Ohtake T, et al. Reduced myocardial flow reserve in non-insulin-dependent diabetes mellitus. *J Am Coll Cardiol* 1997;30:1472–1477.
128. Yokoyama I, Ohtake T, Momomura S, et al. Hyperglycemia rather than insulin resistance is related to reduced coronary flow reserve in NIDDM. *Diabetes* 1998;47:119–124.

129. Di Carli MF, Bianco-Batlles D, Landa ME, et al. Effects of autonomic neuropathy on coronary blood flow in patients with diabetes mellitus. *Circulation* 1999;100:813–819.
130. Nahser PJ Jr, Brown RE, Oskarsson H, et al. Maximal coronary flow reserve and metabolic coronary vasodilation in patients with diabetes mellitus. *Circulation* 1995;91:635–640.
131. Nitenberg A, Valensi P, Sachs R, et al. Impairment of coronary vascular reserve and ACh-induced coronary vasodilation in diabetic patients with angiographically normal coronary arteries and normal left ventricular systolic function. *Diabetes* 1993;42:1017–1025.
132. Lautamaki R, Airaksinen KE, Seppanen M, et al. Insulin improves myocardial blood flow in patients with type 2 diabetes and coronary artery disease. *Diabetes* 2006;55:511–516.
133. Prior JO, Quinones MJ, Hernandez-Pampaloni M, et al. Coronary circulatory dysfunction in insulin resistance, impaired glucose tolerance, and type 2 diabetes mellitus. *Circulation* 2005;111:2291–2298.
134. Campisi R, Czernin J, Schoder H, et al. Effects of long-term smoking on myocardial blood flow, coronary vasomotion, and vasodilator capacity. *Circulation* 1998;98:119–125.
135. Iwado Y, Yoshinaga K, Furuyama H, et al. Decreased endothelium-dependent coronary vasomotion in healthy young smokers. *Eur J Nucl Med Mol Imaging* 2002;29:984–990.
136. Morita K, Tsukamoto T, Naya M, et al. Smoking cessation normalizes coronary endothelial vasomotor response assessed with ^{15}O-water and PET in healthy young smokers. *J Nucl Med* 2006;47:1914–1920.
137. Celermajer DS, Adams MR, Clarkson P, et al. Passive smoking and impaired endothelium-dependent arterial dilatation in healthy young adults. *N Engl J Med* 1996;334:150–154.
138. Celermajer DS, Sorensen KE, Georgakopoulos D, et al. Cigarette smoking is associated with dose-related and potentially reversible impairment of endothelium-dependent dilation in healthy young adults. *Circulation* 1993;88:2149–2155.
139. Zeiher AM, Schachinger V, Minners J. Long-term cigarette smoking impairs endothelium-dependent coronary arterial vasodilator function. *Circulation* 1995;92:1094–1100.
140. Campisi R, Czernin J, Schoder H, et al. L-Arginine normalizes coronary vasomotion in long-term smokers. *Circulation* 1999;99:491–497.
141. Kozakova M, Palombo C, Pratali L, et al. Mechanisms of coronary flow reserve impairment in human hypertension. An integrated approach by transthoracic and transesophageal echocardiography. *Hypertension* 1997;29:551–559.
142. Treasure CB, Klein JL, Vita JA, et al. Hypertension and left ventricular hypertrophy are associated with impaired endothelium-mediated relaxation in human coronary resistance vessels. *Circulation* 1993;87:86–93.
143. Laine H, Raitakari OT, Niinikoski H, et al. Early impairment of coronary flow reserve in young men with borderline hypertension. *J Am Coll Cardiol* 1998;32:147–153.
144. Gistri R, Ebert AG, Palombo C, et al. Effect of blood pressure lowering on coronary vasodilator reserve in arterial hypertension. *Cardiovasc Drugs Ther* 1994;8:169–171.
145. Schneider CA, Voth E, Moka D, et al. Improvement of myocardial blood flow to ischemic regions by angiotensin-converting enzyme inhibition with quinaprilat IV: a study using [^{15}O] water dobutamine stress positron emission tomography. *J Am Coll Cardiol* 1999;34:1005–1011.
146. Akinboboye OO, Chou RL, Bergmann SR. Augmentation of myocardial blood flow in hypertensive heart disease by angiotensin antagonists: a comparison of lisinopril and losartan. *J Am Coll Cardiol* 2002;40:703–709.
147. Schindler TH, Nitzsche EU, Schelbert HR, et al. Positron emission tomography-measured abnormal responses of myocardial blood flow to sympathetic stimulation are associated with the risk of developing cardiovascular events. *J Am Coll Cardiol* 2005;45:1505–1512.
148. Schindler TH, Nitzsche EU, Olschewski M, et al. Chronic inflammation and impaired coronary vasoreactivity in patients with coronary risk factors. *Circulation* 2004;110:1069–1075.
149. Camici PG, Marraccini P, Lorenzoni R, et al. Coronary hemodynamics and myocardial metabolism in patients with syndrome X: response to pacing stress. *J Am Coll Cardiol* 1991;17:1461–1470.
150. Camici P, Cecchi F, Gistri R. Dipyridamole-induced subendocardial underperfusion in hypertrophic cardiomyopathy assessed by positron emission tomography. *Coronary Artery Dis* 1991;2:837–841.
151. Cecchi F, Olivotto I, Gistri R, et al. Coronary microvascular dysfunction and prognosis in hypertrophic cardiomyopathy. *N Engl J Med* 2003;349:1027–1035.
152. Parodi O, De Maria R, Oltrona L, et al. Myocardial blood flow distribution in patients with ischemic heart disease or dilated cardiomyopathy undergoing heart transplantation. *Circulation* 1993;88:509–522.
153. Neglia D, Parodi O, Gallopin M, et al. Myocardial blood flow response to pacing tachycardia and to dipyridamole infusion in patients with dilated cardiomyopathy without overt heart failure. A quantitative assessment by positron emission tomography. *Circulation* 1995;92:796–804.
154. Rajappan K, Rimoldi OE, Dutka DP, et al. Mechanisms of coronary microcirculatory dysfunction in patients with aortic stenosis and angiographically normal coronary arteries. *Circulation* 2002;105:470–476.
155. Rajappan K, Rimoldi OE, Camici PG, et al. Functional changes in coronary microcirculation after valve replacement in patients with aortic stenosis. *Circulation* 2003;107:3170–3175.
156. Burwash I, DeKemp R, Pibarot P, et al. Myocardial blood flow in patients with low flow gradient aortic stenosis: differences between true and pseudo severe aortic stenosis. Results from the multicenter TOPAS study. *Circulation* 2005;112[Suppl 2]:2-718.
157. Rechavia E, Araujo LI, De Silva R, et al. Dipyridamole vasodilator response after human orthotopic heart transplantation: quantification by oxygen-15-labeled water and positron emission tomography. *J Am Coll Cardiol* 1992;19:100–106.
158. Chan SY, Kobashigawa J, Stevenson LW, et al. Myocardial blood flow at rest and during pharmacological vasodilation in cardiac transplants during and after successful treatment of rejection. *Circulation* 1994;90:204–212.
159. Kofoed KF, Czernin J, Johnson J, et al. Effects of cardiac allograft vasculopathy on myocardial blood flow, vasodilatory capacity, and coronary vasomotion. *Circulation* 1997;95:600–606.
160. Bottcher M, Botker HE, Sonne H, et al. Endothelium-dependent and -independent perfusion reserve and the effect of L-arginine on myocardial perfusion in patients with syndrome X. *Circulation* 1999;99:1795–1801.
161. Rosen SD, Uren NG, Kaski JC, et al. Coronary vasodilator reserve, pain perception, and sex in patients with syndrome X. *Circulation* 1994;90:50–60.
162. Muzik O, Paridon SM, Singh TP, et al. Quantification of myocardial blood flow and flow reserve in children with a history of Kawasaki disease and normal coronary arteries using position emission tomography. *J Am Coll Cardiol* 1996;28(3):757–762.
163. Furuyama H, Odagawa Y, Katoh C, et al. Assessment of coronary function in children with a history of Kawasaki disease using (^{15})O-water positron emission tomography. *Circulation* 2002;105:2878–2884.
164. Mahmoud S, Beanlands RS, deKemp RA, et al. Native anomalous left coronary artery from the pulmonary artery in an adult: Evidence of impaired coronary flow reserve by rubidium-82 positron emission tomography quantification. *Can J Cardiol* 2006;22(12):1069–1070.
165. Singh TP, Di Carli MF, Sullivan NM, et al. Myocardial flow reserve in long-term survivors of repair of anomalous left coronary artery from pulmonary artery. *J Am Coll Cardiol* 1998;31(2):437–443.
166. Singh TP, Humes RA, Muzik O, et al. Myocardial flow reserve in patients with a systemic right ventricle after atrial switch repair. *J Am Coll Cardiol* 2001;37(8):2120–2125.
167. Hauser M, Bengel FM, Kuhn A, et al. Myocardial blood flow and flow reserve after coronary reimplantation in patients after arterial switch and ross operation. *Circulation* 2001;103(14):1875–1880.

168. Gambhir SS, Barrio JR, Phelps ME, et al. Imaging adenoviral-directed reporter gene expression in living animals with positron emission tomography. *Proc Natl Acad Sci U S A* 1999;96:2333–2338.
169. Camici P, Chiriatti G, Lorenzoni R, et al. Coronary vasodilation is impaired in both hypertrophied and nonhypertrophied myocardium of patients with hypertrophic cardiomyopathy: a study with nitrogen-13 ammonia and positron emission tomography. *J Am Coll Cardiol* 1991;17:879–886.
170. Chan SY, Brunken RC, Czernin J, et al. Comparison of maximal myocardial blood flow during adenosine infusion with that of intravenous dipyridamole in normal men. *J Am Coll Cardiol* 1992;20:979–985.
171. Lin JW, Sciacca RR, Chou RL, et al. Quantification of myocardial perfusion in human subjects using ^{82}Rb and wavelet-based noise reduction. *J Nucl Med* 2001;42:201–208.
172. Wassenaar R, Beanlands R, Ruddy TD, et al. Three dimensional cardiac positron emission tomography. *Res Adv Nucl Med* 2002;1:51–60.
173. Lortie M, Mostert K, Kelly C, et al. Quantification of myocardial blood flow with rubidium-82 dynamic PET imaging. *J Nucl Med* 2005;46:60P.
174. Campisi R, Nathan L, Pampaloni MH, et al. Noninvasive assessment of coronary microcirculatory function in postmenopausal women and effects of short-term and long-term estrogen administration. *Circulation* 2002;105:425–430.
175. Prior JO, Schindler TH, Facta AD, et al. Determinants of myocardial blood flow response to cold pressor testing and pharmacologic vasodilation in healthy humans. *Eur J Nucl Med Mol Imaging* 2007;34:20–27.
176. Schelbert HR, Wisenberg G, Phelps ME, et al. Noninvasive assessment of coronary stenoses by myocardial imaging during pharmacologic coronary vasodilation. VI. Detection of coronary artery disease in human beings with intravenous N-13 ammonia and positron computed tomography. *Am J Cardiol* 1982;49:1197–1207.
177. Yonekura Y, Tamaki N, Senda M, et al. Detection of coronary artery disease with ^{13}N-ammonia and high-resolution positron-emission computed tomography. *Am Heart J* 1987;113:645–654.
178. Gould KL, Goldstein RA, Mullani NA, et al. Noninvasive assessment of coronary stenoses by myocardial perfusion imaging during pharmacologic coronary vasodilation. VIII. Clinical feasibility of positron cardiac imaging without a cyclotron using generator-produced rubidium-82. *J Am Coll Cardiol* 1986;7:775–789.
179. Marwick TH, Nemec JJ, Stewart WJ, et al. Diagnosis of coronary artery disease using exercise echocardiography and positron emission tomography: comparison and analysis of discrepant results. *J Am Soc Echocardiogr* 1992;5:231–238.
180. Grover-McKay M, Ratib O, Schwaiger M, et al. Detection of coronary artery disease with positron emission tomography and rubidium 82. *Am Heart J* 1992;123:646–652.
181. Laubenbacher C, Rothley J, Sitomer J, et al. An automated analysis program for the evaluation of cardiac PET studies: initial results in the detection and localization of coronary artery disease using nitrogen-13-ammonia. *J Nucl Med* 1993;34:968–978.
182. Simone GL, Mullani NA, Page DA, et al. Utilization statistics and diagnostic accuracy of a nonhospital-based positron emission tomography center for the detection of coronary artery disease using rubidium-82. *Am J Physiol Imaging* 1992;7:203–209.
183. Marwick TH, Shan K, Go RT, et al. Use of positron emission tomography for prediction of perioperative and late cardiac events before vascular surgery. *Am Heart J* 1995;130:1196–1202.
184. Zhou R, Acton PD, Ferrari VA. Imaging stem cells implanted in infarcted myocardium. *J Am Coll Cardiol* 2006;48:2094–2106.
185. Udelson JE, Dilsizian V, Laham RJ, et al. Therapeutic angiogenesis with recombinant fibroblast growth factor-2 improves stress and rest myocardial perfusion abnormalities in patients with severe symptomatic chronic coronary artery disease. *Circulation* 2000;102:1605–1610.
186. Bengel FM, Anton M, Richter T, et al. Noninvasive imaging of transgene expression by use of positron emission tomography in a pig model of myocardial gene transfer. *Circulation* 2003;108:2127–2133.
187. Chang GY, Xie X, Wu JC. Overview of stem cells and imaging modalities for cardiovascular diseases. *J Nucl Cardiol* 2006;13:554–569.
188. Knaapen P, van Campen LM, de Cock CC, et al. Effects of cardiac resynchronization therapy on myocardial perfusion reserve. *Circulation* 2004;110:646–651.

Myocardial Viability

ROB S. B. BEANLANDS, STEPHANIE THORN, JEAN DASILVA, TERRENCE D. RUDDY, AND JAMSHID MADDAHI

Heart failure resulting from impaired left ventricular (LV) function is associated with significant morbidity and mortality. The leading cause of heart failure is coronary artery disease (CAD). Among patients with coronary disease and severe ventricular dysfunction, mortality rates range from 10% to 60% per year (1–5). The inverse relationship of ventricular function with mortality has been well established (3,6). Heart failure is also associated with significant health care costs. The number of hospitalizations from heart failure in North America has risen by 159% from 1990 to 2000 (7). In recent years, advances in medical therapy have improved the outcome for patients with heart failure (7–12). However, even with these advances, mortality rates remain high (9,11), with epidemiological surveys suggesting no significant change in overall death rates (7,13). With limited access to transplantation, revascularization is often considered, as this may improve the clinical outcome in some patients (3,14,15). However, bypass surgery in such patients can have high perioperative risk (16–19). Hence, a need arose for diagnostic techniques that could better define and select the high-risk patients with ventricular dysfunction most likely to benefit from revascularization. The diagnosis of the extent of viable myocardium has become pivotal in this regard. Although several approaches have been developed, the identification of preserved metabolic activity in the myocardium using fluorine-18 [^{18}F]-fluorodeoxyglucose (FDG) positron emission tomography (PET) imaging is the most well-established approach.

GLUCOSE METABOLISM

The primary substrate for energy metabolism in the normal myocardium depends on the substrate that is most available for oxidative metabolism, for which the majority of the time is fatty acids. However, after a glucose load, there is a subsequent increase in insulin levels. This leads to an increase in glucose metabolism and inhibition of lipolysis. Thus, in the fed state, the preferred substrate for cardiac energy metabolism becomes glucose (20,21).

In ischemic myocardium, oxidative metabolism is reduced, and there is a shift from aerobic to anaerobic metabolism. The primary substrate for energy metabolism becomes glucose to support adenosine triphosphate (ATP) production from glycolysis. Thus, the ischemic heart preferentially selects glucose as a substrate regardless of the availability of other fuels (20,21). Imaging techniques that can track myocardial glucose utilization are therefore useful in defining the state of viability in the myocardium.

Glucose is transported across the myocyte membrane by primarily the glucose transporters (GLUTs) GLUT4 and GLUT1 (22,23). Once glucose enters the cell, it undergoes phosphorylation to glucose 6-phosphate, the substrate for glycolysis, glucose oxidation, or glycogen synthesis. FDG is a glucose analogue that enters the myocyte in proportion to glucose uptake and undergoes phosphorylation (24,25). However, unlike glucose, the resulting FDG-6-phosphate becomes metabolically trapped by the myocyte. This allows for FDG uptake to reflect the rate of exogenous glucose utilization and can be used to identify viable myocardium (26,27).

VIABILITY, STUNNING, AND HIBERNATION

When flow is reduced to the myocardium, metabolic cellular changes occur due to ischemia and results in reduced contractile function of the myocardium. When ischemia is acute, severe, and sufficiently prolonged (more than 20 to 30 minutes in the acute setting), infarction may result with irreversible cell injury, cell death, and subsequent myocardial scar formation. Once irreversible cellular damage has occurred, these myocytes are no longer viable and cannot recover even if adequately revascularized.

However, the metabolic derangements in the myocyte after short bouts of ischemia may result in more prolonged reduction in myocardial contractile function than can eventually recover. This postischemic ventricular dysfunction has been termed *stunned myocardium* (28,29). More prolonged sustained or repetitive reductions in flow may also lead to myocardial dysfunction, which some investigators now refer to as *hibernating myocardium* (30,31). Hibernating myocardium can recover if adequate nutrient flow is restored.

Myocardial Stunning

The myocardial dysfunction that can occur after an episode of ischemia (28,29,32) is a form of reperfusion injury that may result from calcium influx, which hinders the myocyte contractile function (33). It has been well described in animal models and in patients, particularly in the setting of acute myocardial infarction after reperfusion therapy, in acute coronary syndromes, and less frequently after severe exercise-induced ischemia (28–30,32,33). When blood flow is restored, the recovery of function may take minutes to days or even weeks depending on the severity of the initial ischemic episode. However, it is considered completely reversible. On the other hand, if repeated episodes of ischemia occur, the resulting postischemic dysfunction may become more persistent. The latter may be an important cause of chronic LV dysfunction in patients with severe ischemic heart disease (32,34–36). This repetitively stunned myocardium is viable and has the potential to recover after adequate revascularization (35,36).

Hibernating Myocardium

Hibernating myocardium is the term applied to dysfunctional myocardium with reduced myocardial perfusion at rest but preserved cell viability (30,31). The resulting reduction in myocardial function has been thought to be a protective chronic down-regulation mechanism to reduce myocardial oxygen utilization and ensure myocyte survival (30–32). The classic perfusion–metabolism mismatch pattern seen on perfusion PET as compared with FDG PET imaging supported this hypothesis of sustained reduction in flow with maintained viability (and therefore, glucose utilization). This perfusion–metabolism mismatch is considered to represent hibernating myocardium.

However, recent data suggest that the pathophysiology may be more complex. Two theories on the pathogenesis of hibernating myocardium have emerged. One suggests it is due to chronic hypoperfusion and secondary down-regulation of function and metabolism (37). Reductions in flow have been demonstrated in some studies but not in others (34,38–45). This, along with progressive histological changes, sequential down-regulation of function, as well as altered gene expression, suggests that other factors contribute to LV dysfunction in these patients (34,42–50). Current evidence points to an alternate mechanism due to repetitive postischemic dysfunction (stunning) that initiates a process of progressive down-regulation. Changes from repetitive stunning with normal resting flow progress to functional hibernation with intact metabolism and contractile reserve; then to structural hibernation without contractile reserve but with preserved glucose uptake on FDG imaging; eventually progressing to irreversible injury with scar formation (34,37,42–52) (Fig. 11.2.1 and Table 11.2.1) Indeed Canty and Fallavollita (45) have observed in a swine model of hibernation

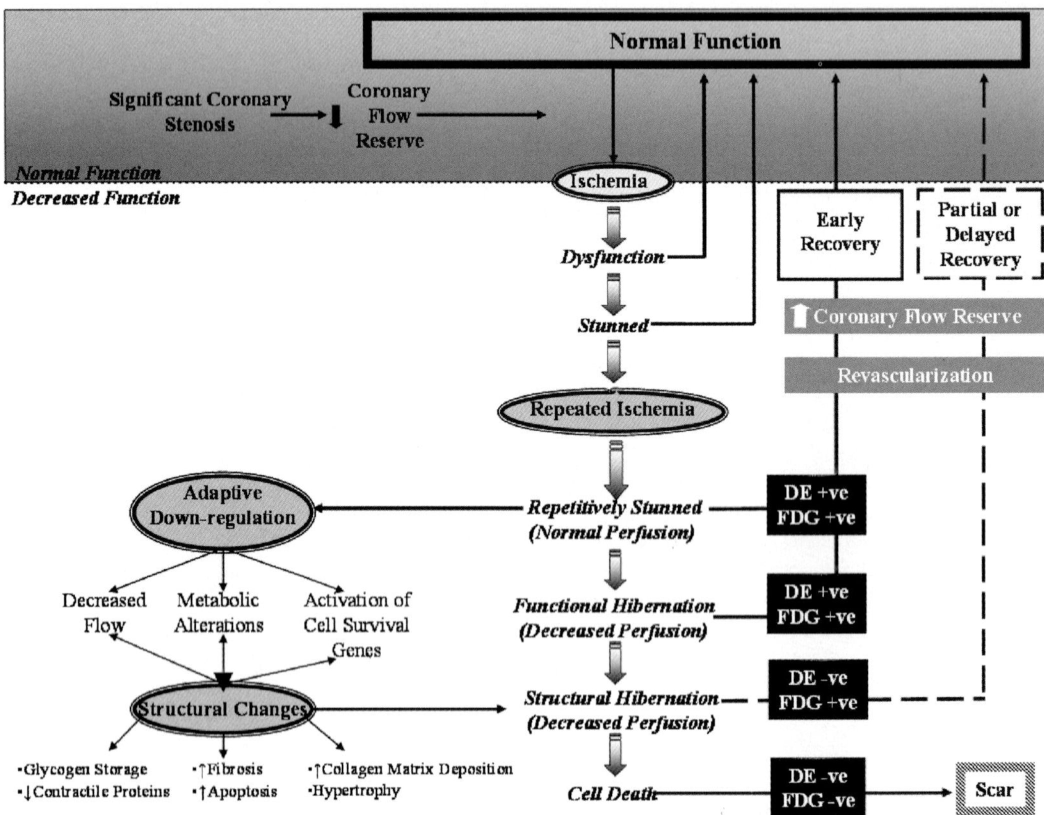

FIGURE 11.2.1. Schematic for pathogenesis of hibernating myocardium: progressive adaptive down-regulation from repetitive stunning to hibernation. CFR, coronary flow reserve; DE, dobutamine echo; FDG, fluorine-18-fluorodeoxyglucose. (Figure adapted from Camici P, Dutka D. Repetitive stunning, hibernation, and heart failure: contribution of PET to establishing a link. *Am J Physiol Heart Circ Physiol* 2001;280:H929–H936; Depre C, Vatner SF. Mechanisms of cell survival in myocardial hibernation. *Trends Cardiovasc Med* 2005;15:101–110; Canty JM Jr, Fallavollita JA. Hibernating myocardium. *J Nucl Cardiol* 2005;12:104–119, with permission.)

TABLE 11.2.1 Features of Hibernating Myocardium

FLOW, METABOLISM, FUNCTION FEATURES
- Reduced perfusion
- Reduced perfusion reserve
- Reduced wall motion
- Wall thinning
- Variable contractile reserve
- Variable oxidative metabolism reserve
- Reduced fatty acid metabolism
- Maintained/Increased exogenous glucose utilization

MECHANISTIC FACTORS
- Ischemia
- Postischemic–repetitive stunning
- Adaptive down-regulation of flow, contractile function, metabolism
- Regional down-regulation of neurohormonal function and responsiveness
- Activation of cell survival genes

MORPHOLOGICAL CHANGES
- Loss of myofilaments
- Loss of sarcoplasmic reticulum
- Increased number of small, circular mitochondria
- Disorganization of cytoskeleton
- Deposition of cellular particles into extracellular space due to atrophy and apoptosis
- Increased matrix and structural proteins
- Increased fibrosis

(Morphological features adapted from Heusch G, Schulz R, Rahimtoola SH. Myocardial hibernation: a delicate balance. *Am J Physiol Heart Circ Physiol* 2005;288:H984–H999, with permission.)

that flow reduction itself is down-regulated secondary to the down-regulation in myocardial function. Other adaptive changes may include reduced high affinity binding sites for β-1 receptors and impaired catecholamine responsiveness. That myocardial hibernation is progressive and may deteriorate to cell death is supported by the repeated observation that *early* revascularization in patients with viable myocardium improves outcomes (53–55) (Fig. 11.2.2). Thus, ischemia from reduction in flow may be only one of multiple factors contributing to the perfusion–metabolic mismatch pattern observed on imaging. Despite this complexity, the accuracy of the PET "mismatch" pattern has been well demonstrated and is associated with recovery after revascularization (5,20,23,32,35,36,56–70).

IMAGE ACQUISITION, ANALYSIS, AND INTERPRETATION

Several approaches for FDG imaging have been developed. However, because myocardial substrate metabolism can be quite variable, most centers use some form of glucose loading and/or insulin protocol to optimize FDG uptake in viable tissue. In addition, because there can also be regional variability, normalization to the perfusion image is often required. Knowledge of the regional perfusion also helps to better characterize the state of the myocardium. Most of the existing accuracy studies have used combined perfusion–FDG uptake imaging protocols using qualitative relative imaging. Accurate detection of myocardial viability, particularly in patients with severely impaired ventricular function, is best achieved by the evaluation of both perfusion and metabolism (5,32,59,71).

Patient Preparation

Oral glucose loading following a 6- to 12-hour fast has become the most widely used approach for preparing patients for FDG imaging. FDG is administered 60 to 90 minutes after a 25 to 100 g (typically 50 g) oral glucose load (5,53,58,59,63,71–75). This switches the primary substrate for myocardial metabolism from free fatty acids to glucose, facilitated by the release of insulin. Thus, viable myocardium will preferentially take up glucose and hence FDG. However, oral glucose loading can result in suboptimal image quality in 2% to 30% of patients (75–79). After the oral load, blood glucose values often unmask glucose intolerance. In such patients and those with frank diabetes, supplemental insulin is necessary (59,71,75). Even with such glucose-loading protocols inclusive of bolus insulin, images are often suboptimal in patients with diabetes (75,79).

In many centers, the hyperinsulinemic euglycemic clamp has been used to improve image quality (43,72,76,79–85). However, this approach can be more time consuming and cumbersome for the patient and staff.

Some centers have modified the hyperinsulinemic glucose clamp with front loading to reduce the time required to reach steady state. However, this clamp approach still requires monitoring of glucose levels every 5 minutes until stable, and then every 5 to 10 minutes. Glucose infusion rates are adjusted accordingly, aiming to maintain baseline glucose levels (85). Patients with diabetes whose blood glucose has not been well controlled before the study may present with high baseline glucose values. In these cases, a supplemental insulin bolus may be required in addition to the clamp, with careful monitoring of glucose. Due to FDG and glucose competition for the same uptake mechanism, lowering blood glucose levels to the normal or near normal range may reduce competition for FDG uptake and improve image quality.

Practically speaking, the oral glucose-loading protocol is technically easier to perform and requires less nursing and technology resources than the insulin clamp approach. The insulin clamp approach is often preferred for patients with diabetes who are likely to have poor imaging quality. Some centers also use modified approaches with intravenous glucose loading with or without intravenous insulin (71).

Newer approaches are utilizing nicotinic acid derivatives (niacin in North America; acipimox in Europe). The antilipolytic effect of these agents leads to a reduction of competing free fatty acids, thereby facilitating glucose utilization by the myocardium. The approach is simple, making it an attractive alternative, although these agents have not been consistently successful in studies for improving image quality (79,86,87). Additionally, there may be some flushing with niacin, but this can usually be minimized by administration of acetylsalicylic acid before the niacin. One study in patients with CAD, *severe* LV dysfunction, and diabetes suggested that only the clamp approach significantly improved uptake of FDG in this patient population (79). Further studies on the role of nicotinic acid derivatives are needed.

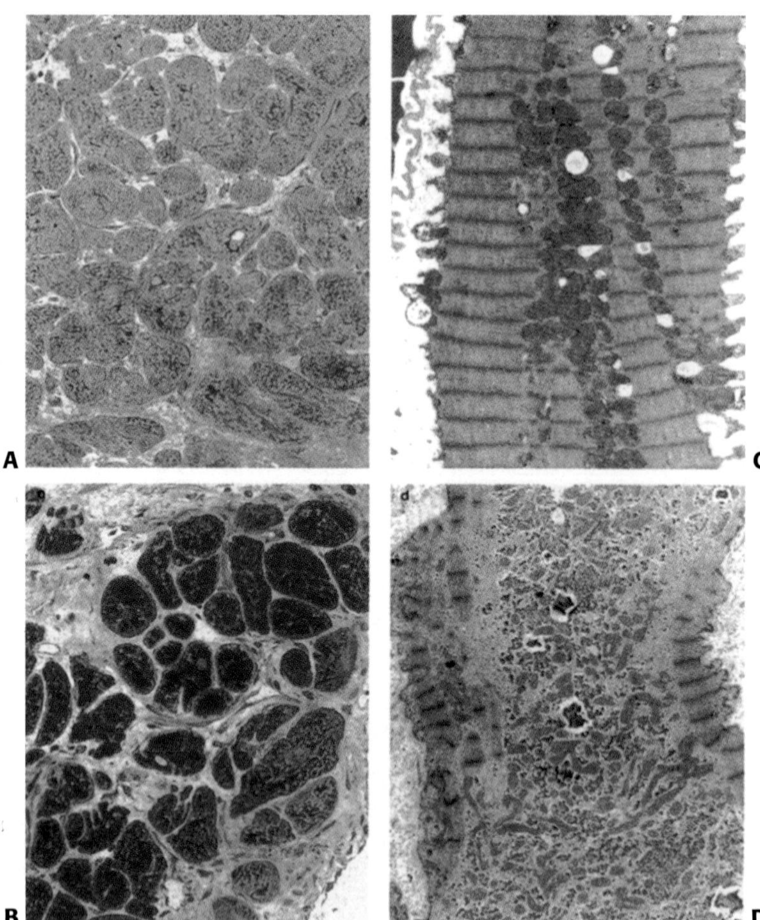

FIGURE 11.2.2. A: Light micrograph of myocardium showing normal cardiomyocytes with virtually no glycogen (Periodic Acid Schiff [PAS] staining in red). **B:** Transmission electron micrograph of normal cardiac myocytes. **C:** Representative light micrograph of a biopsy sample of human hibernating myocardium. Cardiac myocytes are depleted of their contractile material and filled with glycogen (PAS positive staining). **D:** Representative transmission electron micrograph of a hibernating cardiomyocyte. Microcytic cytoplasm is devoid of sacromeres and filled with glycogen. Original magnification: A and C, X320; B, X7100; and D, X7500. (From Vanoverschelde J-LJ, Wijns W, Borgers M, et al. Chronic myocardial hibernation in humans. From bedside to bench. *Circulation* 1997;95: 1961–1971, with permission.)

Because the administration of glucose and insulin can also lead to the influx of potassium (K^+) into cells, hypokalemia could theoretically result. In the authors' experience, the K^+ level may drop by up to 0.5 mEq/L after insulin clamp. Supplemental K^+ may be necessary in rare circumstances. Generally, this is only a problem in patients who already have hypokalemia, often due to the use of diuretics, and those who undergo the insulin clamp or receive multiple insulin boluses.

Cardiac Fluorodeoxyglucose PET Imaging Protocols

Transmission imaging is required to obtain measured attenuation correction. This is particularly important in cardiac studies because of the significant problems of nonuniformity in the thorax. Transmission imaging to measure attenuation correction may be acquired before the perfusion or before FDG (if perfusion is done at a separate time). More recently postemission transmission using computed tomography (CT) attenuation in PET/CT hybrid devices have been used. This can significantly shorten scanner time for the patient by allowing the patient to enter the camera after FDG is injected and just before the image acquisition begins. CT attenuation methods, while quick, may provide challenges as they may not exactly match the position of the PET image acquisition.

Perfusion PET imaging is important to define the relative state of blood flow in the myocardium at rest. This is usually performed at rest and is compared with FDG uptake. Stress perfusion imaging may also be required in the assessment of some patients with ischemic heart disease to rule out stress-induced ischemia.

Several agents have been used as PET perfusion tracers, including rubidium-82 ([^{82}Rb]), nitrogen-13 ([^{13}N])-ammonia, and Oxygen [150]-water (H2[^{15}O]). In centers without access to a cyclotron or strontium-[^{82}Rb] generators, technetium-99m (^{99}mTc)-based agents or thallium-201 (^{201}Tl) single-photon emission computed tomography (SPECT) imaging can be used for the assessment of perfusion (53,61,62, 73,74). This approach carries a limitation of often having perfusion images without attenuation correction (in some centers), while having FDG imaging with attenuation correction. This must be considered when interpreting the images.

FDG imaging can be either static or dynamic. Static imaging typically is a 10- to 30-minute image acquisition, depending on counts, that begin 45 to 60 minutes after injection of 5 to 15 mCi (185 to 555 MBq) FDG (72). This is usually a sufficient time for myocardial uptake to be well visualized while the blood pool activity is low. However later images can also be performed. As FDG clears from the bloodstream over time, it increases the myocardial to blood pool ratio in many patients. Dynamic imaging begins simultaneously with FDG injection and continues for 60 to 70 minutes, such that time activity data for blood pool and myocardium can be determined (e.g., 36 frames: 12 $\times$ 10 seconds, 6 $\times$ 20 seconds, 6 $\times$ 60 seconds, 12 $\times$ 300 seconds). The dynamic data are necessary for quantitative analysis of the rate of myocardial glucose utilization. However, this parameter may not be critical for clinical decision making.

Image Interpretation

Accurate tissue characterization and detection of myocardial viability, particularly in patients with severely impaired ventricular function, is best achieved by evaluation and direct comparison of both perfusion and metabolism (5,35,59). Perfusion FDG imaging has become the standard approach for PET viability imaging and is the focus of the discussion later in this chapter.

After the usual evaluation for image quality control, patient motion, artifacts, and extracardiac activity interpretation should begin with a view of the perfusion images to identify regions of maintained or reduced perfusion. Then FDG imaging should be viewed relative to the maximal zones of perfusion (Fig. 11.2.3) As FDG uptake may actually be greater in ischemic or hibernating zones than the FDG uptake seen in normal well-perfused and functional tissues, it may be necessary to normalize the FDG uptake to the zones of maximal perfusion. This can be achieved by scale adjustments or by semiquantitative analysis (Fig. 11.2.4).

It is also important to consider regional and global ventricular function to identify the regions where viability is in question and to determine the potential impact on overall LV function. Several patterns of uptake may be observed and are discussed.

Reduced Perfusion/Maintained or Increased Fluorodeoxyglucose (Mismatch)

The (low) perfusion (preserved)–metabolism mismatch in a dysfunctional myocardial segment is considered the *sine qua non* of hibernating myocardium (Fig. 11.2.3A). Typically, this has been viewed as representing regions with reduced flow that have been rendered ischemic but are still viable (5,26,32,34,38–41). As the term hibernating implies, this has been viewed as a down-regulation of function and oxidative metabolism, with preservation of glycolysis as a protective mechanism (30,31). However, the pathophysiology of the mismatch pattern may be more complex. Ischemia from reduction in flow may be only one of many contributing factors. Although perfusion tracer uptake appears reduced, absolute flow may or may not be reduced (34,38–43).

Stunning from recurrent stress-induced ischemia may occur and alter the uptake of the perfusion tracer or FDG. Wall thinning and reduced motion may, in part, account for apparent defects on the perfusion image (34). The mixture of ischemic and necrotic tissue may add to the complexity. Reduction in fatty acid oxidation has also been demonstrated in hibernating myocardium (42). Alteration in the GLUT1 and GLUT4 transporter expression has been proposed for hibernating and ischemic tissue (34,88), and glycogen accumulation has been observed, which may not be expected in the presence of ischemia alone (34–36,89,90). In addition, the extensive depletion of sarcomeres, loss of sarcoplasmic reticulum, and the observed cellular sequestration suggest that this is a progressive process that may quickly become irreversible injury if not corrected by adequate revascularization (34–36,47–50,54,55,89,90) (Figs. 11.2.1 and 11.2.2; Table 11.2.1).

Hibernating myocardium may represent the limits of viability when adaptive processes have been exhausted (35,47–50,89)

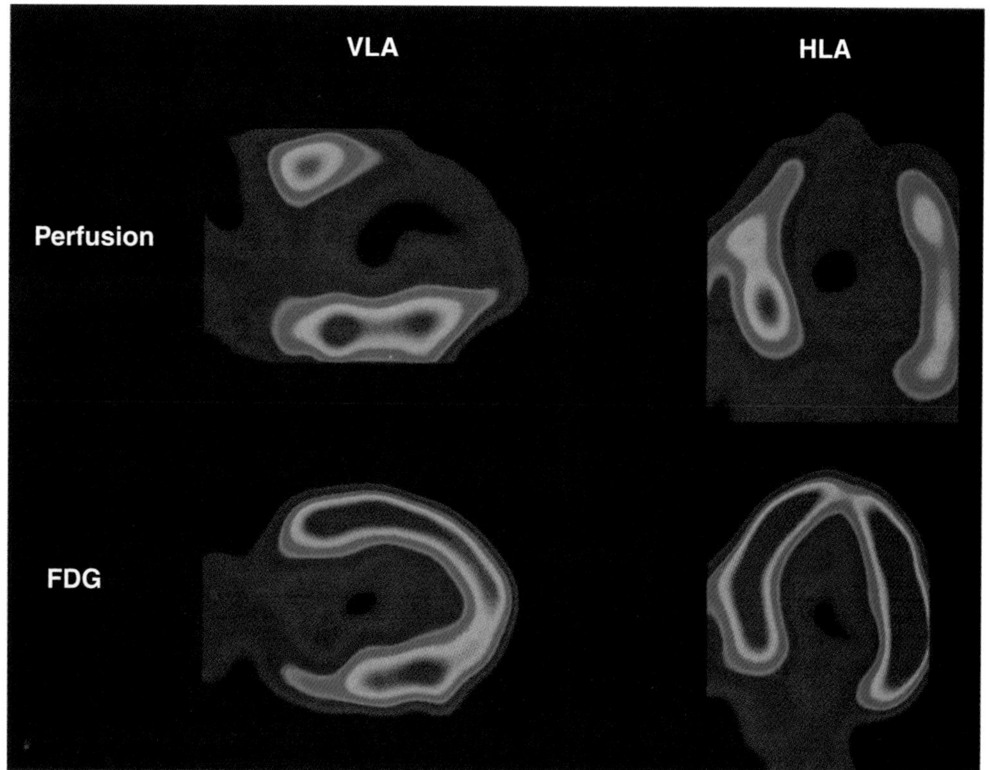

FIGURE 11.2.3. Examples of perfusion fluorodeoxyglucose (FDG) imaging patterns. *Color scale*: lowest to highest radioactivity concentration = black/blue/green/yellow/red (yellow/red are normal). **A:** Perfusion–metabolism mismatch in the anterior, lateral, and anteroseptal regions, indicating extensive hibernating myocardium and high risk. This patient died awaiting revascularization. (*continued*)

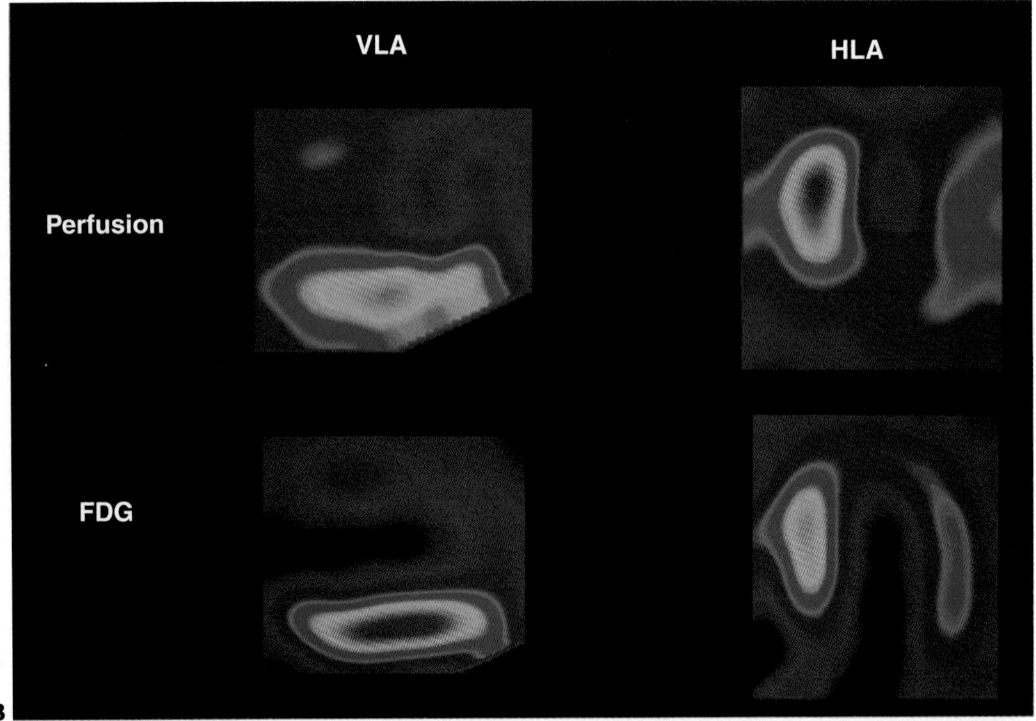

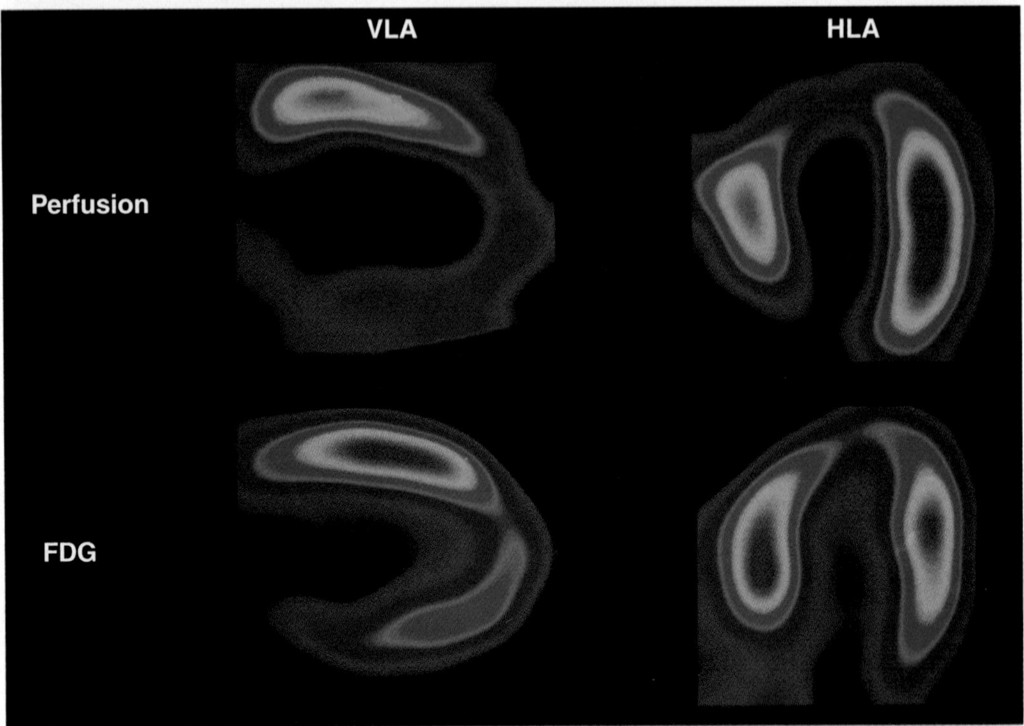

FIGURE 11.2.3. *Continued.* **B:** Perfusion–metabolism matched defect in the anterior, lateral, and apical regions indicating extensive scar. This 45-year-old woman subsequently underwent cardiac transplant. **C:** Partial mismatch in the inferior wall and apex indicating a mixture of nontransmural scar and hibernating myocardium. This patient underwent revascularization and had a modest improvement in ejection fraction from 23% to 28%. (*continued*)

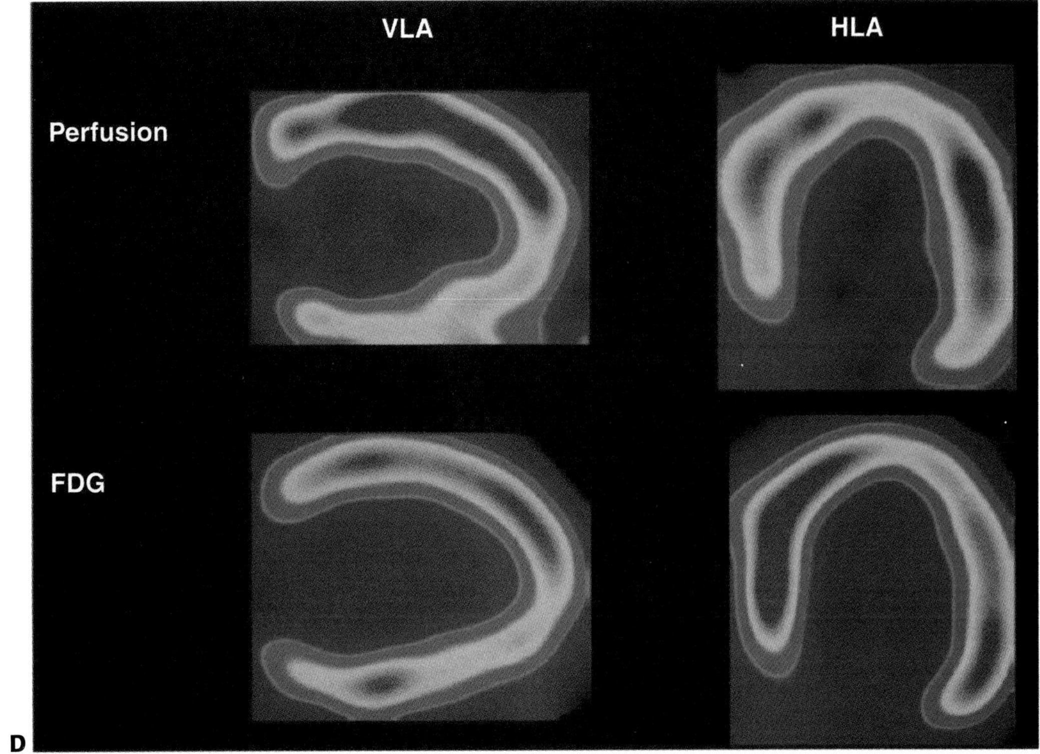

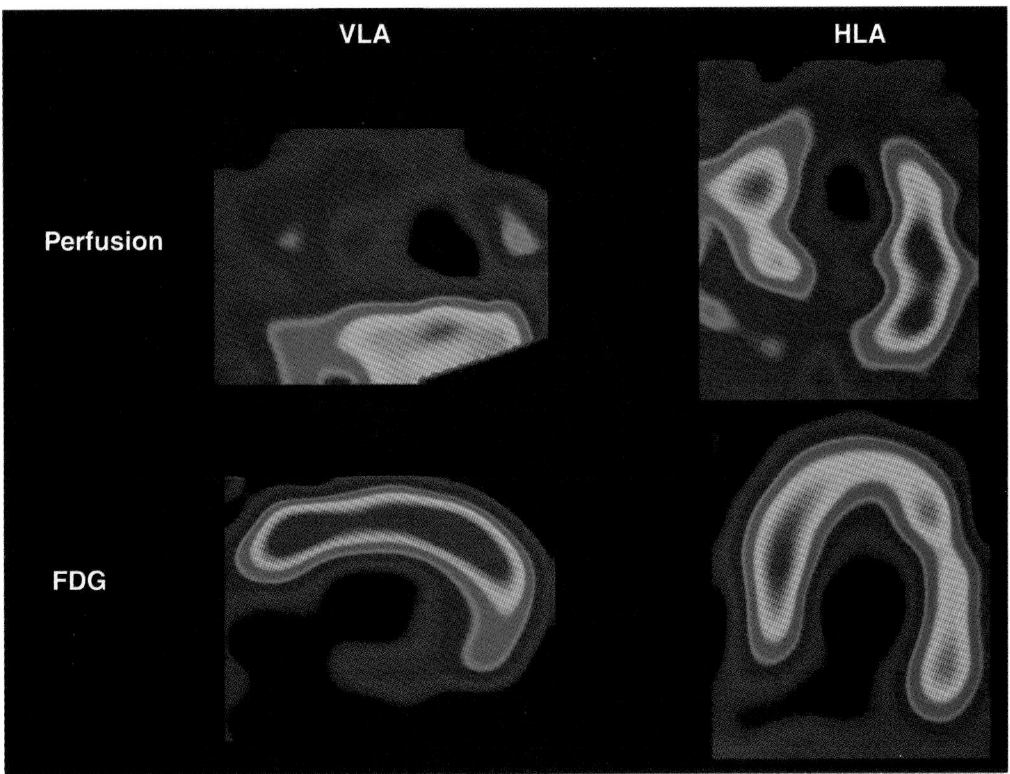

FIGURE 11.2.3. *Continued.* **D:** "Normal" perfusion–metabolism pattern in most of the left ventricle (LV), indicating maintained relative perfusion and metabolism at rest. This patient had severe proximal three-vessel disease and global LV dysfunction. Much of the myocardium was probably "stunned" due to prior ischemic episodes. Ejection fraction improved from 32% to 53% after revascularization. **E:** Reverse mismatch in the inferior wall. There is a large mismatch in the anterior wall and apex. In this case, the reverse mismatch is due to normalization error because of the intense FDG uptake in the contralateral anterior wall. The patient had single-vessel proximal left anterior descending coronary artery disease and underwent successful percutaneous transluminal coronary angioplasty with improvement in heart failure symptoms. VLA, Vertical Long Axis; HLA, Horizontal Long Axis.

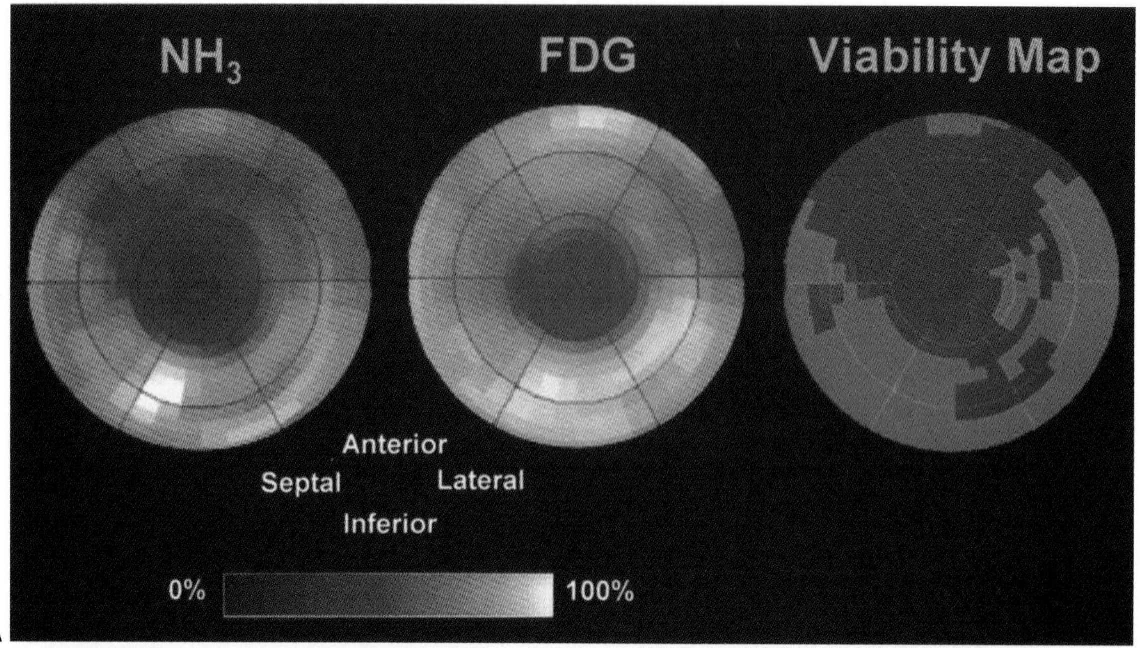

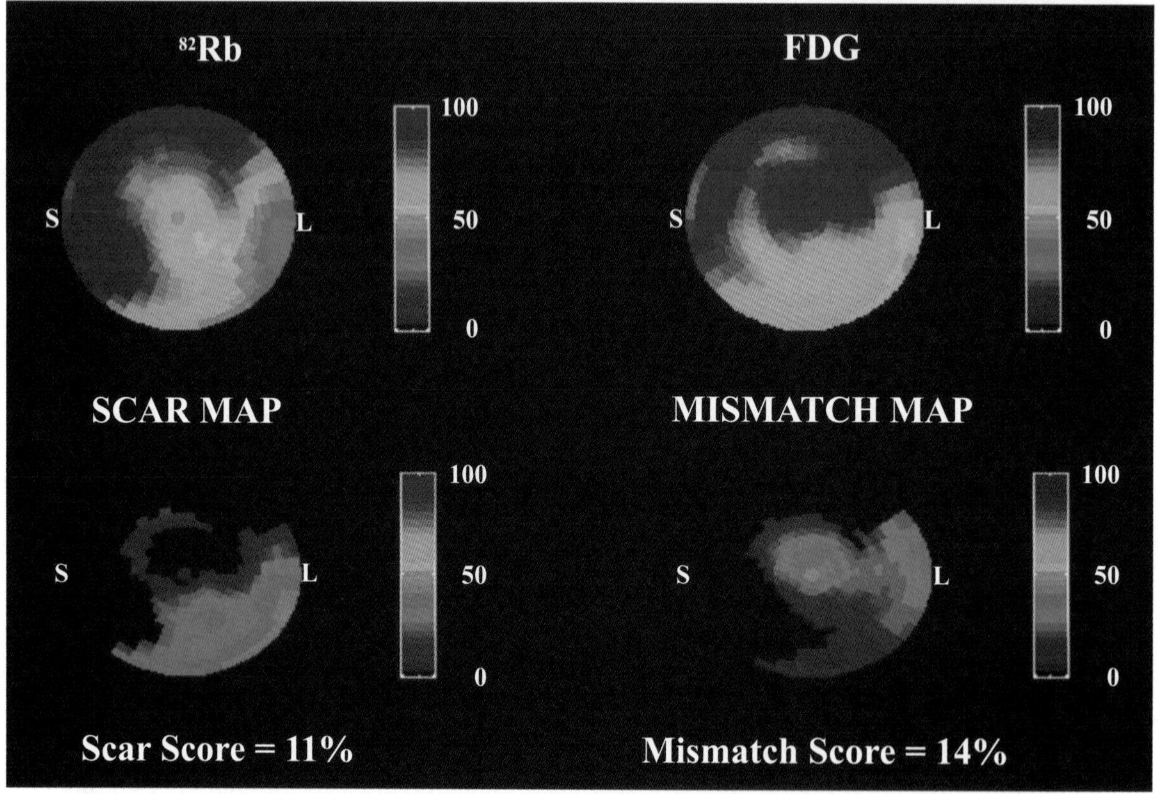

FIGURE 11.2.4. Examples of semiquantitative polar map displays. **A:** Nitrogen-13 ammonia ([^{13}N])-H-ammonia perfusion and fluorodeoxyglucose (FDG) polar maps are shown. The viability map (**right**) shows the percentage of the left ventricular myocardium with "normally" perfused myocardium (*green*), "flow-metabolism mismatch" (*blue*), and "scar tissue" (*red*). (From Haas F, L J, U H, et al. Ischemically compromised myocardium displays different time-courses of functional recovery: correlation with morphological alterations? *Eur J Cardio Thorac Surg* 2001;20:290–298, with permission.) **B:** Rubidium-82 ([^{82}Rb]) perfusion and FDG polar maps are shown. The lower maps are on the same color scale to show the size and extent of the abnormal myocardium expressed as a percentage of the total left ventricle (LV) for both scar tissue and mismatch. The advantage of (**A**) is the ease of interpretation of the parametric map and emphasis on the mismatch in a segment. The advantage of (**B**) is that when there is mixture of scar and mismatch it can be defined in the same segment.

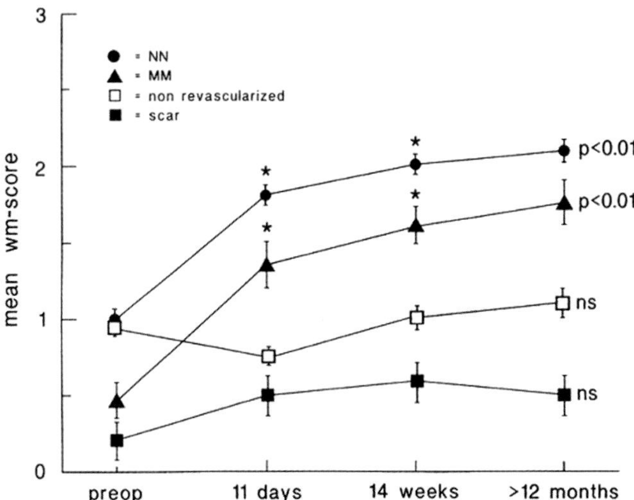

FIGURE 11.2.5. Time course of recovery of regional wall motion (*wm*) scores after revascularization in mismatched myocardium (*MM*), normally perfused myocardium (*NN*), and scar tissue (mean ± SEM). In contrast to viable tissue (MM and NN), no significant changes were observed for scar tissue. ns, not significant. (From Haas F, Augustin N, Holper K, et al. Time course and extent of improvement of dysfunctioning myocardium in patients with coronary artery disease and severely depressed left ventricular function after revascularization: correlation with positron emission tomography. *J Am Coll Cardiol* 2000;36:1927–1934, with permission.)

(Fig. 11.2.1). It may also take several months after revascularization for recovery of function, which may, even then, be incomplete (35,36). This concept of a progressive process of injury is further supported by studies showing increased mortality and impaired recovery of function when revascularization is delayed in patients with viable myocardium (53–55).

Regardless of the mechanism, the accuracy of PET "mismatch" as a marker for hibernating myocardium has been well demonstrated and is associated with recovery after revascularization (5,32,35,36,53,56–64). Furthermore, the extent of mismatch is related to the degree of recovery (5,32,58). Regional recovery may, however, be incomplete or delayed (Fig. 11.2.5) due to the extent of cellular disruption or coexisting subendocardial infarction, ventricular remodeling, or incomplete revascularization (35,36).

Reduced Perfusion/Reduced Fluorodeoxyglucose (Match)

A matched reduction in perfusion and metabolism indicates scar tissue formation. When severe, this usually indicates transmural scar and the absence of any significant viable tissue. Typically, such regions will not recover after revascularization (Fig. 11.2.3B).

When the perfusion FDG defect is mild, this indicates that the scar is "nontransmural." Both scar tissue and viable tissue are in the defect zone, but there is no hibernating tissue. The negative predictive value (NPV) for mild defects is not as high as that for more severe defects (59), probably because of the residual viable myocardium. The dysfunction in such segments is in part related to the nontransmural scar, but if the wall motion abnormality is more severe than expected, there may also be stunned myocardium. Stress perfusion PET imaging may be helpful in defining the presence of stress-induced ischemia, which leads to the recurrent stunning and dysfunction.

Recent data indicate that the extent of scar may be as important in predicting overall LV function recovery as the extent of hibernating myocardium, with a smaller scar predicting a greater degree of recovery (65,92).

Reduced Perfusion/Partly Reduced Fluorodeoxyglucose (Partial Mismatch)

A partial mismatch is observed when FDG uptake is reduced but not as severely as the perfusion defect. This finding indicates the presence of scar mixed with hibernating myocardium. In these defects, the relative extent of the "match" portion and the intensity of the "mismatch" portion may be helpful in predicting the degree of recovery. Recovery would be expected to be incomplete, because there is some scar tissue present (Fig. 11.2.3C).

Normal Perfusion/Normal Fluorodeoxyglucose (Normal Pattern)

In the absence of a wall motion abnormality, such segments are normal at rest and therefore viable. Because the standard perfusion FDG images are acquired at rest, it is still possible that such regions are supplied by a stenotic coronary vessel. Stress perfusion–weighted imaging would be required to rule out stress-induced ischemia.

In the presence of a wall motion abnormality, however, the "normal pattern" may indicate repetitive stunning, which would be expected to improve if adequately revascularized. Clinical information, angiography, and stress perfusion–weighted imaging may all help in this setting (Fig. 11.2.3D).

In dysfunctional segments, the normal pattern is more common than mismatch (70% vs. 24% of dysfunctional segments), has less associated tissue injury, and is more likely to demonstrate complete recovery than mismatched segments (31% vs. 18%, respectively, in one report) (35,36,47) (Figs. 11.2.4 and 11.2.6) Lack of complete

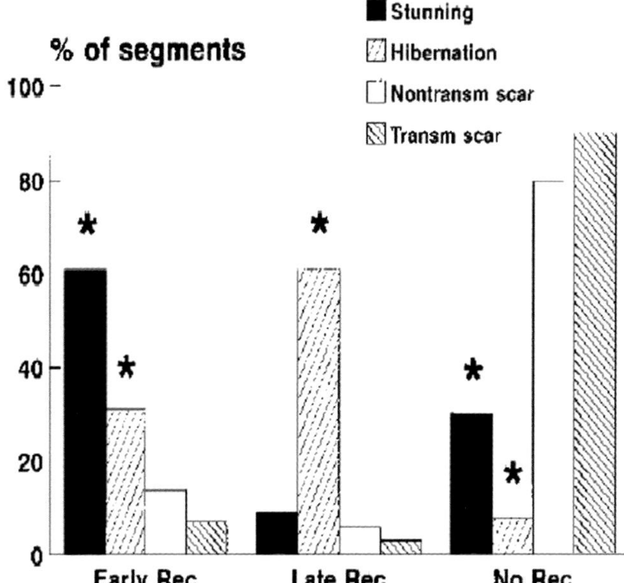

FIGURE 11.2.6. Percentage functional recovery of stunned and hibernating segments after surgical revascularization. (From Bax JJ, Visser FC, Poldermans D, et al. Time course of functional recovery of stunned and hibernating segments after surgical revascularization. *Circulation* 2001;104:I314–I318, with permission.)

recovery in these segments may be due to incomplete revascularization or the effect of remodeling.

When the normal pattern is more global in patients with LV dysfunction, this may indicate a more global process such as a nonischemic dilated cardiomyopathy or balanced severe proximal three-vessel CAD or left main coronary artery disease with right coronary artery disease. In a nonischemic dilated cardiomyopathy, the perfusion and FDG pattern may be patchy, which is consistent with patchy areas of fibrosis (92), while ischemic heart disease often (but not always) has at least one moderate or severe regional perfusion defect. Correlation with coronary angiography may be necessary, because these patients will typically do well if they have coronary disease amenable to revascularization. Recovery will depend on the extent of scar, normal pattern, and mismatch (5,35,36,58,65,91).

Normal Perfusion/Reduced Fluorodeoxyglucose (Reverse Mismatch)

A pattern of normal perfusion with a relative reduction in FDG uptake is often observed with perfusion FDG viability imaging. Some studies have associated this with recent (less than 2 weeks after) myocardial infarction and the presence of multivessel disease (93). In most circumstances, however, this finding should be viewed with caution. Often it is related to a lack of normalization of FDG uptake to the most normal perfusion zone (94).

With severe mismatch where FDG uptake may be greater than normal, a reverse mismatch occurs on the opposite wall if the FDG is not normalized correctly (Fig. 11.2.3E). Increased uptake in the lateral wall relative to the septum may occur in the presence of a left bundle branch block (LBBB), where resting perfusion is maintained but metabolism is decreased because of the decreased workload in the septum. In patients with nonischemic ischemic cardiomyopathy and LBBB this reverse mismatch pattern is very common, occurring in most patients (95,96). However, this phenomenon is not universal in patients with LBBB and ischemic cardiomyopathy, with over 30% of patients not exhibiting septal reverse mismatch. In those without reverse mismatch lateral wall perfusion defects are present in more than 90%. Further studies are needed to elucidate the mechanisms of septal metabolism alterations in patients with LBBB and whether such alterations can help predict the therapeutic response to treatments such as cardiac resynchronization therapy (97). Reverse mismatch in patients who have undergone bypass surgery has been observed, possibly because flow has been restored to regions that have nontransmural scar. This may be due to a mechanism similar to reverse redistribution observed with [^{20}1Tl] imaging (98).

In patients with diabetes, nonischemic viable tissue can have relative reductions in FDG due to impairment of glucose transport. This could lead to regions of reverse mismatch. The use of an insulin clamp may reduce this by increasing glucose uptake in the healthy myocardium in patients with diabetes (79,81,84).

Thus, when reverse mismatch is observed, it is important to consider why it may have occurred, to ensure that a normalization error has not underestimated the degree of mismatch in another territory. Importantly, however, perfusion is usually maintained in these segments. With normal resting perfusion, these regions usually represent viable myocardium that is not ischemic at rest.

Right Ventricular Uptake

With many cardiac radiotracers, when right ventricular hypertrophy develops due to pulmonary hypertension, the tracer uptake in the right ventricle (RV) is increased. FDG is no exception. Normal RV uptake is about 50% of the LV, although this has not been well evaluated (71). Increased RV uptake can be seen with RV pressure or volume overload or may reflect a relative reduction in LV uptake or a combination of the two. The clinical relevance of increased RV uptake in ischemic cardiomyopathy requires further investigation (71). However, in patients with pulmonary hypertension not due to LV dysfunction, a relationship to peak RV wall stress has been demonstrated (99). RV uptake also reduces in response to treatments effective for pulmonary hypertension (99).

Image Reporting

When interpreting and reporting perfusion FDG image results, the patterns of perfusion FDG uptake, the extent of hibernating scar and normal tissue, and the LV cavity size must all be considered. As well, one must understand the clinical information available, angiographic data (if available), and stress imaging results, and one must be in contact with the referring cardiologist or surgeon.

Determining the presence or extent of viable myocardium and whether there is adequate viable tissue to warrant revascularization can be challenging. Imaging can provide very important data to assist clinical decision management in this very difficult patient population. Key management decisions are required, which in any given patient depend on integrating the clinical data with the PET findings. Reporting styles differ for individual physicians and their referral base, but when conveying a message regarding viability, one must characterize all the LV tissue. Reporting only the area of the perfusion defect as scar or mismatch may provide incomplete information and can sometimes be misleading to the referring physician or surgeon. The authors have found that defining all three types of tissue—mismatch (ischemic but viable hibernating myocardium), match (scar), and normal (viable and not ischemic at rest)—their size, and their location can encompass the whole myocardium. This helps to emphasize to the referring physician the true extent of viability and the potential for recoverable tissue.

A note of caution in considering patients early after myocardial infarction. Overestimation of FDG uptake in the myocardium may occur due to uptake from the glycolytic activity of leukocytes in the necrotic zones of the infarct (71). This can lower the predictive accuracy of FDG PET viability imaging (94,100). Alternatively, FDG uptake may appear less than perfusion (reverse mismatch) (93) or uptake may be less than expected in the first week after thrombolysis (101). The accuracy of FDG PET in the subacute phase of myocardial infarction may be impaired compared with the usual patient with chronic CAD in which FDG PET has been much more widely applied (94).

Patients with Poor Image Quality

Image quality may occasionally hinder interpretation. Standard quality control issues should always be considered. Was sufficient glucose administered; was insulin administered if needed; was a sufficient dose of FDG administered; was there patient motion or other technical reasons for poor quality? Poor quality is most often due to poor myocardial FDG uptake. Images may appear as a blood pool image when FDG has not been adequately taken up by the heart. This most often occurs in patients with diabetes or glucose intolerance. When this occurs, several options are available. The perfusion image should be examined to determine whether there is sufficient information about viability to assist in decision making for the patient. If not, FDG imaging can be continued for an additional 20 to 30 minutes to allow for the slower rate of myocardial glucose (and FDG) uptake. If the blood glucose remains elevated, additional insulin can be administered. If this is not successful, the rates of glucose and FDG uptake are even slower. It may be necessary to remove the patient from the camera and have him or her return an hour later. This approach is possible now with postemission transmission imaging and CT attenuation correction. If the study was done with oral loading, repeating the study on a separate day with the clamp approach may be considered. These approaches will solve the poor image quality problem in most patients. For the remaining few, other modalities to assess viability could be considered.

Quantification of the Rate of Myocardial Fluorodeoxyglucose Uptake and Glucose Utilization

The rate of myocardial FDG uptake can be calculated using the Patlak graphical analysis. This mathematic model uses the tissue time–activity curves to determine a combined rate constant, K, for FDG myocardial entry and phosphorylation (102). This approach defines the relationship between (a) myocardial activity, $C_m(t)$, corrected for blood pool activity, $C_b(t)$, and (b) the integral of $C_b(t)$ from time equals 0 to a time t corrected for the blood activity at that time t ($\int C_b dt / C_b[t]$).

This relationship becomes linear after equilibration of tissue FDG (around 5 minutes). K is the slope of the linear portion of this relationship. To determine the rate of myocardial glucose utilization (rMGU), K is multiplied by the mean of three to five blood glucose samples taken after FDG injection and divided by the lumped constant (LC), which corrects for differences in rates of FDG uptake compared with glucose (102) (a value of 0.67 has been used as the LC) (102):

$$\text{rMGU} = K \times [\text{Glu}] \div \text{LC}.$$

In comparison to the standard approach, quantification of the rMGU requires a 70-minute dynamic scan to determine the time activity data for FDG uptake. This technique allows an estimate of myocardial glucose utilization. Because FDG uptake stops at the hexokinase reaction (i.e., FDG 6-phosphate accumulates), the rMGU does not reflect a single metabolic pathway alone, but rather exogenous myocardial glucose utilization.

The rMGU quantification requires the assumption that the LC is fixed. A fixed LC approach has been applied in many previous studies (79,81,83,86,87). However, recent studies (104,105) suggest that the rMGU in nonsteady-state conditions may be less accurate because of a varying LC. Regardless, the rMGU provides a tool to measure exogenous glucose utilization, which reflects FDG uptake. This approach has been extremely useful in understanding myocardial glucose utilization and metabolism. Although some centers have applied this approach to measure viability (52,91), in comparative studies, the quantitative methods have not been shown to improve viability determination but have been shown to add time and complexity to the studies (106).

Gated Fluorodeoxyglucose PET Imaging

Gated FDG PET imaging is now routine in many laboratories (71). Accurate measures of global and regional ventricular function have been demonstrated (Fig. 11.2.7) (66–68,71,107–110). Although the ability to define regional wall motion can sometimes be hindered by the presence of large areas of scar (71), gating of PET images allows better tissue characterization of perfusion, metabolism, and function without the problems of image registration that occur between PET and radionuclide angiography or echocardiography. This approach may also permit evaluation of wall motion and thickening at rest and with dobutamine stress, thus taking advantage of both metabolic and contractile reserve data (107). Advances in image registration between PET and other modalities are ongoing. Coregistration of data from CT coronary angiography using PET/CT or fusion with other modalities such as magnetic resonance imaging (MRI) will allow highly comprehensive tissue characterization with coronary anatomy, flow, metabolism, myocardial structure, and function.

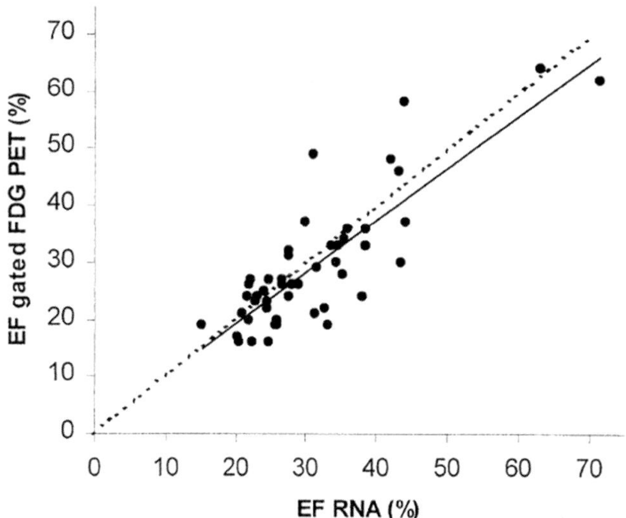

FIGURE 11.2.7. There is excellent agreement between left ventricular ejection fraction measured with QGS(c) analysis of FDG PET versus planar-gated RNA. (From Saab G, de Kemp R, Ukkonen H, et al. Gated 19-fluorine fluorodeoxyglucose positron emission tomography: determination of global and regional left ventricular function and myocardial tissue characterization. *J Nucl Cardiol* 2003;10:297–303, with permission .)

APPLICATION AND UTILITY OF FLUORODEOXYGLUCOSE PET

Ischemic Cardiomyopathy

The clinical utility of FDG PET is well recognized. It is a class I recommendation (level B evidence) for detection of myocardial viability by American College of Cardiology guidelines and a Canadian Cardiovascular Society position statement (111,112). Similar recommendations have been made in Europe (113).

The following clinical end points have been used to assess the utility of FDG PET and to relate it to the recovery of LV dysfunction: (a) recovery of regional LV dysfunction, (b) recovery of LV ejection fraction, (c) improvement in heart failure symptoms, and (d) improvement in survival. Myocardial metabolic imaging with FDG PET is an established method for assessing myocardial viability using these four clinical end points (114). Several additional studies have shown that myocardial metabolic imaging with FDG PET significantly influences management of patients with LV dysfunction. The literature in support of FDG PET myocardial imaging for the assessment of myocardial viability is summarized below.

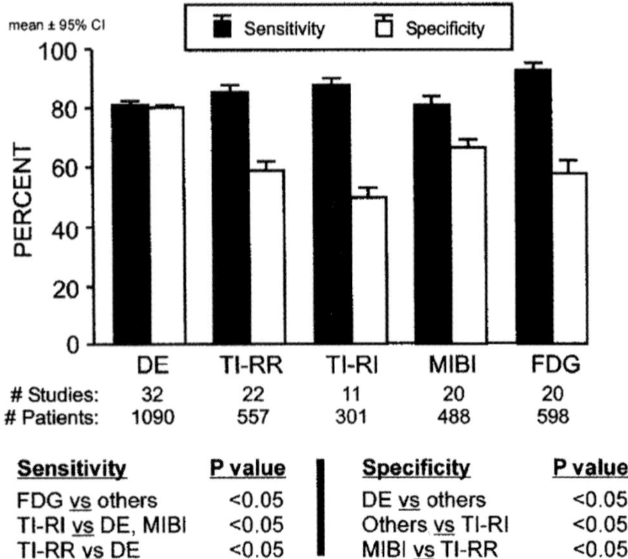

FIGURE 11.2.8. Comparison of the sensitivity and specificity of different noninvasive techniques to identify improvement regional left ventricle function. DE, dobutamine echocardiography; TI-RR, ^{201}TI rest-redistribution; TI-RI, ^{201}TI reinjection; MIBI, ^{99m}Tc-labeled sestamibi; FDG, fluorodeoxyglucose. (From Bax JJ, Poldermans D, Elhendy A, et al. Sensitivity, specificity, and predictive accuracies of various noninvasive techniques for detecting hibernating myocardium. *Curr Probl Cardiol* 2001;26:141–186, with permission.)

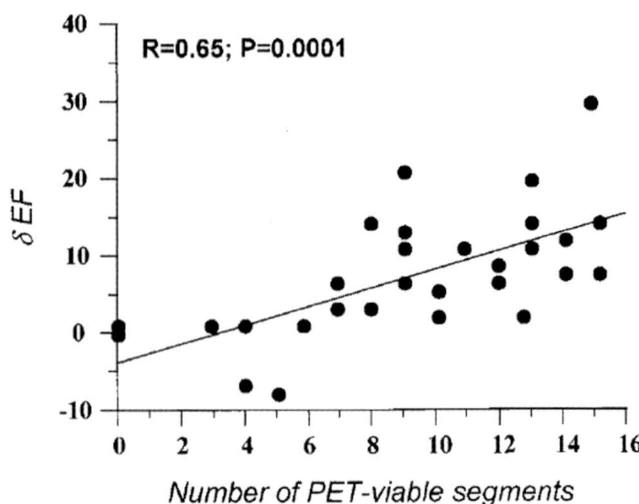

FIGURE 11.2.9. Correlation between the number of viable dysfunctional left ventricular (LV) segments and the absolute change in the LV ejection fraction (LVEF) (δEF) after revascularization. $Y = 1.2X \pm 3.97$. (From Pagano D, Townend J, Littler W, et al. Coronary artery bypass surgery as treatment for ischemic heart failure: the predictive value of viability assessment with quantitative positron emission tomography for symptomatic and functional outcome. *J Thorac Cardiovasc Surg* 1998;115:791–799, with permission.)

Prediction of Recovery of Regional and Global Left Ventricular Dysfunction after Revascularization

FDG PET has become a standard to which other viability methods, including newer approaches such as MRI, are compared (21,52,64,115–118). In 2001, a meta-analysis of all prior viability studies by Bax et al. (64) identified FDG PET as the most sensitive method for predicting wall motion recovery, while dobutamine echo was the most specific (Fig. 11.2.8). Direct comparison studies with dobutamine echocardiography are limited. However, in one study, the high sensitivity of FDG PET appears to be particularly advantageous in the patients with severe LV dysfunction as in the study of Pagano et al. (52), where FDG PET showed high NPV in 30 patients (ejection fraction [EF] = 23 ± 7) (positive predictive values vs. negative predictive values for FDG PET: 66% vs. 96%; dobutamine echo: 68% vs. 55%).

Recently the Canadian Cardiovascular Society, in collaboration with other societies, led a systematic review of advanced cardiac imaging updating the literature since the Bax et al. study (112). The sensitivity and specificity of FDG imaging for postrevascularization LV function recovery were 91% and 61%, respectively, for wall motion or LV function recovery among 1,047 patients with severe LV dysfunction (64,119–126) (Table 11.2.2). The sensitivity of FDG PET is consistently high >80% in all recent studies). Lower specificity likely reflects wider use of FDG PET in patients with more severe impairment of LV function where recovery may be delayed and incomplete. Severe structural hibernating myocardium that lacks contractile reserve but has preserved FDG uptake may take 6 months to 1 year before recovery of function is noted (35,36,47, 48,52). In some patients no recovery may occur. However, in these patients the benefit of revascularization to the viable tissue may be to improve outcome, with or without improved regional LV function (discussed further below).

Many studies have used mismatch as the viability indicator to predict improved function after revascularization. Recent data indicate that total FDG (92) or its inverse (the extent of scar) (65) is also important in predicting recovery (Fig. 11.2.9) (91). In addition, clinical parameters have been incorporated into prediction models along with PET parameters. In one study, extent of scar and extent of mismatch were the important PET predictors, whereas age, diabetes, previous coronary artery bypass graft, and time to surgery were important clinical parameters in predicting recovery of function (65).

Prediction of Improvement in Heart Failure Symptoms after Revascularization

As most patients with poor LV function suffer from symptoms of heart failure, an important goal in assessing myocardial viability is to predict recovery of heart failure symptoms after myocardial revascularization. Improvement in heart failure has been related to the PET pattern (presence or absence of mismatch) and type of treatment (revascularization or medical therapy). Improvement in heart failure symptoms more often occurs in the patients with mismatch who underwent revascularization compared to those without mismatch who were revascularized and to those on medical therapy (127–129). In a study by Di Carli et al. (129), the total extent of a PET mismatch before surgery correlated linearly and significantly, with a percentage improvement in functional state after coronary artery bypass graft ($r = 0.87$; $p < .0001$). A blood flow–metabolism mismatch of more than 18% was associated with a sensitivity of 76% and a specificity of

TABLE 11.2.2 PET Viability Diagnosis (EF <40%)

Authors (ref.)	Year	Number	EF (%)	Method Tracer	Reference Method (F/U)	Sensitivity: Patient/Segments % +ve Test with recovery			Specificity: Patient/Segments % −ve Test without recovery		
Bax (meta-analysis) 20 studies (64)	2001	598	36 ± 8	^{18}FDG ^{13}NH3/^{18}FDG	WM/EF (4.1 m)	751	807	93	417	725	58
Barrington et al. (119)[a]	2004	25	36	uptake+MM ^{201}Tl/^{18}FDG	WM (8 m)	6	6	100	23	25	92
Bax et al. (120)[b]	2001	47	30	SPT MM	WM + EF (3–6 m)	18	21	86	24	26	92
Bax et al. (121)[b]	2002	34	32	$^{13}NH_3$/^{18}FDG MRGR >60%	WM + EF (4–6m)	10	10	100	17	24	71
Bax et al. (122)[b]	2003	47	30	^{18}FDG SPT uptake	EF (6 m)	17	19	89	24	28	86
Gerber et al. (125)[a,b]	2001	178	38	^{18}FDG-MGU % uptake	EF (4–6m)	65	82	79	49	89	55
Korosoglou et al. (123)	2004	41	31	MIBI/FDG uptake	WM (3–6 m)	NR	NR	90	NR	NR	44
Nowak et al. (124)	2003	42	38	TF/FDG MM ^{15}O-water	WM (6–17 m)	32	40	80	23	32	72
Wiggers et al. (126)[b]	2001	35	35	$^{13}NH_3$/^{18}FDG uptake+MM	Pt WM (6.1 m)	14	14	100	14	21	67
Totals + Wt'd Mean		1,047	33.8			913	999	91	591	970	61
Mean weighted by number of patients								90			61

+ve, positive; −ve, negative; WM, wall motion; EF, ejection fraction; ^{18}FDG, fluorine-18-fluorode-oxyglucose; F/U, follow up; MM, mismatch; ^{201}Tl, thallium-201; SPT, single-positron emission computed tomography; $^{13}NH_3$, nitrogen 13 ammonia; MRGR, metabolic rate of glucose (relative); MGU, myocardial glucose utilization; MIBI, methoxyisobutyl isonitrile; NR, not reported; TF, tetrafosmin; Pt, partial.

[a]EF recovery used or patient-based recovery.

[b]Values derived from sensitivity, specificity, and other values provided.

(From Beanlands RS, Chow BJ, Dick A, et al. CCS/CAR/CANM/CNCS/CanSCMR joint position statement on advanced noninvasive cardiac imaging using positron emission tomography, magnetic resonance imaging and multidetector computed tomographic angiography in the diagnosis and evaluation of ischemic heart disease—executive summary. *Can J Cardiol* 2007;23:113, with permission.)

78% for predicting a change in functional state after revascularization. Patients with large mismatches (more than 18%) achieved a significantly higher functional state compared with those with minimal or no PET mismatch (<5%). Similarly, Bax et al. showed that if more than 31% of the LV demonstrated viable segments (normal perfusion or mismatch present), the positive predictive value and negative predictive value for symptom improvement were 76% and 71%, respectively (120).

These data indicate that the PET pattern of myocardial viability not only predicts recovery of regional and global LV dysfunction after myocardial revascularization but also identifies the subgroup of patients with poor LV function and heart failure who are most likely to show relief of heart failure symptoms as a result of revascularization. Furthermore, in patients with ischemic cardiomyopathy, the magnitude of improvement in heart failure symptoms after coronary bypass surgery is related to the preoperative extent and magnitude of myocardial viability as assessed by PET imaging. Patients with large perfusion–metabolism mismatches (i.e., greatest magnitude of ischemic viable myocardium by PET) appear to exhibit the greatest clinical benefit after revascularization.

Prediction of Improvement in Clinical Outcomes after Revascularization

There are now at least nine FDG PET studies that have evaluated clinical outcomes in patients with ischemic cardiomyopathy, comparing those with and without viability and with and without revascularization (112,127,128,130–138) (Fig 11.2.10 is one example). These outcome studies and a 2002 meta-analysis (that included four of the studies) (132) have consistently demonstrated that patients with viable myocardium on FDG PET are at high risk for

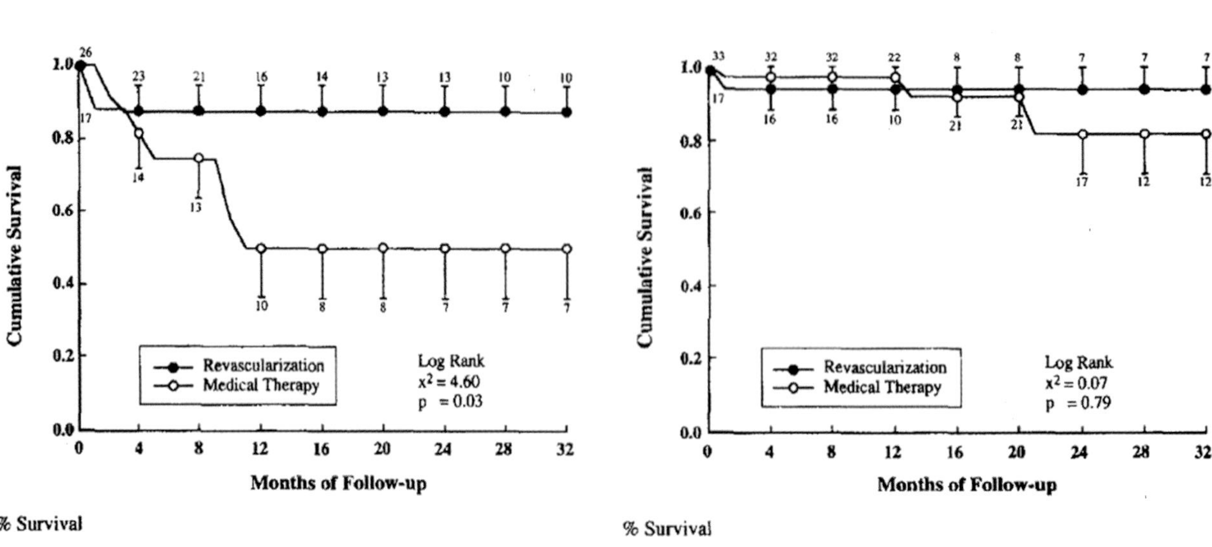

FIGURE 11.2.10. A: Mismatch and (B) no mismatch cumulative survival of patients, by presence or absence of PET mismatch and mode of treatment (i.e., medical therapy or revascularization). (From Di Carli MF, Davidson M, Little R, et al. Value of metabolic imaging with positron emission tomography for evaluating prognosis in patients with coronary artery disease and left ventricular dysfunction. *Am J Cardiol* 1994;73:527–533, with permission.)

death or other cardiac events (myocardial infarction, cardiac arrest, hospitalization) if they do not undergo timely revascularization. For patients with *severe* LV dysfunction (mean EF <30%) and viable myocardium, mortality rates ranged from 21% to 41% without revascularization compared to 0% to 15% for those who undergo revascularization (Table 11.2.3) These data suggest that in patients with ischemic cardiomyopathy, revascularization should be recommended only in those with FDG PET evidence of myocardial viability. These data also corroborate the findings of the above mentioned four studies and indicate that PET perfusion FDG–metabolic assessment of myocardial viability may predict long-term survival as a benefit of revascularization.

Longer term follow-up has also been evaluated. Di Carli et al. (138) followed 93 patients with mean EF equal to 25% for a median of 4 years. Cox survival models identified heart failure class, past myocardial infarction, and PET mismatch as the best predictors of survival. Patients were divided into four groups: (a) mismatch (M/M)(+ve); revascularization (Rev)(+ve); (b) M/M(+ve), Rev(−ve); (c) M/M(−ve) Rev(+ve); (d) M/M(−ve) Rev(−ve). Among patients with PET mismatch, those who underwent revascularization had improved survival compared with those on medical therapy (75% vs. 30%; $P = .007$), those without mismatch, who underwent coronary artery bypass graft, had a trend ($P = .085$) for improved symptoms and survival only if they also had angina. In another study, Sawada et al. (134) demonstrated similar findings in patients with diabetes and severe LV dysfunction (mean EF 29%). Again, for those with mismatch, revascularization improved survival compared to medical therapy at 4 years ($P = .027$). At 8 years, survival was 53% versus 17% ($P = .065$); but when patients with severe LV dysfunction (EF <30%) were considered, survivals were 55% and 0% ($P = .038$), respectively. Patients with viability on medical therapy did worse than those without viability. These data corroborate the findings of the above mentioned nine studies and indicate that PET perfusion FDG-metabolic assessment of myocardial viability may predict long-term survival as a benefit of revascularization.

A study by Tarakji et al. (55) used propensity matching to compare 153 of 230 patients undergoing early (<6 months) revascularization to 153 of 535 patients treated medically. Patients with revascularization did better than the medical group (80% vs. 66% survival at 3 years). The study did not compare those with and without viability but did note that the extent of ischemia and hibernation on PET imaging was predictive of death. The authors indicate that their "findings are consistent with the hypothesis that among patients with evidence of myocardial viability, early mechanical intervention may improve survival." These data are supported by earlier studies also demonstrating the benefits of early revascularization in patients with viability (53–55) (Fig. 11.2.11).

Influence of Fluorodeoxyglucose PET Myocardial Viability Imaging on Clinical Decision Making and Its Cost Effectiveness

A previous study evaluated the influence of PET perfusion FDG–metabolic imaging in the management of 87 patients with low LV ejection fractions (72). Assessment of myocardial viability by PET imaging redirected therapy from transplantation work-up to revascularization in 7 of 11 patients (63%), medical therapy to revascularization in 8 of 18 patients (44%), and from revascularization to medical therapy in 16 of 38 patients (42%); 50 of 87 patients (57%) had their management influenced by PET data. Among the

TABLE 11.2.3 PET Viability Prognosis (EF <40%)

	Patient Population					Mortality Rates			
Authors (ref.)	Year	N	EF	Mean FU (mo)	Test Method Tracer	Viab +ve Rev +ve (%)	Viab +ve Rev −ve (%)	Viab −ve Rev +ve (%)	Viab −ve Rev −ve (%)
Allman (132) (meta-analysis)[a]	2002	3,088	32	25	Tl/DE/FDG	3.2	16.0	7.7	6.2
Allman (PET)[a] (132)		1,029	35	24	perfusion/FDG	6.0	21.0	7.0	8.0
Eitzman et al. (127)	1993	82	33	12	Rb-NH_3/FDG	3.8	33.3[b]	0.0	8.3
Di Carli et al. (128)	1994	93	25	14	NH_3/FDG	11.5	23.5[b]	5.9	18.2
Lee et al. (131)	1994	129	37	17	Rb/FDG	8.2	14.3[b]	5.3	12.5
Beanlands et al. (53)	1998	85	26	17	MIBI/FDG	3.2	28.6[c]	—	18.8
Zhang et al. (132)	2001	123	35	37	MIBI/FDG	0.0	26.7[d]	8.0	3.8
Rohatgi et al. (136)	2001	99	22	25	NH_3/FDG	0.0	34.5[d]	0.0	15.2
Santana et al. (135)	2004	90	26	22	G-Rb/FDG	NR	NR[e]	NR	NR
Desideri et al. (134)[f]	2005	261	29	34	NH_3/FDG	14.5	28.3[d]	10.3	21.5
Sawada et al. (134)[g]	2005	61	29	48	NH_3/FDG	47.4	83.3[d]	57.1	43.8
TOTALS/mean[h]		933	30	26		9.4	30.9[i]	11.8	17.7

EF, ejection fraction; FU, follow up; Viab, viability; Rev, revascularization; Tl, thallium-2001; DE, dobutamine echo; FDG, fluorine-18-fluorodeoxyglucose; Rb, rubidium-82; NH_3, nitrogen 13 ammonia; MIBI, methoxyisobutyl isonitrile; G-Rb, gated rubidium-82; NR, not reported.
[a]Meta-analysis of 24 viability studies; rates reported are for all studies in line 1; line 2 is data for 11 FDG PET studies: 7 of which reported outcomes; 4 of which compared event rates in subgroups and had EF <40%; table data derived from reported values and estimated for 1 year follow-up based on rates and mean follow-up reported.
[b]P<.05 Viab +ve, rev −ve versus rev +ve for total cardiac event rates.
[c]P <.05 delayed versus early revasculuarization.
[d]P < .05 Viab +ve, rev −ve versus rev +ve (also versus other groups [Allman et al. 2002; Zhang et al. 2002]).
[e]Values not reported: 11% survival benefit with revascularization in patients with viability and LV remodeling (End-diastolic volume [EDV] >260).
[f]Values determined from reported percentages.
[g]Patients with diabetes, left ventricle dysfunction, and coronary artery disease.
[h]Totals/mean include eight studies with reported values. Does not include meta-analysis.
[i]P <.05 versus other groups using a Fisher's exact test.
(From Beanlands RS, Chow BJ, Dick A, et al. CCS/CAR/CANM/CNCS/CanSCMR joint position statement on advanced noninvasive cardiac imaging using positron emission tomography, magnetic resonance imaging and multidetector computed tomographic angiography in the diagnosis and evaluation of ischemic heart disease—executive summary. *Can J Cardiol* 2007;23:113, with permission.)

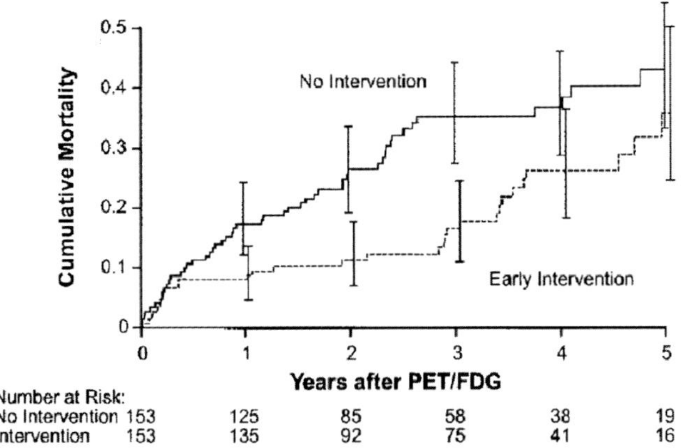

FIGURE 11.2.11. The effects of early intervention of revascularization on mortality rates as predicted by fluorodeoxyglucose (FDG) PET compared to patients with no intervention. (From Tarakji KG, Brunken R, McCarthy PM, et al. Myocardial viability testing and the effect of early intervention in patients with advanced left ventricular systolic dysfunction. *Circulation* 2006;113:230–237, with permission.)

subgroup of patients with an EF less than 30%, 29 of 41 (71%) had their management influenced by PET data. They concluded that the definition of myocardial viability by PET perfusion FDG–metabolic imaging has a significant impact on difficult therapy decisions in patients with impaired ventricular function and CAD.

The impact of FDG PET on therapy decisions may also affect outcome. Haas et al. (139), in a cohort design study of 69 patients, showed that the patients who had FDG PET imaging data used in decisions for surgery had better outcomes after surgical revascularization than patients whose decision was based on coronary angiography and clinical data alone. Mortality rates after revascularization in patients with FDG and without FDG PET were 0% and 11%, respectively, at 30 days. This difference was maintained at 1 year when mortality rates were 3% and 14%, respectively (Fig. 11.2.12)

Although FDG PET imaging appears to impact decision making, studies evaluating its incremental cost in patients with ischemic heart disease and LV dysfunction have been limited. In one study by Jaklin et al. (140), the costs of three approaches were compared: (a) coronary artery bypass grafting for all patients; (b) PET to select those with hibernating myocardium for grafting; and (c) medical

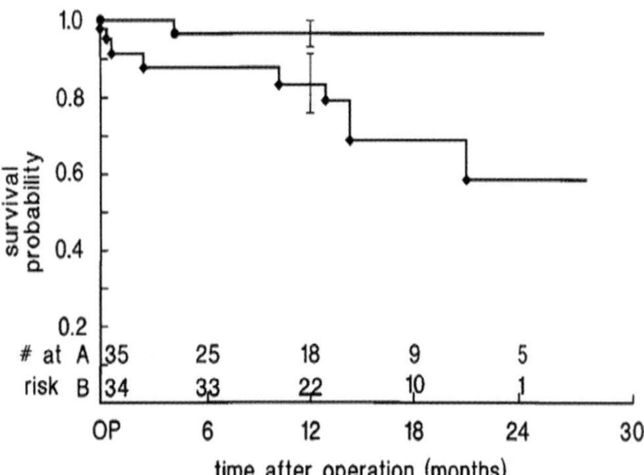

FIGURE 11.2.12. Actuarial survival curve (±SE) with the hospital mortality rate included for patients undergoing surgical revascularization. The decision for surgery was based on coronary angiography and clinical data (group A; *diamonds*) compared with patients in whom the decision was based on coronary angiography, clinical data, and fluorine-18-fluorodeoxyglucose PET viability data (group B; *circles*). Survival was significantly improved in group B ($P < .01$). (From Haas F, Haehnel C, Picker W, et al. Preoperative positron emission tomographic viability assessment and perioperative and postoperative risk in patients with advanced ischemic heart disease. *J Am Coll Cardiol* 1997;30:1693–1700, with permission.)

therapy for all patients. Using a health care perspective, costs and outcomes were considered for 1 year from the time of initial treatment. The study demonstrated that in the selection of patients with LV dysfunction referred for coronary artery bypass graft, the use of FDG PET viability imaging was cost effective. A recent health technology assessment from Quebec also suggested cardiac FDG PET is cost effective (141).

Comparisons to Other Myocardial Viability Imaging Methods

Several modalities have been used clinically for the detection of myocardial viability. Although many of these can be applied in patients with mild or moderate LV dysfunction, FDG PET appears to be preferred in patients with more severe LV dysfunction. Previous studies and reviews have indicated a greater impact of FDG PET over [^{201}Tl] viability imaging (5,142,143). Other studies have shown that severe ^{99m}Tc-methoxyisobutyl isonitrile defects underestimate viability on FDG imaging (144–146). A review of the literature has demonstrated that FDG PET myocardial metabolic imaging is superior to SPECT imaging for the assessment of improvement in regional LV dysfunction after myocardial revascularization (64).

In this same review, FDG PET was found to be significantly more sensitive for predicting regional recovery of function than any of the other viability techniques, whereas dobutamine echocardiography was the most specific (64). However, 45% (9 of 20 patients) of the FDG studies included patient populations with a mean EF less than 35%, while 28% (9 of 32) of dobutamine echocardiography studies included such patients (64).

Direct comparisons between FDG imaging and dobutamine echocardiography are limited (46,52,147,148) and even more limited in severe LV dysfunction. As noted above, a key finding in the study by Pagano et al. (52) was the superiority of FDG PET over dobutamine echocardiography in a group of patients with severe LV dysfunction (EF = 23% ± 7%). This was even greater in the worst functioning (akinetic) segments (positive predictive value vs. negative predictive value of FDG PET: 80% vs. 94%; dobutamine echocardiography: 73% vs. 41%). Another study by Sambuceti et al. (149) reported that dobutamine detected 55% of stunned and only 16% of hibernating myocardium. Recently, two more modestly sized studies in patients populations with mean EF 35% or less also showed significantly increased sensitivity for FDG PET (90% to 100%) compared to dobutamine echocardiography (71% to 83%). However, dobutamine echo had better specificity (44% to 67% vs. 76% to 81%) (123,126).

Many of the current myocardial imaging techniques have clinical value in assessment of viability. However, when considering the patients with severely impaired LV function where viability is most relevant, FDG PET appears to be more useful.

Randomized Controlled Trials

A randomized controlled trial compared FDG PET to ^{99m}Tc-methoxyisobutyl isonitrile-SPECT and observed no significant differences in outcome between the two techniques (150). Unfortunately, the study was probably too small (n = 103) as a prospective outcome study to detect a significant difference. In addition, the patients were a relatively low-risk population with predominately mild to moderate LV dysfunction who waited a long time for revascularization (115 days). Event rates were low, making it too difficult to demonstrate differences (151).

The PARR2 (PET and Recovery following Revascularization-2) Trial has recently completed recruitment. Results of this trial will help to better define the role of viability imaging in patients with severe LV dysfunction (152). Ongoing trials such as the STICH (Surgical Treatment for Ischemic Heart Failure) Trial, the HEART (Heart Failure Revascularization Trial) study and long-term follow-up in PARR2 will continue to add to the data to help define the patient population who would most benefit from FDG PET imaging (152–154).

Cardiac Magnetic Resonance Imaging

Two MRI myocardial viability methods have been used: dobutamine stress MR (DSMR) and late gadolinium enhancement (LGE). Compared to that of dobutamine stress echo, DSMR has similar or improved accuracy for predicting improvement in function postrevascularization. LGE is used to assess infarcted myocardium. Gadolinium, an extravascular contrast agent, accumulates in infarcted tissue due to the large extravascular space compared to normal tissue. LGE demonstrates good correlation with PET and superiority to SPECT in defining viable and nonviable myocardium. The thickness of the scar and viable segment can be also determined. This has been used to improve the predictive accuracy of LGE for recovery after revascularization (112). In one study, segments with less than 25% transmural LGE had a 79% chance of functional recovery postrevascularization compared to 6% when scar thickness was greater than 50% (155).

Much of the data for MRI viability imaging are in patient populations with mild LV dysfunction (mean LV EF >40%) (112). In addition, there are few studies evaluating the impact of DSMR and LGE cardiac magnetic resonance on cardiac outcomes to date, although several studies are under way. This is in contrast to FDG PET where there is a wealth of data in patients with severe LV dysfunction evaluating either LV function recovery or outcomes (112).

In a small study of 19 patients, viable tissue on LGE MRI correlates with FDG uptake. Thick >4.5 mm) and metabolically viable segments ≥50% FDG uptake) recover function in 85% of patients, while thin metabolically nonviable segments improved function in only 13%. Metabolically viable segments with a thin viable rim and thick segments with reduced FDG uptake improved function in only 36% and 23% of segments, respectively. Thus metabolic imaging with FDG PET and tissue composition imaging with MRI provide complementary data that can help discriminate various types of dysfunctional myocardium. Most metabolically viable segments with a thick viable rim on LGE MRI will recover function after revascularization, whereas all other combinations have low recovery rates of contractile function (115). As suggested by Rizzello et al. (156), additional data are often required in patients with intermediate level scar to best predict function recovery. However, as noted above, metabolic activity detected on FDG PET does not always equate to recovery of wall motion or LV function, often because of the delay in recovery and/or the incomplete recovery in these segments, but it does relate to prognosis in patients with severe LV dysfunction. For LGE MRI, further MRI outcome studies are required in the patient population with severe LV dysfunction.

A recently identified complication of gadolinium, *nephrogenic systemic fibrosis*, has led to the recommendation that gadolinium not be used in patients with moderate to severely reduced creatinine clearance (<60 mL/min) (157). This will limit the use of LGE MRI in patients with severe LV dysfunction, many of whom have renal insufficiency.

Other PET Viability Methods

In addition to FDG, other methods using PET perfusion or metabolic imaging have been used to define myocardial viability. The utility of perfusion tracers alone in viability detection is threefold: (a) tracer uptake or kinetics measured at stress and rest can define flow reserve, which provides insight into potential regions of stress-induced ischemia that may contribute to myocardial stunning and possibly hibernation; (b) resting flow provides insight into tissue perfusion, and there is a level of perfusion below which viability may not be sustainable; and (c) as with perfusion FDG imaging, the characterization of viability is often best achieved through techniques that can define both perfusion and cell integrity (5,35,59). The kinetics of some perfusion tracers depends on both delivery to the tissue (or flow) and retention in intact viable cells, and both perfusion and cell viability information can be obtained with one study.

$H_2[^{15}O]$ and the Perfusable Tissue Index

$H_2[^{15}O]$ is freely diffusible with kinetics directly related to flow. This has allowed measurement of the perfusable tissue fraction, which is the fraction of tissue in a given region that can rapidly exchange water (158). Such tissue is presumed to be viable. The method then corrects for the anatomic tissue fraction, which represents the extravascular tissue density defined from transmission data and the $C[^{15}O]$ blood pool images. The perfusable tissue index is the perfusable tissue fraction/anatomic tissue fraction and quantifies the amount of tissue that is freely perfusable with water (and therefore viable) within the given myocardial segment. A normal perfusable tissue index is 1.0, although a perfusable tissue index higher than 0.7 was used to define viable tissue and predicted functional recovery after revascularization in one study (159). In more recent work, perfusable tissue index was correlated inversely with scar defined on contrast-enhanced MRI. However, with increasing quantities of scar, PET tended to overestimate viable tissue. The cutoff value of 0.89 had the best accuracy, with sensitivity and specificity of 75% and 77%, respectively (160).

$[^{13}N]$-ammonia: Flow and Retention

Mathematic modeling of $[^{13}N]$-H_3 kinetics allows quantification of absolute myocardial blood flow. Gewirtz et al. (161) used this approach and demonstrated that there is a threshold blood flow (<0.25 mL/min/g), below which viable recoverable myocardium is unlikely. This finding certainly fits with observations that very severe perfusion defects are less likely to have viable myocardium. However, when flow is reduced but above the threshold, the likelihood of recovery may be less certain. Metabolic or cell integrity information may help tissue characterization in these circumstances.

Nitrogen-13-ammonia retention in the cell is due to conversion to $[^{13}N]$-glutamine, which is an energy-requiring process and therefore depends on cell integrity. In one study, a combined approach of flow data and the volume of distribution of $[^{13}N]$-H_3 was shown to be an accurate measure of viability (118). $[^{13}N]$-H_3 uptake alone has been shown to more accurately predict recovery of function than flow measurements alone (162).

Rubidium-82 Washout Kinetics

As a potassium analogue, $[^{82}Rb]$ uptake is dependent on flow and cell membrane integrity. In the presence of necrotic tissue, $[^{82}Rb]$ uptake may be reduced due to more rapid washout. This differential washout has been used as a marker of viability (163,164). However, studies evaluating recovery postrevascularization and long-term outcome are limited.

Carbon-11-acetate Washout Kinetics

The clearance kinetics of carbon-11 ($[^{11}C]$)-acetate directly correlate with rates of oxidative metabolism and myocardial oxygen consumption. In addition, $[^{11}C]$-acetate PET yields quantitative data on myocardial blood flow. Not surprisingly, it also can be used for defining viability. In experienced centers, it has been found to be a reliable and accurate approach (63,165–168). The addition of dobutamine with $[^{11}C]$-acetate offers some potential for defining metabolic reserve and recovery of function. This approach is discussed in greater detail in Chapter 11.3.

All of these methods have some promise, but studies evaluating LV functional recovery and long-term outcomes are limited. An on-site cyclotron is required for $[^{11}C]$-acetate, $[^{13}N]$-ammonia, and $H_2[^{15}O]$ production that has limited their application in the past in comparison to FDG. Rubidium-82 is generator produced and more widely available in North America but has limited availability in other parts of the world. Accessibility of these tracers will increase with the worldwide growth of PET imaging. Large clinical trials are needed to determine the potential role of these techniques in the determination of viability.

STRESS FLUORODEOXYGLUCOSE IMAGING

Although FDG PET is predominantly used in resting condition to assess myocardial viability, it has also been used in conjunction with stress testing to evaluate transient myocardial ischemia. Several studies have shown that injection of FDG following stress may be used as an "ischemic memory marker" for recent antecedent ischemia. In 1986 Camici et al. (169) injected FDG 5 to 14 minutes following exercise in ten healthy volunteers and 12 patients with chronic stable CAD. In all but one patient, myocardial FDG uptake by ischemic segments was increased in comparison to that in the nonischemic segments. The regions of increased FDG uptake corresponded to the location of perfusion defects that were noted on [^{82}Rb] exercise images. In contrast, FDG uptake by nonischemic areas was relatively unchanged from that in healthy subjects.

In 1991 Marwick et al. (170) injected FDG 30 minutes following exercise in 27 patients with known coronary anatomy. Dipyridamole stress [^{82}Rb] PET perfusion images, on a separate day, were used to identify regions of stress-induced ischemia. They found postexercise FDG PET to be a sensitive indicator of transient ischemia and myocardial hibernation, with a strong correlation between regions of increased FDG uptake compared with ischemic myocardial regions identified by reduced stress [^{82}Rb] uptake and known coronary anatomy. In a subsequent study Araujo et al. (171) injected FDG 20 minutes after the initiation of a 4-minute dipyridamole infusion in 11 patients with chronic stable angina and angiographic evidence of CAD. Poststress FDG PET images were compared with resting FDG PET images obtained on a separate day without prior stress. All patients showed poststress increased FDG uptake in ischemic compared with normal regions, which localized to dipyridamole-induced perfusion defects.

In several other studies, FDG was injected during stress to detect stress-induced ischemia. Abramson et al. (172) injected FDG and ^{99m}Tc-sestamibi 1 minute before peak exercise (in eight patients) or 3 minutes after the completion of the dipyridamole stress (in 11 patients). Eight of the nine patients with angiographically proven CAD showed increased FDG uptake in the myocardial regions supplied by the diseased coronary arteries (sensitivity 89%). Of the ten patients without angiographic evidence of CAD, only one showed increased focal accumulation of FDG (specificity 90%). In a subsequent study, He et al. (173) studied 26 patients with no history of myocardial infarction but with known or suspected CAD. ^{99m}Tc-sestamibi and FDG were injected at peak exercise. Forty to 60 minutes postradionuclide injection, ^{99m}-sestamibi and FDG images were acquired simultaneously using a single crystal SPECT camera with separate energy windows. Rest perfusion images were acquired independently, and all patients underwent coronary angiography. Of the four patients without CAD, FDG uptake was either nonexistent or minimally above the background. Of the 22 patients with angiographic evidence of CAD, 18 demonstrated perfusion abnormalities and 20 showed enhanced myocardial FDG accumulation. Compared with ^{99m}Tc-sestamibi stress images, FDG stress images had increased correlation with known diseased vascular territories (sensitivity of 67% vs. 49%) and the extent of ischemia was greater. Although He et al. found FDG stress images to be of high quality, they discovered that the entire myocardial contour was not always visible. Using perfusion images in conjunction with FDG images for abnormal myocardial localization easily solved this problem. They concluded that combined FDG (^{99m}Tc)-sestamibi stress imaging allows for a more accurate assessment of transient myocardial ischemia than perfusion imaging alone.

Although the studies reviewed here point toward both a high sensitivity and specificity of FDG stress images, several logistical and physiologic limitations remain. From a physiologic standpoint, questions remain as to whether FDG stress imaging is helpful in insulin-resistant patients and whether FDG studies need to be performed in the fasting state or after a glucose load. From a technical standpoint, there is no current validated protocol for FDG stress imaging. Although the biokinetics and blood clearance curves are known for FDG metabolism at rest, they are unknown for FDG metabolism at stress and may differ from those at rest (174). In addition, neither the normal pattern of myocardial FDG accumulation in healthy subjects nor the clinical relevance of increased FDG uptake has been established. Also, the optimal times for FDG injection and imaging have not yet been studied. Finally, some suggest that perfusion imaging is still required to properly interpret the FDG uptake stress images. If so, this approach may be well suited to FDG SPECT imaging, where dual isotope techniques could allow simultaneous measurement of a perfusion tracer and FDG administered during stress (175). All of this underscores the need for further large-scale investigations, which must occur before FDG stress imaging can be commonly utilized.

OTHER APPLICATIONS OF FLUORODEOXYGLUCOSE PET AND FUTURE DIRECTIONS

Recent applications of FDG have extended its potential application beyond viability detection in ischemic cardiomyopathy. Some of these applications include its use (a) as a noninvasive marker of the potential responsiveness to therapy such as β blockade in nonischemic cardiomyopathy (176); (b) as a means to determine and monitor RV metabolic alterations and potential response to therapy in pulmonary hypertension (99); and (c) to define altered septal metabolism and in theory as a means to predict response to cardiac resynchronization therapy (95,97). FDG PET has also been used to define inflammatory disorders, such as sarcoidosis and aortitis with or without myocarditis (177–180).

Recently FDG has been applied to investigate vulnerable plaque in the carotid arteries (181) and more recently has shown early potential as a means to characterize active coronary plaque (182–184). There are potential exciting opportunities in this development. More studies are needed to define the pathogenesis of disease in general and as it relates to the FDG uptake fluctuations, and how these may be used to predict events and/or monitor therapy.

In ischemic heart disease, FDG viability imaging may become useful in conjunction with autonomic imaging with [^{11}C]-hydroxyephedrine as a means to identify patients at risk for sudden cardiac death. This hypothesis is being tested in the ongoing Prediction of Arrhythmic Events with PET Trial (185). As well, FDG PET has been used to monitor and direct new methods of revascularization such as angiogenesis and cellular cardiomyoplasty (use of skeletal myoblasts or stem cells in regions of injury). In these approaches, viable tissue that has potential to recover must be defined so therapy can be targeted to these regions (186). The definition of appropriate target sites for these new therapy approaches is critical to their success and potential future application.

Stem cells have also be labeled with FDG for early tracking human stem cell therapy approaches intended to restore viable tissue in injured or infarct region (187). Although this early tracking may be feasible, it is only a means to define early cell distribution rather than whether there is true cell differentiation. The latter will require techniques to assess changing stem cell function at later time points after delivery with longer half-life tracers or specific means to assess the evolving stem cell function. These approaches are under development (188,189).

SUMMARY

The role of FDG PET viability imaging in patients with poor LV function has been widely evaluated. This approach is an established accurate method for determining the diagnosis of viable myocardium and the prognosis of recovery after adequate revascularization. Although defining mismatch is important, the extent of scar or total viable myocardium is also relevant because stunned myocardium may also play an important role in LV dysfunction. The greatest impact is in patients with severe LV dysfunction, although recovery of the viable myocardium may take several months after revascularization.

FDG PET is now an integral part of clinical cardiology practice in centers where the technology is available. Data from FDG PET images clearly alter clinical decision making, identify patients at high risk of subsequent events who would benefit from revascularization, and do this in a potentially cost-effective manner. Proper identification of such patients for treatment has an impact on optimizing patient outcome. Although FDG PET is an established technique in ischemic heart disease, ongoing studies, including randomized controlled trials, continue to evaluate its evolving role in patients with severe LV dysfunction and heart failure. FDG PET will also be valuable in the future evaluation of new therapies that can improve the integrity and function of the myocardium.

ACKNOWLEDGMENTS

The authors thank Sonja Oxton, Linda Garrard, May Aung, and Rob deKemp for their help in preparing this chapter. Rob Beanlands is a research scientist supported by the Canadian Institute for Health Research.

REFERENCES

1. McKee PA, Castelli WP, McNamara PM, et al. The natural history of congestive heart failure: the Framingham study. *N Engl J Med* 1971;285: 1441–1446.
2. Yateau RF, Peter RH, Behar VS, et al. Ischemic cardiomyopathy: the myopathy of coronary artery disease. Natural history and results of medical versus surgical treatment. *Am J Cardiol* 1974;34:520–525.
3. Alderman EL, Fisher LD, Litwin P, et al. Results of coronary artery surgery in patients with poor left ventricular function (CASS). *Circulation* 1983;68:785–795.
4. Franciosa JA, Wilen M, Ziesche S, et al. Survival in men with severe chronic left ventricular failure due to either coronary heart disease or idiopathic dilated cardiomyopathy. *Am J Cardiol* 1983;51:831–836.
5. Maddahi J, Schelbert H, Brunken R, et al. Role of thallium-201 and PET imaging in evaluation of myocardial viability and management of patients with coronary artery disease and left ventricular dysfunction. *J Nucl Med* 1994;35:707–715.
6. Kojima S, Wu S, Parmley W, et al. Relationship between intracellular calcium and oxygen consumption: effects of perfusion pressure, extracellular calcium, dobutamine and nifedipine. *Am Heart J* 1994; 127: 386–391.
7. Jessup M, Brozena S. Heart failure. *N Engl J Med* 2003;348:2007–2018.
8. Cohn J, Archibald D, Ziesche S, et al. Effect of vasodilator therapy on mortality in chronic congestive heart failure. Results of a veterans administration cooperative study. *N Engl J Med* 1987;314:1547–1552.
9. The CONSENSUS Trial Study Group. Effects of enalapril on mortality in severe congestive heart failure. Results of the Cooperative North Scandinavian Enalapril Survival Study (CONSENSUS). *N Engl J Med* 1987;316:1429–1435.
10. Packer MD, Bristow MR, Cohn JN, et al. The effect of carvedilol on morbidity and mortality in patients with chronic heart failure. *N Engl J Med* 1996;334:1349–1355.
11. Packer M, Coats A, Fowler MB, et al. Effect of carvedilol on survival in severe chronic heart failure. *N Engl J Med* 2001;344:1651–1658.
12. Pfeffer MA, McMurray JJ, Velazquez EJ, et al. Valsartan, captopril, or both in myocardial infarction complicated by heart failure, left ventricular dysfunction, or both. *N Engl J Med* 2003;349:1893–1906.
13. Khand A, Gemmel I, Clark AL, et al. Is the prognosis of heart failure improving? *J Am Coll Cardiol* 2000;36:2284–2286.
14. Evans R, Manninen DL, Garrison LP, et al. Donor availability as the primary determinant of the future of heart transplantation. *JAMA* 1986;255:1892–1898.
15. Baker D, Jones R, Hodges J, et al. Management of heart failure: III. The role of revascularization in the treatment of patients with moderate or severe left ventricular systolic dysfunction. *JAMA* 1994;272: 1528–1534.
16. Louie HW, Laks H, Milgalter E, et al. Ischemic cardiomyopathy: criteria for coronary revascularization and cardiac transplantation. *Circulation* 1991;84:III290–III295.
17. Hochberg MS, Parsonnet V, Gielchinsky I, et al. Coronary artery bypass grafting in patients with ejection fractions below forty percent: early and late results in 466 patients. *J Thorac Cardiovasc Surg* 1983;86:519–527.
18. Kron IL, Flanagan TL, Blackbourne LH, et al. Coronary revascularization rather than cardiac transplantation for chronic ischemic cardiomyopathy. *Ann Surg* 1989;210:348–352.
19. Doenst T, Velazquez EJ, Beyersdorf F, et al. To STICH or not to STICH: we know the answer, but do we understand the question? *J Thorac Cardiovasc Surg* 2005;129:246–249.
20. Opie LH. Substrate and energy metabolism of the heart. In: Sperelakis N, ed. *Function of the heart in normal and pathological states*, 2nd ed. Boston: Kluwer, 1989:327–359.
21. Camici P, Ferrannini E, Opie LH. Myocardial metabolism in ischemic heart disease: basic principles and application to imaging by positron emission tomography. *Prog Cardiovasc Dis* 1989;32:217–238.
22. Kolter T, Uphues I, Wichelhaus A, et al. Contraction-induced translocation of the glucose transporter GLUT4 in isolated ventricular cardiomyocytes. *Biochem Biophys Res Commun* 1992;189:1207–1214.
23. Lopaschuk G, Stanley W. Glucose metabolism in the ischemic heart. *Circulation* 1997;95:415–422.
24. Phelps ME, Hoffman EJ, Selin CE, et al. Investigation of [^{18}F]2-fluoro-2-deoxyglucose for the measure of myocardial glucose metabolism. *J Nucl Med* 1978;19:1311–1319.
25. Choi Y, Brunken RC, Hawkins RA, et al. Factors affecting myocardial 2-[F-18]fluoro-2-deoxy-D-glucose uptake in positron emission tomography studies of normal humans. *Eur J Nucl Med* 1993;20: 308–318.
26. Marshall RC, Tillisch JH, Phelps ME, et al. Identification and differentiation of resting myocardial ischemia and infarction in man with positron computed tomography, ^{18}F-labeled fluorodeoxyglucose and N-13 ammonia. *Circulation* 1983;67:766–778.
27. Schwaiger M, Schelbert HR, Ellison D, et al. Sustained regional abnormalities in cardiac metabolism after transient ischemia in the chronic dog model. *J Am Coll Cardiol* 1985;6:336–347.
28. Braunwald E, Kloner RK. The stunned myocardium: prolonged, postischemic ventricular dysfunction. *Circulation* 1982;66:1146–1149.
29. Bolli R. Myocardial "stunning" in man. *Circulation* 1992;86:1671–1691.
30. Rahimtoola SH. From coronary artery disease to heart failure: role of the hibernating myocardium. *Am J Cardiol* 1995;75:16E–22E.
31. Rahimtoola SH. The hibernating myocardium. *Am Heart J* 1989;117: 211–221.
32. Di Carli M. Predicting improved function after myocardial revascularization. *Curr Opin Cardiol* 1998;13:415–424.
33. Kloner R. Does Reperfusion Injury Exist in Humans? *J Am Coll Cardiol* 1993;21:537–545.

34. Vanoverschelde J-LJ, Wijns W, Borgers M, et al. Chronic myocardial hibernation in humans. From beside to bench. *Circulation* 1997;95: 1961–1971.
35. Haas F, Augustin N, Holper K. et al. Time course and extent of improvement of dysfunctioning myocardium in patients with coronary artery disease and severely depressed left ventricular function after revascularization: correlation with positron emission tomography. *J Am Coll Cardiol* 2000;36:1927–1934.
36. Haas F, Jennen L, Heinzmann U. et al. Ischemically compromised myocardium displays different time-courses of functional recovery: correlation with morphological alterations? *Eur J Cardio Thorac Surg* 2001;20:290–298.
37. Depre C, Vatner SF. Mechanisms of cell survival in myocardial hibernation. *Trends Cardiovasc Med* 2005;15:101–110.
38. Shivalkar B, Maes A, Borgers M, et al. Only hibernating myocardium invariably shows early recovery after coronary revascularization. *Circulation* 1996;94:308–315.
39. Berman M, Fischman AJ, Southern J, et al. Myocardial adaptation during and after sustained, demand-induced ischemia: observations in closed-chest, domestic swine. *Circulation* 1996;94:755–762.
40. Schulz R, Guth BD, Peiper K, et al. Recruitment of an inotropic reserve in moderately ischemic myocardium at the expense of metabolic recovery: a model of short-term hibernation. *Circ Res* 1992;70: 1282–1295.
41. Fallavollita JA, Perry BJ, Canty JM. ^{18}-F-2-deoxyglucose deposition and regional flow in pigs with chronically dysfunctional myocardium. Evidence for transmural variations in chronic hibernating myocardium. *Circulation* 1997;95:1900–1909.
42. Liedtke AJ, Renstrom B, Nellis SH, et al. Mechanical and metabolic functions in pig hearts after 4 days of chronic coronary stenosis. *J Am Coll Cardiol* 1995;26:815–825.
43. Marinho NVS, Keogh BE, Costa DC, et al. Pathophysiology of chronic left ventricular dysfunction: new insights from the measurement of absolute myocardial blood flow and glucose utilization. *Circulation* 1996;93:737–744.
44. Heusch G, Schulz R, Rahimtoola SH. Myocardial hibernation: a delicate balance. *Am J Physiol Heart Circ Physiol* 2005;288:H984–H999.
45. Canty JM Jr, Fallavollita JA. Hibernating myocardium. *J Nucl Cardiol* 2005;12:104–119.
46. Gerber BL, Vanoverschelde J-LJ, Bol A, et al. Myocardial blood flow, glucose uptake, and recruitment of inotropic reserve in chronic left ventricular ischemic dysfunction. Implications for the pathophysiology of chronic myocardial hibernation. *Circulation* 1996;94: 651–659.
47. Bax JJ, Visser FC, Poldermans D, et al. Time course of functional recovery of stunned and hibernating segments after surgical revascularization. *Circulation* 2001;104:I314–I318.
48. Camici P, Dutka D. Repetitive stunning, hibernation, and heart failure: contribution of PET to establishing a link. *Am J Physiol Heart Circ Physiol* 2001;280:H929–H936.
49. Frangogiannis NG, Shimoni S, Chang SM, et al. Active interstitial remodeling: an important process in the hibernating human myocardium. *J Am Coll Cardiol* 2002;39:1468–1474.
50. Yoshinaga K, Katoh C, Beanlands RS, et al. Reduced oxidative metabolic response in dysfunctional myocardium with preserved glucose metabolism but with impaired contractile reserve. *J Nucl Med* 2004; 45: 1885–1891.
51. Doenst T, Taegtmeyer H. Profound underestimation of glucose uptake by [^{18}-F]2-deoxy-2-fluoroglucose in reperfused rat heart muscle. *Circulation* 1998;97:2454–2462.
52. Pagano D, Bonser R, Townend J, et al. Predictive value of dobutamine echocardiography and positron emission tomography in identifying hibernating myocardium in patients with postischemic heart failure. *Heart* 1998;79:281–288.
53. Beanlands RS, Hendry P, Masters R, et al. Delay in revascularization is associated with increased mortality rate in patients with severe LV dysfunction and viable myocardium on fluorine-18-fluorodeoxyglucose positron emission tomography imaging. *Circulation* 1998;98: II51–II56.
54. Bax JJ, Schinkel AF, Boersma E, et al. Early versus delayed revascularization in patients with ischemic cardiomyopathy and substantial viability: impact on outcome. *Circulation* 2003;108[Suppl 1]: II39–II42.
55. Tarakji KG, Brunken R, McCarthy PM, et al. Myocardial viability testing and the effect of early intervention in patients with advanced left ventricular systolic dysfunction. *Circulation* 2006; 113:230–237.
56. Tamaki N, Yonekura Y, Yamashita K, et al. Positron emission tomography using fluorine-18-deoxyglucose in evaluation of coronary artery bypass grafting. *Am J Cardiol* 1989;64:860–865.
57. Tamaki N, Ohtani H, Yamashita K, et al. Metabolic activity in the areas of new fill-in after thallium-201 reinjection: comparison with positron emission tomography using fluorine-018-deoxyglucose. *J Nucl Med* 1991;32:673–678.
58. Tillisch J, Brunken R, Marshall R, et al. Reversibility of cardiac wall-motion abnormalities predicted by positron tomography. *N Engl J Med* 1986;314:884–888.
59. vom Dahl J, Eitzman DT, Al-Aouar ZR, et al. Relation of regional function, perfusion, and metabolism in patients with advanced coronary artery disease undergoing surgical revascularization. *Circulation* 1994;90:2356–2365.
60. Carrel T, Jenni R, Haubold-Reuter S, et al. Improvement of severely reduced left ventricular function after surgical revascularization in patients with preoperative myocardial infarction. *Eur J Nucl Med* 1992;6:479–484.
61. Lucignani G, Paolini G, Landoni C, et al. Presurgical identification of hibernating myocardium by combined use of technetium-99m hexakis 2-methoxyisobutylisonitrile single photon emission tomography and fluorine-18-fluoro-2-deoxy-D-glucose positron emission tomography in patients with coronary artery disease. *Eur J Nucl Med* 1992;19: 874–881.
62. Altehoefer C, Kaiser H-J, Dorr R, et al. Fluorine-18 deoxyglucose PET for assessment of viable myocardium in perfusion defects in 99mTc-MIBI SPECT: a comparative study in patients with coronary artery disease. *Eur J Nucl Med* 1992;19:334–342.
63. Gropler RJ, Geltman EM, Sampathkumaran K, et al. Comparison of carbon-11-acetate with fluorine-18-fluorodeoxyglucose for delineating viable myocardium by positron emission tomography. *J Am Coll Cardiol* 1993;22:1597.
64. Bax JJ, Poldermans D, Elhendy A, et al. Sensitivity, specificity, and predictive accuracies of various noninvasive techniques for detecting hibernating myocardium. *Curr Probl Cardiol* 2001;26:147–186.
65. Beanlands R, Ruddy T, deKemp R, et al. Positron emission tomography and recovery following revascularization (PARR-1): the importance of scar and the development of a prediction rule for the degree of recovery of left ventricular function. *J Am Coll Cardiol* 2002;40: 1735–1743.
66. Saab G, de Kemp R, Ukkonen H, et al. Gated 19-fluorine fluorodeoxyglucose positron emission tomography: determination of global and regional left ventricular function and myocardial tissue characterization. *J Nucl Cardiol* 2003;10:297–303.
67. Willemsen ATM, Siebelink H-MJ, Blanksma PK, et al. Automated ejection fraction determined from gated myocardial FDG-PET data. *J Nucl Cardiol* 1999;6:577–582.
68. Hattori N, Bengel F, Mehilli J, et al. Global and regional functional measurements with gated PET in comparison with left ventriculography. *Eur J Nucl Med* 2001;28:221–229.
69. Hickey KT, Sciacca RR, Bokhari S, et al. Assessment of cardiac wall motion and ejection fraction with gated PET using N-13 ammonia. *Clin Nucl Med* 2004;29:243–248.
70. Germano G, Berman DS. On the accuracy and reproducibility of quantitative gated myocardial perfusion SPECT. *J Nucl Med* 1999;40: 810–813.

71. Machac J, Bacharach SL, Bateman TM, et al. Positron emission tomography myocardial perfusion and glucose metabolism imaging. *J Nucl Cardiol* 2006;13:121–151.
72. Beanlands RSB, deKemp RA, Smith S, et al. F-18-Fluorodeoxyglucose PET imaging alters clinical decision making in patients with impaired ventricular function. *Am J Cardiol* 1997;79:1092–1095.
73. vom Dahl J, Altehoefer C, Sheehan FH, et al. Effect of myocardial viability assessed by technetium-99m-sestamibi SPECT and fluorine-18-FDG PET on clinical outcome in coronary artery disease. *J Nucl Med* 1997; 38:742–748.
74. Fallen EL, Nahmias C, Scheffel A, et al. Redistribution of myocardial blood flow with topical nitroglycerin in patients with coronary artery disease. *Circulation* 1995;91:1381–1388.
75. Rothley J, Weeden A. Clinical PET protocols. In: Schwaiger M, ed. *Cardiac positron emission tomography*. New York: Kluwer, 1996:357.
76. Pirich C, Schwaiger M. The clinical role of positron emission tomography in management of the cardiac patient. *Rev Port Cardiol* 2000; 19:89–98.
77. Arrighi JA, Dilsizian V. Myocardial viability. Radionuclide-based methods. (radionuclide-based methods/nuclear cardiology). In: Pohost GM, et al., eds. *Imaging in cardiovascular disease*. Philadelphia: Lippincott Williams & Wilkins. 2000:213–232.
78. Sandler MP, Bax JJ, Patton JA, et al. Fluorine-18-fluorodeoxyglucose cardiac imaging using a modified scintillation camera. *J Nucl Med* 1998;39:2035–2043.
79. Vitale G, deKemp R, Ruddy TD, et al. Myocardial glucose utilization and the optimization of F-18-FDG PET imaging in patients with NIDDM, CAD and LV dysfunction. *J Nucl Med* 2001;42:1730–1736.
80. vom Dahl J, Herman WH, Hicks RJ, et al. Myocardial glucose uptake in patients with insulin-dependent diabetes mellitus assessed quantitatively by dynamic positron emission tomography. *Circulation* 1993; 88:395–404.
81. Ohtake T, Yokoyama I, Watanabe T, et al. Myocardial glucose metabolism in noninsulin-dependent diabetes mellitus patients evaluated by FDG-PET. *J Nucl Med* 1995;36:456–463.
82. Maki M, Luotolahti M, Nuutila P, et al. Glucose uptake in the chronically dysfunctional but viable myocardium. *Circulation* 1996;93:1658–1666.
83. Knuuti M, Nuutila P, Ruotsalainen U, et al. Euglycemic hyperinsulinemic clamp and oral glucose load in stimulating myocardial glucose utilization during positron emission tomography. *J Nucl Med* 1992;33: 1255–1262.
84. Voipio-Pulkki LM, Nuutila P, Knuuti J, et al. Heart and skeletal muscle glucose disposal in type 2 diabetic patients as determined by PET. *J Nucl Med* 1993;34:2064–2067.
85. DeFronzo R, Tobin J, Andres R. Glucose clamp technique: a method for quantifying insulin secretion and resistance. *Am J Physiol* 1979; 273: E214–E223.
86. Knuuti J, Yki-Jarvinen H, Voipio-Pulkki L, et al. Enhancement of myocardial FDG uptake by a nicotinic acid derivative. *J Nucl Med* 1994;35:989–998.
87. Stone C, Holden J, Stanley W, et al. Effect of nicotinic acid on exogenous myocardial glucose utilization. *J Nucl Med* 1995;36:996–1002.
88. Sun D, Nguyen N, DeGrado T, et al. Ischemia induces translocation of the insulin-responsive glucose transporter GLUT4 to the plasma membrane of cardiac myocytes. *Circulation* 1994;89:793–798.
89. Schwarz E, Schaper J, vom Dahl J, et al. Myocyte degeneration and cell death in hibernating human myocardium. *J Am Coll Cardiol* 1996; 27:1577–1585.
90. Borgers M, Thone F, Wouters L, et al. Structural correlates of regional myocardial dysfunction in patients with critical coronary artery stenosis: chronic hibernation. *Cardiovasc Pathol* 1993;2:237–245.
91. Pagano D, Townend J, Littler W, et al. Coronary artery bypass surgery as treatment for ischemic heart failure: the predictive value of viability assessment with quantitative positron emission tomography for symptomatic and functional outcome. *J Thorac Cardiovasc Surg* 1998;115: 791–799.
92. Mody F, Brunken R, Stevenson LW, et al. Differentiating cardiomyopathy of coronary artery disease from nonischemic dilated cardiomyopath utilizing positron emission tomography. *J Am Coll Cardiol* 1991;17: 373–383.
93. Yamagishi H, Akioka K, Hirata K, et al. A reverse flow-metabolism mismatch pattern on PET is related to multivessel disease in patients with acute myocardial infarction. *J Nucl Med* 1999;40:1492–1498.
94. Schwaiger M, Pirich C. Reverse flow-metabolism mismatch: what does it mean? *J Nucl Med* 1999;40:1499–1502.
95. Nowak B, Stellbrink C, Schaefer WM, et al. Comparison of regional myocardial blood flow and perfusion in dilated cardiomyopathy and left bundle branch block: role of wall thickening. *J Nucl Med* 2004;45: 414–418.
96. Zanco P, Desideri A, Mobilia G, et al. Effects of left bundle branch block on myocardial FDG PET in patients without significant coronary artery stenoses. *J Nucl Med* 2000;41:973–977.
97. Thompson K, Saab G, Birnie D, et al. Is septal glucose metabolism altered in patients with left bundle branch block and ischemic cardiomyopathy? *J Nucl Med* 2006;47:1763–1768.
98. Langer A, Burns RJ, Freeman M, et al. Reverse distribution on exercise thallium scintigraphy: relationship to coronary patency and ventricular function after myocardial infarction. *Can J Cardiol* 1992;9: 709–715.
99. Oikawa M, Kagaya Y, Otani H, et al. Increased [^{18}F]fluorodeoxyglucose accumulation in right ventricular free wall in patients with pulmonary hypertension and the effect of epoprostenol. *J Am Coll Cardiol* 2005;45: 1849–1855.
100. Schwaiger M, Brunken R, Grover-McKay M, et al. Regional myocardial metabolism in patients with acute myocardial infarction assessed by positron emission tomography. *J Am Coll Cardiol* 1986;8:800–808.
101. Maes A, Van de Werf F, Mesotten LV, et al. Early assessment of regional myocardial blood flow and metabolism in thrombolysis in myocardial infarction flow grade 3 reperfused myocardial infarction using carbon-11-acetate. *J Am Coll Cardiol* 2001;37:30–36.
102. Patlak CS, Blasberg RG. Graphical evaluation of blood-to-brain transfer constants from multiple-time uptake data: generalizations. *J Cereb Blood Flow Metab* 1985;5:584–590.
103. Ratib O, Phelps ME, Huang SC, et al. Positron tomography with deoxyglucose for estimating local myocardial glucose metabolism. *J Nucl Med* 1982;23:577–586.
104. Hariharan R, Bray M, Ganim R, et al. Fundamental limitations of [^{18}F]2-deoxy-2-fluoro-D-glucose for assessing myocardial glucose uptake. *Circulation* 1995;91:2435–2444.
105. Botker HE, Bottcher M, Schmitz O, et al. Glucose uptake and lumped constant variability in normal human hearts determined with [^{18}-F] fluorodeoxyglucose. *J Nucl Cardiol* 1997;4:125–132.
106. Knuuti MJ, Nuutila P, Ruotsalainen U, et al. The value of quantitative analysis of glucose utilization in detection of myocardial viability by PET. *J Nucl Med* 1993;34:2068–2075.
107. Yamagishi H, Akioka K, Hirata K, et al. Dobutamine-stress electrocardiographically gated positron emission tomography for detection of viable but dysfunctional myocardium. *J Nucl Cardiol* 1999;6:626–632.
108. Hor G, Kranert WT, Maul FD, et al. Gated metabolic positron emission tomography (GAPET) of the myocardium: ^{18}F-FDG-PET to optimized recognition of myocardial hibernation. *Nucl Med Commun* 1998;19: 535–545.
109. deKemp R, Van Kriekinge SD, Germano G, et al. LV ejection fraction with gated FDG studies on a partial-ring rotating PET scanner. *J Nucl Med* 2000; 41:88P.
110. Schaefer WM, Lipke CS, Nowak B, et al. Validation of an evaluation routine for left ventricular volumes, ejection fraction and wall motion from gated cardiac FDG PET: a comparison with cardiac magnetic resonance imaging. *Eur J Nucl Med Mol Imaging* 2003;30:545–553.
111. Klocke FJ, Baird MG, Lorell BH, et al. ACC/AHA/ASNC guidelines for the clinical use of cardiac radionuclide imaging—executive summary: a report of the American College of Cardiology/American Heart

Association Task Force on Practice Guidelines (ACC/AHA/ASNC Committee to revise the 1995 guidelines for the clinical use of cardiac radionuclide imaging). *J Am Coll Cardiol* 2003;42:1318–1333.
112. Beanlands RS, Chow BJ, Dick A, et al. CCS/CAR/CANM/CNCS/CanSCMR joint position statement on advanced noninvasive cardiac imaging using positron emission tomography, magnetic resonance imaging and multidetector computed tomographic angiography in the diagnosis and evaluation of ischemic heart disease—executive summary. *Can J Cardiol* 2007;23:107–119.
113. Underwood SR, Bax JJ, vom Dahl J, et al. Imaging techniques for the assessment of myocardial hibernation. Report of a Study Group of the European Society of Cardiology. *Eur Heart J* 2004;25:815–836.
114. ACC/AHA Task Force. Guidelines for clinical use of cardiac radionuclide imaging. Report of the American College of Cardiology/American Heart Association Task Force on Assessment of Diagnostic and Therapeutic Cardiovascular Procedures (Committee on Radionuclide Imaging), developed in collaboration with the American Society of Nuclear Cardiology. *J Am Coll Cardiol* 1995;25:521–547.
115. Knuesel PR, Nanz D, Wyss C, et al. Characterization of dysfunctional myocardium by positron emission tomography and magnetic resonance: relation to functional outcome after revascularization. *Circulation* 2003;108:1095–1100.
116. Kuhl HP, Beek AM, van der Weerdt AP, et al. Myocardial viability in chronic ischemic heart disease: comparison of contrast-enhanced magnetic resonance imaging with (^{18})F-fluorodeoxyglucose positron emission tomography. *J Am Coll Cardiol* 2003;41:1341–1348.
117. Klein C, Nekolla SG, Bengel FM, et al. Assessment of myocardial viability with contrast-enhanced magnetic resonance imaging: comparison with positron emission tomography. *Circulation* 2002;105: 162–167.
118. Beanlands RS, deKemp R, Scheffel A, et al. Can nitrogen-13 ammonia kinetic modeling define myocardial viability independent of fluorine-18 fluorodeoxyglucose? *J Am Coll Cardiol* 1997;29:537–543.
119. Barrington SF, Chambers J, Hallett WA, et al. Comparison of sestamibi, thallium, echocardiography and PET for the detection of hibernating myocardium. *Eur J Nucl Med Mol Imaging* 2004;31: 355–361.
120. Bax JJ, Visser FC, Poldermans D, et al. Relationship between preoperative viability and postoperative improvement in LVEF and heart failure symptoms. *J Nucl Med* 2001;42:79–86.
121. Bax JJ, Fath-Ordoubadi F, Boersma E, et al. Accuracy of PET in predicting functional recovery after revascularization in patients with chronic ischemic dysfunction: head-to-head comparison between blood flow, glucose utilization and water-perfusable tissue fraction. *Eur J Nucl Med Mol Imaging* 2002;29:721–727.
122. Bax JJ, Maddahi J, Poldermans D, et al. Preoperative comparison of different noninvasive strategies for predicting improvement in left ventricular function after coronary artery bypass grafting. *Am J Cardiol* 2003;92:1–4.
123. Korosoglou G, Hansen A, Hoffend J, et al. Comparison of real-time myocardial contrast echocardiography for the assessment of myocardial viability with fluorodeoxyglucose-18 positron emission tomography and dobutamine stress echocardiography. *Am J Cardiol* 2004;94: 570–576.
124. Nowak B, Schaefer WM, Koch KC, et al. Assessment of myocardial viability in dysfunctional myocardium by resting myocardial blood flow determined with oxygen 15 water PET. *J Nucl Cardiol* 2003;10: 34–45.
125. Gerber BL, Ordoubadi FF, Wijns W, et al. Positron emission tomography using (^{18})F-fluoro-deoxyglucose and euglycemic hyperinsulinemic glucose clamp: optimal criteria for the prediction of recovery of post-ischemic left ventricular dysfunction. Results from the European Community Concerted Action Multicenter study on use of (^{18})F-fluoro-deoxyglucose positron emission tomography for the detection of myocardial viability. *Eur Heart J* 2001;22:1691–1701.
126. Wiggers H, Egeblad H, Nielsen TT, et al. Prediction of reversible myocardial dysfunction by positron emission tomography, low-dose dobutamine echocardiography, resting ECG, and exercise testing. *Cardiology* 2001;96:32–37.
127. Eitzman D, Al-Aouar Z, Kanter HL, et al. Clinical outcome of patients with advanced coronary artery disease after viability studies with positron emission tomography. *J Am Coll Cardiol* 1992;20: 559–565.
128. Di Carli MF, Davidson M, Little R, et al. Value of metabolic imaging with positron emission tomography for evaluating prognosis in patients with coronary artery disease and left ventricular dysfunction. *Am J Cardiol* 1994;73:527–533.
129. Di Carli MF, Asgazadie F, Schelbert HR, et al. Quantitative relation between myocardial viability and improvement in heart failure symptoms after revascularization in patients with ischemic cardiomyopathy. *Circulation* 1995;92:3436–3444.
130. Yoshida K, Gould KL. Quantitative relation of myocardial infarct size and myocardial viability by positron emission tomography to left ventricular ejection fraction and 3-year mortality with and without revascularization. *J Am Coll Cardiol* 1993;22:984–997.
131. Lee KS, Marwick TH, Cook SA, et al. Prognosis of patients with left ventricular dysfunction, with and without viable myocardium after myocardial infarction: relative efficacy of medical therapy and revascularization. *Circulation* 1995;90:2687–2694.
132. Allman KC, Shaw LJ, Hachamovitch R, et al. Myocardial viability testing and impact of revascularization on prognosis in patients with coronary artery disease and left ventricular dysfunction: a meta-analysis. *J Am Coll Cardiol* 2002;39:1151–1158.
133. Zhang X, Liu XJ, Wu Q, et al. Clinical outcome of patients with previous myocardial infarction and left ventricular dysfunction assessed with myocardial (^{99m})Tc-MIBI SPECT and (^{18})F-FDG PET. *J Nucl Med* 2001;42:1166–1173.
134. Sawada S, Hamoui O, Barclay J, et al. Usefulness of positron emission tomography in predicting long-term outcome in patients with diabetes mellitus and ischemic left ventricular dysfunction. *Am J Cardiol* 2005; 96:2–8.
135. Santana CA, Shaw LJ, Garcia EV, et al. Incremental prognostic value of left ventricular function by myocardial ECG-gated FDG PET imaging in patients with ischemic cardiomyopathy. *J Nucl Cardiol* 2004;11:542–550.
136. Rohatgi R, Epstein S, Henriquez J, et al. Utility of positron emission tomography in predicting cardiac events and survival in patients with coronary artery disease and severe left ventricular dysfunction. *Am J Cardiol* 2001;87:1096–1099, A1096.
137. Desideri A, Cortigiani L, Christen AI, et al. The extent of perfusion-F18-fluorodeoxyglucose positron emission tomography mismatch determines mortality in medically treated patients with chronic ischemic left ventricular dysfunction. *J Am Coll Cardiol* 2005;46: 1264–1269.
138. Di Carli M, Maddahi J, Rokhsar S, et al. Long-term survival of patients with coronary artery disease and left ventricular dysfunction: implications for the role of myocardial viability assessment in management decisions. *J Thorac Cardiovasc Surg* 1998;116:997–1004.
139. Haas F, Haehnel C, Picker W, et al. Preoperative positron emission tomographic viability assessment and perioperative and postoperative risk in patients with advanced ischemic heart disease. *J Am Coll Cardiol* 1997;30:1693–1700.
140. Jacklin PB, Barrington SF, Roxburgh JC, et al. Cost-effectiveness of preoperative positron emission tomography in ischemic heart disease. *Ann Thorac Surg* 2002;73:1403–1409; discussion 1410.
141. Dussault FP, Nguyen VH, Rachet F. La tomographie par emission de positrons au Quebec., 2001. Accessed April 11, 2007. www.aetmis.gouv.qc.ca.
142. Akinboboye O, Idris O, Cannon P, et al. Usefulness of positron emission tomography in defining myocardial viability in patients referred for cardiac transplantation. *Am J Cardiol* 1999;83:1271–1274.

143. Tamaki N, Kawamoto M, Takahashi N, et al. Prognostic value of an increase in fluorine-18 deoxyglucose uptake in patients with myocardial infarction: comparison with stress thallium imaging. *J Am Coll Cardiol* 1993;22:1621–1627.
144. Sawada S, Muzik O, Allman K, et al. Positron emission tomography detects evidence of viability in rest technetium-99m sestamibi defects. *J Am Coll Cardiol* 1994;23:92–98.
145. Soufer R, Dey H, Ng C-K, et al. Comparison of sestamibi single-photon emission computed tomography with positron emission tomography for estimating left ventricular myocardial viability. *Am J Cardiol* 1995;75:1214–1219.
146. Dilsizian V, Arrighi JA, Diodati JG, et al. Myocardial viability in patients with chronic coronary artery disease. Comparison of ^{99m}Tc-sestamibi with thallium reinjection and [^{18}F]fluorodeoxyglucose. *Circulation* 1994;89: 578–587.
147. Baer F, Voth E, Deutsch H, et al. Predictive value of low dose dobutamine transesophageal echocardiography and fluorine-18 fluorodeoxyglucose positron emission tomography for recovery of regional left ventricular function after successful revascularization. *J Am Coll Cardiol* 1996;23: 60–69.
148. Bax JJ, Cornel JH, Visser FC, et al. Prediction of improvement of contractile function in patients with ischemic ventricular dysfunction after revascularization by fluorine-18 fluorodeoxyglucose single-photon emission computed tomography. *J Am Coll Cardiol* 1997;30:377–383.
149. Sambuceti G, Giorgetti L, Corsiglia L, et al. Perfusion-contraction mismatch during inotropic stimulation in hibernating myocardium. *J Nucl Med* 1998;39:396–402.
150. Siebelink H-M, Blanksma PK, Crijns H, et al. No difference in cardiac event-free survival between positron emission tomography–guided and single-photon emission computed tomography–guided management. *J Am Coll Cardiol* 2001;37:81–88.
151. Beanlands R, Ruddy T, Freeman M, et al. Patient management guided by viability imaging. *J Am Coll Cardiol* 2001;38:1271–1272.
152. Beanlands R, Nichol G, Ruddy T, et al. Evaluation of outcome and cost-effectiveness using an FDG PET-guided approach to management of patients with coronary disease and severe left ventricular dysfunction (PARR-2): rationale, design and methods. *Contemp Clin Trials* 2003; 24: 776–794.
153. Joyce D, Loebe M, Noon GP, et al. Revascularization and ventricular restoration in patients with ischemic heart failure: the STICH trial. *Curr Opin Cardiol* 2003;18:454–457.
154. Cleland JG, Freemantle N, Ball SG, et al. The heart failure revascularization trial (HEART): rationale, design and methodology. *Eur J Heart Fail* 2003;5:295–303.
155. Kim RJ, Wu E, Rafael A, et al. The use of contrast-enhanced magnetic resonance imaging to identify reversible myocardial dysfunction. *N Engl J Med* 2000;343:1445–1453.
156. Rizzello V, Poldermans D, Bax JJ. Assessment of myocardial viability in chronic ischemic heart disease: current status. *Q J Nucl Med Mol Imaging* 2005;49:81–96.
157. Sadowski EA, Bennett LK, Chan MR, et al. Nephrogenic systemic fibrosis: risk factors and incidence estimation. *Radiology* 2007; 243:148–157.
158. Iida H, Kanno I, Takahashi A, et al. Measurement of absolute myocardial blood flow with H_2-15-O and dynamic positron emission tomography. Strategy for quantification in relation to the partial-volume effect. *Circulation* 1988;78:104–115.
159. deSilva R, Yamamoto Y, Rhodes CG, et al. Preoperative prediction of the outcome of coronary revascularization using positron emission tomography. *Circulation* 1992;86:1738–1742.
160. Knaapen P, Bondarenko O, Beek AM, et al. Impact of scar on water-perfusable tissue index in chronic ischemic heart disease: evaluation with PET and contrast-enhanced MRI. *Mol Imaging Biol* 2006;8: 245–251.
161. Gewirtz H, Fischman AJ, Abraham S, et al. Positron emission tomographic measurements of absolute regional myocardial blood flow permits identification of nonviable myocardium in patients with chronic myocardial infarction. *J Am Coll Cardiol* 1994;23:851–859.
162. Kitsiou AN, Bacharach SL, Bartlett ML, et al. 13N-ammonia myocardial blood flow and uptake: relation to functional outcome of asynergic regions after revascularization. *J Am Coll Cardiol* 1999;33:678–686.
163. Gould KL, Yoshida K, Hess MJ, et al. Myocardial metabolism of fluorodeoxyglucose compared to cell membrane integrity for the potassium analogue rubidium-82 for assessing infarct size in man by PET. *J Nucl Med* 1991;32:1–9.
164. vom Dahl J, Muzik O, Wolfe E, et al. Myocardial rubidium-82 tissue kinetics assessed by dynamic positron emission tomography as a marker of myocardial cell membrane integrity and viability. *Circulation* 1996;93:238–245.
165. Gropler RJ, Siegel BA, Sampathkumaran K, et al. Dependence of recovery of contractile function on maintenance of oxidative metabolism after myocardial infarction. *J Am Coll Cardiol* 1992;19:989–997.
166. Hata T, Nohara R, Fujita M, et al. Noninvasive assessment of myocardial viability by positron emission tomography with 11-C acetate in patients with old myocardial infarction. *Circulation* 1996;94: 1834–1841.
167. Gropler RJ, Geltman EM, Sampathkumaran K, et al. Functional recovery after coronary revascularization for chronic coronary artery disease is dependent on maintenance of oxidative metabolism. *J Am Coll Cardiol* 1992;20:569–577.
168. Wolpers HG, Burshert W, van den Hoff J, et al. Assessment of myocardial viability by use of ^{11}C-acetate and positron emission tomography. Threshold criteria of reversible dysfunction. *Circulation* 1997;95: 1417–1424.
169. Camici P, Araujo LI, Spinks T, et al. Increased uptake of ^{18}F-fluorodeoxyglucose in postischemic myocardium of patients with exercise induced angina. *Circulation* 1986;74:81–88.
170. Marwick TH, MacIntyre WJ, Salcedo EE, et al. Identification of ischemic and hibernating myocardium: feasibility of post-exercise F-18 deoxyglucose positron emission tomography. *CCD* 1991:100–106.
171. Araujo LI, McFalls EO, Lammertsma AA, et al. Dipyridamole-induced increased glucose uptake in patients with single-vessel coronary artery disease assessed with PET. *J Nucl Cardiol* 2001;8:339–346.
172. Abramson B, Ruddy T, deKemp R, et al. Stress perfusion/metabolism imaging: a pilot study for a potential new approach to the diagnosis of coronary disease in women. *J Nucl Cardiol* 2000;7:205–212.
173. He ZX, Shi RF, Wu YJ, et al. Direct imaging of exercise-induced myocardial ischemia with fluorine-18-labeled deoxyglucose and Tc-99m-sestamibi in coronary artery disease. *Circulation* 2003;108: 1208–1213.
174. Jain D, McNulty PH. Exercise-induced myocardial ischemia: can this be imaged with F-18-fluorodeoxyglucose? *J Nucl Cardiol* 2000;7: 286–288.
175. Sandler MP, Videlefsky S, Delbeke D, et al. Evaluation of myocardial ischemia using a rest metabolism/stress perfusion protocol with fluorine-18 deoxyglucose/technetium-99m MIBI and dual-isotope simultaneous-acquisition single-photon emission computed tomography. *J Am Coll Cardiol* 1995;26:870–878.
176. Hasegawa S, Uehara T, Yamaguchi H, et al. Validity of ^{18}F-fluorodeoxyglucose imaging with a dual-head coincidence gamma camera for detection of myocardial viability. *J Nucl Med* 2000;40:1884–1892.
177. Kaira K, Ishizuka T, Yanagitani N, et al. Value of FDG positron emission tomography in monitoring the effects of therapy in progressive pulmonary sarcoidosis. *Clin Nucl Med* 2007;32:114–116.
178. Takahashi M, Momose T, Kameyama M, et al. Abnormal accumulation of [^{18}F]fluorodeoxyglucose in the aortic wall related to inflammatory changes: three case reports. *Ann Nucl Med* 2006;20: 361–364.
179. Mielniczuk L, DeKemp RA, Dennie C, et al. Images in cardiovascular medicine. Fluorine-18-labeled deoxyglucose positron emission tomography in the diagnosis and management of aortitis with pulmonary artery involvement. *Circulation* 2005;111:e375–376.

180. Meller J, Grabbe E, Becker W, et al. Value of F-18 FDG hybrid camera PET and MRI in early Takayasu aortitis. *Eur Radiol* 2003;13:400–405.
181. Rudd JH, Warburton EA, Fryer TD, et al. Imaging atherosclerotic plaque inflammation with [^{18}F]-fluorodeoxyglucose positron emission tomography. *Circulation* 2002;105:2708–2711.
182. Davies JR, Rudd JH, Weissberg PL, et al. Radionuclide imaging for the detection of inflammation in vulnerable plaques. *J Am Coll Cardiol* 2006;47:C57–C68.
183. Strauss HW, Mari C, Patt BE, et al. Intravascular radiation detectors for the detection of vulnerable atheroma. *J Am Coll Cardiol* 2006;47: C97–C100.
184. Dunphy MP, Freiman A, Larson SM, et al. Association of vascular ^{18}F-FDG uptake with vascular calcification. *J Nucl Med* 2005;46: 1278–1284.
185. Fallavollita JA, Luisi AJ Jr, Michalek SM, et al. Prediction of arrhythmic events with positron emission tomography: PAREPET study design and methods. *Contemp Clin Trials* 2006;27:374–388.
186. Menasche P, Hagege A, Scorsin M, et al. Myoblast transplantation for heart failure. *Lancet* 2001;37:279–280.
187. Hofmann M, Wollert KC, Meyer GP, et al. Monitoring of bone marrow cell homing into the infarcted human myocardium. *Circulation* 2005;111:2198–2202.
188. Shanthly N, Aruva MR, Zhang K, et al. Stem cells: a regenerative pharmaceutical. *Q J Nucl Med Mol Imaging* 2006;50:205–216.
189. Acton PD, Zhou R. Imaging reporter genes for cell tracking with PET and SPECT. *Q J Nucl Med Mol Imaging* 2005;49:349–360.

CHAPTER

11.3 Oxidative Metabolism and Cardiac Efficiency

HEIKKI UKKONEN AND ROB S. B. BEANLANDS

Oxidative metabolism of fuels provides the heart with the energy required for contraction and basal metabolism. Impaired myocardial energy transfer plays an important role in the development of contractile dysfunction in many clinical syndromes, including ischemic heart disease. Positron emission tomography (PET) provides a unique tool for noninvasive quantitative characterization of myocardial metabolic processes *in vivo*, and it has been widely used for the detection of viable myocardium in ischemic heart disease. However, the capabilities of PET to define myocardial metabolism have not been used to their fullest extent. Currently, the efficacy of therapy is monitored primarily by evaluating patients' functional capacity, ventricular function, and hemodynamics. By combining the functional data with PET-derived metabolic data, the treatment effects can be more physiologically assessed. This approach has been applied to measure myocardial efficiency (i.e., myocardial work related to myocardial oxygen consumption) to evaluate cardiac disease and its therapies.

This chapter focuses on myocardial metabolism, particularly the application of oxidative metabolism and oxygen consumption imaging with PET, in cardiac disease and treatment. The role of PET in the determination of myocardial efficiency is also emphasized; application of this methodology in the optimization of therapy is expected to increase as PET becomes more widely available.

MYOCARDIAL METABOLISM

The heart requires a constant supply of energy to sustain contractile function. This energy is supplied by hydrolysis of adenosine triphosphate (ATP), which is primarily derived from aerobic metabolism of fatty acids and carbohydrates and to a significantly lesser extent from aerobic metabolism of amino acids and ketone bodies (Fig. 11.3.1). Although the mechanisms that connect the mechanical work and energy production of the heart are not fully understood, it has been suggested that intracellular calcium plays a regulatory role in the link between cardiac mechanics and energy production (1).

Oxygen is the final electron acceptor in all pathways of aerobic metabolism in the myocardium. Therefore, under steady state conditions, myocardial oxygen consumption provides an accurate measure of overall myocardial metabolism (2). However, the relative utilization of different energy substrates depends mainly on the concentration of these substrates in the afferent blood vessels, on hormonal influences, workload, blood flow, and oxygen demand (3).

ATP is the immediate and quantitatively by far the most important substance that fuels most myocellular processes. Because the myocardium relies predominantly on aerobic metabolism for its energy requirements, myocardial oxygen consumption ultimately reflects the rate of mitochondrial metabolism and ATP production.

The processes of the heart requiring ATP (and therefore oxygen) may be divided into three main categories: basal metabolism, excitation–contraction coupling (ion movements against electrochemical gradients), and force generation by the actin and myosin molecules (4). In clinical terms, the major determinants of myocardial oxygen consumption are basal metabolism of the heart, heart rate, and myocardial wall stress and contractility. Wall stress and contractility are the principal components of "force generation" that results from the actin–myosin interaction.

Approximately 65% to 80% of the total energy produced is converted to heat and the rest is available for force generation and basal metabolism. Basal metabolic energy is required for protein synthesis and maintenance of cellular membrane integrity. The energy needed for excitation–contraction coupling, that is, energy for calcium cycling, is at most 20% to 25% of the total ATP consumption during the isovolumetric contraction phase (5,6).

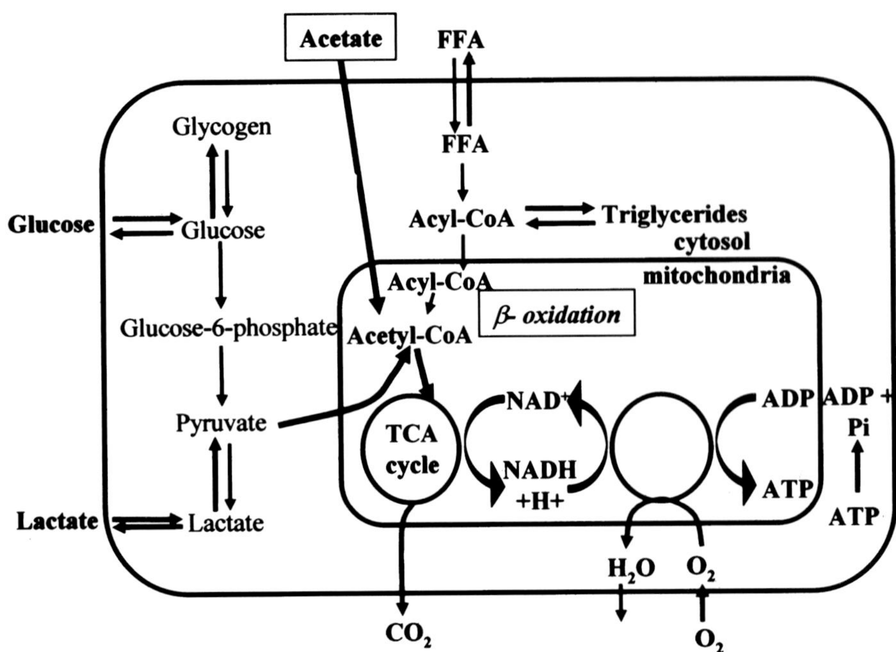

FIGURE 11.3.1. Schematic diagram for myocardial substrate metabolism. The tricarboxylic acid (TCA) cycle is linked to myocardial oxygen consumption via the electron transport chains, which supply most of the energy of the heart. FFA, free fatty acid; acyl-CoA, acyl-coenzyme A; NAD nicotinamide adenine dinucleotide; NADH+ H+ nicotinamide adenine dinucleotide, reduced+proton-ion; H_2O, water; CO_2, carbon dioxide; O_2, oxygen; ADP adenosine diphosphate; ADP+Pi adenosine diphosphate+inorganic phosphate; ATP, adenosine triphosphate.

Cross-bridge activation by actin and myosin molecules (myosin ATP), which leads to myocardial contraction, uses approximately 65% of the energy available for all mechanical processes of the heart.

Fatty Acid Oxidation

Free fatty acids (FFAs) are considered the preferred substrate for myocardial metabolism (7). In the fasted state and after a meal rich in fat, the level of blood FFAs is high and FFAs become the major source of energy, accounting for up to 90% of myocardial oxygen consumption (8). In addition, myocardial workload influences substrate metabolism. FFAs are preferred over glucose up to a moderate level of exercise (9,10). When fatty acids are oxidized, glucose oxidation is inhibited, and the glucose is shuttled into glycogen synthesis (3). Myocardial uptake of albumin-bound FFAs is related to the level of FFA in the blood and to the FFA:albumin ratio. Once inside the myocardial cell, fatty acids are activated to long-chain acyl-coenzyme A (acyl-CoA) by an acyl-CoA synthetase (Fig. 11.3.1). Long-chain acyl-CoA is oxidized to produce acetyl-coenzyme A (acetyl-CoA) (so-called β-oxidation). Each molecule of acetyl-CoA that is oxidized by β-oxidation produces one molecule of NADH (nicotinamide adenine dinucleotide, reduced) and one molecule of $FADH_2$ (flavin adenine dinucleotide, reduced). Acetyl-CoA then enters the tricarboxylic acid (TCA) cycle and produces two molecules of carbon dioxide, three of NADH, and one of $FADH_2$ for each molecule of acetyl-CoA (see later discussion).

Carbohydrate Oxidation (Glucose, Lactate)

Besides FFA, the other main source of acetyl-CoA for the TCA cycle is oxidation of carbohydrates, particularly glucose and lactate. When the organism is in a carbohydrate-fed state, lipolysis is inhibited by insulin and subsequently carbohydrate oxidation increases (11). In this case, carbohydrates can account for 100% of the myocardial oxygen consumption (glucose, 70%; lactate, 30%). During heavy dynamic exercise (65% of an individual's maximal oxygen uptake), the production of lactate increases, and it becomes the major fuel of the heart, accounting for 60% to 70% of the myocardial oxygen consumption (3,12).

During ischemia, the metabolism of glucose to lactate is the main source of energy for the heart. With the lack of a sufficient oxygen supply, glucose uptake, glycogenolysis, glycolytic flux, and ATP hydrolysis are all stimulated (13).

Glucose is transported into the myocardial cell by the glucose transporters GLUT4 and GLUT1 (14). Intracellularly, glucose is rapidly phosphorylated to glucose 6-phosphate, which is further used for glycolysis or glycogen synthesis (Fig. 11.3.1). In glycolysis, glucose 6-phosphate is metabolized to pyruvate. Pyruvate is also formed from lactate taken up by the heart. Under aerobic conditions, most of the pyruvate is converted to acetyl-CoA, which enters the TCA cycle (see later discussion). A minor portion of glucose and lactate is converted to oxaloacetate, which enters the TCA cycle at a different site than acetyl-CoA (13).

Tricarboxylic Acid Cycle

The metabolic pathways for energy substrates transform the major fuels into acetyl-CoA, which then enters the TCA cycle. One molecule of acetyl-CoA produces three molecules of NADH, one of $FADH_2$, and one of guanosine triphosphate (GTP), which is also a high-energy compound. NADH and $FADH_2$ are oxidized in the respiratory electron transport chain and ultimately yield 11 molecules of ATP. Mitochondrial respiration appears to be regulated by nitrous oxide (NO), at least *in vitro*, and thus NO might have a regulatory role in the myocardial metabolic rate of oxygen ($MMRO_2$) *in vivo* (15,16).

The rate at which the TCA cycle operates is the major factor that controls the rate of production of ATP by the heart. The TCA cycle activity increases when myocardial work increases. Reduced

ATP:adenosine diphosphate and NAD:$NADH_2$ ratios may be the major determinants of the rate at which the TCA cycle operates (17), but this has been disputed (18).

Efficiency

In the healthy heart, myocardial metabolism and contraction are closely linked by ATP production and consumption. However, in certain clinical conditions, such as ischemic heart disease, in which oxygen supply is restricted, and in heart failure, this close connection can be lost. The overloaded failing heart is characterized by an imbalance between energy production and utilization (19). The overload itself increases energy expenditure by increasing wall stress in the dilated heart. The energy deficit of the myocardium may further aggravate both systolic and diastolic dysfunction (19).

Myocardial metabolism can be related to myocardial work to further evaluate cardiac physiology. The concept of efficiency has been used for decades for this purpose (20) and was originally described by Starling and Vissher (21) in isolated heart preparations. Efficiency is defined as the ratio between the energy created by a system and the energy put into the system. Because most of the energy (approximately 65% to 80%) consumed by the heart is converted to heat, experimental thermodynamic studies are important for assessing the total efficiency of the heart (22,23). However, *in vivo* (in animal and human studies), efficiency is usually defined as the ratio of mechanical work performed relative to the myocardial oxygen consumption (mechanical efficiency). It has been claimed that the efficiency is maximized under physiologic conditions both in the right ventricle (RV) and in the left ventricle (LV) (20,24). However, the question whether the heart is optimized to operate at maximum efficiency or at maximum stroke work is still a matter of controversy.

In 1979, Suga (25) introduced a comprehensive time varying elastase model. In this model, the area of the pressure–volume relationship (PVA) is a measure of the total work performed by the ventricle during one cardiac cycle. The PVA concept includes both the external or stroke (pressure–volume) work of the heart and an internal component, termed potential energy. The PVA correlates closely with invasively measured $MMRO_2$ per beat (25). The method allows the assessment of contractile efficiency, as well as the cost of basal and activation metabolism. The PVA is the only one of the mechanical variables that can be used to assess myocardial efficiency without a need to separately measure myocardial oxygen consumption. The PVA method to measure oxygen consumption is highly invasive, requiring catheterization with LV micromanometers and conductance catheters. Therefore, the applicability of the method in human studies is limited.

Other approaches require a measure or estimate of both external work and oxygen consumption to determine efficiency. There are several applicable approaches for noninvasive measurement of external cardiac work, which usually employ measurement of blood pressure and heart rate with or without stroke volume (26,27). External work can be assessed with the pressure work index, a product of systolic (or mean) pressure, heart rate, and stroke volume (28), which covers both pressure and flow work. Energy is used for building and maintaining tension, which is needed for contractility and wall stress. Systolic contraction of the ventricle is enhanced by preload and is opposed by afterload, which are both oxygen-requiring processes (29). When related to $MMRO_2$, the pressure work index gives a measure of useful forward mechanical efficiency. The pressure work index and its modifications are readily assessed noninvasively *in vivo*, which improves the applicability of this method in human studies (30–34).

ASSESSMENT OF MYOCARDIAL ENERGY METABOLISM

In Vitro Methods

A common way to study the energy metabolism of the heart is to measure the intracellular levels of metabolic intermediates or the activity of enzymes involved in the various pathways of energy metabolism. With these techniques, the levels of intermediates are measured from frozen or lyophilized tissue samples by spectrophotometry, radiometry, or high-performance liquid chromatography. Although these methods have formed the basis of our understanding of myocardial metabolism, they require tissue samples and are not clinically practical. These methods are also limited in that they can give relevant information about the energy status of the heart, but not information about the rate of the production or utilization of ATP (i.e., oxygen consumption) (35).

Invasive Methods

Percutaneous catheterization of the coronary sinus and blood sampling allow the measurement of cardiac metabolism *in vivo*. Simultaneous measurements of the concentration of energy substrates (carbohydrates, fatty acids) or oxygen in the coronary sinus and in the arterial blood and coronary blood flow allow calculation of net rates of carbohydrate and lipid metabolism and myocardial oxygen consumption (36). The net substrate metabolism can be calculated more accurately if specific substrates labeled with carbon-14 ([^{14}C]) or tritium are used. Despite improved accuracy, *regional* myocardial metabolism cannot be assessed with such methods. Since coronary sinus catheterization is a highly invasive and sometimes difficult procedure, the use of this approach is limited.

Noninvasive Methods

Nuclear Magnetic Resonance

Nuclear magnetic resonance (NMR) spectroscopy allows assessment of molecular structure and substrate concentration. The two most common nuclides measured in studies involving energy metabolism are phosphate-31 ([^{31}P]) and carbon-13 ([^{13}C]). The use of [^{31}P] NMR provides information about the levels of ATP, creatinine phosphate, inorganic phosphate, and sugar phosphates, all of which play a role in the myocardial energy system (35). Various intermediates of metabolism can be labeled with [^{13}C]. NMR spectroscopy allows quantitative detection of these intermediates in the tissue, an approach that has been used to assess TCA cycle activity. Fluorine-19 ([^{19}F])-labeled compounds that bind calcium have been used with NMR to measure intracellular calcium.

Phosphate-31 NMR provides information about the concentration of high-energy phosphate compounds, but not about the rate of ATP production or utilization, which limits the usefulness of this method. Carbon-13 NMR can be used to detect the fate of a predefined substrate in the chain of oxidative metabolism (TCA cycle) (37). However, TCA cycle intermediates and the [^{13}C] label are quickly equilibrated, and as a consequence, [^{13}C] NMR mainly measures incorporation of [^{13}C] into the glutamate pool (37). Carbon-13 NMR is further limited by difficulties in kinetic analysis of metabolite labeling (35).

Magnetic Resonance Imaging

Recent technical advances in cardiac magnetic resonance imaging (MRI) have made it possible to accurately study cardiac morphology and function, as well as myocardial perfusion in healthy volunteers and patients with ischemic heart disease (38–40). T2-weighted fast spin-echo imaging, combined with perfusion-sensitive spin labeling, has also been used to measure myocardial perfusion and oxygen concentration in isolated blood-perfused rabbit hearts (41). However, MRI does not allow quantification of myocardial oxygen consumption.

PET

Regional myocardial metabolism, blood flow, and oxygen consumption can be readily studied with PET using radiolabeled metabolite analogues. The advantages of PET over other radionuclide methods are the unique ability to quantitatively measure tracer concentrations in selected tissue volumes with better spatial and temporal resolution and better sensitivity due to multiple detectors.

Measurement of Glucose and Fatty Acid Metabolism with PET PET can be used to measure the initial steps of glucose metabolism (fluorine-18 [^{18}F]-fluorodeoxyglucose [FDG]) (42) and the rate of fatty acid metabolism ([^{11}C]-palmitate, [^{18}F]-FTHA [6-triaheptecanoic acid]) (43,44). The clearance of [^{11}C]-palmitate represents β-oxidation and oxidation in the TCA cycle. Because the rapid *washout* of [^{11}C]-palmitate from myocardium partly represents the TCA cycle activity, it correlates to some extent with myocardial oxygen consumption. However, the method is sensitive to levels of tissue oxygenation and arterial fatty acids, as well as to the pattern of substrate use (45–48). Fluorine-18-FTHA is a false long-chain fatty acid substrate and inhibitor of fatty acid metabolism. After transport into the mitochondria, it undergoes initial steps of β-oxidation and is thereafter trapped in the cell. The rate of radioactivity accumulation in the myocardium would, therefore, directly reflect the β-oxidation rate of long-chain fatty acids. The uptake rate constant of [^{18}F]-FTHA correlates well with the rate pressure product in healthy volunteers (49).

It has to be kept in mind that the rate of metabolism of one single energy substrate may reflect only a portion of the overall oxidative metabolism of the heart and depends on prevailing metabolic circumstances. Mitochondrial oxidation of intermediary substrates can also be impaired in specific conditions such as myocardial ischemia (50). The overall oxidative metabolism can, however, be quantitatively assessed with [^{11}C]-acetate and oxygen-15 (labeled) oxygen ($^{15}O_2$) PET.

ASSESSMENT OF MYOCARDIAL OXYGEN CONSUMPTION WITH PET

Carbon-11-Acetate PET

FFAs and carbohydrates share the TCA cycle for oxidative metabolism (Fig. 11.3.1). The turnover rate of the TCA cycle reflects the rate of overall oxidative metabolism, and, therefore, it is an ideal site for assessing myocardial oxidative metabolism. Carbon-11-acetate is readily metabolized to carbon dioxide almost exclusively by oxidative metabolism through the TCA cycle.

First-pass extraction of acetate into the myocardium is inversely related to the myocardial blood flow (MBF) (51). In a steady state, the reported myocardial extraction fraction (EF) of radiolabeled acetate in animal models is 60% to 70% for healthy myocardium and up to 95% for ischemic myocardium (52,53). In humans, the EF of acetate is approximately 30% to 40% (54). Acetate is converted to acetyl-CoA in mitochondria, which then enters the TCA cycle. In the TCA cycle, the radiolabel in the carboxyl (C-1) position of acetate undergoes two cycle turns before the label is released as carbon dioxide (or bicarbonate in tissue) (55). Nearly all (80% to 90%) of the acetate extracted by myocardium is oxidized. The major alternative route is transamination of acetate to glutamate and aspartate via the TCA cycle intermediates (56). Therefore, the elimination rate of radiolabeled acetate reflects the overall TCA cycle flux and consequently overall oxygen consumption over a wide range of cardiac workloads (52,56).

Preparation of the Tracer

The production of [^{11}C]-acetate is based on a method developed by Pike et al. (57). In short, [^{11}C]-carbon dioxide is produced by the [^{14}N]-(p,α)[^{11}C] reaction in a medical cyclotron. Methyl magnesium bromide in diethyl ether is carbonated under nitrogen with [^{11}C]-labeled carbon dioxide. After this, hydrochloric acid is added to the reaction during vigorous stirring, and then the phases are allowed to separate. Sodium bicarbonate (10 mL) is added to the solution, and the solution is heated under a stream of nitrogen and finally sterilized by filtration.

Imaging Protocols

The imaging protocol for [^{11}C]-acetate is straightforward. A transmission scan is performed to correct the data for tissue photon attenuation. Carbon-11-acetate is administered as an intravenous bolus over 30 to 60 seconds (30,34). The target dose varies according to camera properties, and the dose is usually 10 to 20 mCi. The length of dynamic scanning in clinical studies varies between 20 and 49 minutes (31,58). To detect the early part of the clearance curve, the early time frames are short and the frames get longer toward the end of the study; for example, 10 × 10 seconds, 1 × 60 seconds, 5 × 100 seconds, 5 × 120 seconds, and 7 × 240 seconds (30).

Analysis of the Data

Regional Analysis

In clinical practice, several different approaches have been used to assess regional myocardial oxygen consumption. Regions of interest (ROIs) can be placed on transaxial slices (Fig. 11.3.2) or short-axis slices (59) of the LV and in some cases on the RV simultaneously (31,60,61).

Regional analysis of the data is of special interest in coronary artery disease (CAD), particularly after a myocardial infarction (MI) when there are likely to be regional differences in myocardial function and metabolism (34). Regional differences can also exist in nonischemic cardiomyopathy (62). An important clinical application of [^{11}C]-acetate PET has been in assessing myocardial viability (58). To facilitate the comparison between PET and echocardiographic studies, one must use the same segmental division in both modalities (30,31,62–65).

Modeling of the Data

In most clinical studies, [^{11}C]-acetate data have been analyzed by monoexponential fitting of the clearance portion of the time-activity curve (TAC) (Fig. 11.3.3) (30,31,33,34,61,66–69).

Biexponential fitting of the data (Fig. 11.3.3) has been used less frequently because the second part of the curve might be less reliable in clinical studies (70). The conventional exponential fitting

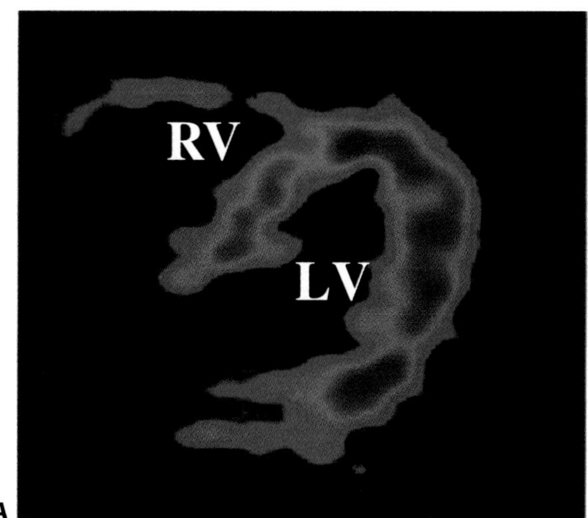

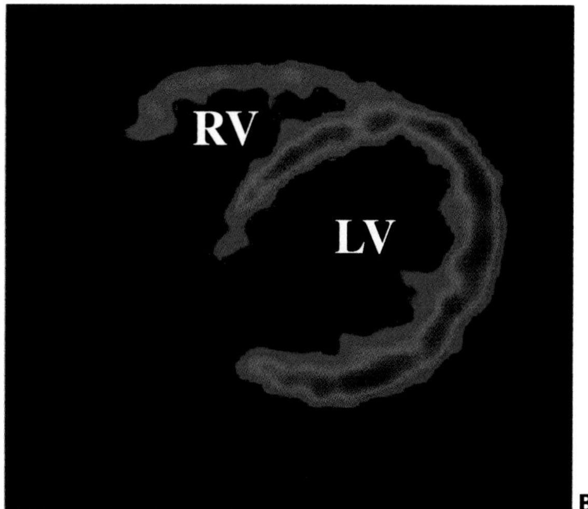

FIGURE 11.3.2. Representative transaxial images showing maximal uptake of carbon-11 ([^{11}C])-acetate in a healthy volunteer (**A**) and a patient with congestive heart failure due to dilated cariomyopathy (**B**). [^{11}C]-acetate uptake is enhanced in the right ventricle (RV) of the patient with heart failure. LV, left ventricle. (From Ukkonen H, Saraste M, Akkila J, et al. Myocardial efficiency during levosimendan infusion in congestive heart failure. *Clin Pharmacol Ther* 2000;68:522–531, with permission.)

analysis does not account for the distribution of arterial input function, the recirculating [^{11}C]-acetate, the spill-over, or the presence of metabolites. Therefore, more sophisticated compartmental and kinetic models have been introduced for estimation of myocardial oxygen consumption with [^{11}C]-acetate PET.

Because only a fraction of injected [^{11}C]-acetate is delivered to the heart during the first pass, a recirculating amount of the tracer can be considerable and may therefore affect the shape of tissue TACs. Using computer simulations, it has been shown that the shape of the arterial input function can significantly alter the monoexponential fitting of the myocardial TAC. Buck et al. (71) introduced a two-compartment model for [^{11}C]-acetate kinetics that accounts for tracer recirculation. The model requires assessment of an input function and correction for tracer metabolites and spill over effects. The model-derived parameter k_2 correlated closely with directly measured $MMRO_2$. This method has been successfully used in patients with congestive heart failure (CHF) (34) and patients with acute MI (72). Raylman et al. (73) were able to improve the accuracy of the fitted k_2 parameter by simultaneously fitting data from multiple ROIs. Sun et al. (74) tested a comprehensive tracer kinetic model (six-compartment model) for [^{11}C]-acetate kinetics in dogs, which takes into account differences in input function. This model yielded accurate $MMRO_2$ measurements compared with invasive measurements. However, this model has not been validated in humans. The same is true for the compartmental model introduced by Ng et al. (75).

Although these models are theoretically more accurate than the traditional fitting methods, their complexity and the need for

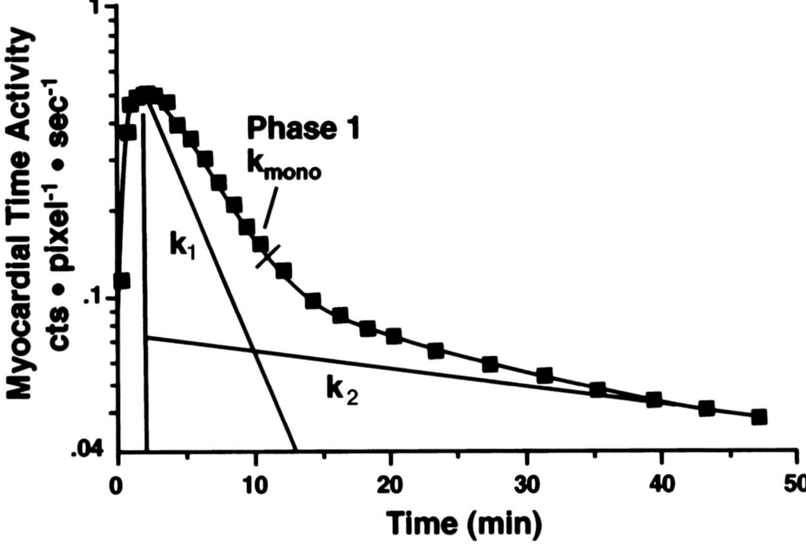

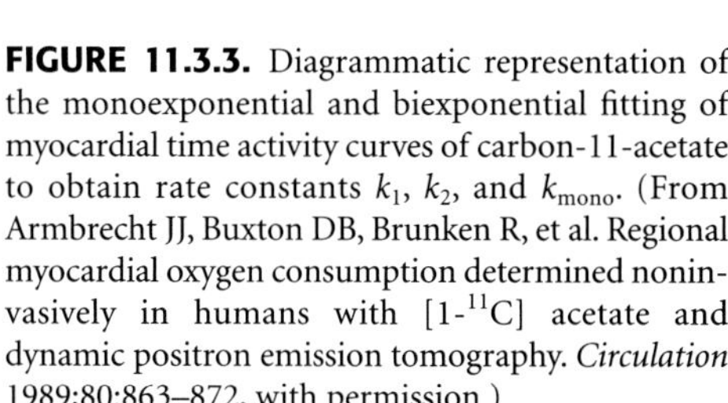

FIGURE 11.3.3. Diagrammatic representation of the monoexponential and biexponential fitting of myocardial time activity curves of carbon-11-acetate to obtain rate constants k_1, k_2, and k_{mono}. (From Armbrecht JJ, Buxton DB, Brunken R, et al. Regional myocardial oxygen consumption determined noninvasively in humans with [1-^{11}C] acetate and dynamic positron emission tomography. *Circulation* 1989;80:863–872, with permission.)

additional assessments, such as arterial blood sampling, limit their feasibility in clinical studies.

Experimental Studies and Validation of the Method

The detected TAC reflecting the clearance of [^{11}C]-acetate from the myocardium can be either monoexponential or biexponential depending on the level of oxidative metabolism. The curve is usually monoexponential at rest, during hypoxia and ischemia, and it is usually biexponential during increased metabolic demands such as during dobutamine infusion (53,70). The decay constant of the initial component of the clearance curve has been shown to be linearly related to myocardial oxygen consumption. The accuracy of [^{11}C]-acetate PET in measuring myocardial oxygen consumption in the LV has been validated in experimental studies in isolated perfused rabbit hearts, rat hearts, and dogs (52,53,56,76) (Fig. 11.3.4). In humans, the elimination rate of [^{11}C]-acetate has been shown to correlate with indirect estimates of myocardial oxygen consumption both in the LV (61,69) and in the RV (60). The elimination rate of [^{11}C]-acetate also correlates well with directly (invasively) measured myocardial oxygen consumption in healthy volunteers (77,78) and patients with dilated cardiomyopathy (34,79). Although variations in the pattern of substrate utilization can alter the ratio of TCA cycle flux to oxygen consumption, the magnitude of the change is insignificant (76).

Potential Sources of Error and Limitations of Carbon-11-Acetate PET

The accuracy of [^{11}C]-acetate PET in assessing $MMRO_2$ may be reduced in specific conditions. In experimental prolonged low-flow ischemia in pigs, the myocardial clearance rate constant (k_{mono}) of [^{11}C]-acetate may overestimate the myocardial oxygen consumption (80). Correction for a decrease in peak [^{11}C] activity and a reduced amino acid pool observed with the prolonged ischemia restores the relationship with $MMRO_2$. The ratio of the [^{11}C]-acetate clearance rate to myocardial oxygen consumption in ischemic canine hearts has also been reported to be higher than that in nonischemic canine hearts (53). It has been suggested that [^{11}C]-acetate could overestimate myocardial oxygen consumption in

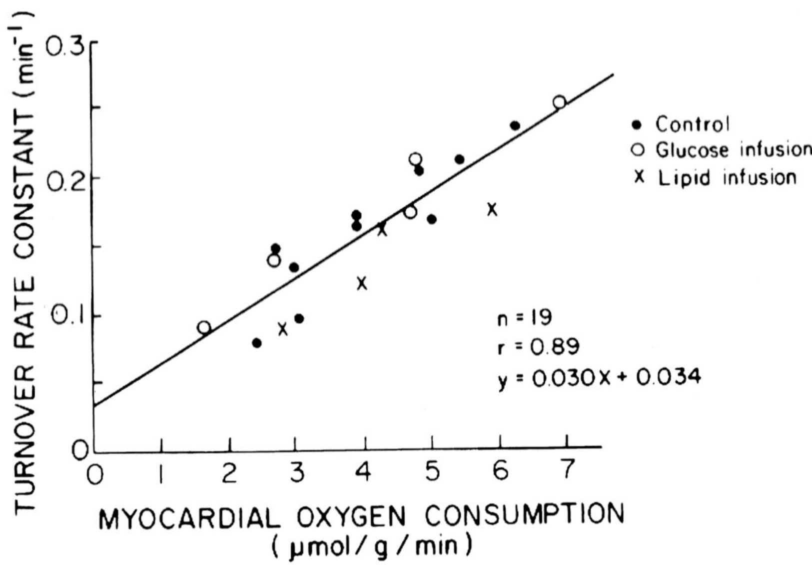

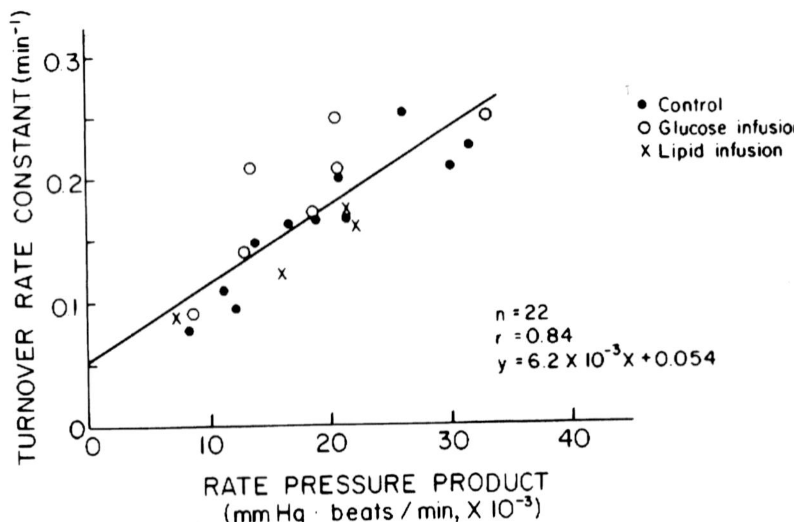

FIGURE 11.3.4. Top: Correlation between the rate constant of the rapid phase of clearance and directly measured myocardial oxygen consumption. There is no significant difference between the control, post-glucose administration, and postlipid administration imaging studies. **Bottom:** Correlation between the rate constant of the rapid phase of clearance and the rate pressure product, which is an index of total myocardial work. There are no significant differences between the control, postglucose administration, and postlipid administration studies. (From Brown MA, Myears DW, Bergmann SR. Validity of estimates of myocardial oxidative metabolism with carbon-11 acetate and positron emission tomography despite altered patterns of substrate utilization. *J Nucl Med* 1989;30:187–193, with permission.)

myocardial segments containing infarcted myocardium, compared with the $^{15}O_2$-based method (81).

To date, the clinical application of [^{11}C]-acetate PET has been established by using the rate constant indices of oxidative metabolism and not absolute quantification of $MMRO_2$. The assessment of treatment efficacy has also been based on relative changes in myocardial oxidative metabolism and not absolute quantification of $MMRO_2$. In clinical practice, it is usually not necessary to correct for the changes in the oxidative metabolism/$MMRO_2$ relationship mentioned above. However, when assessment of absolute myocardial oxygen consumption is needed, correction for these factors should be considered.

$^{15}O_2$ PET

It has been possible to label molecular oxygen with [^{15}O] and to detect the fate of the tracer with PET for over 20 years (82), but the assessment of $MMRO_2$ of the LV with $^{15}O_2$ PET has only recently been achieved in humans. The PET technique employing $^{15}O_2$ inhalation was introduced by Iida et al. (83) for the direct quantification of regional $MMRO_2$ ($rMMRO_2$). This steady-state method takes into account the systematic underestimation of tissue signals caused by the small transmural wall thickness and contractile wall motion (partial volume effect). It also allows the assessment of $rMMRO_2$ in absolute terms (i.e., in milliliters per minute per gram).

Scanning Protocol

The measurement of $rMMRO_2$ with $^{15}O_2$ is based on a series of PET scans that are used for the calculation of functional images. Special attention must be paid to avoid patient movement during the study. The sequence of PET scans does not have any effect on $rMMRO_2$ values, and the sequence can be modified according to the local practice. All PET data are corrected for dead time, decay, and photon attenuation.

To correct for tissue photon attenuation, transmission imaging or computed tomography (CT) attenuation correction is performed before the emission scan. To obtain blood volume data, the patient's nostrils are closed and he or she inhales oxygen-15 carbon monoxide ($C^{15}O$) for 2 minutes through a three-way inhalation flap valve (0.14% carbon monoxide mixed with room air). After the inhalation, 2 minutes are allowed for carbon monoxide to combine with hemoglobin in red blood cells before a static scan for 4 minutes is started. During the scan period, three blood samples are drawn at 2-minute intervals, and blood radioactivity is measured immediately with an automatic gamma counter.

Before the flow measurements, 10 minutes is allowed for $C^{15}O$ radioactive decay. In clinical practice, blood flow is measured either with a slow deuterium [^{15}O] infusion or with slow Oxygen-15 carbon dioxide ($C^{15}O_2$) inhalation (84).

Ten minutes after the infusion of $H_2{}^{15}O$ or inhalation of $C^{15}O_2$, continuous inhalation of $^{15}O_2$ is started for 16 minutes and PET imaging is performed under steady-state conditions (4 × 30 seconds, 6 × 60 seconds, 1 × 600 (or 480) seconds, 9 × 30 seconds) (83). The steady-state image of myocardial $^{15}O_2$ uptake is determined from normalized subtractions of blood volume and lung gas volume from the 10-minute (8-minute) data acquisition obtained during steady-state conditions. Finally, a short 5-minute transmission scan is usually performed at the end to rule out patient movement during the study.

Processing and Modeling of the Data

The measurement of $rMMRO_2$ and regional oxygen extraction fraction (rOEF) with the method described above is based on the inhalation of $^{15}O_2$ gas. The compartmental model describing $^{15}O_2$ behavior in the myocardium is illustrated in Fig. 11.3.5. The model requires a correction for spill over of activity from the vascular pools of the heart chambers and lungs and from the pulmonary airways. The spill over of activity from the vascular pools is corrected by the blood volume measurement using $C^{15}O$, and the spill over of activity from the pulmonary airways is corrected with an indirect measurement of gas volume obtained from the transmission scan.

$^{15}O_2$ is carried as [^{15}O]-hemoglobin by blood and it diffuses to myocardium, where it is converted to water ($H_2{}^{15}O$). This diffusion process is explained by OEF. The $H_2{}^{15}O$ equilibrates instantaneously and its washout rate is proportional to prevailing MBF. The recirculating $H_2{}^{15}O$, produced by other tissues, also contributes to the observed activity in the myocardium, and correction for this is required. Sophisticated mathematic modeling of the data yields the quantified rOEF. Iida et al. (83) described the relationship between rOEF and $rMMRO_2$ as:

$$rMMRO_2 = [O_2]_a \times rOEF \times rMBF,$$

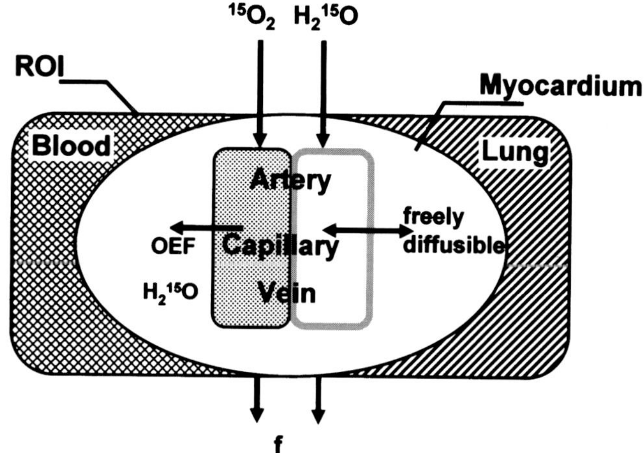

FIGURE 11.3.5. A compartmental model to measure the regional oxygen extraction fraction (rOEF) and the regional myocardial metabolic rate of oxygen by the use of PET and $^{15}O_2$ inhalation. The myocardial region of interest includes radioactivity in the myocardial tissue, spill-over from the radioactivity of blood occupying the cardiac chamber, and spill-over from radioactivity in the lung. The myocardial compartment consists of the tissue component and a vascular component (which includes arterial, capillary, and venous volumes). The hemoglobin-bound $^{15}O_2$ is supplied to the capillary and diffuses into the tissue space, where it is instantaneously converted into labeled water of metabolism ($H_2{}^{15}O$-met). This diffusion process is assumed to be explained by an OEF. There is another input of radioactivity with a different chemical form, circulating $H_2{}^{15}O$, which is assumed to be freely diffusible across the capillary membrane. This radioactivity is assumed to distribute in the same tissue space as $H_2{}^{15}O$-met and is washed out in proportion to the blood flow divided by the partition coefficient of water. ROI, region of interest. (From Iida H, Rhodes CG, Araujo LI, et al. Noninvasive quantification of regional myocardial metabolic rate of oxygen by use of $^{15}O_2$ inhalation and positron emission tomography. Theory, analysis and application in humans. *Circulation* 1996;94:792–807, with permission.)

where $[O_2]_a$ is the total oxygen content of the arterial blood (milliliters of oxygen per milliliter of blood) and rMBF is regional MBF assessed by $C^{15}O_2$ inhalation (85) or $H_2{}^{15}O$ infusion (84). The $[O_2]_a$ is assessed as:

$$[O_2]a = \frac{1.39 \times Hb \times \%Sat}{100},$$

where *Hb* is the hemoglobin concentration of the blood (grams per milliliter), *%Sat* represents the percentage saturation of oxygen in arterial blood, and 1.39 denotes the maximum binding capacity of oxygen per unit mass of hemoglobin (milliliters of oxygen per gram of hemoglobin). The value of 94% was assigned to *%Sat.*

Analysis of the Data

The myocardial ROIs can be placed on extravascular density images according to anatomic segments (81,86–88). To avoid spill-over from the RV, septal ROIs are placed on the LV side of the septum. A large ROI (input function for rMBF) and a small ROI (for calculation of rOEF) are also placed on the LV on blood volume images. A lung ROI, needed for rOEF calculation, is also placed on gas volume images. All the ROIs are projected onto blood and gas volume images and the dynamic $^{15}O_2$ and $H_2{}^{15}O$ data sets to generate arterial and myocardial tissue TACs, which are subsequently used for calculation of $rMMRO_2$ (83).

Validation and Experimental Studies

A linear relationship has been established between $^{15}O_2$ PET-derived and directly measured $MMRO_2$ in animal studies. Studies with dogs (88–90) using various pharmacologic interventions with isoprenaline, adenosine, propranolol, and morphine demonstrated that OEF and $MMRO_2$ values obtained by this technique agreed closely with those obtained by direct measurement of OEF with arteriovenous (AV) sampling (Fick method) and MBF with the microsphere technique (Fig. 11.3.6). There is also a close linear correlation between $^{15}O_2$ PET-derived $rMMRO_2$ and k_{mono} of [^{11}C]-acetate in patients with CAD and old MI ($r = 0.89$; $P < .001$) (Fig. 11.3.7) (81).

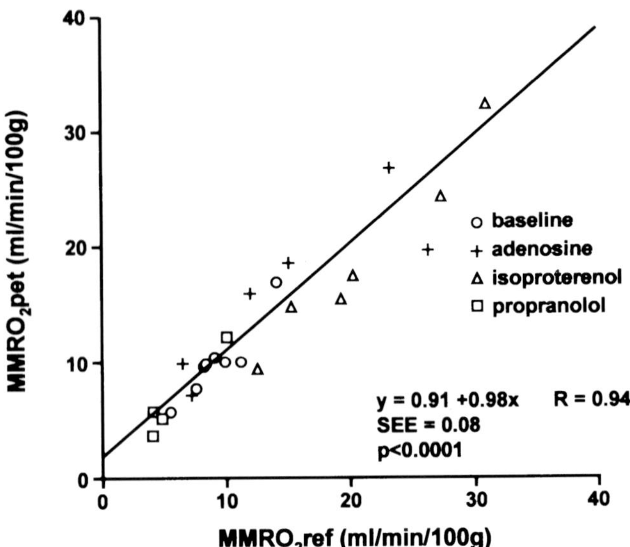

FIGURE 11.3.6. Comparison of myocardial metabolic rate of oxygen ($MMRO_2$) measured by $^{15}O_2$ PET ($MMRO_2$-pet) and invasive arteriovenous sampling and $MMRO_2$ microspheres ($MMRO_2$-ref) shows a close correlation between the two methods despite pharmacologic provocation ($MMRO_2$-pet = 0.98, $MMRO_2$-ref + 0.91; $r = 0.94$). (From Yamamoto Y, de Silva R, Rhodes CG, et al. Noninvasive quantification of regional myocardial metabolic rate of oxygen by $^{15}O_2$ inhalation and positron emission tomography: experimental validation. *Circulation* 1996;94:808–816, with permission.)

Potential Sources of Error and Limitations of $^{15}O_2$ PET

Although $^{15}O_2$ PET has great potential for noninvasive assessment of myocardial oxygen consumption, there are certain limitations to this method (83). Calculation of regional myocardial oxygen consumption with $^{15}O_2$ PET is based on sophisticated modeling, requiring a series of PET studies. The complexity of the scanning procedure increases the vulnerability of the method. The mean

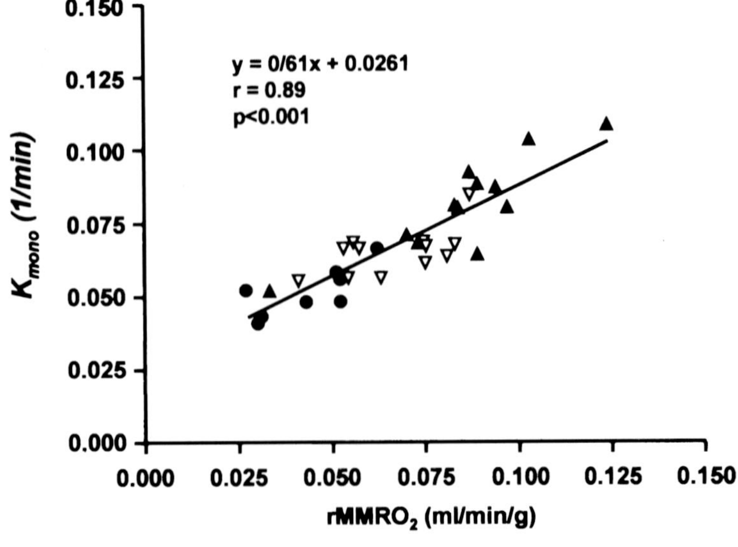

FIGURE 11.3.7. A close linear correlation between k_{mono} and regional myocardial metabolic rate of oxygen ($rMMRO_2$) exists from low to normal myocardial blood flow (MBF) ($r = 0.89$; $P < = .001$; $y = 0.61x + 0.026$). ▲, group A, normal segments; ▽, group B, segments with moderately reduced MBF; ●, group C, segments with low MBF. (From Ukkonen H, Knuuti J, Katoh C, et al. Use of [^{11}C]acetate and [^{15}O]O_2 PET for the assessment of myocardial oxygen utilization in patients with chronic myocardial infarction. *Eur J Nucl Med* 2001;28:334–339, with permission.)

intersubject variability for rMMRO$_2$ has varied from 21% to 32% (83), and this variation is mainly due to the variation in rMBF and to a lesser degree to the variation in rOEF. However, a lower variability and higher reproducibility of the quantitative parameters can be achieved if an iterative reconstruction method based on median root prior reconstruction is used instead of the traditional filtered back projection (FBP) method (91,92).The reproducibility of the septal rMMRO$_2$ values, which have previously been problematic, has significantly improved with the median root prior (MRP) reconstruction method. The main practical problem of the method is the sensitivity of the subject to movement. This can be particularly problematic in critically ill patients. Due to the complex logistics associated with the use of $^{15}O_2$, [^{11}C]-acetate is still preferred for the estimation of rMMRO$_2$ using PET.

Special Features of PET in Assessing Myocardial Oxygen Consumption

The invasive approach to measure cardiac oxygen balance and efficiency carries, apart from an inherent risk to the patient, important methodological drawbacks, particularly if the patient has significant heart disease. Invasively achieved estimates of MMRO$_2$ usually apply only to the left anterior descending coronary artery territory, but they are extrapolated to the entire LV muscle mass. Measurements of myocardial oxygen consumption by PET are necessary to evaluate cardiac efficiency by noninvasive methods. Because cardiac catheterization is not required, this approach facilitates pharmacodynamic studies in both healthy volunteers and patients with disease and makes repeated patient studies more feasible. Moreover, PET allows assessment of myocardial perfusion and metabolism directly at the tissue level. The method assigns accurate topographical data to all vascular beds, even to the RV.

CLINICAL APPLICATIONS

Applications of Carbon-11-Acetate PET in Coronary Artery Disease and Viability Assessment

During ischemia, oxidative metabolism of FFAs is decreased and exogenous glucose becomes the preferred substrate. The production of energy mainly depends on anaerobic glycolysis. In clinical practice, assessment of [^{18}F]-FDG PET has been used as the gold standard in assessing myocardial viability in dysfunctional myocardium. The role of oxidative metabolism in ischemic heart disease, particularly in MI, has been studied with [^{11}C]-acetate PET.

PET has provided evidence of decreased myocardial perfusion reserve in patients with risk factors for CAD before clinical signs or symptoms of ischemia (93). The perfusion reserve is further decreased in territories of stenosed coronary arteries (94). The oxidative metabolism assessed with [^{11}C]-acetate at rest and during dobutamine stimulation is intact regardless of impaired flow reserve, suggesting perfusion-MMRO$_2$ mismatch during myocardial ischemia (95). Oxidative metabolism is also preserved in reperfused but dysfunctional (stunned) myocardium after percutaneous transluminal coronary angioplasty (96).

The natural history of MI has changed tremendously in the era of new revascularization therapies with thrombolysis and stents. Instead of having an infarcted area with only necrotic tissue, there is an area at risk that has a mixture of viable and nonviable tissue. The functional outcome of these regions relies on the amount of the viable tissue within the infarcted area (97).

Carbon-11-acetate PET has been shown to have prognostic value with regard to the recovery of LV function after MI. Maes et al. (72) assessed myocardial oxidative metabolism in 18 patients with acute MI within 24 hours of the onset of symptoms. All the patients received thrombolytic therapy. [^{13}N]-H$_3$ and [^{18}F]-FDG PET were performed on day 5 to assess conventional PET viability. Oxidative metabolism was comparable in PET-viable and -nonviable segments, which is in keeping with previously published data (98). This could be partly due to the inconsistency of NH$_3$ and FDG in defining myocardial viability in the very early stage after infarction and reperfusion therapy. There was a linear correlation between oxidative metabolism and LV ejection fraction at 3 months. Multivariate analysis found the oxidative metabolism of the reperfused myocardium to be the only predictor of LV function at 3 months. This prognostic information concerning LV function could potentially be used to identify the patients with patent infarct-related arteries but poor recovery of LV function (TIMI flow grade 3) who would potentially benefit from more aggressive medical therapy.

Infarcted areas of the myocardium often contain a mixture of viable and necrotic tissue. The recovery of wall motion abnormality after revascularization therefore depends on metabolic activity and amount of scar tissue within the segment. Traditionally, [^{18}F]-FDG PET in combination with a flow tracer has been used to detect viable myocardium. Flow metabolism mismatch accurately predicts functional recovery after revascularization. Preservation of oxidative metabolism is also necessary for recovery of function after revascularization (99). Carbon-11-acetate PET yields quantitative data both on MBF and oxidative metabolism and therefore can be applied for detecting viability.

Gropler et al. (100) studied 34 patients, comparing [^{11}C]-acetate and [^{18}F]-FDG in detecting myocardial viability. Carbon-11-acetate was able to identify viable myocardium in 67% and nonviable in 89% of the cases. The corresponding predictive values for [^{18}F]-FDG were 52% and 81%, respectively. However this FDG accuracy is below the mean predictive accuracies of 71% and 86% reported from a pooled data analysis of 20 previous studies (101). In severely dysfunctional segments, both methods had better predictive accuracy.

Wolpers et al. (59) studied 30 post-MI patients and found the positive predictive accuracy of [^{11}C]-acetate PET to be 62% and negative predictive accuracy to be 65%. It is important to keep in mind, however, that the resting level of myocardial oxidative metabolism can significantly overlap between nonviable and viable segments (58).

The presence of contractile reserve on the dobutamine stress echocardiogram has been shown to be accurate in predicting recovery after reperfusion (102,103). However, the method may have reduced the negative predictive value in certain clinical settings in comparison with conventional metabolic imaging (104–106). Lee et al. (107) studied 19 patients with dysfunctional myocardial segments due to CAD with dobutamine stress echocardiograms, as well as $H_2{}^{15}O$ and [^{11}C]-acetate PET. Myocardial oxidative metabolism reserve and blood flow reserve were lower, both in contractile negative and positive groups compared with normal. In contractile reserve–positive segments, both reserves were higher than in contractile reserve–negative segments. Of the segments defined as viable by PET, 54% were contractile reserve negative and exhibited blunted MBF response to dobutamine. Complementing this work, Yoshinaga et al. (108) showed that segments that had reduced contractile reserve and were viable by FDG imaging demonstrated an impaired oxidative metabolic response. This helps to explain the loss of contractile reserve that likely precedes the loss of glucose utilization. This also explains the greater sensitivity of FDG uptake to detect viability than contractile reserve with dobutamine (108).

Hata et al. (58) validated dobutamine stress [^{11}C]-acetate PET in 28 patients with old Q wave anterior MI. Segmental wall motion assessment was performed after coronary revascularization with echocardiography. The clearance rate constant k_{mono} of [^{11}C]-acetate at rest was significantly higher in viable segments $0.052 \pm 0.010\ \text{min}^{-1}$ versus $0.033 \pm 0.010\ \text{min}^{-1}$. However, there was considerable overlap between the groups. The baseline k_{mono} of the viable segment was 70.7% ± 15.8% and the nonviable segment 43.1% ± 13.0% of that of normal myocardium. The k_{mono} response to low-dose dobutamine was directionally different between the groups, allowing the detection of viable myocardium. In viable segments, normalized k_{mono} increased (70.7% ± 15.8% to 83.2% ± 9.9%) and decreased in nonviable segments (43.1% ± 13.0% to 26.9% ± 10.3%) during dobutamine infusion.

Carbon-11-acetate PET also yields a measure of relative myocardial perfusion. Relative myocardial perfusion was significantly different between the viable and nonviable segments without overlap (67.9% ± 9.6% vs. 32.7% ± 5.8%). During dobutamine administration, relative myocardial perfusion increased slightly in viable segments (to 70.4% ± 7.5%) but decreased significantly in nonviable segments (to 21.1% ± 5.3%) (Fig. 11.3.8).

Myocardial Efficiency

Oxidative metabolism provides the heart with ATP needed for myocardial work and other energy-requiring processes. To understand the overall energy metabolism in different disease states, one should relate myocardial metabolism to myocardial work. Myocardial efficiency can be noninvasively indexed with the work metabolic index (WMI), as follows:

$$\text{WMI} = \frac{SVI \times PSP \times HR}{k},$$

where *SVI* is the noninvasively (usually by echocardiography) assessed stroke volume index, *PSP* is peak systolic pressure, *HR* is heart rate, and *k* is the clearance rate constant of [^{11}C]-acetate (30,31,33,34). *PSP* may be replaced by systolic or mean blood pressure. $^{15}O_2$ PET yields an absolute level of myocardial oxygen consumption and therefore efficiency (%) can be calculated as follows:

$$Efficiency(\%) = \frac{SV \times MAP \times HR \times 0.0136}{MMRO_2 \times c}$$

where *MAP* is mean arterial pressure, *SV* is stroke volume, and $MMRO_2$ is metabolic rate of oxygen of whole heart (87,109). The number 0.0136 represents the constant with units g/m/mL/mm Hg, and *c* is a conversion factor representing energy equivalent per milliliter of oxygen metabolized, equaling 2.059 kg/m/mL oxygen consumed.

Hypertension and Efficiency

Hypertension is a common and well-known risk factor for CAD and heart failure. If hypertension is not well controlled, increased

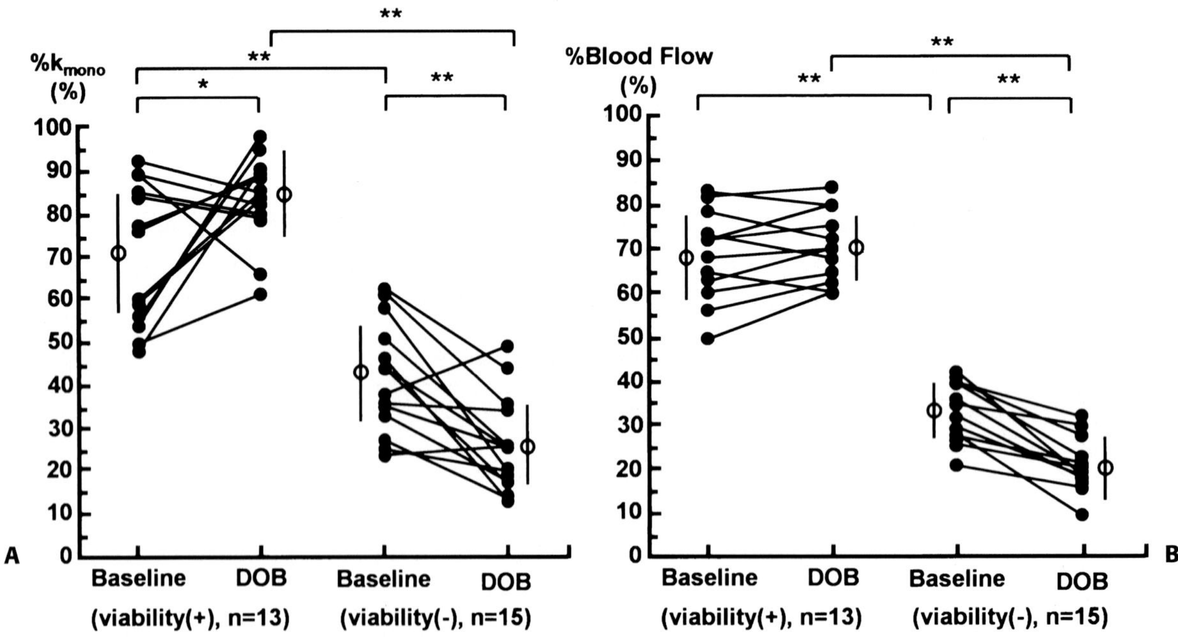

FIGURE 11.3.8. Noninvasive assessment of myocardial viability using carbon-11-acetate in patients with old myocardial infarction. **A:** Changes in normalized oxidative metabolism (%k_{mono}) of the infarct region before and during dobutamine infusion in the two groups. **B:** Changes in normalized blood flow (%blood flow) of the infarct area before and during dobutamine (DOB) infusion in the two groups (*$P < .05$; **$P < .001$). (From Hata T, Nohara R, Fujita M, et al. Noninvasive assessment of myocardial viability by positron emission tomography with ^{11}C acetate in patients with old myocardial infarction. *Circulation* 1996;94:1834–1841, with permission.)

workloads over the years finally result in structural adaptive hypertrophy of the myocardium. The mechanisms that further lead to the development of heart failure are poorly understood. Laine et al. (87) used $^{15}O_2$ PET and echocardiography to study myocardial oxygen consumption and efficiency in nine hypertensive patients with LV hypertrophy and in eight hypertensive patients without hypertrophy and compared the results with the data from ten healthy controls. Myocardial workload, MBF (0.84 ± 0.16 vs. 1.06 ± 0.22 mL/g/min), and oxygen consumption (0.09 ± 0.02 vs. 0.14 ± 0.03 mL/g/min) were increased in patients with hypertension without LV hypertrophy compared with healthy controls. After structural adaptation, LV hypertrophy, workload, MBF, and oxygen consumption were again at the level observed in healthy controls. However, myocardial efficiency was significantly reduced in these patients (13.5% ± 1.9% vs. 18.1% ± 4.1%; $P < .05$). In another study abnormalities in myocardial fatty acid metabolism (as studied with [^{11}C]-palmitate) were apparent in hypertensive LV hypertrophy, and these abnormalities may be responsible, at least in part, for a reduction in myocardial efficiency (110).

In hypertrophic cardiomyopathy, regional myocardial oxidative metabolism and efficiency are also both lower in hypertrophic myocardium compared with nonhypertrophic myocardium (111). These data suggest that structural adaptation in LV hypertrophy is aiming more at preserving the LV oxygen consumption than efficiency. This structural adaptation is known to predict adverse outcome in cardiac patients.

On the other hand, hypertrophy and increased myocardial mass in endurance athletes' hearts are usually considered benign processes. It also appears to be different with regard to the myocardial energetics. Takala et al. (112) studied oxygen consumption in nine endurance athletes and 11 sedentary men with $^{15}O_2$ PET. Athletes had 27% lower $MMRO_2$ than controls (8.8 ± 2.3 vs. 12.0 ± 3.8 mL/min/100 g; $P = .044$). However, myocardial efficiency was comparable between the athletes and sedentary men (16% ± 4% and 14% ± 4%, respectively).

Myocardial Efficiency in Congestive Heart Failure

The level of myocardial oxidative metabolism of the failing LV is often comparable to or even lower than that of the normal LV at rest (31,113). Patients with ischemic heart failure and myocardial scarring due to old MI are expected to have regional heterogeneity in both function and metabolism (114). Heterogeneity of regional function and oxidative metabolism also exists in nonischemic dilated cardiomyopathy (62). Myocardial efficiency, assessed with the WMI, is lower in the failing heart compared with the healthy heart (113,115). Data also indicate that the transplanted human heart is comparable to the healthy heart in terms of myocardial efficiency (116).

Evaluation of Drug Therapy in Heart Failure

In the ideal situation, "mechanism of action" would be the primary basis for decision making in drug development (117). Modern techniques such as gene therapy technology provide numerous new potential mechanisms of action and targets for drug development. Surrogate end points, such as myocardial efficiency, allow the testing of *in vitro* hypotheses in these phase I and II clinical studies before starting large-scale clinical phase III or IV trials. This approach potentially saves both time and research costs (118). The same also applies to devices and other treatment modalities such as cardiac resynchronization therapy or continuous positive airway pressure. In addition, these approaches may allow improved selection of drug therapy for a given patient.

Dobutamine is one of the most commonly used β-adrenergic agonists in the clinical setting. It exerts its inotropic effect mainly through β_1-receptor stimulation. Dobutamine increases contractility in the LV and RV and reduces preload and afterload. It has been used as a reference drug for numerous inotropic agents. On the other hand, sodium nitroprusside can be used as a model agent of vasodilator therapy.

Beanlands et al. (34) noninvasively studied the energetic effects of dobutamine in eight patients with nonischemic cardiomyopathy (mean LV ejection fraction of 22%) and CHF. Myocardial oxidative metabolism was measured with [^{11}C]-acetate PET and myocardial performance by echocardiography during steady-state infusion of dobutamine. The WMI increased by 30%, but this happened at the expense of myocardial oxidative metabolism, because k_2, a clearance rate constant of [^{11}C]-acetate, increased by 48%. Systemic vascular resistance and mitral regurgitation were significantly reduced, which contributed to the observed increase in myocardial efficiency.

The investigators used the same methodology to study the effects of nitroprusside in patients with CHF (119). These patients were characterized by elevated systemic vascular resistance (SVR) and pulmonary capillary wedge pressure (PCWP). As expected, nitroprusside infusion (mean dose of 2.3 ± 1.4 μg/kg/min) resulted in marked reductions in PCWP (48%) and SVR (53%). The k_{mono} of acetate decreased from 0.064 ± 0.012 to 0.055 ± 0.010 min^{-1} (−14%) during nitroprusside infusion. Furthermore, a 61% increase in myocardial efficiency was observed, which highlights the importance of afterload reduction as an energetically favorable treatment modality for CHF. Understanding the energetics with these model drugs provides a framework for understanding the evaluation of new drugs.

Long-term use of β-adrenergic drugs in patients with heart failure has resulted in an increase in mortality. On the other hand, the antagonists of the β-adrenergic system, such as bisoprolol, carvedilol, and metoprolol, have improved the prognosis of patients with heart failure, which further emphasizes the deleterious effect of long-term β-adrenergic activation (120–122). Interestingly metoprolol, a selective β_1-receptor antagonist, has also been shown to improve myocardial energetics after long-term use (33). In this study, patients with LV dysfunction (mean LV ejection fraction of 31% and New York Heart Association [NYHA] functional classification II) were randomized to placebo or metoprolol. In the placebo group (n = 19), there was no change in either k_{mono} (0.061 ± 0.022 vs. 0.054 ± 0.012 min^{-1}; P = n.s.) or efficiency measured as the WMI (5.29 ± 2.46 (10^6 vs. 5.14 ± 2.06 (10^6 mm Hg/mL/m^2; P = n.s.). However, in the metoprolol group (n = 14), a significant decrease in k_{mono} (0.062 ± 0.024 vs. 0.045 ± 0.015 min^{-1}; $P = .002$) and a significant increase in WMI were observed (5.31 ± 2.15 × 10^6 vs. 7.08 ± 2.36 × 10^6 mm Hg/mL/m^2; $P < .001$) (Fig. 11.3.9). Heart rate decreased significantly (from 73 ± 10 to 68 ± 11 beats per minute; $P = .02$) in the metoprolol group, but there were no significant changes in blood pressure or echocardiographic parameters. These improvements in myocardial energetics suggest that β-blockade therapy has an energy-sparing effect in patients with heart failure. This may account for some of the outcome benefits observed in this patient population in other studies.

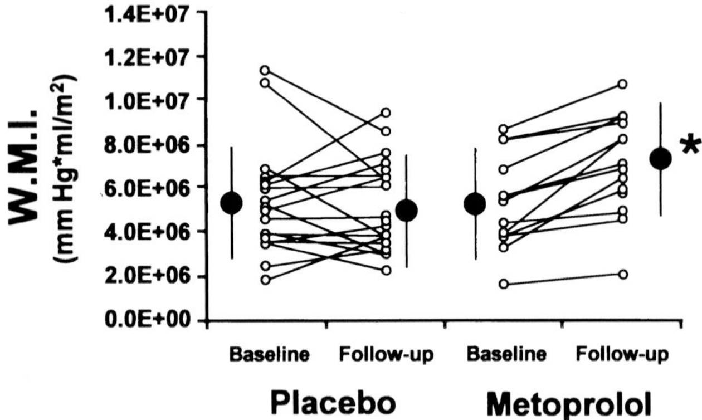

FIGURE 11.3.9. The effect of β_1-blockade on oxygen cost of ventricular work in patients with left ventricular dysfunction. The work metabolic index (W.M.I.) is an estimate of myocardial efficiency in patients receiving placebo (n = 19) or metoprolol (n = 13) (**P* <.02 vs. baseline and placebo). (From Beanlands RSB, Nahmais C, Gordon E, et al. The effects of β_1-blockade on oxidative metabolism and the metabolic cost of ventricular work in patients with left ventricular dysfunction. A double-blind, placebo-controlled, positron emission tomography study. *Circulation* 2000;102:2021–2160, with permission.)

Due to the known problems of the drugs acting via cyclic adenosine monophosphate to increase intracellular calcium (β-agonists and phosphodiesterase inhibitors), other modalities have been tested for the treatment of heart failure. Calcium sensitizers increase myocardial contractility by generating more force for the prevailing level of intracellular calcium, unlike other cardiotonic drugs that simply increase the level of intracellular calcium (123). In theory, this mechanism could result in an energy-saving effect during enhanced contractility.

The myocardial energetics effects of levosimendan, a new calcium-sensitizing drug with vasodilatory properties, were first assessed in healthy volunteers using [^{11}C]-acetate PET and echocardiography (30). The effects of levosimendan on myocardial oxidative metabolism (k_{mono}) and cardiac efficiency were neutral, whereas the hemodynamic profile was consistent with a balanced inotropic effect and vasodilation. Low-dose dobutamine enhanced cardiac efficiency at the expense of an increased oxygen requirement, but the effects of nitroprusside on k_{mono} and cardiac efficiency were neutral. The study also showed the feasibility of PET in phase I pharmacodynamic studies.

In a phase II study, the effects of levosimendan on biventricular energetics were studied in eight hospitalized patients with decompensated (NYHA class III and IV) chronic heart failure (31). In this double-blind crossover comparison (levosimendan vs. placebo), PET with [^{11}C]-acetate was used to assess myocardial oxygen consumption, $H_2{}^{15}O$ to measure MBF, and cardiac performance was assessed by pulmonary artery catheterization. During administration of levosimendan, cardiac output increased by 32% ($P = .002$), mainly because of higher stroke volume. Coronary resistance, pulmonary resistance, and SVR values were significantly reduced. Mean MBF increased from 0.76 to 1.02 mL/min/g ($P = .033$). Levosimendan did not affect myocardial oxygen consumption (LV k_{mono} 0.066 ± 0.003 vs. 0.061 ± 0.004 min^{-1}; $P = .15$ and RV k_{mono} 0.053 ± 0.004 vs. 0.055 ± 0.005 min^{-1}; P = n.s.) and LV efficiency, but it improved RV mechanical efficiency by 24% ($P = .012$) (Fig. 11.3.10). This study suggests that

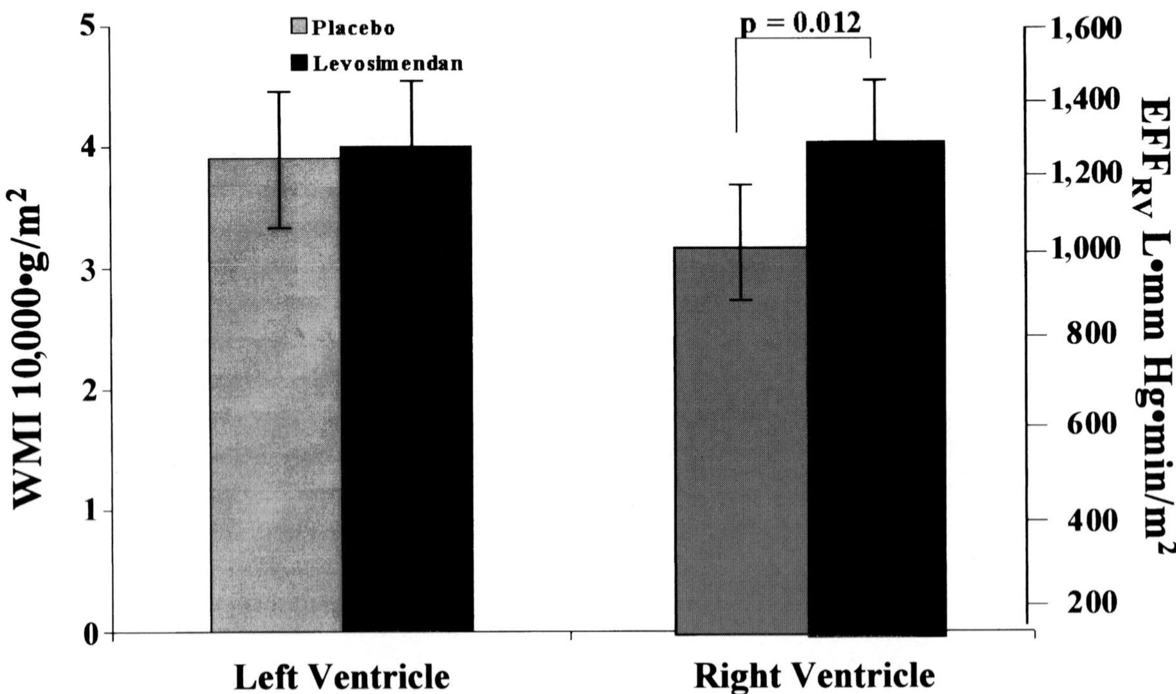

FIGURE 11.3.10. Efficiency (mean ± SEM) of the left and right ventricle during placebo and levosimendan. Levosimendan, a novel calcium sensitizer, had no effect on myocardial efficiency in the left ventricle, but improved right ventricular efficiency by 24% (*P* = .012). WMI, work metabolic index. (From Ukkonen H, Saraste M, Akkila J, et al. Myocardial efficiency during levosimendan infusion in congestive heart failure. *Clin Pharmacol Ther* 2000;68:522–531, with permission.)

levosimendan has an energetically favorable short-term profile in the treatment of CHF because it enhances cardiac output without oxygen wasting, particularly by improving efficiency in the RV.

Metabolic modulators that enhance myocardial glucose metabolism by inhibiting FFA metabolism may improve cardiac function in patients with heart failure. Tuunanen et al. (124) studied the effect of acute FFA withdrawal on cardiac function and energetics in patients with heart failure caused by idiopathic dilated cardiomyopathy. Patients and healthy controls underwent examination of myocardial perfusion ([^{15}O]-water) and oxidative ([^{11}C]-acetate) and FFA ([^{11}C]-palmitate) metabolism, before and after acute reduction of serum FFA concentrations by acipimox, an inhibitor of lipolysis. LV function and myocardial work were echocardiographically measured, and efficiency of forward work (WMI) was calculated. Acipimox decreased myocardial FFA uptake by more than 80% in both groups. Myocardial perfusion remained unchanged, whereas cardiac work decreased similarly in both patients and healthy controls. In the healthy controls, reduced cardiac work was accompanied by decreased oxidative metabolism (k_{mono} from 0.071 ± 0.019 to 0.055 ± 0.016 min^{-1}; $P < .01$). In patients with idiopathic dilated cardiomyopathy, cardiac work fell, whereas oxidative metabolism remained unchanged and efficiency fell (WMI from 35.4 ± 12.6 to 31.6 ± 13.3 mm Hg/L/g^{-1}; $P < .05$).

These data demonstrate that failing hearts are unexpectedly more dependent than healthy hearts on FFA availability. The authors suggest that both glucose and fatty acid oxidation are required for optimal function of the failing heart.

Evaluation of Mechanical Therapies in Heart Failure

Cardiac Resynchronization

In advanced heart failure, myocardial depolarization is often prolonged and contraction dysynchronized. Cardiac resynchronization therapy (CRT) acts by recoordinating ventricular activation using atriobiventricular pacing. This results in increased left ventricular contractility.

The short-term effect of CRT on myocardial oxidative metabolism and efficiency was studied in eight patients with NYHA class III and IV congestive heart failure and left bundle-branch block (LBBB) (125). Patients were studied during atrial pacing (control) and atriobiventricular stimulation at the same rate. Carbon-11-acetate PET was used to assess myocardial oxidative metabolism in the LV and RV. Myocardial efficiency was measured using WMI. The stroke volume index improved by 10% ($P < .011$) with CRT, although both global LV and RV k_{mono} were unchanged compared with control. Septal k_{mono} increased by 15% ($P < .04$), and the septal:lateral wall k_{mono} ratio increased by 22% ($P < .01$) as a result of successful resynchronization. WMI increased by 13% ($P < .024$) with CRT.

The long-term effect of CRT was studied by Lindner et al. (126) using [^{11}C]-acetate PET. They studied 16 patients who had severe heart failure and LBBB, and the patients were evaluated at 4 and 13 months after starting CRT. Thirteen patients with mild heart failure without LBBB served as a comparison group. The clearance rate (k_2) of [^{11}C]-acetate was measured with PET to assess myocardial oxidative metabolism. Stroke volume was derived from the dynamic PET data according to the Stewart-Hamilton principle. WMI was used to assess myocardial efficiency in the LV. After 4 months of CRT, stroke volume index (SVI) increased by 50% (p = .012) and WMI increased by 41% ($P < .001$). Global k_2 remained unchanged but regional k_2 demonstrated a more homogeneous distribution pattern. The parameters showed no significant changes during therapy up to 13 months. Under CRT, cardiac efficiency, SVI, and the distribution pattern of regional k_2 did not differ from patients with mild heart failure without LBBB.

The effect of CRT on right ventricular oxidative metabolism has also studied (see below).

Continuous Positive Airway Pressure

Yoshinaga et al. (127) studied both the short-term and longer-term (6 weeks) effects of continuous positive airway pressure treatment (CPAP) on myocardial energetics in 12 patients with obstructive sleep apnea (OSA). Seven patients with OSA were treated with CPAP, and five patients without OSA served as a control group. Oxidative metabolism was measured using the monoexponential fit of the myocardial [^{11}C]-acetate PET time-activity curve (k_{mono}) and LV function using echocardiography. Myocardial efficiency was derived using WMI, measured at baseline; during short-term CPAP and after 6 ± 3 weeks of CPAP (Fig. 11.3.11). Short-term CPAP tended to reduce SVI and reduced oxidative metabolism. The WMI did not change indicating no change in efficiency. However, longer-term CPAP improved LV ejection fraction (38.4% ± 3.3% to 43.4% ± 4.8%; $P = .031$), tended to reduce oxidative metabolism (0.047 ± 0.012 to 0.040 ± 0.008 min^{-1}; $P = .078$), and improved WMI (7.13 ± 2.82 ± 106 to 8.17 ± 3.06 × 10^6 mm Hg/mL/m^2; $P = .031$). In the control group these parameters did not change. The authors concluded that an energy-sparing effect of longer term CPAP may contribute to the benefits of CPAP therapy. The reduction of transmural pressure, combined with CPAP's effects of eliminating hypoxia and reducing sympathetic nervous activity, likely contribute to a reduction in myocardial energy demand and oxygen consumption. Since heart failure is known to be an energy-depleted state, CPAP could permit repletion of energy stores and more efficient energy transduction to useful work, which is constantly demanded of the failing heart. Bradley and Floras (128) have proposed that the favorable effects of CPAP on the sympathetic nervous system and LV function are similar to β-blockers.

Right Ventricular Oxygen Consumption

The monoexponential elimination rate of [^{11}C]-acetate (k_{mono}) correlates with indirect estimates of myocardial oxygen consumption in the RV (34), which offers an intriguing opportunity to quantitate myocardial oxidative metabolism simultaneously in the LV and RV. This approach has been used in healthy volunteers (61), patients with aortic valve disease (129), and those with CHF (31,130). There are no other practical methods to study RV metabolism *in vivo*.

RV performance is known to have prognostic value in patients with CHF. The RV can also play a significant role in determining patients exercise tolerance. Knuuti et al. (130) studied ten patients with idiopathic dilated cardiomyopathy who had undergone implantation of a biventricular pacemaker. RV and LV oxidative metabolism were measured using [^{11}C]-acetate PET and LV stroke volume by echocardiography. Measurements were done at rest and during low-dose dobutamine (5 μg/kg/min) infusion with CRT on and with CRT off.

CRT had no effect on RV k_{mono} at rest. Dobutamine-induced stress increased RV k_{mono} significantly under both conditions, but oxidative metabolism was more enhanced when CRT was on (0.076 ± 0.026 vs. 0.065 ± 0.027; $P = .003$). In five patients the response to CRT

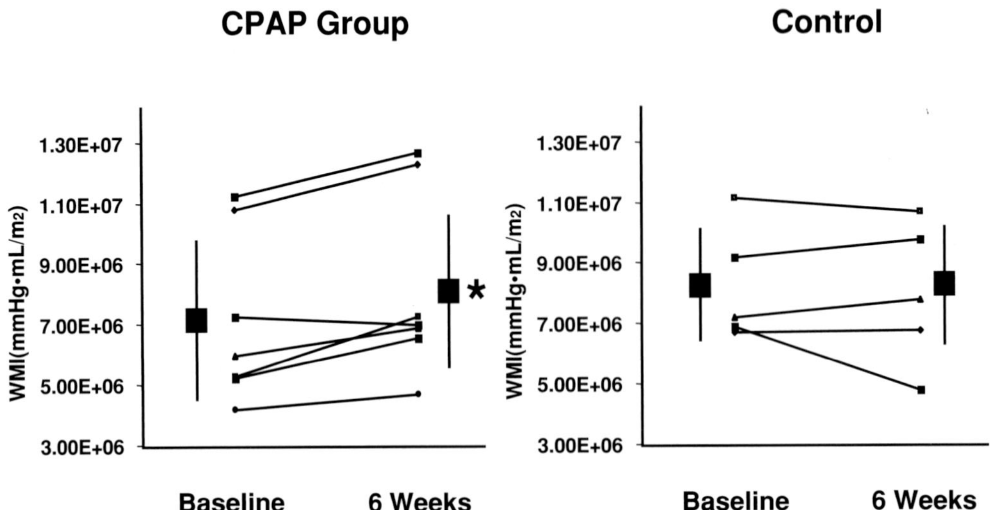

FIGURE 11.3.11. The effect of 6 weeks of continuous positive airway pressure treatment (CPAP) on the work metabolic index (WMI) in patients with heart failure and obstructive sleep apnea (*P = .031 vs. controls). (From Yoshinaga K, Burwash IG, Leech JA, et al. The effects of continuous positive airway pressure on myocardial energetics in patients with heart failure and obstructive sleep apnea. *J Am Coll Cardiol* 2007;49:450–458, with permission.)

was striking (32% increase in mean LV stroke volume, range 18% to 36%), while in the other five patients no response was observed (mean change +2%, range −6% to +4%). RV k_{mono} and LV stroke volume response to CRT correlated inversely ($r = -0.66$; $P = .034$). None of the other measured parameters, including all LV parameters and electromechanical parameters, were associated with the response to CRT. In responders, RV k_{mono} with CRT off was significantly lower than in nonresponders (0.036 ± 0.01 vs. 0.058 ± 0.02; $P = .047$).

In this study CRT appeared to enhance RV oxidative metabolism and metabolic reserve during stress. Also, lower RV oxidative metabolism at rest was associated with greater response to CRT. Measurement of RV metabolism could therefore help to identify patients who would benefit the most from CRT.

Measurement of RV oxidative metabolism is clinically feasible with [^{11}C]-acetate PET. However, the validation of the method is limited and requires further study. Lack of reference methods *in vivo* makes this very difficult.

Measurement of Myocardial Oxidative Metabolism in Other Diseases

Carbon-11-acetate PET has been used to understand the mechanisms of disease in other cardiac conditions. In hypertrophic cardiomyopathy, impairment in regional efficiency has been identified. Ishiwata et al. (111) demonstrated that the septum had reduced oxidative metabolism compared with the lateral wall. There was an increase in the k_{mono}/regional work (effectively the inverse of regional efficiency) for the whole heart in patients with hypertrophic cardiomyopathy. This was greater in the septum. Thus, impaired regional metabolism and reduced regional and overall LV efficiency may play a role in the pathophysiology of hypertrophic cardiomyopathy.

Nony et al. (132) used [^{11}C]-acetate PET and echocardiography to evaluate anthracycline cardiotoxicity. Although the investigators detected a small but significant decrease in LV systolic function, myocardial oxidative metabolism was preserved. They concluded that myocardial oxidative metabolism does not contribute to the mechanism of disease in anthracycline cardiotoxicity.

Carbon-11-acetate PET has also been used to study myocardial involvement in endocrine disorders. Investigators have demonstrated regional heterogeneity in myocardial oxidative metabolism in patients with noninsulin-dependent diabetes mellitus (133). In another study, excessive myocardial oxidative metabolism was observed in hyperthyroid patients despite β-blocker therapy with propranolol (66).

SUMMARY

To date, according to the American College of Cardiology/American Heart Association guidelines, the use of PET in clinical cardiology has primarily focused on myocardial perfusion and viability imaging. Although [^{11}C]-acetate PET can be applied for both flow and viability imaging, its greatest potential probably lies in the evaluation of oxidative metabolism and cardiac efficiency. Both $^{15}O_2$ and [^{11}C]-acetate PET have been demonstrated to be feasible in assessing global and regional myocardial oxygen consumption in healthy volunteers and patients with heart disease of various etiologies. This technique offers a unique opportunity to evaluate the myocardial energetic effects of new and established treatments to better direct therapies in cardiac conditions such as CHF.

ACKNOWLEDGMENTS

The authors are grateful to Linda Garrard, May Aung, and Sherri Nipius for their help in preparing the manuscript and figures.

REFERENCES

1. Kojima S, Wu ST, Parmley W, et al. Relationship between intracellular calcium and oxygen consumption: effects of perfusion pressure,

extracellular calcium, dobutamine and nifedipine. *Am Heart J* 1994; 127:386–391.

2. Braunwald E. Control of myocardial oxygen consumption: physiologic and clinical considerations. *Am J Cardiol* 1971;27:416.
3. Opie LH. Aerobic and anaerobic metabolism. In: Opie LH, ed. *The heart: physiology from cell to circulation*. Philadelphia: Lippincott-Raven Publishers, 1998:295–342.
4. Burkoff D. Introduction—the hierarchy of cardiac function. *Basic Res Cardiol* 1993;88:3–5.
5. Takaki M, Kohzuki H, Kawatani Y, et al. Sarcoplasmic reticulum Ca2+ pump blockade decreases O_2 use of unloaded contracting rat heart slices: thapsigardin and cyclopiazonic acid. *J Mol Cell Cardiol* 1998;30:649–659.
6. Ohgoshi Y, Goto Y, Kawaguchi O, et al. Epinephrine and calcium have similar oxygen costs of contractility. *Heart Vessels* 1992;7:123–132.
7. Neely J, Morgan H. Relationship between carbohydrate and lipid metabolism and energy balance of the heart. *Rev Physiol* 1974;36: 413–459.
8. Wisneski JA, Gertz E, Neese RA, et al. Myocardial metabolism of free fatty acids: studies with ^{14}C labeled substrates in humans. *J Clin Invest* 1987;79:359–366.
9. Schelbert HR, Henze E, Sochor H, et al. Effects of substrate availability on myocardial carbon 11 palmitate kinetics by positron emission tomography in normal subjects and patients with ventricular dysfunction. *Am Heart J* 1986;111:1055–1064.
10. Neely J, Hansen CA, Lopaschuk GD, et al. Substrate utilization in the normal and diseased heart. In: Schelbert HR, Neely J, Phelps ME, et al., eds. *Advances in clinical cardiology: regional myocardial metabolism by positron emission tomography*, vol 3. Mahwah, NJ: Foundation for Advances in Clinical Medicine, 1987:20–31.
11. Knuuti J, Maki M, Yki Jarvinen H, et al. The effect of insulin and FFA on myocardial glucose uptake. *J Mol Cell Cardiol* 1995;27:1359–1367.
12. Heiss HW, Barmeyer SR, Wink K, et al. Studies on the regulation of myocardial blood flow in man. Training effects on blood flow and metabolism of the healthy heart at rest and during standardized heavy exercise. *Basic Res Cardiol* 1976;71:658–675.
13. Depre C, Vanoverschelde J LJ, Taegtmeyer H. Glucose for the heart. *Circulation* 1999:578–588.
14. Lopaschuk GD, Stanley W. Glucose metabolism in the ischemic heart. *Circulation* 1997;95:415–422.
15. Shinke T, Takaoka H, Takeuchi K, et al. Nitric oxide spares myocardial oxygen consumption through attenuation of contractile response to beta adrenergic stimulation in patients with idiopathic dilated cardiomyopathy. *Circulation* 2000;101:1925–1930.
16. Mital S, Loke KE, Chen JM, et al. Mitochondrial respiratory abnormalities in patients with end-stage congenital heart disease. *J Heart Lung Transplant* 2004;23:72–79.
17. Opie LH, Owen P. Assessment of mitochondrial free NAD+/NADH ratios and oxaloacetate concentrations during increased mechanical work in isolated perfused rat heart during production or uptake of ketone bodies. *Biochem J* 1975;148:403–415.
18. Heineman FW, Balaban RS. Effects of afterload and heart rate on NAD(P)H redox state in isolated rabbit heart. *Am J Physiol* 1993;264: H433–H440.
19. Katz AM. Cardiomyopathy of overload. A major determinant of prognosis in congestive heart failure. *N Engl J Med* 1990;322:100–110.
20. Schipke JD. Cardiac efficiency. *Basic Res Cardiol* 1994;89:207–240.
21. Starling EH, Vissher MB. The regulation of energy output of the heart. *J Physiol (London)* 1926;62:243.
22. Denslow S. Relationship between PVA and myocardial oxygen consumption can be derived from thermodynamics. *Am J Physiol* 1996; 270:H730–H740.
23. Backx P. Efficiency of cardiac muscle: thermodynamic and statistical mechanical considerations. *Basic Res Cardiol* 1993;88:21–27.
24. Fourier PR, Coetzee AR, Bolliger CT. Pulmonary artery compliance: its role in right ventricular arterial coupling. *Cardiovasc Res* 1992;26: 839–844.
25. Suga H. Total mechanical energy of a ventricle model and cardiac oxygen consumption. *Am J Physiol* 1979;236:H498–H505.
26. Robinson BF. Relation of heart rate and systolic blood pressure to the onset of pain in angina pectoris. *Circulation* 1967;34:1073–1083.
27. Nelson RR, Gobel F, Jorgensen CR, et al. Hemodynamic predictors of myocardial oxygen consumption during static and dynamic exercise. *Circulation* 1974;50:1179–1189.
28. Rooke GA, Feigl EO. Work as a correlate of canine left ventricular oxygen consumption and the problem of catecholamine oxygen wasting. *Circ Res* 1982;50:273–286.
29. Opie LH. Mechanisms of cardiac contraction and relaxation. In: Braunwald E, ed. *Heart disease*. Philadelphia: WB Saunders, 1997: 360–393.
30. Ukkonen H, Saraste M, Akkila J, et al. Myocardial efficiency during calcium sensitization with levosimendan: a noninvasive study with positron emission tomography and echocardiography in healthy volunteers. *Clin Pharmacol Ther* 1997;61:596–607.
31. Ukkonen H, Saraste M, Akkila J, et al. Myocardial efficiency during levosimendan infusion in congestive heart failure. *Clin Pharmacol Ther* 2000;68:522–531.
32. Beanlands RSB, Muzik O, Hutchins GD, et al. Heterogeneity of regional nitrogen 13-labeled ammonia tracer distribution in the normal human heart: comparison with rubidium 82 and copper 62-labeled PTSM. *J Nucl Cardiol* 1994;1:225–235.
33. Beanlands RSB, Nahmais C, Gordon E, et al. The effects of β_1 blockade on oxidative metabolism and the metabolic cost of ventricular work in patients with left ventricular dysfunction. A double blind, placebo controlled, positron emission tomography study. *Circulation* 2000;102:2021–2160.
34. Beanlands R, Bach D, Raylman R, et al. Acute effects of dobutamine on myocardial oxygen consumption and cardiac efficiency measured using C^{11} acetate kinetics in patients with dilated cardiomyopathy. *J Am Coll Cardiol* 1993;22:1389–1398.
35. Lopaschuk GD. Advantages and limitations of experimental techniques used to measure cardiac energy metabolism. *J Nucl Cardiol* 1997;4:316–328.
36. Ganz W, Tamura K, Marcus HS, et al. Measurement of coronary sinus blood flow by continuous thermodilution in man. *Circulation* 1971;44:181–195.
37. Weiss RG, Gloth ST, Kalik Filho R, et al. Indexing tricarboxylic acid cycle flux intact hearts by carbon 13 nuclear magnetic resonance. *Circ Res* 1992;70:392–408.
38. Koskenvuo JW, Sakuma H, Niemi P, et al. Global Myocardial blood flow and global reserve measurements by MRI and PET are comparable. *J Magn Reson Imaging* 2001;13:361–366.
39. Pärkka JP, Niemi P, Saraste A, et al. Comparison of MRI and positron emission tomography for measuring myocardial perfusion reserve in healthy humans. *Magn Reson Med* 2006;55:772–779.
40. Lee DC, Simonetti OP, Harris KR, et al. Magnetic resonance versus radionuclide pharmacological stress perfusion imaging for flow-limiting stenoses of varying severity. *Circulation* 2004;110:58–65.
41. Reeder SB, Holmes A, McVeigh ER, et al. Simultaneous noninvasive determination of regional myocardial perfusion and oxygen content in rabbits: toward direct measurement of myocardial oxygen consumption at MR imaging. *Radiology* 1999;212:739–747.
42. Gambhir SS, Schwaiger M, Huang S C, et al. Simple noninvasive quantification method for measuring myocardial glucose utilization in humans employing positron emission tomography and fluorine 18 deoxyglucose. *J Nucl Med* 1989;30:359–366.
43. Taegtmeyer H. Energy metabolism of the heart: from basic concepts to clinical applications. *Curr Probl Cardiol* 1994;19:59–113.
44. Maki M, Haaparanta M, Nuutila P, et al. Free fatty acid uptake in the myocardium and skeletal muscle using fluorine 18 fluoro-6-heptadecanoic acid. *J Nucl Med* 1998;39:1320–1327.
45. Schelbert HR, Henze E, Schon HR, et al. Carbon 11 palmitate for the noninvasive evaluation of regional myocardial fatty acid metabolism with positron computed tomography. *In vivo* demonstration of the

effects of substrate availability on myocardial metabolism. *Am Heart J* 1983;105:492–504.
46. Schelbert HR, Phelps ME, Schon HR. Normal alterations in substrate metabolism demonstrated by positron emission tomography. In: Schelbert HR, Neely J, Phelps ME, et al, eds. *Advances in clinical cardiology: regional myocardial metabolism by positron emission tomography*, vol 3. Mahwah, NJ: Foundation for Advances in Clinical Medicine, 1987:205–213.
47. Rosamond TL, Abendschein DR, Sobel BE, et al. Metabolic fate of radiolabeled palmitate in ischemic canine myocardium: implications for positron emission tomography. *J Nucl Med* 1987;28:1322–1329.
48. Fox K, Abendschein DR, Amdos HD, et al. Efflux of metabolized and nonmetabolized fatty acid from canine myocardium. Implications for quantifying myocardial metabolism tomographically. *Circ Res* 1985; 57:232–243.
49. Ebert A, Herzog H, Stocklin G, et al. Kinetics of 14(R,S) fluorine 18 fluoro 6-thia-heptadecanoic acid in normal human hearts at rest, during exercise and after dipyridamole injection. *J Nucl Med* 1994;35:51–56.
50. Liedtke AJ. Alterations of carbohydrate and lipid metabolism in the acutely ischemic heart. *Prog Cardiovasc Dis* 1981;23:321–336.
51. Chan S, Brunken RC, Phelps M, et al. Use of the metabolic tracer carbon 11 acetate for evaluation of regional myocardial perfusion. *J Nucl Med* 1991;32:665–672.
52. Brown M, Marshall DR, Sobel BE, et al. Delineation of myocardial oxygen utilization with carbon 11-labeled acetate. *Circulation* 1987;3: 687–696.
53. Armbrecht JJ, Buxton D, Schelbert H. Validation of [1-^{11}C] acetate as a tracer for noninvasive assessment of oxidative metabolism with positron emission tomography in normal, ischemic, postischemic, and hyperemic canine myocardium. *Circulation* 1990;81: 1594–1605.
54. Lindeneg O, Mellemgaard K, Fabricius J, et al. Myocardial utilization of acetate, lactate and free fatty acids after ingestion of ethanol. *Clin Sci* 1964;27:427–435.
55. Klein LJ, Visser FC, Knaapen P, et al. Carbon 11 acetate as a tracer of myocardial oxygen consumption. *Eur J Nucl Med* 2001;28:651–668.
56. Buxton D, Schwaiger M, Nguyen A, et al. Radiolabeled acetate as a tracer of myocardial tricarboxylic acid cycle flux. *Circ Res* 1988;63: 628–634.
57. Pike V, Eakins M, Allan R, et al. Preparation of [1-^{11}C] acetate—an agent for the study of myocardial metabolism by positron emission tomography. *Int J Appl Radiat Isot* 1982;33:505–512.
58. Hata T, Nohara R, Fujita M, et al. Noninvasive assessment of myocardial viability by positron emission tomography with ^{11}C acetate in patients with old myocardial infarction. *Circulation* 1996;94:1834–1841.
59. Wolpers HG, Burshert W, van den Hoff J, et al. Assessment of myocardial viability by use of ^{11}C acetate and positron emission tomography. Threshold criteria of reversible dysfunction. *Circulation* 1997;95: 1417–1424.
60. Hicks RJ, Kalff V, Savas V, et al. Assessment of right ventricular oxidative metabolism by positron emission tomography with C11 acetate in aortic valve disease. *Am J Cardiol* 1991;67:753–757.
61. Tamaki N, Magata Y, Takahashi N, et al. Oxidative metabolism in the myocardium in the normal subjects during dobutamine infusion. *Eur J Nucl Med* 1993;20:231–237.
62. Bach D, Beanlands R, Schwaiger M, et al. Regional wall motion heterogeneity and myocardial oxidative metabolism in nonischemic dilated cardiomyopathy. *J Am Coll Cardiol* 1995;1256–1262.
63. Marshall RC, Tillisch JH, Phelps ME, et al. Identification and differentiation of resting myocardial ischemia and infarction in man with positron computed tomography, ^{18}F labeled fluorodeoxyglucose and N13 ammonia. *Circulation* 1983;67:766–778.
64. Knuuti MJ, Nuutila P, Ruotsalainen U, et al. Euglycemic hyperinsulinemic clamp and oral glucose load in stimulating myocardial glucose utilization during positron emission tomography. *J Nucl Med* 1992;33: 1255–1262.
65. Czernin J, Porenta G, Brunken RC, et al. Regional blood flow oxidative metabolism and glucose utilization in patients with recent myocardial infarction. *Circulation* 1993;88:884–895.
66. Torizuka T, Tamaki N, Kasagi K, et al. Myocardial oxidative metabolism in hyperthyroid patients assessed by PET with carbon 11 acetate. *J Nucl Med* 1995;36:1981–1986.
67. Ohte N, Hashimoto T, Iida H, et al. Extent of myocardial damage in regions with reverse redistribution at 3h and at 24h on 201Tl SPECT: evaluation based on regional myocardial oxidative metabolism. *Nucl Med Commun* 1998;19:1081–1087.
68. Bach DS, Beanlands RSB, Schwaiger M, et al. Heterogeneity of ventricular function and myocardial oxidative metabolism in nonischemic dilated cardiomyopathy. *J Am Coll Cardiol* 1995;25:1258–1262.
69. Armbrecht JJ, Buxton DB, Brunken R, et al. Regional myocardial oxygen consumption determined noninvasively in humans with [1^{-11}C] acetate and dynamic positron emission tomography. *Circulation* 1989;80:863–872.
70. Henes CG, Bergmann SR, Walsh MN, et al. Assessment of myocardial oxidative metabolic reserve with positron emission tomography and carbon 11 acetate. *J Nucl Med* 1989;30:1798–1808.
71. Buck A, Wolpers G, Hutchins GD, et al. Effect of carbon 11 acetate recirculation on estimates of myocardial oxygen consumption by PET. *J Nucl Med* 1991;32:1950–1957.
72. Maes A, Van de Werf F, Mesotten LV, et al. Early assessment of regional myocardial blood flow and metabolism in thrombolysis in myocardial infarction flow grade 3 reperfused myocardial infarction using carbon 11 acetate. *J Am Coll Cardiol* 2001;37:30–36.
73. Raylman RR, Hutchins GD, Beanlands R, et al. Modeling of C 11 acetate kinetics by simultaneously fitting data from multiple ROI's coupled by common parameters. *J Nucl Med* 1994;35:1286–1291.
74. Sun KT, Chen K, Huang S C, et al. Compartment model for measuring myocardial oxygen consumption using [1-^{11}C] acetate. *J Nucl Med* 1997;38:459–466.
75. Ng C K, Huang S C, Schelbert HR, et al. Validation of a model for [1-^{11}C] acetate as a tracer of cardiac oxidative metabolism. *Am Physiol Soc* 1994:H1304–H1315.
76. Brown MA, Myears DW, Bergmann SR. Validity of estimates of myocardial oxidative metabolism with carbon 11 acetate and positron emission tomography despite altered patterns of substrate utilization. *J Nucl Med* 1989;30:187–193.
77. Gropler R, Shelton ME, Herrero P, et al. Measurement of myocardial oxygen consumption using positron emission tomography and C11 acetate: direct validation in human subjects. *Circulation* 1993;88: I172(abst).
78. Sun KT, Yeatman L, Buxton D, et al. Simultaneous measurement of myocardial oxygen consumption and blood flow using [1 carbon 11] acetate. *J Nucl Med* 1998;39:272–280.
79. Beanlands RSB, Schwaiger M. Changes in myocardial oxygen consumption and efficiency with heart failure therapy measured by ^{11}C acetate PET. *Can J Cardiol* 1995;11:293–300.
80. Schulz R, Kappeler C, Coenen H, et al. Positron emission tomography analysis of [1 ^{11}C] acetate kinetics in short term hibernating myocardium. *Circulation* 1998;97:1009–1016.
81. Ukkonen H, Knuuti J, Katoh C, et al. Use of [^{11}C]acetate and [^{15}O]O_2 PET for the assessment of myocardial oxygen utilization in patients with chronic myocardial infarction. *Eur J Nucl Med* 2001;28:334–339.
82. Parker JA, Beller G, Hoop B, et al. Assessment of regional myocardial blood flow and regional fractional oxygen extraction in dogs, using ^{15}O water and ^{15}O hemoglobin. *Circulation* 1978;42:511–518.
83. Iida H, Rhodes CG, Araujo LI, et al. Noninvasive quantification of regional myocardial metabolic rate of oxygen by use of $^{15}O_2$ inhalation and positron emission tomography. Theory, analysis and application in humans. *Circulation* 1996;94:792–807.
84. Iida H, Takahashi A, Tamura Y, et al. Myocardial blood flow: comparison of oxygen 15 water bolus injection, slow infusion and oxygen 15 carbon dioxide slow inhalation. *J Nucl Med* 1995;36:78–85.

85. Araujo LI, Lammerstma AA, Rhodes CG, et al. Noninvasive quantification of regional myocardial blood flow in normal volunteers and patients with coronary artery disease using oxygen 15 labeled water and positron emission tomography. *Circulation* 1991;83:875–885.
86. Agostini D, Iida H, Takahashi A, et al. Regional myocardial metabolic rate of oxygen measured by $[^{15}O]O_2$ inhalation and positron emission tomography in patients with cardiomyopathy. *Clin Nucl Med* 2001;26: 41–49.
87. Laine H, Katoh C, Luotolahti M, et al. Myocardial oxygen consumption is unchanged but efficiency is reduced in patients with essential hypertension and left ventricular hypertrophy. *Circulation* 1999;100: 2425–2430.
88. Yamamoto Y, de Silva R, Rhodes CG, et al. Noninvasive quantification of regional myocardial metabolic rate of oxygen by $^{15}O_2$ inhalation and positron emission tomography: experimental validation. *Circulation* 1996;94:808–816.
89. Bol A, Melin JA, Bahija E, et al. Assessment of myocardial oxygen reserve with PET: comparison with Fick oxygen consumption. *Circulation* 1991;84:II425(abst).
90. Yamamoto Y, de Silva R, Rhodes CG, et al. Validation of quantification of myocardial oxygen consumption and oxygen extraction fraction using $^{15}O_2$ and positron emission tomography. *Circulation* 1991;84: II47(abst).
91. Alenius S, Ruotsalainen U. Bayesian image reconstruction for emission tomography based on median root prior. *Eur J Nucl Med* 1997; 24:258–265.
92. Katoh C, Ruotsalainen U, Alenius S, et al. Iterative reconstruction based on median root prior in quantification of myocardial blood flow and oxygen metabolism. *J Nucl Med* 1999;40:862–867.
93. Pitkanen OP, Raitakari OT, Ronnemaa T, et al. Influence of cardiovascular risk status on coronary flow reserve in healthy young men. *Am J Cardiol* 1997;79:1690–1692.
94. Uren NG, Melin JA, De Bruyne B, et al. Relation between myocardial blood flow and the severity of coronary artery stenosis. *N Engl J Med* 1994;330:1782–1788.
95. Janier MF, Andre Fouet X, Landais P, et al. Perfusion MVO_2 mismatch during inotropic stress in CAD patients with normal contractile function. *Am J Physiol Heart Circ Physiol* 1996;271:H59–H67.
96. Gerber B, Wijns W, Vanoverschelde J LJ, et al. Myocardial perfusion and oxygen consumption in reperfused noninfarcted dysfunctional myocardium after unstable angina: direct evidence for myocardial stunning in humans. *J Am Coll Cardiol* 1999;34:1939–1946.
97. deSilva R, Yamamoto Y, Rhodes CG, et al. Preoperative prediction of the outcome of coronary revascularization using positron emission tomography. *Circulation* 1992;86:1738–1742.
98. Vanoverschelde J LJ, Melin JA, Bol A, et al. Regional oxidative metabolism in patients after recovery from reperfused anterior infarction. Relation to regional blood flow and glucose uptake. *Circulation* 1992;85:9–21.
99. Gropler RJ, Geltman EM, Sampathkumaran K, et al. Functional recovery after coronary revascularization for chronic coronary artery disease is dependent on maintenance of oxidative metabolism. *J Am Coll Cardiol* 1992;20:569–577.
100. Gropler RJ, Geltman EM, Sampathkumaran K, et al. Comparison of carbon 11 acetate with fluorine 18 fluorodeoxyglucose for delineating viable myocardium by positron emission tomography. *J Am Coll Cardiol* 1993;22:1597.
101. Bax JJ, Poldermans D, Elhendy A, et al. Sensitivity, specificity, and predictive accuracies of various noninvasive techniques for detecting hibernating myocardium. *Curr Probl Cardiol* 2001;26:141–186.
102. Cigarroa CG, deFilippi CR, Brickner ME, et al. Dobutamine stress echocardiography identifies hibernating myocardium and predicts recovery of left ventricular function after coronary revascularization. *Circulation* 1993;88:430–436.
103. LaCanna G, Alfieri O, Giubbini R, et al. Echocardiography during infusion of dobutamine for identification of reversible dysfunction in patients with chronic coronary artery disease. *J Am Coll Cardiol* 1994;23:617–626.
104. Afridi I, Klieman NS, Raizner AE, et al. Dobutamine echocardiography in myocardial hibernation: optimal dose and accuracy in predicting recovery of ventricular function after coronary angioplasty. *Circulation* 1995;91:663–670.
105. Panza JA, Dilsizian V, Laurienzo JM, et al. Relation between thallium uptake and contractile response to dobutamine: implications regarding myocardial viability in patients with chronic coronary artery disease and left ventricular dysfunction. *Circulation* 1995: 990–998.
106. Perrone Filardi P, Pace L, Prastaro M, et al. Assessment of myocardial viability in patients with chronic coronary artery disease: rest 4 hour 24 hour ^{201}Tl tomography versus dobutamine echocardiography. *Circulation* 1996;94:2712–2719.
107. Lee H, Davila Roman VG, Ludbrook P, et al. Dependency of contractile reserve on myocardial blood flow. Implications for the assessment of myocardial viability with dobutamine stress echocardiography. *Circulation* 1997;96:2884–2891.
108. Yoshinaga K, Katoh C, Beanlands R, et al. Reduced oxidative metabolic response in dysfunctional myocardium with preserved glucose metabolism but impaired contractile reserve. *J Nucl Med* 2004;45: 1885–1891.
109. Bing R, Hammond M, Handelsman J, et al. The measurement of coronary blood flow, oxygen consumption, and efficiency of the left ventricle in man. *Am Heart J* 1949;38:1–24.
110. de las Fuentes L, Soto PF, Cupps BP, et al. Hypertensive left ventricular hypertrophy is associated with abnormal myocardial fatty acid metabolism and myocardial efficiency. *J Nucl Cardiol* 2006;13:369–377.
111. Ishiwata S, Maruno H, Senda M, et al. Mechanical efficiency in hypertrophic cardiomyopathy assessed by positron emission tomography with carbon 11 acetate. *Am Heart J* 1997;133:497–503.
112. Takala TO, Nuutila P, Katoh C, et al. Myocardial blood flow, oxygen consumption and fatty acid uptake in endurance athletes during insulin stimulation. *Am J Physiol* 1999;277 [Suppl 4, Pt 1]: E585–E590.
113. Bengel FM, Permanetter B, Ungerer M, et al. Noninvasive estimation of myocardial efficiency using positron emission tomography and carbon 11 acetate—comparison between the normal and failing human heart. *Eur J Nucl Med* 2000;27:319–326.
114. Kalff V, Hicks RJ, Hutchins G, et al. Use of carbon 11 acetate and dynamic positron emission tomography to assess regional myocardial oxygen consumption in patients with acute myocardial infarction receiving thrombolysis or coronary angioplasty. *Am J Cardiol* 1990;71: 529–535.
115. Bengel FM, Ueberfuhr P, Ziegler S, et al. Patterns of sympathetic reinnervation after cardiac transplantation: comparison of the orthotopically transplanted with heterotopically transplanted and autotransplanted heart. *J Nucl Med* 2000;41:168P 773(abst).
116. Bengel FM, Ueberfuhr P, Schiepel N, et al. Myocardial efficiency and sympathetic reinnervation after orthotopic heart transplantation. *Circulation* 2001;103:1881–1886.
117. Frank R. Nuclear bioimaging in drug development and regulatory review. *J Clin Pharmacol* 1999;39:51S–55S.
118. Gradnik R. Drug design in cardiology: the pharmaceutical industry point of view. In: Comar D, ed. *Positron emission tomography for drug development and evaluation.* Dordrecht: Kluwer, 1995:215–218.
119. Beanlands R, Armstrong WF, Hicks R, et al. The effects of afterload reduction on myocardial C 11 acetate kinetics and noninvasively estimated mechanical efficiency in patients with dilated cardiomyopathy. *J Nucl Cardiol* 1994;1:3–16.
120. CIBIS II Investigators and Committees. The Cardiac Insufficiency Bisoprolol Study II (CIBIS II). *Lancet* 1999;353:9–13.
121. MERIT HF Study Group. Effect of metoprolol CR/XL in chronic heart failure: metoprolol CR/XL. Randomized intervention trial in congestive heart failure (MERIT HF). *Lancet* 1999;353:2001–2007.

122. Packer MD, Bristow MR, Cohn JN, et al. The effect of carvedilol on morbidity and mortality in patients with chronic heart failure. *N Engl J Med* 1996;334:1349–1355.
123. Haikala H, Linden IB. Mechanism of action of calcium sensitizing drugs. *J Cardiovasc Pharmacol* 1995;26:S10–S19.
124. Tuunanen H, Engblom E, Naum A, et al. Free fatty acid depletion acutely decreases cardiac work and efficiency in cardiomyopathic heart failure. *Circulation* 2006;114:2130–2137.
125. Ukkonen H, Beanlands R, Burwash I, et al. The effect of cardiac resynchronization on myocardial efficiency and regional oxidative metabolism. *Circulation* 2003;107:28–31.
126. Lindner O, Sorensen J, Vogt J, et al. Cardiac efficiency and oxygen consumption measured with ^{11}C-acetate PET after long-term cardiac resynchronization therapy. *J Nucl Med* 2006;47:378–383.
127. Yoshinaga K, Burwash IG, Leech JA, et al. The effects of continuous positive airway pressure on myocardial energetics in patients with heart failure and obstructive sleep apnea. *J Am Coll Cardiol* 2007;49:450–458.
128. Bradley TD, Floras JS. Sleep apnea and heart failure: part I: obstructive sleep apnea. *Circulation* 2003;107:1671–1678.
129. Hicks RJ, Savas V, Currie PJ, et al. Assessment of myocardial-oxidative metabolism in aortic valve disease using positron emission tomography with C 11 acetate. *Am Heart J* 1992;123: 653–664.
130. Knuuti J, Sundell J, Naum A, et al. Assessment of right ventricular oxidative metabolism by PET in patients with idiopathic dilated cardiomyopathy undergoing cardiac resynchronization therapy. *Eur J Nucl Med Mol Imaging* 2004;31:1592–1598.
132. Nony P, Guastalla JP, Rebattu P, et al. *In vivo* measurement of myocardial oxidative metabolism and blood flow does not show changes in cancer patients undergoing doxorubicin therapy. *Cancer Chemother Pharmacol* 2000;45:375–380.
133. Hattori N, Tamaki N, Kudoh T, et al. Abnormality of myocardial oxidative metabolism in noninsulin dependent diabetes mellitus. *J Nucl Med* 1998;39:1835–1840.

CHAPTER

11.4

Myocardial Neurotransmitter Imaging

MARKUS SCHWAIGER, ICHIRO MATSUNARI, AND FRANK M. BENGEL

The innervation of the heart represents an important aspect for the adaptation of cardiac performance to the hemodynamic requirements in the healthy and diseased human body. The cardiovascular work of the normal heart depends on neuronal input for its adequate response to physiologic stimuli such as exercise and mental stress. The importance of the autonomic nervous system (ANS) in the pathophysiology of various heart diseases, such as congestive heart failure (CHF) (1) and arrhythmias (2), has been increasingly recognized. With the introduction of tracer approaches, noninvasive functional assessment of the cardiac ANS by scintigraphic techniques has become a practical reality and provided important pathophysiologic information in various cardiac disease states.

The catecholamine analogue iodine-123 ([^{123}I]) metaiodobenzylguanidine (MIBG) (3,4) has opened noninvasive assessment of presynaptic neuronal function for broader clinical application using single-photon emission computed tomography (SPECT). Tracers for positron emission tomography (PET) are also available to assess the human sympathetic nervous system with carbon-11 ([^{11}C])-hydroxyephedrine (HED) (5,6), fluorine-18 ([^{18}F])-fluorodopamine (7,8), [^{11}C]-epinephrine (EPI) (9), [^{11}C]-phenylephrine (10), and [^{11}C]-CGP12177 (11). These agents permit the regional quantification of tracer concentration in pre- and postsynaptic sites with high spatial resolution.

DESCRIPTION OF THE AUTONOMIC NERVOUS SYSTEM IN THE HEART

The ANS, referred to as the visceral nervous system, consists of two main divisions: sympathetic and parasympathetic innervation. The two systems have different major neurotransmitters, norepinephrine or acetylcholine (ACh), which define the stimulatory and inhibitory physiologic effects of each system (12). Sympathetic and parasympathetic innervation of the heart facilitates electrophysiologic and hemodynamic adaptation to changing cardiovascular demands. Both sympathetic and parasympathetic activity control the rate of electrophysiologic stimulation and conduction, whereas contractile performance is primarily modulated by sympathetic neurotransmission. This functional characterization is reflected by the anatomic distribution of sympathetic and parasympathetic nerve fibers and nerve terminals.

Sympathetic nerve fibers are characterized by multiple nerve endings that are filled with vesicles containing norepinephrine. Sympathetic nerve fibers travel parallel to the vascular structures on the surface of the heart and penetrate the underlying myocardium in much the same fashion as the coronary vessels. Based on tissue norepinephrine concentration, the mammalian heart is characterized by dense adrenergic innervation with a norepinephrine concentration gradient from the atria to the base of the heart and from the base to the apex of the ventricles (13).

In contrast to sympathetic nerve fibers, parasympathetic innervation is most prevalent in the atria of the heart, the atrioventricular node, and to a lesser degree within the ventricular myocardium. Parasympathetic fibers in the ventricles appear to travel close to the endocardial surface, in contrast to sympathetic innervation.

The enzyme choline acetyltransferase (ChAT) has been used as a reliable marker of cholinergic innervation (14). ChAT concentration is highest in the atria and decreases sharply in both the right and left ventricular myocardium. Fig. 11.4.1 depicts norepinephrine and ACh synthesis in the sympathetic and parasympathetic nerve terminal, respectively.

Sympathetic Nerve Terminal

Norepinephrine, the dominant transmitter in the sympathetic nervous system, is synthesized from the amino acid tyrosine by several enzymatic steps (7). The generation of DOPA from tyrosine is the rate-limiting step in the biosynthesis of catecholamines. After

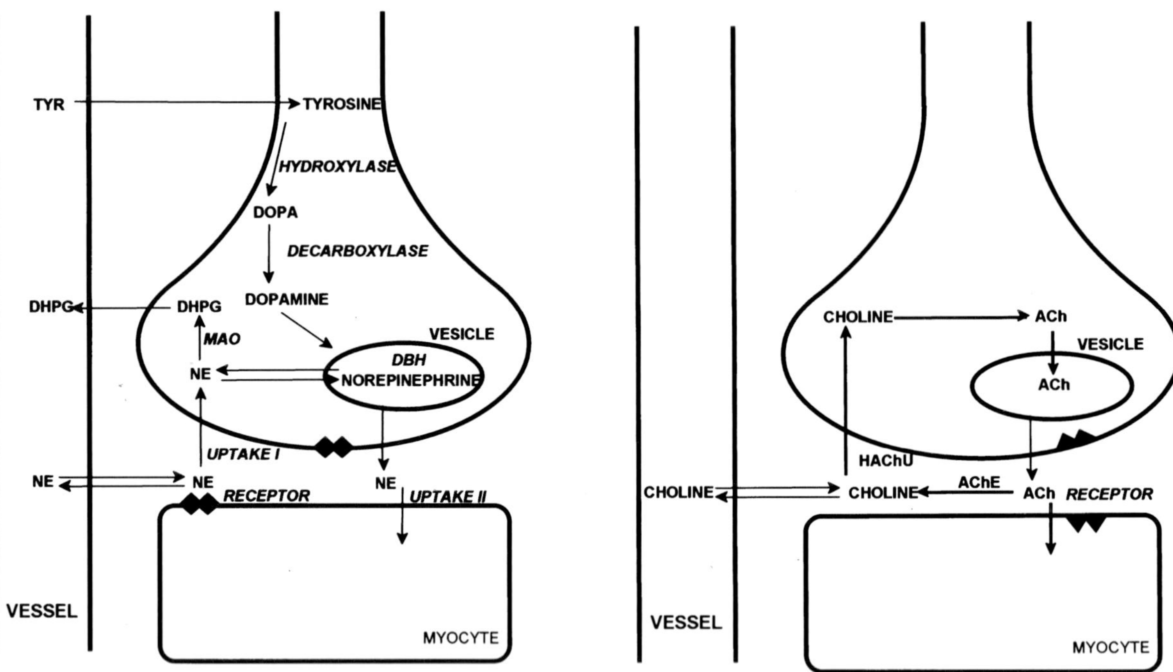

FIGURE 11.4.1. Schematic display of sympathetic and parasympathetic nerve terminals. NE, norepinephrine; TYR, tyrosine; MAO, monoamine oxydase; ACh, acetylcholine; AChE, acetylcholinesterase.

DOPA conversion to dopamine by DOPA decarboxylase, dopamine is transported into storage vesicles by an energy-requiring mechanism. Norepinephrine is synthesized by the action of dopamine β-hydroxylase (DBH) on dopamine within the storage vesicles. Nerve stimulation leads to norepinephrine release, which occurs as the vesicles fuse with the neuronal membrane and expel their contents by exocytosis. Single nerve stimulation, however, leads to exocytosis of only a small fraction of the many thousands of storage vesicles in the sympathetic nerve terminal.

The average adrenergic neuron has approximately 25,000 vesicles. Each vesicle contains approximately 250 pg of norepinephrine (15). Thus, although most norepinephrine is thought to be released by exocytosis, nonvesicular release also occurs. Apart from neuronal stimulation, norepinephrine release is also regulated by a number of receptor systems. The α_2-receptors on the membrane surface are thought to provide negative feedback of the exocytotic process, and thus, the exocytotic release can be inhibited by presynaptic α_2-receptor agonists such as clonidine, guanabenz, and guanfacine (16).

Muscarinic and adenosine receptors have an antiadrenergic effect in the heart. Neuropeptide Y is stored and released together with norepinephrine from the nerve terminal. Neuropeptide Y is thought to inhibit norepinephrine release by the nerve terminal (17). Presynaptic angiotensin II receptors and β-receptors, on the other hand, mediate facilitation of norepinephrine release from sympathetic nerve endings. Therefore, some antihypertensive pharmaceuticals such as angiotensin-converting enzyme inhibitors and nonselective β-blocking agents can inhibit excessive norepinephrine release.

The complex modulation of sympathetic neurotransmission obviously involves many systems including dopamine, prostaglandin, and histamine. Only a small amount of the norepinephrine released by the nerve terminal is actually available to activate receptors on the myocyte surface. Most of the norepinephrine released undergoes reuptake in the nerve terminal (uptake-1 mechanism) and recycles into the vesicles or is metabolized in the cytosol of the nerve terminal. The uptake-1 system is characterized as saturable and sodium, temperature, and energy dependent (18). It can be inhibited by cocaine and desipramine (19). Structurally related amines such as EPI, guanethidine, and metaraminol are also transported by this system.

In addition to neuronal uptake via uptake-1, the uptake-2 system moves norepinephrine into nonneuronal tissue (20). Uptake-2 is characterized as nonsaturable and not sodium-, temperature-, or energy-dependent. It can be inhibited by steroids and clonidine (21). Free cytosolic norepinephrine is degraded rapidly to dihydroxyphenylglycol by monoamine oxidase (MAO). Only a small fraction of the released norepinephrine diffuses into the vascular space where it can be measured as norepinephrine spill over in the coronary sinus venous blood.

Parasympathetic Nerve Terminal

ACh is synthesized within the parasympathetic nerve terminal. Choline is transported into the cytosol of the nerve ending via a high-affinity choline uptake system (22). In the nerve terminal, choline is rapidly acetylated by ChAT and is subsequently shuttled into storage vesicles. In contrast to amine uptake in the sympathetic nerve terminals, the choline uptake system is restrictive. Even choline analogues with very similar structures are poor substrates for this uptake mechanism. Upon nerve stimulation, ACh is released into the synaptic cleft where it interacts with muscarinic receptors. Free ACh is rapidly metabolized by acetylcholinesterase.

RADIOPHARMACEUTICALS FOR NEUROTRANSMITTER IMAGING

Presynaptic Function

Tracers for neurotransmitter imaging have been developed by either direct labeling of the physiologic neurotransmitter or labeling of their structural analogues (Fig. 11.4.2). Table 11.4.1 summarizes currently available radiopharmaceuticals for the scintigraphic evaluation of the presynaptic nervous function. Iodine-123 MIBG was developed as a norepinephrine analogue by Wieland et al. (4); it was first used in the human heart by Kline et al. (3) in the early 1980s. This compound is an analogue of guanethidine and shares a cellular uptake mechanism similar to norepinephrine at the sympathetic nerve terminals. It is transported into cells by uptake-1 and is stored in the vesicles but not catabolized by MAO or catechol-*O*-methyltransferase (COMT). This compound has a low affinity for postsynaptic adrenergic receptors and thus has little pharmacologic action. It has been shown that tissue norepinephrine concentration correlates with MIBG uptake (23).

Because PET has several advantages over SPECT (e.g., quantification of regional tracer uptake with the use of accurate attenuation correction and higher spatial resolution), efforts have been made to develop positron-emitting tracers for neurotransmitter imaging.

Fluorine-18-labeled metaraminol, which also was first synthesized by Wieland et al. (24) at the University of Michigan, is taken up by the sympathetic nerve terminal in a manner similar to norepinephrine but is not catabolized by MAO. Imaging studies in regionally denervated canine hearts indicated sufficient suitability of the tracer to quantitatively assess the integrity of myocardial sympathetic innervation. Transient myocardial ischemia, again in the canine model, resulted in reduced [^{18}F]-metaraminol retention in tissue, which is consistent with neuronal dysfunction in reversibly damaged myocardium (25). Radiopharmaceutical problems associated with low specific activity and potential pharmacologic effects, however, limited its further clinical application.

Carbon-11-HED, also introduced by the Michigan group, emerged as a more promising tracer because it can be synthesized with high specific activity (26). Experimental studies have indicated that there is a highly specific uptake into sympathetic nerve terminals with little nonneuronal binding (27). Carbon-11-HED is currently the most successfully used positron-emitting tracer for cardiac neurotransmitter imaging in humans. More recently, [^{11}C]-EPI has been proposed as a truly physiologic tracer (28). It has been demonstrated that, as with norepinephrine, accumulation of [^{11}C]-EPI by the heart reflects mainly vesicular storage in the sympathetic neuron (29). In contrast to [^{11}C]-HED, free [^{11}C]-EPI is metabolized in the cytosol by the MAO system. Because [^{11}C]-HED is not metabolized, it diffuses out of the nerve terminal and undergoes reuptake.

Myocardial retention of [^{11}C]-HED primarily reflects uptake-1 activity and to a lesser degree the storage capacity of neurons for

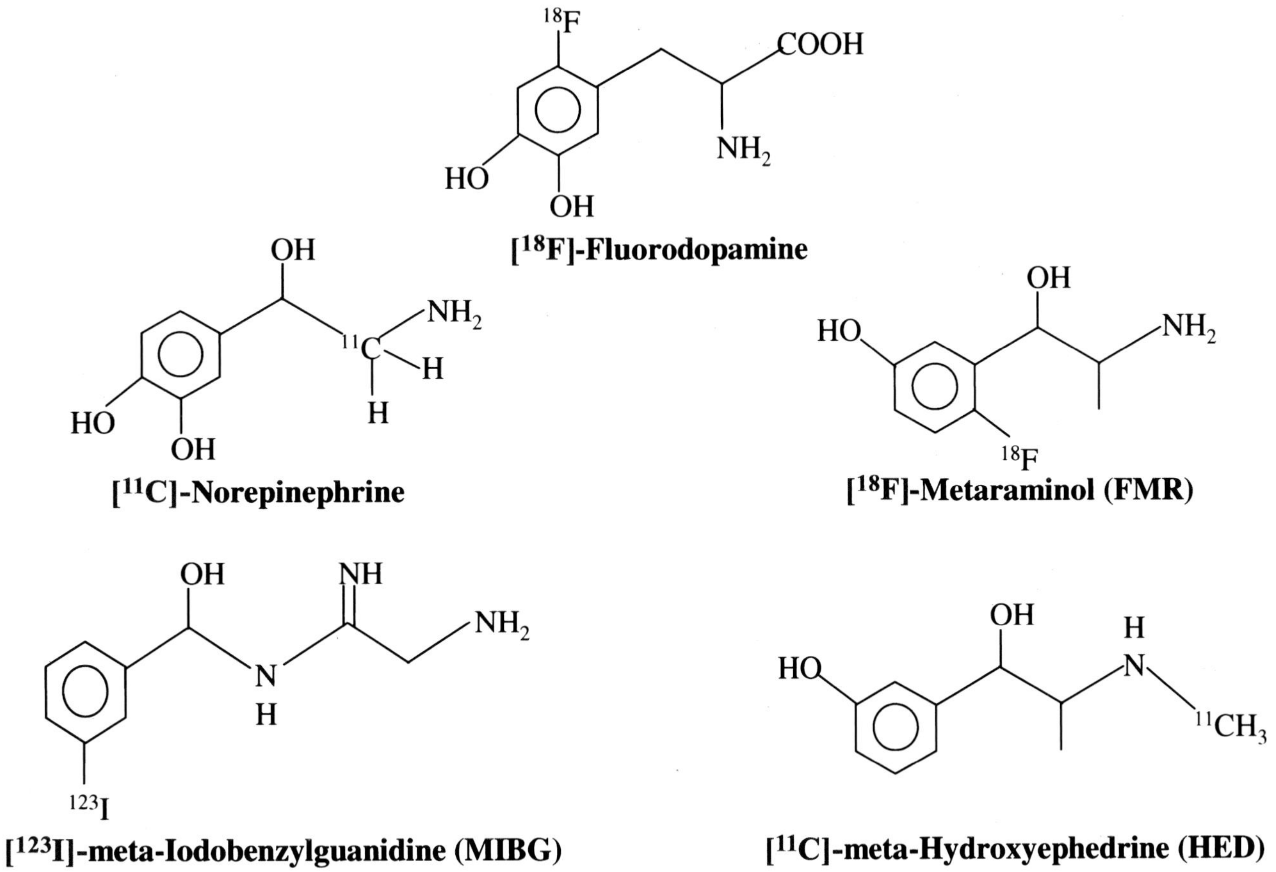

FIGURE 11.4.2. Chemical structures of radiolabeled catecholamine analogues.

TABLE 11.4.1 Radiopharmaceuticals Used for Neurotransmitter Imaging

	SPECT	PET
Sympathetic	^{123}I-metaiodobenzylguanidine (^{123}I-MIBG)	^{18}F-fluorometaraminol ^{11}C-hydroxyephedrine (^{11}C-HED) ^{11}C-epinephrine (11C-EPI) ^{11}C-phenylephrine ^{18}F-fluorobenzylguanidine ^{18}F-fluorodopamine ^{18}F-fluoronorepinephrine
Parasympathetic		^{18}F-fluoroethoxybenzovesamicol

norepinephrine (27,30). Therefore, [^{11}C]-EPI may be the more suitable tracer for the evaluation of sympathetic vesicular function of the heart (29). Because [^{11}C]-EPI is metabolized by MAO and COMT, careful consideration should be given to the influence of metabolic pathways on measurements of [^{11}C] retention attributed to vesicular storage functions.

A further analogue of EPI is [^{11}C]-phenylephrine, which also has been synthesized by Del Rosario et al. (31) at the University of Michigan. This tracer enters the nerve terminal via uptake-1, is stored within vesicles, but is also metabolized by the MAO enzyme system. Carbon-11-phenylephrine, therefore, allows for the evaluation of vesicular and enzymatic integrity of the nerve terminal (10,32). Other potential tracers include [^{18}F]-fluorodopamine (7,33) and [^{18}F]-fluoronorepinephrine (34). Although the available clinical and experimental data for these tracers are still limited, the longer physical half-life of [^{18}F] may allow for washout analysis to assess sympathetic nerve tone. Further PET tracers for assessing sympathetic nerve function, such as bromine-76 ([^{76}Br])-labeled or [^{18}F]-labeled benzyl guanidine (35,36), analogues of MIBG, have also been proposed but did not reach a clinical application.

To date, only a few studies have addressed myocardial parasympathetic neuronal imaging, probably because of a low specificity for neuronal uptake and storage. However, recent studies in the brain in mice (37) and rats (38) have shown that iodine-125 ([^{125}I])-labeled iodobenzovesamicol allowed scintigraphic assessment of cholinergic nerve terminals. Fluorine-18-fluoroethoxybenzovesamicol was developed for parasympathetic neurotransmitter imaging using PET (39). The myocardial retention of the tracer was low because of the low cholinergic neuron density, limiting its potential as an imaging agent. Further efforts in developing tracers for the parasympathetic nervous system are required.

Postsynaptic Receptor Imaging

The sympathetic neurotransmission in the heart primarily involves adrenoceptors of type β_1 and β_2, which are located on myocardial cells. The α-adrenoceptors are primarily associated with vascular structures. The positive inotropic and chronotropic response of the heart is mediated by β-receptors. The neurotransmitters norepinephrine and EPI have a high affinity to these receptors. Adrenoreceptors are linked to a complex second-messenger system that modifies the signal transduction (40,41). The surface density of receptors can be up-regulated and down-regulated in response to the extraneuronal catecholamine concentration (42). This down-regulation of β-receptors, primarily by β_1-receptors, has been described in patients with heart failure. In addition, the treatment of patients with heart failure today includes β-receptor antagonists, which have a beneficial effect on left ventricular function. This has led to an increasing interest in the noninvasive characterization of receptor distribution by tracer techniques.

The most commonly used tracer for postsynaptic imaging is [^{11}C]-CGP12177, which represents a nonselective but hydrophilic β-receptor antagonist. Lipophilic tracers such as [^{11}C]-propranolol and pindolol display a high retention in lung tissue and bind to internalized receptors. They are, therefore, not suitable for cardiac imaging purposes.

Delforge et al. (43) developed a quantitative imaging method that includes two tracer injections with varying specific activity, yielding absolute measurements of β-receptor density in the heart. Merlet et al. (11) applied receptor imaging to various disease groups including patients with dilated cardiomyopathy. This imaging approach has emerged as the most widely used test to visualize β-receptors. The radiochemistry of [^{11}C]-CGP12177 is demanding because of the need for phosgene as a precursor for synthesis. More recently, [^{11}C]-CGP12388 has been proposed as an alternative tracer with similar biologic characteristics, and it is easier to synthesize (44). Animal and clinical results are promising but await further evaluation (45,46).

Law et al. (47) reported the evaluation of [^{11}C]-*N*-desmethyl-GB67 as a specific α_1-receptor ligand in the heart. Rapid plasma clearance, no metabolites, and high myocardial retention yield good image quality. Future studies will have to document the ability of this new tracer to visualize and quantitate α-receptor density in the healthy and diseased heart.

Finally, radioactive-labeled ligands have been used to visualize the muscarinic receptors in the heart. There is a high density of these receptors in both the right and the left ventricles, which yields excellent image quality. This excellent imaging is somewhat surprising given the presence of only very sparse cholinergic presynaptic innervation of both cardiac ventricles. The PET research group at Orsay developed tracer approaches using [^{11}C]-methylquinuclidinyl benzilate (MQNB) for the quantitative assessment of muscarinic receptors (48,49).

IMAGING PROTOCOLS

An [^{11}C]-HED PET imaging protocol typically includes dynamic PET acquisition for 40 to 60 minutes after injection and blood flow imaging using flow tracers such as nitrogen-13 ([^{13}N])-ammonia or rubidium-82 (50–55). For [^{11}C]-EPI PET imaging, with which high levels of [^{11}C] metabolites are detected in the blood, correction for metabolite radioactivity in the arterial input function is required for the calculation of tracer retention in the tissue (9). The use of [^{18}F]-labeled tracers allows a longer imaging time, because of their longer physical half-life (110 minutes) compared with [^{11}C] (20 minutes). The longer half-life of [^{18}F] may obviate the necessity of an on-site cyclotron and thus may potentially allow for more widespread clinical use.

DATA INTERPRETATION

After intravenous injection of [^{11}C]-HED or [^{11}C]-EPI, there is rapid uptake of the tracers into the myocardium and clearance of the [^{11}C] activity from the blood pool. The myocardial time activity curves show a very slow clearance of [^{11}C] activity with a biologic half-life of several hours for HED and EPI (9). In contrast, in the denervated heart, there is very little tracer retention, indicating low nonspecific binding in the human heart (Fig. 11.4.3). Regional myocardial tracer distribution can be visually assessed by summing imaging frames 10 to 20 minutes after tracer injection. Myocardial activity is homogeneous in the healthy heart for both [^{11}C]-HED and [^{11}C]-EPI, yielding excellent image quality (Fig. 11.4.4).

Several approaches have been introduced for the quantification of regional tracer retention (55,56). The most commonly used method includes the calculation of the myocardial retention fraction (percentage per minute), which represents the regional myocardial activity measured between, for example, 30 and 40 minutes after injection. This is normalized to the integral of the arterial input function from 0 to 40 minutes after tracer injection, which is derived by placing a region of interest over the left ventricular cavity (55). The myocardial retention fraction averaged about 0.14 for [^{11}C]-HED and 0.24 for [^{11}C]-EPI in the healthy heart. In patients with recent cardiac transplantation, these values were reduced to 0.04 and 0.05, respectively, consistent with denervation of the heart (9).

The Hammersmith PET research group developed a tracer kinetic model to calculate the distribution volume for [^{11}C]-HED in the myocardium. Because the tissue half-life of HED is long and the physical half-life of [^{11}C] only 20 minutes, this approach is methodologically challenging. Although clinical results are potentially useful, no in-depth validation of this method has yet been published (56–58).

The neuronal extraction of catecholamine analogues is relatively high due to the efficient uptake-1 transport, at least under

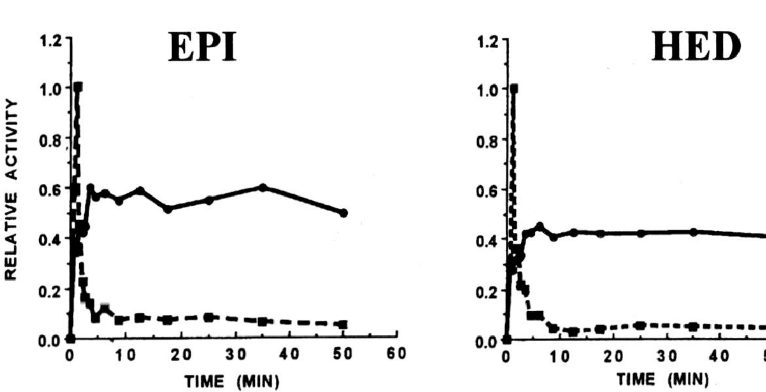

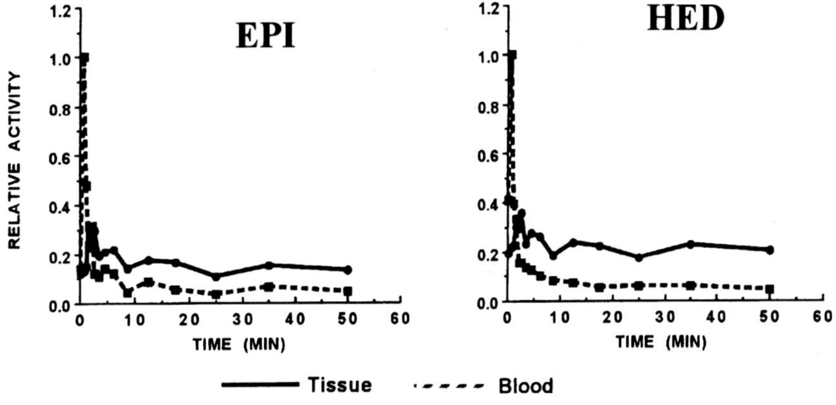

FIGURE 11.4.3. Time-activity curves in blood, as well as myocardial tissue derived from regions of interest placed over the left ventricular cavity and the myocardial walls. A few minutes after injection, there is high retention of both tracers, epinephrine (EPI) and hydroxyephedrine (HED) in myocardial tissue, which remains constant over the imaging time period of 50 minutes. In contrast, the transplanted heart tissue shows very little uptake of both EPI and HED, indicating low nonspecific binding.

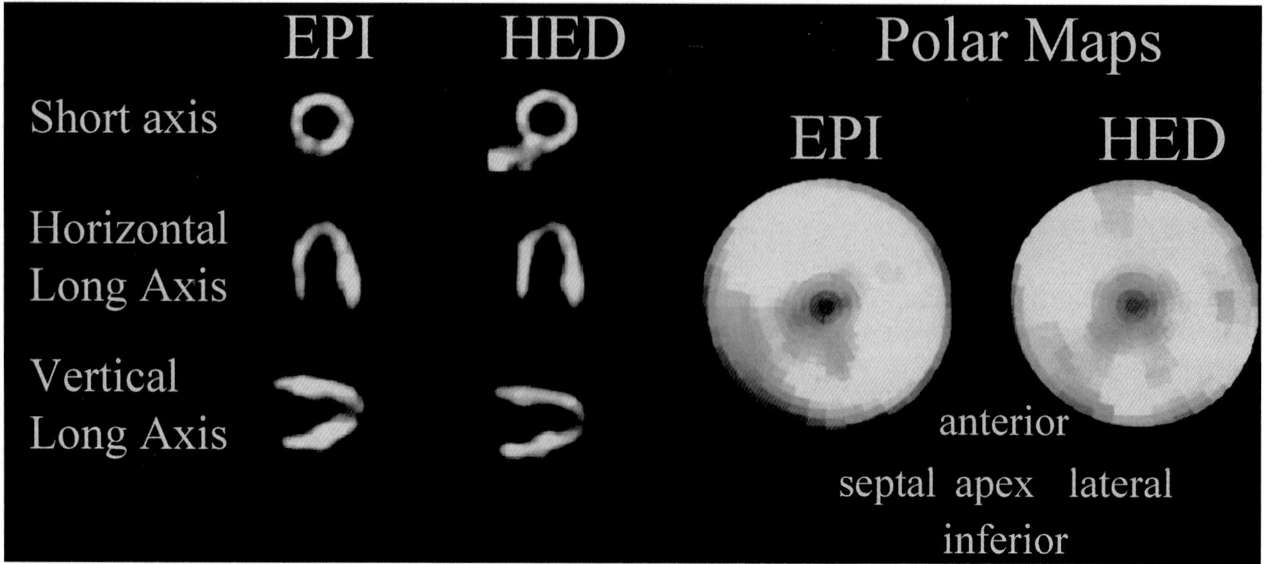

FIGURE 11.4.4. PET images obtained in healthy volunteers after injection of carbon-11 ([^{11}C])-labeled epinephrine and [^{11}C]-labeled hydroxyephedrine. The PET images are displayed in short axis, horizontal long axis, and vertical long axis. Semiquantitative analysis reveals homogeneous distribution of tracer retention throughout the left ventricle, as displayed in the polar maps.

resting conditions, and absolute measurements of myocardial tracer retention must be corrected for blood flow. Although this may not pose a problem for the regional evaluation of relative tracer uptake, it may be of utmost importance for the interindividual comparison of tracer retention fractions. Most PET studies include the measurement of regional myocardial blood flow, which allows for the regional normalization of [^{11}C] activity to, for example, [^{13}N]-ammonia measurements (59,60).

CLINICAL APPLICATIONS

Myocardial Ischemia and Infarction

Myocardial infarction (MI) has been shown to induce cardiac denervation exceeding the area of necrosis and/or scar (61–64). Minardo et al. (63) demonstrated that MIBG images in dogs after transmural MI show perfused but denervated myocardial areas apical to the infarct. Their observation was confirmed by the study of Dae et al. (23). In the latter study, they showed that nontransmural infarction also leads to regional ischemic damage of sympathetic nerves, but with minimal extension of denervation beyond the infarct.

Wolpers et al. (65) showed in the canine model of ischemia/reperfusion that the neuronal dysfunction as defined by decreased [^{11}C]-HED retention correlated closely with the extent and severity of ischemia during coronary occlusion. Another study at the authors' laboratory demonstrated that sympathetic neuronal damage measured by technetium-99m (^{99m}Tc)-methoxyisobutyl isonitrile SPECT is closely related to the risk area in patients with acute MI (66). This supports the notion that sympathetic nerves are more sensitive to ischemia than myocardial tissue. This in turn may explain the mismatch between the extent of denervation and perfusion abnormalities in the experimental and clinical setting. Consistent with this, Bulow et al. (67) observed denervation with [^{11}C]-HED in patients with coronary artery disease but without myocardial infarction.

Although denervation defects extending beyond necrotic regions are commonly observed in patients after MI, the prognostic significance of this scintigraphic information remains to be elucidated. Published studies were based on relatively small patient populations, which may limit the ability to draw conclusions. Further prospective studies involving a larger patient population are necessary to evaluate the clinical impact of autonomic imaging in terms of clinical outcome in patients after MI.

Reinnervation after Myocardial Infarction

Although inhomogeneity of cardiac sympathetic reinnervation may play an important role in the risk of arrhythmias early after MI, it remains controversial whether reinnervation after MI occurs in humans. Cardiac sympathetic reinnervation after MI has been reported in experimental canine studies (63). In humans, Hartikainen et al. (68) showed partial reinnervation in the peri-infarct zone between 3 and 12 months after infarction, and Fallen et al. (69), using flurodopamine PET, showed increased tracer uptake between 2 weeks and 3 months after MI.

Conversely, using serial HED PET imaging, Allman et al. (51) studied the extent and reversibility of neuronal abnormalities in patients with an acute MI. They observed more extensive HED abnormalities than those for blood flow, particularly in patients with non-Q-wave infarction, but they did not observe any change in either the extent of abnormality or the tracer retention 8 ± 3 months later, suggesting persistent neuronal damage without evidence of reinnervation.

Ventricular Arrhythmia

A role for the sympathetic nervous system in the generation of arrhythmias has been suggested (70,71). Different theories are proposed for the induction of arrhythmias, but *in vivo* data are limited.

Therefore, scintigraphic techniques may provide unique information on the pathophysiology of arrhythmogenic heart disease.

Using HED PET, Calkins et al. (53) observed a correlation between reduced HED retention and ventricular refractoriness in patients with a history of sustained ventricular tachycardia. Regional [^{11}C]-HED retention and blood flow were correlated with epicardial electrophysiologic mapping during open heart surgery. Denervated myocardial segments displayed a significant prolonged relative refractory period, suggesting regional dispersion of electrophysiologic properties, which can be imaged with [^{11}C]-HED. Thus, the presence of denervated but viable myocardium, as assessed by scintigraphic techniques, may have important implications for the pathogenesis of ventricular arrhythmias.

Wichter et al. (58) investigated eight patients with arrhythmogenic right ventricular cardiomyopathy using PET. The density of β-receptors was determined and correlated with the distribution volume of [^{11}C]-HED. They reported a significant global decrease of β_{max} (5.9 vs. 10.2 pmol/g of tissue), but no significant decrease of [^{11}C]-HED retention. Myocardial blood flow measured with $H_2[^{15}O]$ was not altered. These PET data contradict to a certain degree MIBG data by the same group (72), which demonstrated regional presynaptic abnormalities and emphasized the need for a better understanding of the differences between MIBG and [^{11}C]-HED pharmacokinetics.

Schafers et al. (57) investigated another group of patients with idiopathic arrhythmias. Eight patients with right ventricular outflow tract tachycardia underwent PET studies with [^{11}C]-HED, [^{11}C]-CGP12177, and $H_2[^{15}O]$. Both the density of β-receptors and the distribution volume of [^{11}C]-HED were reduced, suggesting an abnormality in pre- and postsynaptic function. Surprisingly, no regional differences were reported in this disease group, which had a structural abnormality involving the right ventricle. Myocardial blood flow in these patients was not significantly different from that of a control group of 29 volunteers.

Sympathetic imbalance with decreased right cardiac sympathetic activity has been attributed to the induction of ventricular arrhythmias in long QT syndrome. Decreased HED uptake was reported in genotype patients with long QT syndrome, supporting the "sympathetic imbalance" hypothesis (73). Abnormalities of HED uptake, however, were not observed in a study by Calkins et al. (74), so this issue remains somewhat unclear.

Diabetes Mellitus

Diabetic patients often develop autonomic neuropathy, and autonomic dysfunction may be associated with increased morbidity in these patients (75). Using HED PET, Allman et al. (50) studied diabetic patients with and without autonomic neuropathy and observed regional reductions in cardiac HED retention, predominantly in apical, inferior, and lateral regions, in patients with autonomic neuropathy, compared with healthy subjects, but not in diabetic patients without evident neuropathy (Fig. 11.4.5). They also observed a correlation between the extent of the scintigraphic abnormality and the severity of autonomic dysfunction.

Stevens et al. (76) compared regional [^{11}C]-HED retention with severity of diabetic neuronal dysfunction (i.e., diabetic autonomic neuropathy [DAN]). The sensitivity of the imaging approach was demonstrated by the fact that 40% of DAN-negative diabetic patients displayed an abnormality on their [^{11}C]-HED images. In subjects with mild neuropathy, defects were observed in the distal inferior wall of the left ventricle, whereas with more severe neuropathy, tracer defects extended to involve the distal anterolateral

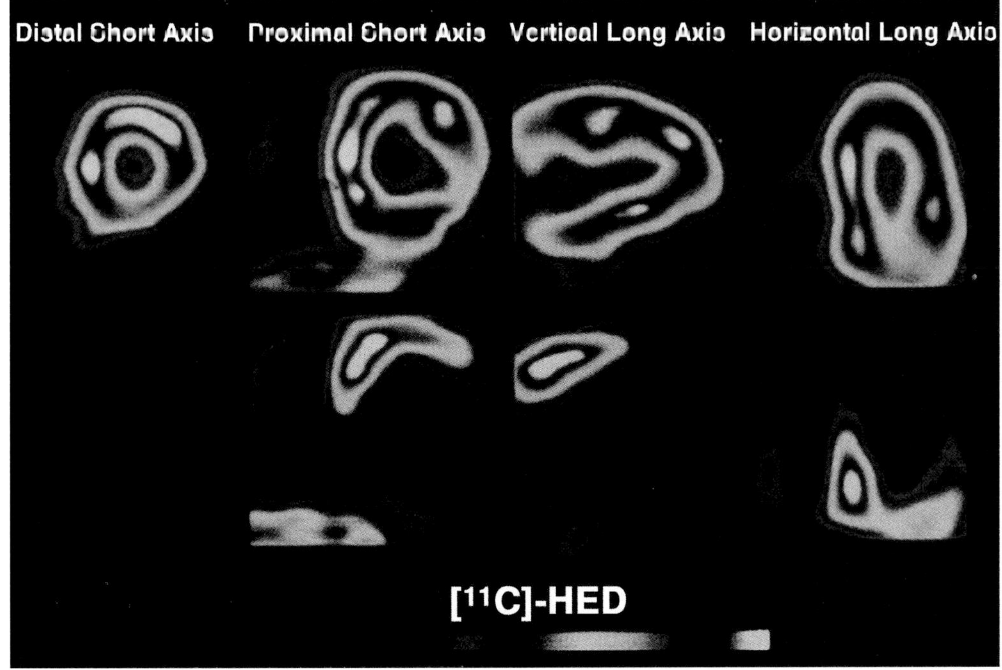

FIGURE 11.4.5. PET images of myocardial perfusion with nitrogen-13-ammonia (**top row**) and sympathetic nerve function (carbon-11-hydroxyephedrine [HED]) in a patient with diabetic cardiac neuropathy. There is maintained myocardial perfusion but decreased HED retention in the inferior and apical wall of the left ventricle.

and inferior walls. The investigators also observed an increased regional blood flow by PET in the denervated myocardial segments of diabetic patients. In a subsequent study, Stevens et al. [77] compared DAN as evidenced by [^{11}C]-HED imaging with measurements of regional coronary flow reserve and demonstrated a decreased vasodilatory reactivity in severely denervated segments.

Reinnervation after Heart Transplantation

Schwaiger et al. (54) described for the first-time scintigraphic evidence of reinnervation in patients after heart transplantation using HED PET. In that study, patients who had undergone transplantation more than 2 years before the PET scan showed partial sympathetic reinnervation in the proximal anterior and septal walls, whereas patients who had recently received a transplant (<1 year) did not show evidence of reinnervation. Fig. 11.4.6 displays a representative patient 8 years after undergoing heart transplantation compared with a healthy subject. These observations were confirmed in a subsequent study by Ziegler et al. (78), who performed HED PET imaging in 48 patients at various times after heart transplantation and reported that sympathetic reinnervation was a time-dependent phenomenon that paralleled electrophysiologic evidence of functional reinnervation such as an increase in heart rate variability.

The functional integrity of sympathetic nerve terminals in the transplanted heart was investigated by the comparison of [^{11}C]-HED uptake and pharmacologically induced norepinephrine release (79). Both measurements were well correlated, indicating the ability of the nerve terminals to adequately respond to tyramine. Bengel et al. (80) performed serial PET studies in patients with orthotopic heart transplantation over a period of several years and observed a continuous increase of reinnervation with time.

It is interesting that the reinnervation process leads only to a partial reappearance of neuronal structures and is limited primarily to the anterior, septal, and anterolateral segments of the left ventricle. In the largest cross-sectional group of transplant recipients studied with PET to date, the largest reinnervated area observed in a patient was 66% of the left ventricle (81). Determinants of reinnervation other than time after transplantation were identified and included the number of prior rejection episodes, donor age, and aortic manipulations at surgery. The regional heterogeneity of innervation within the transplanted heart provides a unique model to study the effect of autonomic innervation on cardiac performance.

Bengel et al. (82) correlated the pattern of innervation in transplant patients with cardiac substrate metabolism as assessed by [^{11}C]-acetate and [^{18}F]-fluorodeoxyglucose and PET. The data suggest that innervation has a significant impact on myocardial substrate utilization. Denervated segments displayed a higher glucose utilization rate, whereas the innervated heart most likely is dependent on free fatty acid oxidation. This observation is important with respect to myocardial energy metabolism in the failing heart, which is often associated with denervation. The clinical impact of

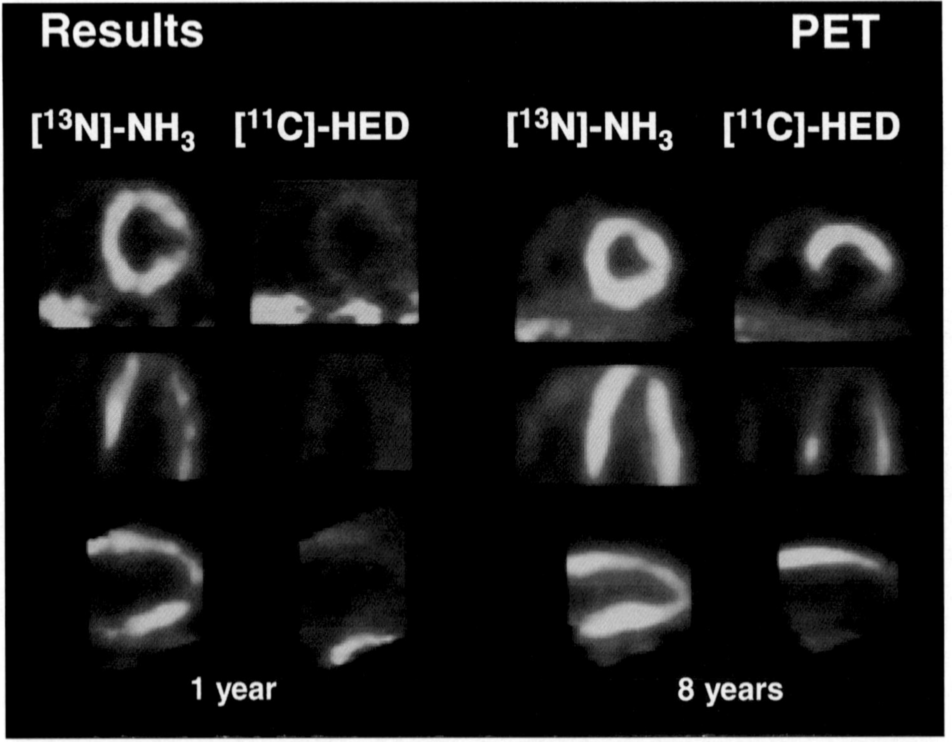

FIGURE 11.4.6. PET images of two patients after cardiac transplantation. Blood flow images were obtained after intravenous injection of nitrogen-13-ammonia and images of sympathetic nerve terminals after injection of carbon-11 ([^{11}C])-hydroxyephedrine (HED). In the patient early after cardiac transplantation, there is maintained myocardial perfusion but no visible myocardial uptake of HED, documenting complete denervation. In contrast, in the patient 8 years after transplantation, there is regional reuptake of [^{11}C]-HED in the anterior wall of the left ventricle, indicating reinnervation.

the reinnervation on hemodynamic and cardiac performance was also investigated. Schwaiblmair et al. (83) showed that transplant patients with PET evidence of reinnervation did exhibit a longer exercise time as compared with denervated patients.

The authors' laboratory also addressed the question whether the reappearance of innervation lead to an improved cardiac performance during exercise (52). Global and regional function was measured by radionuclide ventriculography at rest and during exercise in innervated and denervated transplant patients. The global left ventricular ejection fraction (LVEF) increased significantly during exercise in innervated patients, and the regional response correlated with the [^{11}C]-HED retention pattern in the left ventricle. These data support the importance of the reinnervation process for functional recovery after cardiac transplantation.

Congestive Heart Failure

There is general agreement that increased adrenergic nervous system activity plays an important role in the pathophysiology of CHF (84). Increased plasma norepinephrine levels , increased spill over of norepinephrine, reduced cardiac stores of norepinephrine, and desensitization of β-adrenoreceptors have been reported in patients in heart failure (1). This increased sympathetic nervous system activity is associated with increased norepinephrine turnover and reduced efficiency of norepinephrine reuptake and storage. It has also been suggested that patients in heart failure with high plasma norepinephrine levels have an unfavorable prognosis (85). Plasma norepinephrine, however, is derived from sympathetic activity throughout the body and, thus, does not necessarily reflect cardiac sympathetic activity. Noninvasive scintigraphic techniques, therefore, may provide important knowledge of cardiac sympathetic nervous system activity, which could be of value in understanding the pathogenesis and prognosis of heart failure.

A number of studies have shown that abnormal MIBG findings in the case of heart failure typically include a reduced heart/mediastinum tracer-uptake ratio, heterogeneous distribution of MIBG within the myocardium, and more rapid MIBG washout from the heart (86,87). A reduced heart/mediastinum uptake ratio (<1.2) is reportedly a powerful predictor of poor prognosis in patients with CHF (87). It appears that these scintigraphic findings are independent of the underlying cause of heart failure (88).

Reduced HED retention has been reported in patients with idiopathic dilated cardiomyopathy (89). Using quantitative analysis, the reduction of HED retention correlated with the severity of heart failure as expressed by the New York Heart Association functional classification (59). Vesalainen et al. (90) reported a 30% reduction of [^{11}C] retention in 30 patients with moderate heart failure and correlated these findings with heart rate variability and blood pressure control. There was no significant relation of HED retention with heart rate variability, but a relation was found with blood pressure regulation during the tilt test. The retention of [^{11}C]-HED in the failing heart is heterogeneous with more pronounced abnormalities in distal segments. This neuronal dysfunction is independent of myocardial blood flow, as shown by direct comparison with [^{13}N]-ammonia distribution in the same patients (59). Additionally, reduced sympathetic innervation is correlated with impaired regional contractile function (91) and impaired global myocardial efficiency (92).

Ungerer et al. (60) investigated the relation between scintigraphic findings and myocardial tissue analysis in candidates for cardiac transplantation. Regional [^{11}C]-HED retention correlated with tissue norepinephrine content and the density of catecholamine transport proteins (uptake-1). There was no significant relation between presynaptic scintigraphic measurements and density of β-receptors (42). These quantitative PET data in patients in heart failure indicate the validity of the imaging approach to delineate neuronal dysfunction and to use PET in combination with [^{11}C]-HED to monitor neuronal function during therapy.

Aside from a down-regulation of β-receptor density (11), there are scintigraphic data suggesting an up-regulation of muscarinic receptors in patients in heart failure. Le Guludec et al. (93) reported approximately 30% up-regulation of [^{11}C]-MQNB binding in 22 patients with severe reduction of left ventricular function (mean LVEF of 22%) as compared with 12 healthy controls. The clinical and pathophysiologic significance of this finding remains to be elucidated.

Finally, Pietila et al. (94) published results on the prognostic value of [^{11}C]-HED imaging in patients with advanced heart failure. Forty-six patients with impaired left ventricular function (LVEF of 8% to 35%) were monitored for 55 $\pm$ 19 months after an HED PET study. The patients were divided into two groups based on myocardial HED retention. Below the cutoff value of 0.184 for retention fraction, there was a significantly higher incidence of complications (death, cardiac transplantation) as compared to patients with maintained tracer retention. Myocardial HED retention was independent from peak oxygen uptake and end diastolic volume as a significant predictor for complications. These clinical results with [^{11}C]-HED confirm the prior prognostic experience with MIBG imaging and suggest a potentially important application of PET in patients with heart failure.

SUMMARY

Myocardial neurotransmitter PET imaging allows for the assessment of cardiac autonomic innervation in humans under various clinical conditions. Early detection of abnormalities before the evidence of structural changes is an important goal of these scintigraphic approaches. Monitoring of therapeutic procedures appears to be an additional promising application of neurotransmitter imaging.

Several issues remain to be addressed. First, controversial results have been published for healthy subjects and for various disease conditions using the SPECT tracer MIBG and the most popular PET tracer HED. It is also noteworthy that a number of MIBG studies describe regional abnormalities involving the inferior wall. These differences may be attributed to technical differences between SPECT and PET (e.g., the attenuation correction and higher spatial resolution of PET compared with SPECT) and differences in tracer kinetics and characteristics between MIBG and HED, including differences in specific activity and uptake of the tracer in nerve terminals. Second, the clinical significance and prognostic value of scintigraphic techniques have not yet been fully established. More convincing data involving larger patient populations are required to draw significant conclusions regarding the utility of these scintigraphic techniques in the clinical setting. Finally, future developments aimed at synthesizing new radiopharmaceuticals to discriminate different aspects of autonomic nerve function and to allow for the application of PET on a wider clinical basis (i.e., through a robust [^{18}F]-labeled tracer) will further broaden the experimental and clinical applications of this imaging approach.

PET will provide the opportunity to quantitatively map the pre- and postsynaptic innervation using a combination of tracers. No other imaging technique has the sensitivity or the biologic specificity to rival tracer techniques in the delineation of cardiac neuronal tissue. Thus, PET is and will remain an attractive research tool to investigate the relation between cardiac disease and autonomic innervation. It is hoped that this research will continue to lead to a wider clinical application and potentially new therapeutic strategies.

REFERENCES

1. Cohn J. The sympathetic nervous system in heart failure. *J Cardiovasc Pharmacol* 1989;5.
2. Barron HV, Lesh MD. Autonomic nervous system and sudden cardiac death. *J Am Coll Cardiol* 1996;27:1053–1560.
3. Kline R, Swanson D, Wieland D. Myocardial imaging in man with I-123 meta-iodobenzylguanidine. *J Nucl Med* 1981;22:129–132.
4. Wieland D, Brown L, Rogers W, et al. Myocardial imaging with a radioiodinated norepinephrine storage analog. *J Nucl Med* 1981;22: 22–31.
5. Rosenspire KC, Haka MS, Van Dort ME, et al. Synthesis and preliminary evaluation of carbon-11-meta-hydroxyephedrine: a false transmitter agent for heart neuronal imaging. *J Nucl Med* 1990;31: 1328–1334.
6. Schwaiger M, Hutchins G, Rosenspire K, et al. Quantitative evaluation of the sympathetic nervous system by PET in patients with cardiomyopathy. *J Nucl Med* 1990;31:792(abst).
7. Goldstein DS, Chang PC, Eisenhofer G, et al. Positron emission tomographic imaging of cardiac sympathetic innervation and function. *Circulation* 1990;81:1606–1621.
8. Goldstein DS, Eisenhofer G, Dunn BB, et al. Positron emission tomographic imaging of cardiac sympathetic innervation using 6-[^{18}F]fluorodopamine: initial findings in humans. *J Am Coll Cardiol* 1993;22: 1961–1971.
9. Munch G, Nguyen NT, Nekolla S, et al. Evaluation of sympathetic nerve terminals with [(^{11})C]epinephrine and [(^{11})C]hydroxyephedrine and positron emission tomography. *Circulation* 2000;101:516–523.
10. Raffel DM, Corbett JR, del Rosario RB, et al. Clinical evaluation of carbon-11-phenylephrine: MAO-sensitive marker of cardiac sympathetic neurons. *J Nucl Med* 1996;37:1923–1931.
11. Merlet P, Delforge J, Syrota A, et al. Positron emission tomography with ^{11}C CGP-12177 to assess beta-adrenergic receptor concentration in idiopathic dilated cardiomyopathy. *Circulation* 1993;87:1169–1178.
12. Randall W, Ardell J. Functional anatomy of the cardiac efferent innervation. In: Kulbertus H, Franck G, eds. *Neurocardiology*. New York: Futura Publishing, 1988:3–24.
13. Pierpont G, DeMaster E, Reynolds S, et al. Ventricular myocardial catecholamines in primates. *J Lab Clin Med* 1985;106:205–210.
14. Schmid P, Freif B, Lund D, et al. Regional choline acetyltransferase activity in the guinea pig heart. *Circ Res* 1978;42:657–660.
15. Crout J. The uptake and release of ^{3}H-epinephrine by the guinea pig heart *in vivo*. *Naunyn-Schmiedebergs Arch Pharmacol* 1964;248: 85–98.
16. Francis GS. Modulation of peripheral sympathetic nerve transmission. *J Am Coll Cardiol* 1988;12:250–254.
17. Kilbourn M, Potter E, Mc Closkey D. Neuromodulation of the cardiac vagus: comparison of neuropeptide Y and related peptides. *Reg Pep* 1985;12:155–162.
18. Jaques S Jr, Tobes M, Sisson J, et al. Comparison of the sodium dependency of uptake of meta-iodobenzylguanidine and norepinephrine into cultured bovine adrenomedullary cells. *Mol Pharmacol* 1984;26: 539–546.
19. Schomig A. Catecholamines in myocardial ischemia. Systemic and cardiac release. *Circulation* 1990;82:II13–II22.
20. Russ H, Gliese M, Sonna J, et al. The extraneuronal transport mechanism for noradrenaline (uptake-2) avidly transports 1-methyl-4-phenylpyridinium (MPP+). *Naunyn Schmiedebergs Arch Pharmacol* 1992;346:158–165.
21. Salt PJ. Inhibition of noradrenaline uptake 2 in the isolated rat heart by steroids, clonidine and methoxylated phenylethylamines. *Eur J Pharmacol* 1972;20:329–340.
22. Ducis I. The high-affinity choline uptake system. In: Whittaker V, ed. *The cholinergic synapse*. New York: Springer-Verlag, 1988:409–445.
23. Dae MW, Herre JM, O'Connell JW, et al. Scintigraphic assessment of sympathetic innervation after transmural versus nontransmural myocardial infarction. *J Am Coll Cardiol* 1991;17:1416–1423.
24. Wieland DM, Rosenspire KC, Hutchins GD, et al. Neuronal mapping of the heart with 6-[^{18}]fluorometaraminol. *J Nedicinal Chem* 1990;33: 956–964.
25. Schwaiger M, Guiborg H, Rosenspire K, et al. Effect of regional myocardial ischemia on sympathetic nervous system as assessed by fluorine-18-metaraminol. *J Nucl Med* 1990;31:1352–1357.
26. Rosenspire K, Haka M, Jewett D, et al. Synthesis and preliminary evaluation of ^{11}C-meta-hydroxyephedrine: a false transmitter agent for heart neuronal imaging. *J Nucl Med* 1990;31:1328–1334.
27. DeGrado TR, Hutchins GD, Toorongian SA, et al. Myocardial kinetics of carbon-11-meta-hydroxyephedrine: retention mechanisms and effects of norepinephrine. *J Nucl Med* 1993;34:1287–1293.
28. Chakraborty PK, Gildersleeve DL, Jewett DM, et al. High yield synthesis of high specific activity R-(–)-[^{11}C]epinephrine for routine PET studies in humans. *Nucl Med Biol* 1993;20:939–944.
29. Nguyen NT, DeGrado TR, Chakraborty P, et al. Myocardial kinetics of carbon-11-epinephrine in the isolated working rat heart. *J Nucl Med* 1997;38:780–785.
30. Raffel DM, Chen W, Sherman PS, et al. Dependence of cardiac ^{11}C-meta-hydroxyephedrine retention on norepinephrine transporter density. *J Nucl Med* 2006;47:1490–1496.
31. Del Rosario RB, Jung YW, Caraher J, et al. Synthesis and preliminary evaluation of [^{11}C]-(–)-phenylephrine as a functional heart neuronal PET agent. *Nucl Med Biol* 1996;23:611–616.
32. Raffel DM, Wieland DM. Influence of vesicular storage and monoamine oxidase activity on [^{11}C]phenylephrine kinetics: studies in isolated rat heart. *J Nucl Med* 1999;40:323–330.
33. Goldstein DS, Coronado L, Kopin IJ. 6-[Fluorine-18]fluorodopamine pharmacokinetics and dosimetry in humans. *J Nucl Med* 1994;35: 964–973.
34. Ding Y, Fowler J, Dewey S, et al. Comparison of high specific activity (–) and (+)-6-^{18}F-fluoronorepinephrine and 6-^{18}F-fluorodopamine in baboons: heart uptake, metabolism and the effect of desipramine. *J Nucl Med* 1993;34:619–629.
35. Berry CR, Garg PK, Zalutsky MR, et al. Uptake and retention kinetics of para-fluorine-18-fluorobenzylguanidine in isolated rat heart. *J Nucl Med* 1996;37:2011–2016.
36. Raffel D, Loc'h C, Mardon K, et al. Kinetics of the norepinephrine analog [^{76}Br]-meta-bromobenzylguanidine in isolated working rat heart. *Nucl Med Biol* 1998;25:1–16.
37. Rogers G, Parsons S, Anderson D, et al. Synthesis in vitro acetylcholine-storage-blocking activities, and biological properties of derivatives and analogues of trans-2-(4-phenylpiperidino)cyclohexanol (vesamicol). *J Med Chem* 1989;32:1217–1230.
38. Jung YW, Van Dort ME, Gildersleeve DL, et al. A radiotracer for mapping cholinergic neurons of the brain. *J Med Chem* 1990;33:2065–2068.
39. DeGrado TR, Mulholland GK, Wieland DM, et al. Evaluation of (–)[^{18}F]fluoroethoxybenzovesamicol as a new PET tracer of cholinergic neurons of the heart. *Nucl Med Biol* 1994;21:189–195.
40. Vatner DE, Asai K, Iwase M, et al. Beta-adrenergic receptor-G protein-adenylyl cyclase signal transduction in the failing heart. *Am J Cardiol* 1999;83:80H–85H.
41. Xiao RP, Cheng H, Zhou YY, et al. Recent advances in cardiac beta(2)-adrenergic signal transduction. *Circ Res* 1999;85:1092–1100.

42. Ungerer M, Weig HJ, Kubert S, et al. Regional pre- and postsynaptic sympathetic system in the failing human heart—regulation of beta ARK-1. *Eur J Heart Fail* 2000;2:23–31.
43. Delforge J, Syrota A, Lancon JP, et al. Cardiac beta-adrenergic receptor density measured in vivo using PET, CGP 12177, and a new graphical method [erratum appears in J Nucl Med 1994;35(5):921]. *J Nucl Med* 1991;32:739–748.
44. Elsinga PH, Doze P, van Waarde A, et al. Imaging of beta-adrenoceptors in the human thorax using (S)-[(^{11})C]CGP12388 and positron emission tomography. *Eur J Pharmacol* 2001;433:173–176.
45. de Jong RM, Willemsen AT, Slart RH, et al. Myocardial beta-adrenoceptor downregulation in idiopathic dilated cardiomyopathy measured in vivo with PET using the new radioligand (S)-[^{11}C]CGP12388. *Eur J Nucl Med Mol Imaging* 2005;32:443–447.
46. Momose M, Reder S, Raffel DM, et al. Evaluation of cardiac beta-adrenoreceptors in the isolated perfused rat heart using (S)-^{11}C-CGP12388. *J Nucl Med* 2004;45:471–477.
47. Law MP, Osman S, Pike VW, et al. Evaluation of [^{11}C]GB67, a novel radioligand for imaging myocardial alpha 1-adrenoceptors with positron emission tomography. *Eur J Nucl Med* 2000;27:7–17.
48. Delforge J, Le Guludec D, Syrota A, et al. Quantification of myocardial muscarinic receptors with PET in humans. *J Nucl Med* 1993;34: 981–991.
49. Syrota A, Comar D, Paillotin G, et al. Muscarinic cholinergic receptor in the human heart evidenced under physiological conditions by positron emission tomography. *Proc Natl Acad Sci U S A* 1985;82:584–588.
50. Allman KC, Stevens MJ, Wieland DM, et al. Noninvasive assessment of cardiac diabetic neuropathy by carbon-11 hydroxyephedrine and positron emission tomography. *J Am Coll Cardiol* 1993;22:1425–1432.
51. Allman KC, Wieland DM, Muzik O, et al. Carbon-11 hydroxyephedrine with positron emission tomography for serial assessment of cardiac adrenergic neuronal function after acute myocardial infarction in humans. *J Am Coll Cardiol* 1993;22:368–375.
52. Bengel FM, Ueberfuhr P, Schiepel N, et al. Effect of sympathetic reinnervation on cardiac performance after heart transplantation. *N Engl J Med* 2001;345:731–738.
53. Calkins H, Allman K, Bolling S, et al. Correlation between scintigraphic evidence of regional sympathetic neuronal dysfunction and ventricular refractoriness in the human heart. *Circulation* 1993;88:173–179.
54. Schwaiger M, Hutchins GD, Kalff V, et al. Evidence for regional catecholamine uptake and storage sites in the transplanted human heart by positron emission tomography. *J Clin Invest* 1991;87:1681–1690.
55. Schwaiger M, Kalff V, Rosenspire K, et al. Noninvasive evaluation of sympathetic nervous system in human heart by positron emission tomography. *Circulation* 1990;82:457–464.
56. Schafers M, Dutka D, Rhodes CG, et al. Myocardial presynaptic and postsynaptic autonomic dysfunction in hypertrophic cardiomyopathy. *Circ Res* 1998;82:57–62.
57. Schafers M, Lerch H, Wichter T, et al. Cardiac sympathetic innervation in patients with idiopathic right ventricular outflow tract tachycardia. *J Am Coll Cardiol* 1998;32:181–186.
58. Wichter T, Schafers M, Rhodes CG, et al. Abnormalities of cardiac sympathetic innervation in arrhythmogenic right ventricular cardiomyopathy: quantitative assessment of presynaptic norepinephrine reuptake and postsynaptic beta-adrenergic receptor density with positron emission tomography. *Circulation* 2000;101:1552–1558.
59. Hartmann F, Ziegler S, Nekolla S, et al. Regional patterns of myocardial sympathetic denervation in dilated cardiomyopathy: an analysis using carbon-11 hydroxyephedrine and positron emission tomography. *Heart* 1999;81:262–270.
60. Ungerer M, Hartmann F, Karoglan M, et al. Regional in vivo and in vitro characterization of autonomic innervation in cardiomyopathic human heart. *Circulation* 1998;97:174–180.
61. Barber MJ, Mueller TM, Henry DP, et al. Transmural myocardial infarction in the dog produces sympathectomy in noninfarcted myocardium. *Circulation* 1983;67:787–796.
62. Fagret D, Wolf JE, Comet M. Myocardial uptake of meta-[^{123}I]-iodobenzylguanidine [(^{123}I]-MIBG) in patients with myocardial infarct. *Eur J Nucl Med* 1989;15:624–628.
63. Minardo J, Tuli M, Mock B, et al. Scintigraphic and electrophysiological evidence of canine myocardial sympathetic denervation and reinnervation produced by myocardial infarction or phenol application. *Circulation* 1988;1988:1008–1019.
64. Stanton MS, Tuli MM, Radtke NL, et al. Regional sympathetic denervation after myocardial infarction in humans detected noninvasively using I-123-metaiodobenzylguanidine. *J Am Coll Cardiol* 1989;14:1519–1526.
65. Wolpers H, Nguyen N, Rosenspire K, et al. C-11 hydroxyephedrine as marker for neuronal dysfunction in reperfused canine myocardium. *Coron Artery Dis* 1991;2:923–929.
66. Matsunari I, Schricke U, Bengel FM, et al. Extent of cardiac sympathetic neuronal damage is determined by the area of ischemia in patients with acute coronary syndromes. *Circulation* 2000;101:2579–2585.
67. Bulow HP, Stahl F, Lauer B, et al. Alterations of myocardial presynaptic sympathetic innervation in patients with multi-vessel coronary artery disease but without history of myocardial infarction. *Nucl Med Commun* 2003;24:233–239.
68. Hartikainen J, Kuikka J, Mantysaari M, et al. Sympathetic reinnervation after acute myocardial infarction. *Am J Cardiol* 1996;77:5–9.
69. Fallen EL, Coates G, Nahmias C, et al. Recovery rates of regional sympathetic reinnervation and myocardial blood flow after acute myocardial infarction. *Am Heart J* 1999;137:863–869.
70. Corr PB, Gillis RA. Autonomic neural influences on the dysrhythmias resulting from myocardial infarction. *Circ Res* 1978;43:1–9.
71. Inoue H, Zipes D. Results of sympathetic denervation in the canine heart: Supersensitivity that may be arrhythmogenic. *Circulation* 1987;75: 877–887.
72. Wichter T, Hindricks G, Lerch H, et al. Regional myocardial sympathetic dysinnervation in arrhythmogenic right ventricular cardiomyopathy. An analysis using ^{123}I-meta-iodobenzylguanidine scintigraphy. *Circulation* 1994;89:667–683.
73. Mazzadi AN, Andre-Fouet X, Duisit J, et al. Heterogeneous cardiac retention of ^{11}C-hydroxyephedrine in genotyped long QT patients. A potential amplifier role for severity of the disease. *Am J Physiol Heart Circ Physiol* 2003;285:H1286–H1293.
74. Calkins H, Lohmann MH, Allman K, et al. Scintigraphic pattern of regional cardiac sympathetic innervation in patients with familial long QT syndrome using positron emission tomography. *Circulation* 1993;87: 1616–1621.
75. Ewing DJ, Campbell IW, Clarke BF. The natural history of diabetic autonomic neuropathy. *Q J Med* 1980;49:95–108.
76. Stevens MJ, Raffel DM, Allman KC, et al. Cardiac sympathetic dysinnervation in diabetes: implications for enhanced cardiovascular risk. *Circulation* 1998;98:961–968.
77. Stevens MJ, Dayanikli F, Raffel DM, et al. Scintigraphic assessment of regionalized defects in myocardial sympathetic innervation and blood flow regulation in diabetic patients with autonomic neuropathy. *J Am Coll Cardiol* 1998;31:1575–1584.
78. Ziegler S, Frey A, Überfuhr P, et al. Assessment of myocardial reinnervation in cardiac transplants by positron emission tomography: functional significance tested by heart rate variability. *Clin Sci* 1996;91 [Suppl]:126–128.
79. Odaka K, von Scheidt W, Ziegler SI, et al. Reappearance of cardiac presynaptic sympathetic nerve terminals in the transplanted heart: correlation between PET using (^{11})C-hydroxyephedrine and invasively measured norepinephrine release. *J Nucl Med* 2001;42:1011–1016.
80. Bengel FM, Ueberfuhr P, Ziegler SI, et al. Serial assessment of sympathetic reinnervation after orthotopic heart transplantation. A longitudinal study using PET and C-11 hydroxyephedrine. *Circulation* 1999;99: 1866–1871.
81. Bengel FM, Ueberfuhr P, Hesse T, et al. Clinical determinants of ventricular sympathetic reinnervation after orthotopic heart transplantation. *Circulation* 2002;106:831–835.

82. Bengel FM, Ueberfuhr P, Ziegler SI, et al. Non-invasive assessment of the effect of cardiac sympathetic innervation on metabolism of the human heart. *Eur J Nucl Med* 2000;27:1650–1657.
83. Schwaiblmair M, von Scheidt W, Uberfuhr P, et al. Functional significance of cardiac reinnervation in heart transplant recipients. *J Heart Lung Transplant* 1999;18:838–845.
84. Bristow MR. The autonomic nervous system in heart failure. *N Engl J Med* 1984;311:850–851.
85. Cohn JN, Levine TB, Olivari MT, et al. Plasma norepinephrine as a guide to prognosis in patients with chronic congestive heart failure. *N Engl J Med* 1984;311:819–823.
86. Glowniak J, Turner F, Gray L, et al. Iodine-123 metaiodobenzylguanidine imaging of the heart in idiopathic congestive cardiomyopathy and cardiac transplants. *J Nucl Med* 1989;30:1182–1191.
87. Merlet P, Valette H, Dubois-Rande J, et al. Prognostic value of cardiac metaiodobenzylguanidine imaging in patients with heart failure. *J Nucl Med* 1992;33:471.
88. Imamura Y, Ando H, Mitsuoka W, et al. Iodine-123 metaiodobenzylguanidine images reflect intense myocardial adrenergic nervous activity in congestive heart failure independent of underlying cause. *J Am Coll Cardiol* 1995;26:1594–1599.
89. Schwaiger M, Beanlands R, vom Dahl J. Metabolic tissue characterization in the failing heart by positron emission tomography. *Eur Heart J* 1994;15:14–19.
90. Vesalainen RK, Pietila M, Tahvanainen KU, et al. Cardiac positron emission tomography imaging with $[^{11}C]$hydroxyephedrine, a specific tracer for sympathetic nerve endings, and its functional correlates in congestive heart failure. *Am J Cardiol* 1999;84:568–574.
91. Bengel FM, Permanetter B, Ungerer M, et al. Relationship between altered sympathetic innervation, oxidative metabolism and contractile function in the cardiomyopathic human heart; a non-invasive study using positron emission tomography. *Eur Heart J* 2001;22: 1594–1600.
92. Bengel FM, Permanetter B, Ungerer M, et al. Alterations of the sympathetic nervous system and metabolic performance of the cardiomyopathic heart. *Eur J Nucl Med Mol Imaging* 2002;29:198–202.
93. Le Guludec D, Cohen-Solal A, Delforge J, et al. Increased myocardial muscarinic receptor density in idiopathic dilated cardiomyopathy: an in vivo PET study. *Circulation* 1997;96:3416–3422.
94. Pietila M, Malminiemi K, Ukkonen H, et al. Reduced myocardial carbon-11 hydroxyephedrine retention is associated with poor prognosis in chronic heart failure. *Eur J Nucl Med* 2001;28:373–376.

CHAPTER 12

PET/CT Imaging of Infection and Inflammation

ORA ISRAEL

Nuclear medicine plays an important role in the assessment of a multitude of infectious and inflammatory processes. Functional scintigraphic procedures are part of the noninvasive diagnostic armamentarium for assessment of infection and inflammation and should be viewed by the referring clinicians and the imaging community as complementary to, and not as competing with, anatomic modalities such as x-rays, computed tomography (CT), magnetic resonance imaging (MRI), or ultrasound. A number of radiotracers using single-photon emitting radionuclides have served for decades as infection and inflammation-seeking agents. The widest experience has been gained with gallium-67 ([^{67}Ga]) and leukocytes (white blood cells [WBC]) radiolabeled with either technetium-99m (^{99m}Tc) or indium-111 ([^{111}In]). Immunoscintigraphy using various labeled antibodies has also been introduced in recent years using single photon agents and is in clinical use in many parts of the world

With the increasing use of fluorine-18-fluorodeoxyglucose ([^{18}F]-FDG) for assessment of malignancies, uptake of this positron-emitting tracer in nonmalignant processes has also been described. FDG is a tumor-seeking, but not a tumor-specific, imaging agent. Accumulation of increased FDG uptake in benign, infectious, and inflammatory processes was initially described as an incidental finding, labeled as a pitfall and cited as a cause for false-positive results in imaging cancer patients (1). This initial observation was followed by the understanding that diagnosis and monitoring of infectious and inflammatory processes may represent an additional important indication for FDG positron emission tomography (PET) imaging.

The further technological development of the hybrid PET/CT technology (2,3) has given a new dimension to combined metabolic and anatomic evaluation of infection and inflammation, with a significant impact on patient care as currently demonstrated by an increasing number of publications in ever expanding clinical indications.

MECHANISM OF FLUORODEOXYGLUCOSE UPTAKE AND TECHNICAL ASPECTS OF PET/CT IN INFECTION AND INFLAMMATION

The basis for FDG accumulation in malignant cells has been extensively described in other chapters of this book. However, cancer is not the only process characterized by increased glycolysis and glucose utilization. Inflammatory cells such as activated lymphocytes, neutrophils, and macrophages are present in infectious and inflammatory processes. Similar to malignant cells, they exhibit, high intracellular levels of hexokinase and increased expression of surface glucose transporter proteins with a high affinity for FDG, and sufficient intracellular adenosine triphosphate to allow phosphorylation of FDG to FDG 6-phosphate, and therefore develop a high cytoplasmic concentration of the phosphorylated product (4–6). Activated cells present in inflammatory and infectious processes also have a high capacity for accumulating FDG, probably due to their stimulation by large amounts of cytokines and growth factors among other factors (7).

The initial incidental clinical observation of FDG uptake in nonmalignant processes has been further evaluated in animal models, confirming the affinity of this tracer for benign hypermetabolic processes (6,8,9). Experimental studies have demonstrated increased glucose uptake in inflammatory cells during the acute stage of the process (9,10). Abscess forming bacteria use glucose as their energy substrate (11). Furthermore, FDG uptake in experimental infectious processes, expressed as the lesion to background ratio, was higher when compared to that of [^{67}Ga] (12).

The next step was the implementation of these experimental results to patient studies, specifically challenging the hypothesis that FDG PET may be used in the clinical setting for imaging and evaluation of infection and inflammation in humans. FDG is taken up by most infectious and inflammatory processes in a large variety of organs. This was documented first by case reports appearing in the literature over more than two decades, followed in recent years by studies involving larger number of patients. One of the early papers describing the use of FDG PET for detection of infection evaluated 11 patients with known or suspected infectious processes. FDG PET correctly diagnosed 10 of 11 patients (13).

The development of this field of clinical research and practice has progressed at a relatively slow pace for a number of reasons. Failure, at the time this chapter was written, to reimburse PET studies performed for assessment of infection has limited its use to a few academic centers with a specific research interest in the field. In addition, the relatively long list of differential diagnoses for FDG-avid sites and the low spatial resolution of early stand-alone PET imaging devices have made precise definition of suspicious lesions difficult. This raised concerns about the certainty of the reported findings, their etiology, and localization.

The use of hybrid imaging in general, and PET/CT specifically, in the evaluation of infectious and inflammatory processes, similar to their implementation for cancer imaging, has decreased the overall uncertainty and the number of equivocal readings (3,14). In order to improve the differential diagnosis between malignant and infectious or inflammatory processes, the use of threshold standard uptake value (SUV) measurements have also been recommended by some, as well as dual time point acquisition showing different dynamics of FDG retention in lesions with a different etiology (15,16).

A number of practical advantages make FDG PET/CT one of the procedures of choice for assessment of patients with infection and inflammation. [^{18}F] has good physical properties and FDG has good tracer kinetics with rapid accumulation in infections, better than that of single-photon emitting radionuclides used in this clinical context. The short physical half-life is responsible for lower radiation doses delivered to patients who undergo, as a rule, a large number of imaging procedures using ionizing radiation. The fact that the physical characteristics of the agent require the procedure to be performed within an approximate time of 2 hours should not be viewed as a limitation, but rather represents an additional advantage by providing clinical results within a short time span. In addition, PET devices provide images with better spatial resolution and higher contrast as compared to single-photon emission computed tomography.

Limitations of FDG imaging of infection and inflammation are related in part to the normal tracer biodistribution of FDG. Lesions or suspicious FDG-avid foci located in organs with, or in close vicinity to areas of high physiologic tracer concentration may be misinterpreted as false-positive as well as false-negative findings. The recent addition of a CT component to PET in the form of PET/CT has lead to improvement in the spatial localization of findings and makes this less of a limiting factor both in patients with malignancy and in those assessed for the presence or the suspicion of an infectious process.

Infection is a major and severe complication of patients with diabetes mellitus. FDG imaging may have a lower sensitivity in the presence of high blood glucose levels (17). A decrease in FDG uptake in experimental inflammatory and infectious processes has been found in the presence of high serum glucose levels due to a decreased expression of glucose transporters (GLUT1 and GLUT3) and also due to direct competition with unlabeled glucose for tracer uptake (18). Preliminary patient studies suggest, however, that this factor does not represent a major limitation for assessment of infectious processes in the clinical setting (19,20).

An additional practical issue that has not yet received sufficient evaluation is the potential influence of prior antibiotic treatment on FDG uptake. Although relevant evidence in literature data is still lacking at present, it is suggested that the sensitivity of FDG imaging decreases in partially treated infectious processes.

FLUORODEOXYGLUCOSE PET/CT IMAGING OF MUSCULOSKELETAL INFECTION AND INFLAMMATION

The use of FDG PET for diagnosis and monitoring patients with suspected infectious or inflammatory processes involving the musculoskeletal system is one of the most extensively investigated non-cancer-related areas of research for clinical PET/CT.

Diagnosis of Acute or Chronic Osteomyelitis

For decades, nuclear medicine techniques have played a role in diagnosis of acute and chronic osteomyelitis, mainly with the use of three-phase bone scintigraphy, labeled WBCs with or without bone marrow imaging, and [^{67}Ga] scintigraphy. Although these procedures still are, at present, principal diagnostic tools in routine clinical scenarios, FDG has been shown to accumulate in infectious processes involving the bone. FDG PET imaging has been advocated for the more complicated diagnostic challenges, such as diagnosis of chronic osteomyelitis, frequently resulting from a continuing, insufficiently treated acute infection, vertebral osteomyelitis or discitis, and bone infection in diabetic patients, mainly the diabetic foot.

Chronic osteomyelitis is defined, as a rule, as an infectious process involving the skeleton that requires more than a single episode of treatment and persists for more than 6 weeks (21). Diagnosis is difficult since the prolonged infectious process, as well as previous treatment, can frequently alter the normal regional bone anatomy and physiology and also due to the low-grade nature of the disease (22). A variety of imaging techniques have been used for noninvasive diagnosis of chronic osteomyelitis, including plain x-rays, CT, MRI, general nuclear medicine techniques, and FDG PET.

Among the studies that assess the role of FDG PET for imaging chronic infection of the bone, most have demonstrated a high sensitivity and a specificity ranging between 88% to 92% (23,24). FDG PET was found to be superior to [^{111}In] WBC for assessment of chronic osteomyelitis (25). FDG PET was also assessed in 60 patients with a suspected chronic musculoskeletal infection involving the central or peripheral skeleton. All patients with a final diagnosis of chronic infection were correctly identified. The sensitivity, specificity, and accuracy of FDG PET were 100%, 88%, and 93%, respectively, similar for suspected infections in the axial and appendicular skeleton (26).

A recent meta-analysis provided a systematic review of 23 clinical studies reporting on the accuracy of the different imaging modalities for diagnosis of chronic osteomyelitis (22). The pooled data demonstrated that FDG PET imaging had the highest sensitivity, 96%, compared to 78% for combined bone and WBC scintigraphy, and 84% for MRI. The specificity of FDG PET was 91% as compared to 84% for combined bone and WBC scanning and 60% for MRI. The authors concluded that based on this extensive peer-reviewed data FDG PET surges as the modality with the highest diagnostic accuracy for diagnosis or exclusion of chronic osteomyelitis, in particular in the axial skeleton (22).

Diagnosis of vertebral or disc space infection, with an incidence of 2% to 4% of all cases of osteomyelitis, is another diagnostic dilemma, even with the extensive use of MRI (27). Conventional nuclear medicine infection-seeking tracers also have a lower sensitivity in the vertebrae or spine as compared to other skeletal sites. FDG PET was successfully used in 30 consecutive patients for the differential diagnosis of degenerative spinal disease versus disc-space infection and showed better performance, with a reported 100% sensitivity and specificity as compared to MRI, which had a sensitivity of 50% and a specificity of 96%. Although FDG PET is not recommended as the first-line diagnostic modality in patients with back pain of unclear etiology, the authors suggest its use in cases with equivocal MRI findings (28).

Infectious processes represent a major complication in patients with diabetes. Angiopathy and neuropathy induced by severe diabetes lead to infectious processes that can involve the skin, soft tissues, and bone, mainly in the pedal region. Differential diagnosis of the "diabetic foot" is important for patient management with the goal of defining various pathological processes that require different therapeutic strategies (29). Current treatment of early stage Charcot neuroarthropathy in the diabetic foot includes surgery if it has not been performed previously. In a study of 39 diabetic patients FDG PET successfully diagnosed Charcot joint lesions and was superior to MRI (30).

Clinical diagnosis of osteomyelitis in the feet of diabetic patients is important for further treatment planning, but difficult. Although PET can show the presence of an FDG-avid focus in sites of acute infection, PET/CT has been shown of value for differentiating between osteomyelitis and soft tissue infection (Fig. 12.1) (20). In a preliminary study involving 14 patients, FDG PET/CT correctly localized eight foci of abnormal tracer uptake to the bone and thus enabled the diagnosis of osteomyelitis. A single site of mild FDG activity was falsely interpreted as bone infection, while the final diagnosis indicated a Charcot joint. The precise localization provided by PET/CT with a subsequent correct diagnosis directed further treatment toward surgery in patients with osteomyelitis as compared to conservative treatment in patients with soft tissue infection (20).

Infection Involving Metallic Implants and Joint Prostheses

Pain is common in patients following implant of joint prostheses. The differential diagnosis of a painful joint transplant includes loosening as a result of mechanical failure or, in a smaller percentage of patients, periprosthetic infection (31). In spite of the similar clinical presentation, a preoperative differential diagnosis is essential, since they result in different treatment strategies, revision surgery as compared with long-term antibiotic therapy followed by surgery. Diagnosis of an infected joint prosthesis is made using a variety of laboratory tests, including microbiological cultures, imaging with conventional x-ray radiography, and general nuclear medicine procedures, which could include a combined approach of three-phase bone scintigraphy, an infectious-seeking agent, such as [^{67}Ga] scintigraphy, or labeled WBCs associated at times with bone marrow scintigraphy (32–34). However, this complex battery of diagnostic tests provides suboptimal results with a low sensitivity and specificity (35).

Patients with metallic implants after trauma or bone surgery can also present with a clinical suspicion of infection. Diagnosis of osteomyelitis in the complicated postsurgical bone is important but impaired by the low specificity of laboratory data and the relatively low performance of conventional anatomic imaging and nuclear medicine procedures. MRI, one of the major tools for assessment of musculoskeletal pathology in general, is of limited use in the

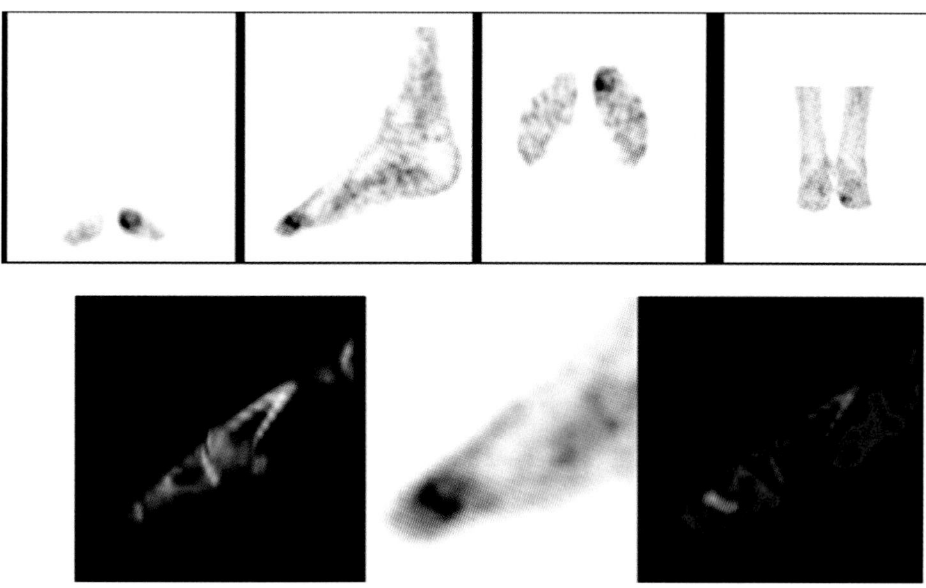

FIGURE 12.1. Diagnosis of osteomyelitis in a patient with local signs of infection involving the left first toe. **Upper row:** Axial, sagittal, and coronal PET slices, respectively, at the level of the toes and maximum intensity projection image of the feet (*far right*) demonstrate the presence of a focus of abnormal fluorodeoxyglucose activity in the left first toe. **Lower row:** Sagittal PET, PET/CT, and CT slices, respectively, localize the suspicious lesion to the distal part of the first left proximal phalanx, consistent with osteomyelitis.

presence of metallic devices due to technical artifacts and also to a variable and nonspecific imaging pattern (36).

Literature data with respect to FDG imaging of suspected infection of prosthetic joints has been accumulating. Initial studies have shown that FDG PET can differentiate loosening from infection of a joint transplant with variable accuracy (37,38). An early feasibility study evaluated FDG PET for diagnosis of 74 hip or knee prostheses suspected of infection. FDG PET had a sensitivity, specificity, and accuracy of 91%, 72%, and 78%, respectively, for assessment of knee prostheses, and 90% for all three indices in cases of hip arthroplasty, with an overall sensitivity of 91% and a specificity of 82% (38). In another study, FDG PET was evaluated and compared to three-phase bone scintigraphy in 92 hip joint prostheses in 63 patients (39). FDG PET had a sensitivity of 94%, and specificity and accuracy of 95%, significantly higher when compared with 68%, 76% and 74% respectively for bone scintigraphy. The authors, however caution that increased periprosthetic FDG uptake may be also found in patients with aseptic loosening due to tracer uptake in granulomatous tissue that develops around the implanted device. Indeed, the authors' own experience and that of other groups has shown that some uptake of radiotracer around joint prostheses is relatively common.

Another recent study assessed the performance of FDG PET in 27 patients prior to surgical revision procedures of hip and knee endoprostheses (40). Aseptic loosening was diagnosed with high (96%) sensitivity. FDG PET diagnosed all cases of infected arthroplasty and approximately half of the cases that showed an aseptic inflammatory reaction. These authors also conclude that, while a negative PET study may spare revision surgery, a positive result cannot give a clear differentiation between a septic process or an aseptic inflammation, caused as a rule by a foreign-body reaction. Thus, it appears that false-positive results represent a current challenge with the FDG PET approach.

Overall, FDG PET has a diagnostic accuracy ranging between 68% to 100% for assessment of patients with prostheses of the hip joint and between 78% to 100% in evaluation of knee arthroplasty (35). Positive FDG PET studies in patients with lower limb joint prostheses should be interpreted with caution. False-positive results occur due to the presence, sometime for decades, of nonspecific increased tracer activity in sites of granulomatotic tissue developing around the implant (41).

The diagnosis of infection in the postoperative spine, as well as in complicated bones following fractures or surgery, remains a diagnostic challenge, and FDG PET imaging has been assessed in this group of patients. Although in most studies these patients are analyzed as part of a larger population with various clinical scenarios, without addressing the performance of FDG imaging in this specific group, authors agree that it represents a promising diagnostic imaging test. A study assessing FDG PET in 29 patients with a suspicion of metallic implant–associated infections after trauma indicated a sensitivity of 100%, specificity of 93%, and accuracy of 97%, higher for lesions in the axial skeleton. Furthermore, the referring physicians reported an impact of FDG PET reports on further patient care in almost two of three patients in this series (42).

Assessment of FDG PET in 57 patients suspected of having spinal infection after previous surgery of the vertebral column showed a sensitivity of 100%, specificity of 81%, and accuracy of 86%, with most of the false-positive studies occurring over a longer postoperative period and in the presence of metallic implants (43). Hybrid PET/CT will further improve the diagnostic capabilities of FDG imaging by reducing the number of false-positive reports (44).

Only a few studies have reported on the use of combined PET/CT devices in suspected infection after arthroplasty. Early studies have described the presence of metal artifacts that can decrease the accuracy of x-ray attenuation correction in the clinical context of assessing patients with arthroplasty (45–47). It is therefore recommend to routinely assess both corrected and uncorrected PET images in order to decrease the rate of false-positive reports related to artifactually increased FDG activity (35).

A recent study evaluated 33 patients after trauma with suspected osteomyelitis in the axial or peripheral skeleton using FDG PET/CT, with 18 of these patients having a metallic implant. The sensitivity, specificity, and accuracy were 94%, 87%, and 91%, respectively. The authors conclude that FDG PET/CT is an accurate method for the evaluation of chronic infection in patients after trauma, regardless of the presence of metallic devices. The use of fused images enables accurate diagnosis with precise anatomical localization of the suspicious site and precise delineation of the extent of the infectious process (48).

Inflammatory Joint Diseases

Inflammatory processes involving the joints, such as rheumatoid arthritis, degenerative diseases, or synovitis, have been reported to show increased FDG activity of moderate intensity (49). The whole-body capability of PET/CT and the ability to detect changes in the degree of metabolic activity make FDG imaging a potentially useful tool for defining the extent of disease and for monitoring response to treatment. If a site of increased FDG uptake is located on PET/CT in the periarticular synovia the potential of an active arthritic process should be raised.

In patients with rheumatoid arthritis the degree and extent of FDG uptake is related to the intensity of clinical symptoms such as pain, swelling, and tenderness (50). A study assessing over 300 joints in 21 patients showed that the degree of synovial FDG uptake is a good and reliable index of disease activity (51). Further studies are needed to define the role of FDG PET/CT imaging in patients with active arthritic processes, for diagnosis of early stage disease, for monitoring response to treatment, or when there is a suspicion of exacerbation with an acute or chronic process.

Increased FDG uptake has been also described in patients with osteoarthritis, mainly as incidental findings during routine assessment of cancer patients (52). PET/CT localization of increased FDG uptake to an intra-articular space is again the clue for exclusion of metastatic disease (Fig. 12.2).

FLUORODEOXYGLUCOSE PET/CT IMAGING OF FEVER OF UNKNOWN ORIGIN AND FOCAL SOFT TISSUE INFECTIONS

Fever of unknown origin (FUO) defines a large number of entities characterized by prolonged (more than 3 weeks) hyperthermia (over 38.3°C/101°F) of no specific etiology in spite of an extensive diagnostic work-up. Although some of the processes defined as FUO are self-limited and resolve without any specific treatment, a variety of diseases that have severe outcome consequences if untreated can present with this clinical picture. This is the reason

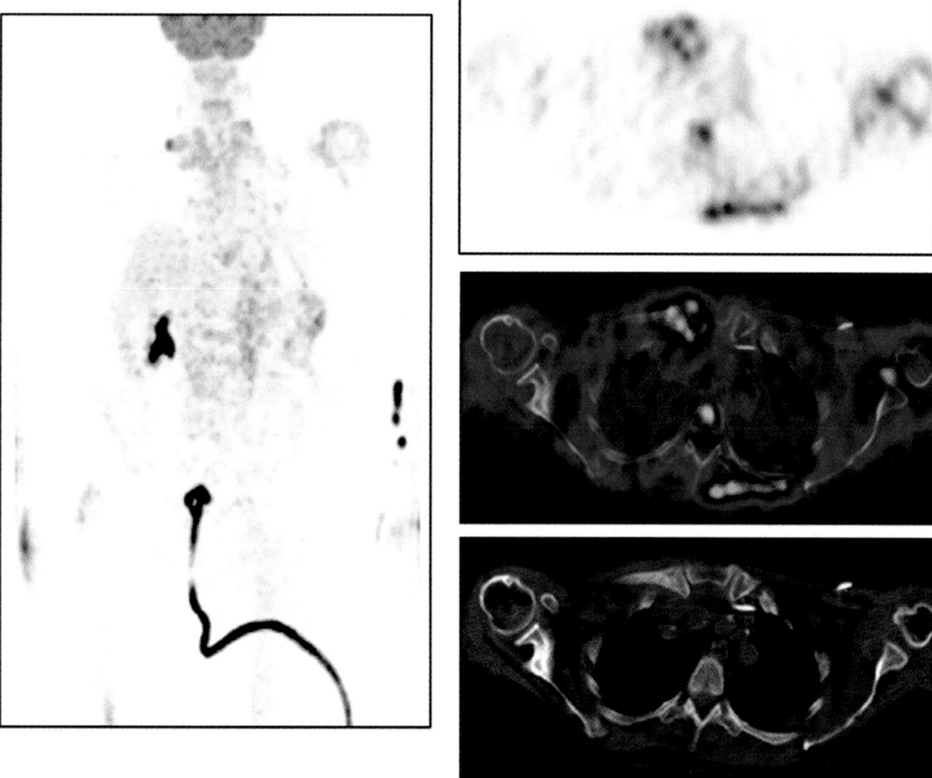

FIGURE 12.2. Localization of multiple infectious foci to bone, soft tissues, and periarticular space in a patient presenting with fever and swelling of the left shoulder and sepsis, 14 days following an epidural block for severe back pain. **Left:** Maximum intensity projection image demonstrates the presence of abnormal fluorodeoxyglucose (FDG) uptake in the upper right and left thorax and left shoulder. **Right:** Axial PET, PET/CT, and CT slices, respectively, at the level of the upper chest indicate the presence of pathological FDG uptake involving the proximal third of the right clavicle, consistent with osteomyelitis, the left paraspinatus muscle, consistent with an abscess, and the intra-articular space in the left shoulder, consistent with septic arthritis.

for the diagnostic effort invested by clinicians in finding the cause for FUO, a work-up that has major impact on patient care and also puts a substantial financial burden on the health system.

The differential diagnosis of FUO includes over 200 causes that have been reported and can be classified into four major categories: infectious, malignant, aseptic inflammatory processes, and miscellaneous (53). Infections represent the main etiology in up to 30% of patients (54,55), mostly of bacterial origin, and include diseases such as tuberculosis, abdominopelvic abscesses, endocarditis or osteomyelitis, and, less frequently, viral infections due to agents such as cytomegalovirus, Epstein-Barr virus, or human immunodeficiency virus (HIV). The second more common cause for FUO are malignancies, mainly lymphoma, leukemia, renal cell carcinoma, or metastatic tumors to the liver, followed by inflammatory processes such as arthritis, arteritis, or other vasculitic processes, inflammatory bowel disease, or systemic lupus erythematosus (54,55). Additional diseases that can cause FUO, include, among others, drug-induced fever and deep vein thrombosis (55).

Although diagnosis of the cause of FUO is difficult, the goal of extensive evaluation of patients with prolonged fever is to reach 90% of patients who should have a recognizable etiology (56). Diagnostic techniques involve a variety of laboratory, imaging, and invasive procedures. Imaging for FUO includes most anatomic modalities, conventional x-rays, ultrasound, CT, and MRI (57,58). General nuclear medicine procedures are also widely performed using tracers such as [^{67}Ga], [^{111}In], or ^{99m}Tc WBC-labeled antibodies, and antibiotics, however, with limited and variable rates of success (59–61).

The potential role of FDG PET in the work-up of patients with FUO was evaluated. FDG is taken up by many infectious processes and inflammatory entities, and imaging of the whole body is of greater importance when the unknown focus of infection can be localized in any region of the body. The overall capability of FDG PET to provide clinically useful information in patients with FUO ranges in the early literature data between 35% to 70% (62–66). The results reported, however, are based on studies performed in a small number of patients, using at times insufficient doses of FDG and imaging devices with variable technical performance capabilities.

One of the early studies reported that FDG PET diagnosed the etiology of prolonged hyperthermia in 11 of 16 patients with FUO, including mainly infectious and connective tissue processes, and one case of malignancy (64). PET was negative in two patients with further diagnosed rheumatic fever and in two patients for whom no final diagnosis could be established and then recovered within 3 months, spontaneously or with nonspecific antibiotic treatment. An additional study assessed the value of FDG PET in a group of 58 patients with FUO (62). In this group the final etiology of prolonged fever was established in only 69% of patients. FDG PET was positive in 79% and helpful for establishing the final diagnosis by correctly identifying the source of fever in 41% of the patients. In the same study the performance of FDG PET was compared and found to have a higher sensitivity than [^{67}Ga] scintigraphy in a subgroup of 40 patients.

The performance indices of FDG PET were also evaluated in a study involving 35 patients with FUO (65). FDG PET had a sensitivity of 93%, specificity of 90%, positive predictive value of 87%, and a negative predictive value of 95% for defining the cause of FUO, with clinically helpful studies in 65% of patients. FDG PET correctly pointed to the source of fever in 13 patients, but was false positive in two patients, including one patient with focal colonic tracer uptake and one patient with increased FDG activity in multiple lymph nodes. Histological tissue sampling was negative and fever resolved in both patients, with no further evidence of disease in the suspected sites. FDG PET was true negative in 94% of patients with no evidence of focal infection, and in those without a known cause of FUO. A study involving 74 prospectively collected patients, with a final diagnosis established in 53% of the group, indicated that FDG PET was positive in 53 of 74 patients (72%) (66). Based on the final diagnosis, 36% of the positive studies were considered to be clinically helpful.

Studies assessing the role of FDG PET in patients with FUO concluded that the potential of this functional imaging modality for guiding further testing required final validation of the PET results with high-resolution anatomic imaging techniques (67). This is now performed in a single step PET/CT acquisition (Fig. 12.3). A study assessing a large group of 118 subjects included a subgroup of patients assessed with PET/CT. In this report FDG PET or PET/CT was clinically contributory in 84% of patients with confirmed positive studies and in 36% of the total study population (68). Although no definite data are presented, the authors suggest that the ability of PET/CT to define and separate physiologic sites of FDG uptake from foci of clinical significance is of major value in the work-up of patients with FUO.

Based on the wide experience gained from assessment of cancer patients with hybrid PET/CT, it is well accepted today that fused data may confirm the presence of disease and localize it to specific organs or regions of the body, and it can exclude disease in areas of physiologic tracer biodistribution. Accordingly, in patients with FUO, PET/CT has the ability to detect sites of disease that may be masked or missed in the presence of intense physiologic tracer uptake, with a subsequent decrease in the number of false-negative studies and an increase in sensitivity, and also to define increased FDG activity as related to clinically nonsignificant processes with a subsequent decrease in the false-positive rate and an increase in specificity for establishing the etiology of FUO.

Studies that have assessed the use of FDG imaging in patients with FUO suffer from some limitations inherent to this specific population, which have also influenced the results of other imaging modalities. In a certain percentage of patients a final diagnosis is never established (i.e., the "unknown origin" remains), while for some of the entities that represent the final diagnosis, FDG does not provide any diagnostic information (69).

FDG PET/CT may have a particularly important role in the detection of small infectious foci that have not yet led to mass effects or other anatomic changes detectable on conventional anatomic imaging modalities such as CT or ultrasound. They may also be located in an anatomic region that is difficult to examine, such as an abscess in the subdiaphragmatic region (69,70). At the present time it is recommended that in patients with suspected intra-abdominal sepsis FDG PET/CT should be performed only if ultrasound and CT have been reported as negative.

At times, retrospective assessment of the CT component of the study in a specific region, guided by a focus of increased FDG uptake detected on the PET component, can diagnose previously missed small foci of intra-abdominal infection. Also, infectious processes involving organs with high normal FDG uptake, such as infected renal or hepatic cysts, as well as diagnosis of pathology in regions of distorted anatomy following surgery can be identified

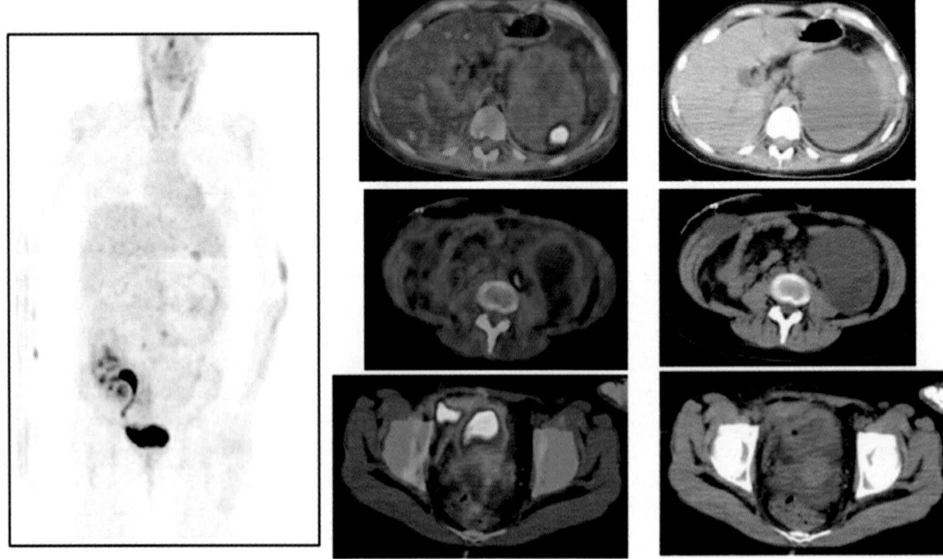

FIGURE 12.3. Diagnosis of multiple infectious foci in a patient with polycystic kidneys, fever of unknown origin, and pain in the left lumbar region, 1 month after renal transplant. **Left:** The maximum intensity projection image demonstrates a focus of increased fluorodeoxyglucose (FDG) uptake in the left upper abdomen and an additional suspicious small lesion of mild intensity in the lower midabdomen. **Right:** Axial slices at the level of the upper abdomen (*top row*) demonstrate that the superior focus of abnormal FDG uptake is located at the posterior aspect of a left infected renal cyst; axial slices at the level of the midabdomen (*center row*) demonstrate that the focus of mildly increased FDG uptake is localized to a slightly increased para-aortic lymph node, most probably representing reactive lymphadenopathy; axial slices at the level of the pelvis demonstrate the presence of a focus of highly intense FDG activity adjacent to the urinary bladder, consistent with an abscess.

with the use of hybrid imaging, thus increasing the sensitivity of this modality (71).

FLUORODEOXYGLUCOSE PET/CT IMAGING VASCULAR INFECTION AND INFLAMMATION

Vasculitis

Vasculitis represents a group of clinical entities characterized by an inflammatory process involving the vascular wall. Vascular wall thickening that is found during the early stages of this process can progress to fibrosis in more advanced stages. Diagnosis is, as a rule, biopsy proven. FDG PET has been used to image increased vascular metabolic activity in patients with vasculitis, and increased tracer uptake has been described in patients with various entities in this group, including giant cell and Takayasu's arteritis, aortitis, or unspecific inflammatory processes involving other large vessels. Its routine clinical use is, however, still controversial (72,73). FDG uptake in vasculitis is considered nonspecific. It appears as a pattern of diffusely increased FDG activity along vascular walls in the large cervical and thoracic vessels and is most probably related to smooth muscle proliferation or to the presence of macrophages within plaques (74,75).

A study comparing FDG imaging and MRI in five patients with Takayasu's arteritis indicated that FDG, although performed with a coincidence camera, was a suitable whole-body screening method in the diagnosis of early disease, mainly when presenting symptoms were not specific (76). The advantages of MRI included its ability to precisely define the presence of pathomorphological changes and to diagnose vascular complications such as stenosis or aneurysmatic transformation.

A study involving 22 patients with giant cell arteritis showed that all patients with positive findings in large arteries on duplex ultrasound showed elevated FDG uptake in the same anatomic location. This was, however, not the case with disease localized to the temporal arteries. They concluded that FDG PET imaging may be used to demonstrate the presence of giant cell arteritis in vessels larger than 4 mm in diameter (77). Case reports have suggested the use of FDG PET for monitoring response to treatment for aortitis, which is otherwise difficult to perform (78). At present, this still represents preliminary evidence of a logical hypothesis that needs large-scale research for confirmation. Since there can commonly be FDG uptake in the aortic wall, believed due to atherosclerosis/inflammation, there is clearly a continuum of activity in vascular wall activity that may reduce somewhat the specificity of this imaging approach in older patients.

Vascular Graft Infection

Graft infection is an uncommon but potentially severe complication following prosthetic vascular reconstruction (79). The clinical presentation is often subtle and nonspecific, and accurate diagnosis is challenging but of utmost significance for further patient care. Delay in treatment is the cause for severe complications such as sepsis or hemorrhage (80). Amputation of the affected limb is performed in a large number of patients with infected vascular grafts (81). CT is considered the diagnostic procedure of choice with a relatively simple diagnosis when it demonstrates the vascular graft surrounded by a soft tissue abscess. This is, however, an uncommon pattern in earlier stages of the infectious process, when findings are mostly nonspecific and impaired by the presence of sites of infection adjacent to, but not involving, the implanted device (82,83).

Following the use of ^{99m}Tc or ^{111}In-labeled WBC for suspected prosthetic graft infection with variable rates of success (84,85), a few studies, mainly case reports, have recently suggested that FDG PET imaging has a potential role in this clinical setting (86–88).

A study involving 33 consecutive patients has assessed the diagnostic accuracy of FDG PET for detection of aortic graft infection. FDG PET had a high sensitivity of 91% but a specificity of only 64%, as compared to CT, which had a lower sensitivity of 64% but a specificity of 86%. Focality of the abnormal FDG uptake increased the specificity of PET to 95%. Therefore, both the presence of increased FDG uptake and the focal pattern should be considered as diagnostic criteria for aortic graft infection on PET (86).

Although functional data obtained by PET are, as a rule, correlated with anatomic information obtained from CT or MRI for accurate localization of the site of disease, this process is difficult to achieve in side-by-side comparison with high accuracy in this particular setting. The close proximity of the evaluated structures and the influence of any, even minimal, positional changes between separately performed imaging studies may be significant for the final report. Also, increased FDG activity may occur in sites of postsurgical inflammatory changes, in scar tissue, and native vessels (89) in addition to high-intensity uptake in foci of soft tissue infection in close proximity of the vascular graft. It is important to differentiate these findings from uptake within the graft itself, and PET/CT may have an incremental value if it can accurately localize the FDG-avid focus to the precise infected anatomic site (Fig. 12.4). Preliminary results in a group of 39 patients show that PET/CT had a specificity of 91% for diagnosis of the infectious process and its precise localization to vascular graft involvement (90).

In patients with a complicated regional anatomy after multiple surgical procedures, PET/CT can also pinpoint the infected implant and differentiate between multiple suspicious findings. When fused images localize the infectious process to soft tissues only, the patient can be spared unnecessary surgery with high morbidity (90). The authors of this study also describe the presence of mild, linear diffuse FDG uptake that is found along noninfected grafts, probably due to a low-grade foreign body–related inflammatory reaction (86,90).

Vulnerable Atherosclerotic Plaque

Ruptures of atherosclerotic plaques and thrombi formation are the primary mechanisms of myocardial infarction or cerebrovascular accident (91), independent of plaque size, but related to the composition of the atheroma. A "vulnerable" plaque can precipitate a clinical event following its rupture (92). Various imaging modalities have been used to discriminate between stable and vulnerable plaques and thus to diagnose high-risk atherosclerotic lesions to risk-stratify patients and to evaluate different therapeutic approaches. Most of these diagnostic techniques are catheter based and can therefore visualize only single atherosclerotic lesions (93,94).

Angiography visualizes the arterial lumen, but cannot define nonprotruding atheromas or plaque composition and cannot differentiate between stable and "vulnerable" lesions. Intravascular ultrasound is currently not widely used because of its invasive nature and the specific expertise it requires. Noninvasive B-mode duplex ultrasound can detect the presence of atherosclerosis in the superficial carotid arteries (95) but is unable to predict plaque rupture. The role of multislice CT

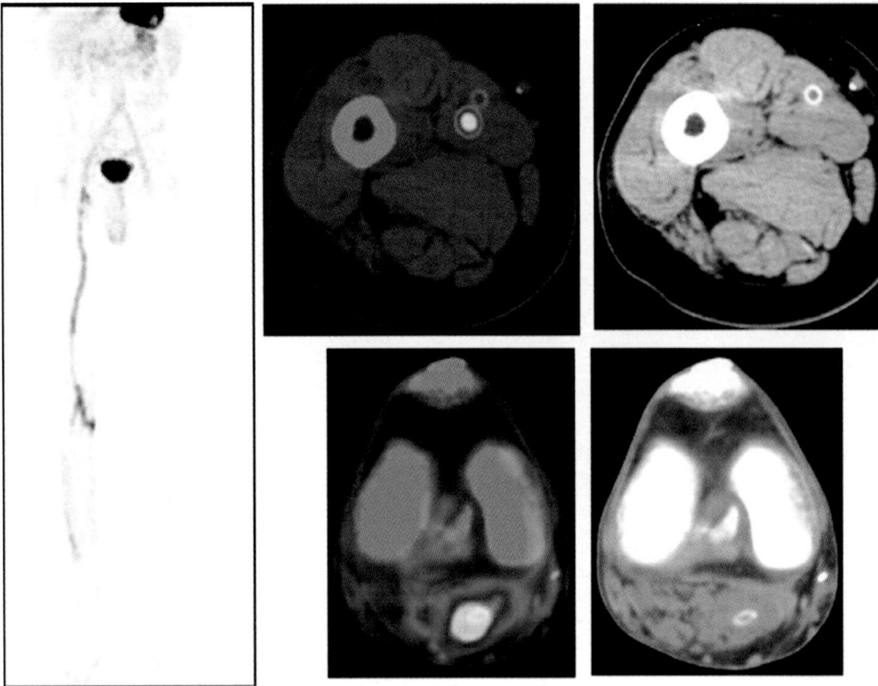

FIGURE 12.4. Diagnosis of vascular graft infection in a patient with peripheral vascular disease who presented with an infected surgical wound at the level of the distal anastomosis 10 months after insertion of a right femoropopliteal GoreTex graft. **Left:** The maximum intensity projection image demonstrates a linear focus of intense fluorodeoxyglucose (FDG) activity along the trajectory of the graft, with some areas of focal tracer uptake. **Right:** Axial images at the level of the upper thigh (*top row*) indicate the presence of increased FDG activity in the muscle, without involvement of the vascular graft. Axial images at the level of the calf indicate the presence of a focus of intense abnormal FDG uptake involving the vascular graft and adjacent soft tissues, consistent with soft tissue and graft infection.

in the detection and serial monitoring of coronary artery calcifications is currently under investigation. MRI has the potential to identify different stages in plaque formation (96) but does not provide, at present, data with respect to inflammatory cell activity.

Overall, these modalities offer high anatomic resolution without providing information on the metabolic status of the lesions (97,98). Attempts to use single-photon emitting tracers such as [^{111}In] or ^{99m}Tc-labeled antibodies against plaque, fibrin, and its degradation products or platelets for targeting the cells or molecules involved in atherosclerotic lesions have not gone beyond the experimental setting (99–101).

FDG is taken up and accumulates in metabolically active cells in direct relationship to their metabolic activity, and PET imaging has been investigated as an alternative modality that could detect inflammatory changes in the arterial wall and thus diagnose early stages of atherosclerosis. Experimental studies in a model of arterial wall injury have shown that the amount of FDG uptake in atherosclerotic lesions corresponds to the presence of intimal proliferation (75,102). Macrophage density can be quantified noninvasively using FDG PET, with more intense uptake reported in the aortas of atherosclerotic rabbits (103). In addition, it has been shown that the amount of FDG uptake decreased significantly in animals by changing from high-cholesterol to a normal diet (91).

In patient studies, FDG has been shown to accumulate in macrophages in atherosclerotic plaques in carotid endarterectomy specimens examined *in vitro*. Foci of increased tracer uptake have also been detected by PET in patients with symptomatic carotid stenosis (104). Increased FDG uptake in the vascular wall of large blood vessels has been noted in 60% of patients over the age of 60 (105). Focal increased FDG uptake in the walls of large arteries has been reported in 31% to 59% of cancer patients 50 years and older, presumably representing atheroma. Increased FDG uptake in the arterial wall was more common with advancing age, as well as in hypertensive and hyperlipidemic patients (106,107).

Hybrid PET/CT imaging optimizes the detectability rate and precise localization of focal vascular wall CT calcifications and FDG uptake (106,107). Three different patterns of CT calcifications and FDG uptake have been described in the wall of large arteries, including vascular wall abnormalities that are either PET negative and CT positive (PET−/CT+), both PET and CT positive (PET+/CT+), or PET positive and CT negative (PET+/CT−) (107).

Abnormal vascular wall FDG activity may be transient, representing the stage of active inflammation. The incongruent PET and CT patterns indicate that focal FDG uptake is not necessarily closely associated with CT calcification and support the hypothesis that there may be a different anatomic and metabolic status in early or active (PET+) versus late or inactive (CT+) atherosclerotic plaques. Incongruent vascular wall (PET+/CT−) abnormalities may progress and change their pattern into PET−/CT+ areas in the chronic stage, when active inflammation is no longer present. Changes in vascular wall abnormalities were indeed more frequent in PET+ sites when compared with CT+ sites (48% vs. 4%) (108). It was therefore hypothesized that FDG-avid mural sites, regardless of the presence or absence of CT calcifications, may potentially predict dynamic changes occurring in the status of the atherosclerotic lesions related to transient episodes of active inflammation. FDG imaging may, therefore, be used in the future as a diagnostic tool for plaques vulnerable to rupture with the help of serial follow-up PET/CT studies.

FLUORODEOXYGLUCOSE PET/CT IMAGING INFECTION IN THE IMMUNE-COMPROMISED PATIENT

Infectious processes in immune-compromised patients represent a severe clinical problem of various etiologies. HIV-positive patients may present with a clinical symptomatology that can be related to a neoplastic or infectious cause (41). FDG PET can demonstrate the presence of acute respiratory tract infections. The whole-body PET imaging technique can also detect intra-abdominal infection, commonly associated with HIV positivity.

Using FDG-PET in cases in which routine clinical, laboratory, and conventional imaging examinations do not reveal the precise etiology of increased FDG uptake has been assessed. SUV measurements have been used to differentiate between malignant lymphoma and a benign process, mainly toxoplasmosis, in 15 patients with AIDS (109). An additional study including 80 patients confirmed the value of measuring the intensity of uptake on FDG PET in the differential diagnosis of lymphoma, toxoplasmosis, or leukoencephalopathy for an overall sensitivity of 92% and specificity of 94% (110).

Patterns of FDG activity in HIV-positive patients have been used for better definition of the stage of infection. A study evaluating 30 patients indicated that healthy HIV-positive subjects had none or only faint FDG uptake in nodal stations, while patients with early and advanced active HIV infection demonstrated increased FDG activity in peripheral lymph nodes (111). FDG PET/CT was found to be superior to [^{67}Ga] for assessment of patients with FUO, and specifically of patients with HIV-associated infections (53).

Diagnosis of superimposed infection in patients with malignancy can be challenging. The role of FDG imaging in diagnosis of infection in 248 patients who underwent PET for staging of multiple myeloma was retrospectively reviewed. FDG PET was true positive for the presence of infection even in neutro- and lymphopenic patients, which represented approximately 20% of events. FDG PET findings in up to 46% of patients were of clinical relevance for further management. The authors conclude that FDG PET may be a useful tool for diagnosing and managing infections even in the setting of severe immunosuppression (112).

Following organ transplantation, patients may be prone to early graft dysfunction due either to infection or rejection. FDG PET imaging has been evaluated for the differential diagnosis of rejection or infection in 15 lung transplant recipients. Abnormally increased FDG uptake was found in patients with proven infection but not in patients with rejection only. The authors suggest that, if confirmed in large-scale studies, noninvasive FDG PET imaging, which also has the advantage that it can be repeatedly used to monitor patients with suspected infection, could reduce the number of transbronchial biopsies required at present for diagnosis and further management of these two entities (8).

FLUORODEOXYGLUCOSE PET/CT IMAGING: MISCELLANEOUS INFLAMMATORY AND INFECTIOUS PROCESSES

Sarcoidosis

Sarcoidosis represents a chronic systemic entity characterized by the presence of an unspecific inflammatory process, leading to activation of macrophages and lymphocytes, which is followed by the formation of granuloma in almost any region or organ of the body. Although most commonly it represents a self-limiting process, severe cases can present with fibrosis and organ dysfunction, more often involving the lungs and mediastinal lymph nodes. The ability to define the presence and degree of an active inflammatory process is therefore of clinical significance, both for deciding if anti-inflammatory therapy should be instituted and to determine its duration. Various laboratory and imaging tests (chest x-rays, [^{67}Ga] scintigraphy) or invasive procedures (bronchial lavage) provide only partial solutions (113).

FDG is taken up by active sarcoidosis (114–116). The typical pattern is characterized by moderately increased tracer activity in multiple sites. The differential diagnosis is difficult in patients with cancer. FDG PET is not consistently included in the routine clinical diagnostic armamentarium for suspected sarcoidosis, and is not, at present, one of the primary modalities at initial diagnosis. The typical pattern for positive FDG PET imaging is similar to that described with [^{67}Ga] scintigraphy and includes mainly bilateral mediastinal and pulmonary hilar uptake, with potential extension into the central region of the lungs, associated at times with increased activity in lacrimal glands and in an enlarged spleen (Fig. 12.5A).

Sarcoidosis, being a systemic disease, can involve multiple organs or systems. Whole-body PET can detect cutaneous, nodal, or musculoskeletal disease involvement (117), but the role of FDG imaging in the diagnosis of cardiac or neurologic manifestations of sarcoidosis is controversial and unclear (118,119). In a study of 18 patients FDG imaging was found to be superior to [^{67}Ga] scintigraphy, mainly for assessment of the extent of extrapulmonary sarcoidosis (120).

Since abnormal FDG uptake in sarcoidosis can mimic malignancy, PET/CT can be a useful tool to guide tissue sampling when needed for final diagnosis, by defining the location of hypermetabolic sites that should be further evaluated (Fig. 12.5B). When anti-inflammatory therapy is considered, and later, during the course of treatment, FDG PET can be a useful tool to monitor the patient's response. The presence and intensity of FDG uptake can provide a visual or semiquantitative index to assess the efficacy of the administered treatment and follow-up of disease activity, identifying the presence of residual active sarcoidosis that would justify further treatment, or, on the other hand, lead to the decision to discontinue drug administration (113,121).

Inflammatory Bowel Disease

Inflammatory bowel disease includes a number of clinical entities, mainly Crohn's disease and ulcerative colitis, and represents a frequent clinical dilemma in terms of diagnosis, defining the extent of disease, determining the need and duration of treatment, and in the differential diagnosis of disease- or treatment-related complications during follow-up. Although initial diagnosis is performed, as a rule, using endoscopic and radiological procedures, these tests are limited in their capability to be performed repeatedly in order to monitor response to treatment.

FDG uptake has been described in sporadic cases of enterocolitis as a sensitive index of metabolic activity (122,123). However, one of the major limitations for the use of this tracer is related to its route of biodistribution, with major gastrointestinal tract excretion, as well as to increased muscular activity due to peristalsis and bowel motility (124). Although focal abnormal FDG uptake is associated in the majority of findings with malignant or premalignant processes (125), patterns of segmental, regional FDG uptake have been described in patients with proctitis and different types of colitis (126).

With PET/CT the diagnostic limitations of FDG imaging can be overcome in part. A site of focal, highly intense FDG uptake localized by PET/CT to a specific segment of the small intestine or colon in a patient with known inflammatory bowel disease should be used for guiding further endoscopic examinations with tissue sampling

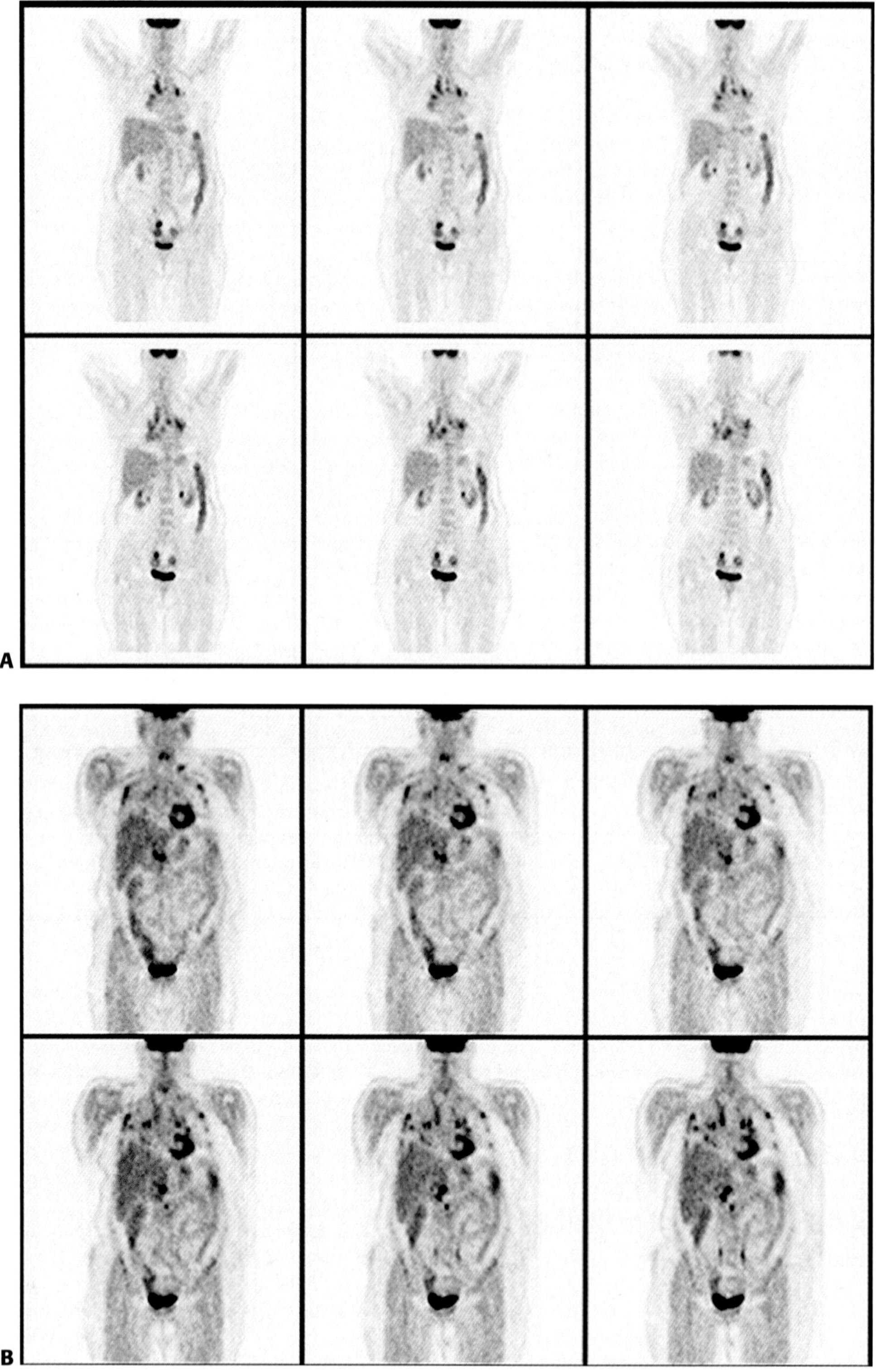

FIGURE 12.5. Patterns of fluorodeoxyglucose (FDG) PET in sarcoidosis. **A:** Increased FDG uptake involving enlarged lymph nodes in the mediastinum and pulmonary hila. **B:** A patient with breast cancer was referred for further assessment of lung nodules on CT, suspicious for metastases. There is increased FDG uptake involving multiple peripheral nodules in both lungs. Additional suspicious FDG-avid foci are located in enlarged supraclavicular, mediastinal, and abdominal lymph nodes. Endobronchial tissue diagnosis indicated the presence of sarcoidosis.

when a localized acute exacerbation of the disease is suspected. Also, uptake in the colon can be separated from uptake in surrounding soft tissues, facilitating the differential diagnosis between a mass on CT that can be fibrotic after treatment, or an abscess complicating an acute episode of inflammatory bowel disease with perforation into the abdominal cavity (127).

A new agent, FDG-labeled WBC, which has been described in recent years for some infection-related clinical indications, can play a potentially promising role in the assessment of patients with inflammatory bowel disease (128). Although only three patients were evaluated in this study, the authors found a promising correlation between the intensity of FDG WBC uptake and the degree of inflammation. Future studies will most probably assess whether this tracer may also represent a good tool for monitoring the therapeutic response of inflammatory bowel disease. Treatment of inflammatory bowel disease involves long-term use of anti-inflammatory and immunosuppressive drugs, known for their severe adverse effects. Tailoring the optimal therapeutic regimen is a major challenge in patient management. It can be hypothesized that the combined use of high-resolution functional PET imaging with landmarks of abdominal and pelvic anatomy provided by the sequential CT acquisition, mainly if enhanced by administration of oral contrast, will optimize FDG WBC imaging for assessment of inflammatory bowel disease even more; however, this area remains under active study.

Cardiorespiratory Infectious Processes

FDG is taken up by the normal myocardium, and diagnosis of focal infectious processes in the heart using FDG PET has been described only in rare cases. Focal cardiac FDG uptake was found in six patients with proven endocarditis (129). With new studies showing that myocardial FDG uptake could be manipulated by certain drugs or a specific diet (130), the use of FDG PET/CT could become of more clinical significance in the future for diagnosis of these entities.

The role of FDG imaging in infectious or sterile inflammatory processes involving the respiratory tract has been assessed mainly through early publications showing the presence of increased tracer uptake in both malignant and benign pulmonary nodules. FDG avidity in pulmonary lesions can be complicated even more since both tumor and infection located in postobstructive atelectasis can take up FDG and can falsely suggest a tumor of larger dimensions than initially thought. The triangular shape and the lower intensity of activity can in some cases suggest the benign etiology of part of these findings (131). FDG uptake by active tuberculosis can also mislead toward the diagnosis of malignancy (132,133). Overall, increased FDG uptake has been described in a large number of nonmalignant pulmonary processes including infection, chronic obstructive lung disease, sarcoidosis, acute lung injury, and acute respiratory distress syndrome (134).

Foreign Body Inflammatory Reaction

It is important here to caution inexperienced (as well as experienced) PET readers about a potential pitfall when interpreting FDG PET/CT studies in cancer patients or when an acute infectious process is clinically suspected. Healing processes, as frequently encountered in postsurgical scars, lead to an inflammatory reaction with leukocyte infiltrates in newly formed granulation tissue. This explains moderate to high-degree of FDG uptake for several months following recent surgery or biopsy (135). In a study of 18 patients, while the sensitivity of FDG PET for detection of infection in the area of a surgical wound was 100%, the specificity was very low, only 56%, as compared with a specificity of 86% outside the operation field (136).

Teflon has been used for decades to treat vocal cord paresis or other velopharyngeal insufficiency but has been shown to be prone to foreign-body granulomatotic reactions. These appear as highly FDG avid and can be falsely interpreted as malignant sites if the clinical details of a former procedure are not known. In the presence of suggestive anamnestic data MRI should be performed prior to invasive tissue sampling (137,138). Focal, intense FDG uptake has also been reported in patients with central venous catheters, related either to the presence of a thrombotic process, infection, or inflammatory reaction (139).

PET/CT IMAGING OF INFECTION AND INFLAMMATION: BEYOND FLUORODEOXYGLUCOSE

Following, or in parallel with, studies assessing the efficacy of FDG for imaging infection and inflammation, there is a quest to provide a more specific agent that would also benefit from the high resolution and improved sensitivity of PET. Evaluating FDG-labeled leukocytes (FDG WBC) was the reasonable approach. Initial studies *in vitro* have demonstrated that FDG can label human granulocytes with rapid incorporation and high efficiency (140,141).

A study in an experimental model in rats compared the imaging properties of FDG WBC and FDG stand alone in sterile and septic inflammation processes and showed a significantly higher uptake ratio of FDG WBC compared with FDG in all sterile and septic inflammation models, further confirmed by micro-PET imaging (142).

Dosimetry estimations have shown that radiation doses from FDG WBC were comparable to those of [^{111}In]-labeled WBC, with less delivery to organs such as the brain and urinary bladder (128,143). Feasibility studies of imaging in humans, addressing also the issue of its normal biodistribution, have shown that only small amounts of FDG WBC are found in healthy gastrointestinal and urinary tracts, as compared to FDG alone, thus the hypothesis that this may be the future tracer of choice when infection in these organs is suspected (128,143).

Two main studies have presented initial clinical data. A study of 23 consecutive patients with suspected or documented infectious processes underwent PET/CT at 3 hours after injection of FDG WBC. The patient-based performance of this new PET agent indicated a sensitivity, specificity, and accuracy of 86% each, and for the lesion-based analysis the sensitivity was 91%, specificity of 85%, and accuracy of 90%. The authors concluded that although this was found in a small number of patients, a negative FDG WBC PET/CT study can reliably rule out the presence of a focal active infectious process (144). The second study involved 51 patients who were assessed mainly for suspected musculoskeletal infections. In addition to evaluating the role of FDG WBC for imaging of infection the authors also prospectively compare the diagnostic accuracy of this tracer to that of [^{111}In]-oxine–labeled leukocytes (145). FDG WBC had a sensitivity of 87%, specificity of 82%, and accuracy of 84% as compared to 73%, 86%, and 81%, respectively, for the [^{111}In]-labeled agent. It remains unclear if FDG WBC is superior to FDG for infection imaging, however. The short half-life of FDG may be less than optimally matched to the localization kinetics of white cells, but more study is needed.

Very preliminary data have also addressed the potential use of [^{68}Ga] stand-alone or [^{68}Ga]-labeled peptides, mainly in an experimental setting (69,146). Based on prior animal data, [^{68}Ga] alone, with its short half-life, may not localize as quickly to infections as needed for it to be a reliable infection imaging agent, although more study is needed.

CONCLUSION

FDG PET and PET/CT imaging is performed soon after the radiotracer is injected, it is fast, it has high resolution and contrast, it is sensitive even for low-grade infectious processes, it delivered a low radiation burden, and, due to the quality of the images, it is likely to have low interobserver variability. FDG PET/CT has become an exciting modality for diagnostic imaging of infection and inflammation in many settings. It appears to have an incremental value over anatomic or other imaging methods in the assessment of both acute and chronic disease entities. Due to the nonspecific uptake mechanism of FDG differentiation between infection, aseptic inflammatory processes, and malignancy, is difficult, and at times, not possible. Most studies assessing FDG imaging in infectious and inflammatory processes include only a small number of patients. Large-scale studies, similar to those available today for most types of malignancy, need to be performed in order to provide the appropriate clinical decision-making tools and cost-effectiveness calculations in this relatively new field. Whether FDG PET/CT or hybrid imaging with new, more infectious-specific tracers will replace standard nuclear medicine procedures or standalone conventional imaging modalities is an evolving issue, but it is probable this approach will continue to grow in clinical importance in the coming years.

REFERENCES

1. Cook GJ, Maisey MN, Fogelman I. Normal variants, artefacts and interpretative pitfalls in PET imaging with 18-fluoro-2-deoxyglucose and carbon-11 methionine. *Eur J Nucl Med* 1999;26:1363–1378.
2. Beyer T, Townsend DW, Brun T, et al. A combined PET/CT scanner for clinical oncology. *J Nucl Med* 2000;41:1369–1379.
3. Bar-Shalom R, Yefremov N, Guralnik L, et al. Clinical performance of PET/CT in evaluation of cancer: additional value for diagnostic imaging and patient management. *J Nucl Med* 2003;44:1200–1209.
4. Fantone JC, Ward PA. Role of oxygen-derived free radicals and metabolites in leukocyte-dependent inflammatory reactions. *Am J Pathol* 1982;107:395–418.
5. Weisdorf DJ, Craddock PR, Jacob HS. Glycogenolysis versus glucose transport in human granulocytes: differential activation in phagocytosis and chemotaxis. *Blood* 1982;60:888–893.
6. KubotaR, Yamada S, Kubota K, et al. Intratumoral distribution of fluorine-18-fluorodeoxyglucose *in vivo*: high accumulation in macrophages and granulation tissues studied by microautoradiography. *J Nucl Med* 1992;33:1972–1980.
7. Zhuang H, Alavi A. 18-fluorodeoxyglucose positron emission tomographic imaging in the detection and monitoring of infection and inflammation. *Semin Nucl Med* 2002;32:47–59.
8. Jones HA, Donovan T, Goddard MJ, et al.Use of ^{18}FDG-PET to discriminate between infection and rejection in lung transplant recipients. *Transplantation* 2004;77:1462–1465.
9. Yamada S, Kubota K, Kubota R, et al. High accumulation of fluorine-18-fluorodeoxyglucose in turpentine-induced inflammatory tissue. *J Nucl Med* 1995;36:1301–1306.
10. Higashi T, Fisher SJ, Brown RS, et al. Evaluation of the early effect of local irradiation on normal rodent bone marrow metabolism using FDG: preclinical PET studies. *J Nucl Med* 2000;41:2026–2035.
11. Anderson RL, Wood WA. Carbohydrate metabolism in microorganisms. *Annu Rev Microbiol* 1969;23:539–578.
12. Sugawara Y, Gutowski TD, Fisher SJ, et al. Uptake of positron emission tomography tracers in experimental bacterial infections: a comparative biodistribution study of radiolabeled FDG, thymidine, L-methionine, ^{67}Ga-citrate, and ^{125}I-HSA. *Eur J Nucl Med* 1999;26: 333–341.
13. Sugawara Y, Braun DK, Kison PV, et al. Rapid detection of human infections with fluorine-18 fluorodeoxyglucose and positron emission tomography: preliminary results. *Eur J Nucl Med* 1998;25: 1238–1243.
14. Bar-Shalom R, Yefremov N, Guralnik L. et al. SPECT/CT using ^{67}Ga and ^{111}In-labeled leukocyte scintigraphy for diagnosis of infection. *J Nucl Med* 2006;47:587–594.
15. Love C, Tomas MB, Tronco GG, et al. FDG PET of infection and inflammation. *Radiographics* 2005;25:1357–1368.
16. Matthies A, Hickeson M, Cuciara A, et al. Dual time point ^{18}F-FDG PET for the evaluation of pulmonary nodules. *J Nucl Med* 2002;43: 871–875.
17. Diederichs CG, Staib L, Glatting G, et al. FDG PET: elevated plasma glucose reduces both uptake and detection rate of pancreatic malignancies. *J Nucl Med* 1998;39:1030–1033.
18. Zhao S, Kuge Y, Tsukamoto E, et al. Fluorodeoxyglucose uptake and glucose transporter expression in experimental inflammatory lesions and malignant tumours: effects of insulin and glucose loading. *Nucl Med Commun* 2002;23:545–550.
19. Zhuang HM, Cortes-Blanco A, Pourdwehnad M, et al. Do high glucose levels have a differential effect on FDG uptake in inflammatory and malignant disorders? *Nucl Med Commun* 2001;22:1123–1128.
20. Keidar Z, Militianu D, Melamed E, et al. The diabetic foot: initial experience with ^{18}F-FDG PET/CT. *J Nucl Med* 2005;46:444–449.
21. Schauwecker DS. Osteomyelitis: diagnosis with In-111-labeled leukocytes. *Radiology* 1989;171:141–146.
22. Termaat MF, Raijmakers PG, Scholten HJ, et al. The accuracy of diagnostic imaging for the assessment of chronic osteomyelitis: a systematic review and meta-analysis. *J Bone Joint Surg Am* 2005;87: 2464–2471.
23. Zhuang H, Duarte PS, Poudehand M, et al. Exclusion of chronic osteomyelitis with F-18 fluorodeoxyglucose positron emission tomographic imaging. *Clin Nucl Med* 2000;25:281–284.
24. Guhlmann A, Brecht-Krauss D, Suger G, et al. Chronic osteomyelitis: detection with FDG PET and correlation with histopathologic findings. *Radiology* 1998;206:749–754.
25. Meller J, Altenvoerde G, Munzel U, et al. Fever of unknown origin: prospective comparison of [(^{18})F]FDG imaging with a double-head coincidence camera and gallium-67 citrate SPET. *Eur J Nucl Med* 2000;27:1617–1625.
26. de Winter F, van de Wiele C, Vogelaers D, et al. Fluorine-18 fluorodeoxyglucose-position emission tomography: a highly accurate imaging modality for the diagnosis of chronic musculoskeletal infections. *J Bone Joint Surg Am* 2001;83:651–660.
27. Modic MT, Steinberg PM, Ross JS, et al. Degenerative disk disease: assessment of changes in vertebral body marrow with MR imaging. *Radiology* 1988;166:193–199.
28. Stumpe KDM, Zanetti M, Weishaupt D, et al. FDG-PET for differentiation of degenerative and infectious end plate abnormalities in the lumbar spine detected on MR imaging. *AJR Am J Roentgenol* 2002;179:1151–1157.
29. Hochhold J, Yang H, Zhuang H, Alavi A. Application of ^{18}F-fluorodeoxyglucose and PET in evaluation of diabetic foot. *PET Clin North Am* 2006;1:123–130.
30. Hopfner S, Krolak C, Kessler S, et al. Preoperative imaging of charcot neuroarthropathy in diabetic patients: comparison of ring PET, hybrid

PET, and magnetic resonance imaging. *Foot Ankle Int* 2004; 25:890–895.
31. Mahomed NN, Barrett JA, Katz JN, et al. Rates and outcomes of primary and revision total hip replacement in the United States medicare population. *J Bone Joint Surg Am* 2003;85:27–32.
32. Spangehl MJ, Younger ASE, Masri BA, et al. Diagnosis of infection following total hip arthroplasty. *J Bone Joint Surg Am* 1997;79:1587–1588.
33. Palestro CJ, Kim CK, Swyer AJ, et al. Total-hip arthroplasty: periprosthetic indium-111-labeled leukocyte activity and complementary technetium-99m-sulfur colloid imaging in suspected infection. *J Nucl Med* 1990;31:1950–1955.
34. Alazraki NP. Diagnosing prosthetic joint infection. *J Nucl Med* 1990; 31:1955–1957
35. Zhuang H, Yang H, Alavi A. Critical role of ^{18}F-labeled fluorodeoxyglucose PET in the management of patients with arthroplasty. *PET Clin North Am* 2006;1:99–106.
36. White LM, Buckwalter KA. Technical considerations: CT and MR imaging in postoperative orthopedic patient. *Semin Musculoskeletal Radiol* 2002;6:5–17.
37. Zhuang H, Duarte PS, Pourdehnad M, et al. The promising role of ^{18}F-FDG PET in detecting infected lower limb prosthesis implants. *J Nucl Med* 2001;42:44–48.
38. Manthey N, Reinhard P, Moog F, et al. The use of [^{18}F]fluorodeoxyglucose positron emission tomography to differentiate between synovitis, loosening and infection of hip and knee prostheses. *Nucl Med Commun* 2002;23:645–653.
39. Reinartz, P, Mumme T, Hermanns B, et al. Radionuclide imaging of the painful hip arthroplasty: positron-emission tomography versus triple-phase bone scanning. *J Bone Joint Surg Br* 2005;87:465–470.
40. Delank KS, Schmidt M, Michael JW, et al. The implications of ^{18}F-FDG PET for the diagnosis of endoprosthetic loosening and infection in hip and knee arthroplasty: results from a prospective, blinded study. *BMC Musculoskelet Disord* 2006;7:20.
41. de Winter F, Vogelaers D, Gemmel F, et al. Promising role of ^{18}-F-fluoro-D-deoxyglucose positron emission tomography in clinical infectious diseases. *Eur J Clin Microbiol Infect Dis* 2002;21:247–257.
42. Schiesser M, Stumpe KD, Trentz O, et al. Detection of metallic implant-associated infections with FDG PET in patients with trauma: correlation with microbiologic results. *Radiology* 2003;226:391–398.
43. de Winter F, Gemmel F, Van de Wiele C, et al. ^{18}-Fluorine fluorodeoxyglucose positron emission tomography for the diagnosis of infection in the postoperative spine. *Spine* 2003;28:1314–1319.
44. Trampuz A, Zimmerli W. Diagnosis and treatment of infections associated with fracture-fixation devices. *Injury* 2006;37[Suppl 2]: S59–S66.
45. Kamel EM, Burger C, Buck A, et al. Impact of metallic dental implants on CT-based attenuation correction in a combined PET/CT scanner. *Eur Radiol* 2003;13:724–728.
46. Bujenovic S, Mannting F, Chakrabarti R, et al. Artifactual 2-deoxy-2-[(^{18})F]fluoro-D-glucose localization surrounding metallic objects in a PET/CT scanner using CT-based attenuation correction. *Mol Imaging Biol* 2003;5:20–22.
47. Heiba SI, Luo J, Sadek S, et al. Attenuation-correction induced artifact in F-18 FDG PET imaging following total knee replacement. *Clin Positron Imaging* 2000;3:237–239.
48. Hartmann A, Eid K, Dora C, et al. Diagnostic value of (^{18})F-FDG PET/CT in trauma patients with suspected chronic osteomyelitis. *Eur J Nucl Med Mol Imaging* 2007;34:704–719.
49. Hustinx R, Malaise MG. PET imaging of arthritis. *PET Clin North Am* 2006;1:131–139.
50. Palmer WE, Rosenthal DI, Schoenberg OI, et al. Quantification of inflammation in the wrist with gadolinium-enhanced MR imaging and PET with 2-[F-18]-fluoro-2-deoxy-D-glucose. *Radiology* 1995; 196:647–655.
51. Beckers C, Ribbens C, Andre B. Assessment of disease activity in rheumatoid arthritis with (^{18})F-FDG PET. *J Nucl Med* 2004;45:956–964.
52. Wandler E, Kramer EL, Sherman O, et al. Diffuse FDG shoulder uptake on PET is associated with clinical findings of osteoarthritis. *AJR Am J Roentgenol* 2005;185:797–803.
53. Knockaert DC, Vanderschueren S, Blockmans D. Fever of unknown origin in adults: 40 years on. *J Intern Med* 2003;253:263–275.
54. de Kleijn EM, Vandenbroucke JP, van der Meer JW. Fever of unknown origin (FUO). A prospective multicenter study of 167 patients with FUO, using fixed epidemiologic entry criteria. The Netherlands FUO study group. *Medicine* 1997;76:392–400.
55. Mourad O, Palda V, Detsky AS. A comprehensive evidence-based approach to fever of unknown origin. *Arch Intern Med* 2003;163: 545–551.
56. Petersdorf RG. Fever of unknown origin. An old friend revisited. *Arch Intern Med* 1992;152:21–22.
57. Abu Rahma AF, Saiedy S, Robinson PA, et al. Role of venous duplex imaging of lower extremities in patients with fever of unknown origin. *Surgery* 1997;121:366–371.
58. Wagner AD, Andresen J, Raum E, et al. Standardised work-up programme for fever of unknown origin and contribution of magnetic resonance imaging for the diagnosis of hidden systemic vasculitis. *Ann Rheum Dis* 2005;64:105–110.
59. Landor M. Clinical problem-solving. A hidden agenda. *N Engl J Med* 1998;338:46–50.
60. Kjaer A, Lebech AM, Eigtved A, et al. Fever of unknown origin: prospective comparison of diagnostic value of ^{18}F-FDG PET and ^{111}In-granulocyte scintigraphy. *Eur J Nucl Med Mol Imaging* 2004; 31:622–626.
61. Peters AM. Nuclear medicine imaging in fever of unknown origin. *Q J Nucl Med* 1999;43:61–73.
62. Blockmans D, Knockaert D, Maes A, et al. Clinical value of [(^{18})F]fluoro-deoxyglucose positron emission tomography for patients with fever of unknown origin. *Clin Infect Dis* 2001;32:191–196.
63. Meller J, Koster G, Liersch T, et al. Chronic bacterial osteomyelitis: prospective comparison of (^{18})F-FDG imaging with a dual-head coincidence camera and (^{111})In-labelled autologous leucocyte scintigraphy. *Eur J Nucl Med Mol Imaging* 2002;29:53–60.
64. Lorenzen J, Buchert R, Bohuslavizki KH. Value of FDG PET in patients with fever of unknown origin. *Nucl Med Commun* 2001;22: 779–783.
65. Bleeker-Rovers CP, de Kleijn EM, Corstens FH, et al. Clinical value of FDG PET in patients with fever of unknown origin and patients suspected of focal infection or inflammation. *Eur J Nucl Med Mol Imaging* 2004;31:29–37.
66. Buysschaert I, Vanderschueren S, Blockmans D, et al. Contribution of (^{18})fluoro-deoxyglucose positron emission tomography to the work-up of patients with fever of unknown origin. *Eur J Intern Med* 2004; 15:151–156.
67. Bleeker-Rovers CP, Corstens FH, Van Der Meer JW, et al. Fever of unknown origin: prospective comparison of diagnostic value of (^{18})F-FDG PET and (^{111})In-granulocyte scintigraphy. *Eur J Nucl Med Mol Imaging* 2004;31:1342–1343.
68. Jaruskova M, Belohlavek O. role of FDG-PET and PET/CT in the diagnosis of prolonged febrile states. *Eur J Nucl Med Mol Imaging* 2006;33:913–918.
69. Oyen WJ, Mansi L. FDG-PET in infectious and inflammatory disease. *Eur J Nucl Med Mol Imaging* 2003;30:1568–1570.
70. Blockmans D, Stroobants S, Maes A, et al. Positron emission tomography in giant cell arteritis and polymyalgia rheumatica: evidence for inflammation of the aortic arch. *Am J Med* 2000;108: 246–249.
71. Vos FJ, Bleeker-Rovers CP, Corstens FH, et al. FDG-PET for imaging of non-osseous infection and inflammation. *Q J Nucl Med Mol Imaging* 2006;50:121–130.
72. Meller J, Strutz F, Siefker U, et al. Early diagnosis and follow-up of aortitis with [(^{18})F]FDG PET and MRI. *Eur J Nucl Med Mol Imaging* 2003;30:730–736.

73. Webb M, Chambers A, Al-Nahhas A, et al. The role of ^{18}F-FDG PET in characterizing disease activity in Takayasu arteritis. *Eur J Nucl Med Mol Imaging* 2004;31:627–634.
74. Belhocrine T, Blockmans D, Hustinx R, et al. Imaging of large vessel vasculitis with 18FDG PET: illusion or reality? A critical review of the literature data. *Eur J Nucl Med Mol Imaging* 2003;30:1305–1313.
75. Vallabhajosula S, Machac J, Knesaurek K, et al. Imaging atherosclerotic macrophage density by positron emission tomography using F-18-fluorodeoxyglucose (FDG). *J Nucl Med* 1996;37[Suppl]:38P.
76. Meller J, Grabbe E, Becker W, et al. Value of F-18 FDG hybrid camera PET and MRI in early Takayasu aortitis. *Eur Radiol* 2003; 13:400-405
77. Brodmann M, Lipp RW, Passath A, et al. The role of 2-^{18}F-fluoro-2-deoxy-D-glucose positron emission tomography in the diagnosis of giant cell arteritis of the temporal arteries. *Rheumatology (Oxford)* 2004;43:241–242.
78. Rozin AP, Bar-Shalom R, Strizevsky A, et al. Fever due to aortitis. *Clin Rheumatol* 2007;26:265–267.
79. Orton DF, LeVeen RF, Saigh JA, et al. Aortic prosthetic graft infections: radiologic manifestations and implications for management. *Radiographics* 2000;20:977–993.
80. Seeger JM. Management of patients with prosthetic vascular graft infection. *Am Surg* 2000;66:166–177.
81. Chang JK, Calligaro KD, Ryan S, et al. Risk factors associated with infection of lower extremity revascularization: analysis of 365 procedures performed at a teaching hospital. *Ann Vasc Surg* 2003;17:91–96.
82. Vogelzang RL, Limpert JD, Yao JS. Detection of prosthetic vascular complication: comparison of CT and angiography. *AJR Am J Roentgenol* 1987;148:819–823.
83. Ramo OJ, Varna M, Lantto E, et al. Postoperative graft incorporation after aortic reconstruction—comparison between computerised tomography and Tc-99m-HMPAO labelled leucocyte imaging. *Eur J Vasc Surg* 1993;7:122–128.
84. Samuel A, Paganelli G, Chiesa R, et al. Detection of prosthetic vascular graft infection using avidin/indium-111-biotin scintigraphy. *J Nucl Med* 1996;37:55–61.
85. Libertadore M, Iurilli AP, Ponzo F, et al. Clinical usefulness of technetium-99m-HMPAO-labeled leukocyte scan in prosthetic vascular graft infection. *J Nucl Med* 1998;39:875–879.
86. Fukuchi K, Ishida Y, Higashi M, et al. Detection of aortic graft infection by fluorodeoxyglucose positron emission tomography: comparison with computed tomographic findings. *J Vasc Surg* 2005;42:919–925.
87. Keidar Z, Engel A, Nitecki S, et al. PET/CT using 2-deoxy-2-[^{18}F]fluoro-D-glucose for the evaluation of suspected infected vascular graft. *Mol Imaging Biol* 2003;5:23–25.
88. Stadler P, Bilohlavek O, Spacek M, et al. Diagnosis of vascular prosthesis infection with FDG-PET/CT. *J Vasc Surg* 2004;40:1246–1247.
89. Cook GJ, Fogelman I, Maiset MN. Normal physiological and benign pathological variants of 18-fluoro-2-deoxyglucose positron-emission tomography scanning: potential for error in interpretation. *Semin Nucl Med* 1996;26:308–314.
90. Keidar Z, Engel A, Hoffman A, et al. Prosthetic vascular graft infection: the role of FDG-PET/CT. *J Nucl Med* 2007;48:1230–1236.
91. Davies JR, Rudd JH, Weissberg PL. Molecular and metabolic imaging of atherosclerosis. *J Nucl Med* 2004;45:1898–1907.
92. Virmani R, Kolodgie FD, Burke AP, et al. Lessons from sudden coronary death: a comprehensive morphological classification scheme for atherosclerotic lesions. *Arterioscler Thromb Vasc Biol* 2000;20:1262–1275.
93. Pasterkamp G, Falk E, Woutman H, et al. Techniques characterizing the coronary atherosclerotic plaque: influence on clinical decision making? *J Am Coll Cardiol* 2000;36:13–21.
94. Siegel RJ, Ariani M, Fishbein MC, et al. Histopathologic validation of angioscopy and intravascular ultrasound. *Circulation* 1991;84:109–117.
95. Eliaziv M, Rankin RN, Fox AJ, et al. Accuracy and prognostic consequences of ultrasonography in identifying severe carotid artery stenosis: North America Symptomatic Carotid Endarterectomy Trial (NASCET) Group. *Stroke* 1995;26:1747–1752.
96. Kooi ME, Cappendijk VC, Cleutjens KB, et al. Accumulation of ultrasmall superparamagnetic particles of iron oxide in human atherosclerotic plaques can be detected by in vivo magnetic resonance imaging. *Circulation* 2003;107:2453–2458.
97. Raggi P. Coronary calcium on electron beam tomography imaging as a surrogate marker of coronary artery disease. *Am J Cardiol* 2001;87: 27A–34A.
98. Helft G, Worthley SG, Fuster V, et al. Atherosclerotic aortic component quantification by noninvasive magnetic resonance imaging: an *in vivo* study in rabbits. *J Am Coll Cardiol* 2001;37:1149–1154.
99. Vallabhajosula S, Paidi M, Badimon JJ, et al. Radiotracers for low density lipoprotein biodistribution studies in vivo: technetium-99m low density lipoprotein versus radioiodinated low density lipoprotein preparations. *J Nucl Med* 1988;29:1237–1245.
100. Fischman AJ, Rubin RH, Khaw BA, et al. Radionuclide imaging of experimental atherosclerosis with nonspecific polyclonal immunoglobulin G. *J Nucl Med* 1989;30:1095–1100.
101. Demacker PNM, Dormans TPJ, Koenders EB, et al. Evaluation of indium-111-polyclonal immunoglobulin G to quantitate atherosclerosis in Watanabe heritable hyperlipidemic rabbits with scintigraphy: effect of age and treatment with antioxidants or ethinylestradiol. *J Nucl Med* 1993;34:1316–1321.
102. Vallabhajosula S, Fuster V. Atherosclerosis: imaging techniques and the evolving role of nuclear medicine. *J Nucl Med* 1997;38:1788–1796.
103. Tawakol A, Migrino RQ, Hoffman U, et al. Noninvasive in vivo measurement of vascular inflammation with F-18 fluorodeoxyglucose positron emission tomography. *J Nucl Cardiol* 2005;12:294–301.
104. Rudd JH, Warburton EA, Fryer TD, et al. Imaging atherosclerotic plaque inflammation with [^{18}F]-fluorodeoxyglucose positron emission tomography. *Circulation* 2002;105:2708–2711.
105. Yun M, Yeh D, Araucho LI, et al. F-18 FDG uptake in the large arteries. A new observation. *Clin Nucl Med* 2001;26:314–319.
106. Tatsumi M, Cohade C, Nakamoto Y, et al. Fluorodeoxyglucose uptake in the aortic wall at PET/CT: possible finding for active atherosclerosis. *Radiology* 2003;229:831–837.
107. Ben-Haim S, Kupzov E, Tamir A, et al. Evaluation of ^{18}F-FDG uptake and arterial wall calcifications using ^{18}F-FDG PET/CT. *J Nucl Med* 2004;45:1816–1821.
108. Ben-Haim S, Kupzov E, Tamir A, et al. Changing patterns of abnormal vascular wall F-18 fluorodeoxyglucose uptake on follow-up PET/CT studies. *J Nucl Cardiol* 2006;13:791–800.
109. Hoffman JM, Waskin HA, Schifter T, et al. FDG-PET in differentiating lymphoma from nonmalignant central nervous system lesions in patients with AIDS. *J Nucl Med* 1993;34:567–575.
110. O'Doherty MJ, Barrington SF, Campbell M, et al. PET scanning and the human immunodeficiency virus-positive patient. *J Nucl Med* 1997;38:1575–1583.
111. Brust D, Polis M, Davey R, et al. Fluorodeoxyglucose imaging in healthy subjects with HIV infection: impact of disease stage and therapy on pattern of nodal activation. *AIDS* 2006;20:985–993.
112. Mahfouz T, Miceli MH, Saghafifar F, et al. ^{18}F-fluorodeoxyglucose positron emission tomography contributes to the diagnosis and management of infections in patients with multiple myeloma: a study of 165 infectious episodes. *J Clin Oncol* 2005;23:7857–7863.
113. Yu JQ, Zhuang H, Mavi A, et al. Evaluating the role of fluorodeoxyglucose PET imaging in the management of patients with sarcoidosis. *PET Clin North Am* 2006;1:141–152.
114. Lewis PJ, Salama A. Uptake of fluorine-18-fluorodeoxyglucose in sarcoidosis. *J Nucl Med* 1994;35:1647–1649.
115. Larson SM. Cancer or inflammation? A holy grail for nuclear medicine. *J Nucl Med* 1994;35:1653–1655.
116. Yasuda S, Shotsu A, Ide M, et al. High fluorine-18 labeled deoxyglucose uptake in sarcoidosis. *Clin Nucl Med* 1996;21:983–984.
117. Aberg C, Ponzo F, Raphael B, et al. FDG positron emission tomography of bone involvement in sarcoidosis. *AJR Am J Roentgenol* 2004; 182:975–977.

118. Ishimaru S, Tsujino I, Takei T, et al. Focal uptake on ^{18}F-fluoro-2-deoxyglucose positron emission tomography images indicates cardiac involvement of sarcoidosis. *Eur Heart J* 2005;26:1538–1543.
119. Kaku B, Kanaya H, Horita Y, et al. Failure of follow-up gallium single-photon emission computed tomography and fluorine-18-fluorodeoxyglucose positron emission tomography to predict the deterioration of a patient with cardiac sarcoidosis. *Circ J* 2004;68:802–805.
120. Nishiyama Y, Yamamoto Y, Fukunaga K, et al. Comparative evaluation of ^{18}F-FDG PET and ^{67}Ga scintigraphy in patients with sarcoidosis. *J Nucl Med* 2006;47:1571–1576.
121. Milman N, Mortensen J, Sloth C. Fluorodeoxyglucose PET scan in pulmonary sarcoidosis during treatment with inhaled and oral corticosteroids. *Respiration (Herrlisheim)* 2003;70:408–413.
122. Meyer MA. Diffusely increased colonic F-18 FDG uptake in acute enterocolitis. *Clin Nucl Med* 1995;20:434–435.
123. Kresnik W, Mikosch P, Gallowitsch HJ, et al. F-18 fluorodeoxyglucose positron emission tomography in the diagnosis of inflammatory bowel disease. *Clin Nucl Med* 2001;26:867.
124. Jadvar H, Schambye RB, Segall GM. Effect of atropine and sincalide on intestinal uptake of F-18 fluorodeoxyglucose. *Clin Nucl Med* 1999; 24:965–967.
125. Israel O, Yefremov N, Bar-Shalom R, et al. PET/CT detection of unexpected gastrointestinal foci of ^{18}F-FDG uptake: incidence, localization patterns, and clinical significance. *J Nucl Med* 2005;46:758–762.
126. Tadlidil R, Jadvar H, Badin JR, et al. Incidental colonic fluorodeoxyglucose uptake: correlation with colonoscopic and histopathologic findings. *Radiology* 2002;224:783–787.
127. Kresnik W, Mikosch P, Gallowitsch HJ, et al. Role of fluorodeoxyglucose PET on inflammatory bowel disease: a review. *PET Clin North Am* 2006;1:153–162.
128. Pio BS, Byrne FR, Aranda R, et al. Noninvasive quantification of bowel inflammation through positron emission tomography imaging of 2-deoxy-2-[^{18}F]fluoro-D-glucose-labeled white blood cells. *Mol Imaging Biol* 2003;5:271–277.
129. Yen RF, Chen YC, Wu YW, et al. Using 18-fluoro-2-deoxyglucose positron emission tomography in detecting infectious endocarditis/endoarteritis: a preliminary report. *Acad Radiol* 2004;11:316–321.
130. Israel O, Weiler-Sagie M, Rispler S, et al. PET/CT effect of patient-related factors on cardiac ^{18}F-fluoro-deoxyglucose uptake. *J Nucl Med* 2007;48:234–239.
131. Bakheet SMB, Powe J, Ezzat A, et al. F-18-FDG uptake in tuberculosis. *Clin Nucl Med* 1998;23:739–742.
132. Bakheet SMB, Powe J, Kandil A, et al. F-18 FDG uptake in breast infection and inflammation. *Clin Nucl Med* 2000;25:100–103.
133. Goo JM, Im JG, Do KH, et al. Pulmonary tuberculoma evaluated by means of FDG PET: findings in 10 cases. *Radiology* 2000;216:117–121.
134. Jones HA. Inflammation imaging. *Proc Am Thorac Soc* 2005;2: 545–548.
135. Rosenbaum SJ, Lind T, Antoch G, et al. False-positive FDG PET uptake—the role of PET/CT. *Eur Radiol* 2006;16:1054–1065.
136. Meller J, Sahlmann CO, Lehmann K, et al. [F-18-FDG hybrid camera PET in patients with postoperative fever] *Nuklearmedizin* 2002; 41:22–29.
137. Truong MT, Erasmus JJ, Macapinlac HA, et al. Teflon injection for vocal cord paralysis: false-positive finding on FDG PET-CT in a patient with non-small cell lung cancer. *AJR Am J Roentgenol* 2004;182:1587–1589.
138. Harrigal C, Branstetter BF 4th, Snyderman CH, et al. Teflon granuloma in the nasopharynx: a potentially false-positive PET/CT finding. *AJNR Am J Neuroradiol* 2005;26:417–420.
139. Bhargava P, Kumar R, Zhuang H, et al. Catheter-related focal FDG activity on whole body PET imaging. *Clin Nucl Med* 2004;29:238–242.
140. Osman S, Danpure HJ. The use of 2-[^{18}F]fluoro-2-deoxy-D-glucose as a potential *in vitro* agent for labelling human granulocytes for clinical studies by positron emission tomography. *Int J Rad Appl Instrum B* 1992;19:183–190.
141. Forstrom LA, Mullan BP, Hung JC, et al. ^{18}F-FDG labelling of human leukocytes. *Nucl Med Commun* 2000;21:691–694.
142. Pellegrino D, Bonab, AA, Dragotakes SC, et al. Inflammation and infection: imaging properties of ^{18}F-FDG-labeled white blood cells versus ^{18}F-FDG. *J Nucl Med* 2005;46:1522–1530.
143. Forstrom LA, Dunn WL, Mullan BP, et al. Biodistribution and dosimetry of [(^{18})F]fluorodeoxyglucose labelled leukocytes in normal human subjects. *Nucl Med Commun* 2002;23:721–725.
144. Dumarey N, Egrise D, Didier B, et al. Imaging infection with ^{18}F-FDG-labeled leukocyte PET/CT: initial experience in 21 patients. *J Nucl Med* 2006;47:625–632.
145. Rini JN, Bhargava KK, Tronco GG, et al. PET with FDG-labeled leukocytes versus scintigraphy with ^{111}In-oxine-labeled leukocytes for detection of infection. *Radiology* 2006;238:978–987.
146. Makinen TJ, Lankinen P, Poyhonen T, et al. Comparison of ^{18}F-FDG and ^{68}Ga PET imaging in the assessment of experimental osteomyelitis due to staphylococcus aureus. *Eur J Nucl Med Mol Imaging* 2005;32:1259–1268.

CHAPTER

13 PET and Drug Development

JERRY M. COLLINS

Development of a drug is a process that depends heavily on knowledge of its distribution in the body and its effects on the body. As phrased in Table 13.1, researchers want to know where the drug goes, what it does there, and if there are apparent relationships between drug localization and drug effects.

With positron emission tomography (PET) imaging it is possible to obtain direct information about both the distribution and the functional effects of a drug. PET can provide unique, value-added contributions to the drug development process. Perhaps even more important than its exquisite sensitivity, PET provides spatial information on drug distribution and drug effects that is virtually never attained in living humans by other means.

There are many similarities between the development of therapeutic agents and probes for PET imaging of *in vivo* functions (the term *probe* is used in this chapter to designate the positron-emitting compound used to image biochemical, molecular, and/or physiologic pathways). Both treatment and imaging approaches attempt to exploit differences between some process within the target and in other tissues. Another very practical characteristic for both therapeutics and probes is that the development process can be viewed as a pipeline or process that stretches over several years. The time at which a novel therapeutic agent enters clinical testing is far too late to decide that it would be useful to pursue imaging of its impact. Once a target for screening of new therapeutics has been identified, it also becomes a target to be considered for imaging. Even if developed from the same screening approach, the ideal probe molecule may or may not be the same as the optimal therapeutic molecule.

One of the major challenges is development of new probes. Fluorine-18 ([^{18}F])-fluorodeoxyglucose (FDG) is the only functional imaging probe readily available at all PET facilities. Pilot trials have been reported for various other potential probes, but a concerted effort is required to prioritize targets and probe development projects. The recent announcement by the U.S. Food and Drug Administration on exploratory investigational new drugs has been especially useful for the initial human experiences with novel PET imaging agents (1).

Although drug development and probe development can be interrelated, they can also be separate processes. At one level, the role of a probe is to support the development of the therapeutic. In some cases, the probe might assist in the choice of doses of the therapeutic for the pivotal trials, leading to marketing approval. In such cases, the approval of the therapeutic is based on the success of the trials, not the imaging studies. The probe itself may never be used again. It is thus to be expected that some highly specialized probes may be used in drug development that does not have an ultimate clinically practical applicability.

In other cases, a general functional probe may be valuable for an entire class of drugs, or even many classes of drugs. The probe itself becomes a diagnostic tool that might be marketed in its own right. Fluorine-18-FDG is the most advanced example of this pattern for PET probes.

As described in the next two sections, useful probes for PET imaging can be obtained by positron labeling of either the therapeutic substance itself or the indicators (ligands, substrates, tracers) of functional status. For drug distribution studies, the most relevant information is obtained when the drug itself can be labeled with a positron-emitting atom.

Functional imaging evaluates processes occurring at the cellular or tissue/organ level: physiologic (e.g., transport carrier system), molecular (e.g., receptor binding), or biochemical (e.g., enzymatic activity). Thus, for functional imaging, the most important factor is a clear concept of the process to be probed. Focus on specific targets at these levels is part of a general shift in the paradigm of clinical diagnosis and treatment.

In addition to the value of imaging for drug development, the same tools could be used for customizing patient-specific treatment. Physicians have long sought tests that could assist in the choice of the most appropriate therapy for the individual patient. Traditional selection of therapy for individuals has relied on prognostic factors derived from large populations. For example, in anticancer therapy, the histology of the tumor is a key factor. Once therapy has been selected, it is generally continued until there is an obvious failure to control disease (e.g., tumor growth) or to control symptoms (e.g., pain).

By shifting emphasis toward underlying targets, functional imaging with PET has the potential to improve the selection and subsequent evaluations of therapy. PET provides the opportunity to

TABLE 13.1 Question-based Drug Development

1. Does the drug reach its target?
2. What does it do there?
   a. Desired impact on target?
   b. Side effects?
3. What is the relationship between questions 1 and 2?

measure several characteristics of a disease target serially and noninvasively.

For some imaging targets (e.g., enzymes, receptors, and transporters), patients can be phenotyped *before* initiation of treatment. The goal is to obtain information that can be used to optimize the match between drugs and the patient-specific characteristics of the target. In addition to the potential for improving efficacy, these procedures would be valuable for avoiding needless toxicity from treatment regimens that are inappropriate for the individual patient being assessed.

Regardless of whether pretreatment phenotyping is feasible, all potential targets should be able to provide therapeutic assessment once treatment is under way. Rather than waiting until overt failure is demonstrated, which could be many months for conditions that are difficult to assess, the goal is to determine as quickly as possible whether the particular therapy is working for a specific patient. The optimal imaging time will depend on the mechanism of action for the therapy, but the ideal situation would be immediately after the first dose so a decision can be made regarding further treatment. Positive findings would be greatly appreciated by all. Negative results would provide the opportunity to explore other therapeutic approaches before further deterioration of the patient's condition and ability to tolerate therapy.

The examples provided in the next two sections elaborate on these concepts. It is important to keep in mind that all of these examples are works in progress. There are currently very few PET imaging probes that are "accepted" for routine use by the nuclear medicine community except [^{18}F]-FDG.

ASSESSMENT OF DRUG DELIVERY WITH PET

The ultimate goal of drug delivery (pharmacokinetics) is to get the active molecule to the target site. In classic drug development, systemic exposure to the drug is assessed by serial measurements of the drug concentration in plasma. Monitoring plasma concentrations to determine the systemic exposure component of drug delivery is certainly helpful, but there remain fundamental questions that can only be addressed by examining the second component of drug delivery, namely, the interaction between systemic exposure and local transport processes. In the preclinical phases of drug development, drug distribution studies are conducted in animal species to gain confidence that the active molecules reach the target sites of interest. In contrast, once human testing begins, researchers no longer have access to invasive sampling of many tissue sites. Without the noninvasive tools of imaging, the second component of local drug delivery is *invisible*, except for the potential effects of the drug on the target, and researchers can only evaluate the systemic component.

Anti-infective Drugs: Penetration to Target

The success of an anti-infective drug depends on its ability to reach bacteria, viruses, fungi, or other parasites wherever they may reside in the body. There is particular concern about delivering adequate concentrations of drugs to so-called sanctuary sites such as the brain or prostatic fluid. Comprehensive testing is conducted to determine the intrinsic sensitivity of various invading organisms, with the results often focusing on concentrations required to achieve 90% kill or 90% inhibition of growth—that is, the IC_{90}. No matter how impressively potent a drug might be in attacking the target in laboratory tests, it cannot be successful in patients unless it is delivered to the target site.

Fig. 13.1 provides an excellent demonstration of the role PET imaging can play in determining if a particular drug is likely to reach the critical tissue of interest. Fischman et al. (2) labeled the antifungal drug, fluconazole, with [^{18}F] and administered it to human volunteers in a phase I study. As illustrated, the time course of distribution for [^{18}F]-fluconazole was followed for 2 hours in eight body areas. Because humans do not metabolize fluconazole, only the parent drug is present. Thus, the absolute quantitation of radiolabel provided by PET imaging can be translated into traditional units of drug concentration (in micrograms per milliliter) that can then be compared against the therapeutic goals defined by IC_{90} testing. In this case, with a single study early in drug development,

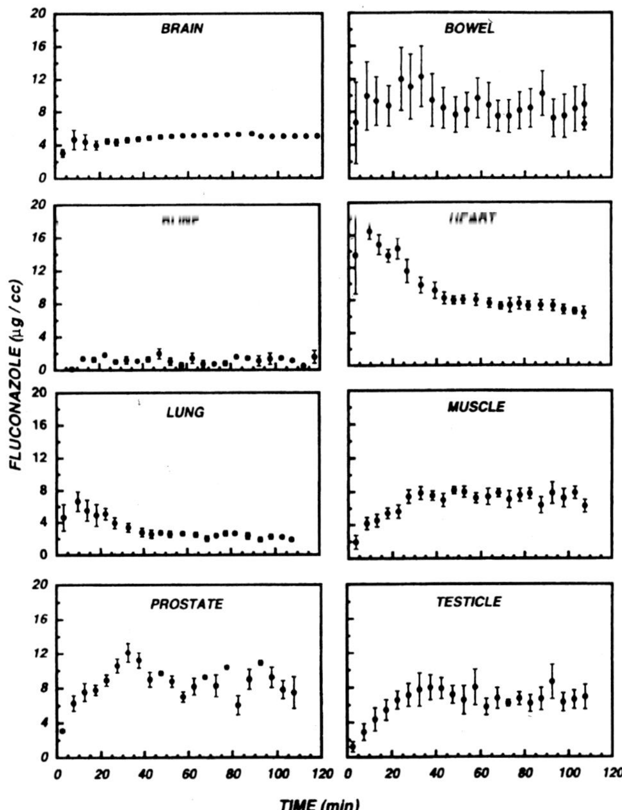

FIGURE 13.1. Fluorine-18-fluconazole distribution over time in 6 healthy volunteers. (From Fischman AJ, Alpert NM, Babich JW, et al. The role of PET in pharmacokinetic analysis. *Drug Metab Rev* 1997;29:923–956, with permission.)

a positive finding can help sustain interest in the lead candidate. Alternatively, the outcome of such a study could definitively show serious obstacles to further development. Although such a result would be disappointing, it is surely better to find out early in development, before clinical efficacy studies in patients are started.

Transporters and Their Modulation

As mentioned at the beginning of this section, local transport processes can control access of a drug to its target. The understanding of these transporters or pumps has blossomed dramatically in the past few years. Several families of pumps have been discovered and classified phenotypically. In addition, the genes have been cloned, and transporters are now recognized as one of the largest categories of expression products of the mammalian genomes.

Because of the key role of these transporters in regulating drug delivery to target sites, development of probes to assess their operation is a major opportunity for PET imaging. Developmental programs for probes of drug uptake into the cell and efflux from the cell are in early stages of development but build on a tradition of monitoring PET probes of the transporters for amino acid entry into the cell (3).

There is movement away from the study of the distribution of a particular drug and toward a general functional probe for a transporter. Some groups have sought a general probe because there are too many drugs to study each of them. With the recent explosion in the catalog of transporters, one might also say that there are too many transporters to have a probe for each of them. The choice of approach not only is philosophical but also should be driven by the specific question under study.

Drug Delivery to Tumors

Although transport processes can influence all categories of drugs, their role is critical for drug delivery to tumors, due to the narrow therapeutic index of anticancer drugs. Efflux pumps can mediate resistance to anticancer drugs. As the drug approaches its target, the tumor may pump it out. Thus, concentrations at the target are very low, making them ineffective and actually promoting the development of further resistance mechanisms. There are a number of efforts under way to develop modulators that block these transport systems.

PET imaging is a tool that can focus directly on drug delivery at the target of interest. Delivery of a drug to the tumor does not guarantee successful therapy. However, if the drug never gets to the target or gets pushed away as soon as it arrives, it certainly will not be effective. The earlier researchers discover the problem, the sooner they can implement strategies for attempting to modulate this pharmacokinetic issue and the sooner they can consider alternative therapy. Many of these concepts are illustrated in Fig. 13.2. Consider the case in which a drug (e.g., paclitaxel) has been selected for treating a patient with a tumor, based on the tumor's histology and other prognostic factors. If paclitaxel is labeled with a positron emitter, it becomes a suitable probe to seek an answer to the question at the top of Fig. 13.2: does the drug accumulate in the tumor? If the answer is no (the drug fails to accumulate in the tumor), one option is to conclude that paclitaxel can only cause toxicity for this patient and another therapeutic approach should be taken. Substantial validation would be required to confirm the logical scheme, but the outline for decision making is clear.

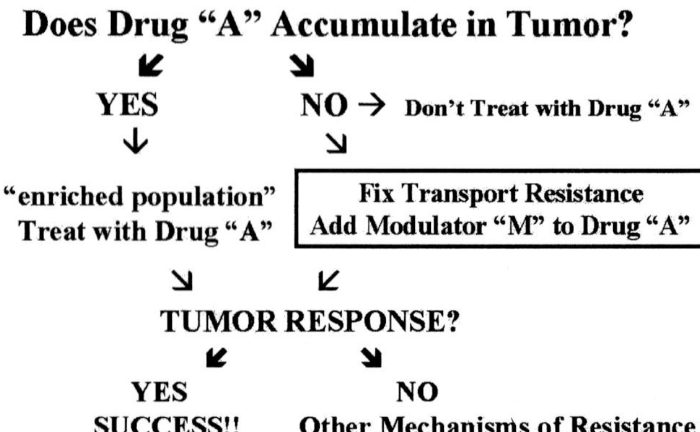

FIGURE 13.2. Decision tree for image-guided assessment of efflux transporter impact.

If the answer is yes (the drug does accumulate in the tumor), there is no guarantee that the tumor will respond to paclitaxel, but the probability of success has been enhanced because at least some nonresponders have been eliminated from the population. Accumulation of drug in the tumor is essential but is not the sole determinant of chemosensitivity. In other words, accumulation is necessary, but not sufficient for response. If the tumor fails to respond despite adequate drug accumulation, one of the most common mechanisms of resistance has been ruled out, and other reasons must be considered.

Patients with tumors that fail to accumulate paclitaxel can become candidates for therapy with drugs that are intended to modulate paclitaxel delivery to tumors—that is, to "fix" resistance due to transport. If the labeled paclitaxel still fails to accumulate in the tumor, then the modulator has failed, at least for the dose and schedule chosen. Once again, it may be desirable to spare the patient the toxicity of paclitaxel and to seek other therapeutic approaches.

If the use of the modulator does permit labeled paclitaxel to accumulate in the tumor, transport resistance has been fixed. Once again, there is no guarantee that transport resistance is the sole mechanism of resistance, but at least a population has been identified with an enhanced probability that the modulator will permit benefit from paclitaxel to be attained. Critical to the success of a radiolabeled drug as a targeting probe is that it is not extensively metabolized. PET only traces the radiolabel but does not indicate to what the radiolabel is attached. For extensively metabolized drugs, the PET imaging approach will be complicated by the distribution *in vivo* of radiolabeled metabolites.

CELLULAR AND MOLECULAR TARGETS FOR PET IMAGING

Some of the major categories of targets for PET probes are shown in Table 13.2. The first two categories—energy metabolism and DNA synthesis—are very general downstream approaches to the determination of tumor functional status. Although the contemporary emphasis is on precise molecular classification of targets, it is still quite desirable to have these "universal" probes as a check on the relevance of hypotheses, as well as for the situations in which an appropriate target-specific or drug-specific probe is simply not available.

As described earlier, FDG is the leading functional PET probe and has remarkable versatility. Evaluation of the rate of DNA

TABLE 13.2 Categories of PET Functional Imaging Targets

1. General energy metabolism (^{18}F-fluorodeoxyglucose)
2. DNA synthesis/cellular proliferation
3. Receptors: signaling/regulation
4. Enzymes: many tumor targets

synthesis and cellular proliferation is another approach toward a general probe. In the laboratory, tritiated thymidine (dThd) has been used for decades to evaluate DNA synthesis in cell culture. In anticancer therapy, the ability to monitor the impact of conventional cytotoxic regimens on DNA synthesis is easily appreciated. In addition, therapeutic approaches of many contemporary targets are ultimately intended to reduce proliferation and may be evaluated using dThd analogues (dThd analogues are discussed in more detail later in this section).

A much more target-specific approach is represented by the last two categories of probes. Receptors and enzymes are well established as drug targets across the full spectrum of disease areas, and they are the cornerstones of modern therapeutic developmental programs in the areas of cell signaling and regulation. Thus, according to the paradigm for probe development, receptors and enzymes are also potential targets for functional imaging. Although the imaging of these targets remains in the pilot stage for most diseases, the feasibility for monitoring *in situ* receptor occupancy and enzyme activity has been solidly established in neuropharmacology, as described below.

The list of targets in Table 13.2 for functional PET probes is not meant to be comprehensive. Also, some targets are in an intermediate position on the scale from "general" to "specific." For example, there are probes for measuring blood flow and capillary permeability, as well as phenomena such as tissue hypoxia.

As noted in Table 13.3, once the ideal (relevant) targets are chosen based on biochemical/molecular/physiologic factors, additional probe-specific parameters are encountered. From the viewpoint of nuclear chemistry, the half-life of the positron-emitting isotope must be matched to the time scale of the process being probed. A rapid synthesis must be feasible, due to the short half-lives of most positron-emitting atoms. From a pharmacokinetic perspective, minimal catabolism is highly desirable because the background signal from accumulating metabolites will interfere with the desired signal from the parent molecule. Finally, the ratio of specific to nonspecific localization within the tumor is critical. Once all other obstacles are overcome and a new probe has entered the clinic, the most common reason that development is abandoned is the finding of a broad and nonspecific distribution of the probe throughout the body, preventing the monitoring of specific target interactions.

TABLE 13.3 Desirable Characteristics for Design of Functional PET Probes

1. Relevant target for interaction
2. Match isotopic half-life to process time scale
3. Rapid synthetic time
4. Minimal interference from catabolites
5. Target localization

The ability to image the response of the target of drug action is fundamental to the advances in the individualization of therapy, as well as enhancements in drug development. These concepts are illustrated by the following examples.

Neuroreceptors: D_2 and 5-HT_2

Applications of PET imaging for drug development are furthest advanced in the field of neurosciences. This progress has been pushed by multiple factors. There is very strong interest in obtaining information about the brain, but it is the least accessible part of the body for invasive sampling. Due to huge investments over the past few decades in building a knowledge base for receptors and their ligands, the selection of targets and probes has been facilitated. Fortuitously, the least accessible part of the body has a major advantage for imaging because the blood–brain barrier tends to preferentially exclude the relatively more hydrophilic catabolites of the probes, thus, reducing the background noise.

The dopaminergic- and serotonergic-receptor systems have been mapped extensively. The work of Farde et al. (1) demonstrated how the impact of a drug can be measured in two separate receptor systems in a single patient. Carbon-11 ([^{11}C])-raclopride is an established probe for the D_2 dopaminergic receptor subtype and [^{11}C]-*N*-methyl spiperone probes both 5-HT_2 and D_2 receptors. Of course, these probes cannot be given simultaneously because the PET camera cannot distinguish which molecule has [^{11}C] attached. However, the short half-life of [^{11}C] is an advantage for taking sequential "snapshots" of each probe individually, with perhaps only 1 or 2 hours between imaging sessions.

The efficacy of receptor blockade is commonly determined by "blocking" studies with unlabeled drug. Similarly, PET can assess the effect of chronic receptor blockade, such as in psychotropic therapies, when the patient is on or off therapy (Fig. 13.3). Fig. 13.3. demonstrates the impact of risperidone on two receptor subtypes in a patient being treated with this drug. The D_2 receptors are almost completely blocked. Although there is a substantial blockage of 5-HT_2 receptors by risperidone, the quantitative extent is lower than the drug's impact on D_2 receptors. The broad pattern of spatial distribution for 5-HT_2 receptors in the human brain can also be identified as quite different from the narrower localization of D_2 receptors.

Researchers are frequently reminded that even the most potent and selective drugs can have multiple effects in the body. In the case of antipsychotics such as risperidone, drug designers intentionally built molecules with dual effects, based on earlier therapeutic experience with blockade of the individual receptors. What is the optimal balance between D_2 and 5-HT_2 effects? At the time of selection of candidates for clinical testing, the answer was unknown, and decisions had to be based on the hypotheses that were available during the developmental phase. After the initial subjects are tested, imaging results can provide rapid feedback regarding the extent of blockade achieved with the two receptors.

It should be recognized that this imaging information does not test the therapeutic hypotheses. Instead, it tests whether the intended balance between relative receptor impact was actually achieved *in vivo.* At this early stage, there is no information about clinical benefit. If the receptor impact meets design criteria, the developer will be encouraged to pursue this drug as a lead candidate. On the other hand, failure to achieve design criteria for receptor impact may push toward a decision to test other candidates before making major investments in therapeutic clinical trials.

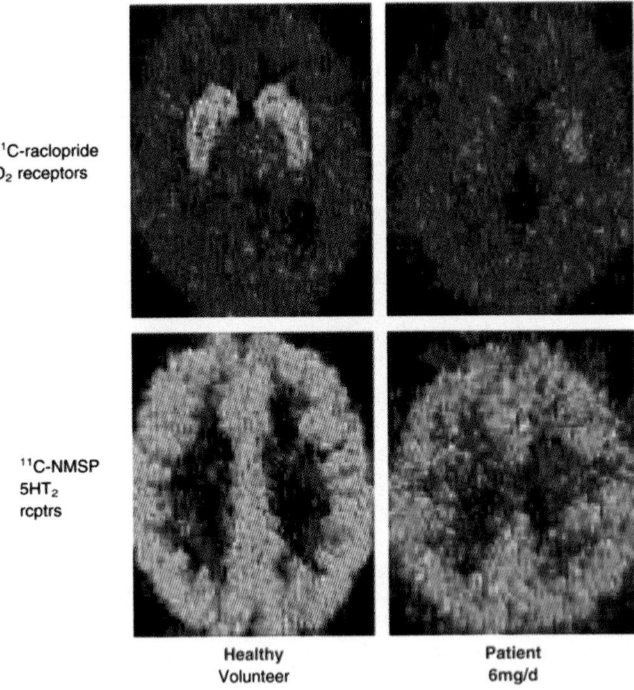

FIGURE 13.3. Impact of the antipsychotic drug, risperidone (6 mg/d), on D_2 and 5-HT_2 neuroreceptors. **Right panel:** Indicates that D_2 receptors are almost completely blocked by this dose of risperidone. **Bottom left panel:** The broad pattern of spatial distribution for 5-HT_2 receptors in the human brain can be identified as quite different from the narrower localization of D_2 receptors **(upper left)**. A substantial blockage of 5-HT_2 receptors by risperidone can be observed, but the quantitative extent is lower than the drug's impact on D_2 receptors. (From Farde L, Nyberg S, Oxenstierna G, et al. Positron emission tomography studies on D_2 and 5-HT_2 receptor binding in risperidone-treated schizophrenic patients. *J Clin Psychopharmacol* 1995;15 [Suppl 1]:19S-23S, with permission.)

Without early feedback from imaging, intermediate decisions cannot be made, the subtype specificity *in vivo* cannot be evaluated, and the developmental program must wait until clinical outcomes provide feedback. Unfortunately, by that time, the resources (e.g., time and labor) have been spent and patient opportunities cannot be recaptured.

If the decision is made to proceed, clinical benefit information will be collected in the usual fashion for such trials. At the end of these trials, the relationship between imaging results and clinical outcomes will be the final test of the hypotheses regarding the nature of optimal receptor blockade.

Estrogen-receptor Blockage by Tamoxifen

For hormone-sensitive tumors such as breast cancer, the established approach to disease management is based on characterization of the hormone receptors (estrogen and progesterone) in biopsies from individual tumors. The ability to noninvasively monitor estrogen receptors with [^{18}F]-fluoroestradiol (FES) is a natural extension of existing practice.

The overall approach is illustrated in Fig. 13.4. Dehdashti et al. (5) injected [^{18}F]-FES into a patient with a large metastasis of breast

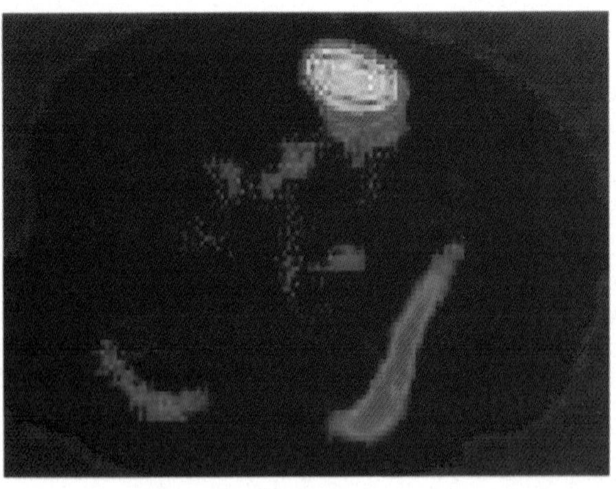

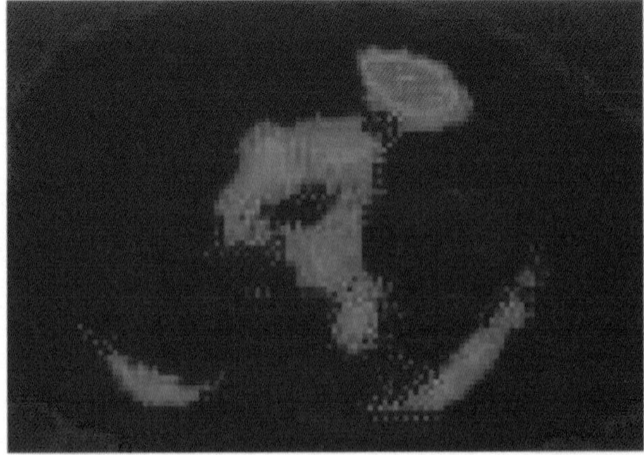

FIGURE 13.4. A patient with estrogen-receptor–positive metastases of breast cancer in the pleural space. Fluorine-18-fluoroestradiol is the radiopharmaceutical. The PET image obtained prior to therapy clearly shows tracer uptake by the tumor (oval at top of **left panel**). The **right panel** is the same image slice after 7 days of tamoxifen therapy. A decrease in tracer uptake is apparent in the lesion. (From Dehdashti F, Flanagan FL, Mortimer JE, et al. Positron emission tomographic assessment of "metabolic flare" to predict response of metastatic breast cancer to antiestrogen therapy. *Eur J Nucl Med* 1999;26:51-56, with permission.)

cancer in the pleural space, which was known to have estrogen receptors. Before therapy, avid binding of [^{18}F]-FES to the receptors on the tumor was observed (in the top of the left panel in Fig. 13.4). Therapy with tamoxifen was initiated, with the intent of occupying estrogen receptors and blocking the uptake of other estrogenic substances. As demonstrated in the PET image (right panel of Fig. 13.4), localization at the tumor site of [^{18}F]-FES has markedly diminished after 7 days of tamoxifen therapy. Although these images do not constitute an index of clinical value, they verify that the specific therapy for this particular tumor is acting as intended.

Tumor Cell Proliferation Probed with Thymidine Analogues

Almost 40 years ago, the first exploration of positron-labeled dThd was reported by the Brookhaven group (6), with the demonstration that [^{11}C]-dThd could be synthesized and injected into mice in a time frame compatible with imaging. During the 1980s through the 1990s, a series of human investigations using [^{11}C]-dThd attempted to build on these murine studies. Some success was obtained, but it is now known that pyrimidine biochemistry in mice is quite different from that in humans. The rapid catabolism of dThd in humans creates an enormous background signal of labeled molecules, and dThd itself is available for labeling of DNA for only a few minutes. Complex mathematic corrections are required for catabolic interference.

The proof of concept for dThd PET was eventually demonstrated with publication by Shields et al. (7) of the first therapeutic assessment images. As illustrated in the left panel of Fig. 13.5, there is extensive uptake of [^{11}C]-dThd both in the primary lung tumor and in the vertebral space before therapy. After a standard regimen of cisplatin on day 1 and etoposide on days 1 to 3, the patient was re-evaluated on day 6. The tumor is still present anatomically, but the image in the right panel indicates that the tumor has stopped taking up [^{11}C]-dThd for DNA synthesis and cellular proliferation.

Although this initial demonstration of the principle has been gratifying, the pool of catabolites of [^{11}C]-dThd in humans creates major difficulties. PET imaging is essentially the detection of total radioactivity, so an extensive search has been under way to find an analogue of dThd that has minimal catabolism but retains the favorable anabolic (DNA labeling) properties of dThd itself. Some candidate structures are shown in Fig. 13.6.

Shields et al. (8) have added [^{18}F] at the 3′ position in the sugar of dThd to yield [^{18}F]-FLT (3′-[^{18}F]-3′-deoxy-dThd) (Fig. 13.6). Images obtained with [^{18}F]-FLT in patients (Fig. 13.7) have demonstrated a similar distribution to dThd itself, despite the inability of phosphorylated FLT to efficiently enter DNA. Shields et al. (9) have also reported initial clinical studies of [^{18}F]-FMAU (2′-[^{18}F]-5-methyl-arabinofuranosyluracil).

Delineation of the differences between information obtained with PET and dThd analogues versus FDG PET will be a key aspect of further clinical investigations. Anecdotal experiences with inflammatory lesions suggest situations that favor dThd analogues. In the initial study of [^{11}C]-dThd (7), the qualitative information obtained from dThd PET was similar to that obtained with FDG PET in the same patients, but the authors report that the quantitative assessment with dThd seemed more closely related to clinical outcome. When compared with computed tomography (CT), dThd PET images obtained before and after therapy also provided an assessment of tumor response more quantitatively related to clinical outcome. However, both FLT and dThd show much more uptake in bone marrow than FDG, which is usually undesirable, and generally showed poorer tumor/background uptake ratios, which may provide sensitivity for disease detection.

For the set of gene therapy protocols that use herpes simplex virus (HSV) thymidine kinase as either a suicide gene or a reporter gene, any of the aforementioned dThd approaches, as well as iodinated analogues, should be able to provide an assessment of whether gene expression was successful (10). In addition, because of their specific affinity for HSV thymidine kinase, a series of analogues of acyclovir or ganciclovir have been shown preclinically, and in early clinical studies, to be successful probes for gene expression (11).

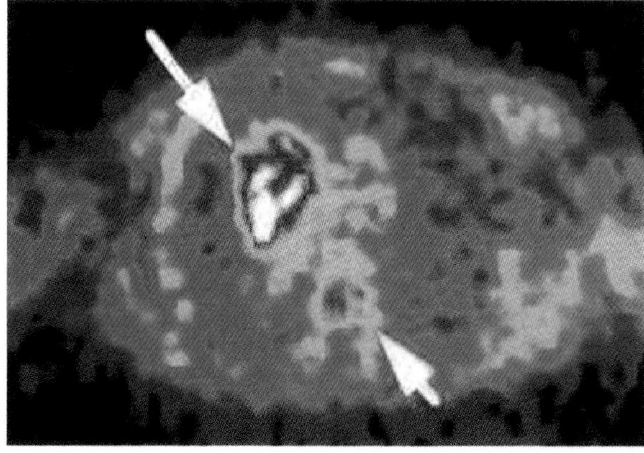

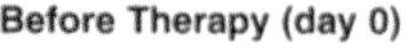

Before Therapy (day 0)

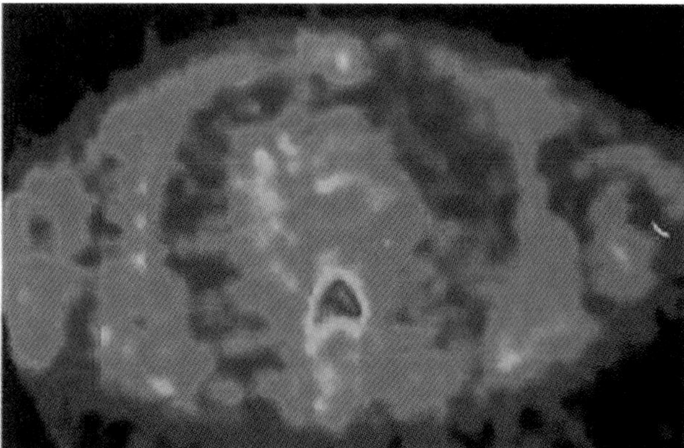

After Therapy (day 6)

FIGURE 13.5. A patient with primary lung cancer was evaluated with carbon-11-thymidine ([^{11}C]-dThd) as the probe. Prior to therapy (**left panel**) transverse PET images show extensive uptake of [^{11}C]-dThd was observed both in the tumor (*large arrow*) and the vertebral space (*small arrow*). In the **right panel**, the same patient was evaluated on day 6 of therapy, after a dose of cisplatin on day 1 and etoposide on days 1 to 3. The tumor was still present anatomically, but it had stopped taking up [11C]-dThd. This tracer is used to image DNA synthesis and cell proliferation. (From Shields AF, Mankoff DA, Link JM, et al. Carbon-11-thymidine and FDG to measure therapy response. *J Nucl Med* 1998;39:1757-1762, with permission.)

dThd **FMAU** **FLT**

FIGURE 13.6. Structures for endogenous thymidine and two of its fluorinated analogues. Thymidine has been labeled for PET imaging with carbon-11 ([11C]) on the pyrimidine base at either the 2-carbon or the 5-methyl carbon. FLT and FMAU have been labeled with fluorine-18 on the 3′ or 2′ position of the sugar. dThd, thymidine; FMAU, 2′-[18F]-5-methyl-arabinofuranosyluracil; FLT, 3′-[18F]-3′-deoxy-dThd.

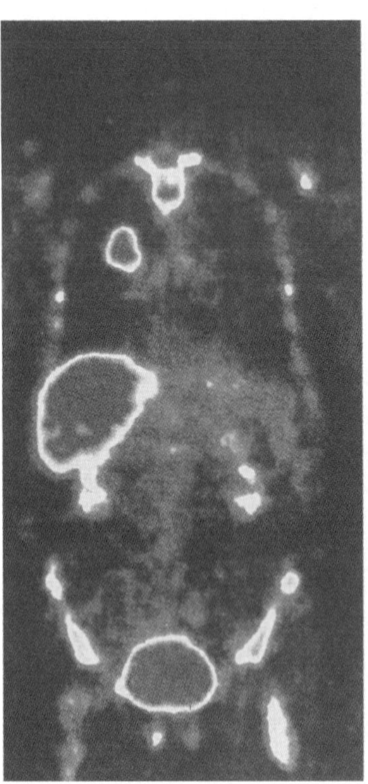

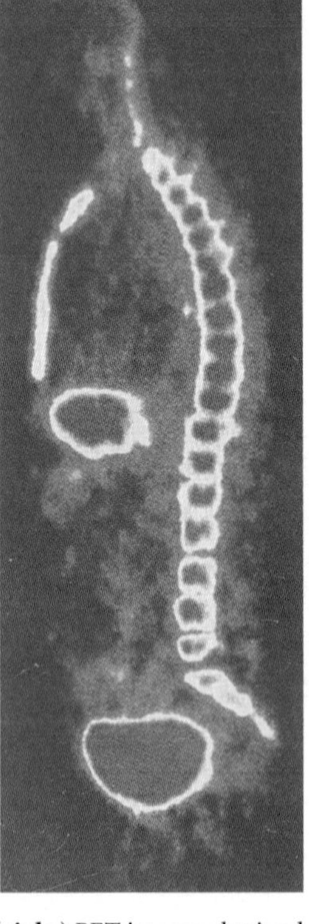

FIGURE 13.7. Coronal (**left**) and sagittal (**right**) PET images obtained using 3′-[18F]-3′-deoxy-dThd, 1.3 mCi, administered to a patient with a lung tumor and imaged at 60 mm. postinjection. Uptake in the right upper lung, liver, bone marrow, and bladder is seen. (Adapted from Shields AF, Grierson JR, Dohmen BM, et al. Imaging proliferation in vivo with [F-18]FLT and positron emission tomography. *Nat Med* 1998;4:1334-1336, with permission.)

Monoamine Oxidase B Enzyme Inhibition

Fowler et al. (12,13), who have reported on the phenotypic expression of monoamine oxidase B (MAO-B) in human brain *in situ*, have solidly established the feasibility for PET monitoring of enzyme activity. Further, they have measured the dose dependence and time course of enzymatic activity for both reversible and irreversible inhibitors. These works are elegant in their own right as a study of the MAO-B enzyme *in vivo*, but they also provide enormous insight into the paradigm for use of target-based imaging in drug development.

During the course of new drug development, the three questions in Table 13.4 can sometimes be answered with clinical observations, but a purely clinical approach is generally very inefficient in the absence of a firm grasp of the complex biochemistry of the targets. As demonstrated by the studies of MAO-B, PET imaging can provide a unique tool to help answer all three of these questions.

The first investigation by Fowler et al. (12), summarized in Fig. 13.8, is probably the best published example of the extraordinary power of PET imaging to guide selection of dose and interval during the earliest phase I evaluation of drugs. The upper left panel shows pretreatment activity of MAO-B in the human brain using an established probe, [^{11}C]-selegiline. When lazabemide, an investigational drug that reversibly inhibits MAO-B, was administered at 25 mg twice a day (upper right panel), almost all MAO-B activity

TABLE 13.4 **Efficacy Issues in Drug Development**

1. Does this treatment affect the presumed target?
2. Do we know the best dose?
3. What is the preferred interval between doses?

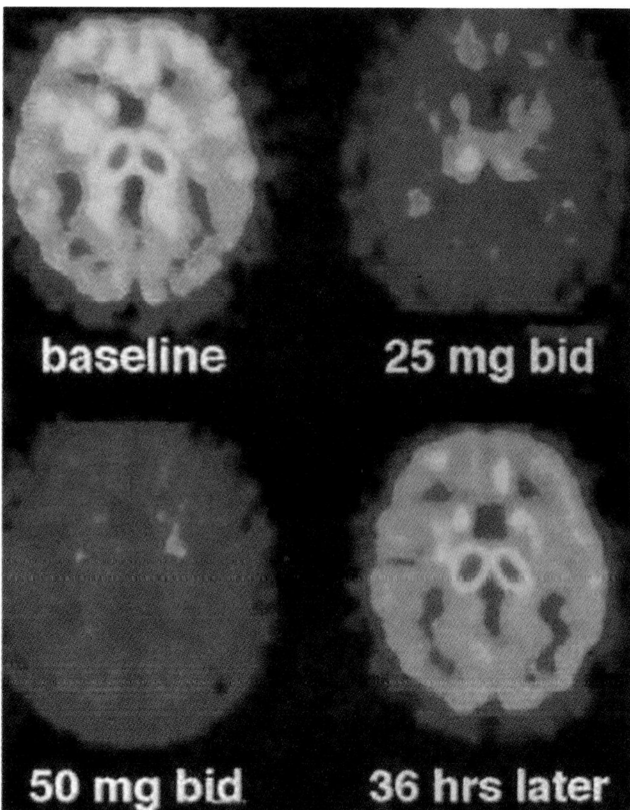

FIGURE 13.8. Reversible dose-dependent monoamine oxidase B (MAO-B) inhibition by lazabemide. (From Fowler JS, Volkow ND, Logan J, et al. MAO B inhibitor therapy in Parkinson's disease: the degree and reversibility of human brain MAO B inhibition by Ro 19 6327. *Neurology* 1993;43:1984-1992, with permission.)

was inhibited. Thus, the first question in Table 13.4 was answered: yes, this drug has an impact on its target.

Doubling the lazabemide dose to 50 mg twice a day (lower right panel) abolished the remaining MAO-B activity. Taken together, the information from the 25- and 50-mg doses helps to answer the second question in Table 13.4: The best dose is unlikely to exceed 50 mg, and lower doses could also be considered.

The lower right panel explores the washout of enzymatic inhibition 36 hours after the last dose. In keeping with the reversible nature of the inhibitory profile of lazabemide, a substantial amount of the baseline activity has been restored. Thus, the answer to the third question in Table 13.4 is that, as studied, twice per day is a usable dose interval. However, these data suggest that once per day could also be a successful dose interval. Because patient adherence to medication is thought to be best at once per day, it would be helpful to obtain imaging information at 24 hours.

Answers to these three questions were readily obtained with PET imaging and can greatly assist the design of definitive clinical activity testing. Nonetheless, it is fair to consider whether such information was truly essential. Fortunately, these same authors conducted a follow-up study with deprenyl (selegiline), which provides some powerful lessons regarding the importance of appropriate dose selection (13). Their deprenyl study was retrospective, because this drug has been marketed for many years.

Using [^{11}C]-selegiline again as the probe, the upper left panel in Fig. 13.9 shows the same pretreatment map of MAO-B activity in human brain as in the previous study. The upper right panel demonstrates that 5 mg twice a day, the dose and schedule listed in the official product brochure, completely abolishes MAO-B activity. Dosing with selegiline was stopped, and the time course for return-to-baseline activity was followed. After 1 week, not much activity was found. Even after 3 weeks, the level of enzymatic activity remained substantially lower than at baseline. Because selegiline is an irreversible inhibitor, this study is actually probing the rate of synthesis of new enzyme in the brain. If the effect of the drug persists for such long periods of time, why is it administered twice a day? Further, the authors estimate from their imaging results that the recommended dose of selegiline is 20-fold higher than that necessary to maintain full inhibition of MAO-B.

These conclusions are readily observed retrospectively, so it should be asked why the original drug development program produced such disparate answers. Selegiline provides modest relief for parkinsonian symptoms, and there are few other therapeutic options. For drugs with only modest activity, it is particularly difficult to choose the optimal dose. As a substitute for the optimal dose, the maximum feasible dose is often used. Thus, the dose is escalated in the hope of generating the most benefit. Of course, if all the benefit is obtained with the first 5% of the dose, then the remaining 95% of the dose can only ensure that a large fraction of patients will suffer side effects. Such an approach to drug development may be expected to improve the safety ratio of therapeutics in which the optimal biological effect is seen at doses much less than the maximum tolerated dose.

SUMMARY

If researchers focus on drug development as a process with enormous dependence on information about drug distribution and effect throughout the body, then its linkage with PET imaging provides a powerful tool for gathering unique data. The design of successful imaging probes is critical and can be a bottleneck that requires broad collaboration among synthetic chemists, pharmacologists, and clinicians from both nuclear medicine and disease-specific areas.

In the broader context of drug development, regulatory approval, and marketing, it is important to classify imaging information properly. In the spectrum of tools from biomarkers to surrogate end points to clinical outcome measures, there are opportunities for new contributions and improvements at all levels. Table 13.5 places the role of imaging into the overall context of drug development.

In the first stage, PET imaging can provide biomarkers that should be particularly useful early in the development of a new

TABLE 13.5 Two Stages of Hypothesis Testing

1. Does the drug impact target as intended?
   (inhibit enzyme; decrease vessel count)
   **Major role for noninvasive images as biomarkers
2. Any clinical benefit?
   (increase survival; improve quality of life)
   **Only controlled clinical trials can evaluate the surrogate end points

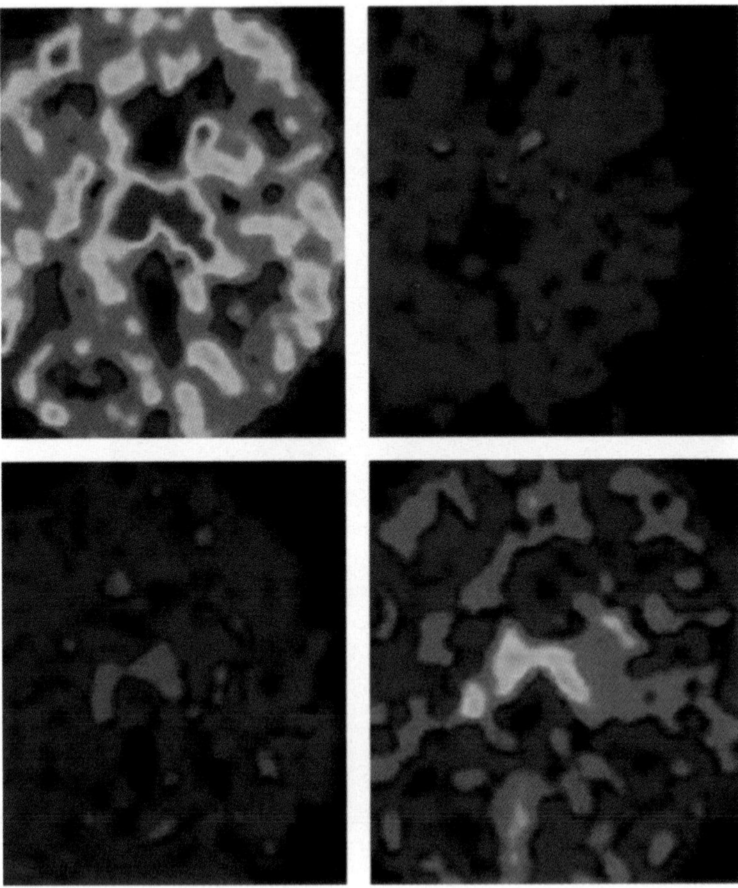

FIGURE 13.9. Irreversible inhibition of monoamine oxidase B (MAO-B) by selegiline. (From Fowler JS, Volkow ND, Logan J, et al. Slow recovery of human brain MAO B after L-deprenyl (selegiline) withdrawal. *Synapse* 1994;18:86-93, with permission.)

drug, and it can guide the selection of dose and schedule of administration for subsequent testing phases. Biomarkers can also contribute to "go, no go" decision making at this stage, based on the presumed mechanism of action for the therapeutic.

As the focus moves forward toward marketing approval of therapeutics, the second stage of the hypothesis is that the drug provides clinical benefit. Biomarkers (such as PET probes) by themselves do not establish quality of life or increased survival. Although imaging data can be highly informative for drug development, drug approval and marketing must be based on a demonstration of clinical value, in the context of the benefit-to-risk ratio applicable to the condition being treated. Controlled clinical trials can evaluate biomarkers to determine if they are candidates to become surrogate end points for clinical benefit, but this is a much larger and somewhat different undertaking than the development of biomarkers.

Increasingly, the linkage between diagnostics (including biomarkers) and therapeutics is changing the way populations are chosen for studies of drugs. Furthermore, the more carefully a drug is studied during the development stages, the more adequate will be the guidance for customizing therapy once the drug enters clinical practice. As imaging is increasingly able to define the molecular phenotype of individual patients, only patients with the appropriate targets will be considered eligible for the therapeutic trials. It is clearly hoped that with such an approach, the probability of the desired response would be increased.

Although the applications of PET in drug development are still in the early stages, the examples provided in this chapter illustrate useful applications across several broad disease areas. These examples also show that proof-of-concept studies have already been successfully conducted for all major categories of targets. A number of emerging events are poised to facilitate further progress including improvements in hardware for imaging (especially PET/CT), rapid expansion in the number of PET centers, and a more favorable regulatory system for early human studies.

With careful consideration of appropriate imaging targets and probe design, as well as the dedicated efforts of skilled professionals from many disciplines, PET imaging is well on its way toward changing the way drugs are developed and successfully using drugs as they enter clinical practice.

ACKNOWLEDGMENTS

I thank Drs. Robert Dedrick, Merrill Egorin, and Carl Peck for keeping me focused on the questions in Table 13.1, and Dr. Anthony Shields for encouraging my interest in PET imaging.

REFERENCES

1. U.S. Food and Drug Administration. *Guidance for industry, investigators, and reviewers: exploratory IND* [investigational new drugs] *studies.* Washington, DC: U.S. Department of Health and Human Services Food

and Drug Administration Center for Drug Evaluation and Research (CDER), 2006. World Wide Web URL: http://www.fda.gov/cder/guidance/7086fnl.pdf. Accessed March 2008.

2. Fischman AJ, Alpert NM, Babich JW, et al. The role of positron emission tomography in pharmacokinetic analysis. *Drug Metab Rev* 1997; 29:923–956.
3. Kubota K, Ishiwata K, Kubota R, et al. Feasibility of fluorine-18-fluorophenylalanine for tumor imaging compared with carbon-11-L-methionine. *J Nucl Med* 1996;37:320–325.
4. Farde L, Nyberg S, Oxenstierna G, et al. Positron emission tomography studies on D_2 and 5-HT_2 receptor binding in risperidone-treated schizophrenic patients. *J Clin Psychopharmacol* 1995;15[Suppl 1]: 19S–23S.
5. Dehdashti F, Flanagan FL, Mortimer JE, et al. Positron emission tomographic assessment of "metabolic flare" to predict response of metastatic breast cancer to antiestrogen therapy. *Eur J Nucl Med* 1999;26:51–56.
6. Christman D, Crawford EJ, Friedkin M, et al. Detection of DNA synthesis in intact organisms with positron-emitting [methyl-^{11}C]thymidine. *PNAS* 1972;69:988–992.
7. Shields AF, Mankoff DA, Link JM, et al. Carbon-11-thymidine and FDG to measure therapy response. *J Nucl Med* 1998;39:1757–1762.
8. Shields AF, Grierson JR, Dohmen BM, et al. Imaging proliferation *in vivo* with [F-18]FLT and positron emission tomography. *Nat Med* 1998;4: 1334–1336.
9. Sun H, Sloan A, Mangner TJ, et al. Imaging DNA synthesis with [^{18}F]FMAU and positron emission tomography in patients with cancer. *Eur J Nucl Med Mol Imaging* 2005;32:15–22.
10. Tjuvajev JG, Finn R, Watanabe K, et al. Noninvasive imaging of herpes virus thymidine kinase gene transfer and expression: a potential method for monitoring clinical gene therapy. *Cancer Res* 1996;56:4087–4095.
11. Wiebe LI, Morin KW, Knaus EE. Radiopharmaceuticals to monitor gene transfer. *Q J Nucl Med* 1997;41:79–89.
12. Fowler JS, Volkow ND, Logan J, et al. Monoamine oxidase B (MAO B) inhibitor therapy in Parkinson's disease: the degree and reversibility of human brain MAO B inhibition by Ro 19 6327. *Neurology* 1993;43: 1984–1992.
13. Fowler JS, Volkow ND, Logan J, et al. Slow recovery of human brain MAOB after L-deprenyl (selegiline) withdrawal. *Synapse* 1994;18:86–93.

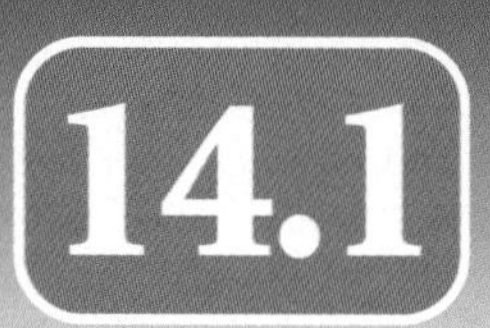

Imaging Gene Expression

UWE HABERKORN

After the identification of new genes, functional information is required to investigate the role of these genes in living organisms. This can be done by analysis of gene expression, protein–protein interaction, or biodistribution of new molecules and may result in new diagnostic and therapeutic procedures. These could include visualization of and interference with gene transcription and the development of new biomolecules to be used for diagnosis and treatment. Recent progress in basic science has delivered a better understanding of the mechanisms of carcinogenesis, tumor progression, and the patients' immune response toward the tumor. The characterization of tumor cell-specific properties allows the design of new treatment modalities as gene therapy, which circumvents resistance mechanisms toward conventional chemotherapeutic drugs. This chapter focuses on imaging cancer-related gene expression (both artificially introduced and endogenous). Although this chapter focuses on cancer, the methods described have potential applicability to a diverse range of diseases such as neurodegenerative, cardiac, and genetically linked metabolic diseases.

Currently, four approaches are evaluated in experimental and clinical studies related to cancer:

1. Protection of normal tissues (as the bone marrow), which are normally targets for cytotoxic drugs. The transfer of the gene for the drug efflux pump P-glycoprotein may achieve this. The presence of this pump in bone marrow cells may regulate the intracellular concentration of chemotherapeutic drugs in bone marrow progenitor cells at a lower nontoxic level and thereby protect these cells selectively.
2. Improvement of the host antitumor response by increasing the antitumor activity of tumor infiltrating immune competent cells or by modifying the tumor cells to enhance their immunogeneity. This approach relies on the introduction of genes that are responsible for the production of foreign surface antigens and elicit a concomitant immune response against the foreign antigen and the otherwise unrecognized tumor antigen. This may result in the elimination of the genetically modified as well as the wild type tumor cells. The expression of cytokines in tumor-infiltrating lymphocytes or in the tumor cells leads to an enhanced intratumoral cytokine concentration, which directs and activates immune-competent cells in the tumor.
3. Reversion of the malignant phenotype either by suppression of oncogene expression or by introduction of normal tumor suppressor genes. The inactivation of oncoproteins may be performed by introduction of genes for intracellular antibodies (intrabodies) against these oncogenes or by the use of antisense oligonucleotides and ribozymes.
4. Direct killing of tumor cells by the transfer of cytotoxic or prodrug-activating genes.

VISUALIZATION OF GENE TRANSFER

For the clinical application of gene therapy, noninvasive tools are needed to evaluate the efficiency of gene transfer. This includes the evaluation of infection efficiency as well as the verification of successful gene transfer in terms of gene transcription (Table 14.1.1). This information can be obtained by imaging methods and is useful for therapy planning, follow-up studies in treated tumors, and as an indicator of prognosis.

ASSESSMENT OF VIRAL VECTOR BIODISTRIBUTION

An understanding of the biodistribution of vectors carrying therapeutic genes to their targets would be helpful to develop strategies for target-specific delivery of these therapeutic agents. Schellingerhout et al. (1) used enveloped viral particles labeled with indium-111 ([^{111}In]), allowing the viruses to be traced *in vivo* by scintigraphic imaging. The labeling procedure did not significantly reduce the infectivity of the herpes simplex virus as evidence by the lack of significant release of the radionuclide within 12 hours after labeling. Sequential imaging of animals after intravenous administration of the [^{111}In]-labeled virus showed a fast accumulation in the liver and a redistribution from the blood pool to liver and spleen. The recombinant adenovirus serotype 5 knob (Ad5K) was also radiolabeled with technetium-99m (^{99m}Tc) (2) and retained specific, high-affinity binding to U293 cells, which shows that the radiolabeling process had no effect on receptor binding. *In vivo* dynamic

TABLE 14.1.1 Genes and Radioisotope Imaging Methods Used for Monitoring Successful Gene Transfer

Gene	Principle	Imaging Method	Tracer/Contrast Agent
ENZYMES			
CD	Enzyme activity	MRS, PET	5-fluorocytosine
HSVtk	Therapeutic effects	MRI, MRS, PET, SPECT	FDG, HMPAO, misonidazole
HSVtk	Enzyme activity	SPECT, PET	Specific substrates
HSVtk mutant	Enzyme activity	PET	Specific substrates
Tyrosinase	Metal scavenger	MRI, SPECT, scintigraphy	^{111}In
NONSUICIDE REPORTER GENES			
SSTR2	Receptor expression	SPECT, scintigraphy	Radiolabeled ligand
D_2R	Receptor expression	PET	Radiolabeled ligand
Transferrin receptor	Receptor expression	MRI	Radiolabeled ligand
CEA antigen	Antigen expression	Scintigraphy	Radiolabeled antibody
Modified green fluorescence protein	Transchelation	SPECT, scintigraphy	^{99m}Tc-glucoheptonate
Human sodium iodide transporter	Transport activity, therapy	Scintigraphy	^{99m}Tc, ^{123}I, ^{131}I
Human norepinephrine transporter	Transport activity, therapy	Scintigraphy	^{123}I-MIBG, ^{131}I-MIBG

CD, cytosine deaminase; MRS, magnetic resonance spectroscopy; MRI, magnetic resonance imaging; FDG, fluorodeoxyglucose; HMPAO, hexamethylpropyleneamine oxime, HSVtk, herpes simplex virus thymidine kinase, ^{111}In, indium-111, CEA, carcinoembryonic antibody; ^{99m}Tc, technetium-99m; ^{123}I, iodine-123; ^{131}I, iodine-131; MIBG, meta-iodobenzylguanidine.

scintigraphy revealed extensive liver binding, with a measured 100% extraction efficiency. The liver uptake corresponded to the results of a biodistribution study where tissues were removed and counted.

SUICIDE GENE THERAPY

The transfer and expression of suicide genes into malignant tumor cells represents an attractive approach for human gene therapy. Suicide genes typically code for nonmammalian enzymes, which convert nontoxic prodrugs into highly toxic metabolites. Therefore, systemic application of the nontoxic prodrug results in the production of the active drug at the tumor site. Although a broad range of suicide principles has been described (Table 14.1.2), two suicide systems are applied in most studies: the cytosine deaminase (CD) and herpes simplex virus thymidine kinase (HSVtk).

Cytosine deaminase, which is expressed in yeasts and bacteria but not in mammalian organisms, converts the antifungal agent 5-fluorocytosine (5-FC) to the highly toxic 5-fluorouracil (5-FU). In mammalian cells no anabolic pathway is known that leads to incorporation of 5-FC into the nucleic acid fraction. Therefore, pharmacologic effects are moderate and allow the application of high therapeutic doses (3–5). 5-FU exerts its toxic effect by interfering with DNA and protein synthesis due to substitution of uracil by 5-FU in RNA and inhibition of thymidylate synthetase by 5-fluorodeoxy-uridine monophosphate, resulting in impaired DNA biosynthesis (6).

Nishiyama et al. (7) implanted CD-containing capsules into rat gliomas and subsequently treated the animals by systemic application of 5-FC. They observed significant amounts of 5-FU in the tumors as well as a decrease in the tumor growth rate and systemic cytotoxicity. This approach for local chemotherapy was expanded by Wallace et al. (8) for application in patients with disseminated tumor. They used monoclonal antibody (mAb)-enzyme conjugates to achieve a selective activation of 5-FC, thereby obtaining a sevenfold higher level of 5-FU in the tumor after administration of mAb-CD and 5-FC compared to the systemic application of 5-FU.

Gene therapy with HSVtk as a suicide gene has been performed in a variety of tumor models *in vitro* as well as *in vivo* (9–16). In contrast to human thymidine kinase, HSVtk is less specific and it phosphorylates other nucleoside analogues such as acyclovir and ganciclovir (GCV) to their monophosphate metabolites (17). These monophosphates are subsequently phosphorylated by cellular kinases to the di- and triphosphates. After integration of the triphosphate metabolites into DNA, chain termination occurs, followed by cell death. Encouraging results have been obtained in rat gliomas using a retroviral vector system for transfer and expression of the *HSVtk* gene (15,16).

Recently, *in vitro* and *in vivo* studies have further demonstrated the potency of the CD suicide system. Tumor cells that had been infected with a retrovirus carrying the cytosine deaminase gene showed a strict correlation between 5-FC sensitivity and CD enzyme activity (18–20). However, although not all of the tumor cells have to be infected to obtain a sufficient therapeutic response, the *in vivo* infection efficiency of currently used viral vectors is low, and repeated injections of the recombinant retroviruses may be necessary to reach a therapeutic level of enzyme activity in the tumor.

A prerequisite for gene therapy using a suicide system is monitoring of the suicide gene expression in the tumor for two reasons: to decide if repeated gene transductions of the tumor are necessary and to find a therapeutic window of maximum gene expression and consecutive prodrug administration (21). Since 5-FC as well as GCV can be labeled with fluorine-18 ([^{18}F]) with sufficient *in vivo* stability (22,23), positron emission tomography (PET) may be applied to assess the enzyme activity *in vivo* (Table 14.1.1). The measurement of therapy effects on the tumor metabolism may also be useful for the prediction of therapy outcome at an early stage of the treatment. PET using tracers of tumor metabolism has been applied for the evaluation of treatment response in a variety of tumors and therapeutic regimens (24–27), indicating that these tracers deliver useful parameters for the early assessment of therapeutic efficacy.

TABLE 14.1.2 Suicide Genes Used for Gene Therapy of Cancer

Enzyme	Prodrug	Active Metabolite
E. coli purine nucleoside phosphorylase (DeoD)	6-methylpurine-2′-deoxyribonucleoside	6-methylpurine
E. coli thymidine phosphorylase	5′-deoxy-5′-fluorouridine, tegafur	5-fluorouracil
E. coli guanosine-xanthine phosphoribosyltransferase (gpt)	6-thioxanthine, 6-thioguanine	6-thioxantine-MP, 6-thioguanine-MP
Carboxypeptidase G2	Benzoic acid mustards-glumatic acid	Benzoic acid mustards
Alkaline phosphatase	Etoposide phosphate, doxorubicin phosphate, mitomycin phosphate	Etoposide, doxorubicin, mitomycin phenol mustard
Cassava linamarase	Linamarin	Aceto cyanohydrin, HCN
Carboxypeptidase A	Methotrexate-alanine	Methotrexate
Cytosine deaminase	5-fluorocytosine (5-FC)	5-fluorouracil (5-FU)
Cytosine deaminase + uracil phosphoribosyltransferase	5-fluorocytosine	5-fluorouracil + 5-fluorouridine-5′-monophosphate
Penicillin amidase	Doxorubicin-phenoxyacetamide	Doxorubicin
	Melphalan-phenoxyacetamide	Melphalan
		Palytoxin
		Palytoxin-4
		Hydroxyphenoxyacetamide
β-glucosidase	Amygdalin	Cyanide
β-glucoronidase	Epirubicin-glucoronide, phenol mustard-glucuronide, daunomycin-glucoronide, adrimycin-glucoronide	Epirubicin, phenol mustard, daunomycin, adriamycin
β-lactamase	Phenylenediamine mustard cephalosporin	Phenylenediamine mustard
E. coli nitroreductase	CB1954 (5-aziridin 2,4-dinitrobenzamidine)	5-aziridin 2,4-hydroxyamino 2-nitrobenzamidine
Cytochrome P450 2B1	Cyclophosphamide	Phosphoramide mustard
Rabbit hepatic carboxylesterase	Irinotecan	SN38 (7-ethyl-10-hydroxycamptothecin)
Human deoxycytidine kinase	Cytosine arabinoside (Ara C), fludarabine	Ara-CMP, fludarabine-MP
Herpes simplex virus thymidine kinase	Ganciclovir (GCV), acyclovir (AVC)	Phosphorylated metabolites
Varicella zoster virus thymidine kinase	6-methoxypurine arabinonucleoside (araM)	Phosphorylated metabolite

MONITORING GENE THERAPY BY MEASUREMENT OF THERAPEUTIC EFFECTS

Monitoring the tumor response to gene therapy using imaging procedures for the assessment of morphological changes has been performed with magnetic resonance imaging (MRI) techniques in rats bearing chemically induced hepatocellular carcinoma, C6 rat glioblastomas and in patients with glioblastoma (28–42) using replication-deficient viral vectors as well as replicating herpes simplex virus mutants (41). In these studies, marked tumor necrosis or growth retardation and regression after induction of HSVtk expression followed by GCV application were observed.

Maron et al. (30) found an initial response to GCV treatment in 90% of the animals and a complete regression in two thirds of the treated rats. Tumor recurrence could also be observed. In a more clinically relevant experimental protocol consisting of late GCV delivery to large tumor formations, the long-term survival of treated rats was improved by 60% (37). MRI demonstrated a complete regression of tumors in the surviving animals. The effects of cytosine deaminase gene transfer and 5-FC administration were evaluated in different tumor models (43–46). The 5-FC sensitivity in 9L cells increased 1,700-fold after infection with an adenoviral vector carrying the CD gene (46). These rats demonstrated a remarkable inhibition of tumor growth by MRI with 70% survival for more than 90 days. The mean tumor diffusion increased by 31% within 8 days of initiating 5-FC treatment. These effects were observed prior to tumor growth arrest and tumor regression (45).

Effects of suicide gene therapy on the tumor vascularization may occur since endothelial cells of the tumor blood vessels may integrate retroviral vectors and thus become sensitive towards ganciclovir. This hypothesis was investigated in the subcutaneous 9L gliosarcoma tumor model using measurements of tumor blood flow with Doppler color-flow and ultrasound imaging (47,48). The tumor vasculature decreased after initiation of ganciclovir therapy in the HSVtk-transduced tumors. Furthermore, early necrotic changes were associated with ultrasonographic signs of scattered intratumoral hemorrhage.

Tumor perfusion, as measured in GCV-treated HSVtk-expressing KBALB tumors after intravenous administration of ^{99m}Tc-HMPAO (hexamethylpropyleneamine oxime), increased twofold during treatment at day 2 (49). Intratumoral hypoxia was changed: the accumulation of tritium-misonidazole decreased to 30% to 40% from day 0 until day 3 after the onset of treatment, indicating that tumor tissue had become less hypoxic.

The measurement of metabolic changes after therapeutic intervention has proven to be superior to morphological procedures for the assessment of early therapy effects. MRI quantitation of changes in intracranial 9L tumor doubling times revealed a significant variation in therapeutic response to gene therapy with HSVtk and GCV. Localized H magnetic resonance spectra of treated 9L tumors showed a dramatic increase in mobile lipids and/or lactate. These changes in intracranial tumor doubling times correlated with changes in H tumor magnetic resonance spectra (50).

Fluorodeoxyglucose (FDG) uptake has been demonstrated to be a useful and very sensitive parameter for the evaluation of glucose metabolism (25,26,51,52). Since the HSVtk/GCV system induces DNA chain termination, additional changes in thymidine incorporation into tumor cell DNA are expected to occur. This may be assessed using carbon-11 ([^{11}C])-thymidine, which has been applied to determine DNA synthesis *in vivo* (53,54). In a HSVtk-expressing rat hepatoma cell line, uptake measurements using thymidine (TdR)-FDG, 3-O-methylglucose, aminoisobutyric acid (AIB), and methionine were performed in the presence of different concentrations of ganciclovir (55,56). In the HSVtk-expressing cell line an increased (up to 250%) thymidine uptake in the acid-soluble fraction and a decrease to 5.5% in the acid-insoluble fraction was found. The decrease of radioactivity in the nucleic acid fraction occurred early (4 hours) after exposure of the cells to GCV and represents DNA chain termination induced by the HSVtk-ganciclovir system.

The phenomenon of a posttherapeutic accumulation of TdR or its metabolites in the acid-soluble fraction was observed in former studies after chemotherapy (24). This effect may be explained by an increase in the activity of salvage pathway enzymes (e.g., of host thymidine kinase activity during repair of cell damage). Therefore, PET measurements with [^{11}C]-TdR may be used to assess the effects of the HSVtk-GCV system on DNA synthesis if quantitation is based on a modeling approach. *In vitro* the AIB uptake decreased to 47%, while the methionine uptake in the acid-insoluble fraction decreased to 17%, which is evidence of an inhibition of protein synthesis as well as of the neutral amino acid transport.

During GCV treatment, the uptake of FDG and 3-O-methylglucose increases up to 195% after 24 hours' incubation with GCV. A high-performance liquid chromatography (HPLC) analysis revealed a decline of the FDG-6-phosphate fraction after 48 hours' incubation with GCV. Consequently, a normalization of FDG uptake was observed after this incubation period, whereas the 3-O-methylglucose uptake was still increased. Experiments performed with different amounts of HSVtk-expressing cells and control cells showed that these effects are dependent on the percentage of HSVtk-expressing cells (55).

Dynamic PET studies of [^{18}F]-FDG uptake were performed in animals shortly after the onset of therapy with 100 mg GCV/kg body weight as well as after administration of sodium chloride (Fig. 14.1.1).

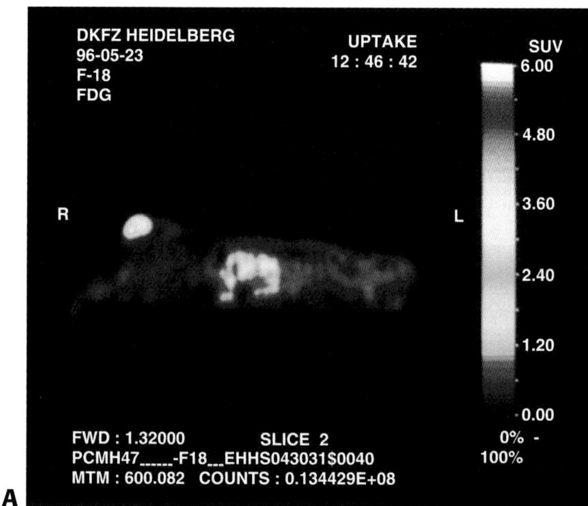

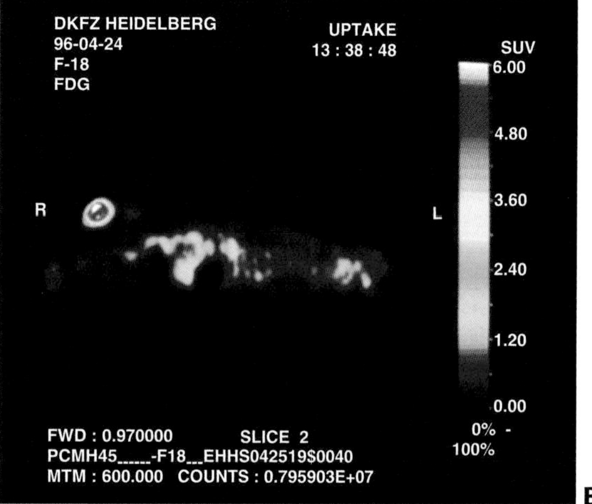

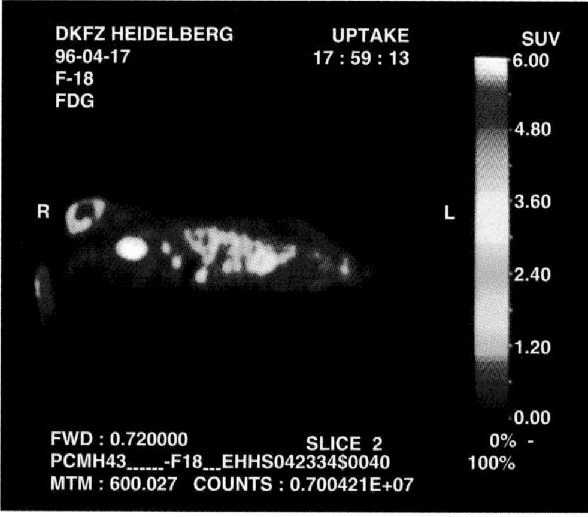

FIGURE 14.1.1. Fluorodeoxyglucose uptake (80 to 90 minutes postinjection) in animals with herpes simplex virus thymidine kinase–expressing tumors after sodium chloride administration of treatment with ganciclovir 100 mg/kg per body weight. The images are standardized to the injected dose and the body weight of the animals. Intense tracer uptake in tumor is seen after sodium chloride administration (**A**) with substantially more uptake apparent at 2 days after treatment likely due to increase in the glucose transport protein levels at the cell membrane (**B**). Central tumor necrosis is apparent by 4 days posttreatment (**C**).

The arterial FDG plasma concentration was measured dynamically in an extracorporeal loop and the rate constants for FDG transport (K_1, k_2) and FDG phosphorylation (k_3) were calculated using a three-compartment model modified for heterogeneous tissues. An uncoupling of FDG transport and phosphorylation was found with enhanced K_1 and k_2 values and a normal k_3 value after two days of GCV treatment (57).

In clinical and experimental studies an increase of FDG uptake early after treatment of malignant tumors has been described (26,51,58,59). Cell culture experiments with rat adenocarcinoma cells under chemotherapy revealed that this effect is predominantly caused by an enhanced glucose transport (58). The underlying mechanism may be a redistribution of the glucose transport protein from intracellular pools to the plasma membrane, and this is observed in cell culture studies as a general reaction to cellular stress (60–63). Since prodrug activation by the HSVtk leads to DNA chain termination and cell damage, the same reactions may also occur with this suicide system in tumor cells under gene therapy. Translocation of glucose transport proteins to the plasma membrane as a first reaction to cellular stress may cause enhancement of glucose transport and represents a short-term regulatory mechanism, which acts independently of protein synthesis.

DETERMINATION OF SUICIDE GENE ACTIVITY BY THE UPTAKE OF SPECIFIC SUBSTRATES

In a rat hepatoma model (55,56,64) uptake measurements were performed up to 48 hours in a HSVtk-expressing cell line and in a control cell line bearing the empty vector using 5-iodo-2′-fluoro-2′deoxy-1-b-D-arabinofuranosyluracil (FIAU), fluorodeoxycytidine (FCdR), 5-fluoro-1-(2′-deoxy-2′-fluoro-β-D-ribofuranosyl)-uracil (FFUdR), and ganciclovir. The FCdR uptake was higher in the HSVtk-expressing cells with a maximum after 4 hours (12-fold and threefold higher in the acid-insoluble and acid-soluble fraction, respectively). After longer incubation periods, the FCdR uptake declined. HPLC analysis showed rapid and almost complete metabolization and degradation in both cell lines (56), which might be due to dehalogenation or the action of nucleosidases. The GCV, FIAU, and FFUdR uptake showed a time-dependent increase in HSVtk-expressing cells and a plateau in control cells. The HPLC analysis revealed unmetabolized GCV in control cells and a time-dependent shift of GCV to its phosphorylated metabolite in HSVtk-expressing cells (56).

The ganciclovir, FFUdR, and the FIAU uptake were highly correlated to the percentage of HSVtk-expressing cells and to the growth inhibition as measured in bystander experiments (56,64,65). Similar results were obtained with genetically modified MCF7 human mammary carcinoma cells (66). However, the rat Morris hepatoma cells revealed a much higher difference between HSVtk-expressing cells and control cells in GCV uptake than MCF7 cells (56). MCF7 cells were not as sensitive to the HSVtk/GCV system as Morris hepatoma cells. This difference in the amount of tracer accumulation and sensitivity may be explained by the slower rate of growth of MCF7 cells as compared to Morris hepatoma cells.

Inhibition/competition experiments were performed to further elucidate the transport mechanism of ganciclovir. The nucleoside transport in mammalian cells is known to be heterogeneous with two classes of nucleoside transporters: the equilibrative, facilitated diffusion systems and the concentrative, sodium-dependent systems. In these experiments competition for all concentrative nucleoside transport systems and inhibition of the ganciclovir transport by the equilibrative transport systems was observed, whereas the pyrimidine nucleobase system showed no contribution to the ganciclovir uptake (56,66).

In human erythrocytes acyclovir has been shown to be transported mainly by the purine nucleobase carrier (67). Due to a hydroxymethyl group on its side chain, ganciclovir has a stronger similarity to nucleosides, and, therefore, it may also be transported by a nucleoside transporter. Moreover, the 3′-hydroxyl moiety of nucleosides has been shown to be important for their interaction with the nucleoside transporter (68). In rat hepatoma cells as well as in human mammary carcinoma cells the GCV uptake was shown to be much lower than the thymidine uptake (56,66). In addition to the low infection efficiency of the current viral delivery systems, slow transport of the substrate and its slow conversion into the phosphorylated metabolite have limited the therapeutic success of the HSVtk/GCV system. Cotransfection with nucleoside transporters or the use of other substrates for HSVtk with higher affinities for nucleoside transport and phosphorylation by HSVtk may improve therapy outcome.

The principle of *in vivo* HSVtk imaging was first demonstrated by Price et al. (69) and Saito et al. (70) for the visualization of HSV encephalitis. Several groups have recently performed *in vivo* studies using different tracers (71–80). Gambhir et al. (71) used 8-[^{18}F]-fluoroganciclovir (FGCV) for the imaging of adenovirus-directed hepatic expression of the HSVtk gene in living mice. There was a significant positive correlation between the percentage of injected dose of FGCV retained per gram of liver and the levels of hepatic HSVtk gene expression. Over a similar range of HSVtk expression *in vivo*, the percentage of injected dose retained per gram of liver was 0% to 23% for ganciclovir and 0% to 3% for FGCV.

Alauddin et al. (72,73) used of 9-(4-[^{18}F]-fluoro-3-hydroxymethylbutyl)-guanine ([^{18}F]-FHBG) and 9-[(3-[^{18}F]-fluoro-1-hydroxy-2-propoxy)-methyl]-guanine ([^{18}F]-FHPG) for combined *in vitro/in vivo* studies with HT29 human colon cancer cells, transduced with a retroviral vector, and they also found a significantly higher uptake in HSVtk-expressing cells as compared to the controls. *In vivo* studies in tumor-bearing nude mice demonstrated that the tumor uptake of the radiotracer is three- and sixfold higher at 2 and 5 hours, respectively, in transduced cells compared with the control cells.

Others used radioiodinated nucleoside analogues such as (E)-5-(2-iodovinyl)-2′-fluoro-2′-deoxyuridine (IVFRU) and FIAU to visualize HSVtk expression (74–77,82). Autoradiography, single-photon emission computed tomograph (SPECT) and PET images after injection of iodine-131 ([^{131}I]) or [^{124}I]-labeled FIAU revealed highly specific localization of the tracer to areas of HSVtk gene expression in brain and mammary tumors (76,77). The amount of tracer uptake in the tumors was correlated to the *in vitro* ganciclovir sensitivity of the cell lines that were transplanted in these animals (76,77).

Haubner et al. (82) studied the early kinetics of [^{123}I]-FIAU in the CMS5 fibrosarcoma model. Biodistribution studies a half hour postinjection showed tumor/blood and tumor/muscle ratios of 3.8 and 7.2 in HSVtk-expressing tumors, and 0.6 and 1.2 in wild type tumors. The tracer showed a biexponential clearance with an initial half-life of 0.6 hours followed by a half-life of 4.6 hours. The highest activity accumulation in HSVtk-expressing tumors was observed at

1 hour postinjection. Scintigraphy showed specific tracer accumulation as early as a half hour postinjection, with an increase in contrast over time, suggesting that sufficient tumor/background ratios for *in vivo* imaging of HSVtk expression with [^{123}I]-FIAU are reached as early as 1 hour postinjection.

Similar results were reported for IVFRU by Wiebe et al. (74,75). Due to low nontarget tissue uptake, unambiguous imaging of HSVtk-expressing tumors in mice is possible with labeled IVFRU. The advantage of iodinated tracers like FIAU may be that delayed imaging is possible. Since [^{18}F]-labeled compounds only allow imaging early after administration of the tracer, these iodinated compounds may prove to be more sensitive in *vivo*. However, quantification with iodine isotopes may be a problem either with [^{131}I], a γ- and β^{-}emitter with a high radiation dose, or with the corresponding positron emitter [^{124}I], which shows only 23% β^{+} radiation with high energy particles and multiple γ rays of high energy, which leads to a high radiation dose.

To improve the detection of lower levels of expression of PET reporter genes, a mutant herpes simplex virus type 1 thymidine kinase (*HSV1-sr39tk*) was used as a PET reporter gene (83). After successful transfer of this mutant gene, the accumulation of the specific substrates [8-^{3}H]-penciclovir ([8-^{3}H]PCV), and 8-[^{18}F]-fluoropenciclovir (FPCV) in C6 rat glioma cells was increased twofold when compared with wild type HSVtk-expressing tumor cells and led to increased imaging sensitivity.

CD was evaluated in human glioblastoma cells. A human glioblastoma cell line was stably transfected with the *Escherichia coli CD* gene (21) and experiments with tritium-FC were performed. Tritium-5-FU was produced in CD-expressing cells, whereas in the control cells only tritium-5-FC was detected (21). Moreover, significant amounts of 5-FU were found in the medium of cultured cells, which may account for the bystander effect observed in previous experiments. However, uptake studies revealed a moderate and nonsaturable accumulation of radioactivity in the tumor cells, suggesting that 5-FC enters the cells only via diffusion (21). Although a significant difference in 5-FC uptake was seen between CD-positive cells and controls after 48 hours' incubation, no difference was observed after 2 hours' incubation and a rapid efflux could be demonstrated. Therefore, 5-FC transport may be a limiting factor for this therapeutic procedure and quantitation with PET would have to rely on dynamic studies and modeling, including HPLC analysis of the plasma, rather than on nonmodeling approaches (21).

To evaluate the 5-FC uptake *in vivo*, a rat prostate adenocarcinoma cell line was transfected with a retroviral vector bearing the *E. coli CD* gene. The cells were found to be sensitive to 5-FC exposure, but lost this sensitivity with time. This may be due to inactivation of the viral promoter (cytomegalie virus) used in this vector. *In vivo* studies with PET and [^{18}F]-FC showed no preferential accumulation of the tracer in CD-expressing tumors, although HPLC analysis revealed production of 5-FU, which was detectable in tumor lysates as well as in the blood of the animals (65).

Finally, the coupling of two genes as a therapeutic gene together with a reporter gene by use of bicistronic vectors (involving the internal ribosomal entry site [IRES] of picornaviruses) may be useful for the evaluation of gene transfer. By the measurement of the PET reporter gene, the assessment of another therapeutic gene (e.g., a cytokine) would be possible (84). Problems could arise from low levels of gene expression, which may be influenced by the number of infected cells and by attenuation of the gene downstream from the IRES.

IMAGING USING NONSUICIDE REPORTER GENES

Reporter genes (e.g., β-galactosidase, chloramphenicol-acetyltransferase, green fluorescent protein, luciferase) play critical roles in investigating mechanisms of gene expression in transgenic animals and in developing gene delivery systems for gene therapy. However, measuring expression of these reporter genes requires biopsy or killing of the animals. *In vivo* reporter genes are genes that allow measurement of gene expression in living animals (Fig. 14.1.2). In this respect, the *HSVtk* gene has been shown to be useful as a noninvasive marker (71–80).

Receptor genes have also been used as reporter genes (85,86). The dopamine D_2 receptor gene represents an endogenous gene that is not likely to invoke an immune response. The corresponding tracer 3-(2′-[^{18}F]-fluoroethyl)-spiperone (FESP) rapidly crosses the blood–brain barrier, can be produced at high specific activity and is currently used in patients. As a SPECT tracer [^{123}I]-iodobenzamine is available. MacLaren et al. (85) used this system in nude mice with an adenoviral-directed hepatic gene delivery system and in stably transfected tumor cells that were transplanted in animals. The tracer uptake in these animals was proportional to *in vitro* data of hepatic FESP accumulation, dopamine receptor ligand binding, and the D_2 receptor mRNA. Tumors modified to express the D_2 receptor retained significantly more FESP than wild-type tumors.

Using a replication-incompetent adenoviral vector encoding the human type 2 somatostatin receptor, Zinn et al. (86) modified non–small cell lung tumors and imaged the expression of the *hSSTr2* gene using a radiolabeled, somatostatin-avid peptide (P829), which was radiolabeled to high specific activity with

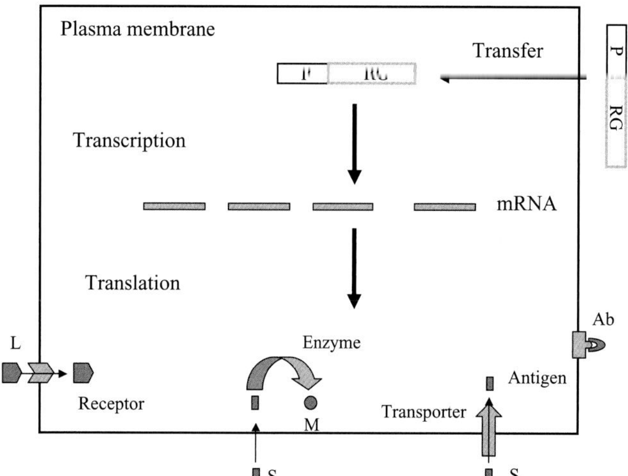

FIGURE 14.1.2. Simplified scheme of gene transfer and visualization of gene expression. As *in vivo* reporter genes (RG) enzymes, receptors, and transporters may be used. After infection and integration (in the case of retroviral particles as transfer vehicles) the expression of the corresponding artificial property of the tumor occurs. Enzyme activity can be assessed by the accumulation of the metabolites (M) of radiolabeled specific substrates (S), receptors by the binding and /or internalization of ligands (L), antigens by binding of antibodies (Ab), and transporters by the uptake of their substrates. This may be combined with specific promoters (P) for the characterization of gene regulation, signal transduction, and so forth.

^{99m}Tc or rhenium-188 ([^{188}Re]). In the genetically modified tumors, a five- to 10-fold greater accumulation of both radiolabeled P829 peptides as compared to the control tumors was observed. Both isotopes are generator produced, which confers advantages concerning the availability, costs, and imaging with widespread existing, high-resolution modalities. The [^{188}Re]-labeled peptide offers the additional advantage of β decay, which may be used for therapy.

Specific imaging can also be obtained by radiolabeled antibodies. To overcome the limitation of low expression of human tumor-associated antigens on target cells, a human glioma cell line was modified to express high levels of human carcinoembryonic antigen using an adenoviral vector (87). In these cells, high binding of a [^{131}I]-labeled anti-carcinoembryonic antibody was observed *in vitro* as well as by scintigraphic imaging.

Another approach is based on the *in vivo* transchelation of oxotechnetate to a polypeptide motif from a biocompatible complex with a higher dissociation constant than that of a dicglycilcysteine complex. It has been shown that synthetic peptides and recombinant proteins like the modified green fluorescence protein (gfp) can bind oxotechnetate with high efficiency (88,89). In these experiment rats were injected intramuscularly with synthetic peptides bearing a GGC motif. One hour later ^{99m}Tc-glucoheptonate was administered intravenously and the accumulation was measured by scintigraphy. The peptides with three metal-binding GGC motifs showed a threefold higher accumulation as compared to the controls. This principle can also be applied to recombinant proteins that appear at the plasma membrane (90). These genes can be cloned into bicistronic vectors, which allow for the coexpression of therapeutic genes and *in vivo* reporter genes. Radionuclide imaging may then be used to detect gene expression.

Tyrosinase catalyzes the hydroxilation of tyrosine to DOPA and the oxidation of DOPA to DOPAquinone, which after cyclization and polymerization results in melanin production. Melanins are scavengers of metal ions such as iron and indium through ionic binding. Tyrosinase transfer leads to the production of melanins in a variety of cells. This may be used for imaging with nuclear magnetic resonance or with [^{111}In] and a gamma camera. Cells transfected with the tyrosinase gene stained positively for melanin and had a higher [^{111}In] binding capacity than the wild type cells (91). A dependence of tracer accumulation on the amount of the vector used could be observed in transfection experiments. The problems with this approach are possible low tyrosinase induction with low amounts of melanin and the cytotoxicity of melanin. These problems may be reduced or eliminated by the construction of chimeric tyrosinase proteins and by positioning of the enzyme at the outer side of the membrane.

PROTEIN–PROTEIN INTERACTION

Protein interaction analysis delivers information about the possible biological role of genes with unknown function by connecting them to other better-characterized proteins. Furthermore, it detects novel interactions between proteins that are known to be involved in a common biological process and to novel functions of previously characterized proteins.

Protein interactions have been deduced by purely computational methods or using large-scale approaches (92,93). Ideally, the characterization of protein interactions should be based on experimentally determined interactions between proteins that are known to be present at the same time and in the same compartment. With the increasing availability of intrinsically fluorescent proteins that can be genetically fused to a wide variety of proteins, their application as fluorescent biosensors has extended to dynamic imaging studies of cellular biochemistry even at the level of organelles or compartments participating in specific processes (94). Fluorescence imaging allows the determination of cell-to-cell variation, the extent of variation in cellular responses, and the mapping of processes in multicellular tissues.

Procedures for noninvasive dynamic *in vivo* monitoring are needed to show whether the protein interactions also work in the complex environment of a living organism such as mice, rats, or humans where external stimuli may affect and trigger cells or organ function. The yeast two-hybrid technique has been adapted for *in vivo* detection of luciferase expression using a cooled charge coupled device (CCD) camera (95). GAL4 and VP16 proteins were expressed separately and associated by the interaction of MyoD and Id, two proteins of the helix-loop-helix family of nuclear proteins, which are involved in myogenic differentiation. In this experimental setting association of GAL4 and VP16 resulted in expression of firefly luciferase, which was under the control of multiple copies of GAL4 binding sites and a minimal promoter.

Drawbacks of the cooled CCD camera are mainly its limitation to small animals with different efficiencies of light transmission for different organs, lack of detailed tomographic information, and lack of an equivalent imaging modality applicable to human studies (96). Therefore, another approach based on the two-hybrid system used a fusion of a mutated *HSVtk* gene and the green fluorescent protein gene for *in vivo* detection of the interaction between p53 and the large T antigen of simian virus 40 by optical imaging and PET. Interaction of both proteins resulted in association of GAL4 and VP16 and reporter gene expression that was visualized after administration of an [^{18}F]-labeled specific substrate for HSVtk (97).

Current approaches are based on intracistronic complementation and reconstitution by protein splicing (Fig. 14.1.3). Complementation does not require the formation of a mature protein. Both parts of the reporter protein are active when closely approximated (98). The complementation strategy can be exploited for a wide range of studies directed at determining whether proteins derived from two active genes are coincident or colocalized within cells. Other applications include transgenic animals expressing complementary lacZ mutants from two promoters of interest, which should identify cell lines in which the products of both genes coincide spatially and temporally. Reconstitution is based on protein splicing in trans, which requires the reassociation of an N-terminal and C-terminal fragment of an intein, each fused to split N- and C-terminal halves of an extein such as a reporter gene like enhanced green fluorescent protein or luciferase (99). Reassociated intein fragments form a functional protein-splicing active center, which mediates the formation of a peptide bond between the exteins, coupled to the excision of the N- and C-inteins. Newer strategies fuse the intein segments to interacting proteins, which results in initiation of protein splicing in trans by protein–protein interaction (100).

The feasibility of imaging interaction of MyoD and Id based on both a complementation and a reconstitution strategy has been demonstrated using a CCD camera and split reporter constructs of firefly luciferase (101). After cotransfection of two plasmids the complementation as well as the reconstitution strategy achieved activities between 40% and 60% of the activity obtained after transfection of a plasmid bearing the full length reporter gene. A cooled CCD camera was applied for visualization of luciferase activity in

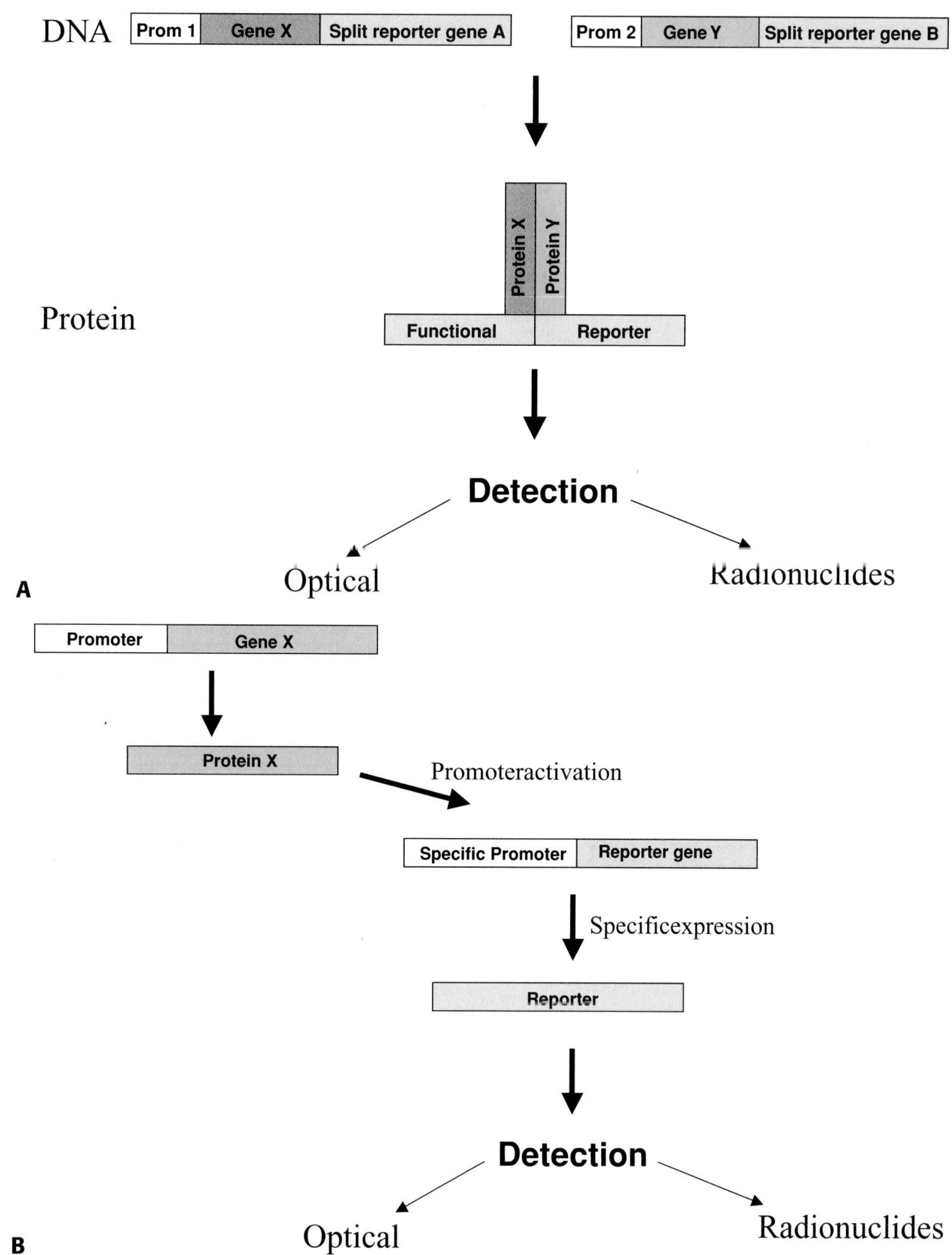

FIGURE 14.1.3. **A:** Differential regulation of split reporter gene expression using different endogenous promoters (Prom). The reporter gene fragments are fused to two physically interacting proteins. Complementation or reconstitution then leads to reporter gene activity. **B:** Characterization of functional interaction by transfer of a potential interactor (protein X) together with a plasmid bearing a specific promoter for another protein that regulates the expression of a reporter gene.

nude mice. This strategy presents a promising tool for the *in vivo* evaluation of protein function and intracellular networks and may be extended to approaches involving combinations of reporter genes and radionuclides. However, MyoD and Id are strong interacting proteins. There may be a weaker *in vivo* signal when systems with a weaker interaction are used.

Protein interactions occur not only as physical interactions but also as functional interactions (Fig. 14.1.3). These may be studied by analysis of promoters or promoter modules (102) or using combinations of specific promoters and reporter genes (103,104).

Tissue-specific transcriptional regulation is often mediated by a set of transcription factors whose combination is unique to specific cell types. The vast majority of genes expressed in a cell type–specific manner are regulated by promoters containing a variety of recognition sequences for tissue-specific and ubiquitous transcription factors. It is the precise functional interaction between these various regulating proteins and the regulatory DNA sequences that enables individual cell types to play their role within an organism.

To date, three transcription factors that specifically regulate thyroid-specific gene expression have been identified: thyroid transcription factor-1 (TTF1) is a homeodomain-containing protein expressed in embryonic diencephalon, thyroid, and lung. Thyroid transcription factor-2 (TTF2), a forkhead domain containing protein is expressed in the pituitary gland and thyroid, and Pax8, which belongs to the Pax family of paired domain containing genes, is expressed in the kidney, the developing excretory system, and in the thyroid. None of these transcription factors is expressed exclusively in the thyroid, but their combination is unique to this organ and is likely to be responsible for differentiation of thyrocytes.

TTF1 and Pax8 directly interact and synergistically activate thyroid-specific transcription and, therefore, represent a promising model system for the visualization of functional protein–protein interaction. These genes were transfected into hepatoma cells to measure functional protein–protein interaction expressed as activation of reporter gene constructs bearing combinations of the human thyroglobulin (hTg), human thyroperoxidase (hTPO), or the sodium iodide symporter (NIS) promoter/enhancer elements with the luciferase gene (105). Low transcriptional activation of these constructs was observed in cells expressing either hPax8 or dTTF1 alone. In contrast, the hTg and hTPO and to a lesser extent the rNIS regulatory region were significantly activated in cell lines expressing both transcription factors.

Imaging the transcriptional activation of the thyroid-specific regulatory regions by Pax8 and TTF1 was possible in nude mice implanted with MHhPax8dTTF1 cells using a cooled CCD camera. Sodium [^{125}I] uptake experiments and reverse transcription-polymerase chain reaction showed no effect of hPax8 and dTTF1 on endogenous thyroid-specific gene expression in genetically modified cells, even when not in the presence of the histone deacetylase inhibitor trichostatin A. A possible explanation is that the endogenous thyroid-specific regulatory regions may be inaccessible to Pax8 and TTF1. The appropriate regulation of gene expression requires the interplay of complexes that remodel chromatin structure and thereby regulate the accessibility of individual genes to sequence-specific transcription factors and the basal transcription machinery.

In vivo reporter systems are promising for the examination of whole organisms. These *in vivo* reporters may be used for the characterization of promoter regulation involved in signal transduction, gene regulation during changes of the physiological environment, and gene regulation during pharmacological intervention. This may be done by combining specific promoter elements with an *in vivo* reporter gene (Fig. 14.1.2). However, specific promoters are usually weak (106). This problem was addressed using a two-step amplification system for optical imaging of luciferase and PET imaging of HSVtk expression (107). In that study tissue specific reporter gene expression driven by the prostate specific antigen (PSA) promoter was enhanced by the transfer of a plasmid bearing a GAL4-VP16 fusion protein under the control of the PSA promoter together with a second plasmid bearing multiple GAL4 responsive elements and the reporter gene. Optical imaging revealed a fivefold signal enhancement in nude mice. Another strategy may be the use of multiple specific enhancer elements upstream of their corresponding promoter.

ENHANCEMENT OF IODIDE UPTAKE IN MALIGNANT TUMORS

Currently used viral vectors for gene therapy of cancer have a low infection efficiency leading to moderate or low therapy effects. This problem could be solved using an approach that leads to accumulation of radioactive isotopes with β emission. In this case, isotope trapping centers in the tumor could create a cross-firing of β particles, thereby efficiently killing transduced and nontransduced tumor cells. The transfer of genes for sodium iodide or norepinephrine transporters or the thyroid peroxidase has also been tried.

The first step in the complex process of iodide trapping in the thyroid is the active transport of iodide together with sodium ions into the cell, which is mediated by the sodium-iodide symporter. This process against an electrochemical gradient requires energy, is coupled to the action of Na+/K+-ATPase, and is stimulated by thyroid-stimulating hormone (TSH) (108–112). Since the cloning of the human and rat cDNA sequences several experimental studies have been performed that investigated the recombinant expression of the *hNIS* gene in malignant tumors by viral transfer of the *hNIS* gene under the control of different promoter elements (113–127, Fig. 14.1.4). Although all of them reported high initial uptake in the genetically modified tumors, differing results have been obtained concerning the efficiency of radioiodine treatment based on NIS gene transfer. Generally, very high doses have been given to tumor-bearing mice.

A rapid efflux of iodide occurred *in vitro* with 80% of the radioactivity released into the medium after 20 minutes (114,119, 121,123–125,128). Since the effectiveness of radioiodine therapy depends not only on the type and amount but also on the biological half-life of the isotope in the tumor, a therapeutically useful absorbed dose seems unlikely for that type of experiment.

A significant efflux was also seen *in vivo* when doses were applied that are commonly administered to patients: only 0.4% ± 0.2 % and 0.24% ± 0.02% of the injected dose per gram were observed in the *hNIS*-expressing tumors at 24 hours after tracer administration (114,119). Similarly Nakamoto et al. (121) found less than 1% of the injected radioactivity at 24 hours after [^{131}I] administration in modified *MCF7* mammary carcinomas, although initially a high uptake was seen (121). This corresponds to a very short half-life of [^{131}I] (approximately 7.5 hours) in rat prostate carcinomas, which has also been described by Nakamoto et al. for human mammary carcinomas with a calculated biological half-life of 3.6 hours. In contrast, differentiated thyroid carcinoma showed a biological half-life of less than 10 days and normal thyroid of approximately 60 days (129, 130).

In vitro clonogenic assays revealed selective killing of NIS-expressing cells in some studies (115,117,126,131). Bystander effects have also been suggested in three-dimensional spheroid cultures (131). *In vivo* experiments in stably transfected human prostate carcinoma cells showed a long biological half-life of 45 hours (126). This resulted in a significant tumor reduction (84% ± 12%) after a single intraperitoneal administration of a very high [^{131}I] dose of 111 MBq (118,126,127). The authors concluded that transfer of the *NIS* gene causes effective radioiodine doses in the tumor and might therefore represent a potentially curative therapy for prostate cancer.

In order to improve therapy outcome, Smit et al. (125) investigated the effects of low-iodide diets and thyroid ablation on iodide kinetics. The half-life in NIS-expressing human follicularly thyroid carcinomas without thyroid ablation and under a regular diet was very short, 3.8 hours. In thyroid-ablated mice kept on a low-iodide diet, the half-life of radioiodide was increased to 26.3 hours, which may be due to diminished renal clearance of radioiodine and a lack of iodide trapping by the thyroid. Subcutaneous injections of 74 MBq in thyroid-ablated nude mice, kept on a low-iodide diet, postponed tumor development. However, 9 weeks after therapy, tumors had developed in four of the seven animals. The estimated tumor dose in these animals was 32.2 Gy (125).

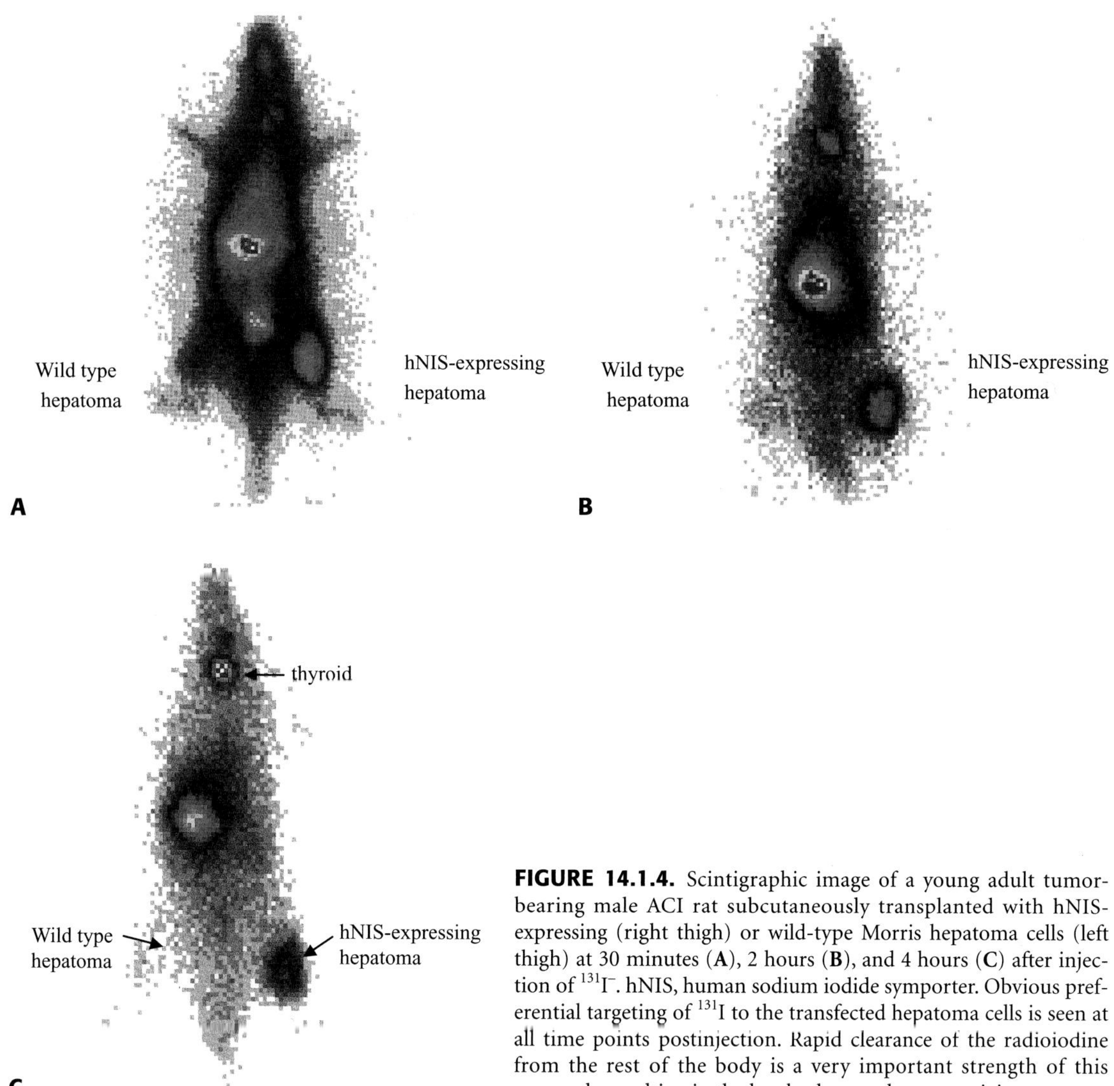

FIGURE 14.1.4. Scintigraphic image of a young adult tumor-bearing male ACI rat subcutaneously transplanted with hNIS-expressing (right thigh) or wild-type Morris hepatoma cells (left thigh) at 30 minutes (**A**), 2 hours (**B**), and 4 hours (**C**) after injection of $^{131}I^{-}$. hNIS, human sodium iodide symporter. Obvious preferential targeting of ^{131}I to the transfected hepatoma cells is seen at all time points postinjection. Rapid clearance of the radioiodine from the rest of the body is a very important strength of this approach, resulting in the low background tracer activity.

These studies used very high doses: in a mouse 74 MBq and 111 MBq correspond to administered doses of 11,100 MBq/m^2 and 16,650 MBq/m^2, respectively. This is far more than the doses used in patients. In rat prostate carcinomas treatment with amounts of [^{131}I] corresponding to those given to patients (1,200 MBq [^{131}I]/m^2 and 2,400 MBq [^{131}I]/m^2) resulted in an absorbed dose of only 3 Gy in the genetically modified tumors (119). Since approximately 80 Gy has been described as necessary to achieve elimination of metastases in patients with thyroid cancer, this is not likely to induce a significant therapeutic effect in the tumors (130). Furthermore, the experiments were performed under ideal conditions with 100% NIS-expressing cells in the tumors. Given the low infection efficiency of currently viral vectors *in vivo* the absorbed dose in a clinical study would be considerably lower.

There are also other differences in these studies: tracer administration, time of treatment, and animal versus tumor models. Differences in the biodistribution of iodide and the biochemical properties of the tumor cells may lead to differences in iodide retention.

In order to prolong the iodine retention time in tumors some researchers tried to transfer the NIS and the thyroperoxidase gene simultaneously (117,128). Boland et al. (117) observed iodide organification in cells coinfected with both the *NIS* and the *TPO* gene in the presence of exogenous hydrogen peroxide (117). However, the levels of iodide organification obtained were too low to increase the iodide retention time significantly. In a variety of different cell lines, including human anaplastic thyroid carcinoma and rat hepatoma cells, researchers were not able to measure TPO enzyme activity or enhanced accumulation of iodide irrespective of very high amounts of hTPO protein after retroviral transfer of the human *TPO* gene (132).

In contrast, Huang et al. (128) observed an increased radioiodide uptake (by a factor of 2.5) and retention (by a factor of 3) and enhanced tumor cell apoptosis after transfection of non–small cell lung cancer cells with both human *NIS* and *TPO* genes. However, a 72 % efflux occurred *in vitro* during the first 30 minutes, indicating very low hTPO activity in the genetically modified cells. Other modulations of iodide retention in tumor cells should be evaluated in future studies.

Lithium has been reported to reduce the release of iodine from the thyroid and, therefore, was used to enhance the efficacy of radioiodine treatment of differentiated thyroid cancer (133). When the biological half-life was less than 3 days, lithium prolonged the effective half-life by more than 50% (133). In FRTL5 rat thyroid cells and in primary cultures of porcine thyroid follicles 2 mM lithium suppressed TSH-induced iodide uptake, iodide uptake stimulated by 8-bromo-cAMP, iodine organification, and *de novo* thyroid hormone formation (134,135). Lithium is concentrated by the thyroid and inhibits thyroidal iodine uptake and iodotyrosine coupling, alters thyroglobulin structure, and inhibits thyroid hormone secretion (134–138). If enhanced iodide trapping in the thyroid by lithium relies on interaction with iodine coupling to tyrosine residues or inhibition of thyroid hormone secretion, an organification process is still needed to obtain sufficient iodine accumulation in the tumor. First experiments in the author's laboratory showed no significant effect of lithium in hNIS-expressing hepatoma cells (123,139).

A further option to increase therapy outcome is the use of biologically more effective isotopes. Dadachova et al. (140) compared [^{188}Re]-perrhenate with [^{131}I] for treatment of NIS-expressing mammary tumors. In a xenografted breast cancer model in nude mice, [^{188}Re]-perrhenate exhibited NIS-dependent uptake into the mammary tumor. Dosimetry showed that [^{188}Re]-perrhenate delivered a 4.5 times higher dose than [^{131}I] and, therefore, may provide enhanced therapeutic efficacy. The high LET-emitter astatine-211 has been suggested as an isotope with high radiobiologic effectiveness (141). First experiments showed that the tracer uptake in NIS-expressing cell lines increased up to 350-fold for [^{123}I], 340-fold for $^{99m}Tc\text{-}O_4^-$, and 60-fold for astatine-211 ([^{211}At]). Although all radioisotopes showed a rapid efflux, higher absorbed doses in the tumor were found for [^{211}At] as compared to [^{131}I] (141).

In conclusion, a definitive proof of therapeutically useful absorbed doses *in vivo* after transfer of the *NIS* gene is still lacking. Further studies will have to examine pharmacologic modulation of iodide efflux or the use of the *hNIS* gene as an *in vivo* reporter gene (104,119).

The question of whether the transfer of the *hTPO* gene is sufficient to restore the iodide trapping capacity in undifferentiated thyroid and nonthyroid tumor cells has been investigated (132). The human anaplastic thyroid carcinoma cell lines C643 and SW1736, the rat Morris hepatoma cell line MH3924A, and the rat papillary thyroid carcinoma cell line L2 were used as *in vitro* model systems. Although a significant expression of the *hTPO* gene was seen, the [^{125}I] uptake was not enhanced in these cells. Moreover, only minimal enzymatic activity of the recombinant hTPO was determined in individual cell lines as shown by low levels of guaiacol oxidation. This suggests that the recombinant gene is either expressed as a functionally inactive protein or that a functional protein becomes inactive in a nonoptimal cellular milieu. In most *in vitro* systems, the hTPO introduced by cDNA-directed gene expression was detected by means of immunohistology, immunoblotting, or autoantibodies of patients with thyroid autoimmune disease. However, the production of catalytically active hTPO was not achieved, irrespective of the expression system and cell culture system employed for the experimental approach (142–145).

The function and activity of hTPO are probably influenced by the multimerization of the protein as well as by additional factors, including the incorporation of heme, the glycosylation the localization of the enzyme, and the thyroglobulin content of the cells (146–150). The transduction of the *hTPO* gene *per se* is not sufficient to induce the iodide accumulation in human anaplastic carcinoma cells, and a low enzymatic activity in the recombinant cell lines is supposed to account for it. Studies are currently being performed to define additional factors required for iodide uptake in undifferentiated thyroid tumor cells.

Another approach of a genetically modified isotope treatment is the transfer of the norepinephrine gene. [^{131}I]-meta-iodobenzylguanidine (MIBG), a metabolically stable false analogue of norepinephrine, has been widely used for imaging and targeted radiotherapy in patients suffering from neural crest derived tumors such as neuroblastoma or pheochromocytoma. In the adrenal medulla and in pheochromocytoma MIBG is stored in the chromaffin neurosecretory granules (151). The transport of MIBG by the human norepinephrine transporter (hNET) seems to be the critical step in the treatment of MIBG-concentrating tumors. The mechanism of MIBG uptake, which is qualitatively similar to that of norepinephrine, has been studied in a variety of cellular systems, and two uptake systems have been postulated. Although most tissues accumulate MIBG by a nonspecific, nonsaturable diffusion process, cells of the neuroadrenergic tissues and malignancies derived from these tissues exhibit an active uptake of the tracer that is mediated by the noradrenalin transporter (152–155). The clinical use of the MIBG radiotherapy is so far restricted to neural crest derived malignancies and, due to insufficient [^{131}I]-MIBG uptake, therapy in these tumor patients is not curative.

The effect of *hNET* gene transfection was investigated in a variety of cells including COS1 cells, HeLa cells, glioblastoma cells, or rat hepatoma cells and a three- to 36-fold increase of [^{131}I]-MIBG or noradrenaline accumulation was achieved (154,156–158). *In vivo* experiments performed with nude mice bearing both the hNET expressing and the wild type tumor showed a 10-fold higher accumulation of [^{131}I]-MIBG in the transfected tumors with respect to the wild type tumors. In rat hepatoma cells when compared to previous studies concerning the efflux of [^{131}I] from hNIS-expressing cells, a longer retention of MIBG in the hNET-transfected cells was observed (158). Nevertheless, 4 hours after incubation with MIBG an efflux of 43% of the radioactivity was determined for the recombinant cells, whereas wild type cells had lost 95% of the radioactivity. For MIBG radiotherapy in nonneuroectodermal tumors, an intracellular trapping of the tracer is required to achieve therapeutically sufficient doses of radioactivity in the genetically modified tumor cells. A positive correlation has been observed between the content of chromaffin neurosecretory granules and the uptake of radiolabeled MIBG (159).

Human glioblastoma cells transfected with the bovine NET gene were killed by doses of 0.5 to 1 MBq/mL [^{131}I]-MIBG in monolayer cell culture as well as in spheroids (157). Accordingly, the authors expected the intratumoral activity in a 70-kg patient to be 0.021%. This corresponds to the range of MIBG uptake usually achieved in neuroblastoma. However, data obtained from *in vitro* experiments cannot be applied to the *in vivo* situation. In contrast to stable *in vitro* conditions the radioactive dose delivered to the tumor *in vivo* differs due to decreasing radioactivity in the serum and due to heterogeneity within the tumor tissue.

In order to calculate the radiation dose in a particular tumor more precisely, an *in vivo* dosimetry is superior. Using 14.8 MBq of [^{131}I]-MIBG in tumor-bearing mice, corresponding to 2,200 MBq/m^2 in humans, a radiation dose of 605 mGy in the hNET-expressing and of 75 mGy in the wild type tumor was calculated (158). For treatment of patients suffering from a nonneuroectodermal tumor transfected by the *hNET* gene this absorbed dose is too low to evoke any tumor response. As with most gene transfer studies, the *in vivo* experiments were performed with animals that had been transplanted with 100% stable hNET-expressing cells. Due to the low *in vivo* infection efficiency of virus particles, infection of tumor cells *in vivo* will result in even lower radiation doses.

Future development should comprise pharmacologic modulation of MIBG retention or interaction with competing catecholamines. Employment of the recombinant *hNET* gene product as an *in vivo* reporter has only been somewhat promising because the images showed high background and relatively faint appearance of the genetically modified tumor (158). The longer retention than seen with hNIS transfected cells remains a strength as well as the "human nature" of the NET system utilized.

ANTISENSE OLIGONUCLEOTIDES

The estimation of gene function using the tools of the genome program has been referred to as *functional genomics*, which can be seen as describing the processes leading from a gene's physical structure and its regulation to the gene's role in the whole organism. Many studies in functional genomics are performed by analysis of differential gene expressions using high throughput methods such as DNA chip technology. These methods are used to evaluate changes in the transcription of many or all genes of an organism at the same time in order to investigate genetic pathways for normal development and disease. The assessment and modification of the mRNA content of single genes is also of interest in functional studies.

Antisense RNA and DNA techniques were originally developed to modulate the expression of specific genes. These techniques originated from studies in bacteria and demonstrated that these organisms are able to regulate gene replication and expression by the production of small complementary RNA molecules in an opposite (antisense) direction. Base pairing between the oligonucleotide and the corresponding target mRNA leads to highly specific binding and specific interaction with protein synthesis. Several laboratories showed that synthetic oligonucleotides complementary to mRNA sequences could down-regulate the translation of various oncogenes in cells (160,161).

Silencing of genes can also be obtained by a mechanism that is based on double-stranded RNA (dsRNA), which is cleaved by a ribonuclease (Dicer) to yield short RNAs of 21 to 25 nucleotide length (siRNA). After interaction of these siRNAs with a complex of cellular proteins to form an RNA-induced silencing complex (RISC) the RISC binds to the complementary RNA and inhibits its translation into a protein. This is known as *RNA interference* (RNAi) and can be used for treatment either by application of synthetic oligonucleotides or after introduction of DNA-bearing vectors that produce RNA hairpins *in vivo* that are cleaved in the cell to the corresponding siRNAs (162–165).

Besides their use as therapeutics for specific interaction with RNA, processing oligonucleotides have been proposed for diagnostic imaging and treatment of tumors. Assuming a total human gene number between 24,000 and 30,000, calculations that take into account alternative polyadenylation and alternative splicing result in an mRNA number between 46,000 and 85,000 (166). It is expected that an oligonucleotide with more than 12 (12-mer) nucleobases represents a unique sequence in the whole genome (167). Since these short oligonucleotides can easily be produced, antisense imaging using radiolabeled oligonucleotides offers a high number of new tracers with high specificity. Prerequisites for the use of radiolabeled antisense-oligonucleotides are ease of synthesis, stability *in vivo*, uptake into the cell, accumulation of the oligonucleotide inside the cell, interaction with the target structure, and minimal nonspecific interaction with other macromolecules. Nuclease resistance of the oligonucleotide, stability of the oligo-linker complex, and a stable binding of the radionuclide to the complex are required for the stability of radiolabeled antisense molecules. Modifications of the phosphodiester backbone such as phosphorothioates, methylphosphonates, peptide nucleic acids, or gapmers (mixed backbone oligonucleotides) result in at least a partial loss in cleavage by RNAs.

Evidence has been presented of receptor-coupled endocytosis as the low capacity mechanism by which oligonucleotides enter cells (168,169). Subcellular fractionation experiments showed a sequestration of the oligonuleotides in the nuclei and the mitochondria of cervix carcinoma (HeLa) cells (169). This phenomenon of fractionation, problems with *in vivo* stability of the oligonucleotides, as well as the stability of the hybrid oligo-RNA structures may prevent successful imaging of gene expression. Binding to other polyanions, such as heparin, based on charge interaction results in unspecific signals.

Successful antisense imaging has been reported in several studies: accumulation of [^{111}In]-labeled c-myc antisense probes with a phosphorothioate-backbone occurred in mice bearing c-myc overexpressing mammary tumors (170). Imaging was also possible with a transforming growth factor β antisense oligonucleotide, an antisense phosphorothioate oligodeoxynucleotide for the mRNA of glial fibrillary acidic protein and a [^{125}I]-labeled antisense peptide nucleic acid targeted to the initiation codon of the luciferase mRNA in rat glioma cells permanently transfected with the luciferase gene (171–174). PET was used for the assessment of the biodistribution and kinetics of [^{18}F]-labeled oligonucleotides (175). Yttrium-90 ([^{90}Y])-labeled phosphorothioate antisense oligonucleotides may be applied as targeted radionuclide therapeutic agents for malignant tumors (176). Although imaging is feasible, the degree of targeting of these methods in their current form suggests translation to the clinic will not be without challenges.

Data obtained from messenger RNA (mRNA) profiling do not faithfully represent the proteome because the mRNA content seems to be a poor indicator of the corresponding protein levels (177–179). Direct comparison of mRNA and protein levels in mammalian cells, either for several genes in one tissue or for one gene product in many cell types, revealed only poor correlations with up to 30-fold variations. This might lead to misinterpretation of mRNA profiling results. Furthermore, mRNA is labile and leads to spontaneous chemical degradation as well as to degradation by enzymes, which may be dependent on the specific sequence and result in nonuniform degradation of RNA. This phenomenon introduces quantitative biases that are dependent on the time after the onset of tissue stress or death. In contrast, proteins are generally more stable and exhibit slower turnover rates in most tissues. A substantial fraction of interesting intracellular events is located at the protein level, for example, operating primarily through phosphorylation/dephosphorylation and the migration of proteins. Proteolytic modifications of membrane-bound precursors also appear to regulate the release of a large series of extracellular signals such as angiotensin or tumor necrosis factor.

Since protein levels often do not reflect mRNA levels, antisense imaging may not be a generally applicable approach for a clinically useful description of biological properties of tissues. Expression profiling data would be more useful if mRNA samples could be enriched for transcripts that are being translated (180). This can be achieved by fractionation of cytoplasmic extracts in sucrose gradients, which leads to the separation of free mRNPs (ribonucleoprotein particles) from mRNAs in ribosomal preinitiation complexes and from mRNAs loaded with ribosomes (polysomes). Since only the polysomes represent actively translated transcripts, this fraction should be directly correlated with *de novo* synthesized proteins.

Polysome imaging with nuclear medicine procedures has not been tried to date, and it may not even be possible. Antisense imaging for the determination of transcription by hybridization of the labeled antisense probe to the target mRNA makes sense in cases where RNA and protein content are highly correlated. Successful imaging was possible in cases where the expression of the protein was proven or the gene of interest was introduced by an expression vector (170–174). In the absence of such a correlation between mRNA and protein content, the diagnostic use of antisense imaging seems questionable. Therapeutic applications may use triplex oligonucleotides with therapeutic isotopes such as Auger electron emitters, which can be brought near to specific DNA sequences to induce DNA strand breaks at selected loci. Imaging of labeled siRNAs makes sense if these are used for therapeutic purposes in order to assess the delivery of these new drugs to their target tissue.

Our rapidly improving understanding of the genetics of cancers and other diseases provides a multitude of pathways for imaging the genes themselves, the messages and proteins they produce, as well as cells transfected with the relevant genes. This area has great promise, but the translation to human trials remains challenging due to the many steps involved, not least of which for therapeutic approaches includes adequate and reasonably long duration expression of the gene targets. These methods of imaging will be of great value as gene replacement therapy grows and in better understanding the expression of genes that are translated to proteins in health and disease.

REFERENCES

1. Schellingerhout D, Bogdanov A Jr, Marecos E, et al. Mapping the *in vivo* distribution of herpes simplex virions. *Hum Gene Ther* 1998;9: 1543–1549.
2. Zinn KR, Douglas JT, Smyth CA, et al. Imaging and tissue biodistribution of ^{99m}Tc-labeled adenovirus knob (serotype 5). *Gene Ther* 1998; 5:798–808.
3. Scholer HJ. Flucytosine. In: Speller DCE, ed. *Antifungal chemotherapy*. New York: John Wiley, 1980:35–106.
4. Polak A, Eschenhof E, Fernex M, et al. Metabolic studies with 5-fluorocytosine-6-14C in mouse, rat, rabbit, dog and man. *Chemotherapy* 1976;22:137–153.
5. Koechlin BA, Rubio F, Palmer S, et al. The metabolism of 5-fluorocytosine-2-^{14}C and of cytosine-1-^{14}C in the rat and the disposition of 5-fluorocytosine-2-^{14}C in man. *Biochem Pharmac* 1966;15:435–446.
6. Myers CE. The pharmacology of the fluoropyrimidines. *Pharmacol Rev* 1981;33:1–15.
7. Nishiyama T, Kawamura Y, Kawamoto K, et al. Antineoplastic effects of 5-fluorocytosine in combination with cytosine deaminase capsules. *Cancer Res* 1985;45:1753–1761.
8. Wallace PM, MacMaster JF, Smith VF, et al. Intratumoral generation of 5-fluorouracil mediated by an antibody-cytosine deaminase conjugate in combination with 5-fluorocytosine. *Cancer Res* 1994;54: 2719–2723.
9. Chen SH, Shine HD, Goodman JC, et al. Gene therapy for brain tumors: regression of experimental gliomas by adenovirus-mediated gene transfer *in vivo*. *Proc Natl Acad Sci U S A* 1994;91:3054–3057.
10. Borrelli E, Heyman R, Hsi M, et al. Targeting of an inducible toxic phenotype in animal cells. *Proc Natl Acad Sci U S A* 1988;85:7572–7576.
11. Barba D, Hardin J, Sadelain M, et al. Development of anti-tumor immunity following thymidine kinase-mediated killing of experimental brain tumors. *Proc Natl Acad Sci U S A* 1994;91:4348–4352.
12. Moolten FL, Wells JM. Curability of tumors bearing herpes thymidine kinase genes transferred by retroviral vectors. *J Natl Cancer Inst* 1990; 82:297–300.
13. Caruso M, Panis Y, Gagandeep S, et al. Regression of established macroscopic liver metastases after *in situ* transduction of a suicide gene. *Proc Natl Acad Sci U S A* 1993;90:7024–7028.
14. Oldfield EH, Ram Z, Culver KW, et al. Gene therapy for the treatment of brain tumors using intra-tumoral transduction with the thymidine kinase gene and intravenous ganciclovir. *Hum Gene Ther* 1993;1:39–69.
15. Culver KW, Ram Z, Walbridge S, et al. *In vivo* gene transfer with retroviral vector-producer cells for treatment of experimental brain tumors. *Science* 1992;256:1550–1552.
16. Ram Z, Culver WK, Walbridge S, et al. *In situ* retroviral-mediated gene transfer for the treatment of brain tumors in rats. *Cancer Res* 1993;53: 83–88.
17. Keller PM, Fyfe JA, Beauchamp L, et al. Enzymatic phosphorylation of acyclic nucleoside analogs and correlations with antiherpetic activities. *Biochem Pharmacol* 1981;30:3071–3077.
18. Huber BE, Austin EA, Good SS, et al. *In vivo* antitumor activity of 5-fluorocytosine on human colorectal carcinoma cells genetically modified to express cytosine deaminase. *Cancer Res* 1993;53:4619–4626.
19. Mullen CA, Kilstrup M, Blaese M. Transfer of the bacterial gene for cytosine deaminase to mammalian cells confers lethal sensitivity to 5-fluorocytosine: a negative selection system. *Proc Natl Acad Sci U S A* 1992;89:33–37.
20. Mullen CA, Coale MM, Lowe R, et al. Tumors expressing the cytosine deaminase suicide gene can be eliminated in vivo with 5-fluorocytosine and induce protective immunity to wild type tumor. *Cancer Res* 1994; 54:1503–1506.
21. Haberkorn U, Oberdorfer F, Gebert J, et al. Monitoring of gene therapy with cytosine deaminase: *in vitro* studies using ^{3}H-5-fluorocytosine. *J Nucl Med* 1996;37:87–94.
22. Visser GWM, Boele S, Knops GHJN, et al. Synthesis and biodistribution of (^{18}F)-5-fluorocytosine. *Nucl Med Comm* 1985;6:455–459.
23. Monclus M, Luxen A, Van Naemen J, et al. Development of PET radiopharmaceuticals for gene therapy: synthesis of 9-((1-(^{18}F)-fluoro-3-hydroxy-2-propoxy)methyl)guanine. *J Label Comp Radiopharm* 1995;37:193–195.
24. Haberkorn U, Oberdorfer F, Klenner T, et al. Metabolic and transcriptional changes in osteosarcoma cells treated with chemotherapeutic drugs. *Nucl Med Biol* 1994;21:835–845.
25. Haberkorn U, Strauss LG, Dimitrakopoulou A, et al. Fluorodeoxyglucose imaging of advanced head and neck cancer after chemotherapy. *J Nucl Med* 1993;34:12–17.
26. Rozenthal JM, Levine RL, Nickles RJ, et al. Glucose uptake by gliomas after treatment. *Arch Neurol* 1989;46:1302–1307.
27. Bergstrom M, Muhr C, Lundberg PO, et al. Rapid decrease in amino acid metabolism in prolactin-secreting pituitary adenomas after bromocriptine treatment: a PET study. *J Comput Assist Tomogr* 1987;11:815–819.
28. Sobol RE, Fakhrai H, Shawler D, et al. Interleukin-2 gene therapy in a patient with glioblastoma. *Gene Ther* 1995;2:164–167.
29. Izquierdo M, Cortés M, de Felipe P, et al. Long-term rat survival after malignant brain tumour regression by retroviral gene therapy. *Gene Ther* 1995;2:66–69.
30. Maron A, Gustin T, Le Roux A, et al. Gene therapy of rat C6 glioma using adenovirus-mediated transfer of the herpes simplex virus thymidine kinase gene: long-term follow up by magnetic resonance imaging. *Gene Ther*1996; 3:315–322.
31. Izquierdo M, Martin V, deFelipe P, et al. Human malignant brain tumor response to herpes simplex thymidine kinase (HSVtk)/ganciclovir gene therapy. *Gene Ther* 1996;3:491–495.

32. Namba H, Iwadate Y, Tagawa M, et al. Evaluation of the bystander effect in experimental brain tumors bearing herpes simplex virus-thymidine kinase gene by serial magnetic resonance imaging. *Hum Gene Ther* 1996;7:1847–1852.
33. Deliganis AV, Baxter AB, Berger MS, et al. Serial MR in gene therapy for recurrent glioblastoma: initial experience and work in progress. *Am J Neuroradiol* 1997;18:1401–1406.
34. Izquierdo M, Cortes ML, Martin V, et al. Gene therapy in brain tumours: implications of the size of glioblastoma on its curability. *Acta Neurochir Suppl Wien* 1997;68:111–117.
35. Klatzmann D, Valery CA, Bensimon G, et al. A phase I/II study of herpes simplex virus type 1 thymidine kinase "suicide" gene therapy for recurrent glioblastoma. Study group on gene therapy for glioblastoma. *Hum Gene Ther* 1998;9:2595–2604.
36. Poptani H, Puumalainen AM, Grohn OH, et al. Monitoring thymidine kinase and ganciclovir-induced changes in rat malignant glioma *in vivo* by nuclear magnetic resonance imaging. *Cancer Gene Ther* 1998; 5:101–109.
37. Bouali-Benazzouz R, Laine M, Vicat JM, et al. Therapeutic efficacy of the thymidine kinase/ganciclovir system on large experimental gliomas: a nuclear magnetic resonance imaging study. *Gene Ther* 1999;6: 1030–1037.
38. Sandmair AM, Loimas S, Poptani H, et al. Low efficacy of gene therapy for rat BT4C malignant glioma using intra-tumoural transduction with thymidine kinase retrovirus packaging cell injections and ganciclovir treatment. *Acta Neurochir Wien* 1999;141: 867–872.
39. Shand N, Weber F, Mariani L, et al. A phase 1-2 clinical trial of gene therapy for recurrent glioblastoma multiforme by tumor transduction with the herpes simplex thymidine kinase gene followed by ganciclovir. GLI328 European-Canadian Study Group. *Hum Gene Ther* 1999;10: 2325–2335.
40. Namba H, Tagawa M, Miyagawa T, et al. Treatment of rat experimental brain tumors by herpes simplex virus thymidine kinase gene-transduced allogeneic tumor cells and ganciclovir. *Cancer Gene Ther* 2000;7:947–953.
41. Markert JM, Medlock MD, Rabkin SD, et al. Conditionally replicating herpes simplex virus mutant, G207 for the treatment of malignant glioma: results of a phase I trial. *Gene Ther* 2000;7:867–874.
42. Gerolami R, Cardoso J, Lewin M, et al. Evaluation of HSV-tk gene therapy in a rat model of chemically induced hepatocellular carcinoma by intratumoral and intrahepatic artery routes. *Cancer Res* 2000;60: 993–1001.
43. Hamstra DA, Rice DJ, Fahmy S, et al. Rehemtulla-A enzyme/prodrug therapy for head and neck cancer using a catalytically superior cytosine deaminase. *Hum Gene Ther* 1999;10:1993–2003.
44. Adachi Y, Tamiya T, Ichikawa T, et al. Experimental gene therapy for brain tumors using adenovirus-mediated transfer of cytosine deaminase gene and uracil phosphoribosyltransferase gene with 5-fluorocytosine. *Hum Gene Ther* 2000;11:77–89.
45. Stegman LD, Rehemtulla A, Hamstra DA, et al. Diffusion MRI detects early events in the response of a glioma model to the yeast cytosine deaminase gene therapy strategy. *Gene Ther* 2000;7:1005–1010.
46. Ichikawa T, Tamiya,T, Adachi Y, et al. *In vivo* efficacy and toxicity of 5-fluorocytosine/cytosine deaminase gene therapy for malignant gliomas mediated by adenovirus. *Cancer Gene Ther* 2000;7:74–82.
47. Ram Z, Walbridge S, Shawker T, et al. The effect of thymidine kinase transduction and ganciclovir therapy on tumor vasculature and growth of 9L gliomas in rats. *J Neurosurg* 1994;81:256–260.
48. Ram Z, Culver K, Oshiro EM, et al. Therapy of malignant brain tumors by intratumoral implantation of retroviral vector-producing cells. *Nature Med* 1997;3:1354–1361.
49. Morin KW, Knaus EE, Wiebe LI, et al. Reporter gene imaging: effects of ganciclovir treatment on nucleoside uptake, hypoxia and perfusion in a murine gene therapy tumour model that expresses herpes simplex type-1 thymidine kinase. *Nucl Med Commun* 2000;21:129–137.
50. Ross BD, Kim B, Davidson BL. Assessment of ganciclovir toxicity to experimental intracranial gliomas following recombinant adenoviral-mediated transfer of the herpes simplex virus thymidine kinase gene by magnetic resonance imaging and proton magnetic resonance spectroscopy. *Clin Cancer Res* 1995;1:651–657.
51. Haberkorn U, Bellemann ME, Altmann A, et al. F-18-fluoro-2-deoxyglucose uptake in rat prostate adenocarcinoma during chemotherapy with 2′,2′-difluoro-2′-deoxycytidine. *J Nucl Med* 1997; 38:1215–1221.
52. Wahl RL, Zasadny K, Helvie M, et al. Metabolic monitoring of breast cancer chemohormonotherapy using positron emission tomography: initial evaluation. *J Clin Oncol* 1993;11:2101–2111.
53. Christman D, Crawford EJ, Friedkin M, et al. Detection of DNA synthesis in intact organisms with positron-emitting (methyl-^{11}C) thymidine. *Proc Natl Acad Sci U S A* 1972;69:988–992.
54. Shields AF, Lim K, Grierson J, et al. Utilization of labeled thymidine in DNA synthesis: studies for PET. *J Nucl Med* 1990;31:337–342.
55. Haberkorn U, Altmann A, Morr I, et al. Multi tracer studies during gene therapy of hepatoma cells with HSV thymidine kinase and ganciclovir. *J Nucl Med* 1997;38:1048–1054.
56. Haberkorn U, Altmann A, Morr I, et al. Gene therapy with herpes simplex virus thymidine kinase in hepatoma cells: uptake of specific substrates. *J Nucl Med* 1997;38:287–294.
57. Haberkorn U, Bellemann ME, Gerlach L, et al. Uncoupling of 2-fluoro-2-deoxyglucose transport and phosphorylation in rat hepatoma during gene therapy with HSV thymidine kinase. *Gene Ther* 1998;5:880–887.
58. Haberkorn U, Morr I, Oberdorfer F, et al. Fluorodeoxyglucose uptake *in vitro*: aspects of method and effects of treatment with gemcitabine. *J Nucl Med* 1994;35:1842–1850.
59. Haberkorn U, Reinhardt M, Strauss LG, et al. Metabolic design of combination therapy: use of enhanced fluorodeoxyglucose uptake caused by chemotherapy. *J Nucl Med* 1992;33:1981–1987.
60. Wertheimer E, Sasson S, Cerasi E, et al. The ubiquitous glucose transporter GLUT-1 belongs to the glucose-regulated protein family of stress-inducible proteins. *Proc Natl Acad Sci U S A* 1991;88:2525–2529.
61. Widnell CC, Baldwin SA, Davies A, et al. Cellular stress induces a redistribution of the glucose transporter. *FASEB J* 1990;4:1634–1637.
62. Pasternak CA, Aiyathurai JEJ, Makinde V, et al. Regulation of glucose uptake by stressed cells. *J Cell Physiol* 1991;149:324–331.
63. Clancy BM, Czech MP. Hexose transport stimulation and membrane redistribution of glucose transporter isoforms in response to cholera toxin, dibutyryl cyclic AMP, and insulin in 3T3 adipocytes. *J Biol Chem* 1990;265:12434–12443.
64. Germann C, Shields AF, Grierson JR, et al. 5-Fluoro-1-(2′-deoxy-2′-fluoro-β-D-ribofuranosyl)uracil trapping in Morris hepatoma cells expressing the herpes simplex virus thymidine kinase gene. *J Nucl Med* 1998;39:1418–1423.
65. Haberkorn U. Monitoring of gene transfer for cancer therapy with radioactive isotopes. *Ann Nucl Med* 1999;13:1999:369–377.
66. Haberkorn U, Khazaie K, Morr I, et al. Ganciclovir uptake in human mammary carcinoma cells expressing herpes simplex virus thymidine kinase. *Nucl Med Biol* 1998;25:367–373.
67. Mahony WB, Domin BA, McConnel RT, et al. Acyclovir transport into human erythrocytes. *J Biol Chem* 1988;263:9285–9291.
68. Gati WP, Misra HK, Knaus EE, et al. Structural modifications at the 2′and 3′ positions of some pyrimidine nucleosides as determinants of their interaction with the mouse erythrocyte nucleoside transporter. *Biochem Pharmacol* 1984;33:3325–3331.
69. Price R, Cardle K, Watanabe K. The use of antiviral drugs to image herpes encephalitis. *Cancer Res* 1983;43:3619–3627.
70. Saito Y, Price R, Rottenberg DA, et al. Quantitative autoradiographic mapping of herpes simplex virus encephalitis with radiolabeled antiviral drug. *Science* 1982;217:1151–1153.
71. Gambhir SS, Barrio JR, Phelps ME, et al. Imaging adenoviral-directed reporter gene expression in living animals with positron emission tomography. *Proc Natl Acad Sci U S A* 1999;96:2333–2338.

72. Alauddin MM, Shahinian A, Kundu RK, et al. Evaluation of 9-[(3-^{18}F-fluoro-1-hydroxy-2-propoxy)methyl]guanine ([^{18}F]-FHPG) *in vitro* and *in vivo* as a probe for PET imaging of gene incorporation and expression in tumors. *Nucl Med Biol* 1999;26:371–376.
73. Alauddin MM, Conti PS. Synthesis and preliminary evaluation of 9-(4-[^{18}F]-fluoro-3-hydroxymethylbutyl)guanine ([^{18}F]FHBG): a new potential imaging agent for viral infection and gene therapy using PET. *Nucl Med Biol* 1998;25:175–180.
74. Morin KW, Knaus EE, Wiebe LI. Non-invasive scintigraphic monitoring of gene expression in a HSV-1 thymidine kinase gene therapy model. *Nucl Med Commun* 1997;18:599–605.
75. Wiebe LI, Morin KW, Knaus EE. Radiopharmaceuticals to monitor gene transfer. *Q J Nucl Med* 1997;41:79–89.
76. Tjuvajev JG, Stockhammer G, Desai R, et al. Imaging the expression of transfected genes *in vivo*. *Cancer Res* 1995;55:6126–6132.
77. Tjuvajev JG, Avril N, Oku T, et al. Imaging herpes virus thymidine kinase gene transfer and expression by positron emission tomography. *Cancer Res* 1998;58:4333–4341.
78. de Vries EF, van Waarde A, Harmsen MC, et al. [^{11}C]FMAU and [^{18}F]FHPG as PET tracers for herpes simplex virus thymidine kinase enzyme activity and human cytomegalovirus infections. *Nucl Med Biol* 2000;27:113–119.
79. Wiebe LI, Knaus EE, Morin KW. Radiolabelled pyrimidine nucleosides to monitor the expression of HSV-1 thymidine kinase in gene therapy. *Nucleosides Nucleotides* 1999;18:1065–1066.
80. Hustinx R, Shiue CY, Alavi A, et al. Imaging *in vivo* herpes simplex virus thymidine kinase gene transfer to tumour-bearing rodents using positron emission tomography and (^{18}F)FHPG. *Eur J Nucl Med* 2001; 28:5–12.
81. Iwashina T, Tovell DR, Xu L, et al. Synthesis and antiviral activity of IVFRU, a potential probe for the non-invasive diagnosis of herpes simplex encephalitis. *Drug Des Del* 1988;3:309–321.
82. Haubner R, Avril N, Hantzopoulos PA, et al. *In vivo* imaging of herpes simplex virus type 1 thymidine kinase gene expression: early kinetics of radiolabelled FIAU. *Eur J Nucl Med* 2000;27:283–291.
83. Gambhir SS, Bauer E, Black ME, et al. A mutant herpes simplex virus type 1 thymidine kinase reporter gene shows improved sensitivity for imaging reporter gene expression with positron emission tomography. *Proc Natl Acad Sci U S A* 2000;97:2785–2790.
84. Yu Y, Annala AJ, Barrio JR, et al. Quantification of target gene expression by imaging reporter gene expression in living animals. *Nature Med* 2000;6:933–937.
85. MacLaren DC, Gambhir SS, Satyamurthy N, et al. Repetitive noninvasive imaging of the dopamine D_2 receptor as a reporter gene in living animals. *Gene Ther* 1999;6:785–791.
86. Zinn KR, Buchsbaum DJ, Chaudhuri TR, et al. Noninvasive monitoring of gene transfer using a reporter receptor imaged with a high-affinity peptide radiolabeled with ^{99m}Tc or ^{188}Re. *J Nucl Med* 2000;41: 887–895.
87. Raben D, Buchsbaum DJ, Khazaeli MB, et al. Enhancement of radiolabeled antibody binding and tumor localization through adenoviral transduction of the human carcinoembryonic antigen gene. *Gene Ther* 1996;3:567–580.
88. Bogdanov A, Petherick P, Marecos E, et al. *In vivo* localization of diglycylcysteine-bearing synthetic peptides by nuclear imaging of oxotechnetate transchelation. *Nucl Med Biol* 1997;24:739–742.
89. Bogdanov A, Simonova M, Weissleder R. Design of metal-binding green fluorescent protein variants. *Biochim Biophys Acta* 1998;1397:56–64.
90. Simonova M, Weissleder R, Sergeyev N, et al. Targeting of green fluorescent protein expression to the cell surface. *Biochem Biophys Res Commun* 1999;262:638–642.
91. Weissleder R, Simonova M, Bogdanova A, et al. MR imaging and scintigraphy of gene expression through melanin induction. *Radiology* 1997;204:425–429.
92. Tucker CL, Gera JF, Uetz P. Towards an understanding of complex protein networks. *Trends Cell Biol* 2001;11:102–106.
93. Marcotte E, Pellegrini M, Ng HL et al. Detecting protein function and protein-protein interactions from genome sequences. *Science* 1999; 285:751–753.
94. Wouters FS, Verveer PJ, Bastiaens PIH. Imaging biochemistry inside cells. *Trends Cell Biol* 2001;1:203–211.
95. Ray P, Pimenta H, Paulmurugan R, et al. Noninvasive quantitative imaging of protein-protein interactions in living subjects. *Proc Natl Acad Sci U S A* 2002;99: 3105–3110.
96. Wu JC, Sundaresan G, Iyer M, et al. Noninvasive optical imaging of firefly luciferase reporter gene expression in skeletal muscles of living mice. *Mol Ther* 2001;4: 297–306.
97. Luker GD, Sharma V, Pica CM, et al. Noninvasive imaging of protein–protein interactions in living animals. *Proc Natl Acad Sci U S A* 2002; 99:6961–6966.
98. Rossi FMV, Blakely BT, Blau HM. Interaction blues: protein interactions monitored in live mammalian cells by β-galactosidase complementation. *Trends Cell Biol* 2000;10:119–122.
99. Mills KV, Paulus H. Reversible inhibition of protein splicing by zinc ion. *J Biol Chem* 2001;276:10832–10838.
100. Gimble FS. Putting protein splicing to work. *Chem Biol* 1998;5: R251–R256.
101. Paulmurugan R, Umezawa Y, Gambhir SS. Noninvasive imaging of protein–protein interactions in living subjects by using reporter protein complementation and reconstitution strategies. *Proc Natl Acad Sci U S A* 2002;99:15608–15613.
102. Werner T. Promoters can contribute to the elucidation of protein function. *Trends Biotechnol* 2003;21:9–13.
103. Haberkorn U, Altmann A. Noninvasive imaging of protein-protein interaction in living organisms. *Trends Biotechnol* 2003;21:241–243.
104. Haberkorn U, Altmann A, Eisenhut M. Functional genomics and proteomics—the role of nuclear medicine. *Eur J Nuc Med* 2002;29: 115–132.
105. Altmann A, Schulz RB, Glensch G, et al. Effects of Pax8 and TTF-1 thyroid transcription factor gene transfer in hepatoma cells: imaging of functional protein–protein interaction and iodide uptake. *J Nucl Med* 2005;46:831–839.
106. Jiang S, Altmann A, Grimm D, et al. Tissue-specific gene expression in medullary thyroid carcinoma cells employing calcitonin regulatory elements and AAV vectors. *Cancer Gene Ther* 2001;8:469–472.
107. Iyer M, Wu L, Carey M, et al. Two-step transcriptional amplification as a method for imaging reporter gene expression using weak promoters. *Proc Natl Acad Sci U S A* 2001;98:14595–14600.
108. Marcocci C, Cohen JL, Grollman EF. Effect of actinomycin D on iodide transport in FRTL-5 thyroid cells. *Endocrinology* 1984;115: 2123–2132.
109. Weiss SJ, Philp NJ, Grollman EF. Iodide transport in a continuous line of cultured cells from rat thyroid. *Endocrinology* 1984;114: 1090–1098.
110. Paire A, Bernier-Valentin F, Selmi-Ruby S, et al. Characterization of the rat thyroid iodide transporter using anti-peptide antibodies. *J Biol Chem* 1997;272:18245–18249.
111. Nakamura Y, Ohtaki S, Yamazaki I. Molecular mechanism of iodide transport by thyroid plasmalemmal vesicles: cooperative sodium activation and asymmetrical affinities for the ions on the outside and inside of the vesicles. *J Biochem* 1988;104:544–549.
112. Nakamura Y, Kotani T, Ohtaki S. Transcellular ioide transport and iodination on the apical plasma membrane by monolayer porcine thyroid cells cultured on collagen-coated fibers. *J Endocrin* 1990;126:275–281.
113. Smanik PA, Liu Q, Furminger TL, et al. Cloning of the human sodium iodide symporter. *Biochem Biophys Res Commun* 1996;226:339–345.
114. Haberkorn U, Henze M, Altmann A, et al. Transfer of the human sodium iodide symporter gene enhances iodide uptake in hepatoma cells. *J Nucl Med* 2001;42:317–325
115. Mandell RB, Mandell LZ, Link CJ. Radioisotope concentrator gene therapy using the sodium/iodide symporter gene. *Cancer Res* 1999;59: 661–668.

116. Cho JY, Xing S, Liu X, et al. Expression and activity of human Na+/I– symporter in human glioma cells by adenovirus-mediated gene delivery. *Gene Ther* 2000;7:740–749.
117. Boland A, Ricard M, Opolon P, et al. Adenovirus-mediated transfer of the thyroid sodium/Iodide symporter gene into tumors for a targeted radiotherapy. *Cancer Res* 2000;60:3484–3492.
118. Spitzweg C, Zhang S, Bergert ER, et al. Prostate-specific antigen (PSA) promoter-driven androgen-inducible expression of sodium iodide symporter in prostate cancer cell lines. *Cancer Res* 1999;59:2136–2141.
119. Haberkorn U, Kinscherf R, Kissel M, et al. Enhanced iodide transport after transfer of the human sodium iodide symporter gene is associated with lack of retention and low absorbed dose. *Gene Ther* 2003;10:774–780.
120. La Perle KM, Shen D, Buckwaiter TL, et al. *In vivo* expression and function of the sodium iodide symporter following gene transfer in the MATLyLu rat model of metastatic prostate cancer. *Prostate* 2002;50:170–178.
121. Nakamoto Y, Saga T, Misaki T, et al. Establishment and characterization of a breast cancer cell line expressing Na+/I− symporters for radioiodide concentrator gene therapy. *J Nucl Med* 2000;41:1898–1904.
122. Shimura H, Haraguchi K, Miyazaki A, et al. Iodide uptake and experimental ^{131}I therapy in transplanted undifferentiated thyroid cancer cells expressing the Na+/I− symporter gene. *Endocrinology* 1997;138:4493–4496.
123. Sieger S, Jiang S, Schönsiegel F, et al. Tumour specific activation of the sodium/iodide symporter gene under control of the glucose transporter gene 1 promoter (GTI-1.3). *Eur J Nucl Med* 2003;30:748–756.
124. Smit JW, Shröder-vander Elst JP, Karperien M, et al. Reestablishment of *in vitro* and *in vivo* iodide uptake by transfection of the human sodium iodide symporter (hNIS) in a hNIS defective human thyroid carcinoma cell line. *Thyroid* 2000;10: 939–943.
125. Smit JW, Shröder-vander Elst JP, Karperien M, et al. Iodide kinetics and experimental ^{131}I therapy in a xenotransplanted human sodium-iodide symporter-transfected human follicular thyroid carcinoma cell line. *J Clin Endocrinol Metab* 2002;87:1247–1253.
126. Spitzweg C, O'Connor MK, Bergert ER, et al. Treatment of prostate cancer by radioiodine therapy after tissue-specific expression of the sodium iodide symporter. *Cancer Res* 2000;60:6526–6530.
127. Spitzweg C, Dietz AB, O'Connor MK, et al. *In vivo* sodium iodide symporter gene therapy of prostate cancer. *Gene Ther* 2001;8:1524–1531.
128. Huang M, Batra RK, Kogai T, et al. Ectopic expression of the thyroperoxidase gene augments radioiodide uptake and retention mediated by the sodium iodide symporter in non–small cell lung cancer. *Cancer Gene Ther* 2001;8:612–618.
129. Berman M, Hoff E, Barandes M. Iodine kinetics in man: a model. *J Clin Endocrinol Metab* 1968;28:1–14.
130. Maxon HR, Thomas SR, Hertzberg VS, et al. Relation between effective radiation dose and outcome of radioiodine therapy for thyroid cancer. *N Engl J Med* 1983; 309:937–941.
131. Carlin S, Cunningham SH, Boyd M, et al. Experimental targeted radioiodide therapy following transfection of the sodium iodide symporter gene: effect on clonogenicity in both two-and three-dimensional models. *Cancer Gene Ther* 2000;7:1529–1536.
132. Haberkorn U, Altmann A, Jiang S, et al. Iodide uptake in human anaplastic thyroid carcinoma cells after transfer of the human thyroid peroxidase gene. *Eur J Nucl Med* 2001;28:633–638.
133. Koong S, Reynolds JC, Movius EG, et al. Lithium as a potential adjuvant to ^{131}I therapy of metastatic, well differentiated thyroid carcinoma. *J Clin Endocrinol Metab* 1999;84:912–916.
134. Urabe M, Hershman JM, Pang XP, et al. Effect of lithium on function and growth of thyroid cells *in vitro*. *Endocrinology* 1991;129:807–814.
135. Lazarus JH. The effects of lithium therapy on thyroid and thyrotropin-releasing hormone. *Thyroid* 1998;8:909–913.
136. Sedvall G, Jonsson B, Petterson U, et al. Effects of lithium salts on plasma protein bound iodine and uptake of ^{131}I in thyroid gland of man and rat. *Life Sci* 1968;7:1257–1264.
137. Temple R, Berman M, Robbins J, et al. The use of lithium in the treatment of thyrotoxicosis. *J Clin Invest* 1972;51:2746–2756.
138. Gershengorn MC, Izumi M, Robbins J. Use of lithium as an adjunct to radioiodine therapy of thyroid carcinoma. *J Clin Endocrinol Metab* 1976;42:105–111.
139. Chen L, Altmann A, Mier W, et al. Radioiodine therapy of hepatoma using targeted transfer of the human sodium/iodide symporter gene. *J Nucl Med* 2006;47:854–862.
140. Dadachova E, Bouzahzah B, Zuckier LS, et al. Rhenium-188 as an alternative to iodine-131 for treatment of breast tumors expressing the sodium/iodide symporter (NIS). *Nucl Med Biol* 2002;29:13–18.
141. Petrich T, Helmeke HJ, Meyer GJ, et al. Establishment of radioactive astatine and iodine uptake in cancer cell lines expressing the human sodium iodide symporter. *Eur J Nucl Med* 2002;29:842–854.
142. Hidaka Y, Hayashi Y, Fisfalen ME, et al. Expression of thyroid peroxidase in EBV-transformed B cell lines using adenovirus. *Thyroid* 1996;6:23–28.
143. Kaufman KD, Filetti S, Seto P, et al. Recombinant human thyroid peroxidase generated in eukaryotic cells: a source of specific antigen for the immunological assay of antimicrosomal antibodies in the sera of patients with autoimmune thyroid disease. *J Clin Endocrinol Metab* 1990;70:724–728.
144. Kimura S, Kotani T, Ohtaki S, et al. cDNA-directed expression of human thyroid peroxidase. *FEBS Lett* 1989;250:377–380.
145. Guo J, McLachlan SM, Hutchinson S, et al. The greater glycan content of recombinant human thyroid peroxidase of mammalian than of insect cell origin facilitates purification to homogeneity of enzymatically protein remaining soluble at high concentration. *Endocrinology* 1998;139:999–1005.
146. Giraud A, Franc JL, Long Y, et al. Effects of deglycosylation of human thyroperoxidase on its enzymatic activity and immunoreactivity. *J Endocrinol* 1992;132:317–323.
147. Giraud A, Siffroi S, Lanet J, et al. Binding and internalization of thyroglobulin: selectivity, pH dependence, and lack of tissue specificity. *Endocrinology* 1997;138:2325–2332.
148. Taurog A, Dorris ML, Yokoyama N, et al. Purification and characterization of a large, tryptic fragment of human thyroid peroxidase with high catalytic activity. *Arch Biochem Biophys* 1990;278;333–341.
149. Ohtaki S, Kotani T, Nakamura Y. Characterization of human thyroid peroxidase purified by monoclonal antibody-assisted chromatography. *J Clin Endocrinol Metab* 1986;63:570–576.
150. Ohtaki S, Nakagawa H, Nakamura M, et al. Thyroid peroxidase: experimental and clinical integration. *Endocrine J* 1996;43:1–14.
151. Smets LA, Loesberg C, Janssen M, et al. Active uptake and extravesicular storage of m-iodobenzyl guanidine in human neuroblastoma. *Cancer Res* 1989;49:2941–2944.
152. Wafelman AR, Hoefnagel CA, Maes RAA, et al. radioiodinated metaiodo-benzylguanidine: a review of IST distribution and pharmacokinetics, drug interactions, cytotoxicity and dosimetry. *Eur J Nucl Med* 1994;21:545–559.
153. Mairs RJ, Livingstone A, Gaze MN, et al. A prediction of accumulation of ^{131}I-labelled meta-iodobenzylguanidine in neuroblastoma cell lines by means of reverse transcription and polymerase chain reaction. *Br J Cancer* 1994;70:97–101.
154. Glowniak JV, Kilty JE, Amara SG, et al. Evaluation of metaiodobenzylguanidine uptake by the norepinephrine, dopamine and serotonin transporters. *J Nucl Med* 1993;34:1140–1146.
155. Lode HN, Bruchelt G, Seitz G, et al. Reverse transcriptase-polymerase chain reaction (RT-PCR) analysis of monoamine transporters in neuroblastoma cell lines: correlations to meta-iodobenzylguanidine (MIBG) uptake and tyrosine hydroxylase gene expression. *Eur J Cancer* 1995;31A:586–590.
156. Pacholczyk T, Blakely RD, Amara SG. Expression cloning of a cocaine- and antidepressant-sensitive human noradrenaline transporter. *Nature* 1991;350:350–354.

157. Boyd M, Cunningham SH, Brown MM, et al. Noradrenaline transporter gene transfer for radiation cell kill by ^{131}I meta-iodobenzylguanidine. *Gene Ther* 1999;6:1147–1152.
158. Altmann A, Kissel M, Zitzmann S, et al. Increased MIBG uptake after transfer of the human norepinephrine transporter gene in rat hepatoma. *J Nucl Med* 2003;44:973–980.
159. Bomanji J, Levison DA, Flatman WD, et al. Uptake of iodine-123 MIBG by pheochromocytomas, paragangliomas, and neuroblastomas: a histopathological comparison. *J Nucl Med* 1987;28:973–978.
160. Zamecnik PC, Stephenson ML. Inhibition of Rous sarcoma virus replication and cell transformation by a specific oligodeoxynucleotide. *Proc Natl Acad Sci U S A* 1978;75:280–285.
161. Mukhopadhyay T, Tainsky M, Cavender AC, et al. Specific inhibition of K-ras expression and tumorigenicity of lung cancer cells by antisense RNA. *Cancer Res* 1991;51:1744–1748.
162. Hannon GJ. RNA interference. *Nature* 2002;418:244–251.
163. Zeng Y, Wagner EJ, Cullen BR, et al. Both natural and designed micro RNAs can inhibit the expression of cognate mRNAs when expressed in human cells. *Mol Cell* 2002;9:1327–1333.
164. Sui G, Soohoo C, Affarel B, et al. A DNA vector-based RNAi technology to suppress gene expression in mammalian cells. *Proc Natl Acad Sci U S A* 2002;99: 5515–5520.
165. Moss EG. Silencing unhealthy alleles naturally. *Trends Biotechnol* 2003;21:185–187.
166. Claverie JM. What if there are only 30,000 human genes? *Science* 2001;291:1255–1257.
167. Woolf TM, Melton DA, Jennings CGB. Specificity of antisense oligonucleotides *in vivo*. *Proc Natl Acad Sci U S A* 1992;89:7305–7309.
168. Iversen PL, Zhu S, Meyer A, et al. Cellular uptake and subcellular distribution of phosphorothioate oligonucleotides into cultured cells. *Antisense Res Dev* 1992;2:211–222.
169. Loke SL, Stein CA, Zhang XH, et al. Characterization of oligonucleotide transport into living cells. *Proc Natl Acad Sci U S A* 1989;86: 3474–3478.
170. Dewanjee MK, Ghafouripour AK, Kapadvanjwala M, et al. Noninvasive imaging of c-myc oncogene messenger RNA with indium-111-antisense probes in a mammary tumor-bearing mouse model. *J Nucl Med* 1994;35:1054–1063.
171. Cammilleri S, Sangrajrang S, Perdereau B, et al. Biodistribution of iodine-125 tyramine transforming growth factor? Antisense oligonucleotide in athymic mice with a human mammary tumor xenograft following intratumoral injection. *Eur J Nucl Med* 1996;23: 448–452.
172. Kobori N, Imahori Y, Mineura K, et al. Visualization of mRNA expression in CNS using ^{11}C-labeled phosphorothioate oligodeoxynucleotide. *Neuroreport* 1999;10:2971–2974.
173. Shi N, Boado RJ, Pardridge WM. Antisense imaging of gene expression in the brain *in vivo*. *Proc Natl Acad Sci U S A* 2000;97:14709–14714.
174. Urbain JL, Shore SK, Vekemans MC, et al. Scintigraphic imaging of oncogenes with antisense probes: does it make sense? *Eur J Nucl Med* 1995;22:499–504.
175. Tavitian B, Terrazzino S, Kühnast B, et al. *In vivo* imaging of oligonucleotides with positron emission tomography. *Nature Med* 1998;4: 467–471.
176. Watanabe N, Sawai H, Endo K, et al. Labeling of phosphorothioate antisense oligonucleotides with yttrium-90. *Nucl Med Biol* 1999;26: 239–243.
177. Anderson L, Seilhamer J. A comparison of selected mRNA and protein abundances in human liver. *Electrophoresis* 1977;18:533–537.
178. Futcher B, Latter GI, Monardo P, et al. A sampling of the yeast proteome. *Mol Cell Biol* 1999,19:7357–7368.
179. Gygi SP, Rist B, Gerber SA, et al. Quantitative analysis of complex protein mixtures using isotope-coded affinity tags. *Nat Biotechnol* 1999;17:994–999.
180. Pradet-Balade B, Boulme F, Beug H, et al. Translation control: bridging the gap between genomics and proteomics? *Trends Biochem Sci* 2001;26:225–229.

CHAPTER

14.2 The Kidneys

ZSOLT SZABO, JINSONG XIA, AND WILLIAM B. MATHEWS

RATIONALE

The successful application of positron emission tomography (PET) in cancer is expected to translate to other diseases. Considerable progress can already be observed in cardiac and neurological PET applications. Other potential nononcological uses of PET imaging may include diseases of the kidneys, lungs, and liver. With its high sensitivity for detection of molecular signatures *in vivo*, PET could be useful for solving many clinical problems. Examples of potential pulmonary applications of PET include the diagnosis, management, and follow-up of cystic fibrosis, α-1 antitrypsin deficiency, idiopathic pulmonary fibrosis, primary pulmonary hypertension, asthma, chronic obstructive pulmonary disease, chemical lung injury, and infections in immune-compromised persons. Potential applications in hepatology would be in the management of viral hepatitis, acute liver failure, and liver transplant complications.

Areas of nephrourology that could benefit from PET include the management of acute or chronic renal failure, proteinuria, kidney stones, urinary tract infections, and polycystic kidney disease. Of increasing importance is the understanding and management of interconnected disorders where strategies of disease management encounter strategies of disease prevention. Areas that could be included are the metabolic syndrome, diabetes, and hypertension, with the complications of renal insufficiency, cardiomyopathy, and cerebrovascular disease. To apply PET in these important clinical areas researchers will have to improve their understanding of the underlying molecular mechanisms and match them with the unique features of PET chemistry and imaging technology.

PET could already replace the gamma camera for imaging renal blood flow or cortical function. The spatial resolution of modern PET scanners is 5 to 6 mm at a counting sensitivity of 30 cps/Bq/mL (1), quite adequate for imaging the kidneys. Image acquisition at 1- to 2-second frame times is now possible for rapid dynamic studies, while static scans of outstanding quality can be obtained in 3 to 5 minutes. The recently evolving technique of list mode acquisition will permit reconstruction of time intervals with the best signal to noise ratios. Iterative reconstruction algorithms are also available that can handle PET scans with high activity gradients attributable to large perfusion differences between the cortex and medulla or to the accumulation of radiopharmaceuticals in the pelvocalyceal system.

At the present time clinical protocols are not available for routine PET imaging of the kidneys. PET has been used occasionally to diagnose renal cancer, but this imaging modality has limited sensitivity for this disease (2). An important area that needs better imaging sensitivity is the diagnosis and follow-up of renovascular hypertension. Although the accuracy of digital subtraction angiography (DSA) and even of computed tomography angiography (CTA) for diagnosis of renal artery stenosis is high (3–5), these methods involve the use of potentially nephrotoxic contrast agents and ionizing radiation. Magnetic resonance angiography (MRA) can also be used for diagnosis of renal artery stenosis. It is considered to be noninvasive and safe and quite accurate in diagnosing renal artery stenosis, yet it is apparently less accurate than, for example, captopril renography in assessment of its hemodynamic significance (6). The experience with captopril enhanced MR is extremely limited (7). Diagnosis of renovascular hypertension, prediction of the outcome of revascularization, detection of reperfusion injury, and early detection of a hemodynamically significant restenosis are important unanswered problems. Another significant problem is the assessment of the hemodynamic significance of arterial stenoses in the presence of duplicated or polar renal arteries (8–10).

PET techniques can be grossly divided into functional and molecular imaging applications. Functional imaging techniques that await immediate clinical application include determinations of regional renal blood flow and glomerular filtration. Molecular imaging of the kidneys is at best in an experimental stage. In this chapter renal imaging techniques will be classified according to the kinetic properties of the radiopharmaceuticals adhering to the following containment hierarchy of terms: (a) tracer: any radiolabeled molecule used for PET or single-photon emission computed tomography (SPECT) imaging; (b) radiopharmaceutical: any drug or druglike organic molecule used as tracer; (c) radioligand: a radiopharmaceutical that binds with high affinity to molecular recognition sites or serves as a substrate or pseudosubstrate of transporters and enzymes. The expression substrate can be used for tracers that in addition to binding to recognition sites also undergo chemical changes (if the target protein is an enzyme) or spatial translocations (if the target protein is a transporter). A pseudosubstrate is one that retains some but not all the characteristics of the substrate, an example is fluorine-18-fluorodeoxyglucose ([^{18}F]-FDG).

TRACER KINETIC MODELS

Tracer kinetic models have been used to understand the biological behavior of radiopharmaceuticals and to derive quantitative parameters of radiopharmaceutical accumulation, binding, and clearance. Ideally kinetic parameters are directly or indirectly related to clinically useful physiological measures of renal blood flow, glomerular filtration, tubular transport, or receptor density. A tracer kinetic model is a simplified representation of the biological behavior of the radiopharmaceutical and serves as a logical link between the PET measurement and its computerized analysis. An algorithm, on the other hand, is the algebraic reformulation of the model optimized for the computational steps needed for derivation of quantitative parameters. Algorithms usually also include the processing tools needed to deal with image noise or error progression and for maximization of the accuracy of the estimated parameters.

There are three basic types of tracer kinetic models: stochastic models, distributed models, and compartmental models (11), and all three models can be applied in renal PET studies. The most complicated one is the distributed model, which typically includes many details of the measured biological process. Due to the large number of parameters needed for process description, distributed models are seldom used (12). Compartmental modeling is much more widespread because it is based on generalizations that permit its application to a large number of pharmacokinetic processes. The third one, the stochastic model (13), makes no assumptions about the inner structure of the kinetic process and treats it as a "black box" with a response function brought forth by an input function. The stochastic model provides the impulse response function, a basic function that can be used to describe the response to any time concentration profile of the radiopharmaceutical that enters the organ via its feeding artery. Stochastic and compartmental models share two fundamental assumptions for tracer kinetics: (a) linearity (doubling the injected dose results in doubling of the organ activity); and (b) time invariance (blood volume, blood flow, and binding processes remain constant during the time of imaging). The stochastic model cannot quantify the exchange between the individual compartments, but it can still provide useful pharmacokinetic parameters. Such parameters are the tracer distribution volume, which is the area under the impulse response function, the mean transit time, which is the first momentum of the impulse response function, or the retention fraction, which is the ratio of a value at a chosen time point and the peak value of the impulse response function.

The operational equation that describes the course of a radioligand in the renal parenchyma, the convolution integral between the arterial input function, and the impulse response function is common to both the stochastic and the compartmental model:

$$C_T(t) = C_A(t) \otimes f(t), \qquad (14.2.1)$$

where, $C_T(t)$ equals the parenchymal tissue activity curve, $C_A(t)$ equals the input function, $f(t)$ equals the tissue impulse response function, and $\otimes$ is the operation of convolution.

$C_T(t)$ is derived from the dynamic PET images of the organ; $C_A(t)$ is most accurately measured by rapid arterial blood sampling, but it is also often approximated by time activity curves derived from the abdominal aorta (or the cardiac blood pools if the myocardium is the organ of interest). The capability to correct the noninvasive input function for confounding physical sources of error, such as partial volume effects, or biological sources of error, such as red blood cell binding or protein binding, will have a direct influence on the accuracy of quantitative analysis. The process of convolution can be reversed by deconvolution analysis if one needs to obtain $f(t)$ from $C_T(t)$ and $C_A(t)$. Since the activity in the renal vasculature is not negligible, total tissue activity also includes intravascular activity $C_A(t)$ weighted by the blood volume:

$$C_{TOT}(t) = BV\, C_A(t) + (1\text{-}BV)C_T(t). \qquad (14.2.2)$$

Blood volume (BV) is typically expressed in units of milliliters blood to milliliters tissue or milliliters of blood to grams of tissue. Equation 14.2.2 represents the first steps leading away from the stochastic model toward the compartmental model. BV can be estimated from the tissue activity curve if included in the compartmental model, or it can be approximated with an arbitrary number, which is approximately 5% in the brain and 15% in the kidneys. This number may even be higher. Although not yet established for the human kidney, in the dog kidney the parenchymal blood volume is about 20% (14). Blood volume in the kidneys depends on the highly variable glomerular volume, which is governed by the tubuloglomerular feedback mechanism (15).

Renal radiopharmaceuticals can be divided into four groups according to their impulse response function (Fig. 14.2.1): freely diffusible tracers, chemical microspheres, tracers with urinary excretion, and radioligands. Fig. 14.2.1 shows the four corresponding impulse response functions. The impulse response function is the simplest time activity curve (also called the primitive or base function) that would be measured in an organ after instantaneous injection of a radioactive bolus into the feeding artery of the organ excluding any subsequent recirculation of radioactivity. The tracer can be trapped in the organ (Fig. 14.2.1B), it can return to circulation rapidly (Fig. 14.2.1A) or slowly (Fig. 14.2.1C,D), but in either of these cases the first point of the impulse response function will always be its maximum value, f_{max}. The shape of the rest of the impulse response function is determined by the degrees of retention, trapping, or washout.

Freely Diffusible Tracers

Radiopharmaceuticals with rapid exchange between blood and renal parenchyma such as oxygen-15 ([^{15}O])-labeled water follow a simple kinetic model with a single parenchymal compartment and two compartmental rate constants, K_1, which describes the uptake and k_2, which describes the washout of the tracer. The parameter K_1 is equivalent to flow x extraction, FE. Extraction of water is considered complete so that K_1 is identical to blood flow. The most exact way to measure the input function involves the use of an automatic blood sampler that propels the arterial blood through a coincidence detector cross-calibrated and synchronized with the PET scanner (16). Even this highly accurate input function suffers from distortions such as the delay and dispersion of the radioactive bolus (17). The parameter k_2 is less affected by delay and dispersion than K_1 and can also be used to estimate renal blood flow since the distribution

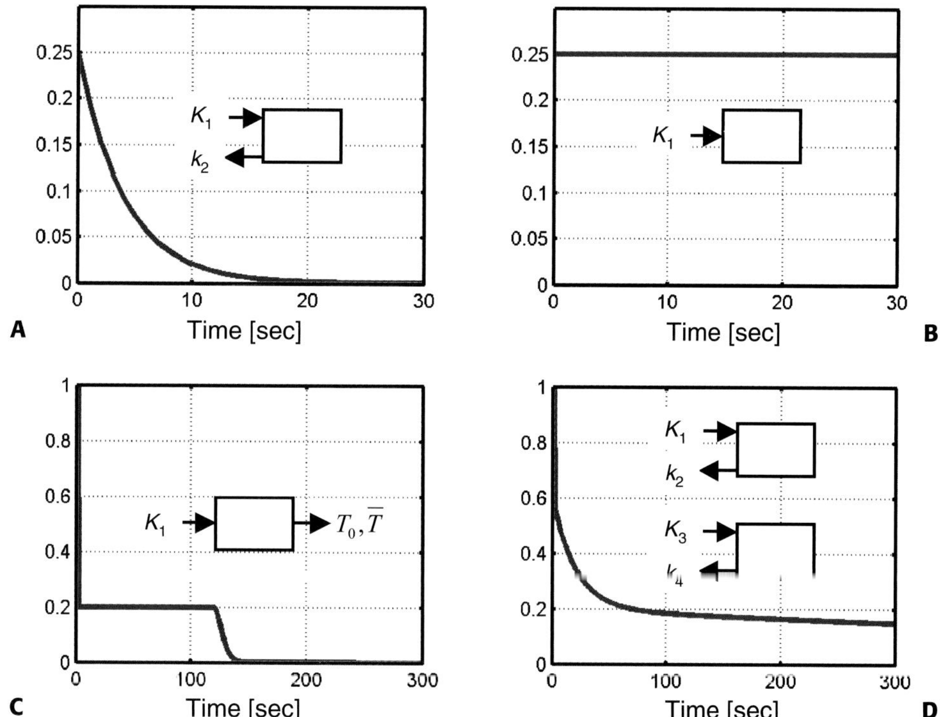

FIGURE 14.2.1. Radiopharmaceutical impulse response functions and compartmental models. **A–C:** Consist of only one parenchymal compartment. **D:** Two parenchymal compartments. **A:** Freely diffusible tracers such as oxygen-15-water demonstrate an uptake and a washout component described by the rate constants K_1 and k_2. **B:** Trapped tracers such as microspheres and chemical microspheres (rubidium-82, nitrogen-13-ammonia) have only one rate constant K_1, which is the product of blood flow and tracer extraction. The tracer extraction of these radiopharmaceuticals can be as high as 80%. **C:** Tracers excreted through the kidneys such as cobalt-55-ethylene-diaminetetraacetic acid are characterized by parenchymal uptake (K_1) and transport into the collecting system. The transport rate is quantified by the minimal transit time (T_0) and mean transit time ($\overline{T}$). **D:** The kinetics of radioligands that bind to nonspecific and specific binding sites is also often described by two tissue compartments. Uptake into these virtual compartments is described by K_1 and K_3, while release from them is described by k_2 and k_4. The purpose of using capital and small letters is to differentiate between perfusion-dependent (K) and perfusion-independent (k) compartmental transfer. In the kidneys, a parallel connectivity tracer kinetic model (**D**) appears more appropriate than the serial connectivity model used for radioligand kinetics of brain receptors.

volume of water $DV = K_1/k_2$ is approximately 1 in this organ (18). Glomerular filtration of 20% of the water entering the kidneys will contribute a slow kinetic process to this rapid washout model first because of the transportation of this water within the tubular lumen and, second, because of partial recycling of water within the loop of Henle. These processes may result in an apparent water distribution volume larger than 1.

As early as in 1971, a positron-emitting radiopharmaceutical, [^{15}O]-labeled water was injected into the renal artery of experimental animals, and its washout was measured with an external radiation detector (19). Using the kinetic model of inert gases, renal blood flow was obtained from the washout rate of the tracer. Fig. 14.2.1A shows the impulse response function of [^{15}O]-water when the volume of interest only contains one tissue type, either the cortex or medulla. Since it is impossible with external detectors and without tomographic imaging capabilities to separate these two tissue components, the time activity curve looked rather like the one shown in Fig. 14.2.1D. A few assumptions were incorrect with those early studies. First, the assumption that [^{15}O]-water behaves in the kidneys like an inert gas such as xenon-133 ([^{133}Xe]) was improper. This was not correct since water is likely the most ubiquitous molecule present in biochemical reactions. Second, an erroneous assumption was that the input function was assumed to be an infinitesimally short bolus (in mathematical terms a δ function). This was incorrect since recirculation of water is significant if the measurement is longer than the renal vascular transit time. No algorithm was provided for solving a convolution integral. The measured time activity curve was fitted with a simple biexponential function whereby, following Fig. 14.2.1D, k_2 described the washout rate from the cortex and k_4 described the washout rate from the medulla. Astonishingly, the measured values were quite realistic and showed a cortical blood flow of 370 mL/min/100 g and a medullary blood flow of 55 mL/min/100 g (19).

With current PET scanners renal perfusion imaging can be performed in dynamic mode, and time activity curves can be analyzed in every voxel of the study. To achieve this in human subjects, 1,110 to 1,850 MBq (30 to 50 MCi) [^{15}O]-water is injected intravenously, and PET scans are acquired at 3-second steps over 90 seconds. In humans the input function is obtained from a region of interest placed in the center of the abdominal aorta and is corrected for partial volume effects. In healthy individuals the estimated renal blood flow with this method is 340 mL/min/100 g, which is similar to the results of probe measurements. Cortical blood flow is significantly decreased in renal diseases (20). Fig. 14.2.2A illustrates the reduced accumulation of [^{15}O]-water in experimental renovascular hypertension.

Chemical Microspheres

Rubidium-82 Chloride

Rubidium-82 ([^{82}Rb]-chloride, and nitrogen-13 ([^{13}N])-ammonia are radiopharmaceuticals with high parenchymal extraction and insignificant washout rates. The kinetic model of these tracers is the most simple one since it includes only an uptake parameter but no washout parameter (Fig. 14.2.1B). This tracer trapping model is identical to the distribution model of radioactive microspheres, which are typically injected into the left atrium or left ventricle of experimental animals (21,22).

Radioactive microspheres are retained in the capillaries of organs according to the distribution of cardiac output (23–26). Chemical microspheres behave similarly to true microspheres since, to a large degree, they also are trapped in the organs, but they accumulate inside the cells rather than within the capillaries. The chemical properties and biological behavior of these radiopharmaceuticals are responsible for their tissue trapping. The Gjedde-Patlak graphical method of irreversible tracer binding has been used for quantification of tracer trapping (27,28). The slope of this plot, K_i is directly related to rate constants of tissue uptake K_1, tissue incorporation k_3, and inversely related to the rate constants of tracer release from the reversible component $k_2 + k_3$:

$$K_i = \frac{K_1 k_3}{k_2 + k_3}. \tag{14.2.3}$$

If washout from tissue (determined by k_2) is negligible, the slope is identical to K_1, which in case of microspheres with 100% extraction becomes equivalent to renal blood flow (29). In reality, the extraction fraction of chemical microspheres is <100% since there is always some tracer backflow before retention is accomplished. If, however, trapping is significant though <100%, the Gjedde-Patlak plot will achieve linearity at the time point when plasma activity and reversible tissue activity reach equilibrium.

Rubidium-82, like thallium-201, is a potassium analogue. Rubidium-82 is a positron emitting radioisotope obtained from strontium-82 ([^{82}Sr]) in a generator and has a physical half-life of 75 seconds and a maximum positron energy of 3.35 MeV. The high positron energy results in a longer positron range, and together with the rapid decay, makes this isotope less optimal for imaging organ perfusion. Despite certain disadvantages, [^{82}Rb] is successfully used for cardiac imaging and can also be used for imaging the kidneys. Rubidium-82 is injected in a dose of 40 to 60 MCi (1,480 to 2,220 MBq). For quantification of split renal perfusion or for detection of regional cortical perfusion defects a single static image can be acquired (Fig. 14.2.2F), but a dynamic PET protocol is needed for detailed quantitative analysis. During dynamic PET imaging, 2- to 3-second frames are acquired (30).

The kinetic model from Fig. 14.2.1A was used to fit the time activity curve of [^{15}O]-water (Fig. 14.2.3A) and the kinetic model from Fig. 14.2.1B was used to fit the time activity curve of [^{82}Rb]-chloride (Fig. 14.2.3B). Assuming a density of renal tissue of 1 g/mL using [^{82}Rb] the renal blood flow in the right (R) kidney was 467 mL/min/100 g and in the left (L) kidney 619 mL/min/100 g with a R/L ratio of 0.75. Measurement with [^{15}O]-water yielded a right kidney blood flow of 222 mL/min/100 g, a left kidney blood flow of 422 mL/min/100 g, and a R/L ratio of 0.53. The input function was obtained from the region of interest (ROI) of the aorta and was not corrected for partial volume effects, which is probably the most

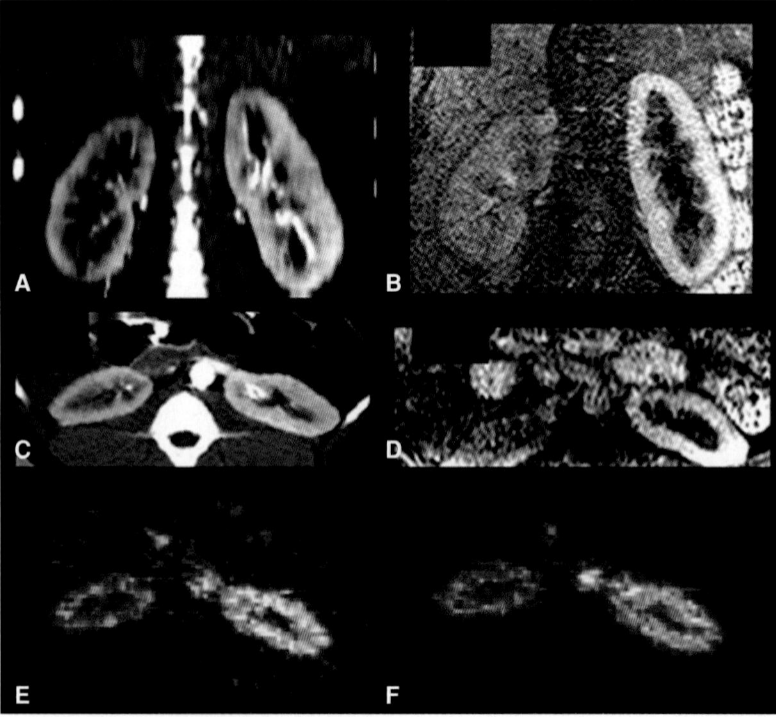

FIGURE 14.2.2. Images of pig kidneys with stenosis of the right renal artery. **A,C:** Computerized tomographic angiography (CTA). **B,D:** Magnetic resonance angiography (MRA). **E:** Oxygen-15 ([^{15}O])-water with PET. **F:** Rubidium-82 ([^{82}Rb]) with PET. Both PET images represent a time window of 20 seconds, starting with peak activity observed in the abdominal aorta. The right kidney is reduced in size and shows reduced accumulation of both CT and MR contrast material as well as reduced accumulation of [^{15}O]-water and [^{82}Rb].

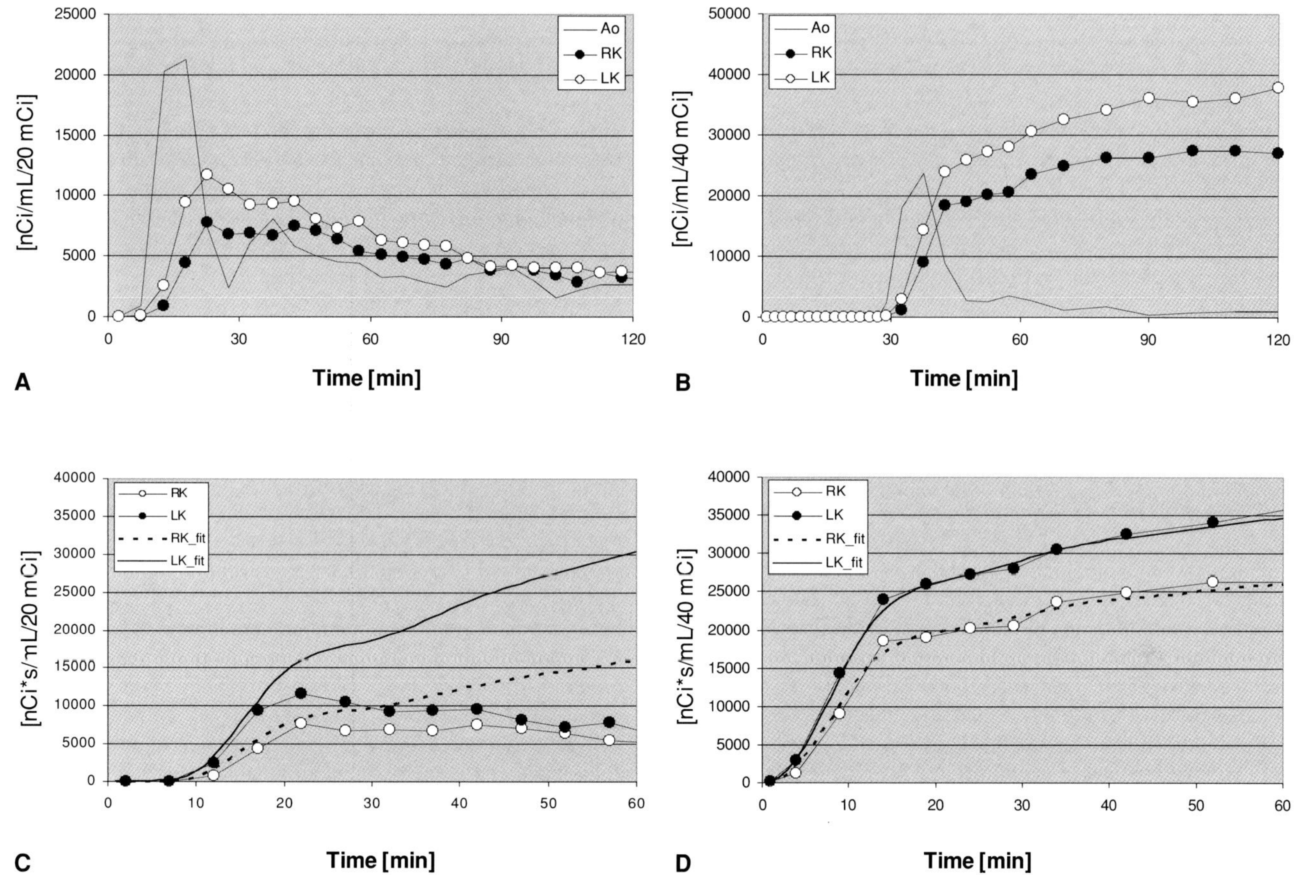

FIGURE 14.2.3. Time activity curves of the kidneys obtained with oxygen-15 ([^{15}O])-water (**A**) and rubidium-82 ([^{82}Rb]) (**B**) in a pig with right-sided renal artery stenosis. Magnetic resonance angiography, computed tomography angiography, and PET images of this same animal are shown in Fig. 14.2.2. The time activity curves were derived using regions of interest of the aorta (Ao), right kidney (RK), and left kidney (LK). Compared to [^{15}O]-water, the renal accumulation of [^{82}Rb] is delayed due to the dead space and prolonged bolus duration of the infusion system. The activity difference between the two kidneys is larger with [^{15}O]-water during the first pass of the tracer, but the difference persists longer with [^{82}Rb], permitting longer imaging times. The integrated input function derived from the abdominal aorta and the tissue time activity curves of [^{15}O]-water are diverging, which is consistent with back diffusion of this tracer into the circulation (**C**). The integrated input function and tissue time activity curves of [^{82}Rb], on the other hand, are nearly identical (**D**), which is consistent with the behavior of this tracer as a chemical microsphere. It is important to emphasize that the integrated input functions are adjusted for each kidney using the renal blood flow values calculated with each tracer.

important factor to explain the high blood flow values. The ROIs were drawn separately for the [^{82}Rb] and [^{15}O] studies which contributed to the different blood flow values obtained with the two isotopes. To establish either one of these two tracers in clinical studies, and [^{82}Rb] is the more likely candidate, it will be important to standardize and validate the procedures of imaging and image analysis.

With [^{15}O]-water the integral of the input function calibrated with the corresponding blood flow showed slightly higher values than the organ time activity curve during the up-sloping phase (Fig. 14.2.3C) and increasing deviation from the organ curve at the peak activity and later time points, which is consistent with the washout of this radiopharmaceutical from the kidneys. On the other hand, with [^{82}Rb], the correspondence between the measured organ time activity curve and the integral of the input function calibrated for blood flow was nearly perfect (Fig. 14.2.3D). This implies that [^{82}Rb] can be used to image and quantify blood flow over a longer time interval with high precision, which will result in good quality images. This may not apply to the accuracy of the measurement since the accumulation of [^{82}Rb] also depends on the parenchymal extraction of the tracer, which may be lower than the extraction of [^{15}O]-water and show a nonlinear regression with organ blood flow. This limitation of [^{82}Rb] was demonstrated by the finding that [^{82}Rb] overestimated the stenotic/nonstenotic kidney blood flow ratios compared to [^{15}O]-water.

For [^{82}Rb] only washin K_1 but no washout k_2 was included in the model. The close fit between the integrated input function and the organ time activity curve confirms the correctness of the assumption on the behavior of [^{82}Rb] as a (nearly perfect) chemical microsphere. The close curve fit confirms the lack of washout but, unfortunately, it does not provide an estimate of the extraction fraction of [^{82}Rb]. The extraction of [^{82}Rb] in the kidneys has been estimated to be over 80% (30).

The zero washout rate (i.e., $k_2 = 0$) of [^{82}Rb] permits the use of a continuous tracer infusion technique and the tissue:blood [^{82}Rb] ratio to assess renal blood flow. The infusion method requires only one blood sample for calibration and is particularly suited for serial measurements of renal blood flow in one experimental setup (31).

Copper-PTSM

Copper(II)-pyruvaldehyde bis (n-4-methylthiosemicarbazone) (Cu-PTSM) also behaves like a chemical microsphere. Its high tissue extraction is explained by the lipid solubility of the copper complex. Washout is slow due to a reductive decomposition of the copper chelate by intracellular sulfhydryl groups (32). PTSM can be labeled with either [^{64}Cu], which is a cyclotron product with a half-life of 12.7 hours, or with [^{62}Cu], a generator product with a half-life of 9.8 minutes. Both copper isotopes are positron emitters. In dogs, renal cortical blood flow determined with Cu-PTSM is 300 to 550 mL/min/100 g (33) and correlates well with renal blood flow determinations with radioactive microspheres (33,34).

Nitrogen-13-Ammonia

Nitrogen-13-ammonia is the third tracer suitable for imaging renal blood flow due to its microspherelike behavior. The renal blood flow determined with this tracer in dogs is 400 mL/min/100 g, which correlates well with renal blood flow obtained with [^{15}O]-water (35). The mechanism of uptake in the kidneys is unknown, but it may be similar to the uptake in the myocardium where the glutamic acid–glutamine pathway has been postulated as the predominant means of tissue extraction. This reaction requires adenosine 5′-triphosphate (ATP) and is mediated by the enzyme glutamine synthetase (36), thus, the uptake of [^{13}N]-ammonia, like the uptake of the potassium analogue [^{82}Rb], depends not only on organ perfusion but also on tissue viability. In pigs, reduced renal blood flow has been documented using [^{13}N]-ammonia in warm ischemia, allograft rejection, and cyclosporine nephrotoxicity (37).

Tracers for Glomerular Filtration

Radiolabeled ethylenediaminetetraacetic acid (EDTA) behaves biologically like technetium-99m (^{99m}Tc) diethylenetriamine pentaacetic acid (DTPA). It is excreted by the kidneys via glomerular filtration. For PET either cobalt-55 ([^{55}Co]) (38) or gallium-68 ([^{68}Ga]) (39) can be used for labeling. Cobalt-55 is obtained in a cyclotron and has a half-life of 17.5 hours and a maximal positron energy of 1.5 MeV. Gallium-68 is obtained from a generator (40), has a half-life of 68.3 minutes, and a maximal positron energy of 1.9 MeV.

The renal kinetics of radiolabeled EDTA can be best characterized with the stochastic impulse response function previously described for ^{99m}Tc DTPA (13,41), which has a vascular and a parenchymal component. The vascular peak value is followed by 20% extraction and transfer of tracer into primary urine within the capsule of Bowman and from there into the tubular lumen. Since the length of the tubules is variable the fate of the tracer is best described by a random pathway distribution model quantitatively characterized by the minimal and mean transit times T_0 and $\overline{T}$ (Fig. 14.2.1C).

Altered tubular transport is a sensitive indicator of altered renal function in renovascular hypertension, obstructive nephropathy, transplant rejection, and other diseases of the kidneys. Planar renal imaging studies with a gamma camera result in a significant overlap of activity from renal parenchyma, collecting system, and adjacent organs such as the liver and spleen. Decomposition of the individual constituents of this curve is achieved by factor analysis (42) or other sophisticated pattern recognition techniques such as neural network analysis (43). One important advantage of PET is an effective separation of these activity components by tomographic imaging. Even so, the tracer may accumulate in the collecting system at high concentrations that could result in image artifacts and may require implementation of iterative image reconstruction algorithms that are less sensitive to effects of high concentration gradients within the field of view.

Radioligands

Small labeled drugs (radiopharmaceuticals) that undergo molecular interactions with larger molecules such as enzymes, transporters, receptors, and other specific tissue binding sites are called radioligands. In inorganic chemistry, ligands are molecules that can share electrons through a covalent bond with another molecule. In organic chemistry, ligands are molecules that can bind to a specific recognition site of a protein. Natural ligands are hormones and neurotransmitters with agonistic effects on their targets. Their interaction with the target permits intercellular communication and initiation of intracellular signal transduction cascades. The role of these intracellular signal transduction cascades is to amplify or, in general, modulate the incoming signal.

Radioligands developed for PET imaging of receptors are usually specific and selective antagonists labeled with [^{11}C] or [^{18}F]. After intravenous injection, these radioligands form specific bonds with the target receptor, transporter, enzyme, or signal transduction protein. Whether an agonist or antagonist is used, it is important that the radioligand be injected in subpharmacological doses to avoid biological effects. This is achieved by injection of radiopharmaceuticals in low drug mass (e.g., at high specific activity). In addition to high specific activity, high ligand affinity will result in high specific-to-total or specific-to-nonspecific binding ratios.

Compartmental impulse response functions have been widely applied to describe the kinetics of radioligands. Each compartment is mathematically defined by a separate monoexponential impulse response function $f(t) = K_{in}e^{-k_{out}(t)}$. If the tracer is distributed in multiple compartments, the resulting impulse response function will be composed of a sum of multiple exponential functions, and the number of the exponentials will equal the number of compartments. This number has been referred to as the model order. For example, if one compartment is present for nonspecific binding and one compartment for specific binding, the model order is 2.

Tracer kinetic models of radioligands used for imaging receptors of the neurons within the brain assume a sequential connection of two compartments. The nonspecific binding compartment is directly related to the uptake of radioligand through the blood–brain barrier K_1. Receptor binding follows at a second step, and, therefore, the two impulse response functions are convolutive in the time space or multiplicative in Laplacian and Fourier spaces. Due to absence of the blood–brain barrier and contemporaneous exposure of the radioligand to both binding sites, a parallel connectivity model is more appropriate for description of radioligand kinetics in the kidneys and organs other than the brain. For these organs the tissue impulse response function can be described as a sum of the two individual exponential functions without a need for convolution. If K_1 and k_2 are the parameters of nonspecific binding and K_3 and k_4 are the parameters of specific binding, it is desirable to have a $K_3 > K_1$. In serial connectivity models it is desirable to have $k_3 > k_2$. The use of a capital K_3 indicates that it describes direct transfer from blood to tissue, while small k_3 indicates exchange between intraparenchymal compartments. If the criterion $K_3 > K_1$ cannot be achieved, one has to wait until nonspecific binding is washed out, and in this case the second criterion to be fulfilled is $k_4 < k_2$. Typically, specific binding has a low capacity and a high affinity (i.e., K_3 is $< k_1$ but k_4 is also $< k_2$). With the parallel connectivity model, the ratios K_1/k_2 and K_3/k_4 describe the distribution volumes of nonspecific and specific binding DV_n and DV_{sp} and their sum $DV_n + DV_{sp}$ represents the total tissue distribution volume of the radioligand. If the ligand has a large distribution volume with a small k_4, better images are achieved if it is labeled with [^{18}F] than if labeled with [^{11}C], which has a much shorter half-life. In terms of pharmacokinetics and molecular interactions, a better term of specific binding is displaceable binding because the radioligand can be displaced from its binding site with a pharmacological dose of a competitive drug.

Since the distribution volume can only be calculated reliably if k_2 and k_4 have nonzero values, the concept of distribution volume is only applicable to radioligands with reversible binding. For freely diffusible tracers such as [^{15}O]-water, reversibility is attained by backflow into the circulation, while reversibility is attained by excretion into the urine for tracers that undergo glomerular filtration, such as [^{55}Co]-labeled EDTA. For radioligands designed for renal receptor imaging it is desirable to have significant specific receptor binding, slow backflow into circulation, and no or negligible urinary excretion.

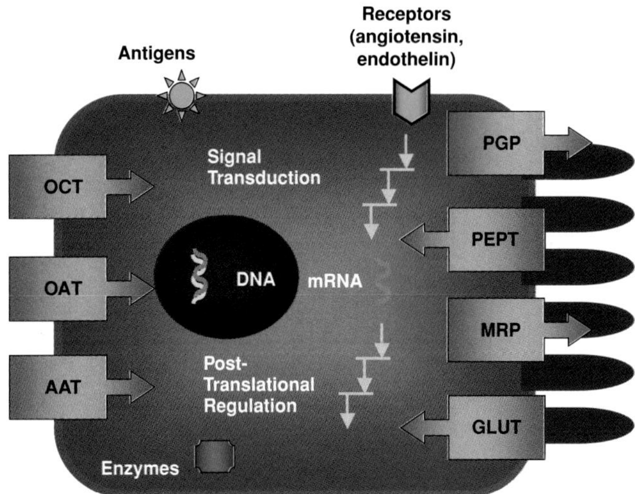

FIGURE 14.2.4. Schematic representation of renal molecular imaging targets in a tubular epithelial cell. The smooth wall on the left side of the cell represents the basolateral membrane. The undulated wall on the right side of the cell represents the luminal brush border. Membrane targets include antigens, receptors, and transporters. The most important membrane transporters are the glucose transporter (GLUT), organic anion transporter (OAT), organic cation transporter (OCT), amino acid transporter (AAT), peptide transporter (PEPT), pg protein (PGP), and multidrug resistance protein (MRP). Intracellular targets are proteins of signal transduction, reporter genes, DNA, mRNA, and components of the posttranslational regulatory cascade.

MOLECULAR IMAGING

The goal of the emerging field of molecular imaging is to develop tools that can be utilized as disease biomarkers. The images and parameters derived from them should permit disease diagnosis and severity assessment and serve as surrogate end points of therapy response. Important general steps for development of PET-based molecular imaging methods include identification of the target molecules or pathophysiological processes of particular clinical interest and subsequently the design, synthesis, preclinical, and clinical validation of the new radioligands. During this process one has to bear in mind the natural variance of the quantified biomarker, the technical variance of measurement, and the variance of the biomarker caused by disease and treatment. In terms of variance analysis, the one caused by disease and treatment should surpass the other to a degree that will permit not only dichotomous decisions required during diagnosis but also gradual assessments required during therapy follow-up.

Molecular imaging targets of interest in the kidneys can be membrane proteins (receptors, antigens, and transporters), intracellular proteins (enzymes and proteins of signal transduction), natural or imported (reporter) genes, or the mRNA (Fig. 14.2.4). Based on their kinetic behavior, specific and selective radioligands can be developed with various degrees of affinity, which usually translates to the degree of reversibility of binding. Radioligands with tight binding permit imaging at delayed time points when nonspecific binding decreases and are preferably labeled with [^{18}F], which makes them eligible for clinical applications. Radioligands with rapid dissociation can also be radiolabeled with a short-lived isotope such as [^{11}C], but their applicability is limited to research studies due to the need of radiochemical synthesis near the imaging site.

Transporters

Substrate transport is an essential task performed by the tubular epithelium. Membrane transport in itself is an essential function of the organ responsible for recycling of water, electrolytes, and nutrients filtered in the glomeruli and excretion of hydrophilic drugs, toxins, and endogenous metabolic products. Membrane transport processes may also play a supportive role in membrane repolarization and tissue signaling. The most important transport pathways include blood-to-cell, cell-to-blood, cell-to-lumen, and lumen-to-cell transport.

Transporters involved in the elimination of xenobiotics are the multidrug resistance transporters, the organic anion and organic cation transporters, and the peptide transporters. P-glycoprotein (multidrug resistance protein 1, MRP1) is expressed in the brush border membranes of proximal tubules where it is involved in the removal of hydrophobic xenobiotics such as digoxin, steroids, and anthracyclines. Multidrug resistance proteins MRP2 to MRP5 belong to the ATP binding cassette transporter family and localize to the apical membrane. Organic anion and cation transporters primarily localize to the basolateral membrane of renal epithelial cells. Along with drug-metabolizing enzymes, these transporters of the kidneys are important determinants of drug effectiveness and toxicity (44). Fig. 14.2.4 shows the schematic representation of the proximal tubular cell with its membrane transporters and other potential molecular imaging targets.

Renal sodium transporters are responsible for some forms of sodium sensitive hypertension, including Gordon and Liddle syndromes and certain forms of hypertension of pregnancy (45). The sodium-hydrogen exchanger (NHE) is involved in several steps of recovery of kidney function after grafting, including tubular epithelium repair and proliferation (46). Other important transporters in the kidney are the nucleoside transporters and water channels (45,47). Despite their functional significance, the role of these transporters in disease is not well known, and none of them have been explored for molecular imaging of the kidneys.

Uptake of organic anions across the basolateral membrane is mediated by the classic sodium-dependent organic anion transport (OAT) system. The apical (brush-border) membrane (BBM) also contains various transport systems for efflux of organic anions into the lumen or reabsorption from the lumen into the cell. Well-known substrates of organic anion transporters in nuclear medicine are iodine-123 ([^{123}I])-ortho-iodo-hippuric acid (OIH) and ^{99m}Tc-mercaptoacetyltriglycine (MAG3). Sun et al. (48) developed 3-monooxo-tetraazamacrocyclic ligands radiolabeled with [^{64}Cu], which have demonstrated excellent accumulation in the renal cortex caused by their binding to the OAT.

In uremia organic anions accumulate in plasma and compete with the excretion of OIH and MAG3. This can result in underestimation of the measured renal clearance values. To minimize this effect, diaminocyclohexane (DACH) has been labeled with ^{99m}Tc as a tracer of the organic cation transporters OCT (49,50). The organic cation transporter systems are responsible for the renal reabsorption or excretion of bioactive cations, including monoamines (dopamine, epinephrine, histamine), cationic toxins, and cationic drugs such as cimetidine and procainamide (51). Cellular uptake of organic cations across the basolateral membrane is mediated by organic cation transporters OCT1, OCT2, and OCT3, while exit of cellular organic cations across the brush border membrane is mediated by P-glycoprotein. PEPT1 and PEPT2 mediate the luminal uptake (in the intestines) or reuptake (in the kidneys) of peptide and peptide-like drugs.

The proton peptide symporters PepT1 and PepT2 are strongly expressed in both the renal cortex and renal medulla and are involved in protein, peptide, and amino acid homeostasis. Peptidelike drugs including angiotensin-converting enzyme (ACE) inhibitors, renin inhibitors, and β-lactam antibiotics are important substrates of these transporters. Peptidelike residues can be linked to other drugs to facilitate their absorption in the intestines or reabsorption in the kidneys. Attachment of a drug to a peptide to improve its absorption in the intestines or reapsorbtion in the kidneys is called peptide transporter associated prodrug therapy. This is just one form of prodrug design. Prodrugs are designed to be readily transported to the site of action, to be selectively cleaved to the active drug at the site, and to stick to their target for a considerable time. The proton peptide transporters are regulated by epidermal growth factor (EGF), insulin, and leptin and are affected by fasting and starvation (52). Development of radioligands for investigation of these transporters would be important both for studying tubular reabsorption and clearance of peptide like drugs (53) as well as for investigation of the kinetics of peptide prodrugs (54). Prodrug-capable peptides that have been radiolabeled for PET imaging of PepT2 include [^{11}C]-glycylsarcosine (Gly-Sar) and its derivative, [^{11}C]-cyclo-(glycylsarcosine) [1-methylpiperazine-2,5-dione]. Carbon-11-glycylsarcosine demonstrates slow clearance from the medulla, while [^{11}C]-cyclo(glycylsarcosine) is rapidly cleared by the kidneys. Salvage of amino acids that would be lost by glomerular filtration occurs by reabsorption in the proximal tubules and is managed by amino acid transporters.

Many amino acid analogues have been radiolabeled that could be employed for investigation of renal amino acid transporters. They include natural amino acids [^{11}C]-methionine or [^{11}C]-tyrosine as well as artificial amino acids such as [^{123}I]-Iodo-L-α-methyltyrosine (IMT), L-3-[^{18}F]-α-methyltyrosine (FMT), O-2-[^{18}F]-ethyl-L-tyrosine (FET), [^{18}F]-L-phenylalanine, [^{18}F]-1-amino- 3-fluorocyclobutane-1-carboxylic acid, [^{18}F]-L-proline, and [^{11}C-methyl]- α-aminoisobutyric acid (55).

There are two major glucose transporter families: the GLUT family is responsible for facilitated transport of glucose and the sodium dependent glucose transporter (SGLT) family for active transport against concentration gradients. [^{11}C]-Methyl-D-glucose has been developed to measure facilitated glucose transport because it enters the intracellular free glucose pool without being utilized for metabolism (56). Fluorine-18-FDG is a substrate of both the GLUT and the hexokinase enzyme but not of the SGLT (57). Its intratubular accumulation is in part responsible for poor delineation of renal cell carcinomas with FDG PET imaging. Glucose transporters that are expressed in the kidneys include the GLUT1, GLUT3, and GLUT4 isoforms. The transport of FDG by GLUT follows Michaelis Menten kinetics: It is saturable in the kidneys and most other organs and is therefore affected in diabetes. Both angiotensin II and EGF are involved in the regulation of GLUT1 expression (58).

The SGLT is an ATP-dependent saturable transporter (59). Glucose transporters have been implicated in the development of nephropathy of non-insulin dependent diabetes mellitus (60–62) and in progressive glomerular injury of glomerular hypertension (63). Plasma glucose filtered in the glomeruli is reabsorbed in the proximal tubules by an SGLT, which has at least three isoforms: SGLT1, SGLT2, and SGLT3 (64). SGLT transporters are expressed in the intestines, kidneys, and the brain. Inhibitors of the SGLT have been developed as antidiabetic drugs. For example, derivatives of phlorizin inhibit glucose uptake in the small intestine and enhance glucose excretion in the kidneys by blocking the reuptake SGLT (65). Methyl-D-glucoside has been recently radiolabeled with [^{11}C] by methylation of glucose as a glucose analogue that is a substrate of SGLT but not of GLUT. β-methyl-D-glucoside accumulates in the kidneys to a greater extent than its α-anomer.

[^{11}C]-methyl-α-D-glucoside is mainly accumulated in the renal cortex that contains S1 and S2 segments of renal proximal tubules. No accumulation of [^{11}C]-methyl-α-D-glucoside has been observed in the outer stripe of the outer medulla because most [^{11}C]-methyl-α-D-glucoside is cleared from the glomerular filtrate in the S1 and S2 segments. Another glucoside, 2′-[^{18}F]-ethyl-β-D-glucoside accumulates in the outer part of the outer medulla, a kidney region that contains the S3 segments of renal proximal tubules where SGLT1 is found. The data suggest that the activity of SGLT1 in humans can be visualized by 2′-[^{18}F]-ethyl-β-D-glucoside, whereas the activity of both SGLT1 and SGLT2 can be visualized by [^{11}C]-methyl-α-D-glucoside (66).

Metabolism

Carbon-11 acetic acid is a general metabolism probe that enters the Krebs cycle after its linkage to coenzyme A. Its final metabolic product [^{11}C]-carbon dioxide is released by exhalation (67). Excellent image quality can be obtained for the kidneys, and the uptake of [^{11}C]-acetate is significantly reduced in renal artery stenosis and other diseases of the kidneys. The impulse response function of this tracer is very simple and only depends on the uptake constant K_1 and the washout constant k_2 (Fig. 14.2.1A). The k_2 of [^{11}C]-acetate is ten times smaller than its K_1 and also much smaller than the k_2 of [^{15}O]-water because of the involvement of the tracer in metabolic processes in addition to its diffusion in and out of tissue. Due to its limited extraction fraction of only 20% to 25% (68), the K_1 of [^{11}C]-acetate, however, is also lower than the K_1 of [^{15}O]-water (i.e., while the uptake of [^{15}O]-water is flow limited, the uptake of acetate, like [^{18}F]-FDG is extraction limited).

The regression of k_2 on K_1 of [^{11}C]-acetate is logarithmic in normal kidneys and diseases such as renal artery stenosis, diabetic nephropathy, hypertensive nephropathy, and membranous glomerulonephritis. On the other hand, the k_2 value is very low and uncoupled from K_1 in renal cell carcinomas, which results in a high tumor to background ratios (68). Carbon-11-acetate has also been used in prostate cancer. Due to its lack of urinary excretion it demonstrated a better tumor-to-nontumor contrast than [^{18}F]-FDG (69) but similar to that of [^{11}C]-choline PET (70).

Enzymes

Farnesyl transferase inhibitors (FTIs) have been proposed as chemotherapeutic agents since they have the potential effect to deactivate the Ras protein (71). FTIs have also been proposed for treatment of proliferative glomerular diseases (72). The FTI (S)-1-(3-fluoromethyl-5-iodophenyl)-4-[1-(4-cyanobenzyl)-5-imidazoyl]-5-[([^{11}C]-methanesulfonyl)-ethyl]-2-piperazinone has been radiolabeled with [^{11}C] for imaging the kidneys (73). It yielded excellent image quality and high specific binding.

The angiotensin converting enzyme of the lungs and kidneys has been imaged in humans with [^{18}F]-captopril (74). Zofenopril is the other ACE inhibitor that has been labeled with [^{11}C] for PET imaging. [^{11}C]-zofenopril also accumulates in the lungs and kidneys, organs that express the ACE (75). Imaging of the ACE may play a role in investigations of the kidneys in renovascular disease and other types of arterial hypertension.

Receptors

There are many membrane receptors involved in the regulation of renal function, but the one that has been examined most extensively in the past few decades is the angiotensin receptor. A literature search with PubMed returned 11,576 citations. Despite its enormous significance, the number of *in vivo* imaging studies is quite limited with less than ten publications reporting the use of single photon or positron tracers.

Angiotensin II elicits its biological actions by binding to specific receptors that activate multiple intracellular transduction pathways (76). Physiological and pharmacological research studies resulted in identification of two major receptor subtypes, AT1R and AT2R. The receptor is expressed in vascular smooth muscle, liver, lung, kidney, and the adrenal and pituitary glands. Only one AT1R subtype is known in humans, and its gene is located on chromosome 3; two subtypes (AT1a and AT1b) have been identified in rodents. The receptor subtype AT2R appears to play a stronger role during fetal development, and its role in the adult organism is less understood. It appears to be involved in the regulation of arterial blood pressure with an antagonistic effect to the stimulation of the AT1R.

In the kidneys, the density of the AT1R is highest in the glomeruli; the receptor is also expressed in the inner stripe of the outer medulla in a more diffuse manner (77). In the adrenal glands AT1R predominates in the zona glomerulosa where >90% of the angiotensin receptors are of the AT1R and <10% are of the AT2R subtype.

AT1R mediates most of the physiological effects of angiotensin II, including renal blood flow, glomerular filtration, sodium and water reabsorption, myocardial contractility, and aldosterone secretion. Expression of the receptor, on the other hand, is affected by many factors, including angiotensin II itself, dietary sodium, testosterone, estrogen, stress, thyroid hormones, and renal hypoperfusion.

PET has been used successfully for studying the regulation of the AT1R in animals *in vivo* (17,78). Important insights into the regulation of the AT1R and its role in sodium sensitive hypertension are also expected to be gained when radioligands for human PET studies become available.

The role of the AT1R in the pathogenesis of arterial hypertension is complex and includes mechanisms that can be schematically divided into acute (vasoconstriction), subacute (sodium retention), and chronic (vascular remodeling). Clear timely separation of these three mechanisms is not possible, and most likely they take place simultaneously in a concerted fashion.

Atrial natriuretic peptide, prostaglandins, and nitric oxide enhance sodium secretion in addition to their vasodilating effects. Angiotensin II and other vasoconstrictors such as norepinephrine and aldosterone, on the other hand, enhance sodium retention. Thus, activation of AT1R by angiotensin II will increase arterial blood pressure both by increasing peripheral as well as renal vascular resistance and by promoting sodium and, consequently, water retention. Chronic stimulation of the AT1R, on the other hand, will mediate inflammatory changes and remodeling of renal blood vessels (glomerulosclerosis) and peripheral blood vessels (deposition of atheromatous plaques) with subsequent further reduction of vessel compliance.

The AT1R is a G protein coupled receptor and its activation by angiotensin II results in its cellular internalization and degradation, an important mechanism needed to reduce the risk of receptor overstimulation under physiological conditions. In disease states, on the other hand, angiotensin II may up-regulate its own receptor (79), although arterial hypertension may also result from an increased responsiveness of the AT1R (80). Overall, more studies are required to understand the status of this important receptor *in vivo*.

At first, the AT1R will most likely be studied in the kidneys with PET, an organ that can be considered as both the victim and the villain of hypertension. In progressive renal diseases, local production of angiotensin II is increased in tubules, glomeruli, as well as interstitial tissues and mediates the pathobiology of renal injury. Overstimulation of the AT1R by intrarenal angiotensin II resets the tubuloglomerular feedback mechanism to higher blood pressure levels, increases the functional expression of the sodium proton pumps in the proximal tubules, and ultimately induces arterial hypertension even in the absence of systemic renin angiotension system (RAS) activation.

Increased activity of the AT1R could result from multiple mechanisms: (a) increased total number of receptors, (b) increased number of physiologically active receptors, (c) inappropriate up-regulation of receptors in response to sodium intake, stress, or altered hormone levels, or (d) increased concentration of circulating renin and angiotensin II. These multiple possibilities of receptor dysregulation prompt one to design three types of PET studies: (a) solitary measurements to assess the status of the AT1R in health and disease, (b) same-day repeat measurements with short-term pharmacological or physiological interventions that can change the occupancy and availability of the receptor, and (c) long-term, longitudinal studies based on perturbations that will result in receptor up- or down-regulation. All three types of experiments have been performed in experimental animals (17,78,81).

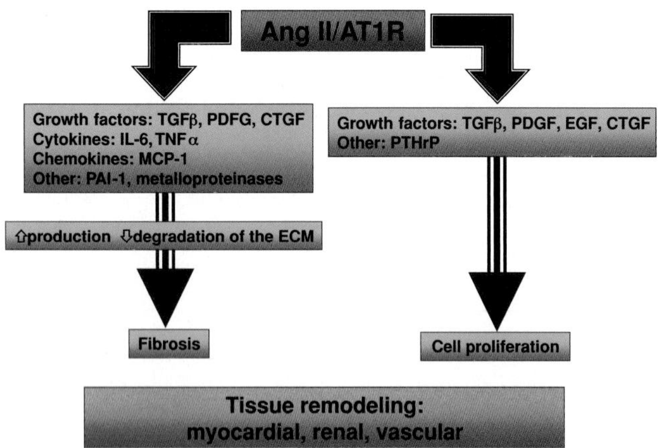

FIGURE 14.2.5. Role of angiotensin II (Ang II) in tissue remodeling. Ang II via its AT1R subtype activates growth factors, cytokines, chemokines, and other mediators of fibrosis and cell proliferation that may help preserve the anatomical integrity but not functional integrity of the organ. TGFβ, tumor growth factor β; PDFG, platelet derived growth factor; CTGF, connective tissue growth factor; EGF, epidermal growth factor; IL-6, interleukin 6; TNFα, tumor necrosis factor α; PTHrP, parathyroid hormone related protein; MCP-1, monocyte chemoattractant protein type 1; PAI-1, plasminogen activator inhibitor type 1; ECM, extracellular matrix.

The AT1R is involved in remodeling processes of the myocardium, kidneys, and blood vessels, and these changes contribute to the development of hypertension and its complications (Fig. 14.2.5). The molecular cascade involves activation of growth factors by angiotensin II and the release of cytokines, chemokines, and metalloproteinases, which ultimately results in increased production and decreased degradation of the extracellular matrix and enhanced cellular proliferation (82). Both arterial hypertension and tissue remodeling can be alleviated with angiotensin receptor blockers (ARBs), drugs that are excellent candidates for the development of radioligands for PET applications.

The first radioligand used for imaging the angiotensin receptors was a derivative of the natural agonist [^{123}I]-Sar1,Ile8-angiotensin II (83). Its use for kidney imaging was hampered by its hepatobiliary excretion. The next generation of radioligands was based on ARBs, small molecules with high affinity and selectivity for the AT1R. The first successful [^{11}C]-labeled ARB was the benzoylsulfonamide-[^{11}C]-MK-996 (also called L-159,282) (84). It was followed by [^{11}C]-L-159,884 (85), a radioligand (Fig. 14.2.6A), which has mostly been used in rodents and dogs (17,86–87). (The International Union of Pure and Applied Chemistry [IUPAC] name for MK-996 is N-[[4′-[(2-ethyl-5,7-dimethyl-3H-imidazo[4,5-b]pyridin-3-yl)methyl][1,1′-biphenyl]-2-yl]sulfonyl]-benzamide. The IUPAC name for L-159,884 is N-[[4′-[(2-ethyl-5,7-dimethyl-3H-imidazo[4,5-b]pyridin-3-yl)methyl][1,1'-biphenyl]-2-yl]sulfonyl]-4-methoxybenzamide.)

Insurmountable ARBs such as candesartan, valsartan, and irbesartan reduce the maximal response to angiotensin II at any pharmacologically active level. Surmountable ARBs such as losartan, eprosartan, and telmisartan cause a rightward shift in the angiotensin II dose-response curve, but they do not reduce the effect when a maximal dose is given. Surmountable antagonists dissociate more rapidly from the receptor than insurmountable antagonists (88). Thus, surmountable antagonists are more practical for rapid organ imaging using the distribution volume for quantitative analysis, while insurmountable antagonists are more practical for slow dynamic or static studies.

Since [^{11}C]-L-159,884 has not shown specific receptor binding in human volunteers, a new radioligand, [^{11}C]-KR31173, was developed (Fig. 14.2.6B). Carbon-11-KR31173 has demonstrated high organ uptake and high specific binding in the kidneys of mice, dogs, and baboons (89,90) (Fig. 14.2.7).

Since the *in vivo* dissociation of [^{11}C]-L-159,884 from the AT1R is very slow, consistent with an insurmountable ligand, time activity curves derived from the renal cortex have been analyzed by the Gjedde-Patlak plot to obtain the influx rate constant K_i of the radioligand (87). The binding of [^{11}C]-KR31173, on the other hand, is more consistent with a surmountable ligand and can be analyzed by the Logan plot, and its binding is quantified by the tissue distribution volume (*DV*) (90).

In addition to pharmacological studies of specific binding, more subtle changes of AT1R binding can also be observed with PET imaging. For example, experiments in dogs showed that increasing dietary sodium increases AT1R binding *in vivo* (17). Conversely, decreasing dietary sodium decreases AT1R binding *in vivo*. These findings have physiological significance regarding regulation of blood pressure. The *in vivo* results have been confirmed by *in vitro* assays including autoradiography, ligand binding, and reverse transcriptase-polymerase chain reaction. A very important finding of the *in vivo* experiments is the negative feedback between angiotensin II and AT1R: when AT1R levels increase, angiotensin II (and plasma renin activity) levels decrease and *vice versa*. This negative physiological feedback has an important role in preventing abnormal receptor responses either in the direction of hypertension or hypotension (17). These studies were performed in dogs, but the

[^{11}C]-L-159,884

[^{11}C]-KR31173

FIGURE 14.2.6. Two carbon-11 ([^{11}C])-labeled radioligands developed for imaging the renal AT1R—[^{11}C]-L-159,884 and [^{11}C]-KR31173.

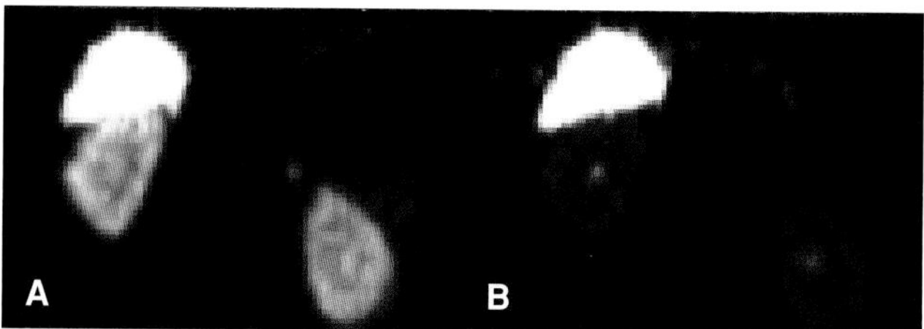

FIGURE 14.2.7. Accumulation of carbon-11 ([^{11}C])-KR31173 in the baboon kidney 35 to 95 minutes posttracer injection at baseline (**A**) and after blocking specific binding with 1 mg/kg SK-1080 intravenous (**B**). There is significant specific binding and minimal nonspecific binding. Urinary excretion is also minimal. Intense tracer uptake in the liver is also noted.

protocols can easily be transferred to humans. Animal studies also demonstrate concordance between expression of the receptor and its messenger RNA (AT1R mRNA). A smaller magnitude of change was observed for the mRNA, indicating the existence of posttranscriptional amplification mechanisms. Independent of the regulatory level, *in vivo* binding may be the best measure of receptor expression and have the closest relationship to its functional consequences.

In another study, the effects of estrogen on the AT1R were investigated. These studies were also performed in dogs and demonstrated that estrogen deficiency increased AT1R levels while estrogen replacement decreased AT1R levels, an important observation that can help elucidate the increased vulnerability to cardiovascular diseases in the menopause (78). These hormonal *in vivo* experiments confirmed the presence of a negative feedback between angiotensin II and AT1R and reinforced the role of PET in simultaneous investigation of the dynamic hormone interplay of multiple components of the RAS *in vivo*. The dog kidney was chosen because it represents a biologically more relevant model than the rodent kidney. The molecular mechanisms governing AT1R regulation of rodent renal hemodynamics are distinct from humans because two AT1R sub types (AT1aR, AT1bR) mediate fluid homeostasis in rodents compared to only one in all other mammalian species.

In the rat, reciprocal mechanisms of glomerular and tubular epithelial receptor regulation exist, which is attributed to the differential regulation of AT1aR and AT1bR. In the canine renal cortex, the majority of AT1R is found in the glomeruli. Thus, PET images of the dog kidney predominantly reflect changes in glomerular AT1R.

Ischemia and Remodeling

One potential application of AT1R imaging would be the diagnosis of renovascular hypertension since animal studies indicate upregulation of the receptor in the affected kidney (91). In renovascular hypertension plasma renin activity and circulating angiotensin II are initially increased (92,93) and may return to normal levels in the chronic phase. Angiotensin II regionally synthesized in the kidney may uncouple from circulating levels of the hormone and contribute to the pathogenesis of hypertension (94). PET imaging would permit investigation of the hypothesis that expression of the AT1R in chronic renal artery stenosis is a cardinal pathogenetic factor of arterial hypertension and intrarenal hemodynamic changes.

Percutaneous revascularization represents an important therapeutic approach to ischemic renal disease. Selection of patients for this partially invasive procedure is difficult, and the prediction of response is limited. Captopril renography has been used, but its accuracy is limited in cases of reduced renal function and bilateral disease (95). An important consequence of renal ischemia and chronic renal disease is tissue remodeling. In embryos and young individuals, injuries are easily repaired and lost tissue can largely be replaced by functional tissue of the same kind. In the adult organism, injuries frequently result in proliferation of an altered tissue, which may provide anatomical compensation but no functional compensation of organ integrity. Fibrosis and tissue sclerosis are components of the remodeling processes in the kidneys, myocardium, and blood vessels. Transforming growth factor-β (TGFβ) is the chief inductor of fibroblasts that synthesize and contract the extracellular matrix. In the kidneys there is a close relationship between interstitial fibrosis on one hand and glomerulosclerosis and tubular atrophy on the other. Increased excretion of proteins or glucose, as happens in diabetic kidneys, is a tubular stimulant that induces the expression of chemokines, which stimulates inflammatory cell infiltration of the interstitium. Apoptosis of tubular epithelial cells in the kidneys is also a hallmark of progressive renal disease that contributes to the release of mediators of inflammation and fibrosis. Thus, progressive renal disease affects multiple tissue components and a cascade of multiple deleterious signaling proteins (96).

Fibroblasts can be recruited from residual embryonal mesenchymal stem cells of renal and extrarenal (bone marrow) origin. Both tubular recovery after ischemic tubular necrosis and regression of diabetic glomerulosclerosis and tubulointerstitial fibrosis have been observed, and the kidneys do have regenerative capacity if the causes of tissue stress are removed before the stage of disease is too advanced. The goal of renal protection is promotion of specific tissue regeneration and inhibition of adverse remodeling. Downstream mediators of TGFβ have been targeted to explore antifibrotic effects (96) since TGFβ is the key mediator of glomerular and tubulointerstitial pathobiology of chronic kidney disease (97). The angiotensin signaling mechanism is strongly involved in renal remodeling, and it has been shown that aggressive treatment with a combination of ARB, angiotensin converting enzyme inhibitor, and aldosterone receptor antagonists can reverse the remodeling process.

Extracellular matrix molecules, matrix-regulating cytokines, and metalloproteinases determined in renal kidney biopsies are powerful indicators of renal tissue injury. Since the AT1R is directly involved and often the chief culprit in these processes (Fig. 14.2.5), quantification of the AT1R *in vivo* can contribute to understanding its role in chronic renal injury, including chronic rejection, which also has a strong inflammatory component. FDG has been used for diagnostic localization of a renal abscess (98), but as of now, no radioligands have been developed for imaging renal inflammation and remodeling.

Specific probes developed for quantitative imaging of the components of the extracellular matrix may be helpful to reduce the number of needed biopsies. Extracellular matrix turnover has been studied with [^{18}F]-proline (99), and specific labels of the matrix metalloproteinases are being developed for PET (100–102). Radiolabeled arginine-glycine-aspartate tripeptides are also being radiolabeled for imaging integrin $\alpha_v\beta_3$, which is an important receptor for the extracellular matrix proteins (103).

The density of AT1R in the myocardium is approximately 50 times less than in the kidneys, although it can be significantly upregulated with myocardial muscle loss and fibroblast proliferation (104). Myocardial infarction leads to impairment in the contractile behavior of the remaining cells and to the activation of AT1R and its effector pathways (105). Remodeling and dysfunction correlate with increased expression of cardiac AT1R mRNA in rats with left ventricle myocardial infarction (106).

The AT1R is also an important mediator of atherosclerosis and a potential candidate for vulnerable atherosclerotic plaque imaging. Components of the RAS, including AT1R, are expressed at strategically relevant sites of human coronary atherosclerotic plaques and contribute to inflammatory processes within the atherosclerotic vascular wall (107).

Nephrotoxic drugs such as amphotericin B, cyclosporine, contrast materials, and cisplatin lead to oxidative stress, perturbations of calcium homeostasis, and activation of stress response proteins, including protein kinases and protein phosphatases (108–111). In the kidneys, as in other tissues, the family of mitogen-activated protein kinases promotes apoptosis, while extracellular signal regulated kinases and protein kinase B facilitate cell survival (112). Stress response signaling pathways and apoptosis have been the focus of imaging research. Radioligands for PET imaging of apoptosis are already being tested (113,114) for applications outside the kidneys. Development of specific ligands for cellular stress proteins could lead to sensitive methods for molecular imaging of renal injury, which could detect and quantify nephrotoxicity in its earliest stages.

Gene therapy continues to be a promising experimental method for treatment of renal diseases that will allow selective targeting of essential molecules with minimal side effects within and outside the kidneys. For example, chronic transplant rejection that is resistant to various types of treatment would benefit from this type of therapy. For *in vivo* transfection, five routes of administration have been investigated: (a) injection through the renal artery, (b) injection through the renal vein, (c) direct intraparenchymal injection, (d) subcapsular injection, and (d) ureteral delivery. Plasmids, liposomes, parainfluenza viruses, adenoviruses, retroviruses, lentivirus, genetically modified monocytes, and mesangial cells have been used as delivery vectors (115). Gene delivery has been enhanced by electroporation, ultrasound-mediated microbubble disruption (116), and laser technology (117).

Hereditary diseases of the kidneys that could benefit from gene therapy include Alport syndrome, which is based on a defective type IV collagen framework of the glomerular basement membrane. Glomerulonephritis and renal fibrosis could be treated with hepatocyte growth factor (HGF) gene transfer. HGF is a multifunctional cytokine, which regulates mitosis, angiogenesis, morphogenesis, cell movement, and apoptosis. HGF administration and HGF gene therapy have been shown to suppress renal fibrosis in the experimental obstructive nephropathy. Experimental ischemia reperfusion injury has been treated successfully with ICAM-1 antisense oligonucleotides and plasmid coding 3ND gene therapy. This resulted in inhibition of acute tubular necrosis and reduced macrophage infiltration (118). The adenoviral vector coding *CTLA4Ig* gene injected into renal artery of transplanted kidneys in rats has alleviated the acute rejection reaction and improved graft survival for more than 50 days by inhibiting the activation of T cells involved in acute rejection (119). Although no experience exists for the kidneys, reporter genes have been developed for PET and SPECT applications in cancer and cardiac diseases.

THE PROSPECTS OF RENAL PET

The continuing development of new treatment options in oncology explains the success of PET/CT imaging in this field. FDG provides images of cancer with very high contrast, and its sensitivity for relatively small malignant foci is very good. The specificity of the technique is much more limited, and interpretation of images is strongly influenced by the clinical context in which they are acquired. The success of renal PET imaging will also be based on three important points: (a) increasing need, (b) improved technology, and (c) availability. Most important, however, is the development of new ideas about how to use molecular imaging to tackle important clinical questions of nephrology and urology. Molecular imaging has a great likelihood of success since it will be less affected by the competing imaging methods, which provide excellent details of renal anatomy and parenchymal perfusion and function. One should not completely ignore functional PET studies, however, since they provide excellent image quality and more accurate quantitative data than other imaging technologies.

Radioligands for molecular imaging of the kidneys have to be developed together with imaging protocols appropriate for them. Since the sensitivity and spatial resolution of PET are already excellent and are likely to improve further, one has to focus on optimizing imaging times. Radioligands with rapid parenchymal turnover times will utilize short dynamic PET studies, pattern recognition procedures, and artificial neural networks (120–122). Radioligands with slow dissociation will require delayed imaging times and methods of data analysis based on static imaging. To diagnose receptor alterations in renovascular hypertension or transplant rejection, delayed images of short duration should be the goal. This would permit time for clearance of any metabolized, or unmetabolized, tracer from the collecting system. For accurate assessment of split renal function such as the glomerular filtration rate, a dynamic study of very short duration of only 5 minutes could be sufficient if started immediately with the injection of the radioligand. Thus, both early postinjection dynamic studies and late postinjection static studies could be obtained in 5 minutes. Renal imaging with PET is likely to grow in the coming decade, with techniques ranging from simple flow/functional assessments to more sophisticated receptor imaging approaches.

ACKNOWLEDGMENTS

This work was supported by the National Institute of Diabetes and Digestive and Kidney Diseases (grant RO1DK050183), and by the National Cancer Institute (grants P50CA103175 and R24CA092871).

REFERENCES

1. Tarantola G, Zito F, Gerundini P. PET instrumentation and reconstruction algorithms in whole-body applications. *J Nucl Med* 2003;44: 756–769.
2. Schoder H, Larson SM. Positron emission tomography for prostate, bladder, and renal cancer. *Semin Nucl Med* 2004;34:274–292.
3. Kaatee R, Beek FJ, de Lange EE, et al. Renal artery stenosis: detection and quantification with spiral CT angiography versus optimized digital subtraction angiography. *Radiology* 1997;205:121–127.
4. Kim TS, Chung JW, Park JH, et al. Renal artery evaluation: comparison of spiral CT angiography to intra-arterial DSA. *J Vasc Interv Radiol* 1998;9:553–559.
5. Carlos RC, Axelrod DA, Ellis JH, et al. Incorporating patient-centered outcomes in the analysis of cost-effectiveness: imaging strategies for renovascular hypertension. *AJR Am J Roentgenol* 2003;181: 1653–1661.
6. Hacklander T, Mertens H, Stattaus J, et al. Evaluation of renovascular hypertension: comparison of functional MRI and contrast-enhanced

MRA with a routinely performed renal scintigraphy and DSA. *J Comput Assist Tomogr* 2004;28:823–831.
7. Prasad PV, Goldfarb J, Sundaram C, et al. Captopril MR renography in a swine model: toward a comprehensive evaluation of renal arterial stenosis. *Radiology* 2000;217:813–818.
8. Ergun EL, Caglar M. Tc-99m-DTPA captopril renography in the detection of renovascular hypertension due to renal polar artery stenosis. *Ann Nucl Med* 2001;15;167–170.
9. Khamanarong K, Prachaney P, Utraravichien A, et al. Anatomy of renal arterial supply. *Clin Anat* 2004;17:334–336.
10. Garel D, Allouch G, Boccon-Gibod L, et al. [Arterial hypertension subsequent to stenosis of the inferior polar artery. Apropos of 2 cases]. *Ann Pediatr (Paris)* 1986;33:211–214.
11. Carson RE. Mathematical modeling and compartmental analysis. In: Harbert JC, Eckelman WC, Neumann RD, eds. *Nuclear medicine diagnosis and therapy*. New York: Thieme, 1996:167–193.
12. Caldwell JH, Kroll K, Li Z, et al. Quantitation of presynaptic cardiac sympathetic function with carbon-11-meta-hydroxyephedrine. *J Nucl Med* 1998;39:1327–1334.
13. Szabo Z, Vosberg H, Sondhaus CA, et al. Model identification and estimation of organ-function parameters using radioactive tracers and the impulse-response function. *Eur J Nucl Med* 1985;11: 265–274.
14. Gibson JG, Seligman AM, Peacock WC, et al. The distribution of red cells and plasma in large and minute vessels of the normal dog, determined by radioactive isotopes of iron and iodine. *J Clin Invest* 1946; 25(6):848–857.
15. Trinh-Trang-Tan MM, Bouby N, Doute M, et al. Effect of long- and short-term antidiuretic hormone availability on internephron heterogeneity in the adult rat. *Am J Physiol* 1984;246:F879–F888.
16. Eriksson L, Bohm C, Kesselberg M, et al. An automated blood sampling system used in positron emission tomography. *Nucl Sci Appl* 1988; 3:133–143.
17. Szabo Z, Speth RC, Brown PR, et al. Use of positron emission tomography to study AT1 receptor regulation *in vivo*. *J Am Soc Nephrol* 2001; 12:1350–1358.
18. Juillard L, Janier MF, Fouque D, et al. Renal blood flow measurement by positron emission tomography using ^{15}O-labeled water. *Kidney Int* 2000;57:2511–2518.
19. Peters PE, Ter-Pogossian MM, Rockoff ML, et al. Measurement of renal blood flow by means of radioactive water labeled with oxygen 15. In: Blaufox MD, Funck-Brentano JL, eds. *Radionuclides in nephrology*. New York: Grune and Stratton, 1971:27–36.
20. Alpert NM, Rabito CA, Correia DJ, et al. Mapping of local renal blood flow with PET and H(2)(15)O. *J Nucl Med* 2002;43:470–475.
21. Chin A, Radhakrishnan J, Fornell L, et al. Effects of tezosentan, a dual endothelin receptor antagonist, on the cardiovascular and renal systems of neonatal piglets. *J Pediatr Surg* 2001;36:1824–1828.
22. Heyman MA, Payne BD, Hoffmann JIE, et al. Blood flow measurements with radionuclide-labelled particles. *Prog Cardiovasc Dis* 1977; 10:55–79.
23. Even GA, Green MA. Gallium-68-labeled macroaggregated human serum albumin, ^{68}Ga-MAA. *Int J Rad Appl Instrum B* 1989;16: 319–321.
24. Brooks DJ, Frackowiak RS, Lammertsma AA, et al. A comparison between regional cerebral blood flow measurements obtained in human subjects using ^{11}C-methylalbumin microspheres, the $C^{15}O_2$ steady-state method, and positron emission tomography. *Acta Neurol Scand* 1986;73:415–422.
25. Turton DR, Brady F, Pike VW, et al. Preparation of human serum [methyl-^{11}C]methylalbumin microspheres and human serum [methyl-^{11}C]methylalbumin for clinical use. *Int J Appl Radiat Isot* 1984;35:337–344.
26. Mintun MA, Ter Pogossian MM, Green MA, et al. Quantitative measurement of regional pulmonary blood flow with positron emission tomography. *J Appl Physiol* 1986;60:317–326.
27. Gjedde A. Compartmental analysis. In: Wagner HN Jr, Szabo Z, Buchanan WJ, eds. *Principles of nuclear medicine*. Philadelphia: Saunders, 1995:451–461.
28. Patlak CS, Blasberg RG, Fenstermacher JD. Graphical evaluation of blood-to-brain transfer constants from multiple-time uptake data. *J Cereb Blood Flow Metab* 1983;3:1–7.
29. Nitzsche EU, Choi Y, Killion D, et al. Quantification and parametric imaging of renal cortical blood flow *in vivo* based on Patlak graphical analysis. *Kidney Int* 1993;44:985–996.
30. Mullani NA, Ekas RD, Marani S, et al. Feasibility of measuring first pass extraction and flow with rubidium-82 in the kidneys. *Am J Physiol Imaging* 1990;5:133–140.
31. Tamaki N, Rabito CA, Alpert NM, et al. Serial analysis of renal blood flow by positron tomography with rubidium-82. *Am J Physiol* 1986; 251:H1024–H1030.
32. John EK, Green MA. Structure-activity relationships for metal-labeled blood flow tracers: comparison of keto aldehyde bis (thiosemicarbazonato)copper(II) derivatives. *J Med Chem* 1990;33: 1764–1770.
33. Shelton ME, Green MA, Mathias CJ, et al. Assessment of regional myocardial and renal blood flow with copper-PTSM and positron emission tomography. *Circulation* 1990;82:990–997.
34. Young H, Carnochan P, Zweit J, et al. Evaluation of copper(II)-pyruvaldehyde bis (N-4-methylthiosemicarbazone) for tissue blood flow measurement using a trapped tracer model. *Eur J Nucl Med* 1994; 21:336–341.
35. Chen BC, Germano G, Huang SC, et al. A new noninvasive quantification of renal blood flow with N-13 ammonia, dynamic positron emission tomography, and a two-compartment model. *J Am Soc Nephrol* 1992;3:1295–1306.
36. Schelbert HR, Phelps ME, Huang S-C, et al. N-13 ammonia as an indicator of myocardial blood flow. *Circulation* 1981;63:1259–1272.
37. Killion D, Nitzsche E, Choi Y, et al. Positron emission tomography: a new method for determination of renal function. *J Urol* 1993;150: 1064–1068.
38. Goethals P, Volkaert A, Vandewielle C, et al. ^{55}Co-EDTA for renal imaging using positron emission tomography (PET): a feasibility study. *Nucl Med Biol* 2000;27:77–81.
39. Madar I, Anderson JH, Szabo Z, et al. Enhanced uptake of [^{11}C]TPMP in canine brain tumor: a PET study. *J Nucl Med* 1999;40:1180–1185.
40. Loc'h C, Maziere B, Comar D. A new generator for ionic gallium-68. *J Nucl Med* 1980;21;171–173.
41. Rutland M. Database deconvolution. *Nucl Med Commun* 2003;24: 101–106.
42. Samal M, Karny M, Penicka P, et al. On the existence of an unambiguous solution in factor analysis of dynamic studies. *Phys Med Biol* 1989:34:223–228.
43. Hamilton D, Miola UJ, Mousa D. Interpretation of captopril transplant renography using a feed forward neural network. *J Nucl Med* 1996;37:1649–1652.
44. Izzedine H, Launay-Vacher V, Deray G. Renal tubular transporters and antiviral drugs: an update. *AIDS* 2005;19:455–462.
45. Capasso G, Cantone A, Evangelista C, et al. Channels, carriers, and pumps in the pathogenesis of sodium-sensitive hypertension. *Semin Nephrol* 2005;25:419–424.
46. Matteucci E, Carmellini M, Mosca F, et al. The contribution of Na+/H+ exchange to postreperfusion injury and recovery of transplanted kidney. *Biomed Pharmacother* 1999;53:438–444.
47. Agre P, Kozono D. Aquaporin water channels: molecular mechanisms for human diseases. *FEBS Lett* 2003;555:72–78.
48. Sun X, Kim J, Martell AE, et al. *In vivo* evaluation of copper-64-labeled monooxo-tetraazamacrocyclic ligands. *Nucl Med Biol* 2004; 31:1051–1059.
49. Sonmezoglu K, Erdil Y, Demir M, et al. Evaluation of renal function in low-dose cyclosporine-treated patients using technetium-99m diaminocyclohexane: a cationic tubular excretion agent. *Eur J Nucl Med* 1998;25:1630–1636.
50. Padhy AK, Solanki KK, Bomanji J, et al. Clinical evaluation of ^{99m}Tc diaminocyclohexane, a renal tubular agent with cationic transport: results in healthy human volunteers. *Nephron* 1993;65:294–298.

51. Inui KI, Masuda S, Saito H. Cellular and molecular aspects of drug transport in the kidney. *Kidney Int* 2000;58:944–958.
52. Nielsen CU, Brodin B. Di/tri-peptide transporters as drug delivery targets: regulation of transport under physiological and patho-physiological conditions. *Curr Drug Targets* 2003;4:373–388.
53. Nabulsi NB, Smith DE, Kilbourn MR. [([11])C]Glycylsarcosine: synthesis and in vivo evaluation as a PET tracer of PepT2 transporter function in kidney of PepT2 null and wild-type mice. *Bioorg Med Chem* 2005;13:2993–3001.
54. Han HK, Amidon GL. Targeted prodrug design to optimize drug delivery. *AAPS Pharmsci* 2000;2:E6.
55. Jager PL, Vaalburg W, Pruim J, et al. Radiolabeled amino acids: basic aspects and clinical applications in oncology. *J Nucl Med* 2001; 42:432–445.
56. Feinendegen LE, Herzog H, Wieler H, et al. Glucose transport and utilization in the human brain: model using carbon-11 methylglucose and positron emission tomography. *J Nucl Med* 1986;27:1867–1877.
57. Phelps ME, Huang SC, Hoffman EJ, et al. Tomographic measurement of local cerebral glucose metabolic rate in humans with (F-18)2-fluoro-2-deoxy-D-glucose: validation of method. *Ann Neurol* 1979;6:371–388.
58. Nose A, Mori Y, Uchiyama-Tanaka Y, et al. Regulation of glucose transporter (GLUT1) gene expression by angiotensin II in mesangial cells: involvement of HB-EGF and EGF receptor transactivation. *Hypertens Res* 2003;26:67–73.
59. Heilig CW, Brosius FC 3rd, Henry DN. Glucose transporters of the glomerulus and the implications for diabetic nephropathy. *Kidney Int Suppl* 1997;60:S91–S99.
60. Baroni MG, Oelbaum RS, Pozzilli P, et al. Polymorphisms at the GLUT1 (HepG2) and GLUT4 (muscle/adipocyte) glucose transporter genes and non-insulin-dependent diabetes mellitus (NIDDM). *Hum Genet* 1992;88:557–561.
61. Tao T, Tanizawa Y, Matsutani A, et al. HepG2/erythrocyte glucose transporter (GLUT1) gene in NIDDM: a population association study and molecular scanning in Japanese subjects. *Diabetologia* 1995;38: 942–947.
62. Grzeszczak W, Moczulski DK, Zychma M, et al. Role of GLUT1 gene in susceptibility to diabetic nephropathy in type 2 diabetes. *Kidney Int* 2001;59:631–636.
63. Gnudi L, Viberti G, Raij L, et al. GLUT-1 overexpression: Link between hemodynamic and metabolic factors in glomerular injury? *Hypertension* 2003;42:19–24.
64. Wright EM. Renal Na(+)-glucose cotransporters. *Am J Physiol Renal Physiol* 2001;280:F10–F18.
65. Tsujihara K, Hongu M, Saito K, et al. Na(+)-glucose cotransporter inhibitors as antidiabetics. I. Synthesis and pharmacological properties of 4'-dehydroxyphlorizin derivatives based on a new concept. *Chem Pharm Bull (Tokyo)* 1996;44:1174–1180.
66. de Groot TJ, Veyhl M, Terwinghe C, et al. Synthesis of ^{18}F-fluoroalkyl-beta-D-glucosides and their evaluation as tracers for sodium-dependent glucose transporters. *J Nucl Med* 2003;44:1973–1981.
67. Klein LJ, Visser FC, Knaapen P, et al. Carbon-11 acetate as a tracer of myocardial oxygen consumption. Eur J Nucl Med 2001;28:651–668.
68. Shreve P, Chiao PC, Humes HD, et al. Carbon-11-acetate PET imaging in renal disease. *J Nucl Med* 1995;36:1595–1601.
69. Oyama N, Miller TR, Dehdashti F, et al. ^{11}C-acetate PET imaging of prostate cancer: detection of recurrent disease at PSA relapse. *J Nucl Med* 2003;44:549–555.
70. Kotzerke J, Volkmer BG, Glatting G, et al. Intraindividual comparison of [^{11}C]acetate and [^{11}C]choline PET for detection of metastases of prostate cancer. *Nuklearmedizin* 2003;42:25–30.
71. Gibbs JB, Kohl NE, Koblan KS, et al. Farnesyltransferase inhibitors and anti-Ras therapy [review]. *Breast Cancer Res Treat* 1996;38:75–83.
72. Khwaja A, O'Connolly J, Hendry BM. Prenylation inhibitors in renal disease. *Lancet* 2003;355:741–744.
73. Szabo Z, Ravert HT, Mathews WB, et al. Kinetic modeling of a farnesyl transferase specific PET radiotracer. *J Nucl Med* 1999;40:228P.
74. Hwang DR, Eckelman WC, Mathias CJ, et al. Positron-labeled angiotensin-converting enzyme (ACE) inhibitor: fluorine-18-fluorocaptopril. Probing the ACE activity *in vivo* by positron emission tomography. *J Nucl Med* 1991;32:1730–1737.
75. Matarrese M, Salimbeni A, Turolla EA, et al. ^{11}C-Radiosynthesis and preliminary human evaluation of the disposition of the ACE inhibitor [^{11}C]zofenoprilat. *Bioorg Med Chem* 2004;12:603–611.
76. Allen AM, Zhuo J, Mendelsohn FA. Localization and function of angiotensin AT1 receptors. *Am J Hypertens* 2000;13:31S–38S.
77. Grone J, Simon M, Fuchs E. Autoradiographic characterization of angiotensin receptor subtypes in fetal and adult human kidney. *Am J Physiol* 1992;262:F326-F331.
78. Owonikoko TK, Fabucci ME, Brown PR, et al. *In vivo* investigation of estrogen regulation of adrenal and renal angiotensin (AT_1) receptor expression by PET. *J Nucl Med* 2003;45:94–100.
79. Braam B, Allen P, Benes E, et al. Human proximal tubular cell responses to angiotensin II analyzed using DNA microarray. *Eur J Pharmacol* 2003;464:87–94.
80. Goodfriend TL. Angiotensin receptors: history and mysteries. *Am J Hypertens* 2000;13:442–449.
81. Aleksic S, Szabo Z, Scheffel U, et al. *In vivo* labeling of endothelin receptors with [^{11}C]L-735,037: studies in mice and a dog. *J Nucl Med* 2001;42:1274–1280.
82. Ruiz-Ortega M, Lorenzo O, Ruperez M, et al. Role of the renin-angiotensin system in vascular diseases: expanding the field. *Hypertension* 2001;38:1382–1387.
83. Gibson RE, Beauchamp HT, Fioravanti C, et al. Receptor binding radiotracers for the angiotensin II receptor: radioiodinated [Sar1, Ile8]angiotensin II. *Nucl Med Biol* 1994;21:593–600.
84. Mathews WB, Burns HD, Dannals RF, et al. Carbon-11 labeling of a potent, nonpeptide, AT1-selective angiotensin-II receptor antagonist: MK-996. *J Lab Comp Radiopharm* 1994;36:729–737.
85. Hamill TG, Burns HD, Dannals RF, et al. Development of [^{11}C] L-159,884: a radiolabelled, nonpeptide angiotensin II antagonist that is useful for angiotensin II, AT1 receptor imaging. *Appl Radiat Isot* 1996;47:211–218.
86. Kim SE, Scheffel U, Szabo Z, et al. *In vivo* labeling of angiotensin II receptors with a carbon-11-labeled selective nonpeptide antagonist. *J Nucl Med* 1996;37:307–311.
87. Szabo Z, Kao PF, Burns HD, et al. Investigation of angiotensin II/AT1 receptors with carbon-11-L-159,884: a selective AT1 antagonist. J Nucl Med 1998;39:1209–1213.
88. de Gasparo M, Catt KJ, Inagami T, et al. International union of pharmacology. XXIII. The angiotensin II receptors. *Pharmacol Rev* 2000; 52:415–472.
89. Mathews WB, Yoo SE, Lee SH, et al. A novel radioligand for imaging the AT1 angiotensin receptor with PET. *Nucl Med Biol* 2004;31: 571–574.
90. Zober TG, Seckin E, Mathews WB, et al. Imaging the AT1 receptor with the radioligand [^{11}C]KR31173 and PET in mice, dogs and baboons. *Nucl Med Biol* 2005;33:5–13.
91. Xia J, Seckin E, Yan X, et al. PET Imaging of the AT1R in Swine Renal Artery Stenosis. *Hypertension* 2008;51:466–473.
92. Anderson WP, Ramsey DE, Takata M. Development of hypertension from unilateral renal artery stenosis in conscious dogs. *Hypertension* 1990;16:441–451.
93. Tsuji Y, Goldfarb DA, Masaki Z, et al. Patterns of renal function in hypertension due to unilateral renal artery occlusion. *Clin Exp Hypertens A* 1992;14:1067–1081.
94. Admiraal PJ, Danser AH, Jong MS, et al. Regional angiotensin II production in essential hypertension and renal artery stenosis. *Hypertension* 1993;21:173–184.
95. Blaufox MD, Fine EJ, Heller S, et al. Prospective study of simultaneous orthoiodohippurate and diethylenetriaminepentaacetic acid captopril renography. The Einstein/Cornell Collaborative Hypertension Group. *J Nucl Med* 1998;39:522–528.

96. Okada H, Kalluri R. Cellular and molecular pathways that lead to progression and regression of renal fibrogenesis. *Curr Mol Med* 2005;5: 467–474.
97. Bottinger EP, Bitzer M. 2002. TGF-beta signaling in renal disease. *J Am Soc Nephrol* 2002;13:2600–2610.
98. Kaya Z, Kotzerke J, Keller F. FDG PET diagnosis of septic kidney in a renal transplant patient. *Transpl Int* 1999;12:156.
99. Jones HA, Hamacher K, Clark JC, et al. Positron emission tomography in the quantification of cellular and biochemical responses to intrapulmonary particulates. *Toxicol Appl Pharmacol* 2005;207:230–236.
100. Zheng QH, Fei X, Liu X, et al. Comparative studies of potential cancer biomarkers carbon-11 labeled MMP inhibitors (S)-2-(4′-[^{11}C]methoxybiphenyl-4-sulfonylamino)-3-methylbutyric acid and N-hydroxy-(R)-2-[[(4′-[^{11}C]methoxyphenyl)sulfonyl]benzylamino]-3-methylbut anamide. *Nucl Med Biol* 2004;31:77–85.
101. Breyholz HJ, Schafers M, Wagner S, et al. C-5-disubstituted barbiturates as potential molecular probes for noninvasive matrix metalloproteinase imaging. *J Med Chem* 2005;48:3400–3409.
102. Sprague JE, Li WP, Liang K, et al. *In vitro* and *in vivo* investigation of matrix metalloproteinase expression in metastatic tumor models. *Nucl Med Biol* 2006;33:227–237.
103. Liu S. Radiolabeled multimeric cyclic RGD peptides as integrin alpha(v)beta(3) targeted radiotracers for tumor imaging. *Mol Pharm* 2006;3:472–487.
104. Lu N, Tian DZ, Zhou L, et al. [Changes in expression of angiotensin subtype AT1A and AT2 receptors in rats during cardiac remodeling following myocardial infarction]. *Sheng Li Xue Bao* 2001;53:128–132.
105. Meggs LG, Coupet J, Huang H, et al. Regulation of angiotensin II receptors on ventricular myocytes after myocardial infarction in rats. *Circ Res* 1993;72:1149–1162.
106. Zhang G, Yang Y, Pu S, et al. Relationship between remodeling and function of left ventricle and angiotensin II AT1 receptor expression after myocardial infarction in rats. *Chin Med J (Engl)* 1999;112: 593–596.
107. Schieffer B, Schieffer E, Hilfiker-Kleiner D, et al. Expression of angiotensin II and interleukin 6 in human coronary atherosclerotic plaques: potential implications for inflammation and plaque instability. *Circulation* 2000;101:1372–1378.
108. Arany I, Safirstein RL. Cisplatin nephrotoxicity. *Semin Nephrol* 2003; 23:460–464.
109. Goldman RD, Koren G. Amphotericin B nephrotoxicity in children. *J Pediatr Hematol Oncol* 2004;26:421–426.
110. Li C, Lim SW, Sun BK, et al. Chronic cyclosporine nephrotoxicity: new insights and preventive strategies. *Yonsei Med J* 2004;45:1004–1016.
111. Oudemans-van Straaten HM. Contrast nephropathy, pathophysiology and prevention. *Int J Artif Organs* 2004;27:1054–1065.
112. van de WB, de Graauw M, Le Devedec S, et al. Cellular stress responses and molecular mechanisms of nephrotoxicity. *Toxicol Lett* 2006;162:83–93.
113. Cauchon N, Langlois R, Rousseau JA, et al. PET imaging of apoptosis with (64)Cu-labeled streptavidin following pretargeting of phosphatidylserine with biotinylated annexin-V. *Eur J Nucl Med Mol Imaging* 2007;34:247–258.
114. Keen HG, Dekker BA, Disley L, et al. Imaging apoptosis in vivo using ^{124}I-annexin V and PET. *Nucl Med Biol* 2005;32:395–402.
115. van der Wouden EA, Sandovici M, Henning RH, et al. Approaches and methods in gene therapy for kidney disease. *J Pharmacol Toxicol Methods* 2004;50:13–24.
116. Imai E, IsakaY. Perspectives for gene therapy in renal diseases. *Intern Med* 2004;43:85–96.
117. Knoll T, Sagi S, Trojan L, et al. *In vitro* and *ex vivo* gene delivery into proximal tubular cells by means of laser energy—a potential approach for curing cystinuria? *Urol Res* 2004;32:129–132.
118. Imai E, Takabatake Y, Mizui M, et al. Gene therapy in renal diseases. *Kidney Int* 2004;65:1551–1555.
119. Tomasoni S, Azzollini N, Casiraghi F, et al. CTLA4Ig gene transfer prolongs survival and induces donor-specific tolerance in a rat renal allograft. *J Am Soc Nephrol* 2000;11:747–752.
120. Szabo Z, Kao PF, Mathews WB, et al. Positron emission tomography of 5-HT reuptake sites in the human brain with C-11 McN5652 extraction of characteristic images by artificial neural network analysis. *Behav Brain Res* 1996;73:221–224.
121. Wang ZJ, Qiu P, Liu K, et al. Model-based quantization analysis for PET parametric imaging. *Proc IEEE Eng Med Biol Conf* 2005:5908–5911.
122. Wang ZJ, Szabo Z, Lei P, et al. A factor-image framework to quantification of brain receptor dynamic PET studies. *IEEE Trans Signal Proc* 2005;53:3473–3487.

CHAPTER 14.3

Imaging the Neovasculature

A. J. BEER, H. J. WESTER, AND M. SCHWAIGER

Angiogenesis, the formation of new blood vessels, is a fundamental process involved in a variety of physiological as well as pathological conditions. Physiologically, it is required for development, wound repair, reproduction, and response to ischemia. Pathologically, it is associated with disease conditions like arthritis, psoriasis, retinopathies, and cancer (1). Especially in oncology, angiogenesis is an essential process for tumor growth and tumor metastasis, since the growth of solid tumors remains restricted to 2 to 3 mm in diameter until supported by the onset of angiogenesis. This concept was first proposed by Folkman (2) in 1971 and initiated intense research efforts and detailed investigations on the biology of angiogenesis, which subsequently have identified more than 20 angiogenic growth factors, their receptors, and signal transduction pathways.

Endogenous angiogenesis inhibitors have been discovered, and the cellular and molecular characterization of the angiogenic phenotype in human cancers has been achieved (2–4). Over the past few years, the concept of antiangiogenic therapy has evolved as a therapeutic strategy for diseases associated with increased angiogenic activity, like arthritis, psoriasis, and especially malignant neoplasms. In clinical oncology, antiangiogenic therapy is aimed at stopping cancer progression by suppressing the tumor blood supply (1).

Although the results of the first clinical trials using angiogenesis inhibitors did not meet the then very high expectations, encouraging results have recently been achieved with the anti–vascular endothelial growth factor (VEGF) antibody bevacizumab (Avastin) in combination with standard cytotoxic chemotherapy in metastatic colorectal cancer, breast cancer, and non–small cell lung cancers (5–8). In part, the disappointing results of the first antiangiogenic agents might be due to the difficulties in designing clinical trials for such drugs, which, unlike traditional chemotherapeutic agents, are not cytotoxic and usually have limited side effects. The concept of looking for the maximum tolerated dose is potentially not appropriate for most antiangiogenic drugs. Another problem in trial design is defining tumor response with these new agents, which are often not primarily cytotoxic in their mechanisms of action.

Clinical trials with conventional cytotoxic chemotherapeutic agents usually use morphological imaging such as computed tomography (CT) or magnetic resonance imaging (MRI) to provide indices of therapeutic response. Linear measurements in one or two dimensions are mainly used to estimate changes in tumor size in response to the investigational therapy as compared with a baseline measure. The introduction of the RECIST (Response Evaluation Criteria for Solid Tumors) criteria in 2000 resulted in considerable progress in standardizing these measurements (9). However, since antiangiogenic agents often lead to a decrease of tumor progression rather than to tumor shrinkage, the assessment of tumor response by conventional imaging methods might take months or years. New biomarkers of early tumor response to noncytotoxic drugs, which predict subsequent clinical response, are badly needed (10). Such biomarkers would not only facilitate clinical trials of new drugs but could also be used to aid in the selection of optimal treatment for individual patients ("personalized medicine").

There is great interest in imaging techniques that can be used as biomarkers and will provide an early indicator or predictor of effectiveness at a functional or molecular level. Currently, changes in hemodynamic parameters such as blood flow, blood volume, or vessel permeability are evaluated as biomarkers for response evaluation in trials with antiangiogenic drugs. Various imaging techniques are used for this purpose, mainly dynamic contrast enhanced MRI (DCE MRI), but also positron emission tomography (PET) (mostly with oxygen-15 [^{15}O]-water), dynamic contrast enhanced CT, and ultrasound (11). For all these techniques, significant correlations with conventional markers of angiogenesis, like microvessel density (MVD) or VEGF expression in immunohistochemistry, have been demonstrated, although the results of different studies are far from being uniform as these techniques vary substantially in their methods from center to center (12–17).

All the techniques mentioned above have their inherent technical problems that limit their general use in clinical routine and make the results difficult to interpret. Although PET with [^{15}O]-water is a truly quantitative method that has been quite comprehensively evaluated with good results for perfusion measurements of the heart and brain, the results in malignant tumors are harder to interpret (18). The reason for this is that vessels in tumors are leaky, tortuous, and have dead ends as well as shunts between the arterial and venous systems. Tumors often have relatively low blood flow, causing a low and variable signal from the tumors. Moreover, the production of [^{15}O]-water with its short half-life requires a cyclotron, which limits the use of this technique to a few PET centers. DCE MRI on the other hand is widely available and uses U.S. Food and Drug Administration–approved contrast agents with reasonably low toxicity like Gd-DTPA (gadolinium diethylenetriamine penta-acetic acid; e.g., Magnevist). However, MRI has several challenges regarding quantitation, and changes in the design of the pulse sequences influence the results and make them difficult to compare between institutions and across different manufacturers of MRI equipment (19).

Until recently, these techniques have shown mixed results. Some studies show no effect at all with DCE MRI in response to therapy. In a phase I study, DCE MRI was used to evaluate the effects of the VEGFR2 inhibitor SU5416 in patients with treatment refractory solid tumors, including soft tissue sarcoma, melanoma, renal cancers, and other entities. No changes in the hemodynamic parameters K^{trans} (rate transfer constant) and v_e (volume of the extravascular extracellular space per volume of tissue) were seen in response to treatment (20). Other studies successfully showed the effects of therapy, but no correlation with the response to treatment.

In patients with inflammatory and locally advanced breast cancer treated with bevacizumab alone for one cycle and subsequently in combination with chemotherapy and examined with DCE MRI at baseline and after cycles one, four, and seven, all hemodynamic parameters showed significant decreases after treatment with bevacizumab alone, and continued to decrease after the start of chemotherapy. However, there was no significant correlation of any of these parameters with clinical response (21). On the other hand, there are also promising results that show a correlation between response to treatment and the results of DCE MRI. One study evaluated DCE MRI in patients with colorectal cancer and metastatic liver lesions who received the VEGF receptor tyrosine kinase inhibitor PT787/ZK222584. Twenty-six patients were examined at baseline and one or more time points during treatment. A significant negative correlation between the DCE MRI pharmacokinetic parameter examined (K_i, which is related to K^{trans}) and both the oral dose and plasma levels of PT787/ZK222584 were found. Correct response evaluation was possible, as significantly greater reductions in K_i were found for responders with complete remission, partial remission, or stable disease according to the RECIST criteria than for nonresponders (22).

These different results emphasize that the role of DCE MRI for response evaluation is complex and still has to be further evaluated in order to define its value as a surrogate end point. In the future, markers at the molecular level might be used for response evaluation of antiangiogenic agents, which hopefully will provide more specific information compared to the functional assessment of hemodynamic parameters.

PET tracers for assessment of glucose metabolism or proliferation like fluorine-18-fluorodeoxyglucose ([^{18}F]-FDG) and fluorine-18-fluorothymidine ([^{18}F]-FLT) have already shown promising results in clinical studies for response assessment of cytotoxic chemotherapies (23,24). In the same way, targeting specific molecular markers of angiogenesis might be used for response assessment of antiangiogenic therapies, like the VEGF pathway or cell surface markers like the integrin $\alpha v\beta 3$.

THE BIOLOGY OF ANGIOGENESIS

Angiogenesis is a very complex process involving a multitude of growth factors, cell surface receptors, enzymes, and so forth. A basic knowledge of the biology of angiogenesis is mandatory for a thorough understanding of the different approaches used for imaging the neovasculature with PET. The cascade of angiogenesis will be discussed in the following section. A detailed review of the processes of angiogenesis can be found elsewhere (25,26), on which the following explanations are based.

The same applies to the different antiangiogenic therapeutic strategies, which are currently being evaluated, because knowing the most promising targets and their ligands for antiangiogenic therapy facilitates understanding of the most common strategies used for imaging these targets with PET (27,28).

The Cascade of Angiogenesis

The lack of access to circulating oxygen, growth factors, and nutrients in early tumor development limits tumor growth because tumors do not have their own blood supply. Consequently, solid tumors initially are composed of only a small population of transformed cells whose growth is controlled by a balance between apoptosis and tumor cell proliferation. To overcome this problem, tumors grow toward pre-existing nearby blood vessels. Tumor cells may then infiltrate these blood vessels regionally and form vessels consisting of normal endothelial cells mixed with infiltrative tumor cells called a "mosaic vessel" (29). Since this process mainly serves the tumor periphery, further tumor expansion leads to increasing central hypoxia. This initial phase of limited tumor growth may persist for months or even years.

The next step in the process of angiogenesis is called the *angiogenic switch*, because the tumor switches to its angiogenic phenotype. It is a phase of rapid tumor growth and involves a multitude of peptide angiogenic factors that are produced in response to tumor hypoxia. These include the VEGF, the acidic and basic fibroblast growth factors (aFGF, bFGF), and platelet-derived endothelial cell growth factor (PD-ECGF) (30). Local angiogenesis inhibitors like thrombospondin-1, endostatin, angiostatin, or antiangiogenic antithrombin III can also be found in tumor tissue.

The angiogenic switch occurs when the tumors produce angiogenic factors in excess of local angiogenesis inhibitors. The angiogenic growth factors diffuse toward nearby pre-existing blood vessels and bind to receptors located on endothelial cells like receptors to VEGF (VEGF-R1/Flt-1, VEGF-R2/KDR/Flk-1, VEGF-R3/KDR, Flt-1, VEGF-R2, VEGF-R3/Flt-4, VEGF-R4/neuropilin-1) (31). The binding of ligands to their receptors leads to activation of endothelial cells by receptor dimerization and activation of various signal transduction pathways, like phosphorylation of tyrosine kinases, protein kinases, and mitogen-activated protein kinases (32–38). Once endothelial cells become activated, the original vessels undergo characteristic morphological changes and form *mother vessels*, which are characterized by basement membrane degradation, a thinned endothelial cell lining, increased endothelial number, decreased pericyte numbers, and pericyte detachment (39). These vessels have an enlarged diameter and are hyperpermeable compared to normal microvessels (40). Consequently, the earliest histopathological features of angiogenesis are microvascular dilatation, hyperpermeability, edema, and extravascular fibrin deposition. This transient process only lasts for a few days and in the next step, mother vessels undergo at least four divergent morphological transformations (40–43).

The first mechanism for tumor vascularization is *sprouting angiogenesis*, which involves the proliferation and migration of endothelial cells from pre-existing blood vessels and the organization of tubular vascular structures (44). This is the most important and best understood process, and it requires the focal dissolution of the basement membrane of surrounding mother vessels. This is achieved by a number of proteolytic enzymes, like matrix metalloproteinases and plasminogen activator, which enable endothelial cells to exit the vessel abluminally (45).

Activated angiogenic endothelial cells proliferate rapidly and migrate into the extracellular matrix toward the angiogenic stimulus (46,47). Important factors in this step of angiogenesis are adhesion molecules known as integrins, such as the $\alpha v\beta 3$ and $\alpha v\beta 5$ integrin, which facilitate migration and vascular survival (48–51). Collagenases such as matrix metalloproteinases are secreted at the sprouting tips of growing vessels by endothelial cells and are responsible for the degradation of the extracellular matrix and facilitate cell invasion (52,53).

Finally, a lumen within an endothelial cell tubule has to be formed to allow for the supply of nutrients and oxygen to the tumor via circulation. This requires interactions between the extracellular matrix and cell-associated surface proteins, such as galactin-2, platelet endothelial cell adhesion molecule-1 (PECAM-1), and VE-cadherin (54–56). The newly formed vessels are stabilized through the recruitment of smooth muscle cells and pericytes. In this process, the angiopoietin family plays a major role, like angiopoietin-1 (Ang-1), which binds to the Tie-2 receptor on angiogenic endothelium (49).

Besides sprouting angiogenesis, various other processes may occur. Mother vessels may retain their large diameter and evolve into medium-sized arteries and veins by acquiring a smooth muscle and internal elastica. This process takes from a few days to several months. Alternatively, the endothelium of a mother vessel may form smaller separate well-differentiated vessel channels by projecting cytoplasmic structures into the lumen, which form transluminal bridges. This takes from several days to 3 weeks.

Another process is called *intussusception*, which involves focal invagination of connective tissue pillars from within the mother vessel and takes from several days to several weeks (41,42). During intussusception, two opposite endothelial cell membranes get in contact with each other and interendothelial junctions develop. The gap between the two newly formed vessels is filled by mesenchymal cells composed of fibroblasts and pericytes to form a pillar or an interstitial or intervascular tissue structure, and extracellular matrix proteins, such as collagen or fibrin, accumulate within the pillar. Intussusception generates vessels more rapidly than sprouting. The molecular mechanism of intussusception is not fully understood, but an increasing rate of blood flow plays a major role, as well as shear stress, which can be sensed by endothelial cells and transduced inside the cell by PECAM-1, resulting in increased expression of angiogenic factors and adhesion molecules.

Antiangiogenic Therapeutic Strategies

Antiangiogenic drugs are classified according to their main mechanism of action. True angiogenesis inhibitors do not destroy pre-existing blood vessels within a tumor, but only stop the formation of neovasculature. The expected effect of true angiogenesis inhibitors is thus disease stabilization rather than tumor regression. Contrary to that, vascular targeting agents also destroy the pre-existing tumor vasculature. Finally, nonselective antiangiogenic agents, which are basically conventional chemotherapeutic agents, show cytotoxic, antiproliferative, or anti-invasive effects on multiple cell types, including angiogenic endothelial cells. Especially at low concentrations, several conventional cytotoxic chemotherapeutic drugs have shown antiangiogenic effects. A multitude of antiangiogenic drugs targeting different steps in the angiogenic cascade have been or are currently being studied in clinical trials, and only a short overview of the most important ones are presented here.

Growth Factor Antagonists and Endothelial Cell Signal Transduction Inhibitors

Several drugs, such as suramin, interferon-α, and Angiozyme (Ribozyme Pharmaceuticals, Boulder, Colorado), suppress production of angiogenic growth factors. Monoclonal antibodies and soluble receptors have been developed against VEGF, with bevacizumab being the most promising agent in this group. Bevacizumab showed encouraging results in metastasized colorectal cancer, breast cancer, and non–small cell lung cancer (5,6). Small molecule drugs that inhibit the endothelial signal transduction caused by specific growth factor-receptor binding are currently being tested in clinical trials. Most of them are tyrosine kinase inhibitors. Both selective (against VEGF or PDGF) and nonselective agents are under evaluation. Two of these nonselective small molecule tyrosine kinase inhibitors, SU11248 (sunitinib [Sutent]) and BAY-43-9006 (sorafenib [Nexavar]) have shown antitumor activity in clinical trials in patients with gastrointestinal stromal tumor refractory to imatinib (Gleevec) and in metastasized renal cell cancer. Due to these encouraging results, they have recently been approved as monotherapy for kidney cancer (5,29).

Inhibitors of Endothelial Cell Proliferation

A variety of antiangiogenic agents, such as TNP-470, thalidomide, squalamine, and captopril, inhibit endothelial cell proliferation. Treatment with TNP-470 has been shown to be more effective in limiting the growth of micrometastases than the growth of established tumors. It has shown some stabilization of disease in clinical trials of patients with Kaposi sarcoma and cervical cancer (28).

Inhibitors of Integrin Activation

Integrins are heterodimeric transmembrane glycoproteins that play an important role in cell–cell and cell–matrix interactions. Among them, the subtypes $\alpha v\beta 3$ and $\alpha v\beta 5$ have been well examined and are expressed on angiogenic endothelial cells and on some metastatic tumor cells, but not on quiescent endothelium. Blocking the $\alpha v\beta 3$ integrin by monoclonal antibodies or cyclic peptides can lead to activation of p53 and endothelial cell apoptosis. Examples of drugs in clinical trial include Vitaxin (MedImmune, Gaithersburg, Maryland; humanized antibody to $\alpha v\beta 3$ LM-609) and EMD-121974 (Cilengitide, Merck, Darmstadt), a cyclic pentapeptide with highly specific binding to $\alpha v\beta 3$ and $\alpha v\beta 5$. These agents are currently being evaluated in phase I through III trials comprised of patients with irinotecan refractory colorectal cancer, patients with glioblastoma in combination with temozolomide, and patients with Kaposi sarcoma, among other trials.

Matrix Metalloproteinase Inhibitors

Matrix metalloproteinases (MMP) are interesting targets for antiangiogenic treatment because their inhibition interferes with both endothelial and tumor cell invasion into the extracellular matrix at primary and metastatic sites. The gelatinases MMP-2 and MMP-9 are closely associated with angiogenesis and are the most promising targets among the family of MMPs, which consists of at least 20 distinct enzymes. Selective and nonselective MMP inhibitors, which include Marimastat (British Biotech, Inc, Oxford, United Kingdom), AG-3340 (Prinomastat, Agouron Pharmaceuticals, Pfizer, San Diego, California), Col-3, Neovastat (Aeterna Laboratories, Quebec City, Canada), and BMS-275291, are in advanced clinical trials. Marimastat demonstrated a survival benefit in patients with metastatic gastric cancer and in patients with glioblastoma treated in combination with temozolomide. However, it is also one of the first antiangiogenic agents that demonstrated dose-limiting side effects, mostly severe inflammatory polyarthritis (28).

IMAGING OF FUNCTIONAL MARKERS OF ANGIOGENESIS

Imaging of functional hemodynamic parameters like blood flow and blood volume with PET are not new techniques. Such methods have been widely applied and thoroughly evaluated in brain and heart tissue. Although there is some experience with using these techniques for assessment of functional parameters in tumors, their use in this respect is still limited and warrants further evaluation. For a good overview of this topic, see the excellent review of Laking and Price (18).

Blood Flow

For assessment of blood flow, one needs a tracer that is freely diffusible and metabolically inert. Water fulfills all these requirements and is therefore an ideal perfusion tracer. [^{15}O]-water can be used for PET imaging, and because it is biologically and metabolically inert and freely diffusible, "tissue water" can be modeled as a single compartment including both tissue and its draining fluids. With a half-life of 123 seconds, [^{15}O]-oxygen is the longest-lived positron emitting isotope of oxygen. Besides reaction with hydrogen to produce [^{15}O]-water, it can be further reacted with carbon to produce [^{15}O]-carbon dioxide or [^{15}O]-carbon monoxide.

Two methods can be used for measuring perfusion with [^{15}O]-water, the steady-state method of Frackowiak, and the [^{15}O]-dynamic water method developed by Lammertsma and Jones (57). The dynamic water method is more commonly used today and is considered to be the current gold standard for imaging perfusion with PET. The tracer is administered by inhalation or by peripheral venous bolus injection. Continuous arterial data are obtained either by image-based arterial input functions (a large vessel like the aorta or the left ventricle) or by peripheral sampling to a well counter device. Arterial blood sampling is the method of choice because an image-based arterial input function might lead to an underestimation of the peak activity. The change in tissue concentration over time is modeled as:

$$\frac{dC_t(t)}{dt} = P * C_a(t) - (P/V_D + \lambda) * C_t(t), \qquad (14.3.1)$$

where V_D equals volume of distribution, the "proportion of the region of interest in which the radioactive water is distributed" mL_{blood}/mL_{tissue}, $C_t(t)$ equals instantaneous tissue concentration of [^{15}O]-water at time t, Bq/mL_{tissue}, $C_a(t)$ equals corrected instantaneous arterial concentration of [^{15}O]-water at time t, Bq/mL_{tissue}, P equals perfusion, $mL_{carrier}$ $*min^{-1}*$ $mL_{tissue}{}^{-1}$, and λ equals radioactive decay constant for [^{15}O], 0.338 Bq/(min*Bq).

The mathematics for solving P and V_D from the dynamic curves depend on convolution of the arterial and tissue data sets. The expression for tissue concentration at each time t is given by the convolution integral:

$$C_t(t) = \int P * C_a(T) * e^{-(P/V_D+\lambda)*(t-T)}dT, \qquad (14.3.2)$$

or

$$C_t(t) = P * C_a(t) \otimes e^{-(P/V_D+\lambda)*t} \qquad (14.3.3)$$

where $\otimes$ is the operation of convolution, $C_t(t)$ describes a biphasic curve with an initial peak followed by a longer tail of decay, and P and V_D can be determined from this curve using nonlinear least-squares fitting.

The dynamic method is less sensitive to tissue heterogeneity than the steady-state model. It is, however, more sensitive to the assumption about free and instantaneous diffusion of [^{15}O]-water out of arterial blood and through the tissues because equilibrium is not reached (58). This means that it is assumed that tissues exhibit neither tracer binding nor concentration gradients, and that the arterial extraction fraction is uniform. However, tumor blood supply on microscopic scales is very heterogeneous due to such phenomena as ischemia, shunts, and necrosis. Therefore, the assumption of a single arterial input and equilibration of arterial and tissue water is not completely physiologic in the context of the tumor microcirculation.

The exact physiological meaning of V_D is not completely clear yet. V_D is expected to reflect tissue water composition, and first results in patient studies corroborate these assumptions as markedly lower V_D values were found in breast, which is a fatty tissue, than in spleen or kidney (59). The validity and reproducibility of this method was initially assessed for the brain and myocardium but subsequently also for tumors of pancreas, brain, breast, and liver. The range of values reported by PET for tumors is within the reported range for PET in other tissues (60,61).

The ultimate test for the utility of perfusion measurements with PET will be to determine if useful conclusions can be drawn from changes in perfusion during antiangiogenic or conventional cytotoxic chemotherapy or radiotherapy. [^{15}O]-water PET has only rarely been used for response evaluation in the past, but first results seem promising. In locally advanced breast cancer blood flow as measured by dynamic [^{15}O]-water PET decreased in the responder group after chemotherapy, whereas it increased in the nonresponder group (62).

Another important topic for future studies will be the comparison of hemodynamic parameters derived from DCE MRI and [^{15}O]-water PET. Currently, DCE MRI is used far more often in clinical trials than [^{15}O]-water PET because of wider availability and easier examination protocols. However, although a DCE MRI examination might seem easy to perform, the interpretation of the data is very complex, probably more so than with [^{15}O]-water PET. First, MRI is not fully quantitative and the results are very dependent on the exact parameters of the pulse sequences used and thus are difficult to standardize between institutions. Second, with conventional DCE MRI using low-molecular-weight contrast agents, blood flow cannot be derived directly from the data outside the brain. Other hemodynamic parameters are used to describe the results, mainly the volume transfer constant K^{trans}, the volume of the extravascular extracellular space per volume of tissue γ_e, and the rate constant for the back flux from the extracellular extravascular space to the vasculature K_{ep} (63). However, the exact physiological meaning of these parameters is complex and not related to a single process such as blood flow or blood volume only.

K^{trans} has several physiologic interpretations, depending on the balance between capillary permeability and blood flow. When capillary permeability is very high, the flux of the contrast agent into the extravascular extracellular space is limited by the flow rate, and K^{trans} is equal to the blood plasma flow per unit volume of tissue. When tracer flux is very low and blood flow is high, the blood plasma can be considered as a single pool and any change in signal is due to the increase in the concentration of the contrast agent in the extravascular extracellular space, which means that K^{trans} is equal to the permeability surface area (64).

Although tumor heterogeneity also impairs interpretation of results of [^{15}O]-water PET as discussed before, blood flow can be derived directly from the data, the examination is truly quantitative and data are comparable between institutions. Prospective studies for response evaluation comparing the parameters derived from [^{15}O]-water PET and DCE MRI will hopefully clarify which method provides useful prognostic information for the patients.

Blood Volume and Vascular Permeability

The technique for blood volume measurements with PET is simple and can be easily combined with blood flow measurements using [^{15}O]-water, combining both functional parameters for angiogenic activity. Oxygen-15-carbon monoxide is produced by reaction of [^{15}O] with carbon and is inhaled at a fixed dose by the patient. Alternatively, carbon-11 ([^{11}C]) can be used for labeling, resulting in [^{11}C]-carbon monoxide, which has the advantage of a longer half-life (65). Both [^{15}O]-carbon monoxide and [^{11}C]-carbon monoxide bind irreversibly with hemoglobin to form [^{15}O]/[^{11}C]-carboxyhemoglobin (CO-Hb), which can be used as a tracer of vascular volume because it remains exclusively within the vasculature. Tissue concentration is measured over 5 to 6 minute and an arterial [^{15}O]-CO-Hb concentration curve is derived from a series of arterial blood samples over the same interval. Tissue vascular volume can be defined as:

$$V_v = \frac{V_t \int C_t}{R * \int C_a}, \tag{14.3.4}$$

where V_v equals volume of vessels, $mL_{vessels}$, V_t equals volume of tissue within region of interest on scan, mL_{tissue}, R equals the ratio of small vessel to large vessel hematocrit (assumed to be 1 in tumors), $C_t(t)$ equals tissue activity, Bq/(mL*min), and $C_a(t)$ equals arterial activity, Bq/(mL*min).

Blood volume data are of great interest for response evaluation of antiangiogenic drugs such as Combretastatin (CA4P, OXiGENE, Waltham, Massachusetts) because they exert their main effect via collapse of blood vessels and not via reduced flow through isovolumetric vessels. It is expected that blood flow will not be influenced, while blood volume may decrease in response to drugs that are mainly for capillary directed antiangiogenic therapies. The value of blood volume measurements is less certain because histological examinations show that capillaries represent only a minor percentage of total tumor blood volume (66).

Another PET tracer for imaging of blood volume is gallium-68 ([^{68}Ga])-DOTA-albumin, which showed favorable results in initial animal studies (67). An advantage is that the radionuclide [^{68}Ga] is generator produced and is therefore continuously available even to centers lacking an in-house cyclotron. By dynamic imaging, leakage of the tracer into the tumor could be measured, and the vascular permeability could be analyzed as well. No results from clinical trials using this tracer have been reported yet.

IMAGING OF MOLECULAR MARKERS OF ANGIOGENESIS

The principle of molecular imaging of angiogenesis is to define a specific target like a receptor or enzyme that is involved in angiogenesis and to use a ligand to this target conjugated with an imaging probe for noninvasive identification. This principle is of course not restricted to PET alone and is successfully used with MRI, ultrasound, and optical imaging as well (68). All of these methods have their inherent advantages and limitations, and none is ideal in every respect.

PET has certain advantages, especially when it comes to translation of preclinical results to the clinical arena, because PET combines high sensitivity with excellent depth penetration. Although optical imaging techniques also have excellent sensitivity, their depth penetration is limited to approximately 10 cm; they are mainly applied in preclinical animal studies or for analysis of superficial tissue and regions accessible to endoscopy. MRI has good depth penetration but a low sensitivity; therefore, comparably high doses of imaging agents are required, which limits their use in humans. The fibrin-specific MRI contrast agent EP2140R is the only MRI molecular imaging agent used in humans so far (69). Ultrasound, while being noninvasive and widely available, is user dependent, and many regions of the body, like the brain in adults, the lungs, and bones, are not accessible for ultrasound.

The main limitation of PET for use in humans is its restricted spatial resolution of 5 to 6 mm in standard clinical scanners. However, considerable progress is being achieved in this field and resolutions of 3 to 4 mm are possible with experimental scanners (70). PET will therefore continue to be one of the main molecular imaging modalities for use in humans and include imaging of molecular markers of angiogenesis. One of the key molecules in angiogenesis, the integrin $\alpha v\beta 3$, has already been successfully imaged with PET and SPECT in humans (71,72).

Integrin Expression

Integrins are heterodimeric transmembrane glycoproteins consisting of different α- and β-subunits, which play an important role in cell–cell and cell–matrix interactions. One important member of the family of integrins is $\alpha v\beta 3$, which mediates the migration of endothelial cells through the basement membrane during blood vessel formation. This receptor is also involved in various other pathological processes including tumor metastasis, restenosis, osteoporosis, and inflammatory processes (73). Several extracellular matrix proteins like vitronectin, fibrinogen, and fibronectin interact with integrins via the amino acid sequence arginine-glycine-aspartic acid (or RGD in the single letter code) (74). Based on these findings, Kessler et al. (75) developed the pentapeptide cyclo(-Arg-Gly-Asp-DPhe-Val-), which shows high affinity and selectivity for $\alpha v\beta 3$ and is the leading structure for the development of molecular imaging compounds for the determination of $\alpha v\beta 3$ expression. The first radioiodinated RGD peptides showed comparable affinity and selectivity to the lead structure and revealed receptor-specific tumor uptake *in vivo*. However, the first compounds also demonstrated predominantly hepatobiliary elimination, resulting in high activity concentration in the liver and intestines, which is unfavorable for patient studies (76).

Improving the pharmacokinetics of radiohalogenated peptides is mandatory for clinical use, and several approaches to achieve this goal have been developed. The glycosylation approach is based on the introduction of sugar derivatives, which are conjugated to the ε-amino function of a corresponding lysine in the peptide sequence. [*I]-Gluco-RGD and [^{18}F]-Galacto-RGD have been developed for PET and single-photon emission computed tomography (SPECT) imaging by conjugating the RGD containing cyclic pentapeptide cyclo(-Arg-Gly-Asp-DPhe-Val-) with glucose- or galactose-based sugar amino acids. Both compounds demonstrated predominantly renal elimination and increased uptake and retention in a murine tumor model compared with the first generation peptides (77).

The conjugation of hydrophilic D-amino acids was also used to improve the pharmacokinetics of peptide-based tracers (78). The tumor uptake of the compound [^{18}F]-D-Asp3-RGD was lower than that found for [^{18}F]-Galacto-RGD, but tumor/background ratios calculated from small animal PET images were comparable due to the even faster elimination. Another way to improve many properties of peptides and proteins is PEGylation (79). Chen et al. (79) conjugated RGD-containing peptides with PEG [poly(ethylene glycol)] moieties with different sizes, using different radiolabeling strategies. The effects of PEGylation on the pharmacokinetics and tumor uptake and retention of RGD peptides was very variable and seem to depend strongly on the nature of the lead structure and perhaps on the size of the PEG moiety.

Radiometallated tracers for $\alpha v\beta 3$ imaging have been developed as well, including peptides labeled with indium-111 ([^{111}In]), technetium-99m (^{99m}Tc), copper-64 ([^{64}Cu]), yttrium-90 ([^{90}Y]), and rhenium-188 ([^{188}Re]). Again, they are mostly based on the cyclic pentapeptide and are conjugated via the ε-amino function of a lysine with different chelator systems, such as DTPA, the tetrapeptide sequence H-Asp-Lys-Cys-Lys-OH, and DOTA. Although they show high receptor affinity, selectivity, and specific tumor accumulation, the pharmacokinetics of most of these compounds still have to be improved before a clinical application seems feasible (80).

A relatively new strategy to improve the properties of radiotracers is the concept of multimerization. Multimeric compounds presenting more than one RGD site have been introduced recently. The groups of Wester and Kessler conducted a systematic study of the influence of multimerization on receptor affinity and tumor uptake with a series of monomeric, dimeric, tetrameric, and octameric RGD peptides. These compounds contain different numbers of c(RGDfE) peptides connected via PEG linkers and lysine moieties, which are used as branching units. They found an increasing binding affinity in a series of monomer, dimer, tetramer, and octamer compounds in an *in vitro* binding assay, which was confirmed by small animal PET studies.

PET studies comparing a tetrameric structure containing four c(RGDfE) peptides with a tetrameric compound containing only one c(RGDfE) and three c(RaDFE) peptides, which do not bind to the $\alpha v\beta 3$ integrin, showed a threefold lower accumulation of activity in the tumor for the pseudomonomeric tetramer than for the "real" tetramer (Fig. 14.3.1). This indicates that the higher uptake in the tumor really is due to multimerization and is not based on other

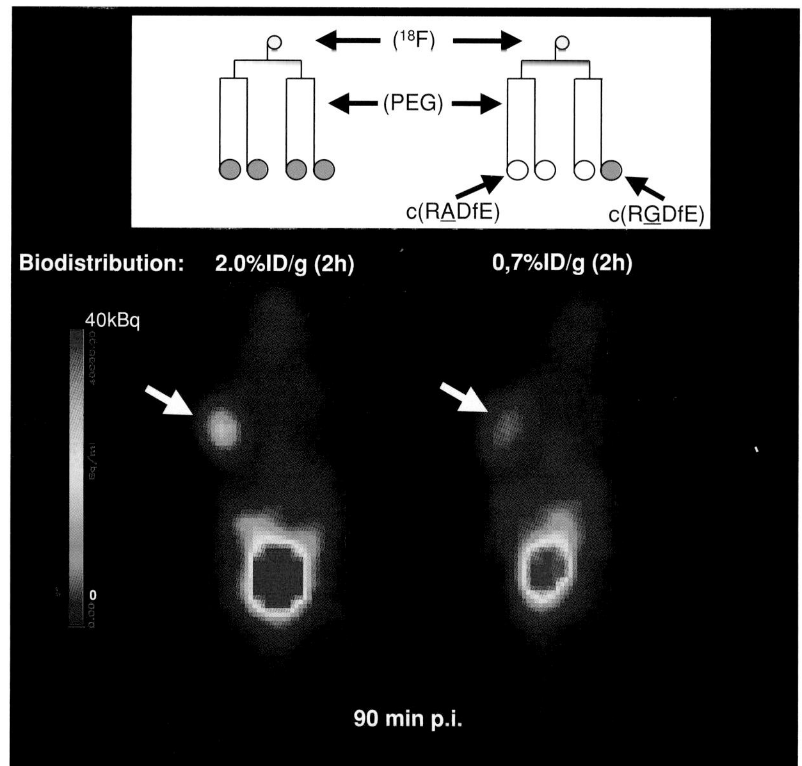

FIGURE 14.3.1. Tumor xenografts of $\alpha v\beta 3$ positive M21 tumors in the right shoulder in a mouse model. In the small animal PET scans, the RGD tetramer with four RGD binding sites clearly shows a much more intense accumulation in the tumor compared to the RGD tetramer with only one RGD binding site and three unspecific RAD sites. ^{18}F, fluorine 18; PEG, PEGylation.

structural effects (81). The multimerization approach thus seems very promising for increasing binding affinity and tumor uptake and at the same time improving the pharmacokinetics of peptide-based tracers.

From the mentioned substances, [^{18}F]-Galacto-RGD has been evaluated most extensively in preclinical tumor models and was the first substance to be used in patients for PET imaging of $\alpha v\beta 3$ expression. In the M21 melanoma tumor, which shows a strong $\alpha v\beta 3$ expression on the tumor cells, specific tracer uptake could be demonstrated, whereas the $\alpha v\beta 3$ negative M21L control tumor showed no substantial tracer uptake (76). The tracer uptake also correlated significantly with the degree of $\alpha v\beta 3$ expression in tumor xenografts containing different amounts of M21 and M21L cells (72). These data were obtained from studies in which the tumor models were already receptor positive. From this study, no information is given on whether $\alpha v\beta 3$ expression on endothelial cells during tumor-induced angiogenesis could be monitored in this situation where the density of $\alpha v\beta 3$ expressing cells is expected to be substantially lower. Therefore, further studies with the A431 squamous cell carcinoma model and the RIP-Tag model were used. A431 cells do not express the $\alpha v\beta 3$ integrin, but induce extensive angiogenesis when subcutaneously transplanted into nude mice. Transaxial images of squamous cell carcinoma–bearing nude mice obtained with a small animal PET scanner showed an intense tracer accumulation in the tumor that was exclusively based on $\alpha v\beta 3$ expression on the tumor vasculature (72).

The RIPTag model was used for evaluation of angiogenesis over time. In this transgenic mouse model of carcinogenesis and angiogenesis, the oncogene SV40 T antigen is expressed under the control of the rat insulin promoter. The advantage of this model is that the tumor arises from normal cells in its natural tissue environment and progresses through multiple stages, like human cancers. Insulin-producing β cells develop into islet cell hyperplasia, adenomas, and finally carcinomas. The angiogenic switch occurs after approximately 7 weeks, resulting in highly vascularized insulinomas. Autoradiographic studies of pancreatic sections of mice sacrificed 2 hours after intravenous injection of iodine-125 ([^{125}I])-gluco-RGD showed high focal activity accumulation in the pancreas in RIP-Tag-positive mice. In contrast, only low activity accumulation corresponding to the background was found in the RIP-Tag-negative mice. Corresponding with the tumor differentiation, there was a clear increase in activity accumulation in the pancreas of RIP-Tag-positive mice between 7 and 9 weeks, whereas tumor accumulation remained low over the whole observation period in RIP-Tag-negative mice.

In summary, preclinical data indicate that $\alpha v\beta 3$ expression on endothelial cells can be monitored during tumor-induced angiogenesis. However, in clinical settings, it is impossible to distinguish between $\alpha v\beta 3$ expression on tumor and endothelial cells by PET, and monitoring tumor-induced angiogenesis may be problematic in tumors known to have a high level of $\alpha v\beta 3$ expression on tumor cells, like melanoma. However, in benign disorders characterized by an imbalance of angiogenesis, this class of radiolabeled peptides may be used for monitoring angiogenic activity. For example, it has been demonstrated that radiolabeled RGD peptides targeting $\alpha v\beta 3$ allow imaging of delayed-type hypersensitivity reaction in a mouse model of chronic inflammation. It was found that the radiolabeled RGD peptides specifically accumulate in the chronic inflamed tissue because of $\alpha v\beta 3$-specific binding, and that this process can be monitored noninvasively with PET and is related to the microvascular density (82).

In the clinical setting, $\alpha v\beta 3$-positive tumors can be successfully imaged with [^{18}F]-Galacto-RGD PET in patients and good tumor/background ratios result. As expected from the preclinical studies, the biodistribution was favorable with predominantly renal elimination of tracer and some hepatic elimination. The tracer was rapidly washed out from the blood pool and background activity in muscle tissue is low (Fig. 14.3.2). There is intermediate tracer retention in the liver, spleen, and intestine, which impairs detection of lesions in these organs with only weak or moderate tracer uptake. All other regions of the body can be well analyzed with [^{18}F]-Galacto-RGD PET.

Dynamic studies of the tumors over 60 minutes showed a similar pattern of tracer accumulation for most of the lesions, with an increase during the first minutes, followed by a plateau phase, mostly with a slight decrease of activity during the last 20 minutes (83). Kinetic modeling studies were consistent with a two-tissue compartment model and suggested slowly reversible, specific tracer binding. As k_4 could be defined, the tracer does not seem to be irreversibly trapped inside the cells (Fig. 14.3.3). However, as k_4 usually was substantially lower than k_3, some amount of internalization of the receptor after tracer binding is possible. These results indicate that a good time point for starting static emission scans would be 40 to 60 minutes after injection, because most tracer activity is already washed out from the blood pool and tracer retention in the tumor is still in the plateau phase or only slightly decreasing during the following scan time.

The effective dose of 18 μSv/MBq is similar to that for [^{18}F]-FDG, with the bladder being the organ with the highest absorbed radiation dose (84). The correlation of tracer uptake and $\alpha v\beta 3$ expression as determined by immunohistochemistry was positive and significant, corresponding to the preclinical results (85).

The pattern of $\alpha v\beta 3$ expression seen in immunohistochemistry depended strongly on the tumor type and showed marked variability. Whereas malignant melanoma showed strong $\alpha v\beta 3$ expression on endothelial as well as on tumor cells in lymph node metastases, distant metastases showed only weak $\alpha v\beta 3$ expression and no uptake of [^{18}F]-Galacto-RGD PET, indicating a dependence of $\alpha v\beta 3$ expression not only according to tumor type, but also according to tumor stage and pattern of metastases. Sarcomas showed staining of neovasculature and tumor cells, whereas squamous cell carcinomas of the head and neck region showed staining predominantly of the neovasculature (Fig. 14.3.4). There was high inter- and intrapatient variability of tracer accumulation, with intense accumulation in the primary tumor, but only weak to moderate accumulation in metastases.

These preliminary results indicate that tumor staging is unlikely to be the primary indication for $\alpha v\beta 3$ imaging. However, [^{18}F]-Galacto-RGD and similar compounds could be used as new noninvasive prognostic markers, as has already been demonstrated for breast cancer using immunohistochemistry (86). In sarcomas, low-grade tumors showed substantially lower tracer accumulation of [^{18}F]-Galacto-RGD than patients with high-grade sarcomas (Fig. 14.3.5).

The assessment of angiogenic activity in tumors with $\alpha v\beta 3$ expression predominantly on the neovasculature is another potential application for response evaluation during antiangiogenic therapy (Figs. 14.3.6 and 14.3.7). Moreover, the pretherapeutic selection of patients amenable for $\alpha v\beta 3$ specific therapies, like with Cilengitide or Vitaxin, might also be feasible. New tracers like multimeric RGD peptides might further improve tumor to background contrast in the future.

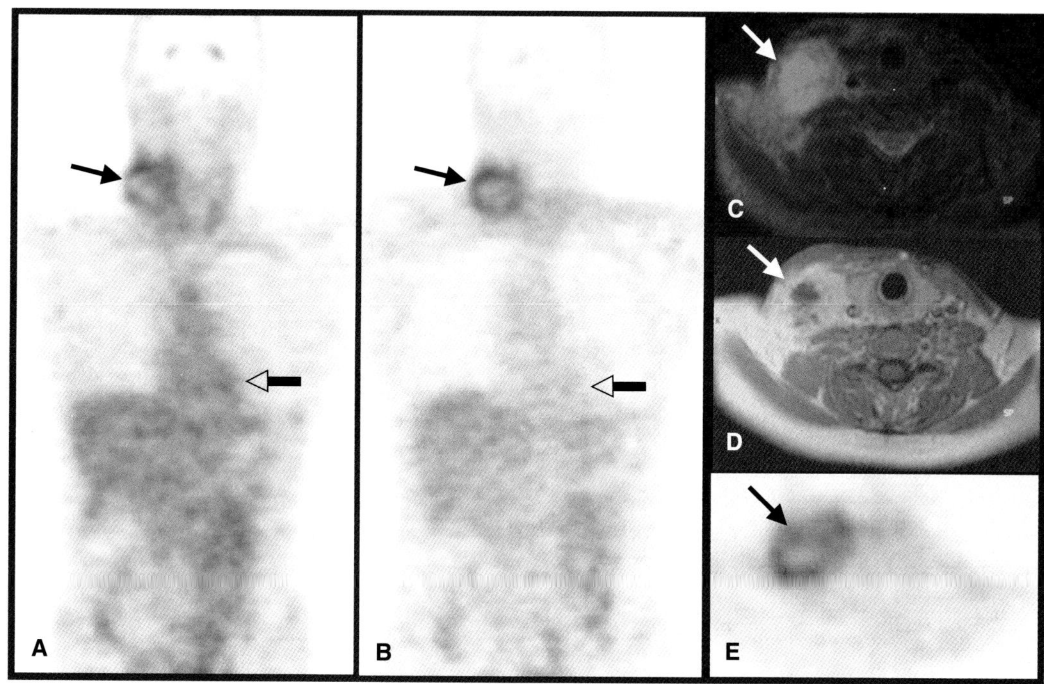

FIGURE 14.3.2. Fluorine-18 ([^{18}F])-Galacto-RGD PET scan of a patient with a large lymph node metastasis in the neck of a squamous cell carcinoma of the uvula on the right side (*arrow, closed tip*). In the coronal slices (**A:** 5 minutes postinjection; **B:** 60 minutes postinjection) the tumor can be clearly delineated with stable tracer uptake over time. Due to rapid tracer elimination from the blood pool (*arrow, open tip pointing to heart*), tumor-to-background contrast becomes better over time. There is intermediate tracer uptake in the liver and intestine. In the axial slices of the corresponding MRI (**C:** fat saturation T2w; **D:** T1w + GdDTPA) the metastasis shows a central necrosis and peripheral contrast enhancement. In the axial slice of the [^{18}F]-Galacto-RGD PET (**E**), the area of necrosis remains cold and the periphery shows variable tracer uptake, suggesting variable levels of angiogenesis.

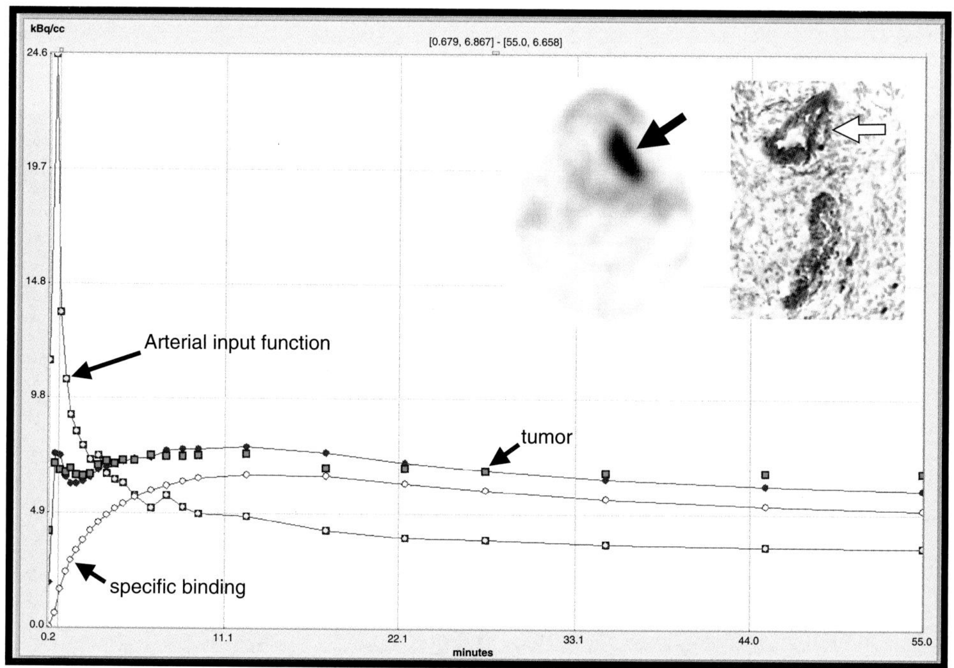

FIGURE 14.3.3. Dynamic study with kinetic modeling using a two-tissue compartment model of a squamous cell carcinoma of the oral cavity (*arrow, closed tip*). There is intense staining of the neovasculature in the immunohistochemistry of $\alpha v\beta 3$ expression (*arrow, open tip*). There is rapid tracer washout in the blood pool, while activity in the tumor increases during the first minutes, plateaus, and finally decreases slightly. The green squares denote the measured data, the blue line represents the modeled curve fit. The blue circles represent data from curve fit. The yellow squares represent arterial input function. The white circles represent the amount of specific binding, which is high and decreases only slightly during the scan period.

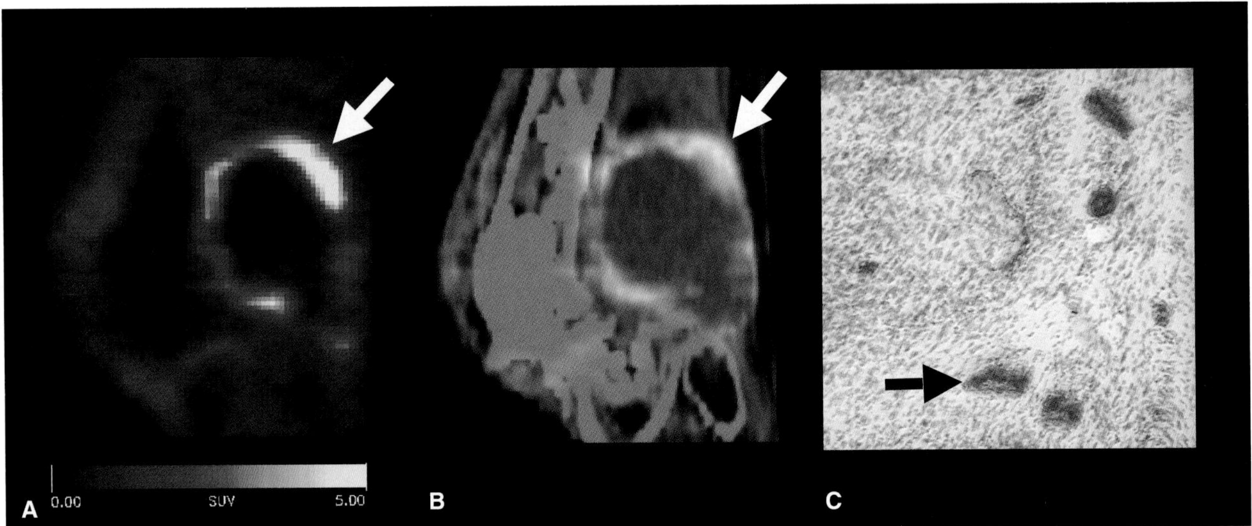

FIGURE 14.3.4. Soft tissue sarcoma of the knee. Note intense tracer uptake in the periphery of the tumor, whereas the necrotic center remains cold (*arrow*; **A:** fluorine-18 ([^{18}F])-Galacto-RGD PET, **B:** [^{18}F]-Galacto-RGD PET/CT image fusion). Immunohistochemistry of $\alpha v\beta 3$ expression shows intense staining predominantly of tumor vessels (**C;** *arrow*).

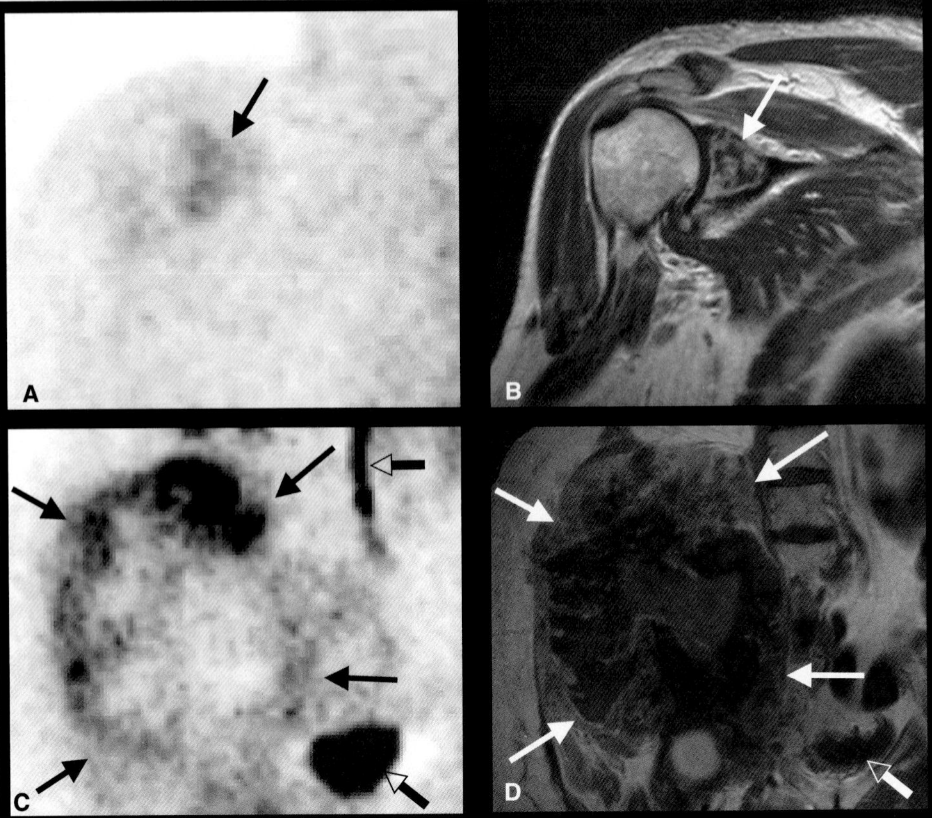

FIGURE 14.3.5. Comparison of a low-grade chondrosarcoma of the glenoid (**A:** Fluorine-18 ([^{18}F])-Galacto-RGD PET, **B:** magnetic resonance image (MRI) T1w + GdDTPA) and a high-grade chondrosarcoma of the iliac bone (**C:** [^{18}F]-Galacto-RGD PET, **D:** MRI T1w + GdDTPA). The tracer uptake in the low-grade chondrosarcoma is only moderate, whereas there is intense uptake in the periphery of the high-grade chondrosarcoma (*arrows, closed tip*). Tracer retention in the ureter and bladder is physiologic due to the predominantly renal elimination (*arrows, open tip*).

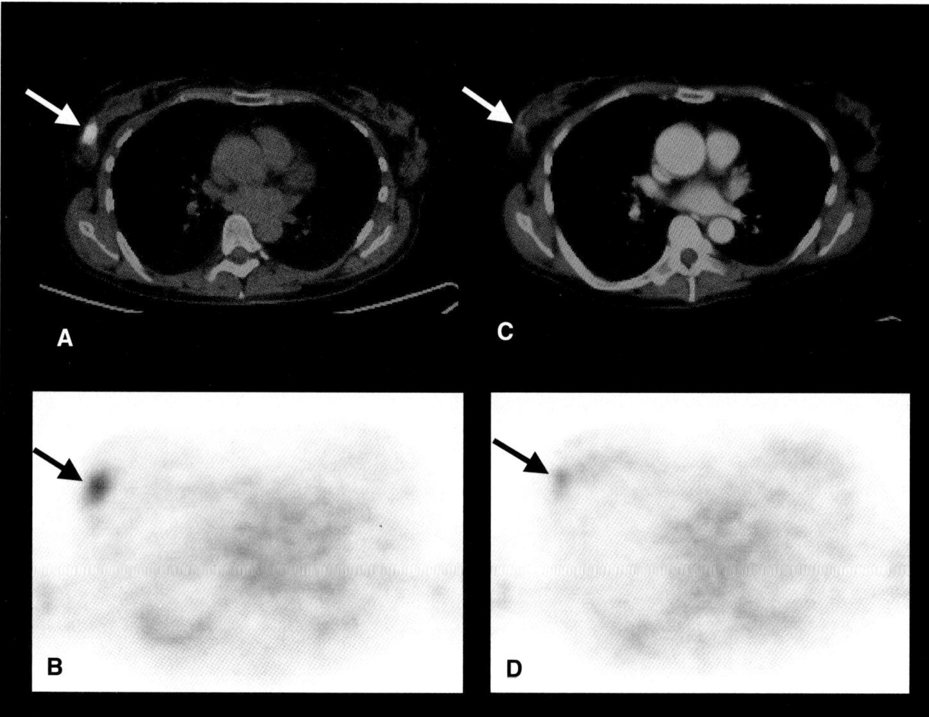

FIGURE 14.3.6. Time course of fluorine-18-fluorodeoxyglucose ([^{18}F]-FDG) PET/CT (**A,B**) and [^{18}F]-Galacto-RGD PET (**C,D**) in a patient with metastatic breast cancer before chemotherapy (**A,C**) and after one cycle of cytotoxic chemotherapy in combination with bevacizumab (**B,D**). There is intense uptake of both tracers before therapy and the decrease of uptake after one cycle of therapy in the primary (*arrows*). Which tracer will finally be better for response evaluation has to be examined in future studies.

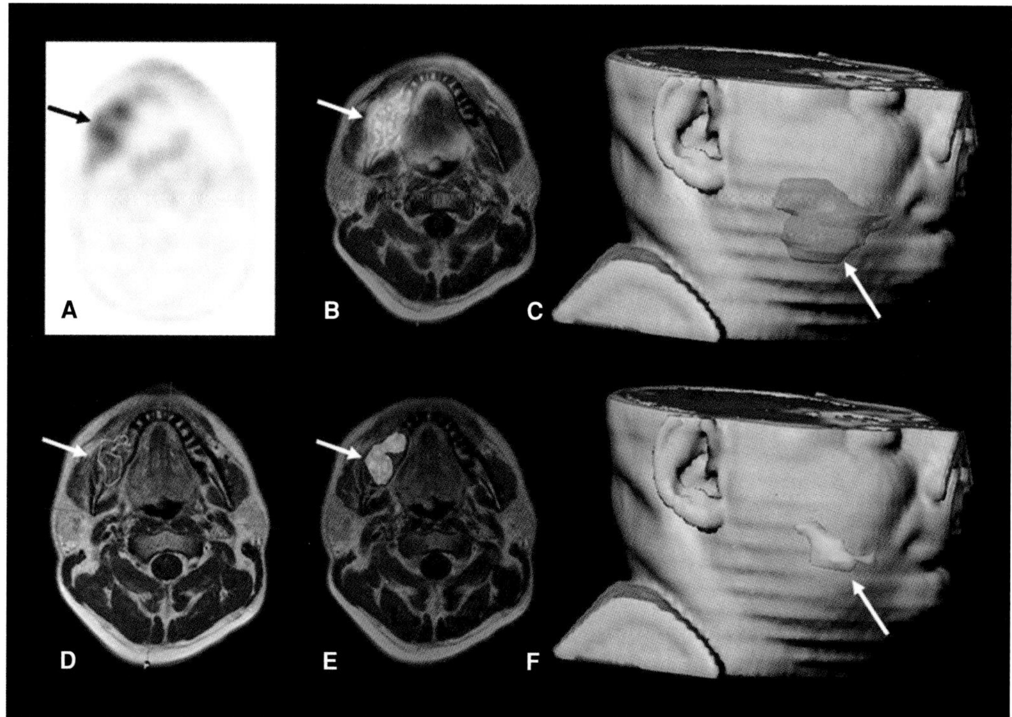

FIGURE 14.3.7. Patient with a squamous cell carcinoma of the right mandible (*arrows*). The fluorine-18 ([^{18}F])-Galacto-RGD PET (**A**) shows intense and heterogeneous tracer uptake in the lesion, which can also be clearly delineated in the image fusion with the corresponding magnetic resonance imaging (MRI) scan (**B**). **C:** Shows the tumor volume in red as defined by MRI in the three-dimensional reconstruction. By applying a threshold of standardized uptake value (SUV) 3.0 and only using pixels with SUVs above this threshold, a subvolume with more intense $\alpha v\beta 3$ expression can be defined (**D:** *blue line*; **E:** blue area), which is shown in the three-dimensional reconstruction in **F.**

Recently, the SPECT tracer ^{99m}Tc-NC100692 was introduced by GE Healthcare (Chalfont St. Giles, Buckinghamshire, England) for imaging $\alpha v\beta 3$ expression in humans and was first evaluated in breast cancer and a PET tracer is supposed to follow. Nineteen of 22 tumors could be detected with this agent, which was safe and well tolerated by the patients (71). It is therefore possible that agents for $\alpha v\beta 3$ imaging may soon be available commercially and that $\alpha v\beta 3$ imaging with PET and SPECT will be performed on a larger scale in the future, although this area continues to evolve rapidly.

Matrix Metalloproteinases

MMPs are zinc endopeptidases responsible for the enzymatic degradation of connective tissue that facilitate endothelial cell migration during angiogenesis. From the more than 18 members of the MMP family, the gelatinases MMP 2 and 9 are most consistently detected in malignancies are therefore interesting for assessment of angiogenesis (87). Many strategies have been used for radiolabeling MMP specific ligands. Via phage display techniques, the MMP specific decapeptide H-Cys-Thr-Thr-His-Trp-Gly-Phe-Thr-leu-Cys-OH was identified and could be labeled via the Iodogen (Thermo Scientific Pierce Protein Research Products, Rockford, Illinois) method by adding a d-Tyr at the N-terminal end of this decapeptide. However, metabolic stability of the compound was low and lipophilicity was high, so this tracer has unfavorable characteristics for *in vivo* imaging.

Another approach is labeling small molecule MMP inhibitors, which are also used as antiangiogenic drugs. Different [^{18}F]- and [^{11}C]-labeled MMP inhibitors have been synthesized and evaluated preclinically with mixed results (88). One of the more promising substances is based on a MMP inhibitor belonging to the family of N-sylfonylamino acid derivatives. A [^{11}C]-labeled analogue was synthesized and showed favorable pharmacokinetics in mice and metabolic stability up to 30 minutes after injection (89). However, mainly due to the pharmacokinetic problems of most tested substances, none of these compounds has been used in patient studies up to now.

Vascular Endothelial Growth Factor and Its Receptors

VEGFs are important in angiogenesis and stand at the beginning of the angiogenic cascade. This has stimulated interest in the use of VEGFs, VEGF receptors, and their complexes as antigens for the targeted delivery of imaging agents to the tumor neovasculature. However, the experience with VEGF-based radiotracers is limited because this fragile molecule is easily inactivated by conjugation with bifunctional chelators such as HYNIC. A new approach has recently been presented by using a C-tagged compound, which could be successfully labeled with ^{99m}Tc. The resulting compound ^{99m}Tc-HYNIC-VEGF could visualize murine mammary carcinoma models, and uptake decreased during low-dose and high-does chemotherapy (90).

Whole-animal PET imaging studies with the human antibody VG76e that binds to VEGF, labeled with [^{124}I], showed high tumor-to-background ratios in VEGF overexpressing tumors (91). However, preliminary results in patients with hepatic and pancreatic cancers and other solid tumors using radiolabeled VEGF165 and the VEGF antibody HuMV833 showed only very faint tumor uptake with very high activities in blood pool and in normal organs (92,93). This tracer uptake could easily be attributed to nonspecific blood pool activity. Before widespread use in patient trials, considerable improvements in the pharmacokinetic properties of these compounds have to be achieved.

Extra-domain B of Fibronectin

Fibronectin is a large glycoprotein, which can be found physiologically in plasma and tissues. The extra-domain B of fibronectin (EDB), consisting of 91 amino acids, is not present in the fibronectin molecule in normal conditions and is essentially undetectable in most normal adult tissues, except for the endometrium in the proliferative phase and some vessels of the ovaries. It is typically inserted in the fibronectin molecules at sites of tissue remodeling by a mechanism of alternative splicing at the level of the primary transcript. What makes EDB interesting as a marker of angiogenesis is its expression in a variety of solid tumors, as well as in ocular angiogenesis and wound healing.

The pattern of EDB expression in tumors either is predominantly perivascular or exhibits a diffuse staining of the tumor stroma (94). The human antibody fragment scFv(L19) binds with subnanomolar affinity to EDB and has been shown to efficiently localize on tumoral and nontumoral neovasculature both in animal models and in cancer patients. In a study of patients suffering from various solid tumors like lung cancer, metastases from colorectal cancer, and glioblastoma, 16 of 20 tumor lesions could be identified by SPECT using [^{123}I]-scFv(L19). It is not clear whether the unidentified tumors were not detected due to the technical limitations of SPECT imaging or because they were in a phase of slow growth with low levels of angiogenesis (95). This compound is also potentially promising for PET imaging, but no reports about PET tracers targeting EDB are available now.

Promising New Targets

The angiogenic cascade involves many more possible targets for molecular imaging than the ones mentioned above. Two of these targets seem to be especially promising and warrant further evaluation as imaging markers of angiogenesis. One is magic roundabout (MR) or ROBO-4. Roundabouts are large transmembrane receptors for ligands known as slits. An endothelial-specific roundabout was discovered, which is highly restricted. In fact, MR is absent from adult tissues except at sites of active angiogenesis, including tumors, which in theory makes it ideally suited to vascular targeting (96). Biodistribution studies with radiolabeled ligands are eagerly awaited to assess the real potential of ROBO-4 as a target for imaging angiogenesis.

Other interesting targets are the tumor endothelial markers (TEMs) 1 through 8, which display elevated expression in endothelial cells isolated from colorectal carcinoma. Further studies showed that TEMs are also up-regulated in endothelial cells undergoing physiologic angiogenesis in humans and mice. TEM 5 belongs to a group of adhesion G-protein coupled receptors, which are involved in cell–cell and cell–matrix interactions. It has recently been shown that a soluble fragment of TEM 5 (sTEM 5) is shed by endothelial cells upon activation by growth factors. When sTEM 5 is degraded by MMP 9, a cryptic RGD containing binding site is revealed, which upon binding to $\alpha v\beta 3$ mediates endothelial cell survival (97). Imaging of activated endothelial cells might be feasible with this compound, and studies with radiolabeled sTEM 5 are awaited in the near future.

PERSPECTIVES

The techniques for imaging the neovasculature at a functional level with PET by measuring blood flow and blood volume are not new, but it is expected that they will be more widely applied for assessment of response to antiangiogenic therapy in the future. The role of specifically targeted tracers for molecular imaging of angiogenesis still has to be further evaluated in patient studies. More research has to be done on a molecular level to fully understand the role of the different angiogenic molecules, because it is unlikely that any one molecule will represent angiogenic activity at every stage of tumor development in every tumor type.

Although most efforts currently focus on the integrin $\alpha v\beta 3$, its variable expression on tumor cells in some tumor types shows that it is sometimes not a marker of angiogenesis alone, but probably also of tumor aggressiveness and metastatic potential. Thus, an *in vivo* signal with this tracer could be from the tumor, the vessel, or both. More specific molecular markers for PET imaging of angiogenesis are eagerly awaited. Finally, by the introduction of combined PET/CT scanners, or even combined PET-MR scanners in the future, the simultaneous acquisition of functional parameters by DCE CT and DCE MRI and molecular parameters by PET with tracers like [^{18}F]-Galacto-RGD in one examination is possible and will probably be more widely used in forthcoming studies.

REFERENCES

1. Folkman J. Angiogenesis in cancer, vascular, rheumatoid and other disease. *Nat Med* 1995;1:27–31.
2. Folkman J. Tumor angiogenesis: therapeutic implications. *N Engl J Med* 1971;285:1182–1186.
3. Ribatti D, Vacca A, Dammacco F. The role of the vascular phase in solid tumor growth: a historical review. *Neoplasia* 1999;1:293–302.
4. Risau W. Mechanisms of angiogenesis. *Nature* 1997;386:671–674.
5. Kerbel RS. Antiangiogenic therapy: a universal chemosensitization strategy for cancer? *Science* 2006;312(5777):1171–1175.
6. Hurwitz H, Fehrenbacher L, Novotny W, et al. Bevacizumab plus irinotecan, fluorouracil, and leucovorin for metastatic colorectal cancer. *N Engl J Med* 2004;350(23):2335–2342.
7. Bergers G, Javaherian K, Lo KM, et al. Effects of angiogenesis inhibitors on multistage carcinogenesis in mice. *Science* 1999;284:808–812.
8. Miller JC, Pien HH, Sahani D, et al. Imaging angiogenesis: applications and potential for drug development. *J Natl Cancer Inst* 2005;97(3):172–187.
9. Jaffe CC. Measures of response: RECIST, WHO, and new alternatives. *J Clin Oncol* 2006;24(20):3245–3251.
10. Tortora G, Melisi D, Ciardiello F. Angiogenesis: a target for cancer therapy. *Curr Pharm Des* 2004;10(1):11–26.
11. Galbraith SM. Antivascular cancer treatments: imaging biomarkers in pharmaceutical drug development. *Br J Radiol* 2003;76:83–86.
12. Oshida K, Nagashima T, Ueda T, et al. Pharmacokinetic analysis of ductal carcinoma in situ of the breast using dynamic MR mammography. *Eur Radiol* 2005;15:1353–1360.
13. Padhani AR, Gapinski CJ, Macvicar DA, et al. Dynamic contrast enhanced MRI of prostate cancer: Correlation with morphology and tumour stage, histological grade and PSA. *Clin Radiol* 2000;55:99–109.
14. Schlemmer HP, Merkle J, Grobholz, R, et al. Can pre-operative contrast-enhanced dynamic MR imaging for prostate cancer predict microvessel density in prostatectomy specimens? *Eur Radiol* 2004;14:309–317.
15. Hara N, Okuizumi M, Koike H, et al. Dynamic contrast-enhanced magnetic resonance imaging (DCE-MRI) is a useful modality for the precise detection and staging of early prostate cancer. *Prostate* 2005;62:140–147.
16. Hawighorst H, Knapstein PG, Weikel W, et al. Angiogenesis of uterine cervical carcinoma: characterization by pharmacokinetic magnetic resonance parameters and histological microvessel density with correlation to lymphatic involvement. *Cancer Res* 1997;57:4777–4786.
17. Hawighorst H, Knapstein PG, Knopp MV, et al. Cervical carcinoma: standard and pharmacokinetic analysis of time-intensity curves for assessment of tumor angiogenesis and patient survival. *Magma* 1999;8:55–62.
18. Laking GR, Price PM. Positron emission tomographic imaging of angiogenesis and vascular function. *Br J Radiol* 2003;76:50–59.
19. Hylton N. Dynamic contrast-enhanced magnetic resonance imaging as an imaging biomarker. *J Clin Oncol* 2006;24(20):3293–3298.
20. O'Donnell A, Padhani A, Hayes C, et al. A phase I study of the angiogenesis inhibitor SU5416 (semaxanib) in solid tumours, incorporating dynamic contrast MR pharmacodynamic end points. *Br J Cancer* 2005;93:876–883.
21. Wedam SB, Low JA, Yang SX, et al. Antiangiogenic and antitumor effects of bevacizumab in inflammatory and locally advanced breast cancer patients. *J Clin Oncol* 2006;24:769–777.
22. Morgan B, Thomas AL, Drevs J, et al. Dynamic contrast-enhanced magnetic resonance imaging as a biomarker for the pharmacological response of PTK787/ZK 222584, an inhibitor of the vascular endothelial growth factor receptor tyrosine kinases, in patients with advanced colorectal cancer and liver metastases: results from two phase I studies. *J Clin Oncol* 2003;21:3955–3964.
23. Pio BS, Park CK, Pietras R, et al. Usefulness of 3′-[F-18]fluoro-3′-deoxythymidine with positron emission tomography in predicting breast cancer response to therapy. *Mol Imaging Biol* 2006;8:36–42.
24. Weber WA, Ott K, Becker K, et al. Prediction of response to preoperative chemotherapy in adenocarcinomas of the esophagogastric junction by metabolic imaging. *J Clin Oncol* 2001;19:3058–3065.
25. Carmeliet P. Mechanisms of angiogenesis and arteriogenesis. *Nat Med* 2000;6:389–395.
26. Auguste P, Lemiere S, Larrieu-Lahargue F. Molecular mechanisms of tumor vascularization. *Crit Rev Oncol Hematol* 2005;54(1):53–61.
27. Mousa SA, Mousa AS. Angiogenesis inhibitors: current and future directions. *Curr Pharmaceut Design* 2004;10:1–9.
28. Albo D, Wang TN, Tuszynski GP. Antiangiogenic therapy. *Curr Pharmaceut Design* 2004;10:27–37.
29. Holash J, Maisonpierre PC, Compton D, et al. Vessel cooption, regression, and growth in tumors mediated by angiopoietins and VEGF. *Science* 1999;284:1994–1998.
30. Nguyen M. Angiogenic factors as tumor markers. *Invest New Drugs* 1997;15:29–37.
31. Veikkola T, Karkkainen M, Claesson-Welsh L, et al. Regulation of angiogenesis via vascular endothelial growth factor receptors. *Cancer Res* 2000;60:203–212.
32. Morabito A, De Maio E, Di Maio M, et al. Tyrosine kinase inhibitors of vascular endothelial growth factor receptors in clinical trials: current status and future directions. *Oncologist* 2006;11(7):753–764.
33. Waltenberger J, Claesson-Welsh L, Siegbahn A, et al. Different signal transduction properties of KDR and Flt1, two receptors for vascular endothelial growth factor. *J Biol Chem* 1994;269:26988–26995.
34. Landgren E, Schiller P, Cao Y, et al. Placenta growth factor stimulates MAP kinase and mitogenicity but not phospholipase C-gamma and migration of endothelial cells expressing Flt 1. *Oncogene* 1998;16:359–367.
35. D'Angelo G, Struman I, Martial J, et al. Activation of mitogen-activated protein kinases by vascular endothelial growth factor and basic fibroblast growth factor in capillary endothelial cells is inhibited by the antiangiogenic factor 16-kDa N-terminal fragment of prolactin. *Proc Natl Acad Sci U S A* 1995;92:6374–6378.
36. Nor JE, Christensen J, Mooney DJ, et al. Vascular endothelial growth factor (VEGF)-mediated angiogenesis is associated with enhanced endothelial cell survival and induction of Bcl-2 expression. *Am J Pathol* 1999;154:375–384.
37. O'Connor DS, Schechner JS, Adida C, et al. Control of apoptosis during angiogenesis by survivin expression in endothelial cells. *Am J Pathol* 2000;156:393–398.

38. Kim I, Kim HG, So JN, et al. Angiopoietin-1 regulates endothelial cell survival through the phosphatidylinositol 3′-kinase/Akt signal transduction pathway. *Circ Res* 2000;86:24–29.
39. Paku S, Paweletz N. First steps of tumor-related angiogenesis. *Lab Invest* 1991;65:334–346.
40. Pettersson A, Nagy JA, Brown L, et al. Heterogeneity of the angiogenic response induced in different normal adult tissues by vascular permeability factor/vascular endothelial growth factor. *Lab Invest* 2000;80: 99–115.
41. Djonov V, Schmid M, Tschanz SA, et al. Intussusceptive angiogenesis: its role in embryonic vascular network formation. *Circ Res* 2000;86:286–292.
42. Patan S, Munn LL, Jain RK. Intussusceptive microvascular growth in a human colon adenocarcinoma xenograft: a novel mechanism of tumor angiogenesis. *Microvasc Res* 1996;51:260–272.
43. Metzger RJ, Krasnow MA. Genetic control of branching morphogenesis. *Science* 1999;284:1635–1639.
44. Ausprunk DH, Folkman J. Migration and proliferation of endothelial cells in preformed and newly formed blood vessels during tumor angiogenesis. *Microvasc Res* 1977;14:53–65.
45. Pepper MS, Ferrara N, Orci L, et al. Vascular endothelial growth factor (VEGF) induces plasminogen activators and plasminogen activator inhibitor-1 in microvascular endothelial cells. *Biochem Biophys Res Commun* 1991;181:902–906.
46. Denekamp J. Vascular attack as a therapeutic strategy for cancer. *Cancer Metastasis Rev* 1990;9:267–282.
47. Zetter BR. Migration of capillary endothelial cells is stimulated by tumour-derived factors. *Nature* 1980;285:41–59.
48. Asahara T, Chen D, Takahashi T, et al. Tie2 receptor ligands, angiopoietin-1 and angiopoietin-2, modulate VEGF-induced postnatal neovascularization. *Circ Res* 1998;83:233–240.
49. Maisonpierre PC, Suri C, Jones PF, et al. Angiopoietin-2, a natural antagonist for Tie2 that disrupts *in vivo* angiogenesis. *Science* 1997;277:55–60.
50. Friedlander M, Brooks PC, Shaffer RW, et al. Definition of two angiogenic pathways by distinct alpha v integrins. *Science* 1995;270:1500–1502.
51. Brooks PC, Montgomery AM, Rosenfeld M, et al. Integrin alpha v beta 3 antagonists promote tumor regression by inducing apoptosis of angiogenic blood vessels. *Cell* 1994;79:1157–1164.
52. Nelson AR, Fingleton B, Rothenberg ML, et al. Matrix metalloproteinases: biologic activity and clinical implications. *J Clin Oncol* 2000;18:1135–1149.
53. Sang QX. Complex role of matrix metalloproteinases in angiogenesis. *Cell Res* 1998;8:171–177.
54. Nangia-Makker P, Honjo Y, Sarvis R, et al. Galectin-3 induces endothelial cell morphogenesis and angiogenesis. *Am J Pathol* 2000;156:899–909.
55. Gamble J, Meyer G, Noack L, et al. B1 integrin activation inhibits in vitro tube formation: effects on cell migration, vacuole coalescence and lumen formation. *Endothelium* 1999;7:23–34.
56. Yang S, Graham J, Kahn JW, et al. Functional roles for PECAM-1 (CD31) and VEcadherin (CD144) in tube assembly and lumen formation in three-dimensional collagen gels. *Am J Pathol* 1999;155:887–895.
57. Lammertsma AA, Jones T. Low oxygen extraction fraction in tumours measured with the oxygen-15 steady state technique: effect of tissue heterogeneity. *Br J Radiol* 1992;65:697–700.
58. Blomqvist G, Lammertsma AA, Mazoyer B, et al. Effect of tissue heterogeneity on quantification in positron emission tomography. *Eur J Nucl Med* 1995;22:652–663.
59. Wilson CB, Lammertsma AA, McKenzie CG, et al. Measurements of blood flow and exchanging water space in breast tumors using positron emission tomography: a rapid and noninvasive dynamic method. *Cancer Res* 1992;52:1592–1597.
60. Anderson H, Price P. Clinical measurement of blood flow in tumours using positron emission tomography: a review. *Nucl Med Commun* 2002;23:131–138.
61. Ruotsalainen U, Raitakari M, Nuutila P, et al. Quantitative blood flow measurement of skeletal muscle using oxygen-15-water and PET. *J Nucl Med* 1997;38:314–319.
62. Tseng J, Dunnwald LK, Schubert EK, et al. ^{18}F-FDG kinetics in locally advanced breast cancer: correlation with tumor blood flow and changes in response to neoadjuvant chemotherapy. *J Nucl Med* 2004;45(11): 1829–1837.
63. Tofts PS, Brix G, Buckley DL, et al. Estimating kinetic parameters from dynamic contrast-enhanced T(1)-weighted MRI of a diffusable tracer: standardized quantities and symbols. *J Magn Reson Imaging* 1999; 10:223–232.
64. Padhani AR. Dynamic contrast-enhanced MRI in clinical oncology: current status and future directions. *J Magn Reson Imaging* 2002;16:407–422.
65. Kurdziel KA, Figg WD, Carrasquilo JA, et al. Using positron emission tomography 2-deoxy-2-[^{18}F]fluoro-D-glucose, ^{11}CO, and ^{15}O-water for monitoring androgen on dependent prostate cancer. *Mol Imaging Biol* 2003;5:86–93.
66. Anderson HL, Yap JT, Miller MP, et al. Assessment of pharmacodynamic vascular response in a phase I trial of Combretastatin A4 phosphate. *J Clin Oncol* 2003;21:2823–2830.
67. Hoffend J, Mier W, Schuhmacher J, et al. Gallium-68-DOTA-albumin as a PET blood pool marker: experimental evaluation *in vivo*. *Nucl Med Biol* 2005;32:287–292.
68. Brack SS, Dinkelborg L, Neri D. Molecular targeting of angiogenesis for imaging and therapy. *Eur J Nucl Med Mol Imaging* 2004;31:1327–1341.
69. Spuentrup E, Botnar RM. Coronary magnetic resonance imaging: visualization of vessel lumen and the vessel wall and molecular imaging of arteriotrombosis. *Eur Radiol* 2006;16:1–14.
70. Matsumoto K, Kitamura K, Mizuta T, et al. Performance characteristics of a new 3-dimensional continuous-emission and spiral-transmission high sensitivity and high resolution PET camera evaluated with the NEMA NU 2-2001 standard. *J Nucl Med* 2006;47:83–90.
71. Bach-Gansmo T, Danielsson R, Saracco A, et al. Integrin receptor imaging of breast cancer: a proof-of-concept study to evaluate ^{99m}Tc-NC100692. *J Nucl Med* 2006;47(9):1434–1439.
72. Haubner R, Weber WA, Beer AJ, et al. Non-invasive visualization of the activated $\alpha v\beta 3$ integrin in cancer patients by positron emission tomography and [^{18}F]Galacto-RGD. *PLoS Med* 2005;2:e70.
73. Ruoslahti E, Pierschbacher MD. New perspectives in cell adhesion: RGD and integrins. *Science* 1987;238(4826):491–497.
74. Haubner R, Finsinger D, Kessler H. Stereoisomeric peptide libraries and peptidomimetics for designing selective inhibitors of the $\alpha v\beta 3$ integrin for a new cancer therapy. *Angew Chem Int Ed Engl* 1997;36:1374–1389.
75. Haubner R, Wester HJ, Reuning U, et al. Radiolabeled $\alpha v\beta 3$ integrin antagonists: a new class of tracers for tumor targeting. *J Nucl Med* 1999;40:1061–1071.
76. Haubner R, Wester HJ, Weber WA, et al. Noninvasive imaging of $\alpha v\beta 3$ integrin expression using ^{18}F-labeled RGD-containing glycopeptide and positron emission tomography. *Cancer Res* 2001;61:1781–1785.
77. Haubner R. $\alpha v\beta 3$-integrin imaging: a new approach to characterise angiogenesis? *Eur J Nucl Med Mol Imaging* 2006;33:54–63.
78. Harris JM, Martin NE, Modi M. Pegylation: a novel process for modifying pharmacokinetics. *Clin Pharmacokinet* 2001;40:539–551.
79. Chen X, Park R, Shahinian AH, et al. Pharmacokinetics and tumor retention of ^{125}I-labeled RGD peptide are improved by PEGylation. *Nucl Med Biol* 2004;31:11–19.
80. van Hagen PM, Breeman WA, Bernard HF, et al. Evaluation of a radiolabelled cyclic DTPA-RGD analogue for tumour imaging and radionuclide therapy. *Int J Cancer* 2000;90:186–198.
81. Janssen MLH, Oyen WJG, Massuger LFAG, et al. Comparison of a monomeric and dimeric radiolabeled RGD-peptide for tumor imaging. *Cancer Biother Radiopharm* 2002;17:641–646.
82. Pichler BJ, Kneilling M, Haubner R, et al. Imaging of delayed-type hypersensitivity reaction by PET and ^{18}F-Galacto-RGD. *J Nucl Med* 2005;46:184–189.
83. Beer AJ, Haubner R, Goebel M, et al. Biodistribution and pharmacokinetics of the $\alpha v\beta 3$ selective tracer ^{18}F Galacto-RGD in cancer patients. *J Nucl Med* 2005;46:1333–1341.

84. Beer AJ, Haubner R, Wolf I, et al. PET-based human dosimetry of ^{18}F-galacto-RGD, a new radiotracer for imaging alpha v beta 3 expression. *J Nucl Med* 2006;47:763–769.
85. Beer AJ, Haubner R, Sarbia M, et al. Positron emission tomography using [^{18}F]Galacto-RGD identifies the level of integrin $\alpha v\beta 3$ expression in man. *Clin Cancer Res* 2006;12:3942–3949.
86. Gasparini G, Brooks PC, Biganzoli E, et al. Vascular integrin $\alpha v\beta 3$: a new prognostic indicator in breast cancer. *Clin Cancer Res* 1998;4: 2625–2634.
87. Hidalgo M, Eckhardt SG. Development of matrix metalloproteinase inhibitors in cancer therapy. *J Natl Cancer Inst* 2001;93(3):178–193.
88. Furumoto S, Takashima K, Kubota K, et al. Tumor detection using ^{18}F-labeled matrix metalloproteinase-2 inhibitor. *Nucl Med Biol* 2003;30(2): 119–125.
89. Fei X, Zheng QH, Liu X, et al. Synthesis of radiolabeled biphenylsulfonamide matrix metalloproteinase inhibitors as new potential PET cancer imaging agents. *Bioorg Med Chem Lett* 2003;13(13):2217–2222.
90. Blankenberg FG, Backer MV, Levashova Z, et al. *In vivo* tumor angiogenesis imaging with site-specific labeled (99m)Tc-HYNIC-VEGF. *Eur J Nucl Med Mol Imaging* 2006;33(7):841–848.
91. Collingridge DR, Carroll VA, Glaser M, et al. The development of [(^{124})I]iodinated-VG76e: a novel tracer for imaging vascular endothelial growth factor in vivo using positron emission tomography. *Cancer Res* 2002;62(20):5912–5919.
92. Li S, Peck-Radosavljevic M, Kienast O, et al. Imaging gastrointestinal tumours using vascular endothelial growth factor-165 (VEGF165) receptor scintigraphy. *Ann Oncol* 2003;14:1274–1277.
93. Jayson GC, Zweit J, Jackson A, et al. Molecular imaging and biological evaluation of HuMV833 anti-VEGF antibody: implications for trial design of antiangiogenic antibodies. *J Natl Cancer Inst* 2002;94(19):1484–1493.
94. Neri D, Carnemolla B, Nissim A, et al. Targeting by affinity matured recombinant antibody fragments of an angiogenesis associated fibronectin isoform. *Nat Biotechnol* 1997;15:1271–1275.
95. Santimaria M, Moscatelli G, Viale GL, et al. Immunoscintigraphic detection of the ED-B domain of fibronectin, a marker of angiogenesis, in patients with cancer. *Clin Cancer Res* 2003;9:571–579.
96. Huminiecki L, Gorn M, Suchting S, et al. Magic roundabout is a new member of the roundabout receptor family that is endothelial specific and expressed at sites of active angiogenesis. *Genomics* 2002;79: 547–552.
97. Vallon M, Essler M. Proteolytically processed soluble tumor endothelial marker (TEM) 5 mediates endothelial cell survival during angiogenesis by linking integrin alpha v beta 3 to glycosaminoglycans. *J Biol Chem* 2006;28(15):31179–31100.

CHAPTER

14.4 Progress in Amyloid Imaging

BRIAN J. LOPRESTI, WILLIAM E. KLUNK, AND CHESTER A. MATHIS

Alzheimer's disease (AD) is the most prevalent form of dementia afflicting the elderly population and is characterized by a progressive loss of memory and cognitive function. AD is one of the leading causes of death in industrialized societies, and afflicts more than 4 million Americans and an estimated 30 million people worldwide (1–4). Presently, a definitive diagnosis of AD can only be made at autopsy when the presence of the pathologic hallmarks of the disease, amyloid plaques, and neurofibrillary tangles (NFTs) can be confirmed (5).

BRIEF SURVEY OF ALZHEIMER'S DISEASE PATHOLOGY

Amyloid plaques are comprised of fibrillar deposits of the amyloid-β (Aβ) peptide, which varies from 40-42 amino acids in length (6). Amyloid plaques can be classified as either diffuse or neuritic, the latter being characterized by a dense central core of Aβ fibrils that stain with dyes such as Congo red or thioflavin-S and are surrounded by glial cells and abnormal neuritic processes. NFTs are comprised of intraneuronal fibrillar deposits of a hyperphosphorylated form of the microtubule-associated protein tau (7), which have a characteristic looplike appearance and are also stained with Congo red and thioflavin-S.

Plaques occur earliest in the neocortex, where they are relatively evenly distributed (8), while NFTs appear first in limbic areas, such as the transentorhinal cortex and progress in a predictable pattern to the neocortex (9). Topological studies of the distribution of neuritic plaques and NFTs in AD brains revealed plaques to be more evenly distributed throughout the cortex than NFTs. The exceptions are the limbic periallocortex and allocortex (including the hippocampal formation), where NFTs are most concentrated and neuritic plaques are much less abundant (10,11). The cerebellum was found to be free of neuritic plaques and NFTs, even in late-stage AD, although it is not uncommon for diffuse cerebellar amyloid deposits to be observed in cerebellum (12,13).

The vast majority of cases of AD can be classified as sporadic, as no clear genetic or environmental causes have been identified. For sporadic AD, the most significant risk factor for developing the disease is age, with prevalence increasing from approximately 5% at age 70 to as high as 45% at age 85 (14). A small fraction of cases of AD (approximately 1%) can be attributed to specific genetic mutations with autosomal-dominant inheritance (15,16). These mutations occur in domains that encode the amyloid precursor protein (APP), the precursor to the 40 to 42 amino acid Aβ peptides that comprise amyloid plaques, or in domains encoding the presenilin proteins PS-1 and PS-2 that are believed to be involved in APP processing. These rare cases, classified as early onset familial AD (eoFAD), result in early AD pathology with 100% penetrance in gene carriers.

Although eoFAD does not represent a dominant public health concern, the study of this small population is particularly interesting as it permits the identification of a pool of subjects (carriers of the mutations) who are ensured of developing AD pathology years or decades before the onset of symptoms. Longitudinal assessments of brain amyloid burden using a noninvasive imaging agent in eoFAD subjects may provide a unique opportunity to elucidate the natural history of brain amyloid deposition.

Mild cognitive impairment (MCI) is a condition characterized by isolated memory impairment or impairments in several cognitive domains. The cognitive impairments are similar to those seen in patients with AD, but they are not severe or pervasive enough to meet the diagnostic criteria for AD (17). Although MCI patients convert to AD at a rate of 10% to 15% per year, 30% to 40% of MCI patients remain stable or do not convert to AD over 5 to 10 years (18). A great deal of effort has been directed toward detecting what clinical characteristics of MCI are predictive of conversion to AD, but a variety of underlying pathologic substrates and the relative mildness and heterogeneity of clinical symptoms have complicated these efforts.

Role of Amyloid in Alzheimer's Disease Target for Therapeutics

Aβ plaques in the brain are a pathologic hallmark of the dementia first characterized by Alois Alzheimer's in 1906, and a considerable body of evidence implicates elevated Aβ levels and the deposition of Aβ plaques as central events in the pathogenesis of AD (19). Perhaps the most compelling piece of evidence supporting this "amyloid cascade hypothesis" is that rare mutations in chromosome 21 result in abnormal processing of APP and cause eoFAD (20). Also compelling is the observation that mutations in the region of chromosome 14 that codes PS-1, which is believed to be an essential component of the γ-secretase complex that cleaves Aβ from APP, are the most common genetic causes of autosomal dominant eoFAD (21). Thus, these rare eoFAD cases have established that altered metabolism of APP results in increased Aβ and clinical AD.

A logical corollary of the amyloid cascade hypothesis is that decreased cerebral levels of Aβ should help prevent or delay the onset of AD. Indeed, the development of antiamyloid therapies is an active area of drug discovery and investigation. Some prospective antiamyloid therapies focus on means to decrease production of Aβ by inhibiting the β- or γ-secretase enzymes, which are responsible for cleaving Aβ from its precursor APP (22). Another antiamyloid approach seeks to increase clearance of Aβ by active immunization with Aβ or passive immunization with anti-Aβ antibodies (23,24).

Given the increasing incidence of AD with age, coupled with the aging of the population, AD threatens to become one of the most significant public health concerns of the 21st century. The economic implications of increased AD prevalence have motivated a vigorous effort to identify potential new treatments for AD. Novel technologies capable of identifying subjects destined to develop AD prior to the onset of clinical symptoms will prove to be invaluable, as therapeutic interventions most likely will be optimally effective in the preclinical phase of the disease prior to irreversible neurological damage. Imaging technologies capable of noninvasively quantifying the hallmark characteristics of AD, amyloid plaques and NFTs in the brain, using positron emission tomography (PET) or single-photon emission computed tomography (SPECT) show promise as potential biomarkers for brain amyloidosis.

Motivation for Amyloid Imaging

A technique able to localize and quantify amyloid deposition in the living brain would represent a major advancement in the study of the pathophysiology and treatment of AD. A logical application for such a tool would be to critically assess the amyloid cascade hypothesis in longitudinal studies of at-risk, presymptomatic subjects (e.g., elderly controls and carriers of mutations causing eoFAD). Amyloid imaging might also provide key information that could help predict which MCI patients would and would not progress to AD. This information could provide a key piece of information that would allow clinicians to identify patients most likely to benefit from intervention with an antiamyloid therapeutic.

A third important application of such a tool would be to accelerate the development of antiamyloid therapies by providing quantitative observations of brain amyloid burden pre- and posttreatment. This would provide rapid feedback regarding the efficacy of candidate therapies, which could streamline efforts by focusing on the rapid development of the most promising therapies.

Although amyloid imaging agents are relative newcomers to the armamentarium of molecular imaging agents, they are beginning to provide some valuable (and sometimes unexpected) information that is helping to elucidate the mechanisms of AD and other dementias. This chapter summarizes what has been learned to date in this short but exciting journey.

TRACERS FOR PET AMYLOID IMAGING STUDIES IN HUMANS

Radiolabeled Monoclonal Antibody Fragments

The earliest documented attempts to image amyloid deposits in the brains of patients with AD using noninvasive imaging techniques employed a monoclonal antibody fragment, 10H3, which was targeted to the first 28 amino acids of the Aβ peptide. Labeled with technetium-99m (^{99m}Tc) for SPECT imaging, [^{99m}Tc]-10H3 exhibited some promising preclinical results, as it was demonstrated to bind significantly to neuritic plaques and cerebrovascular amyloid deposits on autoradiographic sections of human brain (25,26). However, systemic injection of [^{99m}Tc]-10H3 showed negligible brain entry that could not distinguish AD from control subjects (27). It is likely that the relatively large molecular weight of the agent contributed to low brain entry. This was not an altogether unexpected result, as poor blood–brain barrier penetration is a common feature of large molecular weight radiolabeled antibody fragments that limits their utility for molecular imaging of the brain (28). Although it may be possible to achieve detectible brain concentrations of radiolabeled antibody fragments after a protracted period of uptake of several days, the short biological half-life of 10H3 and the relatively short half-life of ^{99m}Tc (6 hours) rendered this approach impractical for visualizing brain amyloid deposits *in vivo*. Subsequent attempts to image amyloid *in vivo* focused on lipophilic small molecules capable of readily penetrating the blood–brain barrier.

Fluorine-18-FDDNP

A radiofluorinated derivative (termed FDDNP; Fig. 14.4.1) of the solvent- and viscosity-sensitive fluorophore 2-[1-[6-(dimethylamino)-2-naphthyl]ethylidene]malononitrile (DDNP) was the first PET agent to be investigated in humans for the purpose of visualizing amyloid *in vivo*. Agdeppa et al. (29,30) reported that FDDNP bound to both amyloid plaques and NFTs *in vitro*, and FDDNP was shown to bind with high affinity (K_d = 0.12 nM) to synthetic Aβ(1-40) fibrils using a fluorescence assay method (29). No binding assays using radioligand binding assay methods or cortical brain homogenates from pathologically confirmed AD subjects have been reported with FDDNP, nor have binding affinities for FDDNP to tau or NFTs been reported to date. Initial human studies of fluorine-18-labeled FDDNP ([^{18}F] FDDNP) in AD patients (n = 9) and controls (n = 7) showed greater retention in frontal, parietal, temporal, and occipital cortices at steady state (60 to 120 minutes postinjection), although this increased cortical retention was shown to exceed the reference region (pons) by only 10% to 15% (31). The area of highest retention at equilibrium was the mesial temporal cortex (MTC), including hippocampus, amygdala, and

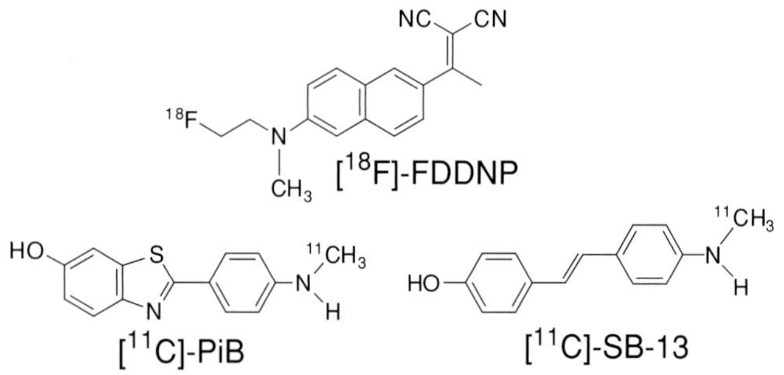

FIGURE 14.4.1. Structures of three PET amyloid imaging agents whose properties in human brain imaging studies have been reported. Radiofluorinated fluorophore 2-[1-[6-(dimethylamino)-2-naphthyl]-ethylidene]malononitrile (FDDNP) is radiolabeled with fluorine-18 (110-minute half-life), while Pittsburgh compound-B (PiB) and stilbene derivative 4-*N*-methylamino-4′-hydroxystilbene (SB-13) are radiolabeled with carbon-11 (20-minute half-life).

entorhinal cortex, and retention of [^{18}F]-FDDNP in the MTC was shown to exceed retention in the pons by 30%. The mesial temporal cortex is a region known to be relatively free of neuritic plaques, but relatively enriched in NFTs compared to cortex (9,32).

Initial analyses of [^{18}F]-FDDNP PET data were performed using a novel kinetic analysis method, termed the relative residence time (RRT), which equates specific binding of radiotracer to the negative net difference between the reciprocal of the tissue clearance constants (k_2) for the reference and amyloid-laden tissues. Although the authors demonstrated significantly longer RRT values for AD patients compared to controls, RRT values appeared to be sensitive to both peak and steady-state levels of [^{18}F]-FDDNP in tissue. (31) This dependence on peak and steady-state radiotracer concentrations may result in an untoward influence of blood flow and transport phenomenon on the overall [^{18}F]-FDDNP outcome measure. RRT estimates differed by a factor of 15 or more in brain regions with identical late-time levels of tracer, such as temporal and occipital cortex, indicating that it was the difference in peak entry levels into these brain areas that was driving the difference in RRT.

The applicability of conventional quantitative analysis methodologies, such as compartmental modeling and graphical analyses, to dynamic [^{18}F]FDDNP PET data remains to be demonstrated, although a recent report employed the noninvasive Logan graphical analysis (33) without demonstrating attainment of steady-state conditions (34). These studies are necessary to fully understand the nature of [^{18}F]-FDDNP retention and to assess the overall sensitivity and specificity of the compound for the detection of AD pathology *in vivo*.

Carbon-11-Pittsburgh Compound-B

A carbon-11-labeled benzothiazole derivative of the amyloid dye thioflavin-T, termed Pittsburgh compound-B (PiB; Fig. 14.4.1), was the second PET agent to be employed in human *in vivo* amyloid imaging studies (35,36). Tritiated-PiB was shown to bind specifically and with high affinity (K_d = 1.4 nM) to frontal cortex brain homogenates from pathologically confirmed AD subjects, while cerebellar and white matter tissue did not bind [^{3}H]-PiB specifically (37). In addition, [^{3}H]-PiB bound to synthetic Aβ(1-40) fibrils with a similar high affinity (K_d = 4.7 nM). The initial human study of [^{11}C]-PiB by Klunk et al. included 16 patients with mild AD (minimental state examination [MMSE] scores of 18 to 28) and nine healthy control subjects. Compared to controls, AD patients showed greater than twofold higher retention of [^{11}C]-PiB in areas of brain association cortex known to contain large amounts of amyloid deposits in AD (P <.002), but the levels of retention in areas known to be relatively unaffected by amyloid pathology (e.g., subcortical white matter, pons and cerebellum; P >.2) were equivalent.

Later investigations built on this proof-of-concept study and aimed to extend these observations to include longer periods of data acquisition (90 minutes), coregistered magnetic resonance images for precise region-of-interest definition, and arterial input function determination. These refinements sought to identify a valid and robust compartmental model that described the *in vivo* kinetics of [^{11}C]-PiB across the spectrum of control and AD subjects. These fully quantitative analyses concluded that the [^{11}C]-PiB PET data were well described by a two-tissue four-parameter (2T-4*k*) compartmental model that assumed reversible *in vivo* kinetics and negligible occupancy of the binding sites by the radiotracer or carrier. These studies also identified the distribution volume ratio (DVR) as the preferred outcome measure, as it provided a reliable nonnegative index of amyloid deposition in both AD and control subjects (38).

Although the 2T-4*k* model was found to best describe [^{11}C]-PiB kinetics *in vivo*, difficulties in estimating small parameter values in regions with little or low signal (i.e., control brain or cerebellum) resulted in spuriously overestimated DVR values and hence higher test-retest variability. For this reason, the Logan graphical analysis (39) using 90 minutes of data (ART90) was investigated as a potential alternative to the 2T-4*k* analysis. ART90 methods showed significantly lower intersubject variability than the 2T-4*k* analysis (generally 10% to 20%), although DVR measures obtained using the two methods were strongly correlated (r ~0.9) across all regions of interest.

ART90 DVR measures were found to be approximately twofold higher in cortical regions of AD subjects, relative to controls. These findings, coupled with an observed test-retest variability of approximately 7% across regions, identified ART90 as the optimum arterial-input–based method for human [^{11}C]-PiB studies and the method against which later simplified methods of analysis would be compared.

Anticipating the widespread use of [^{11}C]-PiB in an elderly demented population, more recent investigations sought to simplify the experimental paradigm for [^{11}C]-PiB assessments of brain amyloid burden to make the procedure more practical and tolerable to the subject. The simplifications examined included (a) a shortened scan duration of 60 minutes; (b) the use of an image-derived arterial input function from the carotid artery and a population metabolite correction; (c) the implementation of cerebellar reference tissue methods; and (d) the use of a single late-scan measure of the radioactivity distribution normalized for injected dose, body mass, and nonspecific retention of [^{11}C]-PiB.

These studies demonstrated that several simplified methods of analysis performed satisfactorily when compared to the benchmark ART90 method identified by Price et al. (38), although there were tradeoffs in methodologic bias, intersubject and intrasubject variability, and ease of implementation that could make the best choice of simplified methods of analysis application dependent (40). The most simplified method examined employed a ratio of regional to cerebellar standardized uptake values (SUVR) determined over the 40 to 60 minutes (SUVR60) and 40 to 90 minutes (SUVR90) postinjection intervals. The SUVR methods showed lower intersubject variability compared to ART90, test-retest variability that ranged from 3.3% to 8.0%, the largest effect sizes (6.9) of any method examined, and excellent agreement with ART90 DVR values ($r^2 = 0.93$). The ease of implementation of the SUVR method and the need to collect as little as 20 minutes of emission data make this method especially attractive for large cross-sectional or multisite trials in human subjects.

Carbon-11-SB-13

The stilbene derivative 4-*N*-methylamino-4′-hydroxystilbene (SB-13; Fig. 14.4.1) is the most recently reported PET amyloid imaging agent to be investigated in human subjects (41). Tritiated-SB-13 was shown to bind specifically and with high affinity ($K_d = 2.4$ nM) to cortical brain homogenates from pathologically confirmed AD subjects, while cerebellar and white matter tissue did not bind [^{3}H]-SB-13 specifically. Film autoradiography of [^{3}H]-SB-13 was shown to label Aβ plaques in sections of human AD cortex, but not in control brain. These favorable *in vitro* properties supported the continued investigation of SB-13 as a potential molecular imaging probe for the noninvasive assessment of brain amyloid deposition in human subjects.

SB-13 was labeled with carbon-11 for PET studies of AD subjects (n = 5) and healthy controls (n = 6) (41). For the purpose of comparison, these subjects also underwent a second PET scan using [^{11}C]-PiB. Following the injection of [^{11}C]-SB-13, the cerebellum exhibited similar retention characteristics between AD patients and controls, although clearance of the nonspecific binding of [^{11}C]-SB-13 was significantly slower than that observed for [^{11}C]-PiB in the same subjects. Increased retention of [^{11}C]-SB-13 was observed in AD subjects compared to controls in cortical areas known to contain significant amyloid deposits in AD, such as the frontal cortex.

Using [^{11}C]-SB-13, SUV values in frontal cortex ranged from a factor of 1.40 to 1.74 times control SUV values, while for the same subjects the ratio of AD to control SUV values for [^{11}C]-PiB ranged from 1.96 to 2.52 times control values. The data suggest that decreased clearance of nonspecific binding resulted in less discrimination between control and AD subject groups. Although the pattern of retention of [^{11}C]-SB-13 in AD subjects appears to mirror that observed for [^{11}C]-PiB, the decreased dynamic range observed using [^{11}C]-SB-13 might result in poorer distinction of AD subjects from controls than [^{11}C]-PiB. Nevertheless, the relative success of [^{11}C]-SB-13 as an amyloid imaging agent suggests that this class of stilbene derivatives has the potential to yield agents that may possess more favorable qualities.

PET AMYLOID IMAGING STUDIES IN HUMANS

Normal Control Subjects (Pittsburgh Compound-B-Negative)

In order to assess the utility of amyloid imaging agents, it is important to characterize such agents in a population of control subjects. Ideally, such investigations would be carried out in young control subjects who are free of brain amyloid deposits, as significant amyloid deposits have been found in postmortem brains from normal elderly subjects with no cognitive impairments at the time of death (11). Young control subjects are also less likely to be affected by comorbid diseases that could impact the delivery and metabolism of the prospective amyloid imaging agent, such as atherosclerosis, hypertension, cardiac disease, impaired liver function, and normal age-related brain atrophy. These investigations provide critical observations of the nonspecific binding properties of the agents that are necessary to interpret subsequent studies in a diseased population.

In the initial proof of concept study of [^{11}C]-PiB (36), data were presented from nine control subjects. Three of these subjects were young control subjects (21 years of age), while the remaining six control subjects were matched in age to the cohort of 16 AD subjects (69.5 ± 11 years of age). The young control subjects showed rapid entry of [^{11}C]-PiB into all cortical and subcortical gray matter regions, followed by rapid clearance from all gray matter regions. Most elderly control subjects showed a nearly identical pattern (see also the section "Normal Control Subjects [Pittsburgh Compound-B Positive]" below). Lower uptake and slower clearance of [^{11}C]-PiB was observed in subcortical white matter and pons, which was emphasized in late-scan SUV images. However, the degree of white matter retention of [^{11}C]-PiB was shown to be identical across young control, elderly control, and AD subjects (36,38,40) and does not confound efforts to assess [^{11}C]-PiB retention in gray matter regions where the vast majority of AD amyloid pathology is confined. The cerebellum, a region known from postmortem studies to be devoid of neuritic plaques, showed identical uptake and retention characteristics in control and AD subjects. No statistically significant differences in the nonspecific retention of [^{11}C]-PiB were observed between young and elderly control subjects in the original [^{11}C]-PiB study (36).

In a more recent study, Lopresti et al. (40) examined the Logan DVR outcome measure for [^{11}C]-PiB with cerebellum as the reference region (33) in the cortical regions (frontal, parietal, temporal, and occipital cortices) of eight elderly control subjects over 90 minutes postinjection (Fig. 14.4.2). The cortical DVR values of [^{11}C]-PiB in the consolidated control subject group ranged from 1.24 ± 0.12 (frontal cortex) to 1.02 ± 0.06 (mesial temporal cortex). DVR values in pons and subcortical white matter were somewhat higher than cortical regions (1.47 ± 0.08 and 1.33 ± 0.06 DVR units, respectively), and this white matter and pons retention of [^{11}C]-PiB is believed to be nonspecific in nature, as few amyloid plaques are found in postmortem white matter tissue in AD subjects. Consistent with this interpretation, DVR values in white matter regions were not significantly different between the control and AD groups ($P > 0.2$). The degree of intersubject variability was shown to vary somewhat across methods of analysis, but in general ranged from 5% to 25% across regions and methods of analysis (40).

A recent report detailing a large study of [^{18}F]-FDDNP included data from a group of 30 elderly control subjects (64 ± 15 years of age) (34). DVR values were estimated using the noninvasive Logan graphical analysis (33) over the 35 to 125 minutes postinjection interval and a cerebellar reference region. The control group showed DVR values (Fig. 14.4.3) that ranged from 1.03 ± 0.03 (frontal cortex) to 1.11 ± 0.03 (mesial temporal cortex), which were in general agreement with [^{11}C]-PiB control DVR values determined in control subjects using the same method of analysis (40). Fluorine-18-FDDNP showed lower intersubject variability in the control group (approximately 3% across regions) than that reported for [^{11}C]-PiB using this method of analysis, and this may

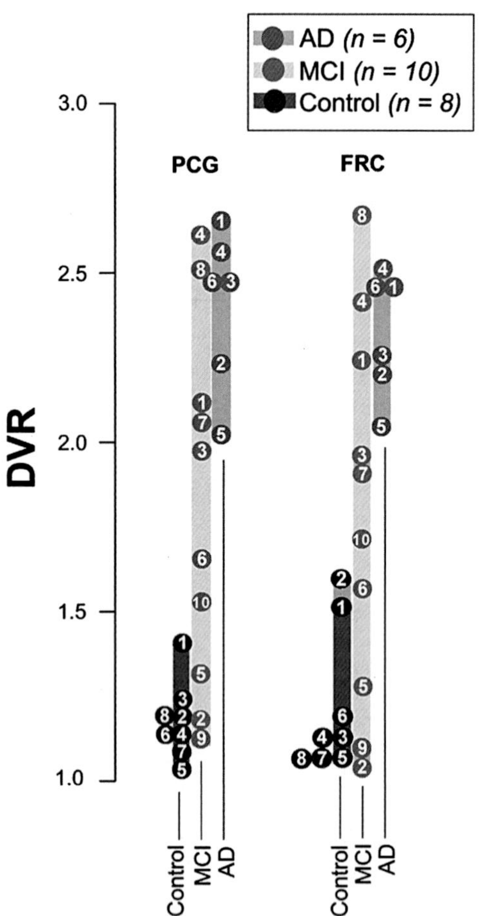

FIGURE 14.4.2. Distribution volume ratio (DVR) outcome measures of [^{11}C]-PiB for individual control (n = 8), mild cognitive impairment (MCI) (n = 10), and Alzheimer's disease (AD) (n = 6) subjects for posterior cingulate gyrus (PCG) and frontal cortex (FRC) regions of interest. The regional DVR outcome measures were determined using the noninvasive Logan graphical analysis method with cerebellum as the reference region over 90 minutes postinjection. The numbered circles represent the individual subjects, while the bars denote the range of values within the group. Subjects with overlapping values are placed adjacent to one another. (Adapted from Lopresti BJ, Klunk WE, Mathis CA, et al. Simplified quantification of Pittsburgh compound B amyloid imaging PET studies: a comparative analysis. *J Nucl Med* 2005;46(12): 1959–1972, with permission.)

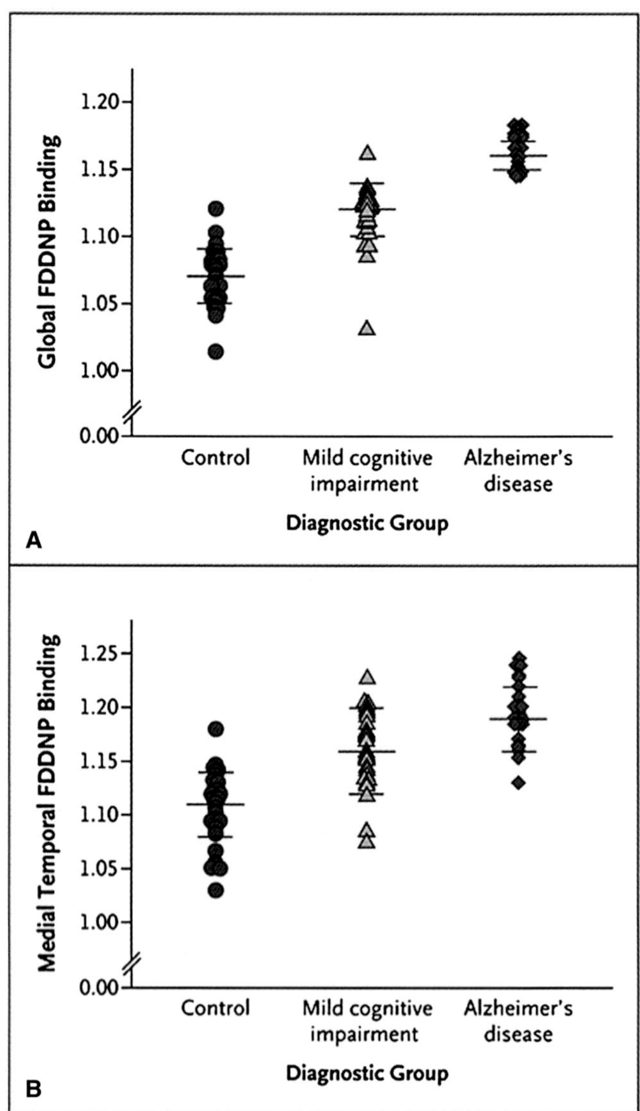

FIGURE 14.4.3. Baseline values for fluorine-18-fluorophore 2-[1-[6-(dimethylamino)-2-naphthyl]ethylidene]malononitrile ([^{18}F]-FDDNP) global cortical binding (**A**) and medial temporal cortex binding (**B**), according to diagnostic group. [^{18}F]-FDDNP binding is expressed in terms of the distribution volume ratio (DVR) derived by the noninvasive Logan graphical analysis using cerebellum as reference region. (From Small GW, Kepe V, Ercoli LM, et al. PET of brain amyloid and tau in mild cognitive impairment. *N Engl J Med* 2006;355(25): 2652–2663, with permission. ©2006 Massachusetts Medical Society. All rights reserved.)

be attributable either to a significantly larger sample size in the case of the [^{18}F]-FDDNP study (n = 30 vs. n = 8 controls) or to the relatively small dynamic range of [^{18}F]-FDDNP DVR values.

Alzheimer's Disease

The initial report of [^{11}C]-PiB in an AD subject showed significantly increased retention of the tracer in cortical regions known from the postmortem literature to contain large amounts of neuritic plaques in AD (35). Although this first indication of the potential utility of [^{11}C]-PiB as an amyloid imaging agent was compelling, more definitive studies were needed to confirm the initial demonstration and characterize the nature of the increased signal observed in the cortex of AD subjects. These subsequent studies showed that retention of [^{11}C]-PiB in AD subjects was approximately twofold higher in amyloid-laden cortical regions than in control subjects (Fig. 14.4.2), while nonspecific retention of [^{11}C]-PiB was not significantly different between groups (36,40–43).

In the 2004 report by Klunk et al. (36), the control and AD subject groups were clearly differentiated in cortical regions (P <0.0001 in frontal cortex), although there were three subjects classified as AD, which showed [^{11}C]-PiB SUV values in the control range (36). Closer examination of these subjects revealed that they had high MMSE scores of 28 to 29 at the time of scanning, and that these scores had not decreased over the previous 2 to 4 years. In addition, these three subjects did not show any discernible parietal [^{18}F]-fluorodeoxyglucose (FDG) PET metabolic defect. It is likely that these three subjects represented cases in which [^{11}C]-PiB correctly identified subjects for which the pathologic diagnosis would not have corroborated the clinical diagnosis of probable AD. Indeed, a 2-year follow-up of these same three subjects continued to exhibit no significant [^{11}C]-PiB retention, normal parietal glucose metabolism, and no progression of cognitive symptoms. They were subsequently reclassified as mild cognitive impairment by clinicians who were blind to the [^{11}C]-PiB PET findings (44).

A recent [^{11}C]-PiB study by Edison et al. (42) in 19 AD subjects found two subjects fulfilling the clinical criteria for AD, but with normal range on [^{11}C]-PiB scans. Careful longitudinal follow-up in these subjects will help determine the accuracy of the clinical diagnosis or the [^{11}C]-PiB scan results.

The 2004 study by Klunk et al. (36) using [^{11}C]-PiB in AD subjects showed that there was some variability in the degree of amyloid present in the brain, although the mild to moderate AD subjects studied were fairly homogeneous in terms of their degree of cognitive impairment (MMSE: 24.9 ± 3.4). A more detailed regional analysis than that included in the initial report of [^{11}C]-PiB in humans revealed that the posterior cingulate/precuneus and frontal cortex regions showed the highest levels of [^{11}C]-PiB binding (38,40). The posterior cingulate gyrus has been considered a critically important region to sample in PET studies designed to facilitate early detection of AD in a presymptomatic population (45,46).

Recently Engler et al. (44) reported the follow-up of 16 patients with AD who were recruited as part of the initial proof of concept study of [^{11}C]-PiB (36). These 16 subjects were re-examined using [^{11}C]-PiB and [^{18}F]-FDG after a mean interval of 2.0 ± 0.5 years from their initial scans. No significant differences in the degree of [^{11}C]-PiB retention were observed between the baseline and follow-up scan, while cortical regional cerebral glucose metabolic rates measured showed an approximately 20% decline over the same interval. MMSE scores also showed a small decline during this period, from 24.3 ± 3.7 to 22.7 ± 6.1, although this decline in cognitive performance did not reach the threshold of statistical significance. Although some technical aspects of the study may have complicated the interpretation of the data, such as the lack of magnetic resonance coregistration and correction for the dilutional effects of brain atrophy (47), the finding that [^{11}C]-PiB retention in AD remained unchanged over a period of observation of 2 years was not surprising. It is well established that postmortem amyloid deposits do not correlate well with cognitive performance (32,48).

Evidence suggests that the process of amyloid deposition is not continually progressive throughout the course of the disease, but rather reaches a maximum point and may decline in the later stages of the disease (49). Interestingly, the subjects in the Engler et al. (44) study who had the most advanced AD at baseline and who showed the most severe cognitive decline at follow-up actually showed a decrease in [^{11}C]-PiB retention over the 2-year interval. These findings are consistent with a model of AD that includes an early phase of initiation of amyloid deposition, followed by a brief period of rapid progression, and finally a period of relative equilibrium that may be punctuated or terminated by periods of regressive amyloid plaque pathology.

This study represents an important first look at the natural history of amyloid deposition, but it is important to consider that it may record only one epoch of that history, and that the most significant changes in brain amyloid burden may occur years before the presentation of clinical symptoms. Indeed, postmortem studies in Down syndrome, a genetic disorder that results from a third copy of chromosome 21 and for which amyloid plaque pathology is typically observed by midlife, indicate that plaque formation may antecede clinical symptoms by a decade or more (50,51).

Although it will take considerably more effort to truly define the natural history of amyloid deposition using amyloid imaging agents, these agents have the power to reveal what could previously only be speculated regarding the pathogenesis of AD. An agent that directly indexed amyloid burden in the brain could be a useful surrogate end point for a clinical trial of an antiamyloid therapeutic.

Fluorine-18-FDDNP studies have also been recently reported in a study that included 25 patients (73 ± 9 years of age) with mild to moderate AD (34). Small et al. (34) showed that global [^{18}F]-FDDNP binding was increased significantly (P <0.001) in AD patients relative to controls (Fig. 14.4.3). Previously, Agdeppa et al. (29) reported that [^{18}F]-FDDNP binds to both amyloid plaques and NFTs *in vitro*, although the relative contribution of each of these components to the [^{18}F]-FDDNP PET signal is unclear. In the 2006 study, Small et al. (34) reported average DVR values in AD subjects that ranged from 1.11 ± 0.02 in the frontal cortex to 1.19 ± 0.03 in the medial temporal region. Average DVR values of [^{18}F]-FDDNP in the control subjects ranged from 1.03 ± 0.03 in the frontal cortex to 1.11 ± 0.03 in the medial temporal cortex. Interestingly, this pattern was opposite to that observed with [^{11}C]-PiB and [^{11}C]-SB-13, and suggests that the retention of [^{18}F]-FDDNP is not driven predominantly by Aβ plaque load.

Based on the finding that FDDNP stains NFTs in postmortem tissue sections at a concentration of 10 μM (approximately 10,000-fold higher than concentrations attained *in vivo* with PET imaging) (29), it has been suggested that [^{18}F]-FDDNP can detect both amyloid plaques and NFTs in human PET studies (34). It is relevant to note that PiB and other benzothiazoles also stain NFTs at these high micromolar concentrations, but do not bind specifically to NFTs at low nanomolar concentrations used in PET studies (52).

Mild Cognitive Impairment

Amyloid imaging of subjects with a diagnosis of MCI is perhaps one of the most important and anticipated applications of these new agents. Although MCI can be considered a prodromal stage of AD in 60% to 70% of the patients diagnosed, the remaining 30% to 40% do not progress to AD over 5 to 10 years of follow-up (53–56). In some of these cases, the cognitive symptoms of MCI can be attributed to other dementias, such as vascular dementia or frontotemporal dementia, which are not characterized by neuritic amyloid plaques. An amyloid imaging agent could be used to identify those MCI patients likely to progress to AD, could improve the clinical management of this heterogeneous class of patients, and also could identify those patients who would most likely benefit from antiamyloid therapies.

The initial report of the use of an amyloid-imaging agent in MCI reflected the expected pathologic heterogeneity of the disorder. In a small sample of five MCI subjects, Price et al. (38) found that three of five subjects showed cortical [^{11}C]-PiB binding measures in the same range as the AD subjects, while the remaining two

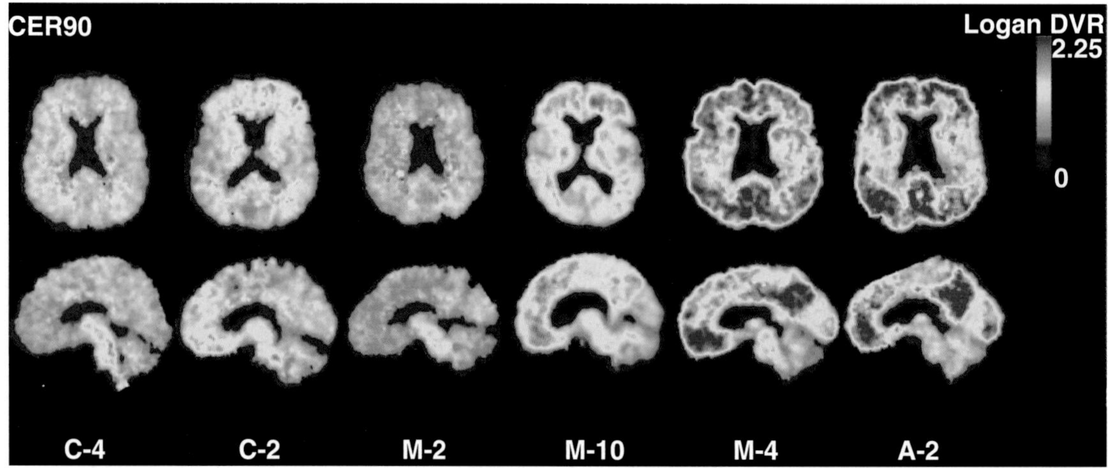

FIGURE 14.4.4. Carbon 11-Pittsburgh compound-B ([^{11}C]-PiB) parametric images of the reference Logan distribution volume ratio (DVR) using cerebellar tissue (CER90) as input. Shown are a young control (*C-4*) ([^{11}C]-PiB-negative), a control with detectable amyloid deposition in frontal cortex (*C-2*) (PiB-positive), a [^{11}C]-PiB-negative mild cognitive impairment (MCI) subject (*M-2*), an MCI subject with intermediate levels of [^{11}C]-PiB retention (*M-10*), a [^{11}C]-PiB-positive MCI subject with levels of [^{11}C]-PiB retention characteristic of AD (*M-4*), and a typical AD subject (*A-2*). (From Lopresti BJ, Klunk WE, Mathis CA, et al. Simplified quantification of Pittsburgh compound B amyloid imaging PET studies: a comparative analysis. *J Nucl Med* 2005;46(12):1959–1972, with permission. © 2005. All rights reserved.)

subjects were indistinguishable from controls. A subsequent report including ten MCI subjects showed the same dichotomization of the MCI subject group. Five of ten MCI subjects were indistinguishable from the AD group in terms of cortical [^{11}C]-PiB binding, while three of ten were indistinguishable from the controls (40). Interestingly, only two of the ten subjects exhibited intermediate values between those of the control group and the AD subjects (Fig. 14.4.4). There appeared to be no correlation between MMSE and [^{11}C]-PiB binding measures within the AD-like subset of MCI subjects. The AD-like subjects with the lowest (23) and highest (29) MMSE scores showed the least amount of cortical amyloid deposits as assessed using [^{11}C]-PiB.

A recent study by Rowe et al. (43) using [^{11}C]-PiB in nine MCI subjects provided similar results, with five MCI subjects (60%) presenting an AD-like [^{11}C]-PiB retention pattern and four MCI subjects presenting a normal pattern of cortical [^{11}C]-PiB retention. These early studies indicate that significant amyloid deposits are present in some MCI subjects and absent in others (Fig. 14.4.4), and longitudinal amyloid imaging studies of all MCI subjects will likely be informative as to the extent and progression of amyloid deposition and the course of AD.

Small et al. (34) recently reported PET imaging studies of [^{18}F]-FDDNP in 28 MCI subjects. The authors found that average global DVR measures of [^{18}F]-FDDNP binding were lower in the control group than in the MCI group (1.07 ± 0.02 vs. 1.12 ± 0.02; P <0.001), and the average global DVR values in the MCI group were lower than the AD group (1.12 ± 0.02 vs. 1.16 ± 0.01; P <0.001). [^{18}F]-FDDNP regional brain differences were greatest between the MCI and AD groups in parietal (1.10 ± 0.03 vs. 1.16 ± 0.03, respectively) and posterior cingulate regions (1.13 ± 0.05 vs. 1.19 ± 0.03, respectively). Overlap of the [^{18}F]-FDDNP DVR values between the MCI group and the control and AD groups were evident (Fig. 14.4.3), and the number of MCI subjects in the AD range (defined as ≥1.13 DVR units in the medial temporal cortex) was reported to be 24 of 28 MCI subjects (86%).

Normal Control Subjects (Pittsburgh Compound-B Positive)

The discovery at autopsy of significant amyloid plaque deposits in individuals without evidence of dementia or cognitive dysfunction is well documented (9,57–59). Although such observations would seem to contradict the amyloid cascade hypothesis, it is quite possible that the time course of the amyloid deposition and its relationship to neurotoxicity and cognitive decline is simply not well understood. Indeed, a corollary of the amyloid cascade hypothesis is that some amyloid deposition precedes the onset of clinical symptoms. The characterization of this relationship was and remains a primary objective of studies employing noninvasive imaging agents in longitudinal studies of normal aging. The study of this particular population is of great interest not only to explore the amyloid cascade hypothesis, but also because these subjects stand to benefit most from intervention with future antiamyloid therapies.

The first glimpse that amyloid imaging agents have the potential to detect amyloid deposition prior to the onset of clinical symptoms came in the initial proof-of-concept study of [^{11}C]-PiB, where Klunk et al. (36) documented levels of [^{11}C]-PiB retention consistent with those observed in cortical regions of AD subjects in one of the six elderly control subjects. Later studies using [^{11}C]-PiB in nondemented subjects showed a similar phenomenon.

Lopresti et al. (40) showed elevated levels of [^{11}C]-PiB retention in cortical areas of two cognitively normal elderly control subjects, although the [^{11}C]-PiB retention measures did not reach the threshold of AD subjects. In a more extensive study using [^{11}C]-PiB in 41 cognitively normal elderly subjects, Mintun et al. (60) documented levels of amyloid deposition in three subjects that were consistent with those observed in other subjects with a diagnosis of probable AD. A fourth cognitively normal subject showed milder increases in cortical [^{11}C]-PiB retention that were more analogous to those reported by Lopresti et al. (40). Rowe et al. (43) obtained similar results in [^{11}C]-PiB studies in 27 elderly controls in which six elderly controls showed cortical uptake and retention of [^{11}C]-PiB despite normal neuropsychological scores.

Interestingly, Small et al. (34) did not report elevated global or regional DVR measures of [^{18}F]-FDDNP in any of 30 cognitively normal elderly control subjects included in their recent study. However, there appears to be overlap of several control subjects with the AD group in the medial temporal cortex region (≥1.13 DVR unit) (Fig. 14.4.3), but the relative amounts of [^{18}F]-FDDNP binding to amyloid plaques and NFTs in this region have not been defined. It is unclear if the narrow DVR range of [^{18}F]-FDDNP binding in control and AD subjects relative to that of [^{11}C]-PiB (Figs. 14.4.2 and 14.4.3) or the relatively young age of the control group in the Small et al. study (64 ± 15) contributed to the different group findings with the two radioligands.

The existing [^{11}C]-PiB studies are insufficient to answer the question as to whether the presence of substantial amyloid deposits in cognitively normal elderly subjects is a feature of preclinical AD or merely a feature of the normal aging process, which may be necessary but not sufficient for developing AD. Carefully controlled longitudinal studies will be needed to characterize the progression of AD *in vivo*. It is anticipated that longitudinal amyloid imaging studies in cognitively normal elderly subjects will help define the natural history of amyloid deposition and help to further evaluate the amyloid cascade hypothesis.

Dementia with Lewy Bodies

Lewy bodies are comprised primarily of deposits of α-synuclein protein (61). Dementia with Lewy bodies (DLB) accounts for about 15% of dementia cases and frequently occurs together with amyloid plaques and NFTs (62–64). Pure DLB, lacking amyloid plaque and NFT deposits, is observed relatively rarely, and amyloid plaques are seen in approximatley 80% of clinically diagnosed DLB cases upon postmortem examination (64–69). Thus, although PiB and other benzothiazoles bind poorly to homogenates from pure DLB brain tissues (52), significant binding of [^{11}C]-PiB in most DLB cases would be expected as a result of the high prevalence of amyloid plaque pathology.

A recent report by Rowe et al. (43) using [^{11}C]-PiB in ten clinically diagnosed DLB subjects reported cortical [^{11}C]-PiB binding to be generally lower and more variable than in AD subjects. Four of ten DLB subjects in this study displayed [^{11}C]-PiB neocortical DVR values in the range of AD subjects, two DLB subjects displayed DVR values in the range of control subjects, and four DLB subjects displayed intermediate DVR values between the DVR ranges of control and AD subjects (Fig. 14.4.5). An additional interesting finding by Rowe et al. (43) in DLB subjects was that high neocortical DVR values correlated inversely with the time between the onset of cognitive impairment recalled by a caregiver and the development of the diagnostic clinical features of DLB ($r = -0.75$; $P = 0.01$). In contrast, there was no correlation in the AD group between neocortical DVR and time from onset of cognitive decline to diagnosis ($r = -0.06$; $P = 0.9$).

Frontotemporal Lobar Degeneration

Frontotemporal lobar degeneration (FTLD), which is most often linked with Pick disease (70), is a progressive dementia that primarily affects frontal and temporal lobe function. Pathologically, Pick disease is characterized by intraneuronal argyrophilic spherical deposits of tau protein. Although the pathologic substrate of FTLD is distinct from AD, overlapping clinical symptoms and age of onset can make the differentiation of AD and FTLD challenging. Currently available symptomatic therapies for AD are frequently ineffective in treating FTLD, and anti-Aβ treatments under development for AD

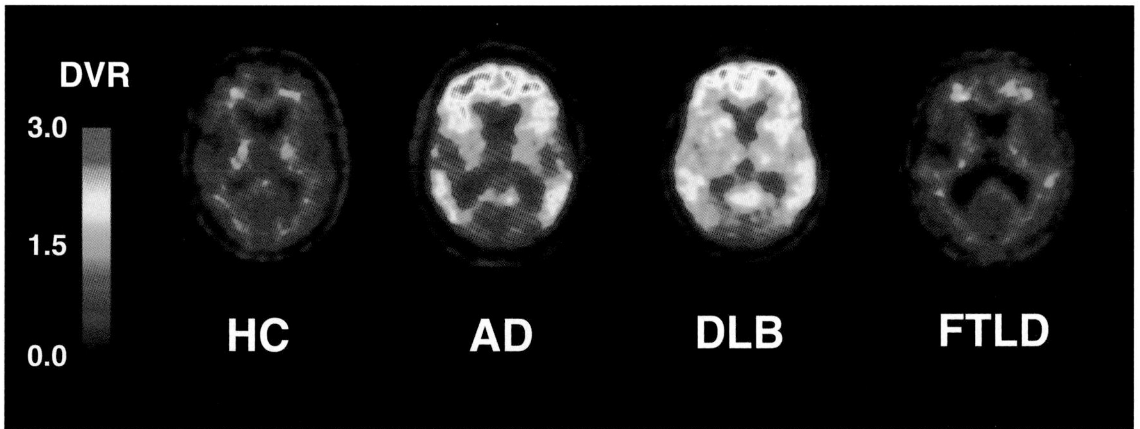

FIGURE 14.4.5. *In vivo* imaging of carbon 11-Pittsburgh compound-B ([^{11}C]-PiB) binding in aging and dementia. Representative parametric PET images of the distribution volume ratio (DVR) of a 73-year-old healthy control (*HC*) subject (MMSE 30), an 82-year-old patient with Alzheimer's disease (*AD*) (MMSE 22), a 78-year-old patient with dementia with Lewy bodies (*DLB*) (MMSE 19), and an 80-year-old patient with frontotemporal lobar degeneration (*FTLD*) (MMSE 25). [^{11}C]-PiB PET DVR images show clear differences when comparing HC or FTLD subjects with DLB or AD patients, with nonspecific [^{11}C]-PiB binding in white matter in the HC and FTLD subjects compared to [^{11}C]-PiB binding in the frontal, temporal, and posterior cingulate/precuneus cortex of the AD and DLB patients. (Images courtesy of Dr. Chris Rowe, Austin Health, University of Melbourne, VIC, Australia.)

are unlikely to be effective in treating FTLD tau deposits. However, AD pathology was found to coexist in about 17% of all patients with an FTLD clinical syndrome (71,72). A clinical tool with the ability to confirm the presence or absence of AD amyloid plaque pathology likely would improve the differential diagnosis of FTLD and AD in most cases.

To examine the clinical utility of [^{11}C]-PiB for the differential diagnosis of FTLD and AD, Rabinovici et al. (73) conducted [^{11}C]-PiB and [^{18}F]-FDG PET studies in 12 patients with clinical diagnoses of FTLD and seven with moderate AD (MMSE = 19.3 ± 7.1). Eight age-matched elderly controls were also included for comparison. Four of 12 FTLD subjects showed patterns and levels of [^{11}C]-PiB retention that were qualitatively indistinguishable from those observed in six of the seven AD subjects. The [^{11}C]-PiB scans of the remaining eight FTLD subjects showed little [^{11}C]-PiB retention, including one pathologically confirmed case of FTLD that came to autopsy. Among the four [^{11}C]-PiB-positive FTLD subjects, two of the four subjects had [^{18}F]-FDG PET scans consistent with AD, while patterns of [^{18}F]-FDG PET retention in the remaining two subjects indicated FTLD. This study indicated that while [^{11}C]-PiB had diagnostic utility in the differential diagnosis of FTLD and AD, postmortem pathological confirmation was needed to determine whether or not the four [^{11}C]-PiB-positive FTLD patients represented false positives, comorbid AD and FTLD, or AD patients with clinical symptoms that were more characteristic of FTLD.

Another recent [^{11}C]-PiB study by Rowe et al. (43) in six FTLD subjects demonstrated controllike levels of [^{11}C]-PiB binding in neocortical areas of all six FTLD patients examined (Fig. 14.4.5). In contrast to the Rabinovici et al. study, Rowe et al. prescreened all the FTLD subjects in their study to ensure they demonstrated frontal or temporal lobe atrophy on magnetic resonance imaging and concordant hypometabolism on [^{18}F]-FDG PET scans. These prescreening procedures or the small number of subjects may account for the different findings in the two studies.

Cerebral Amyloid Angiopathy

Cerebrovascular deposits of Aβ (cerebral amyloid angiopathy [CAA]) are implicated as important contributors to spontaneous hemorrhagic stroke and vascular cognitive impairment (74,75). CAA occurs comorbidly in 80% or more subjects with AD (76). Johnson et al. (77) compared [^{11}C]-PiB binding in six nondemented subjects with probable CAA based on tissue biopsy (n = 4) or multiple lobar bleeds (n = 2) and compared the [^{11}C]-PiB binding pattern to that shown by typical [^{11}C]-PiB-negative normal controls and [^{11}C]-PiB-positive AD patients. Global cortical [^{11}C]-PiB binding was elevated in the CAA group relative to normal controls, but was lower in CAA than in AD. However, the relative occipital [^{11}C]-PiB binding was higher in CAA than in AD, whereas the frontal cortex to global cortical ratio was higher in AD compared to the CAA group. Based on the typical location of CAA pathology and hemorrhages, it was expected that the occipital lobes would be disproportionately affected in CAA. Thus, the authors concluded that [^{11}C]-PiB can detect cerebrovascular Aβ and may serve as a method for identifying the extent of CAA in living subjects.

Early Onset Familial Alzheimer's Disease

As mentioned previously, the rare occurrence of a completely penetrant, autosomal dominant early onset form of AD opens an opportunity to study the disease in ways that would be difficult or impossible in the general population. One way in which this population can facilitate amyloid imaging research is in the study of the presymptomatic phase of the natural history of amyloid deposition. By virtue of their choice to know the results of their mutation carrier status, there is a population of individuals who know with certainty whether they will develop eoFAD and, because the age of onset in a given family is somewhat predictable, the time course of their symptoms can be estimated. Thus, individuals can be studied 10 years or more before they would be expected to develop the first symptoms of AD.

Klunk et al. (78) studied two unrelated kindred, composed of five carriers of the PS-1 C410Y mutation and five carriers of the PS-1 A426P mutation. The most notable finding of the first cross-sectional studies was that amyloid deposition appears to begin focally and intensely in the striatum (caudate and putamen) of the PS-1 mutation carriers. Two subjects as young as 35 years old showed this pattern (Fig. 14.4.6). In the C410Y kindred, none of the five subjects had clinical symptoms (including extrapyramidal symptoms), but all showed an abundant pattern of striatal amyloid deposition.

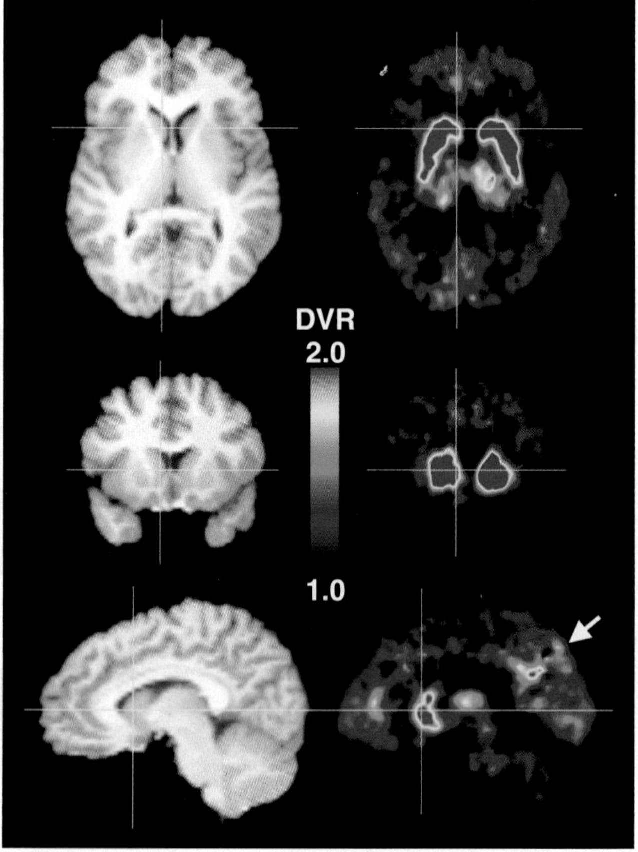

FIGURE 14.4.6. Axial (**top**), coronal (**middle**), and sagittal (**bottom**) views of the magnetic resonance imaging (**left**) and carbon 11-Pittsburgh compound-B ([^{11}C]-PiB) PET (**right**) of a 37-year-old asymptomatic subject who carries the C410Y PS-1 mutation. Intense and focal [^{11}C]-PiB retention is evident throughout the striatum. Much less intense amyloid deposition is evident in the precuneous/posterior cingulate area (seen best on the sagittal slice with an arrow indicating the location of this region).

As the average age of onset in this family was approximately 48, the striatal deposition began at least a decade prior to the expected age of onset. Smaller increases in [^{11}C]-PiB retention were observed in the usual cortical areas (frontal, precuneus/posterior cingulate, parietal and temporal), but these were intermediate between those seen in sporadic AD and control subjects. Postmortem data from older members of the C410Y kindred showed extensive striatal amyloid deposition that appeared to exceed that in the cortical areas. Thus, the [^{11}C]-PiB retention data were consistent with these postmortem findings and appear to reflect true amyloid load as opposed to some possible artifact related to the mutation.

Although the pattern is striking and clear, the cause of this striatal deposition remains unknown. This study points out the potential of *in vivo* amyloid imaging to detect preclinical amyloid. This may become critical for accurately identifying candidates for anti-amyloid therapy at a time when the therapy is likely to have its optimal effect. This study also points out some differences in the natural history of amyloid deposition in eoFAD and the typical late-onset sporadic form of AD.

CHALLENGES AND FUTURE DIRECTIONS

For the most part, PET amyloid imaging studies with [^{18}F]-FDDNP, [^{11}C]-PiB, and [^{11}C]-SB-13 have been cross-sectional in nature. These cross-sectional studies have identified areas of applicability where longitudinal studies will be informative, particularly to follow MCI and [^{11}C]-PiB-positive control subjects over the course of several years. These longitudinal PET amyloid imaging studies will clearly be most informative when augmented with additional and complementary neuropsychological cognitive testing measures, [^{18}F]-FDG brain metabolic studies, and other biomarkers of disease progression, such as cerebrospinal fluid Aβ(1-42) and tau (79,80). Finally, postmortem confirmation of the *in vivo* imaging studies will be most definitive in assessing the accuracy of the PET amyloid imaging methodologies.

The use of PET amyloid imaging technology to enhance the drug discovery process in an effort to develop effective anti-Aβ therapies is ongoing and will likely increase in the coming years. An imaging technology that directly reflects the efficacy of drugs designed to reduce or eliminate the targets of the therapies (i.e., the amyloid plaques deposited in the brains of AD, MCI, or amyloid-positive control subjects) is likely to be a powerful tool in assisting the *in vivo* evaluation of the therapeutic agents.

Finally, progress in developing and applying new and improved ^{18}F-labeled Aβ- and NFT-specific PET imaging agents is needed to assist in identifying the contributions of each of these protein deposits to the pathophysiology of dementing disorders. New ^{18}F-labeled Aβ- and NFT-specific PET amyloid imaging agents should provide a relatively large dynamic detection range of specific binding over which the regional concentration of these protein deposits can be assessed and followed *in vivo*. A comparison of the binding potential (BP) range of [^{11}C]-PiB and [^{18}F]-FDDNP in control, MCI, and AD subjects (Fig. 14.4.7) indicates considerable room for improvement for future ^{18}F-labeled Aβ- and NFT-specific PET imaging agents. The longer-lived ^{18}F radionuclide likely will assist in the production and regional distribution of these Aβ- and NFT-specific PET imaging agents, just as [^{18}F]-FDG has for PET metabolic imaging. Nevertheless the ^{11}C radionuclide will likely continue to play a role in academic PET amyloid imaging research studies, because its short half-life allows several sequential studies of the ^{11}C-labeled amyloid imaging agent and other ^{11}C- or ^{18}F-labeled agents to be performed in a research subject on the same day.

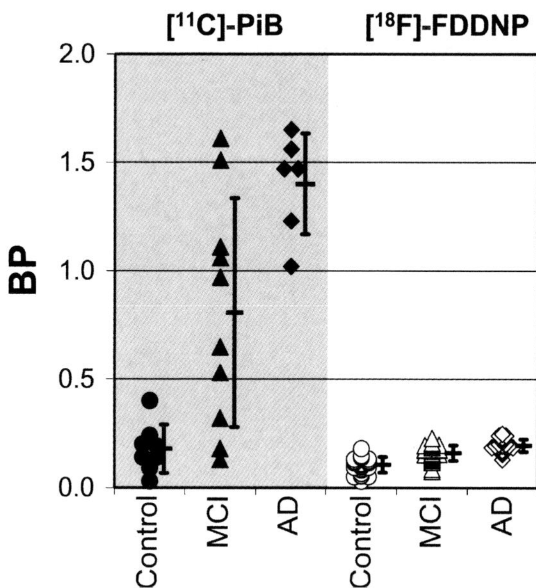

FIGURE 14.4.7. Comparison of the binding potential (BP) values of carbon 11-Pittsburgh compound-B ([^{11}C]-PiB) (**left**) and fluorine-18-fluorophore 2-[1-[6-(dimethylamino)-2-naphthyl]ethylidene] malononitrile ([^{18}F]-FDDNP) (**right**) in the brain regions of highest specific binding (posterior cingulate gyrus for [^{11}C]-PiB and medial temporal cortex for [^{18}F]-FDDNP). The BP values are related to the distribution volume ratio (DVR) values shown in Figs. 14.4.2 and 14.4.3 by the relationship BP = DVR-1. Note the narrow range of BP values for [^{18}F]-FDDNP compared to the larger range of BP values for [^{11}C]-PiB. The BP values were determined from the DVR values shown in Figs. 14.4.2 and 14.4.3. MCI, mild cognitive impairment; AD, Alzheimer's disease. (From Small GW, Kepe V, Ercoli LM, et al. PET of brain amyloid and tau in mild cognitive impairment. *N Engl J Med* 2006;355(25):2652–2663; Lopresti BJ, Klunk WE, Mathis CA, et al. Simplified quantification of Pittsburgh compound B amyloid imaging PET studies: a comparative analysis. *J Nucl Med* 2005;46(12):1959–1972, with permission.)

Over the past 5 years, considerable progress has been made in imaging amyloid in the brains of living human subjects using PET technology. Considering that the imaging field had only *in vitro* data for several attractive candidate agents 5 years ago, research has come a considerable distance in a short time. Much remains to be accomplished with the amyloid imaging agents at hand and with new agents under development. Over the next 5 years it is expected that many of the promising uses of these agents will be further investigated and more exciting progress will be realized.

ACKNOWLEDGMENTS

Financial support for this work was provided by grants from the National Institutes of Health (R01 AG018402, P50 AG005133, K02 AG001039, R01 AG020226, R01 MH070729, R37 AG025516, P01 AG025204), and the Alzheimer's Association (TLL-01-3381). These funding agencies had no role in the design or interpretation of results or preparation of this chapter.

REFERENCES

1. Lobo A, Launer LJ, Fratiglioni L, et al. Prevalence of dementia and major subtypes in Europe: a collaborative study of population-based cohorts. Neurologic Diseases in the Elderly Research Group. *Neurology* 2000;54[11 Suppl 5]:S4–S9.
2. Rice DP, Fillit HM, Max W, et al. Prevalence, costs, and treatment of Alzheimer's disease and related dementia: a managed care perspective. *Am J Manag Care* 2001;7(8):809–818.
3. Selkoe DJ. Alzheimer disease: mechanistic understanding predicts novel therapies. *Ann Intern Med* 2004;140(8):627–638.
4. Terry RD, Katzman R, Bick KL, et al. *Alzheimer's disease*. Philadelphia: Lippincott Williams & Wilkins, 2000.
5. Mirra SS, Heyman A, McKeel D, et al. The Consortium to Establish a Registry for Alzheimer's Disease (CERAD). Part II. Standardization of the neuropathologic assessment of Alzheimer's disease. *Neurology* 1991;41:479.
6. Iwatsubo T, Odaka A, Suzuki N, et al. Visualization of A beta 42(43) and A beta 40 in senile plaques with end-specific A beta monoclonals: evidence that an initially deposited species is A beta 42(43). *Neuron* 1994;13:45.
7. Goedert M. Tau protein and the neurofibrillary pathology of Alzheimer's disease. *Trends Neurosci* 1993;16:460–465.
8. Thal DR, Rub U, Orantes M, et al. Phases of A beta-deposition in the human brain and its relevance for the development of AD. *Neurology* 2002;58(12):1791–1800.
9. Braak H, Braak E. Neuropathological staging of Alzheimer-related changes. *Acta Neuropathol* 1991;82:239.
10. Arnold SE, Hyman BT, Flory J, et al. The topographical and neuroanatomical distribution of neurofibrillary tangles and neuritic plaques in the cerebral cortex of patients with Alzheimer's disease. *Cereb Cortex* 1991;1(1):103–116.
11. Price JL, Morris JC. Tangles and plaques in nondemented aging and "preclinical" Alzheimer's disease. *Ann Neurol* 1999;45(3):358.
12. Joachim CL, Morris JH, Selkoe DJ. Diffuse senile plaques occur commonly in the cerebellum in Alzheimer's disease. *Am J Pathol* 1989; 135:309.
13. Yamaguchi H, Hirai S, Morimatsu M, et al. Diffuse type of senile plaques in the cerebellum of Alzheimer-type dementia demonstrated by beta protein immunostain. *Acta Neuropathol* 1989;77:314.
14. Evans DA, Funkenstein HH, Albert MS, et al. Prevalence of Alzheimer's disease in a community population of older persons. Higher than previously reported. *JAMA* 1989;262(18):2551–2556.
15. St. George-Hyslop PH. Molecular genetics of Alzheimer disease. *Semin Neurol* 1999;19(4):371–383.
16. Tanzi RE, Kovacs DM, Kim TW, et al. The gene defects responsible for familial Alzheimer's disease. *Neurobiol Dis* 1996;3(3):159–168.
17. Petersen RC. Mild cognitive impairment as a diagnostic entity. *J Intern Med* 2004;256(3):183–194.
18. Gauthier S, Reisberg B, Zaudig M, et al. Mild cognitive impairment. *Lancet* 2006;367(9518):1262–1270.
19. Hardy J, Selkoe DJ. The amyloid hypothesis of Alzheimer's disease: progress and problems on the road to therapeutics. *Science* 2002; 297(5580):353–356.
20. Hardy JA, Higgins GA. Alzheimer's disease: the amyloid cascade hypothesis. *Science* 1992;256:184–185.
21. Xia W, Ostaszewski BL, Kimberly WT, et al. FAD mutations in presenilin-1 or amyloid precursor protein decrease the efficacy of a gamma-secretase inhibitor: evidence for direct involvement of PS1 in the gamma-secretase cleavage complex. *Neurobiol Dis* 2000;7(6 Pt B):673.
22. Olson RE, Copeland RA, Seiffert D. Progress towards testing the amyloid hypothesis: inhibitors of APP processing. *Curr Opin Drug Discov Devel* 2001;4(4):390.
23. Bard F, Cannon C, Barbour R, et al. Peripherally administered antibodies against amyloid α-peptide enter the central nervous system and reduce pathology in a mouse model of Alzheimer disease. *Nature Med* 2000; 6:916.
24. DeMattos RB, Bales KR, Cummins DJ, et al. Peripheral anti-A beta antibody alters CNS and plasma A beta clearance and decreases brain A beta burden in a mouse model of Alzheimer's disease. *Proc Natl Acad Sci U S A* 2001;98(15):8850.
25. Friedland RP, Majocha RE, Reno JM, et al. Development of an anti-A beta monoclonal antibody for *in vivo* imaging of amyloid angiopathy in Alzheimer's disease. *Mol Neurobiol* 1994;9(1–3):107.
26. Majocha RE, Reno JM, Friedland RP, et al. Development of a monoclonal antibody specific for beta/A4 amyloid in Alzheimer's disease brain for application to *in vivo* imaging of amyloid angiopathy. *J Nucl Med* 1992;33:2184.
27. Friedland RP, Kalaria R, Berridge M, et al. Neuroimaging of vessel amyloid in Alzheimer's disease. *Ann N Y Acad Sci* 1997;826:242.
28. Mathis CA, Wang Y, Klunk WE. Imaging beta-amyloid plaques and neurofibrillary tangles in the aging human brain. *Curr Pharm Des* 2004; 10(13):1469–1492.
29. Agdeppa ED, Kepe V, Liu J, et al. Binding characteristics of radiofluorinated 6-dialkylamino-2-naphthylethylidene derivatives as positron emission tomography imaging probes for beta-amyloid plaques in Alzheimer's disease. *J Neurosci* 2001;21(24):RC189.
30. Agdeppa ED, Kepe V, Liu J, et al. 2-Dialkylamino-6-acylmalononitrile substituted naphthalenes (DDNP analogs): novel diagnostic and therapeutic tools in Alzheimer's disease. *Mol Imaging Biol* 2003;5(6):404–417.
31. Shoghi-Jadid K, Small GW, Agdeppa ED, et al. Localization of neurofibrillary tangles and beta-amyloid plaques in the brains of living patients with Alzheimer disease. *Am J Geriatr Psychiatry* 2002;10(1):24–35.
32. Terry RD, Masliah E, Salmon DP, et al. Physical basis of cognitive alterations in Alzheimer's disease: synapse loss is the major correlate of cognitive impairment. *Ann Neurol* 1991;30(4):572.
33. Logan J, Fowler JS, Volkow ND, et al. Distribution volume ratios without blood sampling from graphical analysis of PET data. *J Cereb Blood Flow Metab* 1996;16(5):834–840.
34. Small GW, Kepe V, Ercoli LM, et al. PET of brain amyloid and tau in mild cognitive impairment. *N Engl J Med* 2006;355(25):2652–2663.
35. Engler H, Nordberg A, Blomqvist G, et al. First human study with a benzothiazole amyloid-imaging agent in Alzheimer's disease and control subjects. *Neurobiol Aging* 2002;23(1S):S429.
36. Klunk WE, Engler H, Nordberg A, et al. Imaging brain amyloid in Alzheimer's disease with Pittsburgh compound-B. *Ann Neurol* 2004; 55:306.
37. Mathis CA, Wang Y, Holt DP, et al. Synthesis and evaluation of ^{11}C-labeled 6-substituted 2-aryl benzothiazoles as amyloid imaging agents. *J Med Chem* 2003;46:2740–2754.
38. Price JC, Klunk WE, Lopresti BJ, et al. Kinetic modeling of amyloid binding in humans using PET imaging and Pittsburgh compound-B. *J Cereb Blood Flow Metab* 2005;25:1528–1547.
39. Logan J, Fowler JS, Volkow ND, et al. Graphical analysis of reversible radioligand binding from time-activity measurements applied to [N-^{11}C-methyl]-(-)-cocaine PET studies in human subjects. *J Cereb Blood Flow Metab* 1990;10(5):740–747.
40. Lopresti BJ, Klunk WE, Mathis CA, et al. Simplified quantification of Pittsburgh compound B amyloid imaging PET studies: a comparative analysis. *J Nucl Med* 2005;46(12):1959–1972.
41. Verhoeff NP, Wilson AA, Takeshita S, et al. *In vivo* imaging of Alzheimer disease β-Amyloid with [^{11}C]SB-13 PET. *Am J Geriatr Psychiatry* 2004;12(6):584–595.
42. Edison P, Archer HA, Hinz R, et al. Amyloid, hypometabolism, and cognition in Alzheimer disease: an [^{11}C]PIB and [^{18}F]FDG PET study. *Neurology* 2007;68(7):501–508.
43. Rowe CC, Ng S, Ackermann U, et al. Imaging beta-amyloid burden in aging and dementia. *Neurology*. 2007;68(20):1718–1725.
44. Engler H, Forsberg A, Almkvist O, et al. Two-year follow-up of amyloid deposition in patients with Alzheimer's disease. *Brain* 2006;129(pt 11): 2856–66.
45. Buckner RL, Snyder AZ, Shannon BJ, et al. Molecular, structural, and functional characterization of Alzheimer's disease: evidence for a relationship

between default activity, amyloid, and memory. *J Neurosci* 2005;25(34): 7709–7717.

46. Minoshima S, Foster NL, Kuhl DE. Posterior cingulate cortex in Alzheimer's disease. *Lancet* 1994;344(8926):895.
47. Klunk WE, Mathis CA, Price JC, et al. Two-year follow-up of amyloid deposition in patients with Alzheimer's disease. *Brain* 2006;129(Pt 11):2805–2807.
48. Braak H, Braak E. Evolution of neuronal changes in the course of Alzheimer's disease. *J Neural Transm Suppl* 1998;53:127–140.
49. Hyman BT, Marzloff K, Arriagada PV. The lack of accumulation of senile plaques or amyloid burden in Alzheimer's disease suggests a dynamic balance between amyloid deposition and resolution. *J Neuropathol Exp Neurol* 1993;52(6):594–600.
50. Hyman BT. Down syndrome and Alzheimer disease. *Prog Clin Biol Res* 1992;379:123.
51. Hyman BT, West HL, Rebeck GW, et al. Neuropathological changes in Down's syndrome hippocampal formation. Effect of age and apolipoprotein E genotype. *Arch Neurol* 1995;52(4):373.
52. Klunk WE, Wang Y, Huang GF, et al. The binding of 2-(4′-methylaminophenyl)benzothiazole to postmortem brain homogenates is dominated by the amyloid component. *J Neurosci* 2003;23(6):2086–2092.
53. Morris JC, Price AL. Pathologic correlates of nondemented aging, mild cognitive impairment, and early-stage Alzheimer's disease. *J Mol Neurosci* 2001;17(2):101.
54. Petersen RC, Doody R, Kurz A, et al. Current concepts in mild cognitive impairment. *Arch Neurol* 2001;58(12):1985–1992.
55. Petersen RC, Stevens JC, Ganguli M, et al. Practice parameter: early detection of dementia: mild cognitive impairment (an evidence-based review). Report of the Quality Standards Subcommittee of the American Academy of Neurology. *Neurology* 2001;56(9):1133–1142.
56. Yesavage JA, O'Hara R, Kraemer H, et al. Modeling the prevalence and incidence of Alzheimer's disease and mild cognitive impairment. *J Psychiat Res* 2002;36(5):281–286.
57. Hulette CM, Welsh-Bohmer KA, Murray MG, et al. Neuropathological and neuropsychological changes in "normal" aging: evidence for preclinical Alzheimer disease in cognitively normal individuals. *J Neuropathol Exp Neurol* 1998;57(12):1168–1174.
58. Katzman R. Alzheimer's disease as an age-dependent disorder. *Ciba Found Symp* 1988;134:69–85.
59. Tomlinson BE, Blessed G, Roth M. Observations on the brains of nondemented old people. *J Neurol Sci* 1968;7(2):331–356.
60. Mintun MA, Larossa GN, Sheline YI, et al. [^{11}C]PIB in a nondemented population: potential antecedent marker of Alzheimer disease. *Neurology* 2006;67(3):446–452.
61. Spillantini MG, Schmidt ML, Lee VM, et al. Alpha-synuclein in Lewy bodies. *Nature* 1997;388(6645):839–840.
62. McKeith I, Mintzer J, Aarsland D, et al. Dementia with Lewy bodies. *Lancet Neurol* 2004;3(1):19–28.
63. McKeith IG, Dickson DW, Lowe J, et al. Diagnosis and management of dementia with Lewy bodies: third report of the DLB Consortium. *Neurology* 2005;65(12):1863–1872.
64. McKeith IG, Galasko D, Kosaka K, et al. Consensus guidelines for the clinical and pathologic diagnosis of dementia with Lewy bodies (DLB): report of the consortium on DLB international workshop. *Neurology* 1996;47(5):1113–1124.
65. Ballard CG, Jacoby R, Del Ser T, et al. Neuropathological substrates of psychiatric symptoms in prospectively studied patients with autopsy-confirmed dementia with Lewy bodies. *Am J Psychiatry* 2004;161(5):843–849.
66. Del Ser T, Hachinski V, Merskey H, et al. Clinical and pathologic features of two groups of patients with dementia with Lewy bodies: effect of coexisting Alzheimer-type lesion load. *Alzheimer Dis Assoc Disord* 2001;15(1):31–44.
67. Harding AJ, Broe GA, Halliday GM. Visual hallucinations in Lewy body disease relate to Lewy bodies in the temporal lobe. *Brain* 2002;125(Pt 2):391–403.
68. Jellinger KA. Influence of Alzheimer pathology on clinical diagnostic accuracy in dementia with Lewy bodies. *Neurology* 2004;62(1):160.
69. Merdes AR, Hansen LA, Jeste DV, et al. Influence of Alzheimer pathology on clinical diagnostic accuracy in dementia with Lewy bodies. *Neurology* 2003;60(10):1586–1590.
70. Pick A. Über die Beziehungen der senilen Hirnatrophie zur Aphasie. *Prager medicinische Wochenschrift* 1892. 17:165–167.
71. Forman MS, Farmer J, Johnson JK, et al. Frontotemporal dementia: clinicopathological correlations. *Ann Neurol* 2006;59(6):952–962.
72. Kertesz A, McMonagle P, Blair M, et al. The evolution and pathology of frontotemporal dementia. *Brain* 2005;128(Pt 9):1996–2005.
73. Rabinovici GD, Furst AJ, O'Neil JP, et al. [C-11]PIB PET imaging in Alzheimer's disease and frontotemporal lobar degeneration. *Neurology* 2007;68(15):1205–1212.
74. Greenberg SM, Gurol ME, Rosand J, et al. Amyloid angiopathy-related vascular cognitive impairment. *Stroke* 2004;35[11 Suppl 1]:2616–2619.
75. Vinters HV. Cerebral amyloid angiopathy. A critical review. *Stroke* 1987;18(2):311–324.
76. Jellinger KA. Alzheimer disease and cerebrovascular pathology: an update. *J Neural Transm* 2002;109(5–6):813–836.
77. Johnson KA, Gregas M, Becker JA, et al. Imaging of amyloid burden and distribution in cerebral amyloid angiopathy with Pittsburgh compound B. *Ann Neurol* 2007;62(3):229–234.
78. Klunk WE, Price JC, Mathis CA, et al. Amyloid deposition begins in the striatum of Presenilin-1 mutation carriers from two unrelated pedigrees. *J Neurosci* 2007;27(23):6174–6184.
79. Fagan AM, Mintun MA, Mach RH, et al. Inverse relation between *in vivo* amyloid imaging load and cerebrospinal fluid Abeta42 in humans. *Ann Neurol* 2006;59(3):512–519.
80. Fagan AM, Roe CM, Xiong C, et al. Cerebrospinal fluid tau/beta-amyloid(42) ratio as a prediction of cognitive decline in nondemented older adults. *Arch Neurol* 2007;64(3):343–349.

CHAPTER 15

PET Imaging as a Biomarker

WOLFGANG A. WEBER, CAROLINE C. SIGMAN, AND GARY J. KELLOFF

Biomarkers have been defined as "characteristics that are objectively measured and evaluated as indicators of normal biological processes, pathogenic processes, or pharmacologic responses to a therapeutic intervention" (1). In oncology the main focus of research has been to develop biomarkers for prediction of patients' prognosis, selection of therapeutic approaches, and assessment of tumor response to therapy. DNA chips and mass spectrometry now allow simultaneous study of several thousands of genes or proteins expressed by cancer cells that can be used as potential biomarkers. In contrast, the number of biological parameters that can be studied clinically by positron emission tomography (PET) imaging is currently limited (Table 15.1). In other words, modern genomics and proteomics provide a detailed "signature" of the cancer, whereas PET appears, at first inspection, to provide at best a few "dots." Therefore, the obvious question is what can PET add to the huge amount of other, possible biomarkers?

PET differs in several ways from biomarkers derived from tumor biopsies or plasma samples. PET and other imaging biomarkers allow noninvasive serial studies of the whole tumor mass. In contrast, only small parts of the tumor can be evaluated by biopsies. Intratumoral heterogeneity may, therefore, significantly confound the analysis of biomarkers derived from tumor biopsies. This is of particular concern when evaluating changes in a biomarker during treatment, because it is difficult to ascertain that the expression of the biomarker in different parts of the tumor was the same prior to therapy.

Serum biomarker studies are noninvasive and can easily be used to measure changes in multiple biomarkers over time. However, the results may be confounded by the metabolism and excretion of tumor-derived biomarkers. Imaging is likely to complement these biomarker studies by allowing direct assessment of the tumor tissue without the interference of metabolic processes in plasma or normal organs.

Perhaps the most unique characteristic of PET-based biomarkers is that they measure a biological process and not the concentration of a particular cellular protein or of messenger RNA. Thus, PET is generally *not* a noninvasive form of immunohistochemistry. For some applications this may be seen as a disadvantage because the PET signal cannot invariably be attributed solely to the expression of a particular protein and may, therefore, appear to be unspecific. On the other hand, the ability to image a biochemical process in a living organism is probably the biggest strength of PET when compared to nonimaging biomarkers. Although continuous progress is being made, the ability to predict cellular function on the basis of gene or protein expression remains limited (2). Therefore, the best way for PET and other imaging biomarkers to complement gene and protein expression profiles may be to provide information about the functional consequences of certain alterations in these profiles and to monitor functional changes during therapeutic interventions. The other key advantages of PET include, when using fluorodeoxyglucose (FDG), it is quite reproducible and widely available, increasingly standard methods are being applied to assess the intrinsically quantitative images, and it can be used before treatment as well as during and after treatment. The ability to measure noninvasively the effects of a cancer therapy in an individual is a very attractive aspect of PET imaging.

APPLICATIONS OF PET AS A BIOMARKER

The broad definition of biomarkers covers almost all applications of PET in oncology, including differentiation of benign and malignant tumors, tumor staging, and detection of recurrent disease. These aspects of PET imaging are covered in others chapters of this book for individual tumor types. In this chapter the focus is on the evaluation of tissue pharmacokinetics by radiolabeled drugs and assessment of tumor response to therapy.

TABLE 15.1 Overview of PET Imaging Agents that have been Used to Study Malignant Tumors in Patients

Biological Process	PET Imaging Agents
Glucose metabolism	^{18}F-fluorodeoxyglucose
Amino acid transport/ metabolism	^{11}C-methionine, ^{11}C-tyrosine, ^{18}F-fluoroethyltyrosine, and others
Lipid metabolism	^{11}C-acetate, ^{11}C-choline, ^{18}F-choline
Hypoxia	^{18}F-FMISO, *Cu-ATSM
Perfusion	^{15}O-water, ^{13}N-ammonia
Transgene expression (HSV tk1)	^{18}F-FHBG, ^{124}I-FIAU
RECEPTOR EXPRESSION	
Estrogen	^{18}F-FES
Androgen	^{18}F-FDHT
Somatostatin	^{18}F-octreotide, ^{68}Ga-octreotide analogues
$\alpha v \beta 3$ integrin	^{18}F-RGD peptides, *Cu-RGD peptides

C, carbon; Cu, copper; Cu-ATSM, *Cu-labeled diacetyl-bis(N4-methylthiosemicarbazone; Cu-RGD, *Cu labeled peptides with an Arginine, Glycine, Asparate or RGD sequence; F, fluorine; FDHT, 16β-[^{18}F]-fluoro-5α-dihydrotestosteron; FES, 16-fluorine-18-fluoro-17-estradiol; FHBG, 9-[4-[(^{18})F]fluoro-3-(hydroxymethyl)butyl]guanine; FIAU, 5-iodo-1-(2-deoxy-2-fluoro-beta-d-arabinofuranosyl) uracil; FMISO, fluoromisonidazole; Ga, gallium; I, iodine; N, nitrogen; O, oxygen.

Evaluation of the Tissue Pharmacokinetics

Labeling of drugs with positron-emitting radionuclides to study their pharmacokinetics was used in drug development even before PET became available. In 1973 Fowler et al. (3) described a procedure to radiolabel the then relatively new drug 5-fluorouracil (5-FU) with the positron emitter fluorine-18 ([^{18}F]). In 1977 Shani and Wolf (4) demonstrated in a mouse model of leukemia that tumor uptake of 5-[^{18}F]-fluorouracil ([^{18}F]-5-FU) is significantly lower in resistant tumors than in sensitive tumors. They conclude that "non-invasive quantification of tumor/blood ratios following administration of [^{18}F]5FU" may allow "differentiation of those human tumors that are likely to respond to drug therapy from those in which the response will be minimal or nil."

Although this prediction has eventually been found to be correct, quantification of [^{18}F]-5-FU has proven to be extremely complex. Rapid metabolism of injected [^{18}F]-5-FU gives rise to high levels of labeled catabolites, which makes quantitative assessment of the [^{18}F]-5-FU kinetics challenging. Thirty years after the publication of the study of radiosynthesis of [^{18}F]-5-FU, the quantification of the tumor uptake and metabolism of [^{18}F]-5-FU is still the subject of experimental studies.

Unfortunately, [^{18}F]-5-FU is only one example of radiolabeled anticancer drugs with pharmacokinetics that are challenging to measure by PET imaging. Rapid metabolism and/or high unspecific accumulation are common problems when using radiolabeled anticancer drugs as imaging agents. Despite these difficulties, PET imaging with radiolabeled drugs has been successfully used to study tissue pharmacokinetics noninvasively in patients. For example, Saleem et al. (5) were able to quantify the increase of the intratumoral concentration of 5-FU in response to treatment with eniluracil, which inhibits the catabolism of 5-FU. Jayson et al. (6) used PET imaging to demonstrate the variability of tumor uptake of the iodine-124 labeled anti–vascular endothelial growth factor antibody HuMV833. PET has also been applied to study drug efflux by using various radiolabeled substrates of the mdr1 transporter. In animal models tumors with and without mdr1 expression could be differentiated by PET imaging. Furthermore, it was possible to monitor the inhibition of mdr1 function by specific antagonists. However, these encouraging findings still need to be confirmed in systematic clinical trials in patients with malignant tumors (7).

In summary, these studies demonstrate the feasibility of using PET with radiolabeled drugs for noninvasive pharmacokinetic studies. However, it is clear that radiolabeling strategies and techniques for PET image analysis need to be developed early in the course of drug development. Otherwise it is unlikely that a radiolabeled analogue of a drug will be available in time for the clinical testing of a new drug.

Monitoring Tumor Therapy

A significant number of studies have now shown that an abnormal FDG PET scan after completion of chemotherapy or chemoradiotherapy is associated with a high risk for early disease recurrence and poor prognosis. This has been demonstrated most extensively in patients with malignant lymphomas, but similar findings have been reported in a variety of solid tumors, such as cervical, esophageal, and lung cancers. In patients treated with neoadjuvant chemoradiotherapy, residual tumor FDG uptake has been shown to be correlated with the degree of histological tumor regression.

The observation that patients with a favorable response frequently show negative PET scans after completion of therapy, despite significant residual morphological abnormalities, has lead to the hypothesis that measurable quantitative changes in tumor metabolism may already occur *during* therapy, and that these may be used as an early indicator for tumor response. This hypothesis was initially evaluated by Wahl et al. (8) in patients with breast cancer undergoing neoadjuvant chemotherapy. The results of this study indicated that in responding tumors metabolic activity markedly changes within the first weeks of therapy. Subsequent studies by Jansson et al. (9) in breast cancer and by Findlay et al. (10) in colorectal cancer have also suggested that tumor glucose utilization is rapidly decreased by effective therapy. More recently the accuracy of FDG PET to predict response and patient survival has been evaluated in larger studies and other tumor types. The results of these trials are summarized in Table 15.2.

In vitro studies have suggested that chemotherapy and radiotherapy may cause a "metabolic flare phenomenon" (11,12). This phenomenon has been attributed to the activation of energy-dependent cellular repair mechanisms. On the basis of these data it has been recommended that assessment of tumor response should not be performed until several weeks after completion of therapy. In these *in vitro* studies, however, FDG uptake was measured per *surviving* cells, and in Higashi et al. (12) per surviving well and per tissue culture well (mimicking the whole tumor). This parallels the clinical situation, where the change in the PET signal is determined by a combination of decreased FDG uptake due to cancer cell death

TABLE 15.2 Prognostic Relevance of Quantitative Changes in Tumor FDG-Uptake During Chemo- or Chemoradiotherapy

Tumor	Authors (Ref.)	Year	N	Criteria	Median Survival (Months)		*P* Value
					Responder	Nonresponder	
Lymphoma	Kostakoglu et al. (92)	2002	30	Visual	>24	5	<.001[a]
	Haioun et al. (93)	2005	90	Visual	>36	11	<.001[a]
	Mikhaeel et al. (94)	2005	121	Visual	>41	12	<.001[a]
	Hutchings et al. (95)	2006	77	Visual	>36	11	<.01[a]
Esophagus	Weber et al. (96)	2001	40	ΔSUV >35%	>48	20	.04
	Wieder et al. (97)	2004	38[b]	ΔSUV >30%	>38	18	.011
	Ott et al. (98)	2006	65	ΔSUV >35%	:50	18	.01
Gastric	Ott et al. (99)	2003	35	ΔSUV >35%	>48	17	.001
Head and neck	Brun et al. (85)	2002	47	MR <0.14[c]	>120	40	.004
Ovarian	Avril et al. (100)	2005	33	ΔSUV >20%	38	23	.008
Lung	Weber et al. (44)	2003	57	ΔSUV >20%	9	5	.005
	Hoekstra et al. (101)	2005	47	MR <0.13[c]	45	13	.0004

SUV, standard uptake value.
[a]Progression-free survival, otherwise overall survival.
[b]Chemoradiotherapy, otherwise chemotherapy.
[c]MR, metabolic rate for glucose in μmol/g/min.

plus potentially increased FDG uptake by surviving tumor cells. The study differs from the *in vivo* setting in that no inflammatory cells were present nor was delivery of the radiotracer an issue in the tissue culture wells. A metabolic flare phenomenon has been observed clinically in metastatic breast cancer treated with tamoxifen and was associated with a good response to therapy. This initial increase in tumor metabolic activity is likely due to the partial estrogenlike stimulatory activity of this antiestrogen, which is apparent during the initial days of treatment (13).

There are concerns that quantitative assessment of tumor glucose utilization by FDG PET is not reliable in clinical studies, since the measured signal is influenced by a variety of factors such as data acquisition and reconstruction protocols, lesion size, and blood glucose levels. However, for treatment monitoring it is only necessary to perform an intraindividual comparison of tumor FDG uptake. In this situation, many of the confounding factors will cancel out if the baseline and the follow-up scan are acquired and analyzed according to the same protocol. This is confirmed by studies indicating that the test/retest reproducibility of quantitative measurements of tumor FDG uptake in untreated patients is excellent, with a coefficient of variation of approximately 10% in the standard uptake values (SUV) (14,15).

FDG PET is also attractive for monitoring treatment with certain protein kinase inhibitors, since many signaling pathways targeted by protein kinase inhibitors also have a well-established role in regulating tumor glucose metabolism. For example the protein kinase Akt is a central regulator of cellular apoptosis (16,17), but it is also involved in the regulation of glucose utilization (18). Recent experimental data suggest that activation of Akt may be a key factor for the markedly increased glucose utilization of cancer cells (19,20).

FDG PET has already been used in clinical studies to monitor the response of gastrointestinal stromal tumors to treatment with imatinib (21–24). A marked reduction of tumor metabolic activity was noted as early as 24 hours after the first dose of imatinib (21,25). Moreover, extensive anatomical abnormalities observed by computed tomography (CT) persisted at a time when metabolic alterations had already been resolved. This rapid change in FDG uptake appears to be mediated by a translocation of glucose transporters from the plasma membrane to the cytosol and precedes cell death. Similar observations have been made in experimental models for epidermal growth factor receptor kinase inhibitors (26,27). These data suggest that FDG PET may become a valuable tool to monitor treatment with imatinib and potentially other protein kinase inhibitors.

Monitoring Tumor Cell Proliferation and Apoptosis

Despite the encouraging data, it is not clear whether there are similar marked changes for other forms of targeted therapy. For example, recent studies have indicated that antiangiogenic therapy may not significantly affect tumor glucose utilization, despite significant growth inhibition (28). There is considerable interest in techniques that more directly image proliferation and apoptosis, the major processes targeted by anticancer therapy.

The thymidine analogue $[^{18}F]$-fluorothymidine (FLT) has been evaluated in several studies as a marker of tumor cell proliferation (29–32). Following cellular uptake FLT is phosphorylated by the cytosolic thymidine kinase 1 (TK1) and trapped intracellularly as FLT phosphate. In contrast to thymidine, FLT is not incorporated into the DNA. Nevertheless, FLT uptake is a marker of cellular proliferation, since significant TK1 activity is only observed during S phase.

Preclinical and clinical studies in untreated tumors have confirmed that tumor FLT uptake is generally well correlated with histologic markers of tumor cell proliferation. Animal studies have shown that inhibition of cellular proliferation by chemotherapy (33), radiotherapy (34,35), androgen deprivation (36), or ErbB1/2 kinase inhibition (37) leads to a rapid decrease of tumor FLT uptake that is correlated with *ex vivo* measurements of tumor cell proliferation. These data make FLT a promising imaging agent for monitoring the efficacy of cytostatic drugs. However, clinical experience with FLT PET for treatment monitoring is still limited. In patients, tumor FDG uptake is generally significantly lower than FLT uptake, which may make quantitative assessment of tumor cell proliferation challenging in tumors with relatively low baseline proliferative activity as the tumors cannot be clearly imaged distinct from surrounding normal tissue background levels.

Annexin V binds with high affinity to phosphatidyl serine, which is externalized during apoptosis. Single-photon emission computed tomography (SPECT) with technetium-99m-labeled annexin V has been used in small clinical studies to monitor tumor cell apoptosis induced by chemo- and radiotherapy. These studies have shown that the annexin V signal is frequently small and not easily detectable by SPECT imaging (38,39). This is not unexpected since apoptosis is a relatively rapid process. Therefore, even after effective therapy only a fraction of the tumor cells are expected to be in the apoptotic state. PET should provide higher sensitivity and resolution for imaging of annexin V binding than SPECT, and PET also provides the opportunity for quantitative assessment of annexin V uptake. Fluorine-18- or iodine-124-labeled annexin V analogues have been developed and validated in animal models (40,41). However, clinical studies using these PET-imaging agents have not yet been published. Since the time course of detectability of apoptotic cells may be brief, this appears to represent a challenging process to image.

DEVELOPMENTAL PATH FOR QUALIFICATION OF FLUORODEOXYGLUCOSE PET AS A SURROGATE MARKER FOR CLINICAL BENEFIT FROM CANCER TREATMENT AND ITS VALUE IN CANCER DRUG DEVELOPMENT

The data on monitoring tumor therapy suggest that FDG PET has potential for qualification as a surrogate end point for clinical benefit. Once qualified with approved therapies, FDG PET could be employed as a trial end point, both in phase III accelerated approval trials and to support go/no go decisions in phase II clinical trials. As such, FDG PET has the potential to accelerate the drug development process by allowing dosing adjustments or early identification of responders.

The paragraphs below present ten case studies that highlight the outstanding issues and drug development opportunities of employing FDG PET as a surrogate end point biomarker of clinical benefit. Based on existing data, the European Organisation for Research and Treatment of Cancer (EORTC) has published recommendations regarding the use of FDG PET for disease assessment (42). It is anticipated that further insight into the appropriate target-organ-specific cutoffs for changes in tumor FDG uptake and application of FDG PET will be defined using receiver operating characteristic (ROC) analyses from data generated in clinical trials of specific cancers (Table 15.2). Once available, these data will guide the design of definitive prospective qualification studies of FDG PET for clinical benefit. As an example, Fig. 15.1 shows such a prospective qualification study of FDG PET with standard approved chemotherapy. Once qualified, FDG PET could then be incorporated into studies of new therapeutics to accelerate their development and ultimately facilitate progress in the management of cancer patients (Fig. 15.2).

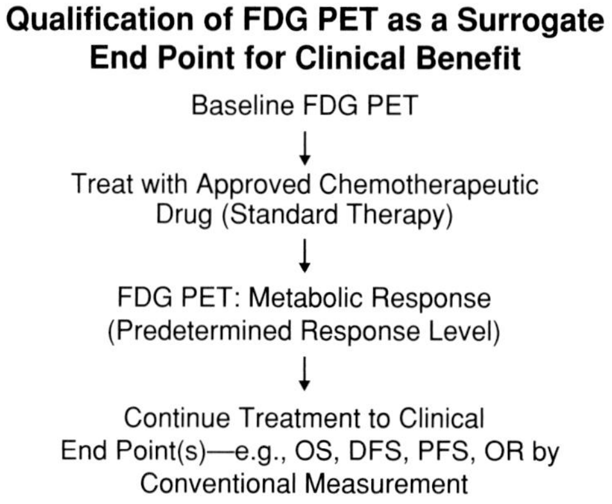

The Oncology Biomarkers Qualification Initiative (OBQI), announced in February 2006, is an agreement among the National Cancer Institute (NCI), U.S. Food and Drug Administration (FDA), and Centers for Medicare and Medicaid Services (CMS) to collaborate on improving the development of cancer therapies and the outcomes for cancer patients through biomarker development and evaluation. The goal of this collaboration is to qualify particular biomarkers so they can be used to evaluate new, promising technologies in a manner that will shorten clinical trials, reduce the time and resources spent during the drug development process, improve the linkage between drug approval and drug coverage, and increase the safety and appropriateness of drug choices for cancer patients.

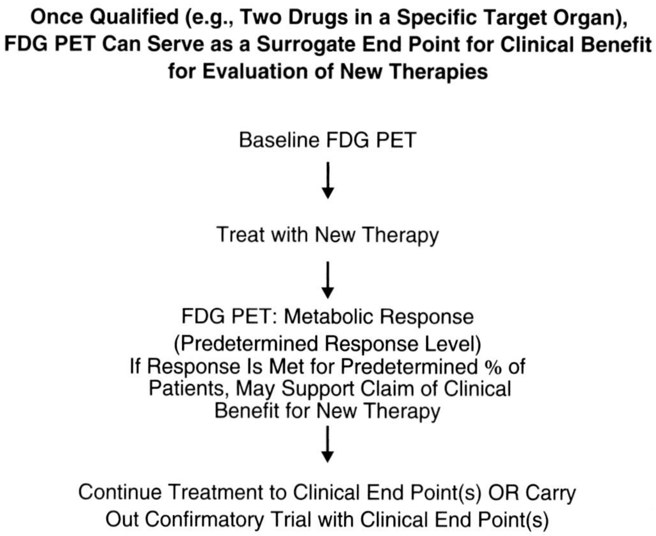

Qualification of FDG PET as a Surrogate End Point for Clinical Benefit

Baseline FDG PET

↓

Treat with Approved Chemotherapeutic Drug (Standard Therapy)

↓

FDG PET: Metabolic Response (Predetermined Response Level)

↓

Continue Treatment to Clinical End Point(s)—e.g., OS, DFS, PFS, OR by Conventional Measurement

FIGURE 15.1. Concept for qualifying fluorodeoxyglucose (FDG) PET as a surrogate end point. DFS, disease-free survival; OS, overall survival; PFS, progression-free survival.

Once Qualified (e.g., Two Drugs in a Specific Target Organ), FDG PET Can Serve as a Surrogate End Point for Clinical Benefit for Evaluation of New Therapies

Baseline FDG PET

↓

Treat with New Therapy

↓

FDG PET: Metabolic Response (Predetermined Response Level) If Response Is Met for Predetermined % of Patients, May Support Claim of Clinical Benefit for New Therapy

↓

Continue Treatment to Clinical End Point(s) OR Carry Out Confirmatory Trial with Clinical End Point(s)

FIGURE 15.2. Application of fluorodeoxyglucose (FDG) PET as a surrogate end point.

The first projects are focusing on standardizing and evaluating FDG PET-based biomarkers through clinical trials. For each cancer setting studied, standardized protocols are being developed for image acquisition, data collection and analysis, and FDG end points using carefully defined SUV measurements (43). Efforts are being made to identify and develop procedures for optimizing reproducibility. For example, scanner-introduced error is reduced by specifying scanner models, and acquisition and reconstruction parameters and end points may be represented by SUV ratios and percentages of change instead of absolute values. In addition to these methods, interobserver variability in multisite studies is being minimized by use of core imaging laboratories for centralized data analysis and review.

Specific questions can be examined in each target organ. These include potentially better care of cancer patients by ceasing ineffective therapies early in the course of treatment, avoiding toxicity, and providing opportunities to evaluate new therapies. Further, new oncology drugs can be compared against standard therapies in multiarm phase II trials. Finally, data qualifying the ability of FDG PET to predict clinical benefit in specific target organs using approved treatments will provide an opportunity for FDG PET to serve as a surrogate end point in phase III trials of new drugs, which should support accelerated approval from the FDA under Code of Federal Regulations Title 21 Part 314.510.

The collaboration of NCI, FDA, and CMS provides an opportunity to comprehensively develop prospectively designed protocols to ask these specific questions, augment drug development, and address unmet medical needs in important cancer target organs. The following sections describe the target organ specific clinical opportunities for FDG PET.

Non–small Cell Lung Cancer

Because treatment failure is closely followed by death in non–small cell lung cancer (NSCLC), it has been possible to correlate FDG PET response after a single cycle of chemotherapy with patient survival (44). Compared with CT imaging, response assessment by FDG PET can be conducted much sooner, and in recent studies FDG PET was superior to CT for predicting survival in 73 patients (45), and in the interim analysis of an ongoing multicenter trial (reviewed in Stroobants et al. [46]). In addition, in a randomized trial with erlotinib, the survival benefit of 2 months was not accounted for solely by the responders identified by anatomic imaging, showing that patients with stable disease contributed to the outcome. This suggests the need to refine classical response criteria by molecular imaging techniques, particularly for cytostatic agents.

One approach to qualify FDG PET for monitoring tumor response in NSCLC is a comparison of FDG PET response with end points used to demonstrate clinical benefit in the approval trials of NSCLC treatments. Following the principles shown in Fig. 15.1, a new trial will evaluate early FDG PET response as a predictor of patient outcome (Fig. 15.3). This trial will also study the test-retest reproducibility of quantitative measurements of tumor FDG uptake. A metabolic response in FDG PET is prospectively defined as a 25% decrease of baseline FDG tumor uptake. If this preselected definition of a response in PET predicts patient outcome (survival), additional protocols evaluating alternative/new therapies will be conducted to determine the generality of the ability of FDG PET to serve as a surrogate end point of clinical benefit. This

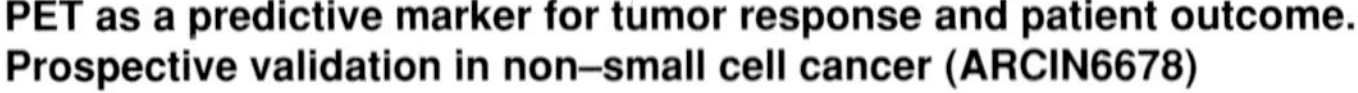

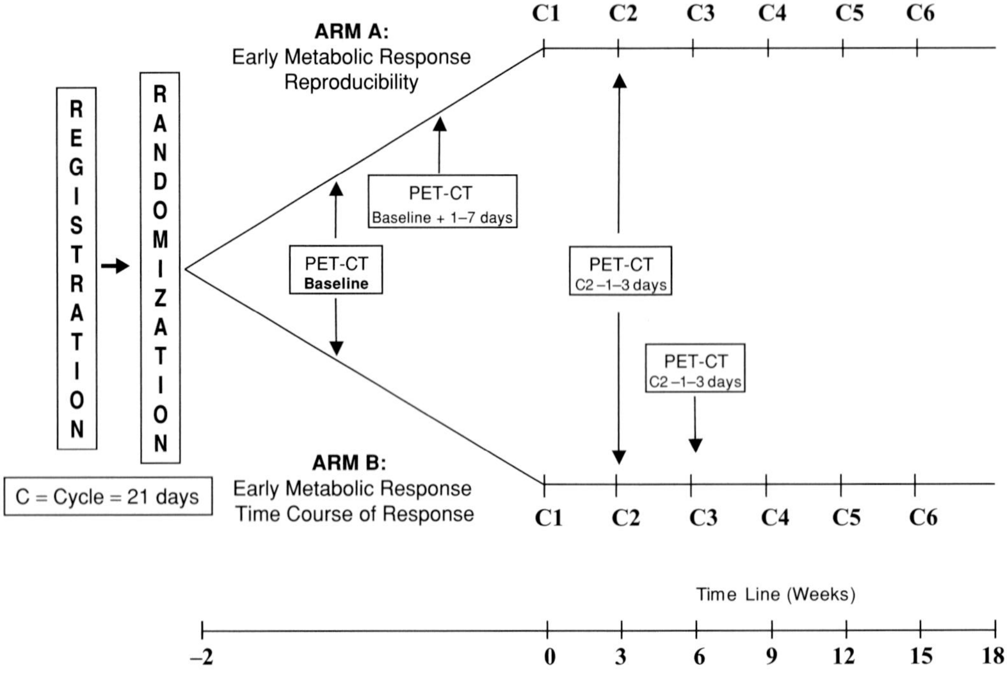

FIGURE 15.3. Validation of fluorodeoxyglucose PET as a predictor for patient outcome in patients with advanced non–small cell lung cancer.

and anticipated studies will also include rigorous ROC analysis to determine any therapeutic agent specificity in optimal cutoff points to predict outcome.

Lymphoma

In lymphoma, complete clinical responses are seen more frequently than in solid tumors; they correlate with, and are accepted surrogates of, survival. However, shorter end points are needed, particularly in phase II trials conducted in relapsed patients and those with refractory disease (47–49). A key issue in lymphoma is the post-treatment characterization of residual masses to discriminate cancerous from necrotic or fibrotic tissue, and several studies have now shown the high predictive value of FDG PET compared with anatomic imaging (49,50). These data suggest that the definition of a clinical response by anatomic imaging should be refined with a confirmatory FDG PET scan to detect residual disease in those patients with normal-sized nodes or to rule out disease in those with enlarged nodes.

Several investigations have found that lack of response using FDG PET criteria (e.g., persistent FDG uptake) correlated with progression-free survival and overall survival in both Hodgkin's and non-Hodgkin's lymphoma (49,50). These data suggest an opportunity to qualify FDG PET as an accurate early measure of response and to refine current standards for assessment of tumor response in patients with lymphoma (51). A new OBQI trial (Fig. 15.4) will develop robust FDG PET measurements to accomplish this qualification. The ability to get an early, accurate assessment of response is an important tool in the management of a patient with lymphoma since prognosis is usually poor in nonresponding and relapsed patients, and early, intensive treatment (e.g., high-dose chemotherapy with autologous stem cell transplant) may be of benefit to selected patients.

Breast Cancer

FDG PET has been approved by CMS to monitor response to breast cancer therapy when a change in therapy is anticipated. A number of studies support its accuracy for assessing response to cytotoxins as well as antiestrogens (52,53). One breast cancer setting for further qualification of FDG PET in assessing new oncologic agents would be to build on existing data in evaluating neoadjuvant therapy in patients with early stage or locally advanced disease who are scheduled for surgery (54,55). Such a trial would provide an opportunity for qualification of FDG PET judged against the histologic end point of the extent of residual disease in the breast tissue at definitive surgery. Once qualified, FDG PET could be employed as an end point in phase II trials assessing response in this neoadjuvant setting as a predictor of systemic benefit and in eradicating micrometastatic disease. Of course, PET cannot directly image micrometastatic disease due to resolution limitations.

Data are emerging that a pathological complete response in the breast following neoadjuvant chemotherapy predicts systemic benefit and a low rate of systemic recurrent disease (56). In addition, FDG PET also has application as a surrogate end point in several other clinical breast cancer settings. In patients with stage IIIA or IIIB disease, FDG PET could be used as an early predictor of drug efficacy, both for local and systemic disease. In such patients, 6-month preoperative anthracycline- and taxane-based chemotherapy is standard. An indication by FDG PET of a lack of antitumor activity could signal discontinuation of toxic, ineffective therapy and initiation of alternative, non–cross-resistant therapies.

Sarcoma

Sarcoma is a relatively rare but deadly disease. Osteogenic and Ewing sarcomas affect mostly children, while both chondrosarcoma

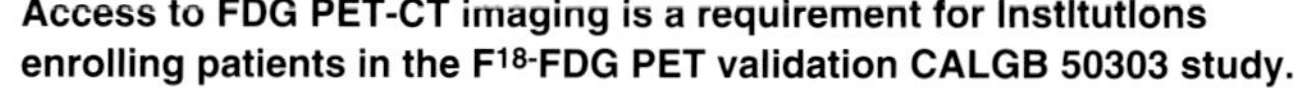

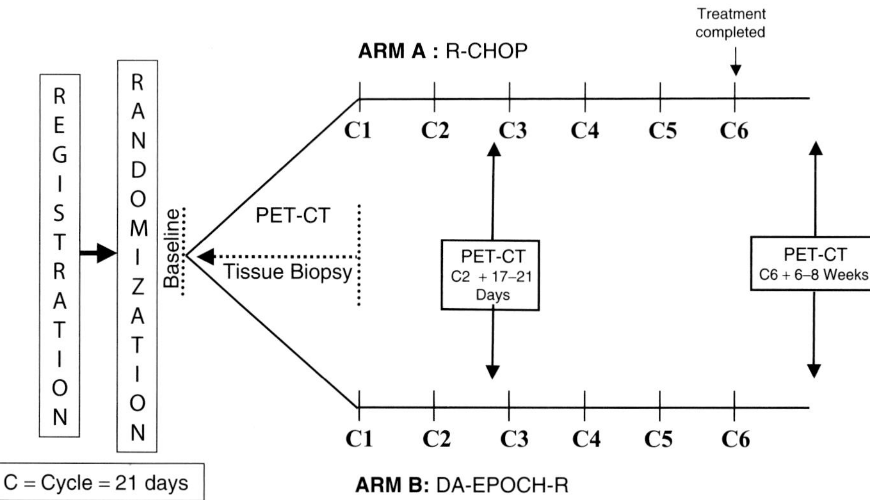

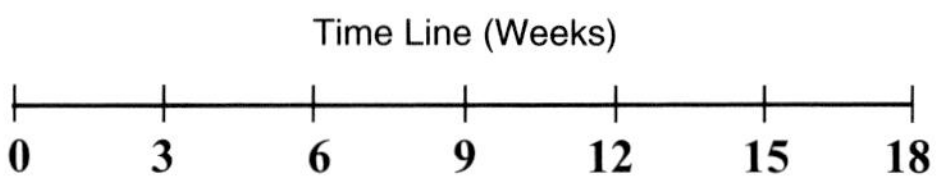

FIGURE 15.4. Validation of fluorodeoxyglucose (FDG) PET for assessment of tumor response in patients with non-Hodgkin's lymphoma. DA-EPOCH-R, a chemotherapy regimen including dose adjusted etoposide, prednisone, vincristine, cyclophosphamide and doxorubicin. R-CHOP, a chemotherapy regimen including rituximab, cyclophosphamide, doxorubicin, vincristine and prednisone.

and soft tissue sarcomas predominantly occur in adults (57). Surgical resection is the primary treatment, but in many clinical situations neoadjuvant chemotherapy and/or radiation therapy are also administered. Sufficiently powered clinical trials using survival as an end point are extremely challenging (58–60), and there is a clear need to assess the early clinical signals of the efficacy of candidate drugs. Despite the rarity of sarcoma, an opportunity to evaluate FDG PET is provided by the frequent use of chemotherapy in the neoadjuvant setting (59). End points that might serve as a surrogate to survival would facilitate identification and early testing of only the most promising novel agents or therapies in large clinical trials.

The histologic response to neoadjuvant treatment correlates with survival in osteosarcoma, Ewing sarcoma, and soft tissue sarcomas (61). As histologic response can only be assessed after surgical excision of a tumor, a noninvasive means is needed to assess ongoing treatment response and to use as a surrogate for survival. Data from single institution studies suggest that the FDG PET signal correlates with tumor response to neoadjuvant treatment and is predictive of survival in both bone and soft tissue sarcomas (62–65). Multicenter trials are needed to confirm these findings in order to qualify FDG PET as a surrogate measure for survival. This would serve to both enable and accelerate needed oncologic drug development for this serious unmet medical need and undoubtedly would facilitate progress in the care of patients with sarcomas.

Prostate Cancer

To date, FDG PET studies in prostate cancer have typically included heterogeneous populations, with mixed findings (66–68). Emerging data have begun to define the disease settings in which FDG PET has value in detecting recurrence and its potential to serve as a short-term indicator of response. In patients with metastatic disease who are to receive androgen deprivation, prostate-specific antigen (PSA) is typically a better (and much less costly) measure of disease; however, FDG PET could potentially be used instead of bone scintigraphy to identify and monitor active, nonproliferating (or at least less glycolytically active) or silent lesions versus those that continue to proliferate (and use glucose) and may be appropriate for consolidation therapy. FDG PET also has utility in patients treated by radiation or radical prostatectomy with primary intent to cure but who subsequently having rising PSA. In this setting PSA doubling time is of prognostic value (69), and FDG PET could provide complementary information, including the identification of metastatic disease sites.

Another avenue is to employ surrogate end points to facilitate assessment of novel agents or new docetaxel combinations in small, comparative phase II trials in which assessment of metastatic bone lesions, even in asymptomatic patients, would represent a key measure of drug efficacy. The promise of FDG PET as an outcome measure in this setting is already being evaluated (70). It is anticipated that, with further prospective validation against survival outcomes, FDG PET could be a valuable early end point to facilitate efficacy assessments in this metastatic disease setting, and, combined with PSA-based end points, provide a reasonably likely measure of clinical benefit.

Colorectal Cancer

In 2005, the FDA Oncologic Drug Advisory Committee accepted disease-free survival as a surrogate end point for clinical benefit (i.e., overall survival) in the adjuvant setting. In metastatic disease, it is not yet clear whether progression-free survival or time-to-progression is an acceptable surrogate of clinical benefit to support drug approvals. In five recent approvals in colon cancer, disease progression has been assessed using standard imaging techniques (e.g., Response Evaluation Criteria in Solid Tumors criteria). Based on its improved sensitivity and specificity for detecting and characterizing recurrent and metastatic disease, FDG PET could improve the sensitivity of time-to-recurrence measures in advanced colon cancer patients. FDG PET data may be applied at shorter intervals than conventional imaging, allowing more immediate assessments of drug efficacy. FDG PET could also refine the determination of eligibility for hepatic resection based on absence of extrahepatic metastatic disease (71,72). Finally, FDG PET could be considered for assessments of rectal cancer, since emerging data suggest the utility of FDG PET for assessing response to therapy in this setting (73,74).

Ovarian Cancer

Emerging data suggest that FDG PET has utility for detecting and measuring recurrent or residual disease, particularly in women with elevated or rising cancer antigen 125 (CA125) (75,76). CA125 has already been suggested as an important surrogate end point for drug development studies in ovarian cancer (77). Just as the initial CMS approval of FDG PET in colon cancer–targeted patients with an unexplained rise in carcinoembryonic antigen, a rising CA125 could be used to select patients for follow-up imaging with FDG PET. This approach could lead to an improved characterization of disease in women with a rising or elevated CA125 and could be valuable as a confirmatory end point in trials. As an example, a trial could be designed using the CA125 Gynecologic Cancer Intergroup progression criteria (77), with patients experiencing an increased CA125 then screened with FDG PET to detect recurrence.

Esophageal Cancer

Histopathological response to neoadjuvant chemotherapy or chemoradiotherapy is one of the most important prognostic factors in locally advanced esophageal cancer (78,79). Studies comprising more than 200 patients support the potential of FDG PET to predict histopathologic response noninvasively within weeks after initiating preoperative therapy and provide evidence that survival is also predicted (see Chapter 8.13 on esophageal carcinoma). If FDG PET could be shown to detect nonresponding patients this early, futile toxic therapies could be discontinued and short-term window of opportunity trials with FDG PET end points could be conducted in these patients for evaluating new treatments.

Head and Neck Cancer

Head and neck cancers are clinically heterogenous, comprising multiple anatomic sites of origin with distinct natural histories and prognoses. Cure rates are low (30% to 50%) in locally advanced disease. In such patients (stage III or IV), the accuracy of FDG PET for detecting residual disease provides particular utility for assessing response to neoadjuvant or definitive treatment. Following treatment, prompt salvage surgery improves local control, but the procedure can be avoided or reduced (i.e., for organ preservation) in responding patients. It may also be possible to limit or avoid neck dissection if lymph nodes are shown to be disease free following treatment. Several studies have demonstrated that FDG PET can assess treatment response and predict outcome (reviewed in Stokkel et al. [62]) in these cancers (80–86). These results suggest that FDG PET-derived biomarkers could serve as end points for phase II studies of new drug regimens.

Cervical Cancer

FDG PET is significantly predictive of response to therapy in cervical cancer because it is relatively accurate for assessing the extent of disease, particularly in lymph nodes that do not change in size following therapy. The extent of lymph node metastases determined by FDG PET predicted 3-year cause-specific survival in 47 treated stage IIIb patients (86). Compared with a 73% survival at 45 months in patients negative for lymph node FDG uptake, those with increased FDG signal from pelvic, plus para-aortic, or plus para-aortic and supraclavicular nodes had reduced survival rates of 58%, 29%, and 0%, respectively ($P = .0005$). In other studies any or no posttreatment FDG uptake in the cervix and lymph nodes correlated with overall survival (87). None of the patients who developed new sites of FDG uptake were alive at 2 years' follow-up. As confirmed in a later report from the same investigators of an expanded population of 152 cervical cancer patients (88), posttreatment positive FDG PET has been found to be the most significant prognostic factor for death from cervical cancer. These data suggest that FDG PET-derived end points potentially could be developed for evaluating new treatments for patients with metastatic disease.

COMBINING ANATOMIC AND FUNCTIONAL TREATMENT MONITORING USING PET/CT

At many institutions, most FDG PET scans are performed as part of a combined PET/CT examination. Several studies have shown that combined PET/CT is superior to PET or CT alone for staging disease, although few studies have used PET/CT for treatment monitoring. As described above for lymphoma, there are settings in which there is already significant evidence that tumor infiltrated lymph node size and metabolic activity can be combined to improve the differentiation between responding and nonresponding lymphomas. The new OBQI trials described above in lymphoma and lung (Figs. 15.3 and 15.4) will use combined PET/CT scanners, and the lymphoma study will specifically evaluate the refinement of standard anatomic imaging response criteria with FDG PET response. In addition to using standard uni- or bidimensional CT measurements of size, there are good theoretical arguments that measurements of total tumor FDG uptake (mean intratumoral FDG concentration times tumor volume, as measured by volumetric CT) may further improve treatment monitoring (89). Such evaluations will be explored in the new lung study described above.

Early Development and Validation of Other PET Probes for Cancer Drug Development

Development and Evaluation of PET Imaging Probes

In addition to FDG, other small molecule PET probes that measure events or specific drug effects associated with cancer occurrence and progression (e.g., proliferation, apoptosis, hypoxia, estrogen receptor and androgen receptor expression, angiogenesis) are of interest in oncologic drug development because of their potential utility in monitoring response to cancer therapy (Table 15.1). None of these is as well studied or developed as FDG, and so additional clinical research is needed to define biomarkers based on measurements of these newer PET probes and to optimize and validate assays based on these probe measurements. Just as for oncology drugs and biologics, the primary mechanism for imaging probe development and testing is the investigational new drug/device application specified in 21 Code of Federal Regulations Title 21 Part 312. FDA guidance relevant to developing imaging drug and biologic products for approval indications was updated in 2005.

Particularly important for probes that are new molecular entities (i.e., previously untested in humans) is guidance for conducting exploratory investigational new drug trials, since traditional preclinical and early clinical development studies are not relevant to the clinical settings in which the probes will be used. The exploratory investigational new drug trials permits early clinical testing without high-dose, long-term preclinical toxicology studies, extensive Chemistry, Manufactoring, and Controls (CMC) requirements, or attendant scale-up synthesis. In addition, because preclinical studies cannot always predict the clinical potential of an imaging probe, early clinical pharmacokinetic and pharmacodynamic studies (including comparisons among multiple related candidates) are critical for go/no-go decisions. Exploratory studies are defined as those of limited duration (e.g., 7 days) and drug exposures that are without therapeutic intent; one example is a study of a novel agent at a microdose (i.e., less than one 100th of the calculated pharmacologic dose, with a maximum of 100 μg). The goals of exploratory studies may include pharmacokinetic or pharmacodynamic evaluation, characterization of a new therapeutic target, or comparative study of several promising candidates designed to interact with a particular target. Importantly, exploratory studies can detect failures early in the development process, thus limiting human exposure to unsuccessful candidates.

Similarly, for imaging agents that are not new molecular entities (i.e., agents with prior human exposure either endogenously or exogenously, such as drugs studied under prior investigational new drugs), basic scientific research questions can be addressed in small clinical studies under FDA-approved Radioactive Drug Research Committee programs. The European Agency for the Evaluation of Medicinal Products has also provided a position paper calling for only limited nonclinical safety studies to support prephase I clinical microdose studies.

Application of PET Imaging Probes in Exploratory Clinical Studies of Oncologic Drug or Biologic Products

After initial characterization, PET imaging agents have significant potential to facilitate the conduct of other types of exploratory studies described in the FDA draft guidance, particularly for the evaluation of oncologic agents. These include exploratory clinical investigations of the mechanisms of action of new oncologic drug or biologic products. Application of imaging probes and technology could facilitate the pharmacologic measures of activity during preclinical testing. Moreover, such use would validate application of the same probes or technology in the exploratory clinical testing of the drug. Simultaneous use of two imaging probes to assess both the drug effect on the molecular target (e.g., epidermal growth factor receptor) and its ultimate effect on the tumor (e.g., proliferation using FLT) would be especially valuable for these early assessments, including comparisons among agents within a given class (90).

SUMMARY AND DISCUSSION

PET-imaging–derived biomarkers for cancer provide several advantages over those derived from tissue biopsy or blood samples. PET allows noninvasive serial evaluation of whole tumors. This contrasts with invasive tissue sampling methods that capture only small parts of the tumor, yielding results possibly confounded by the tumor's heterogeneity. Although noninvasive, blood sampling may also yield confounded results because of metabolism of excretion of the tumor biomarker. Finally, molecular probes used with PET (e.g., FDG, FLT) measure biological processes associated with the tumors. This is unlike most biomarkers derived from biopsies or blood samples, which measure only concentrations and not biological activities of the biomarkers, and is unlike anatomic images, which measure only size and shape. Combining PET with anatomic imaging (CT) should provide more comprehensive information on the status of a tumor.

PET-based biomarkers have applications in oncology drug development. The first is to study the pharmacokinetics of radiolabeled drugs. A second, more promising application is monitoring response to cancer therapy. FDG PET is proving useful for evaluating efficacy of certain classes of drugs that affect glucose metabolism (e.g., some protein kinase inhibitors) as well as efficacy in many cancers. Other probes are in early stages of clinical development.

Accumulating data support the qualification of FDG PET for response assessment in several settings, and future prospective trials in other settings could provide the definitive evidence needed (44,91).

In a number of clinical settings (e.g., NSCLC, lymphoma), FDG PET can also provide an early measure of response to treatment with approved therapies. Understanding the tumor response is an essential consideration in patient management (e.g., discontinuing ineffective therapies or planning additional surgical or therapeutic intervention), and thus FDG PET may significantly affect patient outcome. FDG PET response is well correlated with conventional measures of disease progression and survival, and FDG PET is superior to anatomically based imaging modalities for assessing response and predicting outcome in some studies. These emerging data provide initial qualification of FDG PET as a surrogate end point of clinical benefit in some cases; in others, new prospective or additional retrospective studies (e.g., with ROC analyses) are needed to optimize SUV cutoffs and the anticipated magnitude of response for specific diseases. These data can then be used to design prospective studies that will provide definitive qualification of FDG PET end points.

Once qualified, the application of FDG PET as a surrogate for clinical benefit has the potential to facilitate drug development. For example, the modality may shorten the duration of phase II studies. Phase III trials with an FDG PET end point could serve as the basis for accelerated approval, with full approval contingent on evidence of a survival benefit with longer term follow-up. The case studies (NSCLC, lymphoma, breast, prostate, sarcoma, colon, ovary, esophagus, head and neck, and cervix) presented in this chapter highlight the opportunities for a much expanded use of FDG PET in drug development and in support of drug approvals. These include clinical settings where current measures of treatment efficacy and disease progression are inadequate and in which FDG PET may provide a superior and earlier assessment of drug efficacy.

REFERENCES

1. Biomarkers Definition Working Group. Biomarkers and surrogate endpoints: preferred definitions and conceptual framework. *Clin Pharmacol Ther* 2001;69(3):89–95.
2. Janes KA, Albeck JG, Gaudet S, et al. A systems model of signaling identifies a molecular basis set for cytokine-induced apoptosis. *Science* 2005;310(5754):1646–1653.
3. Fowler JS, Finn RD, Lambrecht RM, et al. The synthesis of ^{18}F-5-fluorouracil. *J Nucl Med* 1973;14(1):63–64.
4. Shani J, Wolf W. A model for prediction of chemotherapy response to 5-fluorouracil based on the differential distribution of 5-[^{18}F]fluorouracil in sensitive versus resistant lymphocytic leukemia in mice. *Cancer Res* 1977;37(7 Pt 1):2306–2308.
5. Saleem A, Yap J, Osman S, et al. Modulation of fluorouracil tissue pharmacokinetics by eniluracil: *in vivo* imaging of drug action. *Lancet* 2000;355(9221):2125–2131.
6. Jayson GC, Zweit J, Jackson A, et al. Molecular imaging and biological evaluation of HuMV833 anti-VEGF antibody: implications for trial design of antiangiogenic antibodies. *J Natl Cancer Inst* 2002;94(19): 1484–1493.
7. Sharma V. Radiopharmaceuticals for assessment of multidrug resistance P-glycoprotein-mediated drug transport activity. *Bioconjug Chem* 2004;15(6):1464–1474.
8. Wahl RL, Zasadny K, Helvie M, et al. Metabolic monitoring of breast cancer chemohormonotherapy using positron emission tomography: initial evaluation. *J Clin Oncol* 1993;11(11):2101–2111.
9. Jansson T, Westlin JE, Ahlstrom H, et al. Positron emission tomography studies in patients with locally advanced and/or metastatic breast cancer: a method for early therapy evaluation? *J Clin Oncol* 1995;13 (6):1470–1477.
10. Findlay M, Young H, Cunningham D, et al. Noninvasive monitoring of tumor metabolism using fluorodeoxyglucose and positron emission tomography in colorectal cancer liver metastases: correlation with tumor response to fluorouracil. *J Clin Oncol* 1996;14(3): 700–708.
11. Haberkorn U, Morr I, Oberdorfer F, et al. Fluorodeoxyglucose uptake *in vitro*: aspects of method and effects of treatment with gemcitabine. *J Nucl Med* 1994;35(11):1842–1850.
12. Higashi K, Clavo AC, Wahl RL. *In vitro* assessment of 2-fluoro-2-deoxy-D-glucose, L-methionine and thymidine as agents to monitor the early response of a human adenocarcinoma cell line to radiotherapy [comments]. *J Nucl Med* 1993;34(5):773–779.
13. Mortimer JE, Dehdashti F, Siegel BA, et al. Metabolic flare: indicator of hormone responsiveness in advanced breast cancer. *J Clin Oncol* 2001;19(11):2797–2803.
14. Minn H, Zasadny KR, Quint LE, et al. Lung cancer: reproducibility of quantitative measurements for evaluating 2-[F-18]-fluoro-2-deoxy-D-glucose uptake at PET. *Radiology* 1995;196(1):167–173.
15. Weber WA, Ziegler SI, Thodtmann R, et al. Reproducibility of metabolic measurements in malignant tumors using FDG PET. *J Nucl Med* 1999;40(11):1771–1777.
16. Blume-Jensen P, Hunter T. Oncogenic kinase signalling. *Nature* 2001;411(6835):355–365.
17. Lawlor MA, Alessi DR. PKB/Akt: a key mediator of cell proliferation, survival and insulin responses? *J Cell Sci* 2001;114(Pt 16):2903–2910.
18. Whiteman EL, Cho H, Birnbaum MJ. Role of Akt/protein kinase B in metabolism. *Trends Endocrinol Metab* 2002;13(10):444–451.
19. Majumder PK, Febbo PG, Bikoff R, et al. mTOR inhibition reverses Akt-dependent prostate intraepithelial neoplasia through regulation of apoptotic and HIF-1-dependent pathways. *Nat Med* 2004;10(6):594–601.
20. Elstrom RL, Bauer DE, Buzzai M, et al. Akt stimulates aerobic glycolysis in cancer cells. *Cancer Res.* 2004;64(11):3892–3899.

21. Van den Abbeele AD, Badawi RD. Use of positron emission tomography in oncology and its potential role to assess response to imatinib mesylate therapy in gastrointestinal stromal tumors (GISTs). *Eur J Cancer* 2002;38[Suppl 5]:S60–S65.
22. Antoch G, Kanja J, Bauer S, et al. Comparison of PET, CT, and dual-modality PET/CT imaging for monitoring of imatinib (STI571) therapy in patients with gastrointestinal stromal tumors. *J Nucl Med* 2004; 45(3):357–365.
23. Gayed I, Vu T, Iyer R, et al. The role of ^{18}F-FDG PET in staging and early prediction of response to therapy of recurrent gastrointestinal stromal tumors. *J Nucl Med* 2004;45(1):17–21.
24. Demetri GD, von Mehren M, Blanke CD, et al. Efficacy and safety of imatinib mesylate in advanced gastrointestinal stromal tumors. *N Engl J Med* 2002;347(7):472–480.
25. Stroobants S, Goeminne J, Seegers M, et al. ^{18}FDG-positron emission tomography for the early prediction of response in advanced soft tissue sarcoma treated with imatinib mesylate (Glivec). *Eur J Cancer* 2003; 39(14):2012–2020.
26. Su H, Bodenstein C, Dumont RA, et al. Monitoring tumor glucose utilization by positron emission tomography for the prediction of treatment response to epidermal growth factor receptor kinase inhibitors. *Clin Cancer Res* 2006;12(19):5659–5667.
27. Dorow DS, Cullinane C, Conus N, et al. Multi-tracer small animal PET imaging of the tumour response to the novel pan-Erb-B inhibitor CI-1033. *Eur J Nucl Med Mol Imaging* 2006;33(4):441–452.
28. Miller KD, Miller M, Mehrotra S, et al. A physiologic imaging pilot study of breast cancer treated with AZD2171. *Clin Cancer Res* 2006; 12(1):281–288.
29. Shields AF, Grierson JR, Dohmen BM, et al. Imaging proliferation in vivo with [F-18]FLT and positron emission tomography. *Nat Med* 1998;4(11):1334–1336.
30. Vesselle H, Grierson J, Muzi M, et al. *In vivo* validation of 3′deoxy-3′-[(^{18})F]fluorothymidine ([(^{18})F]FLT) as a proliferation imaging tracer in humans: correlation of [(^{18})F]FLT uptake by positron emission tomography with Ki-67 immunohistochemistry and flow cytometry in human lung tumors. *Clin Cancer Res* 2002;8(11):3315–3323.
31. Wagner M, Seitz U, Buck A, et al. 3′-[^{18}F]fluoro-3′-deoxythymidine ([^{18}F]-FLT) as positron emission tomography tracer for imaging proliferation in a murine B-cell lymphoma model and in the human disease. *Cancer Res* 2003;63(10):2681–2687.
32. Buck AK, Schirrmeister H, Hetzel M, et al. 3-deoxy-3-[(^{18})F]fluorothymidine-positron emission tomography for noninvasive assessment of proliferation in pulmonary nodules. *Cancer Res* 2002;62 (12):3331–3334.
33. Barthel H, Cleij MC, Collingridge DR, et al. 3′-deoxy-3′-[^{18}F]fluorothymidine as a new marker for monitoring tumor response to antiproliferative therapy in vivo with positron emission tomography. *Cancer Res* 2003;63(13):3791–3798.
34. Sugiyama M, Sakahara H, Sato K, et al. Evaluation of 3′-deoxy-3′-^{18}F-fluorothymidine for monitoring tumor response to radiotherapy and photodynamic therapy in mice. *J Nucl Med* 2004;45(10):1754–1758.
35. Yang YJ, Ryu JS, Kim SY, et al. Use of 3′-deoxy-3′-[(^{18})F]fluorothymidine PET to monitor early responses to radiation therapy in murine SCCVII tumors. *Eur J Nucl Med Mol Imaging* 2006;33(4):412–419.
36. Oyama N, Ponde DE, Dence C, et al. Monitoring of therapy in androgen-dependent prostate tumor model by measuring tumor proliferation. *J Nucl Med* 2004;45(3):519–525.
37. Waldherr C, Mellinghoff IK, Tran C, et al. Monitoring antiproliferative responses to kinase inhibitor therapy in mice with 3′-deoxy-3′-18F-fluorothymidine PET. *J Nucl Med* 2005;46(1):114–120.
38. Belhocine T, Steinmetz N, Hustinx R, et al. Increased uptake of the apoptosis-imaging agent (^{99m})Tc recombinant human annexin V in human tumors after one course of chemotherapy as a predictor of tumor response and patient prognosis. *Clin Cancer Res* 2002;8(9):2766–2774.
39. Haas RL, de Jong D, Valdes Olmos RA, et al. *In vivo* imaging of radiation-induced apoptosis in follicular lymphoma patients. *Int J Radiat Oncol Biol Phys* 2004;59(3):782–787.
40. Yagle KJ, Eary JF, Tait JF, et al. Evaluation of ^{18}F-annexin V as a PET imaging agent in an animal model of apoptosis. *J Nucl Med* 2005;46(4):658–666.
41. Collingridge DR, Glaser M, Osman S, et al. *In vitro* selectivity, *in vivo* biodistribution and tumour uptake of annexin V radiolabelled with a positron emitting radioisotope. *Br J Cancer* 2003;89(7):1327–1333.
42. Young H, Baum R, Cremerius U, et al. Measurement of clinical and subclinical tumour response using [^{18}F]-fluorodeoxyglucose and positron emission tomography: review and 1999 EORTC recommendations. European Organization for Research and Treatment of Cancer (EORTC) PET Study Group. *Eur J Cancer* 1999;35(13):1773–1782.
43. Shankar LK, Hoffman JM, Bacharach S, et al. Consensus recommendations for the use of ^{18}F-FDG PET as an indicator of therapeutic response in patients in National Cancer Institute trials. *J Nucl Med* 2006;47(6):1059–1066.
44. Weber WA, Petersen V, Schmidt B, et al. Positron emission tomography in non–small-cell lung cancer: prediction of response to chemotherapy by quantitative assessment of glucose use. *J Clin Oncol* 2003;21(14):2651–2657.
45. Mac Manus MP, Hicks RJ, Matthews JP, et al. Positron emission tomography is superior to computed tomography scanning for response-assessment after radical radiotherapy or chemoradiotherapy in patients with non–small-cell lung cancer. *J Clin Oncol* 2003;21(7):1285–1292.
46. Stroobants S, Verschakelen J, Vansteenkiste J. Value of FDG-PET in the management of non–small cell lung cancer. *Eur J Radiol* 2003;45(1): 49–59.
47. Cheson BD, Horning SJ, Coiffier B, et al. Report of an international workshop to standardize response criteria for non-Hodgkin's lymphomas. NCI sponsored International Working Group. *J Clin Oncol* 1999;17(4):1244.
48. Juweid ME, Cheson BD. Positron-emission tomography and assessment of cancer therapy. *N Engl J Med* 2006;354(5):496–507.
49. Juweid ME, Cheson BD. Role of positron emission tomography in lymphoma. *J Clin Oncol* 2005;23(21):4577–4580.
50. Mikhaeel NG. Use of FDG-PET to monitor response to chemotherapy and radiotherapy in patients with lymphomas. *Eur J Nucl Med Mol Imaging* 2006;33[Suppl 13]:22–26.
51. Juweid ME, Wiseman GA, Vose JM, et al. Response assessment of aggressive non-Hodgkin's lymphoma by integrated International Workshop Criteria and fluorine-18-fluorodeoxyglucose positron emission tomography. *J Clin Oncol* 2005;23(21):4652–4661.
52. Eubank WB, Mankoff DA. Evolving role of positron emission tomography in breast cancer imaging. *Semin Nucl Med* 2005;35(2):84–99.
53. Cachin F, Prince HM, Hogg A, et al. Powerful prognostic stratification by [^{18}F]fluorodeoxyglucose positron emission tomography in patients with metastatic breast cancer treated with high-dose chemotherapy. *J Clin Oncol.* 2006;24(19):3026–3031.
54. Smith IC, Welch AE, Hutcheon AW, et al. Positron emission tomography using [(^{18})F]-fluorodeoxy-D-glucose to predict the pathologic response of breast cancer to primary chemotherapy. *J Clin Oncol* 2000;18(8):1676–1688.
55. Schelling M, Avril N, Nahrig J, et al. Positron emission tomography using [(^{18})F]fluorodeoxyglucose for monitoring primary chemotherapy in breast cancer. *J Clin Oncol* 2000;18(8):1689–1695.
56. Wolmark N, Wang J, Mamounas E, et al. Preoperative chemotherapy in patients with operable breast cancer: nine-year results from National Surgical Adjuvant Breast and Bowel Project B-18. *J Natl Cancer Inst Monogr* 2001;30:96–102.
57. Enzinger FM, Weiss SW. *Soft tissue tumors*. St. Louis: Mosby, 1995.
58. Bramwell VH. Adjuvant chemotherapy for adult soft tissue sarcoma: is there a standard of care? *J Clin Oncol* 2001;19(5):1235–1237.
59. Wittes RE. Therapies for cancer in children—past successes, future challenges. *N Engl J Med* 2003;348(8):747–749.
60. Scurr M, Judson I. Neoadjuvant and adjuvant therapy for extremity soft tissue sarcomas. *Hematol Oncol Clin North Am* 2005;19(3):489–500.
61. Eilber FC, Rosen G, Eckardt J, et al. Treatment-induced pathologic necrosis: a predictor of local recurrence and survival in patients

receiving neoadjuvant therapy for high-grade extremity soft tissue sarcomas. *J Clin Oncol* 2001;19(13):3203–3209.

62. Stokkel MP, Draisma A, Pauwels EK. Positron emission tomography with 2-[^{18}F]-fluoro-2-deoxy-D-glucose in oncology. Part IIIb: therapy response monitoring in colorectal and lung tumours, head and neck cancer, hepatocellular carcinoma and sarcoma. *J Cancer Res Clin Oncol* 2001;127(5):278–285.
63. Schulte M, Brecht-Krauss D, Werner M, et al. Evaluation of neoadjuvant therapy response of osteogenic sarcoma using FDG PET. *J Nucl Med* 1999;40(10):1637–1643.
64. Schuetze SM, Rubin BP, Vernon C, et al. Use of positron emission tomography in localized extremity soft tissue sarcoma treated with neoadjuvant chemotherapy. *Cancer* 2005;103(2):339–348.
65. Hawkins DS, Rajendran JG, Conrad EU 3rd, et al. Evaluation of chemotherapy response in pediatric bone sarcomas by [F-18]-fluorodeoxy-D-glucose positron emission tomography. *Cancer* 2002;94 (12):3277–3284.
66. Sanz G, Robles JE, Gimenez M, et al. Positron emission tomography with 18fluorine-labelled deoxyglucose: utility in localized and advanced prostate cancer. *BJU Int* 1999;84(9):1028–1031.
67. Hofer C, Laubenbacher C, Block T, et al. Fluorine-18-fluorodeoxyglucose positron emission tomography is useless for the detection of local recurrence after radical prostatectomy. *Eur Urol* 1999;36(1):31–35.
68. Sung J, Espiritu JI, Segall GM, et al. Fluorodeoxyglucose positron emission tomography studies in the diagnosis and staging of clinically advanced prostate cancer. *BJU Int* 2003;92(1):24–27.
69. D'Amico AV, Moul JW, Carroll PR, et al. Surrogate end point for prostate cancer-specific mortality after radical prostatectomy or radiation therapy. *J Natl Cancer Inst* 2003;95(18):1376–1383.
70. Morris MJ, Akhurst T, Larson SM, et al. Fluorodeoxyglucose positron emission tomography as an outcome measure for castrate metastatic prostate cancer treated with antimicrotubule chemotherapy. *Clin Cancer Res* 2005;11(9):3210–3216.
71. Strasberg SM, Dehdashti F, Siegel BA, et al. Survival of patients evaluated by FDG-PET before hepatic resection for metastatic colorectal carcinoma: a prospective database study. *Ann Surg* 2001;233(3):293–299.
72. Fernandez FG, Drebin JA, Linehan DC, et al. Five-year survival after resection of hepatic metastases from colorectal cancer in patients screened by positron emission tomography with F-18 fluorodeoxyglucose (FDG-PET). *Ann Surg* 2004;240(3):438–447; discussion 47–50.
73. Guillem JG, Moore HG, Akhurst T, et al. Sequential preoperative fluorodeoxyglucose-positron emission tomography assessment of response to preoperative chemoradiation: a means for determining long-term outcomes of rectal cancer. *J Am Coll Surg* 2004;199(1):1–7.
74. Calvo FA, Domper M, Matute R, et al. ^{18}F-FDG positron emission tomography staging and restaging in rectal cancer treated with preoperative chemoradiation. *Int J Radiat Oncol Biol Phys* 2004;58(2):528–535.
75. Mangili G, Picchio M, Sironi S, et al. Integrated PET/CT as a first-line re-staging modality in patients with suspected recurrence of ovarian cancer. *Eur J Nucl Med Mol Imaging* 2007;34(5):658–666.
76. Chung HH, Kang WJ, Kim JW, et al. Role of [(^{18})F]FDG PET/CT in the assessment of suspected recurrent ovarian cancer: correlation with clinical or histological findings. *Eur J Nucl Med Mol Imaging.* 2007;34(4):480–486.
77. Rustin GJ, Bast RC Jr, Kelloff GJ, et al. Use of CA-125 in clinical trial evaluation of new therapeutic drugs for ovarian cancer. *Clin Cancer Res* 2004;10(11):3919–3926.
78. Swisher SG, Hofstetter W, Wu TT, et al. Proposed revision of the esophageal cancer staging system to accommodate pathologic response (pP) following preoperative chemoradiation (CRT). *Ann Surg* 2005;241(5):810–817; discussion 7–20.
79. Berger AC, Farma J, Scott WJ, et al. Complete response to neoadjuvant chemoradiotherapy in esophageal carcinoma is associated with significantly improved survival. *J Clin Oncol* 2005;23(19):4330–4337.
80. Kitagawa Y, Sadato N, Azuma H, et al. FDG PET to evaluate combined intra-arterial chemotherapy and radiotherapy of head and neck neoplasms. *J Nucl Med* 1999;40(7):1132–1137.
81. Schoder H, Yeung HW. Positron emission imaging of head and neck cancer, including thyroid carcinoma. *Semin Nucl Med* 2004;34(3):180–197.
82. Greven KM, Williams DW 3rd, McGuirt WF Sr, et al. Serial positron emission tomography scans following radiation therapy of patients with head and neck cancer. *Head Neck* 2001;23(11):942–946.
83. Lowe VJ, Dunphy FR, Varvares M, et al. Evaluation of chemotherapy response in patients with advanced head and neck cancer using [F-18]fluorodeoxyglucose positron emission tomography. *Head Neck* 1997;19(8):666–674.
84. Yao M, Graham MM, Hoffman HT, et al. The role of post-radiation therapy FDG PET in prediction of necessity for post-radiation therapy neck dissection in locally advanced head-and-neck squamous cell carcinoma. *Int J Radiat Oncol Biol Phys* 2004;59(4):1001–1010.
85. Brun E, Kjellen E, Tennvall J, et al. FDG PET studies during treatment: prediction of therapy outcome in head and neck squamous cell carcinoma. *Head Neck* 2002;24(2):127–135.
86. Singh AK, Grigsby PW, Dehdashti F, et al. FDG-PET lymph node staging and survival of patients with FIGO stage IIIb cervical carcinoma. *Int J Radiat Oncol Biol Phys* 2003;56(2):489–493.
87. Grigsby PW, Siegel BA, Dehdashti F, et al. Posttherapy surveillance monitoring of cervical cancer by FDG-PET. *Int J Radiat Oncol Biol Phys* 2003;55(4):907–913.
88. Grigsby PW, Siegel BA, Dehdashti F, et al. Posttherapy [^{18}F] fluorodeoxyglucose positron emission tomography in carcinoma of the cervix: response and outcome. *J Clin Oncol* 2004;22(11):2167–2171.
89. Weber WA. Positron emission tomography as an imaging biomarker. *J Clin Oncol* 2006;24(20):3282–3292.
90. Kelloff GJ, Krohn KA, Larson SM, et al. The progress and promise of molecular imaging probes in oncologic drug development. *Clin Cancer Res* 2005;11(22):7967–7985.
91. Kelloff GJ, Hoffman JM, Johnson B, et al. Progress and promise of FDG-PET imaging for cancer patient management and oncologic drug development. *Clin Cancer Res* 2005;11(8):2785–2808.
92. Kostakoglu L, Coleman M, Leonard JP, et al. PET predicts prognosis after 1 cycle of chemotherapy in aggressive lymphoma and Hodgkin's disease. *J Nucl Med* 2002;43(8):1018–1827.
93. Haioun C, Itti E, Rahmouni A, et al. [^{18}F]fluoro-2-deoxy-D-glucose positron emission tomography (FDG-PET) in aggressive lymphoma: an early prognostic tool for predicting patient outcome. *Blood* 2005;106(4):1376–1381.
94. Mikhaeel NG, Hutchings M, Fields PA, et al. FDG-PET after two to three cycles of chemotherapy predicts progression-free and overall survival in high-grade non-Hodgkin lymphoma. *Ann Oncol* 2005;16:1514–1523.
95. Hutchings M, Loft A, Hansen M, et al. FDG-PET after two cycles of chemotherapy predicts treatment failure and progression-free survival in Hodgkin lymphoma. *Blood* 2006;107(1):52–59.
96. Weber WA, Ott K, Becker K, et al. Prediction of response to preoperative chemotherapy in adenocarcinomas of the esophagogastric junction by metabolic imaging. *J Clin Oncol* 2001;19(12):3058–3065.
97. Wieder HA, Brucher BL, Zimmermann F, et al. Time course of tumor metabolic activity during chemoradiotherapy of esophageal squamous cell carcinoma and response to treatment. *J Clin Oncol* 2004;22(5):900–908.
98. Ott K, Weber WA, Lordick F, et al. Metabolic imaging predicts response, survival, and recurrence in adenocarcinomas of the esophagogastric junction. *J Clin Oncol* 2006;24(29):4692–4698.
99. Ott K, Fink U, Becker K, et al. Prediction of response to preoperative chemotherapy in gastric carcinoma by metabolic imaging: results of a prospective trial. *J Clin Oncol* 2003;21(24):4604–4610.
100. Avril N, Sassen S, Schmalfeldt B, et al. Prediction of response to neoadjuvant chemotherapy by sequential F-18-fluorodeoxyglucose positron emission tomography in patients with advanced-stage ovarian cancer. *J Clin Oncol* 2005;23(30):7445–7453.
101. Hoekstra CJ, Stroobants SG, Smit EF, et al. Prognostic relevance of response evaluation using [^{18}F]-2-fluoro-2-deoxy-D-glucose positron emission tomography in patients with locally advanced non–small-cell lung cancer. *J Clin Oncol* 2005;23(33):8362–8370.

INDEX

I

W

X

Z